DISORDERS

PROFESSIONAL ISSUES IN THE CARE OF THE AGED

THEORETICAL CONCEPTS RELATED TO AGING

NORMAL AGING CHANGES AND HEALTHY AGING

TOWARD HEALTHY AGING

Human Needs and Nursing Response

ABOUT THE AUTHORS

Priscilla Ebersole, Ph.D., R.N., F.A.A.N., has been involved in gerontic nursing for over 25 years. She has conducted nationwide workshops and seminars on aging. Her expertise is in the fields of geropsychiatric nursing, middle age, and aging. She is a graduate of San Francisco State University, the University of California, San Francisco, and Columbia Pacific University and has earned a certificate in gerontologic nursing from the University of Southern California, Los Angeles. Dr. Ebersole has held an appointment in the Applied Gerontology Certificate Program at the university and at the Ethel Percy Andrus Gerontology Center, University of Southern California, and is professor emerita in the School of Nursing, San Francisco State University. From 1981 to 1984 she was on leave of absence to act as the field director of a gerontologic nurse practitioner project funded by the W.K. Kellogg Foundation and administered by the Mountain States Health Corporation in Boise, Idaho. In 1988 Dr. Ebersole was a visiting professor at Case Western Reserve University and occupied the Florence Cellar endowed gerontological nursing chair. In 1987 she was named Educator of the Year by the American College of Health Care Administrators. In 1997 Dr. Ebersole was inducted into The Hall of Fame at San Francisco State University. She currently is editor of *Geriatric Nursing.*

Patricia Hess, Ph.D., R.N., G.N.P.-C.S., N.A.P., has earned certificates in gerontologic nursing from the Ethel Percy Andrus Gerontology Center, University of Southern California, Los Angeles, and Holy Names College, Oakland, California, and is a graduate of Case Western Reserve University, Cleveland, the University of Colorado, Boulder, and Walden University, Naples, Florida. In 1986 she completed the geriatric nurse practitioner program at the University of California School of Nursing, San Francisco. She is also a member of the National Academies of Practice. She has been involved in gerontic nursing for over 35 years and has conducted workshops and seminars on aging. Her expertise is in the areas of health promotion and wellness, dying and death, and education of students and staff to the specific needs of the aged in acute care settings. She is a professor in the School of Nursing, San Francisco State University, and holds an appointment in the Applied Gerontology Certificate Program at the university.

TOWARD HEALTHY AGING

Human Needs and Nursing Response

FIFTH EDITION

PRISCILLA EBERSOLE. Ph.D., R.N., F.A.A.N.

Professor Emerita
San Francisco State University
San Francisco, California

PATRICIA HESS, Ph.D., R.N., G.N.P.-C.S., N.A.P.

Professor of Nursing
San Francisco State University
San Francisco, California

with 240 illustrations

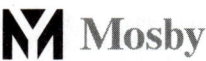 Mosby

A Harcourt Health Sciences Company

St. Louis   London   Philadelphia   Sydney   Toronto

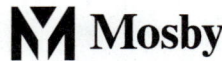
Mosby

A Harcourt Health Sciences Company

Publisher: Nancy L. Coon
Editor: Michael S. Ledbetter
Developmental Editor: Laurie K. Muench
Project Manager: John Rogers
Senior Production Editor: Helen Hudlin
Manuscript Editor: Lois Lasater
Designer: Yael Kats
Cover Design: Sheilah Barrett
Cover, logo art: Sheilah Barrett
Manufacturing Supervisor: Don Carlisle

FIFTH EDITION

Printed in the United States of America

Mosby, Inc.
11830 Westline Industrial Drive
St. Louis, Missouri 63146

Library of Congress Cataloging-in- Publication Data
Ebersole, Priscilla.
    Toward healthy aging: human needs and nursing response/
  Priscilla Ebersole, Patricia Hess.--5th ed.
      p.   cm.
    Includes bibliographical references and index.
    ISBN 0-8151-2879-7
    1.   Geriatric nursing.   2.   Aging.   I.   Hess, Patricia A.
  II. Title.
    [DNLM: 1. Geriatric Nursing.   2. Aging--nurses' instruction.   WY
  152 E16t 1997]
  RC954.E23   1997
  610.73´65--dc21
  DNLM/DLC   97-29887

00   01 / 9   8   7   6   5   4   3

Contributors

JOHN BUFFUM, PharmD, BCPP
Pharmacist Specialist, Psychiatry
Veterans Affairs Medical Center
Associate Clinical Professor, School of Pharmacy
University of California
San Francisco, California

MARTHA D. BUFFUM, RN, DNSc, CS
Associate Chief, Nursing Service for Research
Veterans Affairs Medical Center
Assistant Clinical Professor, School of Nursing
University of California
San Francisco, California

ANNETTE DEVER, RN, MSN
Gerontologic Consultant
Rocky River, Ohio

PHYLLIS GASPAR, RN, PhD
Associate Professor
Winona State University
Winona, Minnesota

SAMUEL LEE, PharmD
Clinical Pharmacy Supervisor
VA Outpatient Department
Oakland, California

GRAHAM McDOUGALL, RN, PHD, CS
Assistant Professor, Gerontologic Nursing
Frances Payne Bolton School of Nursing
Case Western Reserve University
Cleveland, Ohio

HELEN MONEA, RN, BSN, MS
Gerontic Consultant/Nursing Instructor
San Francisco State University
San Francisco, California

ROSEMARY ROTHKOPF, BA, MT, ASCP
Medical Technologist
St. Francis Hospital
Beech Grove, Indiana

Reviewers

LYNNE J. BOUFFARD, RN, MSN
Nursing Faculty
Shepherd College
Shepherdstown, West Virginia

LOUVENIA MCGEE CARTER, PhD, RN, CNA
Assistant Professor
Northwestern State University of Louisiana
Shreveport, Louisiana

JUDITH A. CSOKASY, PhD, RN
Associate Professor
Indiana University
Kokomo, Indiana

JUDITH C. DREW, PhD, RN
Adult Health Department
The University of Texas Medical Branch School of
Nursing
Galveston, Texas

SHIRLEY KALLEN, RNC, BS
Administrative Director of Nursing
Crest Haven Nursing Home
Cape May Court House, New Jersey

FERNE KYBA, RN, MSN, PhD
Adjunct Assistant Professor, School of Nursing
University of Texas
Arlington, Texas

HOLLY EVANS MADISON, RN, MS
Nursing Faculty, Southern Vermont College
Bennington, Vermont
Staff, Rutland Regional Medical Center
Rutland, Vermont

JOAN NEEDHAM, MSEd, BS, RN
Author, Consultant, Educator
DeKalb, Illinois

FRANCES JANE SMITH, RN, MSN, CNS
Assistant Professor, Department of Nursing
Lamar University
Beaumont, Texas

ELAINE E. STEINKE, PhD, RN
Associate Professor, School of Nursing
Wichita State University
Wichita, Kansas

CONNIE M. WALLACE, MSN, RN, CS
Assistant Professor
Nebraska Methodist College
Omaha, Nebraska

For my children and grandchildren who center my existence: Lorraine and Jerry O'Brien, Jason and Laura Kester; Raymond and Janet Ebersole, Priscilla and Anna; Randolph Ebersole; Elisabeth and Ralph Beierly, Paul, Raymond, Benjamin, and Ashley Tanti.

Priscilla Ebersole

To Anselm Strauss, a modern renaissance man, and a model for healthy aging despite chronicity. His soft-spoken presence was a forceful influence on others as a colleague, mentor, and friend.

Patricia Hess

Preface

The fifth edition of *Toward Healthy Aging: Human Needs and Nursing Response* continues to be based on Maslow's conceptual framework of human needs from the basic to the transcendental. The textbook is also organized from the basic to the most complex in terms of understanding the aged and their needs, so students from associate degree programs through graduate programs will find content adapted to their theoretic and intellectual levels. Thus, as one progresses through the text, the concepts and issues of care become less specific and more complex, just as in the Maslovian hierarchy one finds the achievement of each level of satisfaction more personally and idiosyncratically defined. We have used the text in this manner as we teach, and have taught, several levels of nursing students. We have also used it in teaching multidisciplinary courses without the emphasis on nursing process and interventions.

Although content and chapter organization are totally revised, reorganized, and updated, we persist in directing attention toward achieving wellness and healthy aging. Extensive current references, nursing care plans, case studies, student activities, research questions, resources, and useful appendices are included with each chapter. Another feature we think adds enormously to the impact of the text is the actual comments of students and elders as well as vignettes from practice that relate to each of the issues addressed. Key concepts, illustrations, numerous guides, boxes, tables, figures, teaching aids, and attention to the *Federal Guidelines for Healthy People 2000* are features that will assist the student and instructor to rapidly integrate knowledge.

Some of the topics that have emerged with additional emphasis since the fourth edition of the text are the concerns of the Baby Boomers as they approach aging and the great increases in the number of homeless aged and those with AIDS. More attention is given to grandparents who are assuming the role of parents for grandchildren, while there is still great concern for the needs of the caregivers of the aged who provide the majority of all care given. In addition, a completely revised chapter on the use of psychoactive drugs, written by experts in the field, has been added as this has become a critical element of consideration under the Omnibus Reconciliation Act (OBRA) regulations.

We find the wide variances, expected changes, and endless possibilities of healthy aging ever more fascinating. As we continue to work with and study the aged, our conviction is that healthy aging and wellness are within the grasp of every aging person, given reasonable relationship and environmental supports. We do not want to overemphasize the extraordinary elder who, at age 86, jogs across the Golden Gate Bridge daily nor the genetically vulnerable elder who ages much more rapidly than expected at his or her chronologic age. The needs of these exceptional individuals are included in the concepts that are presented. However, there is a greater emphasis on the cultural diversity of the aged as well as on gender and cohort differences. We emphasize the variants, individuality of the aged, and the humanistic and spiritual potential that are the components of continued personal development in late life. The common disorders and disease processes are discussed mainly in the context of healthy adaptation and nursing supports as well as responsibilities in the ongoing aspects of these disorders. This text provides the information needed for holistic care of the aged in the myriad settings in which they are encountered.

Since the first edition was published in 1981, the focus of health care has shifted from the individual provider to the corporate world and the site of delivery has shifted from the bedside to ambulatory care except in the most intensive circumstances. Enormous progress in technologic capabilities has been achieved. Now every part of the human body but the brain can be replaced. Even the unique genetic code of the individual can be exactly replicated through cloning. However, hopes, needs, desires, and personal development are still individually defined and sought while aging remains the one immutable of existence.

In earlier editions we strongly supported Gunter's definition of gerontic nursing as being the most inclusive, and we continue to ascribe to this belief. However, this is a semantic issue rather than a matter of great import. *Gerontic nursing* is an inclusive term and may occur in any setting where nurses use their knowledge, expertise, and caring capacity to assist the aged person toward optimum total function. Traditionally, the roles of the gerontologic nurse and the geriatric nurse have differed in the comprehensiveness of nursing functions and responsibility. A geriatric nurse focuses on illness propensities, and a gerontologic nurse uses a broad scientific base to formulate care. The logic of our choice of the term *gerontic care* is based on a comprehensive understanding of the complex of issues that are important to the aged. Very many of these issues are not medical. A holistic approach, as differentiated from a medical approach, which is implied in the term *geriatric,* or the scientific logical approach, which is implied in the term *gerontologic,* seems to be more inclusive and accurate for the majority of nursing care being provided to the aged. Geriatric nursing has been thought to occur primarily with the ill aged in a medical setting. But given the technologic intensity of the brief care episodes in the hospital, we doubt much of it is really oriented to geriatric care, even though most of the recipients are old. The American Nurses Association has in the past advocated the use of the term *gerontologic nurse* because it implies a broad, research-based understanding of aging. However, the Association has recently shifted to a lifespan focus, family nursing, and has combined the roles of the nurse practitioner and clinical nurse speciality into one—the advance practice nurse. Gerontic nursing is only limited by the expertise and understanding of the nurse and the desires and needs of the client.

This text is unique as a comprehensive major textbook on aging in that it has been authored by us with the assistance of a very few contributors, who were sought because of their particular knowledge in areas where we felt their expertise was absolutely essential to maintain the quality of the text. We wish to thank those contributors for their invaluable additions to the text. We also wish to thank Patricia O'Neill for preparing the *Instructor's Resource Manual and Test Bank.* This manual includes chapter summaries, suggested classroom and clinical activities, critical thinking questions, test questions, and suggested curriculum formats for undergraduate, graduate, and nurse practitioner programs.

In any publication the ultimate quality of the product depends on the commitment of time and resources of the publisher and the entire production team. We have been grateful throughout for the judgment and guidance of Michael Ledbetter, editor, and the expertise, skill, and commitment of developmental editors, Cecily Barolak and Laurie Muench. Dina Shourd provided additional assistance in many of the practicalities of permissions and production as did Helen Hudlin. We would also like to express our appreciation to Rod Schmall for his superb photographic artistry that we have been able to incorporate in this edition. And, of course, our experiences with the aged and our students have brought the text to life.

PRISCILLA EBERSOLE
PATRICIA HESS

Table of Contents

TOWARD HEALTHY AGING

Human Needs and Nursing Response

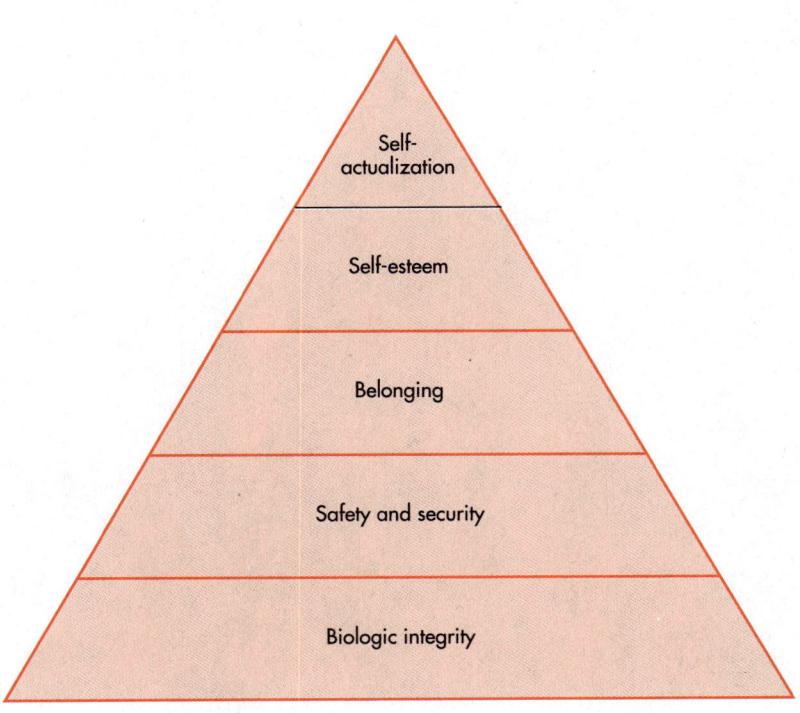

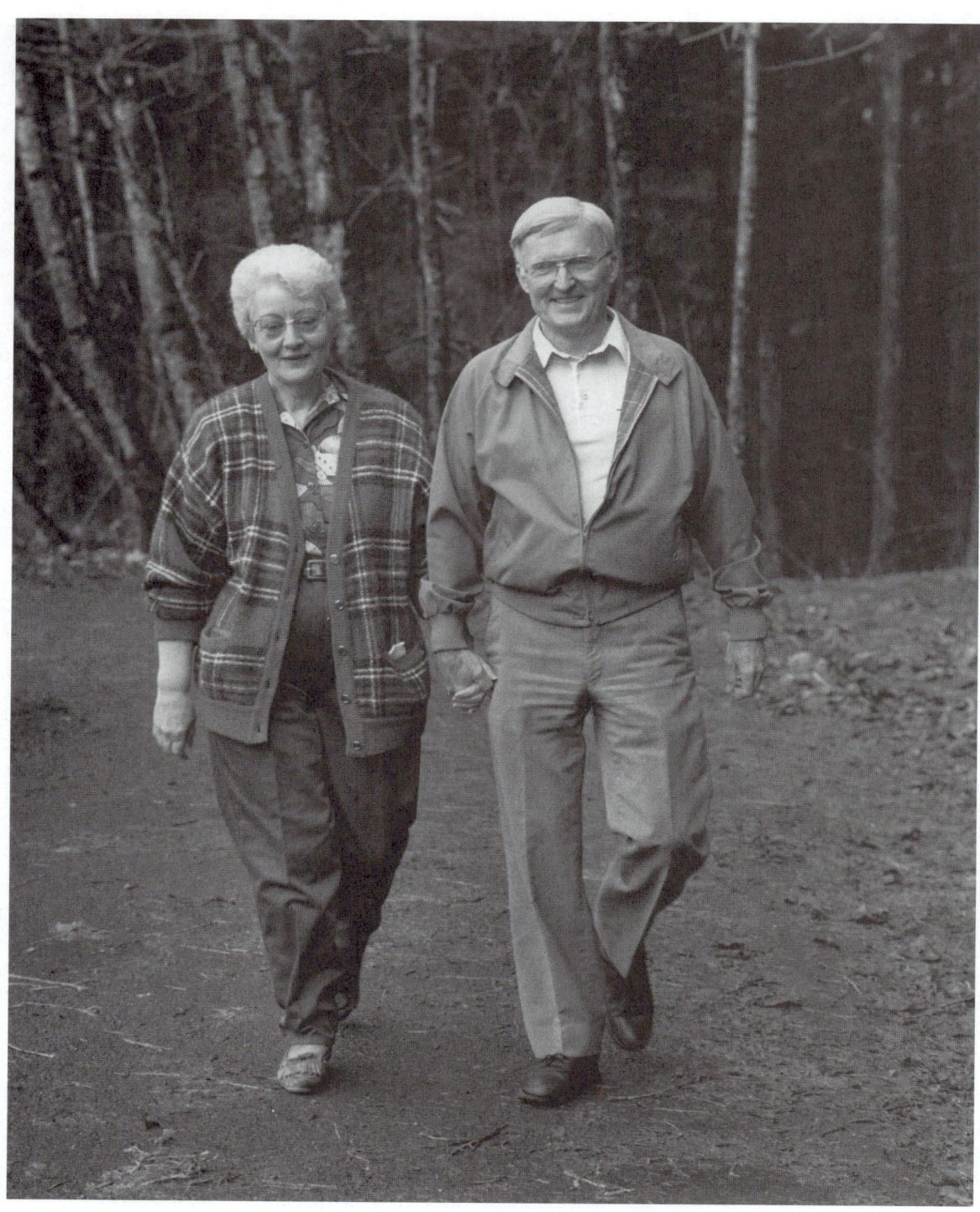

Healthy Aging. (Courtesy Rod Schmall.)

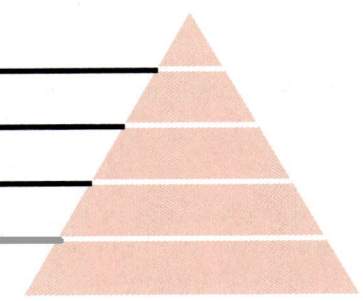

CHAPTER 1
Aging Today

Students speculate

A human life, like a river, meanders through its course, rushing through rapids, flowing placidly over the plains, twisting and turning through countless bends until it spends itself. It is the same river; yet it looks very different from one place to another. So it is with our lives; circumstances vary from one time to another in the course of a life. To impose a semblance of order on this process, people have thought of life as consisting of ages and stages.

Van-Anh Nguyen, age 20

The old, oh, those people: going down the freeway at 45 mph in the fast lane; sitting quietly on a park bench, biding time with nothing to do; sweet little old lady baking cookies for grandchildren; sex-crazed old man chasing a young woman; talking your ear off given half a chance. Oh, you old people, I am each of you.

Catherine Monahan, age 24

Could I possibly be here at age 90? YOU BET I'LL BE HERE! There is no way this old man is leaving this world without a fight. I will be a man that everyone, friends and family alike, will want to be around. I believe we age externally but not internally. Way down deep in our soul we stay the same.

Bill Freedman, age 40

Elders speak

Aging is neither a disease nor a villain that robs one of life's dreams, purpose, or aspirations. It is a growing process, a time for challenges. It is a time to emerge and be centered differently, to move into a new realm of life. Age brings on a new landscape!

Rose Marie Donnelly, age 88

When I was younger I saw the long road into the future narrowing to a thread like the distant perspective in a landscape, but as you move closer the road broadens and new vistas appear.

Barbara Taylor, age 80

LEARNING OBJECTIVES

Upon completion of this chapter, the reader will be able to:

1. Identify several viewpoints that influence the way aging is viewed.
2. Relate own aging processes to those of elders one has known.
3. Identify various perspectives of aging.
4. Specify several demographic changes related to the aging experience in the 20th century.
5. Discuss theoretic concepts of aging.
6. Develop the beginnings of a personal philosophy of aging.
7. Recognize the great diversity of aged individuals.
8. Better understand the many factors that facilitate or hinder the aging process.

WHO IS OLD?

An individual ages biologically, psychologically, sociologically, and spiritually as a unitary being. A disciplinary rather than a humanistic perspective sometimes makes it appear that these are separate components of existence. Whereas in previous editions we have examined disciplinary trends, issues, and contributions to the understanding of aging, we believe that there is now such overlap that disciplinary lines are no longer appropriate in planning care. Multidisciplinary approaches and care programs are essential and are rapidly becoming the method of providing health care. A look at the sections comprising the Gerontological Society of America (GSA) demonstrates this point: Biological Sciences, Clinical Medicine, Behavioral and Social Sciences, Social Research, and Policy and Practice. These sections include individuals from myriad backgrounds and many disciplines who affiliate with a section based on their particular function rather than their educational or professional credentials. Nurses can be found in all sections and occupy important positions as officers and committee chairs in the GSA. The nurses' special interest group which, 20 years ago, met informally in a small hotel suite, now attracts 150 to 200 members and is the most rapidly growing membership contingent. Some nurses argue that the profession should have an established section in GSA. We think not. One of the major benefits of organizations such as GSA is the interdisciplinary contact and multidisciplinary sharing. This mingling of the disciplines based on practice interests is also characteristic of the American Society on Aging (ASA). Other interdisciplinary organizations important to this effort are the Association for Gerontology in Higher Education (AGHE) and the National Council on Aging (NCOA) (Douglass, 1995). In addition, the Veterans Administration has developed Interdisciplinary Team Training Programs (ITTP) and Geriatric Research, Education, and Clinical Centers (GRECCs) throughout the system (Heinemann, 1995). These organizations and others have encouraged the blending of ideas and functions, furthering our understanding of old age and of the integration necessary for optimum care. We respect the complexities of the aging process and intend to present it in this text in a holistic manner while addressing the reality of problems nurses face in working with the aged. The most significant learning regarding the intricacies of aging comes from discussions with elders themselves.

Much has been said and written about the "aged"; some researchers extrapolate from studies of young adults or institutionalized elders, some speculate, some reach conclusions based on substantial research, and some study the aged themselves. In this text we will present and integrate each of these perspectives with the goal of creating better informed nurses and other providers who will use the available knowledge to enhance the later years of clients, friends, family, and, ultimately, themselves. The "aged," although ranging from 55 to 115, are often lumped into a single category. In reality there is little shared experience between the 55-year-old who finds himself or herself first eligible for certain memberships and discounts based on age deference and the 104-year-old residing in a nursing home.

Chronologic Age

Chronology is not the only factor to consider in aging. "Old" is a relative concept based on how one feels physically, mentally, and socially. One can feel old when competing with younger folk or feel young when much healthier or younger looking than age contemporaries. According to a survey by Goldsmith and Heiens (1992), individuals frequently fail to feel their chronologic age. This study surveys the previous literature and points out that age can be biologic, sociologic, subjective, or role referenced. They tested five hypotheses regarding age perception on a random sample of individuals of various ages and geographic origins. Their findings add to our understanding of the concept of age perception. As chronologic age increases, subjective age consistently becomes younger in all respects, although people in their thirties exhibit the greatest variability in their self-perceptions related to age. "Old age," categorically, is very likely to last for 25 additional years if you are healthy at age 65. However, you are likely to be awarded the status of senior citizen when you are 55 years old whether you want it or not and even if you are not a U.S. citizen. Discounts on goods, services, and opportunities may begin as early as age 50 although many more begin at age 60 or 65. In other words, the category of old is arbitrary and varies with time, place, and perception. Generally, we speak of the young-old, the old, the old-old and the elite old; the parameters are variable depending on the particular theorist and possibly how old the definer is, although that has not, to our knowledge, been studied (Boxes 1-1 and 1-2).

AGING AND THE AGED

Special recognition because of one's advancing age is given in many ways, some desirable and some not so welcome. Throughout life there are marker events—physical, social, and psychic—that measure our path through time. However, when these events begin to include more losses than gains, then aging may become an onerous burden, particularly for those who have few social and spiritual resources.

Aging is inextricably tied to history and culture. Views of aging in any era or ethnic group are influenced by expected life span, economic conditions, social expectations, and the way these are dealt with in the media, arts, and literature of the time. We have in our society at present a unique situation. Rapid change and cataclysmic shifts in lifestyles, a shrinking world and expanding universe, and previously undreamed of possibilities and opportunities have created remarkable differences in the life experience of each generation.

Box 1-1	**Categories of Old**	
Pre-elderly	55-64 years	Burnside
Young-old	65-74 years	Neugarten
Middle-old	75-84 years	Atchley
Old	75-84 years	Neugarten
Frail-old	75+ needing protective services	Weber
Frail-old	85+ at risk	Common usage
Oldest-old	85+	National Institute on Aging
Elite-old	95+	Common usage
Centenarians	100+	Common usage

Box 1-2	**Subjective Age Perceptions**		
Percentage with highest age congruence			
Feel	Look	Act	Interests
20s 78%	20s 87%	20s 63%	30s 64%
Percentage with highest younger age perception			
80s 86%	80s 100%	80s 100%	80s 100%
Percentage with highest older age perception			
20s 22%	20s 13%	20s 37%	20s 42%

Modified from Goldsmith R, Heiens K: Subjective age: a test of five hypotheses, *Gerontologist* 32(3):312, 1992.

The Almost-Old

A healthier old age seems to be on the horizon for the population in general and particularly for the segment dubbed baby boomers who are now well into their middle years. They are informed, educated, and have been alerted to the importance of beginning to prepare early for a good old age. They have grown up in a health-conscious environment with the best of medical care and social and recreational services, yet wars and nuclear threats have undergirded and overshadowed their whole lives. They have assiduously cultivated diversity and ethnic integration throughout their lives. They are the "Spock" babies and the "duck-and-cover" children. They blossomed in adolescence, searching for causes and hoping for a peaceful world as the space age dawned. They are now the mature suppliers and consumers of goods and services. Marketing forces are reaching out to them with "adult living" communities and numerous products and services geared especially to their later middle years. Many of them are caregivers to the older members of their family and have a very personal understanding of the needs of elders. These almost-elders are giving us new perspectives on the aging process. They and the numerous longtitudinal studies of aging now in progress are changing the concept of aging and the field of gerontology.

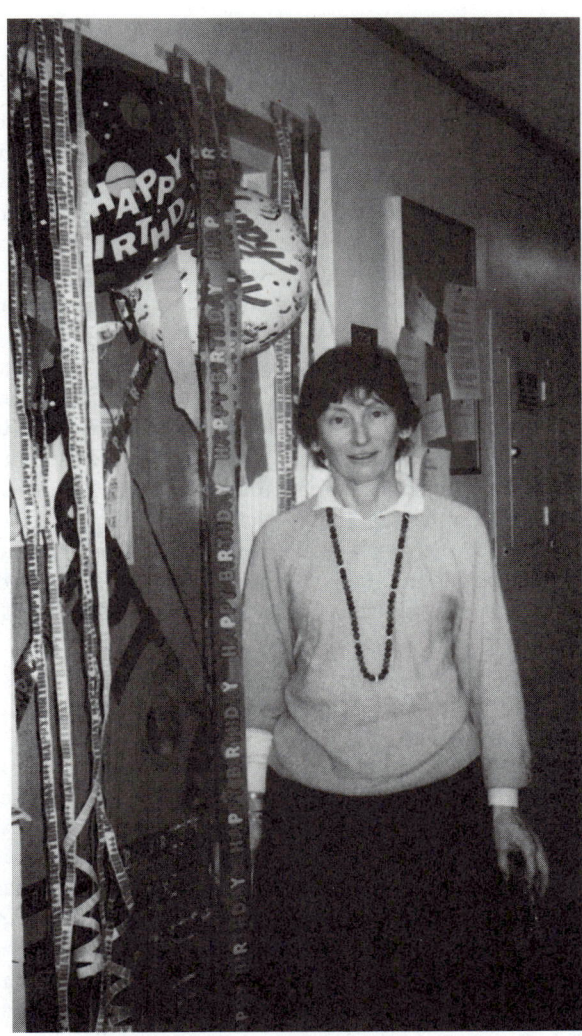

Baby boomer celebrates 50th birthday.

The Already-Old

The parents of the boomers, the children of the "Great Depression," the present old, are fewer in number than the "almost-old" because their parents limited family size as much as it was possible before the advent of birth control pills and legalized abortion. Some immunizations were becoming available in their childhood, but many parents feared them and most children had all of the "childhood" diseases, such as measles, mumps, chicken pox, and whooping cough. Some had tuberculosis, poliomyelitis, and smallpox. There was rampant malnutrition among the poorer people. Dental care was neglected. In areas where the water was "soft," lacking minerals, teeth were soft and cavity prone. "Pigeon chest," a malformation of the ribcage caused by lack of Vitamin D, was common. Goiter and myxedema were less common but were present regionally because of unrecognized iodine deficiencies. These problems were identified and almost eradicated before the next generation, the "baby boomers," came along. The survivors in this "already-old" generation are called the "notch" babies; few in number at birth and even fewer to survive childhood, adolescence, and the World War II. War and patriotism molded their young adulthood. Posttraumatic stress disorder (PTSD), only recently named, is now being recognized among aged veterans who never quite recovered from the traumas of World War II (Buffum, Wolfe, 1995). Most of these elders are fairly sturdy, but their adolescent and young adult lifestyles contributed to many problems that are now evident among the 65- to 80-year-olds. The use and abuse of cigarettes and alcohol were considered sophisticated. A double standard prevailed in the expectations of men and women. Exercise was not valued by most because desirable work was steadily becoming less physically strenuous, and physical exertion was still associated with hard work. Remote memories of poverty and deprivation haunted many of them and propelled them into excesses when such were available and affordable. Few gave much thought to their own aging when in their middle years because most were preoccupied with providing for their children the things they had missed. Saving for children's college education was a high priority (Figure 1-1).

The Very-Old

There is a large group of the very old, those over 85, who remain mobile and active. They are genetically hardy. These are an extraordinarily sturdy group who survived the dangers and diseases of childhood and, with the advancement of medical science, have overcome disorders that may have killed their parents. Some remember well the influenza epidemic of 1918 in which numerous young and vital individuals died within a few hours of developing influenza (Crosby, 1989). One elder, whose father died in the pandemic, said so many died that there were no caskets left and no burial vaults. The dead were put into hastily built pine boxes and burned. Many of our present elders, in spite of or more likely because of the rigorous conditions of survival in their youth, are now living well into their 90s. Yet there are an equal number who are frail and vulnerable; they will be discussed more fully in Chapter 15. This generation raised their families during the height of the "Great Depression." Desperation was prevalent in the country at the time. Few were able to achieve a higher education, and many did not even complete grade school. The bulk of the working population were farmers, agricultural workers, factory workers, miners, and clerks. Unemployment was rampant. Individuals worked very hard for the essentials of existence and felt fortunate if they were employed. Henry Ford became famous for offering wages of $5 a day and producing assembly-line cars that made autos available to the common person. With the availability of autos, the trek to find a better life began. Often it was an ongoing search that lasted a decade or more. These individuals who are the last to remember traveling by horse and wagon have also flown across the nation in supersonic jet airplanes. This generation

has experienced more hardship and more lifestyle disruption and change than any of which we are aware. Federal aid, Social Security, Works Progress Administration, and numerous other New Deal programs were instituted as survival measures during the depths of the Depression. Few of these individuals thought much about old age, and many say they are surprised to have lived so long. This group of elders rarely throw anything away as every scrap has potential value when one has known early deprivation. Many of them arrived in the United States in early childhood as steerage passengers, emigrating with their parents from Europe.

Centenarians, the Elite-Old

The "elite-old" are approached with some awe. They have survived the turning of a century and may yet see the dawn of the new millennium. Many are bright, alert, and have an unequaled personal history. Most, born into an agrarian society, formed the backbone of a society that was faltering. They predate the very old by just a few years and harbored similar concerns in their adulthood. The number of centenarians in the United States has doubled every decade since 1970; in 1970 the Census revealed 4475 people aged 100 or over; in 1990 there were an estimated 54,000 (Poon et al, 1992). Most centenarians are female and come from families in which longevity is common (American Society on Aging, 1995). They are often sought for their opinions on the key to longevity. There is the supposition that because they have lived so long they know the secrets to learning, growing, and thriving. Various ones have recommended such things as a daily highball, hard work, church attendance, healthy diets, or the continuation of sexual activity. Unfortunately, few agree and the myths abound.

Belle Boone Beard, who died in 1984, conducted several thousand interviews with centenarians during a 40-year study. Posthumously, a summary of her findings was published (Wilson and Wilson, 1991) (Box 1-3). Through her study and others', certain interesting things have been discovered about this very elite group of elders. They have been shown to have extremely well developed immune systems and rarely have thyroid autoantibodies that are often increased in the elderly (Franceschi et al, 1995; Pinchera et al, 1995). It appears that a very healthy immune system is one factor that supports extended life. This is obliquely borne out in studies of the cost of their health care. Such studies have shown that hospitalization costs peak for individuals between 70 and 79 years old. While the cost of hospitalization preceding death averaged nearly $17,000 for those 60 to 69 years old, it was one-third that amount for centenarians (Perls, Wood, 1996). Of course, this may only mean that less heroic efforts are exerted toward preserving life in the very old. There are still many questions and conflicting findings regarding both the physiologic and psychologic adaptation of centenarians. Studies are being conducted regarding the importance of past recall and future ambitions in coping with advanced age (Merriam et al, 1995).

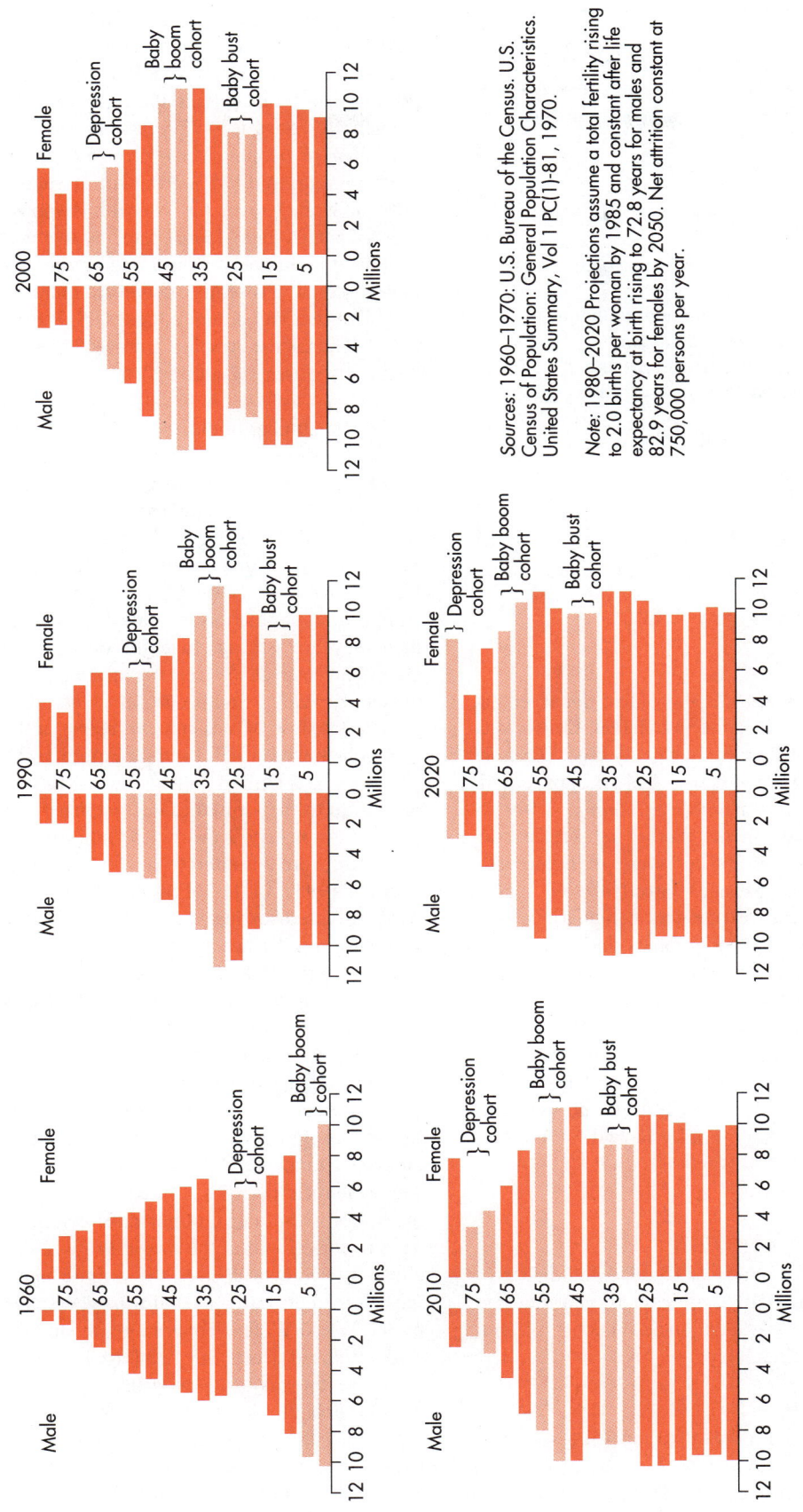

Figure 1-1. Progression of cohorts. (From Pew Commission: *Healthy America: practitioners for 2005: an agenda for action for U.S. health professional schools,* report of the Pew Professions Commission, San Francisco, October, 1992.)

Sources: 1960–1970: U.S. Bureau of the Census. U.S. Census of Population: General Population Characteristics. United States Summary, Vol 1 PC(1)-81, 1970.

Note: 1980–2020 Projections assume a total fertility rising to 2.0 births per woman by 1985 and constant after life expectancy at birth rising to 72.8 years for males and 82.9 years for females by 2050. Net attrition constant at 750,000 persons per year.

Box 1-3	**Characteristics of Centenarians**

Think they are healthy and practice good health habits

Generally optimistic about life

Eat a varied diet and drink coffee, tea, and alcohol in moderation

Have life-long habits of mental and physical activity, enthusiastically enjoy walking

Regardless of educational level, most have good memories and continue to learn

Over 90% say that religion was important to them, though they are tolerant and not dogmatic

Tend to see the positive aspect of situations, are respectful of others and content with own life situation

Continue to have work to do; highly value work and doing things for others

Have broad social contacts and interests

Show tolerance for others and forgiveness of self

Demonstrate integrity and independence

Summarized from Beard BB: *Centenarians: the new generation.* In Wilson NK, Wilson AJE, editors, Westport, CT, 1991, Greenwood Press.

Chris Mortensen at 113 years is the oldest documented living man in the world. He lives in San Rafael, California, in a retirement home and still enjoys a weekly cigar (*Parade Magazine,* 1996). However, Tane Ikai, of Tokyo, Japan, died at age 116 just last year (*San Francisco Examiner,* 1995). Reputedly the oldest person in the world, at 121, Jeanne Calment of Arles, France, retains her sense of humor although blind and barely able to hear (Barrett, 1996).

Recognition of the elitest treatment of centenarians can be found in the awe with which journalists and others approach them. My friend, Catherine, was a curio of the tour given newcomers in the nursing home where she lived. The administrator could often be heard saying as she guided visitors past the room, "And here is our 106-year-old resident." However, we must confront the fact that the numerous centenarians are most likely to be extremely frail and vulnerable both mentally and physically. Frailty is dealt with more completely in Chapter 15.

DEMOGRAPHICS OF AGING

Demographics, the statistical study of the size and distribution of population, is extremely significant in gerontology because, in many cases, it will dictate national concerns and policies as well as future directions.

Aging in the United States

The total population of the United States, according to latest figures in the *U.S. Statistical Abstract* (U.S. Bureau of the Census, 1995) is 248,762,000; of these, 33.2 million persons are over age 65, comprising 12.7% of the population (Table 1-1). About 20 million of these are older women and 13.5 million are older men (AARP, 1996). The average life expectancy for infant girls in the United States is now 79 years whereas for boys it is 72 years. In the United States more than 30% of people over 65 live alone. However, for men over 65 years old, 75% live with a spouse, whereas only 40% of women over 65 live with a spouse. After age 65, 16% of males and 41% of females live alone. Early in the century, the number of rural and urban aged were approximately equal. Presently, however, more than 70% of the aged live in urban communities (U.S. Bureau of the Census, 1995). The fastest growing group of elders are females older than 85 (Figures 1-2 and 1-3).

Variance in Numbers of Aged by State. Numerically, the largest number of elders reside in California (3,346,000), although percentage wise, Florida leads the nation with 18.4% of the population over 65. Other states in which more than 14% of the population are over 65 include Pennsylvania, Rhode Island, Iowa, West Virginia, Arkansas, North Dakota, South Dakota, Connecticut, Massachusetts, Missouri, and Nebraska (AARP, 1996). Clearly, several of these states have a large rural population who may need much more attention than they are getting. In eight states the poverty rate for elders exceeds 20%: Louisiana, Alabama, Arkansas, Tennessee, Kentucky, South Carolina, Georgia; the highest elder poverty rate is in Mississippi with 29%, and most of these are aged, black widows (Table 1-2; Figure 1-4).

Diversity of the Aged in the United States. Peak immigration to the United States occurred between 1901 and 1910 when nearly 9 million people, mostly European immigrants, were admitted to the country (U.S. Bureau of the Census, 1995). In the following 10 years another 5 million were attracted to this "land of opportunity." Today, those who still survive are among the very old. Most have long been assimilated and have produced four and sometimes five generations of descendents—all with varying degrees of attachment to their roots. In addition to varied origins, the old have experienced numerous major historic events and changes in survival patterns. These will be addressed in detail in Chapter 24. The various wars have also brought further mingling of people whose lives would not have otherwise touched. Old folks have been catapulted through socioscientific periods too numerous to mention. Some of the shifts in human thought and technical capacities that have occurred within the single lifetime of the very old include: the industrial age, the atomic age, the space age, the microelectronic age, and the cyberspace age connected by the World Wide Web. A large, unstudied group of older folk, released from the need to keep a work schedule, comprise the majority of cruise travelers, organized tour groups, and globe trotters. Many explore the wonders of the world through educational programs, guided by the Elderhostel organizers. The personal effect of world travel will be considered more fully in Chapter 25, but the effect

Table 1-1   Resident Population, by Age and Sex: 1970 to 1994

[In thousands, except as indicated. 1970, 1980, and 1990 data are enumerated population as of **April 1**; data for **other years** are estimated population as of **July 1**. Excludes Armed Forces overseas. For definition of median, see Guide to Tabular Presentation. See also *Historical Statistics, Colonial Times to 1970*, series A119–134]

Year and sex	Total all years	Under 5 years	5-9 years	10-14 years	15-19 years	20-24 years	25-29 years	30-34 years	35-39 years	40-44 years	45-49 years	50-54 years	55-59 years	60-64 years	65-74 years	75-84 years	85 years and over	5-13	14-17	18-24	Median age (yr.)
1970, total[1]	**203,235**	**17,163**	**19,969**	**20,804**	**19,084**	**16,383**	**13,486**	**11,437**	**11,113**	**11,988**	**12,124**	**11,111**	**9,979**	**8,623**	**12,443**	**6,122**	**1,408**	**36,675**	**15,851**	**23,714**	**28.0**
Male	98,926	8,750	10,175	10,598	9,641	7,925	6,626	5,599	5,416	5,823	5,855	5,351	4,769	4,030	5,440	2,437	489	18,687	8,069	11,583	26.8
Female	104,309	8,413	9,794	10,206	9,443	8,458	6,859	5,838	5,697	6,166	6,269	5,759	5,210	4,593	7,002	3,684	919	17,987	7,782	12,131	29.3
1980, total[2]	**226,546**	**16,348**	**16,700**	**18,242**	**21,168**	**21,319**	**19,521**	**17,561**	**13,965**	**11,669**	**11,090**	**11,710**	**11,615**	**10,088**	**15,581**	**7,729**	**2,240**	**31,159**	**16,247**	**30,022**	**30.0**
Male	110,053	8,362	8,539	9,316	10,755	10,663	9,705	8,677	6,862	5,708	5,388	5,621	5,482	4,670	6,757	2,867	682	15,923	8,298	15,054	28.8
Female	116,493	7,986	8,161	8,926	10,413	10,655	9,816	8,884	7,104	5,961	5,702	6,089	6,133	5,418	8,824	4,862	1,559	15,237	7,950	14,969	31.3
1981, total	229,466	16,893	16,060	18,300	20,541	21,663	20,169	18,731	14,366	12,028	10,985	11,595	11,554	10,359	15,890	7,982	2,349	30,711	15,609	30,245	30.3
1982, total	231,664	17,228	15,958	18,145	19,962	21,682	20,704	18,714	15,566	12,464	11,011	11,414	11,463	10,567	16,147	8,203	2,437	30,528	15,057	30,162	30.5
1983, total	233,792	17,547	16,053	17,869	19,388	21,632	21,141	19,067	16,117	13,150	11,201	11,155	11,457	10,655	16,414	8,429	2,518	30,279	14,740	29,922	30.8
1984, total	235,825	17,695	16,338	17,450	18,931	21,529	21,459	19,503	16,867	13,636	11,429	10,957	11,352	10,803	16,626	8,656	2,595	30,062	14,725	29,461	31.1
1985, total	237,924	17,842	16,665	17,027	18,727	21,265	21,671	20,025	17,604	14,087	11,606	10,854	11,229	10,906	16,858	8,890	2,667	29,893	14,888	28,902	31.4
1986, total	240,133	17,963	17,098	16,474	18,813	20,744	21,893	20,479	18,611	14,398	11,878	10,781	11,135	10,859	17,137	9,127	2,742	30,078	14,824	28,227	31.7
1987, total	242,289	18,052	17,430	16,377	18,698	20,192	21,857	20,984	18,619	15,608	12,294	10,802	10,968	10,783	17,426	9,376	2,823	30,502	14,502	27,694	32.0
1988, total	244,499	18,195	17,759	16,496	18,496	19,655	21,739	21,391	18,993	16,188	12,954	10,995	10,722	10,791	17,626	9,612	2,885	31,028	14,023	27,356	32.3
1989, total	246,819	18,508	17,917	16,797	18,133	19,258	21,560	21,676	19,455	16,960	13,421	11,212	10,534	10,707	17,864	9,850	2,968	31,413	13,536	27,156	32.6
1990, total[3]	**248,718**	**18,757**	**18,035**	**17,060**	**17,886**	**19,135**	**21,328**	**21,833**	**19,846**	**17,589**	**13,744**	**11,313**	**10,487**	**10,625**	**18,046**	**10,012**	**3,022**	**31,826**	**13,340**	**26,950**	**32.8**
Male	121,244	9,599	9,232	8,739	9,175	9,744	10,703	10,862	9,834	8,677	6,739	5,493	5,008	4,947	7,907	3,745	841	16,295	6,857	13,738	31.6
Female	127,474	9,158	8,803	8,322	8,711	9,391	10,625	10,971	10,012	8,912	7,004	5,820	5,479	5,679	10,139	6,267	2,180	15,532	6,482	13,212	34.0
1991, total	252,131	19,195	18,236	17,667	17,185	19,168	20,732	22,158	20,517	18,758	14,097	11,648	10,423	10,584	18,275	10,311	3,179	32,496	13,419	26,341	33.1
1992, total	255,028	19,501	18354	18,098	17,099	19,050	20,179	22,251	21,082	18,801	15,358	12,055	10,485	10,444	18,451	10,527	3,294	33,008	13,653	25,939	33.4
1993, total	257,783	19,691	18,529	18,521	17,267	18,762	19,625	22,251	21,587	19,197	15,931	12,727	10,680	10,242	18,640	10,720	3,413	33,491	13,928	25,661	33.7
1994, total	**260,341**	**19,727**	**18,859**	**18,753**	**17,616**	**18,326**	**19,177**	**22,177**	**21,961**	**19,699**	**16,679**	**13,191**	**10,936**	**10,082**	**18,712**	**10,925**	**3,522**	**33,863**	**14,428**	**25,263**	**34.0**
Male	127,076	10,094	9,657	9,602	9,036	9,311	9,619	11,058	10,920	9,728	8,181	6,410	5,244	4,740	8,290	4,206	980	17,339	7,412	12,856	32.9
Female	133,265	9,633	9,201	9,150	8,580	9,015	9,558	11,119	11,040	9,970	8,498	6,781	5,692	5,342	10,422	6,719	2,542	16,524	7,016	12,407	35.2
Percent																					
1970	100.0	8.4	9.8	10.2	9.4	8.1	6.6	5.6	5.5	5.9	6.0	5.5	4.9	4.2	6.1	3.0	0.7	18.0	7.8	11.7	(X)
1980[2]	100.0	7.2	7.4	8.1	9.3	9.4	8.6	7.8	6.2	5.2	4.9	5.2	5.1	4.5	6.9	3.4	1.0	13.8	7.2	13.3	(X)
1990[3]	100.0	7.5	7.3	6.9	7.2	7.7	8.6	8.8	8.0	7.1	5.5	4.5	4.2	4.3	7.3	4.0	1.2	12.8	5.4	10.8	(X)
1994	**100.0**	**7.6**	**7.2**	**7.2**	**6.8**	**7.0**	**7.4**	**8.5**	**8.4**	**7.6**	**6.4**	**5.1**	**4.2**	**3.9**	**7.2**	**4.2**	**1.4**	**13.0**	**5.5**	**9.7**	**(X)**
Male	100.0	7.9	7.6	7.6	7.1	7.3	7.6	8.7	8.6	7.7	6.4	5.0	4.1	3.7	6.5	3.3	0.8	13.6	5.8	10.1	(X)
Female	100.0	7.2	6.9	6.9	6.4	6.8	7.2	8.3	8.3	7.5	6.4	5.1	4.3	4.0	7.8	5.0	1.9	12.4	5.3	9.3	(X)

X Not applicable.   [1]Official count. The revised 1970 resident population count is 203,302,031; the difference of 66,733 is due to errors found after release of the official series.   [2]See footnote 4, table 1.
[3]The data shown have been modified from the official 1990 census counts. See text, section 1, for explanation. The April 1, 1990, census count (248,718,291) includes count resolution corrections processed through March 1994 and does not include adjustments for census coverage errors.
From U.S. Bureau of the Census: *Current Population Reports*, P25-917 and P25-1095; and Population Paper Listing 21.

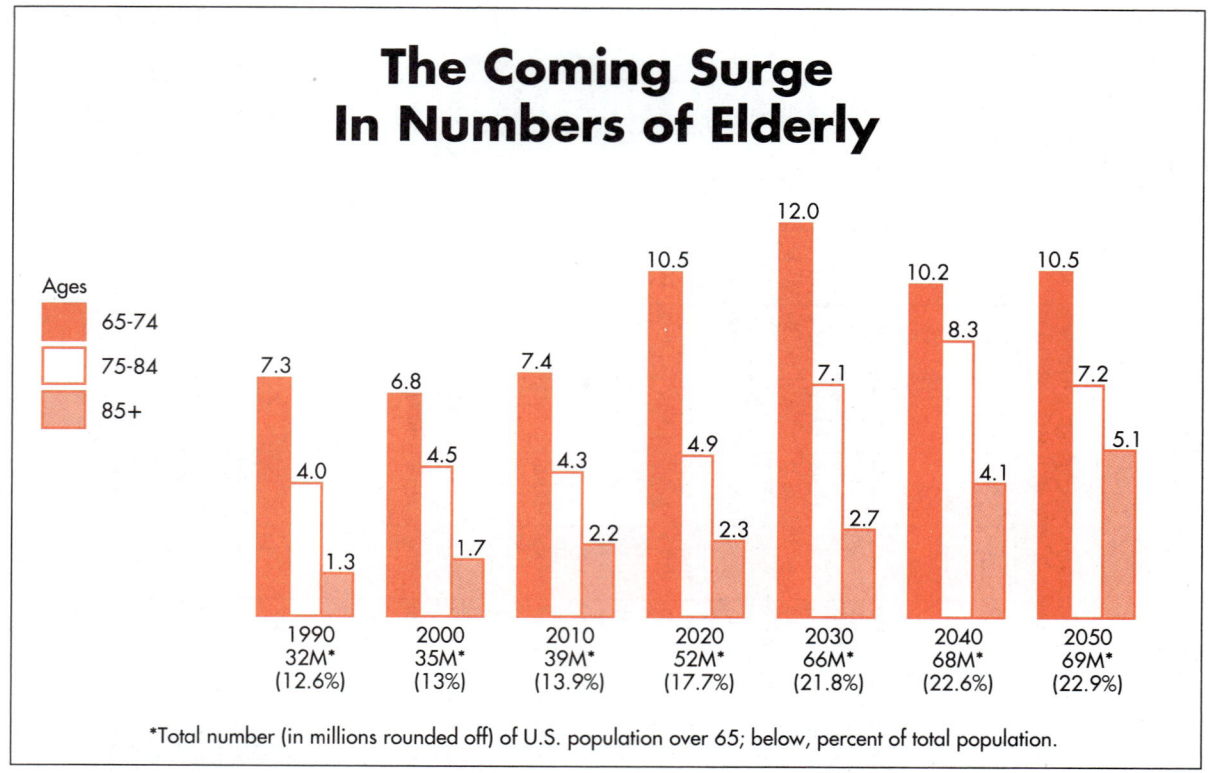

Figure 1-2. The coming surge in the numbers of elderly. (From American Association of Homes and Services for the Aging: states reach out to CCRC resident groups, *Provider News* 10(4):7, 1995.)

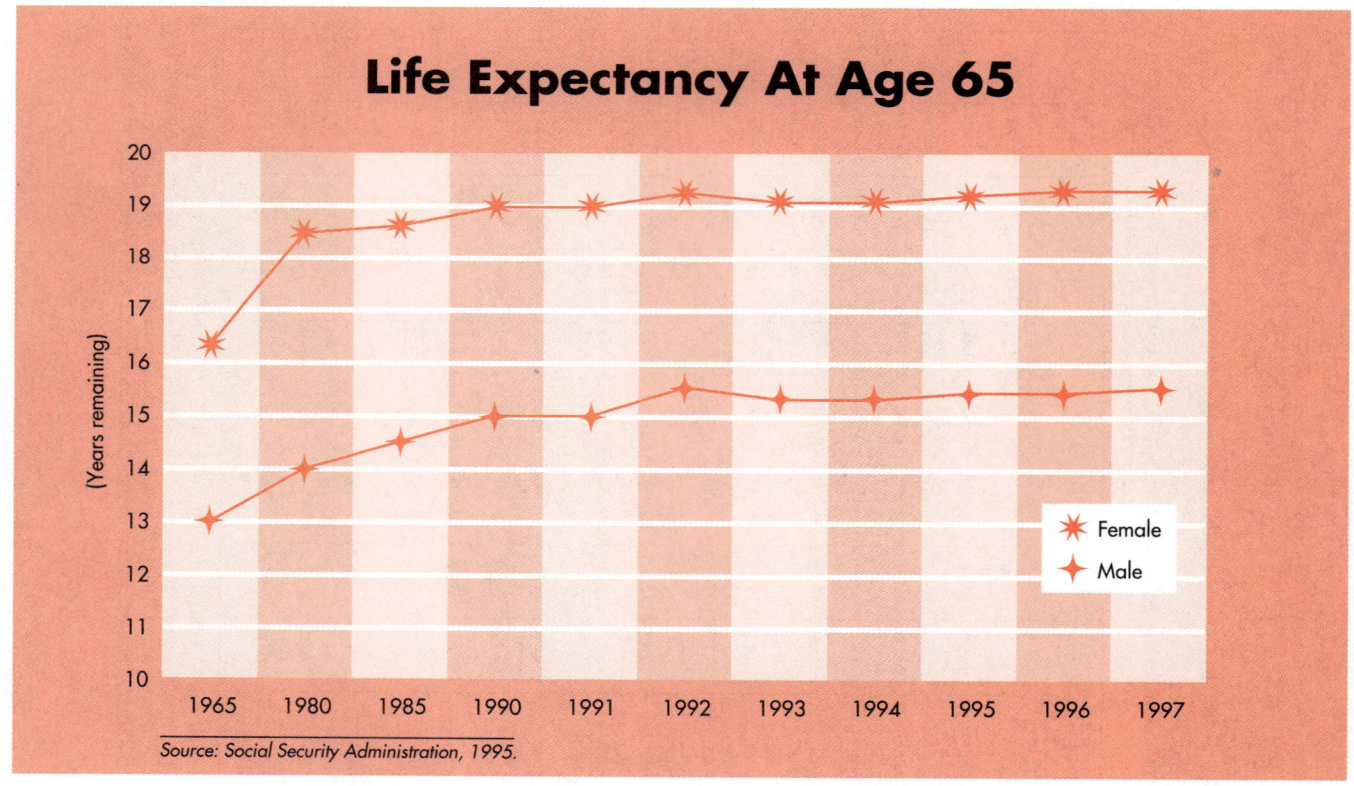

Figure 1-3. Life expectancy at age 65. (From American Association of Homes and Services for the Aging: life expectancy at age 65, *Currents* 11(1):6, 1996.)

Table 1-2 Resident Population, by Age and State: 1994

[**In thousands, except percent.** As of **July 1.** Includes Armed Forces stationed in area. See text, section 1, for basis of estimates. See *Historical Statistics, Colonial Times to 1970,* series A 204-209 for decennial census data]

Region, division and state	Total	Under 5 years	5 to 17 years	18 to 24 years	25 to 34 years	35 to 44 years	45 to 54 years	55 to 64 years	65 to 74 years	75 to 84 years	85 years and over	Percent 65 years and over
U.S.	260,341	19,727	48,291	25,263	41,354	41,659	29,871	21,018	18,712	10,925	3,522	12.7
Northeast	51,396	3,681	8,853	4,711	8,224	8,265	6,077	4,347	4,037	2,411	790	14.1
N.E.	13,270	921	2,274	1,216	2,212	2,182	1,565	1,053	1,007	626	216	13.9
ME	1,240	78	228	115	183	210	150	104	95	57	20	13.9
NH	1,137	80	212	100	190	203	134	83	76	44	16	11.9
VT	580	38	108	57	88	102	72	45	39	23	8	12.1
MA	6,041	423	1,001	566	1,058	972	699	473	460	288	101	14.1
RI	997	71	169	97	161	157	109	77	84	53	18	15.6
CT	3,275	231	557	281	531	538	401	271	253	159	53	14.2
M.A.	38,125	2,760	6,579	3,495	6,012	6,082	4,512	3,295	3,030	1,785	575	14.1
NY	18,169	1,382	3,129	1,702	2,987	2,875	2,147	1,552	1,341	784	268	13.2
NJ	7,904	579	1,352	688	1,264	1,301	966	676	612	356	109	13.6
PA	12,052	799	2,099	1,105	1,760	1,906	1,399	1,066	1,077	644	197	15.9
Midwest	61,394	4,444	11,699	5,940	9,370	9,796	6,992	5,046	4,456	2,716	935	13.2
E.N.C.	43,184	3,157	8,125	4,213	6,665	6,926	4,972	3,557	3,118	1,847	604	12.9
OH	11,102	784	2,070	1,079	1,673	1,773	1,287	945	850	486	155	13.4
IN	5,752	407	1,066	591	878	919	674	483	413	241	80	12.8
IL	11,752	915	2,168	1,128	1,886	1,878	1,341	955	818	499	164	12.6
MI	9,496	701	1,824	932	1,457	1,539	1,101	762	673	385	121	12.4
WI	5,082	350	997	483	771	817	570	412	364	236	84	13.4
W.N.C.	18,210	1,287	3,574	1,727	2,705	2,871	2,020	1,489	1,338	869	331	13.9
MN	4,567	327	914	416	723	757	511	348	300	198	75	12.5
IA	2,829	188	541	274	393	434	316	246	226	152	59	15.4
MO	5,278	376	1,003	498	792	816	600	448	405	249	91	14.1
ND	638	43	129	66	90	99	66	52	47	34	13	14.7
SD	721	54	154	70	97	108	73	58	55	36	14	14.7
NE	1,623	116	326	158	232	253	176	133	119	79	32	14.1
KS	2,554	184	506	247	378	403	278	203	187	120	47	13.9
South	90,692	6,786	16,824	9,076	14,283	14,285	10,440	7,468	6,614	3,749	1,167	12.7
S.A.	46,398	3,345	8,107	4,457	7,475	7,383	5,429	3,872	3,651	2,065	616	13.6
DE	706	51	124	68	120	114	81	58	54	27	8	12.7
MD	5,006	379	884	441	876	861	616	391	330	175	55	11.2
DC	570	43	76	58	114	91	65	46	43	25	9	13.5
VA	6,552	469	1,134	670	1,135	1,098	804	517	426	229	70	11.1
WV	1,822	108	321	190	235	286	225	176	160	92	28	15.4
NC	7,070	510	1,246	733	1,143	1,119	834	599	521	280	83	12.5
SC	3,664	274	678	394	576	576	430	301	262	135	38	11.9
GA	7,055	549	1,344	729	1,207	1,161	830	527	413	228	69	10.1
FL	13,953	962	2,300	1,174	2,069	2,077	1,543	1,256	1,441	873	257	18.4
E.S.C.	15,890	1,135	2,966	1,668	2,388	2,464	1,862	1,374	1,156	662	213	12.8
KY	3,827	261	709	400	577	604	455	333	278	159	52	12.8
TN	5,175	366	931	518	799	822	630	452	375	215	69	12.7
AL	4,219	302	778	446	631	648	491	371	317	179	56	13.1
MS	2,669	207	549	304	382	390	287	219	187	109	35	12.5
W.S.C.	28,404	2,306	5,751	2,952	4,420	4,438	3,148	2,222	1,807	1,022	338	11.1
AR	2,453	172	468	247	343	357	284	219	199	125	40	14.8
LA	4,315	337	898	458	642	663	476	347	287	157	50	11.4
OK	3,258	237	643	328	459	489	374	285	244	147	52	13.6
TX	18,378	1,559	3,742	1,919	2,975	2,929	2,014	1,371	1,078	594	196	10.2
West	56,859	4,816	10,915	5,535	9,478	9,313	6,362	4,157	3,604	2,049	629	11.0
Mountain . . .	15,214	1,229	3,139	1,503	2,294	2,431	1,713	1,180	1,001	561	164	11.3
MT	856	59	179	80	106	141	104	74	62	40	12	13.3
ID	1,133	87	252	120	149	177	125	89	72	46	14	11.6
WY	476	33	104	49	60	82	57	39	30	17	5	11.1
CO	3,656	270	700	344	575	660	453	286	212	117	39	10.1
NM	1,654	140	358	162	238	261	183	131	106	58	17	11.0
AZ	4,075	344	795	392	633	612	436	317	317	180	49	13.4
UT	1,908	181	491	232	283	261	173	118	96	56	17	8.8
NV	1,457	115	261	124	250	238	179	126	106	48	10	11.3
Pacific	41,645	3,587	7,776	4,033	7,184	6,883	4,649	2,977	2,603	1,488	466	10.9
WA	5,343	394	1,014	492	845	929	649	402	345	208	65	11.6
OR	3,086	209	574	278	440	528	386	249	232	145	45	13.7
CA	31,431	2,833	5,844	3,085	5,615	5,109	3,403	2,195	1,921	1,084	342	10.6
AK	606	56	136	61	98	118	73	37	19	7	2	4.4
HI	1,179	95	209	116	186	199	138	94	86	43	12	12.1

From U.S. Bureau of the Census, unpublished data.

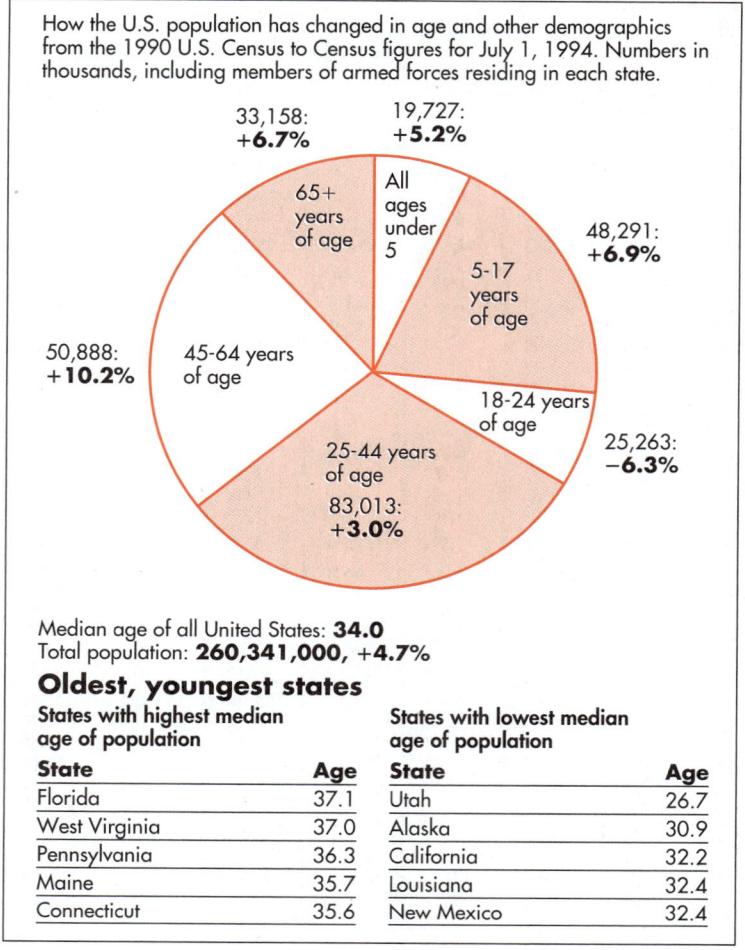

How the U.S. population has changed in age and other demographics from the 1990 U.S. Census to Census figures for July 1, 1994. Numbers in thousands, including members of armed forces residing in each state.

33,158: **+6.7%**

19,727: **+5.2%**

65+ years of age

All ages under 5

5-17 years of age

48,291: **+6.9%**

45-64 years of age

50,888: **+10.2%**

18-24 years of age

25,263: **−6.3%**

25-44 years of age

83,013: **+3.0%**

Median age of all United States: **34.0**
Total population: **260,341,000, +4.7%**

Oldest, youngest states

States with highest median age of population		States with lowest median age of population	
State	**Age**	**State**	**Age**
Florida	37.1	Utah	26.7
West Virginia	37.0	Alaska	30.9
Pennsylvania	36.3	California	32.2
Maine	35.7	Louisiana	32.4
Connecticut	35.6	New Mexico	32.4

Figure 1-4. A shifting profile. (From *San Francisco Examiner*, March 1, 1995, A-13.)

as related to understanding the diversity of the old is of interest here. Exposure to lands and peoples previously unknown have had an important consequence on the perspectives of these elders. Such experiences affect the present aged, whose values and attitudes range from radical to anachronistic. Most amazing is their ability to survive, adapt, and cope with extreme changes, yet retain a fundamental sense of self (Table 1-3).

Global Aging

Numerous international conferences on aging are scheduled each year as gerontologists seek to compare and contrast the needs and strengths of the aged in various developed, developing, and deprived nations. In 1991 there were, worldwide, nearly half a billion persons over 60 years of age. Of those, 50 million (or 1/10th) were over 80 years old (USDHHS, 1992). China has more than twice as many people aged 60 and over as the United States (100 million in China vs. 42,723,000 in the United States). The population age 80 or older, the "oldest old," represents one-tenth of the elderly worldwide. In more developed countries, the oldest old com-

prise a higher proportion of the elderly than in developing countries. Sweden is the world's "oldest" country, both in terms of median population age and the share of its population aged 60 or over (23% versus the United States with 17%). The Japanese continue to experience the longest average life expectancy (76.4 years for males and 82.2 years for females at birth). For the tenth year in a row Japan has the highest life expectancy in the world. In 1994 a female Japanese infant on average could expect to live to be 82 years old and a boy 76 (National Academy on Aging, 1995). There has been a slight but unexplained drop in life expectancy of the Japanese since 1991. These statistics and others issued by the National Institute on Aging in a report on global aging (1992) alert us to worldwide concerns regarding aging populations (Adamchak, 1993). The countries with the oldest average life span are shown in Figure 1-5; see also Table 1-4.

The extent to which longer life is translated into added years of health versus years in a disabled state is becoming an increasingly important question (Davies, 1993). An attempt is under way to produce international standardized measures of "healthy" life expectancy (Office of Demogra-

Table 1-3   Persons 65 Years Old and Over—Characteristics by Sex: 1980 to 1994

[As of **March, except as noted.** Covers civilian noninstitutional population. See headnote, table 49]

Characteristic	Total				Male				Female			
	1980	1985	1990	1994	1980	1985	1990	1994	1980	1985	1990	1994
Total[1] (million)	**24.2**	**26.8**	**29.6**	**30.8**	**9.9**	**11.0**	**12.3**	**12.7**	**14.2**	**15.8**	**17.2**	**18.0**
White (million)	21.9	24.2	26.5	27.6	9.0	9.9	11.0	11.5	12.9	14.3	15.4	16.1
Black (million)	2.0	2.2	2.5	2.5	0.8	0.9	1.0	1.0	1.2	1.3	1.5	1.5
Percent below poverty level[2]	15.2	12.4	11.4	12.2	11.1	8.7	7.8	7.9	17.9	15.0	13.9	15.2
Percent distribution												
Marital status:												
Single	5.5	5.2	4.6	4.5	4.9	5.3	4.2	4.7	5.9	5.1	4.9	4.3
Married	55.4	55.2	56.1	57.0	78.0	77.2	76.5	77.2	39.5	39.9	41.4	42.8
Spouse present	53.6	53.4	54.1	55.1	76.1	75.0	74.2	75.1	37.9	38.3	39.7	41.0
Spouse absent	1.8	1.8	2.0	1.9	1.9	2.2	2.3	2.1	1.7	1.6	1.7	1.8
Widowed	35.7	35.6	34.2	32.9	13.5	13.8	14.2	13.1	51.2	50.7	48.6	46.9
Divorced	3.5	4.0	5.0	5.6	3.6	3.7	5.0	5.0	3.4	4.3	5.1	6.0
Family status:												
In families[3]	67.6	67.3	66.7	67.5	83.0	82.4	81.9	81.3	56.8	56.7	55.8	57.8
Nonfamily householders	31.2	31.1	31.9	31.2	15.7	15.4	16.6	17.1	42.0	42.1	42.8	41.1
Secondary individuals	1.2	1.6	1.4	1.3	1.3	2.2	1.5	1.6	1.1	1.1	1.4	1.1
Living arrangements:												
Living in household	99.8	99.6	99.7	99.9	99.9	99.5	99.9	99.9	99.7	99.6	99.5	99.8
Living alone	30.3	30.2	31.0	30.2	14.9	14.7	15.7	16.0	41.0	41.1	42.0	40.2
Spouse present	53.6	53.4	54.1	55.1	76.1	75.0	74.3	75.1	37.9	38.3	39.7	41.0
Living with someone else	15.9	15.9	14.6	14.6	8.9	9.8	9.9	8.8	20.8	20.2	17.8	18.6
Not in household[4]	0.2	0.4	0.3	0.1	0.1	0.5	0.1	0.1	0.3	0.4	0.5	0.2
Years of school completed:												
8 years or less	43.1	35.4	28.5	22.3	45.3	37.2	30.0	23.3	41.6	34.1	27.5	21.5
1 to 3 years of high school	16.2	16.5	16.1	15.4[5]	15.5	15.7	15.7	[5]14.4	16.7	17.0	16.4	[5]16.0
4 years of high school	24.0	29.0	32.9	34.1[6]	21.4	26.4	29.0	[6]29.3	25.8	30.7	35.6	[6]37.6
1 to 3 years of college	8.2	9.8	10.9	15.8[7]	7.5	9.1	10.8	[7]16.4	8.6	10.3	11.0	[7]15.3
4 years or more of college	8.6	9.4	11.6	12.5[8]	10.3	11.5	14.5	[8]16.7	7.4	8.0	9.5	[8]9.5
Labor force participation:[9]												
Employed	12.2	10.4	11.5	11.9	18.4	15.3	15.9	16.2	7.8	7.0	8.4	8.8
Unemployed	0.4	0.3	0.4	0.5	0.6	0.5	0.5	0.7	0.3	0.2	0.3	0.4
Not in labor force	87.5	89.2	88.1	87.6	81.0	84.2	83.6	83.1	91.9	92.7	91.3	90.8

[1]Includes other races, not shown separately.   [2]Poverty status based on income in preceding years.   [3]Exludes those living in unrelated subfamilies.   [4]In group quarters other than institutions.   [5]Represents those who completed ninth to twelfth grade, but have no high school diploma.   [6]High school graduate. [7]Some college or associate degree.   [8]Bachelor's or advanced degree.   [9]Annual averages of monthly figures. From U.S. Bureau of Labor Statistics: *Employment and Earnings,* January issues. Data beginning 1994 not directly comparable with earlier years. See text, section 13, and February 1994 issue of *Employment and Earnings.*

phy of Aging, 1992, and the U.S. Department of Commerce, Economics and Statistics Administration, Bureau of the Census.) At present, given the current data available, some interesting morbidity and mortality comparisons can be made (Figure 1-6).

It is clear that one's geographic origins remain significant for 95% of the world's population that is physically bound to a particular place. The opportunities, limitations, and culture surrounding the aged are greatly influenced by the geographic conditions and available resources (Kaiser, 1993).

While these issues are very complex, we recognize the need to give such issues more attention worldwide. Even in the comparatively mobile population of the United States, the experience of aging is influenced by where one lives. As the world shrinks and awareness of planetary vulnerabilities increases, understanding of the aging processes and experience must necessarily be expanded. Our consciousness has been raised to the recognition that we are not only of the world but inextricably linked to all that happens in the world.

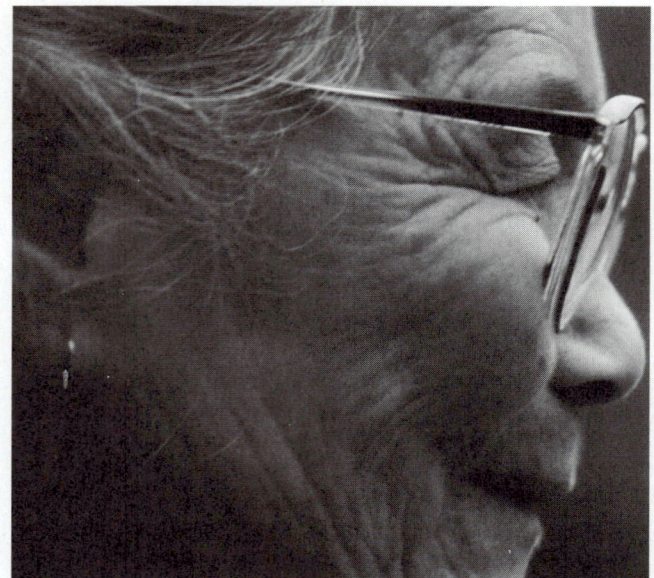
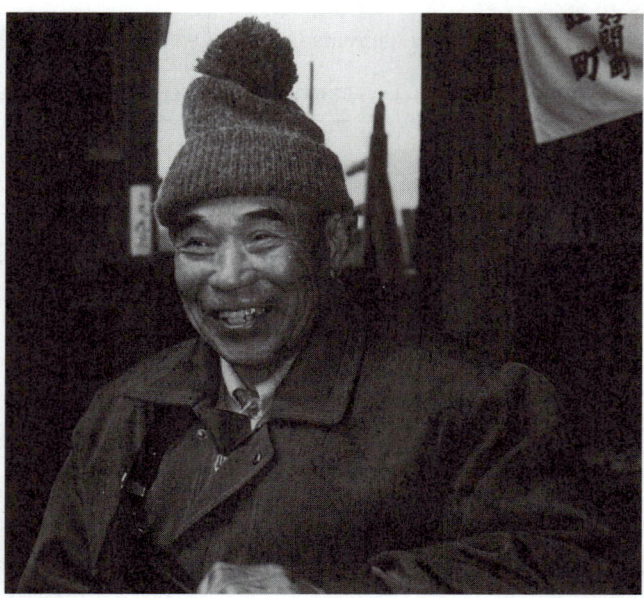

A   B

Aging in Japan.

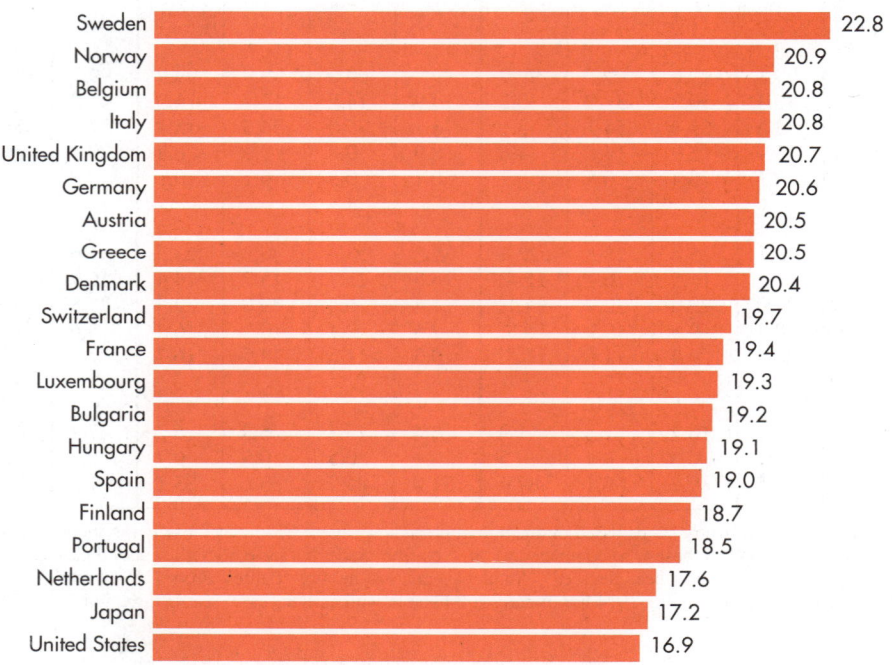

Country	Value
Sweden	22.8
Norway	20.9
Belgium	20.8
Italy	20.8
United Kingdom	20.7
Germany	20.6
Austria	20.5
Greece	20.5
Denmark	20.4
Switzerland	19.7
France	19.4
Luxembourg	19.3
Bulgaria	19.2
Hungary	19.1
Spain	19.0
Finland	18.7
Portugal	18.5
Netherlands	17.6
Japan	17.2
United States	16.9

Figure 1-5. The world's oldest countries: 1991. (From Office of Demography of Aging: *Global aging,* National Institute of Aging [1992], 7201 Wisconsin Avenue, 2C-234, Bethesda, MD 20892, and U.S. Department of Commerce, Economics, and Statistics Administration, Bureau of the Census, Washington, DC.)

ATTITUDES TOWARD AGING

Ageist attitudes may be excessively positive or negative, depending on one's tendency to stereotype individuals based on their age (Figure 1-7). The aged, collectively, have often been seen in negative terms; however, a most striking change in attitudes toward the aged has occurred in the past 20 years. The image of aging held by much of the public has gone from one of a pitiful individual in abject need to one of the elder as excessively affluent (Hudson, 1996). Images of aging presented in the media are becoming increasingly common and more realistically portrayed than in the past. Such images tend to mold and reflect the feelings of the pop-

Table 1-4   Adjusted and unadjusted male and female mortality from all causes by race: selected countries and latest available year

Country and race	Year	Rates per 100,000 population		Country and race	Year	Rates per 100,000 population	
		Adjusted	Unadjusted			Adjusted	Unadjusted
Male *All causes*				**Female** *All causes*			
Japan	1991	803.0	745.3	Japan	1991	463.3	605.4
Hong Kong	1989	828.8	546.9	Hong Kong	1989	493.4	439.1
Greece	1990	903.2	995.0	France	1990	502.0	870.9
Israel	1989	906.5	668.8	Switzerland	1991	524.8	880.1
Sweden	1989	913.5	1,140.7	Canada	1990	551.1	652.7
Switzerland	1991	922.2	966.1	Sweden	1989	560.7	1,029.4
Canada	1990	931.1	793.9	Spain	1989	566.8	769.7
Cuba	1990	948.0	758.2	Italy	1989	571.8	859.4
France	1990	949.2	987.1	Netherlands	1990	581.3	822.4
Spain	1989	958.1	903.1	Australia	1988	593.9	661.6
Italy	1989	973.2	993.1	**United States: White**	**1991**	**598.3**	**847.7**
United States: White	**1991**	**979.7**	**926.2**	Norway	1990	606.2	1,033.3
Australia	1988	984.8	788.2	Greece	1990	609.2	873.4
Netherlands	1990	1,003.3	901.7	**United States: Average**	**1991**	**621.5**	**811.0**
Norway	1990	1,018.4	1,139.0	Finland	1991	634.2	958.8
United States: Average	**1991**	**1,018.5**	**912.1**	Austria	1991	638.2	1,101.4
United Kingdom	1991	1,032.2	1,117.7	Belgium	1987	649.4	1,022.3
Austria	1991	1,037.1	1,028.0	United Kingdom	1991	667.9	1,123.9
Denmark	1991	1,068.6	1,177.4	Germany, Federal Republic of[1]	1990	678.9	1,208.0
New Zealand	1989	1,070.1	866.9	New Zealand	1989	686.1	752.3
Singapore	1990	1,088.0	564.0	Israel	1989	693.6	596.5
Belgium	1987	1,104.4	1,116.1	Denmark	1991	696.3	1,125.2
Costa Rica	1989	1,115.5	431.5	Uruguay	1990	720.1	860.7
Germany, Federal Republic of[1]	1990	1,120.2	1,111.6	Costa Rica	1989	726.9	330.3
Finland	1991	1,144.8	1,009.6	Cuba	1990	728.3	601.0
Ireland	1990	1,193.0	962.3	Singapore	1990	731.1	461.5
Chile	1989	1,198.5	656.2	Ireland	1990	738.1	829.1
Argentina	1989	1,209.1	885.0	Chile	1989	738.7	509.9
Yugoslavia	1990	1,228.5	957.8	Argentina	1989	751.5	687.9
Uruguay	1990	1,250.3	1,098.1	Portugal	1991	755.6	977.4
Portugal	1991	1,251.3	1,147.0	Yugoslavia	1990	807.9	825.1
Bulgaria	1991	1,387.4	1,354.5	**United States: Black**	**1991**	**854.5**	**744.5**
Romania	1990	1,389.5	1,151.4	Poland	1991	862.4	949.2
United States: Black	**1991**	**1,471.0**	**998.7**	Czechoslovakia	1990	873.8	1,083.6
Czechoslovakia	1990	1,537.7	1,268.3	U.S.S.R.	1990	900.0	1,001.0
Poland	1991	1,566.3	1,168.9	Bulgaria	1991	930.8	1,107.8
U.S.S.R.	1990	1,604.3	1,074.1	Hungary	1991	950.1	1,265.0
Hungary	1991	1,665.0	1,545.6	Romania	1990	974.4	980.3

[1]Germany, Federal Republic of, refers to United Germany.
From Zarate AO: *International mortality chartbook: levels and trends, 1955-91,* Hyattsville, Md, 1994, Public Health Service.

ulation at large and as such are important indices of positive change. The aged are less frequently used as a subject of ridicule or as the butt of jokes. Bell (1992) analyzed major prime time television programs, which had central characters who were older and found such characters to be generally portrayed as affluent, influential, and astute. In reality, Ferraro (1992) found that currently many elders feel the media distorts the picture of aging to one more positive than the elders actually experience. However, the impact of media presentation is enormous, and we are gratified to see robust images of aging; fewer aged are portrayed as victims or those to be shunned or made ridiculous by virtue of achieving old age.

Respect

In some countries respect is given in degrees to anyone older than another. The youngest child gets no respect at all but must obey the bidding of all those higher on the chronologic ladder. In these countries individuals will quite unabashedly inquire of others their age in order to establish the hierarchy

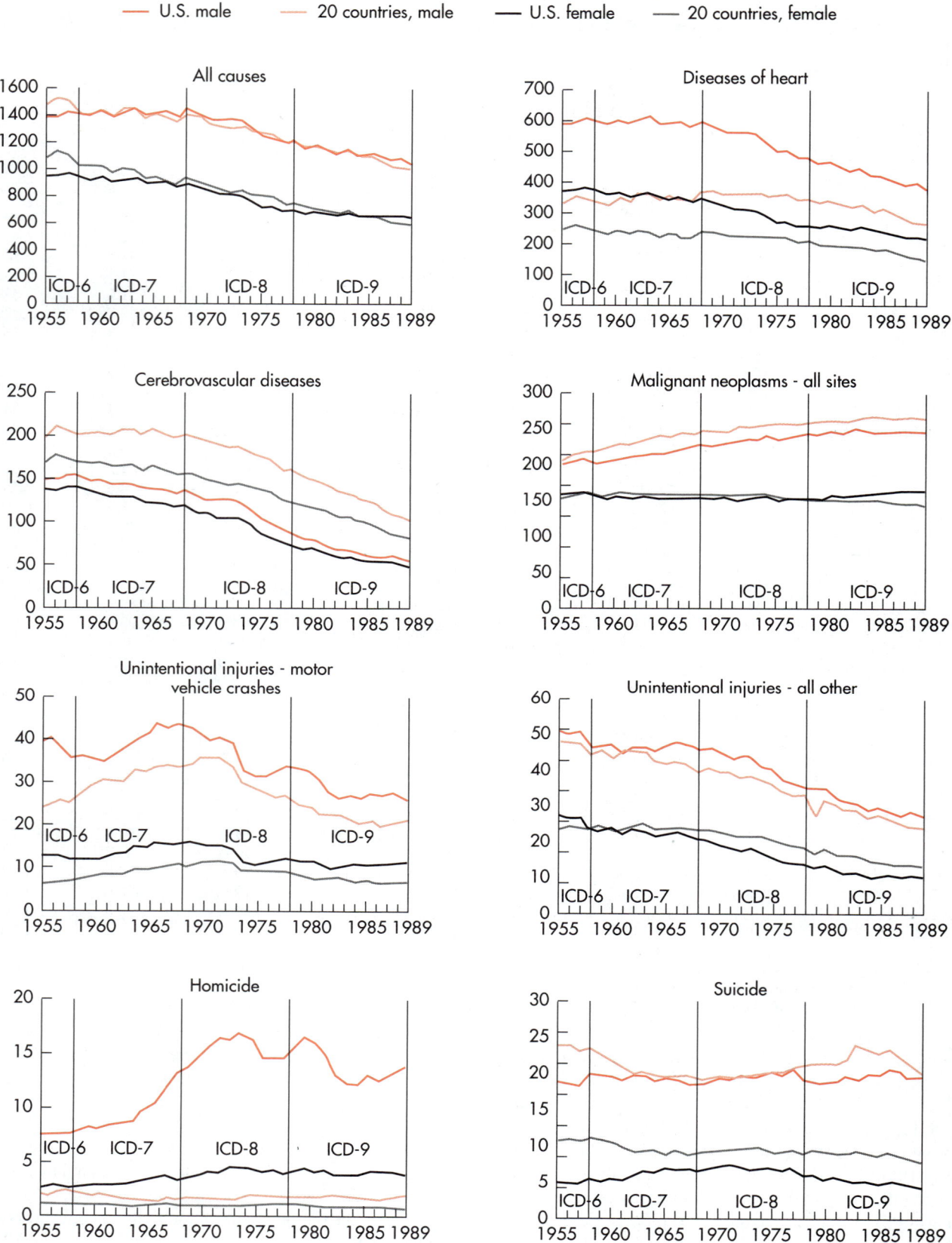

Figure 1-6. World morbidity and mortality. (From Zarate AO: *International mortality chartbook: levels and trends, 1955-91,* Hyattsville, MD, 1994, Public Health Service.)

My Personal View of Aging

Age 50

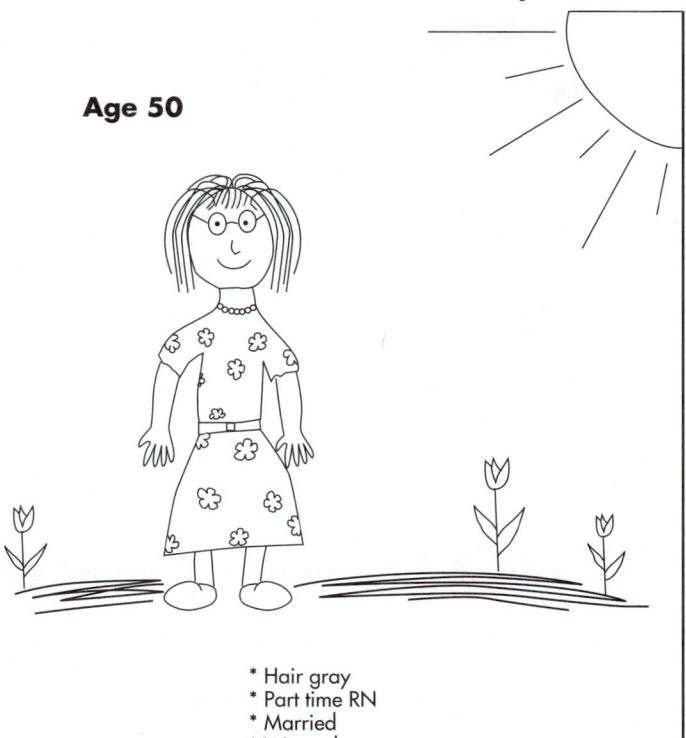

* Hair gray
* Part time RN
* Married
* Wear glasses
* All other systems well

Age 65

* Retirement
* Travel alot
* Vision decreasing more
* Still exercise regularly
* All other systems well

Age 75

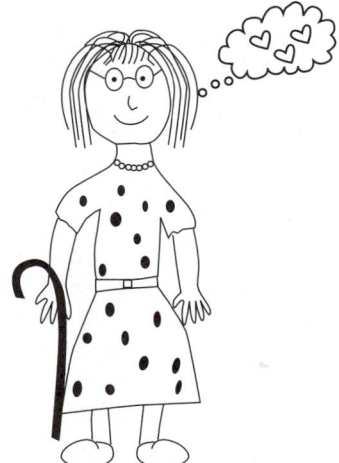

* Still married
* Arthritis in both knees
* Ambulate with cane
* Wear glasses, slight loss in vision
* Breast cancer, removal of L breast

Age 90

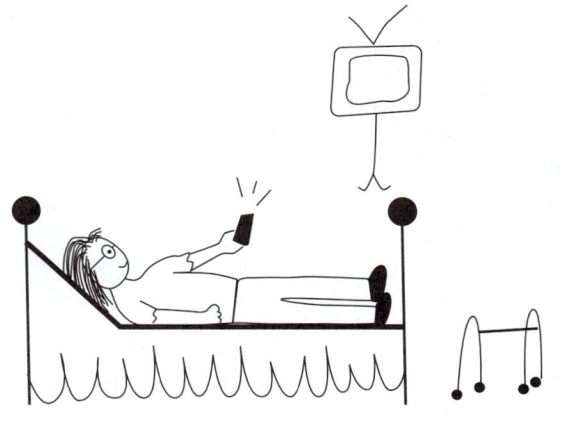

* Widow
* Live in nursing home
* Ambulate with walker
* Significant loss in vision
* Loss in ROM in lower extremities
* Need assistance with ADLs

Figure 1-7. Labaj student view: ages and stages of life.

of respect. In Thailand, a charming recognition of age is celebrated during Songkran, the National New Year holiday. Any person older than oneself may be doused with water to indicate respect. In reality, everyone is doused as the celebration gains momentum. In each society the elders have expectations of appropriate behavior, and youth have proscribed ways of dealing with elders. The more democratic a society, the more variance there is in the potential and expectations of the aged. In all countries in which technologic development has progressed rapidly, where medical care has been available to prolong life and large numbers of elders are surviving, those in advanced old age must be given attention and may be considered a social and economic liability. This is at the root of many negative ageist attitudes, which will be discussed more fully in Chapter 18. This type of collective categorization, or stereotyping, is neither correct nor humane. Elders vary tremendously in age, interests, and capacities.

Attitudes of Elders

Attitudes of the aged toward other elders are often far more rejecting than those of younger persons. The aged with mental disabilities are particularly vulnerable as they represent the fears of healthier elders who are in age proximity and often in the same setting.

Attitudes of Children

Children are able to identify with old persons and feel comfortable with them in direct proportion to their frequency of contact. Those who see elders frequently are more aware of the reality of aging persons. Closeness with grandparents is highly correlated with attitudes young people hold toward older persons. Attitudes of school-aged children and adolescents are generally positive regarding the aged. These tendencies could be sustained and cultivated by giving more attention to aging in public school curricula. To decrease stereotypic notions, students in some schools are given opportunities to work with the elderly. Generally, persons who are younger and better educated and who have contact with the well elderly have the most positive regard for the aged.

DEVELOPMENT OF GERONTOLOGY

Gerontology is the scientific study of the effects of time on human development, specifically the study of the aged. It is at the opposite end of the spectrum from embryology. Embryology deals with the prebirth phenomena of living beings whereas gerontology deals with the predeath. Gerontology, by virtue of the Greek origin of the word "geron" (old man), should mean the study of old men, but many more women than men grow old. Healthy old men and women frequently elude the attention of gerontologists; thus findings regarding illnesses of old age have been extrapolated to the healthier population. In fact, it is not yet certain what healthy old age can be; this will not be known until optimum social and bi-

ologic conditions exist for the aged. Yet elegant and exquisite theories are secondary to the conscious experience of the aged. To learn about aging one must listen to the aged (Kaufman, 1993). A large part of a philosophy of aging comes from listening to the aged and another important part from listening to ourselves and how we perceive our own aging. These two steps are fundamentally important to gerontology. In developing a science and philosophy of aging, one essentially builds on personal experience; ultimately we all do this. How else can we measure the impact of dreams, fantasies, meditation, courage, love, grief, and the phenomena of living?

The Study of Aging

Gerontology began as an inquiry into the characteristics of long-lived people, and we are still intrigued by them. In 1000 B.C. the average life span was 18 years, and people who lived to old age were curiosities, stimulating speculation and myth. Butler (1990) mentions five reasons why the scientific study of aging has become increasingly timely and important:

- Increasing interest in the biology of aging
- A phenomenal shift in life expectancy; even though this more than anything else really reflects infant survival, it makes a significant difference in the social system
- The diseases of affluence, which are abundant in old age and the result of rich diets and sedentary living
- The staggering cost of health care, 30% of which is associated with caring for the old
- Negative attitudes toward the aged that still persist and must be confronted and deactivated

Inquisitions into and curiosity about aging are as old as curiosity about life and death itself. Much that was thought to have been correct about aging has been shown through research to be half-truth, myth, or supposition. Anecdotal evidence had been used in the past to illustrate issues assumed to be universal. It is only in the last 40 years that serious and carefully controlled research studies have flourished. Theoreticians and researchers most commonly interested in the study of aging are sociologists, psychologists, and biologists. Their conceptual bases underlie their perspective regarding survival issues. Nursing draws from all of these disciplines to describe, monitor, protect, and evaluate the quality of life experience among the old. From the gerontic nursing perspective, functional age, or the ability to perform activities of daily living, is a more essential measure of age than chronologic.

Research and Aging

Research and gerontologic knowledge are strongly influenced by federal bulletins that are distributed nationwide to indicate the type of research that is most likely to receive federal funding. In a very real way, the alzheimerization of aging has come about because, since the establishment of the National Institute on Aging (NIA) in 1971, the study of Alzheimer's disease has been awarded the largest share of research dollars for aging. Since the last edition of our textbook was published in 1994, there has been considerable reliable longitudinal research emerging that provides support for some commonly held beliefs regarding aging and refutes some others. The investigators of the Baltimore Longitudinal Studies of the Aged have been collecting data and periodically publishing findings for almost 30 years. These studies were initially restricted to males, but more recently studies of females have been included as well. The Harvard Women's Health Study has now accumulated more than 20 years of data regarding nurses' health. While not specifically focused on aging, quite obviously, the effects of such studies are becoming apparent. Several pharmaceutic companies in consort with universities are currently conducting long-range studies of medications and their potential for alleviating some of the problems that tend to develop in the aged, such as osteoporosis, benign prostatic hypertrophy, coronary artery ischemia, atherosclerosis, and the adverse effects of hormonal depletion. Alzheimer's disease remains a primary area of research concentration with a considerable focus on etiology, prevention, and medications that may halt or slow progress of the disease. Several publications abstract or summarize on an annual basis the major research investigations into aging. The National Institute on Aging, The National Center for Nursing Research, The National Institute of Mental Health, and the Agency for Health Care Policy and Research continue to make significant research contributions to our understanding of the aged. Some recent research focuses on the study of the subtle, progressive diseases that frequently accompany aging, such as hypertension and cardiovascular disease. Of particular interest is the study of noninsulin dependent diabetes mellitus (NIDDM). There is speculation that NIDDM represents a form of accelerated aging and thus may yield important information related to the aging process (USDHHS, 1990). Studies of older women have also assumed greater importance as the preponderance of the very old are females. Their special needs and capacities are slowly being recognized. The studies referred to here are too numerous to summarize, but a few of the interesting findings include those noted in Box 1-4. All of these studies are examples of findings that need further exploration and replication.

In this era quite specific and elegant research in aging is being pursued after several decades of excessive speculation and extrapolation. However, the measurement of anything specific must, by the nature of research methodology, be quite narrow and limited. Aside from study of the physiologic changes of aging measured longitudinally and demographic data, the meaning and experience of aging remains complex and elusive. Phenomenologic studies, therefore, will continue to be some of the richest and the most subject to variable interpretation. Also, in both quantitative and qualitative research the study of the ethnic aged is most

lacking. Federal statistics often include general categories of black and white but seldom more discrete statistics. Nevertheless, a comprehensive collection of data sources, much too extensive to include here, for research into the aged of racial and ethnic groups has been compiled by LaVeist (1995). We would encourage individuals who are interested in gerontology to investigate some of these rich sources.

The Politics of Aging

The actual development of gerontology has probably been more influenced by political expediency than by any other factor, but politics and economics are so intermeshed they can rarely be untangled. In the United States the first real interest in the aged emerged in the 1930s, when a population of aged persons, who were largely impoverished, became demographically significant. Under the Roosevelt administration and the National Recovery Act (NRA) in the mid-1930s, the United States began moving toward a socialistic political control that still persists today although it is often assailed by conservative policy makers. During the 1940s the study of aging was set aside to devote attention to the more pressing problems of national defense and developments in weaponry. However, interest in aging rose rapidly after World War II.

Box 1-4	Interesting Data from Research Studies on Aging

Survival after age 80 is related to adequate physical mobility and high hematocrit and cholesterol control, regardless of levels of other common risk factors (Dontas et al, 1996).

Individuals over 70 years of age who develop bacteremic urinary tract infections (UTI) are often initially diagnosed as having a chest infection. UTI in the elderly frequently presents with repiratory features and patient confusion, and the diagnosis is often delayed (Barkham, Martin, Eykyn, 1996).

The use of oral antidiabetic medication, diuretics, and analgesics is associated with increased daytime sleeping although nightime hypnotics are not associated with daytime sleeping (Asplund, 1996).

Lack of emotional support is a risk factor for mortality in elderly patients who have had a myocardial infarction (Berkman, Leo-Summers, Horwitz, 1992).

Painful and painless ischemic episodes have been found to have a circadian pattern with a peak incidence of ischemia in the early morning (Parmley et al, 1992).

Older women with noninsulin-dependent diabetes mellitus have better bone density than women with normal glucose tolerance (Barrett-Connor, Holbrook, 1992.)

An external hip protector may substantially reduce the risk of fracture, especially in elderly individuals with severe osteoporosis (Lauritzen, Petersen, Lund, 1992).

Today funding for social services is often tied to stringent governmental requirements. Although we hear about shifting the funding responsibility from federal agencies to state agencies, we have yet to see the full effects of this in action. One of the paradoxes that hinders the delivery of services to the aged in the United States is that America is both a capitalistic and a socialistic society, with health care moving rapidly into a highly competitive marketing mode. Therefore, life-sustaining services are now designed for profit although we simultaneously federally subsidize them. See Box 1-5 for a summary of important political developments in the field of aging.

The White House Conferences on Aging (WHCOA). The first WHCOA, in 1961, paved the way for the establishment of the Older Americans Act, the Administration on Aging, and the Medicare Program. Following the second WHCOA, the National Institute on Aging was established with Robert Butler as the first director. The commitment to sustain these programs sometimes seems tenuous although politicians are well aware of the strength of elders' votes. There have been and will continue to be necessary modifications to ensure the viability and continuation of the programs. During the 1995 WHCOA, there was considerable emphasis on the interdependence of the generations, and a large contingent of youthful delegates attended and interacted with the elders. In spite of problems of poor health and inadequate income that many elders still face, we must think in terms of the total population and the distribution of resources and services as equitably as possible. The late Maggie Kuhn, founder of the Gray Panthers, was an eloquent voice for the aged and the necessity of intergenerational support toward health and social services (Box 1-6).

Politicians are likely to enact laws that will accrue votes. The aged, although a large part of the voting population, are highly individualistic and as yet have not formed a political power block except on issues such as erosion of Social Security or reduction of Medicare and Medicaid. The timing of the greatest Congressional threats to these programs, concurrent with the 1995 WHCOA, demonstrated the strength of elders, their diverse opinions, and their collective power on certain issues.

In May of 1995, the Fourth White House Conference on Aging (WHCOA) was held in Washington, D.C., following hundreds of local, state, and regional miniconferences across the United States for the purpose of articulating the needs and desires of elders at the grass-roots level. It was the first WHCOA to be held by a Democratic President and the first to invite the public to suggest themes and agenda items. The conference concurred with the 60th anniversary of Social Security and was focused on four main issues:

- Ensuring comprehensive health care, including long term care
- Promoting economic security
- Increasing housing and supportive services
- Maximizing options for quality of life

Older Americans Act. The Older Americans Act (OAA), instituted following the 1961 White House Conference on Aging (WHCOA), established a vehicle for delivering community-based services through state Area Agencies on Aging (AAA). AAAs have some flexibility in services provided, but they generally include senior centers, nutrition sites, in-home services for frail elderly, elder abuse prevention programs, long-term care ombudsmen, employment services, legal assistance, preretirement counseling, health promotion, and respite care (National Academy of Aging, 1995). Federal appropriations and services have historically increased markedly each year as the numbers of aged have increased (Table 1-5). Now seniors fear that these may not continue. This was one of the major concerns expressed at the 1995 WHCOA. The current political agenda is to transfer much of the responsibility for provision of services to the states, cities, and to the individual. This could mean more individual autonomy in the future. At present the transferring of responsibility has increased the burdens of survival for the least able.

The Business of Aging

Aging is not only a phase of life, a philosophy, or an experience—it is big business. Major marketing attention has been extended to the aged as businesses grasp the market potential of the upcoming young-old. The American Society on Aging published an entire issue entitled "Marketing to the Aged" (ASA, 1995). Even the revered American Association of Retired Persons (AARP) is primarily designed to provide services, education, and conveniences to the well-heeled, well educated young-old, as evidenced by the recent foci of *Modern Maturity* issues. The AARP, relatively affluent, is beginning to gain recognition from many areas. They offer insurance for every purpose, travel and cruise packages, luxurious retirement facilities, and art objects all marketed to the anticipated tastes and needs of vital and prosperous elders. The revival of 1940s memorabilia, music, and nostalgia all reflect market trends that aim toward the active young-elders. In addition to a large market of well elders, there is an enormous market for those needing assistive devices, supplies, and equipment for managment of chronic disorders. *The Maturing Marketplace* is one example of a monthly newsletter providing tips for successfully targeting the elder market (Business Publishers, 1996). Atchley (1995) sees the business world beginning to create niches for gerontologists as they realize the benefits of their special skills as applied to marketing.

The Biomedicalization of Aging

"The medical aspects of aging have been studied since early civilization and have been given various names, such as *Gerocomica* and *Geroncomia.*" (Butler, 1995, p. 411). The term *geriatrics* was coined by an American physician, Ignatz Nascher, around 1900 because he recognized that the medical care of the aged involved special considerations, much as did the field of pediatrics. In fact, he saw many similarities.

Box 1-5	**Political Events Influencing Aging**

1935   Social Security Act signed by Franklin D. Roosevelt.

1937   National Institute of Health established first of the special institutes to study diseases common to older people.

1948   Hospital Construction and Facilities Act (Hill-Burton) provided funds for construction of long-term care facilities.

1950   First National Conference on Aging held in Washington, D.C.

1951   Federal Committee on Aging and Geriatrics created to coordinate Federal programs for the aging.

1952   First Federal-State Conference on Aging held in Washington.

1956   Special Staff on Aging established within U.S. Department of Health, Education, and Welfare. Federal Council on Aging replaced Intradepartmental Working Group on Aging.

1959   Senate subcommittee authorized to consider problems of the aged and aging. Federal Council on Aging reconstituted at Cabinet level.

1960   First appropriation passed for Section 202, Housing Act of 1959, authorizing direct loans for housing for the elderly.

1961   First White House Conference on Aging held in Washington. Senate Special Committee on Aging established as advocate for older Americans. First Annual Conference of State Executives held in Washington.

1962   Federal Council on Aging became President's Council on Aging.

1963   John F. Kennedy sent Congress the First Presidential message on elderly citizens; designated May as Senior Citizens Month. Special Staff on Aging became Office of Aging in HEW's new Welfare Administration.

1965   President Johnson signed Older Americans Act, creating Administration on Aging (AOA). Amendments to the Social Security Act established Medicare program. Foster Grandparent Program initiated by Office of Economic Opportunity and Administration on Aging.

1967   Age Discrimination in Employment Act brightened job outlook for Americans 40 to 65 years old.

1970   Older Americans White House Forums held across the nation to identify problems and issues for upcoming White House Conference on Aging.

1971   Second White House Conference on Aging held in Washington. Cabinet-level Domestic Council Committee on Aging created. ACTION—the Federal volunteer agency—established and given responsibility for senior volunteer programs previously administered by AOA.

1972   New act passed establishing Nutrition Program for the Elderly to be administered by AOA.

1973   Amendments to Older Americans Act called for State agencies on aging to establish area agencies on aging to plan for comprehensive, coordinated service delivery systems for older people at the local level.

Establishment of a National Clearinghouse on Aging and a Federal Council on the Aging with members appointed by the President. Amendments included a separate Older Americans Community Employment Act with responsibility for administering given to Department of Labor. Federal Aid Highway Act of 1973 provided funds for a demonstration program of public transportation in rural areas with an emphasis on the needs of the elderly and handicapped.

1974   Research on Aging Act established National Institute on Aging within National Institute of Health, Robert N. Butler appointed Director. Amendments to Urban Mass Transportation Act of 1964 made funds available to nonprofit private organizations and corporations for transportation vehicles and equipment for the elderly and handicapped. National Mass Transportation Act mandated reduced fares for the elderly and handicapped on all public transportation systems assisted by the Act.

1975   House of Representatives Special Committee on Aging established. Amendments to the Older Americans Act establish four new priority areas under Title IV:
a. Transportation
b. Home Services
c. Legal Services
d. Residential Repair and Renovation

1976   Title V of the Older Americans Act received an appropriation for the first time since inception of the Act in 1965. Five million dollars was appropriated "to pay part of the cost of acquisition, alteration, or renovation of community facilities that will serve as multipurpose Senior Centers."

1977   Title V re-funded at rate of $20 million annually.

1981   Third White House Conference on Aging held in Washington, D.C. Mandatory retirement laws revised.

1982   T. Franklin Williams appointed director of National Institute of Aging.

1983   Diagnostic Related Groups (DRGs) instituted by the Health Care Financing Administration to control costs of Medicare.

1984   Sexual discrimination in pension benefit payments outlawed by U.S. Supreme Court.

1988   Medicare Catastrophic Coverage Act.

1989   Medicare Catastrophic Coverage Act repealed.

1991   Fourth White House Conference on Aging stalled. AOA Funds cut drastically.

1992   Proposals from multiple sources for rescue of health care system.

1995   Fourth WHCOA. Focused on preservation of Medicare, Medicaid, Social Security, and The Older Americans Act (OAA).

1996   Majority of elders moved through Medicare changes to Managed Care Systems.

Box 1-6	History of the White House Conferences on Aging

1950 The National Conference on Aging, the precursor of the White House Conference on Aging, was called under the Truman Administration. It was followed by two Conferences of State Councils on Aging and Federal Agencies, one in 1952 and the other in 1956.

1958 Legislation calling for the first White House Conference on Aging (WHCOA) was introduced in Congress.

1961 Initiated by President Dwight Eisenhower, the first WHCOA focused on the problem of providing health care to the nation's older citizens. The eventual result was the Medicare program.

1971 By the time the second WHCOA took place, the Older Americans Act (OAA) had been enacted. The Conference examined ways of expanding social services and benefits for older people, including the nutrition program and transportation services.

1981 The third WHCOA took place. When the OAA was reauthorized that year, the emphasis was on developing supportive services that could help older people stay independent and in their own homes.

1991 The White House called for a WHCOA to take place in 1993, but the conference never materialized.

1992 Amendments to the OAA authorized the fourth WHCOA. In the legislation, Congress recommended that the conference's primary focus be on fostering public awareness of the interdependence of all generations.

1994 President Bill Clinton called for the fourth conference. Describing the conference as a way of "keeping faith with the senior citizens of this country," the President pledged that the Conference would take place no later than May of 1995.

1995 The fourth WHCOA took place on May 2 to 5. This conference was the first to focus on how to meet the challenges posed by the aging of the "baby boom" generation.

To understand being old, our society has emphasized medical interpretations of old age. Undoubtedly, concrete, measurable physical changes and disorders are easier to define than a concept of aging, but unfortunately such an approach ends up with a "characterization of aging as a debilitating condition of unknown etiology" (Hendricks, 1995, p. 51). Hendricks also emphasizes that this medicalization results in a large amount of social control being given over by the aged to the professions in exchange for some measure of solace and relief from discomfort. Estes and Binney (1989) have also been concerned about this perspective as the only parameter of the aging experience. Aging is increasingly seen as a biomedical problem that must be reversed, eradicated, or held at bay as long as possible. Therefore, the impact of disease, morbidity, and impending death on the quality of life and the experience of aging has provided the impetus for much of the study by gerontologists. In this way, aging has inevitably been seen through the distorted lens of disease. Nevertheless, it is difficult to study such a complex and elusive condition as "healthy aging" without looking at the physical manifestations of function and life-style. Chronic disorders, not amenable to cure but requiring long-term adaptation and management, have not been attractive to medicine or nursing until recently. However, we are finally recognizing that aging and disease are separate entities although frequent companions. One of the dilemmas is a lack of clear understanding of normal aging process. We may never know which changes occur over time because of assaults of the environment and which changes occur because the vital life centers are running out of resources. To complicate the picture, we do know that immunosenescence is a poorly understood factor but one that makes an individual more vulnerable to disease (Williams, 1992; USDHHS, 1990).

Disease vs. Age. There are three ways in which disease and aging intermingle: (1) there are diseases, such as atherosclerosis, which are common, progressive, and irreversible with age; (2) there are those that are more common but not inevitable in the aged, such as cancer; and (3) there are those not necessarily related to age, such as AIDS, that have an extraordinarily high mortality rate when experienced by the aged individual. For a disorder to be truly a factor of the aging process, it must be universal, progressive, and irreversible (Williams, 1992).

Forensics and Age. The effect of medicalization on the study of aging and on public perception has had a widespread influence. NIA funding priorities and RFPs (requests for proposals) have consistently favored the medically defined problems. Because NIA is the largest source of funding for the study of aging, its priorities will influence the selection of research and the nature of our understanding of the aging process. This trend toward medicalization in the study of aging has influenced the general public as well. The biomedical view of the "problem" of aging is reinforced on all sides. Because of this orientation, the old have become the target of anger and resentment. "They" are perceived as the cause of crises in the economy and outrageous medical costs. Unquestioning public acceptance of medical authority is at the root of this dilemma. Truly remarkable life-saving and life-lengthening medical interventions have made it a tempting proposition to give one's life over to the medical establishment. This trend is strengthened and perpetuated by

Table 1-5 OAA Appropriations ($ millions)

Program	Year							
	1966	1971	1973	1976	1981	1986	1991	1995
AOA and FCA	–	–	–	1	2	<1	<1	17
State and community programs								
Supportive services/centers	5	9	68	124	252	254	291	307
Nutrition	–	–	100	156	440	520	599	620
In-home services for frail elderly	–	–	–	–	–	–	7	7
Elder abuse prevention	–	–	–	–	–	–	3	5
Long-term care ombudsman	–	–	–	–	–	–	2	4
Other	–	4	12	26	23	–	–	20
Training, research	2	8	33	42	41	24	27	26
Community service employment	–	–	–	86	277	312	390	411
Native Americans	–	–	–	–	6	7	15	17
Total	7	21	213	436	1,040	1,117	1,334	1,432
Total adjusted for CPI	7	15	142	227	339	302	290	281

From Congressional Research Service and National Association of State Units on Aging

media reporting of remarkable breakthroughs in medicine (Estes, Binney, 1989). Estes and Binney warn that the pitfall of looking for medical solutions to the issues of living in the later years obliterates real concerns and diverts attention from the complex issues that shape these later years. Without a broader focus, we will, in fact, continue to look at this last, most precious, stage of life as nothing more than the playground of research into the biomedical mechanisms of survival at any cost (for example, the biomedical focus on disorders producing dementia such as Alzheimer's disease [Lyman, 1989]). This medicalization viewpoint focuses on the description of the abnormal and pathologic conditions, elements of somatic and organic changes, and precision of diagnosis. However, the real experience of dementing illness for caregivers and for the afflicted individual is a social tragedy that cannot in any way be completely comprehended within biomedical concepts of brain disease (Lyman, 1989).

The interrelationship between rapid decline during the aging process and certain diseases is clear but the mechanism for this relationship is obscure. The relationship between disease, meaning of disease, and behavior may have many variables as yet poorly understood.

Professionalization of Care for the Aged

In the three decades since the institution of Medicare, there has been colossal growth in gerontology as a science, pursuit, and professional specialty. In gerontology, mentoring has played a predominant role (Kastenbaum, 1995). Few students or professionals set out early on to be gerontology specialists. They entered the field most often by accident or because of opportunity. Federal dollars in support of research and research training attracted many to the field of aging. Some were motivated by elders whom they encountered in their personal lives. Often, in nursing, an early serendipitous experience with a physically debilitated or de-

pendent elder who had amazing fortitude and courage was the impression that fostered an interest in the field.

Accreditation. Many individuals have entered the field of aging without any particular professional preparation. At this juncture the issue of institutional accreditation and individual certification for gerontologic practice is being seriously debated. Many individuals and agencies are either strongly in favor of or against such a requirement. The argument against accreditation involves such issues as maintaining curricular flexibility, avoiding elitism or even protectionism, and the very serious charge that accreditation is based in self-interest of the professions as well as the accrediting bodies and tends to guarantee mediocrity because of its inflexibility (Johnson, 1995). It is also costly for an institution to be accredited. The argument for accreditation supports the belief that it would increase reliable quality care, consistency, and assurance that the individuals providing care are properly educated and qualified. Arguments for and against are summarized by Peterson (1995) (Box 1-7).

Underlying these arguments is a type of "compassionate ageism" (Liebig, 1995) or in the other extreme the belief that need, not age-based policies, should be the determinant of special care.

Certification. Certification is a means of ensuring the public that the certified individual has pursued some specialized study in a given area, has successfully demonstrated requisite knowledge, and has been awarded recognition of this achievement. However, although there are numerous groups and institutions that award certificates of achievement, there is no consistency in quality or meaning for this certification.

Medicine. The American Board of Medical Specialties, under the Boards of Family Medicine, Internal Medicine, and Psychiatry, has created a "Certificate in Added Qualifications in Geriatrics." Nearly 4000 physicians took the first

Box 1-7	Arguments For and Against Credentialing in Gerontology

Pro	Con
• Credentialing is the usual form of gaining acceptance and status by other professions • The more than 2 million persons working with the aged owe them assurance of educational preparation • The numbers of elders and proliferation of elder abuse require assurance of ethical behavior from service providers • There are currently 200 degree programs in gerontology; there is a need for assurance of minimal standards of quality in these programs	• Those with degrees in their field are already credentialed and dual credentialing would be costly • Many recognized professions are offering supplemental credentialing, and it soon may be available to all through the traditional professions • Risks to the public through noncredentialed gerontologists is small as all have ethical guidelines within their profession • Practitioners need a degree in an established field because a gerontology degree does not provide the skills needed for practice

certifying examinations, which were given in Spring, 1988. Successful completion allowed them to legitimately claim a subspeciality in geriatrics within their primary specialty (*AGS Newsletter,* 1996; McRae, 1995; Reuben et al, 1994). Although this is encouraging, the number of physicians who are interested and qualified in geriatrics is still far too few. As these are subspecialists, it is not known exactly how many are certified overall or only claim geriatrics as their primary specialty.

Social work. Social workers remain, after decades of practice, polarized regarding the importance of accreditation through the Council of Social Work Education (CSWE) (Lubben, 1995). Some find it costly and draining on time and energy they feel could be better used. The National Association of Social Workers (NASW) administers the Academy of Certified Social Workers (ACSW) credentialing. Many feel that state licensure should be sufficient evidence of expertise. As yet there is no gerontology accrediting body or credentialing available to social workers within their own profession.

Nursing. Although most working nurses are involved in the care of the aged in some manner, there are only 11,081 gerontological nurses certified by the ANA (Adrienne Perry, Certification Division, American Nurses' Association, 9/16/96). In addition there are several thousand advance practice nurses specializing in the care of the aged who are certified as Geriatric Nurse Practitioners, Adult Nurse Practitioners, Family Nurse Practitioners, and Clinical Nurse Specialists.

Unfortunately, nursing educational programs, after 30 years of dabbling with gerontology, may still receive accreditation with only a small part of their curriculum dealing with geriatrics. Lubben (1995, p. 33) states, "the major mission of either accreditation or credentialing should be that of enhancing the status of elderly people and not merely enhancing the status of a new discipline or profession." We believe we owe our elders the best. But (just as Topol said in *Fiddler on the Roof,* "On the other hand . . .") we do believe

certification tends to emphasize profession, territory, and overlapping functions rather than team work, which seems so critical today.

DEVELOPMENT OF GERONTIC NURSING

As early as 1904 the *American Journal of Nursing* published an article on old age and disease. By the 1920s a few visionary nurses called for the development of gerontologic nursing practice as they recognized that a body of nursing knowledge and skills related to nursing care for older persons was distinguishable within the full scope of nursing practice. These nurses also recognized that institutional settings such as old age homes or boardinghouses—all predecessors of today's nursing homes—were settings in which nurses could best provide home-like nursing services for older persons who did not need the acute care services of a hospital. The best of these were truly homes. However, it was not until 1966 that the ANA formed a Division of Geriatric Nursing and in 1970 developed the Standards of Geriatric Nursing Practice. In 1976 the Division of Geriatric Nursing changed its name to the Gerontological Nursing Division to reflect the broad role nurses play in the management of the elderly. In 1984 The Council of Gerontological Nursing was formed and certification in the specialty became available (Box 1-8).

Introduction to the Gerontic Nurse Pioneers

The foundation of gerontic nursing as we know it today was largely built by a small cadre of nurse-explorers between 30 and 40 years ago. Gerontic nursing was defined and shaped by these few nurse-pioneers who saw, early on, that the aged individual had special needs and required the most subtle, holistic, and complex nursing care. Many of these leaders are still available to us to bring the present into focus on the historic continuum.

These gerontic nurse pioneers presented seminal thought and investigated new ideas related to the care of the aged, re-

Box 1-8	**Professionalization of Gerontic Nursing**

1904	First article published in *American Journal of Nursing* (AJN) on care of the aged		ANA Council of Long Term Care Nurses established, group first chaired by Ella Kick
1925	AJN considers geriatric nursing as a possible specialty in nursing	1980	*Geriatric Nursing* first published by AJN; Cynthia Kelly, editor
1950	Newton and Anderson publish first geriatric nursing textbook	1981	ANA Division of Gerontological Nursing issues statement regarding scope of practice
	Geriatrics becomes a specialization in nursing	1983	Florence Cellar Endowed Gerontological Nursing Chair established at Case Western Reserve
1962	ANA forms a national geriatric nursing group		University, first in the nation; Doreen Norton first
1966	ANA creates the Division of Geriatric Nursing		scholar to occupy chair
1970	ANA establishes Standards of Practice for Geriatric Nursing; Committee chaired by Dorothy Moses, included Lois Knowles and Mary Shaunnessey	1984	National Gerontological Nurses Association established
1973	Revised Standards of Practice for Geriatric Nursing		Division of Gerontological Nursing Practice becomes Council on Gerontological Nursing (councils established for all practice specialties)
1974	Certification in geriatric nursing practice offered through ANA; process implemented by Laurie Gunter and Virginia Stone	1986	ANA publishes Survey of Gerontological Nurses in Clinical Practice
1975	*Journal of Gerontological Nursing* published by Slack; first editor, Edna Stilwell	1987	ANA revises and issues *Standards and Scope of Gerontological Nursing Practice*
1976	ANA renames Geriatric Division, "Gerontological"	1989	ANA certifies Gerontological Clinical Nurse Specialists
	ANA publishes Standards for Gerontological Nursing Practice, committee chaired by Barbara Allen Davis	1990	ANA establishes a Division of Long Term Care within the Council of Gerontological Nursing
	ANA begins certifying Geriatric Nurse Practitioners	1992	ANA redefines long term care to include life span approach
	Nursing and the Aged edited by Burnside and published by McGraw-Hill	1994	ANA forms strong Political Action Committee (ANPAC)
1977	First Gerontological Nursing Tract funded by Division of Nursing and established by Sr. Rose Therese Bahr at University of Kansas School of Nursing	1996	ANA officials advise President Clinton regarding Health Care Reforms
1979	*Education for Gerontic Nursing* written by Gunter and Estes; suggested curricula for all levels of nursing education		ANA celebrates centennial in Washington DC; President Clinton gives keynote address

futed mythical tales and fantasies of aging, and found realities through investigation, clinical observation, practice, and documentation; setting under way activities that markedly influenced the course of the aging experience.

These individuals saw new possibilities and a better future for the aged. When interviewed, most were quite matter-of-fact and had not thought of themselves as pioneers. "It was there to be done." "Someone needed to do it." "Well, I wouldn't say I was really a pioneer . . . have you spoken to . . . ?" They saw something that others had not seen before, but because it was self-evident to them it did not seem at all remarkable. One said, "You asked why I established the (gerontology academic) chair and I haven't yet given you a precise answer; I must give that some more thought." Some demonstrated a very personal connection to the aged that involved a certain view of humanity from a more universal and/or spiritual perspective than is commonly held; a stark awareness of the interdependence of generations and individuals. Many of these individuals are

now approaching old age and have been able to add their personal as well as professional perspectives to the field. With humor, grace, and dignity they tell what old age means to them. Who were these individuals that paved the way to the future of gerontic care? There are many to whom we owe the origins of gerontic nursing as a specialty, many unnamed or presently unrecognized. To name only a few and some of their outstanding accomplishments: Sr. Rose Therese Bahr (vitally involved in the development of the National Gerontological Nurses Association); Terri Brower (generated gerontology curriculum and other relevant research); Irene Burnside (mentored numerous nurses interested in geriatric nursing); Florence Cellar (donated funds to establish first gerontologic nursing chair in the nation); Barbara Allen Davis (generated gerontologic interest and foci at American Nurses' Association); Laurie Gunter (established gerontologic certification requirements at ANA); Mary Harper (developed dynamic programs for aged veterans; instrumental in guiding development of geropsychiatric programs);

We need to remind ourselves constantly that the purpose of gerontic nursing is to prevent untimely death and needless suffering, always with the focus of doing with as well as doing for, and in every instance to attempt to preserve personhood as long as life continues. (Doris Schwartz)

Aging individuals are persons, not burdens or problems, and nurses can be educated to a more positive attitude about the older adult and can aid in implementation of professional behaviors to upgrade care of older citizens in America. (Sr. Rose Therese Bahr)

What a fortunate teenager I was!! On September 15, 1946, when I was almost 16, I took a job in a small (25 beds) hospital in a small Ohio community. I was always assigned to the older patients because we got along so well. (Ella Kick)

There is always an interesting person there, sometimes locked in the cage of age. I think I have helped at least a few of my students with this approach, "You see me as I am now, but I see myself as I've always been and all the things I've been—not just an old lady." (Bernita Steffl)

I am less fearful of medical afflictions that befall me in my old age than I am of the system and the professionals to whom my care may be entrusted. (Bernita Steffl)

Among the first lessons that I learned from working with older patients was of patience and perseverance. I found that if they were treated as normal human beings and one took the time to talk to them, and above all listen to what they had to say, they responded normally. (Dorothy Moses)

I believe that one of the most valuable lessons I have learned from those who are older is that I must start with looking inside at my own thinking. I was very guilty of ageism. I believed every myth in the book, was sure that I would never live past my seventieth birthday, and made no plan for my seventies. Probably the most productive years of my career have been since that dreaded birthday, and I now realize that it is very difficult, if not impossible, to think of our own aging. (Mary Opal Wolanin)

I am opposed to anyone going into the field of geriatric nursing until she has experienced the human condition at many points—vicariously through literature and our culture or by close observation. This field demands maturity since recognizing the diversity of aging people is very important in caring for the elderly during acute illness, chronic illness, and wellness. We need a broad knowledge base and a broader mind. (Mary Opal Wolanin)

Cynthia Kelly (first editor of Geriatric Nursing Journal); Ella Kick (developed humanistic care strategies in long term care); Lois Knowles (instrumental in developing first geriatric nursing standards); Barbara Lee (sponsored development of geriatric nurse practitioner programs through Kellogg Foundation funding); Mathy Mezey (Director of the National Teaching Nursing Home Project); Dorothy Moses (developed first gerontology radio/television programs for lay public); Sr. Marilyn Schwab (conceived, developed, and administered national model nursing home); Doris Schwartz (co-authored first textbook related to geriatric nursing care; developed interdisciplinary alliances); Eldonna Shields-Kyle (created staff development curricula for nursing homes); Bernita Steffl (political advocate for aged in Arizona; contributed to understanding of sexuality and aging); Edna Stilwell (editor of *Journal of Gerontological Nursing*); Virginia Stone (developed first graduate program in gerontological nursing); Thelma Wells (numerous research projects and publications relevant to understanding the aged; particular expertise in study of urinary incontinence); and Mary Opal Wolanin (research, mentorship, and seminal work in understanding confusion and aging). Some characteristics apparent in this select group of women are independence and innovation, interpersonal investment, persistence, practicality, assertiveness, strong will, and ability to earn the respect of others both within and outside of nursing profession (Box 1-9).

Mary Opal Wolanin particularly remembers the "pneumonia nurse" as one of the first in the genre of the geriatric nurse (interview, San Antonio, September 1995). These nurses, by sheer nursing skill and devoted care, literally held the life of the pneumonia-stricken elder in their hands. This was in the days before penicillin . . . much less third and fourth generation antibiotics. We are presently relearning respect for the virulence, morbidity, and mortality of many diseases we thought had all but disappeared. We will continue to need pioneering nurses, who can find new and better ways to care for the aged and the young and who can facilitate self-care in the most efficacious manner.

Both practitioners and educators are remiss in developing geriatric knowledge and practice expertise, seemingly finding it difficult to move away from the mother-child-nurse triad that occupied much of nursing attention for the first three-quarters of this century. Although nursing educators have rarely given gerontic care the emphasis in the curriculum that the realities of nursing impose, there has been some progress. In undergraduate nursing, gerontic care is often woven into a "life-span" or "family nursing" course (Morrisey, 1995). (Chapter 28 deals with nursing roles and education for the care of the aged.)

THE FUTURE OF AGING IN THE UNITED STATES

Aging baby boomers will carry their particular energies and expectations into old age and will change the face of aging in America. We have accumulated numerous predictions about their aging. Articles about menopause proliferate, mid-life crises abound, and anxiety about the future is rampant. Will there be income support, adequate retirement, available health care, disability benefits, and all the things the present generation of the old have relied on? There is every reason to believe there will be (Kingson, Quadagno, 1995). The AARP (*Modern Maturity,* Jan/Feb, 1996) recently devoted an entire issue to them. At present the major concerns of Baby Boomers are health, finances, job security, children, and parents. They are the "sandwich generation," trying to meet the needs of college-age children and elderly parents. Some express distrust in the government. Gerontologists, marketing strategists, and the age industry are preparing for the anticipated challenges (Wylde, 1995).

It is predicted that the last member of the celebrated baby boom cohort will die around the year 2080 (National Academy On Aging, 1995), and more than 1.5 million of them will live to reach 100 years of age. There is no typical baby boomer. While it has been fashionable to consider the baby boomers en masse, they are extremely diverse, differing by as much as 19 birth years, separated by race, culture, and socioeconomic status. In order to plan well for their retirement years, we must consider:

- Their diversity
- The uncertain political and economic future
- Potential major shifts in lifestyle expectations
- Radical differences in health care delivery systems
- Progress in technology and medical management of some disorders
- Shifts in values and ethics that will profoundly affect daily life

An AARP study found the fifth decade the most turbulent (AARP, 1996). During that period there are five distinct groups that have special needs:

- The "Continuing Caregivers," responsible for selves, children, and aging parents
- The "Second Chancers," divorced, remarried, and with new families
- The "New Me," survivors of major crises and re-prioritizing life goals
- The "Free Birds," few family obligations and more time
- The "First Families," late starters

The parents of these Baby Boomers continue to plan for their needs in a generational reciprocity. The greatest transfer of assets in history is taking place right now, from elders to their middle-aged children. Those elders in their lifetime have experienced real economic panic and deprivation, and most have saved earnestly to pass something on to their children (Hudson, 1995). Children of the 1940s and 1950s, the golden children, have increasingly had to face the issues of aging parents and are strongly aware of the need for redirection of a system that, for all its extravagances, is not serving them or their parents well.

These adult children are of increasing significance in gerontology. This segment of the population is characterized by its affluence, relative good health, and vitality. The most potent influences on their development are the almost universal opportunities for higher education, inflationary economics, political participation, urban and suburban lifestyles, assimilation of myriad cultures into the mainstream of American life, technologic innovations, youth-centered family life, and now the increasing responsibility for elderly parents. Migratory tendencies and travel opportunities throughout their working lives have led to sophistication and a world focus.

These space-age children can only wonder what the future holds for their own later years. They seem more concerned about healthful life-styles than previous generations, are better educated, have higher expectations of themselves (and others), and are forming the core of the "moral majority." Although formal religion seems to have been supplanted by a sense of personal responsibility, many have sought leadership or inspiration among gurus, charismatic personalities, cults, and mystics.

There remain many uncertainties about the conditions, status, and benefits baby boomers will experience. One of the major concerns is based in the shift of life-styles away from the traditional family. Single parents, blended families, limited parenthood, unmarried parents, and gay parents all represent life-styles that may or may not produce children willing or available to assist parents as they age (Cornman, Kingson, 1996). Yet, in the middle of the 20th century, there was much concern about the break-up of the extended family (Hashimoto, 1993); however, this has not deterred adult children from caring for their elderly parents.

WHAT ARE WE MAKING OF AGING?

Cole (1995) asks, "What have we made of aging?" He contends that visual, symbolic images of aging have much to do with how we conceive the possibilities and problems of the aged. The "sandwich" provides a clear picture of the dilemma of the middle aged. The "machine" conveys how elders suffer wear and tear, even to the analogy of oil in the joints drying up. Often the life course is seen as a "race" that the individual is trying to win or as a "river" that ultimately brings the elder back to the source of all life. The "over the hill" image has been a popular one for decades and is still held by some. If the hill we visualize is somewhat like a bell curve, then attaining the peak of everything good occurs at age 38. "Stages of life" provide a picture of sequential steps toward goodness, wisdom, heaven, or whatever one believes must be achieved in a progressive manner. In all of these symbolic images, there is a model or some type of trajectory that shapes our thoughts (Cirillo, 1993). Literature, theater, and the media contribute to these images (Holstein, 1994). Cole (1995) not only asks what we have made of aging but where we are going now.

In the past, religious as well as secular movements have affected the way individuals viewed aging. Puritans thought the process of aging was a sacred pilgrimage to God and as such the righteous aged were revered. During the Victorian age it was believed that youth was the symbol of growth and expansion. Later, when the need to provide for an expanding population became more pressing, youthful energy, westward migration, and enormous material progress made the aged seem out of touch, and they were viewed with sentimental indulgence. Independence, individual enterprise, and the passion for material wealth characterized the citizens in Jacksonian America, just as wealth, a healthy old age was viewed as needing to be earned by self-care and self-discipline (Cole, 1992). However, the traditions of the elders seemed cumbersome and a hindrance to progress. In the scientific search for longevity, it was thought for awhile that mountain-climbing tribes high in the Andes and the Georgian alps held the secret, lending a picture of reaching ever upward. Now space rockets silhouetted against the sky before launch represent not only phallic symbols of generativity but emblems of our belief in our potential for an ever-expanding universe of possibilities throughout the life course. There seem to be infinite variations on the metaphors of aging throughout the world. What we make of aging, it seems, depends on how we see it. Bernice Neugarten, the foremost gerontologic theorist and editor of the first comprehensive theoretic text, *Middle Age and Aging,* published by the University of Chicago Press in 1968, has recently predicted that we are rapidly moving into an age-irrelevant society.

KEY CONCEPTS

- Although the population as a whole is aging, the greatest categorical increase by group percentage is occurring among those 85 years old and over.
- Old age must be studied as a complex phenomenon with biopsychosocial and spiritual aspects affecting the manner in which an individual ages.
- Each aged cohort is in some ways distinctly different from others, and individual aged persons become more unique the longer they live. Thus one must be careful in attributing any specific characteristics to "old age."
- Normal old age cannot be easily measured as compared to young or middle adulthood.

- It is expected that as the majority of baby boomers become categorically old, in about the year 2010, there will be many changes in the experience of aging in the United States.
- The serious study of gerontology in the United States is comparatively new, with serious study and research going back only about 35 years.
- Centenarians are increasing rapidly, and the study of their lives holds fascination for many scientists and lay persons.
- Political actions and appropriations have had far-reaching influence on the individual experience of aging, chiefly through Medicare, Medicaid, and Social Security.
- With the advance of medical science, there has been a tendency to prolong the lives of the old and to consider their medical needs predominant.
- Nursing has led the field in gerontology because nurses were the first professionals in the nation to be certified as geriatric specialists.

▲ CASE STUDY

Karen began to be aware of her own aging just as she approached menopause. At 47, she occasionally felt stiffness in her joints in the morning on arising. She found herself wishing her grown children would leave the nest, which they showed little inclination to do. Her husband was concerned about his job security as there were numerous companies "downsizing." Karen realized she was depressed and yet continued in the same pattern as she had for a number of years: work as office manager for a small firm 40 hours each week, go to the gym two nights each week after work to exercise, clean house on Saturday, loll about on Sunday and perhaps work in her garden. Then she began to worry about her widowed mother as she saw some of her friends overwhelmed with caretaking responsibilities for parents and adult children. There seemed no end in sight. She was beginning to look forward to a time when she could retire but realistically knew that was a long way off. She became aware that her life offered little adventure and had become routine; that she was rapidly entering the ranks of the "older Americans." She read numerous ads about hormone replacement therapy for older women. She questioned herself—was she fearful of aging? What was it she feared? What did she want from the remainder of her life? Alarmed,

▲ Needs Addressed and Task Strengths	

Need to learn and understand; need for intellectual stimulation (to maintain self-esteem and the sense of belonging)	Experience with aged people in various situations
	   Varieties of friends
	   Ability to communicate well across generations
	   Open and accepting of others

she realized she was thinking of "remainder" rather than "future." She found herself saying, "Is this all there is? Is life just one day after another filled with small and large problems?" "Is there anything I should be doing in preparation for my old age?"

Based upon the case study, develop a nursing care plan using the following procedures:

List comments of client that provide *subjective data*.

List information that provides *objective data*. From these data identify and state, using accepted format, *two nursing diagnoses* you determine are most significant to this client at this time.

List two of Karen's strengths.

Determine and state *outcome criteria* for each diagnosis. These must reflect some alleviation of the problem identified in the nursing diagnosis and must be stated in concrete and measurable terms.

Plan and state one or more *interventions* for each diagnosed problem. Provide specific documentation of source used to determine appropriate intervention. Incorporate Karen's strengths into at least one intervention.

Evaluate success of intervention. Interventions must correlate directly with the stated outcome criteria in order to measure the outcome success.

STUDY QUESTIONS/ACTIVITIES

What do you think are the triggering events that have increased your interest in aging persons?

Name five beliefs you have that are based on your experience with aging people. Discuss these and locate references within the text that either support or refute your belief.

*Students are advised to refer to their nursing diagnosis text and identify possible or potential problems.

What are some of the sociocultural factors that have influenced our present views of the aged?

How has the history of aging influenced our present concerns about aging?

Discuss the meaning and the thoughts triggered by the viewpoints expressed at the beginning of the chapter. How do these vary from your own experience?

SUGGESTED ACTIVITIES

Write an essay about getting old, illustrated with drawings of self at ages 50, 65, 75, and 90. Discuss thoughts and feelings generated.

Participate in *Into Aging: a Simulation Game* available from: Charles B. Slack, Inc., Thorofare, NJ 08086

Develop a collage depicting themes of aging.

Explore literature and identify attitudes toward aging as conveyed.

Make your own audiotapes of a centenarian's memories.

Carefully examine the photograph of an unknown elder. Make up a story about him or her.

Write an essay about the most remarkable elder you have known.

RESEARCH QUESTIONS

Are the changing attitudes toward the aged related in any specific way to ratios of workers vs dependents in society?

At what age or in which circumstances are individuals most likely to begin considering their own aging?

What are the most frequently held assumptions related to the experience of aging?

What effect has the changing intergenerational structure had on attitudes toward aging?

RESOURCES

Name and Address	*Type of Service/Goals/Comments*

AGING

American Society on Aging 833 Market Street San Francisco, CA 94103	To enhance well-being of older individuals, foster unity among those working with the elderly.
Gray Panthers 1424 16th Street, N.W., Suite 602 Washington, D.C. 20036	Consciousness-raising activist group of older adults and young people. Aim: to combat ageism.
National Council on Aging 409 3rd Street, S.W. Washington, D.C. 20024	Cooperates with other organizations to promote concern for older people. National information and consulting center.
National Association of Area Agencies on Aging 1112 16th Street, N.W. Washington, D.C. 20024	Established under provisions of the Older Americans Act. Promotes realistic/reasonable national policy on aging and advocates for needs of older persons at national level.

RESOURCES—cont'd

Name and Address	*Type of Service/Goals/Comments*

AGING

National Center on Rural Aging
c/o National Council on the Aging
409 3rd Street, N.W.
Washington, D.C. 20024

See National Council on Aging.

From Daniels, PK, Schwartz, CA, editors: *Encyclopedia of associations,* ed 28, Detroit, 1995, Gale Research.

GAMES FOR SENSITIVITY TRAINING

The *Road of Life* is a stimulating game board requiring 25 minutes to play that develops awareness of some of the common psychosocial and physical experiences of the elderly.

Write NURSECO, 984 Monument Ave, PO Box 145, Pacific Palisades, CA 90272.

Sex and Aging: A Game of Awareness and Interaction is a game of situations frequently encountered in sexual relationships of the aged. Cost is $18.

Write OREGON STATE UNIVERSITY, Extension Service Stock Room, Ballard Hall, Corvallis, OR 97331, (503)737-4131.

Families and Aging is a simulation game of general problems that families face as they deal with aging parents. Cost is $20.

Write OREGON STATE UNIVERSITY, Extension Service Stock Room, Ballard Hall, Corvallis, OR 97331, (503)737-4131.

Into Aging: Understanding Issues Affecting the Later Stages of Life is played with sets of colorful "Life Event" cards designed to help others experience the daily struggles of the aged.

Write SLACK, Inc., 6900 Grove Rd, Thorofare, NJ 08086, (609)848-1000.

There are several *ELDERGAMES* available. In all cases the intent is to stimulate memory, interaction, and discussion. Players are encouraged to express emotion and wander far from the original question if they wish. Games are of simle but durable construction, are easily printed, and range in price from $6 to $15.

Write ELDERGAMES, 11710 Hunters Lane, Rockville, MD 20852, (301)881-8433.

Generations is a game designed for intergenerational sharing of life experience. Cost is $24.

Write Generations, Inc., PO Box 41069, St Louis, MO 63141.

Communication is a board game to increase interaction and communication skills. Cost is $20.

Write NASCO, Fort Atkinson, WI 53538, (414)563-2446.

REFERENCES

AARP News Release: *Modern Maturity* study finds fifties the most turbulent decade in life: five distinct profiles explode myths long held by marketers, Washington, DC, 1995, American Association of Retired Persons.

AARP: *A profile of older Americans,* Washington D.C., 1996, American Association of Retired Persons.

Adamchak DJ: Demographic aging in the industrialized world: a rising burden, *Generations* 17(4):6-9, 1993.

American Geriatric Society Newsletter: Member response to the AGS membership survey, *AGS Newsletter* 25(2):3-4, 1996.

American Nurses Association: Certification Division, ANA, Washington, DC, 1996.

American Society on Aging: What it means to be a professional in the field of aging, *Generations* XIX(2):whole issue, 1995. (a)

American Society on Aging: Centenarian research: the fountain of data, *Aging Today,* 16(2):1,6, 1995. (b)

Asplund R: Daytime sleepiness and napping amongst the elderly in relation to somatic health and medical treatment, *J Inter Med* 239(3):261-267, 1996.

Atchley RC: Gerontology and business: getting the right people for the job, *Generations* 19(2):42-45, 1995.

Barkham TMS, Martin FC, Eykyn SJ: Delay in the diagnosis of bacteraemic urinary tract infection in elderly patients, *Age Ageing* 25(2):130-132, 1996.

Barrett A: On 121st birthday, she's the world's oldest rapper, World, *San Francisco Chronicle,* A6, February 22, 1996.

Barrett-Connor E, Holbrook TL: Sex differences in osteoporosis in older adults with non-insulin-dependent diabetes mellitus, *JAMA* 268:3333-3337, 1992.

Beard BB: *Social competence of centenarians,* Athens, Ga., 1967, University of Georgia Press.

Bell J: The search of a discourse on aging: the elderly on television, *Gerontologist* 32(3):305, 1992.

Berkman LF, Leo-Summers L, Horwitz RI: Emotional support and survival after myocardial infarction: a prospective, population based study of the elderly, *Ann Intern Med* 117:1003-1009, 1992.

Buffum MD, Wolfe NS: Post-traumatic stress disorder and the World War II veteran, *Geriatric Nurs* 16(6):264-271, 1995.

Business Publishers: *The maturing marketplace. A monthly newsletter,* Silverspring, Md, 1996, Business Publishers, Inc. 1996.

Butler RN: Foreword to second edition. In Cassel CK et al, editors: *Geriatric medicine,* ed 2, New York, 1990, Springer-Verlag.

Butler R: Geriatrics. In GL Maddox, editor: *The encyclopedia of aging,* New York, 1995, Springer.

Cirillo L: Verbal imagery of aging in the news magazines, *Generations* 17(2):91-93, 1993.

Cole TR: *The journey of life: a cultural history of aging in America,* Cambridge, 1992, Cambridge University Press.

Cole TR: What have we "made" of aging? *J Gerontol;* 50B(6):S341-S343, 1995.

Connelly JR: The time for accreditation has come, *Generations* 19(2):25-27, 1995.

Cornman JM, Kingson ER: Trends, issues, perspectives, and values for the aging of the baby boom cohorts, *Gerontologist* 1996;36(1):15-26.

Crosby AW: *America's forgotten pandemic: the influenza of 1918,* Cambridge, 1989, Cambridge University Press.

Davies B: Caring for the frail elderly: an international perspective, *Generations* 17(4):51-54, 1993.

Dontas AS et al: Survival in the oldest old: death risk factors in old and very old subjects, *J Aging Health* 8(2):220-237, 1996.

Douglass EB: Too many doing too little for too few, *Generations* 19(2):35-36, 1995.

Estes C, Binney E: The biomedicalization of aging: dangers and dilemmas, *Gerontologist* 29(5):587, 1989.

Ferraro KF: Cohort changes in images of older adults, 1974-1981, *Gerontologist* 32(3):296-304, 1992.

Franceschi C et al: The immunology of exceptional individuals: the lesson of centenarians, *Immun Today* 16(1):12-16, 1995.

Georges C: Aging is big business, *San Francisco Chronicle,* July 12:8, 1992.

Goldsmith R, Heiens R: Subjective age: a test of five hypotheses, *Gerontologist* 32(3):312, 1992.

Hashimoto A: Family relations in later life: a cross-cultural perspective, *Generations* 17(4):24-26, 1993.

Heinemann GD: In geriatrics, the team approach, *Generations* 19(2):20-22, 1995.

Hendricks J: The social power of professional knowledge in aging, *Generations* 19(2):51-53, 1995.

Holstein M: Taking next steps: gerontological education, research and the literary imagination, *Gerontologist* 34(6):822-827, 1994.

Hudson RB: Giving and getting in contemporary America: the place of age and generation, *Public Policy Aging Report* 7(2):1,9, 1996.

Johnson HR: The foibles and follies of gerontological imperialists, *Generations* 19(2):23-24, 1995.

Kaiser MA: The productive roles of older people in developing countries, *Generations* 17(4):65-59, 1993.

Kastenbaum: Who we are and how we got here, *Generations* 19(2):9-15, 1995.

Kaufman SR: Reflections on the 'ageless self,' *Generations* 17(2):13-16, 1993.

Kingson E, Quadango J: Social security: marketing radical reform, *Generations* 19(3):43-49, 1995.

Lauritzen JB, Petersen MM, Lund B: Effect of external hip protectors on hip fractures, *Lancet* 341:11-13, 1993.

LaVeist TA: Data sources for aging research on racial and ethnic groups, *Gerontologist* 35(3):328-338, 1995.

Liebig PS: Social policy and professional identity, *Generations* 19(2):39-42, 1995.

Lubben J. Claiming boundaries: a reaction to the debate, *Generations* XIX(2):31-32, 1995.

Lyman K: Bringing the social back in: a critique of the biomedicalization of dementia, *Gerontologist* 29(5):597, 1989.

Maslow A: *Maturation and personality,* ed 2, New York, 1970, Harper & Row.

McRae T: Geriatrics as a career, *Generations* 19(2):10-11, 1995.

Merriam SB et al: Centenarians: their memories and future ambitions, *Intl J Aging Hum Dev* 41(2):117-132, 1995.

Modern Maturity: *Boomers: the babies face fifty, entire issue focus,* Washington, DC, 1996, American Association of Retired Persons.

Morrisey S: In nursing, a study in contradictions, *Generations* 19(2):18-20, 1995.

National Academy On Aging: What do people want to know about population aging? *Public Policy Aging Report* 7(1):11, 1995.

National Academy on Aging: Facts on The Older Americans Act, *Gerontology News,* Washington, DC, National Academy on Aging, 7(5):14, 1996.

Parade Magazine. Who is old? *San Francisco Sunday Chronicle,* January 21, 1996.

Parmlee WW et al: Attenuation of the circadian patterns of myocardial ischemia with nifedipine GITS in patients with chronic stable angina, *J Am Coll Cardiol* 19:1380-1389, 1992.

Perls TT, Wood ER: Acute care costs of the oldest old: they cost less, their care intensity is less, and they go to nonteaching hospitals, *Arch Intern Med* 156(7):754-760, 1996.

Peterson DA: Professionals in the field of aging should be credentialed, *Generations* XIX(2):28-30, 1995.

Pinchera A et al: Thyroid autoantibodies and the immune system, *Hormone Research* 43(1-3):64-68, 1995.

Poon LW et al: Biomarkers of aging, *Generations* 16(4):11-14, 1992.

Reuben DB et al: Is geriatrics a primary care or subspecialty discipline? *J Am Geriatr Soc* 42:363-367, 1994.

San Francisco Examiner: Obituaries. Tane Ikai: Japan's oldest person, *San Francisco Examiner.* July 13, 1995:12b.

Theilman SB: The Georgia centenarian study, *Intl J Aging Human Develop* 34(1):1-17, 1992.

U.S. Bureau of the Census: *Statistical abstract of the United States: 1995,* 115th ed, Washington DC, 1995, US Government Printing Office.

U.S. Department of Commerce, *Global aging,* Economics and Statistics Administration, Bureau of the Census, Washington, DC, Government Printing Office, 1992.

U.S. Department of Health and Human Services: *National Institute on Aging: global aging,* National Institutes of Health, Public Health Service, Bethesda, MD, 1992, Government Printing Office.

U.S. Department of Health and Human Services: *National Institute on Aging: special report on aging 1990,* National Institutes of Health, Public Health Service, Bethesda, 1990, Government Printing Office.

Williams TF: Aging versus disease, *Generations* 16(4):21-26, 1992.

Wolanin MO: Personal communication, San Antonio, Texas, 1995.

Wondolowski C, Davis D: *The lived experience of health in the oldest old: a phenomenological study,* unpublished paper, Cleveland, 1988, Case Western Reserve University.

Wylde MA: How to size up the current and future markets: technology and the older adult, *Generations* 19(1):15-19, 1995.

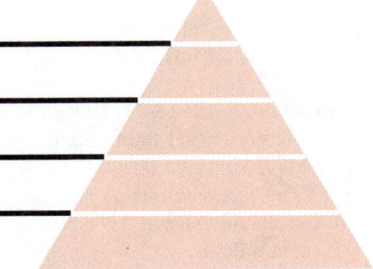

CHAPTER 2

Theories of Aging

A student learns   **Due to the fact that some periods of life are set apart by certain events, it is generally assumed that a period labeled "Old Age" begins with a definite entrance at a certain year or following some outward event which manifests its beginning. However, unless there is a sudden onset of one of the chronic bodily disorders associated with age, we cannot detect an external symbol of entrance into old age.**

Tatyana Urisman, age 30

Elders speak   **Prevention of problems can increase longevity to some degree, but I believe the aging process is genetically passed on as related to the particular genus and species. Being active both socially, through volunteering and organizations, and physically are important. One's peace of mind and ability to accept things as they are has a great deal to do with the progression of the aging process.**

Mary Maguering, age over 70

When I was a young girl Einstein was proposing the molecular theory of matter, and we still believed there were some truths that were beyond dispute. We had never heard of DNA or RNA and only knew of genes in the most rudimentary theoretical sense. Now truth is the greatest of all the theories of relativity, and I hear that scientists believe there is a gene that is controlling my life span. I really hope they find it before I die.

Bessie, age 72

LEARNING OBJECTIVES   Upon completion of this chapter, the reader will be be able to:

1. Name the major theorists who have contributed to theories of aging.
2. Identify some of the historic beliefs about aging that have influenced present-day theorists.
3. Discuss longevity and the beliefs about it that have changed over time.
4. Compare several major theories of aging.
5. Relate some of the problems encountered in attempting to explain aging within one consistent, all-encompassing theory.
6. State a definition of aging that is comprehensive and present it for discussion.
7. Contrast several personality types and how these may influence the aging process.
8. Explain the major biologic, psychologic, and sociologic theories of aging.

EARLY THEORIES OF AGING

This chapter is meant to provide the reader with background on the most prominent and accepted theories of aging—biologic, psychologic, and sociologic. None of the theories are treated in depth but should be investigated in cited original works for a more thorough understanding. The student must keep in mind there are no core theories that all people accept. Ultimately one must consider all aspects of development and attempt to combine them into a holistic view of the individual—personally unique as he or she deals with problems common in the history of the human race.

Buhler (1964) was one of the first humanistic psychologists who saw the uniqueness and potential in each life span. Buhler began in the 1930s to collect biographic and autobiographic material, production and performance records, and biologic and psychologic studies to define three distinct types of adult developmental progression: (1) a type dominated by biophysical performance, (2) by production and achievement, and (3) by contemplative integration. Her approach, followed by Lehman (1953) and Kuhlen (1968), gave a clearer picture of the multifaceted nature of adult development. This approach might be useful in understanding the varied developmental patterns of individuals of different personality types—for example, Jung's introverts and extraverts (1971). The important notion is that individuals may be genetically or socially endowed to follow a unique developmental style within their historic and cultural framework. Newer works, such as Benner's *Interpretive Phenomenology* (1994) are adding further dimensions of understanding to the phenomenon of aging. As she indicates, the study of humans cannot be reduced to a set of procedures or characteristics but must provide an interpretation of the lived experience that is plausible, auditable, and one that offers understanding of practices, meanings, and concerns.

Theories have for the most part emerged from studies of vulnerable populations being served by professionals of one sort or another. The aged are prime targets for medicine and nursing care—thus the biomedicalization of aging. Theories that arise from the study of elderly male veterans or individuals in nursing homes have often been extrapolated, in all sincerity, to explain aging. Some theorists have even speculated that corollaries of the stages of early childhood may be seen in reverse order as one ages. Of course, these presumptions and assumptions have led to gross errors in understanding the mass of aging individuals; in fact, the silent majority of the aged are not available for study. Only recently has serious attention been given to the fact that the aged are composed of two distinctly different genders; this in large part because of pharmaceutical interest in the huge market potential of postmenopausal females. Further discussion of gender issues can be found in Chapter 24.

Many questions about development in old age remain unanswered. How do people change in the later years? What is the reason and purpose of aging? What is one meant to accomplish in the last half of the life span? What are the tasks?

Box 2-1	**Historic Figures and Their Beliefs About Aging**
Aristotle	Disengagement, interiority
Cicero and Montaigne	Self-discovery, pursuit of gentility and complexity
Plato	Development of wisdom
	Metamorphosis of the soul
Galen	Statesmanship and responsibility
Villanova	Moderation and humoral balance critical to vitality
Leonardo da Vinci	Coping with reality of physical decline
Cornaro	Restricted diet and moderation for long life
Sanctorius	Decay of body "spirits" leading to "universal hardness of fibres"
Fothergill	Effects of mind on body
	Positive attitudes recommended
Rush	Importance of heredity
Charcot	Latency periods of disease that only appear in old age

What are the expected internal and external resources? What is the meaning of this last part of the life span? These are not new questions: Theories about them have been debated since the early Greeks; Plato, Aristotle, Cicero, and Montaigne sought the answers (Box 2-1).

LIFE SPAN THEORY DEVELOPMENT

Life span development refers to an individual's progress through time and implies an expected pattern of change. Traditionally, it has been seen as a composite of three elements: biologic, sociologic, and psychologic, expressed through a combination of many variable and some predictable processes. Although linear time and causal relationships are largely a scientifically cultivated and Eurocentric cultural preoccupation, we are aware that many human and biologic processes are time dependent. Some of the conceptual hurdles in determining developmental issues and phases in adult life are the lack of a clear definition of aging and the over-reliance on culturally embedded expectations. Most definitions focus on the gradual decline of cellular replication and function based on either stochastic or nonstochastic theories as discussed later in this chapter. Stochastic theories propose error catastrophes in control mechanisms such as RNA that cannot be predicted but occur randomly. Nonstochastic theories propose changes biologically "intrinsic" to human beings and genetically programmed. "Usual aging" refers to changes in the elderly that are determined by a combination of disease and adverse environmental and life-style factors. "Successful aging" refers to those elderly individuals demonstrating only physiologic decrements uncomplicated by disease, environmental exposures, and life-style factors (Rowe and Schneider, 1990). As usual, it is apparent bodily functions are deemed most significant. We have yet to find a clear definition of biopsychosocial aging that does not involve excessive reliance on the nature of cellular and systemic changes. We believe an integrated understanding of aging remains elusive. However, life span theorists provide some useful ideas.

Two opposing metatheoretic issues have formed the foundations for life span developmental theorists. One is the belief that over time predominant personality characteristics become enlarged and are maintained at the expense of more complex characteristics that simply require energy the aging individual no longer has. The organism eventually runs down and at last becomes chaotic. The contrasting view is that living organisms tend to differentiate and acquire increasing complexity, but ultimately the differentiation becomes disorganization. Birren and Cunningham (1985) suggest that ultimate disorganization begins when the central nervous system control mechanisms lose their effectiveness in maintaining the dynamic equilibrium necessary to adapt to changes in the internal and external environment.

We believe aging is an energy process beginning at conception that is directed by genetic endowment and impelled by perceived phenomenologic events that sustain the process until the biologic mechanism ceases to function. The course of behavior throughout the life span appears to have three major forces: hereditary, cultural, and individual choice (Birren and Cunningham, 1985). In addition, the totality of influences that impinge on any one individual, conceptualized by Kurt Lewin as "life-space," must be considered. To determine the manner in which these influences form patterns that intermingle in some loosely predictable way is the quest of the developmental gerontologist.

Biologic age is the individual's present position with respect to potential life span. Vital organ and functional capacities are as important as elapsed time in applying such a definition. Pure chronologic measure of time since birth tells us little about the vigor of an individual but is usually the primary measure of aging. Although we have been aware of the ebb and flow of vitality in individuals and the significance of biorhythms for several decades, these have stirred renewed interest and study only recently. Circadian rhythms, or day/night shifts in capacity and function, are time and light dependent and regulate many hormonal and enzymatic processes. There is some evidence that biorhythms are altered and become less consistently rhythmic during the aging process. Van Gool and Mirmiran (1986) reviewed the literature on the subject of aging, circadian rhythms, and the metabolic clock. They believe that the human organism can be visualized as a complex of clocks in a clock shop that is located in the suprachiasmatic nucleus of the brain. These numerous "clocks" under ideal circumstances are synchronized but may be desynchronized in the process of aging by some unknown factors. This conceptualization suggests that metabolic age may be a more accurate measure of aging status than chronologic age (Schroots and Birren, 1990). The search for psychosocial rhythms, on the other hand, has never been made explicit because these defy measurement and seem purely conjecture, yet we suspect there are psychosocial waves lapping at the shores of each lifetime that are just as predictable as the more measurable biologic ebb and flow of physiologic juices. We would like to know how behavior becomes organized over the life course in response to intrinsic biologic changes and which psychologic patterns might be common enough to allow some predictablity.

Psychologic age is expressed through the efficiency and control with which one exhibits memory, learning capacity, skills, emotions, and judgment. Maturity and efficacy are indices of the manner in which one is able to adapt psychologically over time to the requirements of the physical and social environment. To complicate this, the satisfactory and effective psychologic adjustment to one's life space may be excellent but totally inappropriate for another place and time. For example, a healthy psychologic adaptation to a nursing home would be entirely different than that of psychologic adaptation to community living; such adaptations may have little chronologic correlation. Thus individuals may demonstrate the psychologic characteristics of maturity or immaturity at any age, totally incongruent with chronologic age. Psychologic time is nonlinear; it is past, present, or future oriented; and may be regressed or progressed by internal and external events. One may be older or younger biologically, functionally, and psychologically than his or her chronologic age.

Social age is measured by age-graded behaviors carrying an expected status and role within a particular culture or society. Transitions are often marked by ritual in stable societies. Type of dress, language, institutional and role participation, and status are all indices of social age that become less distinct or predictable in the course of chronologic aging.

In a divergent, rapidly changing society such as ours where diversity is encouraged, there is less tendency toward age-graded behaviors. Often, it is only wrinkles and gray hair that may provide age categorization because activities, dress, and living situations are not usually predictably based on age in the United States.

Biologically, humans have some influence on their destiny although we have tended to give this undue emphasis in our present era; sociologically, they have considerably more. On a psychological level human potential for adaptation is most clearly apparent. The intimate relationship between biologic, social, and psychologic development that exists through childhood and adolescence does not remain as closely intermeshed in adulthood.

Anthropology and Ethnography of Aging

Anthropologic studies of the aged in remote places have emerged intermittently since the early 19th century as exotic curiosities. They are rarely exclusive studies of the aged but rather are a part of a general cultural study. Tidbits of information about how the aged have been treated in other societies, cultures, and subcultures have sometimes filled us with guilt and/or wonder. It is quite easy to believe that historically less industrialized societies somehow treated their aged better than we, but we must remember there were usually fewer aged and by virtue of attrition only the very hardy and unusual lived to be very old.

It is also important to be aware that anthropologists must cultivate sources in whatever society they study, and these sources are often the aged. These culture bearers will share what they wish and keep secret what they do not care to reveal. There may also be problems with the subtleties of language in translation. Anthropologists often live within a culture for a period of time and win friends and confidants; it is likely that their presence will influence the actions around them, just as our families are usually much different when visitors are present than when alone. There is currently great interest in the care and treatment of the aged in remote times and places as we ferret out the intricacies, meanings, and mysteries of the aged. Geographic pockets of remarkably long-lived people are of particular interest although documentation of births may be unreliable. Additional discussion of longevity is found later in this chapter.

Presently we have the unsound inclination to study blacks and whites as separate ethnographic groups. Federal statistics are often presented in this manner (Bureau of the Census, 1995) as if these were the major and basic ethnographic categories. Clearly, these categories are inaccurate, exclusionary. and perpetuate stereotypic thinking. Divisiveness is promoted when groups are labeled as Mexican American, Black American, Native American or any of the other various contractions that have no implicit meaning except that of distant geography. To understand our aged, it is important to inquire about origins and customs while fully recognizing that socioeconomic status and educational opportunities have had much more to do with present life style than origins of forbears. Chapter 24 deals more fully with cultural issues.

Evolutionary Basis for Aging

An evolutionary perspective of old age implies the emergence of certain characteristics best fitting the individual for survival in changing social and environmental conditions. From that perspective, survival is an end in itself. However, evolutionary theorists tend to view old age as an addendum to the life of sexual maturation and propagation. People usually have raised their children to maturity by the time they are 50 years old. In such cases, seemingly, the last 30 years of life appear meaningless from a species survival perspective. Rosenfeld (1985) postulated a reason for those years of existence unnecessary to species reproduction and nurturance. He proposed the concept of "nature's redundancy," the overassurance that an individual will survive to reproduce and raise progeny to the point of propagation. From a species propagation model, old age has seemed to have little meaning until recently. Now it is becoming more apparent that "nature" has been wise in keeping people alive and vigorous long enough to care for grandchildren. In an increasingly complex, dangerous, and demanding society, many parents simply cannot cope and their capacities for parenting are eroded. Grandparents have become the primary caretakers of 20% of the children in the United States today (Fuller-Thomson et al, 1997). This role will be discussed more completely in Chapter 17.

Perspectives on Aging

All theories and perspectives of aging emerge from underlying premises of the researcher, philosopher, culture, and historic era. A factor of supreme importance in examining old age as a phenomenon is the human inability to be objective about being human and most especially about aging. We are all aging, and, depending on our exposure to and involvement with old persons, we may have a negative, moderate, or positive view of that stage of life. It must be accepted at the outset that we cannot extricate ourselves from the fabric of our own physical, social, cultural, and personal experience. Since the last edition of our textbook, we have observed heightened interest in ethnographic, phenomenologic, and spiritual aspects of aging. The questions reflect a growing interest in the experience of aging as well as its functional parameters. Questions are now being raised more insistently about the meaning of the life experience.

BIOLOGIC THEORIES OF AGING

Scientifically, the architectural basis of a person begins with the cell and cell division. Cell division (meiosis and mitosis) continues to shape the human organism with its varied systems at different rates of generation and regeneration throughout the life span.

Theories of biologic and physiologic aging attempt to explain three in vivo biocomponents: (1) cells that multiply clonally (meiosis) throughout life, such as white blood cells and epithelial cells; (2) cells that are incapable of division and renewal, such as neurons; and (3) noncellular material with little turnover that comes under integrated physiologic control, such as collagen and intercellular substances. These cellular characteristics result in mechanical failure of nonreplaceable parts in organ systems, accumulation of metabolites, depletion or exhaustion of body reserves, and morphologic problems of cell development, which give organs size, shape, and structure.

Various biologic theories of aging have been more persuasive than others at various times. A unifying theory does not yet exist that explains the mechanics and causes underlying the biologic phenomenon of aging. Theories of aging can be addressed from a molecular, cellular, or systems level point of view. It will become apparent that some theories emerge from others and that one or more theories could be superimposed on others. Each theory in its own right provides a clue to the aging process. However, many unanswered questions still remain. Scientists in their continual search for truth persist in piecing together the puzzle of aging. New and exciting data concerning biologic theories of aging have emerged recently through the application of more sophisticated methods of unlocking the secrets of the cell. We are beginning to confirm some of the previous suppositions and to develop a more thorough understanding of the genetic, molecular, and biochemical basis of cellular changes of aging. In time, the student will begin to discriminate and develop an eclectic approach to theories of aging as he or she becomes familiar with the many facets of the aging process.

Stochastic Theories

Stochastic theories suggest that aging events occur randomly and accumulate with time. These theories include the gene theory, the error theory, the somatic mutation theory, the free radical theory, the cross-link theory, the clinker theory, and the wear-and-tear theory.

Gene Theory.
The gene theory suggests that one or more harmful genes in the organism become active in later life, causing failure of the organism to survive. Two variations on this theme exist. One postulates that there are two types of genes: those that mediate youthful vigor and mature adult well-being (juvenescent genes) and those that promote functional decline and structural deterioration (senescent genes). The second variation infers that genes play a dual role: The juvenescent aspects of genes function in early life, and senescent aspects of genes are activated in middle age and thereafter. The second concept is exemplified in female menopause. During the reproductive years estrogen facilitates the normal reproductive cycle. At the point of perimenopause and menopause, the estrogen level declines, increasing the risk of arteriosclerosis and hypertension in women (Hayflick, 1987).

The most important recent discovery in genetics has come from the lowly worm *Caenorhabditis elegans*. One might say the worm has turned and shown one identifiable gene that controls its life span. Researchers are systematically mapping the involved genome with the expectation that it may serve to point the way to a gene controlling the life span in humans (Makinodan, 1990).

Error Theory.
The error theory of aging (sometimes called the Orgel theory or the error catastrophe theory) proposes an accumulation of errors in protein synthesis over time resulting in impaired cellular function. Weakening of organic synthesis produces defective cells. Successive generations of these faulty cells develop and eventually interfere with the ability to maintain biologic function. Two steps are important in normal protein synthesis: (1) An amino acid must be selected by an activating enzyme and then must attach to an appropriate RNA molecule, and (2) an RNA codon must pair with an anticodon. Errors may occur in the RNA synthesis, which, if great enough, will impair cell function. The greater the number of errors accumulated in the macromolecule of the cell, the faster the accumulation of further error. Errors of RNA and DNA synthesis are indistinguishable from each other. The error catastrophe theory, while no longer widely accepted, has spurred a great deal of research.

In fact, some research has shown that the amino acid sequence does not change in young and old animals, nor is there an increase in defective RNA with aging. Age-related changes have not been found in the accuracy of Poly (V)-directed protein synthesis either. Errors have been found to occur more readily in the posttranscription of proteins (Schneider, 1995).

Normal somatic cells may become aberrant through spontaneous and innocent error or through radiation, permitting an undefined life span and errant cell propagation. Similar behavior is seen in cancer cell activity (Figure 2-1).

Somatic Mutation Theory.
The somatic mutation theory is similar to the error theory, but it suggests that when cells are exposed to x-ray radiation or chemicals a cell-by-cell alteration of DNA occurs, increasing the incidence of chromosomal abnormalities. These mutations are a time-dependent accumulation of chromosome aberrations thought to be more frequent in youth. Subsequently, replicated cells are perpetuated and harbored, with the deleterious effects appearing in later life. The ultimate result is a decrease in cellular function and organ efficiency. Those somatic cells that are of the nondividing type and possess a limited life span such as brain and muscle cells are not replaced when injured or dead.

Free Radical Theory.
Free radicals contain unpaired ions that exist momentarily and are highly reactive molecules that can damage membranes of protein, enzymes, and DNA. Their molecular structure differs from ordinary molecules in that they possess an extra electric charge (free electron). This charge instigates a one-time, irreversible, and energy-wasteful reaction that damages or alters the original structure or function of the cell membrane.

The free radical theory, proposed by Harmen (1956), emphasizes the importance of the mechanism of oxygen use by the cell (Hayflick, 1987). The greatest source of free radicals is the metabolism of oxygen, which produces the superoxide radical O_2-. Oxygen is a highly reactive gas both inside and outside the human body. Internally, oxidation of proteins, fats, and carbohydrates results in the free radical formation and unstable end products or compounds. For example, oxidation of polyunsaturated fats forms lipid peroxides that cross-link proteins, lipids, and deoxyribonucleic acid (DNA) (Hampton, 1991).

In the course of normal living, oxidation is continually causing cell destruction and a biologic dichotomy: the need

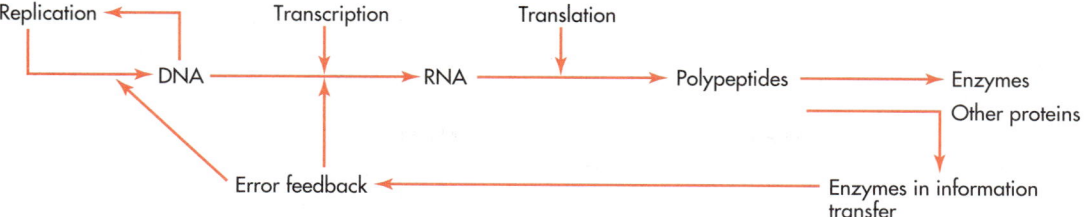

Figure 2-1. Protein synthesis *error* feedback system.

for oxygen for metabolic survival opposed to the gradual self-destruction through the release of free radicals from peroxidation referred to by some as the "oxygen paradox" (Sohal and Weindruch, 1996). Although body cells possess the capacity to eliminate unwanted waste and materials, neutralize by-products, and repair damage, free radical accumulation is thought to be faster than the repair process of the organism.

Scientists who favor the free radical theory consider the cell membrane the key to survival and think that the greatest damage is perpetuated by free radicals at this level. Within the cell, metallic ions, enzymes, and cellular materials combine with oxygen to form free radicals and compounds. Oxidation of cellular waste provides an additional source of radicals and electrons. In arterial walls, oxygen interacts with lipoprotein (a substance in the artery wall), forming free radicals. When DNA, the genetic component of the cell, is irradiated, it responds with free radical formation and establishes aberrant cellular growth and development, which affect aging. Copper, iron, and magnesium in the body increase free radical activity by catalytic action in the oxidation process.

Free radical activity is also introduced into the body from the environment. The best-known source is smog. Other environmental sources thought to cause harmful cumulative breakdown effects in cells are oxidation of gasoline in automobile engines, by-products in the plastic industry, drying linseed oil paints, and atmospheric ozone (Hampton, 1991; Sharma, 1988).

The mitochondria, major site of cellular oxidation, are thought to be protected from the hazards of free radical activity by vitamin E and coenzyme Q or Q10. It is thought that vitamin E provides protection through its antioxidant behavior (Walford, 1983; Hampton, 1991; Scheer, 1996). Studies exploring vitamin E's effectiveness as an antioxidant demonstrate that vitamin E deficiencies increase excessive lipid oxidation. At normal cellular levels of vitamin E, a slower oxidation rate occurs. Research continues into the role of vitamin E as an antioxidant and as a binding agent in the antioxidation process.

The drug COQ (ubiquinone), also known as Co-Enzyme Q, Q10, or COQ10 (Kidd, Huber, Summerfield, and Shallenberger, 1988; Scheer, 1996), is an essential energy carrier and antioxidant that sparks mitochondria energy production and easily gives up its electrons to neutralize oxidants. Q10 exists in many foods, but the ability for an individual to synthesize the nutrient from diet begins to wane in middle age (Scheer, 1996).

Certain enzymes function to degrade, neutralize, or detoxify free radicals that attack the cell membrane. These free radical scavengers include superoxide mutanase, catalase, and glutathione peroxidase. Research at the National Institute of Aging has found that the enzyme dismutase increases proportionally to metabolic rate with increased life span of various species. Individuals who enjoy high levels of protection against oxygen metabolism by-products (free radicals) should live longer than those with lower levels of protection (Walford, 1983). Vitamin A and C and niacin have also been considered to be free radical scavengers because they possess similar properties to mercaptans (free radicals) (Hampton, 1991). Older people generally have decreased blood levels of vitamin A and C. It is thought that these two easily oxidized vitamins form free radical scavengers, binding and neutralizing free radicals in a manner similar to the antioxidant behavior of vitamin E.

The body seems to be bombarded by both internal and external sources of free radicals (oxidative stress). Injection or daily intake of antioxidants, such as vitamin E, selenium, vitamin C, and various food additives (BHT, BHA, and others), has been found to produce a free radical scavenger effect. If the free radical theory is fundamental to aging as proponents believe, monitoring the kind of food consumed and the environment lived in should play an important role toward healthier aging in the future. Food selection might be directed toward intake of items with high antioxidant properties and low potential for stimulating free radical activity (Sawada and Carlson, 1987; Walford, 1986, Agarwal and Sohal, 1996).

Advocates of the free radical theory point to the fundamental microscopic nature of the theory and its relationship to cross-link and chromosomal mutation theories (Hayflick, 1987). Agarwal and Sohal (1996) suggest susceptibility of living animals to experimentally induced O_2 stress increases with age. Research also continues to determine the significance of age pigment, lipofusin, which accumulates in aging tissue (predominantly in heart and brain cells). Lipofusin is thought to be a by-product of lipid and protein fragmentation from perioxidation of the cell membrane. The significance of lipofusin and the role of free radical scavengers and antioxidants continues to be explored in their relationship to the aging process. Figure 2-2 illustrates the dynamics of the free radical theory.

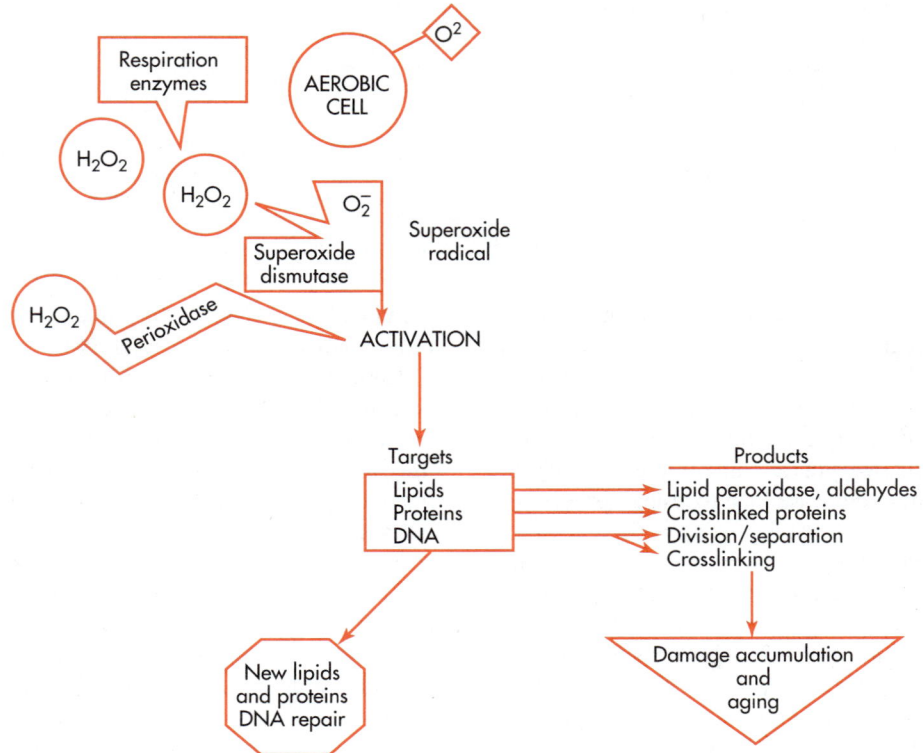

Figure 2-2. Free radical theory of aging.

Cross-Link or Connective Tissue Theory. The cross-link theory is based on the internal and external behavior of collagen, elastin, and ground substance in cells, tissues, and extracellular substances. These materials are widespread and involved in the transport and exchange of material for cell function. The theory is thought to explain some of the age-dependent diseases and disorders (Schneider, 1995).

The theory suggests that chemical reactions create strong bonds between molecular structures that are normally separate. Cross-link agents are so numerous and varied in the diet and in the environment that they are impossible to avoid. Aldehydes, minerals (copper and magnesium), and oxidizing fats serve as biologic reservoirs of cross-link–inducing agents. Lipids, proteins, nucleic acid, and carbohydrates are major body chemicals that exist in repetitive, linear structural patterns and are capable of cross-linking.

Saccharides are important ingredients in collagen, elastin, and DNA. Collagen makes up about 25% to 30% of body protein and is important in physiologic function and in some pathologic processes (Sharma, 1988). Collagen forms the gelatinous cell matrix that is responsible for maintaining structural form, support, and strength of tissues. High concentrations of collagen appear in the skin, tendons, bones, muscle, and such structures as the blood vessels and heart. Discovering the relationship between cross-linkage and aging remains a scientific challenge. Cross-linkage is most

rapid between 30 and 50 years of age but it is not yet known how to prevent cross-links from occurring.

The concept of cross-linkage can best be defined in terms of behavior and characteristics of collagen and elastin, components of connective tissue. Changes in connective tissue indicate that cross-linkage has occurred. Synthesis of new collagen reveals minimum signs of cross-linkage. With age, collagen develops an increased number of cross-links in both intracellular and intercellular structures (Sharma, 1988). Aging collagen becomes increasingly insoluble, chemically stable, and progressively rigid as a result of the cross-link phenomenon. Consider agar or gelatin as an example of what possibly happens in cross-linkage. Gelatin, like collagen, loses its sheen, becomes firmer, cracks, and dries out when exposed to air, heat, or sunlight for several days. Its original resilience and rebound disappear. The sheen turns cloudy dull. Likewise, collagen molecules dehydrate and develop a bonding pattern that links the molecules together.

Elastin in connective tissue mirrors collagen behavior and is equally prone to cross-linkage. Old elastin is frayed, fragmented, and brittle. Extracellular water diminishes and produces a concentration of calcium, sodium, and chloride. Deposits of calcium salts are found throughout the cardiovascular system: in the epicardium and endocardium, in the valves of the heart, and in the major blood vessels. Amino acids are considered to be part of elastin and also cross-link agents. Skin is one of the best examples of what happens in the cross-linkage of elastin. One cannot help but notice the gross change in skin texture and response with age. Skin that was once smooth, silky, firm, and soft becomes drier, saggy, and less elastic.

Cross-linkage of skin tissue has been compared to the changes that occur in the tanning process of animal hides; chemicals applied to hides cause cells or molecules to stick together and transform soft stretchy skin into a shiny stiff leather. The importance of connective tissue cross-linkage in the body with age has numerous implications affecting cell permeability, fibril flexibility of muscles, and heart contractility. The passage of gases, nutrients, metabolites, antibiotics, and toxins throughout the vessels are all affected. Tendons become dry and fibrous, teeth may loosen, arterial walls decline in tensile strength, and the lining of the lungs and gastrointestinal tract decrease in efficiency. Glycolated immunoglobulins, glomerular basement membrane proteins, and glycolate lipoproteins and arterial wall proteins are important in development of age-related kidney and arterial diseases (Schneider, 1995). Glycolated proteins are thought to play a major role in age-dependent opacification of crystalline lens protein, leading to eventual cataract development. Elastin, prominent in connective tissue morbidity and distensibility, affects the function of muscle contraction and all types of tissue pulsation that occur in the matrix of connective tissue. DNA also is capable of cross-linkage (Hayflick, 1987). Linkage is attributed to free radicals that bind DNA molecules together somewhere in their chemical makeup. This raises the question of the possible relationship between the free radical and cross-link theories.

Research continues into what stimulates, depresses, and blocks cross-linkage. Caloric restriction has been able to increase life expectancy and decreases cross-linkage in protein and DNA experiments with rats. Prednisolone, too, has been found to decrease the number of cross-links and prolong life (Walford, 1983). Research has identified chemicals known as lathyrogens that inhibit cross-link formation in collagen (Balazs, 1977). Studies have shown that β-aminopropionotrile (BAPN) and penicillamine produce this antilinkage effect. BAPN, however, causes retardation in the development of young collagen. Penicillamine does not seem to disturb young collagen synthesis but instead affects only mature insoluble collagen (Sacher, 1977).

Clinker Theory. The clinker theory can be considered an independent theory or a variation of the somatic, cross-link, or free radical theories. It assumes that there is an accumulation of time-related deleterious substances in the cells of the body. As chemical by-products of metabolism (lipofusin, hystones, aldehydes, free radicals) accumulate in the cell cytoplasm, there is interference with the normal cell function by displacement. Free radicals denature protein, and lipofuscin accumulates in heart, skeletal muscle, brain, and nervous system.

Wear-and-Tear Theory. A programmed process is the concept considered in the wear-and-tear theory. Cells are ag-

gravated by the harmful effects of internal and external stressors, which include injurious metabolic by-products and increased failure of DNA to repair the organism or replace vital cellular components. These may cause a progressive decline in cellular function or the death of an increasing number of cells. Striated muscle, heart muscle, muscle fibers, nerve cells, and the brain are nonreplaceable when destroyed by wear and tear or by mechanical or chemical injury.

Nonstochastic Theories

The nonstochastic theories consider aging to be predetermined. These theories include the intrinsic pacemaker theories, immune and neuroendocrine theories suggesting genetic programming of a specific time for the life-span of an organism, and programmed senescence, which implies aging of the entire organism.

Programmed Aging Theory. The initial premise of the programmed aging theory, or biologic or genetic clock, begins with an original pool of genetic information that is played out in an orderly manner. Time correlations with this intrinsic process and the development, maturation, and cessation of activity have been made between the beginning of menopause, thymic atrophy, graying of hair, and myriad other changes, all of which are considered normal aging decrements in physical function over time but not pathologic.

In vitro studies of programmed aging (Hayflick, 1968, 1975, 1977, and 1983) are still widely discussed. Experiments with human diploid cell strains have demonstrated that cells double a limited number of times before dying. The number of cell divisions are proportional to the life span of the species. Human cells double 40 to 60 times before the ability to replicate is lost. This in vitro behavior, termed phase III phenomenon by Hayflick, is a gradual and sequential degeneration of cell tissue; the precise moment of its occurrence remains elusive.

Preservation of the cells and subsequent extension of the duration of their existence were achieved by keeping the cells at subzero temperatures for long periods. When thawed years later, the cells continued to double from the point at which doubling action had been interrupted. The total number of doublings remained constant. Continued experimentation showed that cells from embryonic donors underwent more population doublings than those acquired from adult donors. Proponents of the programmed aging theory support the inverse relationship between donor age and number of doublings. Cell death or destruction is a normal part of the morphologic and developmental sequence in animals, particularly mammals. It is one way to shed or eliminate those organs necessary only in the embryonic state of development.

Lockshin and Zakeri (1990) present new thoughts on programmed cell death. They offer the theory that programmed cell death demonstrates (1) that the capacity to self-destruct is common and may be universal among both mitotic cells (lymph system) and postmitotic cells (neurons and muscle fibers), both of which lead to the mechanisms of senescence; (2) that cell death is a response to many factors including stress, changing developmental states, and trophic support with the resultant effect of rapid fragmentation of the cell DNA, also known as physiologic death or apoptosis*; and (3) that initiation of the program can involve the activities of only a handful of genes.

Run-Out-of-Program Theory. A variation of the theory of programmed aging, the run-out-of-program theory, suggests that at the time of ovum fertilization a certain amount of genetic material is allocated. When this material is used up, the cells, tissues, and organs fail. This is reflected in the gradual age-related diminution of activity of certain enzymes and organ functions, such as those in the liver and the brain.

Neuroendocrine Control Theory (Pacemaker). The neuroendocrine control theory focuses on aging as part of the life span program regulated by neurohormonal signals that begin at the time of fertilization and continue until death. Common neurons in the high brain centers act as pacemakers that regulate the biologic clock during development and aging.

Aging is manifested in a slowing down or activity imbalance of the pacemaker neurons, affecting neural, muscular, and secretory function as evidenced in involution, reproduction, loss of fertility, menopause, decreased muscle strength, less ability to recover from stress, and impaired cardiovascular and respiratory activity. Specifically, the performance of an organism is linked to a variety of control mechanisms that regulate the interplay between different organs and tissues. Homeostatic adjustment declines, with consequent failure to adapt, and is followed by aging and death. These results may be considered homeostatic failure. Rudman (1990) demonstrated that there was more than one biologic clock (genetic) for aging. Along with other scientists, Rudman looked for chemicals that directly affect the length of life. Adaptation to stress, both internal (emotions, hormones, immunity, metabolism) and external, depends on control mechanisms of nervous and hormonal systems. The pituitary gland is considered to be in direct control of the thyroid, adrenals, and gonads through the indirect signals of the nervous center, the hypothalamus (Wise, Krajnak, and Kashon, 1996). With age, some signal efficiency of the pituitary-hypothalamus connection is lost or changed, leading to desynchonization and decreased function of the hypothalamus (or the biologic clock) and an increase in pathology of most organ and tissue systems (Wise, et al, 1996). Current thinking suggests that understanding the aging of the reproductive cycle may help us better understand the process of biologic aging because of the interconnectedness of so many neurotransmitters (Wise et al,

---

*Apoptosis means physiologic cell death.

1996). Figure 2-3 provides a visual schematic of the neuroendocrine control theory.

Immunologic Theory. Studies of cell division in numerous vertebrate animals suggest that the cells of the immune system become increasingly more diversified with age and demonstrate a progressive loss of a self-regulatory pattern between the body and the cell (Strehler, 1960; Walford, 1983; Miller, 1996). The result is an autoaggressive phenomenon in which (1) cells normal to the body are misidentified as alien and are attacked by the body's immune system or (2) there is impaired surveillance by antibody cells.

Control of immunity is shared by humoral (B-cell) and cellular (T-cell) systems. In brief, the humoral (B-cell) system provides protection for the body against bacterial and viral reinfection. This function occurs through activity of the plasma cells, tonsillar tissue, abdominal mesentery Peyer patches, and the peripheral lymph system. Cellular immunity (T-cell system) delays hypersensitivity and rejection of foreign tissue cells and organ grafts and provides protection against tumor formation through the activity of the thymus gland and its associated organs (Hershey, 1974). The primary organs in cell-mediated immunity are the bone marrow and the thymus. The spleen and lymph nodes are also important but play a secondary role in cellular immunity. Lymphocytes produced by the thymus and bone marrow serve as precursor cells because they evolve through embryonic development in the organ tissue. Figure 2-4 illustrates the sources and movement of the thymic-independent (B-cell) humoral system and the thymic-dependent (T-cell) cellular immune system. There is presently great interest in the involution of thymic hormonal activity and its relation to aging. Current research suggests that previously thought thymic involution early in adult life may be key in T-cell immune senescence. However, although thymic activity declines by 90% during the first quarter of one's life span, T-cell emigration, proliferation, and removal now strongly indicate the need to look for more evidence to account for the T-cell population changes in adults.

Autoaggression. Lymphocytes generated and released by the lymph nodes are considered to be sensitized to specific antigens. These white blood cells are thought to develop a programmed self-recognition by the time an individual is 1 year old (Hershey, 1974). It has been hypothesized that regulatory cells, particularly the suppressor cells, diminish with age, allowing "previously suppressed clones of autoactive cells to respond" (Birnbaum and Swick, 1981). Any antibodies that are not programmed by this time are identified by the body as foreign and adjudged as invading organisms. Antibodies of the cell-mediated (T-cell) immune system are dispatched from the lymph nodes to surround and devour the invasive antigens by phagocytosis. B and T cells are able to regulate the differential events of humoral and cell-mediated responses. However, the immune response of the cell-mediated system, although major, does receive immune assistance from the humoral system.

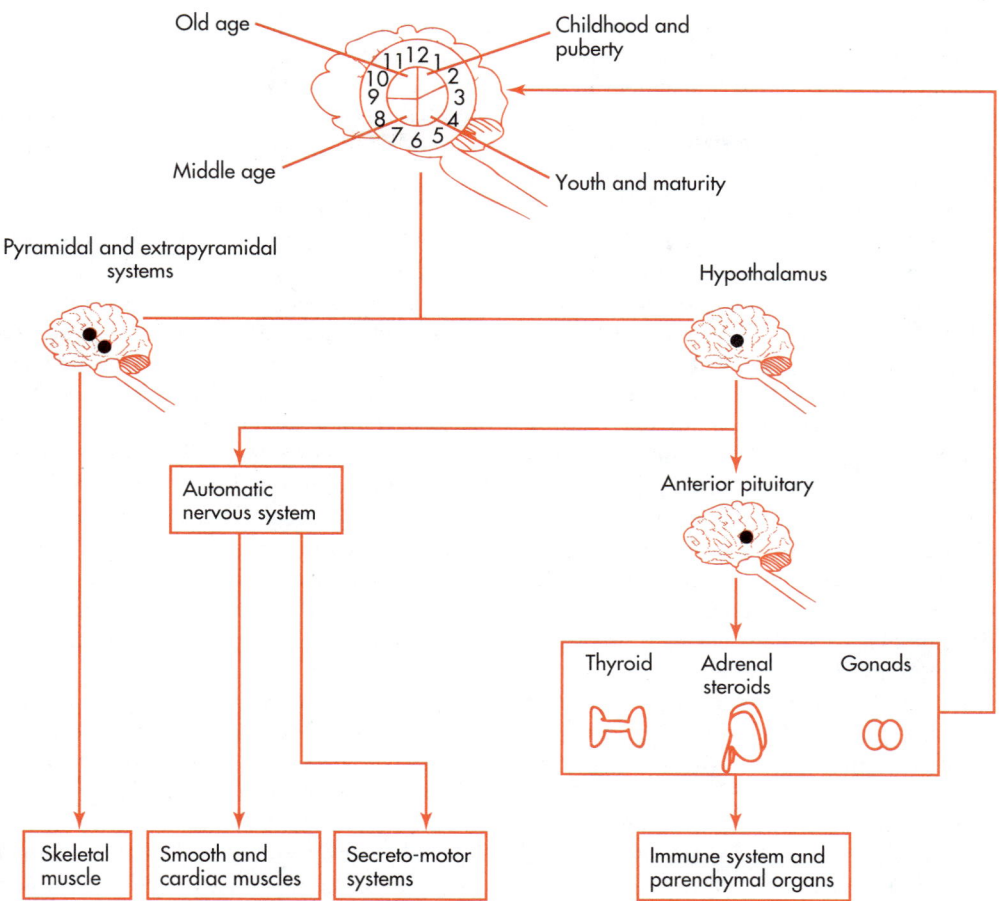

Figure 2-3. The neuroendocrine theory of aging.

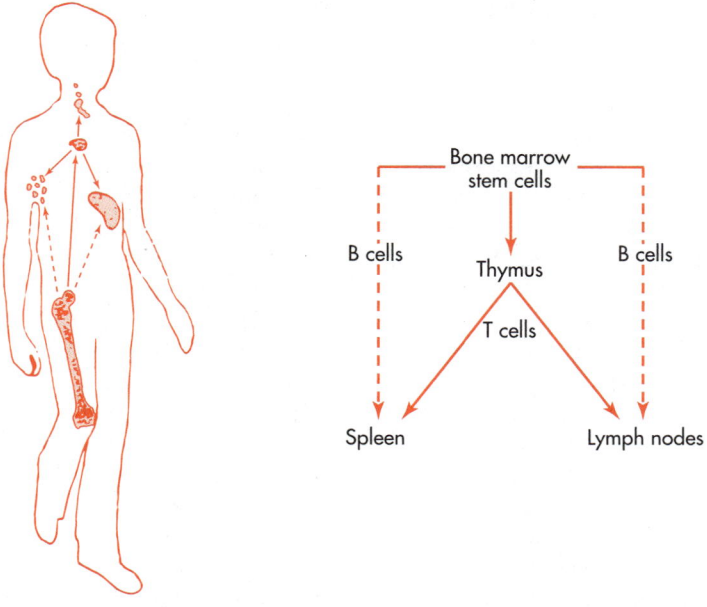

Figure 2-4. Cellular traffic of the immune system. (From Finch C, Hayflick L, editors: *Handbook of the biology of aging,* New York, 1977, Van Nostrand Reinhold.)

Nevertheless, cell-mediated reactions take place before humoral ones. Antibodies of the humoral system (B cells) circulate in the blood and attach themselves to antigens in sufficient numbers to dilute the antigens in a neutralizing effect. Specific B and T cells respond to specific antigenic stimulation by generating functional effector cells (antibodies) or by developing a tolerance so that reexposure does not elicit a destructive reaction. Imbalance of B- and T-cell activity gives rise to an increased production of autoantibodies. Cytotoxic (cellular toxicity) effects occur in host tissue when thymic-deprived lymphoid cells are transferred to the peripheral lymphoid circulation. B- and T-cell imbalance results in a compromise of the humoral mechanism, decreasing the body's immune surveillance capability and causing hypersensitivity to the autoimmune phenomenon. The cell-mediated T cells are responsible for hastening the age-related changes attributed to autoimmune reactions; the body battles against itself. The demonstration of chromosome fragility in T cells provides better understanding of the genetic basis of cellular aging (Makinodan, 1990; Miller, 1996). T cells also pinpoint early deficiencies in transduction that influence the transcription of cellular information and may result in identification of metabolic events that create vulnerability (Makinodan, 1990). Box 2-2 outlines key cell changes that occur in old age.

Haptens (low-molecular-weight compounds) in combination with natural body proteins form hapten-protein units. Antibodies mistake these hapten units for antigen and thus attack their own body protein (Guyton, 1986). The release of abnormal protein products during infectious processes or the release in later life of particular antibodies, which have been dormant or sequestered in various immune system organs from the early development of the individual, is an additional cause for autoimmune responses. Research has shown instances of age-related autoimmune and immune-deficient responses.

Graft-versus-host reaction experiments with mice have demonstrated significantly higher rejection rates of tissue grafts in older mice than in younger mice. This has lead to the postulation that greater cell aberration occurs with age and that cell self-regulation is greatly lacking (Makinodan, 1990). This might be one reason why wound healing and generation of healthy tissue seem to progress more slowly in the aged, despite proper diet, rest, and care.

Immunoglobins, which contain two or more antigen-binding sites and other unique structures, are part of the humoral system and are responsible for antibody activity of globins. There is evidence that gamma globulin, Rh factor, and antithyroid and antiinsulin antibody activity accelerates with increasing age (Rowe and Schneider, 1990). The possibility of immune system exhaustion as a cause of aging has been considered and may eventually explain the number of cases of adult-onset diabetes mellitus and rheumatoid arthritis exacerbations, as well as the development of other conditions among older individuals. Miller (1996) points out that

it is not clear from current in vivo findings whether or not immunodeficiencies are due to expansion of certain T-cell clones at the expense of others, which diminish the functional repertoire of the immune system in old age, thus limiting the ability to respond to new immunogens.

Depletion. Immunodeficient conditions such as infection, autoimmunity, and cancer are thought to be the body's response to several types of events (Hayflick, 1987, Macieira-Coelho, 1987). Studies of newborn mice with slow virus infections showed a suppression of normal immune function. Mice infected with leukenogenic virus also responded with suppression of the immune system. In long-lived mice the onset of the decline of immune function began early in life (Makinodan and Yunis, 1977). Correlations can be made with human responses in similar situations because the responses of laboratory animals generally reflect what might occur in human tissue. The question arises whether all vertebrates harbor slow viruses that can induce the gradual decline in the immune system with advancing age. It would seem reasonable to assume that a decline in immune system function would occur because the function of all systems seems to diminish with age and that age-dependent anatomic and physiologic changes, such as decreased secretions, dry skin, and collagen changes, would add to the disruption of the host's defense mechanisms. The simultaneous decline in the immune system and increase in the autoimmune response would seem to constitute an important consideration. A decline in immunity would allow malfunctioning immune cells to surface or exert themselves. Decreased efficiency of the immune system certainly increases vulnerability to disease and malignancy (Kent, 1977; Makinodan, 1990). Figure 2-5 depicts the immune theory.

Immune system, disease, and aging. Viruses and/or their antigens and corresponding antibodies comprise some of the antigen-antibody complexes. When these lodge in specific body sites, such as kidneys and arteries, factors injurious to the tissue are released and initiate the onset of deterioration. This may be instrumental in triggering or causing normal aging and disease.

Autoimmune disorders and aging may be correlated, as evidenced by several shared characteristics. Both processes exhibit lymphoid depletion and hypoplasia, thymic atrophy, and increased plasma cells in lymphoid organs. The most relevant pathologic change that can be evidenced in the immune system with age is thymic atrophy. T-cell-dependent immunity is probably related to decreased circulating thymic hormone levels (see Figure 2-5). As early as 1969 (Quiniti et al, 1981), thymic transplants, as well as the administration of young thymocytes or thymic extract to patients, were shown to be able to correct several age-dependent immunologic impairments, such as antibody formation. In the aged, if hypergammaglobulinemia is present, the tests for antibodies are positive. However, the alloantigen response (which requires B- and T-cell cooperation) is

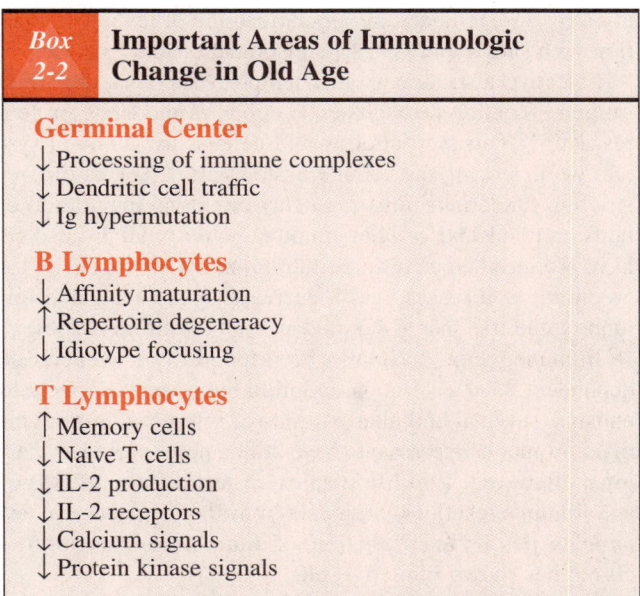

Modified from Miller A: The aging immune system: primer and prospectus, *Science* 273:71, 1996.

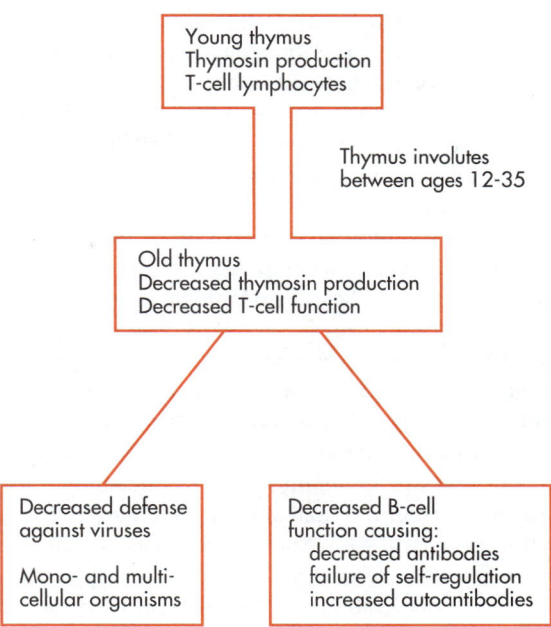

Figure 2-5. Immune system process of aging.

decreased. Two types of autoimmune and immunodeficient diseases exist: those that affect the young person and those that affect the older adult. Autoimmune and immunodeficient diseases in older adults illustrate the impact of the immunologic theory on aging. Cell-mediated immunity decreases in older persons and may be responsible for decreased survival (Wayne, Rhyne, Garry, and Goodwin, 1990).

Decline in the immunologic state is conducive to the development of infections, autoimmunities, and cancer. Amyloidosis, cancer, and adult-onset diabetes mellitus have been considered diseases of aging that emanate from immunodeficiencies. Fibers that appear in amyloidosis are identified as chains of immunoglobulins and are present in various body organs of the aged individual. The islets of Langerhans, for instance, in the pancreas show signs of amyloidosis and complement-fixing antiinsulin antibodies with aging. Cancer appears to be strongly influenced by immunodeficiencies, particularly those associated with immunosuppressant drugs. Individuals who require immunosuppressants are 80 times more vulnerable to cancer than those who do not receive such therapy (Makinodan, 1990). Autoimmune mechanisms also contribute to atherosclerosis, hypertension, and thromboembolism in certain susceptible people. Cardiovascular disease, allergic angitis, and rheumatic heart disease are considered partially the result of immune system dysfunction. Senile plaque, found in aging degenerating human brain tissue, contains a large quantity of amyloid fiber. Studies of aging mice suggest that the cause of neuronal degeneration may lie in the neuron-reactive antibodies in the sera of old mice (Nandy and Bennett, 1983).

There is a growing interest in the effects of aging on the mucosal immune system. Evidence suggests that the secretory immune system may be affected by the aging process. It is known that secretory antibodies play an important role in protection of mucosal surfaces from a variety of pathogens. The complexity of the aging regional immune system suggests that a number of factors (e.g., IgA antibody production) in local ocular, salivary, nasal, and intestinal sites play a pivotal role in the larger immune response (Makinodan, 1990).

The acute antibody response to extrinsic antigens, such as pneumococcal and influenza vaccines, is considerably reduced in the elderly. It is thought possible that lowered circulating immunoglobin levels reflect increased response to intrinsic antigens (autoantibodies) (Nicoletti, Yan, Cerney, 1993).

Cellular immunity most clearly exhibits an age-related decrease in functional ability. The decline of cell-mediated immunity with increasing age correlates with an increasing frequency of reactivation tuberculosis. However, while reduction in the levels of thymic hormones is clearly age related, it is unclear if thymic involution is associated with increased susceptibility to infection (Tockman, 1990).

Challenging the immunologic theory of aging. No theory is without counter arguments. Studies at Duke University have shown through cross-analysis and longitudinal analysis of immune changes that immunoglobins increased with age in about two thirds of the study population (Makinodan and Yunis, 1977).

A correlation was made between low immunoglobin levels in the blood and failure to survive. However, normal to high levels of immunoglobins were noted in the blood of long-lived individuals with various immunodeficiencies. This raised the question, "To what extent do immunoglobins affect aging?" Cell-mediated immunity, presented earlier as a primary factor in immunity, was found to remain relatively intact for the whole life span in long-lived strains of experimental mice (Makinodan and Yunis, 1977).

Early studies suggested a relationship between the immune system and mortality. Researchers continue to attempt to demonstrate the relationship between immune status as an indicator of general health or biologic aging to provide a prognosticator for survival and disease risk. A decline in peripheral blood lymphocyte count has been shown to correlate with diminished 1-year survival in old mice (Bender, Nagel et al, 1986). Correlation between survival and the pace or extent of immune changes has been demonstrated in three studies of immunity in mice. One study illustrated the relatively short life span of mice with high levels of CD8 T-cells (Boersma, 1985). Another study showed the long life span and low tumor generation in a certain type of mouse with high concentrations of induced antibody production (Covelli et al, 1989).

Current research suggests a combination of immune status indices: high T-cell proliferation, high B-cell numbers, and low CD8 to CD4 cell ratio can predict survival over a 2-year follow-up interval in the very old (ages 86-92 [Ferguson, Wikby, Maxson, et al, 1995]). Wayne and associates (1990) suggest that the lack of immunity, anergy, in skin tests for delayed hypersensitivity may also prove a good indicator for subsequent mortality.

Miller (1994) found an associated high risk of early mortality when there was a high number of memory T-cells at 6 months of age. Confounding the analysis of age-related changes in immune competency from a clinical perspective is the comparatively long human life span.

Biologists are looking at the field of immunoengineering for possible approaches to control the decline of the immune system and to retard the aging process. Immunoengineering, the manipulation of some conditions in organ transplants, and the attempt to find a cure for AIDs have opened avenues for exploring aging and the benefits of aging. A number of years ago, it was shown that the complicated immune system was regulated by an aggregate of genes on a single chromosome. Like a super blood grouping system with numerous different types, the cluster of genes was called the major histocompatibility chromosome (MHC). Part of the responsibility of the MHC is self-antiself recognition. Susceptibility to many diseases of aging, such as Alzheimer's disease, is influenced by the MHC type of the affected person, and organ graft survival rate is noted to be better when both donor and recipient have the same MHC type (Walford, 1983). Some of the first evidence that MHC was influential in extending the life span of different mice strains was provided by the research of Smith and Walford (1977) and later confirmed by Williams et al (1981). Two approaches on which immunoengineering is focused are (1) selective alter-

ation by diet, temperature regulation, and drugs in conjunction with surgery and (2) replenishment or rejuvenation.

Selective alteration is an attempt to suppress abnormal immune function through such actions as moderate protein restriction. This restriction would depress the humoral system while leaving the cellular system intact. Severe diet restriction (undernutrition) can delay or extend maturation of both humoral and cellular immune activity. High-fat diets have produced an increase in autoimmunity, a propensity for autoimmune diseases, and a decrease in cell-mediated immunity and life span (Makinodan, 1990; Walford, 1986).

Immune factors have also been found to be temperature dependent. Diet restriction and mild hypothermia appear to enhance survival and alter patterns of immunity in test animals. Immunosuppressants have at this point provided marginal effectiveness in life span extension because of loss of autoimmune reactions. Surgical removal of the spleen in test animals before manifestation of immunodeficiencies occurred has shown limited results.

Replenishment of rejuvenation of the human immune system is based on the idea of injecting immune cells of a compatible young donor into older recipients. The intent is to return the immune system of the aging individual to its normal effective state.

In summary, the immune system responses are thought to produce age-related changes. Accurate accumulated data shows the immune system begins to decline (1) when thymic atrophy occurs and possibly as soon as there is a decrease of thymic hormone (thymosin) in the blood, (2) when there is a significant increase in plasma cell activity, (3) when circulating lymphocytes with an abnormal number of chromosomes are increased, and (4) when there is an increase in immunoglobins in the blood. Research has identified various diseases that may be linked to immunity and aging. Selective alteration and replenishment or rejuvenation are immunoengineering challenges for exerting control and moderating or eliminating the effects of autoimmunity, immunodeficiencies, and perhaps, one day, the aging process.

In summary, although all of these theories provide possible clues to aging, they also raise many questions and stimulate continuing research (Table 2-1). Many symptoms that are attributed to failing circulation in the aged may actually be the effects of nondividing cell death. The frequency of mutations in mammalian aging is influenced by genetic mutation of autoimmune reactions, metabolic rate, genetic background, and environmental factors. In the past few years, the investigation of cellular senescence has expanded to additional cell types, such as endothelial cells and T-lymphocytes. These cells have been combined with immortal cells, which has indicated many or all cell types may have similar pathways. Conversely, as analysis of more cell types are studied, the expression or repression of specific genes are appearing. Hopefully, more research will lead to the discovery of other pathways and key changes in gene expres-

Table 2-1   Summary of Biologic Theories of Aging

Theory	Dynamics	Retardants
Stochastic Theories		
Error	Faulty synthesis of DNA and/or RNA	
Somatic	Alteration in RNA/DNA; protein or enzyme synthesis causes defective structure or function	
Transcription	Failure of transcription or translation between cells; malfunctions of RNA or related enzymes	
Free radical	Oxidation of fats, proteins, carbohydrates, and elements creates free electrons that attach to other molecules, altering cellular function	Improve environmental monitoring; decrease intake of free radical-stimulating foods; increase vitamin A and C intake (mercaptans; increase vitamin E; use of coenzyme Q10)
Cross-link	Lipids, proteins, carbohydrates, and nucleic acid react with chemicals or radiation to form bonds that cause an increase in cell rigidity and instability	Caloric restrictions, lathyrogen-antilink agents
Clinker	Mix of somatic, free radical, and cross-link theories	
Wear and tear	Repeated injury or overuse of cells, tissue, organs, or systems	
Nonstochastic Theories		
Programmed	Biologic clock triggers specific cell behavior at specific time	Hypothermia and diet can delay cell division but not number of divisions
Run-out-of-program	Organism capable of specific number of cell divisions and specific life span	
Neuroendocrine	Control mechanism (pituitary and hypothalamus) regulate interplay between various organs and tissues; efficiency of signals between mechanisms is altered or lost	Treatment with potent hormones such as DHEA (dehydroepiandrosterone) and RU486
Immunologic/autoimmune	Alteration of B and T cells leads to loss of capacity for self-regulation; normal or age-related cells recognized as foreign matter; system reacts by forming antibodies to destroy these cells	Immunoengineering, selective alteration, and replacement or rejuvenation of immune system

sion used by other cells to establish senescence (Smith, Pereira-Smith, 1996). Biogerontologic research has demonstrated that longevity is frequently considered to be related to enhanced metabolic capacity and the response to stress, as well as multiple mechanisms of aging (Jazwinski, 1996).

The biogerontologist has long considered that genes play a part in the aging process, while acknowledging that environmental influences are also important. It is important, however, to realize that life-span is not the same as the action of a genetic program. Aging, according to the biogerontologists, is determined by genetic construction.

More thought is being directed toward the immune function of the body. The work of Yunis and Salazar, (1993) and Salazar et al, (1995) reveal heterozygosity multigene interaction, environmental effects, and longevity in nearly one half of the chromosomes tested. Life span correlates positively with a high-immune responsiveness, both of which were controlled by a small number of gene loci. The inference is that low antibody response has a detrimental effect.

PSYCHOLOGIC ASPECTS OF AGING

Healthy psychologic aging refers to the age-related adaptive capacity of the individual to experience and interpret events in such a way that coping is ensured as one continually seeks greater understanding and higher levels of adaptation. Gerontology has emerged as a subspecialty of psychology within the last quarter century. The first journal devoted exclusively to psychology and aging was published in 1985 by the American Psychological Association. Before that, the psychology of the old was primarily focused on studying cognitive losses or impairments or slowing of various responses.

The psychology of aging is the study of changes in behavior that characteristically occur after young adulthood. Behavior in this sense includes sensation, perception, learning, memory, intellect, motivation, emotion, personality, attitudes, motor movement, and social relationships (Birren and Birren, 1990). The psychology of aging attempts to "discern laws governing the way humankind grows up and grows old" (Birren and Birren, 1990, p. 12) (Box 2-3). Quite naturally, aging psychologists often give more attention to the psychologic development of the aged. Dr. James Birren has been one of the true leaders in the field for 30 years and has with his own aging become increasingly interested in the psychology and metaphysics of aging. His contributions have been broad but his focus on the importance of a developmental autobiography has generated considerable interest

Box 2-3	**Theories of Development**
Maturational	The biologic unfolding according to genetic programming determines development (White, mastery)
Personality	Early formation of responses caused by family and peer influences determine behaviors (Sullivan, interpersonal)
Behaviorist	Learning determines the organization of behavior (tabula rasa)
Cognitive	Development of cognitive capacities provides the basis for differentiation and increasing complexity of goals and behavior (Piaget)
Ecologic	The nature of adult development is quite different from that of children and has yet to be thoroughly articulated (Lewin)
Instinctual	Development of controls of instinctual responses through feedback, based in psychoanalytic thought (Freud)
Psychobiologic	Progress in neuroscience has shown that the balance of 50 or more neurotransmitters may, to a large extent, modulate behaviors, emotions, and thoughts
Dialectic	Crises and transitions release positive and negative forces that lead to developmental progression (Riegel)

in the field. Nursing leaders who have helped us understand the psychologic components of aging include Mary Opal Wolanin and Virginia Stone as they studied the experience and memories of nonagenarians, and May Wykle and Kathleen Buckwalter who established academic programs in psychogeriatric care.

Essential to the concept of psychologic development are the following ideas: (1) the organism is a dynamic system, (2) time is a quantifying element, (3) movement in time is toward complexity of organization, (4) parts are incorporated into the whole, and (5) the highest state of organization is self-regulatory. Little is known about intrinsic psychologic needs and changes that occur as a result of primary aging processes, because we have no such sample of aged persons. All persons are embedded in a cultural matrix that influences every aspect of their lives and that cannot be extricated from the primary and essential components of aging. This is the basis for our firm conviction that we do not yet know the potential of the aged—possibilities are limitless given an enhancing milieu. We, therefore, caution against attributing any particular psychologic change to age alone.

Morality

Obviously, morality must be personally defined within a value context. When values are shaken, the crisis threatens self-view and psychologic distress occurs. Questions about fundamental changes in behavior that occur with age are exceedingly difficult to answer. The classic theory of Kohlberg (1973) proposes that crises and turning points of adult life are moral dilemmas that form structural stage changes analogous to Piaget's cognitive operations in youth. The last stage of moral development is defined as "universal ethical principle orientation." This stage fits nicely into the Eriksonian model of development because integrity is built on morality and ethics. Moral reasoning in later life may take on a very pragmatic function, corresponding to changes associated with one's position in the life span. The nature of moral decisions in old age may be characterized by a shift from purely logical justification to a dialectic resolution between justice and personal caring. Recently, much discussion about the nature of moral aging was centered around the obligations of adults and the old toward future generations (Moody,1988). We believe these discussions will become ever more pressing as world populations grow and as economic and environmental debts increase. Some writers believe that such moral dilemmas can only be effectively dealt with by the aged because the very complexity of situations relies on the wisdom of long experience (Fjelland & Gjengedal, 1994).

Competence

The founders of ego psychology recognize the importance of stimulating experiences and mastery of new situations. According to them, the ego is continually striving for more challenges rather than a state of rest or satisfaction. An invigorating environment is needed to maintain an energized level of stress. Accordingly, individuals do not seek homeostasis (a steady state) but rather stimulation. This has important implications for the elderly. Most old people have had many experiences, and new situations occur with less frequency. Some elders are isolated from the mainstream of life and may deteriorate from boredom and lack of stimulation (Chapter 12). Experiments with sensory deprivation seem to confirm this notion. Perhaps the most challenging stimuli for the aged are maintaining autonomy and independence. Commitment to mastery or competence is critically linked to motivating drives, incentives, needs, and the degree of control one feels. Satisfaction can arise from several channels, although opportunity for mastery relates to social class, health, life stage, and sex. In old age it seems the sense of control is an important precursor of successful coping.

Self-View

Retaining dignity and self-respect in the face of the catastrophes accompanying aging are the poorly understood psychologic components of successful aging (Lenker and Polivka, 1996). Self-efficacy has received some attention as the mediator of behavior (Bandura, 1977). A longitudinal study has shown that social network supports and the availability of financial resources were the strongest factors in maintaining feelings of self-efficacy (McAvay, Seeman & Rodin, 1996). The existential dimensions of "self" reside within the boundaries of a personal moral stance and perceived competence and as such may be vulnerable to internal and external changes. Yet, some individuals maintain a strong sense of self. These are the psychologically "hardy" persons (Bowsher and Keep, 1995). The hardy ones are capable of enduring physical and emotional stressors because they maintain a sense of control and challenge. Each event is seen as an open door on new experience and one that allows for choice (Kobasa, 1979; Ebersole, 1996). As we work with the aged it is important to keep in mind the three cornerstones of hardiness: control, competence, and challenge. Some also add a fourth—compassion. Indeed, it seems those who manage effectively against all odds are those whose central concerns go beyond self to include others. This presupposes some underlying altruism as well as a sense of humor. These topics are considered later in the text. Banks (1996) believes it is also essential to psychological health in later life to be capable of imagining oneself as old. It is a revealing exercise to ask students to imagine themselves as old (see suggested activities, Chapter 1). Our readers will recognize among the student quotes at the beginning of each chapter in this edition of the textbook that some students are very capable of imagining being old and assigning meaning to old age.

Psychologic Tasks of Aging

Theories are the organizing framework from which tasks quite naturally will arise. Box 2-4 and Figure 2-6 summarize some of the concepts, dynamics, issues, and tasks that have been formulated by various life span theorists over the years. Some of the theories give little recognition or attention to the unique characteristics and potential of the aged. The exchange model is one we particularly favor. It implies that with the waning of physical energy one is less inclined to seek more of anything and is more inclined to seek less, but with more emphasis on quality than quantity. According to Lewin (1951), all developmental theories are faulty because childhood development, from which they all arose, is undoubtedly distinctively different in all respects from adult development. G. Stanley Hall's work, in 1922, while largely descriptive, was the first to suggest a science of gerontic development. Jung and Erikson have both written of needs that emerge in the "last half of life." We still rely on their original thought as a starting point for understanding the tasks of the aged. Clark and Anderson (1967) were among the first to identify specific adaptive tasks. These primarily focus on the need to overcome decrements in function and to seize opportunity by substitution, redefinition, acceptance, and reassessment. These all imply that adulthood is the stage of maximum adaptation.

Developmental Tasks and Status

Cynthia Kelly has identified the three Rs that define the tasks of aging as (1) accepting reality, (2) fulfilling responsibility, and (3) exercising rights (1990). Realities have to do with accepting one's capacities in the health, social, and financial realms; responsibilities include planning for one's survivors and for making the best choices regarding the remainder of life; and rights include exercising the right to move at one's own pace, the right to privacy, the right to respect, the right to refuse what one does not desire and to participate in plans and decisions related to one's own life. Developmental tasks, as defined by several theorists are included in Figure 2-7.

We remain convinced that old age is valid in and of itself and that adaptation is toward maximizing and making events meaningful in the last stage of life. Birren and Birren (1990) believe that as more theorists and investigators mature who have their primary training in the field of gerontology we can expect more theories to emerge that are seminal rather than borrowed from other life stages or disciplines.

Establishing Integrity. Erikson is to human development as Maslow is to motivation. Each has framed the depth and clarity of concepts that provide an organizational framework for students and practitioners to categorize behaviors and understand dynamics of individuals. Erikson (1963) described the specific developmental stages and tasks of each age. He saw the last stage of life as a vantage point from which one could look back with integrity or despair on one's life. Erikson believed in a predetermined order of development that proceeded by critical steps, all dependent on timing and sequence. However, he also theorized that individuals return again and again to the stages that have been poorly resolved. His theory does not clearly explain why the organism moves from one state to the next; it is assumed that certain inner biologic and outer sociologic conditions are required (Figure 2-6, model 1). These concepts are quite cultural and class-bound and the centrality of identity achievement reflects Erikson's own need to establish his identity sans any knowledge of his biologic father.

Acknowledging the necessary stages of development proposed by Erikson, Peck (1968) identified discrete tasks of old age that must be addressed in order to establish integrity:

- Ego differentiation versus work role preoccupation: The individual is no longer defined by his/her work.
- Body transcendence versus body preoccupation: The body is cared for but does not consume the interest and attention of the individual.
- Ego transcendence versus ego preoccupation: The "I" becomes less central and one becomes a felt part of the mass of humanity, their struggles, and their destiny.

It is clear that to achieve integrity by Peck's model one must develop the ability to redefine self, to let go of occupational identity, to rise above body discomforts, and to

> **Box 2-4**
>
> ## Summary of Theories of Human Development

I. Life stages model
  A. Jungian (popular)
    1. Anchored in psychoanalytic theory
      a. Mid-life shift—second stage of development
        (1) Anima—female; emergence of in men
        (2) Animus—male; emergence of in women
    2. Issues
      a. Masculinity-femininity
      b. Creativity-destructiveness
      c. Attachment-loss
  B. Eriksonian—psychosexual stages
    1. Organized in sequences of life structures and transitions (6- to 10-year average)
      a. Stability-disruption (1- to 3-year average)
      b. Equilibrium-imbalance
      c. Denial, rebirth (Kübler-Ross)
      d. Socially and personally motivated with genetic and chronologic influence
  C. Levinsonian—mentors (7 to 10 years older) to guide
    1. 35- to 45-year shift
      a. Guided by a dream
      b. Mid-life crises
      c. End of dream
      d. Death of youth
II. Adaptational model (Valliant)
  A. Basic premises
    1. Gradual shifting of self and understanding
    2. Incremental-decremental shifts
    3. Trade-offs
    4. Holding on and letting go—critical
  B. Examples
    1. Sensory decrease/quality of perception increase
    2. Excitement decrease/experience increase
    3. Physical decrease/wisdom increase
  C. Quantity versus quality
    1. What are you willing to let go of or diminish?
    2. What is not worth pursuing?
    3. What are your best assets?
    4. What is possible?
      a. Undiscovered self
      b. New births of self
    5. Stay with growing edge of self
    6. Bargaining is the essence
III. Life structure and transitions (Lowenthal) (based on organizational life cycles)
  A. Family life cycles
  B. Transitions
    1. College
    2. Marriage
    3. Retirement

  C. Premises
    1. Significant others may not be in the same sequence
    2. Evidence from clinical world
    3. Accelerated life structure transitions
      a. Toffler—*Future Shock*
    4. Choice—intolerance of change or creative change
IV. Dialectic/ecologic/systems (Riegel)
  A. Premises
    1. Based on social psychology
    2. No life span approach
    3. Intersection of events produces change by breaking equilibrium
      a. Triggering event
      b. Turning point
      c. Timing of events (Rossi)
    4. Discover self by reaction
    5. Perspective on development by looking backward
    6. Metaphoric conceptualizations
    7. Restoration of balance
    8. Essence in energy exchanges with impact
  B. Examples
    1. World events, trends, culture, milieu
      a. Geography
      b. Ideational
      c. Situational
      d. Micro and macro systems
      e. Health evolution
V. Fielding model—Roger Gould—psychoanalytic consultation
  A. Premises
    1. Become finest self
      a. Give up safety
      b. Creativity reaches beyond myth of safety
      c. Self-actualizing
        (1) Maslow
        (2) Bueler
      d. Past life, future self
      e. Autonomy/control/taking charge
      f. Pilgrimage of the self
        (1) Teleologic
        (2) Future oriented
        (3) Proactive
        (4) Goal oriented
        (5) Shaping one's own world
  B. Agenda for mature adulthood
    1. Individualization
    2. Recreation
    3. Undo the boring—trigger a transition, renewal
    4. Endings and beginnings—the essence of development

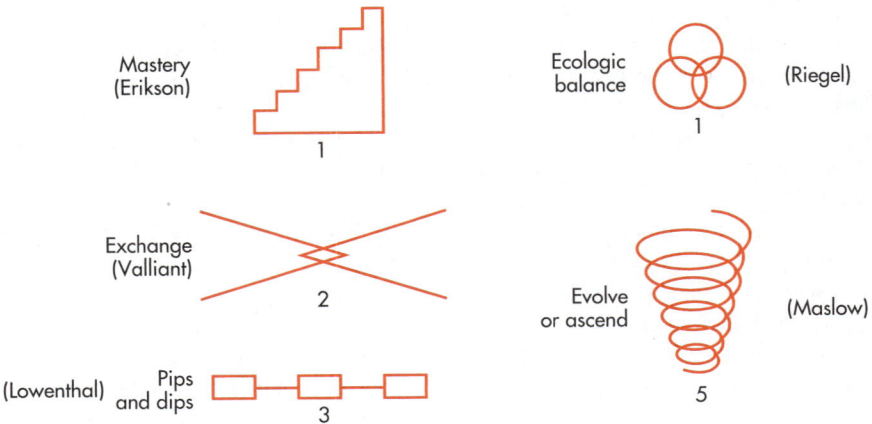

Figure 2-6. Visual models of dynamics of developmental theories. (Developed by Priscilla Ebersole. Extrapolated from Hudson F: Lecture presented at Fielding Retreat, Fielding Institute, Santa Barbara, Calif, 1983.)

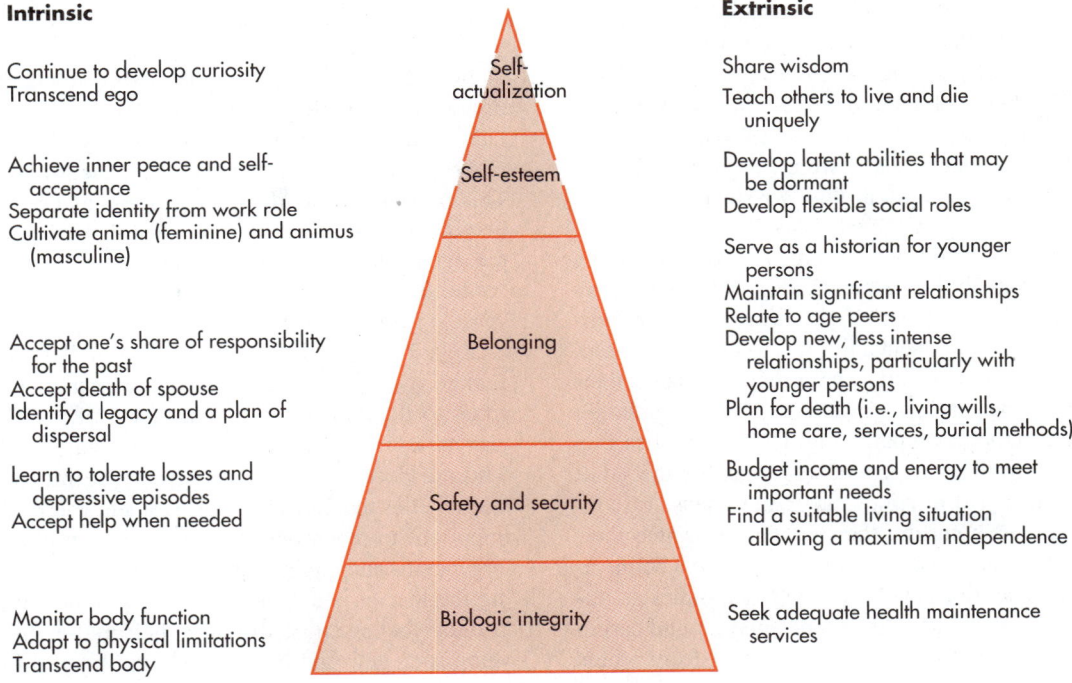

Figure 2-7. Developmental tasks of late life in hierarchic order. (Data from Peck, 1968; Havighurst, 1972; Ebersole, Butler, and Lewis, 1977.)

establish meanings that go beyond the scope of self-centeredness. Although these are admirable and idealistic goals, they place a considerable burden on the aged individual. Everyone may not have the courage or energy to laugh in the face of adversity or surmount all the assaults of old age. There are traces of Aristotelian thought in both Peck's and Erikson's theories.

Interestingly, questions have been raised as to whether integrity is indeed the highest development in old age. Erikson's concept of integrity in old age and the concomi-

tant ego attribute, wisdom, may not be attainable by many elders. The wisdom of old age is an adaptive perception of reality to elicit new meanings from prior experience, but paradoxically this means a mode of knowledge beyond time or age. Unlike ordinary knowledge, wisdom leads to an apprehension of reality in its fullest. The wisdom of old age becomes a crisis of explanation in which the ordinary structures are shaken and the meaning of life is reexamined. It may include the wisdom of questioning assumptions in the search for meaning in the last stage of life.

In later years, Erikson and his wife, Joan, (1986) reconsidered his seminal work from the perspective of their own aging (they were both octogenarians at the time) and from the experience of a select group of their cohort, 29 surviving parents of the children studied in the guidance study of the Institute of Human Development at the University of California in Berkeley. They reframed their presentation of the theoretical framework to focus on a dialectic process of achieving balance at each stage of life. Thus ego integrity is tinged with some regrets, wisdom is balanced with frivolity, and letting go with hanging on. The Eriksons define wisdom as "detached concern with life itself, in the face of death itself. It maintains and learns to convey the integrity of experience, in spite of the decline of bodily and mental functions" (Erikson, Erikson, and Kivnick, 1986, p. 38).

Caring and Continuity. In 1927 Dr. Herbert Stolz established the Institute of Child Welfare under the aegis of the Institute of Human Development and began a longitudinal study of the health and development of every third child born in Berkeley for the ensuing 18 months. The original sample totaled 248 infants. Although they were randomly selected, they nevertheless represented a very select population because Berkeley at that time was an "ivory tower" town. The children are now septuagenarians. Their parents, now mostly nonagenarians, were interviewed by the Eriksons. Their preoccupation at this last stage of life was caring. For many, caring remained focused on children and grandchildren and seemed a vicarious way of continuing vital involvement in living. Others had grown beyond the central focus of the family, and their caring had more universal and altruistic components. For most of these very old, concern for their septuagenarian children dominated their thoughts. Reflecting on the successes of their children seemed to confirm their own parenting. The aspect of caring, so predominant during the generative stages in the adult years, is the quality that provides the greatest sense of continuity. As individuals nurture their young and watch their descendants nurture their young, they experience a connectedness with the repetitious cycles of life and at times an opportunity to redo their youth. As the dialectic around caring is cultivated, the elder is challenged "to accept from others that caring which is required and to do so in a way that is itself caring" (Erikson, Erikson, and Kivnick, 1986, p. 74).

Continuity and vicarious fulfillment are experienced as one sees qualities in grandchildren that were identified in the self, parents, or grandparents of self. As many as six generations may be viewed in continuous progression.

My great-grandmother (Ebersole) left me a watercolor of wildflowers. I am obsessed with the beauty of spring flowers and walk for hours admiring them. Recently my granddaughter bought a field guide to flowers and asked to accompany me on the "flower walks." Although the sixth generation is yet to appear, my granddaughter is in her teens and I in my sixth decade. I expect to see a great-granddaughter before I die, and I will eagerly wait to see

where her interests lie. Although the life history data at the disposal of the Eriksons was rare and of an exceptional longitudinal nature, they did not explore the dynamics of individual lives over time but rather used the collective themes to support conclusions regarding old age, which in their view reiterated the issues of development earlier identified and continued to provide the essence and meaning of life in the later years. They believed that achieving each of the eight stages of psychosocial development produces the necessary strength for extension of one's self in vital involvement with an ever-increasing concern beyond self.

Intimacy and Isolation. The balance between the capacity for intimacy and the need for isolation allows for individual and mutual development in relationships. The elder must reconfirm the joy of being alone with the closeness of supportive and intimate relationships. The capacity for aloneness, the ability to revel in one's own company, may be a developmental requirement of late life. This is not to the exclusion of significant others but only in preparation for the aloneness of loss and the ultimate aloneness of death. Developing the capacity to enjoy being alone has not been identified by developmental theorists as a significant aspect of adaptation in old age, but it seems clear that it may be. In fact, reminiscence may allow one to joyfully relive the past and may be a tool for achieving satisfaction in being alone. This is not to negate the reality of loss and the pain of loneliness, but, just as a child must learn to reach out to others, the aged must learn to value interiority. May Sarton said, "Solitude is the wealth of spirit and loneliness is poverty of spirit" (Sarton, 1979).

Relationships, the most intimate and the most distant, change over time, and the vital older individual learns to adapt to the changes. Although the Eriksons (1986) say it may be easier to think with "fond longing" about friends who are deceased, we think it may be more important to rekindle ties that have lain dormant and unattended. It is also important to reach beyond one's generation to develop intergenerational supports that will tend to be sustaining during the loss of peers and cohorts. Yet Wolanin (1996) says, "I didn't believe that people in their mid-eighties could develop such new and intimate relationships as I have experienced in the last few years." This ability has disproved one of the myths we have held that the old no longer develop new and close relationships with each other.

Achieving a Balance. Erikson and co-workers propose that each of the major stages of development involves a balance of the "syntonic" and "dystonic" modes of coping if one is to remain vitally involved (Erikson, Erikson, and Kivnick, 1986). In other words, trust must be balanced with mistrust to achieve a vital adjustment that proceeds toward higher levels of development. Too much trust results in maladaptation, which is considered neurotic, and too much mistrust results in malignant adaptation, which has the potential for psychoses. Trust is mandatory for development, but it can exist positively only in juxtaposition with a sensible mistrust. The balance of trust versus mistrust results in a sense of hope. The notion of too much and too little is vague and variable, but the contention is that if an appropriate individual balance has been achieved the individual is hopeful. Likewise, for each of the other stage dichotomies the balance must be achieved. "The process of bringing into balance feelings of integrity and despair involves a review of and a coming to terms with the life one has lived thus far" (Erikson, Erikson, and Kivnick, 1986, p. 70). All individuals have a central mental tendency to organize experience, a function of the ego. Erikson and associates found that many informants refrained from mentioning any former discontent with their lives, although the data indicated periods of profound discontent. The researchers speculate that the omissions may result from a desire to construct a satisfactory life view by "pseudo-integration," from the need to maintain privacy, from a lifelong process of recasting and finding new meanings in events, from denial, or from putting traumatic events over the years into perspective. Those who seemed most well adapted were able to draw sustenance from the past but remained vitally involved in the present (Erikson, Erikson, and Kivnick, 1986).

Reviewing and Transmitting. Fitch (1992) points out that when we visit our elder relatives we see the same old house, same old furniture, and sometimes believe the people are as unchanging as their surroundings. Very little is known about the developmental issues and phases of the very old. With encouragement old people will share their understanding of life and forge additional links in the chain of understanding that grows with each generation. Some contend our materialism is a natural outgrowth of our separation from aging and death. We avoid the intimate knowledge and heroism that confrontation with aging and death can cultivate. Fitch says the psychologic tasks of old age are slowing, life-review, transmission, and letting go. However, these describe activities rather than issues of development. Developmental tasks certainly include arrival at a personally acceptable philosophy of existence that transcends the limitations of the aging body and its systems. Butler described the growth potential for aged individuals through the "life-review" process (1963). This process of review and integration of events throughout the mature years is the catalyst for personal growth, integration, and evolving identity. Regrets and disappointments are fuel for reflection and deeper self-awareness. Butler's observations have confirmed Jung's views that reflective activity is intense and healing for many elders. Butler (1975, p. 412) wrote, ". . . the old are not only taking stock of themselves as they review their lives, they are trying to think and feel through what they will do with the time that is left and with whatever emotional and material legacies they may have to give others." The task of transmission may be made more urgent in the presence of vulnerability or recent trauma (Fitch, 1992).

Letting Go and Hanging On. The task of letting go initially sounds deteriorative. We believe it means letting go of the nonessentials, the facades and charades, the need to conform and please, of long held hurts and slights, of the need to brood over injustice. In addition, while letting go, the elder must simultaneously hang on to ideas and objects that are laden with meaning. The pace of this process is unique to each individual and frequently misunderstood by others. Fitch says the last phase of life involves a shift from conceptual thought to a more intuitive, emotional mode. Choices may reflect this in extraordinary ways. She suggests ". . . there is an organic, evolutionary dynamic in the elderly that happens even in the midst of confusion and which is tremendously potent and valid. There is some real victory and celebration possible even in the midst of existential decrepitude. We must do all that we can to see that everyone has that final and crowning opportunity" (Fitch, 1992, p. 106). Facilitating an atmosphere that allows letting go and hanging on in whatever way is significant to the individual can be extremely important. We can support or undermine these developments by the attitudes we hold and the environment we create (Fitch, 1992).

Personality Styles and Phases

The concepts of personality are based on several theoretic viewpoints: (1) neopsychoanalytic, (2) psychometric, (3) behaviorist, and (4) environmental. These viewpoints determine the expectations of personality in old age. From the neopsychoanalytic viewpoint, childhood forms lifelong personality traits. The psychometric view involves testing in order to develop a profile of specific personality traits such as extraversion-introversion, neuroticism, and psychoticism that can be traced through the life cycle; such traits may be genetic, environmental, or nurtured. Descriptive studies of these personality traits at various ages are of considerable interest to psychometricians. The behaviorist concern is focused on that which can be observed and measured in old age, often with the desire to modify. Motivation is not of major interest to behaviorists. The environmentalists contend that traits and situations are both potent predictors of adaptation in later life, and that in some persons personality traits predominate and for others situations are more influential to development. It is difficult to sort out personality traits that are developed or suppressed because of experience rather than age. To further complicate the issue, certain personality traits tend to emerge strongly in particular situations and with particular persons. Personality under ordinary conditions is assumed to remain quite stable across the adult life span. Such personality traits as stability, sociability, imaginativeness, neuroticism, extraversion, and openness to experience do not seem to change when studied longitudinally and cross-sequentially.

Empirically, it would seem that all of these components of personality exist in each individual. Some are nurtured by families and various societies, and some are squelched. Recent studies confirm that even minor personality characteristics may be genetically predetermined or are at least strongly dispositional (McClearn, 1990). Personality stability is a central belief of most life span psychologists.

Interiority. Jung (1971), a contemporary of Freud, was one of the first psychologists to define the last half of life as having a purpose of its own, quite apart from species survival—the development of self-awareness through reflective activity. He strongly believed in the importance of the last half of life, which is characterized by inner discovery, as opposed to the first half, which is oriented to biologic and social issues. Jung's theories contain elements of those of Cicero. The development of the psyche and the inner person is accompanied by a search for personal meaning and the spiritual self. Jung believed that a person who denies the validity of unconscious experience and the existence of the psyche is in self-conflict, consciously denying the relevance of the psyche because it reaches into obscurities beyond understanding. This denial of an aspect of one's nature results in restlessness, uprootedness, disorientation, and meaninglessness. However, many old persons may not be inclined to value psychologic exploration. Nevertheless, spirituality is an important aspect of development in later life and the means by which one becomes whole and develops the integrity described by Erikson. Jung also supports this view of the mature religious sentiment carrying one forward to holistic development in late life. Neugarten (1968) believes increased "interiority" is characteristic of aged persons and also indicates a growing interest in inner development.

Inherent and accumulated personality characteristics influence the adaptation of the individual at any given stage. The following questions need to be investigated in regard to the adaptation of the aged:

- How do the lives of introverts differ from the lives of extroverts?
- Do neuroticism and poor coping styles interfere with an orderly life plan?
- What personality dispositions influence adaptation to stressful life events?

The question that has not been addressed by gerontologists is: what happens to persons who have unstable personalities as they age? Stability of personality over time is in itself a personality characteristic. In other words, some persons will act in very predictable ways throughout their life, and others seem to have a thread of inconsistency in their life patterns and actions. Age as a developmental variable does not appear to be strongly related to most personality traits in healthy, community residents, although serious disease states, brain pathologic conditions, and institutional living may bring about major personality changes. Personality factors, cultural age norms, and expectations interact in undetermined ways to affect the individual life course. In short, the uniqueness, the highly prized fruit of a long life well lived, is the very factor that belies our efforts to predict norms for the later years.

PSYCHOSOCIAL THEORIES OF AGING

The three classic psychosocial theories of aging are essentially behavioristic and examine how one most successfully experiences late life: by disengaging, by maintaining activities of middle age, or by reinforcing personal continuity. These three theories view the processes of aging quite differently, and, because of the controversy arising from the different viewpoints, much research has been stimulated.

Disengagement

The disengagement theory of Cumming and Henry (1961) states that "aging is an inevitable, mutual withdrawal or disengagement, resulting in decreased interaction between the aging person and others in the social system he belongs to" (Cumming and Henry, 1961, p. 2). They contend that when the disengagement is complete a new equilibrium is established between the individual and society that is characterized by increased distance between the individual and society and that the relationship between the two is different than in middle age but mutually satisfactory. High morale is evident at the completion of the process, but the transition is characterized by low morale. The measures of disengagement are based on age, work, and decreased interest or investment. The theory is seen as universal and applicable to the aged in all cultures, although there are expected variations in timing and style. Hultsch and Deutsch (1981) note that when disengagement occurs, it proceeds at variable rates and patterns in various persons with unpredictable psychologic outcomes.

Activity

Activity theory supports the maintenance of regular actions, roles (formal and informal), and solitary as well as social pursuits for a satisfactory old age. Activists began to champion the notion that old age was only an extension of the middle years and could be abolished by keeping active (Maddox, 1963). Longino and Kart (1982) attempted to replicate many of the assumptions of activity theory based on the concepts of Lemon and associates (1972), who articulated an interactionist model of activity, promoting the concept that intimacy and frequency of activity reinforce one's self-concept. Formal activity was deemed less useful than informal activity because it tended to segregate by age, reinforcing a lower self-concept. Longino and associates (1980) found that even average activity levels in retirement community residents resulted in a more positive self-concept than among their counterparts in the general population. The activity theory may make sense when individuals live in a stable society, have access to positive influence and significant others, and have opportunities to participate meaningfully in the broader society if they continue to desire to do so. Attempts at clarifying activity theory as a general concept of satisfactory aging have not been supported.

Continuity

The continuity theory proposed by Havighurst and co-workers (1968) in reaction to the disengagement theory more realistically focuses on the relationship between life satisfaction and activity as an expression of enduring personality traits. Personality is considered the important factor in determining the relationship between role activity and life satisfaction, and personality is seen to be not only enduring but becoming more entrenched and pronounced as one ages. Three ideas important to this perspective, inferred from Neugarten and associates (1968), remain fundamental to beliefs about the aged individual:

- In normal aging personality remains consistent in men and women.
- Personality influences role activity and investment in the same.
- Personality influences life satisfaction regardless of role activity.

Criticisms of the three major theories focus on the obscurities in "life satisfaction" and "morale" and the value-laden term "successful." In addition, it has been found in many studies that self-report is likely to convey a more positive picture than might be reported by an observer and that the aged tend to express dissatisfaction through the "generalized other." For instance, "I am very happy with my life, but other people my age are miserable and complaining all the time." The scales, of which there are many, to measure success, life satisfaction, attitude adjustment, and morale have been questioned both in terms of reliability and validity. None of the three theories can be clearly supported with data. In addition, they have little to do with personal meaning and motivation.

SOCIOLOGIC AGING
Social Gerontology

Social gerontology is a subfield of gerontology that deals with the nonphysical aspects of aging. It focuses on role development and group behaviors of older people, the impact of social phenomena on them, and the impact of older persons on the social system. Essentially, it is the study of how the individual and society adapt to each other. Occasionally a giant in the field, with astute perception, articulates a phenomenon that strikes a responsive chord in enough people to be accepted as a contemporary truth. Social gerontologists tend to see aging as a social problem because our society is not prepared to absorb the ever-increasing number of aged persons into meaningful social roles, particularly those of power and influence. Sociologists often study the disenfranchised members of the population or subcultures: stigmatized individuals and their social status. Some knowledge gaps recognized by social gerontologists include the scant comparisons of cross-national data and the dearth of data on older members of minority groups—particularly of those who are not Black. The tendency to study "white and Black"

is indeed unfortunate as the blending of races and cultures negates the validity of these divisions.

Sociologic aging is a composite of the performance of expected social roles appropriate to one's chronologic age, culture, and capacity. Terms that are associated with sociologic aging are age norms, social time clocks, age-grading, and social time. All of these are descriptive of the place individuals should occupy in a society at any given time in their lives. Socioeconomic status is intrinsically woven into the social roles occupied. Birren and Schroots (1984) developed the concept of "eldering," the process by which elders begin to fill the roles expected of them in their society. Sociologic aging is problematic in societies that have diversified traditional backgrounds, such as United States, and in which flexibility in roles and age-related expectations have become the norm. Age-graded activities were far more reliable in primitive societies from which anthropologists derived these notions. Again, many of the developmental theories are far more applicable to school children or traditional societies than to mature, individualized adults in our era of highly diversified populations. Social scientists have, in the last decade, focused considerably more attention on the interaction of age, period, and cohort in attempts to study the social aspects of aging from a life span perspective. Each issue must be seen as a complex interaction of personal and social variables over time and in culture and subculture. Psychologists often focus on life span development, whereas sociologists speak of life course.

A social psychology of the life course is built on the following assumptions:

- Age structures are necessary for social organization, providing rights and responsibilities and governing rules and expectations.
- Biologic models of the life span are inadequate to account for aging without consideration of social dimensions.
- Continuities and changes in social expectation occur over the entire life course.
- Transformation of identity occurs with each new constellation of social expectation and behaviors.

Life Course

Life course is composed of elements that make up the overall structure and timing of events in one's life from cradle to grave. It must be examined and taken into account to understand the aged individual. This is the basis for longitudinal studies. Life structure is composed of roles (occupational, social, and family), relationships (intimate, personal, and professional), and inner structure (goals, values, motives, and memories). The progress of all these aspects of life can be considered a life course. Change and continuity are the elements that must be examined to understand the progression. Lenker and Polivka (1996) focus on the richness and uniqueness of elders' life course. Helping elders understand the story of their lives preserves identity and feelings of self-worth.

Life Transitions. Transitional periods are a major focus of understanding aging from a sociologic perspective. The transitions throughout the life course include major shifts attributed to age, role, occupation, family, and economics (Cunningham and Brookbank, 1988). Figure 2-8 outlines the distribution of these transitions.

Changes are stressful but often provide opportunities for growth because they require development and application of distinctly different adaptive skills. For many of the major transitions in life, which may be especially traumatic, we receive little preparation. In cases of role accumulation, such as that of grandparent, some previous development will be applicable, with modification, to the new role. Likewise, the shifts in filial relationships are often gradual and do not require complete role deletion or role reversal. Those transitions that make use of past skills and adaptations may be least stressful. Some shifts, such as from functional independence to functional dependence, cut across many aspects of life and require several transitional shifts. Chapters 15, 17, and 21 address some of these issues. From a life course perspective, the transitions and adaptations required produce both stability and change in individual preferences, capacities, expectations, and behavior. Age-related transitions are socially created, shared, and recognized. A transition is socially recognized and entails a reorientation of perceptions and expectations of and by the individual. It is also important to remember that cohort and gender differences are inherent in all of life's major transitions.

Age Norms. Norms are socially shared expectations that present "shoulds" or "oughts" for behavior. Age norms and age constraints are concepts that underscore the need for persons of a given age to conduct their lives in a manner that is socially expected and acceptable at that age. When individuals do not do so it is expected they will feel stressed and perhaps stigmatized. In reality, much depends on the particular social expectation, status of the individual, circumstances, and whether one acts older or younger than one's age. In late life, there are few socially structured expectations and few studies of late life transitions. Some of the difficulty lies in how recently large numbers of cohort members have survived to be extremely old. No investigator seems to have seriously examined the nature of predictable transitions, sequencing of events, or spacing after age 70. Age-graded behaviors at that point are lacking. Issues on which social gerontologists focus most assiduously are (1) social integration, (2) successful adaptation, (3) age variables in social scientific research, (4) society as a succession of cohorts, (5) environment as a variable in understanding behavior, and (6) the search for a unified perspective of aging (Maddox and Campbell, 1985). "The study of the life course is a search for systematic regularities in events of unique meaning" (Back, 1980, p. 2).

Status and Role Changes. Status and role are the concepts around which norms, relationships, conformity and deviance, and stability and change are organized. Rosow

(1985) considers four problems involved in applying role concepts to the aged: (1) is there a role, (2) what are the boundaries, (3) what are the interactions with other roles, and (4) what are the levels of the role performance? When considering the role of the aged in our society, we might examine the regard in which they are held as a measure of role relevance, boundaries, and performance. Rosow refers to an earlier publication (Rosow, 1973) to identify the major issues in role theory as applied to the aged:

- Loss of roles excludes the aged from significant social participation and devalues their contribution.
- Old age is the first stage of life with systematic status loss for the entire cohort.
- Persons in our society are not socialized to the fate of aging.
- Because there is no specified role for the aged, their lives may become unstructured.

Informal and tenuous roles are identified by Rosow (1985) as those lacking structure and stability and not linked to social status. In late life it is expected that institutionalized roles will decrease in number and significance while the tenuous roles will increase in significance if not in number. Tenuous roles are those that embody a definite social position but with vague or insubstantial role expectations (Rosow, 1985).

Social Supports

Social support is derived from the assurance of love, esteem, and belonging to a network involving common and mutual concerns. This certainly sounds like the ideal social support one would wish from intimates and family. However, the social support derived from informal ties may be much less intense but every bit as vital in old age. Friendships, neighbors, and spontaneous social ties may increase in later life. Sociogerontologists are interested in these types of social supports and how such interpersonal ties contribute to the health and well-being of older individuals. See Chapter 17 for further discussion.

Reciprocity

Attitudes of autonomy and independence are highly prized and cultivated within our society and seem to be clung to more ferociously as we see them ebbing away. A single power outage or gas war and we are immediately confronted with our dependency. Unusual life-styles, weddings conducted in hot air balloons, bizarre clothing and haircuts, and the need to be especially assertive about the small details of our lives seem to assume more importance in direct proportion to our increasing dependence on technology for survival. In quite the opposite fashion, our elders, many of whom grew up in a self-sufficient style, were not so in need of symbols of independence but were succored by tradition and other symbols of continuity and collective thought. Undergirding all this is the deep awareness that as humans we must depend on others and be depended on if we are to survive individually and culturally. The concept of reciprocity

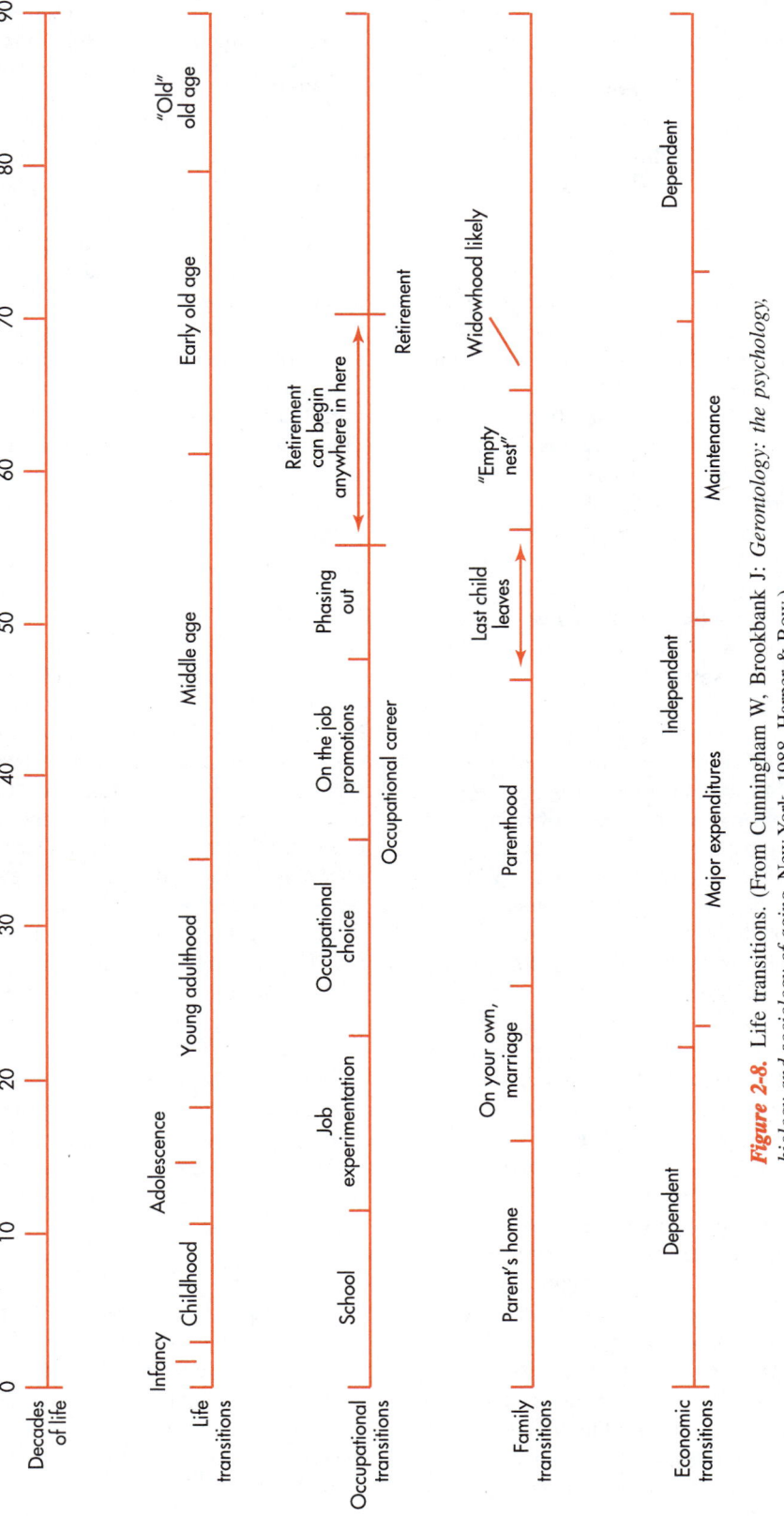

Figure 2-8. Life transitions. (From Cunningham W, Brookbank J: *Gerontology: the psychology, biology and sociology of aging,* New York, 1988, Harper & Row.)

in relationships and society is basic to survival. In old age, as one becomes physically and functionally dependent in various ways, it is important to cultivate the exchange process, reciprocal activities, and interpersonal reliance to avoid erosion of self-esteem. Elders often receive retroactive earnings in the human exchange system. See Chapters 15 and 17 for additional discussion of this concept.

LONGEVITY

The mean life expectancy, or age of survivors within a group born near the same date, has risen almost 40 years (Begley, Hager, and Murr 1990) in this century. A child born in 1994 can now expect to live 25 years longer than his or her counterpart of 1900. However, a person age 65 today can only expect to live 5 years longer than their 1900 counterpart (Downs, 1994). Through postponement of major chronic disorders, we may eventually expect to markedly shorten the period of senescence (Fries, 1980; 1992). However, the attainable maximum life span in the very best of circumstances will remain unchanged (Table 2-2).

There is the popular presumption that elders will live longer and be healthier and happier and that, given continuing advances in technology, we will in the future almost totally conquer mortality. This sort of thinking is stimulated by popular articles such as appeared in *Insight* (1987) purporting to extend life to 180 years by dietary restriction or the scenario offered in *Life* magazine "The war on aging," which describes living 700 years (Darrach, 1992).

Some theorists delving into the processes of aging now contend that perhaps there is no such thing as primary aging. However, most gerontologists today agree that 115 years is a realistic maximum life span (Downs, 1994). Studies of life extension through food restriction have been conducted on rats. Not only do such rats live almost twice as long as the projected life span, but also they do not develop the disorders common to aging rats. The theory is that life is prolonged by restricting food and thus increasing metabolic efficiency. Walford (1986), a renowned and respected gerontologist and theorist in aging research, addresses this approach to life extension in *The 120-Year Diet*.

Others believe that humans may extend their physical and mental capacity in later years by continued use and stimulation. Brain dendrites grow when the brain is stimulated; muscles remain strong and resilient when used. Extensive research into mental function and aging by Schaie (in Steinberg, 1994) indicates mental decline is less in people who learn new things, have a flexible attitude in middle age, adapt to change, and who continue to pursue keen mental interests when they retire. Gradual physical decline begins early in youth but remains gradual if the life-style is not abusive. Better diet, more exercise, and better medical care are usually given credit for elders being in better condition than those of a generation ago.

Even if heart disease, cancer, stroke, and other diseases were eradicated, humans would still be subject to accidents. Cunningham and Brookbank (1988) indicate that after 35 years of age the probability of death doubled every 5 to 8 years. Gompertz mathematically described this phenomenon in 1825. Accidents among those who are 85 years and older, the fastest growing group of elders, are four times more frequent than in other age groups (Darrach, 1992). If accidents could be controlled, longevity would be more attainable (Figure 2-9). Jazwinski (1996) illustrates the physical determinents of aging and longevity in Figure 2-10.

Rudman (1990), in a 6-month experiment, was able to reverse some symptoms of aging in a group of men in their sixties and seventies. A comparable control group was also used. The experimental group injected themselves three times a week for 6 months with a synthetic version of human growth hormone, a potent secretion of the pituitary gland. The dosage used remained within the limits of that naturally secreted in younger men. The variance between the two groups was significant. Those taking the hormone therapy regained 10% muscle mass, 9% skin thickness, and lost 14% of their body fat. While there were some side effects, Rudman indicated that, "the treatment reversed body composition changes that would occur in 10 to 20 years of aging" (Darrach, 1992). Rejuvenation and longevity clinics outside the United States are enticing individuals with the same or similar human growth hormone injections (Humatrope) (Foote, 1994). This "treatment for aging" has not been approved by the Food and Drug Administration for use in the United States on the basis that the dosage is not really known for healthy adults. The doses of Humatrope being used by these rejuvenation and longevity clinics are at levels used for children who have growth defects. Yen (1996), at University of California, San Diego, found that in a group of elders who received DHEA (growth hormone) 75% felt better. The question still remains, what is the role of this steroid hormone in the maintenance of healthy aging? Biologists are beginning to locate genes that govern cellular mortality and they are attempting to identify genes that are responsible for the "on-off switch" (Darrach, 1992). Recently a gene responsible for premature aging (Werner's Syndrome) was identified, causing excitement in biogerontologic circles (King, 1996).

Exceptional Longevity

Data gathered from these groups have been important in pursuit of maximum life span. Common factors influential to longevity were dietary restrictions (low in fat, high in vegetable protein, high fiber, and limited caloric intake), exercise, and sociability. The value of undernourishment as a means of extending life span seems to arise from lifelong patterns of minimum intake. High altitudes and decreased temperature may also be important factors.

Table 2-2	Current and Projected Life Expectancy—1995-2010*		
	Projected life expectancy at birth		
Year	**Men**	**Women**	**Average**
Future life expectancy			
1995	73.7	80.3	77.0
2000	74.3	80.9	77.6
2005	74.9	81.4	78.2
2010	75.6	82	78.8
Current life expectancy			
1995	72.8	79.7	76.3
2000	73.2	80.2	76.7
2005	73.8	80.7	77.3
2010	74.5	81.3	77.9

From Expectation of life at birth and projections 1995-2010, *Statistical Abstracts of the United States 1995,* US Department of Commerce, Economics and Statistics Administration, Bureau of Census, Washington D.C.
*A child born in 1995 has an average life expectancy of 76.3 years

Rosenfeld (1985) indicated that animal studies have shown that a decrease of a few degrees centigrade in body temperature could add approximately 15 to 25 years to human life. One must be careful not to assume that a decrease in measured temperature means a decrease in metabolic rate. It is the core temperature that makes the difference. If the substance that triggers hibernation in animals could be isolated and transferred, researchers might seek ways to trick the human body into periods of torpor or hibernation, thus extending the life span. Drugs, biofeedback, and yoga are other means that are also being explored as methods of lowering body temperature to extend life span.

Heredity

The most provocative studies of the influence of genetics on aging adaptation come from Kallman and Sander (1948, 1949) and the Swedish Adoption/Twin Study of Aging (McClearn et al, 1988). The Kallman/Sander study surveyed cognitive similarities of 1000 pairs of twins over 60 years old residing in the state of New York. Similarities for disease, life span, and time of death were significant for identical twins, more so than for fraternal twins. The authors concluded that genetic influences are primarily responsible for individual differences in aging. The Swedish Adoption/Twin Study on Aging includes a comparison of identical twins reared apart, which has added a strong component to the study of genetics and behavior in late life. This ongoing longitudinal study indicates at this time that, although remaining strong, the significance of genetics on behavior in late life is probably less than in earlier life. However, there is a high correlation of similar life experiences that seems to exist and that may have a genetic basis (Plomin and McClearn, 1990).

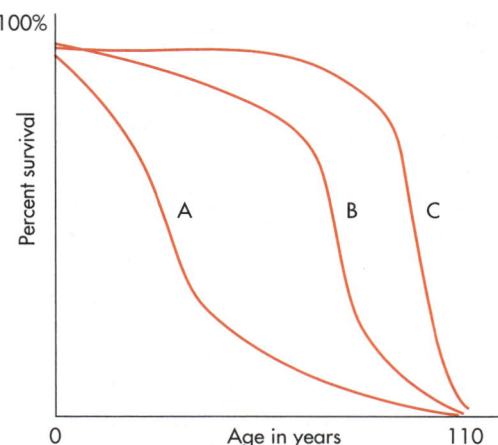

Figure 2-9. When deaths are primarily the result of many random events (disease, accidents, etc.), a curve noting the progressive loss of individuals from a population resembles curve *(A)*. This curve has such a shape because individual deaths are occurring at any time with little regard to age. As deaths occurring in the early years are eliminated, a curve like *(B)* is seen. However, when accident and disease become less and less common, curve *(C)* shows that the mean life span is closer to the maximum life span. The latter is the same regardless of the mean life span, since it is more fully representative of death associated with aging phenomena. (From Hampton J: *The biology of human aging,* Dubuque, Iowa, 1991, Wm C Brown.)

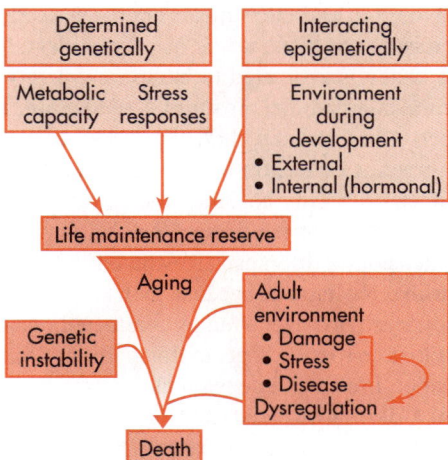

Figure 2-10. Determinants of aging and longevity. Physiologic relations, not molecular mechanisms, are shown. Metabolic capacity, stress responses and environment during development all contribute to the life maintenance reserve, where they interact. Genetic instability is genetically determined, results in genetic alterations, and is influenced by environmental factors. Aging plays itself out at all levels of biologic organization; it is not possible to separate cellular changes from organismal aging. (From The aging immune system: primer and prospectus, *Science,* vol 273(5721): 70, 1996.)

Heredity, once thought to have a great influence on life span, is not considered as important today. An individual born of long-lived relatives may live a very long life, but heredity is only partially influential in this process. The major developmental theorists of aging (Baltes, Reese and Lipsitt, 1980) propose that the older one gets the more influenced one is by nonnormative life events. The last third of life requires very different adaptive capacities than the first two thirds. Ordinarily, one is consumed with and measured by performance until the later years. In older aged, existential issues move to the forefront: losses, transitions to roles not yet understood by society, living in the moment, defining meanings in existence, and learning the measure of one's mettle. In addition, it has always been a problem to sort cohort variances and their influence on adaptation to given situations and life stages (Schaie, 1965).

Nutrition

Nutrition is receiving considerable attention as a major influence on longevity. Americans have become increasingly conscious of the implications and consequences of nutritional status on disease processes and on life span. Even the government now supports nutritional research. Studies as far back as Davis (1975), Benet (1976), and others show distinct differences in the dietary patterns of long-lived populations as compared to the dietary regimens of short-lived populations. Vegetables form the major portion in diets of long-lived people. These foods are high in nutrients and essential trace elements, the latter having been washed into the soil from mineral deposits at higher elevations. Little beef is consumed; mutton and other meats are eaten. Refined sugar does not exist in the diets, nor is obesity evident. The overall caloric intake is estimated to be approximately half that of a typical American diet. Walford (1986), from his ongoing research, advocates the "high/low" diet, a diet that provides the greatest concentration of nutrients with the least amount of calories. In the laboratory, Walford began restricted diets on rats at the time of weaning and found significant extension of life span. Restricted diets at weaning are not feasible for humans because they tend to decrease ultimate body size. However, studies conducted on adolescent rats found that restricting diets at this point in time was just as effective on life span extension as was weaning-initiated restriction. Calorie-restricted diets for rats have received considerable attention in research (Masoro, Katz, and McMahan, 1989; Weraarchakul, Strong, Wood, et al, 1989). The National Institute of Aging (NIA), which began a study on monkeys in 1987 (monkeys being closer to man than rats), so far has shown that reducing caloric intake by 30% leads to lower body temperature in the monkeys. Speculation is that lower body temperature slows body biochemical reactions and lowers levels of pentosidine. Pentosidine has been found to strongly correlate with onset of age-related diseases. Cutting calories may increase monkey life span by 30% to 50% (Ciabattari, 1996).

Findings show that dietary restriction hastens DNA repair. The theory of aging based on the accumulation of DNA damage in somatic cells is an old one, but it was unknown whether repair of DNA was gradually diminished in the aging process. These studies have shown that DNA repair processes are involved in aging and, not only does restricted caloric intake slow DNA error accumulation during aging, but it also facilitates the repair process, resulting in longer lived mice. The success of caloric restrictions on life extension of mice dates back to Cornero, who in 1507, because of illness at the age of 40, limited his food intake to 12 ounces a day and lived another 60 years. Dr. M. Lane of NIA suggests that average life span may be 100 to 110 years with a maximum of a 150-year possibility in the years ahead. He theorizes that if men can reduce daily calorie intake from 3000 calories per day to 2100 calories a day and women reduce their intake from 2500 to 1800 calories per day, life could be prolonged (Ciabattari, 1996).

Environment

Environmental influences affect longevity of an individual in certain obvious ways and many obscure ways not yet fully understood. Environmental factors include the physical, chemical, and thermal environments, humidity, solar radiation, soil and water composition, altitude, various pollutants, and ionizing radiation. Persons living in urban areas are exposed to more pollutants, have more varied economic capacity, and are exposed to more life-threatening situations and psychic stressors than those living in rural settings. Urban mobility is hazardous. The opportunity for exercise, although improved in the past 15 years, is often hampered by one's life-style or chosen work.

Socioeconomic Status

Education, health, and marital status have been considered to have a direct or indirect influence on longevity. Education affects and is affected by social standing, income, occupation, and other factors. The higher the education, the fewer physical hazardous job risks. Individuals who complete college and graduate studies are more often able to select high-paying, low-risk jobs. Higher paying positions afford the individual better opportunity for health care, with health maintenance being a universally recognized important longevity factor. Intelligence, too, is thought to be related to life span. Some researchers believe that those who are intelligent find better ways to survive, and others believe greater intelligence is an obvious index of generalized superior endowment. Intelligence is genetically and environmentally determined. The potential of each of us will be able to surface and be cultivated to its optimum level, given a conducive environment, proper nutrition, and socioeconomic advantages.

Statistics have shown that marital status influences longevity, particularly for men. Whether it is the result of mutual caring by the spouse that occurs in the relationship or because of a more regulated life-style has not been definitely established, but those who are married have a longer life expectancy than those who are single. Social interaction, which is one component of a marital relationship, may reinforce the meaning of life, and attention to the maintenance of self for one's spouse may be a psychologic advantage toward longevity.

The 25-year follow-up of the first Duke University longitudinal study on aging (Palmore, 1982) reaffirms the variables stressed in Woodruff (1977) for the attainment of longevity. Palmore noted that intelligence, health, activities, sexual relations, and life satisfaction were all factors that contributed directly to longevity of the study group.

Jensen and Bellecci (1983) studied a group of nonagenarians in a state veterans' home and found that those very old persons measured up favorably against a group of noninstitutionalized 65- to 75-year-olds. The nonagenarians had few mental health problems or chronic illnesses, took few medications, and were more socially and physically active than their younger counterparts. Their longevity indicates an interplay of many factors as yet poorly defined. Today, increasing numbers of nonagenarians and centenarians provide an ever-increasing group for longevity research. However, biologic theories of aging, which seem more sophisticated than other aspects of longevity research, are still rudimentary. Some of the questions yet to be answered thoroughly in order to understand factors influencing longevity are:

- What factors account for individual longevity?
- How can predisposition for diseases be determined?
- What accounts for the increasing longevity of women as compared to men?
- What are the effects of social class?
- What are the ultimate differences caused by habits of smoking, exercise, diet?
- How are wisdom and creativity cultivated and demonstrated in old age?

The most critical questions do not concern how long we live, but for what reasons and in what conditions. Human progress can be measured by the total percentage of individuals who achieve longevity while maintaining a life of meaning and purpose.

An integrative matrix, drawing from the psychologists, biologists, and sociologists, to organize the voluminous outpouring of data and fragmented bits of information is needed.

In summary, the complexities of aging and the numerous predictable and unpredictable events that occur in an individual lifetime have made many theorists conclude that aging in adulthood is a random process of change with no discernible pattern or undergirding theory. From this viewpoint, the individual organism progresses through the ordered state of programmed development to the chaotic state of later life in which patterns are no longer discernible; when the undefined, and perhaps individually developed, critical thresholds of function are exceeded and incapacity results (Yates, 1988). However, even though at this time there is not sufficient conceptual sophistication to embrace the intricacies of adult development (Schroots, 1988), we continue to try to organize our expectations of the aging process into predictable, or at least expectable, patterns. There are still many areas of adult development and aging that have been minimally explored and may be the essence of development in maturity and old age. The development of love, compassion, creativity, and wisdom are areas that need considerably more attention and may in the future yield specific patterns in the aged. Tentative theories of aging recognize changes in conception of time, self-concept, hope, and future orientation as one grows old. The sense of inner control has important ramifications in terms of how one ages. Being old is an art, a science, and a challenge.

We have attempted to introduce the reader to an overview of oldness as it is seen in our society today. The body of the text will consider the relevance of all these views to health care provision and explore them in depth in further chapters. *Life* magazine featured aging in the October 1992 issue with the question, "Can we stop aging?" The next question, of course, is, "Do we want to?" The notion of a prolonged and perhaps endless life span as a possibility is one that re-emerges in gerontology periodically—just as fads and fashions do in any discipline. Frequently we hear that only 100 years ago life expectancy was 48 years and now it is in the seventies. The implication seems to be that in another 100 years most of us will live to be over 100 years old. However, the figures really mean that far fewer people are dying young, not that the human life span has increased significantly. In 1850, 50% of all deaths occurred in children under age 15. Less than 15% of people lived 60 years or longer. The actual extension of average life span has increased only approximately 0.4% per decade for a century. However, as scientists unlock the genetic code and the secrets of DNA, the next challenge is to confront the master control of death. The question is whether the maximum life span can be extended much beyond the 120 years that has been the scientifically accepted outer limit of individual human survival.

KEY CONCEPTS

- Aging is a gradual process of change over the course of time. Each species has an expected life span and that of the human species as presently understood is limited to approximately 120 years.
- It is unknown at this time what changes over time are due specifically to aging, disease, life-style, or environmental impact. In other words, the changes due purely to the aging process are unknown.
- Studies of the aged in other times and places often lend interest and insight into the present study of the aged.
- There are eight or nine accepted theories of biologic aging, and they are all believed to be true to one extent or another. However, none can stand alone as the explanation of the aging process and why it occurs.

▲	Needs Addressed and Task Strengths	
Need to learn and understand; need for intellectual stimulation (to maintain self-esteem and achieve self-actualization)	Highly observant Analytic thought Interest in knowledge promotion Curiosity	

- The immunologic theory of biologic aging is one of the most coherent and widely accepted.
- Psychologic theories of aging are particularly culture and cohort bound and must be studied with that in mind. Jung and Erikson have made major contributions to our understanding of aging from the psychologic perspective.
- Life-span developmental theorists tend to study the total life course of cohort groups to determine major influences on their development.
- It is becoming more generally accepted that personality characteristics, as well as biologic characteristics, are to some degree inherent in the individual.
- Studies of exceptional longevity in various geographic pockets have shown the importance of diet, exercise, environment, and most importantly adequate documentation of age. Those studies of individuals thought to be over 150 years old have proved to be questionable because of unverified birth records.
- It is expected that within the coming century we will see further "rectangularization" of aging—meaning there will be increased years of healthy aging and a more abrupt and rapid deterioration before death.

▲ CASE STUDY

Jennie attained the remarkable age of 100 the day before Christmas. There were numerous celebrations of her birthday by friends and family. She was delighted and surprised because little had been made of her birthday in the previous years. She always explained it away by the fact it was so near Christmas. Aside from rheumatic aches, difficulty in breathing at times (even though she had never smoked), frequent falls, and limited energy, she considered herself healthy, had rarely been ill enough to see a doctor, and had only recently begun taking digitalis. Jennie sometimes woke during the night with urinary urgency and then had difficulty falling asleep again. At those times she would sip a shot of brandy and read until she fell asleep. During the day she wore a protective pad as she tended to leak urine when she coughed or laughed. Jennie said, "This getting old is like the one-hoss shay: everything falls apart."* Jennie had a large network of friends and an attentive family though she was well acquainted with grief and loss. Her husband of 75 years

*A "one-hoss shay" was a cart drawn by a horse; popular in 1910.

had died 3 years before, and she had left her lovely home and beloved dog when she moved into the retirement center at age 97. She was deeply spiritual but not religious in a ritualized sense. Her granddaughter was majoring in gerontology at the local university and often talked to Jennie about her old age and remarkable adaptation in an attempt to find the key to her longevity.

Based upon the case study, develop a nursing care plan using the following procedure*:

List comments of client that provide *subjective data.*

List information that provides *objective data.*

List two client strengths you have identified from data.

From these data, identify and state, using accepted format, *two nursing diagnoses* you determine are most significant to this client's needs and strengths at this time.

Determine and state *outcome criteria* for each diagnosis. These must reflect some alleviation of the problem identified in the nursing diagnosis and must be stated in concrete and measurable terms.

Plan and state one or more *interventions* for each diagnosed problem. Provide specific documentation of source used to determine appropriate intervention. Plan at least one intervention that incorporates the client's existing strengths.

Evaluate success of intervention. Interventions must correlate directly with the stated outcome criteria in order to measure the outcome success.

STUDY QUESTIONS/ACTIVITIES

What factors would you consider important in determining Jennie's longevity?

Discuss Jennie's physical changes as they relate to theories of aging.

Discuss the factors in longevity that have presently been identified and whether these are evident in the cases of individuals you know, or have heard of, that have attained great old age.

Which of the psychologic and/or sociologic theories of aging seem most relevant in Jennie's case?

What theories of aging seem most plausible to you? Compare the outstanding characteristics of each.

*Students are advised to refer to their nursing diagnosis text and identify possible or potential problems.

Imagine you are Jennie and discuss with your granddaughter your thoughts about your own aging.

Discuss the meanings and the thoughts triggered by the student's and elder's viewpoints as expressed at the beginning of the chapter. How do these vary from your own experience?

Imagine yourself at 90 years old and describe the life style you will have and the factors that you believe account for your long life.

Organize a debate in which each individual attempts to convince others of the logic of one particular concept of aging.

List and discuss the psychologic tasks of aging that you believe will be most difficult for you to accomplish.

Describe in a brief essay the characteristics of the oldest person you have known.

RESEARCH QUESTIONS

What physical changes can be attributed strictly to the aging of an organism?

What environmental factors in our present sociocultural milieu are clearly sources of early mortality?

What factors in relationships contribute to survival?

What variables may affect cell replication patterns?

What are the identifiable factors in extreme longevity?

What caloric distribution of carbohydrates, proteins, and fats actually contributes to longevity?

RESOURCES

Films and Videos

Women of the Georgian Hotel, L. Bloise, Terra Nova Films, Chicago, Ill (20 min.)

This video interviews four women, aged 83-107, who discuss their secrets of longevity, how they cope with adversity, and how they achieve serenity.

REFERENCES

Agarwal S, Sohal RS: Relationship between susceptibility to protein oxidation, aging, and maximum life span potential of different species, *Experiment Gerontol* 31:387, 1996.

Back K: *Life course: integrative theories and exemplary populations,* Boulder, Colo, 1980, Westview Press.

Balazs EA: Intercellular matrix of connective tissue. In Finch CE, Hayflick L, editors: *Handbook of the biology of aging,* New York, 1977, Van Nostrand Reinhold.

Baltes PB, Reese HW, Lipsitt LP: Non-normative developmental events, *Ann Rev Psychol* 31:65, 1980.

Bandura A: Self-efficacy: toward a unifying theory of behavioral change. *Psychol Rev* 84:191-215, 1977.

Banks JT: The sad but instructive case of Virginia Woolf, *J Ident Aging* 1(1):23-36, 1996.

Begley S, Hagar M, Murr A: The search for the fountain of youth, *Newsweek,* vol CXV(10):44-48, 3/5/1990.

Bender BS, Nagel JE, Adler WH, et al: Absolute peripheral blood lymphocyte count and subsequent mortality of elderly men, *J Am Geriatr Soc* 34:649, 1986.

Benet S: *How to live to be 100,* New York, 1976, The Dial Press.

Birnbaum B, Swick L: Human suppressor lymphocyte II: changes in condanava lin A–induced suppressor cells with age, *J Gerontol* 36:410, 1981.

Birren J, Birren B: The concepts, models, and history of the psychology of aging. In Birren J, Schaie K, editors: *Handbook of the psychology of aging,* ed 3, San Diego, 1990, Academic Press.

Birren J, Cunningham W: Research on the psychology of aging: principles, concepts, and theory. In Birren J, Schaie K, editors: *Handbook of the psychology of aging,* ed 2, New York, 1985, Van Nostrand Reinhold.

Birren J, Renner J: Research on the psychology of aging: principles and experimentation. In Birren J, Schaie K, editors: *Handbook of the psychology of aging,* New York, 1977, Van Nostrand Reinhold.

Birren J, Schroots JJF: Steps to an ontogenetic psychology, *Acad Psychol Bull* 6:177, 1984.

Boersma WJA, Steinmeier FA: Age-related changes in the relative number of THy-1 and LyT-2 bearing peripheral blood lymphocytes in mice: a longitudinal approach, *Cell Immunol* 93: 417, 1985.

Bowsher JE, Keep D: Toward an understanding of three control constructs: personal control, self-efficacy, and hardiness, *Issues Mental Health Nurs* 16:33-50, 1995.

Buhler C: The human course of life in its goal aspects, *J Hum Psychol* 4:1, 1964.

Butler RL: Life review: an interpretation of reminiscence in the aged, *Psychiatry* 26:65, 1963.

Butler R: *Why survive? Being old in America,* New York, 1975, Harper & Row.

Ciabattari J: *Parade's* special intelligence report: another reason to diet, *Parade Magazine,* p. 8, August 4, 1996.

Clark M, Anderson PB: *Culture and aging,* Springfield, Ill, 1967, Charles C Thomas.

Clayton V: Erikson's theory of human development as it applies to the aged: wisdom as contradictive cognition, *Hum Dev* 18:119,1975.

Covelli V, et al: Inheritance of immune responsiveness, life span, and disease incidence in interline crosses of mice selected for high and low multispecific antibody production, *J Immunol* 142:1224, 1989.

Cumming E, Henry W: *Growing old,* New York, 1961, Basic Books.

Cunningham W, Brookbank J: *Gerontology: the physiology, biology and sociology of aging,* New York, 1988, Harper & Row.

Darrach B: The war on aging, *Life* 15(10): October, 1992.

Davis D: *The centenarians of the Andes,* New York, 1975, Doubleday.

Downs H: Must we age? *Parade Magazine,* p. 21, August 21, 1994.

Ebersole PR: May your goals never be fully accomplished, *Geriatr Nurs* 17(5):258-259, 1996.

Ebersole JL, Steffen MJ: Aging effects on secretory IgA immune responses, *Immun Invest* 18:59, 1989.

Erikson EH, Erikson JM, Kivnick HQ: *Vital involvement in old age: the experience of old age in our time,* New York, 1986, Norton.

Ferguson FG, Wikby A, Maxson P, et al: Immune parameters in a longitudinal study of a very old population of Swedish people: a comparison between survivors and nonsurvivors, *J Gerontol* 50:B378, 1995.

Fitch V: The psychological tasks of old age, *Naropa Insti J* 8:91, 1992.

Fjelland R, Gjengedal E: The theoretic foundation for nursing as a science. In Benner P, editor: *Interpretive phenomenology: embodiment, caring and ethics in health and illness,* Thousand Oaks, Calif, 1994, Sage Publications.

Foote J: Mexico resorts take shot at eternal youth, *San Francisco Examiner,* p. B-1, March 1, 1994.

Freud S: Introductory lectures on psychoanalysis. In Freud S: *The standard edition of the complete psychological works of Sigmund Freud,* vols 15 and 16, London, 1954, Hogarth.

Fries JF: Aging, natural death, and the compression of morbidity, *N Engl J Med* 303:130, 1980.

Fries JF: *Healthy aging,* Conference sponsored by Institute for Advancement of Human Behavior (IAHB), San Francisco, October 1-4, 1992.

Fuller-Thomson E, Minkler M, Driver D: Grandparents raising grandchildren, *Gerontologist* 37(3): 386-389, 1997.

Georgakas D: The Methuselah factors, *Gerontologist* 22:4, 1980.

Guyton AC: *Textbook of medical physiology,* ed 7, Philadelphia, 1986, WB Saunders.

Hall GS: *Senescence: the second half of life,* New York, 1922, Appleton.

Hampton J: *The biology of human aging,* Dubuque, Iowa, 1991, William C Brown.

Harmen D: Aging: a theory based on free radical and radiation chemistry, *J Gerontol* 11:298, 1956.

Hartmann H: *Essays in ego psychology,* New York, 1964, International Universities Press.

Havighurst R: *Developmental tasks and education,* New York, 1972, David McKay.

Havighurst RL, Neugarten BL, Tobin SS: Disengagement and patterns of aging. In Neugarten BL, editor: *Middle age and aging,* Chicago, 1968, University of Chicago.

Hayflick L: Human cells and aging, *Sci Am* 218:32, 1968.

Hayflick L: Why grow old? *Stanford Mag* 3:36, 1975.

Hayflick L: The cellular basis for biological aging. In Finch CE, Hayflick L, editors: *Handbook of the biology of aging,* New York, 1977, Van Nostrand Reinhold.

Hayflick L: Theories of aging. In Cape R, Coe R, Rossman I, editors: *Fundamentals of geriatric medicine,* New York, 1983, Raven Press.

Hayflick L: Biologic aging theories. In Maddox G, editor-in-chief: *The encyclopedia of aging,* New York, 1987, Springer.

Hedrick M: Immune cells. In Maddox G, editor-in-chief: *The encyclopedia of aging,* New York, 1987, Springer.

Hershey D: *Lifespan and factors affecting it,* Springfield, Ill, 1974, Charles C Thomas.

Hultsch DF, Deutsch F: *Adult development and aging: a life span perspective,* New York, 1981, McGraw-Hill.

Insight: Prolonging lives in the lab, *Insight* 3:15, March 2, 1987.

Jazwinski SM: Longevity, genes, and aging, *Science* 273(5721):54, July 5, 1996.

Jensen GD, Bellecci P: The physical and mental health of nonagenerians (abstract), *Gerontologist* 23:290, 1983 (special issue).

Jung C: *Psychological types,* London, 1923, Routledge & Kegan Paul.

Jung C: The stages of life. In Campbell J, editor: *The portable Jung,* New York, 1971, Viking Press (translated by RFC Hull).

Kallman FJ, Sander G: Swedish twin studies, *Am J Psych* 106:29, 1949.

Kallman FJ, Sander G: Twin studies on aging and longevity, *J Heredity* 39:349, 1948.

Kent S: Can normal aging be explained by the immunologic theory? *Geriatrics* 32:111, 1977.

Kidd PM, Huber W, Summerfield F et al: *CoEnzyme Q10: essential energy carrier and antioxidant,* HK Biomedical Consultants, August, 1988 (monograph).

King W: Scientists find gene link to aging: landmark discovery made in patients suffering from Werner's Syndrome, *San Francisco Examiner,* p. A-18, April 12, 1996.

Kobasa SC: Stressful life events, personality, and health: an inquiry into hardiness, *J Personality Social Psychol* 37(1):1-11, 1979.

Kohlberg L: Continuities in childhood and adult moral development revisited. In Boltes P, Schaie K, editors: *Life span developmental psychology: personality and socialization,* New York, 1973, Academic Press.

Kuhlen R: Developmental changes in motivation during the adult years. In Neugarten B, editor: *Middle age and aging,* Chicago, 1968, University of Chicago Press.

Leaf A: Where life begins at 100, *Nat Geogr* 143(1):93, 1973.

Lehman H: *Age and achievement,* Princeton NJ, 1953, Princeton University Press.

Lemon BW, Bengtson VL, Peterson JA: An exploration of the activity theory of aging: activity types and life satisfaction among in-movers to a retirement community, *J Gerontol* 27:511, 1972.

Lenker LT, Polivka L: Project rationale and history, *J Aging Identity* 1(1):3-6, 1996.

Lewin K: *Field theory in social science,* New York, 1951, Harper, (Theoretical paper selected and edited by Cartwright).

Lockshin RA, Zakeri ZF: Programmed cell death: new thought and relevance to aging, *J Gerontol* 45(5):B135, 1990.

Longino CF, Kart CS: Explicating activity theory: a formal replication, *J Gerontol* 37:713, 1982.

Longino CF, McClelland KA, Peterson WA: The aged subculture hypothesis: social integration, gerontophilia and self-conception, *J Gerontol* 35:758, 1980.

Macieira-Coelho A: Cancer. In Maddox G, editor-in-chief: *The encyclopedia of aging,* New York, 1987, Springer.

Maddox G: Activity and morale: a longitudinal study of selected elderly subjects, *Soc Forces* 42:195, 1963.

Maddox G, editor-in-chief: *The encyclopedia of aging,* New York, 1987, Springer.

Maddox G, Campbell R: Scope, concepts and methods in the study of aging. In Binstock R, Shanas E, editors: *Handbook of aging and the social sciences,* ed 2, New York, 1985, Van Nostrand Reinhold.

Makinodan T: Immunity and aging. In Finch CE, Hayflick L, editors: *Handbook of the biology of aging,* New York, 1977, Van Nostrand Reinhold.

Makinodan T: Gerontologic research. In Beck J, editor: *The year book of geriatrics and gerontology,* 1990, St Louis, 1990, Mosby.

Makinodan T, Yunis E, editors: *Immunology and aging,* New York, 1977, Plenum.

Masoro EF, Katz MS, McMahan CA: Evidence for the glycation hypothesis of aging from the food-restricted rodent model, *J Gerontol* 44(6):B20-B22, 1989.

McAvay GJ, Seeman TE, Rodin J: A longtitudinal study of change in domain-specific self-efficacy among older adults, *J Gerontol* 51B(5):P243-p253, 1996.

McClearn GE, Pederson NL, Plomin R et al: The Swedish adoption/twin study on aging (submitted). Cited in Birren J, Schaie K, editors: *Handbook of the psychology of aging,* ed 3, San Diego, 1990, Academic Press.

Miller RA: The aging immune system: primer and prospectus, *Science* 273(5721):70, July 5, 1996.

Moody HR: *The abundance of life: human developmental policies for an aging society,* New York, 1988, Columbia University Press.

Nandy K, Lal H, Bennett M: *Brain reactive antibodies in aging NZB mice,* Paper presented at annual meeting of Gerontological Society of America, November 21, 1983, San Antonio.

Neugarten B: Adult personality: toward a psychology of the life cycle, In Neugarten G, editor: *Middle age and aging,* Chicago, 1968, University of Chicago Press.

Neugarten B, Havighurst R, Tobin S: Personality and patterns of aging. In Neugarten B, editor: *Middle age and aging,* Chicago, 1968, University of Chicago Press.

Nicoletti C, Yang J, Cerney J: Repertoire diversity of antibody response to bacterial antigens in aged mice, *J Immunol* 150:543, 1993.

Palmore E: Predictors of the longevity difference: a 25-year follow-up, *Gerontologist* 22:513, 1982.

Peck R: Psychological developments in the second half of life. In Neugarten B, editor: *Middle age and aging,* Chicago, 1968, University of Chicago Press.

Piaget J: *Play, dreams, and imitation in childhood,* New York, 1962, WW Norton (translated by C Gattengo and FM Hodgson).

Plomin R, McClearn GE: Human behavioral genetics of aging. In Birren J, Schaie K, editors: *Handbook of the psychology of aging,* ed 3, San Diego, 1990, Academic Press.

Quinti I, Pandolf F, Fiorilli M et al: T-dependent immunity in aged humans: evaluation of T-cell subpopulations before and after short-term administration of thymic extract, *J Gerontol* 36:6, 1981.

Riegel KF: *The psychology of development and history,* New York, 1977, Plenum.

Rosenfeld A: *Prolongevity,* New York, 1985, Alfred A Knopf.

Rosow I: The social context of the aging self, *Gerontologist* 12:82, 1973.

Rosow I: Status and role change through the life cycle. In Binstock R, Shanas E, editors: *Handbook of aging and the social sciences,* ed 2, New York, 1985, Van Nostrand Reinhold.

Rowe J, Schneider E: Aging processes. In Abrams W, Berkow R, editors: *The Merck manual of geriatrics,* Rahway, NJ, 1990, Merck Sharp and Dohme Research Laboratories.

Rudman D (cited in Darrach B: The war on aging, *Life* 15[10]:38, October 1992).

Sacher GA: Life table modification and life prolongation. In Finch CE, Hayflick L, editors: *Handbook of the biology of aging,* New York, 1977, Van Nostrand Reinhold.

Sarton M: *Poetry reading sponsored by Women's Lecture Series,* San Francisco, Calif, 1989.

Sawada M, Carlson JC: Association between lipid perioxidation and life: modified factors in rotifers, *J Gerontol* 42:451, 1987.

Schaie KW: A general model for the study of developmental problems, *Psych Bull* 64:92, 1965.

Scheer JF: Jack of all nutrients: coenzyme Q19, *Better Nutrition* 58(8):48, Aug, 1996.

Schneider EL: Organ systems: introduction. In *The Merck manual of geriatric medicine,* ed 2, Whitehouse Station, NJ, 1995, Merck Research Laboratories.

Schroots JJF: In growing, formative change and aging. In Birren JE, Bengtson VL, editors: *Emergent theories of aging,* New York, 1988, Springer.

Schroots JJF, Birren JE: Concepts of time and aging in science. In Birren J, Schaie K, editors: *Handbook of the psychology of aging,* ed 3, San Diego, 1990, Academic Press.

Sharma R: Theories of aging. In Timiras PS, editor: *Physiologic basis of geriatrics,* New York, 1988, Macmillan.

Smith GS, Walford RL: Influence of the main histocompatibility complex on aging in mice, *Nature* 270:727, 1977.

Sohal RS, Weindruch R: Oxidative stress, caloric restriction, and aging, *Science* 273(5721):59, July 5, 1996.

Strehler B, editor: *The biology of aging, symposium,* no 6, Washington DC, 1960, American Institute of Biological Science.

Swada M, Carlson JC: Association between lipid perioxidation and life modified factors in rotifers, *J Gerontol* 42:451, 1987.

Tockman M: Effects of age on the lung. In Abrams W, Berkow R, editors: *The Merck manual of geriatrics,* Rahway, NJ, 1990, Merck Sharp and Dohme Research Labs.

Van Gool WA, Mirmiran M: Aging and circadian rhythms, *Progr Brain Res* 70:255, 1986.

Walford RL: *Maximum life-span,* New York, 1983, Norton.

Walford RL: *The 120-year diet: how to double your vital years,* New York, 1986, Pocket Books.

Wayne SJ, Rhyne RL, Garry PJ et al: Cell-mediated immunity as a predictor of morbidity and mortality in subjects over 60, *J Gerontol* 45(2):M45, 1990.

Weraarchakul N, Strong R, Wood WG et al: The effect of aging and dietary restriction on DNA repair. In Beck J, Abrass I, Burton JR et al: *Yearbook of geriatrics and gerontology,* Chicago, 1990, Mosby.

White R: Ego and reality in psychoanalytic theory. In *Psychological issues,* vol 3, monograph II, New York, 1963, International Universities Press.

Williams RM et al: Genetics of survival in mice: localization of dominant effects to sub-regions of the major histocompatibility complex. In Serge D, Smith L, editors: *Immunological aspects of aging,* New York, 1981, Marcel Dekker.

Wise PM, Krajnak KM, Kashon ML: Menopause: the aging of multiple pacemakers, *Science* 273(5721):67, July 5, 1996.

Wolanin MO: Personal communication, San Antonio, Tex, Sept 28, 1996, Air Force Village II.

Woodruff D: *Can you live to be 100?* New York, 1977, Chatham Square Press.

Yates FE: The dynamics of aging and time: how physical action implies social action. In Birren JE, Bengtson VL, editors: *Emergent theories of aging,* New York, 1988, Springer.

Yen S: Newsclip, *NBC News,* Sunday, June 18, 1996.

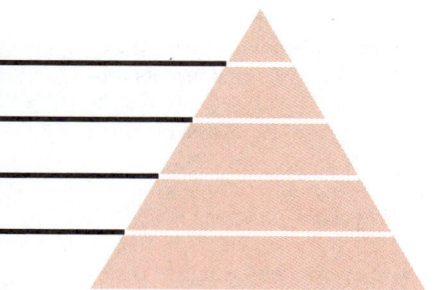

CHAPTER 3

Health and Wellness

An elder speaks   *Wellness covers just about everything, I guess. But, I wonder if you can be well while dying. Maybe that just means you have been happy with your life and can let go with a sense of acceptance. I remember my grandmother saying, "Yes, I'm ready to go anytime . . . but not today, Lord." For me wellness means doing the best you can in whatever situation you are in, but also it means being able to let yourself off the hook sometimes when you don't feel like doing your best.*

Jennie, age 89

LEARNING OBJECTIVES

Upon completion of this chapter, the reader will be able to:

1. Define health and wellness.
2. Compare the difference between the health/wellness concept offered in the health and wellness and medical models.
3. Discuss the five dimensions of wellness.
4. Explain wellness in the context of chronic illness.
5. Identify gender differences that impact on health/wellness and chronic illness.
6. Explain how and if the goals of wellness for elders can be accomplished.

HEALTH

As society approaches the 21st century, the long-existing but ignored concept of illness prevention and health promotion has emerged as if it were a new idea. Only now have the elderly and aging been included in considering health in a positive manner. Elderly individuals now are encouraged to take personal responsibility for their own health through knowledge and behavioral change. Other terms heard in the health arena now are *empowerment of the individual, prevention,* and *health promotion. Healthy People 2000* (1991) offers direction for the achievement of a better quality of life across the life span in the United States through measures that are directed at the reduction and prevention of health risks, unnecessary disease, disability, and death. The goals set forth by this report include: (1) increasing the span of healthy life for Americans, (2) reducing health disparity among Americans, and (3) achieving access to preventive services for all Americans through health promotion, protection, and preventive services. These recommendations will impact 13% of the American population by the year 2000 and 22% by the year 2030. A summary of the *Healthy People 2000* objectives for adults 65 years of age and older appears in Box 3-1. The intent of these goals is not only length of life but, more important, the improvement of functional independence of the aged. Many of those 85 years of age and older are not independent in their physical function, thus impacting their day-to-day living. The ultimate goal for the elderly is to delay illness, prevent the ill from becoming disabled, and assist those who are disabled to function and prevent further disability. In the medical arena, health is considered to exist in the absence of disease. Conformity to physical and mental capacity norms indicates one's health status. Therefore, the more observable the evidence, the more definite the degree of health that can be declared or the diagnosis that can be affixed. In such cases, those biologic and physiologic capacities not considered essential for the performance of "well" activity are less likely to be considered significant.

Box 3-1	Summary Objectives for Adults Age 65 and Older (*Healthy People 2000*)

Health Status

Reduce:

Suicide among white males

Death by motor vehicle accidents (age 70+)

Death from falls and fall-related injury, particularly age 85+

Death from residential fires

Hip fractures

Number of persons who have difficulty performing two or more personal care activities so as to enhance independence

Significant visual impairment

Epidemic-related pneumonia and influenza deaths

Pneumonia-related days of restricted activity

Increase:

Years of healthy life to at least 65 for Blacks and Hispanics

Risk Reduction

Increase:

The percentage of individuals who regularly participate in light-to-moderate activity for at least 30 minutes a day

Immunization levels for pneumococcal influenza among the chronically ill older population

The percentage of older persons who receive, within appropriate intervals, screening and immunization services and at least one counseling service

Services and Protection

Increase:

Percentage of recipients of home food service

Percentage of older adults who have the opportunity to participate yearly in at least one organized health promotion program through senior centers, life care facilities, or community-based settings serving the older adult

Percentage of states in the United States that have design standards for signs, signals, markings and lighting, and other roadway environmental improvements to enhance visual stimuli and protect the safety of older drivers and pedestrians

The proportion of primary care providers who routinely review with their patients prescribed and over-the-counter medications each time a new medication is prescribed

The usage of the oral care system

The proportion who receive clinical breast examinations and mammograms

The number of women age 70+ with uterine cervix who receive Pap tests

Extend:

Long-term institutional facilities, the requirement for oral examinations, and service provided to new admissions no later than 90 days after entering a facility

From *Healthy People 2000*, 1991, US Department of Human Services, US Government Printing Office, Washington, DC, Publ No (PHS) 91-50212.

The dilemma of the nurse and other care givers who attempt to define and apply health to the aged individual is reflected in Kaplan's "law of the instrument."

The more one is trained in one technique of investigation or the more one is trained to look at problems from one perspective the less one is able to think in terms of other perspectives or other techniques (Twaddle and Hessler, 1977, p. 48).

The emergence of the holistic health movement has reintroduced a definition of and an approach to health that operationalizes the definition of "health." The holistic approach has long been in existence but has received little attention. Dunn (1961) saw health in this context and defined it as "an integrated method of functioning which is oriented toward maximizing the potential of which the individual is capable within the environment where he is functioning." Maslow recognized this as self-actualization. The holistic definition does not limit health to just its physical or mental or even social aspects but rather incorporates these facets in the total picture.

Sometimes "health," per se, seems to be a limiting term that does not encompass the breadth that the terms "well-ness" or "well-being" suggest. Spector (1996) indicates that we find it difficult to define health without the use of some form of medical jargon, whereas "Well is a state of being, an attitude . . . it is more than the absence of illness . . . it is an ongoing process" (Travis, 1977). Wellness involves one's whole being—physical, emotional, mental and spiritual—all of which are vital components. Spector (1985) and Markides and Mindel (1987) add the dimension of culture to the holistic health approach. Accordingly, what is considered wellness to the individual must include his or her cultural orientation. Culture cannot be relegated to a subposition under any other health component. It must stand equally so that health care givers can realize and more adequately respond to the significance of culture in the attainment of well-being.

Perhaps Pender (1987) has synthesized this most difficult concept from all the preceding definitions by defining health as "the actualization of inherent and acquired human potential through satisfactory relationships with others, goal-directed behavior and competent personal care while adjustments are made as needed to maintain stability and structural integrity." And yet, no specific definition of health can really convey what it is (Spector, 1996). The meaning that we attribute to health is continuing to change and now the increasing focus is on prevention. Health is now also being seen as a more expansive phenomenon with multiple dimensions: biopsychosocial, spiritual, environmental, and cultural (Pender, 1996). Change in any of these dimensions impacts the health of an individual in a positive or negative manner. A change initiates (triggers) a behavioral change that can lead to empowerment. Empowerment may open many options for improving one's health. A positive approach to health emphasizes strengths, resilience, resources, and capabilities, rather than existing pathology.

Confusion arises when the terms *health, wellness,* and *well-being* are used interchangeably by the general public and medical practitioners when discussing an individual's condition. The wellness model refers to health as one aspect in the achievement of wellness. The wellness approach suggests that every person has an optimum level of functioning for each position on the wellness continuum to achieve a good and satisfactory existence (well-being) (Figure 3-1). *Even in chronic illness and dying there is an optimum level of wellness and well-being attainable for each individual.* Lawton (1983) offers "the good life" concept as useful in considering health of the aged in its broadest context. Well-being in the Lawton model consists of four intersecting yet autonomous segments of life: psychologic well-being, perceived quality of life, objective environment, and behavioral competence. Nurses have been among those care givers who have attempted to provide care using the holistic philosophy, but they continue to struggle to make it an integral part of patient care. In an attempt to weld the broader health-wellness concept together and initiate a more positive ap-

proach to the capacities of the aged, we offer this working definition for the care of the aged individual: *wellness is a balance between one's environment, internal and external, and one's emotional, spiritual, social, cultural, and physical processes.* Figure 3-2 attempts to illustrate the interrelationship of the facets that compose health and successful aging.

Each aspect is like a petal, anchored to the center and overlapping the other petals, each affecting the whole. Alterations in or loss of a petal can change the overall effect or appearance and its wholeness.

To achieve wellness or assist an individual to attain wellness potential, one needs to consider the dimensions of wellness: self-responsibility, nutritional awareness, physical fitness, stress management, and environmental sensitivity (Pender, 1987). Each of these will be discussed later in this chapter.

Measurements of a population's health status rely on life expectancy, morbidity, and death tables. These figures provide information on illness but do not reveal the extent to which the living are affected by these conditions. They do not indicate the health status, only the illness. For example, in morbidity tables people who are actually functioning at a high level of wellness are assigned to illness categories. Persons compiling these tables do not consider that the person with health disorders, malignancies, and other conditions may be able to attain and function at a high level of wellness and be a contributing member of the community. The wellness approach is perhaps the most equitable in the evaluation of the aged individual's potential for maximum functioning.

In the past health values of the young have been used for comparison with the aged, and, if these standards were met

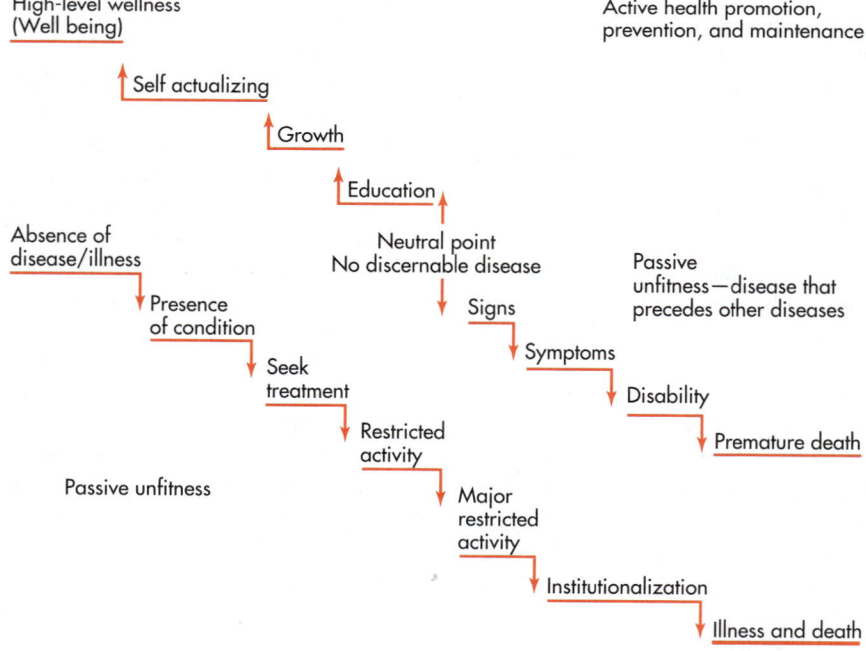

Figure 3-1. Comparison of wellness/health and traditional medical continuum.

by the aged, they were deemed healthy (or remarkable). Society's attitudes are mirrored in those who give care. Attempts are being made through education to change these general attitudes, which present old age as physically and mentally grim and associated with illness.

What are health and wellness for the aged? Are they determined by an individual's health history, a comparison with peers, the population at large, previous generations, or none of these? Barsky (1988) contends that overly worrying about health is often more disabling than incurable illness. When individuals or clients acknowledge disease processes that cannot be cured they are then able to take up their lives and feel better because they are able to cope. Barsky (1988) believes we have learned to take minor symptoms too seriously and are in danger of becoming a nation of hypochondriacs. In other words, those who believe that they are ill, act ill, even in the absence of clinical signs, and those who perceive themselves well will act well.

Cousins (1983) presents a case demonstrating how expectations can induce illness or promote health. Larry went for his annual checkup. After seeing his cardiogram, the physician asked when he had his heart attack. Larry re-sponded that he had never had one. The doctor convinced him he had previously suffered a "silent coronary, of massive proportions." That night Larry experienced severe chest pain, was admitted to the hospital, and collapsed during a treadmill test. An angiogram showed blockage of the major coronary arteries, and he was scheduled for coronary bypass surgery. He was so emotionally devastated, the surgeon called Norman Cousins in to talk with him. Cousins reviewed his chart and suspected he had been frightened into his symptoms. After a week of reassurance, support, making a game of the treadmill exercise, laughing and joking about the machine, and playing music, he exhibited no symptoms at all and the surgery was canceled. Additional evidence that mind influences physiologic responses in an appreciable and measurable way comes from recent endocrinologic studies. A corollary can be drawn to describe interactions between the nurse or other care givers and aged clients; treat the aged as if they are ill and dependent and they will respond with illness and dependence.

The assumption that old age is a downhill course may be realistic from a physiologic point of view. It is also recognized that the overall physical functioning of the body is

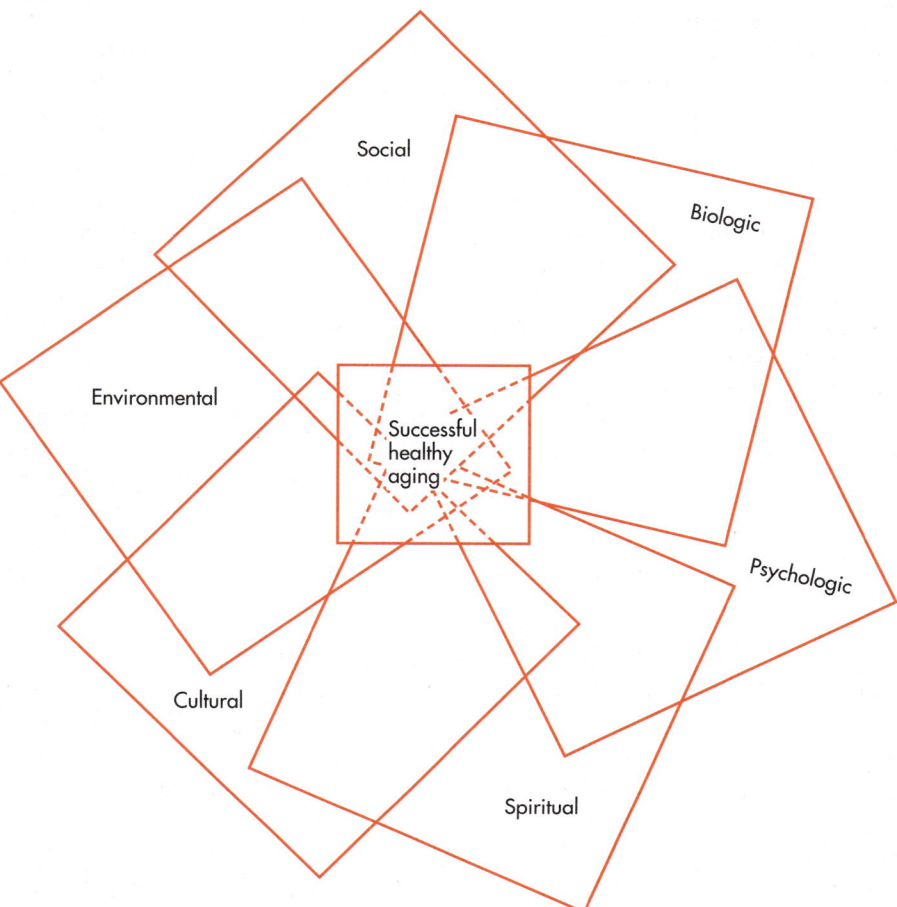

Figure 3-2. Healthy aging. (Developed by Patricia Hess.)

mainly determined by the available energy and adaptive capacities. The conviction by nurses and other care givers that the aged are individuals with declining health generates behavior that includes treating the aged as ill and feeble, or potentially so. It is therefore expected by some that attempts to reverse conditions or situations, maintain a level of ability, or institute preventive health measures are useless for the aged. Nothing could be further from the truth; "all old people are improvable" (Bortz, 1991). Rehabilitation becomes a major part of care of the aged. It may be the key to returning the aged person to a level of independence and functioning on the wellness continuum. Once there, maintenance of health becomes of prime importance.

Rehabilitation involves strengthening weakened muscles, improving endurance, increasing range of motion, improving coordination of movements and skills, restoring a functional gait, and reestablishing activities of daily living that will enable aged persons to regain control over their lives and achieve their own concept of good and satisfactory existence: the attainment of well-being.

In some instances this may be the total return of body function; in other circumstances the individual may not completely recover but is at an acceptable level for himself or herself and others involved. The individual must be allowed to use his or her resources and capacities.

Statistics show that despite the fact that approximately 86% of the aged experience chronic conditions, 95% of these people are able to live in the community (Farquhar, 1992). The image of the poor and sick old has been continuously emphasized by the mass media, despite the fact that it reflects neither the real world of the aged nor the findings of social scientists. Maggie Kuhn, founder of the Gray Panthers and advocate for the aged, in an open letter to the Gerontologic Society of America, pointed out that social gerontology "tends to focus on the individual, to the neglect of the socioeconomic structure and forces that segregate, stereotype, and victimize old people." She went on to state that, as the objects of research, the old, poor, and stigmatized persons are viewed as problems to society, not the victims of that society. The end result is that these aged are then directed to adjust to the situation rather than the society seeking ways to be more humane and making changes that meet the needs of the aging. Well-being for those over 60 years old is strongly related to health but is also affected by socioeconomic factors, degree of social interaction, marital status, and aspects of one's living situation and environment. Needs of the old and the very old differ in kind and degree, just as health behavior differs from one country to another, reflecting a different cultural style and physical and social environment. The aged attempt to be active and self-sufficient in nearly every cultural group. The key words seem to be "productive" and "useful." Admission of illness or incapacity is, to the aged person, a sign of weakness, and to others of that society, it is a sign that the individual cannot carry his or her own weight or be helpful to the

goals of the group. The aged are cognizant that illness leads to dependency and that illness with all its ramifications does not mesh well with modern society and its youth-productivity orientation. Only recently have the aged begun to break out of this mold of illness and dependency. It bears repeating here that every aged person has an attainable optimum level of wellness, which can be achieved independently or with the aid and support of care givers. Dychtwald (1986) and Hey (1996) contend that the aged can achieve high-level wellness through the promotion of productivity, self-actualization, self respect, self-determination, and continued personal growth. In essence, the aged need to make themselves necessary (Bortz, 1991). With limited disability, the aged can still achieve a high level of wellness if the emphasis of care is placed on prevention of the loss of independence and the promotion of function in the least restrictive environment. Box 3-2 presents traits of a healthy person.

HEALTH CONTINUUM

The medical interpretation of the health continuum is that if the individual is in good health or is well, then there is an absence of disease or impairment. Figure 3-1 indicates the progression along the traditional health continuum. When an individual develops a condition, it is expected that treatment will be sought to resolve the ailment. The individual, at this point, begins the descent to dependency, either temporarily or for an extended period. The role of the individual is more passive than active. This dilemma is common in the aged. The individual becomes reliant on the care giver for wellness; the care giver, in turn, tends to foster that dependent position, "the more help older people are given the more help they will come to need . . . well-meaning practitioners undermine autonomy" (Bortz, 1991). With the development of a real or perceived disease or impairment, a restriction of daily activities occurs for a period of time. If one becomes seriously ill, the restrictions result in major limitations of activity. This may lead to the institutionalization and the eventual death of the aged person. Likewise, institutionalization and restriction of major activity are considered prime indicators of poor health.

Health care continues to be based on acute cause and cure, the traditional medical model. In the early 1900s, this was an appropriate approach to health care: individuals contracted diseases that medical science could cure (smallpox, diphtheria, syphilis, tuberculosis, polio, appendicitis, etc.) Today, however, chronic diseases and illnesses are the predominant conditions. Chronic disease or illness does not have a single cause nor does it have a cure (Fries, 1992). Instead it has a universal progression based on risk factors that may begin and remain unseen for decades before the condition surfaces in a pathologic state. Examples include heart disease, diabetes mellitus, arthritis, and cancer.

The aged find themselves more limited in activity because of exacerbations of these chronic problems or because of the effects of multiple conditions. Studies have shown that the number of days spent in the hospital or confined to home increases with age.

Another issue in the medical model is that if the aged person's malady does not fit an already existing disease entity or diagnostic category, it is generally written off as a "sign of old age."

When one uses the wellness or holistic approach, which has been suggested as a more appropriate model for the aged, one regards the health and wellness continuum from a more positive direction and the role of the individual is more active. The traditional or medical model of health questions whether everyone is capable of reaching or maintaining a high level of wellness. The wellness model places wellness within the grasp of all persons, no matter what age. The significance for the aged is a new and positive approach to what the nurse and other care givers call "healthy." Wellness begins with the individual and stimulates the desire for growth and change. This means nurturing the physical self, expressing emotions more freely, improving personal decision-making, becoming more creative with others, staying in touch with the environment despite physical incapacities, and improving health practices (Hey, 1996). The wellness continuum picks up where the traditional medical model leaves off. Instead of a downward negative trajectory for the health of the aged, focused on deterioration, the wellness model rises and moves in a positive direction (see Figure 3-1). The individual may reach plateaus in his or her ascension to higher level wellness. The person may also regress because of an illness event, but the event can be a stimulus for growth potential and a return to moving up the wellness/health continuum (Figure 3-3). The division between the traditional and wellness continuums is a neutral point, where no discernible illness or weakness exists. Wellness is not given to a person; rather it is a state of being and feeling that one strives to achieve through motivation and health practices. An individual must work hard to achieve wellness just as he or she must work hard to perform competently at a job.

It is encouraging to note that some physicians are recognizing the inappropriateness of the traditional medical model for most of the aged within our health care system and are assuming a primary care mode that includes diagnosis and treatment of acute episodic disease, monitoring chronic illness, and controlling the rate of established disease, promoting wellness through vaccination programs, offering behavior modification to decrease health risk factors, and encouraging regular visits to provide psychologic support, counseling, education, and monitoring (Rowe, 1991; Kotthoff-Burrell, 1992; Schmidt, 1994). In addition, some practitioners acknowledge and incorporate alternative therapies such as body work (massage, touch therapy), herbal and nutritional therapies, psycho-neuroimmunology, and acupuncture into their practice (Gillespie, 1996).

Wellness and self-actualization develop through learning and growth. Education for wellness concerns the pursuit of the five dimensions of wellness mentioned earlier in this chapter: self-responsibility, nutritional awareness, physical fitness, stress management, and sensitivity to the environment. All of these dimensions are crucial to one's wellness. Incorporation of these five dimensions into a life-style facilitates individual growth and attainment of Maslow's self-actualization and Erikson's eighth stage of growth and development, integrity. Growth and self-actualization are one's ultimate reward.

Wellness does not mean preventive medicine. Preventive medicine is largely offensive in its approach to illness, employing vaccinations and screenings. Wellness advocates or

---

Box 3-2   Traits of a Healthy Person

Attuned to mind-body signals of pain and pleasure as well as fatigue, anger, sadness.

Can confide one's secrets, traumas, and feelings to others instead of keeping them locked inside.

Exhibits control over own health and quality of life.

Exhibits a strong committment to work, creative activities, or relationships.

Able to see stress as a challenge rather than a threat.

Demonstrates appropriate assertiveness concerning needs and feelings.

Forms relationships based on unconditional love rather than power.

Is altruistically committed to helping others.

Is willing to explore many different facets of own personality, which will provide strength to fall back on if one fails.

Modified from Dreher H: *The immune power personality: seven traits you can develop to stay healthy,* New York, 1995, Dutton.

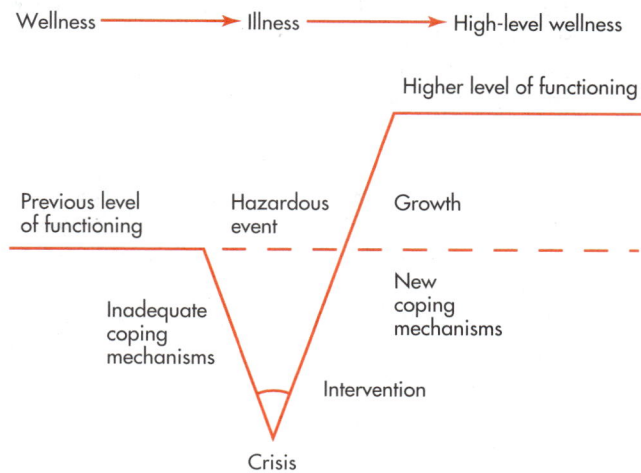

Figure 3-3. Growth potential: crisis as a challenge.

encourages health through health promotion and life enhancement, addressing risk factors that can lead to disease and chronic illness if ignored.

DIMENSIONS OF WELLNESS
Self-Responsibility

Self-responsibility or self-efficacy implies control and places one's wellness in one's own hands. It says to the individual, "Your body is your house; how you maintain your body is your choice." It has a strong effect on one's health behavior. Many aged are not attuned to their body messages nor have knowledge about their health status, while others are attuned to negative rather than positive messages. Often the aged have placed the responsibility for keeping well in the hands of the nurse or others who give care. As a result of abdicating control over their own wellness, dependent behavioral expectations and roles evolve among the family, the care giver, and the client.

Times are changing. The self-help movement for taking care of one's health needs has expanded enormously in the past few years. Governmental agencies are changing their focus to health promotion and disease prevention, necessitating client involvement in health outcomes. Elders and retired workers are teaching each other self-help strategies (Weinrich et al, 1993; Uzelac, 1994). People are responding to these approaches and taking control of their lives. People are learning how to be in touch with their body signals and to take and seek action accordingly. People are now cognizant of wellness through health education and the publicity holistic health has received, but many aged are still functioning within the earlier framework, which is reinforced by Medicare. For the aged to be exposed to new ideas and provided with options or choice, we must have changes in the politics of health care delivery—positive changes rather than an interpretation of self-care as a political solution to the health care problem and an answer to the distribution of resources. Nor should self-care or management be considered a social remedy to the redistribution of power away from the medical profession. Table 3-1 depicts self-management in acute and chronic care models.

In the recent past Senator Inouye and others promoted legislation to establish nurse-managed community clinics for the express purpose of serving individuals vulnerable to institutionalization. These have been piloted successfully at several sites throughout the nation, and nurse-managed community clinics have been established but still are too few in number. In such clinics, the client is a partner in maintaining maximum levels of health and independence in the community.

There is a time lag between change and acceptance of new ideas. The aged today may begin to make inroads to gain control of their lives and bodies, but they need to take the initiative and become empowered through educating themselves or seeking out those who can provide education

about their physical and mental selves, nutrition, and management of stress. Efforts that are most successful build group responsibility and social processes that are intrinsic to the self-health focus of the movement. Publications such as *Take Care of Your Self* (Fries and Vickery, 1990) and *Healthwise for Life* (Kemper and Mettler, 1992) provide the aged with information to make decisions for themselves about health care and teach them how to get their questions answered by physicians. Health Maintenance Organizations (HMOs) are also providing similar publications to their members. In addition to these self-help books, the aged must be taught to communicate clearly with their health care provider to achieve better health. An outline of behaviors needed when the aged interact with their care provider appears in Box 3-3.

Consumer readiness and willingness to adapt new behaviors and learn self-care skills will not lead to increased health or economic benefit unless providers of care simultaneously make adjustments in their own attitudes and responses to the new consumer role (Walker, 1994).

Hirschfeld (1985) cites basic behaviors that must be fulfilled for self-care and responsibility. The individual must initiate the definition of a health care need, define a plan of action, and decide what actual health-related activity steps to take, as well as assume responsibility and accountability for the actions. Another important point made by Hirschfeld is that the individual can act on his or her own behalf or can have a family member or friend act on his or her behalf. The same behaviors apply to groups of elders in the community. Self-care activities can respond to needs along the entire health continuum of promotion, prevention, acute care, chronic conditions, maintenance, and terminal care (Table 3-2).

Change of health care behaviors is difficult for both the aged and the care giver. Dr. James O. Prochaska (1994) outlines five steps toward change: precontemplation, contemplation, preparation, action, and maintenance. An individual may spend months in precontemplation and contemplation

Table 3-1	Comparison of Acute Care (Medical Model) and Chronic Care (Self-Management Model)	
Characteristics	**Acute**	**Chronic**
Onset	Rapid	Gradual
Cause	Generally one thing	Multiple causes
Duration	Short	Indefinite
Diagnosis	Usually accurate	Often uncertain
Treatment	Cure	Cure is rare
Role of professional	Selected and conducted therapy	Teaches and is in partnership with patient
Role of patient	Follows orders	Explains symptoms accurately
		Partnership with professionals for daily management

Box 3-3	**Self-Efficacy for Better Health Through Communication**

- Be proactive about your health by providing as complete information about self as possible and update it regularly
- Be candid about history and symptoms, make a list or log of new aches and pains and changes in body, don't disregard or dismiss symptoms, be aware of physical and mental state
- Answer questions carefully
- Exercise your right to know
- Get help from your family or others familiar with you
- Have regular routine physical examinations and gynecologic examinations (if female)
- Transfer records when changing care provider to ensure continuity of care and complete and accurate records

From Tips for communicating with your health care provider, *NEWSline for Nurse Practitioners,* 1(7):9, 1995; Brothers J: The dream team, *Modern Maturity* 38(5):28.

Box 3-4	**Steps for Health Behavior Change**

Precontemplation
Extended time period
Negative aspects of undesirable behavior stay in the periphery of the mind

Contemplation
Toy with ideas of change
Examine problem behavior
Consider balance between cost and benefit
May take a long time

Preparation
Intention to change unites with plan of action
Concrete steps to be taken within the next month

Action
Actual steps taken to modify behavior
Person feels empowered and in control of life
Frequently relies on support from others
Takes one day at a time

Maintenance
Begins 6 months after action
Prevention of relapse
Lasts a lifetime

From Prochaska JO, et al.: *Johns Hopkins Medical Letter, Health After 50,* Baltimore, 1996, Johns Hopkins Medical Institutions.

before they consider the benefits of action. Once the action occurs, maintenance begins about 6 months later. It is not uncommon and should not be considered failure if an individual has to make several cycles through the stages before the desired effect is achieved. Behavioral researchers have shown that, in the example of smoking, 85% of smokers who eventually quit, recycled back through precontemplation and contemplation stages. However, each relapse taught them something new to try in the next cycle. Box 3-4 outlines the steps in health behavior change.

The nurse can empower, enhance, and support the aged person's movement toward self-responsibility by exploring with the aged the underlying situations that may be creating a wellness imbalance and discussing with the aged the alternatives available to them. Given sufficient unbiased information, the aged can, in most instances, make meaningful decisions.

Nevertheless, some aged persons choose not to be responsible for their wellness. At times people prefer illness because it offers an escape from unpleasantness and responsibility, a means of gaining needed attention, a way of masking inadequacies, and is accepted as a legitimate role for the aged person in society. That choice, although contrary to the wellness concept, is a choice made by the individual. Given the choice of wellness or not, however, most aged will opt to be in control of their bodies, minds, and spirits.

Self-responsibility includes developing a personal health guide for maintaining good health by seeking important health examinations. There is general agreement about what examinations are important for persons 50 years and over, as well as a timetable for such examinations and tests. Table 3-3 lists the suggested preventive examinations that should be sought to maintain good health for those over 50 years old, according to the group involved and the frequency of testing. In addition, self-responsibility incorporates universal self-care requirements (see Box 3-5).

Nutritional Awareness

The nation as a whole overconsumes calories and remains undernourished because of an imbalanced diet. The nutrition of the elderly reflects this current dietary practice of food intake and use. Nutritional awareness involves learning about the foods that will make the body respond in a physically and emotionally healthy way. Heightened awareness is learning about "live" foods (fresh food, not canned or frozen) and nutrient-dense foods.

Economic considerations, mobility, and other factors place the aged in nutritional jeopardy. Eating habits evolve from childhood, and specific dietary preferences and ethnic diets, while favored by an individual, may not provide the best nutrition. The aged frequently depend on fast foods, prepared foods, and soft foods because of their convenience and the ease with which they can be carried and chewed. However, those foods are more expensive and contain many empty calories in addition to high amounts of salt, fats, and

Table 3-2   Theoretic Cells of Self-Care*

Interactional types	Healthy	Acute illness episode	Chronic illness	Bedridden
Self	Engage in physical activity Eat low-calorie diet for weight control Remain active to enhance mental alertness	Take temperature, drink fluids, and rest for a cold Diet and drink herb tea for upset stomach Take aspirin for a headache	Monitor blood pressure Check urine for sugar levels and acetone Perform enemas for colostomy	Exercise to prevent contractions Cough and breathe deeply to prevent pneumonia Continue active decision-making to prevent 'giving up'
Family (significant other)	Include parent in family activities Encourage parent to remain involved Prepare 'healthy' meals for spouse	Provide quiet and comfortable environment Bring medication from pharmacy Give cold sponge bath	Ill demented person Prepare special diet Help with prosthetic devices	Turn to prevent pressure sores Give bed-bath Change bed linen
"Expert" involvement	Initiate doctor visit for health check-up Take course on healthy nutrition Learn accident prevention	Suggest medication to physician and receiving prescription Have ingrown toenail removed Learn from nurse how to treat skin lesions	Learn home kidney dialysis Learn to inject insulin from nurse Go to health professionals for periodic check-ups of health conditions and self-care behaviors	Learn bladder and bowel training from nurse Learn specific ADL from occupational therapist Learn exercises from physiotherapist
Community	Provide income maintenance programs Plan adequate housing Plan work and leisure activities	Establish informal neighborhood organizations to help with errands, shopping etc. Man emergency telephone service (e.g., for suicidal person) Provide courses on how to treat 'simple' illness	Provide public transportation for people with impaired mobility; or wheel chairs Provide environmental adaptation for visually impaired Provide public telephones for hard of hearing	Create family relief services Provide meal services

*Examples of self-care.
From Hirschfeld M: Self-care potential: is it present? *J Gerontol Nurs* 11(8):28, 1985.

sugar. In the aged, caloric needs decrease, but the need for nutrients does not change. Selection of food should be directed toward the highest nutritional density. The problem with nutritional awareness among the aged is the lack of nutritional education. Through reading, counseling, and classes, the aged can learn to select and use "live" food in endless ways. Nutritional education might stimulate creative meal planning and bring to light both the economic benefits and the joy of new discoveries. The aged can be made more cognizant that good nutrition can prevent some of the chronic conditions that occur during old age. Problems such as constipation need not occur if the diet includes sufficient quantities of raw fruits and vegetables and whole wheat grains. Caloric intake for most aged individuals is uncertain; many do not eat the recommended 1200 to 1400 calories per day, whereas others eat well over this amount. The aged may need to take a vitamin supplement. If aged individuals are insecure about their nutrient intake from food, then taking a daily supplement that supplies no more than 100% of the recommended amount of any nutrient will suffice. Beyond that, however, they risk distorting the body's nutrient requirements and suffering toxic effects from nutrient excess.

Those who do not get exposure to sunshine may need vitamin D supplementation.

We are what we eat, and if the aged are to take control of their mind, body, and spirit to provide themselves with the highest level of wellness possible, it is essential that they become active in their nutritional intake. Aged persons who are institutionalized and capable of making food selections should be allowed to do so, not only from the menu offered but also by perhaps forming a dietary selection group to plan menus with the dietitian or the institution's administration.

In summary, few aged individuals eat an adequate diet. Nutrition will be discussed in more depth in Chapter 6.

Physical Fitness

More than 40% of adults over the age of 65 report no leisure time activity; under one third participate regularly in moderate physical activity on a regular basis (walking, gardening), and less than 10% are routinely involved in activity (*Healthy People 2000,* 1991; Fries, 1992). The midcourse review of *Healthy People 2000* (1995) reports little change in this area as it relates to the aged. Inactivity poses serious health hazards to young and old alike. It

Table 3-3	Suggested Examinations for Preventive Health Maintenance for Persons 50 Years Old and Older

Examinations and tests	Population group	Frequency
Complete physical, including cholesterol check	All persons	Every 1-3 years until age 75; then every year thereafter
Pelvic examination and breast examination	Women	Annually
Breast self-examination	Women	Monthly
Clinical breast examination	Women	Yearly
Mammogram	Women	Annually after age 50
Digital rectal examination	All persons	Annually for women with pelvic examination; every 2 years for men
Sigmoidoscopy	All persons	Every 3-5 years after age 50
Stool for occult blood	All persons	Annually
Prostate examination	Men	Every 2 years
Blood pressure	All persons	Every office visit
Eye examination	All persons	Annually after age 50
Glaucoma test	All persons	Every 3 years after 55; every year if family history
Dental examination and cleaning	All persons	Yearly for those with teeth; cleaning every 6 months, every 2 years for denture wearers
Hearing test	All persons	Every 2-5 years
Immunizations		
Flu vaccine	All persons (well and with chronic conditions)	Annually for age 65 and over
Pneumonia vaccine	All persons (well and with chronic conditions)	Once after age 65 or over; ask physician about booster
Tetanus booster	All persons	Every 10 years
Hepatitis B	Those at risk	Complete series

Compiled from AARP strategies for good health; *Healthy People 2000*, 1991, U.S. Government Printing Office, Washington D.C.; Schmidt, RM: Preventive health care for older adults, societal and individual services, *Generations XVIII* (1), 1994; *Healthwise,* Kaiser Permanente, 1994; St. Mary's Medical Center, San Francisco, 1995; *Mayo Clinic Health Letter* 14(1)1996.

can lead to hypertension, coronary artery disease, obesity, tension, chronic fatigue, premature aging, poor musculature, and inadequate flexibility. Many people do not exercise often, but, when they do, it is usually a crash program that ends in injury, failure, or death. Many aged believe that they are too old to begin or participate in an active fitness program, but, even with chronic conditions, a fitness program is possible. The fundamental issue often overlooked is that each individual requires a program of activity that will work best for him or her. No matter how nutritionally aware, practiced in self-responsibility, or able to cope with stress, without physical fitness, one will not be fit or well.

Fitness involves aerobic capacity, body structure, body composition, balance, muscle flexibility, and muscle strength. The rewards are a better self-concept, the ability to cope with stress, decreased depression, improved eating habits, less joint stiffness, a better overall ability to relate to people, and improved balance. The most well-known type of fitness program is aerobic activity. The goal of aerobic activity is to fortify the body against stress. Aerobic activity such as jogging, swimming, and tennis is not out of the reach of the aged. Doing the activity fast is not so important as is sustaining the endeavor long enough to accelerate the respiratory and cardiac rate sufficiently to reap benefits. Regular sustained aerobic exercise of the type and duration that will ben-

efit the heart and blood vessels has been found to produce higher levels of high-density lipoproteins (HDLs) and lower blood triglycerides and cholesterol levels. Exercise also affords more efficient use of carbohydrates and a decreased resistance to insulin. Activity is discussed in greater depth in Chapter 6. Those aged persons who have continued activity and exercise because it is a part of their everyday life-style continue to feel happier and healthier and look younger than those who used to be active and now have abandoned fitness. Those aged who begin physical fitness regimens need to be aware of the benefits but should also seek medical guidance when embarking on an exercise program.

Those who are capable of walking and being relatively active have a number of fitness activities open to them. Brisk walking for a sustained period of 10 to 15 minutes will tone the leg and arm muscles, provide improved oxygen exchange, and increase heart function. Some aged enjoy dancing, which can be as strenuous as programmed exercise; others who enjoy gardening can benefit from this as well (Bortz, 1995; Ulene, 1996). For those aged who are limited in ability or confined to a chair, exercises can be done from a sitting position, which will accomplish many of the same benefits as if the individual were ambulatory.

Body balance is important to prevent falling. Muscle flexibility facilitates full range of motion for life's many

---

Box
3-5
Universal Self-Care Requirements

1. Maintaining sufficient intakes of air, water, food
   a. Taking in that quantity required for normal functioning with adjustments for internal and external factors that can affect the requirement, or, under conditions of scarcity, adjusting consumption to bring the most advantageous return to integrated functioning
   b. Preserving the integrity of associated anatomic structures and physiologic processes
   c. Enjoying the pleasurable experiences of breathing, drinking, and eating without abuses
2. Provision of care associated with eliminative processes and excrements
   a. Bringing about and maintaining internal and external conditions necessary for the regulation of eliminative processes
   b. Managing the processes of elimination (including protection of the structures and processes involved) and disposal of excrements
   c. Providing subsequent hygienic care of body surfaces and parts
   d. Caring for the environment as needed to maintain sanitary conditions
3. Maintenance of body temperature and personal hygiene
   a. Bringing about and/or maintaining internal and external conditions necessary for regulating body temperature processes

   b. Using personal capabilities and values as well as culturally prescribed norms as bases for maintaining personal hygiene
   c. Caring for the environment to maintain a healthy living condition
4. Maintenance of a balance between activity and rest
   a. Selecting activities that stimulate, engage, and keep in balance physical movement, affective responses, intellectual effort, and social interaction
   b. Recognizing and attending to manifestations of needs for rest and activity
   c. Using personal capabilities, interests, and values as well as culturally prescribed norms as bases for development of a rest-activity pattern
5. Maintenance of a balance between solitude and social interaction
   a. Maintaining that quality and balance necessary for the development of personal autonomy and enduring social relations that foster effective functioning of individuals
   b. Fostering bonds of affection, love, and friendship; effectively managing impulses to use others for selfish purposes, disregarding their individuality, integrity, and rights
   c. Providing conditions of social warmth and closeness essential for continuing development and adjustment
   d. Promoting individual autonomy as well as group membership

From Department of Health and Human Services: *Toward a plan for the chronically mentally ill,* report to the Secretary of Health and Human Services, Washington, DC, 1980, The Department.

---

activities that require stretching, bending, and reaching. Muscle strength should be such that one can exert force and control over movement of the body. MacRae (Steinberg, 1994) took 60 residents from 10 California nursing homes who ranged in ages from 80 to 106 (average age 90 years) and put them through a 5-month exercise program. Each of the participants had four chronic conditions and took at least four medications daily. After 5 months the elders were found to regain lost abilities as well as retain what they already had. A study conducted by the Hebrew Rehabilitation Center for the Aged in Roslindale, Massachusetts, used 100 residents age 72 to 98 for an exercise program that included lifting weights. Each person received an individually designed program of regular 45-minute exercise periods. Some in the program needed canes, walkers, and wheelchairs, and more than 60% had fallen in the past year. The results of this physical activity produced a 113% increase in muscle strength and 11% increase in walking speed. Four participants who had used walkers were now able to use only canes (Steinberg, 1994). Easily accessible household objects, such as 1-pound bags of rice or beans or unopened

half pound or pound cans, or partially filled quart or half-gallon water bottles, can be used for weight lifting in sustained continuous repetitions to strengthen arm muscles. It is also possible to purchase variable wrist and ankle weights in sporting goods stores. Ginsberg (1994) reports weights increased older women's muscle strength, bone density and decreased the risk of falls. Individuals who are weak or have poor balance should begin strength training programs before attempting aerobic type programs (*Harvard Health Letter* (1993).

Em, an 84-year-old nursing home resident, jogged every morning in place for about 5 minutes and then briskly walked around the outside of the facility. Although she occasionally had lapses of memory, she was vital, erect, and interested in life around her.

Nellie, 83 years old, began swimming to ease the discomfort of a short left arm, the residual effect of poliomyelitis, and for a frozen shoulder. She became an award-wining synchronized swimmer with 20 gold medals, 12 blue ribbons, and 13 trophies to her credit. Nellie continued to exercise this way despite the need to wear cataract goggles.

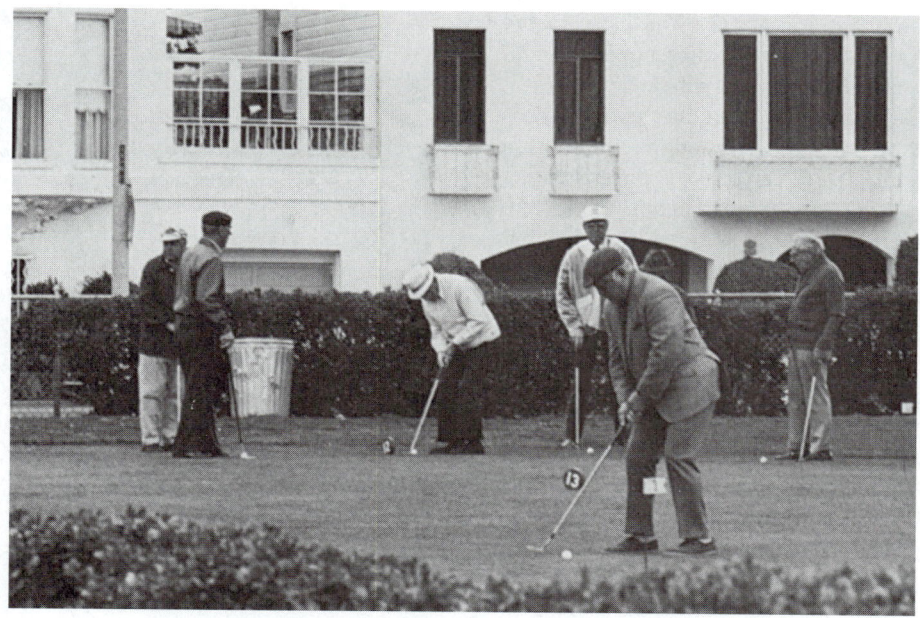

Golf at the putting green. (Photograph by Stewart H. Bloom.)

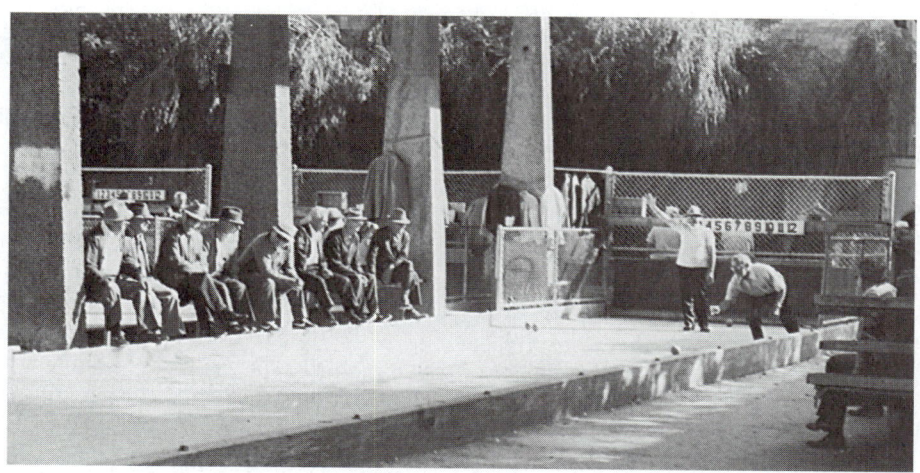

Boccie. (Photograph by Patricia Ryan.)

At 64 years old, Dick became an avid wind surfer.

In 1977, 91-year-old Madame Alexandra Baldina-Kasloff, prima ballerina in the early 1900s with the Bolshoi Theater, Moscow, was still participating in 90-minute workouts with her dance students.

Hans Selye was known to swim for 30 minutes in the morning and ride his bicycle through the McGill University campus and then swim another 30 minutes in the evening and lift weights before his death in 1982 at 75 years old.

Ada, age 82, still runs daily.

Anabel, age 70, just completed her 100th marathon.

Woody, age 83, is a surfer.

The Sun City Aqua Suns, synchronized swimmers, range in age from 68 to 88.

Catherine, who died at 106 years old, walked to the bathroom three times each day; this was her activity. It was difficult for her to do this, but without it she would have no longer walked or been able to sustain herself.

Many programs are designed to reduce premature institutionalization of the elderly and alter the sedentary life-style of the aged by acquainting them with the health benefits of regular physical activity. Nursing homes need to consider exercise programs, such as walking, for their residents even if they are frail. A walking program for frail elders was instituted to promote functional mobility. The outcome was a decrease in falls (Korohnay et al, 1995). The basic theory behind the fitness emphasis is that the better a person's condition, the more oxygen the person can inhale from the air. Although the individual may not need this extra oxygen most of the time, in stress situations he or she will; it is at these times that oxygen reserve can make a difference between health and disease or even life and death.

The nurse who is knowledgeable in aging, age changes, health risk factors, and exercise science can develop and lead exercise programs for older adults. This was demonstrated by Gillett et al (1993) when they worked with overweight women ages 50 to 70 in a health, fitness education, and aerobic training program for a period of 16 weeks. Nurses who were aged 50 to 60 and not athletically inclined were chosen and educated to lead the women. The outcomes proved to be positive. The study suggests that nurses who work with the aged obtain knowledge of exercise science. The aged population would benefit greatly from nurse-led programs designed specifically for the aged, which dealt with their health conditions such as arthritis, diabetes, obesity, hypertension, and low self-esteem.

Stress Management

Attitudes toward various life events determine one's perceptions of pleasure or displeasure. Uncontrollable events in daily life are responsible for many of the stresses experienced by the individual, but the individual also creates many stress situations. Selye (1974) defined stress as "the body's response to any nonspecific demand placed on it, whether pleasant or not."

Any stressor will initiate stimulation and elevation of the enzymes in the adrenal glands to produce the major stress hormones: epinephrine, norepinephrine, and adrenal corticoids. These hormones are responsible for activating biochemical changes in the nervous, endocrine, and immune systems, which in turn affect all organ systems. Stein (1982) and Lazerus and Folkman (1984) investigated the association among psychosocial phenomena, stress, and alterations in the immune system. The findings revealed a significant depression of lymphocyte response following the loss of a spouse, particularly during the first 2 months. The lymphocyte response returned to prebereavement levels by 5 months after the death. These findings support a biologic basis for a link among psychosocial processes, immune function, and health and illness. Sustained stress can lead to such physical consequences as heart disease, hypertension, bowel irritation, and skin disorders (Eliot, 1992). These conditions, when identified with stress as a major factor, are called "stress-related diseases."

Dubos (1965) stated that the mind influences the body and vice versa. Dubos cited the following points: scientific experimentation shows that immunologic and physiologic processes can affect the course or perception of disease. The course of infection depends on the humoral and cellular immunity mechanisms, but these are influenced by the mental

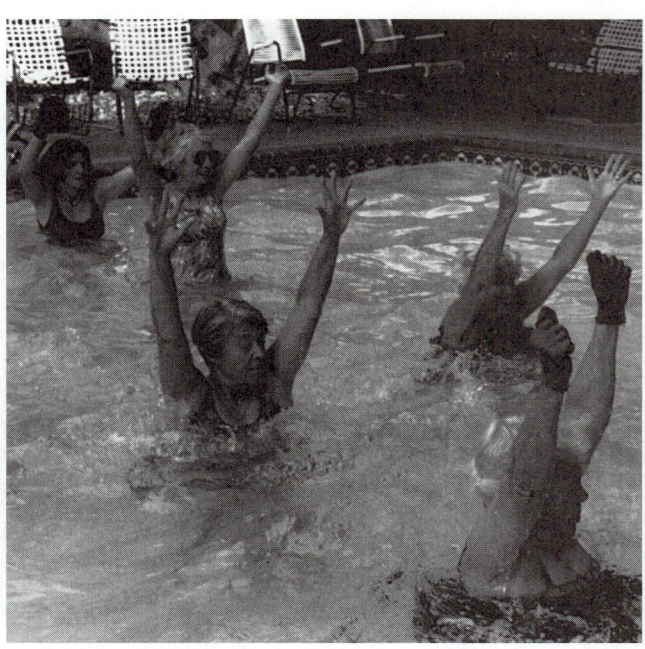

Swim class. (Courtesy Loy Ledbetter.)

state. Digestion can be accelerated or slowed by mental processes. Mental states have long been known to affect secretion of certain hormones, for example, those of the thyroid and adrenal glands. It has been shown that the brain and the pituitary gland contain a class of hormones that are chemically related and collectively called *endorphins*. Their physiologic activity is similar to morphine, heroin, and other opiate substances that relieve pain. Acupuncture can trigger the release of these pituitary hormones that somehow gain access to the cells of the spinal cord and affect the perception of pain. The neuropsychoimmunologic link is associated with both acute and chronic infections as well as cancer (Cacioppo, 1994).

Most people recognize visible manifestations of stress such as increased body movement or language, irritability, sweaty or clammy hands, insomnia, and accelerated heart rate. The body responds to stress through the general adaptation syndrome (fight or flight). Fight or flight is an inborn response and part of the human character. It is frequently referred to as that "extra squeeze of adrenaline." At times it provides the individual with what seems to be superhuman power to escape from danger or the necessary stamina to complete essential detailed information by a deadline.

The general adaptation syndrome (Selye, 1956) is composed of the alarm reaction, the stage of resistance, and the stage of exhaustion. Most stressors produce change only in the first two stages; more serious stressors lead to the exhaustion stage and thus death. However, exhaustion does not always terminate in death; when only part of the body is involved, the exhaustion stage may be reversible. For example, this frequently is the situation in exercise or local or regional

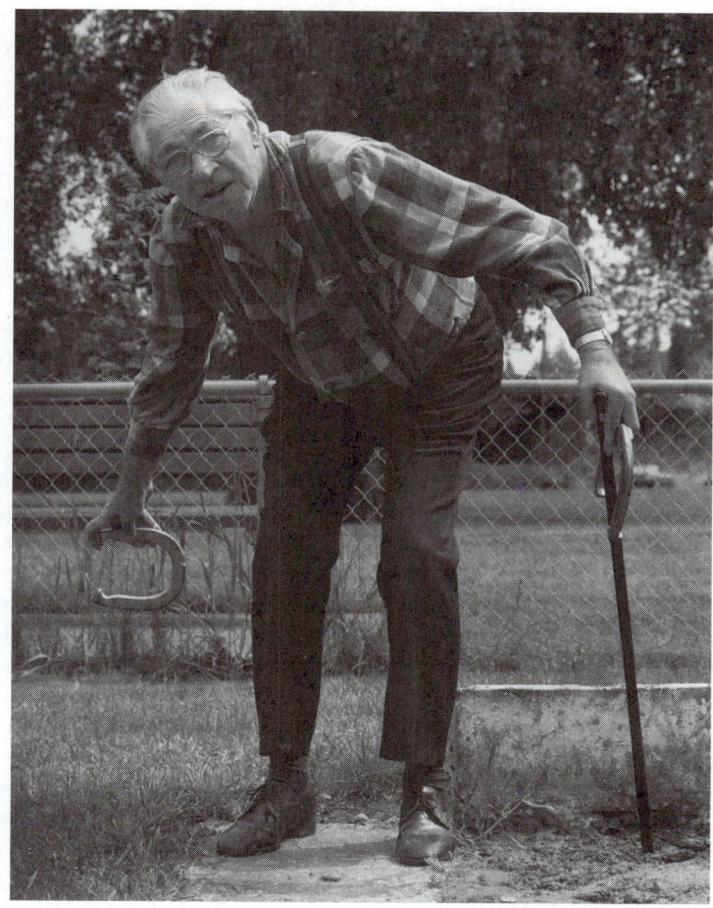

Nothing stops the enjoyment and exercise of horseshoes. (Courtesy Rod Schmall.)

infections. The hormonal activity initiated by the alarm reaction triggers the sympathetic nervous system to respond by elevating the blood pressure, pulse, and respirations and increasing metabolism and blood flow to the muscles. Biochemical changes begin, and the varied defense mechanisms of the body attempt to organize as a united front. At this point, while the body is mobilizing its forces, the individual's resistance is lowered. Once mobilization of defenses is completed, resistance rises to meet the threat. Adaptive capacity of the body is used to establish the individual at a new level of functioning or return the person to the prestress level; in other words, a return to a balanced state.

Adaptive energies are finite. When an individual is stressed over long periods, adaptive capacity is taxed and adaptive reserves depleted. Minor happenings become major events, causing the body to remain mobilized in a ready state. Bortz (1991) refers to this as "too much energy." When stressed again, one is forced to deal with or handle the stress at a lower threshold. Homeostasis remains tenuous and terminates eventually in illness or an irreversible state of exhaustion: death.

The aged are more frequently in a position of decreased ability to cope with daily hassles, cumulative life events, and other stressors because of their waning adaptive capacity. The deficits in adaptability are most evident in neuroendocrine interaction and in the separate responsiveness of the nervous and endocrine systems. It does not make a difference whether stress is physical or emotional; the aged require more time to recover or return to prestress levels than when they were younger. In other words, "The magnitude of displacement is greater, and the rate of recovery slower with increasing age" (Woodruff and Birren, 1983).

Stress inventories are helpful in determining areas and degrees of stress, but it is wise to keep in mind that these tests have flaws. Stress inventories do not weigh individual differences; they relate to generalized stresses. What is stressful to one individual may not be perceived as such by another. It is also important to note that some individuals thrive on stress, and others require peace, quiet, and tranquillity.

Various means of stress reduction exist. Some individuals use one; others use a combination of methods. Most people believe relaxation is best achieved by being in tune with one's feelings. Four basic emotions (anger, fear, enthusiasm, grief) are common to all people. Some cultures place more emphasis on expression of one emotion than on another.

Americans have great difficulty expressing anger. Instead of releasing feelings and thoughts, these are internalized, with such manifestations as muscle tension, voice changes to high tones, cold hands, posturing, and a general feeling of tightness. With an understanding of one's feelings and thoughts, the individual is more able to deal with these emotions and direct them positively to minimize the frequency of stress-involved responses. Exercise is one of the best antistress activities. Other methods include 10 to 20 minutes each day of deep relaxation, yoga, prayer, deep breathing, or fantasizing or daydreaming to remove oneself from stressful situations.

Meditation. Meditation is a form of relaxation and coping with stress. It is an experimental exercise involving the individual's actual attention. There are many forms of meditation. In Eastern tradition, meditation involves working toward a psychologic state termed *transcendental awareness* that restricts the focus or attention to an object of meditation, physiologic process; or internal sensation. Mastery over attention develops an awareness that allows every stimulus to enter into consciousness devoid of our natural selection process; the ordinary cognitive process; is stopped. To truly quiet the mind, practice and perseverance are necessary. Dramatic changes in life-style are not necessarily inherent in effective meditation. Two forms of meditation practiced in Western culture are Zen meditation and transcendental meditation. Both of these induce a state of relaxation.

Biofeedback. Biofeedback is a technique of getting feedback from the body's internal processes. By observing monitoring devices, persons can learn to influence heart rate, circulation, and muscle tension. Biofeedback is a learned skill in stress control and explores the body-mind connection. Biofeedback can be used to treat about 50 different psychosomatic disorders. It is particularly useful in conjunction with a wide variety of relaxation techniques. Machines show the individual the body-mind connection by providing visual or auditory signals to help the person develop awareness and then gain control of a specific autonomic function such as heart rate, blood pressure, muscle tension, or body temperature. Once learned, feelings that evoke the desired responses on the machine are applied by the person to everyday stresses without the aid of the machine. If the skill has been well learned and practiced, the results will be helpful to the person in stressful situations. Pioneer work at the Menninger Foundation demonstrates that individuals can be taught to control such body responses as vascular dilation and constriction to counteract migraine headaches, to lower blood pressure associated with hypertension, and to regulate heart rate in certain cardiac arrhythmias such as premature ventricular contractions.

Autogenic Training. Autogenic training is a system of total body biofeedback or self-regulation without machinery; it is a combination of yoga and autosuggestion. Anyone without excessive hearing impairment or inability to concentrate can learn to regulate involuntary psychologic and physiologic processes through autogenics. Autogenics has been found to be effective in treatment of disorders of the gastrointestinal, circulatory, and endocrine systems, as well as anxiety, irritability, and fatigue. It can be used to increase resistance to stressors, reduce or eliminate sleep disorders, and modify pain. Autogenic training requires motivation. Those without motivation or with severe emotional disorders should not consider autogenics as a means of stress reduction.

Additional Methods of Stress Reduction. There are further methods of stress reduction, which might prove useful.

Progressive relaxation. Relaxation decreases muscle activity and activity in the sympathetic and parasympathetic nervous systems. Relaxation results in decreases in oxygen consumption of the body, metabolic rate, respiratory rate, heart rate, premature ventricular contractions, both systolic and diastolic blood pressure, muscle tension, and an increase in alpha brain waves.

Progressive relaxation can be achieved through the tensing and relaxing of specific muscles or muscle groups or, without tension, through the countdown method, imagery, or recall of pleasant events or experiences.

Arranging one's environment. Arranging one's environment to reduce the potential for stress is also possible. Designing a quiet environment, a place where one can take a momentary break to reenergize, is a way to reduce stress. For the aged, the proximity of familiar belongings and environment can do much to reduce stress. Stress arises not only from worry, anger, expectations, and demands but also from loneliness, noise, and lighting. One should preplan to prevent stress from occurring or, if it does occur, to be ready for it. Application of what one has learned from a previous situation can help to dissipate the intensity of stress. Occasionally getting lost in some creative pursuit is an excellent means of dealing with stress. For some, knitting is helpful, whereas others find that painting a pastoral scene or the side of the house works well. Just stroking a pet or watching fish swim in an aquarium can serve as a tranquilizer to stress. Others enjoy fishing, a game of golf, reading a book, or listening to music. Still others find writing poetry a means of releasing frustration and stress. Physical activity is an appropriate means of handling stress for some individuals. It provides time to revitalize after a stressful incident.

Developing selfishness. It is important to clearly understand what the aged person's goals are and to make sure that those goals are really expressive of self and are not goals that someone else wants fulfilled. Acceptance of someone else's goals can create much stress. Frequently the aged are caught in this situation, when an individual trying to help imposes expectations on the aged person.

Perhaps one of the better ways of handling stress was expressed by Selye in an interview (Cherry, 1978) in which he recommends the practice of altruistic egotism; that is, look out for oneself first and give pleasure to self and others. Eustress, a term coined by Selye, is a balance of selfishness and altruism (altruistic egotism) that facilitates self-care and through which an individual has the desire and energy to care about others. Most individuals who exhibit stress-linked disease tend to be either too selfish or too self-sacrificing.

All methods and means to achieve stress management are open to all ages. Stress management requires education and change, which in itself can be stressful. However, if stress management is taught in the context of eustress, that is, taking stress and making it work positively for you, the individual will gain in ability to control the stress in life.

Environmental Sensitivity

More attention is beginning to be focused on physical, social, and personal environmental spaces and their relationship to stress and health. The physical components of environmental sensitivity (air, water, and land mass) and the social components (government, economics, and culture) are avenues through which the individual's health and wellness can be enhanced or limited. For example, the personal component of environmental sensitivity, one's immediate environs, affects the individual's ability to pursue health and wellness. In mid-life, one creates much of his or her own personal environment by career, job, friends, and life-style choices. However, the individual's influence on physical and social environment is more limited than in the personal sphere. One can consider where to live based on pollution, energy conservation measures, and food sources available, but, if a work situation or a relocation is mandated, there is little one can do. The aged are confronted with social and economic issues that force environmental changes against their wishes.

Energy conservation is an important environmental issue that influences one's health and wellness. Nations would be healthier by economizing their fuel resources. Body heat can adequately be maintained by wearing additional clothing and using extra blankets at night rather than turning the thermostat up. The aged would not find this too difficult despite the concern about their inability to tolerate temperature variations. The variations of temperature that would be of concern would be extreme temperature alterations rather than several degrees one way or other.

Personal space should be designed to include the opportunity for increasing self-development and experience, for receiving helpful feedback, and for establishing roles that are judged important. Personal environment should also facilitate time to be with friends, provide a supportive network, allow for enjoyment of beauty and nature, and provide abundant opportunities to give and receive affection and reinforce wellness behavior. The personal environment of many aged persons living in the community and in institutions is devoid of the ingredients that make and reinforce a state of wellness. Again, instead of watching the aged lan-

guish or by chance discover means of improving their personal spaces, it should be the role of the care giver to help the individual learn about opportunities and ways to design a better, happier, and healthier personal environment. Within confines, this is done in nursing care facilities that allow the aged individual in residential care to bring a limited number of meaningful items.

The sights and sounds confronting the aged person and the opportunities to socialize, to make friends, and to feel wanted and perhaps loved should be important to the care giver. Directly or indirectly, all of one's senses are affected by and affect the environment. Without this fifth dimension, wellness will not be of a high level. All dimensions are interrelated and influence one's state of health and wellness.

States (1986) uses the environmental components of the individual's room, the home, the neighborhood, and the planet at large as a basis of environmental sensitivity. Figure 3-4 provides a graphic view of the interrelation between environment and the four dichotomous elements: sick-well; dependent-independent; immobile-mobile; and malnourished–well-nourished. Environmental sensitivity or "crush" at any one of these levels may determine the individual's response to wellness or illness.

Self-efficacy affects all dimension of health and wellness. Measurement of self-efficacy is a potential predictor of an aged person's "ability to create and recover from new challenges of failure and loss and it should concur with

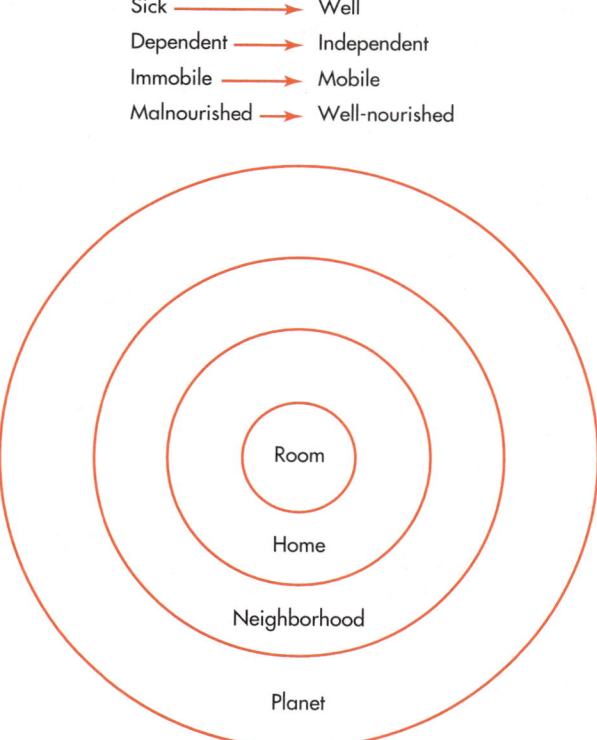

Figure 3-4. Environmental sensitivity. (States, 1986).

individuals' estimate of their ability to deal with complex ambiguous and pressure-filled situations" (Bortz, 1991).

CHRONICITY AND WELLNESS
Chronicity

Chronic illness is the hallmark of aging and the number one health problem for the elderly in the United States. Chronic disorders are difficult to delimit because so many acute disorders have chronic sequelae and, too often, the results of treating acute disorders is a chronic residual disability. Chronic conditions are the accrual of life's earnings, sometimes self-generated, often inherited, or occurring as the result of imposed life-style and environmental hazards. Lubkin (1995) defines chronicity as ". . . the irreversible presence, accumulation, or latency of disease states or impairments that involve the total human environment for supportive care and self-care, maintenance of function, and prevention of further disability" (p. 6).

The prevalence of chronic conditions continues to rise with the decline in mortality, the lengthening of the frail aged life span, and highly technical medical care. The incidence of chronic illness triples after age 45 but decreases markedly in relation to higher socioeconomic status. Although limited in scope, a study of a northern California socioeconomically advantaged community revealed that the individuals in that community lived longer without chronic illness but spent a longer portion of late life in a state of debilitating health (Reed et al, 1995). At times the aggressive treatment of one disorder results in the emergence of additional disabilities iatrogenically induced. (1995).

Certain terms describing the accompaniments of chronic disorders—such as *handicap, impairment,* and *physical limitation*—are used rather indiscriminately. *Decreased function without incapacitation* also needs to be stated consistently because these and other terms are often used interchangeably. Available statistics may be easily misinterpreted if one does not question how these terms are being used.

The explosion of chronic illness is a catalyst for change. Presently two thirds to three fourths of disabled elders are cared for at home with few or no formal services. Because the present approach to health care and health emphasizes symptoms and symptom reduction; society is becoming more malignant in terms of environment, diet, and stress inducers; and health care is becoming economically unavailable to more than 15% of our population, great changes are needed in our philosophy about health and health care. There is a noticeable revival of the American ideal of individualism and self-responsibility with considerable focus on "self-care." It is suggestive of a system failure and adoption of whatever devices one can muster for self-extrication. We believe deeply in self-responsibility, but, as in every situation, if a similar level of responsibility is not exerted in the metasystem one can hardly be successful within the microsystem. For example, an individual intent on a healthy diet may find it impossible to find vegetables and fruits free of pesticides, prepared foods free of preservatives, fish free of toxic waste products, and meat and poultry free of hormones and antibiotics. How can one take appropriate self-care?

The appropriate approach is very individualistic and may involve changing the situation, modifying treatment, or retraining the individual to compensate for the pathophysiologic changes. The impact of chronic illness is also very individual and may include identity erosion, expectations of death, dependency conflicts, and feelings of failure or fatalism or it may mobilize the individual to live life to its fullest.

Wellness in Chronic Illness

A state of wellness may be achieved and maintained quite consistently during chronic illness if the individual feels capable of and motivated to manage the problems with or without assistance. The aged can be supported toward the achievement of wellness and maximizing their life satisfaction when care givers ascribe to a holistic philosophy that incorporates efforts directed toward the maintenance of the aged person's self-care and self-esteem.

Figure 3-5 shows how the wellness continuum and Maslow's hierarchy of needs can complement each other in the attainment of wellness and self actualization. Also Orem's self-care model has grown in popularity based partially on the increased awareness of the individual's direct impact on disease and the impotence of nursing and/or medicine to effect positive change in a depressed, declining individual who no longer cares.

It is clear that a reorganization of thinking is needed by the aged and those associated with them: kin, friends, and care givers. Physical manifestations of chronic illness should not be the sole determinative factor in the establishment of the elder's state of health or wellness. A study by Markides and colleagues (1993), while limited, suggests that one should not always assume that physician assessments represent an objective "gold standard" for validating self-reported measures of health. The greatest factor in establishing wellness is adaptation. To achieve maximization of life satisfaction, adaptation of life-style is necessary whether it is through environmental manipulation, modification of treatment, or retraining the individual to compensate for pathophysiologic changes. Positive coping or adapting to chronic conditions is contingent on the accomplishment of the following tasks:

- Ability to neutralize harmful environmental conditions
- Adjustment to negative events consequent to the illness
- Maintenance of self-image and self-sufficiency
- Maintenance of social relationships
- Coping with emotional reactions of anxiety and depression.

What is wellness in the face of chronic illness? This question produced a lively discussion from the contentious voices of an assertive group of elders. Comments such as, "Let's get real!" "I'm like the old one-hoss shay . . . losing a little something every day. Someday, I'll wake up and find that nothing works." Elders don't graciously accept their chronic disorders—they mourn their losses. They talk about them but not to the exclusion of other events and interests in their lives. They believe competition and conviction undergird their remarkable survival capacity and will always remain important. They also believe in being responsible and responsive to their community.

Nurses can assist and empower the aged toward an enriched capacity for living in the shadow of chronic conditions through the role of resource person, advisor, teacher, and at times assistant to the aged person. It is essential, however, to remember that the aged individual is in control of his or her own adaptation. Nurses can assist by:

- Identifying and stating strengths the individual demonstrates
- Discussing healthy life-style modifications
- Encouraging the reduction of risk factors in the environment
- Assisting the individual to devise methods of improving function, halting disabilities, and adapting life-style to reasonable expectations of self
- Providing access to resources when possible
- Referring appropriately and when needed

It bears repeating that a state of wellness may be achieved and maintained quite consistently if the individual feels he or she is capable of and motivated to manage problems whether it is with or without assistance from others.

Gender and Wellness

The recent upsurge in women's health has brought to the fore differences in health and health care of men and women. There appears to be an innate or philosophical difference in the perception of health between the genders. Implicit in this gender perception of health are cultural and regional factors (Boys, 1994). Differences in health and mortality for men and women are rooted in alterable and unalterable biologic and psychosocial components. Biologic elements include genetics, hormones, and physiologic structure, and acquired risk factors are based on life-style, work hazards, and environmental exposures. Psychosocial factors include how symptoms are perceived, health-reporting behavior, and previous health care (Verbrugge, 1994).

Because women typically live longer than men and more frequently live alone, the issues of management of chronic disorders have a large gender component. The Rand Corporation (Shoben, 1992) released findings from a large study (sample: 11,242) of elders hospitalized with congestive failure (CHF), heart attack, pneumonia, and stroke. The study indicated that elderly men receive more care and more

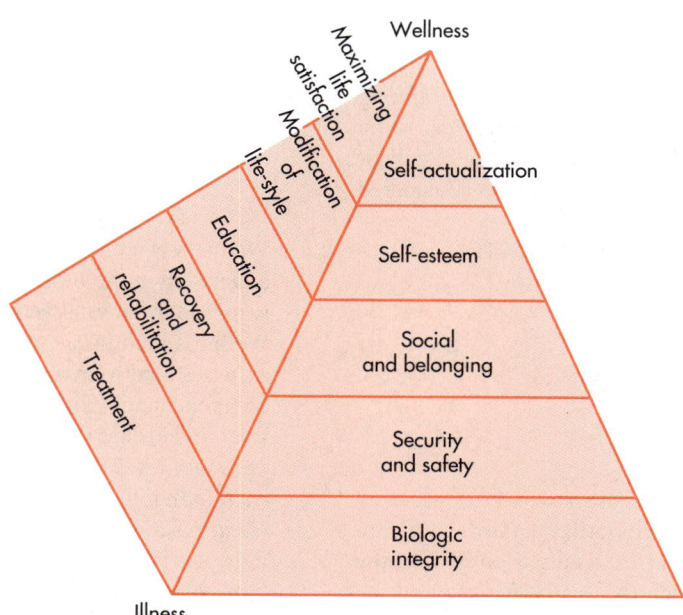

Figure 3-5. Correlation between illness-wellness continuum and Maslow's hierarchy of needs. (Developed by Patricia Hess).

expensive, highly technical services than do women. Whether these findings would be true as the individuals are discharged to home care is unknown and certainly a question for further research. While this study relates only to in-hospital service, one must wonder if there are differences in rehabilitation and chronic care management based on overt or covert attitudes toward older men and women. Much is yet to be done in this potentially fruitful area of research.

Since 1990, the immense knowledge gap related to women's health care is being closed. Under the guidance of Bernadine Healy, Women's Health Initiative, a longitudinal study of women's health needs was launched several years ago.

The most prevalent chronic conditions in individuals over 75 years of age are (in order) arthritis, twice as common in females; hearing impairments, three times as common in females; hypertension, about a third more common in women, heart conditions, about a third more prevalent in women; and cataracts, nearly twice as common in females (U.S. Bureau of the Census, 1995). Of course one must consider the population predominance of females over the age of 75 and the possibility that only the hardier males survive beyond age 75.

Women generally suffer more sickness and dysfunction at any given time and over their whole lifetime. Men, on the other hand, incur life-threatening diseases and because of them die sooner. Nevertheless, men universally see themselves as healthy despite serious problems. It takes a trip to the hospital or the terror of the possibility of dying to motivate most men to doing something about their health. Most of the time it is a wife or a significant female (sister, mother, girlfriend) in the man's life who prods him to seek care and keep physician appointments. Even with an overseer, there is little or no follow through by the man (Boys, 1994). There is no difference in what is considered good health among white collar and blue collar men and ethnic men. Fear is the cause of the inability of men to care for themselves. Fear slows action, and illness is too upsetting to be considered (Doheny, 1993; Boys, 1994).

Men consider good health to be (Boys, 1994):
- The ability to take care of self
- Energy
- Healthy attitude
- Good sex, healthy sex life, good loving
- Having fun in life
- Keep on dreaming—hope
- In good physical condition

Barriers to men seeking health care should be considered if nurses wish to intervene in promoting better health care for men. These include the fear of seeing a physician, the perception of good health when medically this may not be the case, intellectual versus practical outlook (the awareness of poor health but not doing anything about it), and frustration about the mixed messages most men get from

Box 3-6	**Gender Characteristics of Health Consciousness**

Men	**Women**
Know little to nothing about their body	Act on symptoms
Deny health problems and physical pain	Usually see the outcome of therapy
Want problems cleared up immediately	Usually keep appointments
Less likely to take a prescribed medication as directed	Know the system and are not afraid of it
Usually cancel followup appointments	

From Doheny K: Real men don't see doctors, *Modern Maturity,* 36(1):57, Feb/May, 1993; Boys J: *Staying strong,* American Society on Aging annual meeting, San Francisco, March, 1994.

the health community (Boys, 1994). Box 3-6 provides a comparison between the health behaviors of most older men and women.

There are many issues to consider in wellness and chronicity. How these issues apply to the aged is similar yet different from how they apply to the young. It must be remembered that the aged are a population with many chronic conditions, which may only have been thought in terms of decrements rather than looking at potential positive aspects and promoting self-care, self-efficacy, and empowerment. Nurses must learn to guide and support rather than to take over for the aged. Care of the chronically ill is a national issue that deserves a high priority. As the health system changes, nurses need to carve out their role as it relates to supporting the aged and maintaining their highest level of wellness with or without underlying chronic conditions.

KEY CONCEPTS

- Wellness is a concept, not a condition. It is human adaptation at the most individually satisfying level in response to internal and external existing conditions.
- Wellness incorporates the holistic health movement that assumes health involves biopsychosocial and spiritual components of existence.
- Even in chronic illness and the dying process, there is an optimum level of wellness and well-being attainable for each individual.
- *Health* is a term that is subsumed under wellness and indicates behaviors that are preventive of biopsychosocial problems.
- Pender (1987, 1996) states that health is "the actualization of inherent and acquired human potential through satisfactory relationships with others, goal-directed behavior, and

▲ **Needs Addressed and Task Strengths**

Need to maintain all capacities to highest extent possible and to feel self-worth; need to make choices (to satisfy all levels of human need)	Perception of capability
	  Interest in growth and change
	  Ability to take charge of own life-style
	  Self-confidence
	  Functioning at a high cognitive level
	  Strongly held preferences

competent personal care while adjustments are made as needed to maintain stability and structural integrity."

- *Healthy People 2000* is a document developed by the U.S. government to provide measurable goals by which to indicate our population's progress toward health.
- The goal of *Healthy People 2000* for the elderly is to prevent disability, delay illness, and to modify its disabling effects as much and for as long as possible.
- Wellness includes behaviors fundamental to healthy adaptation, such as self-responsibility, physical fitness, stress management, nutritional awareness, and environmental sensitivity.
- The "medicalization" of our society has brought about the common belief that the absence of disease is health.
- The wellness model reinforces the belief that self-care and satisfactory adaptation are uniquely and individually defined.

▲ CASE STUDY

Catherine was 103 years old and had been in a nursing home for several years. She had few friends, no family, and multiple physical limitations. Her sources of emotional support were three old lady friends and her young doctor, whom she trusted and admired. However, once her young doctor tried to have her restrained when she became confused, she said, "I would hate to discharge him but I will if I must. He'd be real upset because he wouldn't get my baby when I die." This was in reference to an ossified fetus she had carried, tumor-like, for 80 years. Her physical support was her cane that she kept with her at all times and used to hobble to the bathroom or, on rare occasions, across the hall to her neighbor in the nursing home. Her psychologic support came from an inculcated reverence for life, respect and love of her progenitors, belief in God, and her absolute belief that in the course of her life history she certainly deserved whatever benefits she could obtain from Medicare and Medicaid. The characteristics that kept her "well" were her sense of humor, personal history, and perspective on the meaning of events in her life. Physical disorders were dealt with to the best of her ability, and she used her depleted energies to keep intact the few relationships that contributed to her survival and peace of mind.

Physically she was filled with pathology. In all other ways she was well. She was at peace with life but was expectant of death.

Based upon the case study, develop a nursing care plan using the following procedure*:

List comments of client that provide *subjective data*.

List information that provides *objective data*.

From these data identify and state, using accepted format, two *nursing diagnoses* you determine are most significant to this client at this time. List two *client strengths* that you have identified from data.

Determine and state *outcome criteria* for each diagnosis. These must reflect some alleviation of the problem identified in the nursing diagnosis and must be stated in concrete and measurable terms.

Plan and state one or more *interventions* for each diagnosed problem. Provide specific documentation of source used to determine appropriate intervention. Plan at least one intervention that incorporates the client's existing strengths.

Evaluate success of intervention. Interventions must correlate directly with the stated outcome criteria in order to measure the outcome success.

STUDY QUESTIONS/ACTIVITIES

What life-style changes might you suggest for Catherine, and what would be your reason for doing so?

Where would you place Catherine in the continuum of wellness? Explain your reasons for doing so.

Construct a definition of health that seems to you to incorporate the essential elements of a holistic perspective.

Discuss your thoughts about wellness as it relates to the medical concerns about old age.

Define wellness for yourself. What would you want to change in your life to achieve a sense of wellness?

Discuss the concept of wellness while dying and your thoughts about this issue.

---

*Students are advised to refer to their nursing diagnosis text and identify possible or potential problems.

RESEARCH QUESTIONS

Which physical conditions are most likely to impede the capacity for wellness?

Do most elders believe there is a state of wellness in spite of physical illness?

What are the factors that indicate one is in a state of "wellness"?

Is the physical deteriorative mode of defining old age related to the medical model or individual perceptions?

What are the variables that indicate a dying person is in a state of "wellness"?

How many people over 50 years old can explain wellness?

What do elders believe about the concept of "wellness"?

RESOURCES

Films and Videos

I Never Planned on This. J. Rowe, Filmmakers Library, New York, NY (46 min.)
This film examines healthy aging, highlighting this gradual biological process that begins at birth.

Age Is No Barrier. J. Rowe, Filmmakers Library, New York, NY (25 min.)
This video celebrates the benefits of developing and maintaining an active lifestyle through the activities of the U. of Agers, a Canadian-based seniors gymnastics team.

Healthy Aging: Model Health Promotion Programs for Minority Elders. ½" videocassette (46 min/color).
Distributor, National Resource Center on Health Promotion and Aging, American Association of Retired Persons, 601 E. Street, N.W., Room B-5, Washington, D.C. 20049. Rent free. Leader's guide included.

How to Live Past 100. ½" videocassette (19 min/color). Distributor, Film for the Humanities and Science, P.O. Box 2053, Princeton, NJ.

The SMILE Program: So much Improvement With a Little Exercise. ½" videocassette (41½ min/color). SMILE Program, The University of Michigan, School of Public Health, Department of Behavior and Health Education, 1420 Washington Heights, Ann Arbor, MI 48109-2029.

Tai Chi for Seniors, Publishers Choice Video, Box 4171, Dept. IS40-PU, Huntington Station, NY 11746

Easy Yoga for Seniors, Publishers Choice Video, Box 4171, Dept. EN90-PE, Huntington Station, NY 11746

Organizations

Check phone directory for local chapters of national associations.

American Cancer Society
1599 Clifton Road NE
Atlanta, GA 30329
1180 Avenue of the Americas
New York, NY 10036-3602
and
Office of Cancer Communications
National Cancer Institute
Bldg 31 Rm 10A16
900 Rockville Pike
Bethesda, MD 20892

Cancer Care Inc.
1180 Avenue of the Americas
New York, NY 10036-3602
212-221-3300
212-719-0263 FAX
e-mail:info@cancercareinc.org
website:http://www.cancercareinc.org

Call Cancer Information Service
(800) 4-CANCER
301-402-5874 FAX
In Alaska (800) 683-6070
In Hawaii (800) 524-1234
In Washington, D.C. (202) 636-5700
e-mail:cancernet@icicb.nci,nih.gov

American Heart Association
7320 Greenville Avenue
Dallas, TX 75231

"E" is for Exercise
Local chapter of American Heart Association

American Lung Association
1740 Broadway, P.O. Box 596
New York, NY 10019-4373
212-315-8700

Office on Smoking and Health
5600 Fishers Lane
Park Building, Room 1-10
Rockville, MD 20857

Alcoholics Anonymous
468 Park Avenue South
New York, NY 10163

The U.S. National Senior Sports Organization
14323 South Outer Forty Road
Suite N-300
Chesterfield, MO 63017
314-878-4900
314-878-9957 FAX

U.S. Masters Swimming Inc.
2 Peter Avenue
Rutland, Maine 01543

Publications

Healthwise for Life. Kemper D, Mettler M, Boise, Idaho, Healthwise Publications, 1992.

Take Care of Yourself. (4th ed) Fries JF, Vickery DM, Menlo Park, Addison-Wesley Publishing Company, 1990.

Exercise and Your Heart
National Heart, Lung, and Blood Institute
NIH Publication No. 81-1677
Department of Health and Human Services
Building 31, Room 4A-21
9000 Rockville Pike
Bethesda, MD 20205

Plain Talk Series—DHHS Publications
Handling Stress
Biofeedback
Mutual Health Groups
U.S. Department of Health and Human Services
Public Health Service
Alcohol, Drug Abuse and Mental Health Administration
5600 Fisher Lane
Rockville, MD 20857

Safety for Older Consumers: Home Safety Checklist
U.S. Consumer Product Safety Commission
Washington, DC 20207

Don't Take It Easy—Exercise
Self-Care and Self-Help Groups for the Elderly: A Directory
National Institute on Aging
Building 31, Room 5C-35
9000 Rockville Pike
Bethesda, MD 20205

Exercise for People with Arthritis
P.O. Box 9782
Arlington, VA 22209

Pep Up Your Life
American Association for Retired Persons
601 E Street NW
Washington, DC 20049

REFERENCES

Barsky A: Doing better, feeling worse, *American Health* VII:105-110, 1988.

Bortz , WM: *Dare to be 100,* New York, 1996, Fireside.

Bortz, WM: *We live too short and die too long,* New York, Bantam Books, 1991.

Boys J: *Staying strong,* presentation, American Society on Aging, annual meeting, San Francisco, Calif, March, 1994.

Cacioppo JT: Social neuroscience: autonomic, neuroendocrine, and immune response to stress, *Psychophysiology* 31:113, 1994.

Cherry L: On the real benefits of eustress, *Psychol Today* 11(10):60, 1978.

Cousins N: How doctors cause disease, *Medical Self-Care,* Winter, 1983.

Doheny K: Real men don't see doctors, *Modern Maturity* 36(1):57, March, 1993

Dubos R: *Man adapting,* New Haven, Conn, 1965, Yale University Press.

Dunn HL: *High-level wellness,* Arlington, Va, 1961, RW Beatty Ltd.

Dychtwald K: *Wellness and health promotion for the elderly,* Rockville, Md, 1986, Aspen Publications.

Eliot SR: Stress and the heart: mechanisms, measurement and management, *Postgrad Med* 92(5):237, 1992.

Farquhar JW: *The future of illness care and health promotion,* Healthy Aging: Challenges and Choices for Health Professionals, conference, San Francisco, Oct 1-4, 1992.

Fries JF, Vickery DM: *Take care of yourself,* ed 4, Menlo Park, Calif, 1990, Addison-Wesley.

Fries JF: *Where in health are we going?* Healthy Aging: Challenges and Choices for Health Professionals, conference, San Francisco, Oct 1-4, 1992.

Gillett PA, Johnson MA, Juretich M et al: The nurse as exercise leader, *Geriatr Nurs* 14(3):133, 1993.

Gillespie L, editor: *Health connection,* St Mary's Medical Center, 1996, Summer, p 7.

Ginsburg M: Weights strengthen older women's bones, *San Francisco Examiner,* December 28, 1994, p A1.

Hall NK: Health maintenance and promotion. In Ham RJ, Sloane PJ, editors: *Primary care geriatrics,* (ed 2), St Louis, 1992, Mosby.

Healthy People 2000: US Department of Human Services, US Government Printing Office, Washington, DC, Publication No (PHS) 91-50212, 1-8; 22-27; 587-591, 1991.

Healthy People 2000 Midcourse Review and 1995 Revisions: US Department of Health and Human Services, Public Health Service, US Government Printing Office, Washington, DC, 1995.

Hey RP: Healthy, wealthy, and wise, *Bulletin-AARP* 37(7):6, July/Aug, 1996.

Hirschfeld M: Self-care potential: is it present? *J Gerontol Nurs* 11(8):28, 1985.

Kemper D, Mettler M: *The senior medical consumer: older adults and medical self-care,* Healthy Aging: Challenges and Choices for Health Professionals, conference, San Francisco, Oct 1-4, 1992.

Koroknay VJ, Werner P, Cohen-Mansfield J et al: Maintaining ambulation in the frail nursing home resident, *J Gerontol Nurs* 21(11):18, 1995.

Kotthoff-Burrell E: Health promotion and disease prevention for the older adult: an overview of current recommendations and a practical approach, *Nurs Pract Forum* 3(4):195, 1992.

Lawton MP: Environment and other determinants of well-being in older people, *Gerontologist* 23:350, 1983.

Lazarus RS, Folkman S: *Stress, appraisal, and coping,* New York, Springer, 1984.

Lubkin IM: *Chronic illness: impact and interventions,* ed 3, Menlo Park, Calif, 1995, Jones and Bartlett.

Markides KS, Mindel CH: *Aging and ethnicity,* vol 163 Newbury Park, Calif, 1987, SAGE Library of Social Research.

Markides KS, Lee DJ, Ray LA et al: Physician's rating of health in middle and old age: a cautionary note, *J Geront Soc Sci* 48(1):s24, 1993.

Pender N: *Health promotion in nursing practice,* Norwalk, Conn, 1987, Appleton-Century-Crofts.

Pender N: *Health promotion in nursing practice,* ed 3, Stamford, Conn, 1996, Appleton & Lange.

Prochaska JO: *Changing for good,* New York, Avon Books, 1994.

Reed D, Satariano WA, Gildengorin G, McMahon K et al: Health and functioning among elderly of Marin County, California: a glimpse of the future, *J Gerontol Med Sci* 50A (2):M61, 1995.

Rowe JW: Reducing the risk of usual aging, *Generations* XV(1):25(99), 1991.

Schmidt RM: Preventive health care for older adults: societal and individual services, *Generations* XVIII(2):33, 1994.

Selye H: *The stress of life,* New York, 1956, McGraw-Hill.

Selye H: *Stress and distress,* New York, 1974, JB Lippincott.

Spector RE: *Cultural diversity in health and illness,* Norwalk, Conn, 1985, Appleton-Century-Crofts.

Spector RE: *Cultural diversity in health and illness,* ed 4, Stamford, Conn, 1996, Appleton & Lange.

States D: Personal conversation, San Francisco, 1986.

Statistical Abstract of the United States, ed 115, Washington, DC, US Department of Commerce, Economic and Statistics Administration, Bureau of Census, 1995.

Stein M: *Stress, brain, and immune function,* paper, meeting of the Gerontological Society of America, Boston, Nov, 1982.

Steinberg D: Senorities: best way to stay young is to stay fit with exercise, *San Francisco Examiner,* July 23, 1994, p. B-5.

Strategies for successful change, *The John Hopkins Medical Letter Health After 50* 8(5):1, July, 1996.

Travis J: *Wellness workbook: a guide to high level wellness,* Mill Valley, Calif, 1977, Wellness Resource Center.

Twaddle AC, Hessler RM: *A sociology of health,* St Louis, 1977, Mosby.

Ulene A: Forever young series, *NBC Today,* July 12, 1996.

Uzelac DG: Keeping fit: put yourself in control, *Golden Age Monthly,* Salt Lake City, Utah, July, 1994, p 16.

Verbrugge LM: *Pathways of health for women and men,* Healthcare for the Older Woman: New Approaches to Old Problems, conference, UCSF/Mount Zion Center on Aging, San Francisco, April, 1994.

Walker SN: Health promotion and prevention of disease and disability among older adults: who is responsible? *Generations* XVIII(1):45, 1994.

Weinrich SP, Weinrich MC, Stromborg MF et al: Using elderly educators to increase colorectal cancer screening, *Gerontologist* 33(4):491, 1993.

Woodruff DS, Birren JE, editors: *Aging: scientific perspectives and social issues,* ed 2, New York, 1983, Van Nostrand.

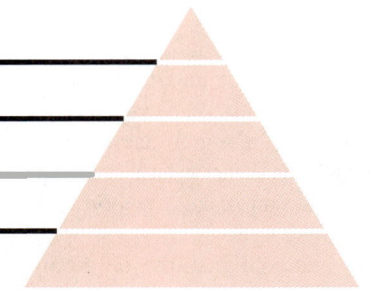

CHAPTER 4

Age-Related Changes

An elder speaks   *Strange how these things creep up on you. I really was surprised and upset when I first realized it was not the headlights on my car that were dim but only my aging night vision. Then I remembered other bits of awareness that forced me to recognize that I, that 16-year-old inside me, was experiencing normal changes that go along with getting old.*

Sally, age 60

LEARNING OBJECTIVES   Upon completion of this chapter, the reader will be able to:

1. Identify and discuss the common age-related changes that occur in the following systems: musculoskeletal, integumentary, cardiovascular, respiratory, gastrointestinal, genitourinary, nervous and special senses, and endocrine.
2. Describe the importance and objective of assessing basic activities of daily living (BADLs) and instrumental activities of daily living (IADLs).
3. Discuss the place of home visits in assessment.
4. Explain what is necessary to consider in obtaining assessment data from an elder of another cultural background.
5. List the essential components in obtaining a health assessment from an elderly person.

PHYSIOLOGIC CHANGES

Physiologic changes have a cumulative effect in the continuum of biologic, psychologic, social, and environmental processes of aging. Goldman (1979) indicates four characteristics of physiologic aging: it is universal, progressive, decremental, and intrinsic. The universality of aging places it outside the realm of pathologic study. The changes that occur are normal for all people but take place at different rates and depend on accompanying circumstances in an individual's life. Normal age changes have usually been studied in concert with pathologic or disease conditions, which has led to the misconception that age changes indicate illness or disease. Progressive and decremental alterations of the whole body often interfere with an aged individual's ability to interact successfully with the environment and increase the risk of death. Age changes of the body as a whole are a matter of daily observation and have been happening for thousands of years. Most of these changes are intrinsic by nature; that is, unmodifiable, whereas other alterations are the result of extrinsic influences specific to one's way of life. Extrinsic factors that affect intrinsic factors are discussed in the biologic theories of aging in Chapter 2.

Interesting approaches to the aging process and age-related changes are proffered by Sloane (1992) and Lakatta (1995). Sloane suggests the "Rule of Thirds," which postulates that one third of age-related changes occur as the result of functional decline due to disease, one third are due to inactivity or disuse, and one third are caused by aging itself. Lakatta places age-related changes into two catagories: usual (average) aging and successful (pure) aging. Usual aging refers to the "combined effects of the aging process, disease and adverse environmental and lifestyle factors" (p. 422). Successful aging refers to "the changes due solely to the aging process uncomplicated by damage from environment, lifestyle, or disease" (p. 422).

To illustrate this, oxygen consumption by sedentary elderly is usually low (usual aging); however, take the sedentary elder and place him or her in a regular aerobic exercise regimen and he or she can achieve oxygen levels equal to sedentary young adults (successful aging). In essence, normal (usual) age-dependent reductions in biofunction reduce compensatory reserve, but with successful aging the age-related changes may not result in clinical symptoms or disease.

Individual variations are enormous at every age and in every part of the body. For many years most research studies of the physical and biologic age changes have based conclusions on the comparison of different age groups in random samples rather than on groups using the longitudinal study approach. This presents an inherent error because the groups used may represent changes as a result of environmental differences (Goldman, 1979). The Baltimore Longitudinal Study (1984), which began in 1958, continues to follow a group of 1000 men as they age, with the objective of identifying normal changes of aging not associated with disease. The Baltimore Longitudinal Study of women began in the 1980s. Table 4-1 provides a summary of selected anatomic and physiologic changes with age of healthy adults.

Changes in body structure and function are lifelong alterations that begin to take on significance internally and externally in the fourth and fifth decades of life. External signs are the clues by which most people judge aging. However, these signs can be deceptive. Skin can become deeply wrinkled or hair become gray early in adult life, even though these features are considered signs of aging. Today individuals have at their disposal cosmetic surgery, hair coloring, makeup, and clothing choices that can make a person look younger than his or her chronologic age.

A study conducted by the National Institute on Aging (Special Report on Aging, 1981) found that people who appear older than their chronologic age may indeed share the characteristics of an older biologic age. Many internal changes mimic disease manifestations and might be interpreted as a pathologic state in need of medical attention. On the other hand, normal changes can mask early signs of disease processes. This dichotomous situation makes it very important for those who care for the aged to carefully explore the changes that do occur rather than immediately categorizing them as pathologic or normal. The individual must be evaluated as a whole being for a correct interpretation of the changes occurring.

Common denominators emerge when one looks at age-related changes. Many changes are effected by a decrease in blood supply to tissues because of the natural deposition of fat and calcium in the vessel intima. Reduced circulation perfusion is also thought to produce the diminished endocrine secretion commonly noted in old age (Costa and Andres, 1986). Finally, lifelong use and abuse of the body through accidents, athletic injuries, and other physical trauma are responsible for some of the changes thought of as wear and tear. When one is young, it is difficult to realize that neglect of skin, teeth, or nutrition will not necessarily produce visible or significant changes until one moves into old age and compensatory reserve becomes limited. At that time the effects of earlier laxness become more apparent and important to a person's health.

Significant changes in structure, function, and biochemistry as well as genetic endowment are responsible for the alterations in tissue elasticity, subcutaneous fat, gastrointestinal function and motility, muscle, bone, immunity, and the sensorium. These changes are not mutually exclusive but rather are synergistic and contribute to alterations in each system and the general evidence of advanced age.

Structure and Posture

One loses 1½ to 3 inches, or 1.2 cm, of height every 20 years as aging occurs (Jacobs, 1981; Cunningham and Brookbank, 1988; Lamb, 1996). Obvious manifestations, which are an interaction of many factors such as age, sex, race, and environment, occur in the fifth decade of life. Long bones take on the appearance of disproportionate size (long arms and legs) because stature decreases. Vertebral disks become thin due to dehydration, causing a shortening of the trunk. Many aged persons assume a stooped, forward-bent posture, with hips and knees somewhat flexed and arms bent at the el-

| Table 4-1 | A Summary of Selected Anatomic and Physiologic Changes with Aging, Healthy Adults |

System affected	Change noted	Age span (yr)
Total body water		
Men	Declines from 60% to 54%	20–80
Women	Declines from 54% to 46%	20–80
Muscle mass	30% decrease	30–70
Taste buds	70% decrease	30–70
Cardiac reserve	Decreases from 4.6 to 3.3 times resting cardiac output	25–70
Maximum heart rate	195 to 155 beats/min	25–70
Lung vital capacity	17% decrease	30–70
Renal perfusion	Reduced by 50%	30–80
Cerebral blood flow	Reduced by 20%	30–70
Bone mineral content	Reduced by 25–30% in women, 10–15% in men	40–80
Brain weight	Reduced by 7%	20–80
Amount of light reaching the retina	Diminished by 70%	20–65
Plasma glucocorticoid levels	No change	30–70

Modified from Kenney RA: *Physiology of aging: a synopsis,* Chicago, 1982, Year Book Medical Publishers, Inc; and Shock NW, Greulich RC, Andres RA et al: *Normal human aging: the Baltimore study of aging,* NIH Publication No 84-2450, Washington, DC, 1984, US Government Printing Office.

bows, raising the level of the arms. To maintain eye contact, the head is tilted backward, which makes it appear that the elderly individual is jutting forward. In addition, shoulder width may narrow due to shrinkage of the deltoid muscles and acromions. Abdominal length also decreases, giving the overall picture of a disproportionate individual who needs to be stretched out a bit. One must keep in mind that these changes involve multiple developmental factors: skeletal, muscular, subcutaneous tissue, fat, and dermal changes.

Bone mass is constantly undergoing cyclic resorption and renewal. Disequilibrium of this process with greater resorption and less calcium deposition is characteristic of aging bone. Posture and structural changes occur primarily because of calcium loss from bone and as a result of atrophic processes of cartilage and muscle. Excessive leaching of calcium from the bone matrix creates the condition called osteoporosis. This type of degeneration is four times more prevalent in women (Lindsay, 1985), becoming apparent as estrogen declines in older women. Maintaining muscle use and bone stress, for example, by walking, can slow the process. (See Chapter 8.) Kyphosis and osteoporosis are two factors that contribute to the shorter stature of the aged. Resorption of the bone leads to poor-fitting dentures and painful sensations when chewing or biting (Coni et al, 1984). Degeneration of underlying cartilage appears to decrease intervertebral distance. The forward-leaning posture is attributed to muscle shrinkage, and breasts that were full and firm begin to sag and become pendulous as the glandular envelope of fat atrophies. Nipples may also invert because of shrinkage and fibrotic changes. Bone demineralization affects the jaw or alveolar bone of the lower jaw, especially in individuals who are edentulous.

Skeletal muscle atrophy occurs because of physical inactivity, a decreased number of neurons to muscle cells, and endocrine factors and is greater in the lower extremities, in much the same manner as that which occurs in long-term muscle inactivity. Abdominal muscles decrease in size and number of fibers, in part because of disuse. Muscle tone or tension of particular muscle groups decreases steadily after 30 years of age. Possible causes are attributed to neuron loss and the loss of sensory and motor elements of spinal nerves of the muscles. Nerve cells in the spinal cord are lost after 80 years of age (Cunningham and Brookbank, 1988; Bartz, 1995). Strength and stamina decrease to 65% to 85% of the maximum strength an individual had at 25 years of age.

Ligaments, tendons, and joints show the results of cellular cross-linkage over time, resulting in hardened, more rigid, less flexible movement and predisposing these structures to tears. Worn-down cartilage around joints produced by continuous flexing over the years coupled with stray pieces of cartilage and diminished lubricating fluid in the joints can lead to slower and painful movement at times.

The fat layer around the orbit of the eye disappears, creating a sunken appearance of the eyes. Landmarks become more prominent, and muscle contours are easily identified.

Skinfold thickness, a measure of subcutaneous fat content, is markedly reduced in the forearm with age. Women over 45 years of age begin to see the skinfolds on the back of their hands rapidly diminish, even if there is a substantial weight gain. Such areas as the pubis, umbilicus, and waist do not change appreciably.

Subcutaneous tissue plays a significant role in the body's adjustment to temperature change. The natural insulation that subcutaneous fat affords is lost, and it is not uncommon to hear aged people mention that they are cold, nor is it unusual to see them wearing a sweater or sitting with a lap blanket. Windy, dry winter weather can accelerate loss of body heat by evaporation, and subsequent hypothermia may lead to death by decreasing body core temperature (Cunningham and Brookbank, 1988). Those elderly living at home tend to keep the room temperature higher than those who are young. Although subcutaneous tissue does not affect the aged's tolerance of heat, it is important to mention that comparable problems exist. The efficiency of sweat glands is reduced through diminished size, number, and activity. Eccrine glands become fibrotic, and surrounding connective tissue becomes avascular. The remainder of the eccrine glands may improperly function. These changes cause a decline in the efficiency of the body's cooling mechanism. The aged person is no longer able to perspire freely and becomes highly susceptible to heat exhaustion and heat stroke, common causes of death during the summer.

Education of the aged about the natural phenomenon of the loss of subcutaneous fat will help them realize why they respond to hot and cold temperature fluctuations so dramatically. In cool or cold weather most elders compensate with sweaters, lap blankets, or other pieces of apparel. In hot weather shade, sufficient fluids, an air conditioned or cool environment, or wet cloths to the head and neck should be considered. It becomes important for the nurse in the institutional setting to be aware of the temperature discomforts of the aged when bathing, dressing, or examining them and to be cognizant of the need for shade, cool temperature, and sufficient fluids in hot weather.

Stengel (1983) studied oral temperature norms in well old persons and found they were significantly lower in women over 80 years than in younger women. Older men consistently had an even lower temperature than women of comparable age. The old old may have a temperature of 96.8° F with an average range of 95° to 97° F. By tympanic membrane thermometer the temperature may be 96° (Hogstel, 1994). These findings emphasize the need to carefully evaluate the basal temperature of aged individuals and recognize that even low-grade fevers in the elderly may signify illness.

Skin, Hair, and Nails

Epidermal cell renewal time increases by one third after 50 years of age. The normal young adult renews epithelium every 20 days, whereas an older person requires 30 or more days because of diminished mitotic epidermal activity. Because of this slow replacement of epidermal cells, wound healing is approximately 50% slower than at 35 years of age (Leyden et al, 1978). The amount of collagen decreases approximately 1% per year, causing the skin to "give" less under stress and tear more easily (Richey et al, 1988). The dermis becomes thinner in the absence of subcutaneous fat (Grove and Kingman, 1983).

Fewer melanocytes are identifiable in the epidermis as skin ages. However, in some areas of aged skin, melanin synthesis is increased. Pigment spots (freckles and nevi) enlarge and can become more numerous with increased exposure to natural and artificial light. Vascular hyperplasia results in more pronounced varicosities, benign cherry angiomas, and venous stars.

Race, sex, sex-linked genes, and hormonal influences determine the maximum amount of hair that one has and the changes that will occur with it throughout life. In both sexes, hair distribution becomes more sparse; hair on the head thins, and leg hair frequently is lacking. This latter finding is often interpreted as a sign of peripheral vascular disease. Other, more conclusive, signs and symptoms should be observed to validate the diagnosis of abnormal hair loss. Orientals and blacks are less hairy than whites, and American Indians have little or no hair on their bodies (Rossman, 1986). Dark, thick, abundant hair becomes lighter, gray, thinner, and less full. At times hair color may turn shades of yellow or yellow-green. Axillary and pubic hair diminishes in quantity and thickness of the hair fibers.

Hair becomes gray because of the decrease in melanin production in hair follicles. Regardless of sex, 50% of the population over 50 years of age has gray or partly gray scalp hair. Body and facial hair becomes gray later. Hair loss is prominent in men, beginning in the second decade for some. Women have less pronounced hair loss. Overall scalp and body hair diminishes with advanced age. By 40 years of age, hair patterns have reached their maximum and begin to recede.

Nails of the fingers and toes develop longitudinal striations and grow at a slower rate than in youth. Toenails grow at a 15% slower rate than fingernails in the aged (Jacobs, 1981; Cornell, 1986). The nail plate may thicken and give the nail a yellow appearance. With age the cuticle becomes less thick and wide. Vigorous manipulation of the cuticle may lead to retardation of the already slowed nail growth.

Facial Changes

Facial changes occur as a result of altered subcutaneous fat, dermal thickness, decreased elasticity, and lateral surface compression of underlying muscle contractions. Loss of bone mass, particularly the mandibular bone, accentuates the size of the upper mouth, nose, and forehead. Indented "loss of lip" appearance of the mouth occurs with tooth loss when uncorrected by dentures or other oral prostheses. Eyelids appear swollen as a result of the redistribution of fat deposits. Conversely, eyes that look sunken are the result of the loss of orbital subcutaneous fat. Loss of elasticity accentuates jowls and elongated ears and contributes to the formation of a "double" chin.

Loss of Tissue Elasticity

Tissue elasticity is most easily observed in skin integrity and reflects the progressive, universal, and intrinsic nature of age

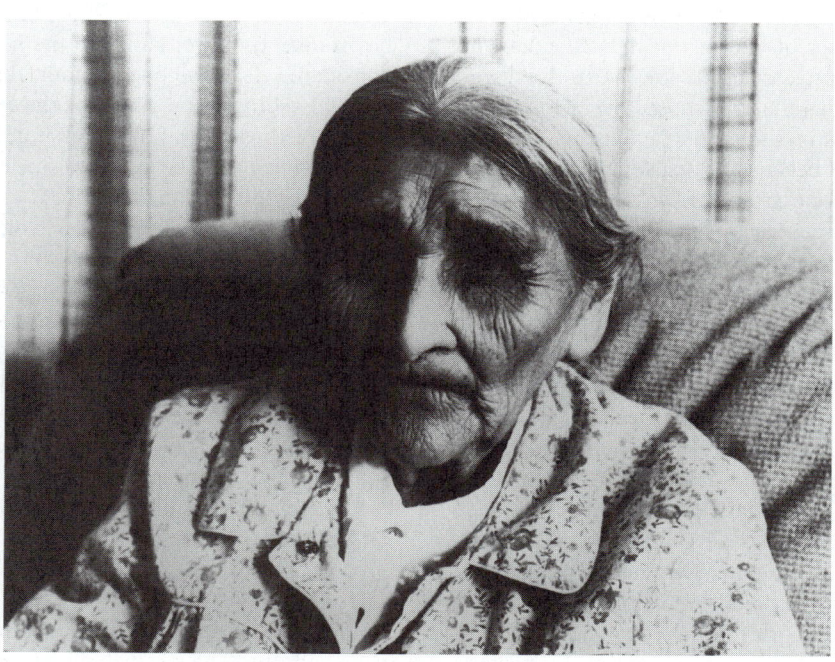

Facial changes.

changes. The aged skin loses resilience and moisture, taking on a characteristic dryness. The epithelial layer thins, and elastic collagen fibers shrink and become rigid. The face and neck wrinkles reflect life patterns of muscle activity in facial expressions, the pull of gravity on tissue, and diminished elasticity in general. Sun exposure accelerates skin tissue changes by hastening collagen fiber alterations. The influence of sun and heat on collagen flexibility has been discussed in the cross-link theory in Chapter 2.

Elasticity affects blood vessel integrity, particularly the arteries. Elastic fibers fray, split, straighten, and fragment. Calcium that leaves the bone is deposited in the vessels. This chemical and anatomic alteration decreases the lumen size of the vessels and causes the blood flow to various organs to become uneven. There is little flow change to the coronary arteries and the brain, but perfusion of the liver and kidneys shows significant changes in the amount of blood brought to these two organs. (Wardell, 1979; Cunningham and Brookbank, 1988; Malasanos et al, 1989). Peripheral resistance in the vessels, which increases in both the systolic and diastolic pressures with advancing age, is a reflection of the elastic changes and calcium deposits. (Refer to cardiovascular changes in this chapter.)

Lung elasticity declines, causing a rigidity in lung tissue. This alone is not responsible for the decrease in oxygen capacity, but it is a contributing factor (Tichy and Malasanos, 1979). (Refer to the discussion of respiratory system changes in this chapter.)

Nursing interventions are limited where tissue elasticity of internal structures is concerned, but retention of tissue moisture can be assisted through the use of body lotion and judicious use of soap in bathing, as well as teaching the aged that overexposure to the sun, heat, and other elements is detrimental to their skin. Chapter 7 will discuss skin integrity and maintenance in more detail.

Body Composition

Body weight changes because of a decline in lean body mass and a loss of body water: 54% to 60% in men; 46% to 52% in women (Kenney, 1982) (Figure 4-1). Fat tissue increases until 60 years of age; therefore body density is lower in youth because of the density of muscle versus the lightness of fat. From 25 to 75 years of age fat content of the body increases by 16%. Cellular solids and bone mass decline; extracellular water, however, remains relatively constant. Cellular sodium increases 20% from 30 to 70 years of age, and there is a need to increase the proportion of protein, calcium, and vitamin D nutritional intake (Gugoz and Munro, 1985; Lakatta, 1995). The intercellular matrix (collagen and elastin) cross-link, reducing resilience. Intracellular concentrations of structural proteins, enzymes, and chromosomal components, including deoxyribonucleic acid (DNA) and ribonucleic acid (RNA), change. Lipofuscin, or "aging pigment," increases in the nervous system and other nonrenewing tissues (for example, the heart).

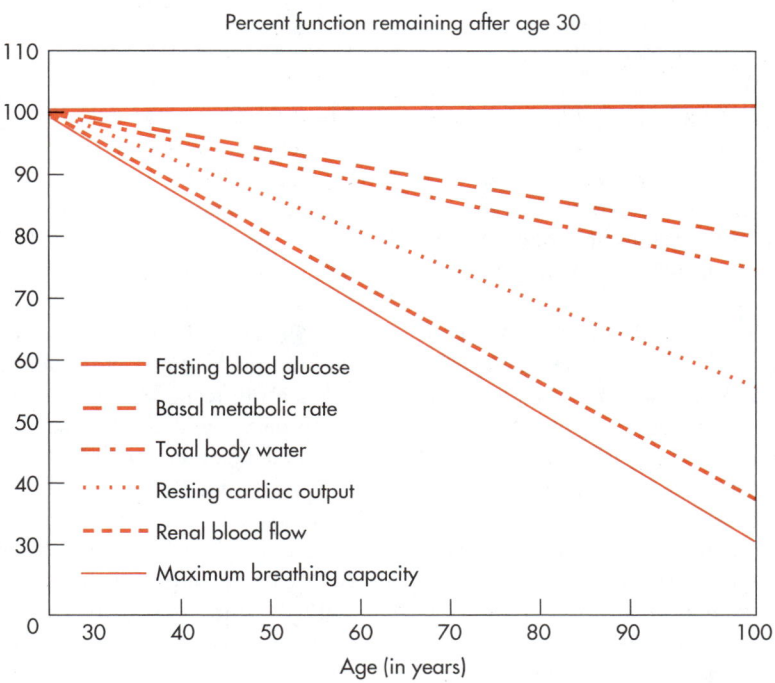

Figure 4-1. Changes in biologic function with age. (Modified from Shock NW. In Carlston LA, editor: *Nutrition in old age,* Tenth Symposium of the Swedish Nutrition Federation, Uppsala, 1972, Almquistand Wilksell.)

Cardiovascular Changes

Heart. For centuries the heart, which must function continuously to maintain life as we know it, was considered the center of life until the technologic redefinition of death included the cessation of brain activity as well as heart function. Cardiovascular disease is a major cause of death worldwide in people age 60 and over. In the United States, one half of all cardiovascular disease occurs in those 65 years of age and older (Johns Hopkins Medical Letter, 1994). One of every two persons age 60 and over may have some severe narrowing of the coronary arteries, but only about 50% of those have clinical signs of coronary artery dysfunction. Screening for this occult manifestation can now be done with magnetic resonance imaging (MRI) (Johns Hopkins Medical Letter, 1994). It is difficult to know whether widespread disease exaggerates functional decline presently considered to be the result of age-related change.

Health professionals are accustomed to caring for aged persons with cardiac-related conditions such as congestive heart failure and hypertension and may be inclined to assume that all aged individuals have enlarged hearts. Studies suggest that the left ventricle wall thickens as much as 30% between ages 25 and 80 due to the increase in myocyte size, but the size remains relatively unchanged in healthy adults. The left atrium also increases about 20% in size between 18 and 93 years of age. This adaptation enhances ventricular filling. In healthy aged a fourth heart sound may be audible due to this atrial enlargement (Lakatta, 1993). Cardiac mass is estimated to increase 1.5 g in women and 1 g in men per year after age 30 (Lakatta, 1993). Radiologic silhouette of cardiac size shows a slight increase but remains within a clinically normal range. (Gersteinblith et al, 1977; Gardin et al, 1979; Lakatta, 1995).

By age 60, the maximum coronary artery blood flow provides the cardiovascular system with 35% less blood than in earlier years. The decline in work response of the left ventricle at rest is a reflection of decreased stroke volume and cardiac output and a delay in heart muscle irritability and contractile recovery. Contraction of the older heart is prolonged, most likely due to the slow release of calcium into the myoplasm during systole. Reduced efficiency and contractile strength of the heart muscle are reflected in (1) a reduced cardiac output that decreases by 1%/yr from the average baseline of 5 L/min and (2) a stroke volume decline of 0.7%/yr (Jacobs, 1981; Kenney, 1982) (see Figure 4-1).

Under normal conditions the aged heart is able to sustain adequate function to maintain an average active life. Under nonstressful conditions the smaller cardiac output is adequate since the mechanisms that determine cardiovascular function depend on the interaction of intrinsic cell performance, heart rate, coronary flow, cardiac filling (preload), and cardiac afterload. All of these are governed by autonomic tone and a negative feedback system. Decreased overall energy demands and a moderate degree of body atrophy place less demand on cardiac function. Diminished cardiac output becomes significant when the aged person is physically or mentally stressed by illness, worry, or excitement. Sudden demands for more oxygen and energy brought on by various physiologic, psychologic, social, and environmental stress result in poor response of heart function attributed to the limited cardiac reserve, or presbycardia. It takes longer for the heart to accelerate to meet the demands placed on it and to return to a normal level. Tachycardia is not as great in the older person but, when occurring, the heart requires a longer time to return to its baseline rate.

The expected increase in the pulse rate when the patient is anxious, is in pain, hemorrhages, or demonstrates the presence of an infectious process is not as evident in the aged as in the young.

General risk factors that can cause stress and strain on the heart include the following:
• Continued intake of high complements of dietary animal fat, salt, and calories
• Obesity and excessive weight
• Long-term cigarette smoking
• Lack of regular exercise
• Internalization of emotions
• Air pollution
• Existing chronic conditions

Other physical conditions that impose added demand on the aged heart or aggravate existing cardiac conditions include infection, anemia, pneumonia, cardiac arrhythmias, surgery, fever, diarrhea, hypoglycemia, malnutrition, avitaminosis, circulatory overload, and drug-induced and noncardiac illnesses such as renal disease and prostatic obstruction.

Circulation time for the adult averages 15 seconds. Diettert (1963) found an average circulation time of 27 seconds to be normal for men in the seventh decade of life. Electrocardiogram changes with age under normal circumstances are minimum. There is a slight lengthening of the PR, QRS, and QT intervals.

Catecholamines and other enzymes that influence the effect of the force and speed of heart contractions diminish in amount, producing a long interval between contractions, a weakened cardiac force, and a greater energy demand on heart muscle. Lower contractile strength, smaller cardiac output, and reduced enzymatic stimulation together cause the heart to respond to the work demand with less efficient performance and greater energy expenditure than would be required when the individual was younger.

Valves. Valves may be thicker and stiffer as a result of lipid deposits, collagen degeneration, and fibrosis. Valvular conditions in the aged are considered residual effects of earlier rheumatic infections and arteriosclerosis. Aortic and mitral valves are most commonly affected and result in slight to moderate regurgitation of blood. Valvular disease in the aged is often misdiagnosed because it is assumed that murmurs are the result of the arteriosclerotic process. Some aged do have aortic and mitral murmurs that were chronicled from childhood, others from the stiffening of the valve leaflets. Generally those murmurs are not as prominent as murmurs that occur in later life. At least 50% of elders have a systolic ejection type of murmur which is a grade 1 or 2 without radiation. Murmurs that are diastolic, however, should always be considered significant since these indicate important alteration in cardiac hemodynamics (Lakatta, 1990).

Conductivity. Sinus rhythm is the expected norm of the aged person's heartbeat. During the third and fourth decade of life pacemaker cells decrease in number as myocardial fat, collagen, and elastin fibers increase. This change affects the sinus (SA) node, which shows evidence of causing an acceleration through the sixth decade. The number of SA cells at age 75 is only 10% of what existed at age 20 (Wei, 1988; Gawlinski and Jensen, 1991; Morgan, 1993). Similarly, the atrioventricular (AV) node and the bundle of His lose a number of conductive cells into the fourth decade and the left bundle between the fifth and seventh decade (Fujino et al, 1983; Miller, 1990). Alteration in the excitation and contraction mechanism is an adaptive rather than a degenerative change because it maintains contractile function of the aged heart. The mean resting rate remains unchanged with age, but the maximum heart rate can be achieved when activity is decreased.

Sinus rate of less than 50 beats/min is common in elderly and does not necessarily indicate SA node disease. Significant interference with the blood flow either by occlusion or by narrowed arteriosclerotic vessels to the SA node can produce arrhythmias.

Arrhythmias may be primary or secondary, but the majority of rate irregularities in the aged are attributed to myocardial damage. The heart muscle is damaged directly by interference with the coronary circulation or indirectly by valvular insufficiency and concomitant interference with circulation to the responsible neurologic mechanisms essential to heart action.

Baroreceptor sensitivity declines, resulting in a decreased ability for compensatory response to hypertensive or hypotensive stimuli. Stiffening of the arteries and a reduced cardiovascular responsiveness to adrenergic stimulation is responsible for the baroreflex (Banaski, 1995).

Accumulation of collagen, mononuclear cells, and smooth muscle cells increases the subintimal areas, and vessel walls thicken due to reorganization of the cellular and extracellular matrix (Cooper et al, 1994).

Vessels. Decreased elasticity of arteries and arterioles is responsible for changes that affect blood flow to body organs such as the heart, liver, kidneys, and pituitary gland. The aorta dilates and elongates as collagen and elastin changes and calcium deposition from degenerating elastin occurs (Lakatta, 1995). Circulation in the coronary arteries diminishes by approximately 35% after the sixth decade; increased resistance to peripheral blood flow occurs at a rate of about 1%/yr. Weakness of vessel walls and varicosities can lead to abnormal swelling when subjected to increased pressure. With normal aging, some atherosclerosis is nor-

mal, but it can be exacerbated to a pathologic state by a diet high in saturated fat (see Appendix 4-A).

Peripheral Vascular Changes

Both arteries and veins exhibit changes as the intima becomes fibrotic and endothelial cell variation increases. The amount of elastin and smooth muscle diminish as collagen and fibrotic tissue increase. The result is loss of flexibility and recoil, an increase in systemic peripheral resistance, and a reduced perfusion to tissues and organs. The stiffening and more rigid structure of the vascular system may lead to the elevation of blood pressure in addition to influencing cardiac and renal changes. Veins lose their elasticity and become less able to store blood volume. Pooling of blood increases the venous pressure, diminishing the effectiveness of peripheral valves and creating tortuous varicosities (Beare and Myers, 1994).

Not more than 20 years ago, it was thought that systolic blood pressure of an aged person was 100 plus the person's age. Thus an individual age 70 was thought to have a normal systolic pressure of 170 mm Hg. Another accepted approach to normal blood pressure was to consider 160/90 as the upper limits of normal for the aged adult. However, The Fifth Report of the Joint National Committee on Detection, Evaluation, and Treatment of High Blood Pressure (1993) states that both young and old have similar blood pressure. The Committee defines hypertension as systolic pressure at or above 140 mm Hg and diastolic pressure at or above 90 mm Hg. It is estimated that 50% of persons over age 65 in industrialized society have blood pressure at or greater than 140/90 mm Hg (Frohlich, 1995).

A form of hypertension seen in elders is isolated systolic hypertension (ISH). This type of hypertension occurs when the diastolic pressure is normal but the systolic pressure is elevated.

The importance of this redefinition of normal blood pressure and hypertension points out the impact that elevated blood pressure has as a risk for cardiovascular disease. Both hypertension and ISH increase during the eight and ninth decades of life.

The incidence of hypertension is higher for the black population than the white population. The National Health and Nutrition Examination Survey (NHANES III), which occurred between 1988 and 1991, confirms this. The survey found that 40% of white men and over 30% of white women ages 50 to 59 had hypertension. The rate was higher for blacks: over one half of the black men ages 50 to 59 were hypertensive and almost half of the black women in that age group were also hypertensive. By ages 60 to 69, the rates increased to over 50% for both white men and women, over 60% for black men, and nearly 80% for black women (Johns Hopkins Medical Letter, 1996).

Weber, Barnard, and Ray (1983) studied older individuals who were on a high–complex carbohydrate, low-fat diet and daily exercise, which involved walking approximately 3.1 miles (5 km) daily, for 26 days. Following this closely monitored program, half of the individuals were able to reduce hypertension, discontinue hypertensive medication, and reduce cholesterol intake. Their work capacity and health status were significantly improved with this dietary program and daily walking. Exercise and diet control remain the mainstay today.

Gardner and Poehlman (1995) looked at age-related increases in blood pressure of men and women. They found a relationship between systolic pressure and age to be stronger in women than in men by the age of 50 to 60 years. This was primarily due to an accelerated increase in systolic pressure that occurred at a greater rate in women. Why is unclear. The age-related increase in men was thought to be related to an increase in body fatness as opposed to a shift in body fat in women. The greater increase in blood pressure in women older than age 62 suggested that the years after menopause might influence this rise. The acceleration was also thought to be related to a reduction in estrogen, but blood pressure changes did not occur until 5 to 10 years later, which is the time required to manifest its effects on blood pressure. It was concluded that the amount of subcutaneous fat deposition and alcohol intake of men were predictors for elevated systolic pressure for men and that the waist-to-hip ratio and aerobic fitness were predictors for systolic and diastolic pressure, respectively, for women.

Even though the death rate from heart and vascular disease is declining, *the aged today still are a reflection of previous health practices.* Some damage can be lessened by modifying behavior.

Continuing education regarding diet, smoking, exercise, activity, and weight control are proving productive in an aging population. The highly complex phenomenon of the blood pressure mechanism within an aging individual is influenced in many ways (Box 4-1). Education for self-care is one facet of the multifaceted condition of hypertension that is receiving increased attention.

Box 4-1	Some Factors Affecting Normotensive/ Hypertensive Blood Pressure

Increased action of adrenergic nervous system
and/or
Catecholamines (norepinephrine is elevated in the elderly)
Increase in renin-angiotensin systemically or autocrine of arteries and other organs (there is a decrease of this in elders with hypertension)
Distensibility of great vessels (affected by atherosclerosis)
Altered fluid and electrolyte balance due to renal, hormonal, humoral factors

---

It is rare but should be acknowledged that a small group of aged persons may have survived to adulthood with small congenital defects such as septal defects. The congenital anomaly in these elders was either missed or did not appear until symptoms presented themselves in later life (Rossman, 1979).

Multiple origins of cardiovascular conditions include disruptions in the heart muscle, the valves, the vessels, or the conductive system or congenital defects. These can cause problems in the function of other structures involved in maintaining cardiovascular performance.

Respiratory Changes

Changes in respiratory and pulmonary performance occur gradually, allowing the elderly to continue to breath effortlessly in the absence of pathologic states. When the elderly are confronted with a little exertion or stress, however, dyspnea and other symptoms usually appear.

It is unclear if respiratory system changes are due to environmental toxins or the progressive subclinical exhaustion of internal respiratory reserve and repair caused by aging itself (Tockman, 1995). Respiratory changes that do occur in structure and function with superimposed consequences of acute illness and chronicity can be sufficiently debilitating to limit life enjoyment.

The prominent effect of age-related changes on the respiratory system is reduced efficiency in ventilation and gas exchange. It is accepted that exercise tolerance declines and that breathlessness leads to varying degrees of fatigue, but under usual or resting conditions the aged have little difficulty accomplishing and participating in customary life activities. However, when the aged are confronted with unusual and stressful circumstances, the demand for oxygen surpasses the available supply and establishes a significant respiratory deficit, which must be resolved. Stable respiratory function is also affected by a lower resistance to infection engendered by a diminished immune system response and less effective self-cleansing action of the respiratory cilia.

The respiratory system includes the nose, pharynx, larynx, trachea, bronchi, bronchioles, alveolar ducts, and alveoli. In addition, an interplay exists with the musculoskeletal and nervous systems.

Nose. The nose is a readily visible appendage, which with age elongates downward. It has been suggested that this age-related change may account for the mouth breathing that occurs while the elder sleeps and thus the lack of saliva production (Saxon and Etten, 1994).

Trachea and Larynx. Stiffening of the larynx and tracheal cartilage occurs as a result of calcification. The cilia that line the trachea and help to push up mucus, debris, and dust into the pharynx are less effective. Cilia decrease in number with the resultant decrease in respiratory epithelium and an increase in bronchial mucous gland hypertrophy (Schumann, 1995). Tockman (1995) suggests the importance of age and mucociliary transport is not fully established but may be clinically significant for the recurrence of respiratory infections.

Voice pitch increases for men and decreases for women, but substantially more so for elders who are in poor health. Breathlessness in speech is the result of less air passing through and incomplete closure of the glottis. Limited mobility of the jaw may also contribute to this.

Chest Wall and Lungs. During one's youth, the chest wall and lungs grow in proportion to the body and correlate with height (Tockmann, 1995). Around age 55, respiratory muscles begin to weaken, chest wall compliance begins to decrease, and there is a loss of elastic recoil. The results of these changes affect ventilation and gas exchange. Normal physiologic changes can resemble pathologic entities. Lillington (1979) relates that the lungs of "healthy" old people who are nonsmokers show evidence of small, scattered areas of lung destruction similar to the manifestations identified in emphysema (Timaris, 1988). Campbell and Lefrak (1978) mention that the normally reduced efficiency of air expulsion found in the general aged population resembles significant findings in those diagnosed with emphysema. In both instances the extent of change is the critical factor in determining normality or pathologic conditions (Kinney, 1989).

Ossification of the costal cartilage and the downward slant of the ribs result in a less compliant, more rigid rib cage, which limits chest expansion. Intercostal and accessory muscles and the diaphragm become more compliant or "floppier" as a consequence of muscle weakness. The potential for greater lung expansion exists but cannot be realized because of structural limitations that develop in the thoracic walls. Skeletal defects such as kyphosis and scoliosis and the generally stooped posture of the aged also contribute to restricting chest expansion by further reducing the size of the chest cavity area in which the lungs can expand. The outcome of these changes increase dead space, decrease vital capacity, and decrease expiratory flow. Collagen remains relatively constant, yet there seems to be an increased amount of vascular collagen as a compensatory response to the decreased number and size of the alveoli (see Appendix 4-A).

Lungs do not shrink in size but do become flabbier and decrease in weight by 20% (Krumpe et al, 1985). The elastin and collagen changes due to cross-linkage and deterioration result in a decrease of outward movement and inward pull with the end result of slightly smaller total lung capacity increased residual capacity, and residual volume, and early airway closure.

After age 30, the alveoli progressively enlarge and thus structurally resemble air sac changes associated with emphysema. The elastin fibers in the alveolar walls are bound to the respiratory and terminal bronchioles, which help to maintain the small airway patency at low lung volumes. The loss of the elastin attachment causes an increase in

compliance, collapse of the small airways, and uneven alveolar ventilation, trapping air and increasing dead space (Schumann, 1995; Tockman, 1995). The alveolar dilation with the loss of alveolar attachments and the increase in the number of collapsed small airways is referred to as "senile lung" and is seen in some individuals over age 60 (Tockman, 1995). Campbell and Lefrak (1978) referred to this physiologic change as "ductectasis" and considered it a normal aging phenomenon, not to be confused with the pathologic findings of emphysema.

Total lung capacity is not significantly altered, but rather it is redistributed. Residual capacity increases with the diminished inspiratory and expiratory muscle strength of the thorax. Incomplete lung expansion does not provide for inflation of the lung bases and leads to basilar lung collapse and hyperinflation of the lung apices.

The changes that have occurred in the anatomic structures of the chest and the altered muscle strength do not lend themselves to the forcefulness needed to expel material that accumulates or causes an obstruction in the airway (Krumpe et al, 1985). Therefore the aged individual has a less effective cough response or cough reflex. However, when other clearing mechanisms are intact, the cough reflex is not essential for respiratory clearance. When there is impairment such as dysphagia or decreased esophageal motility, an intact cough reflex is a necessity (Tockmann, 1995).

The lack of basilar inflation, ineffective cough response, and a less efficient immune system pose potential problems for the aged who are sedentary, bedridden, or limited in activity.

Oxygen Exchange. The aged blood oxygen (Po_2) level is approximately 75 mm Hg, where as the Po_2 level for younger adults ranges from 90 mm Hg to 95 mm Hg (Timaris, 1988). Pierson (1992) suggests Po_2 falls 4 mm Hg per decade. The blood carbon dioxide (Pco_2) level remains constant for both the young and older adult. The blood oxygen (Po_2) tension also remains constant, but the distribution of inspired air to dependent parts of the lung is less sufficient (Timaris, 1988). The absolute lowest normal Po_2 level for an elder is 70 mm Hg.

The transmural gradient that is responsible for holding open airways is diminished. Airway collapse limits the ability of the lungs to empty and decreases the exhalation of Pco_2. This places a greater demand on cardiac function to increase cardiac output to compensate for less oxygen delivery to body tissue. Diminished elastic recoil of the lungs makes gaseous exchange across alveolar membranes more difficult. Aged individuals with Po_2 levels as low as 40 mm Hg have little or no immediate compensatory response in cardiac function. Younger persons with the same blood gas level show a marked increase in cardiac rate as an attempt to compensate and deliver more oxygen to body tissues.

Chemoreceptor function is altered or blunted at the peripheral and central chemoreceptor sites or in the integrating central nervous system pathways. In healthy men ages 64 to

73 response to hypoxia is 51% less and to hypercapnia is 41% less than in younger adults. This response is independent of mechanical lung changes and is attributed to the neuromuscular drive to breath. Maximum inspiration and expiration pressures, which have declined as a result of chest wall inflexibility, reduce functional respiratory reserve and increase risk for respiratory failure. Compensatory responses are significantly hindered when the aged person is experiencing moderate amounts of stress. Decreased physical fitness further limits the availability of adequate gaseous exchange.

Reliable pulmonary function values that depict normal respiratory function of the aged are difficult to obtain. There are few published values on respiratory function tests for the elderly, particularly test values for aged women. Many values considered normal for old people have been derived from studies using small numbers of patients, often highly selected, under specific testing conditions. The absence of reliable pulmonary function values on which to evaluate the respiratory status of the aged requires that the nurse use other methods to assess the aged person's respiratory ability and needs.

Respiratory Problems. It is suggested by Tockman (1995) that airway problems with age are due to repeated inflammatory injuries, disruption of inflammatory mediators and humoral protection (elastase-antielastase, oxidants-antioxidants), neutrophil aggregation, and tissue repair. Diminished immune response, environmental factors, and structural changes are all factors that predispose the aged to respiratory problems. Conditions that affect the respiratory system are among the most common life-threatening disorders experienced by the aged and are considered to be among the leading causes of death.

Pneumonias are the sixth leading cause of death by disease in the United States and the fourth leading cause of death in the elderly (Bartlett, 1995). The old-old (85 years and older) are five times more likely to die of pneumonia than young-old or old adults. Pneumococcal pneumonias are the most common bacterial respiratory infections of the aged. Other less common bacterial pneumonias are *Haemophilus influenzae,* staphylococcus, streptococcus, and *Klebsiella* (Bentley, 1983).

Signs and symptoms of pneumonia manifested in the young are not commonly seen in the aged. The tendency toward atypical responses can easily lead to an incorrect diagnosis or a diagnosis made too late in the progress of the pneumonia. Aspiration pneumonia is a high-risk condition for the obtunded client who is force fed, a client with swallowing difficulties or esophageal disease, a client who regurgitates food, a client with an endotracheal tube or tracheostomy, and a client who is heavily sedated.

Chronic obstructive pulmonary disease (COPD) includes bronchitis, asthma, emphysema, and bronchiectasis. COPD and lung cancer constitute the medical conditions from which respiratory problems develop.

Renal Changes

Kidneys are the primary organs responsible for regulation of the chemical composition of the body and blood and fluid volume. The age-related loss of as many as 50% of the millions of nephrons (each kidney has at least 1 million) leads to little change in the body's ability to regulate its body fluids and the ability to maintain adequate fluid homeostasis in old age.

The size and function of the kidney begins to decrease in the fourth decade and significantly decreases by the middle of the sixth decade, shrinking about 7%, and by the eighth decade by 20% to 30%. This occurs primarily in the cortex. The kidney contour continues to remains relatively smooth. The weight of the kidney of the younger adult is 250 to 270 g; by the age of 80 the weight is 180 to 200 g. This decline in size parallels the general decrease in size and weight of other body organs.

Glomeruli. The number of abnormal glomeruli increases from approximately 5% to 37% between 40 and 90 years of age, but the remaining normal glomeruli increase in size (Rowe, 1995; Richard, 1995). By the eighth decade, 30% of the glomeruli are lost and there is evidence of age-related glomerular sclerosis. Renal tubules develop diverticular changes in the distal portion of the nephron. These manifest as retention cysts common to the elderly. Sclerosis of the glomeruli is unclear, but it is thought that a high protein diet or glomerular ischemia may be responsible (Rowe, 1995). In general, these changes pose little threat to the well-being of the aged unless there is an abrupt reduction in nephron function by an acquired renal disease (Rowe, 1995; Richard, 1995).

Renal vessels. The large renal vessels show evidence of sclerosis with age but do not narrow the vessel lumen. Smaller vessels do not show this change. Only 15% of elders who are normotensive have sclerotic changes in the renal arterioles.

Changes occur in the arterioglomerular units affecting the cortical area (hyalinization and collapse of the glomerular tufts). Preglomerular arterioles become obliterated, resulting in loss of blood flow. The medullary area of the kidney demonstrates sclefrosis of the glomeruli and shrinking between the afferent and efferent arterioles with a loss of glomeruli. The arteriolae rectae verae preserve blood flow to the medullary area. Age does not decrease the number of arterioles in this area.

Glomerular Filtration. Blood flow through the kidney decreases from 1200 ml/min in young adults to 600 ml/min by the age of 80 due to the vascular and fixed anatomic and structural changes described above. Figure 4-1 illustrates the altered renal blood flow. In view of these changes, the glomerular filtration rate (GFR), dependent on the number of glomeruli, steadily declines.

The GFR is measured by the creatine clearance, which also changes with age. It is directly related to muscle mass and a product of muscle metabolism. By age 80, the creatinine clearance is decreased to 100 ml/mm. Urine creatinine, secondary to loss of muscle mass, alters the expected relationship of serum creatinine to the creatinine clearance. A linear decline begins at about age 40 with a rate of 8 ml/min/1.73 m²/decade (Rowe, 1995). Some elders, approximately one third, have been shown not to exhibit a decline in GFR (Lindeman et al, 1985), suggesting that factors other than age-related change may be responsible for altered renal function. Plasma creatinine clearance is constant throughout life. The decline in urine creatinine clearance is an important indicator for appropriate drug therapy in the aged (see Chapter 10).

Renin-Angiotensin. Basal renin is reduced by 30% to 50% even with normal levels of renin substrate (Rowe, 1995). The lower renin levels are associated with a parallel reduction of the same proportions in aldosterone. However, after corticotropin stimulation, aldosterone and corticol responses are not impaired with age. This decreases the kidneys' ability to conserve sodium and delay the response of the acid/base loading.

There is a slight shift in the antidiuretic hormone (ADH). A reduced ability to concentrate urine and conserve water due to medullary loss make the collecting ducts less responsive to ADH. The importance of the age-related kidney changes is that elders are more susceptible to fluid and electrolyte imbalance and renal damage from medications and contrast media of diagnostic tests. Under normal circumstances, kidney function is sufficient to meet the regulation and excretion demands of the body. However, with stress of disease, surgery, or fever, the kidneys have little capacity to respond.

Endocrine Changes

Hormones are responsible for and control reproduction, growth and development, maintenance of homeostasis, and energy production. Two principles must be kept in mind when considering hormonal control and effects: (1) a particular hormone may have an effect on many body systems and functions, and (2) one body function may require the coordinated action of many hormones (Bartz, 1995). Suggested here is that backup and fine-tuning mechanisms adjustments are made to maintain homeostasis or close-to-normal limits. Changes may produce hypoactivity from disease or physiologic down regulating. Serum hormone levels are reflective of changes. Most glands atrophy and decrease their rate of secretion. There is no uniform direction of change; some are less active, slightly active, or not active at all (Solomon, 1995).

Pancreas—Insulin. There is little difference in insulin secretion from the beta cells and glucose metabolism throughout life. The age-related change is in the tissue sensitivity to insulin, thought to be due to a change in the molecular makeup of insulin (Bartz, 1995). In addition, higher levels of circulating proinsulin are found in older adults than in younger adults. Alteration of insulin receptor sites by the

aging process is also considered to render insulin less effective (MacLennan and Peden, 1989). When the pancreas is stressed with sudden concentrations of glucose, blood levels are higher and prolonged (Figure 4-1). Because of this intolerance, increased levels of glucose in the blood make it difficult for physicians to determine if it is a physiologic decline or a genetic trait for which a treatment plan is needed.

Thyroid Gland. Thyroid function remains adequate with age, even though the thyroid gland decreases in mass and becomes fibrotic with an increasing number of colloid nodules. There is also slowing of the metabolic rate and oxygen use by the body. Secretions of thyroid-stimulating hormone (TSH) continue unchanged even with a decrease of 50% between youth and advanced old age. The decrease correlates with a decrease in lean body mass and a decrease in metabolic activity and protein-rich tissue. The serum concentration of T_4 (thyroxin) also remains unchanged (Solomon, 1995; Bartz, 1995). A significant decline in triiodothyronine (T_3) occurs with age, which is thought to reflect reduced conversion of T_4 to T_3 in extrathyroidal locations. Collective signs, such as a slowed basal metabolic rate, thinning of the hair, and dry skin are characteristic of hypothyroidism in the young but are normal manifestations in the aged who have no history of thyroid deficiencies (see Appendix 4-A). Some of the aged do develop hypothyroidism and should be evaluated. This is one instance in which it is difficult, on the surface, to establish the presence or absence of disease.

Adrenal Gland. Cortisol, an important glucocorticoid of the adrenal cortex, although diminished by 25%, does not seem to have an adverse effect. Likewise, the effect of decreased adrenocorticotropic hormone production has not been elucidated. Epinephrine, norepinephrine, and dopamine produced by the adrenal medulla decrease with age, but again the significance is unclear.

Pituitary Gland. The pituitary gland, with its diverse functions and central role in the complex hormone feedback system, decreases in volume by 20%. The significance of this is unclear in light of the maintenance of adequate hormonal secretions.

Adrenogenic, estrogenic, and gonadotropic hormones undergo secretory and stimulatory changes. Diminished hormone levels lead to atrophy of the ovaries, uterus, and vaginal tissue in aged women. Aged men develop firmer testes and a tendency for prostatic hypertrophy, which is a benign condition in most instances. Women lose the ability to procreate. Sexual capacity may diminish as the tissues change and physical and mental health changes, but libido remains present in both sexes. Intercourse may be less frequent and take longer to accomplish, but this does not mean that it is less satisfying to the couple involved.

There tends to be a subliminal belief on the part of nurses and other caregivers that persons (at an arbitrary age) in general no longer are sexually active or possess sexuality. It is true that when one is seriously ill or in poor mental or physical health, the body does not require sexual activity as one of the primary responses. Most institutional care neglects the genital sexual need and the touch, intimacy, and sexuality needs of persons of any age. It behooves the nurse and others to view and care for the aged individual as a totally sexual being. Chapter 16 addresses the touch, intimacy, and sexual needs in greater detail.

Gastrointestinal Changes

The digestive system handles age-related changes better than most systems of the body. The primary functions of the gastrointestinal tract are digestion and absorption, which are accomplished by gastrointestinal secretions and motility. Changes in other organ systems affect gastrointestinal structure and function. Studies have determined that extraintestinal causes, such as diabetes and vascular and neurologic changes, previously may have been mistaken for age-related changes in the gastrointestinal system.

Mouth and Teeth. Dentition is an important adjunct to the gastrointestinal system and can affect digestive activity. Food entering the mouth is prepared for digestion by the action of saliva, which contains ptyalin to break down starch, and mastication by the teeth. Many aged today continue to be edentulous or dependent on dentures. A number of aged who have dentures choose not to wear them; others are unable to afford them.

Normally food is well masticated in the mouth. Due to systemic disorders and their treatment, the saliva level may decline. Recent studies indicate that saliva production is generally unchanged in the aged (Schuster, 1995). In addition, in the presence of few teeth or ill-fitting dentures, the process of preparing the food for swallowing is incomplete with food morsels improperly chewed. The inclination is to place many aged on a pureed diet even though this type of diet lacks the appeal, taste, texture, and appearance needed to stimulate appetite, gastrointestinal motility, eating enjoyment, and the maintenance of adequate nutrition.

In the future, as an effect of better dental hygiene and fluoride in present-day water systems and in dental preparations, the aged may retain their own teeth for the full extent of their lives. The primary problem that will remain and be responsible for tooth loss is periodontal disorders. Gum disease threatens tooth structure and compromises healthy teeth, requiring removal. Many gum conditions can be prevented with proper toothbrushing and oral hygiene. Chapter 7 discusses dental health.

Esophagus. Gastrointestinal muscle strength and motility decrease with a resultant decrease in peristalsis. The esophagus increases the number of muscle movements but does not effectively propel its contents. Decreased peristalic action and the relaxation of the lower esophageal sphincter slow the emptying of the esophagus. Improperly masticated food antagonizes this situation and in part is responsibile for the forceful, emphatic, propulsive contractions that propel the food on its way to further digestion. The sluggish emp-

tying of the esophagus also forces the lower end to dilate, sustaining greater stress in this area and causing digestive discomfort to the aged referred to as *presbyesophagus*. Hiatal hernias also occur in approximatly 60% of those over age 70.

Stomach. The number of parietal and chief cells that produce hydrochloric acid (HCl) and pepsin secretions decreases with the subsequent fall of HCl and pepsin production. The reduction of HCl in the stomach occurs at about age 60. Even with this decline, protein digestion, pancreatic action, and intestinal function seem to compensate for the apparent deficit. The pepsin level begins to fall in about the fourth decade and continues a sharp decline to the sixth decade. At this time the pepsin level evens out and remains at a constant low.

The protective alkaline viscus mucus of the stomach is lost due to the increase in stomach pH. This makes the aged more susceptible to gastric irritation. Loss of smooth muscle in the stomach delays emptying time and also exposes the epithelial lining to extended contact with gastric contents.

Liver, Gallbladder, Pancreas. The glandular secretions of the digestive system come from the liver, gallbladder, and pancreas. The liver is a sturdy organ and continues to function throughout life even with a decrease in volume and weight (mass) of approximately 17% to 28% in those over 65 years of age (Schenker, 1995; Bay,1995). The decrease in mass brings with it a concomitant decrease in liver blood flow of 35%. Protein synthesis and the rate of degradation result in the accumulation of abnormal protein with a corresponding inability to break down protein. Liver regeneration is slow but not greatly impaired. Liver function tests remain unaltered with age.

Bile manufactured by the liver to emulsify fat is stored in the gallbladder. There does not seem to be a specific change in the gallbladder, but the aged 70 years of age and older account for one third of gallbladder surgeries (Tompkins, 1995; Welch, 1995). This is possibly due to the increased lipogenic composition of bile from biliary cholesterol. The decrease in bile salt synthesis increases the incidence of cholilithiasis and cholycystitis (Altman, 1990; Cassmeyer and Blevin, 1993).

The pancreas becomes more fibrotic and shows evidence of ductal hyperplasia, but these changes do not necessarily lead to physiologic dysfunction. There is a decline in pancreatic secretions and enzyme output after the age of 40. This affects fat digestion and may be the reason for increased intolerance of fatty foods with age.

Small Intestine. There is a decrease in smooth muscle, Peyer's patches, and lymphatic follicles of the small intestine. Motility, epithelial membranes, vascular perfusion, and gastrointestinal membrane transport may affect absorption of lipids, amino acids, glucose, calcium, and iron. Calcium use is affected by lack of adequate gastric acid and slow active transport in the body. The tendency toward vitamin and mineral deficiency is caused partly by the faulty absorption of vitamins B_1 and B_{12}, calcium, and iron, and inadequate dietary intake of the aged. Vitamins K, B_1, and B_{12} and minerals such as iron and calcium are the most frequently deficient. Protein consumption is lower than in early life as a result of the cost of dentures or difficulty chewing and digesting meat. For some aged it would be judicious to take a daily vitamin to ensure at least a minimum ingestion and availability of the necessary vitamins and minerals. It might be prudent for the nurse to assist the aged person to learn about inexpensive sources of nutrients and to suggest that better absorption and digestion might be promoted by eating small snack-size meals throughout the day rather than the typical three meals per day. Chapter 6 discusses in depth nutrition for the aged.

Large Intestine. Changes in the large intestine are difficult to determine. There is structural atrophy of the layers and glands and a decrease in mucous secretions. The internal sphincter of the large intestine loses its muscle tone and can create problems in bowel evacuation. The external sphincter, which retains much of its original tone, cannot by itself control the bowels. Slower transmission of neural impulses lessen the awareness of sensations of a forthcoming bowel evacuation. The outcome of this may be either fecal incontinence or constipation. Weakness of the intestinal walls may also lead to outpouching of small segments of the colon (diverticula), which may or may not be symptomatic. The implication for the nurse is to evaluate the elimination pattern of the aged person, which may help avoid embarrassment and provide a positive frame of mind for the aged person. Elimination need is presented in Chapters 6 and 8.

Nervous System Changes

Brain. Nerve cell loss is minimal in the brainstem but more profound in the hippocampus. Brain weight decreases by approximately 10% between the second and ninth decades. The cerebral ventricles enlarge three to four times from the third to the ninth decades.

Lipofuscin, an aging pigment, is deposited in nerve cells, and amyloid deposition occurs in the blood vessels and cells. Senile plaque and, less frequently, neurofibrillary tangles are also found. The latter are usually associated with Alzheimer's disease but they also appear in the brain of elders without evidence of dementia (Joynt, 1995).

Neurotransmitters. Changes in neurotransmitter systems of dopaminergic and cholinergic systems occur with levels of choline acetylase, serotonin, and catecholamines decreasing. Other enzymes such as monoamine oxidase (MAO) increase. Redundancy of brain cells may forstall some changes, but the exact number of cells required for certain functions is not clear.

Nerve Cells. The brain has the ability to compensate for areas of injury or destruction, with compensation more effective in the higher centers. The spinal cord has less ability to do so. Peripheral nerves remain relatively unchanged and will regenerate slowly; however, conduction time of the peripheral nerves decreases in the aged.

As nerve cells gradually deteriorate and die, there is a compensatory lengthening of and an increase in the number of dendrites of the remaining nerve cells. The new connections in the dendrite tree may make up for the lower number of cells. This phenomenon is a normal age change, even though this may be seen to occur with Alzheimer's also.

External factors affect the positive and negative age-related changes. Medical or psychologic stress may result in the elder exhibiting confusion, delirium, or depression. Sleep medication may also affect the elder by creating a confused or delirious state.

Mental Performance. Intellectual performance of the elder without brain dysfunction remains constant into and beyond the 80s; however, the performance of tasks may take longer, an indication that central processing is slowed. Verbal skills continue well into the 70s and beyond. Other subtle changes occur in mentation, such as difficulty learning languages and benign senile forgetfulness. Mental health and cognition are discussed in Chapters 21 and 22.

Sensory Changes

Taste Perception. A number of sensory changes occur with age due to the intrinsic aging process in sensory organs and their association with the nervous system. Other changes are extrinsic and linked to the environment (see Appendix 4-A). One does not totally escape diminution of taste, smell, sight, sound, and touch. Taste buds atrophy, lose efficiency in relaying flavor, and decline in number. The threshold necessary to relay flavors rises for the four primary taste qualities: sweet, salty, bitter, and sour.

Crude taste (sweet and sour) is mediated by the taste buds; fine taste is olfactory mediated. Both taste and smell receptors are replaced. Taste bud receptor cells are in the papillae of the tongue and have a short life span of days. Loss of taste buds begins in the sixth decade and gradually progresses due to neural degeneration (Wilson, 1995). In crude taste there is a decrease in the number of nerve endings, papillae, and taste buds. This is, however, more pronounced when there are protein, estrogen, and protein deficiencies (Wilson, 1995). Smoking may also accelerate the loss.

For many years it was thought that taste declines, but studies have provided strong evidence that this is not so (Bartashuk and Weiffenbach, 1990). Studies support a rise in taste threshold, more for sodium chloride than for sucrose though the threshold of both rises. Changes may be due to dental problems, medications, or illnesses that create background taste and weaken stimuli.

Fine taste mediated by olfactory apparatus is associated with cognition and linguistics. A decrease in this aspect of taste may be due to loss of interest in food and maintaining a proper diet in addition to excess in sugar and salt. Taste changes in the healthy aged are modest and not considered to be significant. The quality of taste may vary, but taste remains robust in the aged.

Smell Perception. Changes in smell are attributed to loss of cells in the olfactory bulb of the brain and a decrease in the number of sensory cells in the nasal lining. In addition, long-term exposure to tobacco smoke and other toxic agents interferes with adequate olfactory function. Age takes the greatest toll on smell perception. There is strong evidence that smell perception declines. Studies find that women were better than men at determining 10 odorants. Nonsmokers also are able to smell better than smokers. Smell deteriorates in about half of the aged in their sixth decade and affects those age 80 and older (Hooper, 1994; Eliopoulos, 1997). In 1986 *National Geographic* magazine surveyed 1.5 million readers of all ages with a scratch test sent out in the monthly magazine. There findings showed that the loss of smell did not occur until one reached 70 but that the intensity and ability to identify specific odors declined earlier. This leaves the question, however, whether this was in relation to the odorants used in the test or all odors.

Pain Perception. At times caregivers have been amazed by the aged person's lack of response to pain. Conditions that are normally painful occur with an absence of pain or create only minor discomfort or a sense of pressure. Life-threatening myocardial and abdominal infarctions are often experienced this way. Another condition that has been missed because of the lack of expected pain response is appendicitis (Anderson, 1976; Rossman, 1986). This does not mean that elders do not experience postoperative pain. The diminution of normal pain signals creates some potentially dangerous situations for the aged and their state of wellness. Persons with limited activity, confined to a wheelchair or to bed, may not feel the pressure on bony prominences or the body messages to change position. Transmission of hot and cold impulses may be delayed just long enough for the aged individual to sustain significant tissue damage to some part of the body. Contact with such items as heating pads, hot water bags, radiators, and iced items can result in serious consequences and lengthy hospitalization for the aged. Issues related to pain and thermal perception are not yet definitive (Timaris, 1988).

Somasthetic and Tactile Perception. Somasthetics, or tactile sensitivity, decreases with age because of skin changes and the loss of a large number of nerve endings. This is particularly striking in the fingertips, palms of the hands, and lower extremities (Whanger and Wang, 1974; Kenshalo, 1979; Verillo, 1980).

Kinesthetic Sense. The kinesthetic sense or proprioception (one's position in space) is altered with age because of the changes in the central nervous system and muscles. Elders have more difficulty orienting their body in space when externally induced changes in body position are made. Slowed movements and altered position in space can lead to considerable difficulty with balance and spatial orientation.

The aged cannot avoid obstacles as quickly in ordinary situations such as those that occur on a crowded street, nor are the aged as able as they once were to prevent an accident from happening to themselves or to others when fast movement might be essential. The automatic response to protect and brace oneself when falling is slower, and one can observe the aged making more precise and deliberate movements, such as placement of the feet when walking. Conditions such as arthritis, stroke, some cardiac disorders, or damage to the structures of the inner ear may affect peripheral and central mechanisms of mobility. Further discussion of sensory alterations appears in Chapter 12.

Eye and Vision Changes

Decline in visual acuity is a progressive change that occurs in the optic compartment (cornea, lens, pupil, aqueous and vitreous humor, retina) of the eye. All persons will eventually experience some decline in visual capacity with age.

Extraocular. *Eyelids* droop (senile ptosis) as a result of the loss of elasticity, and skin atrophy can interfere with vision if the lids sag far enough over the lower lid margin. Decrease in the orbicular muscle strength of the eyes may result in ectropion or entropion. Ectropion may cause the lower lid not to close completely with sleep and lead to corneal dryness. Spasms of the orbicular muscle may cause the eyelashes, particularly of the lower lid, to turn inward, irritating the eyeball with each blink (Kupfer, 1995).

The *conjunctiva* is the thin membrane over the sclera with goblet cells that provide mucin, essential for eye lubrication and movement. Mucin slows the evaporation of tear film. The number of goblet cells decreases resulting in a deficiency of lubrication for the eye. Lack of tear secretions or nonspecific causes contribute to dry eye syndrome (Kupfer, 1995).

Ocular. The *cornea,* which is responsible for refraction of light, is among the first eye structures to be affected by aging. A flatter, less smooth, and thicker cornea is noticeable by its lackluster appearance or loss of sparkling transparency and leaves the aged individual more susceptible to astigmatism. A gray-white ring or partial ring, known as *arcus senilis,* forms 1 mm to 2 mm inside the limbus. It does not affect vision and is composed of deposits of calcium and cholesterol salts. This nonsignificant finding has at times been linked to systemic hyperlipidemia. Almost everyone over the age of 65 will exhibit some degress of arcus senilis, which gives credence to an age correlation of this specific change.

There is some degeneration of endothelial cells lining the inner suface of the cornea. Major changes that become progressive can lead to failure to keep the cornea free of extracellular fluid, causing corneal edema. This is a situation that requires immediate treatment by a physician.

Two sets of *iris* muscles regulate pupil size, affecting the amount of light that reaches the retina and limiting the efficiency of pupillary constriction and dilation. *Pupil* size is smaller in older adults, creating the problem of being dazzled in bright light by sluggish constriction. Slowness to dilate to the dark creates moments when elders cannot see where they are going. Because of the slow ability of the pupils to accommodate to changes in light, *glare* is a major problem for the aged. Glare is a problem created not only by sunlight outdoors, but also by the reflection of light on any shiny object and especially light striking polished or linoleum floors.

The inability of the eyes to accommodate to close and detailed work (presbyopia) begins in the fourth decade and continues throughout the rest of one's life. *Presbyopia* occurs earlier in individuals who live in warm climates and later in individuals who are nearsighted (myopic). Suspensory ligaments, ciliary muscles, and parasympathetic nerves contribute to the decreased accommodation that occurs.

Pupil diameter is also decreased along with the speed at which direct and consentual responses happen. If the pupil response is sluggish or absent, it may be that medication to dilate or constrict the pupils is being taken. Older people require three times as much light to see things as they did when they were in their 20s. There is a need for more light for all visual perception. It is more effective to place high-intensity light on the object or surface that is involved than to increase the intensity of the light in the entire area or room. For example, it would be more effective to focus a light directly on the newspaper a person was reading than to try and increase the light in the whole room.

The extent of the visual field begins to wane, affecting the breadth of vision that is possible. No longer can the aged view things panoramically, but rather the fringes are not as discrete and may be missed (Kupfer, 1995). The decreased ability to respond to rapid eye movement in front of the eyes presents problems for the aged. Rapid blinking or flickering lights or motion cannot be adequately accommodated as in youth.

The anterior chamber of the eye decreases due to the thickness of the lens. The iris becomes paler in color due to pigment loss and increases in the density of collagen fibers. Resorption of the intraocular fluid becomes less efficient with age and may lead to eventual breakdown in the absorption process. This creates the potential for the pathologic condition known as glaucoma.

The constant compression of *lens* fibers with age, the yellowing effect, and the efficiency of the aqueous humor, which provides the lens with nutrition, all have a role in altered lens transparency. Lens cells continue to grow but at a slower rate than previously. The cells on the periphery of the lens regenerate very slowly, while those toward the center are more active. Nearly everyone between ages 40 and 45 begins to discover the need for assistive lenses for reading and accommodation. Those who are nearsighted (myopic) tend to experience reading and accommodation difficulties later in their 50s and 60s.

Lens opacity or cataracts begin to develop around the fifth decade of life. The origins are not fully understood, although ultraviolet rays of the sun contribute with cross-linkage of collagen creating a more rigid and thickened lens structure.

Intraocular. The *vitreous humor,* which gives the eye globe its shape and support, loses some of its water and fibrous skeletal support with age. Opacities other than cataracts can be lines, webs, spots, or clusters of dots moving rapidly across the visual field with each movement of the eye. These opacities, known as *floaters,* are bits of coalesced vitreous that have broken off from the peripheral or central part of the retina. Mostly they are harmless and annoying until they dissipate or one gets used to them. If, however, the person says that he or she sees a shower of these and a flash of light, this requires immediate medical attention, as it might indicate retinal problems (Kupfer, 1995).

The *retina* has less distinct margins and is duller in appearance than in younger adults. Fidelity of color is less accurate with blues, violets, and greens of the spectrum; light colors such as reds, oranges, and yellows are more easily seen. Color clarity diminishes by 25% in the sixth decade and by 59% in the eighth decade. Some of this difficulty is linked to the yellowing of the lens and impaired transmission of light through the retina. The macula may not have as bright fovea reflective light either. Drusen (yellow-white) spots may appear in the macula area. As long as these changes are not accompanied by distortion of objects or a decrease in vision, some pigment deposition is not clinically significant.

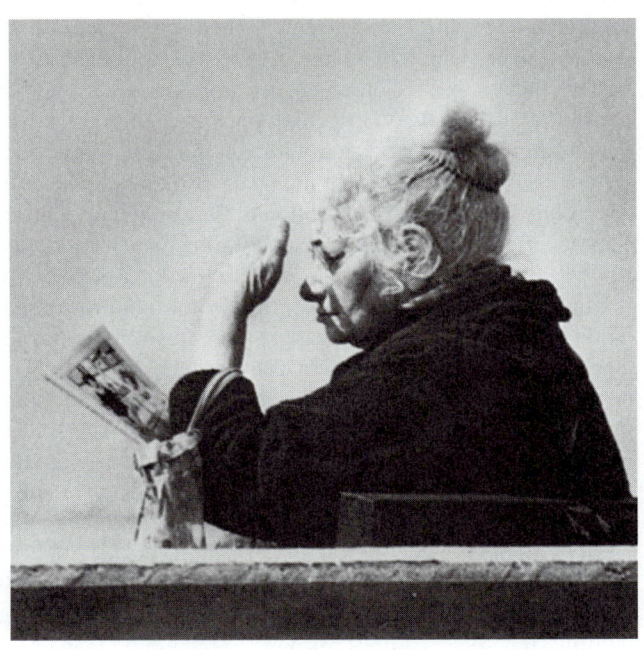

Glare.

Arteries may show atherosclerosis and slight narrowing. Veins may show indentations (nicking) at the arteriovenous crossings.

The lubrication and cleansing action of the lacrimal secretions diminish. Eyes take on a dull appearance, and there is a sensation of dryness, scratchiness, or tightness. Depending on the severity of discomfort of this situation, artificial tears are an available lubricant.

Auditory Changes

External Ear. The *auricle, or pinna,* loses flexibility and becomes longer and wider due to diminished elasticity. The *lobule* sags, elongates, and develops wrinkles. Together these changes make the ear appear larger. The periphery of the auricle develops coarse, wiry, stiff hair in men. The *tragus* also becomes larger in men.

The *auditory canal* narrows, causing inward collapsing. Stiffer and coarser hair lines the ear canal. Cerumen glands atrophy, causing thicker and dryer cerumen, which is more difficult to remove and a substantial cause for hearing impairment.

Middle Ear. The *tympanic membrane* becomes dull, less flexible, retracted, and gray in appearance. The *ossicle* joints between the malleus and stapes develop calcification, causing joint fixation or reduced vibration of these bones and reducing transmitted sound.

Inner Ear. There is a decrease in vestibular sensitivity due to degeneration of the organ of Corti in the cochlea and otic nerve loss. Changes in the efficiency of the cochlea and hair cells of the *organ of Corti* are responsible for the impaired transmission of sound waves along the nerve pathways of the brain and are considered to be the most common cause of presbycusis. Atrophy of the organ of Corti begins in middle age and causes sensory hearing loss. Loss of cochlear neurons occurs in late life, even with the preservation of the organ of Corti, is a neural hearing loss, and is considered to be related to genetic factors. Familial tendencies in middle life associated with electrophysiologic function of the organ of Corti are the basis of metabolic hearing loss (Gulya, 1995). Altered motion of the *cochlear* ducts occurs in middle age and is considered cochlear conductive hearing loss. The role of *basilar membrane* stiffening as a possible cause of this type of hearing loss is not proven. All of these types of loss are presbycusis. Many elders have a combination of causes for their hearing deficit.

Constant or recurring high-pitched *tinnitus* (clicking, buzzing, roaring, ringing, or other sounds in the ear) is usually caused by impairment of the *otic nerve* accompanying the aging process, although it may be caused by medications, infection, cerumen accumulation, or a blow to the head (Gulya, 1995). Tinnitus may be unilateral or bilateral and becomes most acute at night or in quiet surroundings. It is a nuisance that is difficult to combat or treat. The most helpful strategy is to use "masking" techniques that introduce another competing sound. "White noise" (soft static

between FM radio stations) on low volume can be soothing (Harvard Medical School Health Letter, 1983).

The auditory changes occur subtly. Normal decrements in hearing acuity, speech intelligibility, level of auditory threshold, and discrimination of pitch, especially in the speech frequencies, is referred to as presbycusis. *Presbycusis,* "hearing loss of aging," describes the type of loss, not the cause of the loss, and can be classified according to the structural source of impairment (Table 4-2). It is a bilateral and symmetric sensorineural hearing loss associated with age. Excessive wax accumulation in the ear canal will also intensify presbycusis. Men seem to experience more severe presbycusis than women of the same age. High frequency is not interfered with in understandable speech; however, it does begin to affect high-frequency sibilant consonant discrimination, with "z," "s," "sh," "f," "p," "k," "t," and "g" being the most difficult in conversation. Vowels that have a low pitch are more easily heard. Without consonants, the high-frequency-pitched language becomes disjointed and misunderstood. Consider the simple sentence "How are you today?" To the individual with presbycusis it might sound like "hOw arE yOU tOdAy?" The older adult might complain of having difficulty understanding women and children, conversations in large groups, or when there is background noise as in restaurants. Loud music or an intercom or paging system such as those used in hospitals or airports mask conversation with noise. Use of rapid speech when conversing with an older adult will make words sound garbled and unintelligible. Even though this latter problem is related to presbycusis, it is one that can be easily remedied.

Environmental noise, genetic disease, ototoxic agents, and a circulatory deficit to the vital structures of the inner ear are additional factors that contribute to and influence the extent of hearing loss.

Some sort of hearing loss affects about one third of all adults between age 65 and 74 and about one half of those age 75 to 79. More than 10 million elders have hearing impairments (Gulya, 1995). The ability to hear is a major avenue of communication. Hearing loss not only is frustrating to the aged individual, but also is threatening to security and self-esteem. The nurse and others frequently respond with impatience and anger to the aged person's inability to hear clearly, a response that only compounds the hearing problem. Unless there is an injury or a genetic defect, individuals can hear well in the absence of the problems that arise from noise, rapid speech, or varied voice modulation.

Immunologic Changes

"Immune senescense," the lapse of time between exposure and rechallange of pathogens, decreases as does the strength of response with advanced age (Miller, 1990; Hirsh, 1995; Yehuda, 1995). Immunologic responses are mediated by nonspecific, cell-mediated (T cell) and humoral (B cell) immunity.

Nonspecific Immunity provides the first cell interaction with an invading microbe or pathogen, creating the environment for helper T cells to recognize the antigen on the sur-face of invading cells. The T-cell suppressors recognize anti-gens in the nucleated cells (Miller, 1990; Hirsh, 1995; Yehuda, 1995). A chemical, cytokines, is secreted (inter-lukin-2 [IL-2] which helps proliferate T cells and stimulate humoral B-cell growth and antibody production) (Peterson et al, 1995).

Cell-mediated Immunity. Cell-mediated activities in-volve the thymus and T-cell function. The thymus is the or-gan where T-cell maturation and differentiation occur. Be-ginning about age 30, there is a loss of gland mass that continues until age 50. At this time there is approximately 5% to 10% thymus gland function. Whether there is com-plete involution of the thymus at age 60 remains unclear (Peterson et al, 1995).

T cells remain relatively unchanged with age except in the substrate, where helper cells CD4+ increase and CD8+ suppressor cells decrease in number. The thymus loses the ability to differentiate T-cell precursors and T-cell related B-cell differentiation. The result is 25% of healthy adults show evidence of a marked decline in cell-mediated immu-nity, 50% show a moderate decline, and 25% have no de-cline in immunity (Hirsh, 1995; Yehuda,1995).

The loss of functional capacity of the cell-mediated system is demonstrated by a decreased hypersensitivity response to such common skin tests as the tuberculin test. The implications are that the aged are more suscep-tible to reactivation of latent herpes zoster and mycobac-terium. Opportunistic infections such as those associated with *pneumocystis* or *Aspergillus,* which are seen in severely immunosuppressed individuals, are not generally seen in the aged.

Humoral Immunity. Humoral change is reflected in the impairment in T cells. Serum immunoglobulins change little with age, but the distribution changes with increases in IgA and IgG and decreases in IgM and IgD. The decrease in antibody response suggests that to achieve a maximum antibody response a larger dose of antigen is necessary. The effect, however, lasts a shorter period of time due to the decreased IgG production from altered function of cyto-kines stimulation, a response that still is unclear (Miller, 1990).

The decrease in self-tolerance, autoantibodies, to foreign antigens show the dysregulation of the immune system. The decrease in T-cell related B-cell differentiation and B-cell receptors are blocked by specific antigens that cap or patch the receptors, preventing their normal function (Peterson et al, 1995).

In summary, old age brings a decrease in T-cell function due to a decrease in cell-mediated immunity, humoral im-munity, and self-tolerance. The response to foreign antigens decreases, but immunoglobulins increase, creating an au-toimmune response not associated with autoimmune dis-eases, which usually occur before middle age (Miller, 1990). (See Figure 2-4 for a diagram of immunologic changes.)

Biochemical and Genetic Changes

Much interest has been directed at the molecular structure and function of the aging human organism. Investigations designed to reveal the biochemical changes that underlie ag-ing are often directed toward substances that will suppress the phenomenon of aging. Evidence of this emerges from the biologic theories of aging discussed in Chapter 2.

Chromatin, which is involved in the transfer of genetic information, is central in the elaboration of protein and en-zymes and thus has become the focus of interest. Changes in chromatin reflect DNA and associated translation mecha-nisms in aging. Life-span variations among different species of animals and the uncertainty of life span in humans are ex-amples of issues considered in the biochemical and genetic arena. A detailed discussion of longevity and life span oc-curs in Chapter 2.

In summary, many changes that occur with aging have been discussed here and will be elaborated further in subse-quent chapters. Age changes are universal, progressive, decremental, and intrinsic. In addition, it can be concluded that complex functions of the body decline more than sim-ple body processes; that coordinated activity, which relies on interacting systems such as nerves, muscles, and glands, has a greater decremental loss than single-system activity; and that a uniform and predictable loss of cell function oc-curs in all vital organs.

Most aged individuals are able to function within the physical dictates of their body and continue to live to a healthy old age. Aged persons are capable of wisdom, judg-ment, and adding information to already accumulated facts and information.

Table 4-2   Types and Causes of Presbycusis

Types	Description	Cause
Sensory	A sharp hearing loss at high frequencies with little effect on speech understanding	Degeneration of hair cells and atrophy of the organ of Corti
Neural	Hearing loss reduces speech discrimination	Widespread degenera-tion of cochlea nerve fibers and spiral ganglia
Metabolic or strial	Hearing loss that initially reduces sensitivity to all sound frequencies; it later interferes with speech discrimination	Degeneration of the stria vascularis and interruption in essential nutrients
Mechanical	Hearing loss that gradually increases from low to high frequencies and affects speech discrimination when high frequency hearing loss occurs	Mechanical changes in the inner ear

HEALTH ASSESSMENT

Health assessment has been referred to as health appraisal, physical examination, and health screening. Regardless of the nomenclature, it is a process of collecting and analyzing data. This approach is the initial step in the nursing process. Assessment provides information critical to the development of a plan of action that can enhance personal health status, decrease the potential for or the severity of chronic conditions, and assist the individual to gain control over health through self-care.

A comprehensive geriatric assessment requires not only physical data, but also an integration of the biologic, psychosocial, and functional aspects of the aged person. Inquiries into physiologic and anatomic function, growth and development, family relationships, group involvement, and religious and occupational pursuits are essential in a health assessment interview. Questions regarding genetic background, although important, have less significance for the aged because genetic consequences usually appear in earlier phases of life. One cannot entirely eliminate concern for genetic inheritance since latent changes do occur and affect physical and mental well-being.

As part of the health assessment it is most important to include an appraisal of BADLs, the IADLS, also referred to as functional assessment, and advanced activities of daily living, which refer to occupational, recreational, and leisure time activities. These activities are based on choice, not necessity, as are those of the BADLs and IADLs. A functional assessment consists of the fundamental tasks and demands of daily life. The items generally agreed on as constituting a functional assessment are divided into BADLs (those abilities that are fundamental to independent living, such as bathing, dressing, toileting, transferring from bed or chair, feeding, and continence) and IADLs, which include more complex daily activities, such as using the telephone, preparing meals, and managing money (Katz and Barthel in-

dexes; see Appendix 4-B). An evaluation of mental ability is essential. Questions directed at mental intactness are often incorporated into assessment of BADLs and IADLs. Specific tools will be addressed later in this chapter. Psychologic status can be appraised by utilizing such questions as appear in Box 4-2. The physical examination process will not be presented here. Many books provide the essential discussion of examination tools, techniques, and methods.

Health assessment data enable development and implementation of primary, secondary, and tertiary care regimens. Primary care is aimed at prevention of disease and promotion and maintenance of health. Care is directed toward limiting health risks and avoidance of sequelae from common health problems, uncomplicated illness, chronic illness, or mental states induced by a stressful environment, and the individual is usually able to receive the benefits of such care either at home or on an outpatient basis. Secondary care involves specific illness or pathologic conditions and focuses its efforts on the retardation or termination of physical, mental, social, or environmental situations that have induced the condition or situation. Care is provided in a health care setting by professionals who have specific knowledge and skill in the area of concern. Tertiary care deals with restorative measures that will enable the aged individual to achieve an optimum level of function, whatever that might be. Appropriate care requires professionals with specialized knowledge and skill in either an institutional health care setting or in the home or outpatient environment.

Aged persons do not usually seek assistance from health professionals until there is obvious physical or emotional difficulty. Some aged individuals have had adverse experiences with the health care system; others assume that their problems are age related and do not realize that relief and assistance are possible.

The initiation of the health history marks the beginning of the nurse-client relationship and ushers the aged person

---

Box 4-2	Questions to Elicit Information Significant to Health Status*

1. What is the first health problem you can remember? What happened and how was it taken care of? (traumatic expectations)
2. When you were young what did you think about old people? What did you expect to be like when you were old? (ageist attitudes)
3. How old do you feel now? (health status, grief, depression)
4. What was your most gratifying experience? (expression, elaboration, imagination exhibited in description)
5. How did your mother describe you as a child? How did your father describe you as a child? (incorporation, self-evaluation, self-fulfilling prophecies)
6. How would you describe yourself as a child? (identity, self-concept)
7. What is the most important thing that you have done? (values)
8. What is the most difficult thing that you have done? (strength, integrity, endurance, courage)
9. How did you manage to do that? (coping style and patterns)
10. What would you change if you could? (life satisfaction, integrity, acceptance)

*These are only a few thoughts that can be modified or expanded on in any particular situation.

into the health care system. The interview that follows requires skill in establishing client trust and confidence and in avoiding offending the individual. A considerable amount of time is required to complete a health assessment of the aged client, often because of the lack of schooling, the use of English as a second language, or the result of impaired communication skills from previous illness. It is difficult for the interviewer to proceed slowly, one question at a time, and wait for the slow response as a result of perceptive and receptive changes that occur in the nervous system of the aged. The client may find giving certain types of health information stressful and may even decline to discuss changes or problems that might confirm fears of illness, limitations, or old age. Any illness is seen as a threat to independence and viewed as leading to eventual institutionalization (Farquhar, 1992). Sometimes an initial health questionnaire can be completed by the client (if vision and intellectual ability are not problems) before coming to a practitioner's office or while waiting to see the practitioner. The client often feels freer to respond to the printed question, it reduces time needed, and it provides a background from which the interview can develop. In addition, if the aged client can do the questionnaire at home, it often provides time to remember or find the information about his or her health that is requested. The health care giver can clarify questionnaire answers, and the client can elaborate with details.

Many of our present assessment tools do not provide for the attainment of accurate data with the rapidly changing ethnic mix of elders. Assessment must utilize ways to elicit health care beliefs from the ethnogeriatric groups. Cultural/ethnic sensitivity of the care provider is important in order to disentangle cultural normative behavior from behavior that mimics pathology. The tools are very limited that can facilitate this type of assessment data. Pfeifferling and Kleinman both have developed tools that assist a care giver in gleaning pertinent assessment information to provide appropriate health promotion, prevention, maintenance, and interventions. (See Chapter 24 for the health inquiry tool.)

Box 4-3	**Indications for Home Visits**

Lives alone (especially if recently bereaved)
Mental impairment
Major mobility problems
Several risk factors for dependency
History of falls or accidents
Recent hospital discharge (especially if recovery incomplete)
Imminent institutionalization

From Ham RJ: *Geriatrics: I. AAFP home study of self-assessment monograph 89,* Kansas City, MO, American Academy of Family Physicians, 1986.

Assessment of the aged requires special abilities of the nurse: ability to listen patiently, to allow for pauses, to ask questions that are not often asked, to observe the minute details, to obtain data from all available sources, and to recognize normalities of late life that would be abnormal in one who is younger. The quality and speed of the assessment are an art born of experience. The novice nurse should not be expected to do this. According to Benner (1984), it is a task for the expert. Preferably, all initial assessments when an aged individual enters the health care system through any of the doors would be conducted by the most knowledgeable and experienced person available. When this is not possible, it would be useful to have a checklist format that would alert even the novice to pressing concerns.

Any health history form or interview should include a patient profile and social history, a history of current problems, a review of symptoms and systems, a medication history (prescribed and over-the-counter), caregiver stress, family history, ability in activities of daily living, and community services currently provided. Additional data should consider psychologic parameters such as cognitive and emotional well-being, the individual's self-perception, and social parameters such as economic resources and concerns, pattern of health and health care, education, family structure, plans for retirement, and living environment. Areas or problems not frequently addressed by the care provider or mentioned by the aged are sexual dysfunction, depression, incontinence, musculoskeletal stiffness, alcoholism, hearing loss, and dementia (Ham, 1992). Much of this information is obtained orally, but it can also be evaluated by observation of personal grooming, facial expression, responsiveness to the interview, and physical examination. Information about involvement with the surrounding community and group participation should reveal additional information about the emotional state and feelings of self-worth of the aged client. The essentials of a comprehensive geriatric assessment must include functional, physical, social, and mental assessment of the aged and the caregiver (if used) and assessment of the environment in order to plan care and prevent problems.

Home visit assessment complements or provides information that is difficult to gauge in a clinic, physician's office, or other formal settings. Especially difficult to ascertain are such areas as nutrition, alcoholism, actual level of function on a daily basis, and suitability and safety of the environment. Even when the individual is relatively independent, an appreciation for the difficulty encountered in food preparation, use of the bathroom, showering, and heating and cooling the house can be acquired (Boxes 4-3 and 4-4).

The nurse must be cognizant of inherent obstacles and benefits of the health assessment, particularly the potential for developing a stereotyped view of the aged and perceiving the elderly as objects rather than persons. This is especially true when assessment is viewed in terms of potentially meeting the nurse's need for data instead of meeting the needs of the aged person and as a task rather than the basis of care.

<table>
<tr><td>

Box 4-4   **Necessary Home Visit Information**

1. Suitability and safety of home for client's functional level
2. Attitudes and presence of other persons at home
3. Proximity and helpfulness of neighbors and relatives
4. Emergency assistance arrangements
5. Nutritional and alcohol habits
6. Actual and required daily living skills
7. Hygiene habits
8. Safety and convenience modification needed
9. Problems in getting to local community stores and services

</td></tr>
</table>

From Ham RJ: *Geriatrics: I. AAFP home study self-assessment monograph 89,* Kansas City, MO, American Academy of Family Physicians, 1986.

ASSESSMENT TOOLS

An abundance of assessment tools exist that can broadly catagorize motor capacity, manual ability, self-care ability, and more complex or instrumental abilities. Some community agencies and nursing care facilities routinely use health assessment tools designed to obtain specific information needed. Other institutions have developed or modified available tools because the available assessment tools are too complex and too time consuming to be of practical value. Regardless of the method used (established or self-developed), most health forms contain variants of the same basic information (see Appendix 4-B).

Physical Assessment

One assessment tool uses a survival-needs framework with an emphasis on function. The acronym FANCAPES represents fluids, aeration, nutrition, communication, activity, pain, elimination, and socialization and social skills. The information provided is helpful in the appraisal of the aged person's ability to meet his/her needs and the extent to which assistance is necessary (Figure 4-2). FANCAPES is applicable to all types of care environments in which the aged are found, may be used in part or total (depending on the need), and is easily adaptable to the functional pattern grouping of nursing diagnosis. Assessment data obtained from this method are based on the following considerations in each area.

Fluids. Evaluation of fluids requires the functional assessment of the client's state of hydration and those physiologic, situational, and mental factors that contribute to the maintenance of adequate hydration. Attention is directed to the ability of the client to obtain adequate fluids on his or her own, to express feelings of thirst, to effectively swallow, and to evaluate medications that affect intake and output.

Aeration. In considering aeration, one looks at the adequacy of oxygen exchange. Observations include respiratory

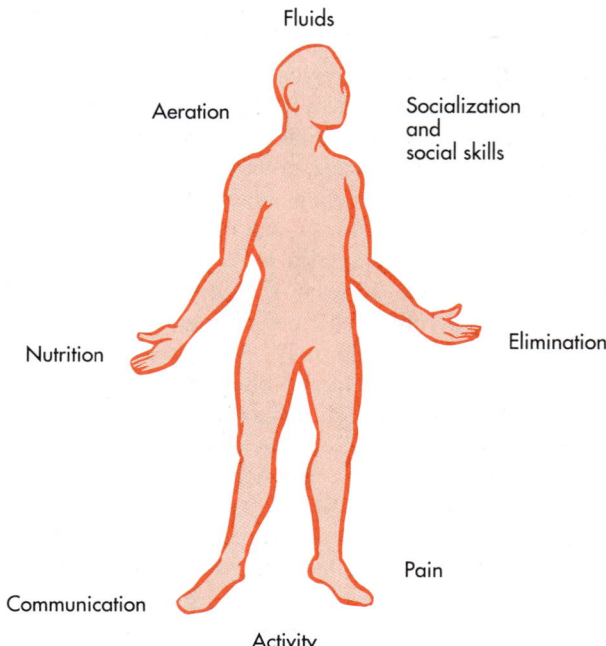

Figure 4-2. Functional assessment of the elderly. Some commonalities are (1) lower levels, needs, tasks, or stages must be met, resolved, or mastered before progression to the next stage; and (2) each stage, part, or need is related to all the others to which the individual responds in a "holistic" way. The initial problem, stress, or stimulus evokes involvement of the total organism.

rate and depth at rest and during activity; talking, walking, and situations requiring added exertion; and the presence or absence of edema in the extremities or abdomen. Breath sounds should be auscultated and medication reviewed to evaluate the effects on aeration.

Nutrition. Nutrition involves mechanical and psychologic factors in addition to the type and amount of food consumed. It is necessary to ascertain the client's ability to bite, chew, and swallow. Edentulous clients may have dentures that fit improperly and are not worn. Alteration in diet because of culture, medical restrictions, available economic resources, and living conditions should be considered. Visual and neurologic impairment, which might interfere with the client's ability to prepare a meal or feed himself or herself, should be noted.

Communication. The sending and receiving of verbal and nonverbal information in the external world and signals in the internal environment of the body require mechanical function of body parts and psychosocial responses from others in the environment. Assessment includes sight and sound acuity, voice quality, and adequate function of the tongue, teeth, pharynx, and larynx. Appraisal of the client's ability to read, write, and understand the spoken language should be ascertained. This is an important issue, since an undetected disability in these skills can lead to erroneous conclusions.

Activity. Activity includes aspects other than exercise. Activities of daily living are an estimate of the individual's ability to maintain self-care and independent living. The nurse looks at the ability to feed, toilet, dress, and groom oneself; to prepare meals; to dial the telephone; and to move around with or without assistive devices. Coordination and balance, finger dexterity, grip strength, and other actions necessary to daily life should also be assessed. Ambulation should be considered a major component in activity. The timed "get up and go," which has the person rise from a chair, walk 10 feet, return to the chair and sit down, correlates with functional dysfunction (Podsiadlo and Richardson, 1991).

Pain. Pain, both physical and mental, is important to consider. The presence and absence of pressure and discomfort are also aspects of pain assessment. Information about recent losses or visible symptoms of anxiety may help determine manifestations of pain. The manner by which a client customarily attains relief from pain or discomfort will provide further sources of information.

Elimination. Bladder and bowel elimination should be investigated for mechanical factors such as evidence of dribbling or incontinence, for use of assistive devices or altered body structures resulting from surgical intervention, and for medications that affect voiding and intestinal peristalsis.

Bowel function can be helped or hindered by what the client uses to purge himself or herself, by how concerned the client seems to be about bowel function, and by the amount of privacy needed for excretory functions. Colloquialisms used by the client must be recognized and used to accommodate obtaining assessment data.

Socialization and Social Skills. Socialization and social skills assess the individual's ability to negotiate in society, to give and receive love and friendship, and to feel self-worth (see Apgar in Chapter 17).

Responses to such influences as hearing and visual losses and approved gestures of friendship are considered under this category. Attention should focus on the individual's ability to deal with loss and to interact with other people in give-and-take situations. Behavioral responses not previously observed may become evident by discussion of the client's feelings of self-worth.

Functional Assessment

The goal of *Healthy People 2000* (1991) is to increase the life span of all Americans. Rather than delay mortality, focus has been directed at the preservation of function and extending active life expectancy. Functional assessment speaks to the "quality of life" in ways medical diagnoses do not (Gallo et al, 1995).

Functional assessment can be defined as the evaluation of a person's ability to carry out basic tasks for self-care and tasks needed to support independent living. It is based on physical, and psychosocial evaluation with the assumption that any clinical condition be diagnosed and properly treated

(Williams, 1995). Additional reasons why functional assessment is so important are that the objective data obtained in a functional assessment accomplish the following:

Define elder's concerns

May indicate a manifestation of disease

Assist in determining a need for service(s)

Assist in determining the type of placement

Assist in determining cost/benefit of treatment/intervention

Assist in realistic goal setting for those with chronic conditions

Decrease fragmentation of care by reviewing goals according to functional status

Assist in ethical/quality-of-life issues

Help track untreated conditions (that is, effects of arthritis)

As can be seen from the value of functional assessment, tools that assess ability in BADLs and IADLs should provide numerically qualified data regarding an individual's capacity to be or remain independent.

The BADLs (eating, toileting, ambulation, bathing, dressing, and grooming) are tasks needed for self-care and are international as well as cross-cultural in nature. Three of these tasks (grooming, dressing, and bathing) require cognitive function. When the BADLs are vertically listed, it is not unusual for the individual who performs an activity to be able to do the activities above it but not below it. Change in or loss of ability occurs in the reverse order of acquisition (Box 4-5).

The IADLs are tasks needed for independent living (Box 4-5). The progression of loss of IADLs begins with cognitive functions, especially finances and shopping. Cooking is least important to community-dwelling elders, even when adjusted for gender differences (Williams, 1995). When the IADLs are arranged in vertical order, performance by a person of one type of activity indicates the person can probably do all the activities below it but not above it (Gallo et al, 1995).

Numerous tools are available that describe, screen, assess, monitor, and predict functional ability. Generally the assessment does not break down a task into its component parts, such as picking up a spoon or cup or swallowing water when assessment of eating is done; instead, eating is seen as a total task. Functional assessment also shows the result, not the cause, of an altered task. This is particularly true with persons who have varying degrees of dementia (Tappan, 1994). The Katz Index (Katz et al, 1963; see Appendix 4-B) provides a basic framework to evaluate a person's ability to live independently and serves as a focal point to provide remedies. Scoring of the Katz Index is based on a 3-point scale and allows one to score client performance abilities as independent, assistive, or dependent. A modification of terms might be independent, semidependent, and dependent.

The value of the Katz Index is that it can be administered by anyone, with minimum training, and it can provide data that identify the abilities of an aged person and the kind

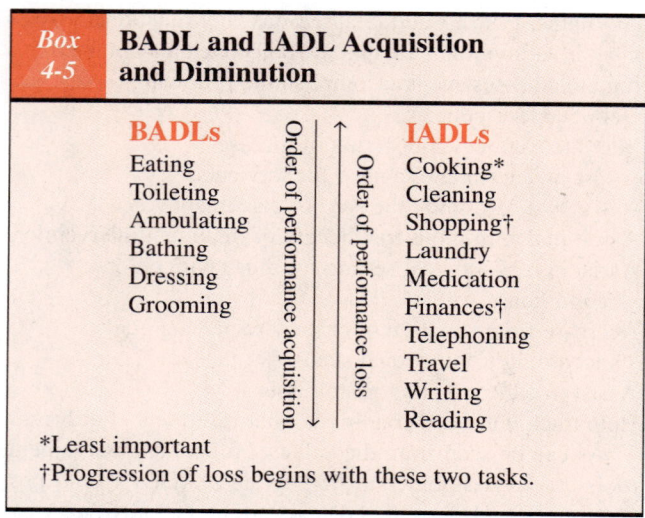

Box 4-5	BADL and IADL Acquisition and Diminution

BADLs
Eating
Toileting
Ambulating
Bathing
Dressing
Grooming

Order of performance acquisition → *Order of performance loss*

IADLs
Cooking*
Cleaning
Shopping†
Laundry
Medication
Finances†
Telephoning
Travel
Writing
Reading

*Least important
†Progression of loss begins with these two tasks.

Modified from Williams M: Contemporary Forums Gerontological Nursing Conference, San Francisco, May 11-13, 1995.

of services that might be needed. The physical self-maintenance scale (PSMS) developed by the Philadelphia Geriatric Institute includes the six functional areas of BADLs and can also be administered without prior training by any health care person.

Another tool used to assess self-care of the elderly is the Barthel Index (1981). This instrument was devised to evaluate the amount of physical assistance required when a person can no longer carry out BADLs. Because it is so detailed, a modified Barthel Index was developed that has proved useful in any setting. It is particularly useful in the home care setting. The index is divided into two categories: independent and dependent. Under each of these headings activities are rated as independent (intact and limited ability) or dependent (requiring a helper or unable to do an activity or activities at all) (see Appendix 4-B).

The Barthel Index provides data to determine the type of support that is needed in BADLs and can serve in rehabilitation settings as a method of documenting improvement of a patient's ability. The ADLs, considered to be more complex activities than the BADLs, assess such abilities as traveling, shopping, preparing meals, doing housework, dialing a telephone, and handling money. Although these tasks may seem more specific to women, the activities are required of most individuals in modern society today (see Appendix 4-B).

Mental Assessment

Many times questionnaires that evaluate mental capacity are combined with BADL and IADL instruments. One such tool is the Functional Dementia Scale (Moore et al, 1983), which can be administered in a written or oral form. This brief assessment tool provides quantification of the presence of dementia and changes in the review of physiologic systems. Whether this tool provides data, over time, of diminished capacity is not evident (Gallo et al, 1995).

The Folstein Mini-Mental State Examination is a short, convenient mental function test composed of two parts: one requires verbal response and assesses orientation, memory, and attention, and the other component requires the ability to write a sentence, draw a complex design, respond to written and oral commands, and name objects. As with other assessment tools, there is a rating scale to quantify ability or disability. Further discussion appears in Chapter 22.

A frequently used mental status examination is the Short Portable Mental Status Questionnaire (SPMSQ) (Pfeiffer, 1979). Its effectiveness as a method for clarifying cognitive function is still undetermined. The questionnaire asks 10 questions that assess the person's orientation, remote memory, and calculation ability; however, there is no task to evaluate short-term memory. Its value as an assessment tool is the ease of administration and the fact that it requires no equipment (Gallo et al, 1995).

Integrated Assessments

The Multidimensional Functional Assessment of the Older American's Resources and Services (OARS) organization is a lengthy and comprehensive tool designed to evaluate ability, disability, and the capacity level at which the aged person is able to function. Five dimensions are considered for assessment: social resources, economic resources, physical health, mental health, and activities of daily living. Each component uses a quantitative rating scale: 1—excellent, 2—good, 3—mildly impaired, 4—moderately impaired, 5—severely impaired, and 6—completely impaired. At the conclusion of the assessment a cumulative impairment score (CIS) is established, which can range from the most fit (6) to total disability (30). This aids in establishing the degree of need. Information considered in each domain includes the following.

Social Resources. The social resources dimension evaluates the social skills and the degree of ability to negotiate and make friends (the number of times friends are seen, the number of telephone conversations). In the assessment interview is the aged person able to ask for things from friends, family, and strangers? Is there a caregiver around in case of need? Who is it, and how long is the person available? Does the individual belong to any social network or group such as a special interest or church group?

Economic Resources. Data about monthly income and sources (Social Security, Supplemental Security Income, pensions, and income generated from capital) are needed to determine the adequacy of income compared to the cost of living and food, shelter, clothing, medications, and small luxury items. This information can provide insight into the client's relative standard of living and point out areas of need that might be alleviated by use of additional resources unknown to the aged person.

Mental Health. Consideration is given to intellectual function, the presence or absence of psychiatric symptoms, and the amount of enjoyment and interaction the aged person gets from life.

Physical Health. Diagnosis of major and common diseases of older persons, the type of prescribed and over-the-counter medications the person is taking, and the aged person's perception of his or her health status are the basis of evaluation. Excellent physical health includes participation in regular vigorous activity such as walking, dancing, or biking at least twice per week. Seriously impaired physical health is the presence of one or more illnesses or disabilities that may be severely painful, be life threatening, or require intensive care.

Activities of Daily Living. The ADLs are divided into two parts for assessment: (1) care of the body, which involves such activities as walking, getting in and out of bed, bathing, combing hair, shaving, dressing, eating, and getting to the bathroom on time by oneself, and (2) IADLs such as dialing the telephone, driving a car, hanging up clothes, obtaining groceries, taking medication, and having correct knowledge of the dosage.

The OARS assessment tool is designed so that each component could be used individually. This enables it to be added to or integrated into self-designed tools. Other comprehensive assessment instruments include PACE (Patient Appraisal and Care Evaluation) and CARE (Comprehensive Assessment and Referral Evaluation) (Kane and Kane, 1981). These methods of appraisal are also very lengthy.

Recording of Data

Problem-oriented medical recording (POMR) is also known as Weed's Problem-Oriented System (Weed, 1971). It was designed primarily by a physician for use by physicians, but it has been adapted to the needs of nurses who care for geriatric clients. The database can be broadened to encompass a multidimensional assessment of a client. The components of the problem-oriented system are database, problem list, initial plan, and progress notes, which assume the SOAP format (subjective data, objective data, assessment or nursing diagnosis, and plan).

The database is usually derived from patient complaints. To obtain an initial database from well elders, however, the nurse should consider obtaining information from the physical, psychologic, social, and economic realms. A database can be obtained through various assessment tools presented in this chapter or from those designed by the agency with which the nurse is affiliated. When there is no tool available, the nurse will need to create one geared to assessment of functional ability or disability in the physical, mental, social, economic, and ADL spheres of the aged person's life.

Once data are collected, one can generate a problem list and a potential problem list that reflects more than the physical arena and will serve as a reference in future encounters with the elder. The initial plan includes diagnosis (if appropriate), treatment (if appropriate), and education, as well as progress notes that emanate from the problem list.

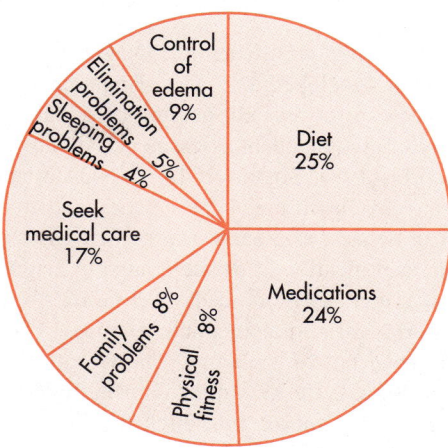

Figure 4-3. Frequency of health counseling topics. (From Furukawa C. In Wells T, editor: *Aging and health promotion,* Rockville, Md, 1981, Aspen.)

The assessment formats in this chapter attempt to provide direction in the development of one's own assessment tool or modification of existing tools that may not fully evaluate the needs of the aged client being assessed. Feeling comfortable with an assessment method requires practice using the tool and refining it so that it will be appropriate to the aged person and the particular setting of the nurse.

Findings and conclusions from the assessment should be discussed with the aged client so that responsibility for the health program can be appropriately delegated. This connotes that the client is an active participant in health care and is encouraged to apply wellness concepts presented in Chapter 3. Given sufficient information, the aged client should be capable of making decisions about his or her health status and needed resources. One must keep in mind that the goal is preventive health care that is aimed at maintenance of the present health status and maximizing function.

Furukawa (1982) found certain recurrent topics requested by the elderly in health counseling sessions (Figure 4-3). If examination findings indicate the client is able to monitor his or her own physical health condition, the client should be taught to do so. Taking one's own blood pressure, cooperation with medications, and conscientious adherence to an exercise program or a nutritional regimen are all examples of self-responsibility and the beginning of wellness, rather than disease, orientation.

Health assessment is appraisal of health status in an attempt to identify latent and obscure conditions, to serve as a screening process, to serve as a follow-up on health care plans, and to serve as the initial establishment of a health baseline. The aim is to help the aged person remain independent and functional at the highest level of wellness regardless of place of residence: in acute or long-term institutional settings or in one's own home.

NURSING DIAGNOSIS AND THE AGED

The North American Nursing Diagnosis Association (NANDA) has developed a system of nursing diagnoses by which nurses can formulate a nursing care plan and initiate interventions based on client assessment (Nursing diagnoses, 1994). Gordon (1987) organized the NANDA diagnostic categories into 11 functional health patterns that are easily learned, can be used as a basis of a holistic assessment, and lead to the identification of possible nursing diagnoses.

Maslow's hierarchy of needs and Gordon's functional health patterns are complementary when used with the elderly who have health problems. The Gordon format provides the nurse with the nursing diagnosis, and Maslow's hierarchy provides a means by which the diagnoses can be prioritized (Figure 4-4).

Many older adults have at least one chronic condition that is amenable to NANDA diagnoses. The present diagnoses, however, are oriented to dysfunction rather than to both functional and dysfunctional health. Although the elderly will usually have some degree of dysfunction, the NANDA guidelines create the mind-set that the aged are always dysfunctional and do not recognize that the aged can be quite functional but still need to be monitored to prevent illness and disease, maintain their present state of wellness, and improve on an existing state of wellness.

Nursing diagnoses for older adults should include wellness, to reflect individual responses that are healthy as well as those that are actually or potentially unhealthy. Interventions must reinforce those that are healthy. A pioneer group of nurses over the last decade has tenaciously advocated for nursing wellness diagnoses because they describe human responses to levels of wellness in an individual that have the potential for enhancement to a higher state despite the presence or absence of a chronic condition or an acute illness. Stolte (1994) believes well nursing diagnoses should focus on wellness patterns, client responses, and strengths that can be accomplished by focusing on progressive attainment of health behaviors or developmental tasks. Houldin et al (1987) produced a manual of wellness diagnoses using functional health patterns.

Stolte (1996) offers a strong argument for the inclusion of wellness nursing diagnoses in all types of health settings. These settings apply not only to elders but all ages. By utilizing wellness nursing diagnoses in addition to NANDA diagnoses, the approach becomes holistic, not dysfunction oriented, and provides the opportunity to draw on strengths and coping abilities inherent in the individual.

Some individuals may argue that these wellness diagnoses are more prescriptive than behavioral, but wellness focuses on prevention, maintenance, and improvement of behavior or physical status from a state of wellness or health. The task of nurses then is to consider wellness diagnoses along with the established dysfunctional diagnoses to generate categories that apply to the practice of gerontic nursing. *This is not to imply that gerontic nursing is elitist and must have separate categories, but it is intended to point out that the aged cannot be measured by the norms of health that are attributed to those who are young and middle aged.* Pathologic states in these age groups are not always pathologic states for the elderly.

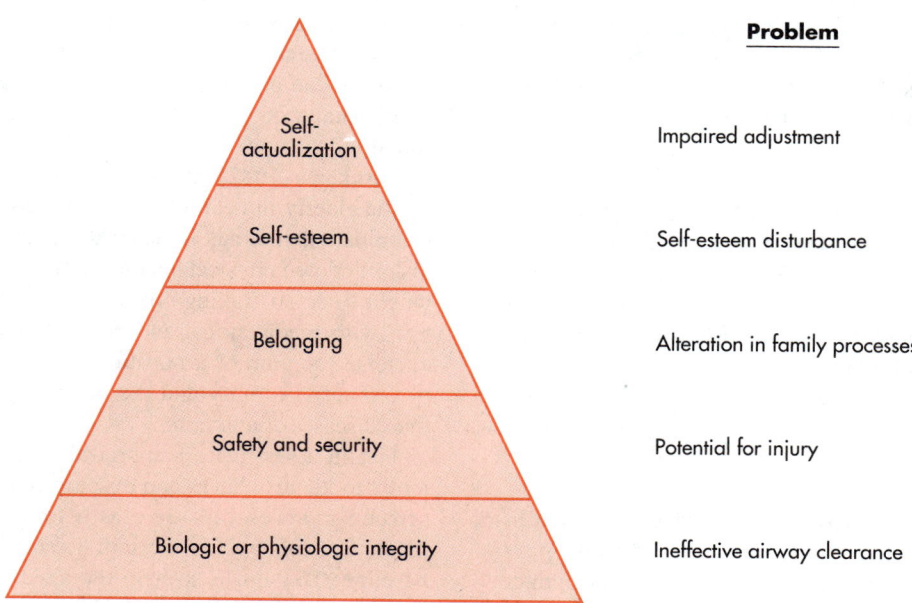

Problem

Self-actualization — Impaired adjustment

Self-esteem — Self-esteem disturbance

Belonging — Alteration in family processes

Safety and security — Potential for injury

Biologic or physiologic integrity — Ineffective airway clearance

Figure 4-4. Correlation between Maslow's hierarchy and Gordon's functional pattern of nursing diagnosis.

When it is considered that a person does not have a "problem," a health-oriented focus could provide encouragement to successfully move through the normal developmental and maturational tasks.

The formulation of wellness nursing diagnoses should reflect positive behaviors (based on the client's strengths), using such action responses as adapting to, reestablishing, adjustment to, assumes responsibility for, participation in, developing a pattern, involvement in, increasing recognition of, improving, and maintaining, which indicate progression and allow the nurse to use interventions that reinforce client response and achieve goals. Goals should facilitate task achievement, provide information, teach or reinforce new skills, foster role attainment, or enhance strengths. Appropriate qualifiers for goals include terms such as attainment, continued, increased, sustained, completion, and acceptance, to mention a few.

For example, an aged individual may be at the optimum level of mobility and activity based on normal cardiac output and respiratory exchange for the person's physiologic age. The wellness diagnosis might be adapting to the present mobility level (if optimal level is now different than before) with the goal of sustaining the present level of mobility and activity. Nursing interventions then are aimed at accomplishing this goal. If the person's responses/strengths are not used to help meet the goal, it is likely that an alteration in mobility and activity may become a diagnosis of dysfunction.

KEY CONCEPTS

- Age-related changes are the observable, measurable, or felt changes that occur in one's being over time and are chiefly focused on physiologic and biologic changes.
- Physiologic aging is universal, progressive, decremental, intrinsic, and unavoidable.
- There are enormous individual variations in the rate of aging of body systems and functions.
- Individuals normally gradually lose bone mass, structural integrity of organs, and specificity of bodily processes in the course of aging.
- Physical appearance inevitably changes with a downward shift of skin and tissues integrity brought about by the pressure of gravity over time.
- Lubrication of joints, elasticity, enzymatic processes, and cellular fluids diminish during aging.

- The changes in the cardiovascular system are most likely to progress toward a disease state in late life.
- Hormonal and endocrine changes are significant in the aging process.
- Nervous system and sensory acuity are diminished in aging and are often compensated by accoutrements or aids.
- Careful assessment of individual aging changes, lifestyle, and desires are fundamental to good nursing care of the old.

▲ CASE STUDY

Fred was 74 years old and had an active and vital life. He was involved in leather tooling and restoration of classic automobiles. He had developed a cadre of acquaintances, worldwide, of similar interests. His retirement from a life-long U.S. Air Force commitment was painful, but he had his hobbies and his friends to sustain him. He would chuckle a little when he often said, "Those years in the war were the best years of my life . . . everything since then has been pale by comparison."

Fred is similar to many of the men who were born in the years between 1920 and 1930. When they arrived at their near majority, there were the "war years;" the male youth of the nation took arms. The females, so often left behind, waited and watched for the return of the heroes. The artificial nature of life at that juncture has resulted in a range of problems that are "unique to that generation." Separating the age-related problems from the generational and environmental ones can be very difficult.

The first difficult problem of growing older that Fred noticed was the diminishment of hearing, especially in situations that were loud and with multiple sources of noise. His nurse friend told him it was likely related to his years in the war when the unnatural noises of shelling had affected his hearing. Then he gradually became aware that his eyesight was impaired so that he could focus only on distant objects but near objects were fuzzy. But the biggest problem he experienced was in his inability to write notes to his acquaintances with the same fluidity he had previously experienced. Sometimes the words were lurking on the tip of his tongue but simply would not come. Another thing that troubled him was the decreasing strength of his grip. Recently it had become more difficult to repair automobiles because of this

Needs Addressed and Task Strengths

Need to adapt to normal changes associated with aging; need for activity; need to feel self-worth (to maintain safety, security, and self-esteem)	Adaptability
	Numerous interests
	Sense of humor
Ability to learn from experience	Assumes active role in health maintenance

decreasing strength. He did not know whether these were normal age-related changes that he must adjust to or whether they were indications of serious pathologic problems that required active medical intervention.

Based upon the case study, develop a nursing care plan using the following procedure*:

List comments of client that provide *subjective data.*

List information that provides *objective data.*

From these data identify and state, using accepted format, two *nursing diagnoses* you determine are most significant to this client at this time. List two *client strengths* that you have identified from data.

Determine and state *outcome criteria* for each diagnosis. These must reflect some alleviation of the problem identified in the nursing diagnosis and must be stated in concrete and measurable terms.

Plan and state one or more *interventions* for each diagnosed problem. Provide specific documentation of source used to determine appropriate intervention. Plan at least one intervention that incorporates the client's existing strengths.

Evaluate success of intervention. Interventions must correlate directly with the stated outcome criteria in order to measure the outcome success.

STUDY QUESTIONS

Which of the changes Fred experienced are the normal concomitants of aging?

Which of Fred's disabilities do you think has created the most distress in his life?

What problem would you address first if Fred asked for your assistance?

What wellness nursing diagnosis(es) could you develop for Fred?

How would you assist Fred to adapt to the changes of aging that he cannot avoid?

What resources would you suggest to Fred to enhance his coping?

Discuss the aging changes you would find most difficult to accept.

RESEARCH QUESTIONS

It is most difficult for elders to cope with which age changes?

Which are the inevitable sensory changes of aging?

Where do individuals seek knowledge of the aging process?

Is chronologic age more significant than physiologic age in determining functional efficacy?

---

*Students are advised to refer to their nursing diagnosis text and identify possible or potential problems.

When does one become aware of changes in function that are related to aging? Which change is likely to appear first? How much influence does environment have on reduced hearing capacity?

How do age-related changes differ in males and females?

RESOURCES

Films and Videos

Resident Assessment Inventory. Presented by Suzanne Doyle Friedman, MS, RN, Program Coordinator for the Geriatric Mental Health Designated Bed Project, consultant in psychiatric-mental health nursing and gerontological nursing. (*Lecture, 23 minutes; Purchase, $300; Rental, $100.*)

To accurately collect data on residents in long-term care, staff must develop skills in describing and defining behaviors. This video program discusses behaviors and conditions that staff need to observe, describe, and document and shows how to develop the necessary skills in this area. The program focuses on developing observational expertise in physical, cognitive, and psychosocial areas. Specific areas addressed include functional status, communication patterns, mood and behavior, nutritional needs, activity participation, and sensory status. Staff working with long-term care residents need training to observe, describe, and document behaviors and conditions in order to provide data that will ensure quality care. *Functional Assessment in the Elderly.* Presented by Jennifer M. Bottomley, MS, PT, Clinical Supervisor, PT Department, Cushing Hospital, Framingham, Mass; Adjunct Faculty for MGH Institute of Health Professions; and Associate, Division on Aging, Harvard Medical School. (19 minutes; Purchase, $200; Rental, $100.)

As an introduction to this program, the medical model and clinical goal for rehabilitation in the elderly is presented. This is followed by a functional assessment of an elderly male with Alzheimer's disease, arthritis, and diabetes. The functional assessment presented is referred to by Jennifer Bottomley as a "quick and dirty" assessment tool, appropriate for use in a clinical or home setting. It is appropriate for use by all members of the health care team.

The patient is asked to do three things—take his shoes and socks off and put them back on again, walk across the room and return to his chair, and feed himself. Observations during these activities include arthritic changes, conditions of the skin and toenail bed, flexibility, strength, endurance, balance, weight shift, presence of contractures, mobility, oral motor functioning, eye-hand coordination, visual acuity, ability to sequence and follow instructions, and cognitive capability.

This tape is of particular importance for training health professionals who will be developing patient care plans for elderly patients with physical limitations, to include the hospital discharge planning team and long-term care staff.

From Video Press, University of Maryland at Baltimore, School of Medicine, Suite 133, 100 Penn Street, Baltimore, MD 21201, (800)328-7450 or (410)328-5497, FAX: (410)328-8471.

REFERENCES

Altman DF: Changes in gastrointestinal, pancreatic, biliary, and hepatic function with aging, *Gastroenterol Clin North Am* 19(2):227, 1990.

Anderson WF: *Practical management of the elderly,* ed 3, Oxford, 1976, Blackwell Scientific Publications.

Baltimore Longitudinal Study of Aging, National Institutes of Health No. 84-2450, Washington, DC, 1984, US Government Printing Office.

Banaski JL: Cardiac function. In Copstead LEC, editor: *Perspectives on pathophysiology,* Philadelphia, 1995, WB Saunders.

Bartashuk LM, Weiffenbach JM: Chemical senses and aging. In Schneider EL, Rowe JW, editors: *Handbook of the biology of aging,* ed 3, San Diego, 1990, Academic Press, Inc.

Barthel Index, *Med Care* 19:491, 1981.

Bartlett JG: Pneumonia and tuberculosis. In *The Merck manual of geriatrics,* ed 2, Whitehouse Station, NJ, 1995, Merck Research Laboratories.

Bartz B: Mechanisms of endocrine control and metabolism. In Copstead LEC: *Perspectives on pathophysiology*, Philadelphia, 1995, WB Saunders Co.

Bay MK: The aging liver. In Abrams WB, Beers MH, Berkow R, editors: *The Merck manual of geriatrics,* ed 2, Whitehouse Station, NJ, 1995, Merck Research Laboratories.

Beare P, Meyers J: *Principles and practices of adult health nursing,* ed 2, St Louis, 1994, Mosby.

Benner P: *From novice to expert,* Menlo Park, Calif, 1984, Addison-Wesley.

Bentley DW: Management of infection in the elderly. In Cape DT, Coe RM, Rossman I, editors: *Fundamentals of geriatric medicine,* New York, 1983, Raven Press.

Campbell EJ, Lefrak SS: How aging affects the structure and function of the respiratory system, *Geriatrics* 33:68, 1978.

Cassmeyer VL, Blevin DB: The patient with biliary and pancreatic problems. In Long BC, Phillips WJ, Cassmeyer VL, editors: *Medical-surgical nursing: a nursing process approach,* ed 3, St Louis, 1993, Mosby.

Coni N, Davison W, Webster S: *Aging: the facts,* New York, 1984, Oxford University Press.

Cooper LT, Cooke JP, Dzau VJ: The vasculopathy of aging, *J Gerontol: Biological Science* 49(5):B191, 1994.

Cornell RC: Aging and the skin: what is normal aging, *Geriatric Med Today,* Part XX, 5:24, 1986.

Costa PT, Andres R: Patterns of age changes. In Rossman I, editor: *Clinical geriatrics,* ed 3, Philadelphia, 1986, JB Lippincott.

Cunningham WR, Brookbank JW: *Gerontology: the psychology, biology, and sociology of aging,* New York, 1988, Harper & Row.

Diettert G: Circulation time in the aged., *JAMA* 183:1037, 1963.

Eliopoulos C: *Gerontological nursing,* ed 4, Philadelphia, 1997, JB Lippincott.

Farquhar JW: *Healthy aging,* Conference, San Francisco, Oct 1-4, 1992.

Fifth Report of the Joint National Committee on Detection, Evaluation, and Treatment of High Blood Pressure, *Arch Inter Med* 153(2):154, 1993.

Frohlich EV: Hypertension. In Abrams WB, Beers MH, Berkow R, editors: *The Merck manual of geriatrics,* ed 2, Whitehouse Station, NJ, 1995, Merck Research Laboratories.

Fujino M, Okada R, Arakawa K: The relationship of aging to histologic changes in the conduction system of the normal heart, *Jpn Heart J* 24:13, 1982.

Furukawa C: Adult health conference: community-oriented health maintenance for the elderly. In Wells T, editor: *Aging and health promotion,* Rockville, Md, 1982, Aspen Systems Corp.

Gallo JJ, Reichel W, Andersen L: *Handbook of geriatric assessment,* ed 2, Rockville, Md, 1995, Aspen Publishers.

Gardin JM, Henry WL, Savage DD et al: Echocardiographic measurements in normal subjects: evaluation of an adult population without apparent heart disease, *J Clin Ultrasound* 7:85, 1979.

Gardner AW, Poehlman ET: Predictors of the age-related increase in blood pressure in men and women, *J Gerontol: Medical Science* 50A (1):M1, 1995.

Gawlinski A, Jensen GA: The complications of cardiovascular aging, *Am J Nurs* 9:221, 1991.

Gerstenblith G, Fredericksen J, Yin FCP et al: Echocardiographic assessment of a normal adult population, *Circulation* 56(2):273, 1977.

Goldman R: Decline in organic function with age. In Rossman I, editor: *Clinical geriatrics,* ed 2, Philadelphia, 1979, JB Lippincott.

Gordon M: *Manual of nursing diagnosis 1986-1987,* New York, 1987, McGraw-Hill.

Grove GL, Kingman AM: Age associated changes in human epidermal cell renewal, *J Gerontol* 38:137, 1983.

Gugoz Y, Munro HN: Nutrition and aging. In Finch CE, Schneider EL, editors: *Handbook of the biology of aging,* ed 2, New York, 1985, Van Nostrand Reinhold Co.

Gulya AJ: Ear disorders. In Abrams WB, Beers MH, Berkow R, editors: *The Merck manual of geriatrics,* ed 2, Whitehouse Station, NJ, 1995, Merck Research Laboratories.

Ham RJ: Assessment. In Ham RJ, Sloane PD: *Primary care geriatrics: a case-based approach,* ed 2, St Louis, 1992, Mosby.

Harvard Medical School Health Letter, Department of Continuing Education, Harvard Medical School 9:5, 1983.

Healthy People 2000: US Department of Health and Human Services, Public Health Service, Washington DC, 1991, US Government Printing Office.

Hirsh B: Normal changes in host defenses: In Abrams WB, Beers MH, Berkow R, editors: *The Merck manual of geriatrics,* ed 2, Whitehouse Station, NJ, 1995, Merck Research Laboratories.

Hogstel MO: Vital signs are really vital in the old-old, *Geriatr Nurs* 15(5):253, 1994.

Hooper CR: Sensory and sensory integrative development. In Border BR, Wagner MB: *Functional performance in older adults,* Philadelphia, 1994, FA Davis.

Houldin AD, Saltstein SW, Ganley KM: *Nursing diagnoses for wellness,* Philadelphia, 1987, JB Lippincott.

Jacobs R: Physical changes in the aged. In Deveraux MO et al, editors: *Elder care: a guide to clinical geriatrics,* New York, 1981, Grune & Stratton.

Johns Hopkins Medical Letter: Health after 50: Important new advice for treating hypertension, 8(2):7, 1996.

Johns Hopkins Medical Letter: Health after 50: The next five years: our experts look ahead, 6(1):1, 1994.

Joynt RJ: Normal aging and patterns of neurologic diseases. In Abrams WB, Beers MH, Berkow R, editors: *The Merck manual of geriatrics,* ed 2, Whitehouse Station, NJ, 1995, Merck Research Laboratories.

Kane RA, Kane RL: *Assessing the elderly: a practical guide to measurement,* Lexington, Mass, 1981, Lexington Books.

Katz S, Ford AB, Moskowitz RW et al: Studies of illness in the aged: the index of ADL, *JAMA* 185:914, 1963.

Kenney RA: *Physiology of aging: a synopsis,* Chicago, 1982, Mosby.

Kenshalo DR: Changes in vestibular and somesthetic systems as a function of age. In Ordey JM, Brizzee KR, editors: *Sensory systems and communication in the elderly,* New York, 1979, Raven Press.

Kinney RA: *Physiologic aging,* ed 2, Chicago, 1989, Mosby.

Krumpe P, Knudson R, Parson G, Reuser K: The aging respiratory system, *Clin Geriatr Med* 1 :143, 1985.

Kupfer C: Ophthalmologic disorders. In Abrams WB, Beers MH, Berkow R, editors: *The Merck manual of geriatrics,* ed 2, Whitehouse Station, NJ, 1995, Merck Research Laboratories.

Lakatta, E: Cardiovascular regulatory mechanisms in advanced age, *Physiol Rev* 73(2):413, 1993.

Lakatta EG: Normal changes in aging. In Abrams WB, Berkow R, editors: *The Merck manual of geriatrics,* Rahway, NJ, 1990, Merck, Sharpe, Dohme Research Laboratories.

Lakatta EG: Normal age changes. In Abrams WB, Beers MH, Berkow R, editors: *The Merck manual of geriatrics,* ed 2, Whitehouse Station, NJ, 1995, Merck Research Laboratories.

Lamb KV: Musculoskeletal function. In Leuckenotte AG, editor: *Gerontologic nursing,* St Louis, 1996, Mosby.

Leyden JJ, Grove GL, Ginley JK: Age-related differences in the rate of desquamation of skin surface in the aging process. In Adelman R, Roberts J, Christofalo VJ, editors: *Pharmacological interventions in the aging process,* New York, 1978, Plenum Press.

Lillington GA: *Diagnosis and arrangement of pulmonary problems in the elderly.* Presentation at Elder Care Workshop, The National Institute of Care of the Elderly, University of Nevada, Reno, October 1979.

Lindemann RD, Tobin JD, Shock NW: Longitudinal studies on the rate of decline in renal function with age, *J Am Geriatr Soc* 33(4):278, 1985.

Lindsay R: The aging skeleton. In Haug M, Ford A, Sheafor D, editors: *Physical and mental health of aged women,* New York, 1985, Springer.

MacLennan W, Peden N: *Metabolic and endocrine problems in the elderly,* New York, 1989, Springer-Verlag.

Malasanos L, Barkauskaus V, Stoltenberg-Allen K: Health assessment, ed 4, St Louis, 1989, Mosby.

Miller RA: Aging and the immune response. In Schneider EL, Rowe JW, editors: *Handbook of biology of aging,* ed 3, San Diego, 1990, Academic Press, Inc.

Moore J, Bobula JA, Short TB et al: A functional dementia scale for assessment, *J Fam Pract* 16:499, 1993.

Morgan S: Effects of age on cardiovascular functioning, *Geriatr Nurs* 14(5):249, 1993.

Nursing diagnoses: definitions and classifications 1995-1996: Philadelphia, 1994, North American Nursing Diagnosis Association.

Peterson FY, Symes J, and Springer P: Alterations in immune function. In Copstead LEC, editor: *Perspectives on pathophysiology,* Philadelphia, 1995, WB Saunders.

Pfeiffer E: *Physical and mental assessment—OARS.* Workshop Intensive, Western Gerontological Society, San Francisco, April 28, 1979.

Pierson DJ: Effects of aging on the respiratory system. In Pierson DJ, Kacmarek RM, editors: *Foundations of respiratory care,* New York, 1992, Churchill Livingstone.

Podsiadlo D, Richardson S: Timed "up & go": a test of basic functional mobility for frail elder persons, *J Amer Geriatr Soc* 39:142, 1991.

Richard C: Renal function. In Copstead LEC, editor: *Perspectives on pathophysiology,* Philadelphia, 1995, WB Saunders.

Richey ML, Richey HK, Fenske NA: Age-related skin changes: development and clinical meaning, *Geriatrics* 43:49, 1988.

Rossman I, editor: *Clinical geriatrics,* ed 2, Philadelphia, 1979, JB Lippincott.

Rossman I, editor: *Clinical geriatrics,* ed 3, Philadelphia, 1986, JB Lippincott.

Rowe JW: Aging process: renal changes and disorders. In Abrams WB, Beers MH, Berkow R, editors: *The Merck manual of geriatrics,* ed 2, Whitehouse Station, NJ, 1995, Merck Research Laboratories.

Saxon SV, Etten MJ: *Physical changes and aging,* New York, 1994, The Tiresias Press, Inc.

Schenker S: The aging liver. In Abrams WB, Beers MH, Berkow R, editors: *The Merck manual of geriatrics,* ed 2, Whitehouse Station, NJ, 1995, Merck Research Laboratories.

Schumann L: Alterations in respiratory function. In Copstead LEC, editor: *Perspectives on pathophysiology,* Philadelphia, 1995, WB Saunders.

Schuster MM: Effects of aging on the GI system. In Abrams WB, Beers MH, Berkow R, editors: *The Merck manual of geriartrics,* ed 2, Whitehouse Station, NJ, 1995, Merck Research Laboratories.

Sloane PD: Normal aging. In Ham RJ, Sloane PD, editors: *Primary care geriatrics: a case-based approach,* ed 2, St Louis, 1992, Mosby.

Solomon DH: Age-related endocrine and metabolic changes: normal and diseased thyroid gland. In Abrams WB, Beers MH, Berkow R, editors: *The Merck manual of geriatrics,* ed 2, Whitehouse Station, NJ, 1995, Merck Research Laboratories.

Special Report on Aging, US Department of Health and Human Services, Public Health Service, NIH Pub No 81-2328, Washington, DC, 1981, National Institute on Aging.

Stengel GB: Oral temperature in the elderly, *Gerontologist* 23:306 (Special Issue), 1983.

Stolte KM: (1994). Health-oriented nursing diagnoses: development and use. In Carroll-Johnson RM, Paquette M, editors: *Classification of nursing diagnoses: proceedings of the 10th conference North American Nursing Diagnosis Association,* Philadelphia, 1994, JB Lippincott.

Stolte KM: *Wellness nursing diagnosis for health promotion,* Philadelphia, 1996, JB Lippincott.

Tappan RM: Development of the refined ADL assessment scale for patients with Alzheimer's and related disorders, *J Gerontol Nurs* 20 (6):36, 1994.

Tichy AN, Malasanos LJ: Physiologic parameters of aging, *J Gerontol Nurs* 5:42, Jan/Feb 1979; 5:38, April/May 1979.

Timaris PS: *Physiologic basis of geriatrics,* New York, 1988, Macmillan.

Tockman MS: The effects of aging on the lungs: lung cancer. In Abrams WB, Beers MH, Berkow R, editors: *The Merck manual of geriatrics,* ed 2, Whitehouse Station, NJ, 1995, Merck Research Laboratories.

Tompkins RG: Surgery: preoperative evaluation and interoperative and postoperative care: surgery of the gastrointestinal tract. In Abrams WB, Beers MH, Berkow R, editors: *The Merck manual of geriatrics,* ed 2, Whitehouse Station, NJ, 1995, Merch Research Laboratories.

Verillo RT: Age-related changes in sensitivity and vibration, *J Gerontol* 35:185, 1980.

Wardell S: *Acute intervention: nursing process throughout the life span,* Reston, Va, 1979, Reston.

Weber F, Barnard RJ, Ray D: Effects of a high-complex carbohydrate low-fat diet and daily exercise on individuals 70 years of age and older, *J Gerontol* 38:155, 1983.

Weed L: *Medical records, medical education and patient care,* Cleveland, 1971, The Press of Case Western Reserve University.

Wei Jy: Cardiovascular system. In Rowe JW, Besdine RW, editors: *Geriatric medicine,* Boston, 1988, Little Brown.

Welch CE: Surgery: Preoperative evaluation and intraoperative and postoperative care: surgery of the gastrointestinal tract. In Abrams WB, Beers MH, Berkow R, editors: *The Merck manual of geriatrics,* ed 2, Whitehouse Station, NJ, 1995, Merck Research Laboratories.

Whanger AD, Wang HS: Clinical correlates of the vibratory sense in elderly psychiatric patients, *J Gerontol* 29:39, 1974.

Williams M: *Functional assessment,* gerontological nursing, Contemporary Forums, San Francisco, May 7-13, 1995.

Wilson WR: Nose and throat disorders. In Abrams WB, Beers MH, Berkow R, editors: *The Merck manual of geriatrics,* Whitehouse Station, NJ, 1995, Merck Research Laboratories.

Yehuda AB: Normal change in host defense. In Abrams WB, Beers MH, Berkow R, editors: *The Merck manual of geriatrics,* ed 2, Whitehouse Station, NJ, 1995, Merck Research Laboratories.

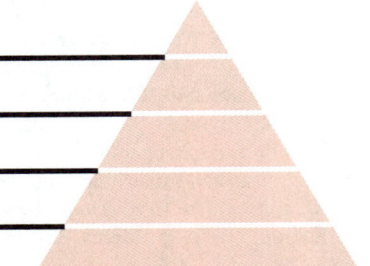

Normal Physical Assessment Findings in the Elderly

Cardiovascular Changes

Cardiac output	Heart loses elasticity; therefore decreased heart contractility in repsonse to increased demands
Arterial circulation	Decreased vessel compliance with increased peripheral resistance to blood flow resulting from general or localized arteriosclerosis
Venous circulation	Does not exhibit change with aging in the absence of disease
Blood pressure	Significant increase in the systolic, at or above 140mmHg suggestive of hypertension, slight increase in the diastolic, at or above 90mmHg suggestive of hypertension, increase in peripheral resistance and pulse pressure
Heart	Dislocation of the apex because of kyphoscoliosis; therefore diagnostic significance of location is lost
	Increased premature beats, rarely clinically important
Murmurs	Systolic murmurs in over half the aged; the most common heard at the base of the heart because of sclerotic changes of the aortic valves
Peripheral pulses	Easily palpated because of increased arterial wall narrowing and loss of connective tissue; feeling of tortuous and rigid vessels
	Possibility that pedal pulses may be weaker as a result of arteriosclerotic changes; colder lower extremities, especially at night; possibility of cold feet and hands with mottled color
Heart rate	No changes with age at normal rest

Respiratory Changes

Pulmonary blood flow and diffusion	Decreased blood flow to the pulmonary circulation; decreased diffusion
Anatomic structure	Increased anterior-posterior diameter
Respiratory accessory muscles	Degeneration and decreased strength; increased rigidity of chest wall
	Muscle atrophy of pharynx and larynx
Internal pulmonic structure	Decreased pulmonary elasticity creates senile emphysema
	Shorter breaths taken with decreased maximum breathing capacity, vital capacity, residual volume, and functional capacity
	Airway resistance increases; less ventilation at the bases of the lung and more at the apex

Data from Ham RJ, Sloane PD, editors: *Primary geriatrics,* ed 2, St Louis, 1992, Mosby; Copstead LEC: *Perspectives on pathophysiology,* Philadelphia, 1995, WB Saunders; Malasanos L et al: *Health assessment,* ed 3, St Louis, 1985, Mosby; and Wardell S, editor: *Acute interventions: nursing process throughout the life span,* Reston VA, 1979, Reston.

Integumentary Changes

Texture	Skin loses elasticity; wrinkles, folding, sagging, dryness
Color	Spotty pigmentation in areas exposed to sun; face paler, even in the absence of anemia
Temperature	Extremities cooler; decreased perspiration
Fat distribution	Less on extremities; more on trunk
Hair color	Dull gray, white, yellow, or yellow-green
Hair distribution	Thins on scalp, axilla, pubic area, upper and lower extremities; decreased facial hair in men, women may develop chin and upper lip hair
Nails	Decreased growth rate
	Healing delayed

Genitourinary and Reproductive Changes

Renal blood flow	Because of decreased cardiac output, reduced filtration rate and renal efficiency; possibility of subsequent loss of protein from kidneys
Micturition	In men possibility of increased frequency as a result of prostatic enlargement
	In women decreased perineal muscle tone; therefore urgency and stress incontinence
	Increased nocturia for both men and women
	Possibility that polyuria may be diabetes related
	Decreased volume of urine may relate to decrease in intake but evaluation needed
Incontinence	Increased occurrence with age, specifically in those with dementia
Male reproduction	
Testosterone production	Decreases; phases of intercourse slower, lengthened refractory time
Frequency of intercourse	No changes in libido and sexual satisfaction; decreased frequency to one or two times weekly
Testes	Decreased size; decreased sperm count; diminished viscosity of seminal fluid
Penis	Smaller; decreased penile sensation
Prostate	Atrophy with hyperplasia
Female reproduction	
Estrogen	Decreased production with menopause
Breasts and Nipples	Diminished breast tissue; decrease breast and nipple size
Uterus	Decreased size; mucous secretions cease; possibility that uterine prolapse may occur as a result of muscle weakness
Vagina	Epithelial lining atrophies; narrow and shortened canal
Vaginal secretions	Become more alkaline as glycogen content increases and acidity declines

Gastrointestinal Changes

Mastication	Impaired because of partial or total loss of teeth, malocclusive bite, and ill-fitting dentures
Swallowing and carbohydrate digestion	Swallowing more difficult as salivary secretions diminish
Esophagus	Decreased esophageal peristalsis (presbyesophagus)
	Increased incidence of hiatus hernia with accompanying gaseous distention
Digestive enzymes	Decreased production of hydrochloric acid, pepsin, and pancreatic enzymes
Fat absorption	Delayed, affecting the absorption rate of fat-soluble vitamins A, D, E, and K
Intestinal peristalsis	Reduced gastrointestinal motility
	Constipation because of decreased motility and roughage
Sphincters	Decrease in anal sphinctor tone

Musculoskeletal Changes

Muscle strength and function	Decrease with loss of muscle mass; bony prominences normal in aged, since muscle mass decreased; more decreased muscle strength in legs than arms; proximal more than distal
Bone structure	Normal demineralization, more porous; shortening of the trunk as a result of intervertebral space narrowing
Joints	Become less mobile; tightening and fixation occur
	Activity may maintain function longer
	Normal posture changes; some kyphosis
	Range of motion limited
Anatomic size and height	Total decrease in size as loss of body protein and body water occurs in proportion to decrease in basal metabolic rate
	Increased body fat; diminished in arms and legs, increased in trunk
	Decreased height from 2.5 to 10 cm from young adulthood

Nervous System Changes

Response to stimuli	All voluntary or automatic reflexes slower
	Decreased ability to respond to multiple stimuli
	Increased time needed to learn and cognition process
	Benign senile forgetfulness
Sleep patterns	Stage IV sleep reduced in comparison to younger adulthood; increased frequency of spontaneous awakening
	Stay in bed longer but get less sleep; insomnia a problem, which should be evaluated
Reflexes	Deep tendon reflexes responsive in the healthy aged, some have decreased or absent ankle jerk, knee, biceps, triceps
Ambulation	Kinesthetic sense less efficient; may demonstrate an extrapyramidal Parkinson-like gait
	Basal ganglions of the nervous system influenced by the vascular changes and decreased oxygen supply
Gait	Women waddle, narrow walking and standing base
	Men small-step, wide base walking and standing
Voice	Decreased range, duration, and intensity of voice; may become higher pitched and monotonous

Sensory Changes

Vision	
Peripheral vision	Decreases
Lens accommodation	Decreases, requires corrective lenses
Ciliary body	Atrophy in accommodation of lens focus
Iris	Development of arcus senilis
Choroid	Atrophy around disk
Lens	May develop opacity, cataract formation; more light necessary to see
Color	Fades or disappears
Macula	Degenerates
Conjunctiva	Thins and looks yellow
Tearing	Decreases; increased irritation and infection
Pupil	May differ in size
Cornea	Presence of arcus senilis
Retina	Observable vascular changes

Sensory Changes—cont'd

Stimuli threshold	Increased threshold for light touch and pain
	Ischemic paresthesias common in the extremities
Hearing	Less perceptible high-frequency tones; hence greatly impaired language understanding; promotes confusion and seems to create increased rigidity in thought processes
Gustatory	Decreased acuity as taste buds atrophy; may increase the amount of seasoning on food
Temperature	Threshold stimulus higher, temperature usually between 96° F to 97° F
	Decrease in thermal regulation heat/cold tolerance
Proprioception	Decreased sense of position and balance
Touch	Decreased sterognosis

Endocrine Changes

Thyroid	Decreased production or clearance of thyroid hormone
Aldosterone	Inactive to active renin
Insulin	Increased levels
Glucagon	Increased levels

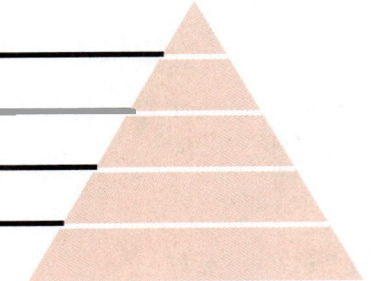

Physical and Functional Assessment Instruments

PREVENTIVE HEALTH HISTORY FORM

1. Name _____ ( ) 2. Sex M _____ F _____ ( )
   Address _____
3. Date _____/_____/_____ ( )
   Month Date Year
4. Age _____ ( ) 5. Place of birth _____ ( )
6. Current doctor:
   Name _____ Phone # _____
   Address _____ ( )
7. Who to contact in case of emergency:
   Name _____ Phone # _____ ( )
   Relationship _____ ( )
   Address _____ ( )
8. Religion _____ ( )
9. Marital status _____ ( )
10. Whom do you live with? Check all that are appropriate:
    Friend _____ Spouse _____ Children _____ Other _____
       ( )   ( )   ( )   ( )
11. How many children do you have? _____ ( )
12. If you have any children, do they live nearby? Yes _____ No _____ ( )
                                                         (1)   (0)
13. Is your mother alive? Yes _____ No _____ ( )
                             (1)   (0)
14. If not, cause of death _____ ( )
15. Is your father alive? Yes _____ No _____ ( )
                             (1)   (0)
16. If not, cause of death _____ ( )
17. Do you have any brothers or sisters? Yes _____ No _____ ( )
                                             (1)   (0)
18. If yes, do they live nearby? Yes _____ No _____ ( )
                                     (1)   (0)
19. If they are no longer alive, please give the causes of their death:
    _____ ( )

From Kopf R, Salamon MJ, Charytan P: The preventive health history form: a questionnaire for use with older patient populations, *J Gerontol Nurs* 8:521, 1982.

20. Have you had any formal education beyond high school? Yes _____ No _____ ( )
21. Your occupation/profession is (was) _____ ( )
22. Are you retired? Yes _____ No _____ ( )
    ₍₁₎   ₍₀₎
23. If not retired, are you working part-time? Yes _____ No _____
    ₍₁₎   ₍₀₎
24. How do you usually get around? _____ ( )
25. Your last medical checkup was _____ /_____ ( )
    Month   Year
26. Rate your general health:
    Excellent _____ Good _____ Poor _____ ( )
27. List any illnesses that seem to run in your family.
    _____

    _____ ( )

28. Have you ever been hospitalized? Yes _____ No _____ ( )
    ₍₁₎   ₍₀₎
    If yes, how many times? _____ ( )
    Give the dates and reasons for your hospitalization:
    Date _____ /_____ ( )   Reason _____ ( )
    Month   Year
    Date _____ /_____ ( )   Reason _____ ( )
    Month   Year
    Date _____ /_____ ( )   Reason _____ ( )
    Month   Year
29. Have you ever had any operations (other than those listed above)?
    Yes _____ No _____ ( )
    ₍₁₎   ₍₀₎
    If yes, give the dates and types of operations:
    Date _____ /_____ ( )   Type of operation _____ ( )
    Month   Year
    Date _____ /_____ ( )   Type of operation _____ ( )
    Month   Year
30. Have you ever had any accidents or injuries (other than listed above)?
    Yes _____ No _____ ( )
    ₍₁₎   ₍₀₎
    If yes, give the dates and kind of accident or injury:
    Date _____ /_____ ( )   Kind _____ ( )
    Month   Year
    Date _____ /_____ ( )   Kind _____ ( )
    Month   Year
31. Do you have any of the following? If yes, check as many as apply.

Heart disease _____	Breathing problems ___	Bladder problems _____
Rheumatic fever _____	Osteoarthritis _____	Kidney problems _____
High blood pressure ___	Rheumatoid arthritis ___	Prostate problems _____
Stroke _____	Tuberculosis _____	Change of life
Leg cramps _____	Diabetes _____	symptoms _____
Bronchitis _____	Cancer _____	Nervousness _____
Angina _____	Thyroid _____	Headaches _____
Heart attack _____	Fever _____	Bleeding _____
Dizziness _____	Ulcers _____	Colitis _____
Asthma _____	Sinus problems _____	Falling _____
Seizures _____	Yellow eyes or skin ___	Other (explain) _____
Sadness _____	Anemia _____	
Gout _____	Diverticulitis _____	

32. Do you have any allergies? If yes, please check as many as apply.
    Food _____ Drugs _____ Pollen _____ Other _____ ( )
    ( )   ( )   ( )   ( )

33. Are there any foods you can't eat? If yes, what are they?
_____ ( )

34. Do you have visual problems? Yes _____ No _____ ( )
(1)   (0)

35. Do you wear glasses? Yes _____ No _____ ( )
(1)   (0)

36. Has there been any change in your vision recently? Yes _____ No _____ ( )
(1)   (0)

37. When was your last examination? _____/_____ ( )
Month   Year

38. Do you wear dentures? Yes _____ No _____ ( )
(1)   (0)

39. Do you have any problems with your teeth? Yes _____ No _____ ( )
(1)   (0)

40. Your last visit to the dentist was _____/_____ ( )
Month   Year

41. How many glasses of wine, beer, or other alcohol do you drink a day? _____ ( )

42. Do you smoke? Yes _____ No _____ ( )
(1)   (0)

43. How many cups of coffee do you drink a day? _____ ( )

44. How many cups of tea do you drink a day? _____ ( )

45. How many cups of cola do you drink a day? _____ ( )

46. Do you take any vitamins? Yes _____ No _____ ( )
(1)   (0)

47. If yes, what kind? _____ ( )

48. Do you exercise regularly? Yes _____ No _____ ( )
(1)   (0)

49. Has your weight changed recently? Yes _____ No _____ ( )
(1)   (0)

50. Do you have any trouble sleeping? Yes _____ No _____ ( )

51. Please list the foods that you eat on an average day, by meal.
Breakfast _____ Lunch _____ Dinner _____
_____   _____   _____
_____   _____   _____
_____   _____   _____

52. Do you take any of the following? If yes, check as many as apply.
Sleeping pills _____   Blood pressure pills _____
Nerve pills _____   Hormones _____
Water pills _____   Heart pills _____
Thyroid pills _____   Laxatives _____
Aspirin/Tylenol _____   Cold/allergy pills _____
Mylanta/Maalox _____   Sugar/diabetic pills _____
Any other? Please list _____

53. Are the medications you take prescribed by your doctor?
Yes _____ No _____ ( )
(1)   (0)

54. What kind of home remedies to you use? _____
_____

55. Please describe what you do on an average day using the times below:
Awakening _____
Morning _____
Afternoon _____
Evening _____

56. Do you feel that your present affection needs are satisfied?
Yes _____ No _____ ( )
(1)   (0)

57. If you wish to make any comment about the questionnaire, please use the remaining space.

Joseph M. Foley Elderhealth Center Self-Assessment Form

BASIC INFORMATION

Name _____

      Last   First   Middle   (Maiden)

Address _____

      City   State   Zip Code

Hospital No. _____   S.S. number _____

Phone no. (____) _____   Birthdate _____

Sex _____ Marital status _____   Religion _____

Next of kin: Name _____   Relationship _____

      Address _____

      Phone no. (home) _____ (work) _____

Person to notify (if other than next of kin) _____

      Address _____

      Phone no. (home) _____ (work) _____

Present physician _____   Telephone _____

      Address _____

Date of last physical exam _____   By whom _____

Date of last visit to physician _____

      Purpose of visit _____

      Name of physician seen _____

Name of person completing this form _____

      Relationship to patient _____

Does anyone have power of attorney for you?   ☐ Yes   ☐ No

Is anyone serving as your guardian?   ☐ Yes   ☐ No

   If yes, please indicate who _____

   Address _____

   Phone no. _____

PURPOSE OF REFERRAL

What is the immediate problem for which the patient, family, or others need help? What event(s) led you to seek help specifically at this time?

_____

_____

_____

_____

_____

Courtesy University Hospitals of Cleveland, Cleveland, Ohio.

INSURANCE INFORMATION
Medicare

Holder's name _____

Medicare no. and letter _____

Effective date (hospital) _____ (medical) _____

Blue Cross

Holder's name _____

Certificate no. _____   Group no. _____

Blue Cross plan _____   Blue Cross service _____

Blue Shield plan _____   Blue Shield service _____

Effective date _____   Additional features _____

Commercial Insurance

Holder's name _____

Policy no. _____   Group no. _____

Insurance to bill _____

Name of company _____

Address _____

_____

HEALTH ASSESSMENT

1. Are you under any unusual stress in the following areas? Mark if "yes."
   - ☐ Financial
   - ☐ Home situation
   - ☐ Transportation
   - ☐ Health
   - ☐ Family or personal relationships
2. Which of the following best describes how you feel?
   - ☐ This is the best time of my life.
   - ☐ While some things are more difficult for me now, my life is usually pleasant and acceptable.
   - ☐ I am just as happy now as when I was younger.
   - ☐ As I age, life has become unpleasant and difficult to tolerate.
   - ☐ I am very unhappy with my present situation.
3. Which of the following best describes your state of health?
   - ☐ My state of health is usually good.
   - ☐ I am in average health.
   - ☐ My health is below average.
   - ☐ I am in very poor health.
4. The following is a list of symptoms or problems which you may have, or have had. Please check any of these which apply to you and indicate when it began or for how long it has been a problem for you.

Check if "yes"   **For how long**

☐   _____   Frequent headaches
☐   _____   Passing out or fainting
☐   _____   Falling or stumbling
☐   _____   Paralysis or leg or arm weakness
☐   _____   Numbness or loss of feeling
☐   _____   Tremor or shaking
☐   _____   Forgetfulness
☐   _____   Problem with memory
☐   _____   Disorientation to time, person, or place
☐   _____   Depression
☐   _____   Agitation
☐   _____   Hallucinations (hearing voices and/or
                                                             seeing things)
☐   _____   Suspiciousness of others
☐   _____   Fearfulness
☐   _____   Unusually high or low moods
☐   _____   Difficulty sleeping
☐   _____   Difficulty speaking
☐   _____   Difficulty understanding what others say
☐   _____   Difficulty swallowing
☐   _____   Hoarseness or other change in voice
☐   _____   Visual or eye problems
☐   Date of last visit to eye doctor _____
☐   _____   Hearing or ear trouble
☐   Date of last hearing examination _____
☐   _____   Dental problems, dental discomfort
☐   Date of last visit to dentist _____
☐   _____   Fever or sweats
☐   _____   Swollen glands
☐   _____   Lumps or sores
☐   _____   Skin trouble
☐   _____   Difficulty breathing
☐   _____   Persistent cough
☐   _____   Chest pain or tightness
☐   _____   Irregular heartbeat
☐   _____   Leg pain when walking
☐   _____   High blood pressure
☐   _____   Poor appetite
☐   _____   Change in weight
☐   _____   Frequent indigestion or stomach ache
☐   _____   Frequent nausea or vomiting
☐   _____   Change in bowel habits
☐   _____   Black bowel movements or rectal bleeding
☐   _____   Frequent diarrhea
☐   _____   Constipation
☐   _____   Urination at night
☐   _____   Painful urination
☐   _____   Difficulty starting or stopping urination
☐   _____   Difficulty holding urine or urine leakage
☐   _____   Sexual difficulties
☐   _____   Back or neck troubles

☐ _____ Joint pain or stiffness
☐ _____ Swelling of feet or ankles
☐ _____ Foot problems

Women only:
☐ Breast lumps or discharge
☐ Vaginal bleeding/discomfort
Date of last Pap test _____

Men only:
☐ Discharge from penis
☐ Swelling/lump in testicle
☐ Ache in lower back or groin

5. Do you have any problem with the following?

Yes No
☐ ☐ Sleeping problems
☐ ☐ Feeling lonely
☐ ☐ Change in sexual interest
☐ ☐ Feeling sad or depressed
☐ ☐ Change in sexual activity
☐ ☐ Thought of "ending it all"
☐ ☐ Feeling tense or anxious
☐ ☐ Change in appetite

6. Past medical history

   Below is a list of medical conditions. Please check which of these you have had in the past and write in the approximate date(s).

☐ Alcoholism
☐ Anemia
☐ Arthritis
☐ Asthma
☐ Bronchitis
☐ Cancer
☐ Cataracts
☐ Depression
☐ Diabetes
☐ Emotional problems
☐ Fractures
☐ Gallbladder problems
☐ Glaucoma
☐ Heart disease
☐ Hernia
☐ High blood pressure
☐ Other _____

☐ Jaundice
☐ Kidney disease
☐ Liver disease
☐ Lung disease
☐ Mental illness
☐ Nervous breakdown
☐ Prostate disease
☐ Phlebitis
☐ Pneumonia
☐ Seizures
☐ Stomach ulcers
☐ Stroke
☐ Thyroid disease
☐ Tuberculosis
☐ Urinary tract infection
☐ Venereal disease

7. Please list *all* of the times you have been in the hospital.

Hospital	Date	Reason

8. Please give the following information about the health of your immediate family. If a family member has or has had any of the following, check and write the person's name and relationship to you (such as mother or father, sister or brother, son or daughter). If the person has died, give age at time of death and cause of death.

☐ Alcoholism _____
☐ Cancer _____
☐ Depression _____
☐ Diabetes _____

☐ Heart disease _____
☐ High blood pressure _____
☐ Kidney disease _____
☐ Memory problems _____
☐ Mental illness _____
☐ Nervous breakdown _____
☐ Speech or language disorder _____
☐ Stroke _____
☐ Other _____

9. Do you now, or did you ever smoke cigarettes/cigar/pipe, or chew tobacco?
   ☐ Yes ☐ No
   How much? _____ For how long? _____
   When did you stop? _____

10. Do you drink alcohol? ☐ Yes ☐ No
    If no, why not? _____
    If yes, how much? _____
       How often? ☐ Less than 3 times a week
                  ☐ More than 3 times a week
                  ☐ Daily
    Has this ever been a problem for you, or has anyone ever told you your drinking
    is a problem for you? ☐ Yes ☐ No

11. Please list all prescription medicines you take.

Medicine	Date	When taken

12. Check any of the following medicines you take in addition to your prescription
    medicines.
    ☐ Aspirin   ☐ Nerve pills
    ☐ Antacids   ☐ Sleeping pills
    ☐ Cold pills/decongestants   ☐ Vitamins/minerals
    ☐ Hormones   ☐ Other _____
    ☐ Laxatives   _____

13. Do you have any allergies to medicine? ☐ Yes ☐ No
    If "yes," please list your allergies: _____
    _____

14. Are doing any of the following activities a problem for you?

Yes	No	If "yes," who helps you?
☐	☐	Shopping for groceries _____
☐	☐	Preparing your own meals _____
☐	☐	Eating _____
☐	☐	Doing housecleaning _____
☐	☐	Writing checks or paying bills _____
☐	☐	Taking medicines _____
☐	☐	Taking sponge or tub bath, or shower _____
☐	☐	Dressing _____
☐	☐	Using the telephone _____
☐	☐	Walking indoors _____
☐	☐	Walking outdoors _____
☐	☐	Going up or down stairs _____
☐	☐	Getting into or out of bed or chair _____
☐	☐	Getting off or on toilet _____

15. Please check which of the following you use:
- ☐ Glasses
- ☐ Hearing aid
- ☐ Cane
- ☐ Wheelchair
- ☐ Contact lenses
- ☐ Dentures
- ☐ Walker
- ☐ Other _____

16. Which of the following describes the place where you live?
- ☐ Apartment (nonpublic)
- ☐ Home (owned)
- ☐ Home (rented)
- ☐ Foster home
- ☐ Public housing
- ☐ Subsidized housing
- ☐ Nursing home
- ☐ Other _____

17. With whom do you live?
- ☐ Alone
- ☐ Children
- ☐ Companion or friend
- ☐ Other _____
- ☐ Husband, wife, or partner
- ☐ Another relative (e.g., grandchild, niece, or nephew)

18. With whom are you in contact? Please list names.
- ☐ Husband, wife, or partner _____
- ☐ Child or children _____
- ☐ Brother(s) or sister(s) _____
- ☐ Other relatives(s) _____
- ☐ Friend(s) _____
- ☐ Neighbor(s) _____

19. Who do you call on for help? _____
_____

20. How often in the past week have you left your home (e.g., going to church, meetings, or other activities)?
Where did you go? _____
_____

21. Please list the interests and activities you most enjoy:
_____
_____
_____
_____

22. Which of the following best describes your employment status?
- ☐ Never fully employed (outside the home)
- ☐ Retired—when? _____
- ☐ Presently working
- ☐ Full-time
- ☐ Part-time

23. What is your present or past occupation?
_____

24. Which of the following best describes your financial status?
- ☐ Comfortably able to afford all necessities (food, clothing, and transportation)
- ☐ Able to afford necessities with careful budgeting
- ☐ Barely able to afford the basic needs
- ☐ Unable to afford the necessities

25. What is your usual form of transportation?
- ☐ Drive my own car
- ☐ Ride with a friend or relative
- ☐ Take a bus
- ☐ Walk
- ☐ Take a cab
- ☐ Don't go out of house or apartment

26. Which of the following services have you used in the past 3 months?
    Check for "yes"   If "yes," who provides the service?
    ☐ Personal care _____
    ☐ Nursing services _____
    ☐ Medical care (physicians) _____
    ☐ Mental health services _____
    ☐ Social services _____
    ☐ Physical therapy _____
    ☐ Occupational therapy _____
    ☐ Hearing or speech testing or therapy _____
    ☐ Sight center _____
    ☐ Rehabilitation services _____
    ☐ Nutritionist _____
    ☐ Transportation _____
    ☐ Day center _____
    ☐ Meal program _____
    ☐ Other _____

27. How many meals a day do you eat? _____

28. How many snacks a day do you eat? _____

29. How many cups of fluids per day do you drink (including tea, coffee, water, juice, milk, soda pop, etc.)? _____

30. Please write down what you have to eat and drink on a usual day. Just fill in the items where they fit in.
    Breakfast _____
    _____
    Morning snack _____
    _____
    Noon meal _____
    _____
    Afternoon snack _____
    _____
    Evening meal _____
    _____
    Evening snack _____
    _____

31. Do you have any questions or concerns about your diet or nutrition?
    ☐ Yes   ☐ No
    If "yes," what are they? _____
    _____

University Hospitals Nursing Assessment Worksheet

Date: _____   Patient: _____   ID: _____
Informant: _____   Relationship: _____
Presenting problem: _____
_____
_____

MENTAL STATUS

Appearance: _____
_____

Mood, affect (including check for depression, orientation): _____
_____

Cognitive function (examples): _____
_____
_____

Communication: _____
_____

SLEEPING

Does patient sleep well? _____   Feel well rested? _____
If not, explain: _____
Ease of falling asleep: _____   Nap pattern: _____
Hours per night/times up during the night: _____
Concerns of patient/family: _____

SENSES

Sight: _____
Hearing: _____
Taste: _____   Smell: _____
Touch: _____

Courtesy University Hospitals of Cleveland, Cleveland, Ohio.

ACTIVITIES OF DAILY LIVING

	Independent	Dependent	
Bathing			Initiation of bath Type of bathing (tub, shower, sponge) Bath preparation Get in/out of tub Ability to wash self Hair washing
Dressing			Clothing selection Putting on garments Doing up buttons, etc. Appropriateness of attire Undressing Laundry
Transfer			From bed to chair From chair to standing
Toileting			Able to find bathroom Able to use toilet appropriately Hygiene
Bowel continence			Frequency and control Constipation
Feeding			Serving self Utensils to mouth Readying food for consumption (buttering, cutting, etc.)

INSTRUMENTAL ACTIVITIES OF DAILY LIVING

	Alone	Assist	Never (N/A)	No longer	
Telephone					Look up number Dial
Medication					Preparation Taking
Outside of home					Organization Getting lost
Driving					Limitations Legal parameters
Housework					Organization Doing (List what able to do.)
Food preparation					Planning Shopping Preparing
Finances					Banking Paying bills Balancing checkbook

URINARY CONTINENCE

Does patient have "accidents"? (If "yes," when?) _____

Patient's knowledge of accidents: _____   Frequency: _____

Urgency: _____   Can patient get to bathroom in time? _____

Does patient wet when coughing or sneezing or at other times? _____

Where is center or concern about wetting (patient, family, both)? _____

Other concerns: _____

_____

MOBILITY

Walking ability (use of assistive devices): _____

Distance able to walk (and frequency): _____

Gait, posture: _____

Stiffness (morning, after inactivity, evening, where?): _____

_____

What does patient do to maximize mobility? _____

Hand dexterity and function: _____

Problems with feet and shoes: _____

Other concerns of patient/family: _____

_____

NUTRITION

No. of meals per day: _____   No. of glasses of fluid: _____

Indigestion, nausea/vomiting, change in bowels: _____

Dentition: _____

Appetite: _____   Weight stability: _____

Concerns of family (need for referral to nutritionist): _____

_____

_____

MEDICATIONS

List medications as prescribed and how they are taken. (Note how long patient has been on medication.)

Patient's knowledge of medications (reason for, side effects, precautions)

_____

_____

_____

_____

_____

Nonprescription medications: _____

_____

Allergies (medications): _____   (other): _____

Person responsible for medication administration: _____

Alcohol intake (past/present): _____   Smoking history: _____

SAFETY

Is patient alone at any time? _____   Gets lost? _____

Kitchen safety: _____

Household safety (rugs, cords, railings, stairs): _____

Other concerns: _____

_____

CARE GIVER

Name of formal care giver: _____   Relationship: _____

Informal care-giving system: _____

Care giver's role/function: _____

_____

Impact of care giving on care giver/family: _____

_____

Assessment of stability/security provided in present care environment:

_____

_____

SUMMARY

Assessment: _____

_____

_____

_____

_____

_____

_____

Problem list: _____

_____

_____

_____

_____

_____

_____

_____

Plan: _____

_____

_____

_____

_____

_____

_____

Completed by: _____

Katz Index of Activities of Daily Living

1. Bathing (sponge, shower, or tub):
   - I: Receives no assistance (gets in and out of tub if tub is the usual means of bathing)
   - A: Receives assistance in bathing only one part of the body (such as the back or a leg)
   - D: Receives assistance in bathing more than one part of the body (or not bathed)
2. Dressing:
   - I: Gets clothes and gets completely dressed without assistance
   - A: Gets clothes and gets dressed without assistance except in tying shoes.
   - D: Receives assistance in getting clothes or in getting dressed or stays partly or completely undressed
3. Toileting:
   - I: Goes to "toilet room," cleans self, and arranges clothes without assistance (may use object for support such as cane, walker, or wheelchair and may manage night bedpan or commode, emptying it in the morning)
   - A: Receives assistance in going to "toilet room" or in cleansing self or in arranging clothes after elimination or in use of night bedpan or commode
   - D: Doesn't go to room termed "toilet" for the elimination process
4. Transfer:
   - I: Moves in and out of bed as well as in and out of chair without assistance (may be using object for support such as cane or walker)
   - A: Moves in and out of bed or chair with assistance
   - D: Doesn't get out of bed
5. Continence:
   - I: Controls urination and bowel movement completely by self
   - A: Has occasional "accidents"
   - D: Supervision helps keep urine or bowel control; catheter is used, or is incontinent
6. Feeding:
   - I: Feeds self without assistance
   - A: Feeds self except for getting assistance in cutting meat or buttering bread
   - D: Receives assistance in feeding or is fed partly or completely by using tubes or intravenous fluids

Adapted from *JAMA* 185:915, 1963.
ABBREVIATIONS: I, independent; A, assistance; D, dependent.

Modified Barthel Index

	Independent		Dependent	
	Intact	Limited	Helper	Null
Feed from dish	10	5	3	0
Dress upper body	5	5	3	0
Dress lower body	5	5	2	0
Don brace or prosthesis	0	0	−2	0
Grooming	5	5	0	0
Wash or bathe	4	4	0	0
Bladder incontinence	10	10	5	0
Bowel incontinence	10	10	5	0
Care of perineum/clothing at toilet	4	4	2	0
Transfer, chair	15	15	7	0
Transfer, toilet	6	5	3	0
Transfer, tub or shower	1	1	0	0
Walk on level 50 yards or more	15	15	10	0
Up and down stairs for one flight or more	10	10	5	0
Wheelchair 50 yards (only if not walking)	15	5	0	0

Adapted from *Medical Care* (19:491), 1981.

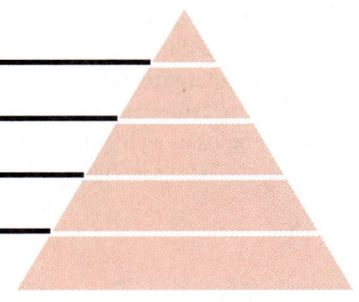

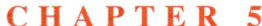

CHAPTER 5

Laboratory Values and Implications for the Aged

Annette Miller Dever
Rosemary Miller Rothkopf

A student speculates

I believe self-care is important and, sure, I watch my cholesterol intake every day and get it checked annually. I worry about my mother as I'm not sure she takes her diabetic diet seriously. Sometimes she forgets to check her blood sugar.

Leslie, age 37

Elders speak

I never thought I would see the day when we would be doing our own lab tests at home. Wouldn't that have been great years ago when we had to sacrifice a bunny to see if we were pregnant!! Most of us didn't want to know any sooner than we had to anyway, sort of an unintended "save the bunny" campaign.

Georgia, age 79

You know, in the old days when my grandfather was practicing he would diagnose by sight, feel, smell, and taste. Yes, taste! But, of course, nobody ever heard of a malpractice suit either.

Daisy, age 82

LEARNING OBJECTIVES

Upon completion of this chapter, the reader will be able to:

1. Identify the laboratory values that increase or decrease with normal aging.
2. Understand the implications and deviations of abnormal laboratory values in the aged.
3. Define cautions the nurse should take when interpreting laboratory values in the aged.
4. Distinguish between clinical findings of hypothyroidism and hyperthyroidism in the elderly.
5. State common causes of hypokalemia and hyperkalemia.
6. Describe symptoms and signs suggestive of diabetes in the elderly.
7. Identify seven laboratory values in the elderly that frequently fall out of the so-called normal range.
8. Discuss several laboratory tests necessary for minimally adequate screening of elderly residents in long-term care institutions.

This chapter is intended to give a background of the importance of laboratory diagnostic findings. Some are exceedingly complex and sophisticated, but each nurse needs a basic knowledge because the review and reporting of laboratory values constitute a significant task of nursing. More frequently now they are reported directly to the client by the nurse, and the nurse will need to explain the significance of findings. Additionally, the gerontologic nurse depends on laboratory values because the ill elderly often present vague clinical signs and symptoms. When reviewing laboratory values seen in the elderly, the nurse questions those values reported outside normal ranges, whether those values reflect illness or normal aging changes (Melillo, 1993).

Normal laboratory values are determined by a random sample of "healthy" individuals, usually aged 20 to 40, obtaining the mean and setting as normal a range of two standard deviations on either side of the mean. It is no longer considered appropriate to refer to *normal laboratory values*. Since the 1970s many studies have been done to establish age-related normal laboratory values. It has been determined that *normal range* is an obsolete term when trying to determine age-related norms in the elderly population. *Reference values* or *reference ranges* are the preferred terms. These are a more accurate explanation of laboratory values of the aged. Geriatric *reference ranges* are those intervals within which 95% of values for persons over 70 years of age will fall. Reference values are arrived at by considering certain population groups, subgroups, and characteristics as to age, sex, race, physiologic and pharmacologic factors, methods of analysis, and statistical methods. *Reference values,* a term recommended by the International Federation of Clinical Chemistry, will be used synonymously with *reference ranges* throughout this chapter. International standards are important because laboratory values for an individual remain extremely stable over time with observed shifts in the median attributed to expected or unexpected changes in the laboratory (Lott et al, 1996). Thus knowledge of reference values, standardized procedures, and individual biologic variations would allow a subject to follow throughout life the evolution of his or her biologic constituents and to detect any deviation suggestive of a pathologic condition (Siest et al, 1995). Solberg (1995) contends that group-based reference values, even when subgrouped according to sex, age, and other criteria, have less sensitivity than comparing the new values against the baseline for the individual.

Another issue is the difficulty of defining a healthy elderly population for the development of normal laboratory values. The majority of elders have one or more disease entities and are taking one or more medications, which may affect laboratory values. In a study of over 5000 participants in a cardiovascular health study, Medicare-eligible, ostensibly healthy individuals residing in the community were used to define a healthy subset of the older population. Blood samples revealed that levels of cholesterol, high-density lipoprotein (HDL) and low-density lipoprotein (LDL) cholesterol, fasting and 2-hour postload glucose and insulin, fibrinogen, factors VII and VIII, potassium, creatinine, albumin, uric acid, white blood count, hematocrit, hemoglobin, and platelet count were all significantly different than the generally accepted reference ranges used in clinical laboratories (Robbins et al, 1995). In longitudinal and cross-sectional studies Beregi et al (1995) found generally similar laboratory values in centenarians and other elders, but there were gender differences in HDL cholesterol. Age and gender differences were observed in hematocrit/hemoglobin values, serum creatinine, total cholesterol, serum IgG, IgA, and IgM levels and in the frequency of the occurrence of antinuclear factor. Lower hemoglobin and hematocrit values, elevated total-cholesterol levels, the presence of antinuclear and rheumatoid factor, and elevated systolic blood pressure were more frequent in aged females than aged males.

This chapter discusses the laboratory values that significantly change with aging. Tables are provided for general reference values for the aged. Since normal reference ranges will vary with institutions, depending on the instrumentation used for performing tests, Table 5-1 should be used as a guideline within institutional laboratory parameters. Also see Table 5-2.

HEMATOLOGY

In the aged, malignancy and disorders of the immune system result in a variety of hematologic abnormalities. Aging itself has less of an effect on hematopoiesis than socioeconomic and physical limitations found in older populations. Inadequate nutrition, sensory deficits, and impaired physical mobility may reduce circulatory red blood cells, granulocytes, and lymphocytes (Lipschitz, 1995).

Red Blood Cells

There is little evidence of age-related differences in red blood cells. There may be changes in red cell enzymes that affect the life span of the cell, but the significance is uncertain. The mean cell diameter may increase slightly after 50 years of age, but blood volume remains constant (Sehy, 1995).

Anemia is a condition indicated by lower-than-normal hemoglobin or hematocrit levels. Signs and symptoms of severe anemia such as apathy, depression, confusion, general fatigue, and pallor may be incorrectly attributed to old age instead of anemia (Nardone et al, 1990). Dizziness and agitation are also commonly observed symptoms of anemia in the elderly. Anemia is a common disease state of the elderly, but it is not a normal aging process. Evaluation of the etiology of any hemoglobin or hematocrit levels below normal is necessary at any age (Freedman, 1995).

Hemoglobin

Hemoglobin is the main component of the red blood cell. It is a conjugated protein whose main function is to transport oxygen and carbon dioxide. In the elderly the hemoglobin concentration in both sexes decreases after 65 years of age. This decrease is more prevalent in men than women and is probably related to the reduction in androgen production in men. In healthy young adults male hemoglobin levels are normally higher than those of females. However, in the elderly the hemoglobin concentrations in both sexes are nearly the same (Freedman, 1995). A decrease in hemoglobin may indicate chronic disease or physiologic changes due to the aging process. When a low hemoglobin level is present, there is lowered oxygen content and a delay in wound healing. Therefore older individuals with pressure sores or any slow-healing wounds should have hemoglobin levels monitored.

Hematocrit

Hematocrit is the ratio of the volume of red blood cells to that of whole blood. Ninety-five percent of elderly men have lower hematocrit levels than younger adult populations

Table 5-1   Laboratory Values for the Elderly

Test	Normal aged	Standard reference ranges*	Implications and deviations†
Hematology			
Hemoglobin	Slight decrease	Male: 14.0-18.0 g/dl Female: 12.0-16.0 g/dl	
Hematocrit	Slight decrease	Male: 40%-54% Female: 38%-47%	
White blood cells	Slight decrease	$4.3\text{-}11.0 \times 10^3/mm^3$	
Erythrocyte sedimentation rate (ESR)			
Minivess method	Slight increase	Male: 0-20 mm Female: 0-20 mm	
Differential lymphocytes			

Neutrophils	Unchanged	46%-82%	Increase:
			    Diabetes mellitus
			    Gout
			    Rheumatoid arthritis
			    Stress
			    Bacterial infections
			    Thyroiditis
			    Hemolytic anemia
			    Rheumatic fever
			    Carcinoma
			    Acute hemorrhage
			    Cushing's disease
			    Increased corticosteroids
			    Lead poisoning
			    Pancreatitis
			Decrease:
			    Vitamin B_{12} deficiency
			    Acute viral infection
			    Folic acid deficiency
			    Bone marrow damage

Lymphocytes	Increased B cells Decreased T cells	11%-45%	

Monocytes	Increased both sexes	2.0%-10.0%	Increase:
			    Tuberculosis
			    Subacute bacterial endocarditis

Eosinophils	Increase or decrease	0%-4.0%	Increase:
			    Parasitosis
			    Allergy
			    Colitis
			    Collagen disease
			    Eosinophilic granulomatosis
			    Eosinophilic leukemia

Basophils	Unchanged	0%-2.0%	Increase:
			    Polycythemia vera
			    Myelofibrosis
			Decrease:
			    Anaphylactic reaction

Serum chemistry			

Iron‡	Decrease 50%-75% of young adult value at about age 71-80 yr	Male: 49-181 μg/dl
		Female: 37-170 μg/dl
			Increase:
			    Pernicious anemia
			    Hemolytic anemia
			    Hemochromatosis
			    Hepatitis
			Decrease:
			    Iron-deficiency anemia

*Standard reference ranges used at St Francis Hospital Laboratory, Beech Grove, IN, 1996.

†The deviations listed are not an all-inclusive list but a helpful guide for many of the frequent deviations seen in the elderly. Modified from Eliopoulos C: *Health assessment of the older adult,* Reading, MA, 1990, Addison-Wesley; and Eliopoulos C: *A guide to the nursing of the aging,* Baltimore, 1987, Williams & Wilkins.

‡Must be differentiated between normal age changes and anemia.

§Garner B: Guide to changing lab values in the elderly, *Geriatric Nurs* 144, 10(3):144, 1989.

Continued

Table 5-1 Laboratory Values for the Elderly—cont'd

Test	Normal aged	Standard reference ranges*	Implications and deviations†
Serum chemistry—cont'd			
B$_{12}$‡	Decrease 60%-80% of young adult value at about age 70+ yr	179-1132 pg/ml	
Folate‡	Unchanged	3.1-12.4 ng/ml	
Thyroid			
T$_4$	Slight functional decrease	4.5-12.0 μg/dl	
T$_3$ by R is	Male decrease after age 70 yr	86-181 mg/dl	
	Female decrease around age 70-80 yr		
TSH		0.49-4.67 μu/ml	
Blood chemistry			
Urea nitrogen (BUN)	Slight increase	Male: 9-20 mg/dl Female: 7-17 mg/dl	Increase: Dehydration Gastrointestinal hemorrhage Intestinal obstruction Renal disease Acute glomerulonephritis Prostatic hypertrophy Burns High protein intake Mercury poisoning Protein catabolism Decrease: Cirrhosis Liver disease Low-protein intake Starvation
Creatinine	Slight increase	Male: 0.8-1.5 mg/dl Female: 0.7-1.2 mg/dl	Increase: Renal dysfunction Chronic glomerulonephritis Tetanus Typhoid fever Salmonella infection Decrease: Anemia Muscular atrophy Leukemia Renal failures
Potassium	Age-related increase after sixth decade	3.6-5.0 mEq/L	Increase: Addison's disease Bronchial asthma Renal disease Tissue breakdown Trauma Anuria Decrease: Steroid therapy Vomiting Cirrhosis Diarrhea Diuretic therapy Diabetic acidosis Cushing's disease Intravenous therapy

Continued

Table 5-1   Laboratory Values for the Elderly—cont'd

Test	Normal aged	Standard reference ranges*	Implications and deviations†
Blood chemistry—cont'd			

Glucose	Increases	70-110 mg/dl	Increase:
			    Diabetes mellitus
			    Emotional stress
			    Hyperthyroidism
			    Infections
			    Thiazide therapy
			    Increased intracranial pressure
			    Pituitary disorder
			Decrease:
			    Hyperinsulinism
			    Hypothyroidism
			    Starvation

Fasting blood sugar	Minimal increase		
1 hour postprandial blood sugar	Increases by 10 mg/dl per decade after age 30		
2 hour postprandial blood sugar	Increases up to 100 plus age after age 40		
CPK	May not be elevated	Male: 55-170 U/L Female: 30-135 U/L	
Alkaline phosphatase	Increases	38-126 U/L	
LDH	1-1$\frac{1}{2}$ times higher, especially in females	313-618 U/L	
SGPT or ALT	Unchanged	Male: 21-72 IU/L Female: 9-52 IU/L	
SGOT or AST	Unchanged	Male: 17-59 IU/L Female: 14-36 IU/L	
Total protein		6.3-8.2 g/dl	
Serum albumin	Decrease	3.9-5.0 g/dl	

Cholesterol (total)	Gradual increase with age	200 mg/dl	Increase:
			    Chronic renal disease
			    Hypothyroidism
			    Diabetes mellitus
			    Liver disease
			    Pancreatic dysfunction
			Decrease:
			    Fasting state
			    Tuberculosis
			    Hypermetabolic states
			    Hyperthyroidism
			    Intestinal obstruction
			    Liver disease
			    Malnutrition
			    Pernicious anemia
			    Hemolytic anemia

HDL	Women consistently higher than men, then difference disappears in elders§	>35 mg/dl	
Triglycerides	Increases	35-160 mg/dl	
Calcium	Men decrease Women increase	8.4-10.2 mg/dl	
Phosphorus	Men decrease Women increase	2.5-4.5 mg/dl	

Continued

Table 5-1	Laboratory Values for the Elderly—cont'd		
Test	**Normal aged**	**Standard reference ranges***	**Implications and deviations†**
Blood chemistry—cont'd			
Uric acid	Males increase more than females Females over 44 years	3.5-8.5 mg/dl 2.5-7.5 mg/dl	Increase: Thiazide diuretic therapy Pneumonia Multiple myeloma Leukemia High salicylate intake Gout Fasting Chronic renal failure Chronic lymphocytic granulocytic leukemia Decrease: Allopurinol therapy
Urinalysis			
Protein	Slight increase	Negative	
Glucose	Unchanged	Negative	
Specific gravity	Decrease	1.005-1.030 o.d. (refractometer)	
Creatinine clearance			
Male	Decrease	85-125 ml/min	Decrease:
Female	Decrease	75-115 ml/min	Renal disease
Arterial blood gases			
PCO_2	Increase or decrease	34-46 mm Hg	Increase: Metabolic alkalosis Respiratory acidosis Decrease: Metabolic acidosis Respiratory alkalosis
PO_2	Decrease	85-95 mm Hg	Increase: Administration of pure O_2 Decrease: Circulatory disorders Decreased hemoglobin Decreased O_2 supply High altitudes Poor O_2 uptake and utilization Respiratory exchange problems

(Lipschitz, 1990.) Studies show that women maintain their hematocrit levels throughout life (Kelso, 1990). Other laboratory tests should always be evaluated along with hematocrit values in making a diagnosis. The hematocrit test is to be used along with other laboratory tests in evaluating the patient with anemia; age-related changes in hematology laboratory values should be defined. Consideration of the serious implications of even a slight decrease in hemoglobin and hematocrit in the older adult is important (Cavalieri et al, 1992; Robbins et al, 1995).

Erythrocyte Sedimentation Rate

When well-mixed venous blood is placed in a vertical tube, erythrocytes will tend to fall to the bottom. The distance the

red blood cells fall in an interval of time is the erythrocyte sedimentation rate (ESR). The changes in plasma constituents in the elderly may possibly increase the ESR. The albumin/fibrinogen and globulin/fibrinogen ratios are relevant in the measurement of the ESR (Jeppesen, 1986). There is considerable evidence of reduced plasma albumin and increased plasma fibrinogen in the aged, which cause the ESR increase. ESR determination may have a limited diagnostic value with the elderly (Lonergan, 1996).

The elders' ESR above the accepted normal range may or may not be an indication of disease and can be consistent with good health. However, ESRs greater than 80 are strongly associated with an underlying disease such as neoplasms, infections, or rheumatic disease (Cavalieri et al,

1992). Elevated ESR is common in patients with connective tissue disease, cancer, and infection (Staab and Hodges, 1996). A thorough history and physical examination is paramount before excluding these diseases by ESR values alone.

White Blood Cells

The formation and development of leukocytes are affected by aging. Susceptibility to infections is enhanced with old age. Since the elderly have a higher incidence of autoimmune disorders, infectious diseases, and lymphoproliferative disorders, it is suggested that tetanus, influenza, and pneumococcal vaccines be considered (Jeppesen, 1986; Kelso, 1990; Cavalieri et al, 1992).

The number of circulating white blood cells may change with age, as cell function and production are weakened. Age alone cannot be the sole explanation for a low white blood count; drug toxicity and sepsis should be considered (Sehy, 1995). Pneumonia and urinary tract infections are two conditions that are frequently seen in the elderly patient. This may be caused by anatomic changes in these organs and changes in leukocyte function . Signs and symptoms that are normally associated with leukocyte abnormality may be different in the elderly. Chronic inflammation, fever, swelling, pain, and lymph node enlargement may be reduced or absent (Sehy, 1995). Often there is no increase in total leukocyte count but a shift to the left called excessive band neutrophils. This shift is a more definitive indication of infection in the aged. White blood cell differential testing is imperative for diagnosis of infection in the aged (Chillag, 1985).

There are five major types of leukocytes in the blood: neutrophils, lymphocytes, monocytes, eosinophils, and basophils. The effects of aging can be seen more clearly by viewing each type of cell separately.

Neutrophils. The largest percentage of white blood cells are neutrophils, which are produced daily in the bone marrow. Neutrophils play an important part in the localization of infections by phagocytizing bacteria. Aging does not appear to change the neutrophil count in older adults. Some data do suggest that the rate of release of neutrophils from the bone marrow may be reduced in older persons. Also, the number of cells being stored in the marrow may be fewer.

Lymphocytes. Lymphocytes are a very heterogeneous population of cells that can cause proliferation of immunoglobulins in response to many antigenic and mitogenic stimuli. These modulate immune responses through cell-cell interactions and secretory products. Lymphocytes are commonly of two types: T cells, which are produced by the thymus and concerned with cell immunity, and B cells, which are bone marrow–related and produce circulating antibodies while working with T cells in the immune process (Thibodeau and Patton, 1993). Normally, 80% of lymphocytes are T cells and most of the remaining cells are B cells. The effect of age on total lymphocyte counts is not evident,

◣ *Table 5-2*	Special Considerations for Laboratory Testing in the Aged
Test	**Cautions***
Hemoglobin	Just because hemoglobin declines with age, do not assume a low hemoglobin is normal in an elder. When hemoglobin and hematocrits are low, look for other signs of anemia: pale skin, pale conjunctiva.
Lymphocytes	Protect elders from infection since they have fewer and weaker lymphocytes with which to fight invading organisms. Immune system changes diminish antibody-antigen response. Encourage elders to have pneumococcal, tetanus, and influenza vaccines.
BUN	A slightly elevated BUN causes no problems unless such stressors as infection or surgery are added.
Creatinine	Consider the creatinine and the creatinine clearance levels to prevent toxicity when giving drugs excreted via the urinary system.
Potassium	Avoid salt substitutes, largely composed of potassium. Teach elders to check food labels for potassium and to learn signs of hyperkalemia.
Glucose	Drugs such as alcohol, MAO inhibitors, and beta blockers can contribute to a rapid fall in glucose. A rise in glucose can quickly precipitate nonketotic hyperosmolar acidosis. A drop in glucose triggers confusion as brain cells are deprived of glucose.
Urinalysis protein	Proteinuria is more common in elders than younger adults. 1+ (30 mg/100 ml) may be of no clinical significance, but renal pathology or a urinary tract infection should be ruled out.
Glucose	Glycosuria may not occur until the plasma glucose exceeds 300 mg/100 ml. Urine glucose checks in diabetic elders are highly unreliable.
Serum albumin	Low serum albumin produces edema. If there is no liver dysfunction, teach the elder to increase protein intake by eating fish, meat, nuts, grains, peanut butter, vegetables, eggs, and milk products. Elders need more protein per kilogram of body weight than does a younger person.
Cholesterol	After menopause, women's risk of cardiovascular problems increases to the male level. Diet high in fiber and in fish oils (e.g., from tuna, salmon, sardines, trout) can lower cholesterol. Weight loss and exercise can raise HDL.

*Garner B: Guide to changing lab values in elders, *Geriatr Nurs* 10(3):144, 1989.

but studies have shown a consistent finding of an increased number of B cells in the elderly and an age-related decline in T-cell function. This decrease in T-cell function is logical because immune functions are known to diminish with age.

Monocytes. Monocytes, like neutrophils, are produced in the bone marrow and perform similarly in fighting infection. Monocytes, unlike neutrophils, have the capacity to become long-lived cells, and an increase in monocytes is seen in both sexes with aging.

Eosinophils and Basophils. Eosinophils are found in response to parasitic infection and immediate hypersensitivity reactions. Studies show adverse results with increases or decreases in both elderly men and women. Basophils also play an important role in hypersensitivity reactions. No data were found to substantiate any age-related changes in this leukocyte.

SERUM CHEMISTRY

Vitamins, minerals, and hormones circulate throughout the body, and these in combination with cellular processes influence individual function in gross and subtle ways.

Serum Iron

The most common cause of anemia in the aged is dietary deficiency of iron, especially among older individuals with low incomes and chronic disease. In addition, Chiari et al (1995) found that in the presence of acute inflammatory responses, the aged present iron-deficiency symptoms, much as those with chronic disease. In both sexes there is a progressive decrease in serum iron levels with age. In the 71- to 80-year age group, the level is 50% to 75% of that of young adults (Lipschitz, 1995). It is important to distinguish between age-related iron level decreases and anemia-related decreases, because anemia is not a normal process of aging. Disease states and dietary deficiencies contribute to anemia. In the elderly, changes in serum iron may reflect blood loss from the gastrointestinal tract, decreased erythropoiesis, overall reduction of hemopoietic reserve, the presence of inflammatory disease, neoplastic disease, or use of anticoagulant, antiinflammatory, or nonsteroidal drugs. Serum iron level appraisal is particularly important for the aged, because inadequate consumption of iron-rich foods, poor appetites, chronic blood loss, and poor absorption of iron are commonly found in elderly patients both in and out of long-term care facilities. This places the older person at risk for developing iron-deficiency anemia. Serum iron values should be interpreted along with total iron binding capacity (TIBC) and the serum ferritin level (Sehy, 1995).

Vitamin B$_{12}$

Vitamin B$_{12}$ deficiency and folic acid deficiency should also be recognized as causes for anemia in the elderly. Sometimes these vitamin deficiencies are overlooked as a cause of anemia even though the clinical signs and symptoms are present. Vitamin B$_{12}$ has been shown to decrease with advancing age (Kane et al, 1994). This implied reduction of B$_{12}$ in tissues is possibly caused by impaired B$_{12}$ absorption with age. This malabsorption might be caused by decreased intrinsic factor secretion from atrophic gastritis and, in fact, low vitamin B$_{12}$ levels (less than 221 pmol/L) following gastric surgery support this supposition (Sumner et al, 1996). In the seventh decade of life, vitamin B$_{12}$ levels are 60% to 80% of those in young adults (Small and Damon, 1996). Although a direct relationship between low vitamin B$_{12}$ values and poor nutrition has been shown (Roe, 1992), long-term studies show age-related decline in vitamin B$_{12}$ values when young and old have comparable dietary intake (Small and Damon, 1996). Undiagnosed pernicious anemia in the aged is thought to afflict as many as 800,000 elders (Carmel, 1996).

Vitamin B$_{12}$ deficiency may create neurologic problems that become irreversible if not promptly treated. Low levels of vitamin B$_{12}$ and folate may be exhibited by clinical signs and symptoms of reversible dementia (Riggs et al, 1996). It is recommended that vitamins B$_{12}$, B$_6$, folate, and homocysteine deficiencies be given more attention as possible contributors to cognitive impairment (Riggs et al, 1996). Vitamin B$_{12}$ deficiency has also been found to depress left ventricular cardiac function (Herzlich, 1996).

Folic Acid

Folic acid deficiency is more commonly dietary in origin than is vitamin B$_{12}$ deficiency. This may result from antifolic agents such as trimethoprim-sulfamethoxazole, alcohol, or anticonvulsants. Other causes of folic acid deficiency are tropical sprue and inflammatory involvement of the bowel. Clinical features of folic acid deficiency include glossitis, organic brain syndrome, and megaloblastic anemia (Rossman, 1986).

Endocrine

The normal aging process causes a number of alterations in hormone production, secretion, and biologic effect. Therefore proper diagnosis and treatment of endocrine problems are especially critical for the aged. Demers (1988) states that the use of age-related reference ranges should facilitate the interpretation of laboratory results in aged persons with subtle manifestations of endocrine disease (Staab and Lyles, 1990) In addition, the normal aging changes in renal, pulmonary, gonadal, gastrointestinal, and hepatic systems complicate endocrine test result interpretation.

Thyroid. The endocrine gland that has been the subject of most studies is the aging thyroid. There is a strong argument for screening for thyroid disease in those elders who visit their physicians for unrelated thyroid reasons and for those admitted to a hospital geriatric unit. Thyroid laboratory tests frequently are the only clinical tool for diagnosing hyperthyroidism and hypothyroidism since the nonspecific symptoms such as mental clouding, cold tolerance, poor appetite, and constipation are features common to the normal aging process. There is much supported evidence of the normal functional decrease of activity in the thyroid in the elderly population. Solomon (1995b) estimated the production rate of thyroid hormone decreased by 50% between 20 and 80 years of age. Laboratory tests play an important role in aiding diagnosis of thyroid function in the elderly. In the interpretation of thyroid function, T_4, T_3, T_3 uptake, TSH, and thyrotropin-releasing hormone (TRH) levels are very useful. The effects of aging should be considered when establishing these reference values, since established values based on a young adult population are inappropriate.

Hypothyroidism. Hypothyroidism is a systemic disorder that results in the decreased secretion of thyroid hormones because of loss of functional cells and metabolic changes. Signs and symptoms of this disorder vary with the severity of the disease. These include lethargy, weakness, dry atrophic skin, poor memory, constipation, and intolerance to cold. The first subtle presentation of hypothyroidism in the elderly may be mild psychic disturbances such as withdrawal, depression, and mild forms of dementia. Other atypical signs and symptoms such as fecal impaction, elevations in plasma, cholesterol, or triglycerides, macrocytic anemia, and congestive heart failure may be clinical indications of hypothyroidism in the older adult (Felicetta, 1987) (Box 5-1). The aged adult may also develop incontinence, decreased mobility, and falls (Solomon, 1995a).

There are a number of causes of hypothyroidism, but the most common is the idiopathic atrophy of the gland. This thyroid gland failure is found more frequently in patients above the age of 50 years and deserves special consideration. At present, idiopathic atrophy is poorly understood.

Hyperthyroidism. Hyperthyroidism is found more frequently in younger populations, but 10% to 15% of hyperthyroid patients are over 60 years of age (Shoback and Jaffe, 1996). This disease occurs when tissues are exposed to excessive quantities of thyroid hormones. Signs and symptoms include lack of energy, easy fatigability, heat intolerance, tachycardia, palpitations, weight loss, weakness, emotional lability, and increased systolic blood pressure. Diagnosis of hyperthyroidism is difficult in the elderly for several reasons: (1) the patient presents fewer diagnostic clues, (2) other existing diseases may mask symptoms, and (3) symptoms that are present in young people with hyperthyroidism may be absent in older adults. Confirmation of the diagnosis of hyperthyroidism relies heavily on laboratory test results.

Thyroxine. Thyroxine (T_4) is quantitatively the predominant thyroid hormone. This hormone level is easily estimated and is the most useful test for thyroid status. Increased levels are found in thyrotoxicosis and hyperthyroidism and decreased levels in hypothyroidism. Hormone studies have shown that circulating T_4 decreases modestly with age as lean body mass declines (Solomon, 1995b). This may lead to reduced use and catabolism of thyroid hor-

mones, with subsequent rise in thyroid hormone levels caused by reduced metabolism of the aging thyroid, where most of T_4 is produced.

Triiodothyronine. Triiodothyronine (T_3) is present in much smaller amounts than T_4 and comes from the peripheral deiodination of T_4. Only about 20% is derived by direct secretion of the thyroid gland. This test, along with a free thyroxine index (FTI), is routinely done for the diagnosis of thyrotoxicosis. T_3 levels are also an important diagnostic tool for the detection of hyperthyroidism. Sometimes T_3 levels are elevated in this disease even when T_4 levels are normal. It is thought that T_3 may really be the primary hormone rather than T_4 since most of T_4 is converted to T_3 and binds more easily with T_4 (Thibodeau and Patton, 1993).

Age-related decrease in T_3 levels average about 20%; this remains within the normal range (Shoback and Jaffe, 1996). This decrease was from 10% to 50%, depending on the study. Rochman (1988) showed that male T_3 levels decreased at age 60 years, whereas females did not show a consistent decrease until 70 to 80 years. This normal decrease in T_3 levels in the aged would make diagnosis of mild hyperthyroidism difficult to detect. This is just one example of the need for age-related values to be carefully considered when diagnosing the elderly.

T_3 uptake tests. The T_3 uptake test alone is not a very useful tool for a patient's thyroid status, but used in conjunction with other thyroid tests, especially FTI, it is beneficial in diagnosis.

Thyroid-stimulating hormone. Thyroid-stimulating hormone (TSH) is involved with the acceleration of metabolism of the thyroid gland. This includes the production and secretion of thyroid hormones. The most sensitive indicator of hypothyroidism is the TSH test (Tal, 1990). In primary hypothyroidism there is a marked elevation of TSH (Solomon, 1995b). Thyroid testing in asymptomatic women over the age of 60 is especially warranted because a high prevalence, an estimated 15%, of these women have an elevated serum TSH concentration (Gallo, Reichel and Anderson, 1995).

Thyrotropin-releasing hormone. When thyrotropin is injected intravenously, it stimulates the release of TSH and prolactin from the anterior pituitary. This stimulation test is used as a discriminating diagnostic assessment for patients with either pituitary or hypothalamic dysfunction. It has been shown that there is a decrease in pituitary secretion of TSH in response to administration of thyrotropin-releasing hormone in healthy elderly men (Rochman, 1988). Since this reaction is commonly found in older men, it may erroneously indicate hyperthyroidism when, in fact, the patient is healthy. Practitioner awareness of age-related values for TSH would help avoid misdiagnosis.

BLOOD CHEMISTRY

Blood chemistry studies form a profile of the characteristics and properties of the circulating plasma, and elements and

Box 5-1	**Standard Clinical Findings of Hypothyroidism and Hyperthyroidism in the Elderly**

Hypothyroidism	**Hyperthyroidism**
General	
Fatigue	Sullen lethargy
Anorexia	Anorexia
Weight loss/gain	Weight loss
Loss of initiative	Goiter*
Confusion	Confusion
Withdrawal	
Nervous system	
Seizures	Nervousness*
Altered cerebellar functioning	Tremulousness
Dementia	Agitation
Mild psychotic disturbance	
Depression	
Gastrointestinal system	
Constipation	Constipation
Fecal impaction	
Musculoskeletal	
Myalgia	Muscle weakness
Decreased mobility	
Falls	
Genitourinary	
Incontinence	
Cardiovascular	
Syncope	Tachycardia*
Congestive heart failure	Palpitations
	Arrhythmias
	Congestive heart failure
	Increased angina
Sensory	
Cold intolerance	Decreased heat tolerance
Reduced aural acuity	Exopthalmos*
Integument	
Dry skin	Moist, flushed skin*
Coarse, dry thickened hair	Fine, smooth hair
Eyebrows sparse, loss of outer $1/3$ margins	
Facial and leg pitting or nonpitting edema	
Laboratory data	
Elevated plasma cholesterol	Thyroxine (T_4) elevated
Elevated triglycerides	Triiodothyronine elevated
Thyroxine (T_4) low	
TSH elevated	

*These symptoms may or may not be present in the aged.

Modified from Solomon DH: Age-related endocrine and metabolic changes: the normal and diseased thyroid gland. In Abrams WB, Beers MH, Berkow R, editors: *The Merck manual of geriatrics,* ed 2, Whitehouse Station, NJ, 1995, Merck Research Laboratories; Staab AS, Hodges LC: *Essentials of gerontological nursing: adaptation to the aging process,* Philadelphia, 1996, JB Lippincott Co.

particles of the blood: glucose, proteins, amino acids, nutritive materials, excretion products, hormones, enzymes, vitamins, and minerals. Those conveying significant diagnostic information will be discussed.

Glucose

Glucose metabolism changes with increasing age (Sehy, 1995). Factors that may contribute to decreasing glucose values in the aged are the increase in adiposity and decrease in lean body mass without significant change in total body weight. Also, physical activity is known to enhance the sensitivity of insulin. Unfortunately, older people tend to have a sedentary lifestyle. It is difficult to form a definitive diagnosis of diabetes in the elderly because of the deterioration in glucose metabolism that occurs with aging. To determine whether or not decreasing glucose values are the result of the aging process or diabetes mellitus of the non–insulin dependent type (type II) creates a dilemma for treatment. This is where the oral glucose tolerance test (OGTT) is helpful for diagnosis. The blood sugar value along with symptoms of thirst, polyuria, and weight loss with glycosuria should be sufficient to confirm the diagnosis of type II diabetes. The signs and symptoms of diabetes in the elderly are seen in Box 5-2.

Oral Glucose Tolerance Test. The OGTT is a standard method used to evaluate individuals by measurement of plasma glucose before and after a specific amount of glucose is given orally. This test produces a high peak at 1 to 2 hours in the older adult. Aging does result in higher "normal" values for OGTT (Sehy, 1995). Possible explanations for increases of the OGTT may be age-related insulin changes: impaired insulin catabolism, insulin may be less active, and the ability of insulin to respond to stress may be reduced. Cavalieri et al (1992) present a general rule of thumb for adopting the 2-hour postprandial blood sugar results for patients over 40 years of age (Box 5-3). "A 2-hour postprandial blood sugar should not exceed 140 mg/dl in patients under age 40 and should not exceed 100 plus the patients' age in patients over age 40" (Cavalieri et al, 1992, p. 69). Sehy (1995) suggests impaired glucose tolerance is present when the 2-hour postprandial blood sugar is 140-200 mg/dL. This, however, is not considered diabetes in the aged. Diabetes is acknowledged when the postprandial blood sugar is greater than or equal to 200 mg/dL on at least two occasions.

Creatine Phosphokinase (Creatine Kinase)

Data on age-related laboratory values are important tools for nurses who are caring for the elderly. Fractionated creatine phosphokinase (CPK; CK) values are especially important in aiding the diagnosis of myocardial infarction in the elderly whose clinical symptoms of intense dyspnea, syncope, and weakness are typically different from those of younger patients (Anderson and Braun, 1995). The current standard for diagnosis of a myocardial infarction for any strata of the

population is the fractionated CK isoenzyme (MB). Increased CPK values are usually seen with myocardial infarctions in younger adults. Total values of CPK may not be abnormally elevated in older adults (Anderson and Braun, 1995). Because their symptoms may be obscure, elders may not seek care within the "time window" in which CPK isoenzyme (MB) will be elevated. This is when CPK isoenzyme separation becomes necessary to confirm myocardial infarction. Age- and sex-adjusted normal ranges should be used when interpreting the older person's CPK values.

Alkaline Phosphatase

Another important enzyme test for aiding diagnosis and identifying treatable bone disease is the serum alkaline phosphatase. Alkaline phosphatase gradually increases with age in both men and women. The increase is more marked in women (Table 5-1). In healthy older adults the normal

---

Box 5-2	**Signs and Symptoms Suggestive of Diabetes in the Elderly**

1. General symptoms such as polyphagia, polyuria, polydipsia, and weight loss.
2. Recurrent infections, particularly, bacterial/fungal origin, that involves the skin, intertriginous areas, or urinary tract and sores/wounds that tend to heal slowly.
3. Neurologic dysfunction including paresthesia, dysethesia or hyperesthesia; muscle weakness and pain (amotrophy); cranial nerve palsies; and autonomic dysfunction of the gastrointestinal tract (diarrhea); cardiovascular system (orthostatic hypotension, arrhythmias), reproductive system (impotence), and bladder (atony, overflow incontinence).
4. Arterial disease (macroangiopathy) involving the cardiovascular, cerebral vascular, or peripheral vasculature.
5. Small-vessel disease (microangiopathy) involving the kidneys (proteinuria, glomerulopathy, uremia) and eyes (macular disease, exudates, hemorrhages).
6. Lesions of the skin, such as Dupuytren's contractures, facial rubeosis, and diabetic dermopathy.
7. Endocrine-metabolic complications, including hyperlipidemia, obesity, and a history of thyroid or adrenal insufficiency (Schmidt's syndrome).
8. A family history of non-insulin or insulin-dependent diabetes and a poor obstetric history (miscarriages, stillbirths, large babies).

From Andres R, Bierman E, Hazzard W: *Principles of geriatric medicine,* New York, 1985, McGraw-Hill; Davidson MB: Diabetes mellitus and other disorders of carbohydrate metabolism. In Abrams WB, Beers MH, Berkow R, editors: *The Merck manual of geriatrics,* ed 2, Whitehouse Station, NJ, 1995, Merck Research Laboratories.

values may be one to one and one-half times the standard normal value (Lonergan, 1996; Kane et al, 1994). This increase is related to extrahepatic sources such as renal insufficiency, bone disorders, and malabsorption.

Lactate Dehydrogenase

Lactate dehydrogenase (LDH) is present in all metabolizing cells but at higher levels in heart, liver, kidney, brain, and skeletal muscle. Damage to any of these tissues will cause release of the LDH enzyme. Highest values are seen with myocardial infarction, hemolytic disorders, and pernicious anemia.

Alanine Aminotransferase/Serum Glutamic Pyruvic Transaminase (ALAT, previously SGPT)

ALAT is found mainly in the liver and is a specific and sensitive index of acute hepatocellular injury. ALAT is also present in the kidney, heart, and skeletal muscles; the release of this enzyme indicates tissue injury.

Aspartate Aminotransferase/Serum Glutamic Oxaloacetic Transaminase (AST, previously SGOT)

Aspartate aminotransferase (AST) is found primarily in heart and skeletal muscle, liver, kidney, pancreas, and red blood cells. Increased levels indicate cellular damage or myocardial infarction, hepatitis, liver necrosis, and skeletal muscle damage.

Laboratory values for LDH, ALAT, and AST may significantly change with normal aging, although additional research is needed in this area. Values of these enzymes are used to determine the functional status of the organs mentioned and the presence of disease. All three of these enzyme levels may need to be appraised to determine the nature of a problem and to rule out hepatic origin of the enzymes.

Serum Albumin

The reduction of serum albumin has been related to decreased liver size, enzyme production, and blood flow in older adults. Albumin concentrations decline in both men and women with increasing age. A recent study by McMurtry and Rosenthal (1995) showed that among elderly veterans on a rehabilitation unit a strong predictor of mortality was a reduced serum albumin level of less than 3.5 g/dL.

A low serum albumin level may be an indicator of malnutrition in the elderly. A serum albumin level of less than 3.5 g/dL is a criterion for justifying a diagnosis of malnutrition serious enough to qualify for Medicare or Medicaid care reimbursement (Gilmore et al, 1995). However, a normal or increased serum albumin level alone does not ensure the nutritional adequacy of an older adult (Kane et al, 1994). A thorough nutritional screening along with laboratory values is essential for assessing the nutritional status of an elder.

Pressure ulcer development and low serum albumin levels have been positively correlated. A diet deficient in protein places the older adult at risk for pressure ulcers, wound infection, and delayed healing. The elderly who have stage II, III, or IV pressure ulcers should have albumin levels monitored routinely to determine effectiveness of the dietary and nursing care therapeutic regimen (Pajk, 1995).

Cholesterol

Cholesterol levels have been reported to gradually increase with age in both men and women. Women have higher levels of HDL in all age groups. Postmenopausal women have a drop in estrogen that triggers a rise in cholesterol (Sehy, 1995). With changes in lipid metabolism, cholesterol rises to a maximum at age 65 and then decreases, but never as low as that of young adults. Total cholesterol is an excellent measure of coronary risk though almost half of the people who suffer myocardial infarcts have a total cholesterol level of 200 mg/dl or less. Fractionization into the dominant hypopolar fractions HDL, LDL, and very low density lipoprotein (VLDL) yield more accurate and sophisticated indices of risk factors that can be monitored and quantitated during therapy. The LDL and HDL fractions in combination with systolic blood pressure are significant in predicting coronary disease risk in the elderly. These levels are used as indicators of risk and may be decreased by diet and exercise (Andres et al, 1985).

Recently questions have arisen regarding the importance, or even the advisability, of pharmacologic intervention in hypercholesterolemia for individuals over 70 years old. Speechley et al (1995) caution that single total cholesterol levels are unreliable for diagnostic purposes. In a study of 142 patients there was a misclassification rate of 22.5%, and for those in the high cholesterolemia group the false-positive rate reached 50%. Misclassification rates did not differ statistically on the basis of sex, blood pressure, smoking history, diabetes, obesity, or the laboratory that was used. The conclusion is that even when subjects are fasting, single readings are insufficient, and the recommendation is that cholesterol readings be taken at different times 1 to 8 weeks apart. These findings add further weight to the emerging interest in the chronotherapeutic approaches to assessment and care. See Chapter 9 for further discussion of chronotherapeutics.

Triglycerides

Triglyceride values gradually increase with age until about middle age. The increase is greater in females than males after age 50. As the male ages, values stay elevated or drop slightly, whereas the female values, which rose slowly until age 50, continue to rise but more rapidly due to the decline in estrogen (Hazzard et al, 1995). With age, women have significantly higher levels than younger females. Abnormal triglyceride levels may indicate alcohol abuse or diabetes; these should be considered when determining a course of action.

Calcium and Phosphorus (Phosphate)

Calcium and phosphorus levels decline in men with age. In women calcium levels remain constant and phosphorus levels seem to increase with age. The effects of postmenopausal estrogen replacement is an important ingredient when deciding on reference values for calcium in women. The age- and sex-related reference values for both phosphorus and calcium remain to be investigated. However, the metabolic companion of calcium, vitamin D, is known to be frequently deficient in the healthy aged and most particularly in the institutionalized aged (Keane et al, 1995; Gloth and Tobin, 1995). Factors such as reduced exposure to sunlight, use of sunscreens, and as yet unknown factors contribute to this deficiency (Pogue, 1995).

Uric Acid

Age-related changes in uric acid show an increase, particularly in women. This change occurs between 40 and 50 years and is related to the hormonal shifts in menopause. Males, at all ages, have higher uric acid levels than females but have a less dramatic increase as they age (McCance and Capriano,1994). It is suggested that the upper limit of reference values for older adults be 7.7 mg/dL (Sack, 1996). Thiazide diuretics are the most common cause for increased uric acid levels in older adults (Jeppesen, 1986). Drugs, obesity, and hypertension have all been associated with significant elevations in uric acid. Attacks of gout have been related to increases in uric acid. Gout is the formation of needlelike monosodium urate crystals in joints. These crystals cause inflammation and discomfort and if not treated will incapacitate the older person (Sack, 1996). Environmental stressors such as trauma, fatigue, cold, and surgery have been associated with acute attacks of gout. Dietary indulgences in foods with glutamic acid must also be considered. Gout becomes a chronic and painful condition in the aged.

Prostate-Specific Antigen

Prostate cancer is the second most common type of cancer found in men, occurring in 50% of those over 70 years of age. Until recently, digital rectal examination was the most accurate diagnostic modality for detection of early stage prostatic cancer. The biochemical markers available to monitor this disease, prostatic acid phosphatase, total alkaline phosphatase, and carcinoembryonic antigen are not specific for prostate cancer.

Prostate-specific antigen (PSA) has been identified as specific for prostatic tissue, both normal and malignant. PSA is not present in any other normal tissue obtained from men. It lacks any acid phosphatase activity and does not react with its antibodies; therefore it is biochemically and immunologically distinct from prostatic acid phosphatase. PSA is a secretion of prostate epithelium and is also produced by prostate cancer cells. Elevated serum PSA concentrations have been reported in patients with prostate cancer, benign prostatic hypertrophy, or inflammatory conditions of other adjacent genitourinary tissues. The PSA test is only 33% specific for early prostate cancer detection, too low to be considered for widespread screening. However, research indicates that PSA may serve as an accurate marker for assessing response to treatment in patients with stages B2 and D1 prostatic cancer. Several measurements of PSA concentrations can be an important test in monitoring patients with prostatic cancer and in determining the potential and actual effectiveness of surgery and other therapies (Bruskewitz, 1995).

Blood Urea and Creatinine

Blood urea has been reported to remain unchanged with age in both men and women (Anderson and Braun, 1995). Hale et al (1983) suggested that blood urea increases with age. Kidney size and volume decrease with age, and values of creatinine increase. Serum creatinine and blood urea follow a similar pattern of increase in the aged, although there is a smaller increase with age but a larger sex-related difference in serum creatinine values. Large increases indicate renal failure. Blood urea and serum creatinine levels are both related to renal function and glomerular filtration rate. Dietary intake of protein, metabolism, and previous physical activity contribute to the increase in these values along with the reduction in lean body mass. Since serum creatinine levels can overestimate renal function in the elderly, serum creatinine values must be related to the creatinine clearance values for a true assessment of renal function.

URINE TESTS

Urine is the fluid that carries waste products from the body as they are filtered from the blood through the kidneys. Abnormal constituents form a picture of aberrant internal processes. A summary of normal values and their clinical significance can be seen in Table 5-3 (Brazier and Palmer, 1995).

Urinalysis

Most urinalysis values do not change with advancing age. Specific gravity is a simple test that measures the density of urine relative to the density of water. This test is helpful in determining the adequacy of the renal concentrative mechanism. Specific gravity declines to 1.024 by the age of 80 (Eliopoulos, 1995; Miller, 1995). This decline has been related to the 33% to 50% decline in the number of nephrons, which impairs the ability of the kidney to concentrate urine (see Chapter 4). Lower maximum values for specific gravity should be evaluated and diets of low sodium and protein restriction instituted when necessary, or the use of diuretics may need to be considered. The limitations of specific gravity testing need to be considered when using this test as a diagnostic tool. "Glucose and protein may contribute substantial increments to the density of urine and semiquantitative

Table 5-3   Urinalysis: A Summary of Normal Values and Their Clinical Significance in the Elderly

Determination	Normal value	Clinical significance
Macroscopic analysis		
Color	Pale yellow to dark amber	Very pale: diabetes insipidus, excess fluid intake, chronic renal disease, nervousness. Very amber: dehydration. Note: Medications may alter color
Appearance	Clear to slightly hazy	Cloudy, turbid: presence of bacteria, WBCs or RBCs
Odor	Faintly aromatic	Fetid odor: bacterial infection Ammonia: Urea breakdown by bacteria
Specific gravity	1.017-1.028	Decreased: over hydration; diabetes insipidus; diet (NA, PRO restriction) Elevated: ↓ fluid intake; fever; diabetes mellitus.♦ Note: lower maximum value in the elderly
pH	4.5-8.0	>8.0: bacterial infection due to *Pseudomonas* or *Proteus,* chronic renal failure <4.5: metabolic/respiratory acidosis, starvation
Protein	Negative	Increased: renal disease, cardiac failure, febrile states, hematuria, amyloidosis
Glucose	Negative	Positive: uncontrolled diabetes mellitus; pituitary disorders; ↑ intracranial pressure. ♦ Renal threshold for glucose rises after age 50, ♀ > ♂.
Ketones	Negative	Positive: uncontrolled diabetes mellitus; prolonged vomiting; fasting
Blood	Negative	Positive: infection, renal calculus
Bilirubin	Negative	Positive: liver dysfunction
Nitrite	Negative	Positive: bacterial infection
Leukocyte esterase	Negative	Positive: pyuria
Microscopic Analysis		
RBCs	Rare per high-power field	Increased: renal genitourinary disorders
WBCs	0-4 per high-power field	Increased: bacterial infection ♦ note always a reliable indicator of infection in the elderly; if clinically asymptomatic, is not significant
Epithelial Cells	0-3	Increased: probable perineal contamination
Casts	Rare per high-power field	Increased: renal disease
Bacteria	<105 colonies/ml	Increased: bacterial infection ♦ significance is dependent upon specimen collection technique and specific gravity of sample

From Brazier AM, Palmer MH: Collecting clean-catch urine in the nursing home: obtaining the uncontaminated specimen, *Geriatr Nurs* 16(5):217, 1995.

determination of these substances is necessary for valid interpretation or correction of urine specific gravity measurements" (Rock et al, 1986, p. 1299). Protein rises slightly with age, and proteinuria is very common in elders but may be of no clinical significance. However, urinary tract infections and renal pathology should be ruled out. Ketones, blood, and glucose should all remain negative at any age.

Creatinine Clearance

Creatinine clearance is a test used to estimate glomerular filtration rate as an indicator of glomerular function. This test is a more reliable measure of renal function than blood urea nitrogen (BUN) or serum creatinine (Anderson and Braun, 1995). Since urine collection is a problem with the elderly and a complete and timed collection is essential for accuracy of this test, catheterization may be necessary. There is a steady decrease in functioning of the kidney despite good health or absence of disease. Anatomic changes in the kidney along with degenerative changes in other organs affect renal function in the aged. Nurses should be aware of the impact of these changes when evaluating laboratory values. Studies of 24-hour urinary creatinine clearance tests show a progressive decline with age, 10% per decade after age 40 (Anderson and Braun, 1995). The average creatinine clear-

ance excretion rate declines from about 24 mg/kg per 24 hours in persons 18 to 29 years of age to about 12 mg/kg per 24 hours in those 80 to 90 years of age.

There are factors that influence accurate measurement of creatinine clearance in the elderly. One is that older persons usually have chronic diseases and are receiving medications regularly. Often the amount of medication prescribed has not been altered to compensate for the decrease in renal function seen with aging. Creatinine clearance values must be considered when deciding medication dosages to avoid miscalculations in drug administration when creatinine clearance values are abnormal. It is always wise to start with the lowest dose and progress slowly according to the elder's response to drug therapy. Another factor is that the amount of creatinine produced per day is changed by the relationship between increased body weight and decreased muscle mass discussed earlier. This may further reduce creatinine clearance.

Bacteriuria

Both men and women are subject to bacteriuria, men due to bladder outlet obstruction from benign prostatic hypertrophy (BPH). In women there is often a decrease due to the decrease in sexual activity, which is a source of bacterial introduction into the bladder (Bruskewitz, 1995). The incidence of bacteriuria in young adults is less than 5% in females and .1% for males. However, from 20% to 50% of women over 80 years old have bacteriuria, and many of those are asymptomatic (Tronetti et al, 1990). Bacteriuria is common in the elderly, especially functionally impaired female nursing home residents (Anderson and Braun, 1995). From 10% to 50% of them have asymptomatic bacteruria. Asymptomatic bacteriuria is defined as having a urine culture with greater than or equal to 10^5 colony-forming units (CFU) per milliliter of urine without clinical signs and symptoms of urinary tract infection (Boscia et al, 1986). Clinicians and researchers agree that typical signs and symptoms of urinary tract infection such as incontinence, urgency, frequency, fever, flank pain, or suprapubic pain are usually nonexistent in the elderly population. This is why urinalysis is an imperative screening test.

Studies investigating the treatment of asymptomatic bacteriuria have not been conclusive. Though antimicrobial therapy is often not recommended, the presence of bacteria must be identified and measures instituted to prevent recurrence (Travis and Lampley-Dallas, 1997). It is not advisable to treat persons with indwelling catheters who have asymptomatic bacteriuria because recolonization rapidly develops after treatment. Therefore it is best to avoid the use of catheters unless it is a medical necessity and to avoid antimicrobial therapy unless necessary to decrease mortality from potential urosepsis (Bruskewitz, 1995; Staab and Hodges, 1996). More research is needed before clinicians can unquestionably know whether to treat or not to treat asymptomatic bacteriuria.

ELECTROLYTES

The elderly are susceptible to electrolyte imbalances because of medications and poor fluid intake. The one of most significance is potassium level (Videback and Ackermann, 1993). Other electrolyte imbalances do not have an age-frequency distribution.

Potassium

Potassium is the electrolyte in highest concentration within cells and is the chief intracellular cation. Serum potassium levels remain constant until the sixth decade, when an age-related increase occurs (Kane et al, 1994; Staab and Hodges, 1996). In addition, up to 30% of patients in geriatric long-term care units may have abnormal potassium levels because of dietary insufficiency, continued use of diuretics or laxatives, or the occurrence of diarrhea or diabetic acidosis (Miller, 1995).

Hypokalemia. Hypokalemia is important to recognize in elderly patients since it is associated with cardiac arrhythmias and may cause glucose intolerance and renal tubular dysfunction. It also potentiates digitalis toxicity (Miller, 1995). Hypokalemia is exhibited at the cellular level by a shift of potassium from the extracellular to the intracellular compartment, which decreases potassium plasma concentration. Apathy, nonspecific weakness, and confusion are symptoms of minor hypokalemia. Chronic hypokalemia may lead to significant renal tubular dysfunction. If discovered early, it may be treated; if not treated quickly, the dysfunction is irreversible.

Hyperkalemia. Hyperkalemia is most commonly exhibited by a shift of potassium from the intracellular to the extracellular compartment, which increases the plasma concentration. A decrease in pH (acidosis) causes potassium to migrate out of cells, resulting in an increase in plasma levels, whereas an increase in pH (alkalosis) causes the potassium to migrate into the cells, resulting in a decrease in plasma levels (Brocklehurst, 1985). A common cause of hyperkalemia in the elderly is the concurrent use of potassium-sparing diuretics with prescribed potassium supplements, nonsteroidal antiinflammatory drugs, angiotensin-converting enzyme (ACE) inhibitors, and beta-blocking drugs (Miller, 1995). Hyperkalemia is found most frequently in renal failure, and there is usually an elevation in blood urea. Marked hyperkalemia produces severe neuromuscular and cardiac dysfunction. For specific causes and clinical manifestations of hypokalemia and hyperkalemia, see Boxes 5-3 and 5-4.

Hyponatremia

In an ambulatory geriatric population of 405 elders it was found that more than 1% demonstrated hyponatremia with serum sodium levels of less than 125 mEq/L. About half of these were very old and had apparently developed the syndrome of inappropriate antidiuretic hormone secretion (SIADH) (Miller et al, 1996). The conclusion from these studies was that aging is a risk factor for the development of SIADH-like hyponatremia in some very old who do not have an apparent underlying etiology.

ARTERIAL BLOOD GASES

Many studies show significant decrease in Po_2 with age. The age-related changes in the lungs—decreased lung elasticity, vascular bed resistance, decreased alveolar surface area, and pulmonary rigidity—along with hematologic changes explicate this decrease of oxygen (Cavalieri et al, 1992). Po_2 decreases approximately 25% between age 30 and age 80. The way to calculate age-appropriate Po_2 levels for the older adult appears in Box 5-5.

LONG-TERM CARE

Admission laboratory tests and regular screening tests are commonly employed when caring for a nursing home resident. Laboratory tests are often viewed positively by both nurses and physicians in long-term care because they are a fast and accurate way to assess the older person's physical status. Older adults and their families view the tests as

Box 5-3	Causes of Hypokalemia and Hyperkalemia

Hypokalemia	**Hyperkalemia**
	Intake
Decreased intake	Increased intake or intravenous administration
Increased secretions	
	Gastrointestinal losses
Vomiting	Active gastrointestinal bleeding
Diarrhea or repeated enemas	
Pyloric and other forms of intestinal obstruction	
Biliary or gastrointestinal fistulas	
Suction or tube drainage	
Laxative use	
	Renal losses
Increased loss	*Decreased excretion*
Renal tubular acidosis (proximal & distal)	Acute renal disease
Thiazide diuretic use	Dyrenium diuretic therapy (triamterene)
Loop diuretic use (furosemide, bumetanide, ethacrynic acid)	Spironolactone therapy
Antibiotic use (gentamycin, penicillins, amphotericin B)	Adrenal insufficiency
Secondary hyperaldosteronism (heart failure, cirrhosis)	ACE inhibitors
Cushing's syndrome	β-Adrenergic blockers
Exogenous glucocorticoids/mineralocorticoids	NSAIDs
Hyperreninemic renovascular hypertension	Tetracycline
Post obstructive diuresis	
Chronic renal insufficiency	
	Transcellular shifts
Alkalosis	Metabolic acidosis
Insulin administration	Hyponatremia (potassium moves out of cell to replace sodium)
β-Adrenergic agonists	Anorexia
	Hemotologic disorders
Vitamin B_{12} treatment of megaloblastic anemia	
Acute myeloid leukemia	
	Miscellaneous
Acidosis of any cause	
Trauma or burns with tissue breakdown	
Intravenous administration of potassium-free liquid	

Adapted from Collins R: *Fluid and electrolyte disorders,* Philadelphia, 1976; JB Lippincott, Miller M: Water and electrolyte disorders. In Abrams WB, Beers MH, Berkow R, editors: *The Merck manual of geriatrics,* ed 2, Whitehouse Station, 1995, NJ, Merck Research Laboratories.

factual presentations of their conditions. Protocols for establishing routine laboratory testing procedures for long-term care vary widely from one institution to the next. Nurses advocate good resident care by encouraging physicians to order and develop protocols to comply with recommended minimal standards for screening and monitoring laboratory tests for elderly in long-term care institutions. Nursing homes generally use laboratory testing to screen for new disease, unsuspected conditions, and to monitor drug effects and chronic conditions (Joseph and Lyles, 1992).

In 1980 the Department of Health and Human Services established guidelines for drug regimen reviews in nursing homes. However, no specific laboratory tests are recommended for screening or monitoring in the new federal regulations under the Omnibus Budget Reconciliation Act of 1987 (Joseph and Lyles, 1992). At least annually we recommend a urinalysis, CBC (complete blood count), serum electrolytes, urea nitrogen, creatinine, glucose, thyroxine levels, and FTI for elderly patients in long-term care institutions. All of these tests are useful in maintaining the maximum health of an elderly population in a long-term

Box 5-4	Clinical Manifestations of Hypokalemia and Hyperkalemia

Hypokalemia	Hyperkalemia
Generalized muscle weakness	Impaired muscle activity
Fatigue	Weakness
Diminished or absent reflexes	Muscle pain/cramps
Decreased GI motility	Increased GI motility
Anorexia	Nausea
Abdominal distention	Diarrhea
Paralytic ileus	Intestinal colic
Vomiting	Oliguria
Hypotension	Dizziness
Dysrhythmias	Bradycardia
Weak pulse	Irritability
Shallow respirations	EKG changes:
Shortness of breath	P wave flattened
Apathy	T wave large, peaked
Drowsiness	QRS broad
Irritability	
Tentany	
Coma	
EKG changes:	
QT interval prolonged	
T wave flattened or depressed	
ST segment depressed	

Modified from: Miller M: Water and electrolyte disorders. In Abrams WB, Beers MH, Berkow R, editors: *The Merck manual of geriatrics,* Whitehouse Station, NJ, 1995, Merck Research Laboratories; Clark JM: Endocrine clinical assessment and diagnostic procedures. In Thelan LA, Davie JK, Urden LD, Lough ME: *Critical care nursing diagnosis and management,* ed 2, St Louis, 1994, Mosby.

Box 5-5	Useful Formulas for Calculating Lab Values in the Elderly

Arterial oxygen

$$PaO \text{ (mm Hg)} = 100.1 - 0.325 \times age$$

Creatinine clearance

$$Cr\ Cl = \frac{(140 - age)\ (\text{weight in Kg})}{72\ (\text{Serum creatinine})}$$

(In women multiply by 0.85)

Two hour postprandial blood sugar (2 hr PPBS) (over 40 yrs)

$$2\ hr\ PPBS = 100 + age$$

From Cavalieri T, Chopra A, Bryman P: When outside the norm is normal: interpreting lab data in the aged, *Geriatrics* 47(5):69, 1992.

g/dl, cholesterol values below 160 mg/dl, and hematocrit levels less than 39% be monitored as strong indications of malnutrition.

Older adults in long-term care institutions may be infrequently seen by a physician and are monitored daily by nursing staff. It is therefore imperative that the nurse be knowledgeable about the importance of routine and specific laboratory tests when vague and atypical signs and symptoms of disease arise.

SPECIMEN COLLECTION

Nurses in long-term care, home care, and hospitals are responsible for obtaining many laboratory specimens. The importance of meticulous specimen collection cannot be overemphasized if accurate laboratory results are to be derived.

The most important step in specimen collection is identification. Institutionalized elders should be identified by full name, and identification bands should be matched to requisition orders. Even if the nurse is familiar with the elder, do not skip the verification process. Obtaining a specimen from the wrong person can have serious, even fatal results. *Standard precautions* must be observed throughout the specimen collection process.

Phlebotomy

The main purpose of phlebotomy is to collect blood for diagnostic testing to assist physicians in establishing the cause and nature of illness. More nurses are performing phlebotomy procedures, especially in home care, health maintenance organization (HMO) clinics, and physicians' offices. This cost-containment strategy is particularly helpful to the elder in the home with limited mobility and lack of transportation to outpatient laboratory facilities (McKenna and Niles, 1995).

setting. We expect that with the upsurge of subacute units in long-term care settings and the efforts in managed care to prevent conditions from fulminating there will be considerably more attention given to monitoring and laboratory values.

Dementia is a widespread problem in long-term care. Laboratory investigators can reveal the cause of reversible dementia. Kane, Ouslander, and Abrass (1994) recommend the following laboratory tests for screening of elders with dementia: CBC, electrolytes, tests for liver and kidney function, BUN, syphilis serology, thyroid function tests, chest x-ray, urinalysis, calcium and phosphorous, serum B_{12}, folate and a Schilling test if pernicious anemia is suspected, and HIV antibodies. Additional tests should be considered when conditions warrant.

Poor dietary intake continues to be a significant problem in long-term care institutions. Protein calorie malnutrition is a major medical problem for long-term care residents (Welch, 1989). It is suggested that albumin levels below 4.0

Venipuncture involves collecting blood by penetrating a vein with a needle and syringe or vacutainer adapter with attached needle and vacuum tube. Most elders tolerate the phlebotomy process with little or no difficulty. Some people become faint at the thought of having blood drawn. There is no way to predict how someone will react to a venipuncture. Always have the individual sitting or lying down before performing the procedure.

There may be complications associated with the phlebotomy procedure. Some complications, such as bruising and hematoma, are unavoidable. Most complications can be minimized by proper collection technique and a knowledgeable nurse. The nurse performing the phlebotomy procedure should be aware of the seven precautions listed in Box 5-6.

Clean-Catch Urine Specimens

Obtaining uncontaminated urine specimens from frail, often incontinent, elders in nursing homes is a difficult task. Their ability to move about and their ability to control urine flow are often impaired. Brazier and Palmer (1995) have given very specific instructions for obtaining urine specimens in these situations. Methods are explained in detail in Tables 5-4 and 5-5.

In summary, nurses are in a primary position to note and interpret laboratory values. The aged person's changing laboratory values reflect normal aging as well as disease states. This presents a challenge for the nurse to make valid interpretations of the changing status of the older individual. The importance of laboratory testing cannot be overemphasized. Laboratory testing can be the major factor in supporting or disproving diagnoses. Many of the age-related laboratory changes are fractional. However, the clinical impact cannot be minimized.

Reference values for the aged are imperative before laboratory test results can guide treatment in the elderly. The variance of values at both ends of the laboratory range could be misinterpreted as abnormal or questionable when they are within normal range for that sex and age group. See Box 5-7 for elderly laboratory values more frequently out of the normal range. The "normal ranges" in the population over 65 years are often different from those of the younger population, and these differences should be and are being established so that we have standards to indicate real pathologic age-related differences (Boxes 5-8 and 5-9). We must not compare those patients over 65 years with those between 20 and 50 years, just as we should not compare infants with children or young adults. Each age group must have its own established norms.

Laboratory values are helpful tools in understanding clinical signs and symptoms, although clinical decisions based on laboratory values alone are not enough for treatment of the elderly. The nurse should perform a comprehensive baseline assessment of the older adult, obtaining information about clinical signs and symptoms, patient history, and psychosocial and physical assessments. The nurse synthesizes this information along with the interpretation of laboratory values to establish appropriate nursing care for the aged. This building block approach to obtaining and synthesizing information about the older adult helps nurses and other health care professionals to provide quality care for the aged.

Box 5-6 **Phlebotomy Collection Guidelines**

Never draw above an intravenous (IV) or indwelling line. There is no exception to this rule. If this is not observed, the specimens will be contaminated with IV fluid, causing erroneous results.

Do not try to obtain a specimen from a damaged or sclerosed vein. These veins are hard, and no specimen can be obtained.

Hematomas are caused by leaking from the vein underneath the skin. If this occurs, release the tourniquet and needle and apply pressure to the site. Never restick the hematoma area.

Edema is caused by abnormal accumulation of fluid in the intracellular spaces, which may be localized or diffused over a large area. Do not stick this area because specimens may be contaminated with tissue fluid.

Do not attempt a venipuncture in an area of a burn or scar. Burns are sensitive and susceptible to infections.

If the patient exhibits petechiae, which are small red spots on the skin, this should alert the nurse that this person has the potential for bleeding problems and special attention should be given to the puncture site.

Reflex sympathetic dystrophy (RSD) is a complication that can occur as a result of injury to a peripheral nerve during the venipuncture/arterial puncture procedure. The patient experiences severe pain, swelling, vasomotor instability, and sweating. This is a severe complication, and a physician should be notified immediately.

Some venipuncture specimens need to be placed on ice after collection; others need to be kept warm. There may also be a time requirement for delivery to the laboratory. Current policies, procedures, ongoing inservice training, and skills verification are necessary for nurses to be competent in obtaining laboratory specimens. The nurse should be familiar with the specimen requirements prior to performing the procedure.

Table 5-4 Technique for Obtaining Clean-Catch Midstream Voided Specimen

A clean-catch midstream specimen is the best clinically effective method of securing a voided specimen for urinalysis. It is not a simple procedure and requires patient education and active assistance of the female patient.

Equipment

Antiseptic solution or liquid soap solution	Disposable gloves for nurse assisting
Sterile water	female patient
4 × 4-inch sponges	Sterile specimen container

Procedure

Nursing action	Rational/amplification
Male patient	
1. Instruct the patient to expose glans and cleanse area around the meatus. Wash area with mild antiseptic solution or liquid soap. Rinse thoroughly.	1. The urethral orifice is colonized by bacteria. Urine readily becomes contaminated during voiding. Rinse thoroughly because these agents can inhibit bacterial growth in a urine culture.
2. Allow the initial urinary flow to escape.	2. The first portion of urine washes out the urethra and contains debris.
3. Collect the midstream urine specimen in a sterile container.	3. The midstream sample reflects the status of the bladder.
4. Avoid collecting the last few drops of urine.	4. Prostatic secretions may be introduced into urine at the end of the urinary stream.
5. Send specimen to laboratory immediately.	5. A culture should be performed as soon as possible to avoid multiplication of urinary bacteria and lysis of cells.
Female patient	
1. Ask the patient to separate her labia to expose the urethral orifice. If no one is available to assist the patient, she may sit backward on the toilet seat facing the water tank or sit on (straddle) the wide part of the bedpan.	1. Keeping the labia separated prevents labial or vaginal contamination of the urine specimen. By straddling the toilet seat/bedpan, the patient's labia are spread apart for cleansing.
2. Cleanse the area around the urinary meatus with sponges soaked with antiseptic/soap solution. Rinse thoroughly. a. Wipe the perineum from the front to the back. b. Do not use sponges more than once.	2. The urethral orifice is colonized by bacteria. Urine is readily contaminated during voiding.
3. While the patient keeps the labia separated, instruct her to void forcibly.	3. This helps wash away urethral contaminants.
4. Allow initial urinary flow to drain into bedpan (toilet) and then catch the midstream specimen in a sterile container, make sure that the container does not come in contact with the genitalia.	4. The first portion of urine washes out the urethra. Have patient remove the container from the stream while she is still voiding.
5. Send the specimen to the laboratory immediately.	5. Too long an interval between collection and analysis causes contaminants to multiply in the urine and cells to lyse.

From Suddarth D, ed, *The Lippincott manual of nursing practice,* ed 5, Philadelphia, 1991, JB Lippincott.
From Brazier AM, Palmer MH: Collecting clean-catch urine in the nursing home: obtaining the uncontaminated specimen, *Geriatr Nurs* 16(5):217, 1995.

Table 5-5 Adaptations to the Standard Guidelines for Obtaining Clean-Catch Urine Specimen in Frail Elders

Tip	Advantage (Rationale)
1. Know the patient's voiding habits by using a bladder log or by consulting the nursing assistant caring for the patient.	1. Decreases time spent in specimen collection.
2. Collect the specimen in the early morning (morning specimens are more concentrated).	2. Assures accuracy of results
3. Avoid collection after giving diuretics.	3. Assures accuracy of results (alters concentration).
4. Perform perineal care on bedridden and/or incontinent patients prior to collection.	4. Decreases risk of contamination.
5. When possible, have patients void in the bathroom, sitting upright	5. Decreases risk of contamination.
6. Use an assistant when the patient is physically impaired.	6. Decreases collection time and increases risk of contamination.
7. Hold the patient's labia apart throughout the procedure	7. Decreases risk of contamination.
8. Use distractionary tactics with the confused or embarrassed patient (speak in calm voice, singing, involve patient in conversation, use assistance of a caregiver more familiar with the patient).	8. May decrease time spent in specimen collection. Facilitates patient cooperation.
9. Ensure good lighting in bathroom with a 75-watt bulb.	9. Increases visibility. Decreases risk of contamination.
10. Prompt resident to increase fluid intake.	10. Decreases time spent in specimen collection.
11. Use physical prompts (running water, spirit of wintergreen).	11. Decreases time spent in specimen collection.
12. Utilize a portable bladder scanner to determine bladder volume prior to specimen collection.	12. Decreases time spent in specimen collection.

From Brazier AM, Palmer MH: Collecting clean-catch urine in the nursing home: obtaining the uncontaminated specimen, *Geriatr Nurs* 16(5):217, 1995.

| Box 5-7 | Lab Values Ordinarily Different from Young Adults |

- Serum alkaline phosphatase (elevations to about 2.5 times the normal)
- Fasting blood glucose (up to 135 to 150 mg/dl)
- Postprandial glucose or oral glucose tolerance test (increased above normal to 10 mg/dl per decade of age)
- Normal serum creatinine with the existence of markedly decreased creatinine clearance
- High erythrocyte sedimentation rates (up to 40 mm/hr)
- Hemoglobin (lowest acceptable level is 11.0 gm/dl in women; 11.5 gm/dl in men)
- Blood urea nitrogen (up to 28 to 35 mg/dl)

From Kelso T: Laboratory values in the elderly: are they different? *Emerg Med Clin North Am* 8 (2):241, 1990.

| Box 5-8 | Summary of Lab Values Unchanged with Age |

Serum bilirubin
AST
ALT
GGTP
PT
PTT
Serum electrolytes
Total protein
Calcium
Phosporus
Serum folate
pH
PaCo
Serum creatinine
T_4
Red blood cell indices
Platelets

Modified from Cavalieri T, Chopra A, Bryman P: When outside the norm is normal: interpreting lab data in the aged, *Geriatrics* 47(5):66, 1992.

Needs Addressed and Task Strengths

| Need to monitor health status (to maintain biologic function within safe limits) | Meticulous in following directions
Inquisitive
Confident in scientific analysis
Interest in comparisons and contrasts |

| Box 5-9 | Summary of Lab Values That Change with Age |

Alkaline phosphatase (increase)
Serum albumin (decrease)
Uric acid (increase)
Total cholesterol (increase)
    HDL
        Male (increase)
        Female (decrease)
    Triglycerides (increase)
Serum B_{12} (decrease)
Serum magnesium (decrease)
Pao (decrease)
Creatinine clearance (decrease)
T_3 (decrease)
T_4 (increase)
Fasting blood sugar (increase)
1-hour postprandial blood sugar (increase)
2-hour postprandial blood sugar (increase)
White blood cell count (decrease)

Modified from Cavalieri T, Chopra A, Bryman P: When outside the norm is normal: interpreting lab data in the aged, *Geriatrics* 47(5):66, 1992.

KEY CONCEPTS

- The range of laboratory values that are considered normal and appear on laboratory reports usually do not make allowance for age differentials.
- The subtle changes in laboratory values that accompany subsets of aging, such as gender, young-old versus old-old, and ethnicity, have not been thoroughly studied.
- The tolerable variance in serum, enzyme, and cellular processes and changes that can occur without causing negative consequences becomes narrower the older one becomes.
- Medications and chronic disorders complicate the measurement of laboratory values in elders because most elders are taking several medications at any given time that may interact to alter the reliability of laboratory measurements.
- Some measurable deficiencies in elders may be due to consistently poor dietary patterns. These deficiencies, when serious, may produce dementia and confusion, mistakenly assumed to be irreversible.
- Thyroid disorders are so common in elders that thyroid screening of all elders is recommended by some pathologists.

- The definitive diagnosis of diabetes in the aged cannot be accurately made based upon decreased glucose tolerance.
- Creatinine phosphokinase values are especially important in aiding the diagnosis of myocardial infarction in the aged.
- Cholesterol levels and their significance in those over 70 is presently being studied.
- Specific protocols and a panel of routine requirements for laboratory tests upon admission to nursing homes have not been developed. It is urged that nurses become active in advocating for these.

▲ CASE STUDY

For several months following an episode of pneumonia, Doris had been experiencing disturbing symptoms such as mental clouding, anorexia, periodic episodes of weakness and unsteadiness of gait, general lethargy, hypertension, sensitivity to cold, and constipation. She was resigned to the inevitability of such problems because she remembered her mother had experienced similar problems in her later years. Doris said, "Oh, this is just part of getting old. Mother had these problems, too." Doris's daughters insisted that she be given a complete medical and laboratory workup though her physician tended to agree with Doris and appeased her with platitudes about adjusting to aging. However, he recognized the daughters' concern and ordered a serum panel SMA 20, a T_4, CBC, and urinalysis. Doris was careful to follow directions regarding obtaining the laboratory specimens even though she did not believe they were needed but would agree there was a problem if it was revealed through the laboratory tests. All were within normal limits as ordinarily expected for adults with the exception of a slightly low serum thyroid hormone concentration (T_4) and an elevated TSH. The physician immediately ordered 0.125 µg of L-thyroxine daily for Doris.

Based upon the case study, develop a nursing care plan using the following procedure*:

List comments of client that provide *subjective data.*

List information that provides *objective data.*

From these data identify and state, using accepted format, two *nursing diagnoses* you determine are most significant to this client at this time. List two *client strengths* that you have identified from data.

Determine and state *outcome criteria* for each diagnosis. These must reflect some alleviation of the problem identified in the nursing diagnosis and must be stated in concrete and measurable terms.

Plan and state one or more *interventions* for each diagnosed problem.

Provide specific documentation of source used to determine appropriate intervention. Plan at least one intervention

*Students are advised to refer to their nursing diagnosis text and identify possible or potential problems.

that incorporates the client's existing strengths.

Evaluate success of intervention. Interventions must correlate directly with the stated outcome criteria in order to measure the outcome success.

STUDY QUESTIONS/ACTIVITIES

Do you believe the physician was justified in ordering replacement thyroid hormone, or is the normal thyroid function reduced during aging?

Are there other laboratory tests that would further clarify Doris's condition, and do you believe they should have been done prior to prescribing L-thyroxine?

Did Doris's symptoms relate in any way to her recent bout with pneumonia?

Refer to a physiology book and list all the symptoms of hypothyroidism and determine which might be considered part of normal aging.

Discuss the meanings and the thoughts triggered by the student's and elders' viewpoints expressed at the beginning of the chapter. How do these vary from your own experience?

Discuss whether you believe mandatory HIV testing should be required for any elder living in a congregate setting.

Discuss how you would proceed with a phlebotomy in an elder's home.

RESEARCH QUESTIONS

What endocrine functions are normally altered as a consequence of aging?

What endocrine functions are altered in response to specific nonendocrine disease states?

What particular laboratory tests are indicative of endocrinopathy?

What differences in laboratory values are characteristic of aged men, and do these differ from those of women of the same age?

What percentage of health professionals are cognizant of the parameters of normal laboratory values for older adults and the variances from those of the young and middle-aged adult?

What is the number of specimens obtained in the client's home that are obtained without proper instruction or precautions?

REFERENCES

Anderson MA, Braun JV: *Caring for the elderly client,* Philadelphia, 1995, FA Davis.

Andres R, Bierman E, Hazzard W: *Principles of geriatric medicine,* New York, 1985, McGraw-Hill.

Beregi E, Regius O, Nemeth J, Rajczy K, Gergely I, Lengyel E: Gender differences in age-related physiological changes and some diseases, *Z Gerontology Geriatrics* 28(1):62, 1995.

Boscia J, Kobaso W, Abrutyn E et al: Epidemiology of bacteriuria in an elderly ambulatory population, *Am J Med* 80:208, 1986.

Brazier AM, Palmer MH: Collecting clean-catch urine in the nursing home: obtaining the uncontaminated specimen, *Geriatr Nurs* 16(5):217, 1995.

Brocklehurst J: *Textbook of geriatric medicine and gerontology,* ed 3, New York, 1985, Churchill Livingstone.

Bruskewitz RC: Disorders of the lower genitiurinary tract: bladder, prostate and testicles, in Abrams WB, Beers MH, Berkow R, editors: *The Merck Manual of Geriatrics,* ed 2, Whitehouse Station, NJ, 1995, Merck Research Laboratories.

Carmel R: Prevalence of undiagnosed pernicious anemia in the elderly, *Arch Intern Med* 156(10):1097, 1996.

Cavalieri T, Chopra A, Bryman P: When outside the norm is normal: interpreting lab data in the aged, *Geriatrics* 47(5):66, 1992.

Chiari MM, Bagnoli R, De Luca PD, Monti M, Rampoldi E, Cunietti E: Influence of acute inflammation on iron and nutritional status indexes in older patients, *J Am Geriatr Soc* 43(7):767, 1995.

Chillag SA: Recognizing atypical geriatric illness, *Geriatric Consultant* 3(6):25, 1985.

Demers L: The aging endocrine system, *Lab Management* 26:24, 1988.

Eliopoulos C: *Manual of gerontological nursing,* St Louis, 1995, Mosby.

Eliopoulos C: *Health assessment of the older adult,* Reading, Mass, 1990, Addison-Wesley.

Felicetta J: Thyroid changes with aging: significance and management, *Geriatrics* 42:86, 1987.

Freedman ML: Age related hematological changes, in Abrams WB, Beers MH, Berkow R, editors: *The Merck manual of geriatrics,* ed 2, Whitehouse Station, NJ, 1995, Merck Research Laboratories.

Gallo JJ, Reichel W, Anderson LM: *Handbook of geriatric assessment,* ed 2, Gaithersburg, Md, 1995, Aspen Publishers.

Garner B: Guide to changing lab values in elders, *Geriatr Nurs* 10(3):144, 1989.

Gilmore S, Robinson G, Posthauer ME, et al: Malnutrition as indicated by serum albumin, *J Am Diet Assoc* 95(9):327, 1995.

Gloth FM, Tobin JD: Vitamin D deficiency in the institutionalized aged, *J Am Geriatr Soc* 43(7):822, 1995.

Hale W, Stewart R, Marks R: Haematological and biochemical laboratory values in an ambulatory elderly population: an analysis of the effects of age, sex, and drugs, *Age Aging* 12:275, 1983.

Hazzard WR, Andres R, Bierman EL, Blass JP, editors: *Principles of geriatric medicine and gerontology,* ed 3, New York, 1995, McGraw-Hill.

Herzlich BC, Lichstein E, Schulhoff N et al: Relationship among homocyst(e)ine, vitamin B-12 and cardiac disease in the elderly: association between vitamin B-12 deficiency and decreased left ventricular ejection fraction, *J Nutr* 126(4 Suppl):1249S, 1996.

Jeppesen M: Laboratory values for the elderly. In Carnevali D, Patrick M, editors: *Nursing management for the elderly,* ed 2, Philadelphia, 1986, Lippincott.

Joseph C, Lyles Y: Routine laboratory assessment of nursing home patients, *Geriatrics* 40:98, 1992.

Kane R, Ouslander J, Abrass I: *Essentials of clinical geriatrics,* ed 3, New York, 1994, McGraw-Hill.

Keane EM, Healy M, O'Moore, Coakley D, Walsh JB: Hypovitaminosis in the healthy elderly, *Br J Clin Pract* 49(6):301, 1995.

Kelso T: Laboratory values in the elderly, *Emerg Med Clin North Am* 8(2):241, 1990.

Lipschitz DA: Aging of the hematopoietic system. In Hazzard WR, Andres R, Bierman EL, Blass JP, editors: *Principles of geriatric medicine and gerontology,* ed 3, New York, 1995, McGraw-Hill.

Lonergan E: Clinical evaluation. In Lonergan E, editor: *Geriatrics: Lange clinical manual,* Stamford, Conn, 1996, Appleton & Lange.

Lott JA, Smith DA, Mitchell LC, Moeschberger ML: Use of medians and "average of normals" of patients' data for assessment of long-term analytical stability, *Clin Chem* 42(6 pt 1):888, 1996.

McCance KL, Capriano PF: Structure and function of the hemolytic system. In McCance KL and Huether SE: *Pathophysiology: the biologic basis for disease in adults and children,* ed 2, St Louis, 1994, Mosby.

McKenna D, Niles SA: Venipuncture: an adjunct to home care services for older adults, *Geriatr Nurs* 16(5):209, 1995.

McMurtry CT, Rosenthal A: Predictors of 2-year mortality among older male veterans on a geriatric rehabilitation unit, *J Am Geriatr Soc* 43(10):1123, 1995.

Melillo KD: Interpretation of abnormal lab values in older adults, *J Gerontol Nurs* 19(1):39, 1993.

Melillo KD: Interpretation of abnormal lab values in older adults, *J Gerontol Nurs* 19(2):35, 1993.

Miller M: Water and electrolyte disorders. In Abrams WB, Beers MH, Berkow R, editors: *The Merck manual of geriatrics,* ed 2, Whitehouse Station, NJ, 1995, Merck Research Laboratories.

Miller M, Hecker MS, Friedlander DA, Carter JM: Apparent idiopathic hyponatremia in an ambulatory geriatric population, *J Am Geriatr Soc* 44(4):404, 1996.

Nardone D, Roth K, Mazur D et al: Usefulness of physical examination in detecting the presence or absence of anemia, *Arch Intern Med* 150:201, 1990.

Pajk M: Pressure sores. In Abrams WB, Beers MH, Berkow R, editors: *The Merck manual of geriatrics,* ed 2, Whitehouse Station, NJ, 1995, Merck Research Laboratories.

Pogue SJ: Vitamin D synthesis in the elderly, *Dermatological Nursing* 7(2):103, 1995.

Riggs KM, Spiro A, Tucker K, Rush D: Relations of vitamin B-12, vitamin B-6, folate, and homocysteine to cognitive performance in the Normative Aging Study, *Am J Clin Nutr* 63(3):306, 1996.

Robbins J, Wahl P, Savage P, Enright P, Powe N, Lyles M: Hematological and biochemical laboratory values in older cardiovascular health study participants, *J Am Geriatr Soc* 43(8):855, 1995.

Rochman H: *Clinical pathology in the elderly,* New York, 1988, Karger.

Rock R, Walker G, Jennings C: Nitrogen metabolites and renal function. In Tietz JA, editor: *Textbook of clinical chemistry,* Philadelphia, 1986, WB Saunders.

Rossman I, editor: *Clinical geriatrics,* ed 3, Philadelphia, 1986, JB Lippincott.

Sack KE: Musculoskeletal diseases. In Lonergan E, editor: *Geriatrics: Lange clinical manual,* Stamford, Conn, 1996, Appleton & Lange.

Sehy Y: Laboratory values in the elderly. In Anderson MA, Braun JV: *Caring for the elderly client,* Philadelphia, 1995, FA Davis.

Shoback DM, Jaffe M: Thyroid disease and disorders of calcium and phosphorous balance. In Lonergan E, editor: *Geriatrics: Lange clinical manual,* Stamford, Conn, 1996, Appleton & Lange.

Siest G, Galteau MM, Henny J: Reference values of laboratory tests: a useful and important epidemiologic contribution of the centers for health tests, *Bull Acad Nat Med* 179(2):235, 1995.

Small EJ, Damon LE: Blood: Macrocytic anemia. In Lonergan E: Clinical evaluation. In Lonergan E, editor: *Geriatrics: Lange clinical manual,* Stamford, Conn, 1996, Appleton & Lange.

Solberg HE: Subject-based reference values, *Scand J Clin Lab Invest Suppl* 222:7, 1995.

Solomon DH: Organ systems: metabolic and endocrine disorders. In Abrams WB, Beers MH, Berkow R, editors: *The Merck manual of geriatrics,* ed 2, Whitehouse Station, NJ, 1995a, Merck Research Laboratories.

Solomon DH: Age-related endocrine and metabolic changes: the normal and diseased thyroid gland. In Abrams WB, Beers MH, Berkow R, editors: *The Merck manual of geriatrics,* ed 2, Whitehouse Station, NJ, 1995b, Merck Research Laboratories.

Speechley M, McNair S, Leffley A, Bass M: Identifying patients with hypercholesterolemia: more than one blood sample is needed, *Can Fam Physician* 41:240, 1995.

Staab AS, Hodges LC: *Essentials of gerontological nursing: adaptation to the aging process,* Philadelphia, 1996, JB Lippincott Co.

Staab AS, Lyles M: *Manual of geriatric nursing,* Glenview, Ill, 1990, Foresman/Little Brown.

Sumner AE, Chin MM, Abraham JL et al: Elevated methylmalonic acid and total homocysteine levels show high prevalence of vitamin B-12 deficiency after gastric surgery, *Ann Intern Med* 124(5):469, 1996.

Tal A: Review of screening for thyroid diseases, *Ann Intern Med* 113(11):896, 1990.

Thibodeau GA, Patton KT: *Anatomy and physiology,* ed 2, St Louis, 1993, Mosby.

Travis SS, Lampley-Dallas V: Nursing management of elderly patients with asymptomatic bacteriuria, *Geriatr Nurs* 18(3):103, 1997.

Tronetti PS, Gracely EJ, Boscia JA: Lack of association between medication use and the presence or absence of bacteriuria in elderly women, *Geriatrics* 38:1199, 1990.

Videbaek A, Ackermann P: The potassium content of plasma and red cells in various age groups, *J Gerontol* 8:63, 1993.

Welch T: Nutrition-related problems in the institutionalized elderly, *Dietetic Currents/Ross Laboratories* 16(1):1, 1989.

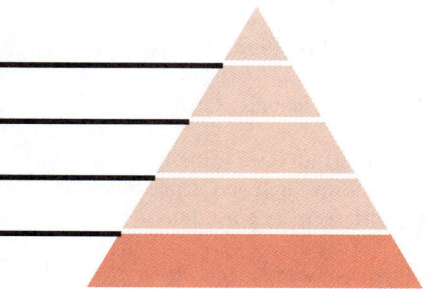

Managing Basic Physiologic Needs

Phyllis Gaspar

An elder speaks

I began thinking how my own sleep patterns have changed. As an active young woman I needed a great deal of sleep. My husband marveled at my ability to sleep 9 and 10 hours a night. Sleep was never a problem unless my mind got locked in high gear over regrets or anticipated disagreeable projects. The mind whirled around getting nowhere like a squirrel in a cage. Instead of sheep I counted lists of people or tried to recall the sequence of events on a trip or in a novel. Still sleepless at 1 or 2 o'clock in the morning, I resorted to warm milk or hot cocoa with Tylenol or cheese and crackers with a slug of brandy.

The years have changed the sleep patterns. Bedtime rituals take longer. Nature wakens me two or three times a night for trips to the bathroom. Sleep returns at once unless my mind turns on and it gets launched on a needless project. The earlier remedies are called on to slow down the activities or the next day is a disaster. My 90-year-old aunt, who slept very little and lightly and lay awake many nights, said she went to the bathroom several times just for something to do instead of just lying there.

Ricarda, 90 years old

LEARNING OBJECTIVES

Upon completion of this chapter, the reader will be able to:

1. Identify age-related changes that affect the basic biologic support needs.
2. List the types of outcomes that occur because of age-related changes in the basic biologic support needs.
3. Describe the nursing assessment relevant to basic biologic support needs.
4. Explain nursing interventions useful in the promotion of the individual's basic biologic support needs.
5. Discuss individualizing nursing care plans for each of the basic biologic support needs.

Life support or survival requirements are no different for the aged than for other human beings. Fluctuations in homeostatic balance of these needs, however, make each of these needs more precarious. Assessing and monitoring survival functions are basic to ensuring the aged person's opportunity to reach his or her highest level of health and wellness.

This chapter addresses these crucial needs in the context of the biologic needs of Maslow's hierarchy. Unless the biologic needs are fulfilled adequately, the individual cannot be expected to ascend to the higher levels of coping.

Attention has been devoted to nutrition, elimination, rest, and activity because these are areas of function in which the nurse can make a significance difference in health and wellness as defined in Chapter 3. Elimination is discussed here with regard to normal function and again in Chapter 8, under chronic problems, as it pertains to urinary and fecal incontinence.

The nurse's role in the maintenance of neurologic, renal, and cardiopulmonary function in the aged is indirect. Nurses cannot directly change the existing physiologic or pathologic conditions of heart, lungs, nervous system, or kidneys, but they can promote and maintain rest, exercise, and nutrition, which affect the function of these systems.

Two important questions should be considered in assessing the life support needs of the aged: What is bothering the client, and what threatens his or her life or health? Keeping these two questions in mind will assist the nurse in providing the most appropriate and realistic approaches to the survival needs of the aged.

NUTRITIONAL NEEDS

Well-being is influenced by the triad of aging, nutrition, and health. Proper nutrition means that all the essential nutrients (carbohydrates, fat, protein, vitamins, minerals, and water) are adequately supplied and used to maintain optimum health and well-being. Detailed discussion of each of these nutrients can be found in textbooks devoted to nutrition.

Proper nutrition provides the energy and building blocks necessary to maintain body structure and function. The variances in nutritional requirements throughout the life span are not well established for the aged. Increased amounts of calcium and vitamins A and C are needed in late life but tend to be deficient in the average diet of the aged or are affected by alterations in storage, use, and absorption. Total caloric intake should decline in response to corresponding changes in metabolic rate and a general decrease in physical activity. Serious nutritional deficits may also be induced by drugs and are discussed in Chapter 10. Nutritional needs of the aged and food sources of required nutrients are provided in condensed form in Table 6-1.

Several approaches in the past several decades were applied to the education and evaluation of the nutritional status of individuals and of nations. Three commonly used approaches are the Food Guide Pyramid, the Recommended Dietary Allowances (RDA), and the United States' Dietary Goals.

Food Guide Pyramid

The Food Guide Pyramid replaces the Basic Four Food Groups. The pyramid provides the types and amounts of food that should be eaten in ascending order of dietary importance. This differs from the original Basic Four, which accorded all the food groups equal importance and emphasized too much fat. Figure 6-1 illustrates the U.S. Department of Agriculture pyramid. With proper instruction the pyramid is an easy and systematic way for a person to evaluate his or her own nutritional intake and independently make corrective adjustments. Pictures can be used to transcend cultural and speech barriers and educational limitations.

The U.S. Department of Agriculture is evaluating the Healthy Eating Index (HEI) as an instrument to monitor changes in dietary intake over time as the basis of nutrition promotion activities for the population. The HEI reflects the food pyramid and includes a 10-component system of five food groups, four nutrients and a measure of variety in food intake (Kennedy et al, 1995).

Recommended Dietary Allowance

Another approach to evaluating nutritional status of individuals is the use of the RDA, established by the National Academy of Science Research Council. Requirements are

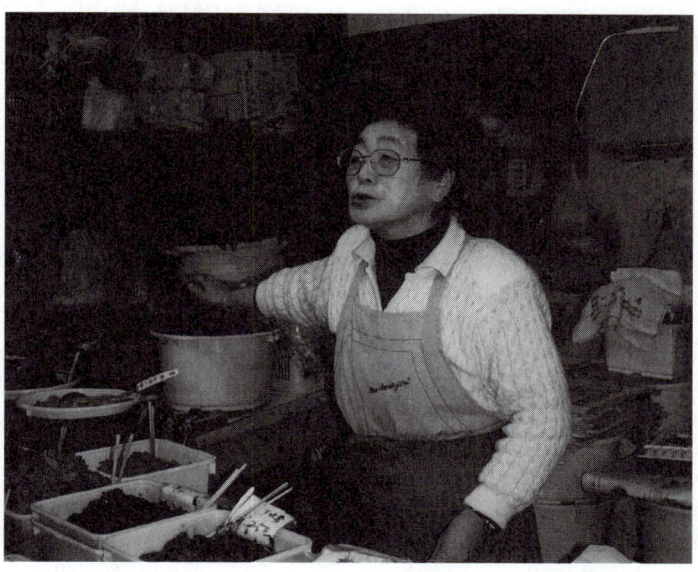

Availability of ethnic foods. (Courtesy Priscilla Ebersole.)

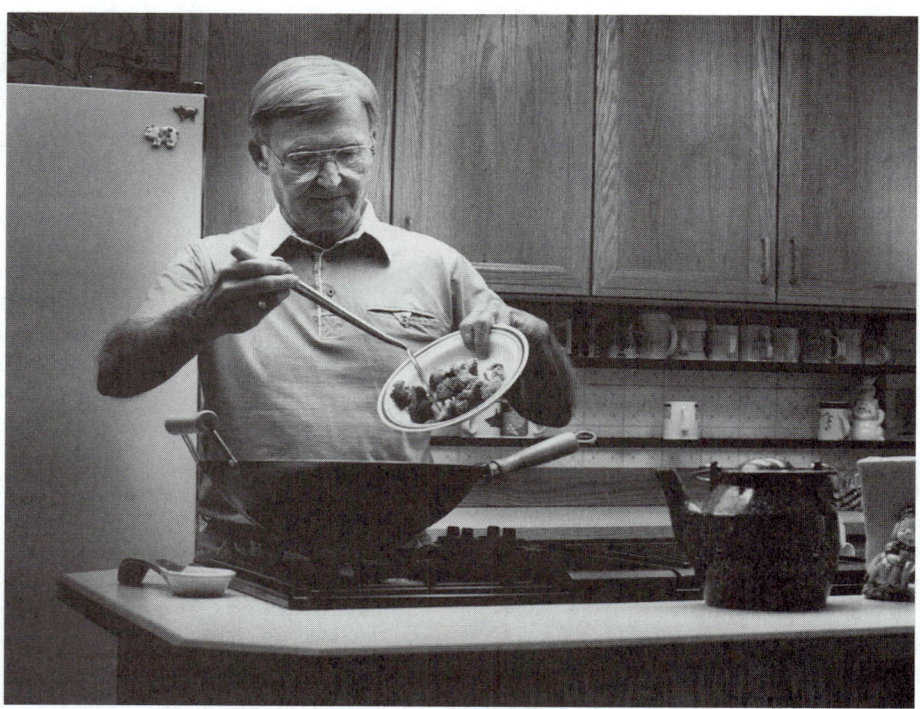

Nutritious home cooking. (Courtesy Rod Schmall.)

revised every 5 years to incorporate new knowledge. The RDA is a guideline for assessing the intake of energy and specific nutrients up to age 50. It establishes the daily minimum amount of vitamins and minerals needed by young and middle-aged healthy individuals based on body size. Some adjustment is required for different individuals. The RDA does not consider requirements for additional nutrients as a result of infection, metabolic disorders, and chronic illness, nor does the RDA address requirements of those older than 65 (Recommended Dietary Allowances, 1989). This is due, in part, to disagreement about the elderly's need for increased amounts of nutrients. Lipske (1993) proposes that the RDA be used to determine "nutritional vulnerability," indicating that calculated nutrient intakes that do not reach RDAs do not necessarily imply a nutritional deficiency but suggest vulnerability.

Studies on nutrient requirements have been carried out on the young, and the estimations for the aged have been based largely on extrapolation. Therefore, inaccuracies exist in the assumption that a 50-year-old and a 90-year-old have similar requirements. Dynamic changes occur between these ages in which nutrients and energy requirements of individuals and population subgroups become more diverse. Certain news items and preliminary research findings alert us to the great amount of information that is still unknown and controversial about geriatric nutrition. For instance, glycine and arginine supplements seem to aid wound healing in older people. Tryptophan, an essential

amino acid, seems to promote better sleep, and tyrosine relieves depression. Interestingly, the National Institute on Aging has found, through a technique called racemization, that chronologic age of individuals can be identified based on structural changes of aspartic acid (amino acid) within their bodies, occurring at a constant and predictable rate over time.

United States' Dietary Goals

The acceleration of malnutrition in the United States and the effects of the eating habits of Americans prompted the U.S. Senate Select Committee on Nutrition and Human Needs to establish dietary goals for the United States (Dietary Goals, 1978). The guidelines attempt to improve eating habits and lower the risk of associated diseases. The goals are caloric consumption that encourages weight control; a program of regular exercise to burn excessive calories; an increased consumption of complex carbohydrates and naturally occurring sugars, which are found in fresh fruits, vegetables, and grains; the elimination of refined and processed sugar, which is present in most prepared and processed food and beverages; and an overall reduction of fat. The final goal is limitation of sodium intake, a difficult undertaking, since considerable amounts of salt are used in processed foods. The dietary goals have since been revised and include seven guidelines for Americans (Box 6-1).

Incorporating the United States' Dietary Goals into the Food Guide Pyramid and supplementing this with the RDA

Table 6-1   Special Nutritional Considerations for the Older Adult

Nutrient	Comments	Major food sources
Essential nutrients		
Fiber	Intakes are often inadequate. Increasing fiber in the diet may aid in preventing constipation.	Whole-grain breads (such as whole wheat, rye, Roman Meal, and pumpernickel); Wheatena, Ry-Crisp, and whole wheat crackers; cereals (such as shredded wheat, oatmeal, four-grain, and seven-grain); whole wheat pastas, and brown rice Fresh fruits and vegetables
Protein	The recommended level for older adults is as high as 1 g/kg body weight. Intakes are usually adequate. (Aged individuals may need to be shown portion sizes that would provide the necessary protein.)	Dried peas, dried or canned beans, lentils (especially in combination with whole grains such as brown rice and whole wheat bread), or peanut butter Cheese, milk, and nonfat dry milk Eggs Canned clams, salmon, sardines, and tuna

Calcium	Intakes are often inadequate. Older women may need generous amounts, 1 to 2 g daily, to protect against demineralization of the bones, leading to osteoporosis.	For those who are lactose intolerant:
		   Tofu (soybean curd)
		   All cheeses except cottage cheese
		   Corn tortillas treated in lime
		   All greens such as turnip, mustard, and collard (except spinach)
		   Sardines
		   Milk in small quantities (may be tolerated by some individuals)
		For those who are not lactose intolerant:
		   All foods listed above
		   Whole, low-fat, skim, evaporated, or dried milk
		   Yogurt, buttermilk, and cottage cheese

Iron	Intakes are often inadequate.	Dried or canned beans Cereals, whole wheat pastas, whole-grain breads, and brown rice Liver Canned oysters
Zinc	Widespread deficiency is found in aged men and women.	Legumes Whole grains Meat
Folic acid	Folic acid deficiency may be linked to dementia.	Leafy green vegetables (such as spinach, collard, mustard, turnip, and kale greens) Dried beans and peas, lentils, and nuts Whole-grain breads, pastas, and cereals Liver
Vitamin A	Intakes are often inadequate.	Green vegetables (such as spinach, turnip, mustard, and collard greens, and broccoli) Carrots, winter squash, and sweet potato Watermelon and cantaloupe Liver
Vitamin B₆ (pyridoxine)	Intakes are sometimes inadequate. Age per se has been shown to influence blood levels, which decrease markedly with age.	Liver Vegetables Nuts and seeds, dried beans and peas Bran and whole grains Bananas, raisins, and cantaloupe
Vitamin C (ascorbic acid)	Intakes are sometimes inadequate, even in nursing home diets. Age per se influences blood levels, which decrease markedly with age. Vitamin C aids in the absorption of iron from vegetable sources.	Oranges, lemons, tomatoes, grapefruit, cantaloupe or other melon, strawberries Broccoli, cabbage, green peppers, fresh chili peppers, and dark, leafy greens Baked potatoes
Vitamin E (tocopherol)	Several researchers have demonstrated that 3-4 months of treatment with vitamin E (300-400 IU—about 30 times the recommended dietary allowance) relieves intermittent claudication (severe cramps in calf muscles during walking).	Fats of vegetable origin Some nuts and seeds Cereal products, especially whole grains Some vegetables

Compiled from *Recommended Daily Allowance,* ed 10, Washington, DC, 1989, National Academy Press; Linder MC: *Nutritional biochemistry and metabolism with clinical application,* New York, 1991, Elsevier; Roe D: *Geriatric nutrition,* ed 3, Englewood Cliffs, NJ, 1992, Prentice Hall.

Continued

Table 6-1	Special Nutritional Considerations for the Older Adult—cont'd	

Nutrient	Comments	Major food sources
Nonestablished nutrients		
Vitamin B_{15} (pangamic acid)*	This is neither a vitamin nor a wonder drug! Promotional claims state that it is effective in treating a wide variety of ailments, including the effects of aging.	
Vitamin B_{17} (laetrile)*	This substance, extracted from apricot pits, is neither a vitamin nor a wonder drug! Promotional claims state that it is effective in treating cancer.	

*Have been claimed to be vitamins. There has been no research that demonstrates the body needs these compounds for metabolism. In fact, large doses of laetrile have led to death in a few cases.

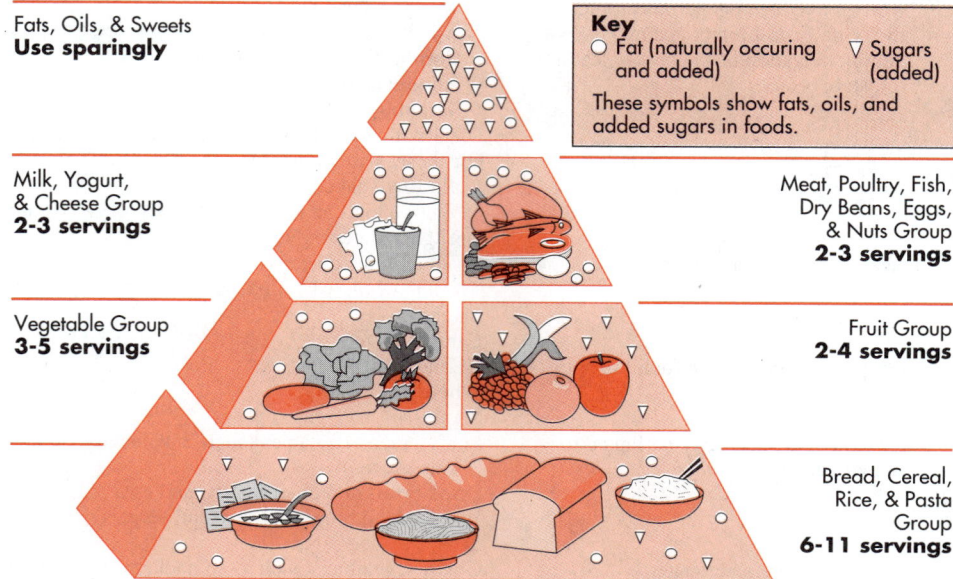

Figure 6-1. Food pyramid. (Courtesy US Department of Agriculture.)

should provide a usable and beneficial means of assessing nutritional needs and planning the diet.

Factors Affecting Fulfillment of Nutritional Needs

Fulfillment of the aged person's nutritional needs is affected by numerous factors, including lifelong eating habits, socialization, income, transportation, housing, and food knowledge.

Lifelong Eating Habits. The nutritional state of a person reflects an individual's dietary history as well as present food practices. Lifelong eating habits are developed out of tradition, ethnicity, and religion, all of which collectively can be called culture. Krebs-Smith et al (1995) found that food habits established since childhood influenced the intake of older adults.

Eating habits do not always coincide with fulfillment of nutritional needs. Rigidity of food habits increases with age as familiar food patterns are sought. Ethnicity determines if traditional foods are preserved, whereas religion affects choice of foods possible. Throughout life then, preferences for particular foods bring deep satisfaction and possess emotional significance. Such foods are called "soul food." Preferences for soul food influence food choices and affect nutrient intake. Foods prepared or served in a special way provide "soul." Rice with every meal or homemade chicken soup given to the individual when ill are examples of what some people consider their soul food. Foods of this nature are not unique to any one group but rather are found all over the world.

Yen (1995b) points out that food habits for various cultures are well documented. Table 6-2 lists cultural food patterns for various ethnic groups and the dietary excesses or omissions associated with the pattern. Yen cautions that lists tend to stereotype individuals and need to be used as background information. Do not assume that elders eat a certain way because they are from a particular ethnic group, or you

---

Box 6-1   **Tips for Following the Dietary Guidelines**

---

1. *Eat a variety of foods.*
   Provide more servings of fruits and vegetables.
   Frequently include dark green vegetables, dried bean dishes, and starchy vegetables.
   Use more grain products.
2. *Maintain ideal weight.*
   Reduce fats, sugars, and alcohol in diet.
   Cut back on size of serving.
   Increase physical activity.
3. *Avoid too much fat, saturated fat, and cholesterol:*
   Select lean hamburger and lean roasts, chops, and steak—trim visible fat.
   Drain meat drippings.
   Limit the amount of margarine or other fat used on bread and vegetables.
   Emphasize low-fat and skim milk and reduce the amount of fat in other foods when whole milk and cheese are used.
   Reduce the amount of fat used in recipes, added to food in cooking, or added at the table.
   Limit the number of fried foods, especially breaded or batter-fried foods.
   Use moderate amounts of organ meats and egg yolk.
   Use fewer creamed foods and rich desserts.
   Limit the amount of salad dressing used.
4. *Eat foods with adequate amounts of starch and fiber.*
   Provide more vegetables and fruits.
   Eat potatoes, sweet potatoes, yams, corn, peas, and dried beans more often.
   Increase consumption of whole-grain cereal products such as brown rice, oatmeal, and whole wheat cereals and breads.
5. *Avoid too much sugar.*
   Avoid or cut down on very sweet foods.
   Reduce the amount of sugar in recipes for baked goods.
   Rely more on fresh fruit and canned fruits packed in juice or light syrup.
   Limit the amounts of sugar, jams, jellies, and syrups.
6. *Avoid too much sodium and salt.*
   Use fewer salty, processed foods.
   Use little or no salt and assume that none is added at the table.
   Make only sparing use of commercially prepared sauces and condiments; these include such foods as catsup, Worcestershire or soy sauce, mustard, relishes and pickles, bouillon cubes, meat tenderizer, MSG, gravy mixes, and canned soups.
   Use more fresh and frozen vegetables than canned or seasoned frozen vegetables, which have added salt.
   Limit the use of salty snack foods such as chips, pretzels, and crackers.
7. *If you drink alcohol, do so in moderation.*
   Provide more fruit and vegetable juice.
   Measure your drink.
   Eat something before drinking.
   Offer nonalcoholic beverages at parties.

---

may find yourself catering to a preferences for rice or some other food when none exists.

Lifelong habits of dieting or eating fad foods also echo through the later years. The aged, in particular, are taken in by food fads that profess to partially or completely cure various ailments or to make one look younger or feel more vital. Skipping meals is another practice that one finds with the aged. The quantity of food eaten diminishes and the adequacy of nutrition becomes questionable. It is very difficult to reach an adequate nutritional intake if the total calories are fewer than 1200 a day. Individuals who are on self-imposed diets of 1000 calories or less a day are inviting malnutrition.

Food Use Patterns. Individuals establish their diets and eating patterns for various reasons. In a study of elder's time perception and food use patterns by Shifflett (1987), five patterns were identified. In the first pattern, physician-prescribed diets, diets are suggested or ordered by the physician as treatment or prevention of disease. These include diets to reduce fat, sodium, weight, or refined sugar. The second pattern is a change in food use due to altered taste, isolation, or income. These seem to be unrelated factors that alter food use, but they actually are linked by one unifying factor: these events are usually beyond the control of the individual and generally result in a reduction of food intake. Self-prescribed diets, a third pattern, are different from a physician-prescribed diet because they are prescribed and implemented by the individual, independent of a physician. These diets may be the same as the prescribed diets above, as well as high-fiber or low-fat diets. Individuals usually adopt these diets because a friend or family member developed or has heart disease, hypertension, diabetes, or cancer. Overall reduction of food intake is a pattern in which there is a change in food habits as a result of a conscious effort by the individual to maintain a healthy body weight and avoid chronic conditions associated with obesity. There is a desire by the individual to enjoy retirement without added medical or health problems. The final pattern, maintenance of life-long food use, is a continuation of a conscientious diet pattern that has incorporated healthy dietary practices, like exercise, long before old age. One may note that three of these patterns reflect self-determination and individual control or self-responsibility. Usually active participation in dietary matters is a determinant in adherence or nonadherence to dietary regimens.

Table 6-2	Ethnic Food Patterns	
Ethnic group	**Cultural food patterns**	**Dietary excesses or omissions**
Mexican (native)	Basic sources of protein—dry beans, flan, cheese, many meats, fish, eggs. Chili peppers and many deep-green and yellow vegetables. Fruits include: zapote, guava, papaya, mango, citrus. Tortillas (corn, flour); sweet bread; fideo; tacos, burritos, enchiladas.	*Limited* meats, milk, and milk products. Some are using flour tortillas more than the more nutritious corn tortillas. *Excessive* use of lard (manteca), sugar. Tendency to boil vegetables for long periods of time.
Filipino (Spanish-Chinese influence)	Most meats, eggs, nuts, legumes. Many different kinds of vegetables. Large amounts of rice and cereals.	May *limit* meat, milk, and milk products (the latter may be due to lactose intolerance). Tend to prewash rice. Tend to fry many foods.
Chinese (mostly Cantonese)	Cheese, soybean curd (tofu), many meats, chicken and pigeon eggs; nuts; legumes. Many different vegetables, leaves, bamboo sprouts. Rice and rice-flour products; wheat, corn, millet seed; green tea. Mixtures of fish, pork, and chicken with vegetables—bamboo shoots, broccoli, cabbage, onions, mushrooms, pea pods.	Tendency among some immigrants to use *excess* grease in cooking. May be *low* in protein, milk, and milk products (the latter may be due to lactose intolerance). Often wash rice before cooking. Large amounts of soy and oyster sauces, both of which are *high in salt.*
Puerto Rican	Milk with coffee. Pork, poultry, eggs, dried fish; beans (habichuelas). Viandas (starchy vegetables; starchy ripe fruits). Avocados, okra, eggplant, sweet yams. Rice, cornmeal.	Utilize *large* amounts of lard for cooking. *Limited* use of milk and milk products. *Limited* amounts of pork and poultry.
Black American	Milk with coffee. Pork, poultry, eggs, dried fish; beans (habichuelas). Viandas (starchy vegetables; starchy ripe fruits). Avocados, okra, eggplant, sweet yams. Rice, cornmeal. Cereals (including grits, hominy, hot breads). Molasses (dark molasses is especially good source of calcium, iron, vitamins B_1 and B_2, and niacin).	*Limited* use of milk group (lactose intolerance). Extensive use of frying, "smothering," simmering for cooking. *Large* amounts of fat: salt pork, bacon drippings, lard, gravies. May have *limited* use of citrus and enriched breads.
Middle Eastern (Greek, Syrian, Armenian)	Yogurt. Predominantly lamb, nuts, dried peas, beans, lentils. Deep-green leaves and vegetables; dried fruits. Dark breads and cracked wheat.	Tend to use *excessive* sweeteners, lamb fat, olive oil. Tend to fry meats and vegetables. *Insufficient* milk and milk products (almost no butter—use olive oil, which has no nutritive value except for calories); deficiency in fresh fruits.
Middle European (Polish)	Many milk products. Pork, chicken. Root vegetables (potatoes); cabbage; fruits. Wheat products. Sausages, smoked and cured meats; noodles, dumplings; bread; cream with coffee.	Tend to use *excessive* sweets and to overcook vegetables. *Limited* amounts of fruits (citrus), raw vegetables, and meats.
Native American (American Indian—much variation)	If "Americanized," use milk and milk products. Variety of meats: game, fowl, fish; nuts, seeds, legumes. Variety of vegetables, some wild; variety of fruits, some wild, rose hips; roots. Variety of breads, including tortillas, cornmeal, rice.	*Limited* quantities of high-protein foods depending on availability (flocks) and economic situation. *Excessive* use of sugar.
Italian	Staples are pasta with sauces; bread; eggs; cheese; tomatoes and vegetables such as artichokes, eggplant, greens, and zucchini. Only small amount of meat is used.	*Limited* use of whole grains; *insufficient* servings from milk group; tendency to overcook vegetables; enjoy sweets.

From Swanson J: *Community health nursing,* Philadelphia, 1993, WB Saunders.

Socialization. Food and eating are behavioral and social symbols. Many aged are forced to remain isolated from the mainstream of life because of impinging factors. When one eats alone, the outcome is often either overindulgence or disinterest in food. Depression, discussed in Chapter 21, is a common problem of aging and a significant inhibitor of appetite.

Some aged spend much of their time in neighborhood bars, the center for social interaction. In seeking this type of fleeting social support, the aged spend money on alcohol that is needed for adequate nutrition. The perception that drinking is a sanctioned way to maintain social contact, which is preferable to not drinking and becoming isolated, is a very powerful consideration, particularly for men who are single-room occupants. Further discussion of this is found in Chapters 18 and 21. Drinking alcohol depletes the body of necessary nutrients and often replaces meals, thus making an individual doubly prone to malnutrition.

There are more constructive means of maintaining social contact and nutritional status. Title VII of the Older Americans Act provides funding for strategically located outreach centers or nutrition sites whose purposes are to provide at least one nutritionally sound meal daily and to facilitate congregate dining to foster social contact and relationships. No one age 60 or over (all spouses are also included) can be denied participation in the nutrition program because of his economic situation. Those who are able to pay for their meal do so according to their ability.

Meals on Wheels is another community program that encourages both the attainment of good nutrition and human contact for those who are unable to prepare meals or go out to obtain them. Most cities and rural areas throughout the United States have such programs. Delivery in the rural areas is usually limited to once or twice a week. Other group feeding programs exist through church and other community auspices such as food cooperatives, home grocery delivery services, and chore services for shopping and meal preparation. In the past, the federal government has awarded grants to the Congregate Housing Services Project to provide meals to elderly residents who needed them to remain independent.

One objective for Healthy People 2000 is to increase to at least 80% the receipt of home food services by people aged 65 and older who have difficulty in preparing their own meals or are otherwise in need of home-delivered meals. In 1991 the data indicated that only 7% of those needing home food services were receiving them (US Department of Health and Human Services, 1995).

The social essence ascribed to eating is sharing and providing a feeling of belonging. All of us use food as a means of giving and receiving love, friendship, or belonging.

Income. Inflation is constantly eroding the purchasing power of the aged, forcing them to buy foods that satiate hunger but provide many empty calories. These foods may or may not be expensive. Some aged eat only once a day in an attempt to make their income last through the month. Aged individuals accustomed to eating meat, fish, and poultry as their main sources of protein have watched the cost climb to heights beyond their purchasing power. Inexpensive alternative protein sources such as tofu (soybean curd) are foreign to the diets of the aged in Western society today but have slowly been making their way into acceptance. At present the development of a taste for alternative protein sources and an understanding of what foods to mix to obtain complete dietary protein requires some knowledge and practice to ensure adequate protein intake and to prevent monotony. If at all possible, the aged should be encouraged to use vegetable protein sources to meet daily needs. This is a more economical form of protein that may help the aged conserve their income for other necessities, unexpected bills, or special treats. Combinations such as milk or cheese with bread or pasta; cereal with milk; rice and cheese or rice and bean casseroles; wheat soy or corn soy bread; wheat bread with baked beans, beans, or pea curry; tortillas and beans; and legume soap with bread are sources of protein.

More nonwhites and women live in poverty than white men (US Bureau of the Census, Statistical Abstracts for 1995). Programs such as the food stamp program have the potential for increasing the purchasing power of the aged who qualify, but these are vulnerable to federal budget cutting. Many aged persons find that the amount of money required to purchase the food stamps is greater than they feel they can afford, or they do not see the benefit to them. Transportation may be limited and the distance too far for the aged to travel to acquire the food stamps, which are sold only at designated locations in cities.

Free food programs, such as donated commodities, are also available at distribution centers (food banks) for those with limited incomes. While this is another valuable option for the aged, use of it is not always entirely feasible. One takes a chance on the types of food available any particular day or week, quantities distributed are frequently too large for the single aged person or the aged couple to use or even carry from the distribution site, and the site may be too far away or difficult to reach. The time of distribution of the food may be inconvenient, too.

Cafeterias and restaurants that provided special meal prices for the aged have had to increase their prices as food costs have risen; thus the previous advantages of eating out have diminished. Yet many single elders rely on them for most meals.

Though rapidly disappearing, "Mom and Pop" stores in the neighborhoods where many elderly live do not have a rapid turnover of fresh products, and this may cause the aged to spend money on partially spoiled items. Those who purchase semispoiled food and discover the spoilage when they return home rarely return the items.

Transportation. Availability of transportation may be limited for the aged. Many small, long-standing neighborhood food stores have been closed in the wake of larger supermarkets, which are located in areas that serve a greater segment of the population. It may become difficult to walk to the market, to reach it by public transportation, or to carry a bag of groceries while using a cane. It is nearly impossible to do this with a walker. Fear is apparent in the elderly's consideration of transportation. They fear walking in the street and being mugged, not being able to cross the street in the time it takes the traffic light to change, and being knocked down or falling as they walk in crowded streets. Despite reduced senior citizen bus fares, the aged remain very fearful of attack when using public transportation. Transportation by taxicab for an individual on a limited income is unrealistic, but sharing a taxicab with others who also need to shop may enable the aged to go where food prices are cheaper and to take advantage of sale items. For the aged, convenience foods, devoid of many essential nutrients, are lighter to carry or pull along in a cart than fresh fruits and vegetables.

Senior citizen organizations in many parts of the country have been helpful in providing the elderly with van service to shopping areas. In housing complexes it may be possible to schedule trips to the supermarket together. Most communities have multiple sources of transportation available, but the aged may be unaware of them. Local departments of aging and senior centers are a good source of information. Additional discussions of transportation can be found in Chapters 11 and 13.

Housing. Poor and near-poor aged are likely to reside in substandard housing. Some live in single rooms that lack storage space for food, a means of refrigeration, and a stove for cooking. At certain times of the year some of the single-room dwellers use the window ledges and fire escapes to keep perishables cool for several days' use. It is difficult for the single-room occupant to prepare adequately nutritious meals unless the individual is aware of other alternatives. Careful planning is a must to ensure that the required amounts of nutrients are obtained.

Ideally, one meal that consists of protein (generally meat, fish, or poultry), potato, vegetable, salad, and dessert should be eaten out daily. Other meals can be prepared and eaten with a minimum of effort in the aged person's room. Pantry-type foods can be safely stored in a heavy cardboard or wooden box with a tight-fitting lid. This box serves not only as a place of storage but can also be used as a table when one is not available. Stored food should be kept in the driest and coolest part of the room. Cookies and crackers should be placed in plastic bags and then in airtight containers. Screw-top jars or coffee cans will accommodate dried fruit, beans, and sugar. Canned food should be purchased in the single-serving size so that there will not be any leftovers. Boxes of edibles should be carefully opened to ensure tight reclosure. Box 6-2 lists items suitable for the single-room occupant's pantry and items that can be purchased to be eaten the same day. Vacuum-packed foods do not require refrigeration, and a greater variety is available than in the past.

The individual's meal patterns and preferences are the foremost concern of the nurse in tailoring an acceptable diet. Additional factors affecting dietary intake include living arrangements, number of meals eaten daily, who cooks and shops, presence of physical impediments affecting cooking and shopping, problems with chewing, use of dentures, alcohol use, and medication use.

Problems in Nutrition

Hydration, adequate fiber, lactose intolerance, osteoporosis, and malnutrition are factors that affect or are affected by the nutritional status of elders.

Adequate Hydration. The aged are vulnerable to fluid and accompanying electrolyte imbalance. Acidosis and alkalosis are potential consequences. Dehydration can also cause confusion because of electrolyte imbalance (Rolls, 1989). Increased amounts of fluid not only prevent confusion associated with dehydration but also are essential for individuals who are receiving specific medications. Lithium, for example, requires that the person drink as much as 3 L of fluid a day. Use of diuretics requires that fluid intake be maintained unless specifically ordered to the contrary. Coffee has a diuretic effect that requires fluid intake to compensate for fluid loss through diuresis. In hot weather increased perspiration and evaporation deplete the individual of needed body fluid. Fever and upper respiratory infections also cause dehydration in the aged. Adequate fluid intake is as important to total nutrition as food. Under normal circumstances a healthy adult needs 1.5 L of oral fluids; an additional 700 ml comes from solid food and 300 ml from oxidation of food during metabolism (Reedy, 1988).

Standard indicators for dehydration among the aged are unreliable. Skin turgor assessment is unreliable, and weight may be impracticable in the nursing home setting. Dry mucous membrane may be misleading because many elderly are mouth breathers. Intake and output charts are generally unreliable. Urine-specific gravity is poorly correlated with serum biochemical parameters of hydration status. Laboratory parameters can be utilized, but other conditions that can occur in elderly can alter these laboratory findings.

Weinberg et al (1995) and the Council on Scientific Affairs, American Medical Association in a review of the published literature regarding dehydration in older individuals formulated a consensus statement. The statement recommends that the OBRA (Omnibus Budget Reconciliation Act of 1987 and 1990) *Dehydration/Fluid Maintenance Triggers*

Box 6-2	**Nonperishable Foods Suitable for Single-Room Occupant**

Milk Products
Box of dry skim or whole milk
Small can evaporated milk
Instant cocoa
Instant pudding to use with dry milk
Small pieces of cheese (if wrapped airtight and kept in cool place)

Meat Products
Small can of tuna fish, sardines, salmon
Canned potted meat
Peanut butter
Cottage cheese
Hard cooked eggs

Fruits and Vegetables
Small cans of any fruits and vegetables
Dried fruit (raisins, apricots, dates)
Fresh apples, oranges, seasonal fruits

Miscellaneous Foods
Instant coffee
Tea
Sugar
Condiments of choice

and Additional Risk Factors for Dehydration among Residents of Long-Term Care Facilities be used for assessment of the elderly in nursing homes as well in the home. The indicators are presented in Box 6-3.

Prevention of dehydration is essential. Nursing staff in a long-term care facility were able to identify dehydration based on poor oral intake (Pals et al, 1995). These authors conclude that observation by staff continues to be the first defense for fever and dehydration detection in residents. Staff education to increase awareness of atypical presentation of dehydration is encouraged.

When dehydration occurs, treatment is based on the type of dehydration experienced—isotonic dehydration, hypertonic dehydration, or hypotonic dehydration. Oral hydration is the first treatment approach if the patient is able to ingest fluids. Sports drinks are recommended over tap water for hypertonic dehydration because they can be easily absorbed by the stomach, are generally palatable to patients, and will more rapidly correct hypertonic states. The last-resort treatment approaches are hypodermoclysis and intravenous therapy (Weinberg et al, 1995).

Gaspar (1988) found that the water intake from food and fluid of rural nursing home residents was inadequate based on the standard of 1600 ml of water per square meter of body surface area. Similar results were found by Gaspar in urban nursing homes and Alzheimer's units. Variables that influence fluid intake of institutionalized elders were identified. It was noted that as age increased fluid intake decreased. Other factors that influence fluid intake are speech, the ability to request fluids, visual impairment, opportunity to obtain water, the amount of time that fluid was in reach, functional ability, and gender. The findings suggest that those who are semidependent are at greater risk for inadequate fluid intake than those who are independent (able to obtain their own fluids) and dependent (care needs are anticipated). In replication studies one additional variable identified was the length of stay in long-term care. The longer the length of stay, the lower the water intake. Gaspar concluded that nursing care plans for those who are semidependent, female, and over the age of 85 should include nursing orders clearly stating the need to increase the number of times water and fluids are offered. Reedy (1988) recommends interventions to prevent dehydration (Box 6-4).

Adequate Fiber. Fiber is an important dietary component that some aged persons do not consume in sufficient quantities. Fiber, the undigestible material that gives plants their structure, is abundant in raw fruits and vegetables and unrefined grains and cereals.

Fiber facilitates the absorption of water, increases bulk, and improves intestinal motility. It prevents constipation, hemorrhoids, and diverticulosis. Fiber also helps reduce caloric intake, aids in the control of obesity, and is thought to play a role in the prevention of "diseases of civilization" such as heart disease and colon cancer. Various types of fiber exist, but all possess the common characteristic of indigestibility. Individuals who can chew foods well could benefit from eating increased amounts of fresh fruits and vegetables daily or combining unsweetened bran with other types of food. Those who have difficulty chewing could sprinkle unsweetened bran on cereals or in soups, meat loaf, or casseroles. The quantity of bran used depends on the individual, but generally 1 to 2 tablespoons daily is sufficient to facilitate intestinal motility. Individuals who have not used bran should begin with 1 teaspoon and progressively increase the quantity until the fiber intake is enough to accomplish its purpose. Otherwise, bloating, gas, diarrhea, and other colon discomforts will initially occur and discourage further use of this important dietary ingredient.

Cooked dried beans are a good source of fiber. Pinto beans, split peas, red beans, and peanuts can be served in casseroles, soups, and dips. These are all relatively inexpensive and nutritious in addition to having high fiber content. See Box 6-5 for fiber choices. The discussion of elimination

---

| **Box 6-3** | **OBRA 1987/1990 Minimum Data Set: Dehydration/Fluid Maintenance Triggers and Additional Risk Factors for Dehydration among Residents of Long-Term Care Facilities** |

Dehydration/Fluid Maintenance Triggers

Deterioration in cognitive status, skills, or abilities in last 90 d
Failure to eat or take medication(s)
Urinary tract infection in last 30 d
Current diagnosis of dehydration (*ICD-9* code 276-5)
Diarrhea
Dizziness/vertigo
Fever
Internal bleeding
Vomiting
Weight loss ($\geq$5% in last 30 d; or 10% in last 180 d)
Insufficient fluid intake (dehydrated)
Did not consume all/almost all liquids provided during last 3 d
Leaves $\geq$25% food uneaten at most meals
Requirement for parenteral (intravenous) fluids

Additional Potential Risk Factors

Hand dexterity/body control problems
Use of diuretics
Abuse of laxatives
Uncontrolled diabetes mellitus
Swallowing problems
Purposeful restriction of fluids
Patients on enteral feedings (need free water in addition to feedings)
History of previous episodes of dehydration
Comprehension/communication problems

From Omnibus Budget Reconciliation Act of 1987 and 1990 (federal). *ICD-9* indicates *International Classification of Diseases, ed 9.*

Box 6-4	Measures to Help Prevent Dehydration of Institutionalized Elderly

- Assure a 24-hour intake of at least 1500 ml of oral fluid. (Food intake and metabolic oxidation should provide additional fluid for hydration.)
- Offer fluids hourly during the day. Include fluids with an evening snack.
- Ask the physician to order intravenous fluids if the elder is not able to take oral fluids.
- Accurately record intake and output on all elders. (The 24-hour urine volume should be 1000 ml to 1500 ml.)
- Note the urine color and specific gravity.
- Listen to bowel sounds. Note any change in activity. (Extra soft or loose stool means losing water, and hard stool means dehydration.)
- Be familiar with tests or examinations that the patient may have had. If they involved enemas or laxatives prior to the tests, there will be a fluid loss.
- Replace fluids when there has been nothing consumed orally or fluids have been lost from test preparation.

- Obtain a drug history.
- Provide cups, glasses, and pitchers that are not too big or heavy for the aged to handle. (Help those who can't help themselves to fluids.)
- Offer other fluids in addition to water. Find out the types of beverages liked and fluid temperature preferred.
- Remember that coffee acts as a diuretic. Fluid loss by coffee should be supplemented to compensate for the fluid loss.
- Note skin turgor and mucous membranes.
- Note increases in pulse and respirations and decrease in blood pressure (suggestive of dehydration).
- Check laboratory values for changes: sodium, blood urea nitrogen, hematocrit, hemoglobin, urine and serum osmolarity, and creatinine. Also check for signs of acidosis.
- Weigh the patient daily at the same time and on the same scale.

From Reedy DF: Fluid intake: how can you prevent dehydration? *Geriatr Nurs* 9:224, 1988.

Box 6-5	High Fiber Choices

Dried beans (kidney, split peas, limas, garbanzo, pinto, black; peas, others: baked beans)
Bran cereals
Whole wheat and other whole-grain products: cereals—rye, oats, buckwheat, stone-ground cornmeal; breads, pastas, pizzas, pancakes, muffins made with whole-grain flour
Dried apricots, figs, prunes
Dates, raisins
Fresh or frozen lima beans; peas
Greens (especially spinach): beet greens, kale, collards, Swiss chard, turnip greens
Sweet corn
Baked potato with skin; also mashed or boiled
Broccoli
Carrots
Green beans
Brussels sprouts
Raspberries, blackberries, cranberries
Bananas
Apples, pears, plums
Strawberries

in this chapter presents recipes for promoting bowel elimination. Each of these recipes has fiber agents.

Milk/Lactose Intolerance. The use of milk and other dairy products is a major and efficient source of protein and calcium for the aged. For many persons, lactose intolerance is a problem that must be considered in nutritional counseling. Lactose intolerance is thought to be a genetic characteristic occurring in blacks, Orientals, American Indians, Eskimos, and other ethnic groups for whom animal milk is not a traditional food. Whites of northern European descent retain the lactase enzyme in adulthood, and other whites begin to experience some degree of intolerance at about age 45. Even low levels of ingested lactose cause such symptoms as gas, bloating, cramping, and diarrhea. Suarez et al (1995) indicate that the problem of lactose intolerance may be less than believed. Of 30 volunteers who believed they were severely lactose intolerant, only 21 subjects actually had some degree of lactose malabsorption in a test of drinking milk. These subjects had only minimal bloating, abdominal pain, diarrhea, and flatulence.

Lactose intolerance resembles milk intolerance. The symptoms displayed are similar and occur when more than 8 ounces of milk are consumed. Intolerance does not occur when other products such as cheese are eaten. It is difficult to know exactly if the milk intolerance is a direct reflection of lactose intolerance or whether it is caused by a lactose intolerance precipitated by disease or superimposed by severe hypoalactasia. To date, however, there has been no systematic investigation to refute or confirm this speculation.

It is thought that those who are lactose tolerant have consistently taken significantly higher quantities of dairy and milk products in their diets over their early and middle years than those who are intolerant. For those who have a low lactose capacity or who have a milk intolerance, diets restricted in lactose are necessary. Chocolate milk has a higher osmolarity than regular milk and may improve tolerance of lactose among malabsorbers. There are over-the-counter products that purport to help improve lactose tolerance. Foods high in calcium, such as greens and dried beans, also can provide essential calcium for those who are lactose intolerant. It may be necessary to supplement the diet with calcium carbonate or calcium lactate, sodium fluoride, and B complex vitamins to maintain skeletal integrity.

Osteoporosis. Osteoporosis is the most common skeletal disorder in the world, second only to arthritis in the elderly. This often debilitating and painful metabolic disorder affects four times as many women as men and has been linked to various causative factors, among which are dietary deficiencies. The bone loss associated with this disease is thought to be due to an inadequate intake of calcium and vitamin D. A more detailed discussion appears in Chapter 8.

The National Institutes of Health (NIH) Consensus Panel (Yen, 1995a) has established a daily maintenance dose of calcium to sustain a neutral calcium balance that prevents the body from drawing on its mineral stores in bone. For the older woman 1000 mg of calcium is recommended and 1500 mg if the woman is not on estrogen therapy. Elderly may also be mildly deficient in Vitamin D due to less sun exposure and a decrease in milk and dietary product intake. The usual dose of Vitamin D, 400 IU, is sufficient, but for those lacking adequate Vitamin D, 800 IU is recommended. It is clear that calcium is the cornerstone to preventing osteoporosis. Calcium can be taken as a dietary supplement (calcium carbonate tablet) (Table 6-3). However, calcium is better absorbed from dairy products and food (Table 6-4). Three to four 8-oz glasses of nonfat or low-fat milk is sufficient to provide the daily requirements. The use of powdered nonfat dry milk sprinkled into sauces, gravies, and soups provides a cheap and effective way to add calcium to the diet. Cheese can also be added to many dishes (Yen, 1995a).

Calcium carbonate supplements are absorbed best when taken with meals mainly due to the lack of sufficient gastric acid in the stomach of older adults between meals. Individuals who have a family history of kidney stones should seek a physician's advice before using calcium supplements. Avoidance of caffeine and nicotine should be encouraged since they stimulate the excretion of calcium. Alcohol affects vitamin D metabolism and also increases the loss of calcium; however, it is not clear how much alcohol must be ingested before these effects occur. Although osteoporosis occurs in men much less frequently than women, elderly men should not be ignored.

Malnutrition. Malnutrition encompasses more than pathologic states that result from a deficiency of essential nutrients and calories. It also refers to significant deviations in dietary patterns, which may produce undesirable risk factors. These can be detected in physical examinations, biochemical studies, and physiologic tests. Included in malnutrition are specific nutrient deficiencies, nutritional imbalances, and obesity. Figure 6-2 provides the malnutrition trajectory.

Table 6-3   Calcium Supplements

Name	Tablet size (mg)	Elemental calcium	Number of pills to = 1000 mg
Calcium carbonate (40% calcium)			
Tums	500	200	5
Tums EX	750	300	$3^1/_2$
OsCal	625	250	4
Oscal 500	1250	500	2
Caltrate 600	1500	600	2
Calcium lactate (13% calcium)			
	325	42	24
	648	85	12
Calcium gluconate (9% calcium)			
	500	45	$21^1/_2$
	650	59	$17^1/_2$
	1000	90	$11^1/_2$

Modified from Knoben JE, Anderson PO, editors: *Handbook of clinical drug data,* ed 7, Hamilton, Ill, 1993, Drug Intelligence Publications.

The occurrence of malnutrition among the elderly has been documented in both institutionalized and community-living elderly. A group of researchers in the Netherlands (van der Wielen et al, 1996) compared the energy and vitamin was intake of four different groups of elderly: institutionalized, community living, and sedentary or not. Dietary intake of the selected vitamins was below the minimum requirements in almost half of the nursing home residents. Intake was low for all the groups but lowest among the most impaired. Low intakes of vitamin, as well as select minerals, were reported by Gaspar (1996) among nursing home residents in the midwestern states. Elderly long-stay hospital patients were found in a study by Lipski et al (1993) to be grossly undernourished, and their dietary intake did not satisfy basal metabolic demands, based on recommended daily allowances. Among this group specific nutrients of concern were calories, vitamins D, E, B_6, and folic acid, magnesium, zinc, and retinol.

Three recent studies have identified malnutrion among community-living elderly. In a study that included rural and urban elderly from 67 communities, 1156 free-living elders underwent in-home assessment for nutritional status. Twenty-eight percent of the elders failed to consume adequate levels (75%) of the RDA for persons 51 years and older for three or more key nutrients. Over 40% of those screened were overweight, and 16% were underweight.

Payette and Gray-Donald (1994) estimated the prevalence of risk of nutritional deficiency in a group of functionally dependent elderly individuals receiving home health care in Canada. Over 65% of the 300 subjects had a low energy intake, and 30% had low body weight with 38% experiencing involuntary weight loss. The mean daily intake of protein, vitamins A, D, and E, folate, calcium, magnesium, and zinc were below recommended levels for more than

Table 6-4	Leading Calcium Sources	
Food	**Amount**	**Milligrams of calcium**
Dairy products		
Low-fat milk, 1% to 2%	1 cup	310
Skim milk	1 cup	300
Whole milk	1 cup	290
Buttermilk	1 cup	290
Nonfat dry milk	2 tablespoons	105
Eggnog	1 cup	330
Ice cream	1 cup	208
Plain yogurt (whole milk)	1 cup	300
Plain yogurt (low fat)	1 cup	400
Mozzarella cheese	1 ounce	210
Parmesan cheese	1 ounce	340
Swiss cheese	1 ounce	270
Cottage cheese, 2% fat	1 cup	160
Vegetables		
Collard greens	1 cup	360
Turnip greens	1 cup	250
Kale	1 cup	200
Bok choy	1 cup	250
Broccoli	1 cup	150
Fish		
Canned sardines (with bones)	4 ounces	500
Canned red salmon	4 ounces	290
Canned mackerel	4 ounces	300
Nuts		
Brazil nuts and hazelnuts	1/2 cup	125
Almonds	1/2 cup	160
Miscellaneous		
Tofu	3 1/2 ounces	128
Chocolate fudge	3 1/2 ounces	100
Light molasses	5 tablespoons	165
Black strap molasses	5 tablespoons	579
Seaweed, kelp, agar	3 1/2 ounces	1093

Compiled from *Reader's Digest:* The hidden health risk most women face, 1985; *Family Circle NBC Special Section:* For women only: your body, your health, 1985; *Kaiser Permanente Fact Sheet,* 1983, Women and calcium; Sardana R: Nutritional management of osteoporosis, *Geriatr Nurs* 13(6):317, 1992.

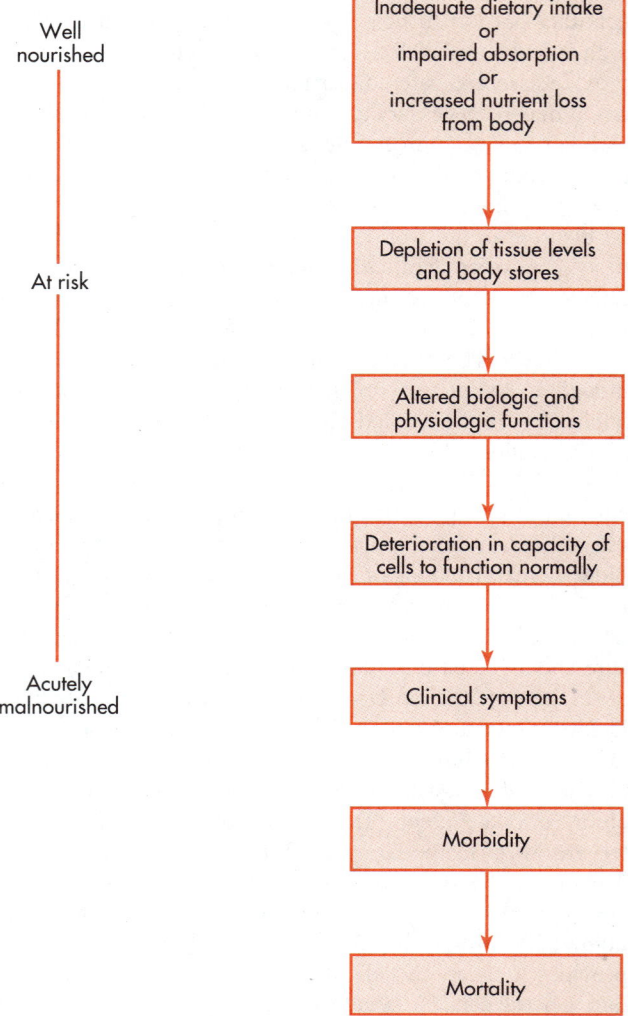

Figure 6-2. A trajectory for malnutrition. (Modified from Prodrabsky M. In Mahan LK, Arlin MT, editors: *Krause's food nutrition and diet therapy,* ed 8, Philadelphia, 1992, WB Saunders.)

50% of the subjects. In 21% of males and 32% of females diet was not adequate to provide two thirds of the recommended amounts for more than four nutrients.

Based on the Nutrition Screening Initiative (NSI) criteria, 30% of a New Jersey sample of elderly were potentially at high risk for nutrition-related problems, and 33% were at moderate risk. The most common nutritional risk factors were eating alone, taking three or more different prescribed or over-the-counter drugs daily, and having an illness or condition that caused a change in the kind or amount of food eaten (Garofalo and Hynak-Hankinson, 1995).

The association of nutritional intake with taste and odor sensation has recently been the focus of several research studies. de Graaf et al (1994) and Griep et al (1995) compared a healthy young group and an elderly group for the effect of odor and taste sensation, respectively, on nutrient intake. There was a significant decline in sensitivity for taste and odors among the older group. Besides the aging changes creating a decline in taste and odor sensation, Yen (1996) lists a number of disorders and factors affecting taste and smell, including Alzheimer's disease, Parkinson's disease, chronic renal failure, upper respiratory infection, smoking, bronchial asthma, diabetes mellitus, certain medications, and deficiencies of zinc, niacin, and vitamin B_{12}.

Duffy et al (1995) found that among a group of older women about half had decreased flavor and odor perception. The intakes of these women with perception alterations were significantly different than the other group with intact taste and odor perceptions. The group with a decline in per-

---

Box 6-6	**Possible Causes of Anorexia**

Social Factors
Poverty
Lack of help with food shopping and preparation
No socialization at meals

Psychologic Factors
Bereavement
Confusion
Depression

Physical Factors
Immobility
Inability to feed self
Bad oral hygiene
Poor dentition or ill-fitting dentures

Physiologic Factors
Decreased metabolic rate
Decreased enjoyment
    Diminished taste, smell, vision
Decreased feeding drive
    Neurotransmitters
    Nutritional factors
Increased satiety
    Peptide hormones
    Stomach emptying
Disease

Box 6-7	**Factors Potentiating Malnutrition in the Aged**

Psychosocial Risk Factors
Limited income
Abuse of alcohol and other central nervous system
    depressants
Bereavement, loneliness, or living alone
Removal from usual cultural patterns
Confusion, forgetfulness, or disorientation
Working toward intentional or subintentional death

Mechanical Risk Factors
Decreased or limited strength and mobility
Neurologic deficits, arthritis, handicap, impairment of
    hand-arm coordination, loss of tongue strength, and
    dysphagia
Decreased or diminished vision or blindness
Inability to feed self
Decubitus ulcers
Loss of teeth, poor-fitting dentures, or chewing
    problems
Difficult breathing
Polypharmacy
Surgery, nothing by mouth (NPO) for extended periods
    of time, or intravenous therapy only

---

ceptions had a lower preference for strongly sour or bitter foods, ate fewer citrus fruits and vegetables, had a preference for sweets, and ate a diet higher in saturated fat.

Schiffman and Warwick (1993) tested the intervention of adding flavor to food to enhance intake. The flavors were added as powders mixed with a small amount of liquid and did not contribute any calories or nutrients to the food. The elderly men and women in a retirement home ate more food and improved their immune function when several foods at each meal were enhanced with either meat, cheese, or maple flavor. It is important to remember that this intervention will work only for those who have some taste sensation left.

Protein calorie malnutrition (PCM) is a commonly misdiagnosed disorder of the elderly. PCM is the inadequate intake of calories and protein because of a high-carbohydrate, low-protein diet (Gupta et al, 1988; Cape, 1990). Symptoms include weight loss; pallor; dry, flaky skin; and loss of muscle mass. Biochemical analysis reveals low serum albumin levels if the malnutrition has been long term. Otherwise there is no evidence of hypoproteinemia. Normochromic or normocytic anemia is present and the elder is susceptible to infections. Elderly clients institutionalized for 2 weeks or more are at high risk for this nutritional problem. PCM also occurs in the presence of poor nutritional intake due to socioeconomic status, loss of dentition, gastrointestinal mal-

absorption, and functional disorders. Generally the elder complains of fatigue, weakness, dyspnea on exertion, and pedal edema. All of these complaints could be attributed to anemia and congestive heart failure when in reality the symptoms may due to PCM. If PCM occurs in the presence of congestive heart failure, one must be concerned with the possibility of digitalis toxicity. The symptoms of anorexia, nausea, and vomiting associated with digitalis toxicity are also precipitators of PCM. Because PCM may coexist with other disorders, it is important to have a medical evaluation and imperative that a complete nutritional history is included. Additional causes of anorexia appear in Box 6-6.

Aged persons who are at high nutritional risk include those who have psychosocial and mechanical difficulty. Wolanin (1976), Cape (1990), Garofalo and Hynak-Hankinson (1995), and Gaspar, (1996) identify situations that potentiate malnutrition in the aged (Box 6-7).

One need not be ill or hospitalized to have or develop one or more mechanical or psychosocial nutritional risk factors. Nutritional deficiencies, according to Roe (1992), develop from diets that are monotonous, destructive, and low in energy and nutrient/caloric ratio. Table 6-5 provides a summary of clinical signs of good and deleterious nutritional states.

Ethics of Nutrition

Fads, megavitamins, feeding, and intentional starvation are ethical issues to be addressed in nutrition of the older adult.

Table 6-5 Clinical Signs of Nutritional Status

	Good	Poor	Signs of malnutrition
General appearance	Alert, responsive	Listless, apathetic, cachectic	
Hair	Shiny, lustrous, healthy scalp	Stringy, dull, brittle, dry, depigmented	
Face			Swollen; dark cheeks and dark areas under eyes; skin on nose and mouth lumpy or flaky; enlarged parotid glands
Neck (glands)	No enlargement	Thyroid enlarged	Thyroid enlarged
Eyes	Bright, clear; no fatigue circles beneath	Dry, signs of infection, increased vascularity, glassiness, thickened conjunctiva	Dull; membranes dry and either too pale or too red; triangular, shiny grape-like spots on conjunctiva; bloodshot ring around cornea
Lips	Good color, moist	Dry, scaly, swollen, angular lesions (stomatitis)	Red, swollen, especially corners of mouth
Tongue	Good pink color, surface papillae present, no lesions	Papillary atrophy, smooth appearance; swollen, red, beefy (glossitis)	Swollen, appears raw, purple; abnormal papillae
Gums	Good pink color; no swelling or bleeding, firm	Marginal redness or swelling, receding, spongy	Same as poor nutritional status; bleed easily
Teeth	Straight, no crowding, well-shaped jaw, clean, no discoloration	Unfilled cavities, caries, absent teeth, worn surfaces, mottled, malposition	Same as poor nutritional status
Skin			
General	Smooth, slightly moist; good color	Rough, dry, scaly, pale, pigmented, irritated, petechia, bruises	
Face and neck	Smooth, slightly moist; good color, reddish pink mucous membranes	Greasy, discolored, scaly	More extensive than in poor nutritional status
Nails			Spoon shaped, brittle, ridged
Physique (musculoskeletal system)	Well developed, firm; no malformations	Flaccid, poor tone; undeveloped, tender	Same as for poor nutritional status but more extensive; muscles wasted; bowlegs, knock-knees, bumps on ribs, swollen joints
	Erect, arms and legs straight, abdomen in, chest out	Bowlegs, knock-knees, chest deformity at diaphragm, beaded ribs, prominent scapulas	
	No tenderness, weakness, or swelling; good color of legs	Sagging shoulders, sunken chest, humped back	
		Edema, tender calf, tingling, weakness of legs	
Weight	Normal for height, age, body build	Overweight or underweight	
Abdomen	Flat	Swollen	
Nervous system	Good attention span for age; does not cry easily, not irritable or restless	Inattentive, irritable	Irritable and confused; burning and tingling sensation of hands and feet; loss of sensation of position, decreased ankle and knee reflexes
Internal function			Heart rate above 100; abnormal rhythm; enlarged spleen and liver; high blood pressure
Gastrointestinal function	Good appetite and digestion; normal, regular	Anorexia, indigestion, constipation, or diarrhea	
General vitality	Endurance high, energetic, sleeps well at night; vigorous	Easily fatigues, no energy, falls asleep during the day, looks tired, apathetic	Absent

Compiled from Russell RM et al: Nutritional assessment. In Calkins E, Davis PJ, Ford AB, editors: *The practice of geriatrics,* Philadelphia, 1986, WB Saunders.; Ebert NJ: Nutrition in the aged and the nursing process. In Yurick AG, Spier BE, Ebert NJ et al: *The aged person and the nursing process,* ed 3, Norwalk, Conn, 1989, Appleton-Lange; Podrabsky M: Nutritional assessment. In Mahan LK, Arlin MT, editors: *Krause's food nutrition and diet therapy,* ed 8, Philadelphia, 1992, WB Saunders.

Food Fads. Aged individuals are not immune to food faddism and fall prey to advertisements that claim specific foods maintain youth and vitality or rid one of chronic conditions. Fad foods are often more costly than a balanced diet and can sometimes be obtained only in health food stores or by mail order. Even if the food is easily obtained in a supermarket, such large quantities may be called for that some nutrients are obtained in excess, while others are excluded.

Megavitamin therapy or the ingestion of large amounts of a specific vitamin or many different vitamins can also be considered a fad. Unless the individual is severely depleted of vitamins, which can usually be obtained in an adequate diet, megavitamin therapy is nonessential and dangerous. Risks exist in megavitamin therapy: bone meal, a source of calcium, may contain lead and thus cause lead poisoning; high doses of zinc causes zinc toxicity; and kelp with its high iodine content can cause goiter in those with preexisting thyroid enlargement. High intake of niacin is discouraged because of a high incidence of cardiac arrhythmias, abnormal biochemical findings, and gastrointestinal problems. Intake of vitamin D has the potential for toxicity, and vitamins C and E have insufficient data to warrant recommendation now (Roe, 1992). The money spent on food fads and unneeded vitamins by the aged could buy more economical foods that benefit the individual's health. Megavitamin therapy has a role in maintaining nutrition when illness, malnutrition, or excessive demands are placed on body function.

Recently attention has been directed toward the lowering of cholesterol in the diet. A soy-containing diet, fatty fish (salmon, herring, mackerel, and anchovies) in the diet at least four times a week and other low-fat diets have been found to decrease total cholesterol and LDL measurements (Siscovick et al, 1995; Anderson et al, 1995; Hubbard, 1995). Fat substitutes such as Olestra are currently appearing in the nation's food stores, but they are fraught with problems, among which are the depletion of fat-soluble vitamins, including A, D, E, and K, and reduction of blood carotenoid levels (even though the substitutes may be fortified with the vitamins to make up for the depletion). Some individuals have noted diarrhea and/or abdominal cramping, and rectal leakage after eating several ounces of food containing the fat substitute. The evidence for potentially adverse effects from the use of the fat substitutes is overwhelming, and the elderly need to be cautioned about their use of foods containing this substance. The FDA is requiring additional studies (Olestra: Just say no, 1996).

Fast foods have become a stable part of the American diet. In a survey of older Americans who attend senior centers in two states, Morris et al (1995) determined the frequency and motivations for eating fast food. Six percent in one state and 11% in the other state reported that they eat at a fast food restaurant once a week. They usually do not eat their main meal there. One-fifth of respondents in both states claimed they frequent fast food restaurants so they will not have to cook. Economics was important to about one quarter of respondents in both states. They visited fast food restaurants for discounts and low food costs. Social reasons for frequenting fast food establishments were cited by 11% of respondents in New Jersey and 18% of the time in Texas.

Snack foods also constitute a substantial component of the American diet. Cross et al (1995) evaluated snacking behavior among 335 noninstitutionalized older adults. They found that the majority of seniors snacked at least once daily, with only 2.1% reporting that they never snack. Evening was the most common time for snacking with the most often reported foods being salty/crunchy foods. When selecting snacks, taste outranked nutrition as a selection criteria.

Feeding the Impaired Aged. It is not uncommon in long-term care facilities to hear over the public address system at mealtime, "Feeder trays are ready." This reference to the need to feed those unable to feed themselves is, in itself, degrading and erases any trace of dignity the aged person is trying to maintain in a controlled environment. It is not malicious intent by nurses or other caregivers but rather a habit of convenience. Feeding the aged who do not respond intelligibly becomes mechanical and devoid of conversation and feeling. The feeding process becomes rapid, and if it bogs down and becomes too slow, the meal may be ended abruptly, depending on the time the caregiver has allotted for feeding the patient. Any pleasure is destroyed that could be derived through socialization and eating, as is any dignity that could be maintained while dependent on others for food. Food should be given with variety throughout the meal, that is, serve a bite of one item, then another, and so forth. This not only eliminates the monotony of eating all of one food before being given another, but also changing textures as one eats, enhances eating enjoyment. When an elder needs encouragement to eat, small, frequent servings of food that he or she likes are better tolerated. In one study of 20 hospitalized elders without severe cognitive dysfunction, touch, verbal cueing and combination of touch and verbal cueing effectively increased nutritional intake (Lange-Alberts and Shott, 1994).

Sidenvall, et al (1994) observed the natural meal situation (in a group setting) of 18 nursing home residents. Lack of eating competence resulted in a lower intake. There was a difference in culture between the staff and the residents. It was a workplace for the staff, and they had broader standards for acceptable table manners than the elderly. The elderly strove to behave in accordance with their standards and suffered because of their own limited eating competence and experience of other patients' problems. Communication was a theme identified. The elderly patients avoided expressing their needs, and the nurses thought they were prying if they asked questions about such issues.

In a group of nursing home residents Thomas (1994) found that the major difference between the malnourished and the nonmalnourished groups was in the acceptance of the diet, that is, the estimated amount of food consumed at each meal expressed as a percentage of the diet taken. The malnourished group consumed 80% of their diet compared with 95% in the nonmalnourished group. The amount of energy offered in the malnourished group tended to be higher than for the nonmalnourished group, but the amount consumed was much less. The degree of assistance required in eating was also correlated with the presence of malnutrition. On admission the groups were equal as to the level of assistance needed, but by the end of the study residents who remained malnourished required more assistance in eating.

Adequate nutrition for the helpless aged depends on the conscientiousness of the individual doing the feeding. It is the nurse's responsibility to ensure that all patients unable to feed themselves not only receive a tray but also are actually fed the food that has been brought to them. Anytime a patient has not eaten a meal or has refused as few as three consecutive meals, it is essential that a nutritional assessment be done to prevent malnutrition and its complications.

In the acute care hospital setting it is equally important to give consideration, care, and attention to the feeding of the dependent aged patient. Sufficient time should be provided to accommodate the aged person who has a slow eating pace.

Intentional Starvation. Refusal of food can be an acceptable means of suicide for the aged person. Some aged truly have given up and wish to die. Not eating is one last bastion of control over life and dignity. It is essential for the nurse to differentiate between the individual who is refusing food because it is unpalatable and the person who is depressed and really wishes to die.

Intentional starvation is easier and more successful when one is not institutionalized. The institutionalized person is often denied this right and is robbed of the option by forced feeding via a nasogastric tube. The American Nurses' Association in 1992 developed a position statement on forgoing artificial nutrition and hydration. The position states: "The decision to withhold artificial nutrition and hydration should be made by the patient or surrogate with the health care team. The nurse continues to provide expert care to patients who are no longer receiving artificial nutrition and hydration."

Watching someone starve is difficult for the nurse, but if intentional starvation is the patient's desire, the nurse should continue to order the tray, take it to the person, and acknowledge that the individual has the right to eat or not eat. It is important to leave the tray so that the person can exercise the option to change his or her mind. If the person is unable to feed himself or herself, check shortly after the first offering of food has been refused to see if the person does wish to eat. An empathetic and nonjudgmental approach by the nurse to the aged person who demonstrates starvation behavior will convey that the individual is still in control, and if for some reason the individual decides to exercise the option to eat again, this too is all right. Either way, the caregiver has provided support and respect for that individual.

Professional team conferences are needed to deal with the client's mental status and ethical issues involved in referral and the right to die. Superficial judgments are not adequate to encompass these profound issues.

Assessment

A position statement on nutrition screening for the elderly by the American Nurses' Association (1992) acknowledges the numerous risks for nutritional deficiencies that are encountered by some older persons. Routine nutrition screening and assessment of elderly individuals on admission into the health care system is supported. Nurses are also urged to collaborate with other professionals in all settings to promote nutritional screening for older adults.

Unless inadequate diet has become an obvious problem, an intensive nutritional assessment is infrequently done. Height and weight may be obtained and compared to standard charts, which are prepared predominantly from normative values of individuals under the age of 55. Several questions are asked regarding food likes and dislikes, the current diet, and other assorted questions pertaining to eating. Weight alone is an inaccurate measurement of nutritional status, since it does not indicate the adequacy of the diet. One can meet the correct weight value for height, but the weight may be the result of fluid retention, edema, or ascites. The adequacy of muscle mass and body fat are not assessed, yet these are the two measurements that can provide accurate information about body nutrition.

The Consensus Conference sponsored by the Nutrition Screening Initiative in 1991 developed nutritional screening materials to promote routine nutritional care in America's health care system. The elderly population was its initial focus in hopes of improving their nutritional state. A basic checklist was developed that has two elements: a self-assessment protocol that helps identify specific eating habits and lifestyles that might put the elder at nutritional risk, and advice to provide basic education on nutritional risk factors to remind the public and professionals of these risk factors (Figure 6-3). A Level I and II screening tool that is more detailed is used by the professional when nutritional risks are identified (see Appendix 6-A). The Nutrition Screening Initiative presents an algorithm for nutritional assessment and approaches (Figure 6-4).

More recently a rapid assessment tool, the Mini-Nutritional Assessment (MNA), has been developed and validated in several populations of elderly (see Appendix 6-B). The results show that the MNA can accurately assess the nutritional status of elderly, differentiating normal or well-nourished subjects from those who are borderline or at risk of malnutrition and from those with the presence of undernutrition. Both normal and malnutrition classifications were the same as those obtained using the nutritional clinical assessment by a physician. This tool was cross-validated in elderly populations from the very frail to the healthy elderly (Guigoz et al, 1994).

A simple screening test for detecting individuals potentially at nutritional risk is called the SCALES (Morley, 1994). The letters of the test stand for the following: S—sadness (Yesavage Geriatric Depression Scale of 15 or greater out of 30); C—cholesterol (less than 160 mg/dl); A—albumin (less than 4 g/dl); L—loss of weight (2 lb in 1 month or 5 lb in 6 months); E—Eat (has problems feeding self either because of physical or cognitive problems); and S—Shopping (sufficient money to buy food and the ability to obtain and prepare it). Laboratory data need to be available for this screening. The importance of depression as a major factor in the etiology of undernutriton is rec-

ognized. A major advantage of the mnemonic is the ease in remembering the categories for assessment (Morley, 1994).

A nutritional assessment that provides the most conclusive data about a person's actual nutritional state consists of four steps: interview, physical examination, anthropometric measurements, and biochemical analysis. The collective results can provide the nurse with data needed to identify the immediate and potential nutrition problems of the client. The nurse can then begin to establish plans for supervision, assistance, and education in the attainment of adequate nutrition for the aged person.

The Warning Signs of poor nutritional health are often overlooked. Use this checklist to find out if you or someone you know is at nutritional risk.

Read the statements below. Circle the number in the yes column for those that apply to you or someone you know. For each yes answer, score the number in the box. Total your nutritional score.

DETERMINE YOUR NUTRITIONAL HEALTH

	YES
I have an illness or condition that made me change the kind and/or amount of food I eat.	2
I eat fewer than 2 meals per day.	3
I eat few fruits or vegetables, or milk products.	2
I have 3 or more drinks of beer, liquor or wine almost everyday.	2
I have tooth or mouth problems that make it hard for me to eat.	2
I don't always have enough money to buy the food I need.	4
I eat alone most of the time.	1
I take 3 or more different prescribed or over-the-counter drugs a day.	1
Without wanting to, I have lost or gained 10 pounds in the last 6 months.	2
I am not always physically able to shop, cook and/or feed myself.	2
TOTAL	

Total Your Nutritional Score. If it's—

0–2 **Good!** Recheck your nutritional score in 6 months.

3–5 **You are at moderate nutritional risk.** See what can be done to improve your eating habits and lifestyle. Your office on aging, senior nutrition program, senior citizens center or health department can help. Recheck your nutritional score in 3 months.

6 or more You are at high nutritional risk. Bring this checklist the next time you see your doctor, dietitian or other qualified health or social service professional. Talk with them about any problems you may have. Ask for help to improve your nutritional health.

These materials developed and distributed by the Nutrition Screening Initiative, a project of:

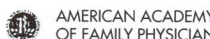
AMERICAN ACADEMY OF FAMILY PHYSICIANS

THE AMERICAN DIETETIC ASSOCIATION

NATIONAL COUNCIL ON THE AGING, INC.

Remember that warning signs suggest risk, but do not represent diagnosis of any condition. Turn the page to learn more about the Warning Signs of poor nutritional health.

Figure 6-3. Warning signs of poor nutrition checklist. (Courtesy The Nutrition Screening Initiative, Washington, DC.)

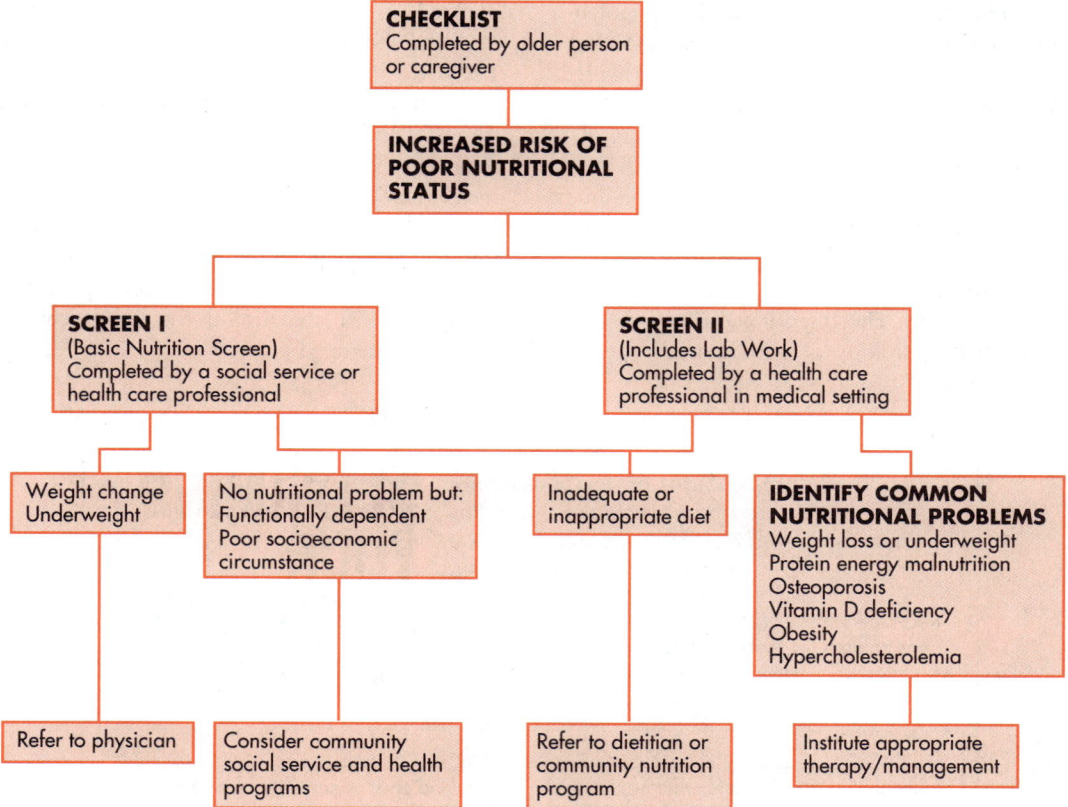

Figure 6-4. Nutritional assessment and approaches. (Courtesy The Nutrition Screening Initiative, Washington, DC.)

Interview. The interview provides background information and clues to the nutritional state and actual and potential problems of the elderly person. Questions about the individual's state of health, social activities, normal patterns, and changes that have occurred should be asked. The nurse must explore the individual's needs, the manner in which food is obtained, and the client's ability to prepare food. Information concerning the relationship of food to daily events will provide clues to the meaning and significance of food to that person. The aged who eat alone are considered candidates for marginal malnutrition. Information about occupation and daily activities will suggest the degree of energy expenditure and caloric intake most correct for the overall activity. One's economic state will have a direct bearing on nutrition. It is therefore important to explore the client's financial resources to establish the income available for food. Knowledge of medications taken should be included in the nutrition history. Discussion in Chapter 10 indicates the effects of medication on one's nutritional status. Additional medical information should be included in the interview. The presence or absence of mouth pain or discomfort, visual difficulty, bowel and bladder function, and food intake patterns should be explored. Frequently a 24-hour diet recall compared with the Food Guide Pyramid or a convenient food grouping format can present an estimate of nutritional adequacy. When the aged person cannot provide all the information requested, it may be possible to obtain data from a family member or another source. There will be times, however, when information will not be as complete as one would like, or the aged person, too proud to admit that he or she is not eating, will furnish erroneous information. The nurse will still be able to obtain additional data from the other three areas of the nutritional assessment.

Keeping a dietary record for 3 days is another assessment tool. Careful recording of when one ate, what was eaten, and amounts eaten must be made. This approach should be attempted only with dependable, cooperative elders. Computer analysis of the dietary records provide information on energy and vitamin and mineral intake. Printouts can provide the elderly and the health care provider with a visual graph of their intake.

Physical Examination. The second step of the nutritional assessment, the physical examination, furnishes clinically observable evidence of the existing state of nutrition. Data such as height and weight; vital signs; condition of the tongue, lips, and gums; skin turgor, texture, and color are assessed, and the general overall appearance is scrutinized for evidence of wasting.

The weight chart in Table 6-6 shows weight averages for older men and women. By adding or subtracting approxi-

Table 6-6   Smooth Average Weights* for Older Men and Women

Height (inches)	Weight (pounds)					
	55-64 yr	65-74 yr	75-79 yr	80-84 yr	85-89 yr	90-94 yr
Men						
62	148	144	133	135		
63	151	148	138	136	133	
64	155	151	143	138	135	
65	158	154	148	141	139	130
66	162	158	154	144	142	133
67	166	161	159	147	145	136
68	169	165	164	150	148	140
69	173	168	169	154	152	144
70	176	171	174	159	156	149
71	180	175	179	164	160	154
72	184	178	184	170	165	
73	187	182	189			
74	191	185	194			
Women						
57	138	132	125			
58	141	135	129	111	110	
59	144	138	132	118	113	
60	149	142	136	121	116	
61	150	145	139	124	120	119
62	152	149	143	128	124	119
63	155	152	146	132	128	120
64	158	156	150	136	133	124
65	161	159	153	140	138	129
66	164	163	157	144	142	
67	167	166	160			
68	170	170	164			

Compiled from weight, height, and selected body dimensions of adults (ages 55 to 79), United States, 1960-1962. Series 11, No. 8, National Center For Health Statistics, Washington, DC; Carnevali D, Patrick M: *Nursing management for the elderly,* Philadelphia, 1979, JB Lippincott.
*Estimated values from regression equations of weights for specific age groups, *Am J Clin Nutr,* 40:63, 1984.

mately 7 kg (14 lb) for men and 6 kg (12 lb) for women, the nurse can establish the optimum weight range for a person of a specific height and in a particular age group. Close inspection of the weight scale shows that there is a gradual decline in weight as age increases. This is different than the values presented on standard weight charts used to assess the weight of most adult people. The standard charts suggest that persons of different ages such as a 20-year-old woman and a 40-year-old woman of comparable height should also weigh about the same. The nurse should be sure that assessment of weight for the elderly is based on schedules specifically developed for the aged (Table 6-6) and not those that were created for individuals under age 51.

Debate continues in the quest to determine the appropriate weight charts for the aged. Weight, however, is not the only issue; fat distribution needs to be considered. Dr. William Castelli, head of the Framingham Heart Study, indicates that fat stored above the waist is associated with hypertension and cholesterol levels. Weight lower on the body (pear shaped) is benign. A man's waist should not exceed the hips at its largest diameter, and a woman's waist should not exceed 80% of her hip diameter (Crowley, 1988).

Anthropometric Measurements. Anthropometric measurements are the third part of the nutritional assessment and should include height, weight, midarm circumference, and triceps skinfold thickness. These include simple body measurement procedures, which take less than 5 minutes to perform. These measurements obtain information about the status of the aged person's muscle mass and body fat in relation to height and weight. In some instances an individual is bedridden or confined to a chair, or the individual has a spinal curvature preventing accurate height measurement. Unlike stature, knee height changes little with age. An estimation of stature can be made using knee height and a sliding broad-blade calipers, similar to the apparatus used to measure the length of an infant. This device consists of an adjustable blade attached to each end at a 90° angle.

While lying supine, the person being measured bends the left knee at a 90° angle. One blade of the sliding, broad-blade calipers is placed under the heel of the left foot; the other blade is placed over the anterior surface of the left thigh, above the condyles of the femur. Computation of stature requires the person's knee height, age (rounded to the nearest whole year), and gender. One formula is used for men and another for women. The following formulas are used to compute stature:

Stature men = 64.19 − (0.04 × age) +

(2.02 × knee height)

Stature women = 84.88 − (0.24 × age) +

(1.83 × knee height)

Chumlea and Guo (1992) indicate that the formulas may be different for men and women that are of a race other than white. Race-specific formulas for black individuals have been developed but not validated at this time.

Muscle mass measurements are obtained by measuring the arm circumference of the nondominant upper arm. The arm hangs freely at the side, and a measuring tape is placed around the midpoint of the upper arm, between the acromion of the scapula and the olecranon of the ulna. The centimeter circumference is recorded and compared with standard values (Table 6-7).

Chumlea and Roche (1986) cite that the combined mid-arm circumference and triceps skinfold calculations provide an estimate of midarm muscle areas that can be a useful indicator for determining protein-calorie malnutrition. These measurements can also be used to monitor interventions and changes in the nutritional status of elders regardless of race. Body fat is assessed by measuring specific skinfolds with Lange or Harpenden calipers. Two areas are accessible for measurement. One area is the midpoint of the upper arm, the triceps area, which is also used to obtain arm circumference. The nondominant arm is again used. The nurse lifts the skin with the thumb and forefinger so that it parallels the humerus. The calipers are placed around the skinfold, 1 cm below where the fingers are grasping the skin. Two readings are averaged to the nearest half centimeter. Results should be compared with standard values such as those cited in Chumlea and Roche (1986). If there is a neuropathologic condition or hemiplegia following a stroke, the unaffected arm should be used for obtaining measurements.

The second and more accurate site is immediately below the tip of the scapula. This area provides uniformity of the fat layer. The skin immediately below the tip of the scapula is grasped with the thumb and forefinger, the calipers applied, and two consecutive readings obtained and averaged in the same manner as the triceps measurement.

A study by Volkert et al (1992) suggests that independent institutionalized well elders age 75 and older reflected anthropometric measurements similar to younger elders but much lower than young adults. Well elders had higher measurements than geriatric patients with overt disease conditions.

Biochemical Examination. The final step in a nutritional assessment is the biochemical examination. This includes an analysis of the pH; the presence or absence of protein, glucose, and acetone in the urine; and the levels of hemoglobin, total protein, serum albumin, and cholesterol and the hematocrit ratio in the blood. Data directly related to the present nutritional state can be gathered and evaluated.

Based on the nurse's assessment, it may be necessary to refer the aged person to a nutritionist for a more intensive evaluation. The nurse in many instances should be able to educate the aged about their nutritional needs and how to effectively meet them.

Intervention

Interventions are formulated around the identified nutritional problem or problems. Perhaps the most significant intervention for the community elder is nutrition education and problem solving with the elder in how to best resolve the potential or actual nutritional deficit. The American Nurses' Association (ANA) Position Statement on Nutrition Screening of the Elderly (1992) supports educational programs focusing on nutrition for older consumers. Knowledge of nutrition has been found to influence intake. Krebs-Smith et al (1995) found that among older adults over 65 years of age only 8% thought they should have five servings of fruits and vegetables a day. The remaining 92% of the sample believed that fewer servings were recommended. In a study conducted by Itoh and Suyama (1995) of healthy elderly Japanese population, participation in nutritional education programs was positively associated with micronutrient intake.

Education in the area of reading nutritional information on labels is needed. Since May 1994 the US Food and Drug Administration (FDA) has required makers of processed foods to list nutrition information based on Daily Values. Daily values represent the maximum amount of nutrients and fiber that are desirable in daily diets of 2000 or 2500

Table 6-7	Anthropometric Measurements		
Percentage of standard		Male	Female
Mid upper arm circumference (in centimeters)			
90		26.33	25.7
80		23.4	22.8
70		20.5	20.0
60		17.6	17.1
STANDARD		29.3	28.5
Triceps skinfold (in millimeters)			
90		11.3	11.9
80		10.0	13.2
70		8.8	11.6
60		7.5	9.9
STANDARD		12.5	16.5

Modified from Keithley JK: Proper nutritional assessment can prevent hospital malnutrition, *Nurs '79* 92:70, Feb 1979.

calories. The nutrients were chosen based on evidence suggesting eating too much or too little of these substances has the greatest impact on your health. FDA defines a "good source" as a food that contains 10% to 19% of the Daily Value per serving. The daily totals for fat, cholesterol, and sodium need to be less than 100%. An emphasis on balance as the key to a healthful diet needs to be promoted (Mayo Clinic Health Letter, April 1995).

Practical suggestions for increasing intake when an older person is experiencing a poor appetite were presented by Yen (1994). Suggestions include the following:

- Add nonfat dry mild powder to just about anything with liquid in it
- Make nourishments part of routine care
- Offer the most food when the patient is most hungry (usually morning)
- Emphasize taste and eye appeal
- Offer finger foods
- Add some fat—margarine—to vegetables, creamed foods and sauces, and cooked cereal
- Use fortified milk
- Conduct calorie counts, because they serve as a useful indicator that progress is being made and show foods that are tolerated

It is important for those elders institutionalized in acute or long-term care facilities to receive appropriate supervision at mealtime so that they are able to eat their food, have their dentures in place and glasses on, have their food cut for them, if necessary, and have any other requirement met that will enable them to meet their nutritional intake needs. It is also important to provide the elder with some degree of social interaction during mealtime. Table 6-8 provides age-related changes, outcomes, and interventions for the gastrointestinal system that directly or indirectly affect nutrition and elimination.

ELIMINATION

The body must remove waste products of metabolism to sustain healthy function, but bladder and bowel activity are fraught with social implications. Bladder and bowel function of the aged, although normally only slightly altered by physiologic changes of age, can develop problems severe enough to interfere with the ability to continue independent living and seriously threaten the body's capacity to function and to survive. The effects of uncontrolled bladder and bowel action are a threat to the person's independence and well-being. Elimination is a private matter not to be

Table 6-8   Age-Related Gastrointestinal Changes, Outcomes, and Health Prevention, Promotion, and Maintenance Approaches

Age-related changes	Outcomes	Health prevention, promotion, and maintenance
Decreased acuity of taste	Dry mouth	Take in adequate high fiber in diet
Decreased saliva production with increased alkalinity	Diminished taste	Adequate exercise
Brittle teeth/retracted gingiva	Pale gums	Bowel training
Less effective chewing	Vermilion border of mouth missing	No or little use of laxative
Decreased esophageal and intestinal motility	Atrophy of gums with loss of teeth or decay	Good oral care
Decrease in gastric secretions	Difficulty chewing	Suck on ice chips or hard candy
Loss of elasticity in intestinal wall	Decreased appetite	Hold cold water in mouth before swallowing
Decreased blood flow to intestines	Thirst	Use sodium-free flavorings
Reduced blood flow to liver	Coughing or choking	Consult dentist once or twice a year
Loss or diminished anal sphincter control	Dysphagia	Use soft bristled toothbrush and dental floss
Weaker neural impulses to lower bowel	Nausea/vomiting	For dentures, brush to clean between teeth
	Heartburn/indigestion	Cut food into small pieces, chew thoroughly
	Diarrhea	Have abdominal pain evaluated
	Constipation	Increase dietary fiber, fluids, and exercise
	Fecal impaction	Have a regular meal pattern
	Malnutrition	Respond promptly to the urge to defecate
	Drug toxicity	Report any change in bowel routine
		Manage diet within budget
		Utilize Meals on Wheels if needed
		Use dietary supplements
		Recognize signs of drug toxicity for drugs taken
Taste		
Fewer taste buds	Food tastes bland	Encourage social dining
	Overseasons food	Nutritional supplementation
		Use herbs for seasoning, lemon, spices (nonsalty)

Nursing Diagnoses

The following potential diagnoses must be considered as well as diagnoses unique to the particular individual:

Alteration in nutrition
 Less than body requirements
 More than body requirements

Risk for fluid volume deficit
Risk for aspiration
Impaired swallowing
Alteration in sensory perception: gustatory

NURSING PROCESS AND NURSING DIAGNOSIS
Alterated Nutrition: Less Than Body Requirements

Etiologies and Related Factors
Biologic changes associated with aging
Illness
Psychologic influences: loneliness, social isolation, living alone
Financial or transportation problems
Physical limitations
Altered mental status
Ethnic/religious eating patterns
Difficulty swallowing

Defining Characteristics
Weight 20% or more below ideal body weight
Lack of interest in food
Aversion to food
Depression
Reported altered taste sensation
Weakness of muscles required to swallow and masticate food
Reported or observed inadequate food intake less than RDA recommendations
Report or evidence of lack of food
Abdominal pain (with or without pathologic conditions)
Anemia
Serum albumin <3 g/dl

Knowledge
Normal anatomic and functional changes with aging
Gastrointestinal disorders common to the aged (pathophysiology)
Independent and dependent nursing management options

Oral cavity problems
Gastrointestinal assessment (illness history, diet history, psychosocioeconomic factors)
Symptoms
Physical examination for normal and abnormal findings
Community screening/teaching

Clinical Judgment and Related Skills
Obtain a complete gastrointestinal interview and history
Conduct a thorough physical examination of face, oral cavity, abdomen
Implement nursing interventions that can prevent and manage altered gastrointestinal function such as proper oral hygiene; medication administration, dietary counseling for adequate intake, constipation; position client for swallowing and elimination; feed clients; cut food in bite size for frail elders; provide food selections, acquisition, and preparation
Maintain an intake and output record; administer enemas or irrigations as needed
Design a home care plan, implement, and evaluate its effectiveness

Evaluation
Weight gain
Enjoys food
Takes an active part in meal planning or choice selection
Laboratory values show improvement or are within normal limits

NEEDS ADDRESSED AND TASK STRENGTHS

Interest in maintaining healthful lifestyle
Attentive to subtle body signals
Able to judge and seek to meet own needs

Respects and provides for current survival needs
Accepts need for others' intervention when necessary

publicized socially. Emphasis is placed on the specific procedures of eliminating and disposing of waste, and the media advertise laxatives to maintain the continued evacuation of fecal matter. Bowel preoccupation costs 250 million dollars in laxative expenditures, mainly to the elderly (Rousseau, 1990). As children, correct behavior in dealing with our own body waste is taught early. Deviations from this are socially unacceptable and can lead to chastisement, ostracism, and social withdrawal (referred to in Chapter 18).

Bowel Function

Attention to bowel function occurs when there is a deviation from what is perceived as normal elimination. The aged are known for their concern with their bowel function and frequently complain to physicians and other health care personnel about problems, particularly constipation. Whatever the complaint, one needs to know exactly what the individual means when he or she says there is a problem. Bowel function problems that the nurse will encounter among aged clients are constipation, fecal impaction, and fecal or bowel incontinence. Bowel incontinence is discussed in Chapter 8.

Constipation. Constipation has different meanings to different people. Some individuals consider constipation infrequent bowel action; others perceive it as difficulty in passing feces, and others consider both to be indicative of constipation. To the health professional, constipation occurs when there are less than three bowel movements a week (Rousseau, 1990).

Normal elimination should be an easy passage of feces, without undue straining or a feeling of incomplete evacuation or defecation. The urge to defecate occurs when the distended walls of the sigmoid and rectum, which are filled with feces, stimulate pressure receptors to relax the sphincters for the expulsion of stool through the anus. Evacuation of feces is accomplished by relaxation of the sphincters and contraction of the diaphragm and abdominal muscles, which raise intraabdominal pressure. When one strains at stool, pressure is elevated in the colon, which causes the formation of pouches, or diverticula, in the colon wall. Increased intraabdominal pressure pushes the stomach against and through the diaphragm, creating hiatal hernias. Downward pressure is transmitted to veins and can cause varicose veins and hemorrhoids.

Constipation appears to be a problem of the old because they use more laxatives than the young and because the advertisements are overwhelmingly directed toward the aged. It is perhaps more correct to consider the extensive use of laxatives by the aged as a cultural habit. During their formative years, weekly doses of rhubarb, cascara, castor oil and other types of laxatives were consumed to promote health. This belief that cleaning out the colon was paramount to maintaining good health still persists with many of the elderly.

Constipation is a symptom. It is a reflection of poor habits, postponed passage of stool, and a misunderstanding of the real definition of constipation. Most people believe that an individual must have a bowel movement daily, when in fact normal bowel function for 98% of the population varies from three movements daily to only three per week (Harari et al, 1993). In a survey of 209 elderly community-dwelling people (Whitehead et al, 1989) 30% of the men and 29% of the women reported that they experienced constipation at least once a month. Yet only 2% of women and 3% of men reported that their average stool frequency was less than three per week.

There are numerous precipitating factors for constipation, which can be categorized as physiologic, functional, mechanical, psychologic, systemic, pharmacologic, and other. A list of these factors is provided in Table 6-9.

Studies have shown that diet plays a significant role in problems with intestinal motility and constipation. Some authorities believe delayed passage of stool facilitates the action of carcinogenic chemical buildup caused by bacteria in the

---

Table 6-9   Precipitating Factors for Constipation

Physiologic	Psychologic
Dehydration	Avoidance of urge to defecate
Insufficient fiber intake	Confusion
Poor dietary habits	Depression
	Emotional stress

Functional	Systemic
Decreased physical activity	Diabetes mellitus
Inadequate toileting	Hypercalcemia
Irregular defecation habits	Hyperparathyroidism
Irritable bowel disease	Hypothyroidism
Weakness	Hypokalemia
	Pheochromocytoma
	Porphyria
	Uremia

Mechanical	Pharmacologic
Abscess or ulcer	Aluminum-containing antacids
Cerebrovascular disease	Anticholinergics
Defective electrolyte transfer	Anticonvulsants
Fissures	Antidepressants
Hemorrhoids	Bismuth salts
Hirschsprung's disease	Calcium carbonate
Neurological disease	Calcium channel blockers
Parkinson's disease	Diuretics
Postsurgical obstruction	Laxative overuse
Prostate enlargement	Iron salts
Rectal prolapse	Nonsteroidal antiinflammatories
Rectocele	Opiates
Spinal cord injury	Phenothiazines
Strictures	Sedatives
Tumors	Sympathomimetics

Other

Lack of abdominal muscle tone	Obesity
Recent environmental changes	Poor dentition

From Allison OC, Porter ME, Briggs GG: Chronic constipation: assessment and management in the elderly, *J Am Acad Nurse Practitioners* 6(7):311, 1994.

bowel. The delayed evacuation of feces permits higher concentrations of these chemicals to remain in contact with the colon wall for longer periods (Burkitt, 1982; Brocklehurst, 1986). However, it has been suggested that constipation in elders might be related to loss of colonic cells that determine water content of stool.

Assessment. The precipitating factors of constipation (Table 6-9) need to be included in the assessment of the client to shed light on the possible cause or causes of altered bowel function. A review of these factors will also determine if a client is at risk for altered bowel function. It is recognized that the elderly at high risk for constipation and subsequent impaction are the aged who have hypotonic colon function, who are immobilized and debilitated, or who have central nervous system lesions. Specific questions for initial assessment of constipation with the rationale for obtaining the assessment data appear in Box 6-8. A review of food and fluid intake may be necessary to determine the amount of fiber and fluid ingested. It is also important to remember that confusion, increased agitation, incontinence, and elevated temperature and/or unexplainable falls can be the only presenting clinical symptoms of constipation in the elderly (Allison et al, 1994).

A physical examination is needed to assess conditions such as dry skin and poor skin turgor, decubitus ulcer, abdominal distention, masses, bowel sounds, flatus, and mobility. Light palpation of the abdomen can detect tenderness and muscular resistance associated with chronic constipation (Allison et al, 1994).

A rectal examination is important to reveal painful anal disorders such as hemorrhoids or fissures that will impede the evacuation of stool and to evaluate sphincter tone. Biochemical tests should include calcium, and potassium levels, complete blood count, and thyroid studies.

Intervention. Nonpharmacologic interventions for constipation that have been implemented and evaluated can be grouped into four areas: (1) fluid/fiber, (2) exercise, (3) environmental manipulation, and (4) a combination of the first three areas. As early as 1977, Wichita noted that prevention and correction of constipation could be obtained if the nursing home residents ate two slices of whole wheat bread daily and had 2 teaspoons of bran in their diet every day. The wheat and bran were capable of increasing stool weight and transit time through the colon and seemed to end constipation in about 3 weeks.

Rodrigues-Fisher et al (1993) evaluated efficacy of fiber and fluid nursing intervention on the maintenance of bowel movements along with the withdrawal of pharmacologic elimination aids in long-term care residents. The number of laxatives and stool softeners needed by the residents decreased significantly as the fiber and fluid intervention was implemented in the 6-month study.

Kovach (1992) promotes the use of bran fiber rather than fruit and vegetable fiber since bran fiber will not degrade as readily in the intestinal tract. Bran fiber results in a functioning colon with higher fecal bulking action and less constipation. Yet Kovach suggests that fruit and vegetable fiber are still important as the products of their degradation could be essential for other physiologic and metabolic actions.

In a well-designed study Gibson et al (1995) found that the use of the "standard recipe" of prune juice, applesauce, and bran was effective in decreasing the use of laxatives

Box 6-8	Constipation Assessment Questions and Rationale	
Question	**Rationale**
When did constipation begin?	Lifelong history of constipation is likely to be a functional disorder; sudden change may be an organic lesion such as carcinoma.
Has anything in bowel function recently changed?	A sudden change even in constipation may signal an underlying disorder.
How often do bowel movements occur?	Frequency of defecation may actually be normal. The question may also unknowingly let clients describe their cathartic use.
Is the urge to defecate lacking or the stool difficult to expel?	Absent urge may indicate chronic suppression of normal function or neurologic disorder. Difficult passage of stool may be due to fiber or fluid deficit, medication use, or thyroid disorder.
Is pain associated with defecation?	Pain implies fecal impaction of rectum, anorectal fissures, or intestinal obstruction.
Is blood evident in bowel movement?	Witnessed, usually is hemorrhoid bleeding, tear, or fissure.
What medications are taken, including over-the-counter drugs?	Multiple drugs are capable of causing constipation.

Modified from Rousseau P: Aging and chronic constipation, *Geriatr Med Today* 9(3):35, 1990.

among elderly rehabilitation patients. Yet the researchers caution that the mixture is not effective for everyone and monitoring is essential. The recipe is used routinely in numerous long-term care facilities. Other dietary alternatives have been implemented to increase acceptance by the elderly. A mixture of dried fruit was found by Beverly and Travis (1992) to be a cost-effective alternative to laxative use. It was well accepted by the elderly in a long-term care facility and was considered easy to administer. A cost analysis comparing laxative use with the use of the fruit mixture revealed an anticipated savings of more than $4,500 per year with the use of the fruit mixture. A "power pudding" was evaluated by Neal (1995) in a group of homebound elderly. The pudding, similar to the standard recipe with the addition of whipped topping, was reported by the elderly to be effective and very acceptable. A selected list of recipes is presented in Box 6-9.

Besides the addition of bran to the diet, other dietary adjuncts have been found to be effective by individuals in promoting bowel elimination. These dietary adjuncts include prunes, rhubarb, apples, oranges, bananas, carrots, cabbage, greens, potatoes with the skin, oatmeal, whole-grain cereals, and seeds (sunflower and sesame). Those with poor dentition can benefit from the same food if it is chopped, not pureed, and with the addition of extra chopped vegetables in soup. Persons with swallowing difficulties need foods that are mashed, not pureed, and additional liquids. The acceptance, tolerance, and the effectiveness of these dietary adjuncts need to be considered on an individual basis.

Increasing fiber intake has been found to be effective for prevention and management of bowel elimination problems. Yet the specific amount and type of fiber utilized in the intervention studies has varied.

One other dietary consideration besides fiber is senna tea. It is still a good laxative and is nontoxic unless used in a manner that produces prolonged overdoses. Senna tea is slightly absorbed systemically, is effective in small doses, and has a local action that increases colon peristalsis. A cup taken in the morning and in the evening is sufficient. Taken in the evening with a bran muffin, raisin whole-wheat cookies, or a piece of whole-wheat toast, it will naturally facilitate regularity (Pearson and Kotthoff, 1979).

Exercise is important as an intervention to stimulate colon motility and bowel evacuation. Daily walking, pelvic tilt exercises, and range of motion (passive or active) exercises are beneficial for those who are less mobile. Exercise and abdominal massage was utilized as an intervention by Resende et al (1993) for 12 immobile, long-stay patients for 12 weeks to prevent and relieve constipation. Episodes of fecal incontinence were significantly decreased with a significant increase in the number of bowel movements. The number of enemas given was reduced, and just one patient took one laxative during the study.

Simple environmental manipulation can facilitate the elimination of constipation. Sometimes placing the feet on a foot stool aligns the colon in the normal anatomic position for passing stool, a position closer to a squat. This may ease the evacuation if there is difficulty and straining. Clients should be encouraged to establish a regular bowel routine that includes attempting defecation after the morning meal. The gastrocolic reflex, the mass propulsion of material through the large intestines that occurs after a meal is strongest after the morning meal. Adequate time and privacy needs to be provided to promote a relaxing environment.

The combination of these approaches (dietary, exercise, and environmental modification) has been found to be effective. Hall et al (1995) established a protocol intervention for constipation that included fiber, fluids, exercise and abdominal exercises, and hygiene measures. The protocol was

---

Box 6-9   Natural Laxative Recipes

Fruit Spread*
2 lbs raisins
2 lbs currants
2 lbs prunes
2 lbs figs
2 lbs dates
2-28 oz containers undiluted prune concentrate

Put fruit through a grinder. Mix with prune concentrate in large mixer (mixture will be very thick). Store in large-mouthed plastic container. Refrigerate. Any dried fruit can be added.

Power Pudding†
$1/2$ cup prune juice
$1/2$ cup applesauce
$1/2$ cup wheat bran flakes
$1/2$ cup whipped topping
$1/2$ cup prunes (canned stewed)
(diabetics may use "no added sugar" applesauce and "light" whipped topping)

Blend ingredients, cover, and refrigerate, and keep as long as 1 week. Take $1/4$ cup portions of recipe with breakfast. Regulate dose as needed.

Standard Recipe
1 cup bran
1 cup applesauce
1 cup prune juice

Mix and store in refrigerator. Start with administration of 1 oz per day. Increase and decrease dosage as needed.

*From Beverley L, Travis I: Constipation: Proposed natural laxative mixtures, *J Gerontol Nurs* 18(10):5, 1992.
†From Neal LJ: "Power pudding": natural laxative therapy for the elderly who are homebound, *Home Healthcare Nurse* 13(3):66, 1995.

evaluated over a 3-year period in a group of hospitalized immobile vascular surgery patients. The incidence of constipation was reduced from 59% to about 9%, and the incidence of impaction was eliminated. Requests for laxatives and enemas were reduced from 59% to about 8%.

Gaspar and Hughes (1994) and Gaspar and Hobus (1996) have reported on the use of nonnutritive sucking on frequency and consistency of bowel elimination. The physiologic basis for this intervention is the parasympathetic effect of increased gut motility by sucking. In the pilot studies paraffin suckers were used for 10-minute periods once or twice daily. The intervention was effective in increasing bowel elimination and decreasing laxative use for some subjects. Further research in identifying how this cost-effective intervention will be effective needs to be conducted.

Pharmacologic measures can be instituted if nonpharmacolgic measures have been tried and have failed. The least aggressive therapy needs to be used first. The bulk-forming agents are generally tried first because they are the most physiologic. An adequate intake of fluids is necessary with the use of bulk-forming agents. Stool softeners need to be used if the patient is having hard, pelletlike stools or if straining needs to be avoided. Saline or osmotic laxatives are recommended if the prior-mentioned agents are not effective. The stimulant or irritant agents are recommended for occasional use only. Long-term use of these agents can result in the risk of electrolyte disturbances and damage to the colon (Allison et al, 1994).

Mantle (1992) developed a decision-making model for interventions to facilitate optimal bowel elimination. The model was based on assessment of the bowel record of each individual and included the use of pharmacologic agents. Following the testing of the model, several clinical implications were stated. One was the effective use of enemas if ½ cup or less of soft stool was eliminated for 2 to 3 days. The administration of the enema in this situation resulted in more complete elimination. They also suggested that the usual report mechanism of a simple "yes" or "no" as a record of bowel movements is inadequate. The amount of the bowel movement is as important as the frequency if optimal health is to be promoted.

A program to prevent as well as treat constipation that incorporates a high-fiber diet, liberal fluid intake, daily exercise, and environmental modifications that promote a regular pattern of bowel elimination needs to be developed for each client. The interventions for clients in any setting are based on a thorough assessment.

Fecal Impaction. Anyone can experience fecal impaction, but it is especially common in the incapacitated and institutionalized elderly. The causes are similar to constipation. Unrecognized, unattended, or neglected constipation eventually leads to fecal impaction and incontinence or paradoxical diarrhea, which results from a ball-valve effect that allows liquid stool to seep around the obstructing fecal mass during normal colon contractions. Removal of a fecal impaction is at times worse than the misery of the condition. Box 6-10 lists the causes and complications of fecal impaction.

Intervention. Management of fecal impactions requires the digital removal of the hard, compacted stool from the rectum after application of an anesthetic and use of lubrication with lidocaine jelly. Generally this is preceded by multiple enemas or an oil-retention enema to soften the feces in preparation for manual removal. Use of suppositories is not effective, since their action is blocked by the amount and the size of the stool in the rectum as compared with the capacity of the sphincter to dilate. Suppositories do not facilitate the removal of stool in the sigmoid, which may continue to ooze once the rectum is emptied.

Several sessions or days may be required to totally cleanse the sigmoid colon and rectum of impacted feces. Once this is achieved, attention should be directed to planning a regimen that includes adequate fluid intake of at least 2 L or more a day, increased dietary fiber in the form of unsweetened bran, fresh fruits and vegetables with the skins, administration of stool softeners, and many of the suggestions presented for prevention of constipation. The provision of privacy and time to attend to defecation without feeling rushed will facilitate easy and regular bowel function.

Box 6-10	**Common Causes and Complications of Fecal Impaction**

Causes
Medications
Diet
Lack of mobility
Illness
Habits

Complications
Fecal incontinence
Large bowel obstruction
Ischemic necrosis of colon wall (stercoral ulcer)

Modified from Wrenn K: Fecal impaction, *N Engl J Med* 321(10):658, 1989.

REST AND SLEEP

The human organism needs rest and sleep to conserve energy, prevent fatigue, provide organ respite, and relieve tension. Sleep is an extension of rest, and both are physiologic and mental necessities for survival. Rest depends on the degree of physical and mental relaxation. It is often assumed that lying in bed constitutes rest, but worries and other related stressors cause muscles throughout the body to continue to contract with tension even though physical activity has ceased. Attainment of rest depends on this interrelationship of psyche and soma. Body functions possess refractory

Nursing Diagnoses

The following potential diagnoses must be considered as well as diagnoses unique to the particular individual:

Perceived constipation
Colonic constipation
Diarrhea
Risk for fecal impaction

NURSING PROCESS AND NURSING DIAGNOSIS
Constipation

Etiologies and Related Factors
Inadequate activity
Immobility
Stress
Hemorrhoidal or fissure pain
Decreased dietary fiber
Decreased fluid intake
Laxative dependence
Medication side effects
Surgery
Decreased peristalsis
Depression
Metabolic dysfunction (thyroid, hypokalemia, hypocalcemia)
Physiologic age changes
Defective or deteriorated innervation

Defining Characteristics
Hard formed stool
Defecation occurring less than three times a week
Abdominal distention
Palpable impaction
Straining and pain on defecation
Report of feeling rectal fullness and/or rectal pressure
Decreased bowel sounds

Knowledge
Normal anatomic and functional changes of the aging gastrointestinal system
Physiology of constipation
Contributing factors to constipation: diet, fluids, medication, sociocultural, timing, position, related diseases
Effect of polypharmacy on bowel elimination

Effect of multiple chronic diseases as contributors to constipation
Constipation assessment
Causes of constipation
Nursing interventions to prevent and manage constipation
Standard bowel program (protocols)

Clinical Judgment and Related Skills
Obtain a bowel elimination history
Conduct an assessment of bowel sounds, abdominal palpation, and inspection of stools
Implement nursing interventions that can manage and prevent constipation; dietary management, fluids/hydration, exercise, privacy, position, administration of medication/enemas, patient teaching
Design a bowel retraining program for an individual whose bowel function is affected by disease/multiple chronic diseases, polypharmacy
Individualize a home care plan
Family/community teach for prevention and management of constipation

Evaluation
Normal bowel movements one to three days apart
Absence of straining or pain with passage of stool
Maintain a regular bowel routine
Intake of dietary fiber and fluids is adequate
Decreased use or dependence on laxatives

NEEDS ADDRESSED AND TASK STRENGTHS

Interest in maintaining healthful lifestyle
Attentive to subtle body signals
Able to judge and seek to meet own needs

Respects and provides for current survival needs
Accepts needs for others' intervention when necessary

times and rest periods in the continuous cycle of activity (biorhythms). Drastically or continually altered sleep and rest cycles disrupt homeostatic balance and create physical or mental aberration.

Rest "par excellence" (Henderson and Nite, 1978) is sleep that occurs for sustained unbroken periods. Sleep is restorative and recuperative and is necessary for the preservation of life.

Biorhythm and Sleep

Our lives are a series of rhythms that influence and regulate physiologic function, chemical concentrations, performance, behavioral responses, moods, and the ability to adapt. The most obvious rhythm is the day-night cycle known as the diurnal or circadian rhythm.

Studies of age-related changes in biorhythms have not been found. The most important and obvious biorhythm is the circadian sleep/wake rhythm that is endogenous. Abnormalities of this cycle may be responsible for some of the difficulties of old age. Gerontologists are beginning to seriously study the relevance of age-related changes in circadian rhythms to health and the process of aging. It is clear that body temperature, pulse, blood pressure, neurotransmitter excretion, and hormonal levels change significantly and predictably in a circadian rhythm. In old age there is a reduction in the amplitude of all of these circadian endogenous responses.

Cycles also exist that are less than 24 hours, infradian, and longer than 24 hours, ultradian. Rhythms can be disrupted by time zone changes, varying work schedules, and physical conditions. Alterations in the usual sleep-wake cycle, sleeping during the day and wakeful at night, can signal serious illnesses.

Institutions that provide care for the aged adhere to specific time schedules, which may not correspond to the biorhythm of the aged person and which may place the individual out of synchronization with his or her body functions. Attention to biorhythms can help establish the normal sleep-wake pattern of the aged person and identify the best times to introduce activities, periods of rest, and therapeutic measures.

Normal Sleep Pattern

The mystery of sleep has been researched for more than 30 years. Scientists such as Jouvet (1967), Kleitman (1960), and others have established that the normal sleep pattern consists of rapid eye movement (REM) sleep and non-REM sleep. One third of life is spent in sleep; REM sleep consumes 20% to 25% of the time; stage I sleep, 5%; stage II, 50% to 55%; stage III, 10%; and stage IV, 10% (Henderson and Nite, 1978). Webb (1982) estimates the amount of wake time for the aged after sleep onset to be about two and one-half times greater after age 60 for stage I sleep with little change in REM and stage II sleep time. Lerner (1982) indicates that stage IV sleep time is reduced 50% by age 50. The number of awakenings increased from one or two to six per night (Webb, 1982; Bixler and Vela-Bueno, 1987).

Two phases of sleep, REM and stage IV, have received the most attention and study. Sleep begins with a nodding or dropping off to sleep (stage I, non-REM), which is characterized by easy arousal by noise, touch, or other varied stimuli. If awakened, the individual does not realize that dozing has occurred and would describe the state as being similar to daydreaming. At times as stage I is entered the individual is awakened by muscle jerks or by the sensation of falling, which is a phenomenon attributed to initial muscle relaxation. If undisturbed, stage II is quickly entered, followed by stage III, a period of medium deep sleep; stage IV deep sleep, from which arousal is extremely difficult, soon follows. From the stage of deepest sleep, the individual ascends to the level of REM sleep, which resembles the sleep pattern of stage I. REM sleep occurs four or five times each night but is most prominent in the early morning hours; it is a more wakeful and active form of sleep, in which mounting excitement and tension are discharged.

Healing Sleep Studies. Early sleep studies have shown the following:

1. Stoyva et al (1970) monitored increased REM activity when volunteers were experiencing learning, memorization, and situations that required adaptation during their waking hours.
2. Mandell (1969) concluded that REM sleep facilitated the discharge of the drive centers and served to nourish and aid metabolism of the central nervous system, a necessity for well-being.
3. Deprivation of REM sleep was shown to produce irritability, anxiousness, and, on occasion, truly disturbed behavior.
4. Stage IV non-REM sleep is a nightly occurrence that has an essential restorative physiologic role in well-being. This sleep period is characterized by the depth of sleep and the difficulty of arousal. Individuals deprived of stage IV sleep have reported feelings of depression, general body malaise, apathy, and general lethargy.
5. Stage IV (considered the restorative stage) sleep is markedly reduced in the aged, but the significance of this has not been clearly established.
6. Research of Takashi et al (1968) has shown that growth hormone level is a key factor in stage IV sleep and correlates with the sleep rhythm. Only now is this research beginning to find its way into medical application.
7. Weitzman and Luce (1969) correlate hormonal activity to sleep. Their correlations find hormonal activity affecting REM sleep. Weitzman and Luce noted that levels of certain corticosteroids of the adrenals (17-hydroxycorticosteroids) are elevated during REM sleep. Perhaps this elevation is a response to activity that takes place during this sleep phase or is responsible for the activity that has been observed.

These studies, though conducted some time ago, all need replication and corroboration. Non-REM sleep is predominantly a quiet period when body secretions in the nose, mouth, throat, eyes, stomach, and bile tract are minimal; small intestine motility is reduced; heart rate slows and systolic pressure is diminished; basal metabolic rate is low; there is generalized muscle relaxation; body temperature falls; breathing is slower and more shallow; and there is no definite eye position, just notable constriction of the pupils.

A list of the characteristics of each stage of sleep appears in Box 6-11.

Sleep in the aged is generally characterized by numerous awakenings, periods of subdued respiration, marked temperature drops, less resilience in response to jet-lag conditions or other biorhythmic disturbances, and very little slow wave sleep (stage III and stage IV sleep). This slow wave activity is three to four times greater in a 13 year old than a 64 year old. A small but significant number of females continue to display sustained periods of stage IV sleep, but males over 60 years of age show very little. The work of Bliwise et al (1989) suggests that slow wave sleep decline may be a close correlate of the aging process in the central nervous system across the adult life span. This would explain significant differences observed in old persons. Ordinarily the amount of REM sleep remains appreciably the same throughout adulthood until extreme old age, but it has been found that REM sleep declines follow the trend of reduced intellectual function and is implicated in the presence of dementia and reduced cerebral function. (See sundowning, p. 190.) When REM sleep is decreased, the physiologic concomitants, such as muscle twitching, increased respirations, heart rate, and blood flow are also suppressed. It appears that the integrity of sleep patterns not only is indicative of central nervous system status but also may conversely be significant in the maintenance of central nervous system integrity. Persons with pulmonary and cardiac disorders may be severely compromised during REM sleep.

Research on normal sleep patterns continues. One recent study that contributes to the understanding of sleep was reported by Sherin et al (1996). Biologic markers were used to track the activity of rat brain cells during sleep. It was found that the ventrolateral preoptic area (VLPO) is the only neuron structure in the brain that becomes very active during sleep. The VLPO acts as a "slumber switch." The next step is to find the specific natural chemicals that cause the VLPO to command the brain to sleep. Because there are many phases of sleep, it is probably only one element of the complex process.

Quality of Sleep

"Good" or "poor" sleep is a subjective judgment based on body position, movement, and personal opinion. One may appear to sleep "well," as nurses' notes frequently record based on closed eyes and no movement in the bed, but other factors are significant in determining sleep quality.

Good sleepers have been described as registering a normal body temperature on awakening and less of a temperature drop in stage IV sleep than do poor sleepers. Those who sleep poorly have body temperatures that do not rapidly return to normal by the time the individual awakens. The question arises whether those who are poor sleepers have a different time sequence or rhythm, that is longer than the established circadian rhythm. Those with a physiologic rhythm not synchronous with the local time clock may sleep longer and arise later than is socially

---

Box 6-11   Characteristics of Sleep Stages

Stage I (Light Sleep)

Drops off to sleep
Relaxed
Fleeting thoughts
Easily awakened
Remembers being drowsy but not asleep

Stage II (Medium Deep Sleep)

Enters within minutes of stage I
More relaxed
Vague, dreamlike thoughts (fragmentary dreams)
Can observe the eyes moving slowly under the eyelids
Unmistakably asleep, but easily aroused

Stage III (Medium Deep Sleep)

About 20 minutes after stage I
Muscles relaxed
Slower pulse
Decreased body temperature
Undisturbed by moderate random stimuli (doors closing, etc.)

Stage IV (Deep Sleep)

Restorative sleep
Very relaxed
Rarely moves
Awakens only with vigorous stimuli
Period during which most sleepwalking, screaming, nightmares, and bedwetting occurs
Lasts 10 to 20 minutes

REM Sleep (Active Sleep)

Relieves tensions
Drifts up from stage IV every 90 to 100 minutes (REM sleep resembles stage I by electroencephalogram monitoring)
Rapid eye movement
Head and neck lose tonus, body feels flaccid
Increased and fluctuating pulse, blood pressure, and respirations
Most dreaming and sleep talking occurs
When medical crisis occurs (i.e., angina, dyspnea), most often because of anxiety or fear induced by dreams

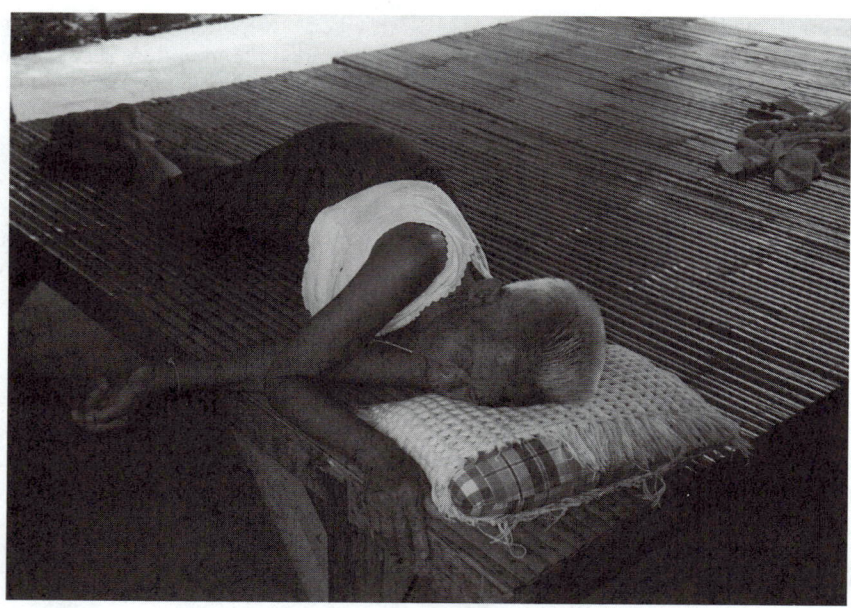

Napping.

convenient. This is true in institutional settings that have specific schedules; thus an individual's body time may lag behind clock time. Ancoli-Israel et al (1989b) found that nursing home patients' sleep is more fragmented and averaged an hour longer than that of independently living elders. Sleep patterns can be disturbed when REM sleep is altered or stopped through the administration of sedatives and hypnotics or by repeated awakening, such as monitoring vital signs and administration of nighttime procedures and medications.

The quality of sleep deteriorates with age. Most older people do not have a problem falling asleep but experience difficulty in staying asleep. According to Anderson (1976) there is a gradual breakdown and consolidation of the polycyclic pattern of the sleep-wake cycle. Often when asked about the quality of sleep, the aged respond with remarks or complaints that they hardly slept the night. Sleep of the aged is more fragmented than that of the young. Frequent and long periods of wakefulness occur during the night. These interruptions may be a result of nocturnal micturition, leg cramps (usually in men), nightmares (characteristic of women), and mental stimulation through worry, bereavement, or extraneous noises in the environment. Women tend to go to bed earlier than men, but both rise later than younger adults in the morning. Monk et al (1991) noted that elders had an earlier habitual time of awakening and a circadian orientation associated with longer sleep in the morning. Older people spend more total time in bed to achieve the same amount of restorative sleep that they had in their younger years. Ancoli-Israel et al (1989b) found that institutionalized elderly spent substantially more time in bed to obtain the same amount of sleep as independent elders. There is scarcely an hour that

goes by without the elder awakening, with the subsequent loss of deep restorative sleep (Lerner, 1982).

Sleep complaints of the elderly are numerous. Evans and Rogers (1994) examined the sleep-wake patterns of 14 healthy elderly persons. Subjects did not have trouble falling asleep, but once asleep, had trouble remaining asleep. Over two thirds of 100 community-dwelling women reported that they had prolonged sleep onset, two or more nocturnal awakenings, and/or awakening earlier than 6 A.M. (Johnson, 1988). In Italy the sleep problems reported by community-living elderly were similar in nature to those found by Johnson, yet the occurrence rate was lower (Frisoni et al, 1993). The majority of the studies describing the sleep problems of the elderly obtain the data through questionnaires. Using a qualitative approach to study sleep complaints of the elderly, Floyd (1993) identified four themes of factors contributing to sleep problems: (1) physical pain or bodily discomfort, (2) external environmental factors—noises, poor quality air, or uncomfortable room temperature, (3) emotional discomforts, and (4) sleep pattern changes—longer time to fall asleep, awakening after falling asleep, difficulty in returning to sleep, or awakening in the morning earlier than desired. Floyd found that the qualitative findings were similar with quantitative results of the study.

Figure 6-5 compares the normal sleep patterns across the life span. The amount of stage IV sleep is less prevalent or absent in the aged. It was thought at one time that the aged needed more sleep, but this is not necessarily true. The aged seem to sleep less. If one sleeps more, it is usually because of boredom, sedation, or symptoms of disease conditions such as uremia and cardiac and renal failure (Prinz et al, 1990). Long periods of sedation can reverse sleep patterns,

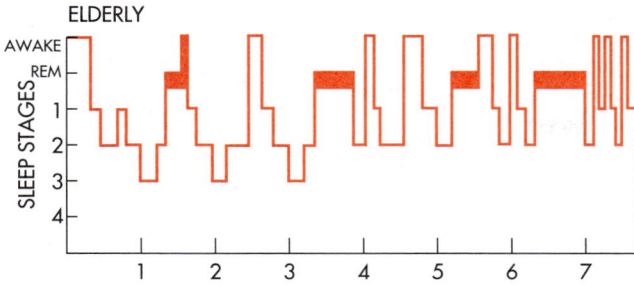

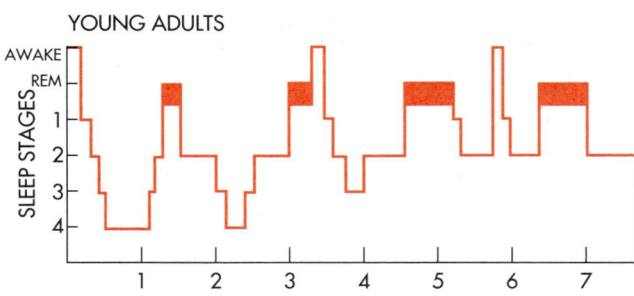

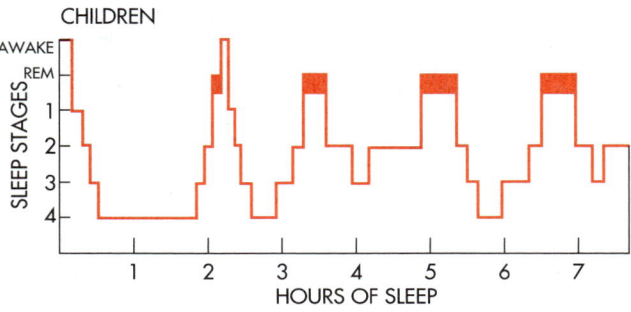

HOURS OF SLEEP

Figure 6-5. Comparison of sleep patterns across the life span. (From Kales JC, Carvell M, Kales A: Sleep disorders. In Castell CK, Riesenberg DE, Sorensen LB et al, editors: *Geriatric medicine,* ed 2, New York, 1990, Springer-Verlag.)

causing the aged to sleep during the day and be awake at night. Discontinuation of sedation can reestablish the aged person's sleep pattern. Often the aged are lonely, cold, and bored and go to bed about 6:00 or 7:00 in the evening. When they awaken in the early morning hours, they do not understand why sleep does not return. To them this constitutes insomnia. The changes that occur with aging are summarized in Box 6-12.

Disorders of Initiating and Maintaining Sleep

Insomnia. One in three persons age 65 and older complain of insomnia (Spiegel et al, 1990). Old people with minimum environmental stimulation or who doze for extended periods of time during the day are prone to insomnia. The prevalence of insomnia is difficult to document because insomnia has a number of definitions, depending on who is

---

Box 6-12	**Age-Related Sleep Changes**

Total sleep time decreases until age 80, then increases slightly.

Time in bed increases after age 65.

Onset to sleep is lengthened (>30 minutes in about 32% of women and 15% of men).

Awakenings are frequent, increasing after age 50 (>30 minutes of wakefulness after sleep onset in over 50% of older subjects).

Naps are more common, although only about 10% report daily napping.

Sleep is subjectively and objectively lighter (more stage I, less stage IV, more disruptions).

Frequency of abnormal breathing events is increased.

Frequency of leg movements during sleep is increased.

---

defining it. Generally, insomnia is considered to be the inability to sleep despite the desire to do so (Prinz and Vitello, 1993).

Elderly are particularly susceptible to insomnia because of changing sleep patterns, particularly in stage IV, or deep sleep. Complaints concerning insomnia include the inability to fall asleep, frequent awakenings, inability to return to sleep, and early morning arousal. Insomnia is a symptom. Successful resolution depends on understanding and addressing the individual's special mix of contributing factors, including biologic, medical, emotional, or bad habits.

Three types of insomnia are short term, transient, and chronic. Short-term insomnia results from environmental changes, stress, anxiety, or depression. Resolution occurs without medical intervention when the individual adapts to the changes or removes them. Transient insomnia is similar to short-term insomnia but generally lasts 1 to 3 weeks. Chronic insomnia is sleep problems lasting more than 3 weeks or recurring throughout one's life. Chronic insomnia occurs most frequently in persons with psychiatric disorders, chronic drug and alcohol dependency, dementia, or serious physical illnesses or conditions. This form of insomnia requires concentrated medical and/or psychiatric attention.

One of the most persistent and troublesome problems of the aged is age-related sleeplessness. Some of the numerous medical conditions, the related reasons for sleep alterations in the elderly, and possible interventions are listed in Table 6-10.

The discovery of a biochemical link between deep sleep and immune response suggests yet another vulnerability of the aged insomniac. Kruger (Moffat, 1988) found that small proteins called muramyl peptides (MPs) not only induce deep sleep but also trigger the production of interleukin-1, a key component of the body's immune system. However, no studies were found that investigated these phenomena in aged subjects.

Table 6-10 Causes, Reasons, and Potential Interventions for Sleep Alterations in the Aged

Causes	Reasons	Potential interventions
Arthritis	Pain builds; joints stiffen during periods of activity; pain relief medicine may wear off	Provide comfortable pillows; offer pain medication before pain becomes too intense
Angina pectoris	Pain likely to occur during REM sleep	Keep nitroglycerine at bedside
Chronic obstructive pulmonary disease	Abnormal increases in alveolar tension; decrease in oxygen saturation; prone position causes dyspnea and stasis of mucus	Patient education regarding self-care Toilet before bedtime; use bronchial dilators; prevent fatigue; rest during day; no diuretics in late afternoon; caution to avoid cola, coffee, tea, chocolate; use sedatives and OTC medication with caution
Heart failure	Nocturnal dyspnea Nocturia	Appropriate cardiotonic regimen; extra pillows; do not take diuretics late in day or in the evening
Diabetes	Inadequate regulation of blood sugar may lead to glycosuria and nocturia; overly tight control of blood sugar	Control by diet, insulin, or oral medication Adjust diabetic regimen
	Hypoglycemic attacks (can mimic anxiety attacks)	Teach regular, adequate caloric intake; bedtime snack
Disturbed sensory perception	Poor environmental lighting; visual difficulties; nocturnal hallucinations; alterations in REM-NREM cycle	Modify environment; check hearing aid; put glasses nearby; reduce noise at home or in hospital; reassure frequently
Alzheimer's disease (AD)	AD patients' sleep shows reduction in stages III and IV sleep early in disease; late in AD these stages disappear; daytime sleepiness increases as disease progresses	Assist staff and family with wandering behavior and sundowning syndrome; major tranquilizers may be needed; be sure person has comfortable chair in which to rest; strict scheduling of nighttime bed hours, day naps, and activity periods and needs; for wanderers and behavior problems, stop all drug treatment to see if normal sleep rhythm returns
Depression	Disturbed sleep pattern: problem falling asleep, early morning awakening, decreased total sleep time; barbiturate use can cause fragmented sleep and nightmares	Assess sleep; check for recent discontinued drugs; frequent reassurance; have same caregiver relate to client; tricyclic antidepressants if depression diagnosed
Congestive heart failure	Fluid buildup produces symptoms	Restrict fluids at bedtime; prop up on pillows
Peptic ulcers	Gastric juices and stomach acid increases during REM sleep	Provide nightly ulcer medicine
Alcoholism	Abnormal EEG pattern results; as effects wear off, sleeper may awaken with withdrawal symptoms and a hangover	No alcoholic beverages; explain that reformed alcoholics may experience insomnia for a year or so after withdrawal of alcohol
Parkinsonism	Total wake time increases, decreased REM	L-Dopa at bedtime may help decrease rigidity that occurs during the night
Surgical procedures	Premature arousal related to blood drawn at 5 AM or 6 AM; anxiety and worry about outcome; pain	Analyze rituals and routines in place. Can they be changed? Keep pain free; monitor vital signs frequently, and promote rest
Cardiac	Discomfort due to environment (noise, temperature, lights); postoperative psychosis (usually follows 24-day lucid interval)	Modify environment Establish therapeutic rapport early; instruct patient preoperatively; orient frequently when postoperative; elicit family support
Situational insomnia	On admission to institution; after visit by relative; after move to new residence; after recent loss or death	Establish one-to-one relationship; provide short-term use of hypnotic

Data from Wagner D: On sleep and Alzheimer's disease, *Alzheimer's Disease and Related Disorders Newsletter* 5(1), 1985; Pacini C, Fitzpatrick J: Sleep patterns of hospitalized and nonhospitalized aged individuals, *J Gerontol Nurs* 8(6):327, 1982; de Brun S: Insomnia: the common sense approach, *Occupational Health Nursing* 29:36, 1981; Hemenway J: Sleep and the cardiac patient, *Heart Lung* 9(3):453, 1980; Raskind M, Eisdorfer C: When elderly patients can't sleep, *Drug Therapy* 7(8):44, 1977.

Hypersomnia. Persons who have hypersomnia routinely sleep more than 8 to 9 hours in a 24-hour period and complain that they sleep excessively. The individual may state or the family or nurse may observe that the person exhibits persistent daytime drowsiness, appears in a drugged state, has sleep "attacks," or seems to be in a comatose state or experiences postencephalitic drowsiness (Dement et al,

1982). The client complains of weakness, fatigue, and learning and memory difficulties.

Sleep Apnea. Sleep apnea syndrome is a disorder characterized by repetitive cessation of respiration during sleep. Sleep apnea is considered widespread among those over age 60. According to Kotagal and Dement (1985), approximately 35% of adults over age 60 experience sleep apnea.

Of nursing home residents, 42% have 5 or more apneas per hour of sleep; 4% of 427 elders at home had 20 or more apnea episodes per hour (Ancoli-Israel et al, 1989a).

Recognition of this disorder is usually through the symptoms of snoring, interrupted breathing of at least 10 seconds, and unusual daytime sleepiness. Medical illness such as congestive heart failure raises incidence of patients with 10 or more apneas per hour to 21% of hospitalized elders over age 65. Sleep apnea has been linked with high relative risk of nonhemorraghic cerebral infarction, angina pectoris, congestive heart failure, pulmonary hypertension, and hypertension. It is recognized as a significant factor for mortality among the elderly. McGinty et al (1988) studied events associated with sleep apnea that may alter nocturnal circulatory function among the elderly. Hypotensive episodes were found to occur among subjects and were associated with hemoglobin desaturation below 80%, secondary to sleep-related breathing disorders, and elevated supine nasopharyngeal airway resistance. These researchers suggest that sympathetic reflexes may be impaired, permitting hypotension and risk of circulatory failure in some elderly.

Sleep apnea may occur in individuals who may not have any respiratory problem while awake. During sleep, breathing may be interrupted as many as 300 times and apneic episodes may last from 10 to 90 seconds (Oesting and Manza, 1988). It is thought that sleep apnea occurs for two reasons:

1. Central nervous system mechanisms in which thoracic breathing movements cease cause a complete absence of ventilatory effort and a constant intrathoracic pressure. Respiration resumes when a person is aroused. Central apnea is associated with brainstem disorders and bulbar damage or is idiopathic.

2. Oropharyngeal membranes collapse or are obstructed by excess tissue. Individuals make increasingly greater attempts to breathe against the obstruction until air is forced through the upper airway with a loud snorting sound. Obstructive apnea is associated with hypertrophy of adenotonsillar or buccal tissue or may be idiopathic.

Persons most likely to have sleep apnea are adult men with a long history of loud, intermittent snoring. Hypertension and cardiac arrhythmias are common, and persons who have had a stroke may be at increased risk. Commonly these individuals are obese and have short, thick necks (Oesting and Manza, 1988).

Another group of patients at risk for sleep apnea are individuals diagnosed with Alzheimer's disease. These patients have been found to have a significantly higher proportion of sleep apnea than healthy elderly (Hoch et al, 1987). Those Alzheimer's patients with sleep apnea had significantly more awake time during the course of the night than Alzheimer's patients who did not experience apnea. Hoch et al (1987) also found that the higher the level of dementia,

the greater the severity of apnea experienced by the Alzheimer's patients. One wonders if the long-range effects of cerebral anorexia during apneic attacks contributes to the dementia.

Symptoms of sleep apnea include loud and periodic snoring, broken sleep with frequent nocturnal waking, unusual nighttime activity such as sitting upright, sleepwalking, and falling out of bed. It seems that additional symptoms such as memory changes, depression, excessive daytime sleepiness, morning headaches, nocturia, and orthopnea result from sleep apnea.

Assessment includes information from the sleeping partner as well as observation of signs and symptoms noted above. Assessment of patients during sleep is important. Emphasis should be placed on describing the respiratory rate, the number of apneic episodes, the length of apneic periods, and the effect of central nervous system depressants of sleeping pills. Sleep assessment will be detailed later in this section.

Specific treatment of sleep apnea may involve weight loss, surgery to remove redundant tissue, or medical management. Persons are counseled to avoid drugs with analeptic effects, particularly alcohol. Anything that interferes with the arousal response is exceedingly dangerous. Extra pillows or sleeping in a chair are sometimes helpful. Ordinarily the individual has quite spontaneously made compensatory adjustments during sleeping hours.

Naps. Napping is a sequence of sleeping and waking from less deep sleep. It is a normal pattern that seems to increase with age and is indicative of a different distribution of sleep, and one should not worry about napping.

There tends to be a correlation between age and the length of napping: the older the person, the longer the nap (Hayter, 1985). An increased frequency of daytime napping in elders may indicate a change in circadian rhythm (Buysse et al, 1992). Naps tend to peak in late afternoon. In a pilot study of geriatric patients in a rehabilitation hospital Creighton (1994) found that afternoon drowsiness was decreased by a nap, making therapy more effective.

Napping is not an attempt to compensate for sleep lost at night. Sleep and napping are independent of each other (Hayter, 1985). Naps augment sleep and increase the total amount slept. Afternoon naps provide deep sleep, a necessity for physical rest. It is speculated that the individual may need napping to restore energy. Napping may be based more on physical health, psychologic health, and volitional factors, which may mediate daytime sleepiness (Buysse et al, 1992).

The average nap lasts from 15 to 60 minutes; this usually occurs several times a day. In a study of 14 healthy elderly subjects, Evans and Rogers (1994) found that all took one or more naps during the daytime. Yet napping time composed only a small fraction of their total sleep time, an average of 60 minutes. These subjects took frequent yet short naps, less than 10 minutes.

Nocturnal Myoclonus. The syndrome of periodic leg jerks or movements in sleep is nocturnal myoclonus. It is diagnosed when the number of periodic leg jerks or movements is equal to or greater than five per hour of sleep (Ancoli-Israel and Kripke, 1986; Herrera, 1990). As many as 40% of persons over 65 experience this disorder. The stereotypical movements consist of flexion of the hip, knee, and ankle with extension of the toes, which occurs sometimes as often as every 40 seconds during sleep (Johnston, 1994).

Because of the repeated awakenings from this condition, complaints of insomnia and excessive daytime sleepiness occur. It is thought that nocturnal myoclonus is associated with sleep apnea. It is, however, more common in association with chronic renal failure, sleep apnea, and tricyclic antidepressants (Kales et al, 1990). Johnston (1994) indicates that individuals with signs and symptoms of this condition should be referred to a sleep disorder clinic for specific diagnosis.

Restless Leg Syndrome. The major difference between this syndrome and nocturnal myoclonus is when the leg movement occurs. Restless leg syndrome is characterized by a nonpainful dysethesia of the lower leg, described as a pulling sensation that is often noticeable only at rest. The discomfort interferes with sleep onset. Relief is obtained by movement of the legs. Research support is lacking for the use of a medication regimen. Exercise during the day may relieve the movements (Johnston, 1994).

Sundown Syndrome. Sundown syndrome describes behavior; it is not a disease. Sundowning is recurring confusion and exacerbation of disruptive behavior and agitation in late afternoon or early evening. It has also been called nocturnal delirium (Duckette and Scotto, 1992). Sundowning is a temporary condition but is disruptive and dangerous when it occurs. Elderly persons may wander out of a home or a facility, or the caregiver may become sleep deprived trying to cope with the night behavior. This presents a major problem to nursing staff in acute-care and long-term care facilities. As the name applies, sundown syndrome is generally associated with an occurrence in the late afternoon and early evening. Yet limited research has documented the time of occurrence. In a pilot study conducted by Beel-Bates and Rogers (1990) the activity of patients with dementia (n = 4) and those without dementia (n = 2) was quite different between 4:00 and 6:30 P.M. Demented subjects increased their activity, whereas the nondemented subjects decreased their activity.

The causes of sundowning, based on the limited research in this area, have been grouped by Duckett (1993) as psychologic, environmental, and physiologic. A combination of variables in these three groups is supported. Karl et al (in Duckette and Scotto, 1992) argue that psychosocial stressors in conjunction with impaired cognitive function may account for sundowning. Evans (1985) presents the idea that sundowning is the result of brain hypoxia due to biologic or biochemical factors such as the effects of drugs, cardiovascular disorders, or dehydration; sensory overload or deprivation; circadian rhythm disruption; psychologic stress; isolation; fear; influence of the lunar cycle; and the weather.

Satlin et al (1992) found that pulsating bright light ameliorated the sundowning behavior of some Alzheimer's patients. The study speculated that the pulsating bright light changed the sleep-wake cycle disturbance. The effect may be attributed to mediation in the chronobiologic mechanism.

Assessment of an individual for risk factors include age, history of delirium or sundowning, cardiovascular disease or dementia, polypharmacy, and electrolyte imbalance. Nursing measures might include providing environmental-orienting cues, minimizing the relocation of a person within a nursing facility, frequent nighttime monitoring, turning on the lights before dark, and offering soft music or social stimulation in the late afternoon. Wallace (1994) studied the outcome of providing specialized training of nurse's aides that incorporated a background understanding of the syndrome and approaches to deal with it. The total number of sundowning behaviors decreased after the educational program. Although the study was limited by sample size, the findings do support the need for interventions.

Duckett (1993) presents a decision-making flow chart for intervening with the sundowning patient based on the research to date. The first questions to be answered are related to the existence of dementia and reversible medical condition(s). Staff-patient conflict is next evaluated. Then the physical environment, social environment and psychologic status of the patient is assessed and interventions planned.

Vitiello et al (1992) suggest restriction of daytime sleep, which may lead to better night sleep, and exposure to bright light. If all else fails, the use of neuroleptics such as haloperidol, or thioridazine is recommended. However, long-term use of these drugs has major sequelae, and monitoring of the individual's reponses is needed.

Sleep and Drugs

Institutions and the aged themselves disrupt sleep quality and patterns and attempt to counteract this by administering sleeping medications. People age 60 and older consume the majority of sleep medications. Often nurses think they are helping the aged person who is awake most of the night to get a "good night's rest" by giving medication. Few hypnotic drugs are compatible with the normal sleep cycle. Instead, these drugs depress the REM sleep necessary for the relief of tension and anxiety. When medication is discontinued, normal sleep patterns usually return, but dreaming and nightmares are increased until natural sleep cycles are reestablished. Some researchers believe this compensates for dreams that have been depressed or obliterated by REM sleep suppression.

Drug tolerance, physical dependence, daytime delirium, drowsiness, and depression of mental alertness occur with chronic use of bedtime hypnotic agents. Some major tranquilizers and sedatives are responsible for loss of equilibrium. Hypnotic drugs often induce night terrors, hallucinations, and such paradoxical responses as agitation instead of relaxation, hangover, depression, and changes in memory, balance, and gait. If hypnotic drugs are necessary, those that are the least disruptive to the sleep cycle should be employed.

A number of prescribed and over-the-counter agents have effects on sleep even if the agent is being taken for an unrelated condition. Table 6-11 presents the effects on sleep of the top 10 prescribed drugs for elderly.

Patients should be treated nonpharmacologically before any medication is prescribed. Jenkins's classic study (1976) reported that elderly patients in her facility were not given routinely prescribed sleeping medication, and nursing actions were substituted. Since that time many facilities have also done so quite successfully. Few patients needed sleep medication if attention was given to specific bedtime needs and rituals.

A natural substance, L-tryptophan, has received publicity as a sleep agent. L-tryptophan is a component of protein foods such as meat, beans, green leafy vegetables, peanuts, and dairy products and was reported to be an effective alternative to sleeping pills. The American Medical Association (AMA) concluded that 1 g or less decreased the latency sleep period for those with difficulty falling asleep; however, in 1989 the FDA recalled L-trytophan because it was linked to a serious and fatal neurologic syndrome, eosinophilic myalgia. Eventually the cause of the sudden outbreak of this condition was traced to contaminated L-tryptophan powder from a foreign manufacturer, which was purchased by U.S. companies and sold in tablet and capsule form in health food stores, grocery stores, and other places of distribution under various brand names (L-tryptophan, 1990). Warm milk, cocoa, and other ordinary food preparations that contain L-tryptophan continue to be prescribed by health care professionals to aid the aged person to fall asleep without the use of hypnotic and sedative preparations.

Melatonin, which is classified as a dietary supplement, has been the topic of talk shows and numerous popular magazines the past several years. It has been cited not only as a sleep aid, but also as an age-reversing, disease-fighting and sex-enhancing hormone. Research supporting the use of melatonin, a hormone secreted by the pineal gland, has been conducted. Haimov et al (1994) examined whether sleep disorders in old age were associated with changes in concentration of 6-sulphatoxymelatonin, the major urinary measure of melatonin. Elderly with and without sleep complaints were compared to a sample of young men without sleep complaints. All patients with insomnia had a significantly lower sleep efficiency and a higher activity level during sleep; their 6-sulphatoxymelatonin excretion was characterized by a lower peak, with delayed onset and peak times. Peak excretion in the elderly subjects was 49% lower than that in young subjects, although the peak in elderly subjects without sleep disorders did not differ significantly from that in the young subjects. The data suggest a relation between deficiency of melatonin or disruption of its rhythms and an increased prevalence of sleep disorders with advancing age. The researchers suggested that lack of exposure to bright light in institutions may lead to diminution of melatonin excretion in old age.

Although no side effects have been found from the use of melatonin, the long-term use and its effect on cycles, especially seasonal and lifetime events, have not been studied (Murray, 1995). If melatonin is utilized, 1 to 5 mg of melatonin at bedtime is recommended, with effective doses varying among individuals. Advise client to begin with 1 mg at bedtime. If unable to fall asleep within 30 minutes, take another 1 mg. Continue to take 1 mg every 20 to 30 minutes up to 5 mg. If unable to go back to sleep, take 1 to 3 mg to fall back asleep. It is also important to remember

Table 6-11   Sleep-Related Effects of the Top 10 Prescribed Drugs for the Elderly

Drug	Indication	Sleep-related effect(s)
Digoxin	Heart failure	Apathy, psychosis
Ranitidine	Ulcers, gastroesophageal reflux disorder (GERD)	Malaise, somnolence, insomnia
Conjugated estrogens	Moderate to severe motor symptoms of menopause	Headache, migraine, depression
Alprazolam	Anxiety disorders	Drowsiness, depression, headache, confusion, insomnia, nervousness, tiredness/sleepiness
Diuretic combinations	Hypertension or edema	Nocturia
Diltiazem HCl	Angina	Depression, hallucination, insomnia, nervousness, paresthesia, somnolence, tinnitus, tremor
Enalapril maleate	Hypertension, heart failure	None
Atenolol	Hypertension, angina, acute MI	Tiredness, drowsiness, depression, excessive dreaming
Nifedipine	Angina, hypertension	Headache, fatigue, insomnia, nervousness, paresthesia, somnolence
Captopril	Hypertension, heart failure	Ataxia, confusion, depression, nervousness, somnolence

Modified from The Top 200 Rx Drugs of 1990, *American Druggist* 203(2):56, 1991.

that as a dietary supplement the manufacture of melatonin is unregulated and there are no standards for quality, purity, or dosage. The quality of the inactive fillers to form tablets and the amount of melatonin actually used in the pills may vary widely. A call to the manufacturer to inquire if the product has been tested by an independent laboratory is advised.

Assessment

Nurses are in an excellent position to assess sleep, to improve the quality of the aged person's sleep, and to study sleep or assist in sleep research by being available at customary sleep times. Sleep history interviews are important and should be obtained from all elderly clients. The nurse should learn how well the person sleeps at home, how many times the aged person is awakened at night, what time the person retires, and what rituals occur at bedtime. Rituals include bedtime snacks, watching television, listening to music, or reading, which, unless carried out, interfere with the individual's ability to fall asleep. Other assessment data should include the amount and type of daily exercise, favorite position when in bed, room environment, temperature, ventilation, illumination, activities engaged in several hours before bedtime, and sleep medications, as well as other medications taken routinely. Some medications taken regularly produce side effects that interfere with the ability to sleep. Information about involvement in hobbies, life satisfaction, and perception of health status are also important to establish possible depression. The history should be cross-checked with the caregiver and/or family members.

A nursing standard-of-practice protocol for sleep disturbances in elderly patients was developed as part of the Nurses Improving Care of the Hospitalized Elderly (NICHE) Project supported by a grant from the Hartford Foundation. Assessment standards are presented in Table 6-12. The assessment is focused to elicit information relative to indicators or defining characteristics of sleep disturbance.

The sleep diary or log is noted as an important part of assessment. This information will provide an accurate account of the person's sleep problem and identify the sleep disturbance. Usually a family member or the caregiver, if the aged person is institutionalized, records specific behaviors on a flow sheet. Two to four weeks is required to obtain a clear picture of the sleep problem. Important items to record are the following:

1. The number of times a call for assistance to the bathroom, pain medication, or subjective symptoms of inability to sleep, such as anxiety, occur
2. If the person is out of bed
3. Whether the person appears to be asleep or awake on rounds
4. Episodes of confusion or disorientation
5. If sleep medication was given and if repeated
6. Time the person awakens in the morning (approximation)

Intervention

Interventions begin after a thorough sleep history has been recorded. Interventions for sleep disturbances among the elderly has been the focus of several research studies in the past five years. Mornhinweg and Voignier (1995) tested the effect of music on promotion of sleep. Subjects listened to classical and New Age music before bedtime when a sleep disturbance was identified. All but one of the 25 subjects reported improved sleep using this self-administered intervention. The majority believed that the music helped them fall asleep, return to sleep quicker if awakened during the night, or sleep longer in the morning. Music allowed them to "turn off" their mind so that they could relax enough to fall asleep.

The use of light has been found to be beneficial. Campbell et al (1993) evaluated the efficacy of bright light exposure in the treatment of sleep maintenance insomnia among 16 elderly men and women who had experienced a sleep disturbance for at least a year. Exposure to bright light resulted in substantial changes in sleep quality. Waking time within sleep was reduced by an hour, and sleep efficiency improved from 77.5% to 90%, without altering time spent in bed. Exposure to 2 hours daily of sunlight was investigated by Castor et al (1991) among 12 elderly institutionalized demented patients. Overall beneficial effects from exposure to sunlight were shown by increased mean sleep hours, increased uninterrupted night sleep hours, decreased night wake hours, and decreased daytime sleep hours. Disrupted sleep patterns resumed in the first 24 hours after sunlight deprivation in week 3 of the study.

Bedtime routine was found by Johnson (1991) as a factor related to sleep patterns of the elderly. Fewer sleep complaints were recorded among the elderly that maintained a bedtime routine. It is important to remember that the bedtime routine is that which is established by the individual, not by the institution.

Noise was found by Alessi et al (1995) to be at a very high level at night in the nursing home. An intervention study is being conducted at UCLA that is designed to promote sound slumber in two ways—through a nighttime-incontinence management program coupled with noise-abatement intervention (UCLA News, April 10, 1995). Incontinence care is provided primarily during time periods that the residents are awake. Nurse aides check incontinent residents hourly during nighttime hours. Those residents who happen to be awake are either helped to the toilet, if they desire, or are checked and changed, if necessary. Residents found sleeping after several consecutive checks are awakened for incontinence as precaution against pressure-sore development. There is also an in-service training for the staff to heighten their sensitivity to sleep and noise. Feedback on noise levels twice per nighttime shift is provided to the staff. The noise level of telephones, buzzers, and intercom systems are reduced after 9 P.M. each night. Preliminary results after two years of testing suggests that the intervention increased residents' average length of sleep time at night.

Table 6-12 Nursing Standard of Practice Protocol: Sleep Disturbance in Elderly Patients

Assessment	Health promotion and maintenance intervention	Evaluation
Sleep-wake patterns	**Maintain normal sleep pattern**	**Objective evidence**
Inquire about usual times for retiring and rising, time for falling asleep, frequency and duration of nighttime awakenings; frequency and duration of daytime naps; daytime physical and social activity	Maintain usual bedtime/wake time	Time required to fall asleep; should fall asleep within 30-45 minutes
	Avoid staying in bed beyond waking hours	Time for awakening, at usual reported time
	Encourage to get up at regular time even if did not sleep well	Behavior, alertness, attention, ability to concentrate, reaction time
	Schedule nightime activities to provide uninterrupted periods of sleep of at least 2-3 hrs	Observe duration of sleep: patient should remain asleep for at least 4-hour intervals
Have person provide a subjective evaluation of the quality of sleep	Balance daytime activity and rest	
Have person complete sleep log for 2 wks	Encourage keeping daytime naps to a minimum	
	Promote social interaction	
	Encourage exercise prior to evening	
Bedtime routines/rituals	**Support bedtime routines/rituals**	**Subjective evidence**
Inquire about activities performed by the individual before bedtime (e.g., personal hygiene, prayer, reading, watching TV, listening to music, snacks)	Offer a bedtime snack or beverage	Verbalizations about the quality and quantity of sleep; e.g. statements of difficulty falling asleep, frequent awakenings; having slept well, feeling well-rested/refreshed; of an increased sense of well-being
	Enable bedtime reading or listening to music	
	Assist with aspects of personal hygiene at bedtime (e.g., bath)	
	Encourage prayer or meditation	
	Assist to establish a relaxing bedtime routine	
Medications	**Avoid/minimize drugs that negatively influence sleep**	
Obtain information relative to all prescribed and self-selected over-the-counter medications used by person, especially, sleep aids, diuretics, laxatives	Pharmacologic treatment of sleep disturbances is treatment of last resort	
	Discontinue or adjust the dose or dosing schedule of any/all offending medications	
	Consider drug-drug potentiation	
Determine types of medications and length of time used by person	Administer meds to promote sleep; i.e. give diuretics at least 4 hours before bedtime	
Diet effects	**Minimize/avoid foods that negatively influence sleep**	
Obtain information about the consumption of caffeinatted and alcoholic beverages	Discourage use of beverages containing stimulants (e.g., coffee, tea, sodas) in afternoon and evening	
	Encourage use of food naturally containing L-tryptophan	
	Provide snacks according to patient preference	
	Generally discourage use of alcoholic beverages	
	Decrease fluid intake 2-4 hours before bedtime	
	Encourage to have lighter meal in evening	
Environmental factors	**Create optimal environment for sleep**	
Evaluate noise, light, temperature, ventilation, bedding	Keep noise to an absolute minimum	
	Set room temperature according to preference	
Inquire about distance of bathroom from bedroom	Provide blankets as requested	
	Use night light as desired	
Inquire about use of night lights	Provide soft music or white noise to mask noise	
	Encourage bed and bedroom for sleep and not other activities	
	Use light exposure during day and evening to maintain wakefulness	
Physiologic factors	**Promote physiologic stability**	
Evaluate breathing pattern with sleep, with attention to pauses	Elevate head of bed as required	
Observe for periodic movement or jerking during sleep	Provide extra pillows per preference	
Inquire about sleeping position	Administer bronchodilators, if prescribed, before bedtime	
Note diagnoses of sleep disorder	Use medical therapeutics (e.g., continuous positive airway pressure machine) as prescribed	
Note diagnoses of specific health problems that adversely affect sleep (e.g., CHF, COPD)		

Modified from Forman MD, Wykle M: Nursing standard-of-practice protocol: sleep disturbances in elderly patients, *Geriatr Nurs* 16(5):238, 1995.

Continued

| Table 6-12 | Nursing Standard of Practice Protocol: Sleep Disturbance in Elderly Patients—cont'd |

Assessment	Health promotion and maintenance intervention	Evaluation
Illness factors	**Promote comfort**	
Inquire about pain, affective disturbances (e.g., depression, anxiety, worry, fatigue, and discomfort)	Provide analgesia as needed 30 minutes before bedtime (Note that some over-the-counter analgesics may have caffeine) Massage, back or foot, to help relax Warm and cool compresses to painful areas as indicated Use relaxation methods—deep breathing, progressive relaxation, mental imagery Encourage to urinate before going to bed Keep path to bathroom clear/provide bedside commode	

Johnson (1993) found that progressive whole body relaxation using controlled breathing and alternation contractions improved the self-reported sleep patterns of noninstitutionalized elderly. There were stronger relationships between improvement in sleep patterns and younger aged individuals. It may be that older subjects had more difficulty using this technique or that they needed more instruction and practice than younger subjects.

Intervention standards are a part of the nursing standard-of-practice protocol (see Table 6-12) for sleep disturbances in elderly patients that was developed as part of the NICHE Project. The interventions were developed based on the principles that to be effective the intervention, first, must be individualized, considering the specific characteristics of the patient and the nature of the sleep disturbance; and second, pharmacologic treatment should be considered an intervention of last resort. Additions were incorporated into the protocol based on a review of the literature.

Drugs should be a last resort and are not intended for long-term treatment. Rebound insomnia as well as episodes of confusion and nightmares are common when sleep medications are withdrawn. The key to selection of a hypnotic is to consider the half-life and the adverse effects of the agent. For example, flurazepam (Dalmane) has active metabolites, some of which have a half-life of 50 to 100 hours. Considering this half-life and the adverse effects of confusion, dizziness, and ataxia, it is not a good choice. Triazolam (Halcion), which has an intermediate onset and rapid elimination, is frequently recommended. Yet there is controversy surrounding this drug because of the adverse effects observed in the elderly. A newer drug of the imidazopyridine class is Zolpidem. It has been found to be as effective as triazolam, yet with less confusion resulting. A high risk of hangover has been reported. Evaluation of this drug continues (Johnston, 1994). Table 6-13 presents the characteristics of selected medications used as hypnotics in treatment of elderly patients.

Evaluation

The nursing standard-of-practice protocol presented in Table 6-12 includes an evaluation component. Observation of the person when awake and asleep is necessary. Physiologic changes observable for each stage of sleep reviewed previously can be evaluated to give clues to the phases of sleep cycle experienced. It is essential to obtain the subjective evidence of the quality and quantity of sleep.

ACTIVITY

Activity is a direct use of energy in voluntary and involuntary physical and mental ways that alter the microenvironment and macroenvironment of the individual. The focus of this section will be on physical activity because mental activity is covered primarily in Chapters 21 and 22. The NIH-sponsored Consensus Development Conference on Physical Activity and Cardiovascular Health (1995) defined physical activity as "bodily movement produced by skeletal muscles that requires energy expenditure and produces progressive healthy benefits." Exercise, a type of physical activity, was defined as "a planned, structured, and repetitive bodily movement done to improve or maintain one or more components of physical fitness." Activities of daily living are another type of physical activity.

Physical activity is often the barometer by which an individual's health and wellness are judged. The inability to exercise, perform physical work, and complete activities of daily living are among the first indicators of decline. Research in gerontologic exercise physiology is relatively young, but in general, results indicate that maintenance of a physically active lifestyle arrests or significantly delays age changes associated with cardiovascular, respiratory, and musculoskeletal function.

Public perceptions of the aged and how they spend their time continue to reflect the belief that retirement ushers in the pursuit of sedentary, private, isolated activity and the assumption of a passive role in society. The prevalence estimates for leisure activity among those age 65 years or older in the United States are low. Thirty percent exercise regularly, and fewer than 10% exercise vigorously (Barry and Eathorne, 1994). Siegel et al (1995), based on the data of the 1990 Behavioral Risk Factor Surveillance System, found

Table 6-13   Characteristics of Selected Medications Used as Hypnotics in Treatment of Elderly Patients

Medication	Class	Hypnotic efficacy	Risk of hangover	Risk of tolerance or dependence	Other complications
Diphenhydramine	Antihistamine	Unpredictable	High	Low	Anticholinergic
Amitriptyline	Tricyclic	Unpredictable	High	Low	Anticholinergic
Trazodone	Triazolopyridine	High	High	Low	Priapism
Flurazepam	Benzodiazepine	Very high	High	High	Falls, worsens obstructive sleep apnea
Temazepam	Benzodiazepine	Very high	Low	High	Falls, worsens obstructive sleep apnea
Triazolam	Benzodiazepine	Very high	Low	High	Memory disturbance
Zolpidem	Imidazopyridine	Very high	Low	Low	Unknown

From McCall WV: Management of primary sleep disorders among elderly persons, *Psych Services* 46(1)49, 1995.

 Nursing Diagnoses

The following potential diagnosis must be considered as well as diagnoses unique to the particular individual:

Sleep pattern disturbance (refer to etiologies and related factors)

NURSING PROCESS AND NURSING DIAGNOSIS
Sleep Pattern Disturbance

Etiologies and Related Factors
Physical discomfort or pain
Illness
Personal/family stress
Medications
Immobility due to cast, traction, etc.
Boredom
Lack of exercise
Environmental and habit changes
Travel

Defining Characteristics
Verbal complaints of difficulty falling asleep, awakening earlier or later than desired, interrupted sleep
Change in behavior or performance
Irritability
Restlessness
Progressive disorientation
Lethargy
Dark circles under eyes
Frequent yawning
Posture change

Knowledge
Normal sleep cycle
Alterations of sleep cycle with age
Sleep promoting methods: relaxation, meditation, environmental
Pharmacologic preparations to induce sleep

Clinical Judgment and Related Skills
Obtain a sleep history
Assess elder's sleep pattern
Consider a variety of interventions appropriate to sleep problem (refer to sleep section of chapter) and discuss with client
Teach client about sleep pattern changes
Listen to and discuss client's stresses, anxieties, and fears
Knowledgeable about community referrals/support and make referrals as necessary, sleep apnea

Evaluation
Verbalization of having slept, feels rested, able to function in daily pursuits without difficulty

NEEDS ADDRESSED AND TASK STRENGTHS

Interest in maintaining healthful lifestyle
Attentive to subtle body signals
Able to judge and seek to meet own needs

Respects and provides for current survival needs
Accepts need for others' intervention when necessary

that leisure-time activity of those 65 years or older was less than that of younger age groups. Yet regular walking (20 minutes 3 times per week) was higher for the older age groups, with 31% of those 65 to 74 years and 24.3% of those 75 years or older reporting regular walking. A similar finding was reported by Uriri and Thatcher-Winger (1995). Among a group of 68 volunteers who were enrolled in a community seniors health service and took the Healthier People Health Risk Appraisal, 38% exercised 20 minutes three times a week on a regular basis prior to the initiation of the project. The aged underestimate their own capacity to engage in activity, using the justification that vigorous activity is a great risk and emphasizing that light and sporadic exercise is physiologically better, or that they garden, shop, and do household chores, which are adequate activity.

Physical inactivity is a risk factor for many conditions experienced by the elderly, including obesity, diabetes, and cardiovascular, respiratory, and musculoskeletal diseases. These conditions and aging changes generally attributed to aging may in fact be due to inactivity. Functional changes that are associated with inactivity include the following: (1) reduced aerobic fitness, (2) loss of postural reflexes, (3) altered lipid metabolism, (4) negative nitrogen balance, (5) loss of muscle mass, and (6) calcium extraction (Barry and Eathorne, 1994). Rather than attributing much of the functional decline seen among the elderly to the aging process, Barry and Eathorne (1994) propose a model that depicts a cycle of aging and reduced physical activity. Deconditioning, weakness, and fatigue result from the reduced physical activity. With the addition of disease, disability, and injury there is an even greater tendency toward inactivity and further physical decline. A deterioration in sense of wellness resulting in poor self-esteem, anxiety, and depression occurs. Poor motivation and a further reduction in physical activity results. This model reveals the complexity of physical activity and aging.

The benefits of exercise are well known and for the aged include the maintenance of a level of functional capacity and strength to enhance self-sufficiency and independence; an improvement of general lifestyle; maintenance of mental functional integrity; self-confidence; decreased depression; and decreased risk of medical problems. Physical benefits include improved cardiac muscle tone, decreased blood pressure, decreasing percentage of body fat, improved ability to breath deeply and effectively, reduced tension, favorable bowel control, and appetite control. Exercise is also

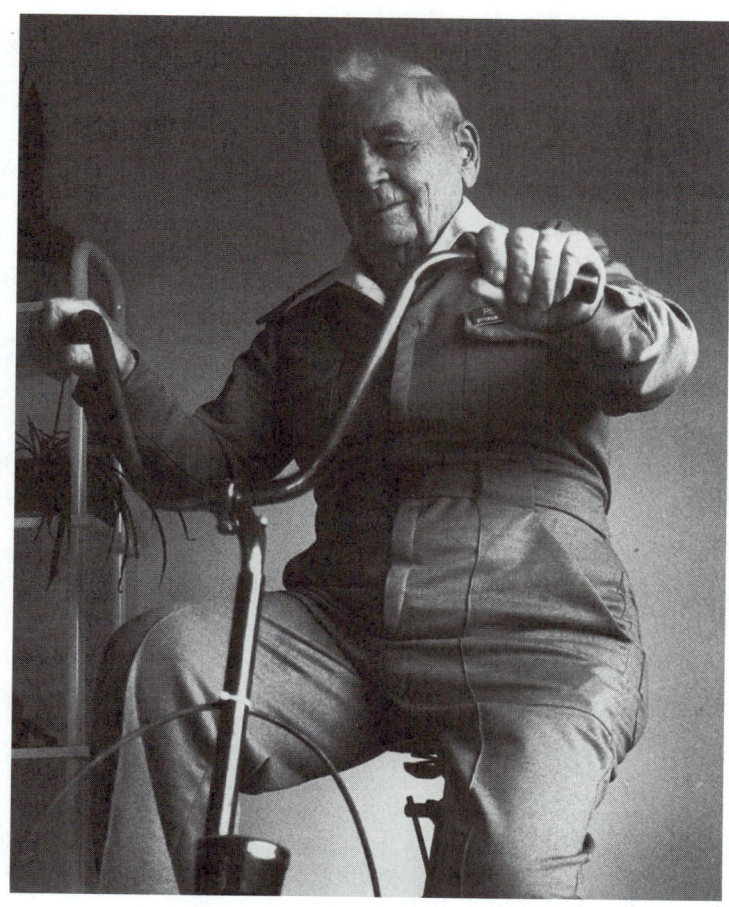

Exercise. (Courtesy Rod Schmall.)

credited as a factor in the retardation of the progress of de-generative conditions and some diseases. Donahue et al (1988) found that in those persons 64 years or older, the rate of definite coronary heart disease in active men was less than half the rate experienced by those who led more seden-tary lives. This study upholds earlier observations that phys-ical activity is beneficial to middle-aged and elderly men.

The majority (75%) of the 215 overweight older women involved in a nurse-led exercise group reported various types of improvements as a result of the exercise (Gillett et al, 1993). The improvements reported were in range of mo-tion, mobility, strength, sleep, bowel function, ability to manage stress, and posture. They also reported decreased lower back and joint pain and marked increases in energy and endurance. The perception of improvements in physio-logic and psychosocial areas have been found in research through objective measurements.

The San Diego Adult Fitness Program, one of the few longitudinal studies on exercise and aging to date, found that maintenance of conditioning over time results in the mainte-nance of fitness. Also, conditioning will increase the health of low-fitness, sedentary individuals to the level of moder-ately active persons.

Psychosocial benefits of exercise were demonstrated as early as 1975 when DeVries found that the elderly who walked and maintained a heart rate of 100 beats per minute had a better degree of anxiety control than a group of aged given meprobamate to control their anxiety.

Goldberg and Fitzpatrick (1980) found that movement therapy increased the morale and self-esteem of older per-sons. They defined movement therapy as the use of body motion and language to meet therapeutic goals of a support-ive group. The goals included increased body awareness, improved breathing patterns, increased attentiveness, in-creased periods of relaxation and stimulation, increased physical mobility and flexibility, increased sense of individ-uality, and increased socialization. Emery and Blumenthal (1990) demonstrated that adults ages 60 to 83 perceived pos-itive changes in their lives as well as improved physiologic outcomes following a 4-month aerobic training program.

Range of motion was found to improve among the el-derly who participated in an exercise program. Kinion et al (1993) implemented the Sit and Get Fit program for seden-tary older adults in a long-term care facility. There was sig-nificant improvement in shoulder, hip, and elbow range of motion among the exercisers. Community-living elderly were the subjects in studies conducted by Mills (1994) and Misner et al (1992). Both found increased range of motion of select joints after involvement in exercise. Misner et al (1992) reported that the increase in range of motion was long term (5 years) with regular exercise.

Improved quadriceps strength and reduced body sway among the elderly subjects resulted from a 20-week exer-cise session that included a walking component and a gentle exercise component (Lord and Castell, 1994), and from a 9-week water exercise program (Lord et al, 1993).

Koroknay et al (1995) reported an improvement in ambula-tory status and a decrease in falls after nursing home resi-dents participated in a walking program. Yet no significant difference in balance was found after exercise programs be-tween exercise and nonexercise groups in studies conducted by Mills (1994) and Topp et al (1993) among community-dwelling elderly.

Benedict and Freeman (1993) studied both physical and psychosocial aspects of aquatic exercise among community-living elderly. Those who exercised regularly in the water had significantly better bone mineral densities of the hips and spines than those who did not exercise. They also found that the exercisers expressed more positive attitudes toward their bodies and had higher morale than the nonexercisers. Depression levels among the two groups were not signifi-cantly different. Happiness and well-being were signifi-cantly improved for a group of 15 community-dwelling women who participated in an exercise program, whereas there was no improvement for the control group (Moore and Bracegirdle, 1994).

Molloy et al (1988) inferred that acute exercise bene-fits aspects of neruopsychologic performance. Dawe and Moore-Orr (1995) looked at the effect of a single session of mild exercise in a group of 20 cognitively unimpaired insti-tutionalized elderly patients on tests of cognitive perfor-mance (set test). Results indicated that nonstrenuous exer-cise of low-intensity (range-of-motion type) does improve the ability to recall immediately following exercise and for at least a half an hour.

In a group of 30 nursing home residents with moderate or severe cognitive impairment due to Alzheimer's disease, Friedman and Tappen (1991) studied the effect of walking and talking on the communication of the subjects. Residents were randomly assigned to either a group that walked 30 minutes 3 times a week while talking with an investigator or a group that spent the same amount of time in conversation. The investigators postulated that because the neurons that control the physical activities of communication and walk-ing are located in the motor cortex, walking would "prime" the motor circuitry involved in communication, and com-munication would improve. After 10 weeks the walking-and-talking group improved on two tests of communication whereas the talking-only group did not.

Benefits in both physical and psychosocial aspects of function have been found for community-living and institu-tionalized elderly. The frail and the healthy independent el-derly have both benefited from various forms of exercise programs.

Assessment

An assessment should be initiated before allowing an older adult to participate in an exercise program. The assess-ment needs to include a medical history, knowledge of the individual's physical activity level and/or physical limita-tions, current medication regimen, and emotional, psycho-logical, and social needs.

In addition to the medical history, a physical examination with emphasis on cardiovascular, pulmonary, musculoskeletal, and neurologic systems should be done. The examination should focus on those aspects that may have an impact on functional status and that may give clues to potential risk. Attention should be focused on joint range of motion, flexibility, and strength. Previous injuries and the presence of active inflammation need to be assessed

Laboratory analysis should include a hematocrit ratio and a hemoglobin level. A low hematocrit ratio and hemoglobin level will increase the workload on the heart to maintain an adequate oxygen supply. In addition, analysis of electrolyte and fluid balance are necessary to evaluate conductivity and contractility of the cardiac muscle and its ability to function adequately.

The American College of Sports Medicine recommends exercise tolerance testing (ETT) for the elderly prior to recommending a moderately intense or vigorous exercise program. This test provides information regarding metabolic equivalents and target heart rate of the older person. Yet ETT for the frail elderly is not recommended. A frail elder's functional impairments may hinder the ability to perform an adequate test. The strength required for ETT may exceed the aerobic capacity of a frail elder. ETT is not essential for the elderly who desire to start a simple walking program or perform a level of exercise as a means to improve mobility and performance of activities of daily living. The patient's exercise goals and functional capacity need to be considered in the decision to use ETT (Barry and Eathorne, 1994).

Tobis (1979) reported that activity tolerance could be monitored through pulse rate. The American Heart Association suggests that this is the quickest way to monitor one's activity tolerance. An accurate resting pulse is the baseline for activity and should increase to approximately 60% to 80% of the cardiopulmonary capacity (Kligman and Pepin, 1992). Those individuals 65 years old and over who are certified medically healthy can safely attain a pulse rate as high as 165 beats per minute during sustained activity for a training effect (Hagberg, 1987). The sustained pulse rate of 99 to 132 beats per minute is the expected (Tobis, 1979). Individuals with a resting pulse of 100 beats per minute and who after a rest period maintain a pulse of 120 beats should have activity carefully chosen. A pulse rate over 130 beats per minute indicates excessive stress to the cardiac system. In severe cardiac conditions the heart should not be stressed more than 20 beats above the baseline pulse and should return to normal in 5 minutes.

The nurse can establish the safe activity pulse of the healthy by two methods or formulas:

$$\text{Safe Cardiac Function} = 200 - \text{Age} \times 60\% \text{ (lower heart rate)}$$
$$\times 80\% \text{ (upper heart rate)}$$
$$\text{or}$$
$$\text{Resting Pulse} + 160\%$$
$$+ 180\%$$

If a resting pulse is 72, multiply by 60% and add the result (43) to the resting pulse for the lower limit (115). Then multiply 72 by 80% and again add the result (57) to the resting pulse for the upper limit (129) of safe cardiac function. In this instance the activity should be kept so that the heart rate is between 115 and 129 beats per minute. Above this limit, excessive demands on the cardiopulmonary function of the person could be deleterious.

A rule of thumb is the ability to talk while doing exercise. The nurse should consider the increase of pulse from the baseline before, during, and at 3-, 5- and 10-minute intervals after activity. Baseline values can be obtained anytime during a resting state except in REM sleep, when physiologic activity is erratic. It is important to remember that there is variation in maximum heart rate and that variability increases with age. Therefore the standard of 60% and 80% of cardiopulmonary capacity may be too high for the older person. Gillett et al (1993) recommend 40% to 70%.

The respiratory system indicates intolerance to activity when dyspnea is evident or when a decrease in respiratory rate occurs during the activity. The cheeks, lips, and nailbeds become red (flushed), pallid, or cyanotic with intolerance. Fatigue, tiredness, and requests to sit down are additional signs of inability to tolerate the activity. Obviously tightness and heaviness in the chest and tightness in the legs are indicative of diminished capacity for activity. If nothing occurs within the expected tolerance level, but the nurse notices that the aged person is slowing down, shows signs of decreased dexterity or coordination, and needs frequent rests, then that aged person is not able to tolerate that level of activity.

A rating of perceived exertion can be used to assess tolerance to exercise. The Borg scale has been used successfully to measure perceived exertion among elderly individuals (Table 6-14). The scale ranges from 6 to 20 points with a rating of 6,7, or 8 for very, very light intensity, 13 and 14 for somewhat hard intensity, up to 19 and 20 for very, very hard intensity. Gillett et al (1993) recommend that a rating of perceived exertion be used rather than a pulse rate for monitoring exertion during exercise.

Intervention and Evaluation

The Centers for Disease Control and Prevention and the President's Council on Physical Fitness and Sports, in collaboration with the American Council of Sports Medicine (1993), have proposed that "Every American adult should accumulate 30 minutes or more of moderate intensity physical activity over the course of most days of the week." Yet exercise is not commonly recommended or incorporated into health prevention care of most elderly persons (Kligman and Pepin, 1992). The benefits of activity on the health of elderly persons support the need for incorporation of activity into the plan of care. The nurse's role has implications for knowledge about fitness and approval of exercise programs in which the aged may participate. Attention should be paid to the simplicity, effectiveness, and adaptability of a program for the aged in whatever setting they may live. Acceptable exercise programs for the aged should have realistic objectives and provide for improvement and maintenance of endurance, strength, flexibility, balance, and coordination while minimizing the risk of injury.

Exercise Programs

Participation in exercise programs is influenced by a number of factors. Fitzgerald et al (1994) found that participation of African American and white females is influenced by their perception of obstacles, specially the amount of time required for exercise and the time they have available. Among a group of mall walkers those told to exercise by their physician perceived significantly greater susceptibility and severity of health problems if they did not walk than those not told by their physician to walk. The mall walkers had more cues and fewer barriers to walk (Sommers JM et al 1995).

Schuster et al (1995) predicted the intentional exercise among postretirement adults using the Social Cognitive Theory. Based on the results, a successful exercise program needs to address perceived barriers to exercise (dispel misconceptions about exercise as dangerous, uncomfortable, exhausting, or embarrassing, and address poor weather and lack of facilities and transportation), tailor the exercise to the current fitness status and abilities of each individual, provide various forms of social support (leader, class members, family, friends and assigned partners), use a decision balance-sheet procedure that has participants contrast potential benefits with barriers to exercise, cue exercise participants to focus on how they feel during exercise, and agree on appropriate exercises. The use of goals was stressed as an important point in planning an exercise program.

Motivating the elderly to change their behavior is not always easy. Among a group of 67 sedentary women in a weight reduction program only 39% adhered to the intervention (Dornealas et al 1994). The 26 subjects who participated in the program had significantly higher self-efficacy of exercise, psychologic well-being, and more positive general health perceptions and affect than did the nonexercisers. Nonexercisers were likely to report feeling depressed and fearful about their health.

The variables identified in the reported research are reflected in the following *critical* characteristics of exercise programs that improve long-term compliance:

1. Low probability of musculoskeletal injury (low to moderate intensity, duration, and frequency)
2. Group participation
3. Emphasis on variety and pleasure (use of games as exercise)
4. Set personal goals, development of contracts
5. Assess response to training
6. Recruit friends, family, or spouse for support
7. Monitor progress (use charts to display changes visually)
8. Use music
9. Provide positive feedback
10. Provide enthusiastic leadership and role models

Gillett et al (1993) incorporated these guidelines into an exercise program and had 88% of the 244 women who entered the program complete it.

Kinion et al (1993) evaluated the effects of the Sit and Get Fit program for sedentary older adults in a long-term care facility. The program was designed so that it could be implemented by paraprofessional caregivers with minimal supervision. The uniqueness and positive regard for each participant were incorporated into the protocol. They concluded that the importance lies not only in the development of an effective exercise program, but also in creating an atmosphere that stimulates engagement and breaks down the barriers erected by the apathetic outlook many elderly persons have learned.

Enjoyment and individualization of the program to meet individual goals and needs are key factors in improving long-term participation. Another consideration for many older adults is the expense associated with the exercise program. Many elderly have limited financial reserves for recreational purposes.

It is also important the individuals who conduct aerobic exercise programs and classes consider differences between the abilities of young and old. Classes are generally taught by young and fit persons who become so involved in what they are doing that they are unaware that the elderly may not be able to do the number of repetitions they consider necessary for toning muscles. These programs can damage the muscles, tendons, ligaments, and joints of the older adult. Gillett et al (1993) trained nonathletic female nurses between the ages of 50 and 60 years as group leaders for exercise classes for the elderly. Bonding with the leaders was apparent the first 2 weeks of the programs. The participants repeatedly mentioned the effectiveness of the leaders.

A variety of exercise programs exist for the elderly. The existing programs need to be evaluated on an individual basis to determine if they are appropriate.

Table 6-14   Borg Scale of Perceived Exertion

Rating	Perceived intensity
6, 7, 8	Very, very light
9, 10	Very light
11, 12	Fairly light
13, 14	Somewhat hard
15, 16	Hard
17, 18	Very hard
19, 20	Very, very hard

From Barry HC, Eathorne, SW: Exercise and aging issues for the practitioner, *Med Clin North Am* 78(2):357, 1994.

Three programs have been developed by the Administration of Aging. Each program is accompanied by pretest exercises to establish the correct starting level in a program. Instructions are carefully stated for starting positions, sequence of exercises, and precautions when doing the exercises. These exercises include jog-walking, walking, bending, head rotation, leg raising, walking a straight line, knee push-ups, and the stork stand. Some require incremental participation to assure individual safety.

Senior Games

Senior centers throughout the United States have instituted physical fitness programs, which include Ping-Pong, boccie, golf, horseshoes, and many other activities enjoyed by the aged. These activities incorporate rhythmic action and stretching and provide improvement in or maintenance of cardiopulmonary function, muscle tone, and mental stimulation.

Nearly all of the states of the United States promote "Senior Games" in collaboration with public service and private corporations. These are Olympic-style competitions for men and women 55 years of age and older (Neville, 1988). Some companies have established par courses or 1-mile exercise fitness trails for the older adult.

A sustained brisk walk is one of the most popular and accessible forms of activity for the aged. Those who have done little walking are encouraged to start slowly by first walking to the corner of the block and eventually being able to develop the capacity for distance walking of several miles. Those limited to institutional facilities should also be encouraged to increase the amount of walking. First it may be only from the bed to the bathroom, then with time down the hall, and eventually around the total facility. If the person can go outside, walking around the block might be a long-term goal. Siegel et al (1995) found that the elderly had more regular walking habits than younger adults.

Dancing

For those accustomed to it, ballroom, folk, or square dancing should be encouraged. This form of activity done properly can have as much aerobic benefit as workouts to music videotapes. Dancing is kind to the joints and can burn as many calories as swimming, biking, or walking. However, it should not be done as the only form of activity since it does not develop upper body strength. To enhance cardiovascular and respiratory fitness, one would have to engage in 20 to 30 minutes of sustained dancing (Social dancing, 1990). Dancing provides another means of obtaining pleasant, sociable, vigorous exercise, which tones the body and benefits cardiopulmonary and mental health.

Swimming

Swimming, one of America's most popular sports, or water exercise facilitates muscle tone, and improves circulation, muscle strength, endurance, flexibility, and weight control, and in addition it can be relaxing and a mood elevator. The benefits of aquatic activity or exercise therapy are that arm and leg movements against water are less painful and do not seem to require as much effort because of the buoyancy of the water. Some aged maintain a swimming program begun earlier in life; others enjoy this as a relaxing new way to get activity and socialize. Those who are nonswimmers or who do not swim well might benefit from water exercise classes held in the shallow end of the pool. The YMCA, YWCA, and the American Red Cross offer classes in these types of activities. Some areas of the country have "senior splash" aerobic swim classes or arthritic aquatic programs, which conform to guidelines set by the Arthritis Foundation. Swimming, however, may be hazardous to those with ischemic heart disease because horizontal water immersion can increase central blood volume, thus stressing the limited cardiac reserve of the individual. Those with ischemic heart disease who want to swim should be under a physician's care.

Isotonic and Isometric Exercises

Yoga is another form of exercise that can be practiced regardless of one's condition. It can foster mental alacrity, independence, and good health in the aged through simple exercise, relaxation, meditation, and nutritional education.

Isotonic exercises train the cardiovascular and skeletal muscles. Isometrics mainly work with the cardiovascular system. Persons who are confined to a bed or chair or who are ambulatory can do these rhythmic tasks or calisthenics. Exercise should be aerobic in nature, easily attained, and not produce an oxygen debt. Numerous programs have been developed in which simplicity and flexibility of the program make it easily adaptable to a variety of settings.

The following guidelines for developing an exercise program and/or modifying an existing program for the elderly have been developed by Marsigilio and Holm (1988) and Gillett et al (1993):

Base program on individual assessment data (underlying conditions, medications, present activity level).

Establish mutual goals.

Teach to use correct body mechanics, appropriate clothing (layer so can change to environment), exercise-specific shoes (supportive), and sufficient hydration (drink water prior, during, and after).

Begin at a very slow level (40% to 50% maximum predicted heart rate) and very gentle exercise progression.

Teach to avoid sudden twisting movements, rapid movements, and rapid transitions from one movement to the next.

Avoid exercises that tax vision and balance.

Avoid sustained isometric contractions of greater than 10 seconds.

Assess ability to tolerate low-level activity without signs and symptoms of muscle fatigue, shortness of breath, angina, arrhythmias, abnormal blood pressure, or intermittent claudication.

Stop exercising if cardiac arrhythmias, angina, or excessive breathlessness occur.

Instruct to avoid exercise during acute viral infections.

Increase activity slowly by intensity (workload), duration (time), and frequency (time interval or length of time).

Monitor exercise intensity by perceived exertion and exercise heart rate.

Perform a gradual, extended exercise warm-up (that is, 15 minutes) to maximize flexibility and decrease muscle injury

Perform cooldown until heart rate returns to resting level to decrease postural hypotension and cardiac arrhythmias.

Modify exercise program based on individual's responses.

Special Needs of the Elderly

It is also important to address special needs of the elderly when initiating an exercise program. The elderly are less able to adapt to the environment during exercise. They should dress in layers to adjust to different environmental temperatures. Well-fitting footwear and stockings are essential to prevent injury because of impaired foot sensation. Blisters and friction injuries may occur without the elderly person knowing it. Maintaining hydration is essential. Total body water is decreased in the elderly. Consumption of fluid before exercising and regularly while exercising is recom-

mended. Environments with poor air quality should be avoided for exercise, including areas near roadways.

Often when beginning a physical exercise program muscles will be sore. Warm, not hot, baths or soaks are excellent. Another way to minimize muscle soreness is a 5- to 10-minute cooldown period of slow walking or stretching to keep the primary muscle groups active, to decrease venous pooling and increase venous return to the heart, and to prevent vagal responses.

When planning activities for the elderly, the age-related changes of the musculoskeletal system need to be considered. Table 6-15 addresses age-related changes of the musculoskeletal system with outcomes and management approaches. Musculoskeletal function is essential to activity.

Nurses should capitalize, more than they do, on activities of daily living, such as providing the aged with bath brushes to wash their own backs in the shower or bathtub and encouraging the aged to dry body parts or rub the back dry with a towel. Reaching for objects while cleaning house can be included in an activity program, as can washing dishes in warm water to provide finger exercises. Warm water aids in the relief of stiffness and enables the fingers to move more easily without discomfort. Various exercises for bed, chair, and standing are presented in Figure 6-6. This does not cover the numerous maneuvers that exist but rather gives a sampling of possible movements.

Housekeeping activities can be utilized for strength and flexibility. Community-dwelling elderly can be taught simple approaches in utilizing household chores for activity.

Table 6-15   Age-Related Musculoskeletal Changes, Outcomes, and Health Prevention, Promotion, and Maintenance Approaches

Age-related changes	Outcomes	Health prevention, promotion, and maintenance
Bones become more porous (osteoporosis)	Dowager's hump (kyphosis)	Have good lighting, dry floors, nonskid rugs
Demineralization of vertebral trabecular bone	Risk of hip fracture	Diet high in calcium
Intervertebral discs dehydrate and narrow	Tremors	Calcium supplements as necessary
Reduced height	Back pain	Do moderate exercise: walking or swimming
Erosion of cartilage through exposure and wearing	Joint swelling	Use assistive devices: cane, walker, if needed
	Ankylosis	Do range of motion activity
Subchondral bone becomes hyperemic and fibrotic	Crepitation	Seek medical evaluation of back pain
Synovial membranes become fibrotic	Decreased range of motion	Wear shoes with low heels, nonskid soles, and support
Synovial fluid thickens	Stiffness	Use leg muscles rather than back muscles when lifting
Muscle wasting of hand dorsum	Muscle wasting	Rest joints when pain occurs
Diminished protein synthesis in muscle cells	Reduced muscle strength	Lose weight when necessary
Glucose mobilizes slowly in response to exercise	Night leg cramps	Develop an appropriate exercise program
Diminished muscle mass decreases glucose stores	Gait problems	Pace activities
Bone and muscle weakness changes the center of gravity	Smaller steps	Allow for rest periods
	Wider stance base	Break big jobs into small parts
	Poor posture	Adjust activities to periods of day when energy is high
		Remove scatter rugs
		Use nonskid rubber mats in tub and shower
		Take stretch breaks
		Eat more potassium and calcium rich foods
		Coordinate and balance exercise

LYING DOWN

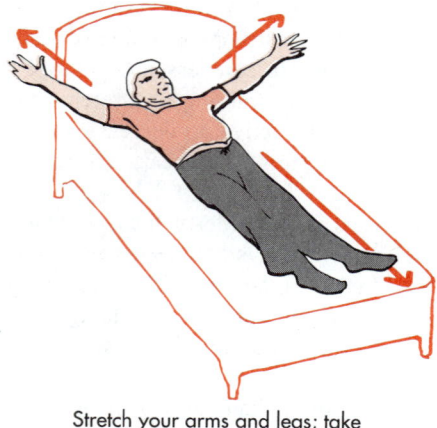

Stretch your arms and legs; take a deep breath.

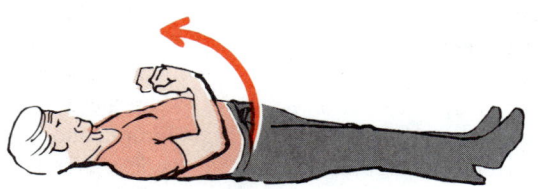

With your arm at your sides, bend at the elbow and curl your arms as if "making a muscle."

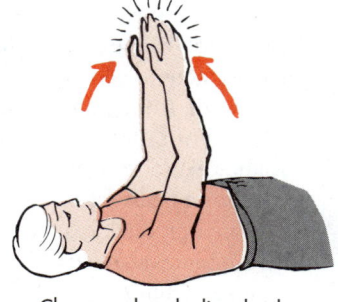

Clap your hands directly above your head.

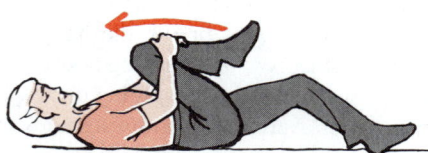

Grab each leg with both hands below the knee and pull toward your chest slowly.

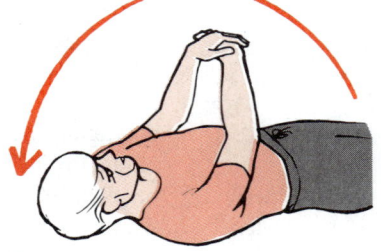

Fold your hands on your stomach; raise your arms over your head toward the headboard.

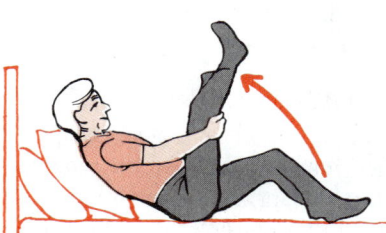

Lift each leg off the bed, but try not to bend your knee. Use an arm to help.

SITTING

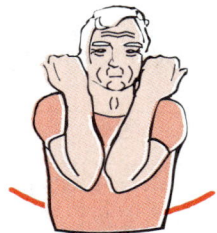

Touch your elbows together in front of you.

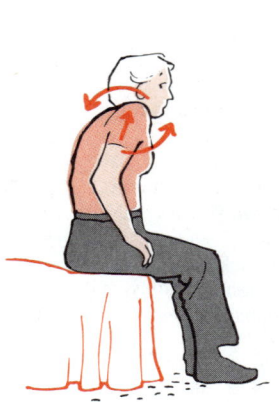

Shrug your shoulders forward, then move them in a circle, raising them high enough to reach your ears.

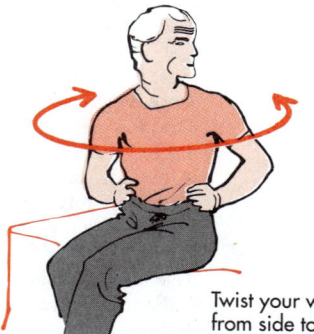

Twist your whole upper body from side to side with your hands on your hips.

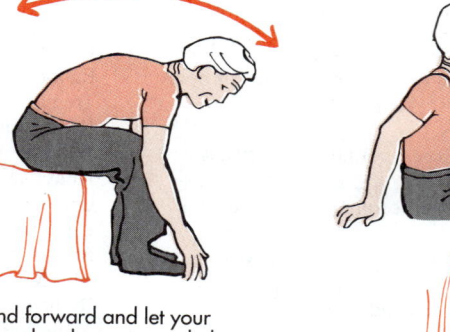

Bend forward and let your arms dangle; try to touch the floor with your hands.

While still sitting, move each of your knees up and down as if you are walking; each time your right foot hits the ground, count it as one. Lift your knee high.

Figure 6-6. Exercises: lying down, sitting, standing up, and walking places. (From Johnson-Paulson JE, Kosher R, *Geriatr Nurs*, 1985, pp 322-325.)

STANDING UP

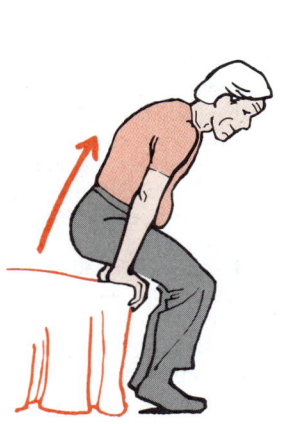

Using your arms, push off from the bed and stand up; if you get dizzy, sit down and try again.

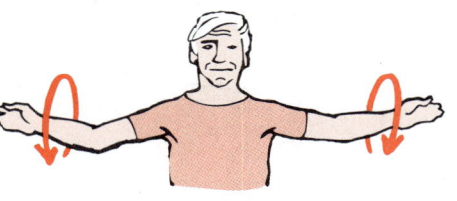

Hold your arms out and turn them in big circles.

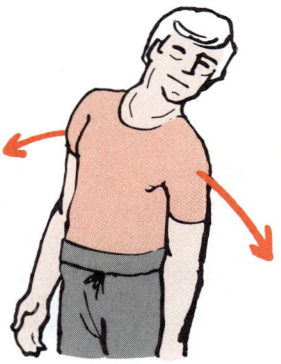

With hands at your side bend at the waist as far as you can to the right side, then to the left.

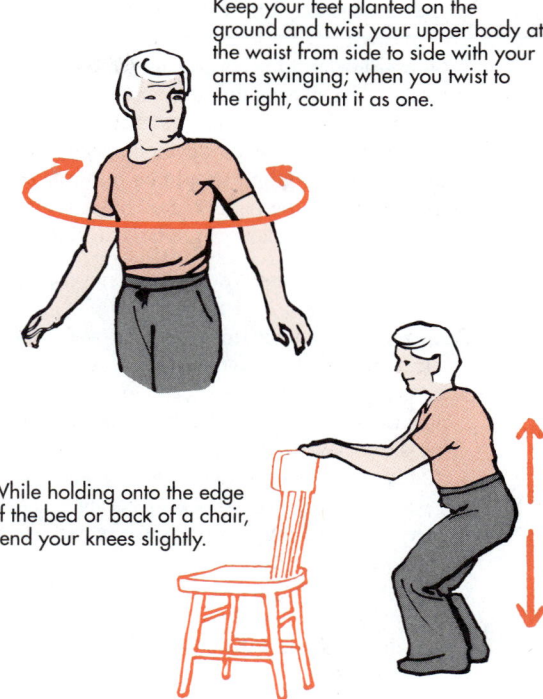

Keep your feet planted on the ground and twist your upper body at the waist from side to side with your arms swinging; when you twist to the right, count it as one.

While holding onto the edge of the bed or back of a chair, bend your knees slightly.

WALKING PLACES

Walking is good exercise. It helps in toning muscles, maintaining flexibility of joints, and also is good exercise for the heart and circulatory system. Walking briskly for 20 minutes a day, 3 times a week can be as effective a heart conditioner as jogging, but it does take a longer time to achieve the same effect as jogging. For those who cannot walk rapidly for long periods, walking to the point of muscular fatigue also helps maintain good muscle tone.

There are signs your body may give you to indicate you are overdoing exercise. Stop, rest, and if necessary call your physician if you experience any of these symptoms:

- SEVERE SHORTNESS OF BREATH
- CHEST PAIN
- SEVERE JOINT PAIN
- DIZZINESS OR FAINT FEELING
- HEART FLUTTERS

In all walking exercises, go only as fast as you are able to walk and still carry on a conversation. If you cannot, slow down.

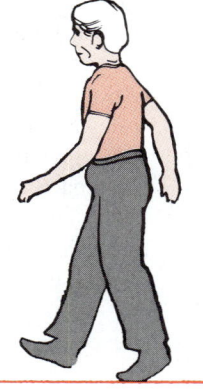

INSIDE

It is important to maintain walking ability. Determine how far you can walk and each day walk to ¾ of that distance, building endurance. Wear supportive shoes and use whatever aids are necessary.

OUTSIDE

Wear soft-soled shoes with good support, i.e., jogging shoes. When walking, push off *from* your toes and land on your heels. Swing arms loosely at your sides. Begin with 10-minute walks and build to 20 to 30 minutes.

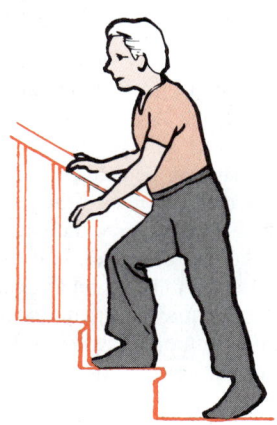

Walking upstairs requires effort. Place one foot flat on a step, push off with the other and shift your weight. Use a railing for balance if necessary.

Figure 6-6, cont'd. For legend, see opposite page.

<table>
<tr><td>

Box 6-13

Movements for Geriatric Patients

The progression should be from smaller, more personal movements to larger ones that may involve communication with the rest of the group. Movements should begin slowly and later develop speed. The amount of balance required should be minimal at first and more later when the patients feel more secure and uninhibited. A sample class might be as follows:

1. Scratch the small of your back againt the chair. Now, try your upper back, too.
2. Begin by pretending to wash your face, then your arms and shoulders and neck.
3. Stretch up as high as you can; now sink down as low as you can. Now try to reach as far forward as possible, now out to each side.
4. Can you nod your head up and down as if to say "yes?" Now try "no"—an even stronger *"no!"*
5. Let's try marching in place to the music. You may use one or both feet.
6. Let's try making circles with different parts of our body. Start with one shoulder. Try both shoulders. Try one hand, now the other hand. Can you reverse directions?
7. How about kicking one leg at a time up in the air as the music gets louder?
8. Let's have one half of the group kick while the other half stomps. Now let's reverse.
9. Can you now reach out as if you're trying to shake hands with the person across the circle from you?
10. Now try actually shaking hands with the person next to you. How about the person on the other side?
11. Now, let's all take a huge deep breath and stretch as tall and as long as possible. Now let the air out slowly and let your head, back, and arms deflate slowly as a balloon. Try it again, take in even more air. Now deflate even more slowly.

The above is a simple example of what can be done with a small group of 6 to 10 patients. It is advisable, if possible, to have one aide present to help encourage patients and monitor safety.

The goals that may be achieved are many and varied. They include increased range of motion and strength, increased balance and coordination, and increased cardiovascular function if the class takes place for at least 20 minutes on a regular basis. Nonphysical goals may be greater social interaction, communication with others who are limited in function or disabled in the same or different ways, and greater self-awareness.

From Fond D: Group movement class model for geriatric patients, *The Coordinator* 2:30, March, 1983.

</td></tr>
</table>

Table 6-16   Benefits of Exercise on Chronic Conditions

Condition	Types of exercise	Benefits
Chronic lung disease	Aerobic	Improve diaphragmatic breathing
		Reduce reliance on accessory muscles
Cognitive dysfunction	Aerobic	Improve cerebral function
		Increase cerebral perfusion
		Increase beta-endorphin secretion
Coronary heart disease	Aerobic	Reduce blood pressure
	Endurance type	Increase HDLs and reduce body fat
		Increase maximal oxygen consumption
Diabetes mellitus	Aerobic	Fat loss
	Endurance type	Increase insulin sensitivity
		Decrease glucose intolerance risk
Hypertension	Aerobic	Decrease systolic blood pressure
	Endurance type	
	Leisure-time activity	Decrease total peripheral resistance
Osteoarthritis	Resistance stretching	Maintain range of motion; muscle mass
	Endurance type	Increase muscle strength
Osteoporosis	Resistance	Strengthen postural muscles
	Weight-bearing	Stimulate bone growth
		Decrease rate of bone loss

Data compiled from Kligman EW, Pepin E: Prescribing physical activity for elder patients, *Geriatrics* 47(8):33, 1992; Edward K, Larson EB: Benefits of exercise for older adults, *Clin Geriatr Med* 8(1):35, 1992; Barry HC, Eathorne SW: Exercise and aging: Issues for the practitioner, *Med Clin North Am* 78(2):357, 1994.

The elderly in long-term care who respond to the work ethic can be encouraged to push wheelchairs, clean tables, and run errands.

Other activities that can be done while watching television or whenever there are a few spare minutes during the day are rolling a pencil between the hand and a hard surface, exaggerating the chewing motion of the jaw, holding the stomach in, tightening the buttocks, flexing the fingers, and rotating the head and the ankles. Benison and Hogstel (1986) elaborate on specific total body exercises for the older immobile patient.

Activity, in general, should be paced and occur regularly every day. Activities that will help eliminate stiffness should be planned for the morning, when stiffness is most prevalent. Relaxation exercises should be considered before bedtime to help induce sleep. With any activity in which the aged are involved, sufficient intermittent rest periods should be provided. An example of a small-group exercise program is presented in Box 6-13.

Safety Considerations

Those who are frail should not engage in strenuous activity nor should their joints be forced past the point of resistance

Nursing Diagnoses

The following potential diagnoses must be considered as well as diagnoses unique to the particular individual:
Risk for activity intolerance
Risk for disuse syndrome
Impaired physical mobility

Fatigue
Social isolation

NURSING PROCESS AND NURSING DIAGNOSIS
Activity Intolerance

Etiologies and Related Factors
Generalized weakness
Sedentary lifestyle
Imbalance of supply and demand of oxygen
Exertional dyspnea
Chronic diseases

Defining Characteristics
Shortness of breath
Dyspnea on exertion
Use of accessory muscles
Verbal report of fatigue or weakness
Abnormal heart rate and/or blood pressure
Exertional discomfort
Decreased flexibility/ability/balance
Limited muscle strength and endurance

Knowledge
Normal anatomic and functional changes with aging
Activity/fitness assessment
Normal laboratory/diagnostic values
Exercise techniques
Measures to conserve energy
Community resources
Rehabilitation concepts and programs
Medication interactions

Clinical Judgment and Related Skills
Interview client regarding prior lifestyle, environmental factors/influences; medication regimen; and utilize a standardized tool to identify activity tolerance/intolerance
Conduct a physical examination with particular attention to energy level; vital signs; functional ADL capacity
Implement nursing actions that prevent and manage activity intolerance:
    Exercise programs prescribed by physical therapy
    Range of motion
    Activities that support cardiac, respiratory, musculoskeletal, and neurologic function
    Teaching parameters for rest and exercise
    Teaching activities
Develop a home care plan to improve activity tolerance or maintain present level of tolerance (if acceptable), evaluate its effectiveness
Conduct group exercise activities for individuals with varying abilities
Teach family/community health maintenance

Evaluation
Individual performs activities without adverse symptoms such as shortness of breath, pain, excessive acceleration of heart rate
Exhibits a more positive attitude toward self
Evidence of incorporation of activity/exercise into lifestyle
States feels better than before beginning activity/exercise program
Develops improvement in one or more areas: endurance, strength, flexibility, balance, coordination

NEEDS ADDRESSED AND TASK STRENGTHS

Interest in maintaining healthful lifestyle
Attentive to subtle body signals
Able to judge and seek to meet own needs

Respects and provides for current survival needs
Accepts need for others' intervention when necessary

or discomfort. If the frail have regularly participated in activity that the nurse deems too stressful to their skeletal systems, it is important to keep in mind that an activity done for many years is not as difficult as if it were just introduced. When the activity is new, serious consideration should be given to levels of stress produced.

Many aged are fearful of falling because of altered balance or the inability to reach or bend. Some fear if they get down on the floor they will not be able to get up again. Sometimes all that is necessary to alleviate this fear is to ensure that the aged person has his or her glasses or other appliances that provide security, stability, and mobility. Mental activity should be planned as carefully as physical activity. These activities should be consistent with the individual's interests. New hobbies may develop; involvement in raising or keeping pets may foster caring and affection for others and a rebirth of socialization. Chapters 21 and 22 deal more completely with mental activity of the aged.

Activity should not be thought of as something to keep the aged busy but should be purposeful to enhance their physical and mental well-being. Table 6-16 shows how exercise can benefit those with chronic conditions.

In summary, this chapter has looked at the life support needs individually. It is apparent that each area influences the function of others. The aged would not continue to survive if these needs could not be met independently or with assistance of others. The quality and the overall perception of life can be augmented when the nurse monitors these specific functions and provides support or assistance according to identified problems.

KEY CONCEPTS

- Interruptions in the basic requirements for nutrition, fluids, elimination, activity and rest may trigger exacerbations of subclinical and chronic disorders.
- When basic needs are out of balance it is common for the very old to demonstrate the deficiency by becoming confused.
- Recommended dietary patterns for the aged are similar to those of younger persons with some reduction in caloric intake based on decreased metabolic requirements. Adequacy of nutrition is affected by lifelong eating habits and patterns, accessibility of food, mood disorders, capacity for food preparation, and income.
- Medications may interfere with adequate food intake, absorption, digestion, and elimination. A common nutritional deficiency is a lack of sufficient calcium, especially for women.
- Making mealtimes pleasant and attractive for the aged who are unable to eat unassisted is entirely a nursing challenge; mealtimes **must** be made enjoyable.
- Elimination is often a preoccupation of the aged,

signifying sluggishness of involuntary responses or a loss of control. Nursing attention to these function is critical for client satisfaction and comfort.

- Deep, stage IV sleep, is not attained by the aged. They tend to be easily aroused. The nursing focus is to help them understand the changes and their sleep pattern and that their individual needs to obtain sufficient rest will vary.
- Sleep apnea is an interruption in breathing during sleep that has been linked to excess pharyngeal tissue, cardiac problems, cerebral infarction, and hypertension. It is often demonstrated by long periods without inspiring and loud snoring on expiration. The long periods of anoxia may have effects, over time, on cerebration.
- Physical activity and the ease with which it is performed is often the barometer by which an individual's health and wellness are judged.

▲ CASE STUDY

Nutrition

Genevieve, 70 years old, had dieted all her life—it seemed. She often chided herself about it. "After all, at my age who cares if I'm too fat? I do. It depresses me when I gain weight and then I gain even more when I'm depressed." At 5′ 1″ and 140 lbs her weight was ideal for her height and age, but Genevieve, as so many women of her generation, had incorporated Donna Reed's weight of 105 lb as ideal. She had achieved that weight for only a few weeks three or four times in her adult life. She had tried high-protein diets, celery and cottage cheese diets, fasting, commercially prepared diet foods, and numerous fad diets. She always discontinued the diets when she perceived any negative effects. She was very invested in maintaining her general good health. Her most recent attempt at losing 30 lbs on an all-liquid diet had been unsuccessful and left her feeling constipated, weak, irritable, mildly nauseated, and experiencing heart palpitations. This really frightened her. Her physician upbraided her regarding the liquid diet but seemed rather amused while reinforcing that her weight was "just perfect" for her age. In the discussion the doctor pointed out how fortunate she was that she was able to drive to the market, had sufficient money for food, and was really able to eat anything with no dietary restrictions. Genevieve left his office feeling silly. She was an independent, intelligent woman; she had been a very successful manager of a large financial office uptown. Prior to her retirement 2 years ago her work had consumed most of her energies. There had been no time for family, romance, or hobbies. Lately, she had immersed herself in reading the Harvard Classics as she had promised herself she would when she retired. Unfortunately, now that she had the time to read them she was losing interest. She knew that she must begin to "pull herself together" and "be grateful for her blessings" just as the doctor had said.

Based upon the case study, develop a nursing care plan using the following procedure*:

List comments of client that provide *subjective data.*

List information that provides *objective data.*

From these data identify and state, using accepted format, two *nursing diagnoses* you determine are most significant to this client at this time. List two *client strengths* that you have identified from data.

Determine and state *outcome criteria* for each diagnosis. These must reflect some alleviation of the problem identified in the nursing diagnosis and must be stated in concrete and measurable terms.

Plan and state one or more *interventions* for each diagnosed problem. Provide specific documentation of source used to determine appropriate intervention. Plan at least one intervention that incorporates the client's existing strengths.

Evaluate success of intervention. Interventions must correlate directly with the stated outcome criteria in order to measure the outcome success.

STUDY QUESTIONS/ACTIVITIES

What factors may be involved in Genevieve's preoccupation with her weight?

What are some of the reasons that fad diets are dangerous?

Discuss how you would counsel Genevieve regarding her weight.

If Genevieve insists on dieting, what diet would you recommend, considering her age and activity level?

What lifestyle changes should Genevieve make?

What lifestyle changes would you suggest to Genevieve?

What are the specific health concerns that require attention in Genevieve's case?

RESEARCH QUESTIONS

What are the ideal weights for older men and women?

What are the dietary patterns of older career women living alone?

What percentage of women over 60 are satisfied with their weight? Men?

What eating disorders are most common among aged men? Women?

What is the compliance rate in regard to major dietary changes suggested for elders by dietitians or physicians?

What percentage of men and women over 80 years old are overweight and/or obese?

▲ CASE STUDY

Elimination

Maud, at 80 years old, could truthfully say she had never had problems with her bowel movements. They had been regular—each morning about 30 minutes after breakfast. In fact, she hardly thought of them at all as they had been so consistent. Following a hospitalization for a fractured hip last year she had never regained her reliable pattern of bowel function. She was greatly distressed by this as bowel function was a symbol to her of good health. Admittedly, she did not move about as much now and used a walker when she did. And she had heard that pain medications sometimes made one constipated, but she tried to use them very sparingly. She had even reestablished her pattern of attempting a bowel movement every morning after breakfast. She began to worry considerably about her constipation and to use laxatives almost routinely. She said, "This constipation really upsets me. I just don't feel like myself if I don't have a bowel movement every day."

Based upon the case study, develop a nursing care plan using the following procedure*:

List comments of client that provide *subjective data.*

List information that provides *objective data.*

From these data identify and state, using accepted format, two *nursing diagnoses* you determine are most significant to this client at this time. List two *client strengths* that you have identified from data.

Determine and state *outcome criteria* for each diagnosis. These must reflect some alleviation of the problem identified in the nursing diagnosis and must be stated in concrete and measurable terms.

Plan and state one or more *interventions* for each diagnosed problem. Provide specific documentation of source used to determine appropriate intervention. Plan at least one intervention that incorporates the client's existing strengths.

Evaluate success of intervention. Interventions must correlate directly with the stated outcome criteria in order to measure the outcome success.

STUDY QUESTIONS/ACTIVITIES

What information will you need to obtain from Maud to help her isolate the causes of her constipation?

What advice will you give her regarding the use of laxatives?

What dietary changes will you suggest, and how will you do this in order to cultivate compliance?

---

*Students are advised to refer to their nursing diagnosis text and identify possible or potential problems.

*Students are advised to refer to their nursing diagnosis text and identify possible or potential problems.

What information regarding the relationship of medications to constipation will be useful to Maud?

When you are constipated, how do you feel?

Do you know any elders that focus a lot of their conversation on elimination? How do you handle that?

RESEARCH QUESTIONS

What are the specific concerns elders harbor related to constipation?

Is concern with constipation a sociocultural artifact?

Do childhood training experiences affect one's eliminatory functions in late life?

What are the remedies for constipation most often deemed effective as perceived by elders?

Does fecal impaction affect urinary incontinence?

▲ CASE STUDY

Rest and Sleep

Jesse had a sleep disorder and consequently was torpid during the day and lonely at night. His wife of 35 years had recently insisted on moving into the guest room as she could no longer cope with his loud snoring and periods of interrupted breathing. Jesse suffered from obstructive sleep apnea. In recent years, he often wakened abruptly with a feeling of drowning and gasping for air. However, he simply tolerated it because he thought nothing could be done about it. Now that it had become a threat to his marriage he became more motivated to investigate possible solutions. Jesse said, "This doesn't amount to anything, but it bugs my wife." Though he did not admit it, he was also worried because he was beginning to feel rather sleepy during the day. Upon consulting the clinic nurse he found that there were some very practical means of dealing with sleep apnea and if not effective there were additional medical interventions that could be helpful.

Based upon the case study, develop a nursing care plan using the following procedure*:

List comments of client that provide *subjective data*.

List information that provides *objective data*.

From these data identify and state, using accepted format, two *nursing diagnoses* you determine are most significant to this client at this time. List two *client strengths* that you have identified from data.

Determine and state *outcome criteria* for each diagnosis. These must reflect some alleviation of the problem identified in the nursing diagnosis and must be stated in concrete and measurable terms.

Plan and state one or more *interventions* for each diagnosed problem. Provide specific documentation of source

used to determine appropriate intervention. Plan at least one intervention that incorporates the client's existing strengths.

Evaluate success of intervention. Interventions must correlate directly with the stated outcome criteria in order to measure the outcome success.

STUDY QUESTIONS/ACTIVITIES

What lifestyle factors may be increasing Jesse's episodes of sleep apnea?

In what circumstances is sleep apnea particularly dangerous to health?

Compose a list of 10 questions you would ask Jesse to obtain a clear picture of factors contributing to his sleep apnea. Discuss the rationale behind each.

Look up and discuss the terms hypnagogic and hypnopompic and relate any episodes you may have experienced and how these affected you.

RESEARCH QUESTIONS

How do sleep patterns correlate with various disease states?

How do sleep patterns change with each decade after age 60?

How are hypnagogic and hypnopompic states related to sleep patterns of the aged?

What is the average time of the total sleep cycle as experienced by a healthy individual over 70 years of age?

RESOURCES

Nutrition

National Dairy Council (Dairy and Nutrition Council)
6300 North River Road
Rosemont, IL 60018-4233

"To your health . . . In your second fifty years"

"For mature eaters only: guidelines for good nutrition"

"Sticks and stones can break your bones . . . and so will too little calcium"

"The all-American guide to calcium rich foods"

American Association of Retired Persons (AARP)
Health Advocacy Sercies (HAS)
601 E Street NW
Washington, DC 20049

Sleep

A to Zzzz Guide to Better Sleep
Better Sleep Council
PO Box 13
Washington, DC 20044

Sleep Disorders
Association of Professional Sleep Society

---

*Students are advised to refer to their nursing diagnosis text and identify possible or potential problems.

604 Second Street SW
Rochester, MN 55902

National Sleep Foundation
1367 Connecticut Ave NW, Suite 200
Washington, DC 20036

Activity

Local YMCA/YWCA activity programs
  Swimming
  Aquatic exercises
  Stretch/flexibility/strengthening
  Square dancing
  Specific activities for seniors

National Senior Sports Organization
14323 South Outer Forty Road
Suite N-300
Chesterfield, MO 63017

Pep Up Your Life: A Fitness Book for Seniors
AARP
1909 K Street NW
Washington, DC 20049

Armchair Fitness Video Programs
CC-M Productions
7755 16th Street NW
Washington DC 20012
(301) 588-4095

REFERENCES

Alessi CA, Schnelle JF, Traub S, Ouslander JG: Psychotropic medications in incontinent nursing home residents: association with sleep and bed mobility, *J Am Geriatr Soc* 43(7):788, 1995.

Allison OC, Porter ME, Briggs GC: Chronic constipation: assessment and management in the elderly, *J Am Acad Nurse Practitioners* 6(7):311, 1994.

American Nurses' Association: *Position statement on foregoing artificial nutrition and hydration,* Washington DC, 1992, The Association.

American Nurses' Association: Position statement on nutrition screening for the elderly, Washington, DC, 1992, The Association.

Ancoli-Israel S, Klauber MR, Kripke DF, Parder L, Cobarrubias M: Sleep apnea in female patients in a nursing home, *Chest* 96(5):1054, 1989a.

Ancoli-Israel S, Kripke D: Sleep and aging. In Calkins E, Davis PJ, Ford AB, editors: *The practice of geriatrics,* Philadelphia, 1986, WB Saunders.

Ancoli-Israel S, Parker L, Sinaee R et al: Sleep fragmentation in patients from a nursing home, *J Gerontol* 44(1):M18, 1989b.

Anderson JW, Johnstone BM, Cook-Newell ME: Meta-analysis of the effects of soy protein intake on serum lipids, *N Engl J Med* 333(5):276, 1995.

Anderson WF: *Practical management of the elderly,* ed 3, Oxford, 1976, Blackwell.

Barry HC, Eathorne SW: Exercise and aging: issues for the practitioner, *Med Clin North Am* 78(2): 357, 1994.

Beel-Bates CA, Rogers AE: An exploratory study of sundown syndrome, *J Neurosci Nurs* 22(1):51, 1990.

Benedict A, Freeman R: The effect of aquatic exercise on aged person's bone density, body image, and morale, AAAA 17(3):67, 1993.

Benison B, Hogstel MO: Aging and movement therapy: essential interventions for the immobile elderly, *J Gerontol Nurs* 12:8, 1986.

Beverley L, Travis I: Constipation: proposed natural laxative mixtures, *J Gerontol Nurs* 18(10): 5, 1992.

Bixler EO, Vela-Bueno A: Normal sleep: physiological behavior and clinical correlates, *Psych Annals* 17:437, 1987.

Bliwise DL, Bliwise NG, Partinen M et al: Sleep apnea and mortality in an aged cohort, *Am J Public Health* 78(5):544, 1989.

Brocklehurst JC: Incontinence. In Ham, RJ, editor: *Geriatric medical annals,* Oradell, NJ, 1986, Medical Economics Books.

Burkitt D: Dietary fiber: is it really helpful? *Geriatrics* 37:119, 1982.

Buysse DJ, Browman KE, Monk TH et al: Napping and 24-hour sleep/wake patterns in healthly elderly and young adults, *J Gerontol* 40(8):779, 1992.

Campbell SS, Dawson D, Anderson MW: Alleviation of sleep maintenance insomnia with timed exposure to bright light, *J Am Geriatr Soc* 41(8):829, 1993.

Cape RDT: Obesity. In Abrams WB, Berkow R, editors: *The Merck manual of geriatrics,* Rahway, NJ, 1990, Merck Sharpe & Dohme Research Laboratories.

Castor D, Woods D, Pigott K et al: Effect of sunlight on sleep patterns of the elderly, *J Am Acad PA* 4(4):321, 1991.

Chumlea WC, Guo S: Equations for predicting stature in white and black individuals, *J Gerontol* 47:192, 1992.

Chumlea WC, Roche AF, Mukherjee D: Some anthropometric indices of body composition for elderly adults, *J Gerontol* 41(1)36, 1986.

Creighton, C: Effects of afternoon rest on the performance of geriatric patients in a rehabilitation hospital: a pilot study, *Am J Occup Ther* 49(8):775, 1995.

Cross AT, Babicz D, Cushman LF: Snacking habits of senior Americans, *J Nutr Elderly,* 14(2/3): 27, 1995.

Daily values: new numbers make healthful eating easier, *Mayo Clin Health Letter* 13(4):6, 1995.

Dawe D, Moore-Orr R: Low-intensity, range-of-motion exercise: invaluable nursing care for elderly patients, *J Adv Nurs* 21(4):675, 1995.

De Graaf C, Polet P, Sraveren WA: Sensory perception and pleasantness of food flavors in elderly subjects, *J Gerontol* 49(3):P93, 1994.

Dement WC, Miles LE, Carskadon MA: White paper on sleep and aging, *J Gerontol* 30:25, 1982.

deVries HA: Physiology of exercise and aging. In Woodruff DS, Birren JE, editors: *Aging, scientific perspectives, and social issues,* New York, 1975, Van Nostrand Reinhold.

Dietary goals for the United States, Oakland, Calif, 1978, Alameda County Chapter American Heart Association.

Donahue R, Abbott R, Reed D et al: Physical activity and coronary heart disease in middle-aged and elderly men: the Honolulu program, *Am J Pub Health* 78:683, 1988.

Dornealas EA, Swencionis C, Wylie-Rosett J: Predictors of walking by sedentary older women, *J Women's Health* 3(4):283, 1994.

Duckett S: Managing the sundowning patient, *J Rehab* 59(1):24, 1993.

Duckette S, Scotto M: An unusual case of sundown syndrome subsequent to a traumatic head injury, *Brain Inj* 6(2):189, 1992.

Duffy VB, Backstand JR, Ferris AM: Olfactory dysfunction and related nutritional risk in free-living, elderly women, *J Am Diet Assoc.* 95: 879-84, 1995.

Emery CF, Blumenthal JA: Perceived change among participants in an exercise program for older adults, *Gerontologist* 30(4):516, 1990.

Evans BD, Rogers AE: 24 hour sleep/wake patterns in healthy elderly persons, *Appl Nurs Res* 7(2):75, 1994.

Evans LK: Sundown syndrome in the elderly: a phenomenon in search of exploration, University of Pennsylvania Center for the Study of Aging, 7:7, 1985, Newsletter.

Fitzgerald JT, Singleton SP, Neale AV, Prasad AS, Hess JW: Activity levels, fitness status, exercise knowledge, and exercise beliefs among healthy, older African American and White women, *J Aging Health* 6(3):296, 1994.

Floyd JA: The use of across-method triangulation in the study of sleep concerns in healthy older adults, *Adv Nurs Sci* 16(2)L 70, 1993.

Friedman R, Tappen RM: The effects of planned walking on communication in Alzheimer's disease, *J Am Geriatr Soc* 39:650, 1991.

Frisoni GB, DeLeo D, Rozzini R, Bernardini M, Dello Buono M, Trabucchi M: Night sleep symptoms in an elderly population and their relation with age, gender, and education, *Clin Gerontologist* 13(1): 51, 1993.

Garofalo JA, Hynak-Hankinson MT: New Jersey's Nutrition Screening Initiative: activities and results, *J Am Diet Assoc* 95(12):1422-4, 1995.

Gaspar PM: Fluid intake: What determines how much patients drink? *Geriatr Nurs* 9:221, 1988.

Gaspar PM: Nutritional intake of nursing home residents and minimum data set variables. Presentation at the ANA Council for Nursing Research Scientific Session, Washington, DC, 1996.

Gaspar PM: Nutritional intake of nursing home residents: development of an at-risk scale. Presentation at the 20th Annual Research Conference of the Midwest Nursing Research Society, 1996, Detroit, Mich.

Gaspar PM, Hobus R: Nonnutritive sucking: Effect on bowel elimination among nursing home residents. Presentation at the American Nurses' Foundation Research Poster Session, American Nurses' Association Conference, Washington, DC, 1996.

Gaspar PM, Hughes M: Non-nutritive sucking: Effect on bowel elimination. *New Horizons* 5(14):5, 1994.

Gibson CJ, Opalka PC, Moore CA, Brady RS, Mion LC: Effectiveness of bran supplement on the bowel management of elderly rehabilitation patients, *J Gerontol Nurs* 21(10):21, 1995.

Gillett PA, Johnson M, Juretich M, Richardson N, Slagle L, Farikoff K: The nurse as exercise leader, *Geriatr Nurs* 14(3):133, 1993.

Goldberg WG, Fitzpatrick JL: Movement therapy with the aged, *Nurs Res* 29:339, 1980.

Griep MI, Mets TF, Vercruysse A et al: Food odor threshold in relation to age, nutritional and health status, *J Gerontol* 50A(6):B407, 1995.

Guigoz Y, Vellas B, Garry PJ: Mini-Nutritional Assessment: a practical assessment tool for grading the nutritional state of elderly patients, *Facts and Research in Gerontology* (Supplement: Nutrition):15, 1994.

Gupta K, Dworkin B, Gambert SR: Common nutritional disorders in the elderly: atypical manifestations, *Geriatr Nurs* 43:87, 1988.

Hagberg JM: Effects of training on the decline of VO-2 Max with aging, *Fed Proc* 46:16, 1987.

Haimov I, Laudon M, Zisapel N et al: Sleep disorders and melatonin rhythms in elderly people, *Br Med J* 309(6948):167, 1994.

Hall GR, Karsten M, Rakel B, Swanson E, Davidson A: Managing constipation using a research-based protocol, *MEDSURG Nursing* 4(1):11, 1995.

Harari D, Gurwitz J, Minaker K: Constipation in the elderly, *J Amer Geriatr Soc* 41(10):1130, 1993.

Hayter J: To nap or not to nap, *Geriatr Nurs* 6:104, 1985.

Henderson V, Nite G: *Principles and practice of nursing,* ed 6, New York, 1978, Macmillan.

Herrera CO: Sleep disorders. In Abrams WB, Berkow R, editors: *The Merck manual of geriatrics,* Rahway, NJ, 1990, Merck Sharpe & Dohme Research Laboratories.

Hoch CC, Reynolds CF, Houck PR: Sleep apnea in Alzheimer's patients and the healthy elderly, *Scholarly Inquiry for Nurs Pract* 1(3):221, 1987.

Hubbard L: In search of 40 winks, *Mod Maturity* 25:72, 1982.

Itoh R, Suyama Y: Sociodemographic factors and life-styles affecting micronutrient status in an apparently healthy elderly Japanese population, *J Nutr Elderly* 14(2/3):39, 1995.

Jenkins BL: A case against sleepers, *J Gerontol Nurs* 2:10, 1976.

Johnson JE: Effect of benzodiazepines on older women, *J Community Health Nurs* 5(2):119, 1988.

Johnson JE: A comparative study of the bedtime routines and sleep of older adults, *J Community Health Nurs* 8(3):129, 1991.

Johnson JE: Progressive relaxation and the sleep of older men and women, *J Community Health Nurs* 10(1):31, 1993.

Johnston, JE: Sleep problems in the elderly, *J Am Acad Nurs Practitioners* 6(4):161, 1994.

Jouvet M: The state of sleep, *Sci Am* 216:62, 1967.

Kales JD, Carvell M, Kales A: Sleep disorders and their management. In Cassel CK, Riesenberg DE, Sorensen LB et al, editors: *Geriatric medicine,* ed 2, New York, 1990, Springer-Verlag.

Kennedy ET, Ohls J, Carlson S, Fleming K: The Healthy Eating Index: design and applications, *J Am Diet Assoc* 95(10):1103, 1995.

Kinion ES, Christie N, Willella AM: Promoting activity in the elderly through interdisciplinary linkages, *Nursing Connections* 6(3):19, 1993.

Kleitman N: The nature of dreaming. In Walslenholme GEW, O'Conner M, editors: *CIBA Foundation symposium on the nature of sleep,* Boston, 1960, Little, Brown & Co.

Kligman EW, Pepin E: Prescribing physical activity for older patients, *Geriatrics* 47(8):33, 1992.

Koroknay VJ, Werner P, Cohen-Mansfield J, Braun JV: Maintaining ambulation in the frail nursing home resident: a nursing administered walking program, *J Gerontol Nurs* 21(11):18, 1995.

Kotagal S, Dement W: Overview of sleep apnea and its prevalence in the elderly, *Consultant* 25:86, 1985.

Kovach T: Managing geriatric chronic constipation, *Home Healthcare Nurse* 10(5):57, 1992.

Krebs-Smith SM, Heimendinger J, Patterson BH, Subar AF, Kessler R, Pivonka E: Psychosocial factors associated with fruit and vegetable consumption, *Am J Health Promotion* 10(2): 98, 1995.

L-tryptophan: *Mayo Clin Health Letter* 8(1):6, 1990.

Lakatta EG: Normal changes of aging. In Abrams WB, Berkow R, editors: *The Merck manual of geriatrics,* Rahway, NJ, 1990, Merck Sharpe & Dohme Research Laboratories.

Lange-Alberts ME, Shott S: Nutritional intake: use of touch and verbal cueing, *J Gerontol Nurs* 20(2):36, 1994.

Lerner R: Sleep loss in the aged: implications for nursing research, *J Gerontol Nurs* 8:323, 1992.

Linder MC: *Nutritional biochemistry and metabolism in clinical application,* ed 2, New York, 1991, Elsevier.

Lipski PS, Torrance A, Kelly PJ, James OF: A study of nutritional deficits of long-stay geriatric patients, *Age Ageing* 22():244, 1993.

Lord S, Castell S: Effect of exercise on balance, strength and reaction time in older people, *Aust J Physiotherapy* 40(2):83, 1994.

Lord S, Mitchell D, Williams P: Effect of water exercise on balance and related factors in older people, *Aust J Physiotherapy* 39(3):217, 1993.

Mandell AJ: Sleep transmitters, *Biopsychiatry* 1:13, 1969.

Mantle J: Research and serendipitous secondary findings, *Canadian Nurse* 88(1):15, 1992.

Marsiglio A, Holm K: Physical conditioning in the aging adult, *Nurse Pract* 13:33, 1988.

McCall WV: Management of primary sleep disorders among elderly persons, *Psych Services* 46(1):49, 1995.

McGinty D, Beahm E, Stern N et al: Nocturnal hypotension in older men with sleep-related breathing disorders, *Chest* 94(2):305, 1988.

Mills EM: The effect of low-intensity aerobic exercise on muscle strength, flexibility, and balance among sedentary elderly persons, *Nurs Res* 43(4):207, 1994.

Misner JE, Massey BH, Bemben M et al: Long-term effects of exercise on the range of motion of aging women, *J Orthop Sports Phys Ther* 16(1):37, 1992.

Moffat A: Immunity booster: "get a good night's rest," *American Health* VII, 54, 1988.

Molloy DW, Beerschoten DA, Borrie MJ, Crilly RG, Capes RDT: Acute effects of exercise on neruopsychological function in elderly subjects, *J Am Geriatr Soc* 36:29, 1988.

Monk TH, Reynolds CF, Buysse DJ et al: Circadian characteristics of healthy 80-year-olds and their relationship to objectively recorded sleep, *J Gerontol* 46(5):M171, 1991.

Moore C, Bracegirdle H: The effects of a short-term, low-intensity exercise programme on the psychological well-being of community-dwelling elderly women, *Br J Occup Therapy* 57(6):213, 1994.

Morley JE: Nutrition assessment is a key comonent of geriatric assessment, *Facts and Research in Gerontolgly* (Supplement: Nutrition): 5, 1994.

Mornhinweg GC, Voignier RR: Music for sleep disturbance in the elderly, *J Holistic Nurs* 13(3):248, 1995.

Morris, Schnelders D, Macey S: A survey of older Americans to determine frequency and motivations for eating fast food, *J Nutr Elderly* 15(1):1, 1995.

Murray F: Awakening to a better life with melatonin, *Better Nutrition for Today's Living* 57(12):50, 1995.

National Institutes of Health Concensus Development Conference on Physical Activity and Cardiovascular Health: *Development Conference Statement Draft,* NIH Consensus Programs, Information Service, Kensington, Maryland, 1996.

Neal LJ: Power pudding: natural laxative therapy for the elderly who are homebound, *Home Healthcare Nurse* 13(3):66, 1995.

Neville K: Promoting health for seniors, *Geriatr Nurs* 9:42, Jan/Feb 1988.

New guides to healthy eating, *Mayo Clin Health Letter* 10(7):3, 1992.

Oesting H, Manza R: Sleep apnea, *Geriatr Nurs* 9:232, July/Aug, 1988.

Olestra: just say no, *University of California at Berkeley Wellness Letter* 12(5): 1, 1996.

Pals JK, Weinberg AD, Beal LF, Levesque PG, Cunningham RJ, Minaker KL: Clinical triggers for detection of fever and dehydration: implications for long-term care nursing, *J Gerontol Nurs* 21(4):13, 1995.

Payette H, Gray-Donald K: Risk of malnutrition in an elderly population receiving home care services, *Facts and Research in Gerontology* (Supplement:Nutrition):71, 1994.

Pearson LJ, Kotthoff ME: *Geriatric clinical protocol,* Philadelphia, 1979, JB Lippincott.

Posner BM, Jette A, Smigelski C, Miller D, Mitchell P: Nutritional risk in New England elders, *J Gerontol* 49(3):M123, 1994.

Prinz PN, Vitello MV, Raskind MA, Thorpy MJ: Geriatrics: Sleep disorders and aging, *N Engl J Med* 323:520, 1990.

Prinz PN, Vitello MV: Sleep loss in aging: sleep disorders and insomnia in the elderly. *Facts and Research in Gerontology* 7:55, 1993.

Recommended dietary allowances, ed 10, Washington, DC, 1989, National Academy Press.

Reedy DF: Fluid intake: how can you prevent dehydration? *Geriatr Nurs* 9:224, 1988.

Resende TL, Brocklehurst JC, O'Neill PA: A pilot study on the effect of exercise and abdominal massage on bowel habit in continuing care patients, *Clin Rehab* 7(3):204, 1993.

Rodrigues-Fisher L, Bourguignon C, Good BV: Dietary fiber nursing intervention: prevention of constipation in older adults, *Clin Nurs Res* 2(4):464, 1993.

Roe D: *Geriatric nutrition,* Englewood Cliffs, NJ, 1992, Prentice-Hall.

Rolls BJ: Regulation of food and fluid intake in the elderly, *Ann N Y Acad Sci,* 561, 1989.

Rousseau P: Aging and chronic constipation, *Geriatr Med Today* 9(3):35, 1990.

Satlin A, Volicer L, Ross V et al: Bright light treatment of behavior and sleep disturbance in patients with Alzheimer's disease, *Am J Psych* 149(8):1028, 1992.

Schiffman SS, Warwick ZS: Effect of flavor enhancement of foods for the elderly on nutritional status: food intake, biochemical indices, and anthropometric measures, *Physiol Behav* 53: 395, 1993.

Schuster C, Petosa R, Petosa S: Using social cognitive theory to predict intentional exercise in post-retirement adults, *J Health Ed* 26(1):14, 1995.

Sherin JE, Shiromani PJ, McCarley RW, Saper CB: Activation of ventrolateral preoptic neurons during sleep, *Science* 271(5246):216, 1996.

Sidenvall B, Fjellstrom C, Ek AC: The meal situation in geriatric care—intentions and experiences, *J Adv Nurs* 20(4): 613, 1994.

Siegel PZ, Brackbill RM, Heath GW: The epidemiology of walking for exercise: implications for promoting activity among sedentary groups, *Am J Public Health* 85(5):706, 1995.

Siscovick DS, Raghunatgan TE, King I et al: Dietary intake and cell membrane level of long-chain n-3 polyunsaturated fatty acids and the risk of primary cardiac arrest, *JAMA* 274(17): 1363, 1995.

Social dancing: *Mayo Clin Nutr Letter,* 3(11):5, 1990.

Sommers JM, Andres FF, Price JH: Perceptions of exercise of mall walkers utilizing the Health Belief Model, *J Health Ed* 26(3):158, 1995.

Spiegel R, Azcona A, Morgan K: Sleep disorders. In Pathy MS, editor: *Principles and practice of geriatric medicine,* ed 2, New York, 1990, John Wiley and Sons.

Stoyva J, Zimmerman J, Metcalf D: *Distorted visual feedback and augmented REM sleep,* Santa Fe, NM, 1970, Association for the Psychophysiologic Study of Sleep. Suarez FL, Savalano DA, Levitt MD: A comparison of symptoms after the consumption of mild or lactose hydrolyzed milk by people with self-reported severe lactose intolerance, *N Engl J Med* 333:1, 1995.

Sullivan M: Atrophy and exercise, *J Gerontol Nurs* 13:26, 1987.

Takashi Y, Kipnis DM, Daughaday WH: Growth hormone accretion during sleep, *J Clin Invest,* 47:2079, 1968.

Thomas DR: Outcome from protein-energy malnutrition in nursing home residents, *Facts and Research in Gerontology* (Supplement:Nutrition):87, 1994.

Tobis JS: Rehabilitation of the geriatric patient. In Rossman I, editor: *Clinical geriatrics,* ed 2, Philadelphia, 1979, JB Lippincott.

Topp R, Mikesky A, Wigglesworth J, Holt W Jr, Edwards JE: The effect of a 12-week dynamic resistance strength training program on gait velocity and balance of older adults, *Gerontologist* 33(4):501, 1993.

UCLA News: *UCLA study aims to improve sleep in nursing homes,* April 10, 1995, p. 1-3 (Newsletter).

Uriri JT, Thatcher-Winger R: Health risk appraisal and the older adult. *J Gerontol Nurs* 21(5):25, 1995.

US Bureau of the Census: *Statistical Abstract of the United States,* 1995, ed 115, Washington, DC, 1995.

US Department of Health and Human Services, Public Health Service, Centers for Disease Control: *Healthy People 2000: review 1994,* DHHS Pub No (PHS) 95-1256-1, Hyattsville, Md, 1995.

Van der Wielen RPJ, de Wild GM, de Groot LC, Hoefnagels WH, van Staveren WA: Dietary intakes of energy and water-soluble vitamins in different categories of aging, *J Gerontol* 51A(1):B100, 1996.

Vitiello MV, Bliwise DL, Prinz PN: Sleep in Alzheimer's disease and the sundown syndrome, *Neurology* 42(7 suppl 6):83, 1992.

Volkert D, Frauenrath C, Micol W et al: Nutritional status of the very old: anthropometric and biochemical findings in apparently healthy women in old people's homes, *Aging Clin Exp Res* 4(1):21, 1992.

Wallace M: The sundown syndrome: will the specialized training of nurse's aides help elders with sundown syndrome? *Geriatr Nurs* 15(3):164, 1994.

Webb WB: Sleep in older persons: sleep structures of 50- to 60-year-old men and women, *J Gerontol* 37:581, 1982.

Weinberg AD, Minaker KL, and the Council on Scientific Affairs, American Medical Association: Dehydration: evaluation and management in older adults, *JAMA* 274(19): 1552, 1995.

Weitzman ED, Luce G: Biological rhythms: indices of pain, adrenal hormones, sleep and sleep reversal, *Mental Health Program Report 3,* National Institute of Mental Health, Public Health Service Pub No 1876, Washington, DC, 1969, US Government Printing Office.

Whitehead WE, Drinkwater D, Cheskin LJ, Heller BR. Schuster MM: Constipation in the elderly living at home: definition, prevalence and relationship to lifestyle and health status, *J Am Geriatr Soc* 37(5):423, 1989.

Wichita C: Treating and preventing constipation in nursing home residents, *J Gerontol Nurs* 3:35, 1977.

Wolanin MO: Nursing assessment. In Burnside IM, editor: *Nursing and the aged,* New York, 1976, McGraw-Hill.

Wrenn K: Fecal impaction, *N Engl J Med* 321(10):658, 1989.

Yen P: Boosting intake when appetite is poor, *Geriatr Nurs* 15:284, 1994.

Yen P: Maximizing calcium intake, *Geriatr Nurs* 16(2): 92, 1995a.

Yen P: What elders think about food, *Geriatr Nurs* 16(4):187, 1995b.

Yen P: When food doesn't taste good anymore. *Geriatr Nurs* 17(1):44. 1996.

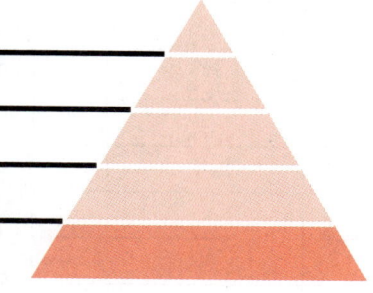

Nutritional Screening of Assessments

LEVEL I SCREEN

To Be Completed by a Social Service or Health Care Professional or Other Trained Personnel

	Value	Measurement Abnormal	
		Yes	No
Height (In.)			
Weight (Lbs.)			
% Desirable Body Weight			
Weight Loss/Gain in 6 Months			

	Yes	No
Dietary Data		
Does not have enough food each day		
Number of days per month without any food		
Poor appetite		
Usually eats alone		
Difficulty chewing or swallowing		
Problems with mouth, teeth, or gums		
Housebound		
Eats milk or milk products daily		
Eats fruits and vegetables daily		
On a special diet		

Continued

	Yes	No
Usual Daily Food Intake (Optional)		
Less than 2 servings of milk or dairy products		
Less than 2 servings of meat/poultry/fish/eggs		
Less than 2 servings of fruit/juice		
Less than 3 servings of vegetables		
Less than 6 servings of bread/cereals/grains		
More than 2 ounces of alcohol for men		
More than 1 ounce of alcohol for women		
Living Environment		
Income less than $6000/year/person		
Lives alone		
Concerned about home security		
Inadequate heating or cooling		
No stove or refrigerator		
Unable or prefers not to spend money on food		
Functional Status		
Needs assistance with:		
Bathing		
Dressing		
Continence		
Toileting		
Eating		
Ambulation		
Transportation		
Food preparation		

Identified problems should be referred to the appropriate health care professional such as physician, nurse, social worker, dietitian, dentist, case manager, etc.

Refer to a Physician if:

An involuntary increase or decrease in weight of greater than 10 lbs in the past 6 months.
A body weight that is 20% above or below desirable body weight.

Refer to a Dietitian for Food-Related Problems.

Repeat This Screen Yearly or if a Major Change in Status Occurs.

LEVEL II SCREEN

In-depth assessment (performed in medical settings)

Additional Information to Be Obtained Following Referral to a Physician or Other Qualified Health Care Professional

	Value	Measurement Abnormal	
		Yes	No
Height (In.)			
Weight (Lbs.)			
% Desirable Body Weight			
Body Mass Index			
Weight Loss/Gain in 6 Months			

	Yes	No
Dietary Data		
Does not have enough food each day		
Number of days per month without any food		
Poor appetite		
Usually eats alone		
Special dietary needs		
Self-defined		
Prescribed		
Problems with compliance/meeting special needs		
Multiple diet prescriptions		
Other unusual dietary practices		
Usual Daily Food Intake		
Less than 2 servings of milk or dairy products		
Less than 2 servings of meat/poultry/fish/eggs		
Less than 2 servings of fruit/juice		
Less than 3 servings of vegetables		
Less than 6 servings of bread/cereals/grains		
More than 2 ounces of alcohol for men		
More than 1 ounce of alcohol for women		

Continued

	Yes	No
Laboratory and Anthropometric Data		
Serum albumin less than 3.5 gm/dl		
Serum cholesterol less than 160 mg/dl		
Serum cholesterol greater than 240 mg/dl		
Triceps skinfold thickness below 10% of desirable		
Midarm muscle circumference below 10% of desirable		
Clinical Features		
Difficulty chewing or swallowing		
Problems with mouth, teeth, or gums		
Skin changes suggest malnutrition		
Angular stomatitis		
Glossitis		
History of bone pain		
Bone fractures		
Living Environment		
Income less than $6000/year/person		
Lives alone		
Concerned about home security		
Inadequate heating or cooling		
No stove or refrigerator		
Unable or prefers not to spend money on food		
Functional Status		
Needs assistance with		
Bathing		
Dressing		
Continence		
Toileting		
Eating		
Ambulation		
Transportation		
Food preparation		
Shopping		

	Yes	No
Mental/Cognitive Status		
Mini-mental examination indicates impairment (score <26)		
Depression Scale suggests depression (Beck <15, GDS >5)		
Drug Use		
More than 3 prescription drugs		
More than 3 nonprescription drugs		
Vitamin and mineral supplements		

CRITERIA FOR THE RECOGNITION OF COMMON PROBLEMS FROM COMPLETION OF THE SCREEN

Is there weight loss or is the patient underweight?
- Weight loss greater than 10% in last 6 months.
- Body weight less than 80% of desirable weight.
- Triceps skinfold thickness below the tenth percentile.
- Midarm muscle circumference below tenth percentile.

Is there evidence of protein energy (hypoalbuminemic) malnutrition?
- Serum albumin less than 3.5 g/dl.

Is there evidence suggesting osteoporosis or mineral deficiency?
- History of bone pain or bone fractures.
- Patient housebound.

Is there evidence of hypovitaminosis or mineral deficiency?
- Angular stomatitis, glossitis, or bleeding gums.
- Inadequate intakes of fruit and vegetables.
- Pressure ulcers.

Is there evidence of obesity or hypercholesterolemia?
- Weight greater than 120% of desirable weight.
- Serum cholesterol greater than 240 mg/dl.

Should the patient be referred to a dietitian or community nutrition program?
- Food intake inappropriate, inadequate, or excessive.
- Problems complying with specialized diet.
- Need for nutrition specific counseling or education, related to specific diseases.
- Functionally dependent for eating or food-related activities of daily living.

Identified Problems Should be Referred to the Appropriate Health Care Professional Such as a Physician, Nurse, Social Worker, Dietitian, Dentist, Case Manager, etc.

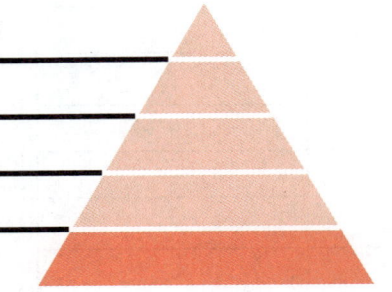

Mini-Nutritional Assessment (MNA)

ID# _____

Name: _____

First Name: _____

Sex: _____

Date: _____

Age: _____

Weight, kg: _____

Height, cm: _____

Knee height (cm): _____

If height applicable

I. ANTHROPOMETRIC ASSESSMENT

1. BMI (weight/height)^2 in kg/m^2
   0 = BMI < 19
   1 = 19 ≤ BMI < 21
   2 = 21 ≤ BMI < 23
   3 = BMI ≥ 23 ☐
2. Mid-arm circumference (MAC in cm)
   0,1 = MAC < 21
   0,5 = 21 ≤ MAC ≤ 22
   1,0 = MAC > 22 ☐,☐
3. Calf circumference (CC in cm)
   0 = CC < 31   1 = CC ≥ 31 ☐
4. Weight loss during last 3 months
   0 = weight loss >3kg
   1 = does not know
   2 = weight loss between, 1 and 3 kg
   3 = no weight loss ☐

II. GLOBAL EVALUATION

5. Does the patient live independently in contrast to a nursing home?
   0 = no   1 = yes ☐
6. Does the patient take more than 3 prescription drugs (per day)?
   0 = yes   1 = no ☐
7. In the past 3 months has the patient suffered psychological stress or acute disease?
   0 = yes   2 = no ☐
8. Mobility
   0 = bed or chair bound
   1 = able to get out of bed/chair but does not go out
   2 = goes out ☐

9. Neuropsychological problem
   0 = severe dementia or depression
   1 = mild dementia
   2 = no psychological problems ☐
10. Pressure sores or skin ulcers
    0 = yes   1 = no ☐

III. DIETETIC ASSESSMENT

11. How many full meals does the patient eat daily?
    0 = 1 meal   1 = 2 meals   2 = 3 meals ☐
12. Does he consume:
    - At least one serving of dairy products (milk, cheese, yogurt) per day?   yes ☐   no ☐
    - Two or more servings of beans or eggs per week?
                                        yes ☐   no ☐
    - Meat, fish or poultry every day?
                                        yes ☐   no ☐
    0.0 = if 0 or 1 yes
    0.5 = if 2 yes
    1.0 = if 3 yes ☐,☐
13. Does he consume two or more servings of fruits or vegetables per day?
    0 = no   1 = yes ☐
14. Has the patient food intake declined over the past three months due to loss of appetite, digestive problems, chewing or swallowing difficulties?
    0 = severe loss of appetite
    1 = moderate loss of appetite
    2 = no loss of appetite ☐

From Guigoz Y, Vellas B, Garry PJ: Mini-Nutritional Assessment: a practical assessment tool for grading the nutritional state of elderly patients, *Facts Res Gerontol* (Supplement: Nutrition):15, 1994.

15. How many cups/glasses of beverages (water, juice, coffee, tea, milk, wine, beer,...) does the patient consume per day?
    0.0 = less than 3 glasses
    0.5 = 3 to 5 glasses
    1.0 = more than 5 glasses   □,□

16. Mode of feeding
    0 = fed requiring assistance
    1 = self-fed with some difficulty
    2 = self-fed without any problem   □

IV. SUBJECTIVE ASSESSMENT

17. Does the patient consider to have any nutritional problems?
    0 = major malnutrition
    1 = does not know or moderate malnutrition
    2 = no nutritional problem   □

18. In comparison with other people of the same age, how would the patient consider his/her health status?
    0.0 = not as good
    0.5 = does not know
    1.0 = as good
    2.0 = better   □,□

Total (maximum 30 points):   □□,□

Score:

≥24 points: well-nourished
17 to 23.5 points: at risk of malnutrition
<17 points: undernutrition

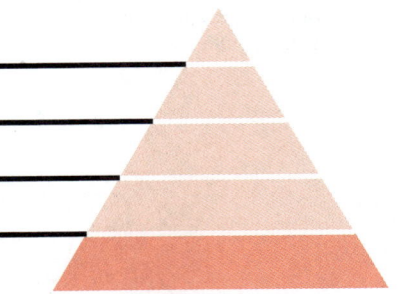

CHAPTER 7

Biologic Maintenance Needs

An elder speaks **Thin skinned, long in the tooth, and ready to bite nails. I guess that pretty well describes my condition right now.**

Jeannette, age 74

LEARNING OBJECTIVES

Upon completion of this chapter, the reader will be able to:

1. Describe health promotion components of maintenance needs.
2. Identify normal age changes of the buccal cavity, feet, and skin.
3. Identify common dental, foot, and skin problems of the elderly.
4. Use standard assessment tools to assess buccal cavity, feet, and skin.
5. Identify preventive, maintenance, and restorative measures for dental, foot, and skin health.
6. Establish selected nursing diagnoses on the basis of assessment for dental, foot, and skin health and care.
7. Make a plan of care for prevention and maintenance of dental, foot, and skin health.

Maintenance needs are adjuncts to life-support needs. The maintenance needs discussed in this chapter also have a direct and indirect effect on the psychosocial well-being of the aged. For some unexplainable reason, patients are well cared for from neck to ankles, instead of from head to toe. Under normal circumstances, teeth and feet receive cursory or minimum attention in the overall care of the client. When care is rushed because of "a busy day" or "a heavy assignment," the care of the teeth and feet is most frequently omitted. Skin care fares better. Much attention is directed to alleviating pressure, but other important integumentary influences such as friction, shearing force, moisture, and nutrition are not addressed as carefully.

DENTAL HEALTH

Dental health of the aged is a basic need that is increasingly neglected with advanced age, debilitation, and limited mobility. One reason for this neglect may be the general assumption that older people are edentulous. The aged, themselves, believe that losing their teeth is a natural consequence of growing old. The problem with this attitude is that it fosters neglect of an essential body part: the mouth. It is no less important to maintain the teeth in old age than it is to maintain teeth in the young. Oro-dental status can affect well-being in a variety of ways. Acute dental problems can put the older person at risk for systemic disease. The mouth is an important zone for communication between people through speech, but much of socialization and pleasure is derived from food and drink (Epstein, 1987). Oro-dental health is integral to general health. Poor oral function, hygiene, and chronic oral problems can lead to loss of life satisfaction and raise concern with self-presentation and fear of embarrassment that affects socialization and self-esteem (Karuza et al, 1988; Watson and Pennebaker, 1989; Marino, 1994).

The percentage of edentulous persons over 65 years of age has decreased, with approximately 58% retaining their natural teeth (Schwab and Pavlatos, 1991). This trend is expected to continue due to advances in gerodontal knowledge and use of fluorides, better nutrition, more mechanical techniques and oral hygiene practices, and improved dental health education. However, the caregiver should realize that whether with natural teeth or full or partial dentures, the teeth need care. In the existing health care system dental care is a low priority, reflected by the inadequacy of third-party reimbursement for the type of dental care needed by the aged. Dental insurance generally terminates at 65 years of age or is too expensive for the aged to continue the premium payments. Average out-of-pocket dental expenses are higher for the retired aged than the working population because national programs such as Medicare and Medicaid do not provide adequate reimbursement for tooth and dental repair. Although some states include certain dental services under Medicaid, those elderly in nursing homes who are eligible for dental treatment often do not receive it. Elders are finding that even with insurance their past employers and health maintenance organizations (HMOs) are paying less of the premiums and the policy holder is paying more (Kingston et al, 1995). Dental services should be more readily available if the aged are to use them. Nurses could render a valuable service to older persons by referring them to a specific dentist who will encourage the development of an ongoing relationship with the older patient.

Tooth loss is not a natural part of the aging process, but rather it is a problem that accrues over time and is most evident in the aged. One cannot forget that there are aged who still have teeth and that it is their right to have help in the maintenance and preservation of their remaining teeth. It cannot be stated too strongly that a functional and healthy mouth has strong psychologic implications all through life. Its role dominates the first orientation to life through sucking and continues to influence such activities as smiling, eating, drinking, and sexual pleasure throughout adulthood. These activities contribute directly or indirectly to one's self-esteem. The ability to communicate, socialize, and maintain adequate nourishment depends on dental health, which concerns the whole buccal cavity: teeth, gums, lips, tongue, and mucous membranes. Fulfillment of dental needs as a physiologic requirement influences the attainment of successive levels of Maslow's hierarchy of needs.

Lack of teeth alters articulation of speech, jaw alignment, and general appearance. Persons without teeth rarely smile; they feel embarrassed and cover their mouths or withdraw from social contacts. The type and consistency of food chosen to eat becomes limited and monotonous. Frequently, food eaten by those who are edentulous is inadequate and deficient in nutritive value.

Teeth seem to be taken for granted until one begins to lose them. In early childhood there is the reprieve of a second set, the permanent teeth, but if dental habits established in early childhood are inadequate, these habits will continue to affect the care of the permanent teeth.

Changes in Buccal Cavity During Aging Process

Aging teeth become brittle, drier, and darker in color; may lose some of the enamel covering; and may loosen from bone loss (resorption) or breakdown of the supporting tissue and gum recession. Years of crushing and grinding wear down the chewing surfaces (attrition), causing teeth to become uneven, fracture, and develop jagged edges.

Vascularity of the gingivae (gums) is reduced, limiting or decreasing the ability of the tissue to heal after injury. Gum recession occurs in part from the loss of tissue elasticity or the periodontal tissue, atrophy of the alveolar bone, and periodontal disease. This process affects the fit of dentures and necessitates periodic dental relining. Box 7-1 lists more changes that occur.

Periodontal changes should be minimum in the healthy aged, but the attention given to oral care by health care professionals and by the aged themselves is inadequate. Inattention to periodontal conditions results in inflammation, swelling, pain of dental structures, and discomfort from mouth taste and odors. Periodontal disease does not appear to be a specific disease of the elderly but the result of chronic periodontitis from young and middle age adulthood. Box 7-2 presents a number of factors that contribute to periodontal disorders in the aged.

"Almost pandemic in the older population, gingivitis may affect up to 80% of all teeth" (Feldman, 1986, p. 5). The most prevalent cause of gingivitis, gum inflammation and disease, is inadequate removal of plaque and calculus. This may be exacerbated by partial dentures, overhanging ledges

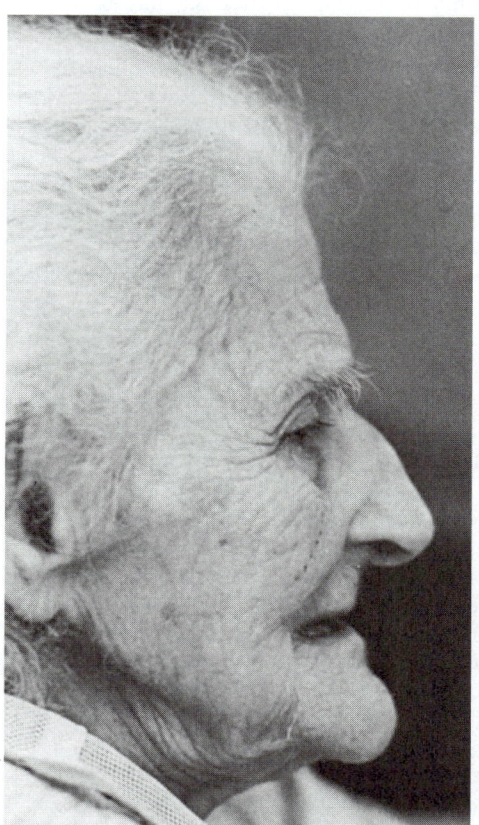

Edentulous profile exaggerting normal elongation of nose that occurs with aging. (Photograph by Stewart H. Bloom.)

of fillings, and faulty bridges that allow the plaque to accumulate between teeth. A predisposition to gingivitis may also occur when the mucous membranes are irritated by dryness of the mouth. Systemic problems such as endocrine dysfunction, chronic airflow limitation (CAL or COPD), medications and nutritional deficiencies may influence the development of the disease.

A study by the Harvard School of Dental Medicine and the New England Research Institute (1992) found 86% of elders studied had at least moderate periodontal disease (Douglass et al, 1993). Dental experts concur that most tooth loss results from periodontal disease. The advent of fluoridation and overall dental health improvements have helped. People are keeping their teeth longer, but additional factors contribute to tooth loss, including excessive wear (attrition) and loosening of the teeth by night grinding (bruxism); habitual consumption of abrasive foods, which accelerates wear and loss of tooth height; diminished salivary secretions; functional wear enhanced by environment or occupation such as among confectionery workers, blasters, or carpenters; various mechanical habits such as biting sewing thread, clenching a pipe stem between the teeth, or brushing the teeth too vigorously. Chemical erosion by substances such as fruit acids, particularly lemon juice and soft drinks, also affects the condition and retention of teeth.

Friability of the buccal mucosa may be caused by the shift of intracellular and intercellular fluid. This is seen in progressive dehydration or decreasing kidney function in the aged. The transitional mucosal border is not covered with keratinizing cells and is vulnerable to mild stress. Since 90% of all oral cancer occurs in individuals 45 years and over, the average being in their sixties, it is significant that the mucosa be maintained intact and free from chronic irritation. Smoking or chewing tobacco insults the oral cavity. Alcohol use has been shown to have a synergistic effect on the development of oral and laryngeal cancer when combined with tobacco. Even though all mucous membranes are susceptible to cancer, the lips and the sides of the tongue are particularly vulnerable.

Diminished vascularity may lead to nutritional deficiencies of the cells. Dietary deficiencies of vitamins A, B, and C, folic acid, and zinc are added factors that affect tissue integrity and susceptibility to periodontal disease. Insufficient vitamin A reduces the cohesion and intactness of the epithelial layer; lack of vitamin B interferes with cell metabolism; an inadequate amount of vitamin C, folic acid, and zinc is responsible for poor differentiation of the connective and fibrous tissue, thus delaying the healing process by prolonging the period of gum edema after tooth extraction. A deficiency of calcium, which is usually related to osteoporosis of bones, can be seen in the mandible and maxilla. Calcium deficiencies with resorption of the alveolar bone ridges may be the first area affected (Palmer, 1991).

Box 7-2   **Contributing Factors in Periodontal Problems in the Aged**

Anatomic
Tooth malalignment
Thinning gingival mucosa

Bacterial
Plaque accumulation
Invasion of organisms at or below gumline
Food impaction

Drugs, Metallic Poisons
Allergic responses
Phenytoin
Cytotoxins
Heavy metals (lead, arsenic, mercury)

Emotional and Psychomotor
Bruxism (grinding of teeth)
Cerebral vascular accident
Mental impairment

Intrinsic (Systemic)
Endocrine
Metabolic
Altered immune system

Mechanical
Calculus
Retention of impacted food
Moveable and spreading teeth
Ragged edged fillings and crown overhangs
Poorly designed or poorly fitting dentures

Data compiled from Zach L, Trieger N: In Rossman I: *Clinical geriatrics,* ed 3, Philadelphia, 1986, Lippincott; Odslehage JC, Magilvey K: *Geriatric nursing* 7:238, 1986; and Papas AS, Niessen LC, Chauncey HH: *Geriatric dentistry, aging and oral health,* St Louis, 1991, Mosby.

Box 7-1   **Age Changes of the Buccal Cavity**

Decrease in the cellular compartment
Loss of submucosal elastin in oral mucosa
Loss of connective tissue (collagen)
Increase in thickness of collagen fibers
Decrease in function of minor salivary glands
Decrease in number and quality of blood vessels and nerves
Attrition on occlusive contact surfaces
Enamel less permeable—teeth more brittle
Tooth color change
Excessive secondary dentin formation
Decrease in rate of cementin deposition
Decrease in size of pulp chamber and root canals
Decrease in size and volume of the tooth pulp
Increase in pulp stones and dystrophic mineralization

Abnormal taste and burning sensation of the tongue occur in about 80% of menopausal women and are thought to be an effect of a low estrogen level or a vitamin B deficiency.

Candida albicans formation under full dentures has also been linked to vitamin B deficits.

Minor salivary gland activity diminishes in response to age changes and to the effects of systemic medication and conditions. There are over 400 medications that are thought to create dry mouth (xerostomia) and that can predispose to caries and irritation of sensitive mucous membranes. These xerostomic categories are antihistamines, antipsychotics, tricyclics, antidepressants, antiparkinsonian drugs, antianxiety agents, antihypertensive drugs, and diuretics (Richter, 1995). Most aged persons experience some dryness of the mouth, which interferes with adequate oral moisture to wet food in chewing. It is for this reason that many aged "dunk" toast, cookies, or other hard and dry foods in liquids such as soup, gravy, coffee, tea, and milk before eating them. An increase in mucin causes saliva to become thicker and ropy in texture and reduces the natural cleaning and washing action of saliva present in earlier years. Inadequate saliva is also responsible for diminished action to protect the gums from irritation. Alterations in the pH acidity or alkalinity seem to be influenced by the number of natural teeth the individual has. The more natural teeth the elderly person retains, the better the pH acidity and the maintenance of its protective properties (Kaplan, 1971).

Common Dental Problems

Xerostomia. Dry mouth is a condition often found in the elderly as a result of salivary gland dysfunction, although salivary gland output remains stable in healthy persons (Ship et al, 1995). The possible causes of this annoying and uncomfortable condition include medication use (at least 400 prescription medications can cause xerostomia), radiation therapy of the head and neck for tumors, chemotherapeutic agents for cancer and immunosuppression therapy, physiologic disorders, blockage of salivary ducts, fibrosis of the parotid glands, and primary or secondary Sjögren's syndrome, defective sensory receptors, or impaired cognition.

Depending on the severity of dry mouth, the elder may complain about a burning sensation or difficulty chewing, swallowing, speaking, or retaining upper dentures. Decreased taste perception, which occurs with dry mouth, leads to disinterest in food, and the lack of saliva results in an increase in caries and tooth sensitivity. When necessary, a variety of prescription and over-the-counter saliva substitutes are available. The commercially available substitutes contain a lubricant-sweetener such as glycerine or sorbitol, salt ions, and a flavoring agent; a few contain fluoride. Saliva substitutes come as sprays, rinses, or swishes and can be used as often as the individual wants.

Root Caries. Root caries occur on any tooth surface where periodontal attachments are recessed from the cementoenamel junction (CEJ). Most root caries are found on the proximal and buccal surfaces of the teeth (Banting, 1991), appearing initially as small, round, shallow, pigmented defects at the root surface. As these caries advance, they usually spread laterally along the CEJ and may undermine the tooth crown. Figure 7-1 illustrates root caries and Table 7-1 lists factors associated with root caries.

Gingivitis and Periodontitis. The increased retention of teeth by today's elderly population is creating concern about the increase in periodontal conditions. Periodontal conditions affect the tissue supporting the teeth, the cementum, periodontal ligament, alveolar bone, and the gingiva. Resulting problems cause loss of tooth anchorage and eventually the loss of teeth from bacterial sources.

Elders today are more aware of facial aesthetics, self-esteem, and the desire to maintain a high quality of life. Brown and Meskin (1990) found that people ages 65 to 69 with higher incomes experience less severe tooth loss than older adults with lower incomes but economics have less influence with increasing age. Half the people in the study over the age of 80 had no teeth. Kingston et al (1995) found that age, urban living, education, and financial resources were predictors of dental service use by elders in the New England Elders Dental Survey (NEEDS). Figure 7-2 illustrates the progression of gingivitis to periodontitis. Box 7-2 outlines factors that contribute to periodontal disease in the elderly, and Box 7-3 lists the signs of periodontal disease. Routine periodontal and screening and recording (PSR),

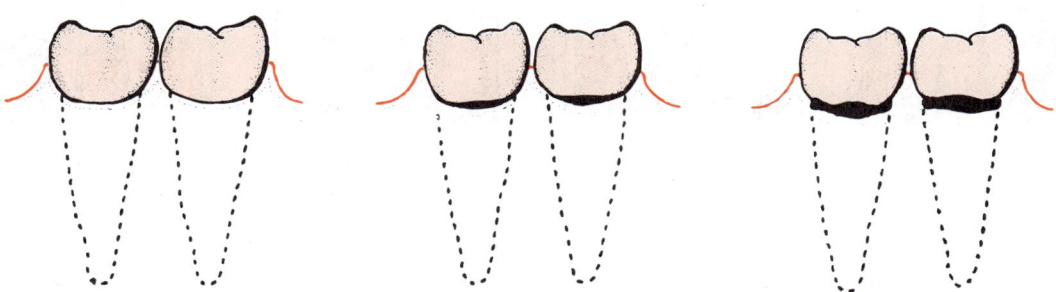

Figure 7-1. Gingival and root decay. (Courtesy Karen L. Merrill, Wellesley, Mass.)

recommended by the American Academy of Periodontology in 1992, has been incorporated by only about one third of dentists into their practice (Health after 50, 1995).

Oral Cancers. Oral cancers are more frequent in the aged. Detailed discussion of these lesions will not be addressed here since numerous texts discuss them in detail. A brief description of several types of lesions that occur on the lips, tongue, and mucous membranes will be presented.

Leukoplakia. Leukoplakia is a precancerous lesion that presents as a slightly raised, slightly circumscribed patch or patches. It is generally found on the lips, tongue, gums, or buccal mucosa. It may also appear as a velvety red patch that does not rub off (erythroplakia). Most lesions begin with erythroplakia. Leukoplakia is generally caused by pipe smoking, ill-fitting dentures, or smokeless tobacco.

Basal cell carcinoma. Basal cell carcinoma is a malignant tumor that begins as a papule and enlarges peripherally. It develops a central crater that erodes, crusts, and bleeds.

Local invasion destroys the underlying and adjacent tissue and if ignored can be very disfiguring. A common site for this type of cancer is the upper lip.

Assessment

Assessment of the oral cavity should be a regular part of dental hygiene. It is much better preventive care to periodically inspect the aged person's mouth than wait until there is a problem. All aged persons with or without dentures should have their gums, tongue, teeth (natural or dentures), and mucous membranes inspected and palpated at least every 6 to 12 months.

Gums should be inspected for color and palpated for lesions and swelling. Ill-fitting dentures are responsible for ulcerations, which resemble cancerous lesions. Generalized inflammation, or sore mouth, is demonstrated by a reddened mucosa and a granular-looking outline of the denture bases along the gingival borders. Papillary hyperplasia is a warty papular type of condition of the palate created by the suction of the upper denture. Ill-fitting dentures can also cause a breakdown at the angle of the mouth. Skinfolds at the mouth corners can overlap causing lesions that resemble lesions seen in vitamin deficiencies such as riboflavin or an infectious process such as candidiasis. It is important not to overlook this possibility.

Teeth, if present, should be checked for jagged edges, fractures, lost fillings, caries, the number of teeth, and adequate occlusion. Dentures, if partial or full, should be removed and inspected for excessive wear, breakage, and rough spots. It is also necessary to learn when dentures were last checked by a dentist for relining, rebasing, and replacement, which is necessary whenever denture fit is too loose or causing pressure sores on the gums. This is frequently very difficult for the aged person to understand or to accept. Equally difficult to accept is that no dentures will ever fit or feel exactly like one's own teeth because the mouth is always changing, especially when there is weight loss or weight gain.

Table 7-1 Factors Associated with Root Caries by Type

Type	Factors
Antecedent	Oral hygiene and plaque
	Gingivitis
	Periodontal disease
	Coronal caries experience
	Root caries experience
	Number of teeth
	Systemic fluoride
Intervening	Diet
	Saliva secretion rate
	Saliva pH
	Saliva buffering capacity
Moderating	Age
	Sex
Causal	*Streptococcus mutans*
	Lactobacillus

From Papas AS, Niessen LC, Chauncey HH: *Geriatric dentistry, aging and oral health,* St Louis, 1991, Mosby.

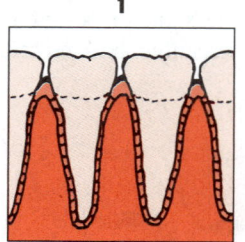 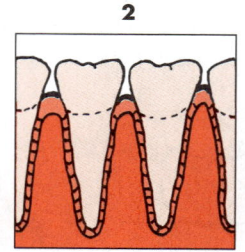 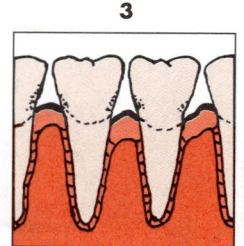 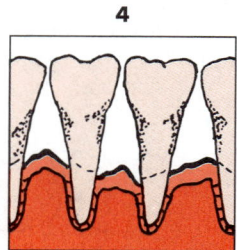

Figure 7-2. Progression of periodontal disease. (1) **Normal, healthy gingivae (gums):** Healthy gums and bone anchor teeth firmly in place. (2) **Gingivitis:** Plaque and its byproducts irritate the gums, making them tender, inflamed, and likely to bleed. (3) **Periodontitis:** Unremoved, plaque hardens into calculus (tartar). As plaque and calculus continue to build up, the gums begin to recede (pull away) from the teeth, and pockets form between the teeth and gums. (4) **Advanced periodontitis:** The gums recede farther, destroying more bone and the periodontal ligament. Teeth—even healthy teeth—may become loose and need to be extracted. (Courtesy Karen L. Merrill, Wellesley, Mass.)

The tongue should be inspected for color, swelling, and lesions and palpated on all surfaces for tenderness and lesions. The mucous membranes, in general, should be observed for color, moistness, smoothness, and the appearance of lesions. Box 7-4 lists the important points of an oral assessment. Assessment should also consider and utilize the positive strength phenomena of the older adult when developing appropriate nursing diagnoses and subsequent interventions for oral care. These strengths include maintenance of self-pride, maintenance of dignity, increased socialization, the desire to be well-groomed and well-dressed, and taking an active role in self–health maintenance.

It cannot be emphasized too strongly how vital dental care is to the well-being of the aged individual. For too long, health care givers have been too naive, unconcerned, or remiss in the maintenance of this important need, which influences so many other equally and more important physiologic, psychologic, and social needs. It is heartening to note that dental schools include dental care of geriatric patients in their curricula, and students receive practice by going into the community with mobile dental vans to senior centers and to visit homebound and institutionalized elders.

A Brief Oral Health Status Exam (BOHSE) developed by Kayser-Jones et al (1995) can be used by most health care providers to assess the oral health of elders in community and institutional settings. In-service education from a professional dentist is necessary before implementing the tool (Figure 7-3). Most BOHSE items use observation and palpation. Some items require verbal responses regarding the length of time a condition has existed. When the elder cannot relate this information, a caregiver/family member may need to answer. The total score as well as the individual score of the BOHSE is important. An overall score may be within normal but an item score may be significant and require immediate referral to a dentist or physician (Kayser-Jones et al, 1995).

Interventions

Care of the Teeth. Generally, the aged are seen by the dentist when it is too late to salvage the teeth. It is therefore imperative to conscientiously include appropriate dental care to maintain and preserve the existing teeth of the aged person. Dental care begins at home and should be reinforced by the caregiver when the aged person requires assistance in meeting this activity of daily living. Prescribed oral hygiene for the individual with some or all teeth is to brush daily and floss or use interdental stimulators to aid in the removal of debris that collects around the teeth and soft tissue. It is best if individuals can brush their teeth after each meal. However, most individuals brush their teeth in the morning and at night before they go to bed. The night brushing is the most important to reduce dental caries and should be followed with an antibacterial mouthwash.

Mechanical plaque removal. A soft, round-bristled toothbrush minimizes the chance of causing trauma to the gums yet stimulates the gums to retain firmness and adequate circulation. Dental experts recommend inclining the toothbrush at a 45-degree angle to the gum line and using a gentle scrubbing motion of short back-and-forth strokes over one or two teeth at a time. All surfaces—inner, outer, and chewing—should be brushed accordingly. It may be easier for the aged to use a child's toothbrush rather than an adult brush. A brush of this size and type is generally made of soft bristles and is a third smaller than the adult brush. It is easier to brush individual teeth and into the back angles of the mouth. Figure 7-4 demonstrates the correct toothbrushing method.

Disclosure tablets or drops will stain the plaque that collects at the gum line and tooth appositions red or deep pink.

Box 7-3	**Signs of Periodontal Disease***

Gums bleeding when teeth are brushed. Even a little bleeding is not normal. If you have a "pink" toothbrush, see your dentist.
Red, swollen, or tender gums
Detachment of the gums from the teeth
Pus that appears from the gum line when the gums are pressed
Teeth that have become loose or change position
Any change in the way your teeth fit together when you bite
Any change in the fit of partial dentures
Chronic bad breath or bad taste

*Not limited to elders alone.

Box 7-4	**Important Points of Oral Assessment**

Salivation
Tongue
   Texture
   Moisture
   Coloring
Palates
Gingival tissues (gums)
Teeth
Dentures/bridgework
Soft tooth debris
Lips
   Texture
   Moisture
   Coloring
Voice
Swallowing ability

*Modified from Danielson KH: Oral care and adults, *J Gerontol Nurs* 14(11):6, 1988.

KAYSER-JONES BRIEF ORAL HEALTH STATUS EXAMINATION

Resident's Name _____
Examiner's Name _____

Date _____
TOTAL SCORE _____

CATEGORY	MEASUREMENT	0	1	2
LYMPH NODES	Observe and feel nodes	No enlargement	Enlarged, not tender	*Enlarged and tender**
LIPS	Observe, feel tissue, and ask resident, family or staff (e.g. primary caregiver)	Smooth, pink, moist	Dry, chapped, or *red at corners**	*White or red patch, bleeding or ulcer for 2 weeks**
TONGUE	Observe, feel tissue, and ask resident, family or staff (e.g. primary caregiver)	Normal roughness, pink and moist	Coated, smooth, patchy, severely fissured or some redness	*Red, smooth, white or red patch; ulcer for 2 weeks**
TISSUE INSIDE CHEEK, FLOOR, AND ROOF OF MOUTH	Observe, feel tissue, and ask resident, family or staff (e.g. primary caregiver)	Pink and moist	*Dry, shiny, rough red, or swollen**	*White or red patch, bleeding, hardness; ulcer for 2 weeks**
GUMS BETWEEN TEETH AND/OR UNDER ARTIFICIAL TEETH	Gently press gums with tip of tongue blade	Pink, small indentations; firm, smooth and pink under artificial teeth	*Redness at border around 1-6 teeth; one red area or sore spot under artificial teeth**	*Swollen or bleeding gums, redness at border around 7 or more teeth, loose teeth; generalized redness or sores under artificial teeth**
SALIVA (EFFECT ON TISSUE)	Touch tongue blade to center of tongue and floor of mouth	Tissues moist, saliva free flowing and watery	Tissues dry and sticky	*Tissues parched and red, no saliva**
CONDITION OF NATURAL TEETH	Observe and count number of decayed or broken teeth	No decayed or broken teeth/roots	*1-3 decayed or broken teeth/roots**	*4 or more decayed or broken teeth/roots; fewer than 4 teeth in either jaw**
CONDITION OF ARTIFICIAL TEETH	Observe and ask patient, family or staff (e.g., primary caregiver)	Unbroken teeth, worn most of the time	1 broken/missing tooth, or worn for eating or cosmetics only	*More than 1 broken or missing tooth, or either denture missing or never worn**
PAIRS OF TEETH IN CHEWING POSITION (NATURAL OR ARTIFICIAL)	Observe and count pairs of teeth in chewing position	12 or more pairs of teeth in chewing position	8-11 pairs of teeth in chewing position	*0-7 pairs of teeth in chewing position**
ORAL CLEANLINESS	Observe appearance of teeth or dentures	Clean, no food particles/tartar in the mouth or on artificial teeth	Food particles/tartar in one or two places in the mouth or on artificial teeth	Food particles/tartar in most places in the mouth or on artificial teeth

Upper dentures labeled: Yes _____ No _____ None _____   Lower dentures labeled: Yes _____ No _____ None _____
Is your mouth comfortable? Yes _____ No _____ If no, explain: _____
Additional comments: _____

Italic*-refer to dentist immediately

Figure 7-3. Kayser-Jones Brief Oral Health Status Examination. (With permission of Jeanie Kayser-Jones, RN, Ph D, School of Nursing, University of California, San Francisco.)

It can help the person see the areas of plaque accumulation that otherwise are not visible on inspection. Brushing teeth routinely for approximately 2 minutes each time should adequately remove debris and stimulate the gums.

Interproximal plaque removal. Dental flossing is an integral part of the cleaning process; once a day is sufficient if done properly. The person should use about a 46-cm length of lightly waxed or unwaxed floss; a seesaw motion places the floss between the tooth surfaces; removal of plaque requires up-and-down movement under the gum line and side surfaces of teeth. Figure 7-5 shows the correct method of flossing. Many people floss just between the teeth but forget to include under the gum line and the single surface of the last molar.

Use of a commercial floss handle may provide the leverage and ease necessary for the aged person to continue flossing (Figure 7-6). If the floss handle is too delicate to grasp, the section on adaptive aids suggests modifications. Persons with sensitive or ulcerated gums might find a Water Pik device appropriate. The Rotadent is a device that cleans teeth and provides a gentle massage to the gums. Its operation is

similar to an electric toothbrush, but it has several small attachments for the rotating scrubbing motion, similar to that used in the dentist's office. One disadvantage is that the aged person must have fine finger dexterity to remove and replace the attachments (Wylde, 1988).

Rinses. There are two types of rinses that individuals use: cosmetic and therapeutic. Cosmetic rinses primarily function to refresh the mouth, but there are major disadvantages. Depending on the brand, cosmetic rinses contain 6% to 29% alcohol by volume, which can be an oral tissue irritant and can exacerbate or create xerostomia. Secondly, alcoholism is a major problem in the elderly, so caution is advised in the use of alcohol-containing rinses. A third disadvantage of cosmetic rinses is that the effect of the mouth-flushing rinse is transient and may mask underlying causes of oral disease such as halitosis.

Therapeutic rinses contain an agent that is beneficial to the surface of the teeth and the oral environment. Some therapeutic rinses require a prescription such as Peridex (chlorhexidine), which contains alcohol but is also a broad-spectrum antimicrobial agent that helps control plaque. Listerine, which is

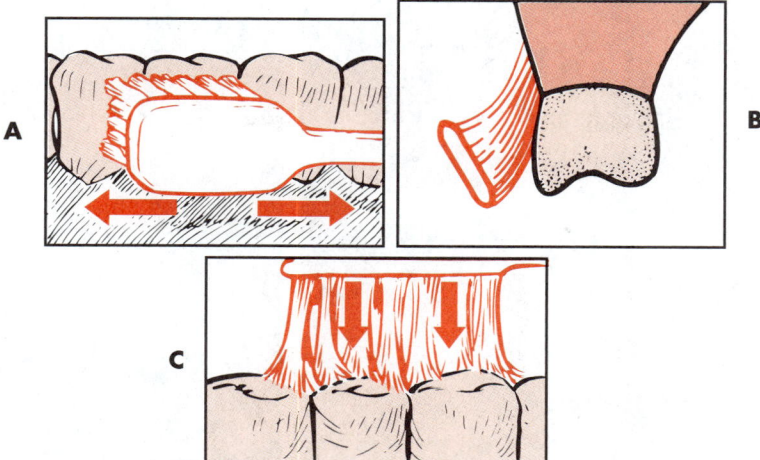

Figure 7-4. Correct toothbrushing routine. **A,** Brush sides of teeth. **B,** Angle brush to clean along gum line. **C,** Brush chewing surface.

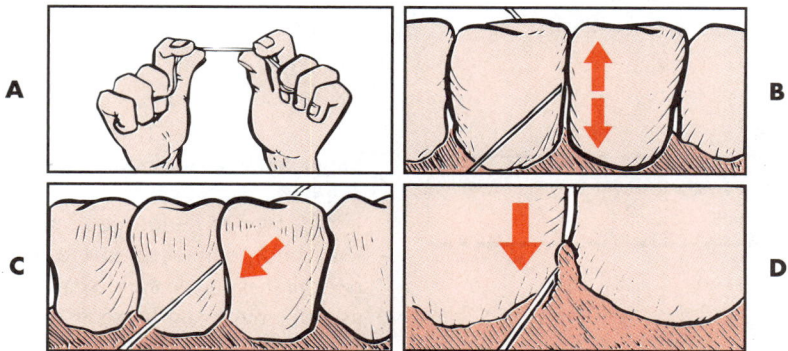

Figure 7-5. Effective flossing technique. **A,** Take a 46-cm piece of floss. **B,** Slide floss between teeth. **C,** Move floss up and down. **D,** Make sure floss goes below gum line.

in this same category, is an over-the-counter product that carries the American Dental Association approval, but it should not be used by persons on Antabuse or who have severe oral mucositis. Listerine also contains a high quantity by volume of alcohol (26.9%). Fluoride rinses such as the over-the-counter ACT and Fluorigard act to prevent caries development by incorporating into developing enamel, enhancing or increasing remineralization of enamel, and by antibacterial action. Remineralizing rinses are used to replace calcium and phosphate lost from enamel or cementum during the caries process.

Electronic devices. Plaque control toothbrushes may be useful for the aged person because they have large handles for easier grasp, require little or no arm or wrist movement, and provide a consistent motion and are relatively lightweight. Some plaque removal devices even stop when too much pressure is applied.

Adaptive aids for oral care. The handle of a toothbrush or floss holder can be easily customized for elders with a grasp weakened by arthritis, stroke, or other conditions. En-

listing the elder's assistance and creativity in designing the home care device is important because he or she is the best judge of what works well. Box 7-5 and Figure 7-7 provide possible adaptations.

Assisting Dependent Elders

It is essential to provide oral care daily regardless of whether the elder is severely disabled, physically handicapped, comatose, or mentally incapable of carrying out their own oral hygiene. Debilitated elders are at a greater risk of developing oral disease. They take more medications; they have decreased saliva production, they lack resistance to bacterial toxins that cause periodontal disease, and they eat softer foods, more liquids, and foods higher in sugar, which tend to remain in their mouths longer, than elders who are healthier.

Homebound

Daily oral home care should be a part of general hygiene care. Having the proper equipment and using the appropriate

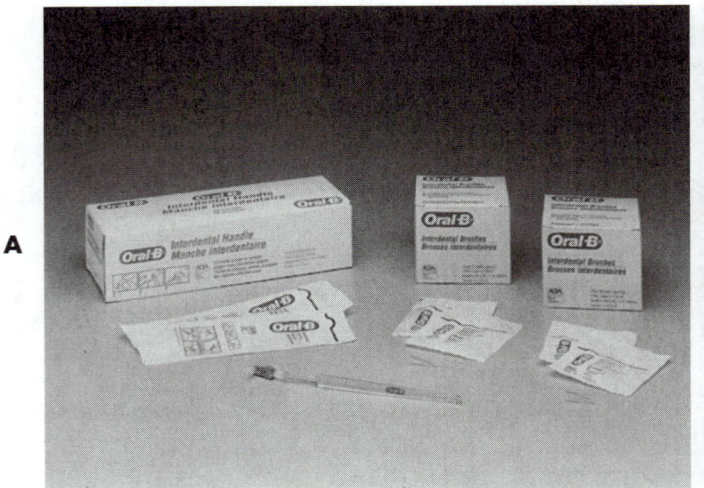 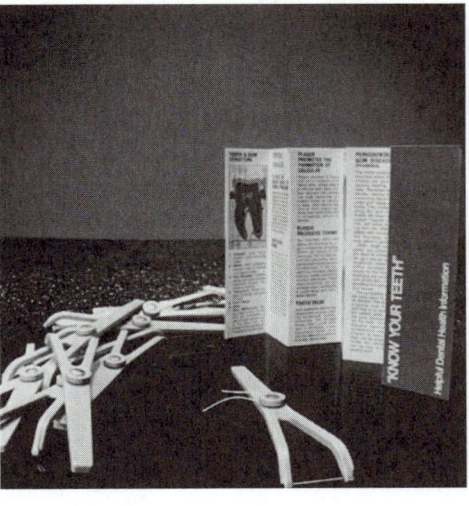

Figure 7-6. **A,** Oral-B interdental handle with extra-fine, tapered, and cylindrical brush refills. **B,** Flossaid dental floss holder. (**A** courtesy Oral-B Laboratories, Redwood, Calif; **B** courtesy Flossaid Corporation, Santa Clara, Calif.)

Box 7-5	Toothbrush and Floss Holder Adaptations

Wrap Handle with:
- Washcloth
- Aluminum foil
- Thin foam sheets

Insert Handle into:
- Sponge ball
- Sponge hair roller
- Plastic bicycle handle grip

Secure to Handle:
- Velcro or elastic strap to handle to slip over hand
- Attach handle to curved handle of nail brush with bristles removed, slip over fingers

techniques can greatly simplify the task and ensure better results. Caregivers should be shown and provided with written instructions to reinforce the verbal instructions and actual demonstration. Box 7-6 provides directions for caregivers.

To make oral hygiene complete, the tongue should be brushed. With age a white coating is formed on the tongue by mouth organisms, and this coating must be brushed or scraped off. This can most easily be done at the time of brushing teeth. It is preferable to brush the tongue or wipe it with a gauze when brushing the teeth in the morning and just before retiring (Jarvik and Small, 1988). Cleaning the tongue may be difficult for some people because it elicits the gag reflex.

The type of dentifrice is not as important as the mechanical action employed in the teeth-cleaning process. Some persons have used mild soap and water, while others have used a simple and inexpensive homemade tooth powder of equal parts bicarbonate of soda and table salt, which is sold commercially in tooth powder or paste form. This is no problem unless an individual's sodium intake is restricted. Today, too, with the discovery of the beneficial effects of fluoride in reducing gum line and root caries and preventing bacterial invasion of teeth, the use of a commercial fluoride toothpaste might be beneficial.

Reduced dexterity of the aged person may necessitate some modification of usual dental care aids to lessen the difficulty of brushing the teeth. A lightweight, rechargeable type of electric toothbrush may be useful because of the automatic action and the large handgrip. Toothbrush handles, in general, can be enlarged to facilitate easier grasp: pierce a soft rubber ball and push the toothbrush handle through; glue a piece of short plastic tubing to the handle; build up the handle with self-curing acrylic resin (plastic); take a rubber bicycle handlebar grip, fill it with plaster of paris, put the handle in the center, and hold until it hardens. If there is limited shoulder movement, an extension handle might be used.

When the aged person with natural teeth is unable to carry out his or her own dental regimen, it is the responsibility of the caregiver to do so. In the institutional setting it may not be possible to brush a person's teeth three or four times each day, but if the teeth are thoroughly brushed for

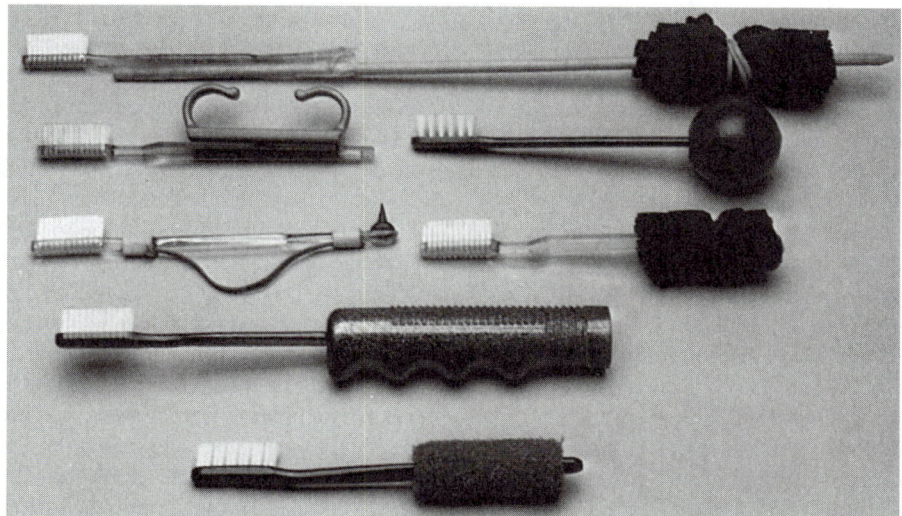

Figure 7-7. Adaptive aids for brushing. (From Papas AS, Niessen LC, Chauncey HH: *Geriatric dentistry, aging and oral health,* St Louis, 1991, Mosby.)

2 minutes and flossed at least once in 24 hours, the integrity of the mouth can be maintained.

A curved-bristle toothbrush for those in nursing homes who need assistance allows greater access to harder-to-reach dental surfaces. These are readily available commercially. They remove more plaque than straight-bristle brushes. The benefit to the caregiver is reduction in time and degree of difficulty in giving oral care. Use of disclosure liquid or chewing tablets would help the caregiver identify whether proper brushing and flossing was actually accomplished.

Good brushing and flossing cannot be emphasized enough. The aged ingest large quantities of refined carbohydrates and no longer have the effective washing and cleaning benefit of saliva. These factors combined with the lack of proper attention to oral hygiene encourage the detrimental effect of plaque formation, the precursor of periodontal disease.

To ensure that the aged person receives thorough oral hygiene, O'Laughlin (1986) suggests it might be necessary to write it as a routine part of the nursing care plan, which can be evaluated daily.

Care of the Dentures

A significant number of elders are edentulous and wear complete dentures. Dentures help maintain adequate nutrition and psychological aid to preserve appearance, social contacts, and relationships that a person has cultivated. Persons with dentures seem to stand more erect, smile more, and be willing to socialize more than edentulous persons (Epstein, 1976).

Many elders believe that once they have dentures there is no longer a need for oral care. Older adults with dentures

---

Box 7-6   Dental Care: Instructions for Caregiver

1. If the patient is in bed, elevate his or her head by raising the bed or propping it with pillows and have the patient turn his or her head to face you. Place a clean towel across the chest and under the chin, and place a basin under his or her chin.
2. If the patient is sitting in a stationary chair or wheelchair, stand behind the patient and stabilize his head by placing one hand under his chin and resting his head against your body. Place a towel across his or her chest and over the shoulders. (It may be helpful to secure it with a safety pin.) The basin can be kept handy in the patient's lap or on a table placed in front of or at the side of the patient. A wheelchair may be positioned in front of the sink.
3. If the patient's lips are dry or cracked, apply a light coating of petroleum jelly.
4. Brush and floss the patient's teeth as you have been instructed (sulcular brushing, if possible). It may be helpful to retract the patient's lips and cheek with a tongue blade or fingers in order to see the area that is being cleaned. Use a mouth prop as needed if the patient cannot hold his or her mouth open. If manual flossing is too difficult, use a floss holder or interproximal brush to clean the proximal surfaces between the teeth. Use a dentifrice containing fluoride.
5. Provide the conscious patient with fluoride rinses or other rinses as indicated by the dentist or hygienist.

From Papas AS, Niessen LC, Chauncey HH: *Geriatric dentistry, aging and oral health,* St Louis, 1991, Mosby.

should be taught the proper home care of their dentures and oral tissue (Box 7-7), which prevents odor, stain, and plaque buildup, and removes debris under dentures that causes pressure and shrinkage of the underlying support structures. Dentures and other dental appliances such as bridges should be cleaned after each meal and anytime they are removed (Box 7-7).

Dentures must be worn constantly. They should be removed at bedtime and replaced in the mouth in the morning to allow relief of the compression on the gums (Rounds and Papas, 1991). If the elder prefers to sleep with dentures in place, he or she should be encouraged to remove them for at least 4 hours during the day. See Box 7-8 for tips on proper care of dentures.

If cleaning must be done by the caregiver, brushing with a denture brush or a medium-firm toothbrush should be done on all surfaces of the dentures. If there are removable bridges or other wires (or prong-type attachments), these should be thoroughly cleaned to remove any debris and food. When cleaning dentures, fill the sink over which the washing will be done one third or half full of water; hold the dentures close to the water so that if the dentures do slip, the water will break the fall and no damage will result. Adaptation by caregivers can be made from Box 7-8.

Some immersion (soaking) cleaners assist in cleaning dentures. These products should be nonabrasive to the denture material, require little handling of the dentures, and reach all parts of the dentures. If used daily in conjunction with brushing, this should be sufficient to keep dentures clean. The elder or caregiver should always brush and rinse the dentures before and after the immersion soak. The gums, tongue, and palate should be cleansed by using a soft-bristled brush or by wiping the soft tissue with a gauze-wrapped finger. It does little for tissue integrity to clean the dentures and leave a residual film of debris on the gums. Gums, too, should be cleansed with a gloved finger wrapped in gauze or with a soft toothbrush to remove the film and residual food particles caught under dentures. This is an opportune time to massage the gums to increase circulation and inspect them for irritations.

Dentures are very personal and expensive possessions. In communal living situations of nursing homes, hospitals, and other care centers, dentures have been misplaced or mixed up. Dentures should be marked; in fact, it should be a mandatory procedure for all persons who wear dentures to have their name, initials, or an identification number, such as their social security number, imprinted on the denture plates.

Box 7-7   Instructions for Denture Cleaning

1. Rinse your denture or dentures after each meal to remove soft debris.
2. Once a day, preferably before retiring, brush your denture according to the method described below. Then place it in a denture-cleaning solution and allow it to soak overnight or for at least a few hours. (Acrylic denture material must be kept wet at all times to prevent cracking or warping.)
3. Remove your denture from the cleaning solution and brush it thoroughly.
   a. Although an ordinary *soft* toothbrush is adequate, a specially designed denture brush may clean more effectively. (CAUTION: Acrylic denture material is soften than natural teeth and may be damaged by being brushed with very firm bristles.)
   b. Brush your denture over a sink lined with a facecloth and half-filled with water. This will prevent breakage if the denture is dropped.
   c. Hold the denture *securely* in one hand, but do not squeeze. Hold the brush in the other hand. It is not essential to use a denture paste, particularly if dentures are soaked before being brushed to soften debris. Never use a commercial tooth powder because it is abrasive and may damage the denture materials. Plain water, mild soap, or sodium bicarbonate may be used.
   d. When cleaning a *removable partial denture,* great care must be taken to remove plaque from the curved metal clasps that hook around the teeth. This can be done with a regular toothbrush or with a specially designed clasp brush.
4. After brushing, rinse your denture thoroughly and insert it into your mouth.

From Papas AS, Niessen LC, Chauncey HH: *Geriatric dentistry, aging and oral health,* St Louis, 1991, Mosby.

Box 7-8   Take Care of Your Dentures

1. When your denture is out of your mouth, it should be stored in a water-filled container. This will prevent the denture material from drying out.
2. Place the container in a secure location where it will not be knocked onto the floor or disturbed by pets or children.
3. Never place your denture in hot water—use only cool or lukewarm.
4. Never soak dentures with metal parts in bleach.
5. Never try to adjust or repair your denture. Let an expert do it.
6. Never use abrasive powders or a hard toothbrush to clean your denture.
7. Never soak your denture in a product that contains alcohol, such as mouthwash, or clean it with regular toothpaste.
8. *ALWAYS rinse your denture thoroughly* under running water before inserting it into the mouth.

From Papas AS, Niessen LC, Chauncey HH: *Geriatric dentistry, aging and oral health,* St Louis, 1991, Mosby.

Dentists, laboratory technicians, or dental hygienists are now marking dentures. Some states require all newly made dentures to contain the client's identification mark (Rounds and Papas, 1991). If dentures have not been marked, the caregiver can write the name, initial, or appropriate identification number on the dentures either on the buccal flange or on the palate and cover it with two coats of clear nail varnish (nail polish). This is a temporary measure, which needs to be repeated after 1 or more years. This is not ideal, but it is better than not having dentures marked at all. A commercial denture marking system called Identure, produced by 3-M Company, provides a simple, efficient, and permanent means of marking dentures. It contains a special marking pen to mark the denture base and a permanent transparent film to cover the marking.

Broken or damaged dentures are a common problem for the aged. This generally happens when dentures are accidentally dropped during cleaning because of poor neuromuscular coordination or because they are slippery to handle. Do-it-yourself fix-it kits are not advisable. Dentures should be correctly repaired by a dentist.

Figure 7-8 shows normal first dentures; with time resorption; and why dentures need relining and at times replacement. Relining of dentures is usually a temporary measure; rebasing dentures is more successful. A new impression is made of the remaining dental ridge. The teeth are removed from the original pink denture and used in the new better-fitting denture base that has been adjusted to the changes in the dental ridges. This is less costly than a new denture because the original teeth are used (Fah, 1981). Prosthetic failure generally results from tissue changes in the mouth. These alterations can develop from the prostheses themselves, from the physical and emotional status of the aged person, or from significant weight fluctuations.

Dentures should be checked once a year. The average time a denture base will be able to support the denture is 20 years. Many lose as much as 50% of supporting bone in 5 to 10 years. Rapid bone loss occurs with ill-fitting dentures (loose dentures). Denture adhesive helps only temporarily.

During the past 20 years several new approaches to dealing with missing teeth have been devised, such as dental implants.

Dental Implants

There are diverse reasons for the cause and inability of elders to wear dentures. Current research indicates that providing a stable prosthetic may be the single most important determinant in fulfilling client aesthetic expectations (Zarb and Schmitt, 1990, 1991). Osseointegrated dental implants have become reliable and safely provide long-term prosthetic stability for edentulous clients of all ages. Dental implants are not an appropriate treatment for all persons. The basic objective of dental implantation is to provide an attachment mechanism for teeth or dentures. Dental implants can anchor lower or upper dentures, provide a method to replace partial or full dentures with fixed bridgework, provide a method of replacing a single tooth, improve chewing function and restore the feeling of natural tooth function, and improve the quality of life by removing the frustration associated with using dentures or removable bridgework.

The procedure is done in several steps, which cover approximately 3 to 5 months from start to completion. Elderly candidates for dental implantations must be fit enough to undergo minor oral surgery and have a jaw that can accommodate the implant system. A major problem for implants is the lack of jaw bone that occurs in 10% of prospective patients. Research is under way to find bone stimulators. These include hormones and the use of Gore-Tex, which encourages bone growth by blocking other cells from filling empty spaces in bone (Ubell, 1992). In addition, the candidate for implants can have no history of drug abuse (potential for misuse of pain management drugs) and must possess realistic expectations of the outcome. Cost of implants range from $1000 for one anchor to $5000 and up per denture, a potential deterrent to elders on a fixed income. Figure 7-9 demonstrates the various types of implant supports.

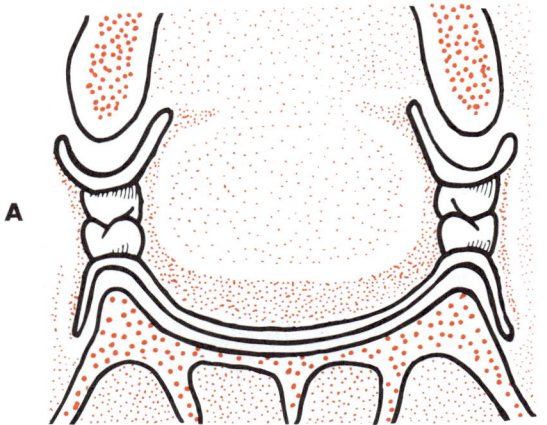 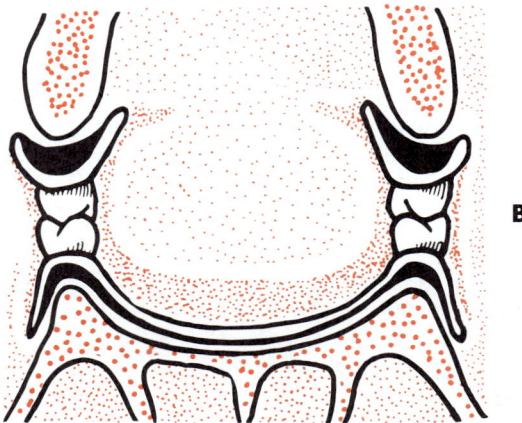

Figure 7-8. Denture fit. **A,** Denture fit before resorption. **B,** Denture fit after resorption.

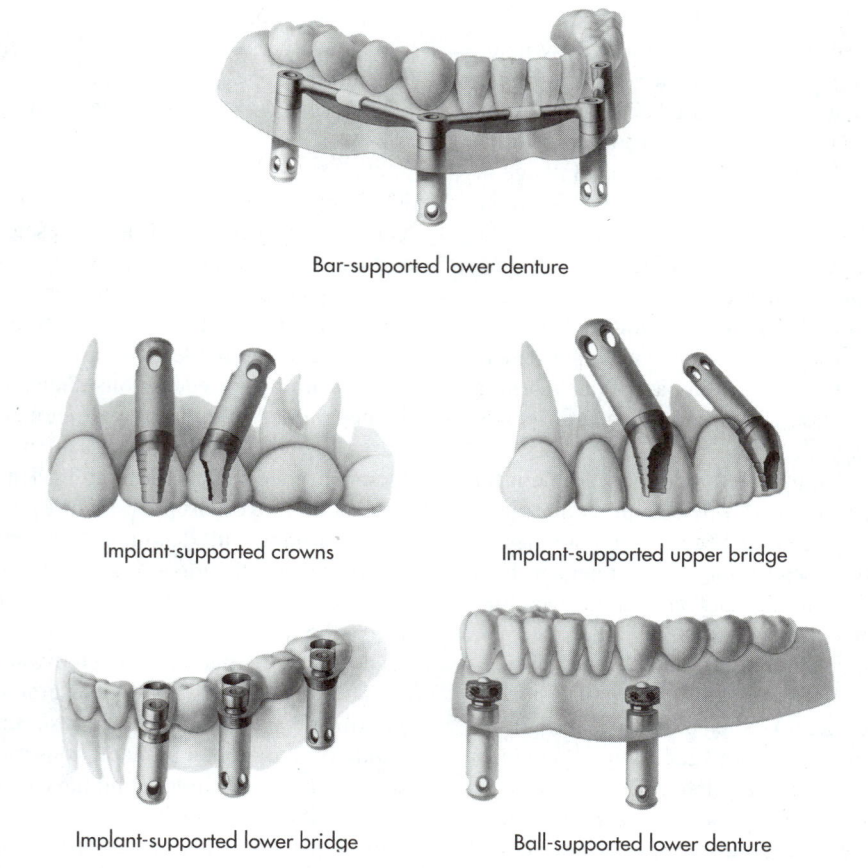

Bar-supported lower denture

Implant-supported crowns

Implant-supported upper bridge

Implant-supported lower bridge

Ball-supported lower denture

Figure 7-9. Type of dental implant supports. (Courtesy Sulzer Calcitek, Inc., Carlsbad, Calif.)

FEET

The feet undergo a great deal of use, trauma, misuse, and neglect as a part of everyday living. Most aged accept foot problems as an inescapable accompaniment of aging. Nurses and people in general have a fairly strong negative reaction to having contact with the feet. It is aesthetically unpleasing (Pelican et al, 1990). Yet, adequate care of the feet can alleviate disability, pain, and the propensity for falling. It is for these reasons that the importance of feet to the well-being of the aged is emphasized more extensively in this chapter than in most texts.

Feet influence the physical, psychologic, and social well-being of the individual. Feet carry one's body weight, hold the body erect in an upright and stationary position, coordinate and maintain balance in walking, and must be rigid yet loose and adaptable enough to conform to the surfaces underfoot (all the while holding the legs and body in an upright position). Little attention is given to these valuable appendages until the feet interfere with ambulation and the ability to maintain independence.

Feet have been symbolically significant from biblical times, when respect and concern were shown by washing the feet, particularly of religious leaders and those held in esteem. We contend that the symbolic significance of the feet is present today and attending to the feet is a gesture of response to the total individual.

Feet often reflect systemic disease conditions or give clues to physical ailments before their actual appearance (Echevarria et al, 1988; Burning feet, 1992). Sudden or gradual changes in nail or skin condition of the feet and/or appearance of recurring infection may be the precursors of more serious health problems. Feet have a significant effect on one's productivity, amiability, and mobility. The effect is comparable to the influence that the automobile has had in our society. Like the automobile, if there is something wrong, it is difficult to get around and the routine of the day is upset. Feet, like the automobile, are taken for granted and accorded little attention as long as they work. Unlike the automobile, though, the feet do not have easily replaceable parts. Neglect of the feet throughout one's active years results in painful conditions later (Collet, 1995).

Uncomfortable and painful feet may force the elderly person to become sedentary and deprived of social contacts. Foot discomfort can cause irritability, fatigue, and chronic complaints. Socrates is thought to have said, "To him whose feet hurt, everything hurts" (An assessment, 1977, p.102). This sums up the essence of foot problems.

The aged person's feet are subjected to functional and physical neglect and traumatic stresses over the years. The residual effect from these varied stresses, compounded by a decreased ability of the aged to clearly see their feet (because of visual impairment) and to bend to give their feet routine care often results in conditions that need not exist or at least could be controlled (Box 7-9).

Mobility for the aged may mean the difference between an independent, active community life, self-respect, motivation, and responsibility for one's health vs. institutionalization. Even in an institution, foot problems may mean the difference between confinement to bed or wheelchair and the ability to ambulate in the protective setting.

Foot Problems in Old Age

The foot begins to change shape in females soon after birth, but in males changes in shape begin in about the fourth decade. There is a gradual loss of fat padding of the adult foot, resulting in greater stress on feet and the potential for the development of musculoskeletal disorders (Echevarria et al, 1988; Helfand, 1989a).

Fifty percent of the general population have foot problems. The number and severity of the problems increase with age. Almost 80% of persons over the age of 50 will have at least one significant foot problem. Three of every four persons 65 years and over complain of foot pain. Individuals over 55 years (88% of women and 83% of men) demonstrate arthritic changes in the foot on roentgenograms. Of these older adults, 25% have symptoms of foot problems (Gudas,1986; Perspectives, 1993).

Major abnormalities occur gradually with discomfort, not with pain. Without proper care and treatment these conditions become disabling and a threat to the person's independence.

Diseases also endanger the foot. Osteoarthritis can cause pain in the feet. Rheumatoid arthritis may lead to hammer toes and dislocated toes. Peripheral vascular disease can lead to infections of the feet, pain due to decreased circulation, and amputation. Gout creates difficulty in walking due to the pain of uric acid crystal accumulation and swelling of toe joints, particularly the joint of the great toe (Figure 7-10). Diabetes with the development of peripheral neuropathy predisposes the foot to injury, infection, and in some instances amputation.

Corns, the conical shaped layers of compacted skin usually on toes, occur as a result of friction and pressure on the skin rubbing against bony, protuberant areas of the toes when shoes are worn. Once the small, hard, white corn is established, continued pressure elicits pain. Unless the cause of the corn is removed, it will continue to enlarge and cause increasing pain. Soft corns form in the same manner but occur between opposing surfaces of the toes. Both corns and calluses interfere with the ability to walk comfortably and wear shoes. These conditions are symptomatic of underlying problems of feet that are subjected to prolonged or recurrent friction and pressure. Most individuals have attempted do-it-yourself remedies for corns and calluses. The aged usually follow what they have done for years to correct their foot discomfort. Over-the-counter preparations for corns, in par-

Box 7-9	**Age-Related Foot Changes**

Skin becomes drier, less elastic, cooler.
Subcutaneous tissue on dorsum and sides of foot thins.
Plantar fat pad shrinks and degenerates.
Toenails become brittle, thicken, and are less resistant to fungal infections.
Degenerative joint disease decreases range of motion.

ticular, damage normal tissue as well as remove the corn. Chemical burns and ulcerations can result in the loss of toes or a leg for the aged person with diabetes, neurologic impairment, or poor circulatory function to the lower extremities. Some elderly use razor blades and scissors to remove corns and calluses. In light of the aforementioned problems with vision and flexibility, this is a dangerous solution.

Oval corn pads, which seem to aid in the relief of corns, actually create greater pressure on the toes and can decrease circulation to the tissue within the oval pad in much the same manner as a rubber ring at the coccyx for a pressure ulcer will damage surrounding tissue. The intent is to relieve pressure, which it does, but at the same time it compresses the tissue around the opening and decreases the amount of circulation in the open space. Oval corn pads can be adapted for effective use. Instead of using the oval pad as it is, the upper or lower section of the corn pad can be cut out so that the pad resembles the letter U. This can be placed around three aspects of the corn, protecting it from pressure without restricting circulation to healthy tissue. Spot adhesive bandages or mole skin are also useful to protect corns from additional friction, but they do not have enough padding to guard against pressure. Irritation from soft corns between the toes can be eased by loosely wrapping small amounts of lamb's wool around the involved toe.

Calluses are also layers of compacted skin that usually occur on the soles and heels of the feet because of chronic irritation and friction from shoes. Calluses can be eased with mole skin applied to those areas that receive undue friction. Mole skin adheres for several days or longer but should be removed when it becomes wet or excessively soiled. Removing mole skin from the feet of the elderly should be done slowly to prevent tearing of skin.

The nurse should be very careful when using adhesive tape on the aged foot. Older foot skin is thinner and more delicate and does not tolerate adhesive tape well (Jahss, 1979).

Decreased sebaceous activity, dehydration of the horny layer, and environmental influences are responsible for the majority of dry and scaly foot problems the elderly exhibit. Metabolic or nutritional alterations and dysfunctions of keratin formation are considered other possible causes of dry feet problems. Dryness leads to fissures in the soles of the feet, particularly the heels. Feet itch and are scratched to

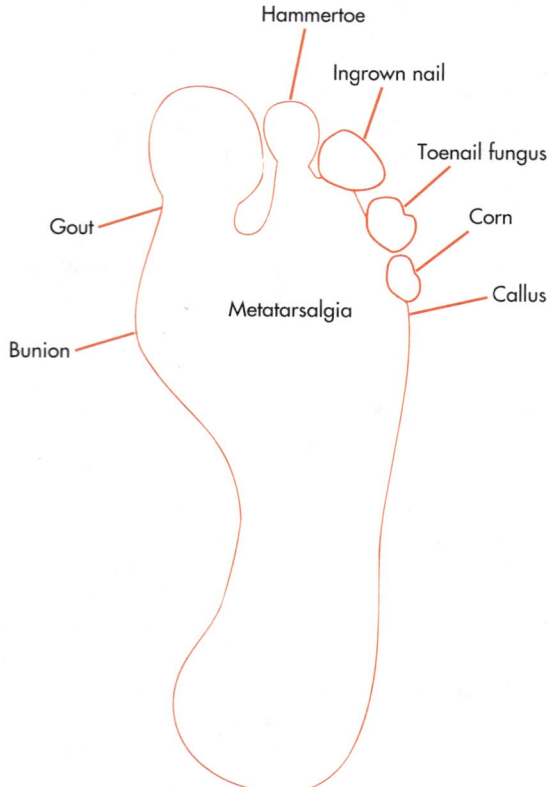

Figure 7-10. Common foot problems.

relieve the discomfort. It is necessary to lubricate the feet with lotion at least twice each day to retain the tissue hydration. Lotion helps keep water in the tissue rather than letting it evaporate and causing dryness (Figure 7-9). Besides the standard over-the-counter lotions, inexpensive and effective substitutes are vegetable and mineral oils. Lotion or oil should be applied and massaged into the foot tissue and the excess removed, particularly between the toes.

Bunions, clinically called hallux valgus, are bony prominences that occur over the medial aspect of the first metatarsal head (the joint of the great toe) and, at times, at the lateral aspect of the fifth metatarsal head (the joint of the little toe), often called the tailor bunion or a bunionette. Bunions are long-standing residual effects from occupational activity and the influence of shoe styles. Women's shoes, which draw the toes together, and the improper weight transmission and restrictive hose all contribute to the problem. Bunions may also be hereditary in nature (Perspectives, 1993).

The nurse should focus on obtaining shoes that properly support, protect, and provide comfort for the foot and encourage the client to wear them. Shoes that provide enough forefoot space laterally and dorsally, such as running shoes, generally have a wide toe box and fit well. Depth inlay shoes made by the Alden Shoe Company, Middleborough, Mass, 02346, have been cited as providing significant relief. Extra

depth in shoes for women is offered by Miller Shoes, now owned by Drew Shoe Company, 252 Quarry Rd, Lancaster, OH, 43130.

Shoe stores have devices that will stretch the shoe at the pressure area, but the customer must purchase the shoe before this easement is made. Shoe repair shops have shoe stretching devices and charge a reasonable fee for stretching a shoe. At home, leather shoes can be eased while they are being worn by wetting the shoe with alcohol. This allows the leather to stretch to the shape of the feet but will not leave a permanent watermark because the alcohol evaporates. Custom-made shoes, although expensive, are available to the aged person with bunions. Less expensive are ultralight walking shoes and running shoes. Fabric shoes, (not recommended for diabetic persons), are perhaps the most comfortable for the aged person with a bunion because the fabric stretches more than leather and synthetic materials. Cloth shoes should have a good quality walking surface. Protective pads are also available to cushion bunion joints. Ingrown toenails will be discussed with care of toe nails on p. 238.

Hammer toe is a permanently flexed and rotated toe or toes that have a clawlike appearance, the result of muscle imbalance and aggravated by poor-fitting shoes. Over time the toe, usually the second toe, is pushed by the bunioned great toe slanting toward and under the toe. The toe then contracts leaving a bulge on top of the joint. Balance and comfort are affected. Treatment includes professional orthotics, properly fitting, nonconstricting shoes and/or surgical intervention to rectify this problem (Perspectives, 1993).

Metatarsalgia is pain in the ball of the foot caused by a narrow high-arched foot, which focuses stress on the ball of the foot; legs that are unequal in length, thus adding stress to the metatarsal joints of the shorter leg; rheumatoid arthritis; stress fractures; fluid accumulation; muscle fatigue; flat feet; and overloaded feet as in the case of obesity. Bunions or tender calluses under the metatarsophalangeal joint or a Morton's neuroma may also be responsible for this foot problem. Relief is often obtained with foot freedom, that is, when the foot is not restricted by shoes, or with adequate shoe length and width. Orthotics and the use of nonsteroidal antiinflammatory medications are also helpful. Orthotics can be a reasonably priced alternative (rather than custom-made shoes) for the elder with foot problems (*Mayo Clinic Health Letter*, 1991).

Burning feet, though usually temporary, are a common problem with the aged. This annoyance occurs due to irritating fabrics, poorly fitting shoes, fungal infections, or contact with toxic substances such as poison ivy or poison oak. Generally, burning feet are not serious but can be symptomatic of such underlying diseases as diabetes mellitus, alcoholism, poor nutritional state (folic acid, B_{12} deficiency), chronic kidney failure, or liver disease. In addition, medications and exposure to such poisons as arsenic and lead may cause burning feet.

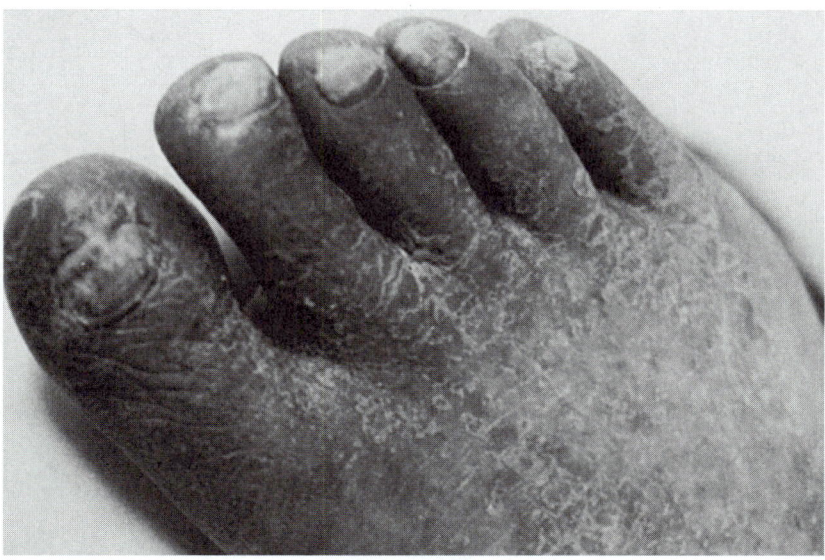

Figure 7-11. Dry scaly foot with toenail fungus. (Photograph by Stewart H. Bloom.)

Self-help measures that can help alleviate burning feet include wearing cotton or cotton blend socks. Shoes made of natural materials that breathe, provide a good fit, and have fitted insoles can help greatly to reduce the burning sensation. Cold tap water foot baths 15 minutes twice a day to cool the feet, in conjunction with rest and avoidance of activities that aggravate the problem, can reduce burning. The use of prescribed and over-the-counter preparations also can bring relief.

Fungal and bacterial infections are common in the aged foot. These conditions usually develop because the foot is encased in a warm, dark, and moisture-holding shoe. Nail fungus is characterized by dirty yellow streaks or total nail discoloration. The nail becomes opaque, scaly, and hypertrophied. A fine powdery substance forms under the center of the nail and pushes it up, causing the sides of the nail to dig into the flesh like an ingrown toenail (Figure 7-11). Culturing is the only definitive way to identify onychomycosis (Tosti, 1995). Hands should be washed each time the feet of a patient with a fungus infection are handled. Feet, especially between the toes, should be dry and exposed to sun and air. If prone to fungal and bacterial conditions, a daily dusting with antifungal powder or spray is appropriate. This condition requires a podiatrist to control and eliminate it. Itraconazole, marketed under the name Sporanox is the first drug to be approved by the U.S. Food and Drug Administration (FDA) that is available to treat and cure most nail fungal infections. It causes fewer side effects than previous oral drugs and provides for a shorter treatment time (UCSF to Our Neighbors, 1996).

Care of the Feet

Foot care is a prime factor in determining mobility and the quality of existence in retaining independence. Elders with painful foot problems and resultant activity limitations are usually forced to remain within the boundaries of their homes.

Nursing care of the aged foot should be directed toward maintaining comfort and function, removing possible mechanical irritants, decreasing the likelihood of infection, and helping to enhance and preserve maximum function. These goals are consistent with podiatric goals.

The nurse has the important function of assessing the feet of the aged person for clues to well-being and functional ability, not just bathing and applying lotion to the feet. Nurses can identify potential and actual problems and refer or seek podiatric assistance for the foot problems of the patient.

Assessment

Nursing care of the feet should include a thorough assessment (Pelican et al, 1990). King (1978, 1980) developed an assessment tool for the lower extremities of the aged, that any caregiver can learn to use. As can be seen in Figure 7-12, it provides illustrations of some of the important aspects to look for and evaluate and simple explanations of specific items to ensure uniform evaluation regardless of who performs the assessment. Until the nurse is familiar with this tool, it will take about 20 minutes or more to complete, but with increased proficiency, the time required can be reduced. The assessment itself includes the essentials of foot care: inspection of feet for irritation, abrasions, and other lesions; determination of functional and other acquired deviations; checks for hazards to the maintenance of adequate circulation to the lower extremities and the existing circulatory status; and observation of the individual's mobility.

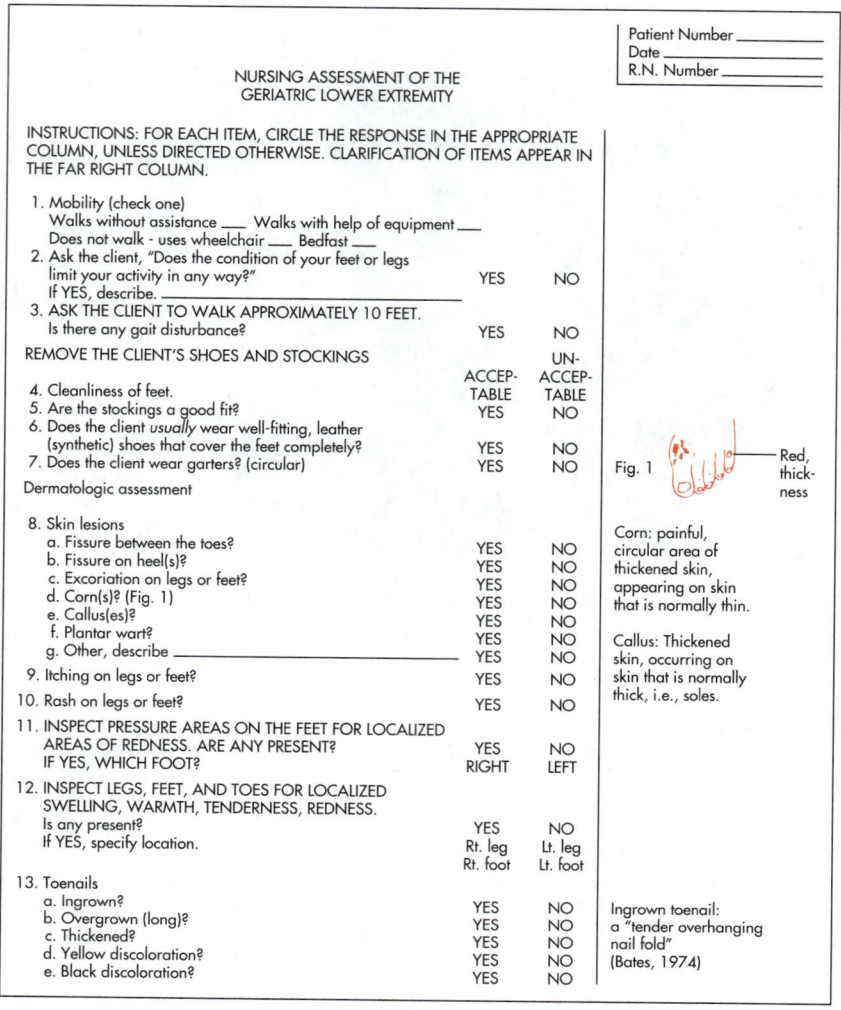

The form reads:

Patient Number _____
Date _____
R.N. Number _____

NURSING ASSESSMENT OF THE
GERIATRIC LOWER EXTREMITY

INSTRUCTIONS: FOR EACH ITEM, CIRCLE THE RESPONSE IN THE APPROPRIATE COLUMN, UNLESS DIRECTED OTHERWISE. CLARIFICATION OF ITEMS APPEAR IN THE FAR RIGHT COLUMN.

1. Mobility (check one)
   Walks without assistance ___ Walks with help of equipment ___
   Does not walk - uses wheelchair ___ Bedfast ___
2. Ask the client, "Does the condition of your feet or legs limit your activity in any way?"   YES   NO
   If YES, describe. _____
3. ASK THE CLIENT TO WALK APPROXIMATELY 10 FEET.
   Is there any gait disturbance?   YES   NO

REMOVE THE CLIENT'S SHOES AND STOCKINGS

	ACCEPTABLE	UN-ACCEPTABLE
4. Cleanliness of feet.		
5. Are the stockings a good fit?	YES	NO
6. Does the client *usually* wear well-fitting, leather (synthetic) shoes that cover the feet completely?	YES	NO
7. Does the client wear garters? (circular)	YES	NO

Fig. 1 — Red, thickness

Dermatologic assessment

8. Skin lesions
   a. Fissure between the toes?   YES   NO
   b. Fissure on heel(s)?   YES   NO
   c. Excoriation on legs or feet?   YES   NO
   d. Corn(s)? (Fig. 1)   YES   NO
   e. Callus(es)?   YES   NO
   f. Plantar wart?   YES   NO
   g. Other, describe _____   YES   NO
9. Itching on legs or feet?   YES   NO
10. Rash on legs or feet?   YES   NO
11. INSPECT PRESSURE AREAS ON THE FEET FOR LOCALIZED AREAS OF REDNESS. ARE ANY PRESENT?   YES   NO
    IF YES, WHICH FOOT?   RIGHT   LEFT
12. INSPECT LEGS, FEET, AND TOES FOR LOCALIZED SWELLING, WARMTH, TENDERNESS, REDNESS.
    Is any present?   YES   NO
    If YES, specify location.   Rt. leg   Lt. leg
    Rt. foot   Lt. foot
13. Toenails
    a. Ingrown?   YES   NO
    b. Overgrown (long)?   YES   NO
    c. Thickened?   YES   NO
    d. Yellow discoloration?   YES   NO
    e. Black discoloration?   YES   NO

Corn: painful, circular area of thickened skin, appearing on skin that is normally thin.

Callus: Thickened skin, occurring on skin that is normally thick, i.e., soles.

Ingrown toenail: a "tender overhanging nail fold" (Bates, 1974)

Figure 7-12. Nursing assessment of the geriatric lower extremities. (From King PA: *J Gerontol Nurs* 4:47, Nov/Dec 1978.)

Other tools for foot assessment have been developed. The Kelechi and Lukas (Kelechi, 1991) assessment tool is a form for regular and follow-up assessment and care. It is divided into five sections, each with a list of data to obtain either by question or through direct observation. An intervention list is included that provides a list of what action was taken and the results. The final section of this tool is completed with the follow-up plan and appointment, then signed by the person who provided the care. Pelican et al (1990) used a shorter form for assessing the feet. They listed those observations that should be part of a plan of care. These assessment tools and that of King (1978, 1980) seek the same information but in different formats (Box 7-10). Only Kelechi and Lukas list the types of interventions that might have been done and a section for follow-up. The variety of tools available speaks to the need for individualization to the client population with whom one is working and to the expertise of the individual who is doing the assessment and giving the care. Ruscin et al (1993) provide a foot assessment tool that incorporates age-related changes, skin and toenail condition, vascular status, and range-of-motion limitations (Figure 7-13). This tool may be helpful in identifying specific problems that require attention for the elder who needs assistance as well as for the independent elder.

Assessment is the key to maintenance of the aged person's highest level of function and mobility. Elderly persons with diabetes mellitus; cardiac, hyperthyroid, and kidney conditions; and pernicious anemia are naturally prone to foot problems. Those individuals with residual foot and leg impairment from strokes may develop foot ulcers from pressure exerted by their shoes or braces and from pressure and persistent friction and irritation caused by altered walking patterns.

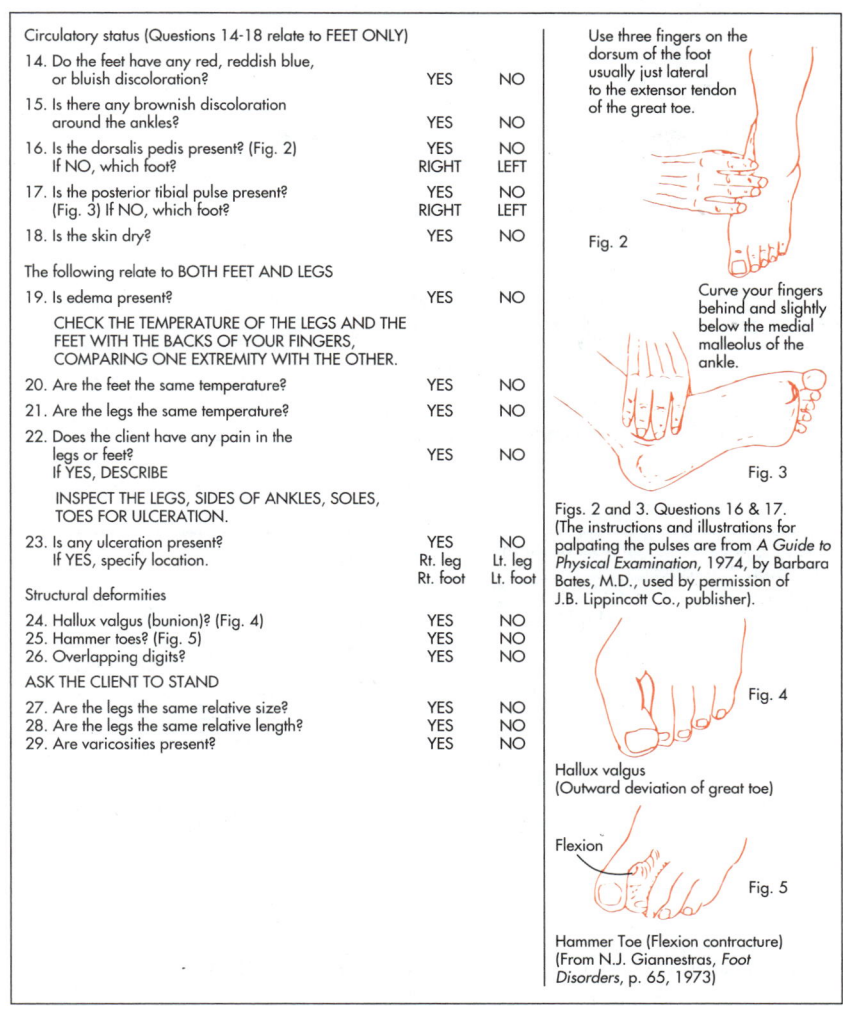

Circulatory status (Questions 14-18 relate to FEET ONLY)

14. Do the feet have any red, reddish blue, or bluish discoloration?	YES	NO
15. Is there any brownish discoloration around the ankles?	YES	NO
16. Is the dorsalis pedis present? (Fig. 2)	YES	NO
If NO, which foot?	RIGHT	LEFT
17. Is the posterior tibial pulse present? (Fig. 3) If NO, which foot?	YES	NO
	RIGHT	LEFT
18. Is the skin dry?	YES	NO

The following relate to BOTH FEET AND LEGS

19. Is edema present?	YES	NO

CHECK THE TEMPERATURE OF THE LEGS AND THE FEET WITH THE BACKS OF YOUR FINGERS, COMPARING ONE EXTREMITY WITH THE OTHER.

20. Are the feet the same temperature?	YES	NO
21. Are the legs the same temperature?	YES	NO
22. Does the client have any pain in the legs or feet? IF YES, DESCRIBE	YES	NO

INSPECT THE LEGS, SIDES OF ANKLES, SOLES, TOES FOR ULCERATION.

23. Is any ulceration present? If YES, specify location.	YES	NO
	Rt. leg	Lt. leg
	Rt. foot	Lt. foot

Structural deformities

24. Hallux valgus (bunion)? (Fig. 4)	YES	NO
25. Hammer toes? (Fig. 5)	YES	NO
26. Overlapping digits?	YES	NO

ASK THE CLIENT TO STAND

27. Are the legs the same relative size?	YES	NO
28. Are the legs the same relative length?	YES	NO
29. Are varicosities present?	YES	NO

Use three fingers on the dorsum of the foot usually just lateral to the extensor tendon of the great toe.

Fig. 2

Curve your fingers behind and slightly below the medial malleolus of the ankle.

Fig. 3

Figs. 2 and 3. Questions 16 & 17. (The instructions and illustrations for palpating the pulses are from *A Guide to Physical Examination*, 1974, by Barbara Bates, M.D., used by permission of J.B. Lippincott Co., publisher).

Fig. 4

Hallux valgus (Outward deviation of great toe)

Flexion

Fig. 5

Hammer Toe (Flexion contracture) (From N.J. Giannestras, *Foot Disorders*, p. 65, 1973)

Figure 7-12. cont'd. For legend see opposite page.

Box 7-10

Essential Data of Foot Assessment

Observation of Mobility

Gait
Ambulation
Foot hygiene
Footwear

Past Medical History

Systemic diseases
Musculoskeletal problems
Vascular/ulcerations/peripheral vascular disease
Vision problems
Falls
Trauma
Smoking history
Pain

Bilateral Assessment of

Color
Circulation
Pulses
Structures (hammer toe, bunion, overlapping digits)
Temperature
Dermatologic aspects
    Skin lesions (fissures, corns, calluses, warts, excoriation)
    Edema
    Itching
    Rash
Toenails
    Long, thick
    Discoloration

ASSESSMENT

Medical history

_____ Arthritis
_____ Diabetes
_____ Peripheral vascular disease
_____ Smoking
_____ Vision problems
_____ Falls in past year
Does client do a daily foot inspection? _____ yes _____ no, comments:
Footwear

                          Does client ever go barefoot? _____ yes _____ no, comments:
_____ Canvas or leather shoes
_____ Shoes fitted properly
_____ Socks
_____ Restrictive leg wear
_____ More than one pair of shoes
                          Appearance of footwear: _____
_____
_____
                          Type of footwear most often worn: _____
_____
Ambulation _____ with _____ without assistance.
Type of device used if assisted: _____
Color and temperature of extremity: _____
Presence of pedal pulses: Right _____   Left _____
Structure
Presence of: Location/remarks
_____ Bunions   _____ Spurs   _____
_____ Corns   _____ Ulcerations _____
_____ Callus   _____ Cracks   _____
_____ Edema   _____ Dry skin   _____
_____ Hammertoes   _____ Blisters   _____
Description of toenails: _____
_____
Skills performed: Foot soak
                  Nail trim
Follow-up date:

Figure 7-13. Foot assessment tool. (From Ruscin C, Cunningham G, Blaylock A: Foot care protocol for the older client, *Geriatr Nurs* 14(4):211, 1993.)

Interventions

Care of Toenails. The inability of the aged to care for their toenails is influenced by poor vision, hand tremors, the inability to bend, obesity, or increased nail thickness. Nails that are neglected or do not receive treatment may become unusually long and curved. This type of nail is known as ram's horn because of its appearance. Hard, thickened nails indicate inadequate nutrition to the nail matrix from trauma or poor circulation. Once the nail becomes thickened, it will remain so. These conditions should be brought to the attention of the podiatrist. Any attempt by the nurse or other caregiver to cut these nails may result in further damage to the matrix or precipitate an infection.

Normal nails that become too long or begin to interfere with stockings, hose, or shoes should be cut straight across and even with the top of the toe (Turner, 1996) (Figure 7-14).

Nails that are hard can easily split, causing trauma to the matrix, pain, and possibly infection. Feet should be soaked in warm water to soften the nails before they are clipped. Ideally, toenails should be trimmed after the bath or shower, but if this is not appropriate, soaking the feet for 20 to 30 minutes will facilitate the procedure. Box 7-11 provides suggestions for a variety of foot soaks for specific aspects of foot care. Foot soaks are not recommended for diabetics. The summary of good foot care, on p. 242, also includes additional foot care measures for persons with diabetes.

An *ingrown toenail* is a fragment of nail that pierces the skin of the nail lip. Often this problem is the consequence of improper cutting of the nail. An additional cause is pressure exerted on the toes by short or supportive hose. This problem, too, should be seen by the podiatrist, but as a temporary measure it is simple enough for the nurse to insert a wisp of

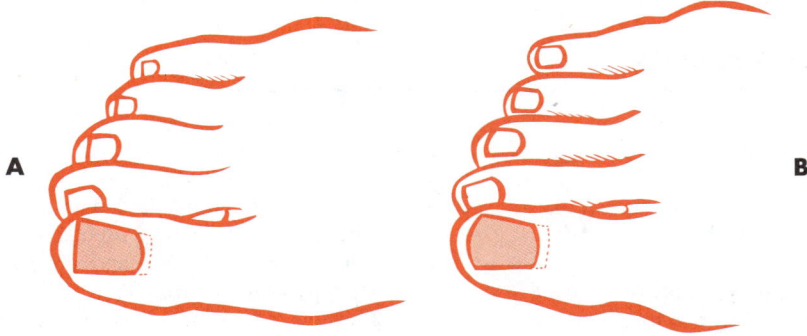

Figure 7-14. Cutting of toenails. **A,** Correct method. **B,** Incorrect method.

cotton under the section of the nail that is growing into the nail lip, which will lift it and reduce the pressure and pain. Cutting a V or wedge in the middle of the nail to cause the nail to grow toward the center and allow the edges to grow properly is totally ineffective. The only result will be that it will take 4 months or more for the V to grow out of the nail. The nail grows from the matrix to the tip of the toe in 120 days; aged nails take approximately 4 to 10 months (Helfand, 1989b).

Shoes. Shoes should be worn that cover, protect, and provide stability for the foot, maximize toe space, and minimize the chance of falls. In essence, shoes should be considered as clothing and be functional (Box 7-12). Slip-on shoes are helpful for those aged who are unable to bend or lace shoes. Velcro closures are also useful to those who have limited finger dexterity. Low-heeled shoes with a wide toe box and a ridged sole minimize falls, place less stress on the legs and back, and are ideal for comfort. The proverbial "thumb's width" is the correct space between the big toe and toe of the shoe. One should also be able to pinch the leather or fabric across the widest part of the upper shoe.

Dependent Edema. Circulatory efficiency in the lower extremities, especially the feet, is sluggish. Edema of the ankles and feet is evident after periods of prolonged sitting and standing. It is helpful if the aged do not wear constricting circular garters, socks with snug bands, or support hose, which constrict the feet. Sitting with the feet elevated on a footstool or hassock is helpful in reducing edema and facilitating better venous circulation. Foot exercises, too, are a means of reducing edema by encouraging more efficient venous return. Exercises can be done anytime. It would be good to develop the habit of doing foot exercises on rising and going to bed. Other times would be during television commercials.

The exercises are simple, and in addition to helping reduce edema, they facilitate foot flexibility. Toe bends, or curling and relaxing the toes, should be done at least five times on each foot. These can be done one foot at a time or both feet together followed by rotating the feet at the ankles

Box 7-11	**Foot Soaks**
Cleansing	Add several drops of mild liquid soap or detergent to warm water
Callus softening	Add ¹/₂ cup vingear or ¹/₄ cup baking soda to 1 quart warm water.
Dry skin	Use warm water only.
Wound or mild infection	Add 2 tablespoons Epsom salts or 1 teaspoon table salt to 1 quart warm water.

Modified from Kaiser Permanente patient information sheet.

clockwise and then counterclockwise 5 to 10 times, and finally, bringing the knees to the chest 5 to 10 times. These exercises can be done consecutively or with short rest periods in between, depending on the stamina of the individual.

Two areas of the foot in older persons may appear to be edematous. The upper outer aspect near the ankle (Figure 7-15) is actually muscle. This can usually be identified by wiggling the toes; it will move. The other area is below and in front of the ankle bone (Figure 7-15). This occurs in some, but not all, women and is a fat pad. Its size remains constant. Singly or together these may look like edema, but they are not. Awareness of these anatomic phenomena will help in assessing edema correctly.

Foot Massage. Foot massage is another useful means of reducing edema, stimulating circulation, and improving pedal flexibility. Not only does massage aid in accomplishing these things, but also it relaxes the feet and stimulates relaxation of the rest of the body. However, *not all elderly are candidates for foot massage.* Individuals with foot lesions or vascular problems of the lower extremities should be seen by the physician for a definitive decision before massage is considered.

Foot massage requires little lubrication and can use the lotion or oil applied after the bath or shower, if done at that

Box 7-12	Buying Comfortable Shoes	
Hint		**Rationale**
Take time to find a good fit		Comfort—it's well worth it
Buy in afternoon		Feet tend to swell during day
Never buy without trying on both shoes		Buy the pair that fits the longer and wider foot
Raise and lower heel of foot in shoe		Heel should fit snugly, instep should not gape
Check soles of shoes		Soles should be flexible and move when foot does
Choose shoes that grip slippery surfaces		Help prevent falls from slips
Allow $1/4$ to $1/2$ inch of room between longest toe and tip of shoe		Prevents cramping, friction, and toe trauma
Look inside shoe for cushioning devices		Helps ease pressure on feet

Modified from Helfand AE: *Focus on geriatric care and rehabilitation,* Rockville, Md, 1989, Aspen.

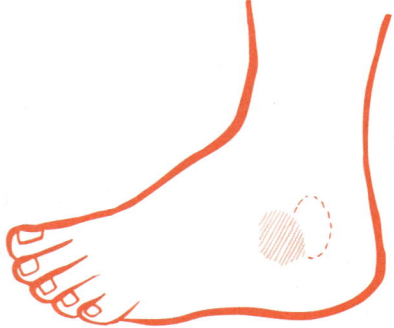

Figure 7-15. Muscle and fat pad mistaken for ankle edema.

time. To give a foot massage, the nurse should be positioned so that the client's feet are easily accessible; sit at the foot of the bed, if the client is reclining, or opposite the client, if seated, with the foot to be massaged cradled between the nurse's knees or resting on something comfortable for support.

Steady the foot to be massaged with one hand, and with the knuckles of the other hand make small, firm circles over the entire sole of the foot including the heel (Figure 7-16). Light touch tends to tickle, firmness does not; however, the feet of the aged may be more sensitive to pressure than those of the young, so the nurse must modulate the firmness of the massage accordingly. There is an overpowering urge when about to touch someone's feet to say "I hope you aren't ticklish." Stifle that urge! The power of suggestion is tremendous! Use firm smooth movements, and you should have satisfying results. You may also find the person seems to spontaneously come forth with conversation. Continue to massage the foot; support the foot with the fingers of both hands while the thumbs repeat the small circles over the entire sole of the foot. As you move your thumbs from the toes you may find that the fingertips are less awkward when you massage around the ankle and the heel (Figure 7-16, *B* and *C*). When your fingers reach the heel, take one hand and gently lift the foot under the ankle, and with the other hand

use the fingertips and thumb to firmly make circles on the heel. More pressure will be required here because of the thicker horny layer of skin (Figure 7-16, *D*).

On the top of the foot, starting at the ankle, look at the long tendons that run from the base of the ankle to each toe. Support the heel of the foot with one hand, and with the tip of the thumb on your other hand firmly but gently run your thumb between each tendon groove and off between the toes (Figure 7-16, *E*). (This can be uncomfortable, so adjust your pressure.) Next grasp the foot between both hands; fingers should be touching on the sole of the foot, heels of the hands touching on the top of the foot (Figure 7-16, *F*). Press the heels of your hands firmly downward on the foot and push up on the sole of the foot with your fingers (like breaking a cracker in half). At the same time slide your hands toward the edges of the foot. Repeat this motion three times. With one hand, steady the foot, and with the thumb and forefinger of the other hand grasp the base of the big toe. Gently stretch and rotate it from side to side, using a corkscrew motion, until your fingers slide off the tip of the toe. Do this to each toe in sequence (Figure 7-16, *G*). To finish the massage, place the foot between your hands; hold the foot gently for several seconds (Figure 7-16, *H*); replace it next to the other foot; gently pick up the other foot, and repeat the massage sequence. The nurse will find that foot massage can be easily modified to incorporate range of motion exercises for the toes and ankles. In addition to foot massage, lukewarm oil (baby, mineral, or vegetable) applied to the feet followed by wrapping in warm moist towels and elevation for 10 to 15 minutes not only facilitates a few minutes of relaxation but aids in improving integrity of the skin of the feet. Feet are then washed in sudsy warm water, dried thoroughly, and dusted with powder.

Diabetic foot care is very similar to that suggested for good foot care. A summary of good foot care and diabetic foot care, identifying the similarities and differences, is presented in Table 7-2. One can basically say that if an individual follows the recommendations for diabetic foot care, feet would be maintained in comfort.

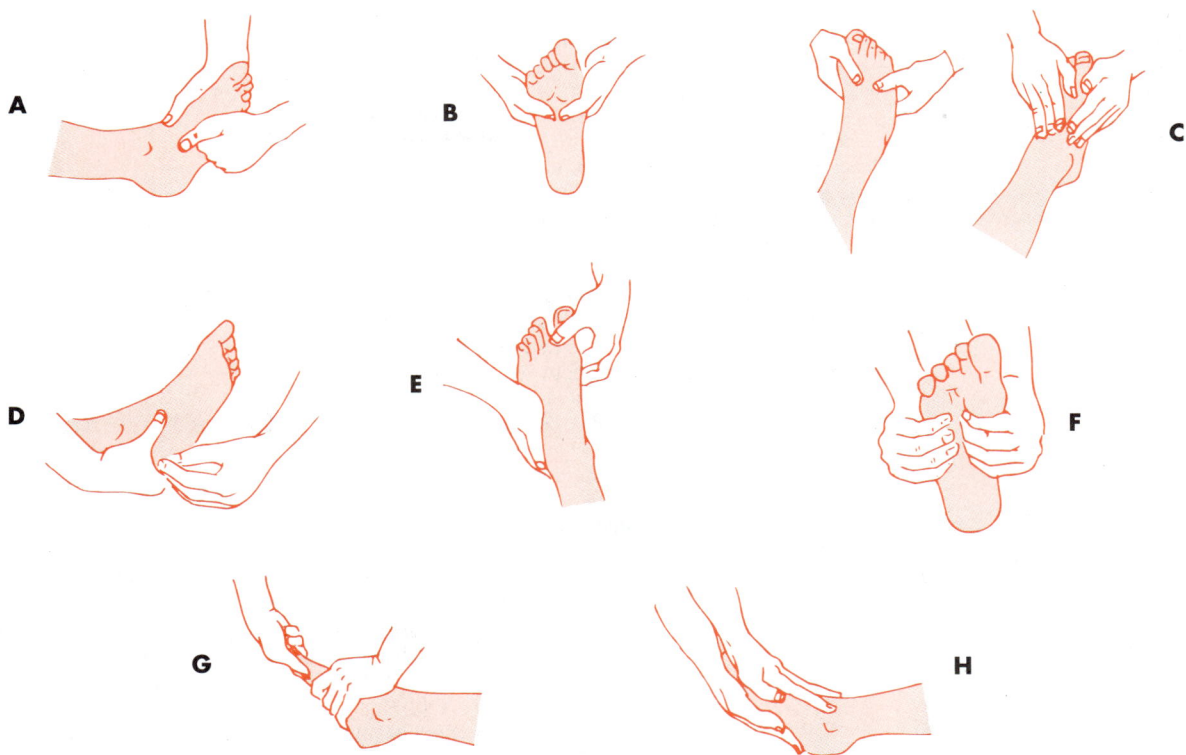

Figure 7-16. Foot massage. **A,** With knuckles make small circles over sole of foot. **B** and **C,** With thumbs and fingers make circles over entire foot. **D,** With tips of fingers make circles on heel. **E,** Gently run thumb between tendon grooves from ankle to toes. **F,** As if breaking a cracker, move the foot back and forth. **G,** Gently stretch and rotate each toe. **H,** End by placing foot between hands.

INTEGUMENT

The skin is looked on as having aesthetic and cosmetic appeal. Artists have portrayed its delicate, flawless qualities, and poets have extolled its virtues through descriptive phrases. Today art, poetry, and conversation still include similar depictions.

The integument does more than keep the skeleton from falling apart. As the largest, most visible organ of the body (Gilchrest, 1986a), its various layers mold and model the individual to give much of his or her identity; glands and hair provide recognizable characteristics and sexual orientation. Skin is important both in health and illness. It provides clues to hereditary, racial, dietary, physical, and emotional conditions. It is also an important means of communication. The integument provides at least seven physiologic functions. It protects underlying structures, serves as a heat-regulating mechanism, serves as a sense organ, is involved in the metabolism of salt and water, and stores fat. The skin facilitates two-way gaseous exchange and converts sunshine into the antirachitic vitamin D (Saxon and Etten, 1994). When the integument malfunctions or is overwhelmed by outside trauma, discomfort, or disfigurement, death may ensue. Despite exposure to heat, cold, water trauma, friction, and pressure, it maintains a homeostatic environment. The skin is durable, pliable, and strong enough to protect the body by absorbing, reflecting, cushioning, and restricting various substances and forces that might enter and alter its function. Yet it is sensitive enough to relay messages to the brain.

The epidermis, dermis, and subcutaneous layers of the skin have specific functions that will affect nursing assessment and intervention. Figure 7-17 outlines the layers of the integument, their structures and functions, and the conditions that frequently occur in the aged. The aged epidermis produces varying cell shapes and sizes. The previously textured skin becomes thin, fragile, shiny, and flat, resulting from the loss of conelike projections called rete ridges. The dermis, lying beneath the epidermis, is a supportive layer of connective tissue composed of a matrix of yellow elastic fibers that provide stretch and recoil, white fibrous collagen fibers that provide tensile strength, and an absorbent gel between the two fibers. The dermis also supports hair follicles, sweat and sebaceous glands, nerve fibers, muscle cells, and blood vessels. With age the dermis elasticity and suppleness is lost because of cross-link changes of the elastin and collagen components (see Chapter 2). Recent studies (1995) have posed the hypothesis that estrogen replacement therapy (ERT) slows skin aging (Wallis, 1995; Wasaha and Angelopoulos, 1996). Though the findings remain controversial, the study found that ERT slowed collagen loss in the

Table 7-2   Essentials of Good Foot Care: Standard and Diabetic

Standard foot care	Applicable to both	Diabetic foot care
	Inspect feet daily for cuts, blisters, reddened areas, and scratches. Use a magnifying glass or mirror to inspect the feet or have someone else do it for you if you can't reach or see well.	
Wash feet daily (if unable to do by self, ask someone else)		Wash feet daily but DO NOT soak feet daily (causes excessive dryness)
	Blot dry rather than rub dry to avoid injury to sensitive skin. Pay particular attention to between toes.	
	Use emollients, cocoa butter, lanolin lotion, mineral oil, or vegetable oil to soften dry skin to help retain moisture and prevent cracking. DO NOT put between toes; it may contribute to fungal infections.	
		Dust lightly with a nonscented powder between toes (can prevent excessive perspiration)
	Soak toenails 10-15 minutes in warm water only on day you trim your toe nails. Cut toenails straight across using a toenail clipper. Never cut down the corners.	
Seek help if unable to trim toenails alone.		Have a podiatrist cut toenails if they are too thick to cut yourself, or if you are unable to cut your toenails alone. DO NOT cut corns or calluses. Have a podiatrist treat them. DO NOT apply harsh chemical corn and wart removing products to the toes and feet. These can remove tissue as well as the corn or wart. DO NOT apply heating pads, chemical or battery operated, to feet.
	Wear clean socks, hose, stockings daily. Cotton socks absorb perspiration for feet that sweat. Keep feet warm with thick fleecy insoles inside slippers to protect from cold or wear cotton socks with comfortable slippers.	
		DO NOT walk barefooted at any time. Sandals for the beach protect the feet from hot sand, sharp objects, etc. At home wear shoes or slippers.
	Wear comfortable well-fitting shoes with broad toe space and low heels.	
Avoid shoes that do not feel comfortable or need to be "broken in."		Good quality athletic shoes, while expensive, outlast regular shoes and are less expensive in the long run. Shake out shoes before putting them on to remove foreign objects that might cause injury. Carefully break in new shoes. Begin by wearing shoes an hour a day, gradually increase the time worn.
	DO NOT pop blisters. Infections can occur	
If blister breaks, wash area, apply antiseptic, keep covered during the day, uncovered at night.		See physician immediately.
	Avoid wearing tight fitting hose, tight stockings, stockings, or garters; DO NOT sit with crossed legs. All of these constrict blood flow to the lower extremities	
	Review the condition of your orthotics regularly. Mark a date with a laundry marker as a reminder for the podiatrist to reevaluate the effectiveness of the device.	
	Stop smoking. Smoking constricts blood vessels, reducing blood flow to the lower extremities.	
	Report foot injuries promptly to the physician.	
		Call physician for any problems such as tenderness, redness, warmth, drainage, ingrown toenail, athlete's foot, pain in the feet or calves.

Modified from Jarvik L, Small G: *Parent care,* New York, 1988, Crown; Helfand AE, issue editor: *The aging foot: focus on geriatric care and rehabilitation,* 2(10):1, 1989; Dellasega C, Yonushonis MEH: Diabetes mellitus in the elderly. In Stanley M, Beare PG: *Gerontological nursing,* Philadelphia, 1995, FA Davis Co.

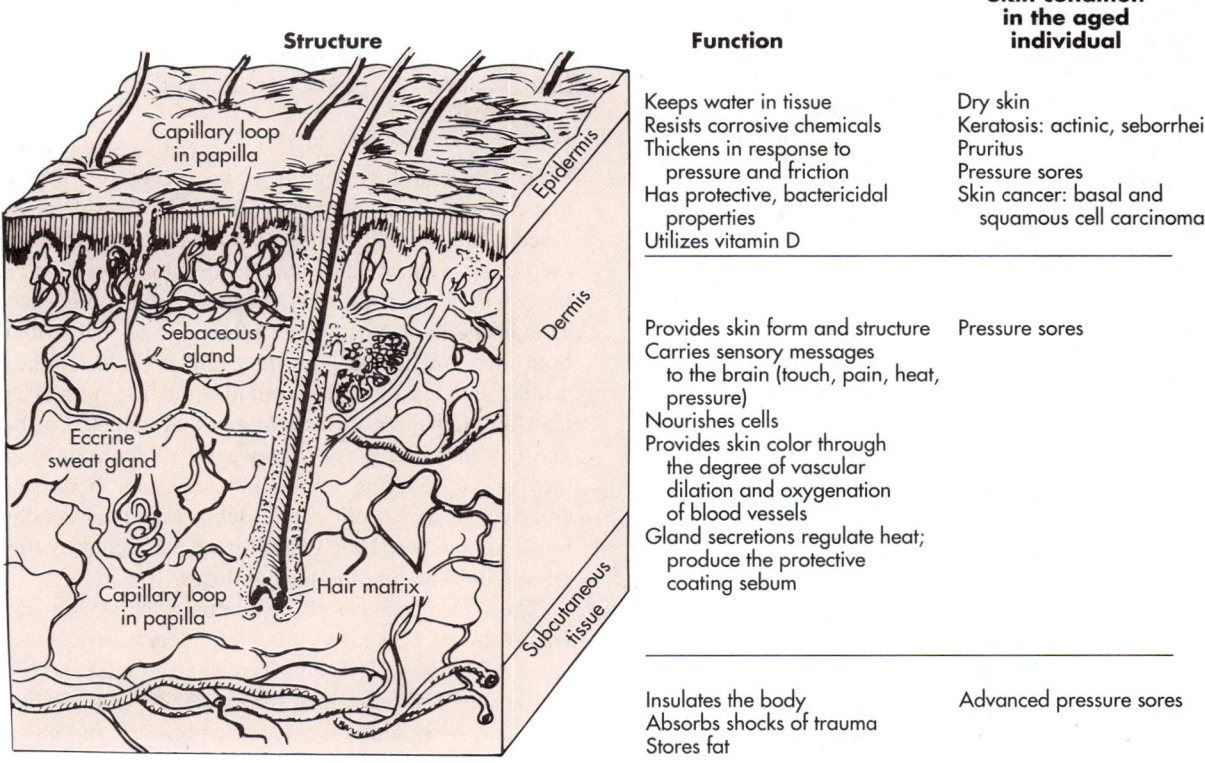

Structure	Function	Skin condition in the aged individual
Epidermis (Capillary loop in papilla)	Keeps water in tissue Resists corrosive chemicals Thickens in response to pressure and friction Has protective, bactericidal properties Utilizes vitamin D	Dry skin Keratosis: actinic, seborrheic Pruritus Pressure sores Skin cancer: basal and squamous cell carcinoma
Dermis (Sebaceous gland, Eccrine sweat gland, Capillary loop in papilla, Hair matrix)	Provides skin form and structure Carries sensory messages to the brain (touch, pain, heat, pressure) Nourishes cells Provides skin color through the degree of vascular dilation and oxygenation of blood vessels Gland secretions regulate heat; produce the protective coating sebum	Pressure sores
Subcutaneous tissue	Insulates the body Absorbs shocks of trauma Stores fat	Advanced pressure sores

Figure 7-17. Correlation of structure and function of integument with some associated conditions.

first few years of menopause. It was also apparent that estrogen deprivation caused alteration of skin elastic fibers. Blood flow diminishes, dermal cells are replaced more slowly, and sensory receptors do not transmit sensations as rapidly (Box 7-13).

The rate at which skin ages is proportional to the degree of exposure to environmental factors such as wind and the irradiation of the sun. The face and hands are the most constantly exposed areas of the body; thus aging is considerably faster in these areas than in those that are rarely exposed. Visible changes of the skin—quality of color, firmness, elasticity, and texture—affirm that one is aging. Skin coloration varies with blood flow. Paleness is apparent with diminished blood blow; conversely, flushing occurs when blood flow increases. Decreased hemoglobin in capillary blood flow that has lost most of its oxygen produces cyanosis. Circulatory disorders affect skin coloration; skin loses its color, and blood vessels become more fragile. Although the aged may appear less attractive physically, like most people they take pride in their appearance and should not be slighted because of wrinkles and saggy tissue.

Pigmentation

Pigmentation changes occur in response to hormone activity. Melanin is affected by the melanocyte-stimulating hormone (MSH), which is similar to adrenocorticotropic hormone (ACTH). Melanocytes increase in size but decrease in number over time; it is the degree of activity that creates the uneven pigmentation. In darker-pigmented races the melanocytes work harder than in light-skinned races. If pigmentation is lacking or insufficient, it is thought that epinephrine, a known MSH antagonist, may have blocked melanin synthesis.

Pigmented moles and nevi are thought to be benign neoplasms, or melanocytes. Freckles are the result of the inability of the melanocytes to produce even pigmentation of the skin. Lentigines, called "age spots" or "liver spots," are similar to freckles. They, too, can occur at any age. In those under 40 or 50 years of age, there does not seem to be a correlation with sun exposure. However, from the sixth decade on, they are thought to be sun related (Lombardo, 1979). The development of lentigines is also thought to be from uneven melanin production. Lentigines are dramatically seen on the back of the hands and wrists of light-skinned races (Porth and Kapke, 1983).

Glands

Eccrine, apocrine, and sebaceous gland activity is influenced by the hormonal and nervous systems; thus if the effectiveness of hormonal and nervous stimulation decreases, glandular activity diminishes significantly.

The sweat glands, or eccrine glands, which are located all over the body, respond to thermostimulation and

Box 7-13	**Structural and Functional Changes of the Aging Skin**

Altered cell proliferation
 Flattened demo-epidermal junction
 Decreased pigmentation (melanocytes)
 Cytoarchitectural disarray
Altered wound healing
Altered immune responsiveness
 Reduced Langerhans cells
Decreased barrier function
Greater tensile strength (less give of tissue)
Elastic fiber changes (wrinkles, lax skin)
Decreased vascularity
Decreased density
Altered thermoregulation
Decreased subcutaneous tissue
Decreased sweat production
Nail changes
Graying of hair (loss of melanocytes)
Decreased sensory perception

Compiled from Richey ML, Richey HK, Fenske NA: Aging-related skin changes: development and clinical meaning, *Geriatrics* 43:49, 1988; Phillips TJ, Gilchrest BA: Skin changes and disorders. In Abrams WB, Berkow R, editors: *The Merck manual of geriatrics*, Rahway, NJ, 1990, Merck, Sharp & Dohme Research Laboratories.

neurostimulation. The usual body response to heat is to produce moisture or sweat from these glands and thus cool the skin by evaporation. Since sweating is diminished in the aged, overheating and heat intolerance are important problems. The aged should avoid spending long periods in the heat, both indoors and outdoors. The summer, in particular, poses a major threat in areas in which there is persistent high humidity and heat. In these areas the death rate among the aged from heat is high. The aged should be encouraged to wear a hat when in the sun, to wear light, cool clothing, and to drink sufficient amounts of fluid.

Apocrine glands are associated with hair follicles and are located in the axillary, genital, and perianal areas and in the external ear canal. These glands are larger than the eccrine glands, depend on hormones, and are responsive to emotions. Their activity begins at puberty but diminishes slightly with advanced age and is responsible for characteristic body odors that occur under stress or excitement (Marks, 1987; Ferrell and Osterwell, 1989). The secretions are odorless until bacteria begin to act on the moisture to produce odors. Deodorants and antiperspirants are often used to suppress odors from the appocrine glands. Dusting powder with baking soda is a natural, inexpensive substance that can keep the axilla dry and free from odor.

Sebaceous glands, which secrete sebum, depend on hormonal stimulation. Because of a decrease in androgen levels and blood supply to sebaceous glands, sebum production decreases with age. Sebum protects the skin by preventing the evaporation of water from the keratin, or horny, layer of the epidermis; it possesses bactericidal properties and contains a precursor of vitamin D. When the skin is exposed to sunlight, vitamin D is produced and absorbed into the skin.

Hair

Hair, as part of the integument, has a biologic, psychologic, and cosmetic value for both men and women. Hair is tightly fused horny cells that arise from the dermal layer and obtain coloration from melanocytes. Hair coloration usually correlates with skin coloration; however, there are exceptions. The hormone testosterone influences hair distribution in both men and women. Axillary and pubic hair tends to diminish with age in women and in some instances disappears. Hair on the head becomes thinner and depleted of melanin, giving it the characteristic gray color. Older women discover they are developing chin and facial hair because of decreased estrogen production. Men become bald or develop a receding hairline. Hair growth is also affected by diet, radiation, physical conditions, and drugs.

The various races have definite hair characteristics, which should be kept in mind when caring for or assessing the aged. Almost all Asians have sparse facial and body hair that is dark, straight, and silky. Blacks have slightly more head and body hair than Asians; however, the hair texture varies widely. It can be fragile and range from long and straight to short, spiraled, thick, and kinky. Whites have the most head and body hair, with an intermediate texture and form ranging from straight to curly and fine to thick and coarse (Giger and Davidhizar 1991; Seidel et al, 1995; Jarvis, 1996). For care of hair and its effects on self-esteem see Chapter 19.

Nails

The aged often complain about the splitting and breaking of their nails. The aged nail becomes harder and thicker, more brittle, dull, and opaque. It changes shape, becoming at times flat or concave instead of convex. Vertical ridges appear because of decreasing water content, calcium, and lipid content. The blood supply decreases as well as the rate of nail growth. The half moon (lunule) of the fingernail may entirely disappear and the color of the nails may vary from yellow to gray (Staab and Lyles, 1990; Gilchrest, 1995).

Photoaging

Solar elastosis, or photoaging, is the result of environmental damage to the skin by ultraviolet sun rays. Many of the changes associated with photoaging are preventable. Ideally, preventive measures should begin in childhood, but clinical evidence has shown that some improvement can be achieved by avoidance of sun exposure and regular use of sunscreens, even after actinic damage has occurred.

Sunscreens offer protection from harmful ultraviolet A and B rays. Effectiveness of sunscreens is measured in terms of the sun protection factor (SPF). The formula, minimal erythema dose (MED), the amount of time it takes to cause the skin to become red, times the SPF provides the length of time, in minutes, that an individual can be in the sun without burning.

Sun-induced damage varies with skin type. Individuals who always burn, never tan, or minimally tan, or who burn moderately and tan to a light brown should be considered to have sensitive to very sensitive skin, which requires SPF 15 or more. Indiviudals who minimally burn and always tan to a moderate brown should use a sunscreen with an SPF 6 to 10. Those individuals who rarely burn and tan to a dark brown require a sunscreen with an SPF of only 4 to 6. The use of sunscreens should not be limited to summer use or sunny days. Damaging ultraviolet rays penetrate clouds and overcast skies.

It must be remembered that the normal skin changes, such as fragility and diminished melanocyte activity, that occur in older adults may not coincide with the level of SPF protection that was adequate when they were younger. The aged individual may require a higher SPF sunscreening preparation. Box 7-14 offers sun protection recommendations.

Preliminary studies have suggested that topical tretinoin (all-*trans*-retinoic acid) has practically reversed the structural damage caused by excessive sun exposure. New capillary formation, collagen synthesis, and regulation of epidermal melanin distribution and the disappearance of premalignant actinic keratoses have been noted with use of tretinoin over a period of 6 to 9 months. However, individuals who apply this topical medication may initially experience erythema and peeling of the treated area. There tends to be more improvement in individuals with slight to moderate sun damage than those with severe photoaging (Phillips and Gilchrest, 1990).

Skin Problems

Consensus in the literature is that the common skin problems of the aged are dry skin, pruritus, seborrheic and actinic keratosis, skin cancer, and pressure sores (Phillips and Gilchrest, 1990). Pressure sores will be discussed in Chapter 8.

Dry Skin. Dry skin (xerosis) is perhaps the most common problem of the aged and is poorly understood. The theory that it results from lack of water in skin tissue has been disproved. Xerosis is probably a reflection of abnormalities in epidermal maturation through lifelong minor cumulative injuries to the skin (Gilchrest, 1986b; Gudas, 1986). Diminished amounts of sebum, secreted by the sebaceous glands, lessen the availability of the protective lipid film that retards the evaporation of water from the horny layer, or stratum corneum. The thinner epidermis allows more moisture to escape from the skin. Inadequate fluid intake has a systemic effect; it pulls moisture from the skin to assist in overall hydration of the body.

Exposure to environmental elements, decreased humidity, use of harsh soaps, frequent hot baths, nutritional deficiencies, smoking, stress, and excessive perspiration con-

---

Box 7-14	**Sun Protection Recommendations**

Avoid getting sunburned. Persons of all skin types and races can sunburn, but fair-skinned persons burn more easily.

Do not consider tanning healthy. Do not try to get a suntan, and avoid tanning booths.

Avoid the midday sun (10 AM to 3 PM) when the ultraviolet radiation is most intense.

Wear protective clothing such as a broad-brimmed hat, long sleeves, long pants; however, be aware that clothing alone does not provide complete protection.

Use sunscreen daily (if going outside), even on a cloudy day because clouds do not block ultraviolet radiation.

Select and use a broad-spectrum sunscreen appropriate for your skin type. Apply to sun-exposed areas 45 minutes before going outside and reapply periodically after perspiring heavily or swimming. If using cosmetics on face, apply sunscreen first.

Use a lip balm that contains a sunscreen. Beware of reflection from sand, snow, and water, which will intensify the radiation.

Avoid sun if using photosensitizing drugs.

Avoid para-aminobenzoic acid (PABA) sunscreens if allergic to procaine, sulfonamides, or hair dyes because of cross sensitization.

Adapted from Hogstel MO: *Clinical manual of gerontological nursing,* St Louis, 1992, Mosby.

---

tribute to skin dryness and dehydration of the stratum corneum. Hospital care promotes dry skin through routine bathing, use of soap, prolonged bedrest, and the action of bed linen on the patient's skin. Repeated wetting and drying of the skin layer cause subsequent swelling and tissue drying. Chapping, drying, and major skin changes occur more slowly and later in those individuals who routinely use emollient skin care products that afford good skin protection. These skin care items are more apt to contain moisturizers and sun-screening agents. Based on the number of commercial skin preparations on the market today, it is obvious that dry skin and protection from ultraviolet rays are recognized problems.

Treatment of dry skin in the aged is focused on the relief of symptoms; the underlying problem cannot be cured. The nurse should be alert to signs of rough, scaly, flaking skin on the face, neck, hands, forearms, sides of the lower trunk, and the exterior and lateral aspects of the thighs. Itching frequently accompanies dryness and may be evident as skin irritation or scratch marks in those areas. Dry skin may be just dry skin, but it may also be a symptom of more serious systemic disease, of which diabetes mellitus, hypothyroidism, and renal disease are examples.

The treatment of dry, itchy skin is to rehydrate the epidermis, especially the keratin, or horny layer. The skin's only moisturizer is water. Substances may be used to enhance water's ability to stay on the skin. This is accomplished with binders (bind water to the skin) and humectants (attract moisture from the air to the skin). Other products such as oils, Vaseline, and zinc oxide serve to keep moisture that is already in the skin from evaporating. Oils and ointments also are designed to coat the skin and replace the skin's natural oil barrier (sebum) (Motta, 1992). Use of superfatted soaps without hexachlorophene are most effective in help to restore the protective lipid film to the skin surface. Basis, Dove, Tone, and Caress are the most common of the superfatted soaps used (Hardy, 1996).

Incorporation of bath oils and other hydrophobic preparations into the bathing routine temporarily helps hold moisture and retards its escape from the skin. However, bath oil poured into the bathtub creates the potential for falls. It is safer and more effective to have the aged person bathe or shower, lightly towel dry, and apply the oil directly onto the moist skin; mild, water-laden emulsions are best. Light mineral oil as a bath aid is equally as effective as commercial brands and is less costly.

Application of lotion or emollients to the body several times each day is another way to keep the epidermal layer lubricated and hydrated; vegetable oil is an inexpensive emollient but may smell or stain clothing. Emollients applied to nonhydrated skin act by trapping the water, which constantly enters the subcutaneous layer from below. "Heavy" (very greasy) emollients have an additional ability to coat the skin, providing a smooth surface film. This seems to be a better barrier against evaporation than cosmetic preparations. Lubricants are most effective when applied to the skin immediately after bathing. Most skin products are effective in the pH range of 6.0 to 7.0 even though the skin pH ranges from 4.5 to 6.0. Cleansing agents with a pH of 7.0 are mild and will cleanse the skin better than cleansers with a lower pH. A moisturizing lotion with a pH range of 6.0 to 7.0 will have a softening effect on the skin. The skin absorbs beneficial ingredients more easily when a product has a neutral pH (Renaissance Medical Inc, 1992).

Maintaining an environment with 60% humidity, alleviating mechanical irritation caused by clothing, encouraging baths and showers with water temperatures at 90° to 105° without limiting bathing, and applying mineral oil after bathing helps to control dry skin (Hardy, 1996). Boxes 7-15 and 7-16 offer tips for healthy skin and care of dry skin.

Pruritus. Pruritus (itching), that "unpleasant cutaneous sensation" (Montagu, 1992), is a symptom, not a diagnosis or a disease, and is an additional threat to skin intactness. Pruritis is the most common complaint of the elderly (Elewski, 1990). It is aggravated by heat, sudden temperature changes, sweating, contact with articles of clothing, fatigue, and emotional upheavals and may accompany such systemic disorders as chronic renal failure, biliary or hepatic disease, and iron-deficiency anemia. Box 7-17 lists the various causes of pruritus in the elderly.

The urge to scratch is an ineffective response to the urge to remove the irritant itch from the skin. When one scratches, a counterstimulus is introduced, which is stronger than the original itch stimulus. The nerve messages become confused or eliminate the itching sensation by the intensity of the scratch stimulus. Itching is akin to pain. The nerve endings that produce cutaneous pain also respond to itching. When rehydration of the stratum corneum is not sufficient to control itching, cool compresses of saline solution or oatmeal or Epsom salt baths may be indicated. Use of a lotion such as Lubriderm or Nutraderm is helpful. Vigorous towel drying intensifies pruritus by overstimulation of the skin and by removing the needed water from the stratum corneum. Guidelines for the treatment of pruritus appear in Box 7-18.

Keratoses. *Seborrheic keratosis* is a benign growth that appears mainly on the trunk, face, and scalp as single or multiple lesions. One or more benign lesions is present on nearly all adults over the age of 65. Most elderly individuals have dozens of benign lesions (Elewski, 1990). It is a superficial, circumscribed, raised area that thickens and darkens in color over time. The greasy, dry-to-rough appearance resembles a "blob of wax." Because the growth gets its coloration from melanin, some individuals fear that it will become malignant. When there is concern about this type of lesion, a biopsy may be necessary to definitively establish that it is benign, not a melanoma. Sebaceous keratotic lesions can at times be picked off with a fingernail, but the lesion soon returns. Generally, this neoplasm is removed by a dermatologist, solely for cosmetic purposes.

Actinic or solar keratosis, unlike the benign seborrheic keratosis, is a precancerous lesion. It is the result of years of overexposure to the sun and is found on sun-exposed areas such as bald heads, hands, faces, ears, and noses. Actinic keratosis is characterized by a localized thickening of the skin eventually becoming crusty which begins as a reddish or brownish, scaly patch or patches on superficial areas. Early recognition, treatment, and removal of this lesion are important to prevent serious problems later.

Skin Cancers. *Squamous cell carcinoma* is the second most common skin cancer, which is more prevalent in fair-skinned, elderly men who live in sunny climates. Other causes that may lead to the development of this type of skin cancer include chronic stasis ulcers, scars from injury, chemical carcinogens such as topical hydrocarbons, exposure to arsenic, and radiation exposure. It begins as a flesh-colored nodule and later becomes reddened and scaly, much like actinic keratosis. It may be hard and wartlike with a gray top and horny texture, or it may be ulcerated and indurated with raised, defined borders. Individuals in their

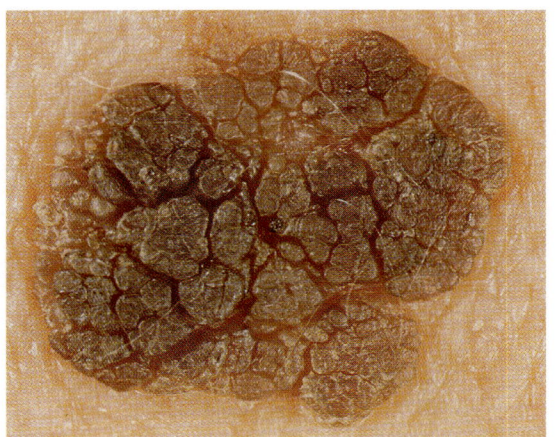

Unn Figure 1. Seborrheic keratosis in older adult. (From Habif TP: *Clinical dermatology: a color guide to diagnosis and therapy*, ed 3, St Louis, 1996, Mosby.)

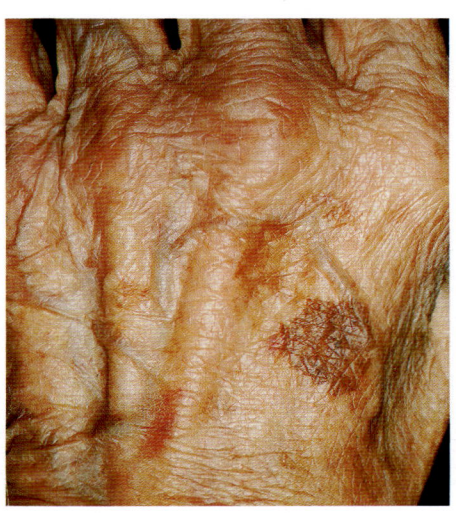

Unn Figure 2. Lentigo, a brown macule that appears in chronically sun-exposed areas. (From Habif TP: *Clinical dermatology: a color guide to diagnosis and therapy*, ed 3, St Louis, 1996, Mosby.)

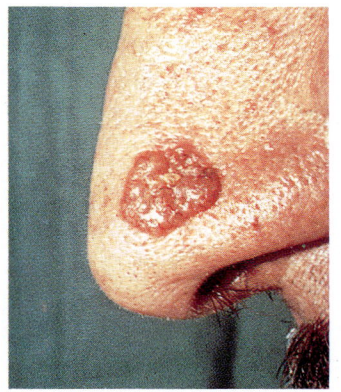

Unn Figure 3. Basal cell carcinoma, the most commonly occurring skin cancer. (Courtesy Gary Monheit, MD, University of Alabama at Birmingham School of Medicine.)

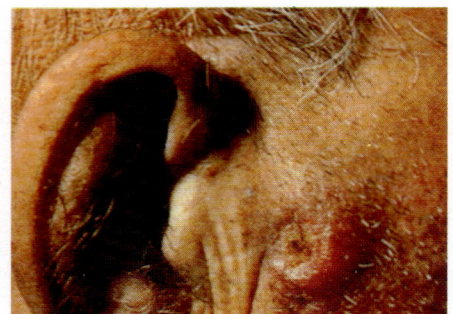

Unn Figure 4. Squamous cell carcinoma. (Courtesy Gary Monheit, MD, University of Alabama at Birmingham School of Medicine.)

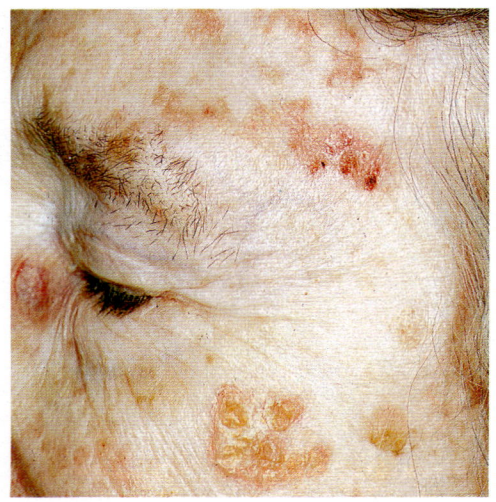

Unn Figure 5. Actinic keratosis in older adult in area of sun exposure. (From Habif TP: *Clinical dermatology: a color guide to diagnosis and therapy*, ed 3, St Louis, 1996, Mosby.)

Box 7-15	Tips for Healthy Skin

Pay attention to any break in the skin.

Use a humidifier if necessary to keep room humidity above 40%.

Bathing every 2 to 3 days is sufficient.

Use a nondeodorant mild soap with lanolin or other creams in its base.

Add bath oil to water—**there is a risk of slipping.**

Use a moisturizer that applies easily, leaves no greasy film, and does not stain clothing.

Apply moisturizers as often as necessary to maintain continuous coverage.

Choose clothing made of soft cotton or other nonabrasive materials.

Drink several glasses of pure water every day.

In cold and windy weather, wear a warm hat, gloves, and scarf to protect extremities.

Wear a brimmed hat to shade from the sun.

Use a sunscreen lotion with the appropriate SPF (usually SPF 15 or higher) on all exposed areas.

Avoid direct sunlight for extended periods.

Box 7-16	Care of Dry Skin

To soften dry skin and keep it soft, do as little as possible to break the skin's natural protective oils; do as much as possible to maintain and replenish them.

- Take fewer and faster soaking baths. In winter, one tub or shower per week is plenty. None is OK too, for the person with dry skin. Sponge bathe armpits, groin, and perianal areas and any other parts of the body that need daily (or more frequent) care.
- Use warm water rather than hot to bathe, whether in the tub or shower. The hotter the water, the more natural oils are washed away.
- Limit the use of soap. One lathering is enough to cleanse most of the normally moist body areas; a damp cloth without any soap is sufficient to clean extremities and body areas that stay dry. Consider using superfatted soap: it need not be expensive— Dove, Tone, and others are superfatted and relatively inexpensive. A soap made of cocoa butter or olive or coconut oil (castile soaps) may be preferred.
- If skin is both dry and itchy, apply a bland cream or lotion freely and often. Do not use rubbing alcohol or rubs containing alcohol: these destroy natural oils on the skin and make it dry out faster.
- Use hand or body cream or lotions that work on all of the dry areas and be sure to apply immediately after bathing, while the skin is moist.
- Avoid long periods in the sun. When going out in the sun or when staying in the sun is unavoidable, use a sun barrier cream. Be sure to reapply protective cream/lotion after swimming.
- Use a cream or lotion that is easily affordable. The most expensive is not necessarily the best. Hydrogenated shortening (Crisco or Spry) or the least expensive cold cream or mineral oil will do a good moisturizing job.
- If dry skin is a problem only in winter, consider installing an efficient, whole house humidifier in the home heating system. Not only will it help the skin hold its natural moisture (less evaporation into dry air), but it will help lower heat costs. Moist air feels warmer than dry; the same degree of comfort at lower temperatures will be experienced.
- If living or working in air-conditioned areas, try to keep the temperature high enough for the air to stay moist. Most air-conditioning systems reduce humidity as well as temperature, and air cooled much below 21° C (about 75° F) is likely to be too dry for dry skin.

---

midsixties who are fair skinned and have been or are chronically exposed to the sun are prime candidates for this type of skin cancer. Squamous cell carcinoma is more aggressive than basal cell carcinoma; it has a higher incidence of metastasis and cannot be ignored.

Basal cell carcinoma begins to appear in about the fifth decade and is the most common malignant lesion of epithelial tissue. It is precipitated by extensive sun exposure, chronic irritation, and chronic ulceration of the skin. It is more prevalent in light-skinned races. This is a slow-growing neoplasm, which appears as a pearly papule with prominent telangiectasis (blood vessels) or as a scarlike area where no history of trauma has occurred. Basal cell carcinoma is also known to ulcerate. Early detection and treatment are advisable, even though metastasis is rare; however, it can occur and be quite disfiguring.

Melanoma. Melanoma is a neoplasm of melanocytes that can spread throughout the body through lymph and blood. It is becoming more prevalent, but it is still less common than squamous cell or basal cell carcinomas. Melanoma has a high mortality rate and also can be a result of sun exposure. Blistering sunburns before the age of 18 are thought to damage the Langerhans cells, which affect the immune response of the skin. The legs and backs of women and backs of men are the most common sites for this neoplasm. Two thirds of the melanomas develop from preexisting moles; only one third arise from new moles. In addition, nonexposed areas of the body are not exempt from the appearance of melanoma (Elewski, 1990; Mayfield, 1992).

Box 7-19 gives the ABCDs for identifying melanomas. Additional identifying features of Melanoma include *E* for elevation (Flory, 1992) and the S factor, or shadow around the lesion. The shadow is a slight erythematous haze extending beyond the normal margins of the mole or suspected lesion (McGrann, 1994).

Box 7-17   Causes of Pruritus in the Elderly

Dermatitis
Eczema
Contact
Seborrhea
Lichen simplex chronicus (neurodermatitis)
Xerosis (dry skin)
Microvascular (stasis dermatitis, erythema)

Papular Scaling Disorders
Psoriasis, Lichen planus

Drug Reactions
Drug withdrawal (delerium tremens)
Erythema multiforme
    Antidepressants, opiates
    Acetylsalicylic acid, idiosyncratic responses

Metabolic Responses
Liver and biliary disorders
Renal failure (uremia)
Diabetes mellitus
Hypothyroidism

Neoplastic Disorders
Benign (seborrheic keratosis)
Malignant (central nervous system tumors)

Hematopoietic Responses
Iron deficiency anemia
Leukemia, lymphoma

Psychogenic Etiologies
Involutional psychoses
Hallucinatory aberrations (dementias)

Infections and Infestations
Bacterial (impetigo, chlamydia)
Viral (herpes zoster)
Yeast infections (candidiasis, monilial intertrigo)
Parasitic (scabies, pediculosis)

Box 7-18   Guidelines for Dealing with Pruritus

Tepid baths using bath oil so as not to further dehydrate skin.
Apply soothing creams or emollients several times daily, especially hands, feet, face.
Wear soft absorbant clothing such as cotton.
Be careful of and use with caution:
    Topical steroid creams (unpredictable absorption)
    Low-dose systemic steroids (likely to result in complications)
    Do not use antihistamines with persons over age 75 (experience sudden, severe side effects).

Box 7-19   The ABCD Rules of Melanoma

A. *Asymmetry:* One half does not match the other half.
B. *Border irregularity:* The edges are ragged, notched, or blurred.
C. *Color:* The pigment is not uniform in color—shades of tan, brown, or black, or a mottled appearance with red, white, or blue areas.
D. *Diameter:* The diameter is greater than 6 mm (size of a pencil eraser) or an increase in size.

From Hogstel MO: *Clinical manual of gerontologic nursing,* St Louis, 1992, Mosby.

KEY CONCEPTS

- Physical adaptation is immeasurably enhanced by good dentition, well cared for and comfortably shod feet, and soft, lubricated skin.
- The appearance, alignment, and anchoring of teeth are subject to negative effects during aging.
- Routine dental care, foods requiring vigorous chewing, and thorough brushing and flossing after meals is helpful in preventing periodontal disease.
- The enjoyment of food and pride in personal appearance are enhanced by care of the teeth and mouth.
- Caring for the feet and toenails is important to maintain mobility, and mobility is fundamental to independence. Foot care should not be neglected.
- Feet often reflect systemic disease or give clues to physical ailments before their actual appearance.
- Foot massage with a good lubricating lotion reduces edema, stimulates circulation, improves pedal flexibility and tends to relax the entire body.
- Individuals with foot lesions or vascular problems of the extremities should have a qualified podiatrist care for their feet routinely. Massage only with the doctor's approval.
- The skin is the largest and most visible organ of the body; the direct mediator with the environment.
- Showering is best for elders and then only 2 or 3 times weekly, followed by the use of moisturizing lotion. Avoid prolonged direct exposure to sunlight.

Nursing Diagnoses

The following potential diagnoses must be considered as well as diagnoses unique to the particular individual:

Impaired skin integrity

Altered health maintenance

Risk for impaired skin integrity: prolonged sun exposure, immobility, decreased natural oils, pressure sores, disruption of skin surface

Risk for impaired skin integrity

NURSING PROCESS AND NURSING DIAGNOSIS
Impaired Skin Integrity: Dry Skin

Defining Characteristics

Flaking skin

Itching skin

Chapped skin

Leathery skin

Scaly skin

Fissures

Erythema (not always present)

Etiologies

Inadequate environmental humidity

Inadequate skin hydration

Dehydration

Exposure to strong soaps

Normal age changes

Knowledge

Normal integument changes with aging

　Anatomic

　Functional

Integument assessment

　Brief history

　Physical examination

Integument disorders (pathologic: common to the aged)

Clinical Judgment and Related Skills

Obtain an integument history using a standardized assessment tool.

Obtain further data about:

　Systemic diseases

　Drug history

　Nutrition

　Environmental factors

Conduct a brief physical examination

　Inspection

　Palpation

Implement nursing interventions to manage and prevent additional problems with dry skin

Teach client/family prevention and self-care and self-maintenance measures (refer to Tips for Healthy Skin; Sun Protection Recommendations; Types and Purposes of Ingredients in Skin Preparations)

Design a home care plan

Evaluate and reassess

NEEDS ADDRESSED AND TASK STRENGTHS

Need to care for self (to maintain biologic function)

Diligent in self-care habits

Has a routine for care of feet, teeth and skin

Monitors own condition

Seeks information on improving aspects of self-care

Continued

The following potential diagnoses must be considered as well as diagnoses unique to the particular individual:
Maintenance of teeth
Alteration in nutrition
Self-esteem disturbance
Altered oral mucous membrane
Altered verbal communication
Social interaction impaired
Risk for social isolation
Body image disturbance

NURSING PROCESS AND NURSING DIAGNOSIS
Altered Oral Mucous Membrane

Defining Characteristics
Oral pain/discomfort
Coated tongue
Xerostomia
Lack of salivation
Oral lesions/ulcers
Leukoplakia
Vesicles
Oral plaque
Dental caries
Halitosis

Related Factors
Pathophysiologic
  Diabetes mellitus
  Oral cancer
  Periodontal disease
  Infection
Treatment-related
  NPO more than 24 hours
  Radiation to head and neck
  Prolonged use of steroids/immunosuppressives
  Antineoplastics
Situational (personal and environmental)
  Chemical trauma
    Acid foods
    Drugs
    Alcohol
    Tobacco
    Noxious agents
  Mechanical trauma
    Jagged/broken teeth
    Ill-fitting dentures
Lack of knowledge
Malnutrition
Dehydration
Mouth breathing
Inadequate oral hygiene

Knowledge
Common changes with age of mucous membranes
  Anatomical
  Functional
  Medication interactions
  Community resources
Mucous membrane assessment
  Brief history:
    Chewing
    Appetite
    Dental history
  Symptoms
  Physical examination
  Nursing interventions to keep mucous membrane intact

Clinical Judgment and Related Skills
Obtain a brief history utilizing a standardized assessment tool
  Dental history
  Nutrition
Conduct a brief physical assessment
  Inspection:
    Mucous membranes
    Teeth
    Saliva
  Observe:
    Nutritional intake
Implement nursing interventions to:
  Prevent and maintain mucous membrane such as:
  Hygiene
  Saliva stimulation
  Diet considerations
  Humidity/lubrication
  Dental advocacy
Patient teaching
  Proper oral care
  Cleaning natural teeth/dentures
  Need for yearly dental examination
Family/community teaching
  Screening
  Prevention
  Self-care
  Health maintenance

▲ CASE STUDY

For two reasons Andrew's teeth, like many others of those 75 years old or over, had loosened and deteriorated. He had ignored regular care, and he smoked a pipe. His teeth were stained and detracted markedly from his appearance and, because they were loosening, his ability to chew was affected. He stubbornly ignored them even though he was fastidious about his appearance and his health in every other respect. Why did he neglect his teeth? Andrew grew up in a time when the dentist had a most amazing array of torture tools and knew exactly how to use them to produce the strongest reaction. Dentists were to be feared. Secondly, it seemed to be in God's plan that all folk lose their teeth around age 70; his parents had, his relatives had, and several of his friends had. He was, in fact, fortunate to still have his teeth and with only one bridge. He had not been to a dentist in more than a decade. He said, "Well, I'm waiting until I get these eyeglasses fitted and the hearing aids taken care of . . . then I'll go to the dentist." When the two lower front teeth loosened to the point he feared swallowing them, he went to the dentist armed with the idea that dental implants would remedy the problem. After thorough discussion of the procedures and alternatives he opted for having all his teeth removed. It seemed to him the best solution, because all his teeth and gums were ravaged by periodontal disease. There was little problem extracting the teeth. Dentures had been made prior to the extractions and were immediately placed in his mouth. The swelling subsided, 2 or 3 weeks elapsed, and the dentures were physically more comfortable—then the psychosocial aspects of the situation began to predominate. Andrew was adamant that he could not adapt to these horrible devices for eating. They would not stay in place, and food strayed beneath them and felt uncomfortable. He couldn't taste his food or enjoy the texture and feel of chewing. He lost interest in food and lost 15 pounds. His socialization had often been around dining, especially going to lovely restaurants. Now he was ashamed to eat in public and thought everyone was aware of how difficult it was for him to chew. He insisted the removal of his teeth was the most devastating thing that had ever happened to him. He did not think it amusing when one of his insensitive friends suggested he was much better off than George Washington had been with his wooden teeth. He returned to the dentist, insisting on implants. The dentist assured him they would consider the possibility if he was unable to adapt to the dentures within a few months. His speech was affected, and articulation was slurred. Sometimes he sounded as if he had imbibed a bit too much. He called friends who had dentures and sought their advice and support. They assured him he would, in time, become unaware of the dentures, and they would feel very natural. They seemed not to understand that the loss of teeth was the first and most undeniable evidence that his body parts were wearing out. He was confronted many times a day with his loss of youth.

Factors to consider: eating was a very important social aspect of Andrew's life; Andrew had been remarkably free from health problems and this was his first confrontation with loss of bodily capacity; Andrew's friends were unable to provide empathetic support; and Andrew felt guilty/angry that he had not taken care of his teeth; and Andrew took great pride in his appearance.

Based upon the case study, develop a nursing care plan using the following procedure*:

List comments of client that provide *subjective data.*

List information that provides *objective data.*

From these data identify and state, using accepted format, two *nursing diagnoses* you determine are most significant to this client at this time. List two *client strengths* that you have identified from data.

Determine and state *outcome criteria* for each diagnosis. These must reflect some alleviation of the problem identified in the nursing diagnosis and must be stated in concrete and measurable terms.

Plan and state one or more *interventions* for each diagnosed problem. Provide specific documentation of source used to determine appropriate intervention. Plan at least one intervention that incorporates the client's existing strengths.

Evaluate success of intervention. Interventions must correlate directly with the stated outcome criteria in order to measure the outcome success.

STUDY QUESTIONS/ACTIVITIES

How do you think this physical change has affected Andrew's self-view? Self-esteem?

How can you assist Andrew to identify and determine previous coping capacities that can assist him to get through this present identity crisis?

Discuss ways you can assist Andrew to avoid a disturbance in nutritional intake.

Develop a teaching plan that you would like to initiate with individuals prior to getting dentures.

What anticipatory guidance might have reduced the stress in the situation?

What preventive strategies can you suggest to avoid loss of teeth and consequent need for dentures?

RESEARCH QUESTIONS

How frequently do older clients see their dentist?

How many old people have access to a specialist in geriatric dentistry, and how many would use these services?

*Students are advised to refer to their nursing diagnosis text and identify possible or potential problems.

Do most elders believe that dentures are an inevitable outcome of aging?

What are the common podiatric problems for which elders seek attention?

How many elders regularly have pedicures?

What percentage of elders have mobility problems related to correctable podiatric problems?

What do elders know about precancerous skin lesions?

Which ingredients in skin cleansing agents (lotions, creams, soaps) facilitate the retention of moisture in the skin and eliminate dry skin and pruritus?

RESOURCES

Skin

Quick Reference Guide for Clinicians No 3
Pressure Ulcers in Adults: Prediction and Prevention

U.S. Department of Health and Human Services
Public Health Service
Agency for Health Care Policy and Research
Summarizes the guidelines and a patient's guide.
AHCPR Publications Clearinghouse
PO Box 8547
Silver Springs, MD 20907
(800)358-9295

American Cancer Society
Slides: *Good News About Skin Cancer* #P72
Video: *A Report on Skin Cancer,* by Dr. Frank Field (13 minutes)
Fry Now, Pay Later #901
Facts on Skin Cancer #825
Melanoma/Skin Cancer—Can You Recognize the Signs #904
Why You Should Know About Melanoma #922
Early Detection of Malignant Melanoma #1523
The Diagnosis and Management of Common Skin Cancers #2558

National Cancer Institute
(800) 4-CANCER
Video loan: *Prevention of Malignant Melanoma; A Program for Melanoma Prone Families*
(Professional Education)
Slides of normal and dysplastic moles

Posters on moles and melanoma
What You Need to Know About Skin Cancer #89-1564
What You Need to Know About Melanomas #89-1563
Progress Against Cancer of the Skin #88-310
The Wellness Way, Skin Health

Krames Communications
312 90th Street
Daly City, CA 94015-1898
Brochure briefly explaining how to examine your skin, conditions to look for, prevention, and risk factors.

Teeth

American Board of Oral Implantology/Implant Dentistry
6900 Grove Road, Dept P
Thorofare, NJ 08066-9447

Local chapter of The American Dental Association
University Dental Schools/Clinics

Oral Care for the Dependent Patient (1/2" videocassette, 20 minutes, color, 1991)
Producer and Distributor, West Virginia Health Science Center
School of Dentistry
Department of Community Dentistry
Morgantown, WV 26506
Sale $39.95; no rental

Feet

Local podiatric society
Local and regional podiatry referral service
Podiatric college/clinic

REFERENCES

An assessment of foot health problems and related health utilization and requirements (abstract), *J Am Podiatr Assoc* 69:102, 1977.

Banting DW: Management of dental caries in the older patient. In Papas AS, Niessen LC, Chauncey HH, editors: *Geriatric dentistry, aging and oral health,* St Louis, 1991, Mosby.

Brown LJ, Meskin HT: *New understanding is gained on patterns of tooth loss,* Rockville Pike, Md, 1990, National Institutes of Dental Research.

Burning feet: *Mayo Clinic Health Letter,* 10(1):1, 1992.

Collet BS: Foot problems. In Abrams WB, Beers MH, Berkow R, editors: *The Merck manual of geriatrics,* ed 2, Whitehouse Station, NJ, 1995, Merck Research Laboratories

Common foot problems: prevention and treatment, *Perspect Health Promo Aging.* 8 (2): 1-3, 1993.

Danielson KH: Oral care and older adults, *J Gerontol Nurs* 14(11):6, 1988.

Dental outlook, keeping a healthy mouth: tips for older adults, Chicago, 1989, American Dental Association.

Dellasega C, Yonushonis MEH: The endocrine system and its problems in the elderly. In Stanley M, Beare PG, editors: *Gerontological nursing,* Philadelphia, 1995, FA Davis Co.

Douglass CW, Jette AM, Fox CH et al: Oral health status of the elderly in New England, *J Gerontol: Medical Science* 48(2): M39, 1993.

Echevarria KH, Bezon J, Black JR et al: A team approach to foot care, *Geriatr Nurs* 9(6):338, 1988.

Elewski BE: Dermatologic disorders of aging. In Bosker G, Schwartz GR, Jones JS, Sequeira M, editors: *Geriatric emergency medicine,* St Louis, 1990, Mosby.

Epstein S: Dental care and the aging, *Perspect Aging,* p 14, Nov/Dec, 1976.

Epstein S: Importance of psychosocial and behavioral factors in food ingestion in the elderly and their ramifications on oral health, *Geriodontics* 3(1):23, 1987.

Fah D: Accessible dental care in an extended care facility, *J Gerontol Nurs* 7:21, 1981.

Feldman RS: Update on geriatric dentistry, *University of Pennsylvania Center for Aging Newsletter* 10:7, 1986.

Ferrell BA, Osterweil D, issue editors: *Aging skin. Focus on geriatric care and rehabilitation,* 2(9): 1989.

Flory C: Skin assessment: perfecting the art, *RN* 55(60):22-260.

Giger JN, Davidhizar RE: *Transcultural nursing,* St Louis, 1991, Mosby.

Gilchrest BA: Dermatologic disorders in the elderly. In Rossman I, editor: *Clinical geriatrics,* ed 3, Philadelphia, 1986a, Lippincott.

Gilchrest BA: Skin disease in the elderly. In Calkins E, Davis PJ, Ford AB, editors: *The practice of geriatrics,* Philadelphia, 1986b, WB Saunders.

Gilchrest BA: Skin changes and disorders, In Abrams WB, Beers MH, Berkow R, editors: *The Merck manual of geriatrics,* ed 2, Whitehouse Station, NJ, 1995, Merck Research Laboratories.

Gudas CJ: Common foot disorders. In Calkins E, Davis PJ, Ford AB, editors: *The practice of geriatrics,* Philadelphia, 1986, WB Saunders.

Hardy MA: What can you do about your patient's dry skin? *J Gerontol Nurs* 22 (5), 1996.

Health after 50: The new tooth saving test, *Johns Hopkins Medical Letter* 7 (8):6, 1995.

Helfand AE, issue editor: *The aging foot: focus on geriatric care and rehabilitation* 2(10):1, 1989a.

Helfand AE: Nail and hyperkeratotic problems in the elderly foot, *AFP* 39(2):101, 1989b.

Jahss MH: Geriatric aspects of the foot and ankle. In Rossman I, editor: *Clinical geriatrics,* ed 2, Philadelphia, 1979, Lippincott.

Jarvik L, Small G: *Parent care,* New York, 1988, Crown.

Jarvis C: *Physical examination and health assessment,* Philadelphia, 1996, Saunders.

Kaplan: The oral cavity in geriatrics, *Geriatrics* 26:96, 1971.

Karuza J, Miller WA, Thines T et al: Psychosocial antecedents and consequences of periodontal disease: a new agenda, *Geriodontology* 7:117, 1988.

Kayser-Jones J, Bird WF, Paul SM, Long L, Schell ES: An instrument to assess the oral health status of nursing home residents, *Gerontologist* 35 (6), 1995.

Kelechi T: Clinical outlook: nursing foot care for the aged, *J Gerontol Nurs* 17 (9):40, 1991.

King PA: Foot assessment of the elderly, *J Gerontol Nurs* 4:47, 1978.

King PA: Foot problems and assessment, *Geriatr Nurs* 1:182, 1980.

Kingston R, Rogowski J, Lillard L: Dental expenditures and insurance coverage among older adults, *Gerontologist* 35(4), 1995.

Lombardo PC: Dermatological disorders in the elderly. In Rossman I, editor: *Clinical geriatrics,* ed 2, Philadelphia, 1979, Lippincott.

McGrann GE: Diagnosis and management and preventing skin cancers, *Ad Nurse Pract* 2(7):36, 1994.

Marino R: Oral health of elderly: reality, myth, and perspective, *Bulletin of PAHO* 28 (3): 1994.

Marks R: *Skin disease in old age,* Philadelphia, 1987, Lippincott.

Mayfield P: Skin. In Hogstel MO, editor: *Clinical manual of gerontological nursing,* St Louis, 1992, Mosby.

Merry JA: Take your assessment all the way down to the toes, *RN* 51(1):60, 1988.

Metatarsalgia: *Mayo Clinic Health Letter,* 9(2): 1991.

Montagu A: *Touching,* ed 2, New York, 1992, Harper & Row Publishers, Inc.

Motta G: *Care of mature skin,* Unpublished manuscript, 1992.

New drugs cure most nail infections, *UCSF to our Neighbors.* 21 (1):1, 1996.

O'Laughlin JM: A dental program for nursing home residents, *Geriatr Nurs* 7:248, 1986.

Palmer CA: Nutrition and oral health of the elderly. In Papas AS, Niessen LC, Chauncey HH, editors: *Geriatric dentistry, aging and oral health,* St Louis, 1991, Mosby.

Papas AS, Niessen LC, Chauncey HH: *Geriatric dentistry, aging and oral health,* St Louis, 1991, Mosby.

Pelican P, Barbieri E, Blair S: Toe the line: a nurse-run well foot care clinic, *J Gerontol Nurs* 16(12):6, 1990.

Phillips TJ, Gilchrest BA: Skin changes and disorders. In Abrams WB, Berkow R, editors: *The Merck manual of geriatrics,* Rahway, NJ, 1990, Merck Sharp & Dohme Research Laboratories.

Porth C, Kapke K: Aging and the skin, *Geriatr Nurs* 4:158, 1983.

Renaissance Medical Inc: Dana Point, Calif, 1992.

Rounds MC, Papas AS: Preventive dentistry for the older adult. In Papas AS, Niessen LC, Chauncey HH, editors: *Geriatric dentistry, aging and oral health,* St Louis, 1991, Mosby.

Richter JE: Functional disorders of the gastrointestinal tract, In Abrams WB, Beers MH, Berkow R, editors: *The Merck manual of geriatrics,* ed 2, Whitehouse Station NJ, 1995, Merck Research Laboratories.

Ruscin C, Cunningham G, Blaylock A: Foot care protocol for the older client, *Geriatr Nurs* 14 (4): 210, 1993.

Saxon SV, Etten MJ: *Physical changes and aging,* ed 3, 1994, Tirasias Press.

Schwab D, Pavlatos CA: The geriatric population as a target market for dentists. In Papas AS, Niessen LC, Chauncey HH, editors: *Geriatric dentistry, aging and oral health,* St Louis, 1991, Mosby.

Seidel HM, Ball JW, Dains JE, Benedict GW: *Mosby's guide to physical examination,* St Louis, 1995, Mosby.

Ship JA, Nolan NE, Pucket SA: Longitudinal analysis of parotid and submandibular salivary flow rates in healthy different-aged adults, *J Gerontol* 50A (5) M 285, 1995.

Staab A, Lyles M: *Manual of geriatric nursing,* Glenview, Ill, 1990, Scott, Foresman/Little Brown Higher Education.

Tosti A: Onychomycosis is often misdiagnosed on clinical exam: culture is the key, *Modern Medicine* 63 (12):3, 1995.

Turner C: Toenail management in the elderly, *Geriatr Nurs* 17(6), 1996.

Ubell E: They can give you a smile that lasts, *Parade Magazine,* 18, March 15, 1992.

Wallis C: The estrogen dilemma, *Time* 145(26):46, June 26, 1995.

Wasaha S, Angelopoulos T: What every woman should know about menopause, *AJN* 96(1):25.

Watson D, Pennebaker J: Health complaints, stress, and distress: exploring the central role of negative affectivity, *Psychol Rev* 96(2):234, 1989.

Wylde M: Finally: a low-tech tooth fairy, *The Aging Connection* 9:3, 1988.

Zarb GA, Schmitt A: The longitudinal clinical effectiveness of osseointegrated dental implants: the Toronto Study. I. Surgical results, *J Prosthet Dent* 63(4):451, 1990.

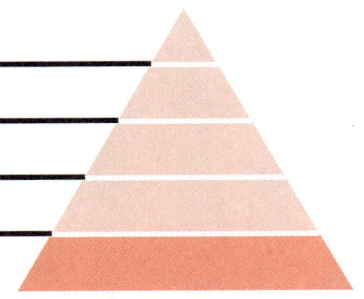

CHAPTER 8

Common Chronic Problems and Their Management

A student learns

Aging has taken on a new meaning for me. I always viewed aging as a new time in life, a time to enjoy and do everything you always wanted to. All of a sudden people would drop dead, not knowing what hit them—no illness, no suffering. The problem is that all the elderly people I have known were financially well off and healthy. But, after taking the course in aging I don't look forward to it anymore. There are inevitable changes that will take place. Disease processes can start that can make you dependent on care and drain you emotionally, physically, and financially. This doesn't include what it does to your family. Aging is an inevitable process that can be good under the right circumstances. However, all it takes is one thing to destroy the remaining years of your life.

Cheryl Pollock, age 27

Elders speak

In living with a chronic illness one is always in danger of a major flare-up over some minor change. Because of this vulnerability, older people become obsessed with everything that might trigger an exacerbation and consequently relate their concerns to anyone who will listen. They become boring and thus are shunned at a time when they most need someone. I have to continually try not to let my disabilities define me, not to present them to others as my identity. It is almost instinctual to use them to seek sympathy. I avoid groups that will continually remind me of my disabilities rather than my remaining abilities.

Fred, age 88

I find an unwillingness to talk about illness in any positive way. I have an incurable disease that will ultimately cause my demise, but I treasure the time I have left. When my friends say, "But you look so well," I feel gratified that for that day I have tamed the illness and it has not got the upper hand.

Lyn, age 85

Coping with the results of a stroke that occurred in 1989 has meant an adjustment to a movement-restricted life. I have had to regard progress in microimprovements and learn to live in this day, sometimes in this moment. It's been important to develop patience and to find the many ways that I can help and support others. Holding off depression and discouragement have become intensely important.

Aveline, over 70

LEARNING OBJECTIVES

Upon completion of this chapter, the reader will be able to:

1. Identify several most common chronic disorders of the aged and their sequelae.
2. Relate strategies that have been used successfully to maintain maximum function and comfort in the client with a chronic disorder.
3. Complete a nursing care plan appropriate to the care of an individual with a chronic disorder.

4. Explain lifestyle factors that frequently exacerbate chronic disorders.
5. Discuss activities of daily living (ADLs) and instrumental activities of daily living (IADLs) in relation to chronicity.
6. Describe some of the effects on self-concept of chronic disorders.
7. Explain the trajectory concept and its relationship to chronicity.

CHRONICITY

Lubkin (1995) provides the most cogent, inclusive, and appropriate definition for chronic illness that we have found: "Chronic illness is the irreversible presence, accumulation, or latency of disease states or impairments that involve the total human environment for supportive care and self-care, maintenance of function and prevention of further disability" (p. 8). Though we particularly ascribe to Lubkin's definition, in 1956 Mayo provided a good definition as well: "All impairments or deviations from normal which have one or more of the following characteristics: are permanent, leave residual disability, are caused by non-reversible pathological alteration, require special training of the patient for rehabilitation, and may be expected to require a long period of supervision, observation or care." Those disorders that truly fit Lubkin's and Mayo's definitions are ongoing, poorly recognized, and largely ignored by everyone except those directly affected by them.

Healthy People 2000: National Health Promotion and Disease Prevention Objectives is a historic document developed in 1991 by the U.S. Department of Health and Human Services (1991) for the express purpose of moving forward into a preventive, wellness attitude toward health and and to decrease the "wait and see what develops and then diagnose and treat" approach to health care. For the elderly this is a significant change in perspective because most of the disorders of aging are chronic ones that must be treated within a framework of lifestyle changes, living situation adaptations, and attention to the whole person coping with a disorder (Burggraf and Barry, 1996). Thus *Healthy People 2000: Midcourse Review and 1995 Objectives* (US Department of Health and Human Services, 1995) measures progress toward specific target goals for older adults that have been defined as desirable and hopefully will be achieved before the year 2000. Some of these are specific to the reduction of the incidence and degree of chronic impairment. We will not reach the desired outcomes in the short time remaining in this decade, century, and millenium, but the shift in direction is significant. In 1985 111/1000 elders (over 65 years old) had difficulty in performing two or more personal care activities. Presently this has been reduced to 100/1000. This is a small but important movement toward health. The greater present concern we have is that those who are now coping with chronic illness be provided sufficient support, assistance, accoutrements, and comforts to enjoy the extended life span that is more and more possible for the aging population. This text and particularly this chapter are devoted to those ends.

We recommend that nurses or students unfamiliar with the specific illnesses of their clients, and the medical managment, review the excellent *Merck Manual of Geriatrics,* second edition (Abrams et al, 1995). *The Merck Manual* is the most widely used medical text in the world. Now in its sixteenth edition, it has been the Bible of diagnosis and therapy since 1899 when the first one was published "expressly designed to meet the needs of general practitioners . . . to make him at once master of the situation and enable him to prescribe exactly what his judgment tells him is needed for the occasion" (Berkow, 1992). In 1990, in response to the massive increases in the aged population, Merck issued the first edition of *The Merck Manual of Geriatrics* (Abrams and Berkow, 1990). They soon realized the necessity of nursing input, and that perspective is included in the second edition of *The Merck Manual of Geriatrics,* published in 1995 (Abrams et al, 1995).

Why do we recommend a medical text in addition to the healthy aging text we are presenting? We believe it is essential that nurses be extremely well grounded and that one nursing text cannot give sufficient guidance in illness and wellness, both of importance to elders. Given the degree of knowledge necessary today and the level of nursing responsiblility for client management, it is imperative that the nurse be thoroughly prepared for each case. The nurse is often the primary care manager and must lay the foundation for all other services. Chronic illnesses create limitations, and when we consider the physiology of the disorder as it affects the quality of life, we implicitly accept the reality of illness.

Chronic disorders and acute illness cannot really be separated, because so many conditions are intricately intertwined; acute disorders have chronic sequelae and many of the commonly identified disorders tend to intermittently flare up and then go into remission. Many elders have several chronic disorders simultaneously and have great difficulty managing the complexity of these overlapping and often contradictory demands. The management of chronic illness largely relies upon the client and caregiver. Health care coverage is usually limited and available only when a particular improved outcome is expected.

Physical disabilities are often multiple and serious but need not kill the spirit or define the person. However, Hwu

(1995) found that psychologic functioning was often more affected than physical or social functioning. The diagnosis, duration of the disease, and economic status were the factors most influential in psychologic adjustment. The challenge to the aged individual with multiple disabilities and chronic problems may simply become overwhelming. Heidrich (1996) found that women with arthritis were as psychologically distressed as those with breast cancer and that strong social networks had more positive effects on both conditions than any other factors. Additionally, Hwe (1995) found that social functioning may mediate psychologic adjustment, but that is largely dependent upon education and occupation as well as age, sex, marital status, and economic status. In Hwe's study, the least affected aspects of a patient's functioning were related to performing ADLs.

One of the earliest geriatric nurse pioneers, Eldonna Shields, once said, "Old age is a losing game when focused on function" (Shields, 1990). Our culture values independence, and winning is among our most revered goals. We, as nurses, are challenged to authenticate necessary dependency and to respect those who have the courage to let go of function when necessary. The things nurses "do" and the order in which they are done is probably far less important in chronic disease management than how they are done and with what attitude.

Carrie (a home health nurse) knelt on the carpet while applying dressings to open, nonhealing leg wounds that were a result of impaired circulation in an elder. She laughed and chatted, sharing some of her own interests and concerns as she worked. She had brought a book of hummingbird

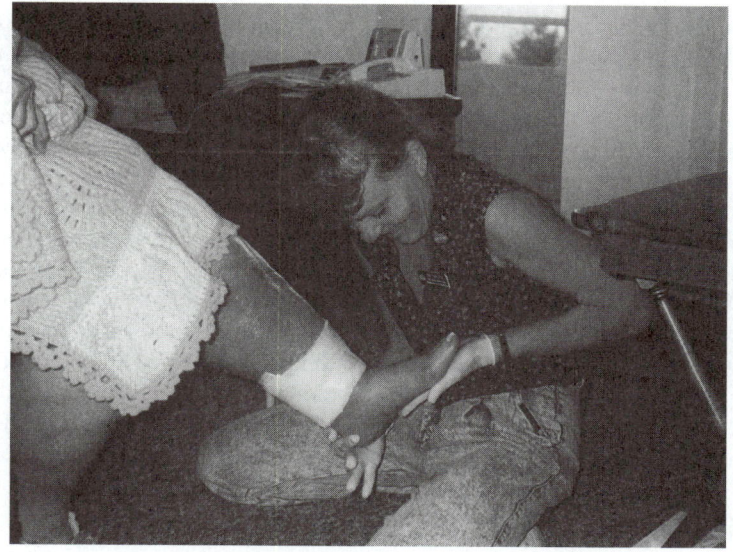

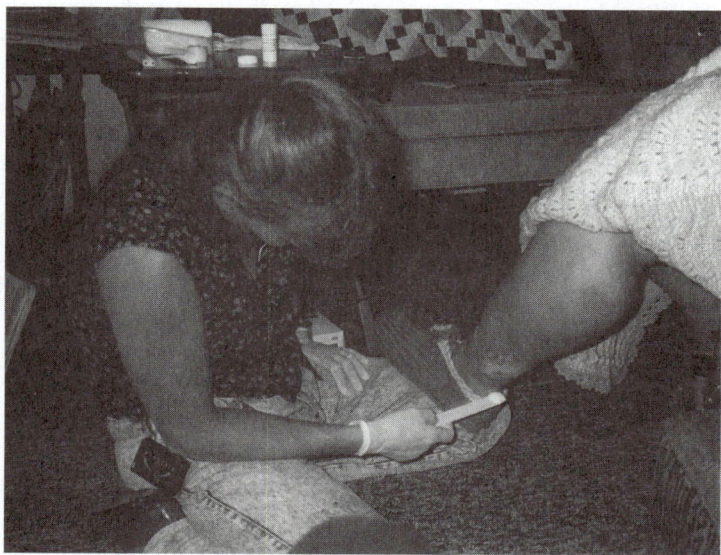

Care of venous statis ulcer. (Courtesy Priscilla Ebersole.)

photographs for the client to enjoy. She said, "I practice down on my knees." This, from our perspective, was nursing in its highest sense. It is symbolic of much of our practice with elders: conducted "down on our knees," pleading to powers beyond our understanding to restore health and function.

The nurse's greatest challenge in working with the chronically ill is to assist them to maintain hope, to sustain interest in their own welfare, and to develop the capacity to view the restrictions imposed by the disorder as having the potential for personal enrichment. Sacks's (1995) work with the neurologically disabled provides insight into a humanistic and expansive manner of dealing with functional deficits: ". . . I am sometimes moved to wonder whether it may be necessary to redefine the very concepts of 'health' and 'disease,' to see these in terms of the ability of the organism to create a new organization and order, one that fits its special, altered disposition and needs, rather than in the terms of a rigidly defined 'norm'" (p. xviii). Nurses must resist the urge to "educate" the client. The giving of information by one who has not experienced the particular condition and knows not the outcome or the subjective resources of the individual is presumptuous at best and often becomes insulting. The good and helpful intentions of the nurse must be in the direction of supplementing, and enhancing when possible, the individual's knowledge of resources, both objective and subjective. Knowledge of the client and caring about the client are crucial, and in the case of chronic disorders the client must educate the nurse before a plan of care can be developed.

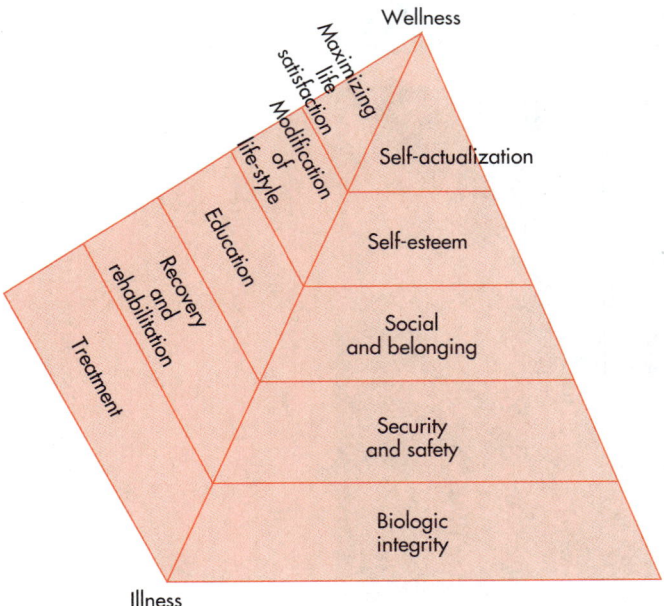

Figure 8-1. Correlation between illness-wellness continuum and Maslow's hierarchy of needs. (Developed by Patricia Hess.)

Wellness in Chronic Illness

The aged with one or more chronic conditions can be supported toward the achievement of wellness and maximization of life satisfaction by caregivers who ascribe to a holistic philosophy that incorporates efforts directed toward the maintenance of the elderly person's self-care and self-esteem. Figure 8-1 shows how the wellness continuum and Maslow's hierarchy of needs can complement each other in the attainment of wellness and self-actualization. It is clear that a reorganization of thinking is needed by the aged and those associated with them: kin, friends, and caregivers. Physical manifestations of chronic illness should not be the sole determinative factor in the establishment of the elder's state of health or wellness. The greatest factor in establishing wellness is adaptation. The illness-wellness continuum illustrates this well (see Chapter 3). To achieve maximization of life satisfaction, adaptation of lifestyle is necessary.

What is wellness in the face of chronic illness? This produced a lively discussion from the contentious voices of an assertive group of elders. Comments such as, "Let's get real!" "I'm like the old one-hoss shay* . . . losing a little something every day. Someday, I'll wake up and find that nothing works." Elders don't graciously accept their chronic disorders—they mourn their losses. They talk about them, but not to the exclusion of other events and interests in their lives. They believe competition and conviction undergird their remarkable survival capacity and will always remain important. They also believe in being responsible and responsive to their community. They are an elite group with plenty of past laurels, but it is doubtful they will ever feel it is time to sit back and rest on them. Although they argue about wellness in illness, we believe they are the epitome of wellness.

Chronic Illness and Aging

Chronic illness is the hallmark of aging. It is the accrual of life's earnings, sometimes self-generated, often inherent or as a result of imposed lifestyles and environmental hazards. Too often, the results of treating acute disorders is a chronic residual disability. The thought has been, "It's a small price to pay for staying alive." For years, individuals with strokes or intractable pain of arthritis were simply told, "You must just learn to live with it." But, finally, chronic disorders are being taken seriously as we confront the individual, social, and economic costs of chronic impairment. The development of geriatric nursing has been largely based on caring for those with persistent disorders that kill slowly but erode joy and function.

In this chapter we consider ways in which nurses may assist their clients toward an enriched capacity for living in the shadow of chronic disabilities, so many of which are common to the aged. Arthritis is almost universal but more trou-

---

*One-hoss shay is a horse drawn cart commonly used for transportation in the early 1900s.

blesome for some than others; often there is some mild to severe cardiovascular problem; breathing becomes more difficult; digestive disorders and nutritional problems go hand in hand, often including elimination problems; and diabetes is common and sometimes out of control, creating many other problems. Several of these disorders may intermingle to put a damper on the vitality of all but the most mentally robust. However, a state of wellness may be achieved and maintained quite consistently if the individual feels capable of and motivated to manage the problems, with or without assistance.

Scope of the Problem

There is a growing recognition that chronic illness is the major area of health concern and that health care professionals and the lay public have inadequate knowledge of chronic illness, its management, and the priorities and economics that have dictated inadequate policies and services. The prevalence of chronic diseases continues to rise with the lengthening of frail aged life span and highly technical medical care. There has been an overall average 9% increase in chronic disorders since 1980, with the greatest increase (26%) in orthopedic impairments. However, these statistics may be inaccurate because the system to collect data and to provide support and care for individuals with chronic problems is both chaotic and ineffectual. Dr. Robert Butler, director of the International Longevity Center, predicts, "We won't get a solution until angry families demand services they haven't had. There'll be a whale of a splash when the baby boomers hit Golden Pond, starting in 2011. Then you wouldn't be elected dog-catcher if you didn't respond to chronic care needs (Ingram, 1996, p. 7).

In 1990 the direct medical cost for treating chronic conditions was $425 billion, 61% of the entire United States' health care costs (Ingram, 1996). It is estimated that 90 million people in the United States were afflicted by chronic disease and the comorbidity. The National Chronic Care Consortium based in Bloomington, Minnesota, notes that these conditions plunder the personal bank accounts of elders. The average Medicare enrollee will spend about $3000 annually out-of-pocket on these disorders. In the past the predominance of short–term cure oriented conditions consumed most health resources. This balance is shifting (Ingram, 1996), though we still do not have a full grasp of the problems of chronic disorders because data is collected only in certain places and by specific groups. Medicare stringently limits home care support for chronic disorders. Verbrugge and Patrick (1995) analyzed seven chronic conditions, three nonfatal (arthritis, visual impairment, and hearing impairment) and four fatal (ischemic heart disease, chronic obstructive pulmonary disease, diabetes mellitus, and melignant neoplasms), for impact on activity levels and use of medical services. The nonfatal conditions limited functioning considerably more than the fatal conditions but received far fewer health services.

Chronic illnesses tend to be composed of multiple diseases, are long term, unpredictable, and expensive, intrude into life course and self-concept, and require extensive palliative care. The incidence of chronic illness triples after 45 years of age but is thought to decrease markedly in relation to higher socioeconomic status. However, Reed et al (1995) studied a large sample of affluent elderly in Marin County, California, to obtain information about health status of an advantaged population. They found few differences in health and function from those with few socioeconomic advantages other than the Marinites having lower mortality and depressive rates and better memory performance. While death was somewhat postponed, the prevalence of disease and disability were not. This shows that some of the suppositions we have about chronic disease and care in the home have simply never been thoroughly investigated. We do know that declines in mortality result in increased morbidity and numbers of individuals with multiple chronic disorders. At times the aggressive treatment of one disorder results in the emergence of additional disabilities, iatrogenically induced.

Certain terms describing the accompaniments of chronic disease, such as handicap, impairment, and physical limitation, are used rather indiscriminately. Decreased function without incapacitation also needs to be stated consistently. Because these and other terms are often used interchangeably, available statistics may be easily misinterpreted if one does not use caution. The most prevalent chronic conditions in individuals over 75 years in rank order are arthritis (58% incidence, nearly twice as common in females), hearing impairments (36% incidence, 75% more common in females), hypertension (39% incidence, slightly more common in females), heart conditions (33% incidence, slightly more prevalent in females), cataracts (28% incidence, nearly twice as common in females), and orthopedic impairments (21%) (U.S. Bureau of the Census, 1995). Of course, one must consider the population predominance of females over the age of 75 and the possibility that only the hardier males survive beyond age 75. Interestingly, individuals between 65 and 74 years old have a higher incidence of dermatitis, sinusitis, ulcers, and asthma than those over 75.

At some point, even in the face of devoted family caretakers, it is highly likely that a very old woman, and about 10% as many very old men, will require care in a nursing home as a result of numerous, ongoing chronic problems that have become devastatingly disabling. It is also likely that resources of family and individual will by then have become exhausted. Elders and others with disabilities make up 27% of Medicaid beneficiaries but account for 59% of the total Medicaid spending, most of it on long-term care (Riley, 1996). Recent figures show that annual spending of Medicaid dollars per capita for elders averages $9,293. This leaves many recipients extremely vulnerable to legislation that is quite rapidly shifting responsibility entirely to states. Numerous governors of poorer states may need to make very difficult choices. The long-term care industry, chiefly represented by the American Health Care Association (AHCA) and American Homes and Services for the Aged (AAHSA) are mounting extensive and expensive campaigns to prevent this shift for fiscal reasons. Ideally, long-term care would be an undergirding service, a benefit of citizenry, that could be relied upon at minimal cost when needed by individuals and their families in late life. However, at present it is not a social service but an enormous profit-making endeavor that will remain so in the foreseeable future. There remain numerous abuses and federal regulations. However, the progress in quality of nursing home care is visible. Primarily nurses, and some other health care providers, have managed in the face of almost insurmountable challenges, through sheer courage and tenacity, to bring the quality of care in nursing homes ever higher. This will continue, with or without federal regulations, because of the commitment of numerous nurses and others.

Chronic Illness Trajectory

In considering an appropriate conceptual framework for the study of chronic illness we have tried to blend Corbin and Strauss with Maslow. The trajectory model of chronic illness, originally conceptualized by Anselm Strauss (Strauss and Glaser, 1975), has aided health care providers to better understand the realities of chronic illness. Later, Corbin and Strauss (1988) presented a view of chronic illness as a trajectory that traces a course of illness through eight phases, which may be upward, downward, or plateaued. In its entirety, a chronic illness may include a preventive phase, a definitive phase, a crisis phase, an acute phase, a comeback, a stable phase, an unstable phase, deterioration, and death. Key points of the model are based on the theoretical assumptions in Box 8-1.

Maslow's concept of five major levels of need that affect function and self-perception fit nicely with the Corbin/Strauss model (see Figure 8-1). The patient's perceptions of needs met and basic biologic functional limitations are paramount to predicting movement within the illness trajectory (Woog, 1992a). In this respect, our wellness approach largely hinges on assisting the elder to meet as many of the Maslovian defined needs as possible at any given time. These efforts enhance the individual's potential for remaining on a plateau or gaining ground in any of the trajectory phases (Table 8-1).

It is significant to note that Corbin and Strauss (1988) focused a great deal of attention on the impact of chronic illness on self-concept and self-esteem. There ". . . are a host of biographical consequences, which in turn cycle back to affect to some degree the trajectory work and the illness itself. These include the changing relationships of body, self, and sense of biographical time" (Corbin and Strauss, 1988, p. 2). The trajectory of chronic illness varies with the individual and the disorder. It may progress slowly, relentlessly, or unpredictably through exacerbations and remissions,

or the superimposition of other disorders and treatments may change the projected course of the disability. It is being found that the diagnosis itself is significant in coping. Women with arthritis perceived their illness to be more severe and less controllable than those with breast cancer, and this had profound effects on their psychologic well-being (Heidrich, 1996). One wonders if there is less concern and sympathy exhibited for arthritis, or fewer secondary benefits.

In 1988, Strauss and Corbin emphasized the changing nature of health care needed for an aging population in which chronic disorders are by far the most prevalent forms of illness. The incidence of chronic disease is increasing in proportion to life-saving technologies. Until the late 1930s, prevailing illnesses were predominantly caused by bacteria or parasites. With the advent of antibiotics and immunizations these diseases decreased markedly in the industrialized nations. Instead, cancers, arthritis, and cardiovascular conditions have become the most common health problems. Recently, cancers and cardiovascular conditions have decreased somewhat, and infectious diseases are returning with a vengeance. Since the last edition of this text we have seen enormous restructuring of the health care system in ways that are beginning to more realistically serve the large numbers of chronically ill. In many ways the acquired immunodeficiency syndrome (AIDS) epidemic has been the catalyst for change. As the society becomes more unhealthy in terms of environment, diet, infectious agents and stress inducers, more attention is being paid to seeking a healthy lifestyle. Strauss, a pioneer in conceptualizing chronic illness, died in September, 1996. We believe he accomplished much toward achieving some of the goals of understanding chronic illness that we are advancing toward at present.

Perceived Uncertainty of Illness Trajectory. Wineman et al (1996), grounded in the theories of illness trajectory, have proposed that there is a relationship between effectiveness of coping and the degree of perceived uncertainty in chronic disease and functional disability. They have shown in previous research that the types and quality of social supports and the perception of purpose in life influence one's adaptation to chronic disorders (Mishel and Braden, 1988). While research is progressing in untangling and understanding the relationships among these apparently critical factors, nurses are the most likely health care providers to be cognizant of these issues and to encourage clients' expression of perceptions related to uncertainty, quality, and durability of support networks and purpose in life. Given the uncertainty of future resources and the numerous concerns about the stability of the health care system, uncertainty is pervasive even in the best of circumstances.

Knowledge of disease processes may help in coping with even those diseases that have an unpredictable course. Many disabilities require organizing and maintaining physical and social arrangements involving space, time, work, and other persons. One's knowledge of personal strengths and needs and careful monitoring of body signs must guide an individual's decisions. Symptoms are signposts. Assisting clients to become alert to subtle bodily signs and symptom changes can be extremely beneficial in reaching a healthier level of existence. Body awareness and management of symptoms that cause acute distress are essential in the process. The comeback phase of illness is a period of rehabilitation that is an uphill course. It may be long and difficult with small setbacks, periods of improvement, and plateaus of unpredictable duration. During this period the client raises many questions that may not have answers:

- How reversible is this illness?
- Which of my previous activities will I be able to pursue?
- How long will I remain on a plateau?
- How much will my actions affect the outcome, and what actions should I take?
- Will the fluctuations in function always be a part of my life?

Box 8-1   Theoretical Assumptions Regarding Chronic Illness Trajectory

- The prevalent form of disease at this time is chronic illness.
- These presumably incurable illnesses may appear at any time in the life span but are most frequent in late life.
- Chronic illnesses are life-long and entail lifetime adaptations.
- Those with chronic illnesses are likely to experience the trajectory phases identified by Strauss and Corbin (1988).
- The acute phase of illness management is designed to stabilize physiologic processes and promote a comeback from the acute phase.
- Other phases of management, except the severely deteriorating, are primarily designed to maximize and extend the period of stability in the home with the help of family and augmented by visits to physicians or clinics.
- Maintaining stable phases is central in the work of managing chronic illness.
- Chronic illness and its management often profoundly affect the lives and identities of the afflicted and the family members.
- The *management in the home by the family, self, or significant other is central to care and is not peripheral to medical management* (Strauss and Corbin, 1988).
- Recommended actions require appropriate timing and patience of the family and the practitioner.
- A primary care nurse able to coordinate multiple resources may be needed.
- Finally, creativity and ability to use what is available are essential to successful management.

The nurse's function is to encourage the client to express these questions and, together, to seek answers and resources.

Special Considerations

Regardless of the nature of chronic problems, there are special considerations that almost universally need attention and must be addressed actively by nurses. It is not sufficient to wait until the client brings up the topic.

Table 8-1   Definitions of Phases and Goals

Phase	Definition
1. Pretrajectory	Before the illness course begins, the preventive phase, no signs or symptoms present
2. Trajectory onset	Signs and symptoms are present, includes diagnostic period
3. Crisis	Life-threatening situation
4. Acute	Active illness or complications that require hospitalization for management
5. Stable	Illness course/symptoms controlled by regimen
6. Unstable	Illness course/symptoms not controlled by regimen but not requiring hospitalization
7. Downward	Progressive deterioration in physical/mental status characterized by increasing disability/symptoms
8. Dying	Immediate weeks, days, hours preceding death

Examples of goals that nurses might establish include:

1. To assist a client in overcoming a plateau during a comeback phase by increasing adherence to a regimen so that he or she might reach the highest level of functional ability possible within limits of the disability.
2. To assist a client in making the attitudinal and life-style changes that are needed to promote health and prevent disease.
3. To assist a client who is in a downward trajectory make the adjustments and readjustments in biography and everyday life activities that are necessary to adapt to increasing physical deterioration.
4. To assist the client who is in an unstable phase to gain greater control over symptoms that are interfering with his or her ability to carry out everyday activities.
5. To assist a client in maintaining illness stability by finding a way to blend illness management activities with biographical and everyday life activities.

Goals can be broken down into specific client-oriented objectives. Built into the objectives are the criteria that will be used to evaluate the effectiveness of each intervention. What is important here is to look at what takes place in the process (the steps) of working toward a goal, as well as the end to be reached, and to be realistic about what can be achieved in what time period, taking into consideration the desires, wants, and abilities of the client and family.

From Woog P: *The chronic illness trajectory framework: the Corbin and Strauss nursing model,* New York, 1992, Springer.

Gender and Chronic Illness. Because women typically live longer than men and more frequently live alone, the issues of management of chronic disorders have a large gender component. The Rand Corporation (Shoben, 1992) found from a large study (sample of 11,242) of elders hospitalized with congestive heart failure (CHF), heart attack, pneumonia, and stroke that elderly men receive more care and more expensive, highly technical services than do women. Several studies since have shown similar findings (Blumenthal, 1995; O'Connor et al, 1996; Nease et al, 1995; Harvard Women's Health Watch, 1994; Pittman and Kirkpatrick, 1994). Whether there is also an unconscious discriminatory practice in chronic care and home care is unknown. Certainly we hope to understand this question better upon the completion of the Womens' Health Initiative. Much is yet to be done in this potentially fruitful area of research. Under the guidance of Bernadine Healy, appointed in 1990 to head the National Institutes of Health, some of the "vast knowledge gap" related to women's health care is being closed. Her concern underlies the award of over one-half billion dollars in grants to the Women's Health Initiative, a longitudinal study of women's health needs. More serious even than the knowledge gap is the lack of caregivers for numerous old women. This is currently not addressed in any systematic way. Peg, one of these very old women who has survived husband, sons, and daughter, said, "I've taken care of people all my life and now there is no one to take care of me. Now, I ask you, is that fair?"

Fatigue from Living with Chronic Disorders. Fatigue from living with chronic disorders is seldom considered in its full significance. It is a variable and unpredictable condition that is often ignored or relegated to an insignificant and incidental aspect of growing old. It may occur in the presence or absence of any other disorder but cannot be ignored. The lassitude that one experiences is often evidence of depression as well as chronic illness. Zest for life is gone, and every action seems to involve an inordinate amount of energy, hardly worth the effort. Nurses confronted by this attitude tend to become either impatient or caught up in the feeling of futility. The most important intervention is undoubtedly to validate the reality and debilitating effects of the disorder. Discussing patterns of fatigue and identifying the precipitants are important. If the elder can be engaged in keeping a log of the low points of energy, it may prove useful. It is also helpful to emphasize the wisdom of the body and the assumption that it is presently necessary for the individual to move in "low gear." Permission to rest periodically and engage in brief periods of mild activity may reassure elders that they can indeed cope with this overwhelming inertia.

Wells (1986) has observed the tendency for individuals to make decisions about where to expend energy and in which situations to conserve it. For instance, an individual may wish to have assistance in dressing in order to save the energy for playing the piano or to use a wheelchair rather than a walker to avoid fatigue during dinner. Nurses, alert to this, will not expect an individual always to be using maximum strength for each activity. Energy to enjoy life's activities becomes more precious with advancing age. Chronic problems tax this existing energy level. Direct assistance by caregivers or families may be necessary to aid the aged person in exploring lifestyle adaptations that decrease energy expenditure and permit continued involvement in valued interests. Throughout the process, the aged disabled person must remain involved in decision making on every level of need. The aged often have different priorities than the caregiver. Elderly clients may relegate their health needs to a lower priority to fulfill other needs or life demands. One must understand and respect the priorities established by the elder.

When caregivers work with the aged who have disabling chronic conditions, the concept of time is important. More time is required. A slower pace of activity and large segments of time for direct care are needed. The slower movements of the aged and the response to physiologic stress require more time for care activities with rest periods in between.

Pain and Chronic Illness. The reader is advised to review Chapter 9 carefully while keeping in mind that chronic disorders usually involve not only certain painful physical impairments but frequently depressed moods that exacerbate pain perception. There is great variance in cohorts in the relationship between pain and depression. The older one becomes, the more likely it is the correlation between pain and depression will exist (Turk et al, 1995). It has been common for these individuals to be told, "You must learn to live with it." Very often an antidepressant is needed in combination with analgesics. However, our attachment to the belief that only Western medicine really works and all else is adjunctive has limited our thinking about pain management. "Alternative" strategies can be extremely effective, especially when sought and managed by the individual. We do not suggest that they are always effective, but in many cases therapeutic benefits are obtained from a combination of scientifically undefined qualities, personal idiosyncrasies, placebo effects, and individual control. However, chronic conditions can and often do produce penetrating pain. Most adjunctive therapies are just that and not adequate for management of extreme pain without medication as well. In fact, one elder got very angry when asked to visualize to relieve his pain. It seemed to him a superficial dismissal of him and his very real problem. Chronicity and pain often go hand in hand, and one of the major management issues is the control of pain. In Chapter 9 this aspect of chronicity is covered quite thoroughly.

Substance Abuse and Chronic Problems. It is thought that nearly half of the elderly hospitalized for unstable chronic medical problems are abusing alcohol and that many others consume enough alcohol to affect their health negatively (Miller, 1992). Successful screening of a patient's alcohol use involves addressing the chronicity of a disease as well as the degree to which the patient is affected by alcohol consumption. Alcohol use should always be considered when looking for factors associated with unstable chronic health problems (Miller, 1992). Methods for determining alcohol overuse include the Michigan Alcoholism Screening Test (MAST), the CAGE questions (need to cut down, easily annoyed, feel guilty, and need eye opener), and laboratory serum analysis for elevated gamma-glutamyltransferase (GGT) (see Chapter 5). For additional discussion of alcoholism see Chapter 21.

Many elders attempt, some quite successfully, to manage their disorders with over-the-counter medication combinations, doctor shopping, or simply by years of habitual codependency with a particular physician. Any of these methods can result in addiction and leave the elder vulnerable. Recently, old Dr. M. retired. He had a pleasant practice and numerous clients whom he had patiently served as they grew old together. Joe needed his medication refilled, so, went to young Dr. J., who had taken Dr. M.'s practice. Dr. J. refused to renew the tranquilizer that Joe had taken for years to combat his sleeplessness. Joe is now busily doctor shopping. We must at some level admire Joe for his tenacity and self-care whether or not we agree with his methods.

Sexuality and Chronic Illness.

Sexual problems and misinformation are pervasive in society in spite of generally high levels of exposure to knowledge about sex and near toxic exposure to sexuality in media, schools, and politics. In spite of this, little attention is paid to those who are living daily with chronic disorders that interfere with sexual intercourse and the fundamental feelings of sexual attractiveness. In addition, individuals with chronic disorders are not immune to the sexual problems that occasionally beset most individuals. Various disorders may produce mechanical problems, erectile problems, decreased libido, and decreased lubrication. Certain disorders involving ostomies and incontinence may produce revulsion in the partner and sexual anxiety in the afflicted. Discussing and assessing medication regimens, the expected dysfunctions that accompany particular diseases, and the individual's expectations are all important. A sexual history may provide important clues regarding the individual's needs and desires. The nurse's responsibility is toward an open, accepting discussion of the patient's sexuality and the provision of information and resources appropriate to the client's situation. PLISST is an acronym that is helpful in reminding us of a useful format for discussing sexuality (Box 8-2). Refer to Chapter 16 for additional discussion of sexuality.

Grieving the Lost Self.

Grieving the loss of appearance, function, independence, and comfort may occupy much of one's time initially when adapting to a chronic disorder, particularly if the onset has been abrupt and the loss interferes directly with a major source of one's pleasure. As the mother with a handicapped newborn mourns the loss of the visualized "perfect" infant, the elder may begin to memorialize the "perfect" self that no longer exists. In fact, the perfection of the earlier image of the self may grow far beyond the reality that existed. The nurse's function is to encourage verbalization, talk with the elder about the lost self, and recognize the stages of grief that may be occurring. Clearly, grief reactions will be highly individual, depending upon the significance of the loss to the individual and the number of additional losses with which they are attempting to cope. The number and recency of other losses in the life of the individual may have depleted psychic reserves.

Moral Dimensions of Living with a Chronic Illness.

van Hooft (1995), a colleague of Jean Watson (the mother of caring theory in nursing), explores caring as fundamental to moral action. He developed a model, from Aristotelian roots, that surmises four levels of caring: the biologic/environmental interactive level, the perceptual/cognitive interpretive level, a proactive level in which we define our world by purposive design, and a spiritual level where our highest hopes, faith, and loves have meaning. He contends we must understand deep caring in order to be truly moral. Those with chronic illnesses will, ideally, gradually recognize and integrate all four levels of caring into an integrated moral sense of wholeness.

There often seems to be a subversive sense of failure or weakness in individuals who have developed a chronic disorder, as if they could will it away by strength of mind, determination, and courage. Suffering a chronic illness is compounded by the sense of responsibility for being healthy, especially in the current wellness climate (Benner et al, 1994). There is often the persistent thought that hard work and adherence to a strict treatment regimen will bring about cure, and when that does not occur, a sense of shame develops, and the person wishes to hide from others (Doolittle, 1994). This is a serious problem, deeply rooted in the work ethic that has been so cultivated in the older generation.

Four stances were observed in the Benner studies: acceptance (26%), transitional (15%), nonacceptance (35%), and adversarial (17%). Acceptance was characterized by an objective view of the illness, rather than a view of illness as an internalized failure, and was accompanied by statements such as, "It's like having a child; a responsibility you must take care of." In the transitional situations elders feel in the process of learning to accept the illness as part of

Box 8-2	**PLISST**

*P*ermission to masturbate, fantasize, and claim feelings
*L*imited *I*nformation related to problem being experienced
*S*pecific *S*uggestions—only when nurse is clear about the problem
Intensive *T*herapy—referral to professional with advanced training if necessary

themselves. The largest group, those who refused to accept the illness, either ignored the need to respond to the demands of the illness or felt it was "all in my mind." The adversarial group was angry and saw the illness as an enemy that must be conquered. Both of the last two positions made the disease an entity outside of the self. Acceptance was gradual and came in small increments as the individual began to accept the altered needs of the self. Given these tendencies, it is imperative that the nurse not overtly or covertly reinforce the client's sense of personal failure. It is not helpful to suggest, "Well, have you tried. . . ." Living with a chronic illness is a process, continually changing as one adapts to the grief of the lost self and learns to embrace the needs of the emerging self. Unfortunately, health care providers often reinforce the notion that the individual is responsible for the illness and is in some way defective in allowing it to occur.

ASSESSMENT

Assessment of the elderly involves selection of appropriate tools, repeated testing, careful observation, periodic monitoring, alert watchfulness and most importantly, discussion and corroboration with elders of their perceptions and the meaning their illness has for them. In the case of chronic illness and the great variability in presentation and impact on individual lifestyle, adequate assessment is critical.

Activities of Daily Living: ADLs and IADLs

It is difficult if not impossible to estimate the number of individuals with functional disabilities. Estimates vary enormously from one study to another and from one agency to another (Figure 8-2). Many of the needs for assistance are going unmet. The crux of adaptation and life satisfaction are the ADLs and those that go beyond basic bodily tasks necessary to daily life, the IADLs. ADLs include eating, bathing, dressing, toileting, walking, and transferring. IADLs include shopping, using the telephone, paying bills, obtaining medical and dental attention, preparing meals, and light housework. ADLs and IADLs are the major thrust of any type of chronic care. The goal is to sustain or improve all functions as much and as long as possible with a minimum of discomfort. Chronic disorders become problems only when they involve pain or self-care deficits in ADLs.

Assessment of capacity for self-care in both ADLs and IADLs can be accomplished through the use of the Barthel Index and the Lawton, Brody IADL Index (see appendixes). Reuben, et al (1993) suggest an algorithmic model of functional assessment that is focused on the goal of compensation for any impairments (Figure 8-3).

Chronic disorders and the qualification for home care are defined by the degree of impairment in ADLs. The more complex and higher level functions are categorized as IADLs. It is apparent that ADLs are largely mechanical, and IADLs are largely cognitive. In order to qualify for Medicare

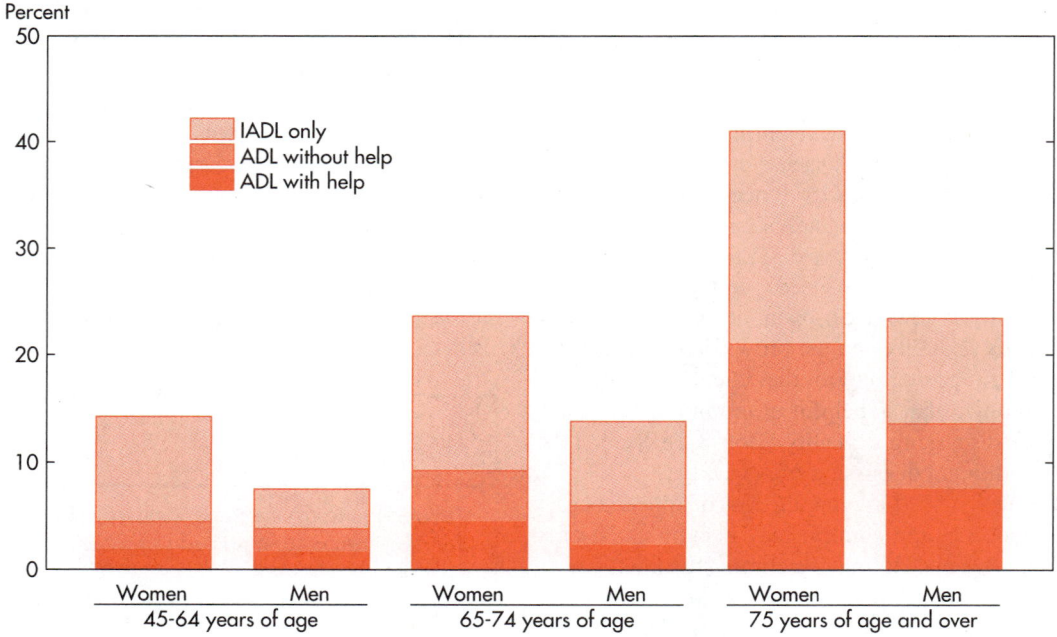

Figure 8-2. Disability status among noninstitutionalized persons in United States 45 years of age and over by sex and age, 1991. (From Centers for Disease Control and Prevention, National Center for Health Statistics, *National Health Interview Survey,* Hyattsville, Md, 1994, DHHS Publication.)

coverage of home care one must be homebound, expected to improve with treatment, have a signed order from a physician, and require the services of a professional. Impairment in ADLs is not sufficient to receive Medicare reimbursement (Rice and Rappl, 1996). However, it is useful to assess the level of ability of an individual for self-care. There are many tools designed to accomplish this. One of the simplest and most used is the previously mentioned Barthel Index. The scale, which measures ADLs and IADLs with values weighted toward difficulty/complexity, is a useful assessment of a person's capacity to manage with or without assistance.

According to the U.S. Bureau of the Census (1995), assistance needs of elders receiving home health care were as follows: bathing (40%), dressing (33%), transferring (29%), taking medications (25%), light housework (24%), toileting (20%), and meal preparation (16%). The primary source of payment for home care of these individuals was Medicare (85%) (Table 8-2).

Chronotherapeutics

Nursing chronotherapeutics is a term used to describe the temporal and rhythmic aspects of internal and external

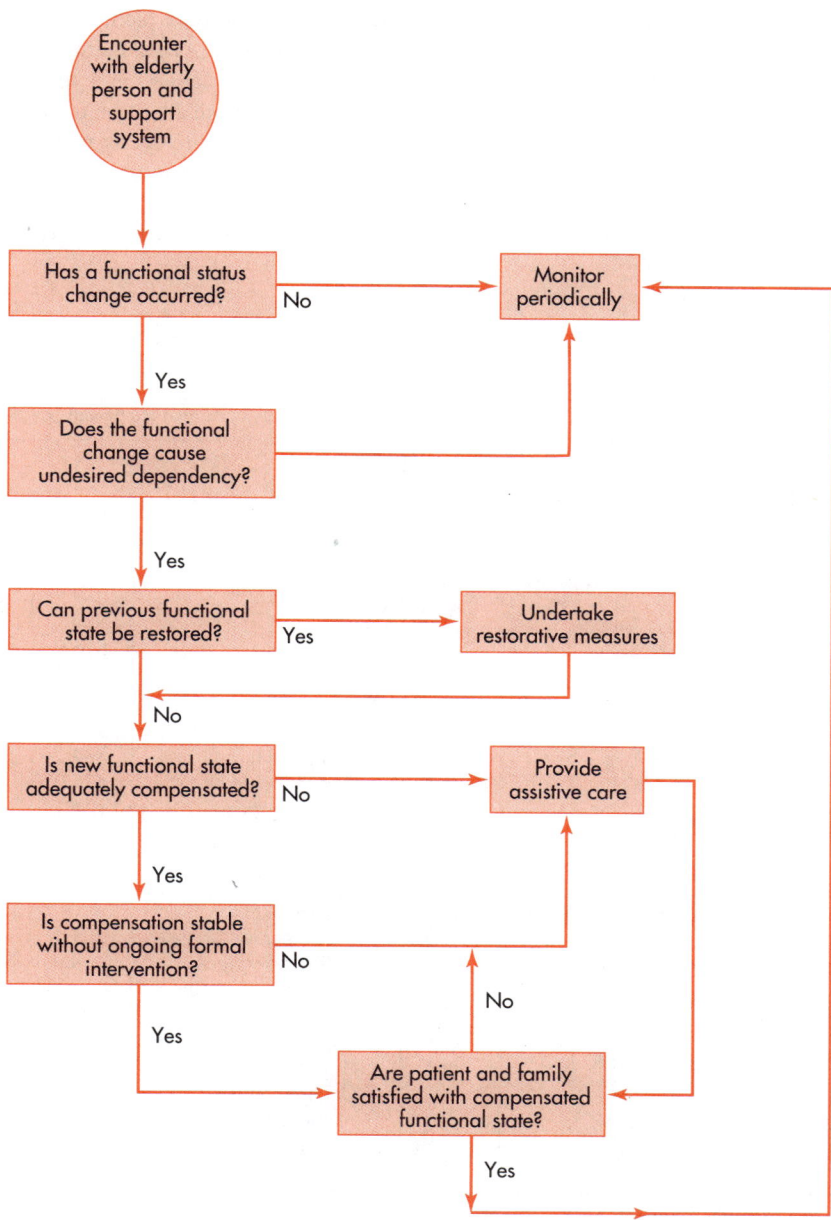

Figure 8-3. Functional status, methodologic issues. (From Reuben DB, Wieland DL, Rubenstein LZ: Functional status assessment of older persons: concepts and implications. In Vellas B, Albarede JL, Garry PJ: *Facts and research in gerontology,* New York, 1993, Springer, p. 237.)

forces that must be considered in therapeutic interventions. Most recently it has been embraced by pharmacologists, who are beginning to realize that the time of day or night makes a considerable difference in the therapeutic results of certain medications. We are all well aware of the diurnal and lunar rhythms that exert controls on everyday life and individual adaptation. A rhythm is a "sequence of events" that repeats through time in the same order and at the same interval. Thus knowing rhythms, patterns, and timing will significantly affect the efficacy of care. Though this is now well known, there has been little practical response to this knowledge. It has been said many times and in many ways with little impact. To conceptualize the whole macrouniverse and microuniverses as pulsating energies is to know that it matters greatly when interceptions occur. The most impact will be at the lowest ebb. In assessing capabilities and in planning therapeutics one may tap the lowest energy levels or the highest, depending upon the nature of desirable results. Timing focuses on determining when an action will provide the optimal benefit and the least harmful impact. For example, medication regimens seldom consider the biorhythmic im-

pact, but it is clearly significant. In chronic disease processes new patterns and rhythms must be established and energies must be more carefully monitored and more judiciously used. We do not yet know just how all these rhythms affect and are affected by health and disease, but we do suspect that individuals have times when they are more vulnerable, based upon the data we now have. Westfall (1992) proposes a model of factors to consider, such as light-dark, noise-quiet, food and fluid consumption patterns, atmospheric pressure, electromagnetic field differences, activity-rest patterns, both internal and external temperature fluctuations, and social actions.

Age in combination with multiple chronic disorders presents a very complex picture when planning therapeutic interventions. It is thought that in old age the rhythms are considerably more labile. We suggest that nurses give this considerably more attention in care planning and that nurse-researchers begin to focus more attention on the rhythmic variabilities of response in the aged, individually and collectively. Impingement upon the internal, self-generated rhythms, sensory receptor integrity, internal pacemaker, age,

Table 8-2   Elderly Home Health Care Patients

[Covers the civilian noninstitutionalized population 65 years old and over who are home health care patients. Home health care is provided to individuals and families in their place of residence. Based on the 1993 National Home and Hospice Care Survey]

Item	Current patients* Number (1,000)	Current patients* Percent distri-bution	Discharges† Number (1,000)	Discharges† Percent distri-bution	Item	Current patients* Number (1,000)	Current patients* Percent distri-bution	Discharges† Number (1,000)	Discharges† Percent distri-bution
Total 65 years old and over	**1,080.2**	**100.0**	**2,622.7**	**100.0**	Medicare	816.9	75.6	2,235.9	85.3
Received help with—					Medicaid	97.7	9.0	74.0	2.8
Bathing or showering	589.0	54.5	1,059.8	40.4	Services rendered last billing period				
Dressing	508.6	47.1	873.2	33.3	Skilled nursing	894.2	82.8	2,203.4	84.0
Eating	132.2	12.2	227.8	8.7	Personal care	475.9	44.1	842.6	32.1
Transferring in/out of a bed or chair	378.0	35.2	782.9	29.9	Social services	124.1	11.5	299.3	11.4
Using the toilet	286.6	26.5	533.2	20.3	Counseling	44.2	4.1	117.7	4.5
Doing light house work	412.1	38.2	631.1	24.1	Medications	63.5	5.9	176.3	6.7
Managing money	22.4	2.1	21.4	0.8	Physical therapy	188.8	17.5	822.9	31.4
Shopping for groceries or clothes	146.9	13.6	196.7	7.5	Homemaker/ companion services	201.1	18.6	274.4	10.5
Using the telephone	36.7	3.4	35.2	1.3	Referral services	19.9	1.8	52.4	2.0
Preparing meals	274.8	25.4	429.1	16.4	Dietary and nutrition services	27.4	2.5	71.2	2.7
Taking medications	278.7	25.8	650.7	24.8	Physician services	17.0	1.6	39.8	1.5
Primary source of payment of last billing:					High tech care	12.8	1.2	50.5	1.9
Private insurance	32.7	3.0	128.1	4.9	Occupational/ vocational therapy	39.5	3.7	132.5	5.1
Own income	25.1	2.3	39.5	1.5	Speech therapy/ audiology	14.5	1.3	41.3	1.6

From U.S. National Center for Health Statistics, unpublished data.
*Patients on the rolls of the agency as of midnight the day prior to the survey.
†Patients removed from the rolls of the agency during the 12 months prior to the day of the survey. A patient could be included more than once if the individual had more than one episode of care during the year.

and chronotype can be significantly detrimental when one's adaptive reserves are depleted. A daily routine is often cited as a powerful synchronizer; given this understanding, it is suggested that an individual's customary and current rhythms provide a base for the planning of nursing actions that are as mildly disruptive as possible. Customary patterns should correlate as closely as possible with planned care. Environmental stimuli that are not patterned or expected may sap energy quickly.

Chronotherapy. Chronotherapy is an idea that has been around for a long time but has been approached as the effect of biorhythms on function. Little real attention had been given to it until 4 or 5 years ago. It is now considered an integral aspect of medication management. In this chapter we suggest it should be given more consideration in terms of chronic care management in general. When is the individual functioning at peak? When are some treatments and activities most acceptable (Figure 8-4)? Circadian rhythms are the most easily recognized, but lunar rhythms, seasonal rhythms, and many other micropulses and macropulses affect each of us at all times. Although we yet understand little about them, we must be cognizant of the variances we are likely to encounter in metabolism and function. Presently it is particularly recognized in the giving of steroids, asthmatics, cardiac disorders, cardiac event vulnerability, cancer chemotherapy treatments, and diabetic management (Long, 1996).

INTERVENTIONS
Caring

Caring, continuity, commitment, competence . . . a litany of *C*s have historically formed the foundation of nursing care. Today, in the face of information overload, pandemics, media irresponsibility, ethical confusion, and the ever-growing capability to technologically accomplish things that are humanely questionable, caring may be fundamental to the continuance of civilization. Caring and compassion form the difference between civilization and corruption. Compassion has been seen as a distinguishing aspect of being human. Although *caring* forms a cornerstone of nursing, it could be found in the index of only two current nursing texts (Lubkin, 1995; Benner et al, 1994), and *compassion* was not found in any.

Numerous definitions of caring in nursing have been presented in the past. One recent and most commonly accepted is Watson's (J. Watson, 1988): "The moral idea of nursing consists of transpersonal human-to-human attempts to protect, enhance, and preserve humanity" (p. 54). It is helpful to understand the roots of the term *care* in order to find its place in nursing. We have often heard that care is the nurse's domain and cure belongs to the physician. Of course, these delineations have weakened considerably in the overlapping roles, managed care, and advanced practice nursing models. However, it is enlightening to look into the origins of the

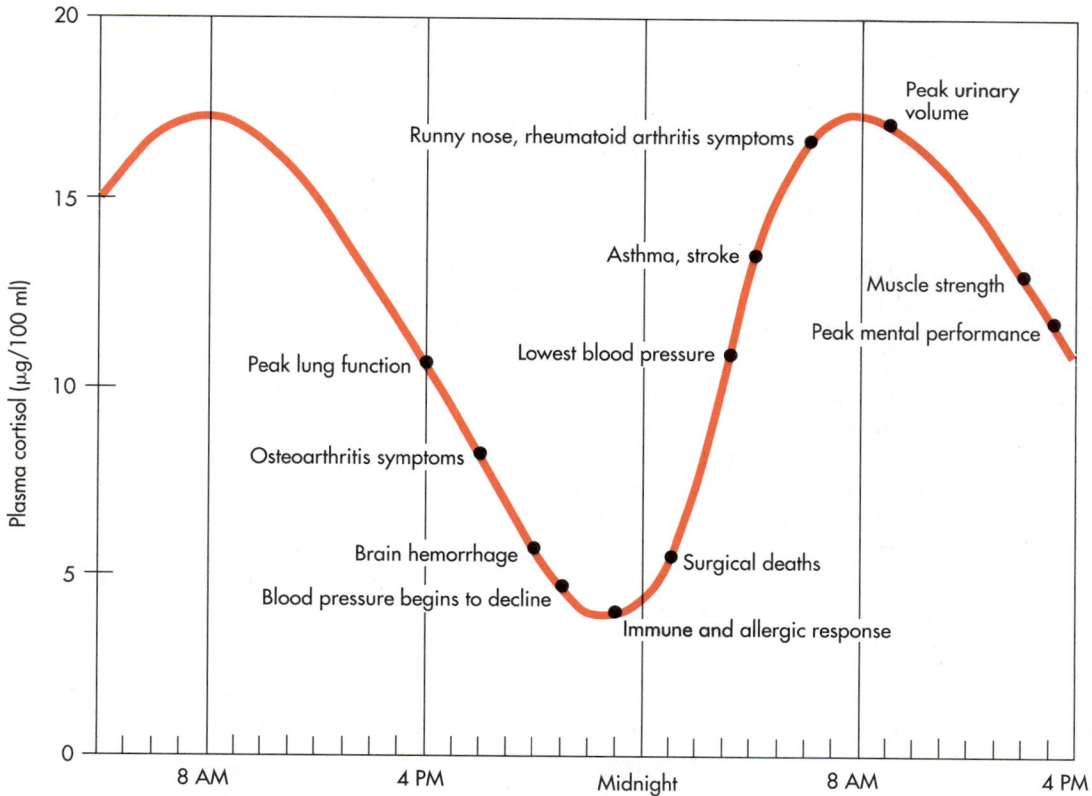

Figure 8-4. 24-hour circadian rhythm of corticol secretion.

words. *Care* is derived from the Old English word of the commoners, *carian,* meaning to trouble oneself for another, whereas *cure* is of high Latin derivation, meaning priest. Dunlop (1994) believes this class difference has influenced medicine and nursing, in that the lower orders cared while the higher orders cured. Although this digression is not a central point in caring, it is significant to nursing in general. In our present system "caring time" is a rare commodity. Milne and McWilliam (1996) surveyed doctors, nurses, and nurse managers and found that they understood caring primarily as "spending time with," "being with," and "doing for." They concluded that there was insufficient time and they must take leadership roles in achieving promotion and allocation of "caring time" within each of their agencies.

Self-Care

In chronic care, self-care is of the greatest importance and must be cultivated beyond all else. The very nature of chronicity demands it. It is important in understanding the self-care movement to know its origins. As it became more apparent that the present system was incapable of providing ongoing care for most of the conditions of elders, self-care as an idea grew in popularity. McElmurry et al (1994) help us understand that the self-care movement is rooted not only in the economic imperative of self care but also in the primacy of the biomedical ethical principle of respect for autonomy and self-governance. This has been a radical change in perspective. Less than 20 years ago the prevailing ethical principle was that of beneficience, conferring good upon others—sometimes against their desires. Orem's self-care movement (1980) in nursing has grown popular based partially on the increasing awareness of the individual's direct impact on disease and the impotence of nursing and/or medicine to effect positive change in a depressed, declining individual who no longer cares.

According to Carpenito (1989), a self-care deficit is experienced when an individual is unable to carry out basic functions without assistance. These deficits are primarily the result of pathophysiologic disorders that impinge upon neuromuscular, musculoskeletal, or sensory integrity. The interruption in function may also stem from situational conditions or treatment sequelae. Thus, when all three situations coalesce, it may require more adaptive capacity than an individual has at the time. The appropriate approach is very individual and may involve changing the situation, modifying the treatment, or retraining the individual to compensate for the pathophysiologic changes. The impact of chronic illness is very individual and may include identity erosion, expectation of death, dependency conflicts, and feelings of failure and fatalism. Interestingly, many of the largest HMO providers are now offering reimbursement for alternative medicine therapies such as massage, touch therapy, acupuncture, chiropracty, biofeedback, homeopathy, and naturopathy (*San Francisco Chronicle,* October 7, 1996). This trend arises from studies showing that alternative med-

icine is less expensive, demands fewer hospitalizations, and tends to be used by individuals who are more concerned about managing their own health in a holistic manner. Now it is possible for individuals to direct their own care, order their own special supplies without physician approval (see resources), and in many cases, purchase their medications over the counter. Although this is an important trend, it places even greater responsibility on the client for making wise decisions, sometimes with insufficient information or education. Nursing will be more often called upon to assist clients in obtaining background and sorting out options in health management.

Maintaining a Health Diary. The health diary has multiple purposes in the assessment and management of chronic disorders (see earlier section on assessment). Its most important function is probably to serve as a mechanism by which an elder may develop self-awareness regarding perception and management of a chronic disorder. It has no recommended form or structure and is thus designed according to individual preference. The entries may be lengthy, with much embellishment, or brief, precise descriptions of daily activities and body responses. Some persons make daily entries, whereas others do so only occasionally. Kept over time, the health diary reveals progression or remission of the condition and provides concrete longitudinal assessment data that may long since have been forgotten by the diarist. It also reveals something of the individual's personality style in the way perceptions are recorded and most importantly, it serves as a coping mechanism. A diarist is able to convey, at will, any thoughts or feelings and have full freedom of expression. The act of expressing brings control and solace. The intended, or unintended, recipient of the information becomes incidental to the process when it is considered as a therapeutic mode of self-care, personal integration, and release. Gerontic nurses might encourage clients with prolonged disorders to keep a health diary. It is extremely useful in many ways, the most important being the acute awareness in the nurse of the true meaning of "wellness" and courage.

Another method used to assist elders to become aware of the body and its signals was developed in Idaho. Elders in a senior center wrote about their bodies, aches, and pains in both poetic and prose forms. They were able in doing so to get a new perspective on an ailing heart, an aching shoulder, and feet that had lost their spring. The collective effort and publication of their small book gave substance to their efforts and built a feeling of community that helped objectify their distress as well as develop a new appreciation for the body.

Small-Group Approaches to Chronic Illness

Group meetings are among the most effective and economic ways of assisting clients to meet informational and psychosocial needs. They can also be designed to provide family support and counseling. Self-help groups can be seen as support systems, consumer participant systems, expressive-social influence groups, or homogeneously identified therapeutic groups. Facilitating adjustment to new roles and activities and redefinition of self and meanings constitute a large part of working with the physically challenged in groups.

The first meeting should set the tone and expectations for the group and also make clear any necessary ground rules. It is important to involve the group in identifying topics and issues they wish to focus on during the groups. These ideally should be planned sufficiently in advance to allow the group facilitator to gather information, brochures, and other resources that may be valuable to the group members. In addition to information there are many psychologic issues to be addressed, such as the following:

1. Fears about incapacitation, pain, abandonment, isolation, and death
2. Expressions of low self-esteem and loss of confidence
3. Feelings of helplessness and uselessness; a desire to be whole and well again
4. A desire to fit into the family system once again
5. Willingness to redefine role relationships with significant others
6. A desire to face and handle public situations without fear or embarrassment

Group Support by Telephone. Organized telephone group therapy may counteract feelings of isolation and loneliness experienced by persons housebound by various degrees of immobility or functional impairment. This mode of intervention has not been thoroughly explored in relation to effectiveness, but telephone support is readily available and conceivably could be very useful.

Adaptive Devices

Seventy-one percent of all assistive devices are used by individuals over 65 years of age. The most common devices used by the aged are (in rank order) handrails (65%), canes (49%), hearing aids (38%), raised toilets (30%), hospital beds (24%), and walkers (24%). Overall, 63% of the payment for these items is out-of-pocket (Adams and Marano, 1995). Many varieties of adaptive feeding and homemaking devices are available to compensate for deficits in function. Gerontologic experts have identified many useful products that can help people deal with problems caused by arthritis, stroke, reduced hearing or vision, diminished strength, and other impairments (Figure 8-5).

An occupational therapist should be contacted for assistance solving individual adaptive needs. At present this is a highly specialized field. High technology has been used to provide assistive devices, computerized training programs, programmed pillboxes, patient distance monitoring, and robotic aids for the handicapped. Voice-activated computer programs are now highly developed and can assist elders who are completely disabled to accomplish many things.

As the effects of computer applications impact the delivery of care for the elderly, new difficulties are created. Computer-assisted retraining can be applied to stroke rehabilitation, aphasia, and cognitively impaired clients. Speech synthesis and telecommunication devices are available for the verbally and orally handicapped. Electronic monitoring of status, activity, and location of hospital and nursing home clients is increasingly feasible. Pocket-sized computer notebooks would be useful for the mildly memory impaired. Electronic monitors can locate the wandering individual. The many potential applications of computer technology must be surveyed and correctly applied for maximum benefit. Given the possibilities, it is imperative that health care providers become educated regarding potentials and serve as advocates for the elderly who could benefit from assistive devices (Pousada, 1995).

Each year more training is required for families and professionals simply to use the equipment; in addition, as these become more sophisticated they often become too expensive for most elders. The challenge of the future is to use computer advances to enhance the quality of life for the elderly while lowering the ultimate cost. At this time, the challenge is to provide some of the many assistive devices that should be made generally available. Arras and Dubler (1995) note that we must begin to focus on the ethical and social implications of these developments and ask how high-tech home care can best serve "the needs of a compassionate but prudent society" (p. 30).

Chronic Disorders and Assistive Devices

Today people are living longer and with more disabilities. The compression of morbidity predicted by many has simply not occurred as yet, and with the continual advances in life-saving methods we doubt that it will ever occur. Unfortunately, disability is usually treated as a medical problem rather than a life adaptation. Therefore health insurance and managed care tend to cover only those things that directly affect morbidity or mortality (Torres-Gil, 1995). For the majority of those coping with disabilities the goal is not just survival but maintaining a quality of life that is gratifying and prolonging independence as long as possible. Disabilities that interfere with the valued activities of one's life must be compensated to the greatest extent desirable by personal or equipment assistance.

Verbrugge et al (1993) found that assistive devices were much preferred by most individuals. Those individuals with impairments seek to increase their physical and mental coping capacities through the use of various devices or to reduce physical, mental, and emotional demands. "Intrinsic disability" is that which is unassisted, whereas "actual disability" is that which remains after appropriate assistance is obtained.

Verbrugge et al (1993) investigated the efficacy of various means of assistance with 28 everyday activities and found that for upper extremity problems personal assistance is more common than equipment assistance; for lower

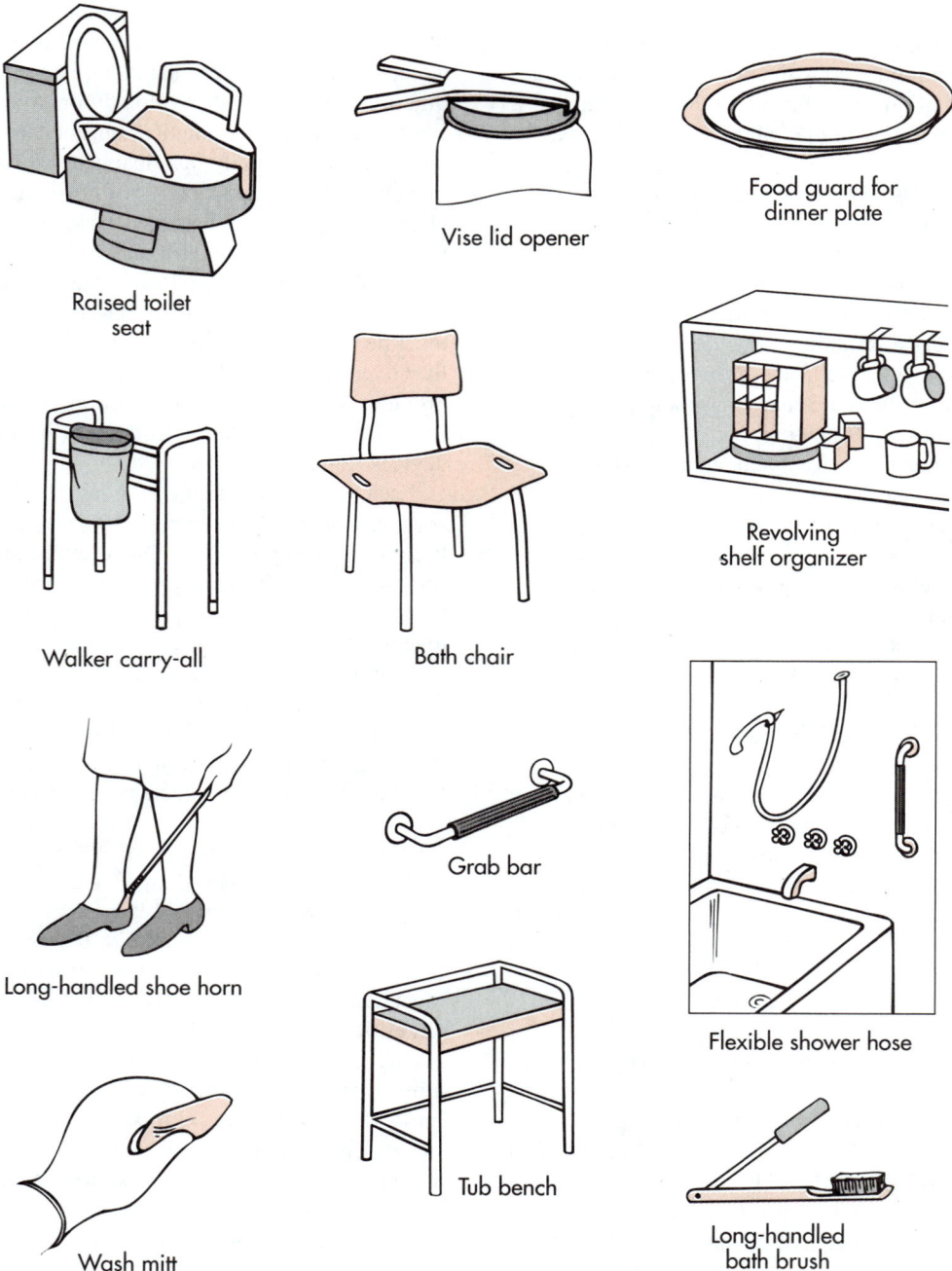

Raised toilet
seat

Vise lid opener

Food guard for
dinner plate

Walker carry-all

Bath chair

Revolving
shelf organizer

Long-handled shoe horn

Grab bar

Flexible shower hose

Wash mitt

Tub bench

Long-handled
bath brush

Figure 8-5. Adaptive equipment commonly used in the home.

extremities the opposite is true. Age differentials in need are great, though gender differences are insignificant. With assistance, either personal or mechanical, 25% of individuals say their difficulty is entirely resolved. The 12 activities in which help was most often needed are listed in Box 8-3.

Assistive devices include mobility aids, vehicle modifications, aids for vision, speech, and hearing impairments, prosthetics and orthotics, bathing devices, environmental control systems, computer access devices, and many others.

The resources section at the end of the chapter lists several sources where information about assistive devices and their use is readily available.

Substitute Activities. Mrs. J bemoaned the fact that with her advanced arthritis she no longer could knead bread. Because she had built a reputation as an excellent bread baker, she not only lost an enjoyable activity but some of her personal recognition. The home health nurse suggested to the family that they purchase a bread-making machine and one of the nu-

Box 8-3	**Activities in Which Help is Most Often Needed**

ADL Tasks
Bathing
Bed/chair transfer
Dressing
Feeding
Toileting
Walking

IADL Tasks
Doing housework
Getting about the community
Handling money
Preparing meals
Shopping
Using the telephone

Data from Division of Medical Expenditure: *Intramural research highlights,* vol 7, Rockville, Md, 1992, Agency for Health Care Policy and Research, Public Health Service.

Box 8-4	**Common Iatrogenic Disorders of the Old Due to Hospitalization**

Loss of mobility due to insufficient ambulation
Temporary incontinence due to inattention when needed; sometimes becoming a permanent problem
Confusion due to medications, treatments, anesthesias, translocation
Pressure sores due to infrequent changes of position
Dehydration due to limited access to fluids
Fluid overload due to improper use of intravenous fluids
Nosocomial infections due to infectious agents in surroundings
Urinary tract infections due to improper pericare care and catheter usage
Upper respiratory tract infections due to immobility and shallow breathing; pneumonia
Fluid and electrolyte imbalances due to medications, treatments
Falls due to unfamiliar environment and instability
Impaired sleep due to treatments and environment
Malnutrition due to anorexia, insufficient assistance in eating

merous bread-making books (see resources for additional information). This is only one substitute activity that could be suggested for an individual with special skills or interests.

PREVENTION OF IATROGENIC DISTURBANCES

In this era of rapid patient turnaround and numerous treatments compressed into a few days, nurses are well aware of the deleterious iatrogenic effects of hospitalization superimposed upon the acute illness that required treatment (Box 8-4). Hospitalized individuals with some functional disabilities often rapidly regress into a helpless state. Simple interventions, noted time and again, have actually proved helpful in retaining functional status during episodic illness (Wanich et al, 1992). A geriatric clinical specialist facilitated the following interventions that were found most helpful: staff education regarding special needs of the hospitalized elder, daily orientation cues for the patient and reassurance regarding the probability of transient delirium, getting the patient up and out of the room at least once daily, using physical and occupational therapy daily for particular therapeutic exercises, environmental modifications, personalization of environment, minimal use of medications, and interdisciplinary discharge planning with frequent revisions. (Box 8-5 includes specifics.)

Telephone Follow-up after Discharge

Recent emphases on cost savings and what often seem to be precipitous discharges of individuals from acute care hospitals have revived interest in telephone follow-up after treatment. Although it is geared to individuals rather than groups and those in the hospital for acute care, it has shown that in-

dividuals have numerous questions when contacted, although they rarely initiated contact themselves even though encouraged to do so (Bostrom et al, 1996). Their most common concerns were not directly related to the disorder or illness for which they were treated but rather dealt with comfort and daily living.

For those individuals with frequent exacerbations of chronic disorders, a consistent follow-up telephone link to the primary provider for general discussion and problem solving seems an excellent idea. Guy (1995) considers the significance of telephone follow-up after discharge and ways to increase its effectiveness. She finds that attentiveness to possible sensory impairments and interpersonal, cultural, and educational factors are important and gives particular suggestions for increasing effectiveness (Box 8-6). She also cautions that proper documentation is a significant aspect of telephone care and counseling.

REHABILITATION AND RESTORATIVE CARE

Restorative care is rehabilitative care within a humanistic framework provided under the guiding assumption that the care and services are thoughtfully designed to capitalize on the individual client's needs and strengths in a manner that will help him or her achieve the "highest practicable level of function" (Klusch, 1995). We prefer the term restorative because it implies the capability of individual renewal whereas rehabilitative seems to focus on restoration of function. This is actually a moot point that we bring out only because of

---

Box 8-5	Minimizing the Effects of Hospitalization on Functional Capacity

Staff Education

Mental and functional status assessment
Management of sensoriperceptual function
Mobility
Environmental modifications

Orientation and Communication

Use of cues and repetition
Discussion of condition
Providing anticipatory guidance regarding procedures
Reassurance regarding likelihood of delerium

Mobilization

Getting patients up, out of bed, and out of room
Involving physical and occupational therapy in exercise

Environmental Modifications

Glasses and hearing aids available and working well
Calendars
Favorite programs on radio and TV available
Increased lighting, night lights from dusk until dawn

Caregiver Education and Consultation

Families asked to bring in significant items; photos

Medication Management

Daily medication review; discouraged use if not clearly necessary; particularly discouraged neuroleptics and anticholinergics, which tend to exacerbate delirium

Discharge Planning

Weekly, or more frequent, case conferences with primary nurse, social worker, PT, OT, nutritionist, and discharge planner

---

Box 8-6	Telephone Communication Tips

1. Cultivate the skill of active listening for spoken and unspoken messages.
2. Use clear, slow speech at low pitch.
3. Speak clearly and directly into the telephone.
4. Eliminate or reduce background noises such as music or talking.
5. Maintain focus.
6. Remain open to cues.
7. Engage in complete assessment and avoid premature diagnosis.
8. Verify the elder's understanding of information
9. Demonstrate sensitivity to and respect for racial–ethnic and cultural differences.
10. Provide telephone care with discretion and competence.
11. Terminate the call in a pleasant, cordial manner.
12. Document care.

From Guy DH: Telephone care for elders: physical, psychosocial and legal aspects, *J Gerontol Nurs* 21(12):27, 1995.

---

our personal interpretation of meanings and because we always lean toward the elusive and away from the mechanical aspects of aging.

Considerations in Planning Rehabilitation Care

Rehabilitation is long term. During acute hospitalizations rehabilitative plans should begin. The following issues are important to consider:

1. The client is in a crisis when admitted to the hospital, and personal strengths are not always visible or easily assessed.
2. Client anxiety impairs learning during hospitalizations, yet clients are more motivated toward change when physical status is threatened.
3. Early discharge to home or a nursing home may impede continuation of rehabilitative efforts.
4. Multidisciplinary discharge planning must begin on admission, and a nurse/case manager should be assigned to each client who will need rehabilitation.

5. Twenty-four hour rehabilitative focus is necessary; it is insufficient to consider physical therapy two or three times per day as "rehabilitation."

Medicare requirements influence inpatient hospital stays for rehabilitative care. A client's medical or surgical needs alone may not warrant inpatient hospital care, but hospitalization may nevertheless be necessary because of the client's need for rehabilitative services. A hospital level of care is required by a client needing rehabilitative services if that client needs a relatively intense program that requires a multidisciplinary coordinated team approach to upgrade ability to function. There are two basic requirements that must be met for inpatient hospital stays for rehabilitation care to be covered by Medicare:

1. The services must be reasonable and necessary (in terms of efficacy, duration, frequency, and amount) for the client's condition.
2. It must be reasonable and necessary to furnish the care on an inpatient hospital basis, rather than in a less intensive facility such as a skilled nursing facility or on an outpatient basis.

Preadmission screening requires a review of the client's condition and previous medical record to establish that significant benefit can be gained from an intensive hospital program or extensive inpatient evaluation. Inpatient assessment of an individual's status and potential for rehabilitation is essential. Assessment is not merely a paperwork review but includes an on-site professional review of the client's condition by all the necessary disciplines. Inpatient assessment conducted by a rehabilitation team through examination of the client usually requires 3 to 10 days, while the client is also receiving therapies in addition to screening.

The fact that an individual has some degree of mental impairment would not per se be a basis for concluding that a multidisciplinary team evaluation is not warranted. Many individuals who have had cerebrovascular accidents (CVAs) suffer both mental and physical impairments. The mental impairment often results in a limited attention span and reduced comprehension with a resultant problem in communication. An intensive rehabilitation program may make it possible to correct or significantly alleviate both the mental and physical problems.

Comprehensive nursing assessment is critical. Nursing assessment includes a comprehensive biopsychosocial history and a client care plan with long- and short-term goals. Weekly interdisciplinary team conferences are held to evaluate client progress and revision of goals. Discharge goals and family conferences are a part of these weekly conferences. The following services should be available to patients in acute rehabilitation programs:

1. Rehabilitation nursing
2. Physical therapy
3. Occupational therapy
4. Speech therapy
5. Social service
6. Discharge planning
7. Psychologists
8. Prosthetist and orthotist services
9. Audiology
10. Physician
11. Consultation with vocational rehabilitation specialists

Rice and Rappl (1996) explain that when assessing individual needs it is important to focus on loss of function rather than the specific disease because therapeutic treatments will be designed to improve funtion. Rice and Rappl provide a list of conditions and diagnoses appropriate for home health rehabilitation referrals (1996) (Box 8-7).

Legislation. The landmark Rehabilitation Act of 1973 was originally intended to provide rehabilitation services regardless of whether or not the disabled recipient could be expected to return to gainful employment. The legislation also required alterations to provide access for the disabled to all institutions receiving any federal funding. Amendments in 1985 gave the National Council on the Handicapped independent status, which in effect gave it more strength and influence. The American Disabilities Act of 1990 went beyond that of 1973 to require physical and vocational access to private as well as federally funded businesses and vocational and educational institutions.

Three subgroups of disabled elderly are increasingly using rehabilitative medicine. The first two are those who are developmentally disabled and those who were traumatically disabled in childhood, who because of medical advances, are for the first time in history remaining alive into old age. The third group, and by far the largest, is composed of individuals who suffer stroke or injury in later life and have been

---

Box 8-7	**Common Conditions and Diagnoses Appropriate for Home Health Rehabilitation Referrals**

1. Patients who have sustained fractures or dislocations
2. Patients who have undergone orthopedic surgeries, including joint replacements or reconstructive surgeries
3. Patients suffering from degenerative joint or disc disease
4. Patients suffering from rheumatoid arthritis
5. Patients who have undergone amputations or require prosthetic training
6. Patients who have sustained burns with joint involvement or have physical impairment with an associated decrease in function
7. Patients who have suffered cerebral vascular accidents
8. Patients who have suffered head injuries or spinal cord injuries
9. Patients with multiple sclerosis
10. Patients with amyotrophic lateral sclerosis
11. Patients with Parkinson's disease
12. Patients with a decrease in function as a result of neuropathies and/or myopathies
13. Patients with chronic obstructive pulmonary disease who require postular drainage and teaching
14. Patients with cardiac impairment requiring cardiac rehabilitation
15. Patients with severe immobility as a result of any disease process requiring instruction to the caregiver in hoyer lift transfers or any assistive device
16. Patients suffering from newly diagnosed blindness
17. Patients with head/neck cancer resulting in partial or total laryngectomies or glossectomies
18. Patients whose underlying disease process, illness, or injury has resulted in dysphagia
19. Patients suffering from a hearing loss

Health Care Financing Administration: *Health insurance manual,* No. 11-T273, Washington, DC, rev 3/95, US Department of Health and Human Services.

---

left with residual impairment following treatment or lack of treatment. The aged with long-standing physical disabilities to which they have adapted quite well may find that the adaptation sustained earlier may be more difficult in late life because of generally decreased functional ability and coping energy. The normal changes of aging must be incorporated into life patterns. It is important to recognize that the issues of the disabled elderly are quite distinct from those of the young (Box 8-8).

There is a fourth group, sometimes difficult to identify as such, those who have iatrogenically induced disabilities. These may be the result of aggressive, passive, or neglectful

Box 8-8	Comparison of Disability Issues of Young and Old

Youth	Aged
Loss of attractiveness	Loss of role/status
Anxiety regarding future	Anxiety regarding dependency
Interference with social life	Fear of institutionalization
Loss of friendships	Loss of mobility
Rapid recuperation	Prolonged recuperation
Traumatic disabilities	Secondary incapacitation
High energy reserves	Diminished endurance
Resistance to infection	Compromised resistance
Lack of health care coverage	Fragmented benefits

Summarized from Frengley MB, Murray P, Wykle ML: Policy and philosophic issues. In *Practicing rehabilitation with geriatric clients,* New York, 1990, Springer.

treatment patterns. Recent observations emphasize the need for intense and immediate rehabilitation efforts during acute illnesses to avoid prolongation, iatrogenic responses, and chronic sequelae. No longer is it appropriate to withhold rehabilitation procedures until the client is medically stable, particularly since diagnosis related groups–incited (DRG-incited) early discharge patterns may then preclude rehabilitation in some settings. Thus professionals dealing in the early phases of an individual's disorder must be able to provide both necessary medical support and rehabilitation services to achieve maximum wellness potential (Melvin, 1988).

Rehabilitation Services. It is estimated that there are 5 million severely disabled persons over 65 years old in the United States today. Many could live independently with rehabilitative and supportive services, but since a return to employability is one driving force in rehabilitation, there may be little assistance available when there is no expectation of improvement. In fact, there is great variation among Medicare, Medicaid, HMOs, and private insurance regarding coverage for various services (Lubkin, 1995). Rehabilitation facilities are reimbursed through Medicare under the Tax Equity and Fiscal Responsibility Act (TEFRA) of 1982 at a flat rate regardless of diagnosis, length of stay, or other variables. Over half of those units are losing money (Ross, 1992). Given managed care and subacute developments, as well as numerous Health Care Financing Administration (HCFA) state waivers, it appears that the excellent rehabilitation units financed through TEFRA that flourished in the 1980s may be destined for abandonment.

The best of the geriatric rehabilitation units being developed now under various funding mechanisms are specially designed to foster function and teach individuals how to influence their environment to adapt to whatever their disability may be. These are also the units where health care

providers become most acutely aware of the need for interdisciplinary teamwork and planning. Resnick (1993) reports on a "supportive care unit" developed by the Department of Medicine at the University of Maryland that is designed to bridge the gap between acute care and home care. In the 6 years of the unit's existence, they have found that orthopedic procedures are the major reason for admission to the unit. Individuals with joint replacements, fractures, stroke, amputations, and arthritis make up most of their clientele. More than 86% of the individuals are discharged to home, and 80% of those are able to remain there for 2 years or longer. We expect many more to emerge along the lines of this model. The National Council on the Handicapped recognizes the increasing problem of secondary and iatrogenically induced disabilities such as pressure sores, contractures, and cognitive impairment as important issues that must be considered in any future rehabilitation models.

Problems in Rehabilitation. Staff members who have worked intensively with the aged in acute rehabilitation settings have noted the following problems occurring frequently (Highland Hospital, Nursing Staff, 1988):

- The aged are reluctant to engage in activities that employ objects that are childish or seemingly irrelevant to daily tasks.
- Individuals suffering traumatic injury early in life are now living until old age; however, the problems they experience are exacerbated by the normal aging changes, such as bowel and bladder atonia. This subject has been addressed thoroughly by Treischmann (1987).
- Individuals who have taken care of others much of their lives and are then stricken with a chronic disorder seem prone to develop excess disability reactions and lose motivation to participate in their own care. It seems as if they feel they have earned the right to be taken care of.
- Frustration, agitation, and irritation are often the overt expressions of the functionally impaired. Rather than focusing entirely on the visible symptoms, it may be more productive to establish groups to teach ways to enhance function. Memory training groups, sensorimotor skill training, and physical therapy are some of the methods of restoring the maximum potential of impaired persons. Remodeling of the environment for ease of adaptation and function should also be considered (Lapp, 1987).

Rehabilitation and the Future. Lack of education in rehabilitation among health care professionals in acute care settings results in inadequate care and even further disabilities. The potentials of rehabilitation are poorly understood by most health care professionals. Better education, appropriate policies and protocols, and definitions of roles in rehabilitative care for allied health professionals are needed to bring rehabilitative care into the mainstream of the health care system. Services to Medicare beneficiaries with chronic diseases provide more than half the revenues of rehabilitation units and hospitals. Other sources of revenue are from the Disability Insurance Program (SSI), Medicaid, workers' compensation programs, and private disability insurance plans. These need to be more extensive and inclusive.

Rehabilitative care providers often have difficulty demonstrating precise outcomes, since services are provided through multiple disciplines: medicine, physical and occupational therapy, speech therapy, nursing, and psychology. Consequently, outcome measures are extremely difficult to develop.

In the future Melvin (1988) expects wider acceptance of rehabilitation by all professionals and increased integration of its principles into all medical and social activities. Greater accountability will be expected of all professionals and institutions. This accountability will seek a balance between the resources expended and the practical outcomes achieved. Effective rehabilitation for aged disabled persons is consistent with the philosophy that all persons should have the opportunity for optimum personal development and function. The penalty for lack of accessibility to appropriate rehabilitation is increased dependence on family, nursing homes, or other care providers at an even greater cost to society (England et al, 1987). The agenda for rehabilitation into the twenty-first century includes increased numbers of rehabilitation hospitals, reimbursement, and rehabilitation educational programs.

Nurses advocating for the needs of the aged and disabled, armed with clinical examples, anecdotal evidence, and empirical research findings, have the power to affect the character of legislation proposed in the U.S. House of Representatives and Senate, as has been shown by the responsiveness of Congress to the lobbying power of nurses in Washington, D.C. (Schumacher, 1996). Cost-effectiveness is the strongest argument in today's political climate. The increased number of disabled elders who will be alive because of technologic advances but will require decades of rehabilitative services is an extremely important issue. How will their care be financed, and will services generally be available? What will happen to Medicare after 2010, and will exorbitant home care costs be sustainable? Numerous questions need answers very soon.

COMMON CHRONIC DISORDERS

Individual common chronic conditions will be the focus of the remainder of this chapter. Numerous textbooks on geriatric diseases and chronic illness are available as references. We look beyond the diagnosis to the broader implications of chronic illness to the aged and their families. Given support, many elders with chronic disabilities can transcend the physical and emotional adversity of chronicity to maintain feelings of self-esteem and self-fulfillment. Expecting and reckoning with episodes of depression in all involved parties, claiming discouragement at times, and grieving for the

lost capacities are all legitimate responses that should be expected in the search for meaning. Many persons have found meaning in suffering and have transcended physical limitations to discover values that those of us without physical disabilities cannot understand.

Certain disorders are encountered frequently enough among the old to merit special attention. Diabetes mellitus, incontinence, congestive heart failure, stroke, pulmonary problems, and pressure wounds are among the most common chronic disorders. Osteoarthritis and osteoporosis are dealt with in Chapter 11, rather than in this chapter, because they so often impair mobility. Parkinson's disease primarily produces problems with mentation and movement, so these are dealt with in Chapters 11 and 22. We do not intend to include comprehensive medical management of these disorders, but they will be addressed individually to focus on the holistic needs and nursing responses.

For medical management refresher and review we refer the reader to the excellent, detailed, and comprehensive *Merck Manual of Geriatrics,* second edition (Abrams et al, 1995). We also refer readers to the Agency for Health Care Policy and Research series of practice guidelines. These provide algorithmic decision-making protocols for incontinence, heart failure, unstable angina, urinary incontinence, pressure ulcers, acute low back pain, and several other common conditions. They have been developed by panels of experts, including nurses, and can be obtained free of charge (see resources at the end of the chapter).

Diabetes Mellitus

Of individuals 65 years and over, 19% are diabetic; women are diabetic only slightly more often than men (U.S. Bureau of the Census, 1995). Diabetes is a complex disorder of metabolism that is primarily a result of a relative or complete lack of insulin secretion by the beta cells of the pancreas or of defects of the insulin receptors. There are two major types of diabetes mellitus: a metabolically complex insulin-dependent disorder (IDDM, type I) and the non–insulin dependent (NIDDM, type II), which is a deficiency disorder (Meneilly and Tessier, 1995). The vast majority of older individuals with diabetes mellitus are afflicted with NIDDM type II, associated with insulin deficiency, acquired later in life, and often well controlled with diet, exercise, stress management, and good health habits.

While there are many bothersome aspects to diabetes, the destructive aspects are the secondary changes that occur systemwide in response to uncontrolled or poorly controlled diabetes: visual, vascular, and neurologic changes occur gradually and insidiously until the end stages when the individual is blind, demented, suffering from cerebrovascular accidents and often has amputations of the feet or legs. Diabetes is truly a chronic disease, which, even in the best of circumstances, slowly and unremittingly progresses.

Holding back progression of the disease is the major goal. Good control of diabetes leads to significant prevention of microvascular complications and slows the progression of the disorder (Fonseca and Wall, 1995) As might be expected, poor perceptions of one's health, anxiety, and depression are frequent accompaniments of a diagnosis of diabetes (Bailey, 1996), and these may dishearten and discourage the individual from consistent self-management. Social support, mastery, and self-esteem were the chief ameliorators of the depression and anxiety (Bailey, 1996). "Locating" the patient on the Corbin/Strauss trajectory may be useful in projecting a more realistic evaluation of the incremental changes that can be expected. Small gains and progress toward change are then seen as significant. This approach could result in a holistic, qualitative approach to diabetes and more depth and breadth in nursing practice related to the care of the diabetic patient. However, Okada et al (1996) found that among Japanese elders there was great diversity in the clinical characteristics and progression of the neuropathies that accompany NIDDM.

Diabetes often hampers sexual function in men, and this presents a great psychologic problem for some. Fifty percent of men with diabetes develop erectile impotence because of reduction in vascular flow, peripheral neuropathy, and uncontrolled circulating blood sugar. Orgasmic and ejaculatory capacity usually remain unchanged. The client may need counseling regarding sexual activity modifications to provide satisfaction by alternative methods. Women ordinarily seem to retain their sexual responsiveness and orgasmic capacity when diabetic.

Assessment. Risk factors for diabetes include medications that affect blood glucose concentration, hypertension, atherosclerosis, smoking, obesity, hyperlipidemia, stress, diet, low socioeconomic factors, being female, and family history of diabetes (Box 8-9) (Meadows, 1995; Bueno et al, 1995; Fonseca and Wall, 1995).

Physiologic and psychologic stressors have been given far too little attention as precipitants and fulminating factors of diabetes type II. The monitoring of blood sugar is the easiest and perhaps the most helpful assessment tool in the management of diabetes. Persistent elevation of blood sugar increases morbidity and mortality (Miller, 1996). Clients should be taught to routinely self-monitor blood glucose (SMBG). Subungual (under a fingernail or a toenail) hemorrhages have been observed as a first manifestation of type II diabetes mellitus in some previously undiagnosed cases. In all these cases, on further examination, the clients were found to have diabetic retinopathy as well (Iglesias et al, 1996). Warning signs of diabetic foot problems include cold feet and intermittent claudication (vascular); burning, tingling, hypersensitivity, or numbness (neurologic); gradual change in shape or sudden painless change without trauma (musculoskeletal); and infections, skin color and texture changes, slow healing, exquisitely painful or painless wounds (dermatologic) (Scardina, 1983). Another major type of evidence of the progression of diabetes is the deteri-

---

Box 8-9	**Medications That May Affect Blood Glucose Levels**

Increase Blood Glucose Levels
Corticosteroids
Diazoxide
Estrogens
Furosemide and thiazide diuretics
Glucagon
Lithium
Phenytoin
Rifampin
Sympathomimetics (antihistamines, decongestants, bronchodilators)
Thyroid

Decrease Blood Glucose Levels
Alcohol
Anabolic steroids
Beta-blockers (antihypertensives)
Salicylates (high doses)

Interactions with Sulfonylureas (Oral Hypoglycemics)

Increased Effects (Lowers Blood Sugar Further)
Allopurinol
Beta-blockers

Clofibrate
Histamine antagonists
Imidazole antifungals
Low-dose salicylates
Monamine oxidase inhibitors
Probenecid
Tricyclic antidepressants

Drugs Not to Be Taken in Combination with Sulfonylureas
Azapropazone
Chloramphenicol
Dicumarol
Oxyphenbutazone
Phenylbutazone
Salicylates (high dose)
Sulfonamides

Decreased Effects (Hinders Hypoglycemic Action)
Barbiturates
Corticosteroids
Diuretics
Estrogens
Rifampin

Summarized from unidentified source: handout at workshop, *Chronic disorders of the aged,* sponsored by Arizona State School of Nursing, Phoenix, Ariz, Sept 1992.

oration of vision as retinopathy progresses. With increased diabetic retinopathy there is increased corneal epithelial fragility, which correlates with the severity of the disease (Saini and Khandalavla, 1995). The advancement of retinopathy also correlates with neuropathy and peripheral neuropathy (Delcourt et al, 1996).

Management of Diabetes. "The sine qua non of good diabetes therapy is to persuade, encourage, cajole, coach, and equip patients to develop the knowledge, tenacity, courage, and optimism necessary for the long-term successful management of their diabetes." Catolico (1995) found that the barriers to self-management of diabetes among older adults were being female and having more complex management regimens, less education, and more severe complications. Those who fared the best were the older clients and those with high self-esteem. Through management of diet, weight reduction, exercise, and drug therapies, blood glucose levels can usually be kept near normal levels (Miller, 1996). Experiential teaching, encouragement, and reinforcement of mastery are important factors that promote successful self-management. Konen et al (1996) found that symptoms of depression, anxiety, panic, and forgetfulness

were unexpectedly common among elder diabetics and affected their ability to comply with therapy. These findings alert nurses to the need to recognize these deterrents when attempting to teach diabetic management.

Maintaining blood glucose at acceptable levels is a major goal of diabetic management, though many physicians now question the value of strict glycemic control in the elderly (Froom, 1990; Colwell, 1994). In older individuals the determination of acceptable levels is not generally agreed upon. Most adults maintain blood sugar between 60 mg/dl and 130 mg/dl. For elders the norms are higher because the pancreas simply does not produce as much insulin, even in the nondiabetic. The issue is to maintain levels that do not harm the blood vessels. Rather than become overly concerned about occasional blood glucose surges, it is recommended that glycosylated hemoglobin be monitored because it reflects the average blood-glucose level over several weeks (Fonseca and Wall, 1995). Focusing on maintaining normal ranges of weight, blood pressure, and lipids is also important. Elders need to know that during times of illness or stress they may temporarily need insulin even though they usually manage quite well through nutritional control. Figure 8-6 shows the management of diabetes mellitus from a wellness perspective.

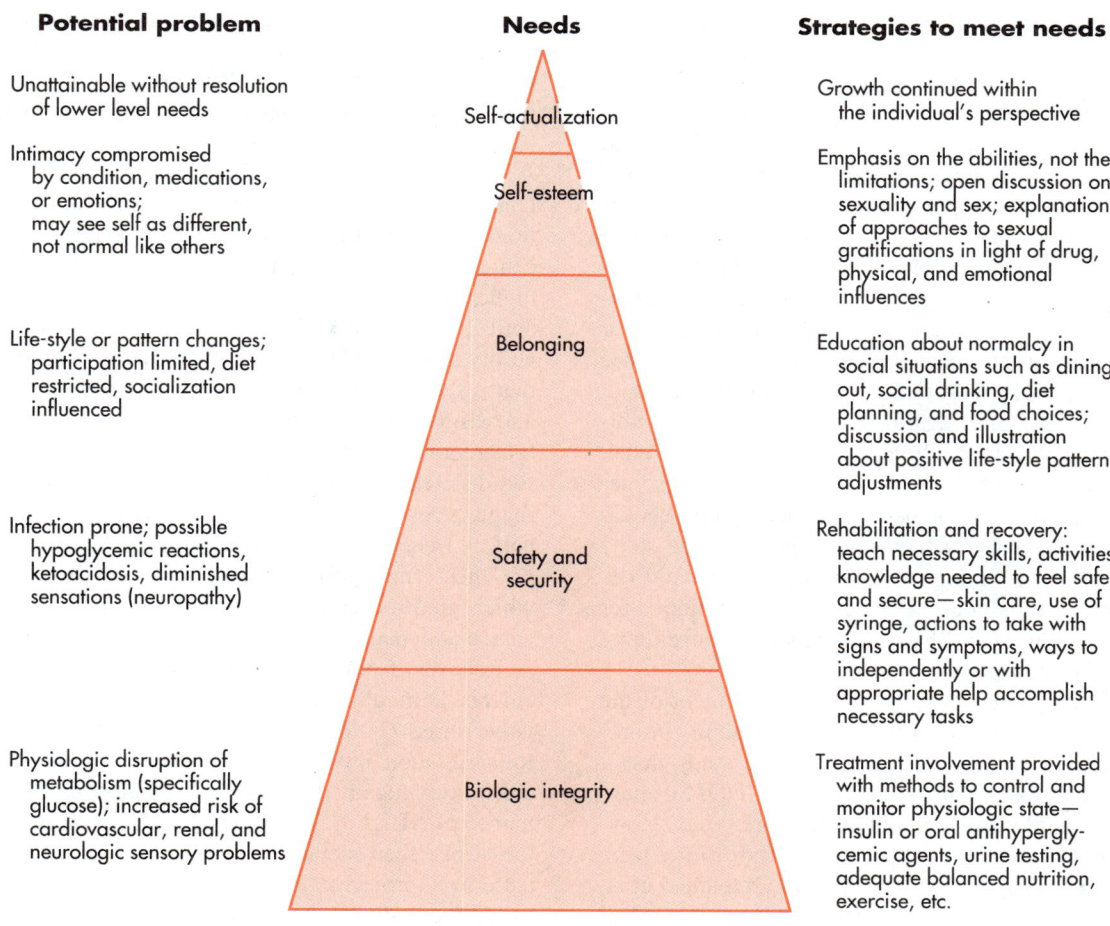

Potential problem	Needs	Strategies to meet needs
Unattainable without resolution of lower level needs	Self-actualization	Growth continued within the individual's perspective
Intimacy compromised by condition, medications, or emotions; may see self as different, not normal like others	Self-esteem	Emphasis on the abilities, not the limitations; open discussion on sexuality and sex; explanation of approaches to sexual gratifications in light of drug, physical, and emotional influences
Life-style or pattern changes; participation limited, diet restricted, socialization influenced	Belonging	Education about normalcy in social situations such as dining out, social drinking, diet planning, and food choices; discussion and illustration about positive life-style pattern adjustments
Infection prone; possible hypoglycemic reactions, ketoacidosis, diminished sensations (neuropathy)	Safety and security	Rehabilitation and recovery: teach necessary skills, activities, knowledge needed to feel safe and secure—skin care, use of syringe, actions to take with signs and symptoms, ways to independently or with appropriate help accomplish necessary tasks
Physiologic disruption of metabolism (specifically glucose); increased risk of cardiovascular, renal, and neurologic sensory problems	Biologic integrity	Treatment involvement provided with methods to control and monitor physiologic state—insulin or oral antihyperglycemic agents, urine testing, adequate balanced nutrition, exercise, etc.

Figure 8-6. Diabetes wellness perspective.

Recommended dietary requirements for diabetics have changed considerably over the years. Early on there was carbohydrate restriction, then an increase in carbohydrates and reduction in fat intake. Now the American Diabetes Association (1994) recommends 10% to 20% protein in the diet but no specific limitations on carbohydrates and fats. An individualized dietary plan is recommended, including occasional indulgences in small amounts of sucrose.

The effects of drugs on blood sugar must be given serious consideration in the management of diabetes because a number of medications commonly used for elders affect blood sugar in adverse ways. A drug profile for the diabetic should be developed with this in mind.

Medical management of diabetes is very poor in many cases (Weiner et al, 1995; Kerr, 1995). Johns Hopkins School of Hygiene and Public Health examined the Medicare claims records of over 100,000 elders with diabetes and found that 84% had not received proper testing for glycohemoglobin (GHC), 54% had not had a thorough eye examination, and 54% had not received adequate cholesterol monitoring. These are the three most important evaluations recommended by the American Diabetes Association. Individuals with type II diabetes require at least two office visits per year, lipid profiles annually, a glycohemoglobin (GHB) A_{1c} test twice yearly, and a thorough ophthalmology exam annually. *Nurses must advocate for elders and encourage them to demand quality care to prevent the devastating end results of poor management.*

The long-term incidence of lower extremity amputation in the elder diabetic is over 7% and is higher in those who have a history of leg ulcers, higher diastolic pressure, elevation of glycosolated hemoglobin, proteinuria, and a 10-year history of diabetes (Moss et al, 1996). In one study of over 300 people, 43% of elders with diabetes had peripheral neuropathy, which impairs sensation and may result in unattended foot injury. Nurses are well aware of the need for routine examination and care of the feet of diabetics (see Chapter 7). Turner (1997) found that some nurses are reluctant to provide foot care regardless of the patient's condition. Plummer and Albert (1996) say that any individual, with or without diabetes, who has foot deformities, peripheral vascular disease, or peripheral neuropathy should be followed routinely by a foot care specialist. One study (Eckman et al, 1995) suggests that physicians should debride the foot and institute a course of oral antibiotics for any individual with NIDDM who appears to be developing osteomyelitis of the foot.

There are many questions about the management of the ongoing and complex needs of the elder diabetic in our present health care system. It appears from one study that it matters little in terms of outcomes whether NIDDM is managed by a private physician or a managed care group. However, outcomes regarding foot ulcers and infections were better when treated by an endocrinologist (Greenfield et al, 1995). Expert management of diabetes may forstall some of the disorders that frequently accompany diabetes. Stegmayr and Aspland (1995) found hypertension, atrial fibrillation, heart failure, and myocardial infarction all significantly more common in diabetic than nondiabetic persons.

Standards of Care for Patients with Diabetes Mellitus. Meticulous management of the diabetic is required to reduce the risk of long-term complications and avert acute problems. The following evaluation is recommended:

- History should include dietary habits, weight patterns, previous treatment programs, current treatment regimen, exercise and activity levels, infections, illnesses, and complications of diabetes.
- Physical examination should include blood pressure; eye ground examination; thyroid palpation; auscultation of pulses; foot, periodontal, and skin examination (see Chapter 7), and neurologic examination.
- Laboratory tests should include fasting plasma glucose; glycosylated hemoglobin; fasting lipid profile; serum creatinine if proteinuria present; and urinalysis, including microalbuminuria, urine culture, thyroid function (T_4 or TSH) and electrocardiogram (ECG).

Interventions include patient education regarding medications, nutrition, exercise, foot care, stress management, serum glucose monitoring, symptoms of hypoglycemia and hyperglycemia, and signals of complications (American Diabetes Association, 1991). Prevention of disease progression, disability, and stroke is of the highest priority

Stroke and Its Aftermath

Diabetes, hypertension, atherosclerosis, and atrial fibrillation are primary risk factors for stroke. When compared with a nondiabetic population, the risk of stroke is four times higher in diabetic men and nearly six times higher in diabetic women. Stroke is the leading cause of long-term disability among adults in the United States. Strokes are CVAs that affect cerebral circulation through occlusive thrombi and emboli or hemorrhagic incidents occurring in the intracerebral or subarachnoid space. These variations account for differences in severity and symptomatology. Hemorrhagic strokes are most life-threatening, but they are only half as frequent as thrombotic strokes. Thrombotic strokes are most frequently a consequence of atrial fibrillation, which predisposes one to systemic emboli. Recent studies advise anticoagulant therapy (Laupacis et al, 1992).

Recovery from stroke is affected by the severity of the accidents. Difficulties and handicaps following stroke often involve three *C*s: communication, continence, and control. Rehabilitation involves timing. Most patients with stroke disabilities regain the maximum toward prestroke performance of ADLs by 9 months later. At 18 months following the stroke there actually tends to be a small decline. The pattern of projected functional improvement is dominated by the severity of the disability 1 month after the stroke

(Anderson, 1992). The inverse relationship between functional improvement and advanced age, social isolation, and emotional distress is clear. Up to one third of stroke victims become profoundly depressed in the year following stroke. Surprisingly, few patients seem to isolate themselves or feel ostracized due to stroke residual disabilities. Improvements in functional performance tend to be seen mainly in the severely and moderately disabled patients. Some of the methods of measuring characteristic functional disorders of the poststroke patient can be seen in Box 8-10.

Nurses are becoming much more aware of the devastation a stroke produces because some of them have experienced it and have written about stroke from a personal perspective. One nurse said, "There are so many things one is confronted with, such as the inability to cross the street before the light turns red." Another nurse, "Suddenly, me who had never even been sick, I became old." "I was unable to do the most basic things." "I have no grand truths to offer—we need breathing room—time and space to respond."

Assessment of Needs. Nowhere in the care of elders is the multidisciplinary team more essential than in the evaluation of the needs of an elder following stroke. We know now that this must be done as soon as the individual is physiologically stabilized in order to maximize the benefits of interventions. The assessment of needs following stroke are extremely complex and require evaluation by neurologists, physiatrist, speech therapist, ophthalmologist, rehabilitation

specialists, psychologists, and environmental planners. Caretakers of the patient must be included at every stage of planning, as well as the elder to every extent possible. The nurse's most important role is in documenting clearly and in detail all the functional capacities that are retained and those that are impaired. The assessment must be redone routinely to carefully evaluate and document areas of progress and areas of need.

Stroke Support Groups. Small-group support for victims of stroke can provide an environment for problem solving and feedback, support, acceptance, and encouragement from others with similar limitations and struggles to relearn. When members have great difficulty verbalizing, it may be useful and relieve some tension to have part of each group designed toward nonverbal expressions such as art, music, or psychomotor activities. Pierce and Salter (1988) note that the success of a stroke group largely depends on the group facilitator. They suggest using a family health nurse with neurosurgical, gerontologic, and rehabilitation experience. When such specialized nurses are not available, it may be best to have cofacilitators whose combined skills most closely align with members' biopsychosocial needs.

Use of art in stroke therapy group. Adsit and Lee (1986) found art an excellent medium of expression for stroke patients. It allowed them to communicate feelings and moods when verbal articulation was impaired. In addition, it provided movement integration and a visible

---

| Box 8-10 | **Tests of Specific Disabilities That Commonly Follow Stroke** |

Hemianopia (Loss of Part of Visual Field)

Sitting opposite patient, hold up simultaneously two pens of different colors 30 cm in front of patient and 30 cm apart; patients with hemianopia will be unable to see one of the pens or may turn head toward hemianopic side in an effort to see.

Proprioception (Awareness of Body in Space)

The wrist of the affected arm is held between the thumb and forefinger of the examiner; patient's hand is raised and lowered and patient, with closed eyes, is asked the position of the hand; this exercise can also be done with fingers to determine even more specific loss of proprioception.

Sensation (Feeling Generated by Sensory Receptors)

With patient's eyes closed the examiner strokes the back of the unaffected hand and then the affected hand and in both cases asks the patient to describe the sensation. The affected side may have varying degrees of loss of sensation or total loss of feeling.

Balance (Bodily Poise)

Patient asked to sit on side of bed with feet off floor and maintain balance and sit unaided for 1 minute; it is usually readily apparent if individual has a problem maintaining balance.

Arm Function (Range of Motion and Control)

Patient asked to lift affected arm to shoulder height and press against examiner's upheld hand:

Complete paralysis = inability to move arm
Severe weakness = can move arm but not lift up or push
Moderate weakness = able to lift arm but unable to push
Slight weakness = able to do task requested but cannot push as hard as with unaffected arm
No weakness = no difference in abilities of either arm

Data summarized from Anderson R: *The aftermath of stroke: the experience of patients and their families,* Cambridge, 1992, Cambridge University Press.

personal accomplishment. It is accepted at face value without judgment. Whether or not one is interested in the unconscious imagery or symbolism it is undoubtedly an important component of these artistic expressions. The overall objective for these groups is to provide an opportunity for the client to express himself or herself emotionally and physically through different media.

Adsit and Lee (1986) suggest the following: ideally keep group size under 10; tape paper to tables to prevent sliding; provide constant verbal and physical cueing to compensate for lapses in attention; and, if they are able, have clients discuss their art. This avenue of expression seems to hold promise as an adjunct means of communication for those clients who find verbal communication frustrating. Ideally speech and art therapy would best provide the client with opportunities for self-expression.

Pressure Sores (Pressure Ulcers)

Pressure sores, or pressure ulcers as they are often called, tend to be a chronic disorder of debilitated elders who are largely bed-bound. They are the consequence of skin breakdown, pressure, friction, shearing, and maceration. They can develop anywhere on the body and are most frequently seen from the waist down. The prevalence is as high as 23% in long-term care settings (Bergstrom et al, 1994) and 30% in acute care settings (Anderson and Braun, 1995). It is often extremely difficult to predict, even with the use of the highly reliable Braden Scale, individuals who will develop pressure ulcers, and it is even more difficult to restore skin integrity once they have developed (Vandenbosch et al, 1996).

Pressure sores are the consequence of ischemia and anoxia to tissue. Tissues are compressed, blood diverted, and blood vessels forcibly constricted by persistent pressure on the skin and underlying structures; thus cellular respiration is impaired, and cells die. The sequence of events in pressure sore formation begins with erythema, then edema, blister formation, and finally, ulceration if the blister sloughs (Figure 8-7).

Intervention at any point in the developing process can stop the advancement of the pressure sore. Figure 8-8 illustrates the development of pressure sores. Anyone can develop pressure sores, but the aged have more friable tissue and more of the predisposing factors that lead to the development of pressure sores: poor nutritional status such as anemia, hypoproteinemia, and vitamin deficiencies; impaired sensory feedback systems; lack of fat padding over bony prominences; corticosteroid therapy; and immobilization by restraint or sedation. All of these contribute to tissue breakdown. Tissue breakdown is aggravated by heat, moisture, and decomposing and irritating substances on the skin. Those 70 years of age and older are particularly vulnerable (Pajk, 1995) to these conditions and situations.

Certain particularly high risk groups include those hospitalized for femoral fractures (66% incidence), critical care patients (33% incidence), quadriplegics (69% incidence) and those in skilled nursing facilities (23% incidence) (U.S. Department of Health and Human Services, 1995). Caution must be used when interpreting these statistics because the timing involved is critical: how long have they been developing, and what grade of pressure sore is being reported? Therefore when a 9.2% incidence is reported for acute care, it must be realized that a developing pressure sore may often go unreported in its earliest stages.

Pressure sores are not limited to those confined to bed. Individuals in wheelchairs or who sit in one place for a long time are equally vulnerable. In the recumbent position, the shoulders, lower back, and heels are susceptible to pressure breakdown. If one is lying on the abdomen, the knees, shins,

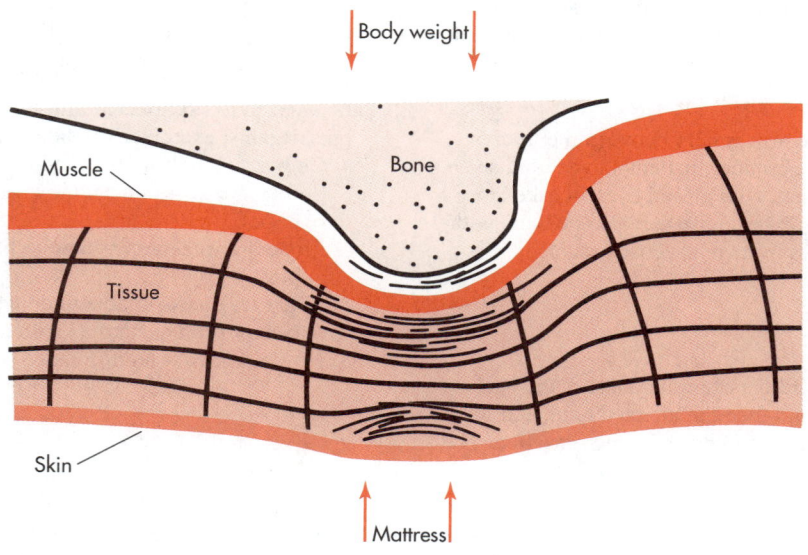

Figure 8-7. Tissue under pressure.

and pelvis sustain undue pressure. The hips or trochanter receive undue pressure when in the side-lying position and the buttocks when the person is in a sitting position. On occasion the pinna of the ear can break down it if is pressed firmly against the side of the head for prolonged periods. It is particularly important to consider the underside of the scrotum and inspect it for pressure and excoriation. This area is subject to the friction and shearing force of the sheets without the benefit of a pull sheet. The warm, moist tissue is particularly susceptible to bacterial action from sustained moisture and soil.

Two tools, the Braden Scale (Bergstrom et al, 1987) and the Norton Scale (Norton et al, 1962), are being used more frequently in the clinical setting in predicting individuals at risk for pressure sores. Since development of pressure sores is a dynamic process, it requires constant vigilance and repeated assessment (Kresevic and Naylor, 1995). Not clearly understood by nurses, physicians, and other caregivers is that it may take as long as 2 weeks of non–weight bearing or total pressure relief to heal a pressure area completely (Pires and Muller, 1991). The use of either the Braden or Norton

assessment tools provides the means for a systematic evaluation and periodic reevaluation of a person's risk for pressure sores. Six subscales are sensory perception, skin moisture, activity, mobility, friction and shearing, and nutritional status. Each category is rated with 1 (least favorable) to 4 (most favorable). The maximum score possible is 24 points; thus the lower the score, the more at risk a patient is for pressure sores and the greater the need for preventive interventions.

A more recent tool, the Pressure Sore Status Tool (PSST) (Bates-Jensen, 1992) provides a framework for assessment of the actual pressure sore, once developed. The revised *Treatment of Pressure Ulcers* (Bergstrom et al, 1994) suggests that this tool "with further research may prove useful for monitoring and reassessment" (p. 26). The PSST focuses on 13 macroscopic parameters, which allows the tracking over time of the status of the pressure sore. This is a dynamic method that is research based and reliable (Bates-Jensen et al, 1992; Bates-Jensen, 1996). The 13 indexes include pressure ulcer staging (1-4) (Figure 8-8), wound size, edges, undermining, type and amount of necrotic tissue,

Stage I

Erythema not resolving within thirty (30) minutes of pressure relief. Epidermis remains intact. REVERSIBLE WITH INTERVENTION.

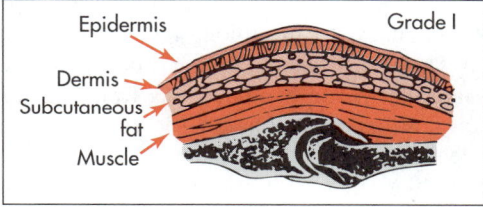

Stage II

Partial thickness loss of skin layers involving epidermis and possibly penetrating into but not through dermis. May present as blistering with erythema and/or induration; wound base moist and pink; painful; free of necrotic tissue.

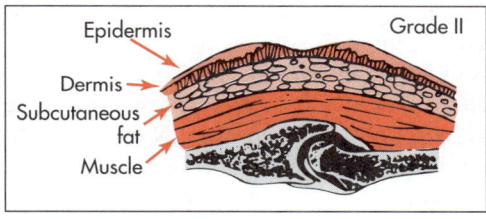

Stage III

Full-thickness tissue loss extending through dermis to involve subcutaneous tissue. Presents as shallow crater unless covered by eschar. May include necrotic tissue, undermining, sinus tract formation, exudate, and/or infection. Wound base is usually not painful.

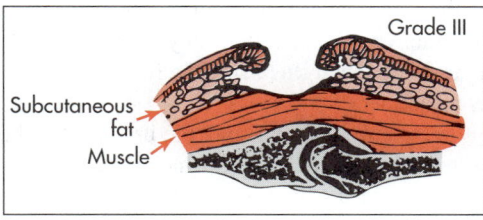

Stage IV

Deep tissue destruction extending through subcutaneous tissue to fascia and may involve muscle layers, joint and/or bone. Presents as a deep crater. May include necrotic tissue, undermining, sinus tract formation, exudate and/or infection. Wound base is usually not painful.

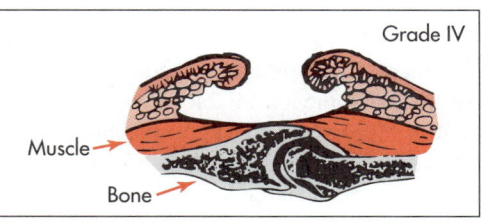

Figure 8-8. Pressure sore development.

type and amount of exudate, characteristics of surrounding tissue, granulation tissue, epithelialization, and an identification of the healing process (Appendix 8-A).

The advantages of the PSST include validity, reliability, sensitivity to wound status, objectivity, quantifiability and subjective impression of wound status, wound-healing parameters, and potential help in prescribing therapy.

The disadvantages of the PSST revolve around the fact that people do not know about the PSST tool. There is a learning curve that occurs with first use, and the tool is valid only with pressure sores, not other wounds (Bates-Jensen, 1996).

It has become apparent that a combination tool to address presssure sores is needed. Use of both the Braden Scale risk factor assessment and the PSST (actual pressure sore assessment) could provide a comprehensive and reliable approach to pressure sore risk and monitoring (Figure 8-9).

Nurses play a vital role in the prevention of pressure sores. They must be able to identify early signs and initiate appropriate interventions to prevent further skin breakdown and to promote healing. Failure to do this jeopardizes the health and life of the elderly person. Pressure sores are costly to treat and may require extended separation from friends and loved ones. For many it can prolong recovery and extend rehabilitation. The acquisition of iatrogenic complications such as pressure ulcers and complications from them such as the need for grafting or amputation, sepsis, or even death may lead to legal action by the individual or his or her representative against the caregiver. Box 8-11 lists the associated complications of pressure sores. Clinical practice guidelines for the prediction and prevention of pressure ulcers have been developed by a multidisciplinary panel of experts under the auspices of the Agency for Health Care Policy and Research (AHCPR) of the U.S. Department of Health and Human Services (1992, and Bergstrom N et al, 1994). They provide essential information and recommendations about predicting, preventing, and caring for pressure ulcers and were developed to help professional and nonprofessional caregivers become knowledgeable about pressure sores and establish a baseline of care. Though they do not endorse any one particular approach at this time, the recommendations provide the guidelines.

Assessment of Pressure Sores. Visual and tactile inspection is essential to establish a normal skin characteristic baseline for a particular patient or client. Inspection is best achieved when performed in nonglare daylight or, if not possible, under the illumination of a 60-watt lightbulb (Giger and Davidhizar, 1991; Seidel et al, 1995; Jarvis, 1996). We also highly recommend Polaroid photographic recording. With the present sophisticated equipment available, accurate documentation is absolute (Morey, 1996). Photographic documentation and inspection should include actual and potential areas for breakdown with special attention directed to specific areas when an individual uses orthotic devices such as corsets, braces, protheses, postural supports, splints,

slings, and casts. Visual inspection should look for hyperemia, and if present, the area should be rechecked in an hour. Even though it is more difficult to see hyperemia in dark-skinned people, a red tone can be detected no matter how dark the skin may be (Giger and Davidhizar, 1991).

Blisters or pimples with or without hyperemia and scabs over weight-bearing areas in the absence of trauma should be considered suspicious. Location, color, and size of area or areas should be noted. Tactile inspection should test hyperemic areas for blanching and palpate for induration, noting hardness and temperature, and comparing this to surrounding skin. Use of a risk assessment tool should be an integral part of any skin assessment. A nutrition assessment should be obtained and if possible a serum albumin value obtained. It has been demonstrated that a serum albumin below 3.5 g/dl has a positive correlation with the severity of the pressure sore (Hanan and Scheele, 1991). Malnutrition ranks second only to excessive pressure in etiology, pathogenesis, and nonhealing of pressure sores. Refer to Box 8-12 for general skin assessment guidelines. The goal of nurses is to help maintain skin integrity against the various environmental, mechanical, and chemical assaults that are potentials for skin breakdown. For those elders who are independent, mobile, and active, an appropriate nursing diagnosis would be health maintenance of skin integrity. For those in dependent-care situations not only is the nursing diagnosis of actual impaired skin integrity pertinent, but a nursing diagnosis of potential for impaired skin integrity is also germane.

Interventions. A wound of a person over 60 years of age takes approximately 100 days to heal. The estimated cost of treating a pressure sore is more than $20,000, not considering the emotional and physical discomfort that results. Miller and Delozier (1994) estimate the cost to the health care system exceeds $1.3 billion. Nursing interventions should focus on *prevention*: actions that eliminate friction and irritation to the skin by lifting, turning, placing, and rolling (using two or more persons) the patient; reducing moisture so tissues can breathe and do not macerate; and displacement of body weight from prominent areas to facilitate circulation to the skin. Adequate nutritional intake should be monitored, as well as the serum albumin level, hematocrit, and hemoglobin. Diets high in protein, carbohydrates, and vitamins are necessary to maintain and promote tissue growth. If appetite is lacking, thyroid hormone is sometimes recommended to stimulate appetite. Supplements of vitamin B help in the metabolism of carbohydrate, and pyridoxine and vitamin C assist in protein use.

Prevention of pressure ulcers in acute care situations has been successful through the consistent use of a mentored nursing practice pressure ulcer protocol (Kresevic and Naylor, 1995). The implementation of the skin protocol began with an educational program for all nurses in the setting followed by clinical specialists assigned to various units for monitoring and mentoring skin care.

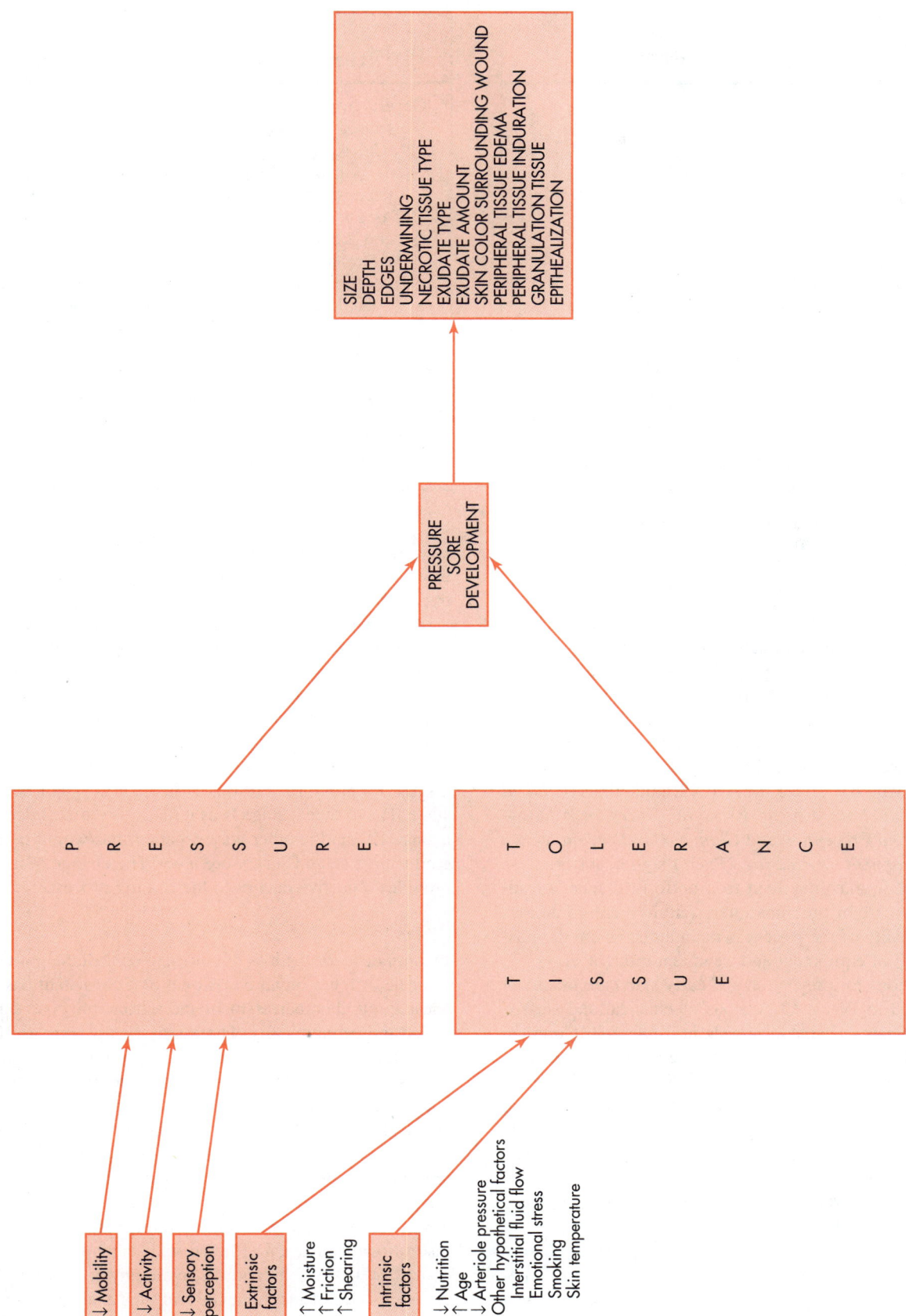

Figure 8-9. Comprehensive risk assessment and pressure sore monitoring.

Box 8-11	Complications of Pressure Sores

Amyloidosis
Endocarditis
Heterotopic bone formation
Maggot infestation
Meningitis
Perineal-urethral fistula
Pseudoaneurysm
Septic arthritis
Sinus tract or abscess
Squamous cell carcinoma in the ulcer
Iodine toxicity or uncover subclinical hyperthyroidism
   (from use of iodine based cleansing)
Hearing loss from use of topical aminoglycosides
Osteomyolitis
Bacteremia
Advanced cellulitis

Modified from Bergstrom N, Allman RM, Alvarez OM et al: *Treatment of pressure ulcers. Clinical practice guidelines,* No 15, US Department of Health and Human Services, Public Health Service, Agency for Health Care Policy and Research, Pub No 95-0652, 1994.

Box 8-12	General Skin Assessment Guidelines

General inspection
   Exposed body parts
      Color: generalized with regard to light- and dark-skinned individuals; variations
      Unexposed parts (if individual is inactive, confined to bed or chair)
General palpation
   Texture, temperature, moisture, turgor, edema
   Inspection and palpation of lesions
      Size, location, mobility, consistency, pattern, type (primary/secondary)
   Hair: Inspection and palpation
      Color, amount, distribution, texture, parasites
   Scalp: Inspection and palpation
      Texture, lesions
   Nails: Inspection and palpation
      Color, shape, texture, condition of nail bed

Once ulcers have developed, treatments include debridement of necrotic tissue and debris, wound cleansing, appropriate dressings and cultivating the growth of granulation tissue (US Department of Health and Human Services, 1994). The number of treatments that exist for pressure sores indicates that no one approach has been entirely successful. However, through the collaborative efforts of the consultants who developed the AHCPR guidelines (*Clinical Practice Guidelines No. 3: Pressure Ulcers in Adults— Prediction and Prevention* and *Clinical Practice Guidelines No. 15: Treatment of Pressure Ulcers*) significant progress has been made that may lead to a uniform manner of addressing the care of pressure sores. Within these guidelines the individuality of the patient is maintained as are the possible choices of equipment and treatment modalities.

Interventions for prevention and early skin care treatment are presented in Box 8-13. Various mechanical and surface support apparatus available appear in Table 8-3. Common types of topical agents and dressings used in the treatment of pressure sores are presented in Table 8-4. It should be remembered that solutions such as alcohol, certain soaps, and hydrogen peroxide are damaging to newly formed fragile skin. Povidone iodine placed on an open sore can be absorbed by tissues and is also a drying agent. It should also be noted that wounds heal best in their own natural environment (clean, moist, normal pH). Never occlude an infected wound.

Realistically, it is not always possible to prevent pressure sores from occurring because of the physiologic or psychologic condition of the patient. Tissue injury is proportional to the amount and duration of the pressure exerted on the

area. Obese people exert more pressure per square inch on tissue than do those who are thin. The deeper the sore penetration, the longer it will take to heal.

It is important to note that reverse staging of pressure ulcers as descriptive of healing is only appropriate as an indication of the depth of tissue involvement. Pressure ulcers as they heal are filled with granulation tissue composed of endothelial cells, fibroblasts, collagen, and an extracellular matrix. Muscle, subcutaneous fat, or dermis is not replaced. A pressure sore retains its initial stage rating. For example, a stage IV pressure sore that is healing does not become a stage III and then a stage II as it heals. It remains defined as a stage III, said another way, a patient has/would be recovered from a stage III pressure ulcer. The change in its status provides objective data as to the healing process.

Incontinence

Incontinence, or the loss of ability to control the elimination of urine or feces on an occasional or a consistent basis, has caused untold embarrassment and astronomic costs both socially and economically. There may be as many as 10 million adults affected at a cost of 3.3 billion dollars. Estimates of costs and numbers of individuals enduring incontinence vary widely as many people isolate themselves and keep silent about the problem unless institutionalized, when it may become apparent, or episodes of incontinence may be present only during a hospitalization, lifestyle change, or physiologic disruption. Elders in rural settings and small towns are more likely than those in metropolitan areas to be institutionalized when afflicted with incontinence (Coward et al, 1995). Many individuals avoid physical activity to reduce episodes of incontinence and thus exacerbate physical debility and further reduce muscle tone and control. In one

Interventions by Risk Factor

Bed or Chair Confinement

Inspect skin at least once daily.
Bathe when needed for comfort or cleanliness.
Prevent dry skin.

Bed confinement

Change position at least every 2 hours.
Use a special mattress that contains foam, air, gel, or water.
Raise head of bed as little and for as short a time as possible.

Chair confinement

Change position every hour.
Use foam, gel, air, cushion to relieve pressure.
Reduce friction by:
    lifting rather than dragging when repositioning.
    using corn starch on skin.
Avoid use of donut shaped cushions.
Participate in a rehabilitation program.

Inability to Move

Bed confinement

Place pillow under legs from midcalf to ankles to keep heels
    off bed.

Chair confinement

Reposition every hour *if unable* to do by self.
Shift weight and position at least every 15 minutes *if able*
    to do by self.
Use pillows or wedges to keep knees or ankles from
    touching each other.

Loss of Bowel and Bladder Control

Clean skin as soon as soiled.
Assess and treat urine leaks.
If moisture cannot be controlled:
    Use absorbant pads and/or briefs with a quick-drying surface.
    Protect skin with a cream or ointment.

Poor Nutrition

Eat a balanced diet.
If a normal diet is not possible, talk to health care provider about nutritional supplements.

Lowered Mental Awareness

Choose preventive action that applies to person with lowered mental awareness. For example: if person chairbound, refer to
    specific prevention action as outlined in the above risk factors.

From *Clinical practice guidelines, preventing pressure ulcers, a patient's guide,* U.S. Department of Health and Human Services, Public Health
Service, Agency for Health Care Policy and Research, Rockville, Md, 1992.

study it was shown that fewer than 23% of primary care physicians routinely ask elderly patients about urinary incontinence, and 62% of those physicians felt they were inadequately prepared to evaluate the condition (Branch et al, 1995). Therefore, continence must be routinely addressed in the initial assessment of every aged person in the nurse's care. Initial and periodic assessments are necessary to maintain an individualized nursing care plan.

Bladder Function in Old Age.   Nocturnal frequency is common in two thirds of women and men over age 65 who do not take medication and over 80% in those elders with three chronic diseases (Wasson and Bruskewitz, 1990). Normal bladder function requires an intact brain, spinal cord, a competent bladder, and active sphincters that will sustain maximum urethral pressure against rising bladder pressure.

A full bladder increases pressure and signals the spinal cord and the brainstem center the desire to micturate. Social training then dictates whether micturition should be attended to or should be postponed until there is an appropriate opportunity to seek out toilet facilities. However, when the bladder contents reach 500 ml or more, the pressure is such that it becomes more difficult to control the urge of micturition. As volume increases, emptying the bladder becomes an uncontrollable act. The bladder of the aged retains its tonus, but the volume that it can hold decreases. If cerebral vascular disease is present, dementia being the most severe form, the changes are exaggerated and bladder control becomes diminished.

Many healthy aged are annoyed by frequency and some degree of urgency. The warning period between the desire

Table 8-3   Mechanical Loading and Support Apparatus

Apparatus	Indications	Advantages	Disadvantages
Convoluted foam pad (high density, solid, 3 to 4-in foam pad)	Those patients whose activity limitation is short lived (postoperative; those in OR undergoing lengthy procedures)	Inexpensive, lightweight, comfortable	Minimum pressure relief, may cause retention of body heat (increasing moisture; possible maceration); fire hazard—many emit lethal fumes if ignited
Vinyl air-filled mattress (inflates and deflates air cells at regular intervals by electric pump)	Those at high risk for skin breakdown; those with stage I or II pressure sores	Mechanically alters the points of pressure against body; provides a moderate degree of protection against pressure; decreases maceration if mattress has air vents; lightweight; easily cleaned if wet or soiled	Minimizes but does not prevent pressure; uncomfortable because feels lumpy; costly because of electric pump operation
Water mattress (heavy vinyl, water-filled mattress placed on top of bed mattress)	Those at high risk for stage I, II, or III pressure sores; those who already have stage I, II, or III pressure sores	Distributes patient's weight evenly; provides moderate protection against pressure; comfortable; easy to maintain; easy to clean if wet or soiled	Minimizes but does not prevent pressure; heavy when filled (130-150 lb) costs approximately the same as an air mattress
Air-fluidized bed (Clinitron, Fluid Air, Mediscus Heavy Duty System)	Those patients with any stage of pressure sore, especially stage III or IV; those undergoing graft or flap surgery	Supports patient at subcapillary closing pressure (<15 to 33 mm Hg); maximum protection against pressure, shearing, friction, maceration; comfortable	Has fixed height; immovable head; patient transfer from bed difficult; unable to maintain a semi-Fowler's position to eat or if there are pulmonary problems; equipment heavy (1800 lb); circulating warm air may dehydrate patient and wound; turning of patient difficult (bed moves and molds) claim is that less turning is necessary; however, it creates risks of immobility; respiratory, mobility, and renal problems, and flexion contractures if not turned or range-of-motion exercises done frequently; rental equipment—expensive fee/day; difficult to adapt to home care
Low-air loss bed (Flexicair, Mediscus Air Support System) (air-filled cushions arranged in segmented configuration that fit into hospital bed)	Same as above	Exerts lowest pressure for patient's weight, height, and body type; uniformly supported over a maximum area with little pressure on bony prominences; bed may be raised or lowered; easy patient transfer in and out of bed; provides low pressure; decreases friction and shearing; prevents moisture buildup; reduces dehydration; patient can sit in semi-Fowler's position	Expensive rental fee
Adjunctive devices			
Sheepskin	Those who may be predisposed to skin breakdown from friction, i.e., under heels		
Heel and elbow protectors (pads of sheepskin)	Those needing protection from friction		
Trapeze	Those who have upper arm strength and the ability to grasp	Allows patient to move or shift weight independently or assist with moving	

Compiled from Bergstrom N, Allman RM, Alvarez OM: *Treatment of pressure ulcers, clinical practice guidelines,* No 15, US Department of Health and Human Services, Public Health Service, Agency for Health Care Policy and Research 1994, Pub No 95-0652; Pajk M: Pressure sores. In Abrams WB, Beers MH, Berkow R, editors: *The Merck manual of geriatrics,* ed 2, Whitehouse Station, NJ, 1995, Merck Research Laboratories.

Table 8-4   Dressings and Topical Agents in the Treatment of Pressure Sores

Type	Description	Action	Guidelines	Advantages	Disadvantages
Liquid barriers, e.g., United Skin Prep, Bard Protective Barrier Film	Contains plasticizing agents and alcohol applied as spray, wipe, or roll-on	Protective waterproof coating over affected areas; reduces maceration and shearing	Gently clean, rinse, and dry skin; apply and allow to dry for one minute; (will sting momentarily excoriated skin)	Do not irritate skin and are not affected by urine, perspiration, or digestive acids; dissolvable by soap solution	High alcohol content makes it sticky when dry; fragile skin may be inadvertently pulled
Film dressings, e.g., Bioocclusive, Tegaderm, Op-Site	Polyurethane; permeable to gases and vapors but not to fluids	Healing occurs more quickly in a moist environment; maintains wound exudate against the wound surface, promoting epithelial cell migration across wound	Wound and surrounding tissue cleansed and dried to enable dressing to adhere; dressing needs at least a 1-inch margin around the wound; do not stretch dressing tightly over wound, this creates shearing against tissue	Oxygen can get to tissue but contaminated fluid cannot; can be left on wound for 5-7 days if wound is not infected	
Hydrocolloid dressings, e.g., DuoDerm, Comfeel Ulcer Care Dressing, Restore	Inert hydroponic polymers containing fluid-absorbing hydrocolloid particles	When hydrocolloid particles contact wound exudate, they swell and form moist gel; optimal wound healing occurs in a closed, moist environment	Cleanse and dry wound and surrounding skin; dressing to extend 1 1/2 inches beyond the wound	Promotes cell migration, cleaning, debridement, and granulation; dressing may be left in place 7 days unless leakage occurs	Not usable if infection is present; may initially enlarge the wound because of debridement properties
Debriding enzymes, e.g., Travase, Elase, Santyl	Protolytic and fibrolytic agents	Act against devitalized tissue	Enzymes must be in contact with wound substrate; some enzyme preparations must be reconstituted every 24 hours (Elase powder) for each use; providone-iodine, hexachlorophene, silver nitrate, and hydrogen peroxide inhibit action of Travase	Chemical debridement	Not effective on hardened or dry eschar; useful as an adjunct to mechanical or surgical debridement
Absorption dressings, e.g., Debrisan, Bard Absorption Dressing, HydraGran	Hydrophilic beads, grains, flakes	Reconstituted per directions; packed into wound; covered with dry dressing	Absorb excess exudate and necrotic debris; deodorizes wound; keeps wound moist		Need to change once or twice a day
Hydrogels, e.g., Vigilon, Gel-Syte	Polymers	Cleanse and dry wound; hydrogel may be refrigerated for patient comfort; dressing should extend 1 1/2 inches beyond wound	Absorbs exudate to form water-soluble gelatinous substance; provides a moist environment for wound healing	Dressing may be left on 1-3 days if remains intact	Occasionally causes maceration of surrounding tissue
Calcium alginate dressings, e.g., Sorban, Kaltostate	Natural polysaccharides from brown seaweed; high-quality textile fiber pad; provides a moist environment	Wound irrigated with normal saline; dry dressing	Absorbs 20 times its weight in exudate; on contact with wound exudate forms a soft gas-permeable gel	As wound heals can be left on longer for up to several days	Alginate as forms gel emits an unpleasant odor (a charcoal pad can be placed over outer gauze dressing to absorb odor)

Compiled from Ostomy/Wound management. In Abrams WB, Berkow R, editors: *The Merck manual of geriatrics*, Rahway, NJ, 1990, Merck Sharp & Dohme Research Laboratories; Pajk M: Pressure ulcers. In Abrams WB, Beers MH, Berkow R, editors: *The Merck manual of geriatrics*, ed 2, Whitehouse Station, NJ, 1995, Merck Research Laboratories.

to micturate and actual micturition is shortened or lost. Severe illness, difficulty in walking or handling the bedpan or urinal, problems manipulating clothing, and emotional disturbances (such as occurs during a change in living situation or resentment, anger, or bereavement) may be responsible for some incontinence. In some instances micturition is uncontrolled as a deliberate means to gain attention or demonstrate anger. Drugs that increase urinary output and sedatives, tranquilizers, and hypnotics, which produce drowsiness or confusion, facilitate incontinence by dulling the transmission of the desire to micturate.

Urinary Incontinence. Urinary incontinence is one of the most prevalent symptoms encountered in the care of the aged. Many families cannot cope with incontinent relatives. It is therefore not surprising that incontinence is judged to be the second leading precipitating cause of institutionalization of the aged (Ouslander, 1992). Among the approximately 28 million elders in the community, 15% to 35% have urinary incontinence (Fantl et al, 1996). Incontinence is present in 53% or more of nursing home residents. This translates into 1.5 million elders. The annual cost for incontinence is $7 million in the community and $3.3 million in nursing homes (U.S. Department of Health and Human Services, *Clinical Practice Guidelines,* 1992), and $15 billion for care of incontinence of all persons, young and old (Fantl et al, 1996).

The current definition of incontinence, "involuntary loss of urine that is sufficient to be a problem (Fantl, 1996 et al, p. 1) varies little from the International Continence Society definition that urinary incontinence is "a condition in which involuntary loss of urine is a social or hygenic problem and is objectively demonstrated" (National Institutes of Health Panel, 1989). Incontinence is *not* a result of advancing age,

---

Box 8-14	**Risk Factors for Incontinent Older Adults**

Immobility of chronic degenerative diseases
Diminished cognitive status, dementia
Delirium
Medications including diuretics
Smoking
Fecal impaction
Low fluid intake
Environmental barriers
High-impact physical exercise
Diabetes
Stroke
Estrogen dificiency
Pelvic muscle weakness

From Fantl JA, Newman DK, Colling J et al: Managing acute and chronic urinary incontinence. In *Clinical practice guideline: quick reference guide for clinicians,* No 2, 1996 update, Rockville Md, US Department of Health and Human Services, Public Health Service, Agency for Health Care Policy and Research, AHCPR, Pub No 96-0686, 1996.

---

nor is it a disease. It is a symptom of existing environmental, psychologic, drug, or physical disturbances and can become a catastrophic event when it interferes with mobility, sociability, and the ability to remain in one's home. Box 8-14 enumerates risk factors associated with incontinence.

Incontinence ushers in dependence, shame, guilt, and fear. The aged who are aware of a problem of continence are mortified by their state. If it is assumed that all aged eventually become incontinent, a resolution of the problem will not be sought, and it will become a self-fulfilling prophecy. A study by Goldstein et al (1992) points out that elders generally did nothing about incontinence because they considered it a normal part of aging, did not realize that treatment existed, did not think that treatment would help, worried about the cost, or were too embarrassed to discuss it. Staff will not attend to the aged person's request for assistance, and the aged will withdraw because no one seems to care.

Health care personnel must begin to change their thinking about incontinence and acknowledge that incontinence can be cured. If it cannot be cured, it can be treated to minimize its detrimental effects. The nurse who cares for the incontinent person needs sensitivity, insight, patience, and understanding. Reassurance rather than guilt should be promoted. The AHCPR increased awareness and knowledge about incontinence and continues to disseminate factual information through the publication in 1992 of the clinical practice guideline, *Urinary Incontinence in Adults,* and the updated version in 1996. This information attempts to improve reporting, diagnosis, and treatment of the ambulatory and nonambulatory individual and to educate health professionals and consumers about urinary incontinence (U.S. Department of Health and Human Services, 1992, 1996).

Urinary Problems. National Institutes of Health Panel 1989 (US Department of Health and Human Services, 1992) identified the most common types of urinary incontinence in older adults as stress incontinence, urge incontinence, and overflow incontinence. Mobley et al (1991) added iatrogenic, functional, and mixed incontinence to the list.

Stress incontinence occurs when intraabdominal pressure exceeds urethral resistance. A number of causes are rooted in anatomic damage to the urethral sphincter and weakened bladder neck supports. This phenomenon may occur when an individual sneezes, coughs, bends over, or lifts a heavy object. The amount of urine leakage is small, and the volume would be low if a postresidual urine were obtained.

Urge incontinence is caused by central nervous system lesions such as stroke, demyelinating diseases, and local irritating factors such as bladder tumors or urinary tract infections. Individuals sense the urge to void but cannot inhibit urination long enough to reach a toilet. The volume of urine lost is moderate, and episodes occur every few hours. Postresidual urine would reveal a low volume.

Overflow incontinence is a result of neurologic abnormalities of the spinal cord that affect the contractility of the detrusor muscle of the bladder. Any factor disrupting detrusor stability such as drugs, tumors, strictures, and prostatic hypertrophy will cause the bladder to become overdistended, leading to frequent or constant loss of urine.

Functional incontinence refers to a situation in which the lower urinary tract is intact but the individual is limited by musculoskeletal disability or severe cognitive impairment. Urine is lost because the individual is unaware of the need to void or is unable to reach a toilet because of arthritis, Parkinson's disease, or for hospitalized patients, their condition or raised bed rails. Environmental conditions and prescribed drug use are additional examples of factors that can create functional incontinence.

Iatrogenic incontinence is associated with medication side effects. This can be managed by decreasing the dosage of medication to maintain the primary drug effect but eliminate the secondary effects. It may be necessary to change a drug to another class of medication that is not associated with incontinence. Other iatrogenic causes of incontinence include expanded extracellular fluid compartmentalization with the development of nocturia and polyuria, as occurs in CHF, chronic venous insufficiency, and in metabolic states such as polyuria with increased glycosuria or increased calcemia.

More than one urinary incontinence problem may exist in the same individual, which is called *mixed incontinence.* These conditions can be caused by anatomic, physiologic, or pathologic factors (internal factors), or by outside factors such as mobility, dexterity, motivation, and environment. Box 8-15 summarizes the types of urinary incontinence and associated causal factors.

Assessment. Nurses are often the ones to identify urinary incontinence, but neither nurses nor doctors have been particularly aggressive in its treatment. Assessment is multidimensional. It includes a health history, physical examination, and a urinalysis. More extensive examinations are considered after the initial findings are assessed. A thorough health history should focus on the medical, neurologic, and genitourinary history, medication review of both prescribed and over-the-counter drugs, a detailed exploration of the symptoms of the urinary incontinence and associated symptoms and other factors (Boxes 8-16 and 8-17), which can assist the physician or advanced practice nurse in accurate diagnosis and treatment. Data should include the duration, frequency, and volume of the incontinence.

The type of incontinence should be validated and described with a voiding diary (Figure 8-10). Accurate notations should be made of significant burning, itching, or pressure. The character of the urine (odor, color, sedimentary, or clear) and difficulty starting and stopping the urinary stream should be recorded. Activities of daily living such as ability to reach a toilet and use it and finger dexterity for clothing manipulation should be documented.

Use of medications such as sedatives, hypnotics, anticholinergics, and antidepressants should be assessed (Table 8-5). Furosemide (Lasix), diazepam (Valium), amitriptyline (Elavil), and phenothiazines are among the common drugs prescribed. In addition, the nurse should not forget to ask about vaginal discharge and/or constipation or fecal impaction. The nurse may also do all or part of the physical examination, which includes evaluation of mental status; mobility; dexterity; and a neurologic, abdominal, rectal, and pelvic examination.

Box 8-15	**Types of Incontinence and Associated Causal Factors**
Type	**Causal Factors**
Stress	Obesity
	Estrogen deficiency
	Pelvic floor muscle weakness
	Radiation or prostate surgery
	Urethral sphincter weakness
	Drugs
Urge	Stroke
	Dementia
	Parkinsonism
	Urinary tract infection
	Detrusor overactivity or instability
	Drugs
Overflow	Fecal impaction
	Enlarged prostate
	Diabetic neuropathy
	Severe pelvic prolapse
	Drugs
Functional	Mobility limitations
	Cognitive impairment
	Depression
	Bipolar/schizophrenic disorders
	External factors:
	Restraints
	Caregiver inattention
	Drugs
	Environmental barriers
Iatrogenic	Extracellular fluid compartment
	Congestive heart failure
	Chronic venous insufficiency
	Metabolic states:
	Glycosuria
	Calcemia
	Drugs

Adapted from Resnick NM: Urinary incontinence. In Abrams WB, Beers MH, Berkow R, editors: *Merck manual of geriatrics,* ed 2, Whitehouse Station, NJ, 1995, Merck Research Laboratories; Staab AS, Hodges LC: *Essentials of gerontological nursing,* Philadelphia, 1996, JB Lippincott; Palmer MH: *Urinary incontinence,* Gaithersberg, Md, 1996, Aspen Publishers, Inc; Miller CA: *Nursing care of older adults,* ed 2, Philadelphia, 1995, JB Lippincott; Fantl JA, Newman DK, Colling J et al: Managing acute and chronic urinary incontinence. In *Clinical practice guideline: quick reference guide for clinicians,* No 2, 1996 update, Rockville, Md, US Department of Health and Human Services, Public Health Service, Agency for Health Care Policy and Research, AHCPR, Pub No 96-0686, 1996.

Box 8-16	Elements of an Incontinence Assessment

History

Duration and characteristics of urinary incontinence
Most bothersom symptom(s) for the aged person
Frequency, timing, and amount of continent and
    incontinent episodes
Other urinary tract symptoms
Daily fluid intake
Bowel habits
Alteration in sexual function because of urinary
    incontinence
Amount and type of perineal pads or protective devices
    used
Previous treatment and effect on urinary incontinence
Expectations of treatment

Mental Evaluation

Cognition
Motivation to self-toilet

Functional Assessment

Manual dexterity
Mobility:
    Observe toileting
        Unaided
        Chemical or physical restraints being used

Environmental

Access and distance to toilet or toilet substitute
Chair/bed allows ease of getting up

Social Factors

Relationship of urinary incontinence to activities
Living arrangements
Identified caregiver and degree of caregiver involvement
Lives alone

Bladder Records (refer to Figure 8-10)

Frequency, timing, and amount of voids
Number of incontinence episodes

Activity associated with urinary incontinence
Fluid intake

Physical Examination
General

Edema
Neurological abnormalities

Abdomen

Diastasis rectii
Organomegly
Masses
Peritoneal irritation
Fluid collection

Rectal examination

Perineal sensation
Resting and active sphinctor tone
Fecal impaction
Masses
Consistency and contour of prostate (males)

Genital examination

Male:
    Skin condition
    Abnormalities of foreskin, penis, perineum
Female:
    Pelvic examination
    Skin
    Genital atrophy
    Pelvic organ prolapse
    Pelvic masses
    Perivaginal musculature

Direct observation of urine loss

With a full bladder under cough stress test
Estimate of post void residual volume

Urinalysis

From Fantl JA, Newman DK, Colling J et al: Managing acute and chronic urinary incontinence. In *Clinical practice guideline: quick reference guide for clinicians,* No 2, 1996 update, Rockville, Md, US Department of Health and Human Services, Public Health Service, Agency for Health Care Policy and Research, AHCPR, Pub No 96-0686, 1996.

Laboratory tests should include urinalysis; serum creatinine or blood urea nitrogen; post void residual (PVR), which can be done by abdominal palpation, percussion, bimanual examination, or bladder ultrasound; and as necessary, urine culture, blood sugar, and urine cytology. Based on these findings, a decision can be made on how to treat the incontinence or the need for additional tests such as urodynamic testing (cystometrogram, electrophysiologic sphincter testing, ultrasound of kidney and bladder, cystourethroscopy, and/or uroflowmetry).

In summary, assessment of urinary incontinence can identify incontinence as either transient—the result of tem-porary conditions that are amenable to medication, surgery, or psychologic intervention—or established—the result of neurologic damage to the urinary system. Transient incontinence is curable; established incontinence is treatable or controllable but not curable.

Intervention.   When there is sufficient understanding of the problem, various therapeutic modalities and concomitant nursing interventions can be initiated. Selection of a modality and interventions will depend on the type of incontinence and its underlying cause and whether the outcome is to cure or to minimize the extent of the incontinence. Box 8-18 lists the numerous modalities available in the treatment of incon-

"URO-Log" (Voiding Diary)

To be completed before your doctor's appointments.

Name _____   Date _____

Time of day	Type and amount of fluid intake	Type and amount of food eaten	Amount voided (in ounces)	Amount of leakage (small, medium, large)	Activity engaged in when leakage occurred	Was urge present?

Figure 8-10. Example of voiding diary. (From HIP, Union, SC).

tinence. Nursing interventions focus primarily on the therapeutic modality of supportive measures. However, the nurse is involved and must remain aware of the prescriptions, implications, and outcomes associated with the other therapeutic modalities. Advanced practice nurses may also be involved in designing restorative therapeutic modalities.

Attitude. An appropriate attitude is most important when providing nursing care to an incontinent individual. Caregivers are often unaware of the many causes of incontinence and passively accept a client's urinary incontinence and feel that it is an inevitable part of aging, only adding to the elder's feelings of low self-worth, dependence, and social isolation (Long, 1985; Wyman et al, 1990). Caregivers who regard incontinence as an unpleasant and demanding hygienic problem emphasize only keeping the patient clean and dry with little consideration of what causes the problem. Ouslander et al (1987) studied an incontinent nursing home population and found that the incontinence was not associated with most clinical conditions or medications, except for bacteriuria. The fact that incontinence is curable and that the nurse and other health care providers will work with the elder to resolve the incontinence is an important idea to foster in the elder who is not cognitively impaired. The role of the nurse in the community is to give the older adult information and tools that will allow the individual to maintain body control.

Toilet accessibility. Accessibility to the toilet is an intervention that is often not considered in providing assistance for the incontinent patient. Environmental circumstances can contribute to incontinence. If the distance the aged person must either walk or travel by wheelchair to reach the toilet is longer than the time between the onset of the desire to

Box 8-17	**Elements of a Supplemental Urinary Incontinence Assessment**

Use of a voiding record
Evaluation of environmental and social factors
Observing voiding
Blood tests
Urine cytology
Urodynamic tests
Endoscopic tests
Imaging tests of upper tract and/or lower tract with and without voiding

From *Clinical practice guidelines: urinary incontinence in adults,* 1992, Rockville, Md, US Department of Health and Human Services, Agency for Health Care Policy and Research, AHCPR, Pub No 92-0038.

micturate and actual micturition, incontinence is certain to occur. Using this formula, the nurse can predict some episodes of incontinence.

$$\frac{D}{T_2} > T_1 = \text{Incontinence}$$

where

T_1 = Time between onset and desire of micturition and uncontrolled micturition
T_2 = Rate at which individual can walk
D/T_2 = Distance individual must walk to reach toilet

An absolute last resort in dealing with incontinence is the use of urinary appliances.

Table 8-5 Medications Potentially Affecting Urinary Continence

Drug type or class	Associated UI type	Mechanism of action
Antispasmodics	Stress	Increase muscle relaxation and sphincter incompetency
α-Blockers	Stress	Relax smooth bladder muscle, decrease urethral closing pressure
Narcotics/sedatives	Stress	Relax bladder muscle
Hypnotics		Depress sensorium and need to void
Diuretics		Increase urine volume and frequency
Anticholinergics	Overflow	Inhibit bladder contraction
Antipsychotic/anticontraction	Overflow	Inhibit bladder contraction
Antihistamines	Overflow/urge	Inhibit bladder contraction; urine retention can occur
Calcium-channel blockers	Overflow	Decrease detrusor contractions; urine retention can occur
α-Stimulants	Overflow	Increase urethral closing pressure; urine retention can occur

From Colling J: Noninvasive techniques to manage urinary incontinence among care-dependent persons, *J WOCN* 23:302, 1996.

Box 8-18 Therapeutic Modalities in the Treatment of Incontinence

Support Measures

Appropriate attitude
Accessible toilet substitutes (bedpan, urinal, commode)
Avoidance of iatrogenic complications (urinary tract infections, excessive sedation, inaccessible toilets, and drugs adversely affecting the bladder or urethral function)
Protective undergarments
Absorbent bed pads
Behavioral techniques (bladder training, toilet scheduling, conditioning, biofeedback, Kegel exercises)
Good skin care

Drugs

Bladder relaxants
Bladder outlet stimulants

Surgery

Suspension of bladder neck
Prostatectomy
Prosthetic sphincter implants
Urethral sling
Bladder augmentation

Mechanical and Electric Devices

Catheters

External (condom or "Texas" catheter)
Intermittent
Suprapubic
Indwelling

Toilet substitutes. Toilet substitutes for the infirm and ill have been around for hundreds of years. Four types are used; commodes for the bedside, overtoilet chairs for transport, bedpans for beds or commodes, and urinals for both men and women that can be used in bed, chair, or a standing po-

sition. The criteria for use of a commode is that the toilet is too far for the elder's mobility or it requires too much energy for the elderly person to get to the toilet. A commode can also substitute for an inadequate number of available toilets (Wells and Brink, 1980). Overtoilet chair criteria are similar to that for a commode. However, it cannot be used as a substitute for available toilets. Urinals are generally used by men; however, bottle-shaped urinals have been designed for women and are used on occasion. They can be obtained from a surgical supply store or various mail order catalogues.

Protective undergarments. A variety of protective undergarments or adult briefs are available for the incontinent older adult (Box 8-19). Disposable types come in several sizes determined by hip and waist measurement, or one size may fit all. The lining of these disposable pants may be fiberfilled or made with an absorbent polymer or gel substance. Polymer and gel substances are more absorbent and tend to keep a protective layer between the skin and wet material. Washable garments with inserts also do a reasonable job of containing urine. However, they tend to be made of plastic or rubber and therefore are hot and cause skin discomfort. If pants are going to leak, they will do so at the groin. It is important to fit them firmly but comfortably around the leg (Figure 8-11).

Protective padding. A variation of the standard drawsheet is a protective washable pad used along with a plastic sheet. The Australian Kylie pad is a sophisticated version of the drawsheet that is successful in keeping both the bed and the incontinent person dry. It is composed of two layers, with a water repellent layer next to the individual. Urine is absorbed by the liner. Disposable protective pads are available in the United States, but it is important to know the amount and type of fill in the pads. A polymer gel is more economical. It is unwise to purchase pads because they are inexpensive if it means using several more per day than if more expensive and more absorbent pads were bought (Figure 8-12).

Behavioral techniques. Behavioral techniques such as scheduled toileting, habit training, bladder training, biofeed-

<table>
<tr><td>

Factors to Consider for Use of Absorbent Products

</td></tr>
<tr><td>

Functional disability of person
Type and severity of incontinence
Gender
Availability of caregivers
Failure with previous treatment program
Client preference
Comorbidity

</td></tr>
</table>

back, and conditioning focus on improving the person's awareness of their lower urinary tract (Box 8-20). These techniques are usually effective in urge and stress incontinence. In some instances the goal is not to regain a normal voiding pattern but to decrease the number of wetting episodes, to decrease laundry costs and use of absorbent protection, and to improve the quality of life and social activity. The methods are free of side effects and do not limit future options. However, they do require time, effort, practice, and an individual who is cognitively intact and highly motivated.

Scheduled toileting consists of a fixed toileting schedule, such as every 2 hours, with techniques to trigger voiding and emptying the bladder completely (National Institutes of Health Panel, 1989; Newman, 1992; Palmer, 1996).

Habit training uses frequent checks (every 1 to 2 hours) for dryness. The client is reminded to void and praised frequently when successful. The objective of habit training is to allow the person to regain a normal voiding pattern and continence. It involves cognitive function, mobility, dexterity, and motivation (Newman, 1992; Rousseau and Fuentevilla-Clifton, 1992; Palmer, 1996).

Bladder retraining uses an interplay of methods. It teaches the individual to void at regular intervals and attempts to lengthen these intervals between voidings. Bladder training has been effective in reducing the frequency of urge and stress incontinence (National Institutes of Health Panel, 1989; Newman, 1992; Palmer, 1996).

Conditioning or pelvic muscle exercises employs use of the Kegel exercises. Conditioning also refers to improving mobility. Pelvic floor exercises strengthen the periurethral and pelvic floor muscles. The contractions exert a closing force on the urethra. Kegal exercises are one approach to the problem of stress incontinence. They can be either slow or rapid. The muscle contraction is held for 3 seconds then relaxed. This is repeated 10 times working up to 20 times. The exercise is repeated five times a day. Quick Kegel exercises begin with tightening and relaxing the pubococcygeal muscle without a pause between. These are done as fast as possible beginning with a count of 15 seconds and working up to 2 minutes. Initially it is difficult to identify, tighten, and relax this muscle but with repeated work becomes easier.

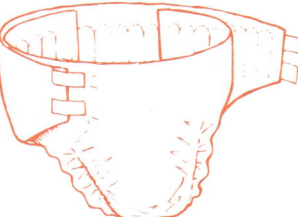

Adult diaper

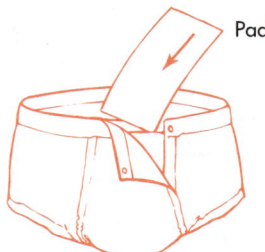

Pad

Adult undergarment

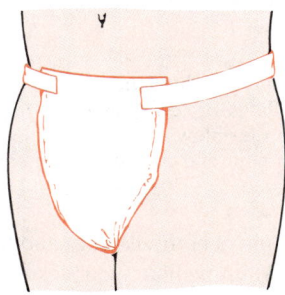

Adult undergarment

Figure 8-11. Disposable and reusable incontinence garments for men and women. (From Gray M: *Genitourinary disorders,* St Louis, 1992, Mosby.)

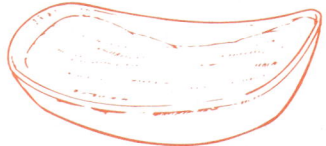

Adult absorbent pad

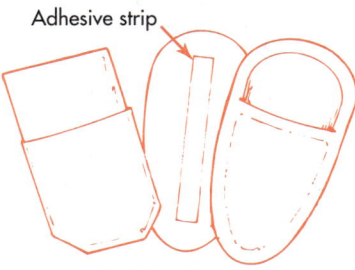

Adhesive strip

Male drip collector

Figure 8-12. Disposable incontinence pads. (From Gray M: *Genitourinary disorders,* St Louis, 1992, Mosby.)

<table>
<tr><td>**Box 8-20**</td><td>**Forms of Behavioral Management**</td></tr>
</table>

Diet modification
Bowel retraining
Behavioral interventions
  Habit training
  Prompted voiding
  Bladder training
  Pelvic floor exercises (Kegel)
Used in conjunction with behavioral interventions
  Vaginal cones
  Biofeedback
  Electrical stimulation

(National Institutes of Health Panel, 1989; Jette et al, 1990; U.S. Department of Health and Human Services, 1992; Palmer, 1996). Mandelstam and Robinson (1977) describe the following exercise routine to improve perineal and sphincter muscle control:

Standing, sitting, or lying, tighten the anal sphincter (as if to control the passage of flatus or feces) and then the urethra/vaginal muscles (as if to stop the flow of urine). This should be done at least four times each hour and can be done in any position or any place.

Biofeedback employs both visual or auditory instruments to give the individual immediate feedback on how well he or she is controlling the sphincter, the detrusor muscle, and/or abdominal muscles. Those who are successful learn to contract the sphincter and/or relax the detrusor and abdominal muscles automatically. Complete continence can occur in 20% to 25% of individuals and improvement in an additional 30%. Biofeedback requires sophisticated equipment (Newman, 1992; US Department of Health and Human Services, 1992). Table 8-6 provides a summary of behavioral modalities, the type of incontinence, outcomes, and appropriate populations for these approaches.

Skin care. Skin care maintains the first line of defense against infection. Skin that is in contact with urine should be washed with mild soap and warm water, then dried thoroughly. Application of a skin lubricant or an ointment such as A & D provides a thin protective layer to skin repeatedly exposed to urine. It is tempting to neglect an individual who wears protective pants, but it is important that the person be checked every few hours for wetness in order to maintain skin intactness. To minimize the episodes of incontinence, it is prudent to establish the incontinence pattern and place the individual on a toilet or commode before voiding.

Drugs. Drugs to eliminate or improve incontinence include bladder relaxants and bladder stimulants. Bladder relaxants include anticholinergic agents that delay, decrease, or inhibit detrusor muscle contractions, especially the involuntary contractions, and may increase bladder capacity. The most commonly used drug is propantheline (Pro-Banthine).

Undesirable side effects such as dry mouth, dry eyes, constipation, confusion, or the precipitation of glaucoma may occur with high doses of this drug. Smooth muscle relaxants such as flavoxate (Urispas), oxybutynin (Ditropan), and dicyclomine (Bentyl) work directly on the bladder detrusor muscle. These drugs exert mild anticholinergic side effects. Calcium channel blockers, also used for cardiovascular problems, have a depressant effect on the bladder. More study is needed to determine if there is a significant benefit for their use in urge incontinence. Imipramine (Tofranil), a tricyclic antidepressant, exerts both anticholinergic and direct relaxant effects on the detrusor muscle, as well as a contractile effect on the bladder outlet, thus enhancing continence. Two important side effects to be aware of in the elderly are hypotension and sedation. Bladder outlet stimulants include alpha-adrenergic agonist agents and estrogen replacement preparations. Alpha-adrenergic agonists, pseudoephedrine and ephedrine, cause contractions of smooth muscle at the bladder outlet and improve stress incontinence. Estrogen replacement therapy, while not definitively used for stress incontinence, has been effective in improving postmenopausal urgency, frequency, and urge incontinence.

Surgery. Surgical intervention is appropriate for some conditions of incontinence. Surgical suspension of the bladder neck in women has proved effective in 80% to 95% of persons electing to have this surgical corrective procedure. Outflow obstruction incontinence due to prostatic hypertrophy is generally corrected by prostatectomy. Sphincter dysfunction due to nerve damage following surgical trauma or radical perineal procedures is 70% to 90% repairable through sphincter implantation. Complications for this type of surgery are greater than 20% and may require an additional surgery. A urethral sling of fascia increases urethral elevation and compression. Continence is restored in approximately 80% of clients who have this surgery. Currently periurethral bulking has been added to the number of surgical procedures that address urinary incontinence. Collagen or polytetrafluoroethylene (PTFE) is injected into the periurethral area to increase pressure on the urethra. This adds bulk to the internal sphincter and closes the gap that allowed leakage to occur (Mayo Foundation for Medical Education and Research, 1994; Palmer, 1996). Bladder augmentation is more specific and limited to neurologic disorders such as a contracted bladder. A segment of the bowel is used to increase bladder capacity and to facilitate release of excess pressure (Rosenberg, 1992).

Nonsurgical devices. The Food and Drug Administration (FDA) has approved two devices, available through prescription, to manage stress incontinence. The Miniguard is about the size of a postage stamp and fits over the urethral opening. It is contoured with an adhesive-foam backing. The other device, the Reliance Urinary Control Insert, is designed for moderate to severe incontinence in women. The device is a balloon tipped plug, about one-fifth the diameter of a tampon, which is inserted by applicator. The force of the insertion inflates the balloon, so that the neck of the bladder

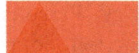

Behavioral Intervention Options for Incontinence

Type of incontinence	Intended population	Behavioral intervention	Purpose of intervention	Expected outcome
Urge, stress, mixed	Cognitively intact; able to discern urge sensation; able to understand or learn how to inhibit urge; able to toilet themselves with or without assistance	Bladder training	Restore normal pattern of voiding and normal bladder function Inhibit involuntary destrusor contractions	↓ Number of wet episodes ↓ Amount of urine lost ↓ Number of voidings ↑ Bladder capacity ↑ Quality of life
Urge, functional	Cognitively impaired; functionally disabled; incomplete bladder emptying; caregiver dependent	Scheduled toileting	Timed with individuals voiding habits Decrease wet episodes; no attempt to regain normal voiding pattern	↓ Number of wet episodes ↓ Laundry costs and/or use of absorbent devices ↑ Life quality ↑ Social activity
Functional, urge, mixed	Same as above	Habit training	Develop a pattern for voiding	↓ Frequency of incontinent episodes ↑ Comfort ↑ Quality of life
Urge, functional	Functionally able to use toilet or toileting device; able to feel urge sensation; able to request toileting assistance; caregiver is available	Prompted voiding	Heighten individual awareness of need to void	↑ Interaction between caregiver and individual ↓ Wet episodes
Stress, urge, mixed	Able to identify and contract pelvic muscles; able and willing to follow instructions and committed to actively participate	Pelvic floor training	Strengthen pubococcygeus muscle efficient urethral closure during sudden increases in intravesical pressure	↑ Strength and size of pubococcygeus ↑ Duration of muscle contraction with increased urethral pressure ↓ Urine loss ↑ Ability to stop urine flow once initiated Self-report of ↓ urine loss ↑ Self-esteem; enhance quality of life ↓ Reliance on pads, pantyliners, or absorbent products
Stress, urge, mixed	Cognitively intact Compliant with instructions Able to stand Sufficient muscle strength to contract muscle and retain the lightest weight No pelvic organ prolapse	Vaginal weight training	Same as above	Same as above
Stress, mixed	Ability to understand analog or digital signals using auditory or visual display Motivated, able to learn voluntary control through observation of biofeedback A health care orivuder who can appropriately assess the incontinence problem and provide behavior interventions	Biofeedback	Same as above	Same as above
Stress, urge, mixed	Ability to discern stimulation	Electrical stimulation	Reeducation of pelvic muscle; inhibit bladder instability and improve striated sphincter and levator anti contractility and efficiency	↑ Resistance of the pelvic floor; block uninhibited bladder contractions

Adapted and compiled from Fantl JA, Newman DK, Colling J et al: Managing acute and chronic urinary incontinence. In *Clinical practice guideline: quick reference guide for clinicians,* No 2, 1996 update, Rockville Md, US Department of Health and Human Services, Agency for Health Care Policy and Research, AHCPR, Pub No 96-0686, 1996; Staab AS, Hodges LC: *Essentials of gerontological nursing,* Philadelphia, 1996, JB Lippincott; Palmer MH: *Urinary incontinence,* Gaithersburg, Md, 1996, Aspen Publishers, Inc; Anderson MA, Braun JV: *Caring for the elderly client,* Philadelphia, 1995, FA Davis Co.

is then obstructed. The device must be removed by pulling a string before urination or intercourse. Trials of both of these devices have been on a limited number of women at present. Women using the devices gained complete or limited continence but also experienced urinary tract infections (UTIs), particularly with the Reliance Control Insert. However, it was felt that as the women gained skill in use of the devices, the UTIs and urethral irritation would decline (Harvard Women's Health Watch, 1996).

Catheters. As a last resort, appliances may need to be used. Too frequently, abuse of appliances occurs because they are convenient for the caregivers. Foley and condom catheters, diapers, and rubber pants carry with them inherent hazards of iatrogenic infection and skin irritation and breakdown. Psychologically the aged person feels and is treated differently, no longer as an adult but rather as a dependent and, perhaps, childlike individual. The aged person who has an indwelling catheter soon loses awareness of the sensa-

tions of bladder pressure and the habit of toileting. Persons with catheters often lose the micturition function completely. Women have fewer appliance options than men. In addition to the Foley catheter, men can use condom and sheath catheters, which are soft and pliable.

Catheter care is important regardless of the type of catheter used. The condom catheter should be removed daily to allow the penis to be scrupulously cleansed, dried, and aired to prevent irritation, maceration, and the development of pressure areas and skin breakdown. Foley catheter care should be performed at least twice a day. Cleansing of the external urethral meatus with a gentle cleanser, maintaining a closed system with unobstructed flow, maintaining an acid urine (Box 8-21), and meticulous care of equipment is essential in acute care or long-term care facilities as well as at home if a Foley catheter is used. Regular Foley catheter care ensures cleansing and removal of secretions and fecal matter, which can become the media for bacterial growth in the perineal area.

Box 8-21   Foods That Do and Do Not Acidify Urine

Do	Do Not	Do	Do Not
Juices		*Beverages*	
Prune	Citrus:	Coffee	Flavored sodas
Plum	Orange	Tea	Fruit ades
Cranberry	Lemon		
	Lime	*Soups*	
	Tomato	Bouillon	
		Meat broths	
Dairy products		Soup with allowed foods	
No more than 8 oz milk			
3 oz cheese:	Avoid excesses of	*Concentrated sweets*	
Cottage	milk as in milk-	White sugar	Molasses
Cream	shakes, malts, etc.	Corn syrup	Almonds
Cheddar		Cranberry sauce	Chestnuts
Swiss		Plum jelly	Coconut
Gruyère		Candy	
Vegetables		*Cereal, breads, potato substitutes*	
Small servings (3)	Potatoes	2 or more servings white/brown	
Corn	Lima beans	rice	
Lentils	Soybeans	Noodles/macaroni/spaghetti	
White beans	Beet greens	Barley	
	Parsnips	1 or more servings dry or cooked	
	Spinach	cereal (whole grain/enriched	
	Dried vegetables	preferred)	
Fruits		4 or more slices whole grain/	
2 or more servings except those	Cantaloupe	enriched bread	
listed to the right—prunes,	Raisins		
plums, cranberries eat freely	Dates		
	Dried fruits (except		
	prunes)		
	Citrus fruits		

Adapted from Newman DK: The treatment of urinary incontinence in adults, *Nurse Pract* 14(6):32, 1989.

Constant use of condom catheters is not a safe practice with elders. Skin under the catheter is prone to the development of fungal skin infections, irritation, edema, fissures, contact burns from urea, UTIs, and septicemia (Wells and Brink, 1980). Long-term use of indwelling catheters should be discouraged because of the complications that can occur. These include fever, bacteremia, acute and chronic pylonephritis, urethral abscesses, bladder or renal stones, renal failure, and possibly death (Greengold and Ouslander, 1986). Some helpful steps that can be taken by noninstitutionalized elders to stem incontinence are listed in Box 8-22. Box 8-23 outlines complications of long-term catheter use and nursing actions.

UTIs are common in the aged. Changes in the acid-base balance, ability of the defense mechanism of the bladder to deal with bacteria, and inefficient micturition are thought to be responsible. Women using estrogen for more than 1 year have an increased incidence of UTIs. The increase was observed only in women with intact uteri. Hysterectomized women had no increased risk. Controlling for diabetes, neurologic deficit, atrophic vaginitis, incontinence, and age did not affect these observed associations (Orlander et al, 1992).

Bacteria thrive in an alkaline urine environment. To increase acidity of urine, drinking a glass of cranberry, plum, or prune juice daily is helpful. These juices do not change from their acid state as they pass through the kidney; however, in some instances it has been noted that the acid nature of cranberry juice contributes to the development of a certain type of renal stones. This might lead to problems in some of the aged, particularly because they do not take in enough fluid to keep urine adequately diluted. A variety of foods also are acidifying to urine. Box 8-21 lists some foods to eat and to avoid. Medication may be needed to overcome UTIs, but the use of acid juices or vitamin C can be an adjunct to the therapy and continued as a preventive measure after therapy is concluded.

When in the hospital, the old person who previously has been able to toilet independently may find siderails at night confining and the administration of hypnotic medication immobilizing. In some instances the aged person has not been oriented to the location of the toilets or may be confused by the darkened room. The response to the call light of the person confined in bed may be slow. These constraints precipitate incontinence in persons who under usual circumstances are not incontinent.

Evaluation.   The success of interventions in urinary incontinence is measured against phased accomplishment:

1. The individual voids when placed on the toilet.
2. The individual drinks at least 2000 ml of fluid daily.
3. The individual remains continent 25% of the time.
4. The individual has fewer accidents in each successive phase.
5. The individual is continent all the time.

Indications for urologic referral are listed in Box 8-24. To develop a nursing care plan related to urinary incontinency, use box on p. 313 for guidance.

Fecal or Bowel Incontinence.   Fecal incontinence is defined as the inability to control the passage of stool or gas via the anus (Basch, 1992) or involuntary loss of stool from the rectum at inappropriate times (Staab and Hodges, 1996). The prevalence of fecal incontinence is approximately 3% to 4% of the community-dwelling elders, and approximately 16% to 60% of the institutionalized aged have some fecal incontinence (Richter, 1995). Often fecal incontinence is associated with urinary incontinence. Fecal incontinence is a relatively benign condition, but like urinary incontinence it has devastating social ramifications to the individuals and families who experience it. Factors affecting fecal incontinence are intestinal transit time, rectal factors (sensory), pelvic floor and sphincter tone, pelvic musculature, medications, muscular flaccidity, and the inability to get to the toilet when the urge to eliminate is present. This translates into such causes as sphincter dysfunction, anatomic

---

Box 8-22	**Helpful Interventions for Noninstitutionalized Elders to Control or Eliminate Incontinence**

Empty bladder completely before and after meals and at bedtime.

Urinate whenever the urge arises, never ignore it.

A schedule of urinating every 2 hours during the day and every 4 hours at night is often helpful in retraining the bladder. An alarm clock may be necessary.

Drink $1\frac{1}{2}$ to 2 quarts of fluid a day before 8 PM. This helps the kidneys to function properly. Limit fluids after supper to $\frac{1}{2}$ to 1 cup (except in very hot weather).

Drink cranberry juice or take vitamin C to help acidify the urine and lower the chances of bladder infection.

Eliminate or reduce the use of coffee, tea, brown cola, and alcohol since they have a diuretic effect.

Take prescription diuretics in the morning upon rising.

Limit the use of sleeping pills, sedatives, and alcohol since they decrease sensation to urinate and can increase incontinence, especially at night.

If overweight, lose weight.

Exercises to strengthen pelvic muscles that help support the bladder are often helpful for women.

Make sure the toilet is nearby with a clear path and good lighting, especially at night. Grab bars or a raised toilet seat may be needed.

Dress protectively with cotton underwear, sanitary pads for women, and protective pants or incontinent pads if necessary.

disarrangement, neurologic impairments, and musculoneural dysfunction (Hanauer and Sable, 1991, Basch, 1992; Wald, 1995). Other factors distinct to bowel evacuation problems are long-term dependence on laxatives, lack of sufficient bulk in diet, insufficient fluid intake, lack of exercise, hemorrhoids, and depression. Many instances of fecal incontinence result from fecal impaction, unless there is a neurologic origin. Serious illness accompanied by delirium and excessive doses of iron, antibiotic, and digitalis preparations may precipitate incontinence. Sedatives, too, can account for incontinence through depression of cerebral awareness and control over sphincter response. Box 8-25 provides causes of fecal incontinence.

Assessment. Assessment should include a complete client history (Box 8-26), as in urinary incontinence described earlier in this chapter. The following questions should be included in a bowel incontinence assessment.

1. What is the availability of the toilet or commode and the time required to get to them?
2. What medications, if any, is the aged person taking that influence peristaltic action, lucidity, or fluid balance?
3. How much bulk is provided in the food? (Pureed food does not help.)
4. What is the manual dexterity required to remove clothing once the aged person is in the bathroom?
5. Is there any neurologic or circulatory impairment of the cerebral cortex?

Box 8-23 Complications of Long-Term Catheter Use

Irritation/pain/discomfort
Inadvertant dislodgement
Obstruction
Erosion of bladder wall
Catheter irritation
Infection
Encrustation/sedimentation/stones

From Friers S: Indwelling catheters and devices: avoiding the problems, *Urol Nurs* 14(3):143, Mosby–Year Book, 1994; Jeter K, Faller N, Norton C: *Nursing for continence,* Philadelphia, 1990, WB Saunders.

Box 8-24 Indications for Urologic Referral

Unexplained incontinence
Surgical failure
Pharmacologic failure
Overt neurologic disease
Uninfected hematuria
Urosepsis
Difficult catheterization
Recurring urinary tract infections

Box 8-25 Causes of Fecal Incontinence in the Aged

Fecal impaction

Functional impairment
Mental
    Dementia
    Mental retardation
    Confusion
Physical
    Weakness
    Immobility

Decreased Reservoir Capacity
Aging
Radiation
Proctitis
Tumor
Ischemia
Surgical resection

Decreased Rectal Sensation
Diabetes mellitus
Megacolon
Fecal impaction
Central nervous system
    Stroke
    Multiple sclerosis
    Meningomyelocele
    Degenerative diseases
    Severe B_{12} deficiency
Peripheral nervous system
    Diabetes mellitus
    Shy-Drager syndrome
    Toxic neuropathy
    Perineal descent syndrome
Drug reaction/intoxication

Impaired Anal Sphincter and Puborectal Muscle Function
Idiopathic
Trauma (disruption of nerves and musculature)
Surgery
Spinal cord or pudendal lesions
Diabetes mellitus

Abnormal Delivery of Feces to Rectum
Drug-induced
Diarrhea
Blind loop syndrome
Inflammatory bowel disease
Infectious disease
Celiac sprue

Adapted from Hanauer SB, Sable KS: Pathology of fecal incontinence. In Doughty DB: *Urinary and fecal incontinence: nursing management,* St Louis, Mosby, 1991; Wald A: Lower gastrointestinal tract disorders. In Abrams WB, Beers MH, Berkow R, editors: *The Merck manual of geriatrics,* ed 2, Whitehouse Station, NJ, Merck Laboratories, 1995.

> ### Box 8-26   Fecal Incontinence Assessment
>
> **History**
> Characteristics of incontinence
> Relevant medical history
> Medication review
> Diet history
> Activity patterns
> Client/caregiver perception
> Environmental characteristics
>
> **Physical Examination**
> Abdomen
> Neurologic
> Rectal
>
> **Functional Assessment of Mobility Status**
>
> **Bowel Record (1 Week)**
>
> **Laboratory and Other Tests as Needed**

Intervention. The nurse's attitude in assisting the person who is incontinent of feces should be the same as for the individual with urinary incontinence. Fecal incontinence is a symptom. It requires that the patient be accepted as a person, that the incontinence problem not be advertised or ridiculed, and that the person is not made to feel ashamed or guilty. A great deterrent to successful intervention in incontinence is inconsistency in implementing the planned strategy and unrealistic expectations of rapid, full recovery. Time and patience are essential ingredients of success. Nursing interventions should include several days' surveillance of the patient's bowel function. A chart similar to that used to monitor urinary incontinence can be constructed.

Nursing intervention should work to manage and/or restore bowel continence. Therapies used in treating urinary incontinence are effective with fecal incontinence such as environmental manipulation, diet alterations, bowel training, sensory reeducation, sphincter training exercises, biofeedback, electrical stimulation, medication, and/or surgery to correct underlying defects (Wald, 1995). Box 8-27 provides a bowel training program for persons with altered

---

> ### Box 8-27   Bowel Training Program
>
> 1. Obtain bowel history and establish a schedule for the bowel training program that is normal and comfortable for the patient and conforms to his or her lifestyle.
> 2. Ensure adequate fiber and fluid intake (normalize stool consistency).
>   Fiber
>   Add high-fiber foods to diet (dried fruit, dried beans, vegetables, and wheat products).
>   Suggest adding 1 to 3 tbsp bran or Metamucil to diet one or two times a day. (Titrate dosage based on response.)
>   Fluid
>   Two to 3 liters daily (unless contraindicated)
>   Four ounces of prune, fig, or pear juice (or a warm fluid) may be given daily as a stimulus (for example, 30 minutes to 1 hour before the established time for defecation).
> 3. Encourage exercise program.
>   Pelvic tilt, modified sit-ups for abdominal strength
>   Walking for general muscle tone and cardiovascular system
>   More vigorous program if appropriate
> 4. Establish a regular time for the bowel movement.
>   Established time depends on patient's schedule.
>
>   Best times are 20 to 40 minutes after regularly scheduled meals, when gastrocolic reflex is active.
>   Attempts at evacuation should be made daily within 15 minutes of the established time and whenever the patient senses rectal distention.
>   Instruct patient in normal posture for defecation. (The patient normally sits on the toilet or bedside commode; for the patient who is unable to get out of bed, the left side-lying position is best.)
>   Instruct the patient to contract the abdominal muscles and "bear down."
>   Have patient lean forward to increase the intra-abdominal pressure by use of compression against the thighs.
>   Stimulate anorectal reflex and rectal emptying if necessary.
>   Insert a rectal suppository or mini-enema into the rectum 15 to 30 minutes before the scheduled bowel movement, placing the suppository against the bowel wall, or
>   Insert a gloved, lubricated finger into the anal canal and gently dilate the anal sphincter.

From Basch A, Jensen L: Management of fecal incontinence. In Doughty DB: *Urinary and fecal incontinence: nursing management,* St Louis, 1991, Mosby.

sensory awareness or poor sphincter control. Instituting a diet adequate in dietary fiber, 6 to 10 g per day (Ellickson, 1987), will add bulk, weight, and form to the stool and improve colon evacuation of the sigmoid and rectum rather than producing a continuous or intermittent oozing of fecal material. This may assist in the attainment of more controlled and complete bowel movements.

When the incontinence has a cerebral neurologic cause, it is often necessary to identify triggers that initiate incontinence. For example, eating a meal stimulates defecation 30 minutes following the completion of the meal, or defecation occurs following the morning cup of coffee. If the fecal incontinence is only once or twice a day, it can be controlled by being prepared. Placing the individual on the toilet, commode, or bedpan at a given time following the trigger event facilitates defecation in the appropriate place at the appropriate time.

When incontinence is continual, as often happens in nursing homes and hospitals, it may be necessary to develop a plan that controls the specific time of day when the individual has a bowel movement or movements. Generally this is accomplished by establishing constipation for several days and evacuating the bowel, for example, every fourth day by enema or suppository. Diet plays a role in this also. Creating the proper diet will affect intestinal motility and help flow evacuation. Bowel training of this type allows for predictability of colon evacuation and more freedom and less embarrassment for the aged person. If protective garments are necessary, they will allow the patient more opportunity to participate actively in events and to be more mobile in the institutional community.

The effectiveness of interventions in fecal incontinence will be self-evident but will take time. As in treatment of urinary incontinence, goals must be realistic. It cannot be stated too often or too strongly that the nurse must always provide immaculate skin care to the incontinent aged because self-esteem and skin integrity depend on it.

Coronary Problems and Rehabilitation

Coronary problems are the major cause of morbidity, disability, and mortality of the aged. Cardiovascular disease is the most prevalent of the disorders of the aged. Coronary problems are likely to produce a "cardiac cripple" when an individual believes any exertion burdens the overtaxed heart and may potentiate heart attack and death. In reality, few elders develop activity-induced ischemia. They are much more likely to trigger an attack by complicating illnesses that increase myocardial oxygen demand, such as infections and bleeding episodes.

A decline in activity actually makes individuals with cardiac problems more vulnerable to decompensation (Well Taken, 1994). Because of this, cardiac exercise rehabilitation programs must be encouraged for the physical and mental health of the individual. It has been found that exercise training of elderly coronary patients increases work capacity and vagal tone and decreases resting heart rate, body weight, and percentage of body fat (Wenger, 1990). Typical programs begin with light activity and progress to moderate activity under the supervision of a nurse or physical therapist.

The level of activity may be expressed in metabolic equivalents (METS). For example, light to moderate housework is equivalent to 2 to 4 METs; heavy housework or yard work is equal to 5 to 6 METs. A person would be tested for a baseline ability of between 4 and 5 METs. Results of the testing can guide a prescriptive physical activity program at home or in a structured rehabilitation program (Itoh, 1995).

Appropriately designed exercise programs take into account the need for building in longer periods for the exercise heart rate to return to its resting level and low-level activity between components of exercise training. Postexercise orthostatic hypotension is more likely to occur in the aged due to decreased baroreceptor responsiveness. Thermoregulation is impaired, and therefore exercise intensity must be reduced in hot, humid climates. These factors must be considered. A recommended training heart rate ranges from 50% to 70% of maximal heart rate achieved at exercise testing and does not result in discomfort during exercise. Perseverance and consistency are the key to success and benefits.

Cardiac rehabilitation programs for the elderly should emphasize activities that build endurance and self-reliance to facilitate self-care and quality of life (Rhodes et al, 1992). For the more impaired clients it is necessary to help them identify energy conservation measures applicable to their daily tasks. Risk reduction programs should be instituted with a clear understanding of the difficulties these present when attempting to alter harmful lifestyles such as smoking, overeating, habitual anger or irritation, and sedentary lifestyle with sporadic bouts of excessive activity. These are often deeply embedded in the personality structure and are not easily eradicated by "education." Begin by discussing this with the individual—nonjudgmentally. The nursing role is to provide acceptance, encouragement, resources, knowledge, and affirmation of the individual and their right to choose. Group programs focused on these issues have shown that some members' motivation and perceived health status improve (Wenger, 1990).

Gender is a factor in the outcome of cardiac rehabilitation. In a study of men and women participating in a structured or home cardiac rehabilitation program Schuster et al (1995) found that men in the structured programs knew more about heart disease and supportive treatment than women. The women failed to increase their understanding of their cardiac disease whether they were in a structured or home cardiac rehabilitation program. Women also demonstrated the poorest exercise adherence. With the increasing number of postmenopausal women, it is important for the nurse to consider this type of finding. It seems from the conclusions of Schuster that women need the reassurance that they already have some knowledge and that they can build on this knowledge to ensure better cardiac health. Because patients with cardiac disorders ordinarily take several medications to control heart rate, strength of beat, hypertension, and angina, these must be carefully and routinely monitored. Many of these drugs have serious toxic side effects, and when an individual decompensates, a medication assessment is the first order of the day.

One of the major ways that cardiac care differs from that for other chronic problems is that most exacerbations require acute hospitalization and intensive treatment, whereas many of the other chronic disorders are essentially managed at home the majority of the time. Onset of illness or exacerbation of chronic disorders may be quite different in older clients. For those with cardiac and other problems, the following events should always trigger investigation:

- Lightheadedness or dizziness
- Disturbances in gait and balance
- Loss of appetite or unexplained loss of weight
- Inability to concentrate or shortened attention span
- Changes in personality
- Changes in grooming habits
- Unusual patterns in urination or defecation
- Emotional incontinence
- Vague discomfort, frequent bouts of anxiety
- Excessive fatigue, vague pain
- Withdrawal from usual sources of pleasure

Congestive Heart Failure. CHF simply defined is the inability of the heart to pump a sufficient amount of blood to supply the metabolic needs of the body (oxygenation of lungs, blood pressure regulation, and control of electrolyte and water excretion). CHF has been recognized as the prototype disease of the twentieth century. Many medical clinicians describe it as "the pathological end point where all of modern society's bad habits—smoking, excessive dietary fat, obesity, lack of exercise—finally meet to produce the chronic, ultimate focal deterioration of our most vital organ" (Seng, 1992). Congestive failure is the number one admitting diagnosis of persons 65 years of age or older to the hospital (Kannel, 1989). It is estimated that 1% of the population 50 to 59 years of age has CHF. Every decade this figure doubles until it reaches a peak of 10% among those in their late eighties (Kannel and Belanger, 1991).

The Framingham Heart Study revealed that less than half the participants diagnosed with CHF survived 5 years or more (Kannel, 1989). Usually CHF is a slow killer, but it can also be quite sudden. Nearly a quarter of the men and 13% of the women in the study died of the disease. This is six to nine times greater than sudden deaths in the general population (Kannel and Belanger, 1991). People do not recover from heart failure; once the heart muscle is damaged it does not regenerate nor can it be repaired. The lost pumping capacity can never be regained (Smith et al, 1992; Braunwald, 1992).

Heart failure is best characterized by its related diseases, which are well documented in medical and nursing texts. The most common are coronary artery disease, by far the greatest single cause of heart failure, valvular disease, and hypertension. The commonality between these conditions and CHF is the substantive and irreversible damage to the heart muscle (Box 8-28). The damage occurs insidiously over time because of poor control of hypertension and atherosclerosis, which initiate the chain of adverse events leading to coronary artery disease, heart failure, and end-stage heart disease. Such factors as bad diet, smoking, and lack of exercise aggravate the disease, especially for those who happen to have a family history of heart disease and the genetic makeup.

Clinical heart failure is categorized as left heart, right heart, or biventricular heart failure. The left is the most common form and in turn is responsible for eventual right heart failure (Braunwald, 1992). There is also a formal classification of CHF established by the New York Heart Association, though this classification does not speak to the pathogenesis,

---

Box 8-28	**Causes of Heart Failure**

Impeded Forward Ejection

Systemic arterial hypertension or elevated systemic vascular resistance
Aortic valve stenosis
Coarctation of Aorta
Subaortic stenosis
Obstructive hypertropic cardiomyopathy
Pulmonary hypertension

Impaired Cardiac Filling

Ventricular hypertrophy
Prolonged myocardial relaxation time (diastolic dysfunction)
Pericardial constriction or tamponade
Restrictive endocarditis or myocardial heart disease
Ventricular aneurysm

Volume Overload

Valvular regurgitation
Increased intravascular volume
Metabolic demands: thyrotoxicosis; anemia
Arteriovenous shunts/fistulas

Myocardial Failure

Loss of muscle function (myocardial infarction; ischemia)
Cardiomyopathy
Myocarditis
Drug induced
Systemic disease (hypothyroid)
Chronic overload

its progression, or treatment (Braunwald and Grossman, 1992). Box 8-29 lists these classifications. Box 8-30 provides assessment guidelines.

Interventions will vary with the degree of congestive failure. They range from teaching the client about lifestyle changes in diet, activity, and rest to acute measures such as administration of oxygen if congestive failure is acute (Box 8-31). In general, interventions about which the nurse should be knowledgeable include the following:

1. Activity tolerance
2. Prescribed exercise program
3. Medication administration and the evaluation of medication effects
4. Monitoring for signs and symptoms of CHF
5. Monitoring intake and output
6. Monitoring client's weight
7. Checking for jugular distention
8. Auscultating heart and breath sounds
9. Noting laboratory values
10. Client education: low-sodium diet; medication regimen; signs and symptoms to report to the physician, such as weight gain of 2 to 3 lb in a few days, increased nocturia, increase in shortness of breath, a persistent cough, and ankle and leg swelling

Incorporate wellness information from Figure 8-13 into nursing care plans. Evaluation of the client reflects an absence or minimum of symptoms and interference with the individual's usual activity pattern. The client might comment that he or she is feeling well or that the symptoms have improved. For those with severe pathology the fact that the condition has not worsened is often all that is possible.

Vascular Insufficiency. Vascular insufficiency includes both arterial and venous systems. Each presents specific and differentiating signs and symptoms (Table 8-7).

Arterial insufficiency of the lower extremities often requires surgical intervention if the circulation can not be improved adequately with vasodilating medication. Not infrequently arterial insufficiency leads to gangrene and amputation of all or a portion of the extremity.

Venous insufficiency affects approximately 500,000 Americans, most of whom are older than 60 years of age (Mayo Clinic Health Letter, 1995). Fortunately, venous insufficiency and stasis ulcers respond to conservative treatment, though it takes many weeks and months to resolve, depending on the extent of tissue involvement.

The microvascular changes that occur with age often leave the vein walls weakened and unable to respond to increased venous pressure. This pressure is due to poor venous flow, vasculitis (inflammation), or thrombophlebitis (venous blood clot), which add to the weakening of vein walls. Heredity and obesity are additional factors that contribute to the altered venous integrity of the lower extremities. Weakened vein walls are also responsible for varicose veins. The backflow that occurs from venous pressure occurs in the small veins in the feet and ankle area, causing leakage of fluid into the tissues with subsequent foot and ankle edema. If the congestion is sufficient, the lower leg also becomes involved. Skin tissue becomes vulnerable to

---

Box 8-29   Classification of CHF

Class I   *Basically asymptomatic*
Cardiac disease without resulting limitations of physical activity

Class II   *Mild heart failure*
Slight limitation of physical activity
Comfortable at rest
An increase in activity may cause fatigue, palpitations, dyspnea, or anginal pain

Class III   *Moderate heart failure*
Marked limitation in physical activity
Comfortable at rest
Ordinary walking or climbing of stairs can quickly bring on symptoms of fatigue, palpitations, dyspnea, or anginal pain
Substantial periods of bed rest required

Class IV   *Severe heart failure*
Almost permanently confined to bed
Inability to carry on any physical activity without discomfort or severe symptoms
Some symptoms occur at rest
Chronic shortness of breath is common

Box 8-30   Assessment for Clients with CHF

Brief history of onset and course of condition
Vital signs
Cardiac and respiratory inspection and auscultation of heart and breath sounds
Mental status check
Activity capabilities
Lifestyle
Genitourinary: nocturia; oliguria
Weight change
Client's perception of condition, reaction to diagnosis, and treatment
General laboratory values: electrolytes, hemoglobin, hematocrit, coagulation

Compiled from Saunders SA: Atherosclerotic heart disease: heart failure. In Rogers-Seidl FF, editor: *Geriatric nursing care plans,* St Louis, 1991, Mosby; Havens LL, Weaver JW: Cardiovascular system. In Hogstel MO: *Clinical manual of gerontological nursing,* St Louis, 1992, Mosby.

insignificant trauma such as an insect bite or snug elastic topped ankle socks. Either of these or other events could precipitate the beginning of venous ulcer formation.

Usually symptoms begin with pruritus, edema, and stasis dermatitis or ulceration from a minor trauma. An ulceration will generally appear on the medial aspect of the tibia above the malleolus. Evidence of previously healed ulcers can be identified by brown or tannish discoloration over the skin.

A conservative treatment approach is usually taken, and the elder is generally treated at home with the intent of maintaining his or her activities (in some instances increasing the activity) Box 8-32 details information and treatment strategies for venous ulcers. Treatment usually consists of one or a combination of therapies such as leg elevation whenever sitting, topical antibiotics when an ulceration is present, use of wet to moist compresses and soaks, debridement with medications that contain fibrinolysin and desoxyribonuclease enzymes, or if necessary, surgical debridement. Elastic support stockings are frequently prescribed to enhance the efficiency of venous circulation. For the aged individual, it can be energy depleting to bend over and pull and tug on the elastic hose. It is sometimes helpful for both men and women with this problem to put on knee-high nylon stockings (not pantyhose) under the elastic hose. This method achieves minimum energy expenditure and might permit the aged person who needs assistance with part of dressing to become independent. A few minor annoyances do exist: the legs tend to get hot in warm weather, women find themselves wearing two (or three) pairs of hose, and men may be reluctant to wear women's stockings. In winter, however, it does have the benefit of keeping the legs warm, particularly for those aged who live in cold climates.

Treatment and resolution of venous stasis ulcers is not the only role for the nurse. Education of the aged person is essential as a means of preventing further episodes or minimizing the severity should ulceration recur. Box 8-33 provides education guidelines and a resource to develop an information sheet that elders can refer to when they need reminders of what to do.

Chronic Obstructive Pulmonary Disease.   Chronic obstructive pulmonary disease (COPD) is a major concern in old age. As a category that includes chronic bronchitis, asthma, and emphysema, it is responsible for 7 deaths per 1000 individuals 65 years of age and over (US Bureau of the Census, 1995). COPD is the result of a combination of factors, including genetic predisposition, environment, and smoking (Terry, 1995). In advanced age, normal age-related physiologic (senile) emphysema compounds any existing pathologic condition. This also increases an elder's risk of bronchitis.

The progressive nature of COPD can lead to malnutrition because energy is consumed by the tremendous effort expended in breathing. Eating requires further effort and is often neglected. Individuals and their families may be so concerned with the breathing difficulties they are hardly aware of the diminished caloric intake. Anxiety is a characteristic symptom when one has difficulty breathing. The role of the nurse is to help the individual determine a baseline of reasonable functional independence in the expenditure of energy and to avoid complications.

Box 8-31

Topics for Patient, Family, and Caregiver Education and Counseling on Heart Failure

General Counseling

Explanation of heart failure and reasons for symptoms
Cause or probable cause of heart failure
Expected symptoms
Symptoms of worsening heart failure
What to do if symptoms worsen
Self-monitoring with daily weights
Explanation of treatment/care plan
Clarification of patient's responsibilities
Importance of cessation of tobacco use
Role of family members or other caregivers in the treatment/care plan
Availability and value of qualified local support group
Importance of obtaining vaccinations against influenza and pneumococcal disease

Prognosis

Life expectancy
Advance directives
Advice for family members in the event of sudden death

Activity Recommendations

Recreation, leisure, and work activity
Exercise
Sex, sex difficulties, and coping strategies

Dietary Recommendations

Sodium restriction
Avoidance of excessive fluid intake
Fluid restriction (if required)
Alcohol restriction

Medications

Effect of medications on quality of life and survival
Likely side effects and what to do if they occur
Coping mechanisms for complicated medical regimens
Availability of lower cost medications or financial assistance

Importance of Adherence with the Treatment/Care Plan

Modified from Konstam MA, Dracup K, Baker DW et al: *Heart failure: evaluation and care of patients with left-ventricular systolic of dysfunction,* Clinical practice guideline No 11, Rockville, Md, 1994, US Department of Health and Human Services, Public Health Service, Agency for Health Care and Policy Research. AHCPR, Pub No 94-0612.

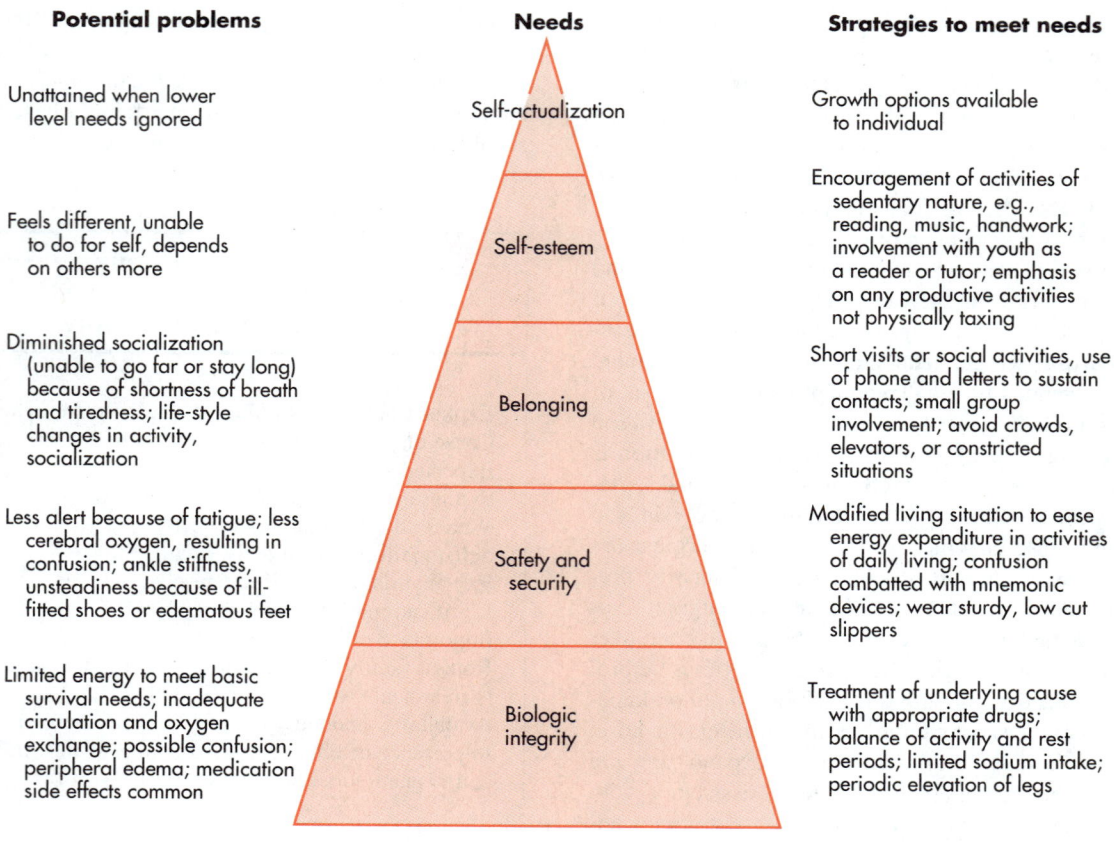

Potential problems

Unattained when lower level needs ignored

Feels different, unable to do for self, depends on others more

Diminished socialization (unable to go far or stay long) because of shortness of breath and tiredness; life-style changes in activity, socialization

Less alert because of fatigue; less cerebral oxygen, resulting in confusion; ankle stiffness, unsteadiness because of ill-fitted shoes or edematous feet

Limited energy to meet basic survival needs; inadequate circulation and oxygen exchange; possible confusion; peripheral edema; medication side effects common

Needs

Self-actualization

Self-esteem

Belonging

Safety and security

Biologic integrity

Strategies to meet needs

Growth options available to individual

Encouragement of activities of sedentary nature, e.g., reading, music, handwork; involvement with youth as a reader or tutor; emphasis on any productive activities not physically taxing

Short visits or social activities, use of phone and letters to sustain contacts; small group involvement; avoid crowds, elevators, or constricted situations

Modified living situation to ease energy expenditure in activities of daily living; confusion combatted with mnemonic devices; wear sturdy, low cut slippers

Treatment of underlying cause with appropriate drugs; balance of activity and rest periods; limited sodium intake; periodic elevation of legs

Figure 8-13. Congestive heart failure wellness perspective.

Table 8-7   Comparison of Arterial and Venous Insufficiency of the Lower Extremities

Characteristics	Arterial	Venous
Pain	Sudden onset with acute; gradual onset with chronic Exceedingly painful Claudication relieved by rest Rest pain relieved by dependency (with total occlusion, no position will give complete relief)	Deep muscle pain with acute deep vein thrombosis Relieved by elevation
Pulses	Absent or weak	Normal (unless there is also arterial disease)
Associated changes in leg and foot	Thin, shiny, dry skin Thickened toenails Absence of hair growth Temperature variations (cooler if there is no cellulitis) Elevational pallor Dependent rubor Atrophy or no change in limb size	Firm ("brawny") edema Reddish brown discoloration with postphlebitic syndrome Evidence of healed ulcers Dilated and tortuous superficial veins Swollen limb Increased warmth and erythema with acute deep vein thrombosis
Ulcer location	Between toes or at tips of toes Over phalangeal heads On heels Over lateral malleolus or pretibial area (for diabetic patients) over metatarsal heads, on side or sole of foot	"Garter area" around ankles (rich in perforator veins), especially the medial malleolus
Ulcer characteristics	Well-defined edges Black or necrotic tissue Deep, pale base Nonbleeding	Uneven edges Ruddy granulation tissue Superficial Bleeding

<table>
<tr><td colspan="2">

Box 8-32   **Treatments for Venous Stasis Ulcers**

</td></tr>
</table>

Conservative

Dressings	
Wet	To absorb weeping fluid
	Prevent tissue drying out
Change daily initially	Decreases risk of infection
	Keeps clean and protected from bacteria
(If not infected, an adhesive film or absorbant gel or foam is possible.)	
Application of fibrinolytic agents	
Cleaning	Mild soap and water
	Mechanically removes loose tissue without additional trauma
	Removes creams/lotions/
	Medications applied
Compression wrap	Increases venous flow
	Should continue to wear even after lesion is healed
Elevation of legs	Decreases swelling
	Improves venous return
Ambulation	Improves venous return

Treatment for Severe Ulcers

Mechanical pump compression	Provides intermittent compression for several hours daily
Elastic stockings or wrap	
Surgery	
Skin graft	For large ulcers
Vein stripping	

Chronic Recurring Stasis Ulcers

Growth factor from human blood platelets applied to ulcer in combination with other treatment	Stimulates new skin formation over ulcer, enhances healing
Cultured skin grown in laboratory (under FDA review)	To cover ulcer and enhance healing

Assessment focuses on obtaining a history and a physical examination that includes respiratory, cardiac, and mental status and on identifying knowledge gaps. Assessing airway clearance, breathing patterns, fatigue, mobility, fear, and socialization are all necessary to establish a reasonable functional expectation. Box 8-34 provides a model for respiratory assessment. Additional information on respiratory assessment can be found in physical assessment texts.

When assessment data have been gathered, the plan of action (interventions) should be designed to maintain or restore an acceptable quality of life for the elder with COPD and to minimize the number of hospitalizations through the interventions related to education, diet, medications, exercise. An older adult with COPD would be considered a candidate for pulmonary rehabilitation as long as he or she does not have severe COPD without pulmonary reserve, unstable heart disease, or psychiatric illness (Terry, 1995). The following interventions are designed to improve the quality of life: education about rest and activity, breathing and coughing techniques, adequate nutrition, anxiety and stress reduction measures, adjustment of ADLs to respiratory tolerance, therapeutic regimen, energy conservation, and signs of respiratory infection.

Interventions

Education. Education should be considered in every aspect of pulmonary care. The older adult should be taught to recognize the signs and symptoms of respiratory infection, how to maintain adequate nutrition, how to use a nebulizer/inhaler, how to clean it, the use of oxygen and oxygen safety, the type of exercise that is beneficial, how to pace activities, coping strategies, and other issues such as sexual function. Each of these areas requires teaching and has specific interventions that will be helpful to older adults and their family or their appointed caregiver.

Diet education should address the reason for monitoring weight and the signs of malnutrition. Weight loss can occur rapidly because of the energy expenditure needed to breathe. Dyspnea interferes with eating. In addition, satiation results from the intake of small amounts of food because of congestion in the abdomen by a flattened diaphram. Anorexia or decreased appetite occurs due to sputum production

Box 8-33	Guidelines for Patients with Venous Insufficiency

Give Legs a Rest

Elevate the feet above heart level while sleeping and several times a day. If necessary, elevate the foot of the bed or mattress.

Change Positions Frequently

Avoid activities that require standing or sitting with feet on the ground for long periods of time.

Give Legs Support

Wear professionally made compression stockings that apply even pressure from ankles to knees.

Learn how to put them on correctly.

Have at least two pairs of the compression hose available so they can be changed daily. After laundering, hang up to dry. DO NOT PUT IN DRYER

Buy new compression hose every 6 months; after that period of time the elastic is stretched.

Put hose on early in the morning; wear all day; remove at bedtime.

Avoid elastic bandages, i.e. ACE. They are difficult to wrap and exert even pressure.

If a compression pump has been prescribed by the physician, follow the instructions.

Take Care of the Skin

Wash lower legs and feet regularly with mild soap and water to avoid buildup of lotion.

Use moisturizing cream and emollients after washing.

Do NOT use lanolin- or petroleum-based creams when wearing support hose made with latex.

Avoid activities that can injure the legs or feet.

Pay attention to skin changes:

Swelling—stays when lying down

Discoloration—especially around ankles and lower legs

Dryness and/or itching—around ankles and lower legs

Any bruises or wounds that do not go away in one week

Apply Dressings

Follow ulcer care directions as prescribed.

Modified from San Francisco Wound Care Center, Seton Medical Center, Daly City, Calif, 1995; Staab AS, Hodges LC: *Essentials of gerontological nursing,* Philadelphia, 1996, JB Lippincott.

Box 8-34	COPD Assessment

History

Respiratory diseases
Smoking history
Symptoms

Physical Examination

Inspection*
  Posture
  Chest symmetry, shape expansion
  Respirations
  Skin color
  Capillary fill
  Sputum (color, amount, consistency)
Palpation
  Tenderness
Percussion
  Areas of hyperinflation, consolidation
Auscultation*
  Breath sounds

Functional Activity Mobility

Levels of activity before dyspneic
Interferences from sensory impairments

Knowledge

Educational attainment
Understanding of disease processes in COPD

*Most important of the four assessment techniques.

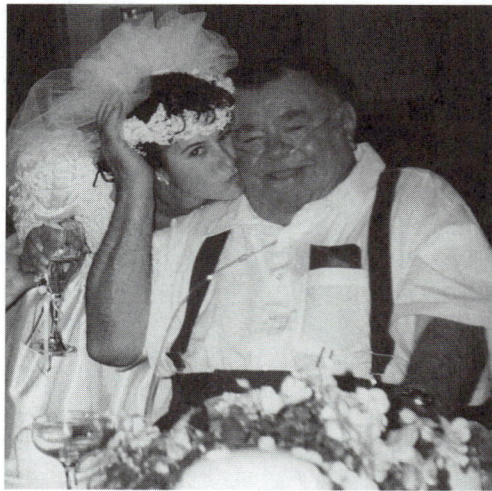

Living with a chronic disorder. (Courtesy Joanne Kayser.)

and gastric irritation from the use of bronchodilators and steroids. The interventions that might lessen these problems appear in Box 8-35.

Exercise tolerance should be assessed by the physician and activities prescribed to increase activity tolerance and improve respiratory status. Exercise may be done with or without oxygen as a supplement to control symptoms so that the older adult can spend enough time in exercise to gain benefit from it.

Medications are used to control dyspnea, cough, and sputum production (Terry, 1995). Older adults generally do better with inhalers/nebulizers than with oral medication be-

| Box 8-35 | **Interventions for COPD** |

Nutrition

Eat small, frequent, nutrient-intense meals.
Eat foods with high protein and calories.
Serve meals on small plates (servings will not look overwhelming).
Select foods that don't require a lot of chewing.
Have food cut in bite-size pieces to conserve energy.
Establish a plan for fluid intake; drink 2-3 L of fluid daily (pineapple juice helps cut secretions; keep a liter of water in the refrigerator or on the kitchen counter to be consumed each day in addition to other fluids).
Weigh at least twice a week.

Exercise

(Based on an established plan suggested by physician or rehabilitation team)
Walk daily all year round (in good weather, outdoors; in bad weather, go to the mall and walk indoors).
    Walk up and down stairs in home (if present).
Use a stationary bicycle.
*When buying shoes for activity and everyday wear, avoid shoes that require bending over to tie; instead get slip-on type and use a long-handled shoe horn to assist the heel into shoe.

Activity Pacing

Avoid high levels of exertion in early morning.
Arrange rest periods throughout day.
Allow plenty of time to complete activities; don't hurry.
Schedule activities in advance to reduce pressure and anxiety.
Obtain and follow prescribed exercise program for maintenance of heart/lung capacity.

ADLs

Allow ample time for bathing and dressing. Have a chair in bathroom for bathing.
Arrange toiletries in easy reach
Wear shoes that slip on or have Velcro closures, not ties.
Select clothing with elasticized waistbands; avoid constrictive clothing; use suspenders rather than belts.
Select and wear clothing that is easy to put on and remove.

Safety

Attempt to keep a dust-free environment.
Minimize or eliminate use of aerosol sprays, fumes, contaminants, dander.
Place plastic covers over mattresses, use hypoallergenic pillows and blankets.
Avoid carpet and rug floor coverings.

Emotional Support

Accept/encourage expression of emotions.
Be an active listener.
Be cognizant of conversational dyspnea; don't interrupt or cut off conversations.

Education

Teach breathing techniques:
    Pursed-lip breathing
    Diaphragmatic breathing
    Cascade coughing (series)
Teach postural drainage.
Teach *medications:*
    What, why, frequency, amount, side effects, and what to do if side effects occur
Use and care of inhalers
Teach signs and symptoms of respiratory infection.
Teach about *sexual activity:*
    Sexual function improves with rest.
    Schedule sex around best-breathing time of day.
    Use prescribed bronchidilators 20 to 30 minutes before sex.
Stay away from the use of alcohol or eating large quantities of food.
Use a position that does not require pressure on the chest or support of the arms.

General Instructions

Listen to weather reports.
    Avoid going out in inclement weather.
    Wear scarf over nose and mouth in cold and windy weather; wear a hat.
    Avoid going out when air pollution is high.
Use air conditioner to filter air and make it drier.
Avoid situations where you may encounter individuals with influenza or upper respiratory infections.
Obtain an annual flu shot if not allergic.
Obtain one-time multivalent pneumococcal immunization.
Notify physician of any temperature above 99° F.
Examine sputum; recognize and report changes to physician.
Do not use over-the-counter drugs unless physician approves.

cause of their more rapid onset, local efficiency, and fewer side effects. The older adult should learn about the medication he or she is taking, its side effects, and what to do if side effects occur. Instruction on the use of the inhaler is also very important if the maximum benefit is to be gained. In-

halers may be troublesome for an older adult with manual dexterity problems such as arthritis. The metered-dose inhaler may be a better choice for that individual because these inhalers have adapters which may aid in easier use of the device. Those with visual problems may also benefit from the metered-dose inhaler, which works on breath activation. Interventions also include explanation of how to use the inhaler, with a return demonstration by the older adult. Box 8-36 provides guidelines for metered-dose inhaler use.

Sexual information for the older adult who wishes to remain active but is consumed by dyspnea and anxiety; the client should be informed that sex is still possible. Box 8-35 provides education and counseling information that should aid the nurse in helping the older adult and the caregivers.

Rehabilitation programs for older adults with COPD consist of drug therapy, reconditioning exercises, and counseling. A multidiciplinary team of health professionals works collectively to help the aged adult achieve the following goals:

Increase the level of independence

Maintain individuality and autonomy

Improve function of the individual in his or her environment

Decrease the number of hospitalizations and need for hospitalization

Increase exercise tolerance

Increase self-esteem

Improve the quality of life

Outcomes of intervention and rehabilitation measures do not suggest a cure and may be elusive. It may not appear that physiologic changes have been effected, but the individual may feel and function better. This, however, is dependent on concomitant conditions that the older adult may have. All the efforts of professionals, family caregivers, and the older adult are directed to create a safe and comfortable environment that will maximize individual function and attainment of the highest level of wellness, with or without direct assistance.

Tuberculosis

Tuberculosis is a chronic pulmonary and extrapulmonary infectious disease characterized by particular symptoms, though these may be modified or not apparent in the very old. In the United States today there are 22,860 reported cases (Centers for Disease Control, 1996). This number has steadily decreased from the 37,100 reported in 1970 (US Bureau of the Census, 1995). However, there has been an upsurge since 1985. In the population over 65, incidence is highest among male Asians/Pacific Islanders (225/100,000) and lowest among white females (6/100,000). In all cultures reported, males had a much higher incidence than females (Centers for Disease Control, 1996).

Tuberculosis has been thought to be a malady of the Victorian Age or of those deprived by the circumstances of poverty and overcrowding. It has lain dormant and quiescent for decades in those previous victims who were actively treated, only to rise quietly as a phoenix from the ashes, stronger and more virulent than ever. Identified cases have increased 60% since 1985, and some have a particularly strong multiple drug–resistant type (MDR). *Mycobacterium tuberculosis* (M.tb) was ostensibly conquered in the 1950s by the development of isoniazid (INH). Many of our present elders were treated following their acquisition of the disease during World War II. Many others contracted the disease in childhood. As they become immunocompromised due to chemotherapy, extreme old age, or human immunodeficiency virus (HIV) infection, the bacterium is reactivated.

Our chief concern is the management of tuberculosis in congregate living situations. Elders living in nursing homes or congregate settings are particularly at risk and have an incidence nearly four times that of the general population (Hopkins and Schoener, 1996). In long-term care facilities the percentage of tuberculosis cases reported varies tremendously depending upon diligence in monitoring and numbers of long-term care residents under surveillance. Though not as contagious as once believed, the tubercle bacillus that is becoming resistant to combinations of drugs (MDR) is tenacious. Therefore prevention is of high priority, especially so among groups in close contact who have compromised immune systems, such as the very old in nursing homes. It is becoming a public health problem of real concern to elders and health care workers who may be exposed to it.

Currently it is recommended that Mantoux skin testing should be conducted routinely regardless of whether the individual was vaccinated in the past with BCG (bacille Calmette-Guérin) (Centers for Disease Control, 1996). The test should be read within 48 to 72 hours. A positive test is the measure of induration of 10 mm or more. When the test is

---

Box 8-36	**Use of a Metered-Dose Inhaler**

- Shake inhaler to mix contents.
- Inhale through nose, then breath out slowly and completely.
- Hold the inhaler 1 to 2 inches outside of open mouth (or use spacer device), and breathe out slowly but naturally.
- Place the mouthpiece in mouth.
- Activate the inhaler by pressing down on the inhaler while simultaneously inhaling slowly and deeply. Breathe in air from around the mouthpiece while inhaling.
- Close mouth and hold breath for 5 to 10 seconds.
- Exhale through nose.
- Rest at least 2 minutes (go by manufacturer's instructions).
- Repeat as prescribed.
- Rinse mouth with water and swallow.

Note: Some older adults with asthma may experience bronchoconstriction after using the inhaler. If tightness in the chest occurs after use of the inhaler, you may be reacting to the propellent used to deliver the medication. Report this to your primary care provider or pharmacist immediately.

positive, INH prophylaxis should be instituted. Further information regarding the resurgence and management of M.tb may be obtained in a free brochure from the American Nurses' Association by calling (800)274-4ANA (Hughes and Gillen, 1993).

Persons over 55 years of age account for 50% of the new cases. The aged and others with compromised immune systems are particularly vulnerable, especially those in collective living situations or institutions. The Centers for Disease Control have identified residents of long-term care facilities and health care workers as being at particular risk. Tuberculosis surveillance for the vulnerable old must be systematic (Wright and Staats, 1992). Recommendations are summarized in Box 8-37. While these suggestions are specifically designed for nursing home residents, nurses working with the frail or vulnerable old in any setting would be wise to inquire regarding purified protein derivative (PPD) testing, history of tuberculosis or exposure to it, and to recommend a preventive/therapeutic regimen when indicated.

Musculoskeletal Impairments

The common occurrence of musculoskeletal decrements as one ages is an important cause of physical disability. Loss of lower extremity and hand strength are particularly disabling. These prevalent and chronic complaints deserve increased attention because they impinge on many factors of daily living and life satisfaction (Jette et al, 1990). In-depth discussion of these can be found in Chapter 11 because in the majority of cases mobility and movement are affected by these disorders.

HEALTH BELIEFS AND ADHERENCE IN CHRONIC ILLNESS

Nonadherence to recommended therapeutic regimens is considered a major problem for persons with chronic disorders. Origins and concepts of health from the clients' and professionals' perspectives are important factors to consider. It also may be worth noting that the lack of "recovery" from the disorder may precipitate client-blaming strategies such as, "Well, if they would follow the recommendations, they would surely get better." Individuals who adapt lifestyle to health deviations are often motivated by fear of death, disability, pain, and social consequences such as effects on work, activities, and family. Adherence is influenced by numerous factors such as complexity of the regimen, duration, amount of change imposed, inconvenience of obtaining necessary care, dissatisfaction with the system, and health beliefs. The health belief model investigated by Redeker (1988) was developed to explain response to preventive health behaviors. The major belief factors are the value to the individual of a particular outcome and the individual's estimate of the likelihood of a particular outcome associated with compliance or noncompliance. Belief in the efficacy of an action implies belief that that action will reduce the threat to health. The requirements of compliance must not out-

weigh the benefits, or the client will rarely feel it is worth the effort. Careful assessment of the client's belief in outcomes and energy needed to comply with the regimen is essential. Questions that need to be addressed are as follows:

- Do health beliefs remain stable over time?
- Is there a difference between the responses of individuals recently diagnosed and those of clients with a long history of chronic disorders?
- How important is symptom severity in compliance?
- What relationship exists between social support and maintenance of health benefits?

Emphasis on the importance of the client's perception of health is consistent with Orem's concept (1980) that education, experience, attitudes, and knowledge all color one's response to health requirements.

Compliance

Compliance has been defined as the extent to which a person's behavior coincides with medical or health advice. If this is viewed traditionally, it essentially means the client becomes a passive respondent to the authoritarian demands of the health care providers. Compliance is one of the dilemmas of the chronically ill. Noncompliance is a nonspecific symptom that may be caused by numerous factors. Given this assumption, we must not expect any one method of intervention to be particularly successful. Physicians treating elderly persons with chronic diseases are often unaware that the compliance rate is less than 50% (De-Nour, 1986).

Box 8-37	**Tuberculosis Testing of Residents Living in Long-Term Care Facilities**

Tuberculin skin test on all admissions to facility unless known to test positive.
Annual retesting of all persons who are negative.
Annual testing of all employees.
If converted to positive:
    Obtain chest X-ray to exclude active disease
    Treat unless specific clinical reason not to treat
    Annual examination for all positive reactors (chest x-ray or physical examination and/or sputum culture)
Record positive and negative results in a specific section of the medical record for easy access of information.
Designate person to be responsible for monitoring TB infections in facility.
Total and document the number of conversions to figure annual conversion rate.
Total and document the number of conversions who are unable to tolerate or complete prophylactic course of Tb medication and reason.

From Wright BA, Staats DO: Tuberculosis surveillance program: a nursing home experience, *Geriatr Nurs* 13 (5):257, 1992; Centers for Disease Control and Prevention: *National Center for HIV/STD and TB Prevention Report,* 1996.

Often, the demands of long-term illness conflict with values and needs developed over a lifetime. Nurses must appreciate the interpersonal, cultural, situational, and other factors that underlie what may appear to be simple resistance and negativity. Noncompliance is a complex, multideterminated phenomenon that may involve indirect self-destructive tendencies, quality-of-life issues, family deterrents, or the quality of the client-physician relationship. In many cases society itself contributes to noncompliance by imposing regulations, policies, insurance restrictions, and medical constraints that reward noncompliance. For example, in recent years individuals who were receiving Supplemental Security Income (SSI) for disability were often dropped from the rolls if they demonstrated any increasing capacity for self-care.

Chronic illness is increasing because of endemic risk factors, deeply ingrained cultural values, and the medical advances that keep people alive longer. The task of living with these chronic illnesses for years by following increasingly restrictive regimens has not been given enough consideration. Knowledge of a medical condition does not significantly affect compliance; however, knowledge of the regimen, a therapeutic alliance with the physician, and higher levels of education all seem to significantly relate to greater levels of compliance. The longer a condition exists, the less one is able or willing to continue complex regimens. Positive coping with chronic illness is contingent on the accomplishment of the following tasks:

1. Ability to neutralize harmful environmental conditions
2. Adjustment to negative events consequent to the illness
3. Maintenance of self-image and self-sufficiency
4. Maintenance of social relationships
5. Coping with emotional reactions of anxiety and depression

Compliance is often directly related to the degree of hope one has for recovery—or maintenance. When this is lost, the hopeless individual may have a cavalier attitude toward any medical or nursing interventions that may be suggested. Researchers are becoming more interested in the impact of self-rated health on compliance and the expectation of recovery. To some extent it appears that an individual's self-ratings prior to illnesses become predictive of outcomes and changes in functional abilities (Idler and Kasl, 1995; Wilcox et al, 1996). If this is a common phenomenon, then we might expect individuals with negative self-appraisals of their health to become apathetic or fatalistic.

Some types of noncompliance are healthy, in that they may demonstrate an individual's acceptance of responsibility and taking charge, even though in some cases not in the best possible manner. Therefore noncompliance must be carefully evaluated before we conclude that it is helpful or harmful.

Compliance is considered to be the extent to which an individual adheres to medical and health advice. Sustaining compliance is a dilemma of the chronically ill. As the aged become increasingly vulnerable to illness and in spite of their best efforts may actually lose ground physically, they often lose motivation to continue a regimen that does not produce anticipated results. That, in addition to misunderstandings and lack of sufficient information regarding medications and treatments, results in a low rate of compliance among the aged as a group. Estimates of noncompliance vary considerably, depending on the disorder and treatment being reported. Low motivation and feelings of defeat are often compounded by physical and environmental hindrances to compliance.

For some there may be an element of self-destruction present or subliminal suicide intent. The biomedicalization of our society has often resulted in medical interference in matters that really should be in the domain of the individual. The nurse needs to assess the knowledge base of the client related to the regimen prescribed and keep on balance an awareness that resistance to direction may be a form of autonomy and personality strength.

CHRONIC PROBLEMS AND LONG-TERM CARE

Problems that impair one's ability to maintain basic ADLs with intermittent support and assistive devices will most often require institutionalization. Though family caregivers, particularly aging spouses, bear the brunt of this care, there comes a time when the burden simply cannot be borne by the family member. This is discussed thoroughly in Chapter 17. In this chapter it is important to focus on the kind and quality of support one may see and find in long-term care institutions. Today the traditional nursing home seldom exists. Most provide several levels of care and have moved steadily toward the hospital model of care, particularly with the numerous subacute units that provide sophisticated medical treatments. It is important for the individual needing assistance for chronic impairments to seek a setting that provides the level of independence and the home atmosphere that is most supportive of comfort, satisfaction, appropriate levels of independence, and dignity. Although in the past it was difficult to locate such accomodations, it can be done with appropriate planning.

First, one must consider the eventual need for this sort of support and make plans prior to the need. The prospective client's name must be on the list for potential admission prior to need, sometimes a year or more in advance. Individuals rarely want to take this step, but it should be reinforced that top-rated facilities simply are not available on an immediate basis. When the name reaches the top of the list, it will move down again until the client is ready for admission. At this writing, a 3-day hospital stay is still required prior to nursing home admission. The long-term care providers throughout the nation are promoting legislative changes that will delete this requirement. It is no longer necessary in terms of client assessment because thorough and adequate assessment, in a holistic manner quite different from that in a hospital, is now assured when the Minimum Data Set (MDS 2.0) is completed. This is required by the federal government within 14 days of admission. See Appendix 8-D for a model of the MDS 2.0 and special strategies for implementing it (Klusch, 1995).

CHRONIC FUNCTIONAL DISABILITY AND HOME CARE

The elderly population with chronic functional disabilities primarily reside in their homes. Schnack (1995) notes that nurse-owned community health care agencies are proliferating and assuming an ever-larger share of this $31 billion dollar industry. In a 1990 study Stone and Murtaugh found that nearly half a million elders need assistance in ADLs, and only one tenth of these individuals, potentially eligible for home care benefits, could meet the very restrictive disability criteria. Since that time the field has changed considerably, and it is now estimated that more than 7 million persons annually receive medical care in the home.

More than a million elders indicate they need and receive active assistance with bathing. Those unable to carry out ADLs most frequently needed active assistance with bathing, dressing, and toileting. For those able to manage basic ADLs, most needed active and standby assistance with grocery shopping, money management, and laundry. Short and Leon (1990) reported that those who use home and community services are most frequently over age 85, female, living alone and having difficulty with several activities, or covered by Medicaid.

Kemper (1992) found that on average disabled persons with a spouse or adult child receive 23 hours more care per week than those with neither. This raises the question of how public home care benefits should be distributed. Strauss and Corbin (1988) suggest that assisting individuals and their support persons to view chronic disorders as having a "trajectory" may help them cope with the ups and downs and the acute exacerbations that may require hospitalization. If they are able to better understand the phases of a disorder, they are likely to weather the difficult periods without undue discouragement. Often it must be seen as a lifetime situation that passes through stages in which resources must be tailored accordingly. In summary, they suggest the following points that practitioners must consider:

1. Chronic illness must be seen through the eyes of the persons experiencing it.
2. The illness is often a lifelong course that passes through many phases.
3. Biographic, medical, spiritual, and everyday needs must be considered.
4. Collaborative rather than purely professional relationships may be most effective.
5. Lifelong support may be necessary, although the type, amount, and intensity of such support will vary.

Effects of Chronic Illness on the Family

Often the ill individual feels like a burden to the family and engages in numerous compensatory behaviors to reduce this feeling of guilt. Home care is inconsistently provided and financed, and caregiver burdens are enormous. These have been explored and described endlessly (see Chapter 17 for additional discussion). Most often, families are found to extend themselves far beyond their own limits in attempting to deal with a member with a chronic disorder.

Effects of Chronic Illness on the Individual

In summary, management of chronic problems of the aged becomes an issue of the individual and the family. Nurses are resource persons, advisors, teachers, and at times assistants, but the individual is in control of his or her adaptation. Nurses will assist by performing the following functions:

- Identifying and stating strengths the individual demonstrates
- Discussing healthy lifestyle modifications
- Encouraging the reduction of risk factors in the environment
- Assisting the individual to devise methods of improving function, halting disabilities, and adapting lifestyle to reasonable expectations of self
- Providing access to resources when possible
- Referring appropriately and when needed
- Organizing interdisciplinary case conferences
- Informing the individual of insights gained in management of disorders.

The goal of care of the chronically ill may be to slow decline, relieve discomfort, and support preferred lifestyle with as few restrictions as possible (Strauss and Glaser, 1975) (Box 8-38). Not all chronic conditions require nursing

---

Box 8-38	**Goals in Management of Chronic Problems**

Stabilize the primary problem
Prevent and manage medical crises
Control symptoms
Encourage compliance with regimen
Prevent secondary disabilities
Prevent social isolation
Treat functional deficits
Promote adaptation
    Person to disability
    Environment to person
    Family to person
Adjust to changes in progression of problems
Normalize interactions

Compiled from Brummel-Smith K: Geriatric rehabilitation, *Generations* 16(1):27, 1992; Corbin JM, Strauss A: *Unending work and care: managing chronic illness at home,* San Francisco, 1988, Jossey-Bass.

service. The ability of the aged individual and the family to manage and cope with the problems encountered determines the need. It is necessary for those who care for the aged with chronic conditions to be reoriented and resocialized to care norms and to recognize a different system of rewards. The basics of the care process emphasize improving function, managing the existing illness, preventing secondary complications, delaying deterioration and disability, and facilitating death with peace, comfort, and dignity (Wells, 1982). Progress is not measured in attempts to achieve cure but rather in maintenance of a steady state or regression of the condition while remembering that the condition does not define the person. This thinking is essential if realistic expectations for the caregiver and the aged are to be achieved. Beyond that, the individual will in some manner seek to understand the meaning of the intrusive non-self of ongoing impairment and struggle to incorporate it in some manner into the perceived total self. The nurse's involvement in this process is to ask about the meanings of the illness and to listen and learn.

KEY CONCEPTS

- Lubkin states: "Chronic illness is the irreversible presence, accumulation or latency of disease states or impairments that involve the total human environment for supportive care and self care, maintenance of function and prevention of further disability."
- Declines in mortality, increasing medical expertise, and sophisticated technologic developments have resulted in a great increase in the survival of the very old with multiple chronic disorders.
- Statistics regarding chronic disease are suspect because they often reflect only those who have come for medical care. In addition, decreased function without incapacitation is rarely reported.
- Women live longer than men and for that and other unknown reasons tend to have a higher incidence of chronic disease.
- One of the most difficult aspects of chronic disease is the unpredictability of the trajectory.
- The management in the home by the family, self, or significant other is central to care and is not peripheral to medical management (Strauss and Corbin).
- Adaptations and assistance with ADLs and IADLs are the crux of chronic disease management.
- The most prevalent chronic problems of the aged are arthritis, hearing impairment, heart conditions, and hypertension.
- The most frequent assistance needed by those with chronic disorders is with bathing, dressing, and ambulation.
- The goals of rehabilitation for the aged are to ensure opportunity for optimum personal development and function. Though rehabilitation legislation is chiefly

designed to return individuals to productive employment, this is not at this time a goal for most of the aged.

▲ CASE STUDY

Diabetes

Ms P, an 82-year-old single lady, lives in a life-care community in her own apartment but has the reassurance of knowing her medical and functional needs will be taken care of regardless of the extent of these needs. This is the primary reason she chose to sell her home and live in the tiny apartment in the life-care complex. She is at present independent though she is diabetic (managed with diet, exercise, and oral medications), suffers CHF, and is having serious problems with her vision. She has also noticed that her toes are cold and somewhat numb. The great toe on her left foot seems to be discolored. Because of the lack of feeling, she often walks around her apartment barefoot because it seems to increase the sensation in her feet. She has also been gaining weight steadily since she moved into the life-care community and attributes that to the fact that she eats much better now that she joins others in the congregate dining room for meals. It is hard for her at times to ignore the delicious desserts that the chef so wonderfully prepares. Overall, she feels quite good and is grateful that she has no severe pains—some mild arthritis but nothing serious. She has not needed to use the health care center and goes to the clinic only to pick up her medication. She sees no reason to bother them with anything else. Her niece stopped by last week to borrow money for her car payment. Ms P seemed a little confused and lethargic. Her niece asked if she had been sleeping well, and Ms P responded that, indeed, she slept too well and too much. The niece encouraged her to go to the clinic for a checkup, but Ms P declined. This week when Ms P went to the clinic for her medication and they checked her blood sugar, it was 280 mg/dl. She said, "Oh, I don't think it is anything to worry about. I ran out of medication and didn't take it for 2 days and I ate two pieces of fudge after lunch."

Based upon the case study, develop a nursing care plan using the following procedure*:

List comments of client that provide *subjective data.*

List information that provide *objective data.*

From these data identify and state, using accepted format, two *nursing diagnoses* you determine are most significant to this client at this time. List two *client strengths* that you have identified from data.

Determine and state *outcome criteria* for each diagnosis. These must reflect some alleviation of the problem identified in the nursing diagnosis and must be stated in concrete and measurable terms.

*Students are advised to refer to their nursing diagnosis text and identify possible or potential problems.

Nursing Diagnoses

The following potential diagnoses must be considered as well as diagnoses unique to the particular individual:
Incontinence: functional, reflex, stress, total, and urge

Motivation for bladder control
Knowledge deficit regarding causes of incontinence
Social isolation

NURSING PROCESS AND NURSING DIAGNOSIS
Urinary Incontinence: Functional

Etiologies and Related Factors
Altered environment
Decreased ability or inability to communicate
Time between urge to void and voiding
Physical mobility, strength, balance
Visual/perceptual deficits
Inability to recognize or use familiar articles
Difficulty finding way to toilet
Memory deficit
Inability to interpret bladder cues
Relationship between food, fluid intake, activity, sleep, and voiding schedule
Anger
Frustration
Motivation (lack of)
Confusion/disorientation

Defining Characteristics
Loss of urine or voiding before reaching an appropriate receptacle

Knowledge
Normal anatomic and functional age changes
Predisposing factors
Bladder/urinary assessment
Medication administration
Medication side effects and interactions
Rehabilitation concepts
Bladder training programs
Community resources

Clinical Judgment and Related Skills
Obtain a complete urinary incontinence history with available assessment tools; include prior lifestyle, environmental influences and factors, effect of medication, chronic illness, activity on incontinence
Conduct a physical examination to include vital signs, functional activities of daily living necessary in maintaining continence
Implement nursing interventions for the appropriate type of incontinence
Monitor medication and fluid intake
Evaluate medication impact and interactions
Design, implement, and evaluate program to resolve or decrease functional incontinence
Conduct support groups for clients/families
Refer client/family to appropriate resources

Evaluation
Client is dry
Number of episodes of incontinence decreases
Number of incontinent episodes is eliminated (resolved)

NEEDS ADDRESSED AND TASK STRENGTHS

Need to adapt to fluctuations of function and comfort: need for self-monitoring (to achieve safety and security)
Capacity for adaptation to changes
Lifestyle flexibility

Strong sense of personal identity
Ability to tolerate physical changes
Attentive to subtle body signals
Takes active role in health maintenance
Assertive in obtaining services and assistive devices

Plan and state one or more *interventions* for each diagnosed problem. Provide specific documentation of source used to determine appropriate intervention. Plan at least one intervention that incorporates the client's existing strengths.

Evaluate success of intervention. Interventions must correlate directly with the stated outcome criteria in order to measure the outcome success.

▲   CASE STUDY

Incontinence

Jenny, at 82 years old, was hospitalized for an abdominal hysterectomy to remove large benign fibroid tumors. When she awoke from anesthesia, she was quite disoriented and had the illusion that something was crawling into her vagina. She tried repeatedly to pull it away, mildly disoriented and highly agitated because of the presence of a Foley catheter to drain her bladder. She said, "What have you done to me that I can no longer pee normally? This is ridiculous and you didn't have permission to do this." The third day following surgery she developed a temperature of 99 degrees. Nevertheless, she was eager to be released to her home. Everything there was so orderly and predictable. Her home was integral to her self-concept. She found that coping with the hospitalization seemed to make her weaker each day even though she ambulated three times daily and scrupulously followed whatever directions she was given regarding her care and recovery. The morning of the fourth day following surgery the Foley was discontinued and her temperature had returned to 98.6 degrees. She was released and her daughter took her home. She found that she was dribbling urine everywhere, seemingly having totally lost control. She attributed this to the trauma of surgery and began wearing disposable pads. When she went to the clinic for her postsurgical check, she told the nurse she felt fine except for her inability to control her urine and her fear that her odor repulsed people.

Based upon the case study, develop a nursing care plan using the following procedure*:

List comments of client that provide *subjective data.*

List information that provide *objective data.*

From these data identify and state, using accepted format, two *nursing diagnoses* you determine are most significant to this client at this time. List two *client strengths* that you have identified from data.

Determine and state *outcome criteria* for each diagnosis. These must reflect some alleviation of the problem identified in the nursing diagnosis and must be stated in concrete and measurable terms.

Plan and state one or more *interventions* for each diagnosed problem. Provide specific documentation of source used to determine appropriate intervention. Plan at least one intervention that incorporates the client's existing strengths.

Evaluate success of intervention. Interventions must correlate directly with the stated outcome criteria in order to measure the outcome success.

STUDY QUESTIONS/ACTIVITIES

What are the most plausible reasons for Jenny's incontinence?

From data available what would you surmise are important aspects of Jenny's personality?

Discuss your thoughts about the effects of being incontinent on Jenny's self-concept.

What would you say to Jennie about her situation?

What might you recommend to Jennie?

Would pelvic floor exercises be beneficial to Jenny? Explain your reasoning.

RESEARCH QUESTIONS

What percentage of women develop urinary incontinence related to disorders of the reproductive organs?

What are the reasons women refrain from seeking treatment for urinary incontinence?

What are the effects of various systemic diseases on continence; for example, diabetes, hypothyroidism, arthritis, CHF?

What are the most frequent reasons men experience urinary incontinence? Do they seek treatment more readily than do women?

How closely does the loss of urine control correlate with feelings of loss of control in other aspects of life?

What percentage of elders curtail social activities purely because of incontinence?

How often is urinary incontinence identified as the trigger event that precedes institutionalization?

Do correlations exist among age, decreased tissue elasticity, and the formation of pressure ulcers?

Do individuals at high risk for pressure ulcer development who never develop ulcers have a protective characteristic or factor?

Which risk assessment factors best predict pressure ulcer development in selected subgroups of high risk patients; i.e., frail elderly or critically ill?

Are the parameters used in risk assessment tools common or different in acute care, long-term care and home care?

How does documentation of pressure ulcers affect prevention of pressure ulcers?

RESOURCES

Film and Audiovisual Programs

COPD: Care in the Geriatric Patient. Through the use of case discussion the program provides a practical multidisciplinary approach to assessment and management of COPD. Available from Geriatric Video Productions, PO Box 1757, Shavertown, PA 18708-0757 (800) 621-9181.

---

*Students are advised to refer to their nursing diagnosis text and identify possible or potential problems.

Prevention and Treatment of Pressure Ulcers directs specific attention to prevention, assessment, and management. Available from Geriatric Video Productions, PO Box 1757, Shavertown, PA 18708-0757 (800) 621-9181.

COPD Is Manageable is an educational video for patient/family, staff or public use. Produced by Progress Products, 5074 Masheena Lane, Colorado Springs, CO 80917-2675, (719) 637-0811, (cost $59.95), 45 minutes, VHS.

Adapting Successfully to Parkinson's Disease. Film West Associates, 287 Kingsway Garden Mall, PO Box 1102B, Edmonton, Alberta T5J 3K3, (403) 474-1936.

The following are available from New Harbinger Publications, 5674 Shattuck Ave, Oakland, CA 94609, (800) 621-0851:

Arthritis. Fifteen-minute 16-mm color film emphasizing the importance of proper diagnosis and treatment to minimize pain and disability (free loan).

Eating for Your Health. Color slide and audiocassette presentation of planning, shopping, reading labels, and eating wisely (cost: $22.00).

Treating Yourself with Care. Color slides and audiocassette presentation that explain how best to use nonprescription drugs (cost: $22.00).

Adaptive Devices

The World of Assistive Technology and other videos explaining various devices to enhance function; training modules, technical reports, books, and journals are available from the Center for Assistive Technology, 515 Kimball Tower, University of Buffalo, Buffalo, NY 14214-3079, or call Thomas Burford, (716) 829-3141.

ABLEDATA, a database containing information on 20,000 assistive technology products, (800) 227-0216.

National Rehabilitation Information Center: newsletters, research updates, publications, (800) 346-2742.

Gadgets for easier living include devices such as talking clocks, stocking pullers, sound-operated light switches, and jumbo-size push-button telephones.

Tub benches assist a person into and out of the bathtub and are designed according to individual needs and degree of mobility.

Reachers assist in grasping items when bending is difficult. There are many other useful items to compensate for deficits in function.

Eye-controlled computer system allows the user to control the computer by visually selected options. This revolutionary computer operates by means of an infrared high speed video camera that focuses on the user's eye and an image processor that determines where on the screen the user is looking. For information, contact LC Technologies, Inc, 4415 Glenn Rose Street, Fairfax, VA 22032, (703) 425-7509.

Sears health care catalog includes products designed for health maintenance, adaptation to disabilities, and rehabilitation. Sears, Roebuck and Co, PO Box 804203, Chicago, IL 60680-4203, toll-free number, 24 hours a day, 7 days a week: (800) 326-1750.

Adaptability: Designs for Independent Living offers products to enhance ADLs for those with deficits. PO Box 515, Colchester, CT 06415-0515, Toll free number: (800) 243-9232.

The Gadget Book (available from AARP Books), Scott, Foresman & Co, Dept ASA, 4005 Edward Street Mt Prospect, IL 60056 (Cost: $9.70).

Dr. Leonard's Health Care Catalog, 74 20th Street, Brooklyn, NY 11232, features assistive devices such as grab bars, folding canes, and automatic seat lifters.

AliMed Direct to You Catalog, C & B Associates, 297 High Street, Dedham, Massachusetts 02026, features aids to ADLs.

Hand, Foot, and Face Prostheses

Life Like Laboratory (Division of Marmich, Inc)
European Crossroads
2829 W Northwest Highway, No. 7001
Dallas, TX 75220

Alternative Strategies for Health and Wellness

Visualization for Change is a concise account of visualization techniques to promote wellness; provides directions for healing (cost: $8.95).

The Chronic Pain Control Workbook is a comprehensive guide to coping with, controlling, and overcoming pain (cost: $12.50).

The Relaxation and Stress Reduction Workbook provides theory and instruction for numerous stress reduction techniques (cost: $12.50).

Clinical Guidelines

Available from the Agency for Health Care Policy and Research, AHCPR Center for Research Dissemination and Liaison, AHCPR Clearing House, PO Box 8547, Silver Spring, MD 20907, (800) 359-9295:

Heart Failure: Evaluation and Care of Patients with Left-Ventricular Systolic Dysfunction

Unstable Angina: Diagnosis and Management

Urinary Incontinence in Adults

Acute Low Back Problems in Adults

Benign Prostatic Hyperplasia: Diagnosis and Treatment

Quality Determinants of Mammography

Treatment of Pressure Ulcers

Evaluation and Management of Early HIV Infection

Acute Pain Management: Operative or Medical Procedures and Trauma

Management of Cancer Pain

Cataract in Adults: Management of Functional Impairment

Incontinence

American Foundation for Urologic Disease, PO Box 8306, Spartanburg, SC 29305-8306, 803-579-7900.

Resource Guide of Continence Aids and Services, Help for Incontinent People (HIP), PO Box 544, Union, SC 29379, (cost: $4.00).

Society of Urologic Nurses and Associates, E Holly Ave, Box 56, Pittman, NJ, 08071-0056, 609-256-2335.

Wound Ostomy and Continence Nurses Society, 2755 Bristol St, Suite 110, Costa Mesa, CA, 92626, Web: http://www.wocn.org.

Managing Incontinence: A Guide for Living with Loss of Bladder Control, Simon Foundation, Box 835, Wilmette, IL 60091, (800) 23SIMON (cost: $12.95).

Organizations

American Diabetes Association
National Center
PO Box 25757
1660 Duke Street
Alexandria, Virginia

Asthma and Allergy Foundation of America
1125 15th Avenue NW, Suite 502
Washington, DC 20004

American Cancer Society
1599 Clifton Road, NE
Atlanta, GA 30329

American Paralysis Association
500 Morris Avenue
Springfield, NJ 07081

American Parkinson's Disease Association
60 Bay Street, Suite 401
Staten Island, NY 10301

American Stroke Association
300 #00 E Hampden Avenue, Suite 240
Englewood, CO 80110-2654.

Amputee Shoe and Glove Exchange
PO Box 27067
Houston, TX 77227

Amyotrophic Lateral Sclerosis Association
2021 Ventura Boulevard, Suite 321
Woodland Hills, CA 91364

AFTER Rehabilitation and Training Center for Limb Deficiencies/Amputations
2559 Fairway Island Drive
Willington, Florida

American Association of Cardiovascular and Pulmonary Rehabilitation
7611 Elmwood Avenue, Suite 201
Middletown, WI 53562

American Disability Association
2121 8th Avenue, N, Suite 1623
Birmingham, AL 35203

National Rehabilitation Association
633 S Washington Street
Alexandria, VA 22314

REFERENCES

Abrams WB, Beers MH, Berkow R, editors: *Merck manual of geriatrics,* ed 2, Whitehouse Station, NJ, 1995, Merck Research Laboratories.

Abrams WB, Berkow R, editors: *Merck manual of geriatrics,* Rahway, NJ, 1990, Merck Sharp & Dohme Research Laboratories.

Adams PF, Marano MA: Current estimates from the national health interview survey, 1994, National Center for Health Statistics, *Vital Health Stat* 10(193), 1995.

Adsit J, Lee R: Art for stroke therapy, *Rehab Nurs* 11(3):120, 1986.

American Diabetes Association: Standards of medical care for patients with diabetes mellitus, *Diabetes Care* 14(2):10, 1991.

American Diabetes Association: Nutrition recommendations and principles for people with diabetes mellitus, *Diabetes Care* 17:519, 1994.

Anderson MA, Braun JV: *Caring for the elderly client,* Philadelphia, 1995, FA Davis.

Anderson R: *The aftermath of stroke: the experience of patients and their families,* Cambridge, 1992, Cambridge University Press.

Arras JD, Dubler NN: Ethical and social implications of high tech home care. In John Arras, editor: *Bringing the hospital home: ethical and social implications of high tech home care,* Baltimore, 1995, Johns Hopkins Press.

Bailey BJ: Mediators of depression in adults with diabetes, *Clin Nurs Res* 5(1):28, 1996.

Basch A, Jensen L: Management of fecal incontinence. In Doughty DB: *Urinary and fecal incontinence,* St Louis, 1991, Mosby.

Bates-Jensen BM: *Why and how to assess pressure ulcers.* The Ninth Annual Symposium on Advanced Wound Care, Atlanta, April 20, 1996.

Bates-Jensen BM, Vredevoe DL, Brecht ML: Validity and reliability of the pressure sore status tool, *Decubitus* 5(6):20, 1992.

Benner P, Janson-Bjerklie S, Ferketich S, Becker G: Moral dimensions of living with a chronic illness: autonomy, responsibility, and the limits of control. In Benner P, editor: *Interpretive phenomenology: embodiment, caring and ethics in health and illness,* Thousand Oaks, Calif, 1994, Sage Publications.

Bergstrom N, Allman RM, Alvarez OM et al: *Treatment of pressure ulcers,* Clinical practice guideline No 15, Rockville, Md, USD-HHS, PHS, Agency for Health Care Policy and Research, AHCPR Publication No 95-0652, 1994.

Berkow R, editor: *Merck manual of diagnosis and therapy,* ed 16, Rahway, NJ, 1992, Merck Research Laboratories.

Blumenthal SJ: *Older women's health fact sheet,* Office on Women's Health, US Public Health Service, DHHS, Washington DC, April 28, 1995.

Bostrom J, Caldwell J, McGuire K, Everson, D: Telephone follow-up after discharge from the hospital: does it make a difference? *Appl Nurs Research* 9(2):47, 1996.

Branch L, Resnick N, Dubeau C: Knowledge, attitudes and practices of physicians regarding urinary incontinence in persons aged >65 years—Massachusetts and Oklahoma, 1993, *MMRW Morb Mortal Wkly Rep* 44(40):747, 1995.

Braunwald E: Pathophysiology of heart failure, *Heart Disease* 14:1992.

Braunwald E, Grossman W: Clinical aspects of heart failure, *Heart Disease* 16:444, 1992.

Burggraf V, Barry R: *Gerontological nursing: current practice and research,* Thorofare, NJ, 1996, Slack, Inc.

Carpenito LJ: *Nursing diagnosis: application to clinical practice,* Philadelphia, 1989, JB Lippincott.

Catolico JT: *Assessment of barriers to diabetes self-management in older adults.* Thesis submitted to Faculty, School of Nursing, San Francisco State University, July 1995.

Centers for Disease Control and Prevention: *National Center for HIV/ STD & TB Prevention report,* Tammy Nunnally, Office of Communications, October 9, 1996, Atlanta.

Colwell JA: DCCT findings: applicability and implications for NIDDM, *Diabetes Reviews* 2:277, 1994.

Corbin JM, Strauss A: *Unending work and care: managing chronic illness at home,* San Francisco, 1988, Jossey-Bass.

Corbin JM, Strauss A: A nursing model for chronic illness management based upon the trajectory framework. In Woog P: *The chronic illness trajectory framework: the Corbin and Strauss nursing model,* New York, 1992, Springer.

Coward R, Horne C, Peek D: Predicting nursing home admissions among incontinent older adults: a comparison of residential differences across six years, *Gerontologist* 35(6):732, 1995.

Delcourt C, Villatte-Cathelineau B, Vauzelle-Kervroedan F, Papoz L: Clinical correlates of advanced retinopathy in type II diabetic patients: implications for screening, *J Clin Epidemiol* 49(6):679, 1996.

De-Nour A: Foreword. *Compliance: the dilemma of the chronically ill,* New York, 1986, Springer.

Doolittle ND: A clinical ethnography of stroke recovery. In Benner P, editor, *Interpretive phenomenology: embodiment, caring and ethics in health and illness,* Thousand Oaks, Calif, 1994, Sage Publications.

Dunlop MJ: Is a science of caring possible? In Benner P, editor: *Interpretive phenomenology: embodiment, caring and ethics in health and illness,* Thousand Oaks, Calif, 1994, Sage Publications.

Eckman MH, Greenfield S, Mackey WC: Foot infections in diabetic patients: decision and cost-effectiveness analysis, *JAMA* 273(9):712, 1995.

Ellickson EB: Bowel management plan for the homebound elderly, *J Gerontol Nurs* 14(1):16, 1987.

England B, Amkraut C, Lesparre M: *An agenda for medical rehabilitation: 1987 and into the 21st century.* Paper prepared for Section for Rehabilitation and Programs, American Hospital Association, Chicago, and Washington Business Group on Health, Institute for Rehabilitation and Disability Management, Washington, DC, 1987.

Fantl JA, Newman DK, Colling J et al: Managing acute and chronic urinary incontinence. In *Clincal practice guideline: quick reference guide for clinicians,* No 2, 1996 update, Rockville, Md, 1996, Agency for Health Care Policy and Research, US Department of Health and Human Services, Public Health Service, Pub No 96-0686.

Fonseca V, Wall J: Diet and diabetes in the elderly, *Nutrition, Aging and Age-Dependent Diseases* 11(4):613, 1995.

Froom J: Glycemic control in elderly people with diabetes, *Clin Geriatr Med* 6:933, 1990.

Giger JN, Davidhizar RE: *Transcultural nursing,* St Louis, 1991, Mosby.

Goldstein M, Hawthorne ME, Engeberg S et al: Urinary incontinence: why people do not seek help, *J Gerontol Nurs* 18(4):15, 1992.

Greenfield D, Rogers W, Mangotich M: Outcomes of patients with hypertension and non-insulin-dependent diabetes mellitus treated by different systems and specialties, *JAMA* 274(18):1436, 1995.

Greengold BA, Ouslander JG: Bladder retraining, *J Gerontol Nurs* 12:31, 1986.

Guy DH: Telephone care for elders: physical, psychosocial and legal aspects, *J Gerontol Nurs* 21(12):27-34, 1995.

Hanan K, Scheele L: Albumin vs weight as a predictor of nutritional status and pressure ulcer development, *Ostomy/Wound Management* 33:22, 1991.

Hanauer SB, Sable KS: Pathology of fecal incontinence. In Doughty DB: *Urinary and fecal incontinence.* St Louis, 1991, Mosby.

Harvard Women's Health Watch: Coronary heart disease, *Harvard Women's Health Watch* 1(6):1, 1994.

Heidrich SM: Mechanisms related to psychological well-being in older women with chronic illnesses: age and disease comparisons, *Res Nurs Health* 19(3):225, 1996.

Highland Hospital, Nursing Staff, Personal communication, 1988.

Hopkins ML, Schoener L: Tuberculosis and the elderly living in long term care facilities, *Geriatr Nurs* 17(1):27, 1996.

Hughes MN, Gillen M: Home study CE: tuberculosis—part 1, *California Nurse* 10:2, Nov/Dec 1992.

Hughes MN, Gillen M: Home study CE: tuberculosis—part 2, *California Nurse* 10:4, Jan/Feb 1993.

Hwe YJ: The impact of chronic illness on patients, *Rehabilitation Nursing* 20(4):221, 1995.

Idler EL, Kasl SV: Self-ratings of health: do they also predict change in functional ability? *J Gerontol* 50B(6):S344, 1995.

Iglesias P, Olmos O, Sastre J, Diez JJ, Fernandez ML, Borbujo J: Subungual hemorrhages: a primary manifestation of diabetes mellitus, *Arch Fam Med* 5(3):169, 1996.

Ingram B: New data reveal national costs of chronic conditions, *Aging Today* 17(5):1, 1996.

Itoh M: Rehabilitation. In Abrams WB, Beers MH, Berkow R, editors: *Merck Manual of Geriatrics,* ed 2, Whitehouse Station, NJ, 1995, Merck Research Laboratories.

Jarvis C: *Physical examination and health assessment,* ed 2, Philadelphia, 1996, Saunders.

Jette AM, Branch LG, Berlin J: Musculoskeletal impairments and physical disablement among the aged, *J Gerontol* 45(6):M203, 1990.

Jetter K, Faller N, Norton C: *Nursing for continence,* Philadelphia, 1990, WB Saunders.

Kannel WB: Epidemiological aspects of heart failure, *Cardiol Clin* 7(1):1, 1989.

Kannel WB, Belanger AJ: Epidemiology of heart failure, *Am Heart J* 121(3):951, 1991.

Kemper P: The use of formal and informal home care by the disabled, *Health Serv Res* 27(4):421, 1992.

Kerr CP: Management of diabetes, *J Fam Pract* 40(1):63, 1995.

Klusch L: *Solutions in restorative caregiving,* Des Moines, Iowa, 1995, Briggs Health Care Products.

Konen JC, Curtis LG, Summerson JH: Symptoms and complications of adult diabetic patients in a family practice, *Arch Fam Med* 5(3):135, 1996.

Konstam MA, Dvacup K, Baker DW et al: *Heart failure: evaluation and care of patients with left-ventricle systolic dysfunction. Clinical guideline #11,* Rockville, Md, USDHHS, PHS, Agency for Health Care Policy. Research, AHCPR, Pub No 94-0612, 1994.

Kresevic DM, Naylor M: Preventing pressure ulcers through use of protocols in a mentored nursing model, *Geriatr Nurs* 16(5):225, 1995.

Kunkel SR, Applebaum RA: Estimating the prevalence of long-term disability for an aging society, *J Gerontol* 47(5):S253, 1992.

LaPlante MP, Hendershot GE, Moss AJ: Assistive technology devices and home accessibility features: prevalence, payment, needs, and trends, *Advance Data* from Vital and Health Statistics of the Centers for Disease Control No 217, Sept 16, 1992, National Center for Health Statistics, US Department of Health and Human Services.

Lapp D: Practical demonstration of cognitive training techniques, (abstract). *Proceedings of the Third Congress of the International Psychogeriatric Association* 3:84, Chicago, 1987.

Laupacis A, Albers G, Dunn M et al: Antithrombotic therapy in atrial fibrillation, *Chest* 102:4265, October supplement, 1992.

Long K: Perfect timing: an overview of chronotherapy, *Nurse Practitioner Forum* 7(1):7, 1996.

Long ML: Incontinence, *J Gerontol Nurs* 11:30, 1985.

Lubkin IM: *Chronic illness: impact and interventions,* ed 3, Boston, 1995, Jones and Bartlett, p 8.

Mandelstam D, Robinson W: Support for the incontinent patient, *Nurs Mirror* 144(15):xix, 1977.

Mayo Clinic Health Letter: Leg ulcers. *Mayo Clinic Health Letter* 13:1, 1995.

Mayo Foundation for Medical Education and Research: Incontinence: collagen injections offer a new solution to bladder control problems, *Mayo Clinic Health Letter* 12(1):1, 1994.

Mayo L: *Guides to action on chronic illness,* New York, 1956, National Health Council, Commission on Chronic Illness.

McElmurry BJ, Harris B, Misner S, Olson L: Nursing ethics and chronic illness. In Benner P, Janson-Bjerklie S, Ferketich S, Becker G: Moral dimensions of living with a chronic illness: autonomy, responsibility, and the limits of control. In Benner P, editor: *Interpretive phenomenology: embodiment, caring and ethics in health and illness,* Thousand Oaks, Calif, 1994, Sage Publications.

Meadows P: Variation of diabetes mellitus prevalence in general practice and its relation to deprivation, *Diabetic Medicine* 12(8):696, 1995.

Melvin J: *Rehabilitation in the year 2000.* Paper presented at the 10th International Congress of Physical Medicine and Disability, Milwaukee, 1988.

Meneilly GS, Tessier D: Diabetes in the elderly, *Diabetic Medicine* 12(11):949, 1995.

Metz R: Overture: the patient and the provider. In Metz R, Benson J, editors: *Management and education of the diabetic patient,* Philadelphia, 1988, WB Saunders.

Miller CA: *Essentials of gerontological nursing: adaptation and the aging process,* Philadelphia, 1996, Lippincott.

Miller H, Delozier J: *Cost implications of the pressure ulcer treatment guideline,* Center for Health Policy Studies, Columbia, Md, Contract No 282-91-0070, 1994.

Miller J: Helping the aged manage bowel function, *J Gerontol Nurs* 11(2):37, 1985.

Miller MA: Is alcohol affecting your elderly patient's medical status? *NCGNP Newsletter* 36:4, Summer 1992.

Milne HA, McWilliam CL: Considering nursing resource as "caring time," *J Adv Nurs* 23(4):809, 1996.

Mishel M, Braden C: Finding meaning: antecedents of uncertainty in illness, *Nurs Res* 37:98, 1988.

Mobley D, Goldberg K, Wilson S: Management of urinary incontinence, *Geriatr Med Today* 10(9):18, 1991.

Morey SE: The HealthCam 2 in use: photos supplement written documentation, *Developments in Photo Documentation* 1(1):1, 1996.

Moss SE, Klein R, Klein BE: Long-term incidence of lower-extremity amputations in a diabetic population, *Arch Fam Med* 5(7):391, 1996.

Nease RF, Kneeland T, O'Connor GT et al: Variation in patient utilities for outcomes of the management of chronic stable angina: implications for clinical practice guidelines, *JAMA* 273(15):1185, 1995.

Newman D: *Continence control: vision for the future,* Senior Focus, Mills-Penninsula Hospitals Conference, San Francisco, Oct. 26-27, 1992.

National Institutes of Health Panel: Reaching a consensus on incontinence, *Geriatr Nurs* 10:78,1989.

Norton D, McLaren R, Exton-Smith AN: *An investigation of geriatric nursing problems in the hospital,* London, 1962, National Corporation for the Care of Old People.

O'Connor GT, Plume SK, Olmstead EM et al: A regional intervention to improve the hospital mortality associated with coronary artery bypass graft surgery, *JAMA* 275(11):841, 1996.

Okada S, Tanokuchi S, Ishii K et al: Diversity of neuropathies in patients with non-insulin-dependent diabetes mellitus, *J Intern Med Res* 24(1):122, 1996.

Orem D: *Nursing: concepts of practice,* ed 2, New York, 1980, McGraw-Hill.

Orlander JD, Jick SS, Dean AD et al: Urinary tract infections and estrogen use in older women, *J Am Geriatr Soc* 40:817, 1992.

Osteoporosis, *Mayo Clin Health Letter* 8:5, 1990.

Ouslander JG, Marishita B, Blaustein J et al: Clinical, functional, and psychosocial characteristics of an incontinent nursing home population, *J Gerontol* 46:631, 1987.

Ouslander J: *Continence control: vision for the future,* Senior Focus. Mills-Penninsula Hospitals Conference, San Francisco, Oct. 26-27, 1992.

Palmer MH: *Urinary continence assessment and promotion,* Gaithersburg, Md, 1996, Aspen.

Pierce L, Salter J: Stroke support group: a reality, *Rehab Nurs* 13(4):189, 1988.

Pires M, Muller A: Detection and management of early tissue pressure indicators: a pictorial essay, *Progressions* 3(3):3, 1991.

Pittman DA, Kirkpatrick M: Women's health and the acute myocardial infarction, *Nursing Outlook* 42:207, 1994.

Plummer ES, Albert SG: Focused assessment of foot care in older adults, *J Am Geriatr Soc* 44(3):310, 1996.

Pousada L: High-tech home care for elderly persons. In John Arras, editor: *Ethical and social implications of high tech home care,* Baltimore, 1995, Johns Hopkins University Press.

Redeker N: Health beliefs and adherence in chronic illness, *J Nurs Scholarship* 29(1):31, 1988.

Reed D, Satariano W, Gildengorin G, McMahon K, Fleshman R, Schneider E: Health and functioning among the elderly of Marin County, California: a glimpse of the future, *J Gerontol Medical Sciences* 50A(2):M61, 1995.

Resnick B: Geriatric rehabilitation. In Abrams WB, Beers MH, Berkow R, editors: *The Merck manual of geriatrics,* ed 2, Whitehouse Station, NJ, 1995, Merck Research Laboratories.

Resnick NM: Urinary incontinence. In Reuben DB, Wieland DL, Rubenstein LZ: Functional status assessment of older persons: concepts and limitations. In Vellas B, Albarede JL, Garry PJ, editors: *Facts and research in gerontology,* vol 7, 1993, New York, 1993, Springer.

Reuben DB, Wieland D, Rubenstein LZ: Functional status assessment of older persons: concepts and implications. In Vellas B, Albarede JL, Garry PJ, editors: *Facts and research in gerontology,* New York, 1993, Springer.

Rhodes R, Morrissey MJ, Ward A: Self-motivation: a driving force for elders in cardiac rehabilitation, *Geriatr Nurs* 13(2):94, 1992.

Rice R, Rappl L: The patient receiving rehabilitation services. In Rice R, editor: *Home health nursing practice: concepts and application,* St Louis, 1996, Mosby.

Richter JE: Functional disorders of the gastrointestinal tract. In Abrams WB, Beers MH, Berkow R, editors: *Merck manual of geriatrics,* ed 2, Whitehouse Station, NJ, 1995, Merck Research Laboratories.

Riley T: The future of Medicaid—the states see hard choices, *Aging Today* 17(5):9,12, 1996.

Rosenberg A: *Continence control: vision for the future,* Senior Focus. Mills-Penninsula Hospitals Conference, San Francisco, Oct 26-27, 1992.

Ross B: The impact of reimbursement issues on rehabilitation nursing practice and patient care, *Rehabilitation Nursing* 17(5):236, 1992.

Rousseau P, Fuentevilla-Clifton A: Urinary incontinence in the aged, part 1 and part 2, *Geriatrics* 47(6):22, 1992.

Sacks O: *An anthropologist on Mars,* New York, 1995, Alfred A. Knopf.

Saini JS, Khandalavla B: Corneal epithelial fragility in diabetes mellitus, *Can J Ophthalmol* 30(3):142, 1995.

San Francisco Chronicle: HMOs are starting to offer alternative medicine coverage, *San Francisco Chronicle,* p. A7, October 7, 1996.

Scardina RJ: Diabetic foot problems: assessment and prevention, *Clin Diabetes* 1(2):42, 1983.

Schnack M: Who's running home health? *Advanced Nurs Pract* 8(4):10, 1995.

Schumacher K: Rep Schroeder featured at ANA-PAC leader's luncheon, *Capital Update* 14(9):8, 1996.

Schuster PM, Wright C, Tomich P: Gender differences in the outcomes of participants in home programs compared to those in structure rehabilitation programs, *Rehabilitation Nursing* 20(2):93, 1995.

Seidel HM, Ball JW, Dains JE et al: *Mosby's guide to physical examination,* ed 2, St Louis, 1995, Mosby.

Seng J: Interscience Communications, Ltd, Washington, DC, Personal communication, Nov 1992.

Shields E: Personal communication, Sept 23, 1990, Vermillion, Ohio.

Shoben A: Hospitals provide similar care to elderly women, men: Rand study finds differences in quality very small, *Rand News Release,* October 14, 1992.

Short P, Leon J: *Use of home and community services by persons ages 65 and older with functional difficulties,* US Department of Health and Human Services Publication No. (PHS) 90-3466, Rockville, Md, 1990, Agency for Health Care Policy and Research.

Smith TW, Braunweld E, Kelly R: The management of heart failure, *Heart Dis* 17:464, 1992.

Staab A, Hodges LC: *Essentials of gerontological nursing,* Philadelphia, 1996, Lippincott.

Staab A, Lyles M: *Manual of geriatric nursing,* Glenview, Ill, 1990, Scott, Foresman/Little Brown Higher Education.

Stegmayr B, Asplund K: Diabetes as a risk factor for stroke: a population perspective, *Diabetologia* 38(9):1061, 1995.

Stein E, Margolin T, Lieff J: High technology and psychogeriatrics (abstract). *Proceedings of the Third Congress of the International Psychogeriatric Association* 3:69, Chicago, 1987.

Stone RI, Murtaugh CM: The elderly population with chronic functional disability: implications for home care eligibility, *Gerontologist* 30(4):491, 1990.

Strauss A, Corbin J: *Shaping a new health care system,* San Francisco, 1988, Jossey-Bass.

Strauss A, Glaser B: *Chronic illness and the quality of life,* St Louis, 1975, Mosby.

Terry PB: Chronic obstructive pulmonary disease (COPD). In Abrams WB, Beers MH, Berkow R, editors: *The Merck manual of geriatrics,* ed 2, Whitehouse Station, NJ, 1995, Merck Research Laboratories.

Torres-Gil F: Disability and aging: tools design and policy, *Aging Today* 16(6):7, 1995.

Treichsmann R: *Aging with disability,* New York, 1987, Demos Publications.

Turk DC, Okifuji A, Scharff L: Chronic pain and depression: role of perceived impact and perceived control in different age cohorts, *Pain* 61(1):93, 1995.

Turner C: Nurses' knowledge, assessment skills, experience and confidence in toenail management of elderly people, *Geriatr Nurs* 17(6):273, 1996.

US Bureau of the Census: *Statistical abstract of the United States: 1995,* ed 115, Washington, DC.

US Department of Health and Human Services: *Healthy people 2000: national health promotion and disease prevention objectives,* US Department of Health and Human Servies Pub. No (Public Health Service) 91-50212, Washington, DC, 1991, US Government Printing Office.

US Department of Health and Human Services: *Healthy people 2000: midcourse review and 1995 objectives,* Washington, DC, 1995, National Institutes of Health.

US Department of Health and Human Services: *Health: United States chartbook, 1995,* Department of Health and Human Services Pub No (Public Health Service) 96-1232-1, 6-0364 (6/96), Centers for Disease Control and Prevention, National Center for Health Statistics, Hyattsville, Md.

US Department of Health and Human Services: *National home and hospice care survey: 1993 summary,* Series 13: data from the National Health Care Survey No 123, US Department of Health and Human Services, Hyattsville, Md, Pub No (PHS) 96-1784.

US Department of Health and Human Services: *Pressure ulcers in adults—predictions and prevention,* Clinical practice guideline No 3, Washington, DC, 1992, AHCPR.

US Department of Health and Human Services: *Treatment of pressure ulcers,* No 15, 1994, Washington, DC, 1995, AHCPR Pub No 95-0652.

US Department of Health and Human Services: *Urinary incontinence in adults: acute and chronic management,* Clinical practice guideline No 2, 1996 update, Washington, DC, 1996, AHCPR 96-0682.

US Department of Health and Human Services: *Urinary incontinence in adults. Clinical practice guidelines,* Agency for Health Care Policy and Research, Public Health Service, USDHHS, Rockville, Md, 1992, AHCPR, Pub No 92-0038.

University Hospitals of Cleveland: *Adaptive devices—a source of independence,* Cleveland, 1988, University Hospitals.

Vandenbosch T, Montoye C, Satwicz M, Durkee-Leonard K, Boylan-Lewis B: Predictive validity of the Braden scale and nurse perception in identifying pressure ulcer risk, *Appl Nurs Res* 9(2):80, 1996.

van Hooft S: *Caring: an essay in the philosophy of ethics,* Niwot, Colo, 1995, University Press of Colorado.

Verbrugge L, Jette J, Rumple C, Madans J: *The great efficacy of personal and equipment assistance.* Paper presented at the meeting of the Gerontological Society of America, New Orleans, November 1993.

Verbrugge LM, Patrick DL: Seven chronic conditions: their impact on US adults' activity levels and use of medical services, *Am J Public Health* 85(2):173, 1995.

Wald A: Lower gastrointestinal tract disorders. In Abrams WB, Beers MH, Berkow R, editors: *The Merck manual of geriatrics,* ed 2, Whitehouse Station, NJ, 1995, Merck Research Laboratories.

Wanich K, Sullivan-Marx EM, Gottlieb GL et al: Functional status outcomes of a nursing intervention in hospitalized elderly, *Image* 24(3):201, 1992.

Wasson JH, Bruskewitz RC: Disorders of the lower genitourinary tract: bladder, prostate, testes. In Abrams WB, Berkow R, editors: *The Merck manual of geriatrics,* Rahway, NJ, 1990, Merck Sharpe & Dohme Research Laboratories.

Watson J: *Human science and human care: a theory of nursing,* New York, 1988, National League for Nursing.

Well Taken: Heart failure sounds final, It's not. *Well Taken, San Francisco,* 1994, p 2, Saint Francis Memorial.

Wells T, Brink C: Helpful equipment, *Geriatr Nurs* 1:264, 1980.

Wells TJ: Incontinence care. In Calkins E, David P, Ford A: *The practice of geriatrics,* Philadelphia, 1986, WB Saunders.

Wenger NK: Rehabilitation of the elderly coronary patient. In Frengley JD, Murray P, Wykle M, editors: *Practicing rehabilitation with geriatric clients,* New York, 1990, Springer.

Westfall UE: Nursing chronotherapeutics: a conceptual framework, *Image* 24(4):307, 1992.

Wilcox VL, Kasl SV, Idler EL: Self-rated health and physical disability in elderly survivors of a major medical event. *J Gerontol* 51B(2):S96, 1996.

Wineman NM, Schwetz KM, Goodkin DE, Rudick RA: Relationships among illness uncertainty, stress, coping, and emotional well-being at entry into a clinical drug trial, *Appl Nurs Res* 9(2):53, 1996.

Woog P: *The chronic illness trajectory framework: the Corbin and Strauss nursing model,* New York, 1992a, Springer.

Woog P: Introduction. In Woog P, editor: *The chronic illness trajectory framework: the Corbin and Strauss nursing model,* New York, 1992b, Springer.

Wright BA, Staats DO: Tuberculosis surveillance program: a nursing home experience, *Geriatr Nurs* 13(5):257, 1992.

Wyman JF, Hawkins SW, Fantl JA: Psychosocial impact of urinary incontinence in the community dwelling population, *J Am Geriatr Soc* 38:282, 1990.

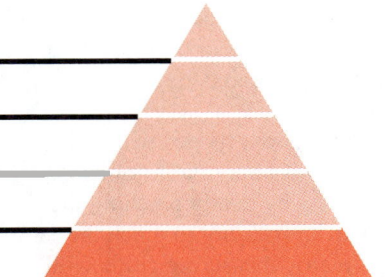

Pressure Sore Status Tool

INSTRUCTIONS FOR USE
General Guidelines

Fill out the attached rating sheet to assess a pressure sore's status after reading the definitions and methods of assessment described below. Evaluate once a week and whenever a change occurs in the wound. Rate according to each item by picking the response that best describes the wound and entering that score in the item score column for the appropriate date. When you have rated the pressure sore on all items, determine the total score by adding together the 13-item scores. The HIGHER the total score, the more severe the pressure sore status. Plot total score on the Pressure Sore Status Continuum to determine progression of the wound.

Specific Instructions:

1. Size: Use ruler to measure the longest and widest aspect of the wound surface in centimeters; multiply length × width.
2. Depth: Pick the depth, thickness, most appropriate to the wound using these additional descriptions:
   1 = tissues damaged but no break in skin surface.
   2 = superficial, abrasion, blister or shallow crater. Even with, and/or elevated above skin surface (e.g., hyperplasia).
   3 = deep crater with or without undermining of adjacent tissue.
   4 = visualization of tissue layers not possible due to necrosis.
   5 = supporting structures include tendon, joint capsule.
3. Edges: Use this guide:
   Indistinct, diffuse = unable to clearly distinguish wound outline.
   Attached = even or flush with wound base, *no* sides or walls present; flat.
   Not attached = sides or walls *are* present; floor or base of wound is deeper than edge.
   Rolled under, thickened = soft to firm and flexible to touch.
   Hyperkeratosis = callous-like tissue formation around wound & at edges.
   Fibrotic, scarred = hard, rigid to touch.

4. Undermining: Assess by inserting a cotton tipped applicator under the wound edge; advance it as far as it will go without using undue force; raise the tip of the applicator so it may be seen or felt on the surface of the skin; mark the surface with a pen; measure the distance from the mark on the skin to the edge of the wound. Continue process around the wound. Then use a transparent metric measuring guide with concentric circles divided into 4 (25%) pie-shaped quadrants to help determine percent of wound involved.
5. Necrotic Tissue Type: Pick the type of necrotic tissue that is *predominant* in the wound according to color, consistency and adherence using this guide:
   White/gray non-viable tissue = may appear prior to wound opening; skin surface is white or gray.
   Nonadherent, yellow slough = thin, mucinous substance; scattered throughout wound bed; easily separated from wound tissue.
   Loosely adherent, yellow slough = thick, stringy, clumps of debris; attached to wound tissue.
   Adherent, soft, black eschar = soggy tissue; strongly attached to tissue in center of base of wound.
   Firmly adherent, hard/black eschar = firm, crusty tissue; strongly attached to wound base and edges (like a hard scab).
6. Necrotic Tissue Amount: Use a transparent metric measuring guide with concentric circles divided into 4 (25%) pie-shaped quadrants to help determine percent of wound involved.
7. Exudate Type: Some dressings interact with wound drainage to produce a gel or trap liquid. Before assessing exudate type, gently cleanse wound with normal saline or water. Pick the exudate type that is predominant in the wound according to color and consistency, using this guide:
   Bloody = thin, bright red
   Serosanguinous = thin, watery pale red to pink
   Serous = thin, watery, clear
   Purulent = thin or thick, opaque tan to yellow
   Foul purulent = thick, opaque yellow to green with offensive odor

8. Exudate Amount: Use a transparent metric measuring guide with concentric circles divided into 4 (25%) pie-shaped quadrants to determine percent of dressing involved with exudate. Use this guide:

None   = wound tissues dry.

Scant   = wound tissues moist; no measurable exudate.

Small   = wound tissues wet; moisture evenly distributed in wound; drainage involves <25% dressing.

Moderate = wound tissues saturated; drainage may or may not be evenly distributed in wound; drainage involved >25% to <75% dressing.

Large   = wound tissues bathed in fluid; drainage freely expressed; may or may not be evenly distributed in wound; drainage involves >75% of dressing.

9. Skin Color Surrounding Wound: Assess tisssues with 4 cm of wound edge. Dark-skinned persons show the colors "bright red" and "dark red" as a deepening of normal ethnic skin color or a purple hue. As healing occurs in dark-skinned persons, the new skin is pink and may never darken.

10. Peripheral Tissue Edema: Assess tissues within 4 cm of wound edge. Non-pitting edema appears as skin that is shiny and taut. Identify pitting edema by firmly pressing a finger down into the tissues and waiting for five seconds; on release of pressure, tissues fail to resume previous position and an indentation appears. Crepitus is accumulation of air or gas in tissues. Use a transparent metric measuring guide to determine how far edema extends beyond wound.

11. Peripheral Tissue Induration: Assess tissues within 4 cm of wound edge. Induration is abnormal firmness of tissues with margins. Assess by gently pinching the tissues. Induration results in an inability to pinch the tissues. Use a transparent metric measuring guide with concentric circles divided into 4 (25%) pie-shaped quadrants to determine percent of wound and area involved.

12. Granulation Tissue: Granulation tissue is the growth of small blood vessels and connective tissue to fill in full-thickness wounds. Tissue is healthy when bright, beefy red, shiny and granular with a velvety appearance. Poor vascular supply apppears as pale pink or blanched to dull, dusky red color.

13. Epithelialization: Epithelialization is the process of epidermal resurfacing and appears as pink or red skin. In partial thickness wounds it can occur throughout the wound bed as well as from the wound edges. In full-thickness wounds it occurs from the edges only. Use a transparent metric measuring guide with concentric circles divided into 4 (25%) pie-shaped quadrants to help determine percent of wound involved and to measure the distance the epithelial tissue extends into the wound.

PRESSURE SORE STATUS TOOL

NAME _____

Complete the rating sheet to assess pressure sore status. Evaluate each item by picking the response that best describes the wound and entering the score in the item score column for the appropriate date.

Location: Anatomic site. Circle, identify right (**R**) or life (**L**) and use "X" to mark site on body diagrams:

_____ Sacrum & coccyx	_____ Lateral ankle	_____ Trochanter
_____ Medial ankle	_____ Ischial tuberosity	_____ Heel _____ Other Site

Shape: Overall wound pattern; assess by observing perimeter and depth. Circle and *date* appropiate description:

_____ Irregular	_____ Linear or elongated	_____ Round/oval
_____ Bow/boat	_____ Square/rectangle	_____ Butterfly _____ Other Site

Item	Assessment	Date Score	Date Score	Date Score
1. Size	1 = Length × width <4 sq cm 2 = Length × width 4-16 sq cm 3 = Length × width 6.1-36 sq cm 4 = Length × width 36.1-80 sq cm 5 = Length × width >80 sq cm			
2. Depth	1 = Non-blanchable erythema on intact skin 2 = Partial thickness skin loss involving epidermis and/or dermis 3 = Full-thickness skin loss involving damage or necrosis of subcutaneous tissue; may extend down to but not through underlying fascia; and/or mixed partial & full thickness &/or tissue layers obscured by granulation tissue 4 = Obscured by necrosis 5 = Full-thickness skin loss with extensive destruction, tissue necrosis or damage to muscle, bone or supporting structures			
3. Edges	1 = Indistinct, diffuse, none clearly visible 2 = Distinct, outline clearly visible, attached, even with wound base 3 = Well-defined, not attached to wound base 4 = Well-defined, not attached to base, rolled under, thickened 5 = Well-defined, fibrotic, scarred or hyperkeratotic			
4. Undermining	1 = Undermining <2 cm in any area 2 = Undermining 2-4 cm involving <50% wound margins 3 = Undermining 2-4 cm involving >50% wound margins 4 = Undermining >4 cm in any area 5 = Tunneling and/or sinus tract formation			
5. Necrotic Tissue Type	1 = None visible 2 = White/grey non-viable tissue &/or non-adherent yellow slough 3 = Loosely adherent yellow slough 4 = Adherent, soft, black eschar 5 = Firmly adherent, hard, black eschar			
6. Necrotic Tissue Amount	1 = None visible 2 = <25% of wound bed covered 3 = 25% or 50% of wound covered 4 = >50% and <75% of wound covered 5 = 75% to 100% of wound covered			
7. Exudate Type	1 = None or bloody 2 = Serosanguinous: thin, watery, pale red/pink 3 = Serous: thin, water, clear 4 = Purulent: thin or thick, opaque, tan/yellow 5 = Foul purulent; thick, opaque, yellow/green with odor			
8. Exudate Amount	1 = None 2 = Scant 3 = Small 4 = Moderate 5 = Large			
9. Skin Color Surrounding Wound	1 = Pink or normal for ethnic group 2 = Bright red and/or blanches to touch 3 = White or grey pallor or hypopigmented 4 = Dark red or purple and/or non-blanchable 5 = Black or hyperpigmented			
10. Peripheral Tissue Edema	1 = Minimal swelling around wound 2 = Non-pitting edema extends <4 cm around wound 3 = Non-pitting edema extends ≥4 cm around wound 4 = Pitting edema extends <4 cm around wound 5 = Crepitus and/or pitting edema extends ≥4cm			
11. Peripheral Tissue Induration	1 = Minimal firmness around wound 2 = Induration <2 cm around wound 3 = Induration 2-4 cm extending <50% around wound 4 = Induration 2-4 cm extending ≥50% around wound 5 = Induration >4 cm in any area			
12. Granulation Tissue	1 = Skin intact or partial thickness wound 2 = Bright, beefy red; 75% to 100% of wound filled &/or tissue overgrowth 3 = Bright, beefy red; <75% & >25% of wound filled 4 = Pink, &/or dull, dusky red &/or fills ≤25% of wound 5 = No granulation tissue present			
13. Epithelialization	1 = 100% wound covered, surface intact 2 = 75% to <100% wound covered &/or epithelial tissue extends >0.5 cm into wound bed 3 = 50% to <75% wound covered &/or epithelial tissue extends to <0.5 cm into wound bed 4 = 25% to <wound covered 5 = <25% wound covered			

TOTAL SCORE _____

SIGNATURE _____

PRESSURE SCORE STATUS CONTINUUM

```
 0    10    13    15    20    25    30    35    40    45    50    55    60    65
 |    |     |     |     |     |     |     |     |     |     |     |     |     |

  Tissue      Wound                                                     Wound
  Health      Regeneration                                             Degeneration
```

Plot the total score on the Pressure Sore Status continuum by putting an "X" on the line and the date beneath the line. Plot multiple scores with their dates to see-at-glance regeneration or degeneration of the wound. ©1990 Barbara Bates-Jensen

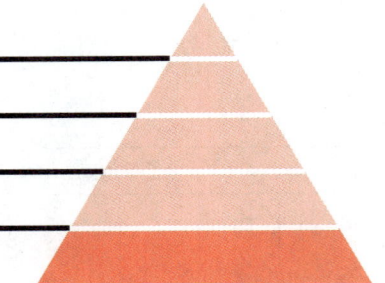

Braden Scale for Predicting Pressure Sore Risk

Patient's name		Evaluator's name
Sensory Perception Ability to respond meaningfully to pressure-related discomfort	**1. Completely Limited:** Unresponsive (does not moan, flinch, or grasp) to painful stimuli, due to diminished level of consciousness or sedation, OR limited ability to feel pain over most of body surface.	**2. Very Limited:** Responds only to painful stimuli. Cannot communicate discomfort except by moaning or restlessness, OR has a sensory impairment which limits the ability to feel pain or discomfort over $\frac{1}{2}$ of body.
Moisture Degree to which skin is exposed to moisture	**1. Constantly Moist:** Skin is kept moist almost constantly by perspiration, urine, etc. Dampness is detected every time patient is moved or turned.	**2. Moist:** Skin is often but not always moist. Linen must be changed at least once a shift.
Activity Degree of physical activity	**1. Bedfast:** Confined to bed.	**2. Chairfast:** Ability to walk severely limited or nonexistent. Cannot bear own weight and/or must be assisted into chair or wheel chair.
Mobility Ability to change and control body position	**1. Completely Immobile:** Does not make even slight changes in body or extremity position without assistance.	**2. Very Limited:** Makes occasional slight changes in body or extremity position but unable to make frequent or significant changes independently.
Nutrition Usual food intake pattern	**1. Very Poor:** Never eats a complete meal. Rarely eats more than $\frac{1}{3}$ of any food offered. Eats 2 servings or less of protei (meat or dairy products) per day. Takes fluids poorly. Does not take a liquid dietary supplement, OR is NPO and/or maintained on clear liquids or IV for more than 5 days.	**2. Probably Inadequate:** Rarely eats a complete meal and generally eats only about $\frac{1}{2}$ of any food offered. Protein intake includes only 3 servings of meat or dairy products per day. Occasionally will take a dietary supplement, OR receives less than optimum amount of liquid diet or tube feeding.
Friction and shear	**1. Problem:** Requires moderate to maximum assistance in moving. Complete lifting without sliding against sheets is impossible. Frequently slides down in bed or chair, requiring frequent repositioning with maximum assistance. Spasticity, contractures, or agitation leads to almost constant friction.	**2. Potential Problem:** Moves feebly or requires minimum assistance. During a move skin probably slides to some extent against sheets, chair, restraints, or other devices. Maintains relatively good position in chair or bed most of the time but occasionally slides down.

From Braden B, Bergstrom N: 1988.
NPO: Nothing by mouth; IV: Intravenously; TPN: Total parenteral nutrition.

	Date of assessment				

3. Slightly Limited:

Responds to verbal commands but cannot always communicate discomfort or need to be turned,

OR

has some sensory impairment which limits ability to feel pain or discomfort in 1 or 2 extremities.

4. No Impairment:

Responds to verbal commands. Has no sensory deficit which would limit ability to feel or voice pain or discomfort.

3. Occasionally Moist:

Skin is occasionally moist, requiring an extra linen change approximately once a day.

4. Rarely Moist:

Skin is usually dry; linen requires changing only at routine intervals.

3. Walks Occasionally:

Walks occasionally during day but for very short distances, with or without assistance. Spends majority of each shift in bed or chair.

4. Walks Frequently:

Walks outside the room at least twice a day and inside room at least once every 2 hours during waking hours.

3. Slightly Limited:

Makes frequent though slight changes in body or extremity position independently.

4. No Limitations:

Makes major and frequent changes in position without assistance.

3. Adequate:

Eats over half of most meals. Eats a total of 4 servings of protein (meat, dairy products) each day. Occasionally will refuse a meal, but will usually take a supplement if offered,

OR

is on a tube feeding or TPN regimen, which probably meets most of nutritional needs.

4. Excellent:

Eats most of every meal. Never refuses a meal. Usually eats a total of 4 or more servings of meat and dairy products. Occasionally eats between meals. Does not require supplementation.

3. No Apparent Problem:

Moves in bed and in chair independently and has sufficient muscle strength to lift up completely during move. Maintains good position in bed or chair at all times.

	Total Score				

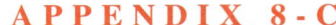

Barthel Index

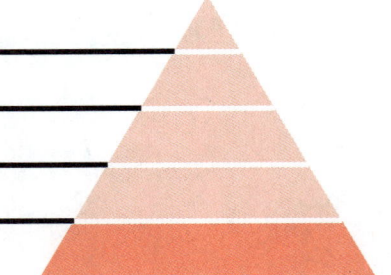

The Barthel Index

	"Can do by myself"	"Can do with help of someone else"	"Cannot do at all"
Self-Care Subscore			
1. Drinking from a cup	4	0	0
2. Eating	6	0	0
3. Dressing upper body	5	3	0
4. Dressing lower body	7	4	0
5. Putting on brace or artificial limb	0	−2	0 (N/A)
6. Grooming	5	0	0
7. Washing or bathing	6	0	0
8. Controlling urination	10	5 (accidents)	0 (incontinent)
9. Controlling bowel movements	10	5 (accidents)	0 (incontinent)
Mobility Subscore			
10. Getting in and out of chair	15	7	0
11. Getting on and off toilet	6	3	0
12. Getting in and out of tub or shower	1	0	0
13. Walking 50 yards on the level	15	10	0
14. Walking up/down one flight of stairs	10	5	0
15. If not walking: propelling or pushing wheelchair	5	0	0 (N/A)

Barthel total: Best score is 100; worst score is 0.

Note: Tasks 1-9, the self-care subscore (including control of bladder and bowel sphincters), have a total possible score of 53. Tasks 10-15, the mobility subscore have a total possible score of 47. The two groups of tasks combined make up the total Barthel index with a total possible score of 100.
From Granger C, Gresham O: *Functional assessment in rehabilitation medicine,* Baltimore, 1984, Williams & Wilkins, p 74.

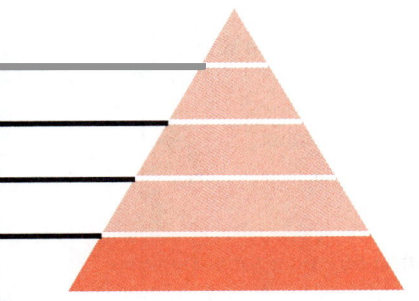

Minimum Data Set (MDS) Version 2.0 (Condensed) for Nursing Home Resident Assessment and Care Screening

IDENTIFICATION INFORMATION	Name, gender, birthday, Social Security and Medicare numbers, provider number, reasons for assessment
BACKGROUND INFORMATION	Assessment reference date, date of entry, marital status, payment sources, responsible person, advance directives
DEMOGRAPHIC INFORMATION	Date of entry, situation prior to admission, occupation, education, language, mental health history and conditions related to MR/DD status
CUSTOMARY ROUTINE	Usual cycle of daily events, eating patterns, functional ability in activities of daily living, social involvement
COGNITIVE PATTERNS	Consciousness, memory, recall ability, decision-making skills, delerium, disordered thinking, changes in cognitive status
COMMUNICATION/ HEARING PATTERNS	Hearing, communication devices/techniques, modes of expression, speech clarity, ability to understand, changes in communication or hearing
VISION PATTERNS	Vision, specific limitations/difficulties, visual appliances
MOOD AND BEHAVIOR PATTERNS	Indicators of depression, anxiety, sad mood, mood persistence, mood changes, behavioral symptoms, changes in behavioral symptoms
PSYCHOSOCIAL WELL-BEING	Sense of initiative/involvement, unsettled relationships, past roles
PHYSICAL FUNCTIONING AND STRUCTURAL PROBLEMS	Activities of daily living (ADL) self-performance: bed mobility, transfer, walking/locomotion, dressing, eating, toileting, personal hygiene, bathing, range of motion, modes of transfers, modes of locomotion, functional and rehabilitation potential, changes in ADL function
CONTINENCE IN LAST 14 DAYS	Self-control categories, bowel continence, bladder continence, bowel elimination pattern, appliances and programs, changes in urinary continence
DISEASE DIAGNOSES	Diseases, infections, other diagnoses
HEALTH CONDITIONS	Problem conditions, pain symptoms, pain site, accidents, stability of conditions
ORAL/NUTRITIONAL STATUS	Oral problems, height and weight, weight changes, nutritional problems, nutritional approaches, parenteral or enteral intake
ORAL/DENTAL STATUS	Oral status and disease prevention, tooth decay, disintegration; buccal cavity exam; dentures, bridges, missing teeth
SKIN CONDITION	Ulcers, type of ulcers, history of unresolved ulcers, other skin problems or lesions, skin treatments, foot problems and care
ACTIVITY PURSUIT PATTERNS	Time awake, time involved in activities, preferred activity settings, general activity preferences, prefers change in daily routines
MEDICATIONS	Number of medications, new medications, injections, days received the following medications (antipsychotic, antianxiety, antidepressant, hypnotic, diuretic)
SPECIAL TREATMENTS AND PROCEDURES	Treatments, procedures and programs; intervention programs for mood, behavior, cognitive loss, nursing rehabilitation/restorative care, devices and restraints, hospital stays, emergency room visits, physician visits, physician orders, abnormal lab values
DISCHARGE POTENTIAL AND OVERALL STATUS	Discharge potential, overall change in care needs
RESIDENT PARTICIPATION IN ASSESSMENT	Resident, family members, significant other

SECTION V. RESIDENT ASSESSMENT PROTOCOL SUMMARY   Numeric Identifier _____

Resident's Name:	Medical Record No.:

1. Check if RAP is triggered.
2. For each triggered RAP, use the RAP guidelines to identify areas needing further assessment. Document relevant assessment information regarding the resident's status.
   - Describe:
     - Nature of the condition (may include presence or lack of objective data and subjective complaints).
     - Complications and risk factors that affect your decision to proceed to care planning.
     - Factors that must be considered in developing individualized care plan interventions.
     - Need for referrals/further evaluation by appropriate health professionals.
   - Documentation should support your decision-making regarding whether to proceed with a care plan for a triggered RAP and the type(s) of care plan interventions that are appropriate for a particular resident.
   - Documentation may appear anywhere in the clinical record (e.g., progress notes, consults, flowsheets, etc.).
3. Indicate under the *Location of RAP Assessment Documentation,* column where information related to the RAP assessment can be found.
4. For each triggered RAP, indicate whether a new care plan, care plan revision, or continuation of current care plan is necessary to address the problem(s) identified in your assessment. The Care Planning Decision column must be completed within 7 days of completing the RAI (MDS and RAPs).

A. RAP Problem Area	(a) Check if Triggered	Location and Date of RAP Assessment Documentation	(b) Care Planning Decision—check if addressed in care plan
1. DELIRIUM	☐		☐
2. COGNITIVE LOSS	☐		☐
3. VISUAL FUNCTION	☐		☐
4. COMMUNICATION	☐		☐
5. ADL FUNCTIONAL/ REHABILITATION POTENTIAL	☐		☐
6. URINARY INCONTINENCE AND INDWELLING CATHETER	☐		☐
7. PSYCHOSOCIAL WELL-BEING	☐		☐
8. MOOD STATE	☐		☐
9. BEHAVIORAL SYMPTOMS	☐		☐
10. ACTIVITIES	☐		☐
11. FALLS	☐		☐
12. NUTRITIONAL STATUS	☐		☐
13. FEEDING TUBES	☐		☐
14. DEHYDRATION/FLUID MAINTENANCE	☐		☐
15. ORAL/DENTAL CARE	☐		☐
16. PRESSURE ULCERS	☐		☐
17. PSYCHOTROPHIC DRUG USE	☐		☐
18. PHYSICAL RESTRAINTS	☐		☐

B. _____   2. ☐☐ – ☐☐ – ☐☐☐☐
   1. Signature of RN Coordinator for RAP Assessment Process   Month   Day   Year

_____   4. ☐☐ – ☐☐ – ☐☐☐☐
   3. Signature of Person Completing Care Planning Decision   Month   Day   Year

TRIGGER LEGEND

1	- Delirium	7	- Psychosocial Well-Being	13	- Feeding Tubes
2	- Cognitive Loss/Dementia	8	- Mood State	14	- Dehydration/Fluid Maintenance
3	- Visual Function	9	- Behavioral Symptoms	15	- Dental Care
4	- Communication	10A	- Activities (Revise)	16	- Pressure Ulcers
5A	- ADL-Rehabilitation	10B	- Activities (Review)	17	- Psychotropic Drug Use
5B	- ADL-Maintenance	11	- Falls	18	- Physical Restraints
6	- Urinary Incontinence and Indwelling Catheter	12	- Nutritional Status		

Modified from *Minimum Data Set (MDS)—Version 2.0 for Nursing Home Resident Assessment and Care Screening,* Form 1728HH, Des Moines, IA, 1995, Briggs Corporation.

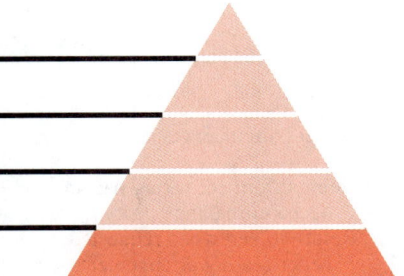

CHAPTER 9

Pain and Comfort

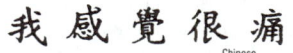 У МЕНЯ СИЛЬНАЯ БОЛЬ _{Russian} ខ្ញុំឈឺ ចាប់ ខ្លាំងណាស់ _{Khmer} 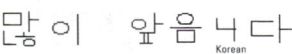 TÔI ĐANG BỊ ĐAU NHIỀU LẮM _{Vietnamese}

我 感 覺 很 痛 _{Chinese}　　많이 앓음ㄴ다 _{Korean}　　ຂອຍເຈັບປວດຫລາຍ _{Laotian}

Napakasakit _{Tagalog}　　Ua tigā ou tino _{Samoan}　　Teńgo mucho dolor _{Spanish}　　*It's very painful!*

Not only degrees of pain, but its existence, in any degree, must be taken upon the testimony of the patient.

Peter Mere Latham [1789-1875]
Diseases of the Heart, Lecture XI

LEARNING OBJECTIVES

Upon completion of this chapter, the reader will be able to:

1. Define the concept of pain.
2. Identify factors that affect the elders' pain experience.
3. Differentiate between acute and chronic pain.
4. Describe data to include in a pain assessment.
5. Identify barriers that interfere with pain assessment and treatment.
6. Discuss comfort measures.
7. Discuss pharmacologic and nonpharmacologic pain management therapies.
8. Discuss the goals of pain management for the elderly.

Comfort seems to be an intrinsic balance of the physiologic, emotional, social, and spiritual essence of the individual and can be perceived as an integral component of wellness. By definition comfort is "a state of ease and satisfaction of the bodily wants and freedom from pain and anxiety." The absence of physical pain is not always sufficient to provide comfort. The aged may have their biologic or bodily needs satisfied but be emotionally distressed. Conversely, physical needs may be the priority and no comfort is possible until need fulfillment is accomplished.

Nurses use the word comfort to describe goals and outcomes to nursing measures, but the meaning remains vague and essentially abstract to the person who is the recipient of the nursing intervention. Hamilton (1989) studied the meaning and attributes of comfort from the point of view of the chronically ill elderly hospitalized in a geriatric setting. The questions explored were the elderly's definition of comfort, contributors to and distractors from comfort, and how to increase elders' comfort. The findings identified several themes: disease process (pain, bowel function, and disability); self-esteem (feelings, adjustment, independence, usefulness, faith in God); positioning (if elders could carry out activites in bed, chair, or wheelchair); approach and attitude of staff (relationships, encounters); and hospital life (surroundings and environment—feeling at home, well fed, pleasant surroundings). Table 9-1 summarizes each of these themes and includes contributors to and distractors from comfort and elders' suggestions for facilitating more comfort.

The International Association for the Study of Pain and the American Pain Society define pain as "an unpleasant sensory and emotional experience associated with actual or potential tissue damage, or described in terms of such damage" (1979, 1992). Hamilton (1989) explains comfort as multidimensional "and meaning many things to different people." This description parallels McCaffery's definition of pain, which states: "Pain is whatever the person experiencing pain says it is" (McCaffery and Beebe, 1989). From these interpretations of pain and comfort the question can be raised as to whether there is a way to identify comfort-discomfort zones outside acute or chronic pain in a manner similar to the pain assessment measures presently used. This is definitely a fruitful area for research.

Table 9-1   Summary of Comfort Findings

Comfort themes	Contributors to comfort	Distractors to comfort	Adds to comfort
Disease process	Achieving relief from pain; regular bowel function	Physical disabilities; being in pain most of time	Better pain management
Self-esteem	Faith in God; being independent; feeling relaxed; feeling useful	Adjust to change; being afraid	Being informed; taking part in decision-making
Positioning	Individually adjusted seating; sitting correctly; independent movement in chair	Unsuitable wheelchairs; sitting too long; sliding down in chair; being in unfavorable position in bed	Return to bed when requested; better seating arrangements
Staff approach and attitudes	Friendly, kind people; empathetic nurses; reliable nurses	Lack of caring and understanding; inaccessible nurses	Caring and understanding encouraging patients to help themselves
Hospital life	Homelike surroundings; social and family contacts; informal pastimes; occupational and physical therapy	Fragmented care; tolerate the system; boredom with activities; lack of privacy Unpleasant meal atmosphere	Staff continuity New content in activities; continuation of personal pastimes; improved patient mealtimes; some privacy

Modified from Hamilton J: Comfort and the hospitalized chronically ill, *J Gerontol Nurs* 15(4):28, 1989.

In this chapter physical pain will be the primary focus. Psychologic pain is addressed in Chapters 19, 20, 22, and 24 and throughout other segments of the text.

Pain, whatever its sources, is one of the most common complaints of the elderly. It erodes personality, saps energy, and manifests itself in an ever-intensifying cycle of pain, anxiety, and anguish until the cycle is broken. Pain can evoke depression, sleep disorders, decreased socialization, impaired mobility, and increased health care costs (Sarvis, 1995). The nurse has a definition or interpretation of pain as does the patient to whom the nurse ministers. These interpretations are formulated from experiences and are influenced by the unique history of the individual and the meaning ascribed to the pain.

Meinhart and McCaffery (1983) cite two factors that influence nurses' and other caregivers' responses to a client's pain and discomfort: (1) one's ability to sympathize with another person, which depends on one's ability to identify imaginatively with the person, and (2) whether one is responsive to hurt in individuals that one does not know. It is also important to realize that an individual responds in a certain way to pain because he or she has been taught that this is correct and normal. Likewise, nurses and other caregivers respond based on their own pain experiences. In addition, repeated exposure to the pain of others desensitizes and may make it seem commonplace (Box 9-1).

Ethnically diverse responses based on years of social modeling, group-pressure influence on pain tolerance, and the influence of the family on pain can be observed (Bates, 1996). Thus social learning is extremely influential in the development of the meaning of and attitude toward pain, something older adults have had many years to internalize. In American culture a dichotomy exists for some: the prac-

tice of self-inflicted pain (in a sense) is seen in professional and amateur sports activities. This infliction of pain is expected and is a rite of passage, so to speak. Equally significant is that until experiencing body discomfort such as aches and pains, an older person does not perceive himself or herself as old. However, when these manifestations do occur, they become a rite of passage into perceived old age (Box 9-2).

ACUTE AND CHRONIC PAIN

Acute, temporary pain has been controlled easily by analgesic preparations for many years. Almost everyone has experienced this type of pain and knows that it is a temporary, time-limited situation with attainable relief. Chronic pain is not that simple. It has no time frame; it is continually persistent at varying levels of intensity, and it manipulates the individual and can manipulate the person attempting to give care (Portenoy, 1995; Salerno and Willens, 1996). Table 9-2 provides a comparison of acute and chronic pain. Meinhart and McCaffery (1983) note that chronic pain can manifest itself as depression, eating disturbances, or sleep disturbances. Chronic pain is categorized as (1) caused by uncontrolled neoplastic disease, (2) benign pain (nonneoplastic), which usually lasts over 6 months and is coped with adequately, and (3) intractable benign pain, which is the most common pain in elders and erodes an individual's coping ability.

Chronic pain may be due to the following:

1. Muscle and joint pain, which includes low back pain, arthritis, and bursitis
2. Causalgia, a searing type of pain, comparable to placing a lighted cigarette to the skin, that is experienced after sudden systemic shock and lasts

<table>
<tr><td>

Box 9-1   Nurses' Misconceptions about the Pain Experience

Patients should expect to have pain in hospital

Obvious pathology, test results, and/or type of surgery determine the existence and intensity of pain

Patients who are in pain always have observable signs

Chronic pain is not as serious a problem for patients as acute pain

Patients are not the experts about their pain—health professionals are

Patients will report that they are in pain and will use the term "pain"

From Watt-Watson JH, Donovan MI: *Pain management: nursing perspective,* St Louis, 1992, Mosby.

</td><td>

Box 9-2   Factors Influencing Clients' Response to Pain

Past pain experience

Culture

Gender

Significance of pain

Depression

Fatigue

Physiologic age changes

Altered pain stimulus transmission

Decrease in inflammation response

Modified from Eland JM: Pain management and comfort, *J Gerontol Nurs* 14(4):10, 1988.

</td></tr>
</table>

Table 9-2   Comparison of Acute and Chronic Pain

Characteristics	Acute pain	Chronic pain
Experience	An event	A situation, state of existence
Source	External agent of internal disease	Unknown, or if known changes cannot occur or treatment is prolonged or ineffective
Onset	Usually sudden	May be sudden or develop insidiously
Duration	Transient (up to 6 mo.)	Prolonged (months to years)
Pain identification	Pain verses nonpain	Pain verses nonpain
	Areas generally well identified	Areas less easily differentiated
		Intensity becomes more difficult to evaluate (change in sensations)
Behavior	Typical response pattern with more visible signs:	Response patterns vary, few overt signs (adapation):
	Facial expressions	Sleeping
	Crying, guarding	Sleep disturbances
	Guarding, moaning	Confusion
	Groaning, restlessness	Rubbing
	Clinching teeth	Stoicism
	Biting lower lip	Depression
	Tight shut eyes	Combativeness
	Open somber eyes	Inactivity
	Involuntary movements	
	Immobility of body part	
	Puposeless body movements	
	Rhythmic body movements, rocking, rubbing	
	Change in speech and vocal pitch (anxiety)	
	Slow monotone (severe pain)	
	Fetal position	
Clinical signs	Elevated blood pressure	No change in vital signs
	Tachycardia	
	Talking	
	Diaphoresis	
Meaning	Meaningful (informs person something is wrong)	Meaningless, person looks for meaning
Pattern	Self-limiting or readily corrected	Continuous or intermittent
		Intensity may vary or remain constant
Course	Suffering usually decreases over time	Suffering usually increases over time
Action	Leads to action to relieve pain	Leads to action to modify pain
Prognosis	Likelihood of eventual complete relief	Complete relief usually not possible

Modified from Karb V: Pain. In Phipps W, Long B, Woods N, editors: *Medical-surgical nursing: concepts and clinical practice,* ed 4, St Louis, 1991, Mosby; Forrest J: Assessment of acute and chronic pain in older adults, *J Gerontol Nurs* 21:10, 1995.

6 to 12 months, but which 25% or more elders experience for longer periods of time

3. Neuralgia arising from peripheral nerves, which is similar to the pain that occurs in conjunction with shingles (herpes zoster) and whose most devastating type is tic douloureux
4. Phantom pain, which arises from an amputated part and begins as a pins-and-needles sensation, possibly developing into cramping, burning, or shooting pains that last for years, similar in type to the sensations experienced by persons paralyzed with spinal cord injuries
5. Vascular pain which is most dramatically evident in migraine headaches
6. Terminal cancer pain, which produces fear and anxiety in the patient and distress in the staff

Peripheral vascular occlusion in people with advanced diabetes often produces a constant burning pain, similar to the pain of frostbite, to the extremities. The aged person who suffers a paralyzing or weakness-inducing stroke with loss of complete sensation on the affected side often experiences deep boring, crushing sensations, or burning and cold sensations in the face, neck, trunk, leg, or generally over the entire affected side. Movement of the affected side and other sensations such as touch, sound, bright light, and air increase this kind of pain. Feeling in the affected extremity may be perceived as similar to a person being squeezed or twisted. Often the extremity is held in a strange position by the patient. For nursing diagnosis, see p. 348.

Pain in the Aged

The prevalence of pain in the elderly who live in the community is known to be twice that of the young and is considered to be extremely high in the long-term care setting. Ferrell (1991) suggests that the incidence of pain in the community is 25% to 50% and as much as 85% in long-term care due to the presence of conditions that cause chronic pain such as arthritis, gout, and peripheral vascular disease.

In the aged, fear and anxiety generate negative effects that emanate from thoughts that pain will result in crippling, forced dependency or that it will be of such intensity that the ability to cope will be inadequate. Pain weakens and interrupts the individual's ideas of relations to self, to others, to the environment, and in time and space.

The aged are at high risk for pain-inducing situations. They have lived longer and have a greater chance of developing degenerative and pathologic conditions through disease or injury. Several conditions may be present simultaneously, so a single pain-producing condition is overlooked in the complexity of health management. Increased susceptibility to accidents because of medications, cognitive function, or illness impacts functional abilities, which further contributes to such accidents as falls. The resultant hip fractures, sprains, and hematomas require longer periods of time to heal and prolong the pain experience. Loneliness through loss of a spouse, a job, independence, and friends and the presence of boredom and depression decrease the ability to cope with pain. These psychosocial aspects of an elder's life are rarely self-reported because of the associated stigma. Chronic pain experienced by a number of elders often results in dramatic lifestyle changes such as altered family relationships and the inability to visit friends. In a study by Ferrell and Ferrell (1990) of 65 elder patients, 54% experienced impairment of enjoyable activities; 53% impaired ambulation; 49% impaired posture; and 45% and 32% experienced sleep disorders and depression, respectively. In this sample it was apparent that lowered pain tolerance exists.

Clinical speculations that pain decreases with age remain inconclusive. Portenoy (1995) reports such pain reduction at organ and tissue sites except the joints. The literature has revealed instances of serious abdominal and cardiac conditions that should elicit severe pain but have produced little or no pain in the aged. It is not uncommon for acuity of symptoms or severity of pain to be less dramatic than in younger persons (Witt, 1989). In addition, the elderly often underreport pain because they consider it a normal part of the aging process. Meinhart and McCaffery (1983) cite behavioral changes or manifestations such as confusion and restlessness as possible indicators of painful stimuli in the aged. The elderly often suffer in silence or attempt to relieve pain with inadequate measures because of the high cost of medical care, consultation, equipment, diagnostic tests, hospitalization, and medications. In addition, the perceptions of pain by others, including caregivers, influence the elder's pain (Hofland, 1992; Sarvis, 1995). Studies of pain threshold among elders have been difficult to conduct because of methodological problems and the refusal of relatives to allow the patient to participate in a study. In addition, questions continue to arise about how to discern pain in the cognitively impaired and nonverbal elderly. Nurses must be extremely observant of subtle cues such as guarding a part of the body, wincing, or favoring certain movements rather than internalizing and projecting their own pain experience on others (Box 9-3).

Pain management and interventions for pain in the elderly often differ from those of other age groups due to the concerns of cognitive function, use of such therapies as transcutaneous electrical nerve stimulation (TENS), antidepressants, or relaxation techniques (Fulmer, et al, 1996). In addition, medications are affected by the increase and decrease of absorption time, depending on what other medications are being taken and the individual illness. The ability of elders to swallow pills easily may be impaired due to a dry mouth or ill-fitting dentures. Injectable medication may also be unreliable due to the inadequacy of the elder's circulation. (Refer to Chapter 10 for pharmacokinetics and pharmacodynamics of medications). A viable alternative to provide pain relief might be rectal administration of pain medication. New forms of medication administration are being developed, among them medication in lollipop form

---

Box 9-3   **Fact and Fiction about Pain in the Elderly**

MYTH:	Pain is expected with aging.
FACT:	Pain is not normal with aging. The presence of pain in the elderly necessitates aggressive assessment, diagnosis, and management similar to that of younger patients.
MYTH:	Pain sensitivity and perception decrease with aging.
FACT:	This assumption is dangerous! Data are conflicting regarding age-associated changes in pain perception, sensitivity, and tolerance. Consequences of this assumption are needless suffering and undertreatment of both pain and underlying cause.
MYTH:	If a patient doesn't complain of pain, there must not be much pain.
FACT:	This is erroneous in all ages but particularly in the elderly. Older patients may not report pain for a variety of reasons. They may fear the meaning of pain, diagnostic workups, or pain treatments. They may think pain is normal.
MYTH:	A person who has no functional impairment, appears occupied, or is otherwise distracted from pain, must not have significant pain.
FACT:	Patients have a variety of reactions to pain. Many patients are stoic and refuse to "give in" to their pain. Over extended periods of time, the elderly may mask any outward signs of pain.
MYTH:	Narcotic medications are inappropriate for patients with chronic nonmalignant pain.
FACT:	Opioid analgesics are often indicated in nonmalignant pain.
MYTH:	Potential side effects of narcotic medication make them too dangerous to use in the elderly.
FACT:	Narcotics may be used safely in the elderly. Although elderly patients may be more sensitive to narcotics, this does not justify withholding narcotics and failing to relieve pain.

From Ferrell BR, Ferrell BA: Pain in the elderly. In Watt-Watson JH, Donovan MI, editors: *Pain management: nursing perspective,* St Louis, 1992, Mosby.

(oral transmucosal) and skin patches (Managing pain, 1996). No data is available for use with the elderly at this time.

Another issue in pain management of the elderly is their fear of losing self-control and fear of addiction. The Agency For Health Care Policy and Research (AHCPR) guidelines (Acute pain management, 1992) were an outstanding contribution to pain intervention, but they did not provide direction for those who care for elders who need pain relief (Fulmer et al, 1996).

PAIN CONTROL

Pain control for elders is challenging. Several pain theories have been used to explain pain phenomenon and interventions for pain control (Box 9-4).

The specificity theory was among the first explanations as to why an individual experienced pain. In essence, the specific theory proposed that single specialized peripheral nerve fibers were responsible for pain transmission. The discovery of delta-A and C fibers lent credence to this theory (Duff 1988; Salerno and Willons, 1996).

The pattern theory, also an early theory, stated that excessive stimulation of all nerve endings produces a pattern that is interpreted as pain by the brain cortex. In phantom limb pain, for example, the pain experienced before amputation of the limb leaves a memory tracing that is recalled after amputation. However, this theory does not provide concepts useful for interventions.

Box 9-4   **Four Stages of Pain Phenomenon**

Activation or nociception*—The stimulation of nerve endings

Pain—The mind's perception of nerve impulses

Suffering—One's emotional reaction to pain, such as alarm, anxiety, frustration, or depression. Varies from person to person based on self-esteem, memory of past pain, family, social and cultural factors

Pain behavior and psychologic changes—Decreased self-worth: invalid, sick role

*The process of pain transmission; usually related to a receptive neuron for painful sensations.
Modified from Chronic pain: medical essay, *Mayo Clinic Health Letter,* June 1996.

The gate theory, introduced by Melzack and Wall (1965) and among the most readily accepted, integrated the specific and pattern theories and proposed that an anatomic gate modulates the pain experience. Simply stated, the peripheral nerve fibers carrying pain impulses to the spinal cord can have their input modified at the spinal cord before the impulses are transmitted to the brain. Stated another way, the gate theory suggests that pain impulses that travel up the spinal cord can be blocked before reaching the brain by a mechanism that acts like a gate closing. This latter theory helps explain why such interventions as rubbing the skin, acupressure, and acupuncture relieve certain types of pain. The theory also suggests that complex physiologic, psychologic, and cognitive processes, such as anxiety, past experiences, and the meaning of pain, are heavily influenced by sociocultural learning. These experiences affect human pain perception and response, which can influence the opening and closing of the gates (Bates, 1996). Neural memory, however, is not explained within the context of the gate theory. The gate control theory is relevant to pain management of the elderly.

Pharmacologic Pain Control

Generally pain relief is accomplished by medication aimed at altering sensory transmission to the cerebral cortex. Various analgesics (nonnarcotic and narcotic agents) are available for use. Nonnarcotic preparations are effective for mild to moderate pain, whereas narcotics should be reserved primarily for moderate to severe pain. General principles of pain control for the aged are the same as for the young, but dosage adjustment is sometimes required.

The use of meperidine (Demerol) should be avoided with the elderly because of pharmacokinetic changes that occur with aging metabolism and excretion (refer to Chapter 10). Reduced metabolism and excretion of Demerol metabolites can produce confusion, psychotic behavior, and seizure ac-

tivity. The same can be said for pentazocine (Talwin) and methadone. Various morphines and codeines are considered safer drugs for use with the elderly (Portenoy, 1995; Watt-Watson and Donovan, 1992). It is important to be aware of equianalgesic doses so that oral pain and parenteral pain medication doses possess pain relief power equivalent to another narcotic drug (Box 9-5).

The patient's misbeliefs about pain and its control include the following (Watt-Watson and Donovan, 1992):

- Pain is to be expected with treatment and diagnoses such as cancer.
- I have no control over my pain.
- Surgery or a pill will fix me up.
- I should not ask for anything for pain unless I'm desperate.

In addition, Davies (1996) and Sarvis (1995) point out that professionals may not ask the elder about their pain for the following reasons:

- The professional may assume that the individual will spontaneously report pain.
- The elder does not want to bother the physician with pain complaints, considering all the other medical problems he or she may have.

Box 9-5 **Guidelines to Use of an Equianalgesic Chart**

An eqianalgesic chart is helpful when (1) switching from one drug to another or (2) switching from one route of administration to another.

Equianalgesic means approximately the same pain relief.

Individual responses must be observed. Dose and interval between doses are then titrated according to the individual's response.

Based on clinical experience, the intravenous (IV) dose is approximately the same as an intramuscular (M) dose. Dose adjustments are then made to the individual's response. Some clinicians suggest approximately half the IM dose equals the IV dose.

Equianalgesic Chart Approximate Equivalents to 10 mg Morphine for Analgesic Effect

	Route		
Analgesic	**IM**	**Oral (PO)**	**Comments**
Morphine-like agonist			
Morphine sulfate	10 mg	60 mg (30)	
Dilaudid	1.5 mg	7.5 mg	
Oxycodone	—	30 mg	
Methadone	10 mg	20 mg	
Levorphanol	2.0 mg	4.0 mg	
Fentanyl	0.1 mg	—	Transdermal patch equivalent to 30 mg sustained-release morphine Q 8 hr
Oxymorphone	1.0 mg	—	
Meperidine	75 mg	300 mg	Not recommended
Mixed agonist/antagonist			
Nalbuphine	10 mg	—	
Butorphanol (Stadol)	2.0 mg	—	
Dezocine	10 mg	—	
Partial agonist			
Buprenorphine	0.4 mg	—	

- Many older adults consider pain an expected part of aging.
- Clinicians are hesitant to prescribe analgesics for the elderly because of concern for troubling side effects with polypharmacy.
- Gray (1996) notes that under managed care, the ability to provide appropriate pain relief is limited by removal of more effective but more costly analgesics from the hospitals' formularies.
- Use of opioids causes too many problems, such as addiction and associated stigma. Other medications that the physician may prescribe for the elderly may be as effective but less problematic.

When acute pain is severe, as in postoperative recovery, it is prudent to combine a nonnarcotic and a narcotic preparation to achieve maximum pain relief. This combination affects pain response at both the peripheral nerve and central nervous system levels.

When a person is allowed nothing by mouth (NPO), a nonnarcotic analgesic can be given by suppository along with the injectable narcotic. An important point to remember is that the dose of the nonnarcotic analgesic must be sufficiently strong to work synergistically with the narcotic preparation. In addition, medication should be given at the point of beginning discomfort, not at the height of pain intensity. Around-the-clock (ATC) medicating schedule has been in the literature since about 1989. It has not been implemented in many instances. This is unfortunate because it is a viable way to provide a more stable therapeutic plasma level of drug and eliminate the extremes of overmedication and undermedication. With this approach to pain control, breakthrough pain allows for a PRN (pro re nata; as needed) dose of medication (McCaffery and Ritchey, 1992; Sarvis, 1995). Narcotic use for long-term chronic pain control in the elderly should be convenient, easy to administer, and short acting for ease of dose adjustment; there is less drug accumulation in the body and low incidence of side effects. Box 9-6 lists preferred narcotics and those to be avoided for use with the elderly.

Mild and moderate pain relief may be achieved with nonnarcotic analgesics such as the nonsteroidal antiinflammatory drugs (NSAIDs) or acetaminophen. The NSAIDs bind with proteins and may induce toxic responses in elders if serum albumin levls are low. In addition, other drugs that elders routinely take compete for the same protein receptor sites and may be displaced by the NSAID, creating unstable therapeutic effects. Drugs that cause central nervous system (CNS) effects should be used with caution in elders sensitive to CNS effects. Box 9-6 identifies preferred NSAID drugs and those to be avoided for use with elders. The following are guidelines for the selection and use of NSAIDs:

- Weigh risks versus benefits in selection.
- Start with a low dose to determine the patient's reaction; for example, side effects. Increase gradually to a dose that relieves pain, not to exceed the maximal daily dose. The dose may need to be increased 1 to 2 times the starting dose.
- If maximal antiinflammatory effect is desired in addition to analgesia, allow adequate trial before discontinuing or switching. With regular doses for 1 week or longer, pain relief may increase.
- If one drug becomes ineffective, but the pain is about the same, try a drug from a different chemical class.
- If the NSAID does not relieve pain when used alone, combine with PO, IM, or IV narcotics for added analgesic effect (McCaffery M, and Beebe A, 1989).

Sharp, shooting, dull, aching, or burning pain that is not responsive to NSAIDS or narcotics may respond to adjuvant drug therapy. Some adjuvant drugs help control symptoms and signs associated with pain. Adjuvant drugs are not analgesics; in combination with analgesics they may potentiate or enhance overall analgesic effects. Elders frequently respond well with adjuvant pain regimens. However, it is important to remember that many adjuvant drugs have a very long half-life, which increase the plasma concentration in elders. This can lead to adverse or toxic effects.

Box 9-6 lists preferred adjuvant drugs and those to be avoided for elderly use. Some guidelines for the administration of adjuvant drugs to the elderly include the following:

- Avoid those drugs with potent anticholinergic effects. These may result in urinary retention and subsequent urinary tract infection; constipation; blurred vision, which increases the chance for injury; dry mouth, affecting the ability to eat; and confusion.
- Neuroleptics, if used, should have the least sedating, cardiotoxic, and hypotensive effects.
- Avoid drugs that precipitate or potentiate extrapyramidal symptoms.
- Tranquilizers that produce sedation and have a long half-life should be avoided. Drugs with a short half-life are more suitable.
- Drugs that can cause othostatic hypotension should be used with caution, especially when there is preexisting cardiac condition.

Box 9-6	Elder Pain Relief Drugs to Use and Avoid	
Type of Drug	**Preferred**	**Avoid**
OPIOIDS	Tylenol with codeine	Pentazocine
	Oxycodone	Meperidine
	Dilaudid	Methadone
NSAIDs	Ibuprofen	Indomethocin
	Acetaminophen	Aspirin
	Salsalate	Feldene
	Dolobid	Phenylbutazone
Adjuvant	Trazodone	Amitriptylene
	Prozac	Phenothiazines
	Desipramine	

- Interactions with other drugs must be monitored carefully since elders take many medications (polypharmacy).

A summary of pharmacologic principles in pain management of the elderly appears in Box 9-7.

Nonpharmacologic Pain Control

Nursing staff are often afraid of inducing iatrogenic addiction and thus give the minimum dosage ordered, which may not be effective. Indeck (1977) considers pain control in the aged to be more effective through the use of various alternative means such as biofeedback, acupuncture or acupressure, behavior modification, hypnosis, meditation, or a combination of these modalities.

In many instances nurses will find a combination of pharmacologic and nonpharmacologic interventions effective to relieve acute or chronic pain.

Cutaneous Nerve Stimulation. Deep and superficial stimulation of the skin by direct, proximal, or distal application for the purpose of pain relief has been practiced for centuries. Massage, vibration, heat, cold, and ointments have been a part of nursing interventions for years. Heat is effective for musculoskeletal disorders such as rheumatic conditions. It is contraindicated with occlusive vascular disease and in the presence of cancer. In nonexpansive tissue such as bursae, heat may even increase pain. Intermittent cold packs are helpful in low back pain and radicular disturbances.

Box 9-7	**Principles of Pharmacologic Pain Management in Elderly Patients**

1. Use a combination of pharmacologic and non-pharmacologic pain management strategies.
2. Give adequate amounts of drug at the appropriate frequency to control pain based on constant assessment.
3. Use around-the-clock dosing; avoid PRN (as needed) drug administration.
4. Use a combination of drugs that potentiate each other, such as a nonsteroidal anti-inflammatory in combination with a narcotic for bone cancer pain.
5. With narcotic analgesic drugs, start low and increase dose slowly.
6. Anticipate and prevent side effects common in elders:
   a. Give anti-inflammatory drugs with food.
   b. Begin a bowel regimen early to prevent constipation.
   c. Be prepared to give an anti-nausea medication with narcotic analgesic drugs.
   d. Anticipate some impaired balance and cognitive function with narcotic analgesic drugs.
7. Consult an equianalgesic potency table when changing medications.

From Glickstein JK, editor: Managing chronic pain, *Focus Geriatr Care Rehab* 10(3):6, 1996.

They serve to negate or delay the transmission of pain impulses to the cerebral pain center. Pathophysiologic conditions should be taken into consideration when using heat and cold with the elderly. Care must be taken when applying heat and cold to the skin of the aged to prevent skin damage from extended periods of heat and cold applications.

Transcutaneous Electrical Nerve Stimulation. Another method of cutaneous stimulation is TENS or dorsal column nerve stimulation (DNS). Electrodes, applied and taped to the skin over the pain site or on the spine, emit a mild electric current that is felt as a tingling, buzzing, or vibrating sensation. The patient operates the stimulator and starts the electric impulses, which then activate the large nerve fibers that transmit impulses to close the hypothetic gate in the spinal cord and prevent pain signals from reaching the brain. TENS has been helpful in phantom limb pain, postherpetic neuralgia, and low back pain.

Touch.   Touch is a natural comfort modality, although its therapeutic properties are still not clearly understood. Sometimes considered a cutaneous stimulation technique, "therapeutic touch" used in experimental laboratory and clinical settings showed that placing hands on or near the body might result in healing or improvement (Kreiger, 1992). Relaxation and proper sensory stimulation decrease anxiety, reduce muscle tension, and help provide distraction from pain and thereby relieve pain. Petrie (1975) found that perceptual tendencies and sensory dimensions influence pain reactions and tolerance. Persons who were sensory deprived exhibited low pain tolerance, but those who received adequate or a high degree of sensory stimulation possessed a high pain tolerance. Laying on hands employed by Kreiger (1975) and the Touch for Health Movement proved to be beneficial, but the reasons behind its effectiveness have not been fully established.

Fakouri and Jones (1987) demonstrated the positive effects of a 3-minute, slow-stroke back rub on both sides of the spinous processes from the crown of the head to the sacrum as a means of promoting relaxation in the aged. Physiologic effects that occurred were a decrease in heart rate and blood pressure and an increase in skin temperature. Meek (1993) found that slow-stroking back massage increased relaxation as evidenced by decreases in blood pressure and heart rate and an increase in body temperature of hospice patients. No mention was made of its effect on pain. However, it is known that tension and anxiety reduction can contribute to an increase in pain tolerance. Mackey (1995) describes the use of therapeutic touch for pain relief and admits that it was not successful as the sole therapy for pain relief but does suggest its value as an adjunct to pharmacologic therapy.

The Touch Research Institute at the University of Miami is engaged in numerous projects to determine the effects of massage. Massage is a powerful modality of therapeutic touch. It can induce muscle relaxation, increase circulation, decrease swelling, soften and stretch scar tissue, reduce adhesions, and relieve pain (Kastner, 1994). Implications for pain reduction through touch therapy deserve additional research.

Acupuncture and Acupressure. Acunpunture is an alternative to electric stimulation. Small nerve fibers are stimulated by the twirling of the needles. Acute pain is registered as pain impulses pass through the gate of the spine. The acute pain registers in the brain and signals the central mechanism of the brain to return counterimpulses, which close the gate. Acupuncture points are located near clusters of nerve cell endings. It is thought that acupuncture stimulates these nerves and causes the gate to close or that it triggers the release of the body's own opiate substances, enkephalins (endorphins).

Acupressure is acunpuncture without needles. Pressure applied to the traditional acupuncture points with the thumbs, tip of the index finger, or palm of the hand or pinching and squeezing as means of applying pressure stimulate the nerves and close the gate or trigger the release of the body's natural endorphins.

Biofeedback. An individual can learn voluntary control over some body processs and alter them by changing the physiologic correlates appropriate to them. Response to certain types of pain can be controlled. Boczkowski (1984) found that biofeedback decreased chronic pain of rheumatoid arthritis. Other studies demonstrated no appreciable effect of biofeedback on migraine headaches in the elderly (Hamm and King, 1984). Training and often time and equipment of some type are needed to learn how to alter one's body response. Biofeedback results have provided conflicting data. In some instances it has proved successful in the reduction or elimination of pain.

Distraction. Distraction lessens the perception of pain by drawing the person's attention away from pain. In some instances the individual is completely unaware of the pain. The success of distraction can be explained by the Gate Theory. Pain messages are slower than diversional messages, therefore the gate closes before the pain signal arrives, and less pain is felt.

Mild to moderate pain responds well to distraction. At times, if an individual concentrates intently on another subject, the acute pain may be relieved. The most common forms of distraction include slow rhythmic breathing, slow rhythmic massage, rhythmic singing or tapping, active listening, and guided imagery (Kosier et al, 1995). Box 9-8 lists the various forms of distraction.

Relaxation, Meditation, and Imagery. Relaxation enables the quieting of the mind and muscles, providing the release of tension and anxiety. It may increase the effectiveness of other pain-relieving measures. Meditation and imagery are two methods of promoting relaxation.

Imagery uses the client's imagination to focus on settings full of happiness and relaxation rather than on stressful situations. Several studies using guided imagery have shown that there was a decrease in pain perception in foot pain and abdominal pain. It was suggested that a strong image of a pain-free state effectively alters the autonomic nervous systems' responses to pain (Hamm and King, 1984; Griffin, 1986; Pearson, 1988; McCaffery and Beebe, 1989).

Hypnosis. Hypnosis has been used to help to alter pain perception through positive suggestions. Research has demonstrated hypnotic analgesia reduces what are called "overreactions" to pain when apprehension and stress are apparent.

Some people have the ability to induce self-hypnosis, and some do not. Most of the population, however, has some capacity for hypnosis and with training can increase their control in this area. There are three recognized modes of hypnosis: (1) spontaneous, which is what most of us do when we daydream; (2) the self-induced trance; and (3) formal hypnosis, which requires the services of a hypnotist.

Intense concentration is required for hypnosis. Hypnosis can be used to alter pain perception, thus blocking pain awareness; to substitute another feeling for a painful one; to displace pain sensation to a smaller body area; or to alter the meaning of pain so that it is viewed as less important and less debilitating (Thomas, 1990; Sarvis 1995). Table 9-3 illustrates the advantages and disadvantages of specific nonpharmacologic pain relief measures.

Placebo

When the word *placebo* is mentioned, one immediately thinks of the use of fake pills and saline injections in place of narcotic analgesics, of an attempt to fool the patient into thinking that he or she is getting the "real thing." Some

---

Box 9-8	**Forms of Distraction**

Visual Distraction
Reading
Watching TV
Watching a sports game
Guided imagery

Auditory Distraction
Humor
Listening to music

Tactile Distraction
Slow rhythmic breathing
Massage
Holding or stroking a pet

Intellectual Distraction
Crossword puzzles
Card games
Hobbies

Modified from Kosier B, Erb G, Blais K et al: *Fundamentals of nursing,* Redwood City, Calif, 1995, Addison-Wesley.

	Table 9-3	Advantages and Disadvantages of Nonpharmacologic Measures

Therapy	Advantage	Disadvantage
Cutaneous Nerve Stimulation TENS DNS Touch Acupuncture/Acupressure	Pleasurable sensations make it popular with elders Relaxation and distraction from pain May be feasible for elders with limited income Requires limited energy expenditure Self-administration provides a sense of control Family participation for those elders unable to do for self	Some elders perceive stimulation as intolerable; objectionable odors from creams and ointments such as menthol Improper use of heat, cold, etc., may do tissue damage

Distraction
  Tactile, auditory,
    visual, kinesthetic
	Sense of control over pain
	Improve mood
	Relaxation
	Increase tolerance to pain
		Choices may be limited by cognitive and sensory impairment

Relaxation	Decreases skeletal muscle tension Decreases anxiety Useful with chronic pain, muscle spasms, sleep loss due to pain	Must be able to understand instructions Takes time and energy to learn Ineffective with depressed or very fatigued
Biofeedback	Decrease chronic pain	Requires equipment (moderate to expensive) Takes time and energy to learn Must be cognitively intact Takes time and energy to learn
Imagery	Very simple, uses elders' imagination; may enhance relaxation and distraction; may feel control over pain; may perceive as an escape from pain Always available Little to no economic or social impact for elderly	Not viewed as a credible technique Must be cognitively intact
Hypnosis	Pain relief on a long-term basis without side effects; Useful for elders unable to tolerate pharmacologic measures; Does not alter mental functioning (a fear of the elderly)	May not be viewed as a credible therapy Feel loss of mental control Must be cognitively intact Requires trained personnel May not be available in remote or small settings

Developed by Patricia Hess.

caregivers consider this dishonest and unethical, destroying the trust established between patient and caregiver. This interpretation became more prominent in the 1960s at the time when many scientific advances created more effective agents, when the emergence of informed consent and patient autonomy occurred, and when no one was interested in just how placebos worked. Few paid attention to those who were placebos responders, nor did anyone wonder whether these responders' pain relief mechanism was different from others. Patients whose pain or illness was relieved by placebo were considered "crocks or complainers." Research suggests a placebo activates one's internal biochemical pain relief mechanism. The placebo can work for anybody in the right circumstances; that is, if the patient believes that someone is trying to help him or her, relief of pain can occur. It is important to note that "A placebo is never justified to determine the existence of pain" (McCaffery and Ritchey, 1992; Fox, 1994).

As a nontraditional approach, one should look at the placebo effect or its concept rather than at the placebo as only a pill or an injection. McCaffery & Ritchey (1992) define placebo as "any treatment or procedure that produces a response in a patient because of its intent, and not because of any actual physiologic or therapeutic properties" (p. 9).

There is a general misunderstanding about the use and effect of placebos. The "pure" placebo is a sugar pill or saline injection or some other inert substance. "Impure" placebos are active drugs with pharmacologic effects unrelated to the condition being treated; for example, giving vitamin B_{12} injections for fatigue.

Despite the fact that a placebo is generally thought to be inert and therefore harmless, reports of adverse effects such as rash, nausea, and thirst have been noted (Todd, 1987). The most common side effects are headaches, depression, or CNS stimulation. This could be considered a nocebo effect. The nocebo effect can occur when one thinks that the outcome of a particular medication, treatment, or intervention will be negative (University of California Berkeley Wellness Letter, 1996).

A caregiver administering a placebo need not be deceptive. Templin et al (1984) state the following:

First explain to the patient that some people are able to mobilize their own pain responses without the help of pharmacologically active analgesics. Then, tell the patient that using placebos can help you find out if he's one of those fortunate people.

Acceptance of placebos and the placebo effect is becoming more widely approved. The American Holistic Nurses'

Association refers to the placebo effect in its Standards for Holistic Nursing: "The placebo effect is evidence of the mind's role in disease and healing, and therefore evaluated as a valid healing event. Spiro (1996) reinforces this idea by suggesting that recognition of the placebo effect as a useful tool has reemerged as a result of interest in mind, body, and spirit integration. "A letter in the *Annals of Internal Medicine* (Preston, 1982) suggested that "all treatments including surgery and patient drugs have placebo effects," which most physicians do not recognize but attribute to the biologic effect of treatment. Research by Spiro (1996) hypothesizes that perhaps placebos "turn the mind, or the brain, away from recognizing the pain, even while the C fibers are still firing their torment" (p. 7).

Nurses foster positive placebo effects by being specific with their patients about expected drug actions; for example, "this is a pain reliever" or "you'll feel warm as it begins to work." Even patient teaching about medications employs a placebo effect. If, for example, a nurse explains that the patient will experience a dry mouth from the medication, when the side effect is experienced, it reinforces the patient's expectations that the drug is working.

A positive response most likely creating a beneficial placebo effect for the elderly is one that can make the illness or pain experience more understandable, that lets the elder know someone cares, and that allows the elder a sense of self-mastery and control over causes of his or her condition.

PAIN CLINICS

Pain center experience with elders has been limited; however, referral for elders with significant and psychologic impairment in most instances is appropriate when the usual standard measures to relieve pain (particularly chronic pain) are unsuccessful.

Pain center programs may be inpatient, outpatient, or both. Pain centers are generally one of three types: syndrome oriented, modality oriented, or comprehensive. *Syndrome-oriented centers* focus on a specific chronic pain problem such as headache or arthritis pain. *Modality-oriented centers* focus on a specific treatment technique such as relaxation or acupuncture/acupressure. The *comprehensive centers* include many services, which begin with an initial assessment and include treatment and follow-up. Staff are usually a coordinated, multidisciplinary team of some or all of the following staff members: physician, nurse, physical therapist, occupational therapist, massage therapist, rehabilitation specialist, and social worker. Treatment includes a variety of approaches; medical treatment may be oral, injectable, or topical medication. Because long-term use of potent medications can be habit forming or addicting when one has chronic pain, medication adjustment is considered. Medication is used only when absolutely necessary in the management of the patient's pain. Physical modalities, including massage, heat and cold applications, exercise,

acupuncture/acupressure, to name a few, are used to reduce or alleviate chronic pain during and after the pain center program. Psychologic techniques such as biofeedback, self-hypnosis, relaxation, and behavior modification are a few of the methods used and taught to individuals to control the pain situation. Even though older adults may find these therapies foreign to them, they are good candidates for these treatment programs and may be able to benefit from them (Saxon and Etter, 1994).

The nurse should be familiar with the several types of clinics that exist so as to provide the patient or the family of the patient with the necessary information to make a knowledgeable decision concerning this approach and what to look for.

NURSE'S ROLE

There is a dilemma in providing comfort. Because bureaucratic policies limit staff, the time that staff spend with patients is confined to the basic needs of treatment, medications, and physical care. The quality of physical care suffers when the paraprofessional is discouraged from taking time to fulfill comfort needs such as providing a back rub or discussing the patient's concerns. If the caregiver could spend 5 minutes massaging and talking with the older person after a bath or treatment, anxiety, pain, and depression would be reduced. The nurse is in a very influential position to make a meaningful contribution to pain relief. Although this text does not discuss the various pain theories in depth, it would be expected that nurses providing care to the aged would have sufficient knowledge of the physiologic condition of pain and the theories currently accepted by the medical community.

The ability to assess pain of another becomes complicated because of differing attitudes and the multidimensional aspects that pain projects. There are no easy answers of how to evaluate, differentiate, or judge the uniquely personal estimates of the quality of pain. Pain experiences are highly individualized, but there is much yet to learn about pain.

Nurses are most familiar and comfortable with acute temporary pain because it is short lived and amenable to expedient relief. Chronic pain presents a frustrating situation for the nurse and an intolerable situation for the patient. Nurses expect patients suffering from chronic pain to display behavior characteristics of acute discomfort; an organic basis for pain makes it legitimate. Nurses tend to undermedicate patients with chronic pain because they fear that they will foster addiction. Often nurses caring for the patient with chronic pain, especially in long-term care situations, become so familiar with the pain that they ignore it as a means of protecting themselves from feeling overwhelmed and powerless in what seems an insurmountable, futile situation. Frequently patients with chronically painful conditions are told they must "just learn to live with it." To the individual experiencing pain, that is a dismal pronouncement and implies a withdrawal of interest and concern.

Assessment

Observe the patient for physical and psychologic signs (Table 9-2). Acute pain precipitates restlessness, grumbling, and audible moans, groans, and crying, to mention a few manifestations. The individual in chronic or acute pain decreases movement; movements are quiet, controlled, and deliberate. Vital signs may be unstable, or there may be an increase in pulse rate and an elevation in blood pressure; however, if pain persists for some time, vital signs stabilize and are not a reliable indicator of pain. Ask questions and discuss the situation you observe.

Assessment of pain in the elderly is important for several reasons: pain is the most common symptom of disease; an accurate assessment will lead to an accurate diagnostic; assessment facilitates evaluation of the effects of therapy; assessment can help differentiate acute, endangering pain from long-standing chronic pain; and successful pain management begins with an accurate assessment (Watt-Watson and Donovan, 1992). Box 9-9 lists the consequences of unrelieved pain.

The characteristic of pain can be described as sharp and throbbing or as sensations of pressure, dullness, and aching. It can manifest itself in acute physical signs. Psychosocial pain or discomfort was identified as occurring from unkindness by caregivers or while awaiting new procedures.

Jacox (1979) noted that 70% of patients studied did not like to discuss their pain with others or were ambivalent when they did talk about it. Two thirds of patients remained calm and did not show their pain experience. No verbal communication occurred until the pain was severe. Accurate assessment includes questioning the patient about pain. Do not rely on the word "pain" alone; use other synonyms: dis-

comfort, sore, ache, hurt, and so on (Watt-Watson and Donovan, 1992). Jacox (1979) found that 80% of patients considered itching (a form of pain) as discomfort.

The cognitively impaired and nonverbal patient is the most difficult to assess and requires astute observation. Marzinski (1991) studied five patients with dementia and pain. She found significant behavior changes during painful experiences. It is not wise to extrapolate on such limited data, but the findings might be helpful. Individuals who moan and groan may become withdrawn and quiet; disjointed verbalization may turn into an accurate description of the location of pain; the quiet and nonverbal person may be observed rapidly blinking with slight facial grimacing; and the friendly outgoing individual might become agitated and combative. The person who is easily involved in activities may cry easily and withdraw from activities, or the elderly may rhythmically rock back and forth (Matteson et al, 1995). It is important to remember that the inability to interpret or detect pain in elders who cannot and do not communicate can lead to undertreatment of pain (Sengstaken and King, 1993). At present, the assessment tools for assessing pain in those who are nonverbal are inadequate (Saxon, 1991; Marzinski, 1991). The development of new methods of pain appraisal is an inviting area for research.

Culture and gender are additional factors that make pain assessment more difficult and complex. Box 9-10 highlights some culturally oriented responses to pain. Study of gender responses to pain is a relatively new area of research. Nurses until now have thought that women should receive smaller

---

Box 9-9	**Consequences of Unrelieved Pain**

- Stress hormone response: tissue breakdown, increased metabolic rate, increased blood clotting, water retention, impaired immune function
- Muscle tension
- Decreased mobility
- Shallow breathing and cough suppression
- Retention of pulmonary secretions
- Pneumonia
- Delayed return of gastric and bowel function
- Alteration in quality of life
- Depression
- Suicidal thoughts

Modified from *Clinical practice guideline: acute pain management,* US Department of Health and Human Services, Public Health Services Agency for Health Care Policy and Research, #920032, 1992, Rockville, Md.

Box 9-10	**Culturally Oriented Responses to Pain**

- Minimizes pain with significant others
  or
  Uses pain to elicit sympathy and support from others
- Carefully controls the expression of pain (calm and unemotional)
  or
  Is vocal about pain (cries or moans, complains)
- Withdraws and wants to be alone when pain is severe
  or
  Seeks attention and presence of others
- Willingly accepts pain-relief measures
  or
  Avoids pain-relief measures in the belief that they indicate weakness
- Wants and expects quick pain relief
  or
  Accepts pain for long periods before requesting help

Modified from Bates MS. *Biocultural dimensions of chronic pain,* 1996, State University of New York Press; Kosier B, Erb G, Blais K et al: *Fundamentals of nursing,* Redwood City, Calif, 1995, Addison-Wesley; Salerno E, Willens JS: *Pain management handbook,* St Louis, 1996, Mosby.

doses of narcotic analgesics than men. Nurses believed that gender differences affected sensitivity to pain (Ferrell and McCaffery, 1992). It is now thought that gender-related variations in pain perception may be physiologic rather than psychologic differences in willingness to report pain (Vallerand, 1995).

Assessment tools have been developed to help both clinicians and researchers measure, document, and communicate clients' pain experience more accurately when patients can communicate their pain. Qualitative tools attempt to describe the client's pain using such tools as pain diaries, pain logs, pain graphs, and observation. The diary and graph are particularly helpful in determining adequacy of pain management. The pain log or diary is a record written and kept by the client. For these methods to be effective the client should carry a notebook and pencil to record pain as soon as possible after the pain episode. Such items as activity, intensity, and duration of the pain during daily activities, medications taken, and when they were taken should be recorded. The diary should be reviewed with the caregiver to assess the relationship between pain, medication use, and activity. The pain graph provides a visual picture of the highs and lows of the client's pain. The caregiver can assist the client when necessary in the plotting of the pain experience.

Quantitative assessment tools include pain rating, visual analog scales (VAS), and verbal descriptor scales (VDS) help to measure pain severity. The McGill Pain Assessment Questionnaire (Melzack, 1975) is a comprehensive tool that is useful for initial intake pain assessments, if the client is not in acute distress. The questionnaire asks about past pain experience, medications used, other treatments tried, current pain episode, pain effect on activity and work, and quality and location of pain. The tool relies heavily on verbal and cognitive capacity and task a long time to administer.

McCaffery and Beebe (1989) present an initial pain assessment tool that can be completed by the client or with the help of the caregiver (Figure 9-1). It obtains information similar to that on the McGill questionnaire but uses a different format. There are several versions of the VAS that can be used. The scale utilizes a 10-cm line that at the left end has a zero (no pain) and at the right end a 10 (worst pain). Clients are asked to indicate where on the line they would place their pain. The numeric version of the VAS places the numbers 0 to 10 along the baseline at the intervals 1 cm apart. Zero indicates no pain, 5 is labeled moderate pain, and 10 remains the worst pain. The Descriptive Pain Intensity Scale uses the same principle and graduates the description of pain from no pain to mild, moderate, severe, very severe, to worst possible pain. Elders do better with a vertical rather than a horizontal VAS scale. Figure 9-2 illustrates the VAS scale and its variations.

A pain color scale is another approach to learning a client's quantity of pain. Stewart (1977) designed a color variation for children that can be used with adults and elders as well. The scale goes from yellow-orange to red-black with verbal descriptors of no pain at the yellow end and worst pain at the black end. Providing a body outline and colored markers is another approach to learning the intensity of a client's pain. Four marker pens or crayons are used to pinpoint the pain on a body outline (Eland, 1981). Each color represents a degree of pain; none, mild, moderate, worst pain. This is a useful tool for an individual who has difficulty with language. Using these tools, the nurse can obtain a fairly accurate idea of the degree of discomfort or pain. The existing tools for pain assessment should be adapted for the elderly, based on their verbal, physical, and cognitive capabilities. When the client is unable to tolerate lengthy questioning, a quick assessment should be done, illustrated by the example presented in Box 9-11.

Ascertain the location, quality, intensity, and chronology of the pain. Rather than ask questions, have the patient describe the pain. Leading questions often give the nurse inaccurate information. Patients often answer according to what they think the nurse expects to hear. Elements of a complete pain assessment include an accurate history, physical examination (attention to musculoskeletal system and nervous system; palpation of trigger points), functional assessment (one of several available evaluations of activities of daily living), and psychologic assessment (mini mental status examination) (Box 9-12).

Nurses must seek answers to the following questions to intervene most effectively:

1. Is the elder concerned about the pain sensation itself or about the future implications of pain?
2. Is the elder afraid the pain indicates fatal illness or that the pain does or will deprive him or her of some specific pleasures of life?
3. Does the elder want to be asked about the pain or not be reminded of it?
4. Does the elder want to be alone for fear of showing an emotional response, or does he or she want to be alone because of having one's own method of handling pain?
5. Does the elder want visitors to share the pain or to use visitors as a distraction?
6. Does the elder expect to obtain relief immediately or to suffer a while?
7. Does it matter to the elder if relief is palliative or curative?
8. Does the elder believe drugs are unnatural pain-relief measures or fear the consequences of addictive drugs?
9. Does crying mean the elder wants immediate pain relief or sympathy, or is it a desire for a demonstration of technical skill?
10. Does the elder view the expression of pain as natural, serving a particular purpose, or indicative of defeat?

In addition, assessment should consider how the pain interferes with the patient's ability to meet needs of security,

INITIAL PAIN ASSESSMENT TOOL   Date _____

Patient's name _____   Age _____ Room _____

Diagnosis _____   Physician _____

                                             Nurse _____

I. LOCATION: Patient or nurse mark drawing.

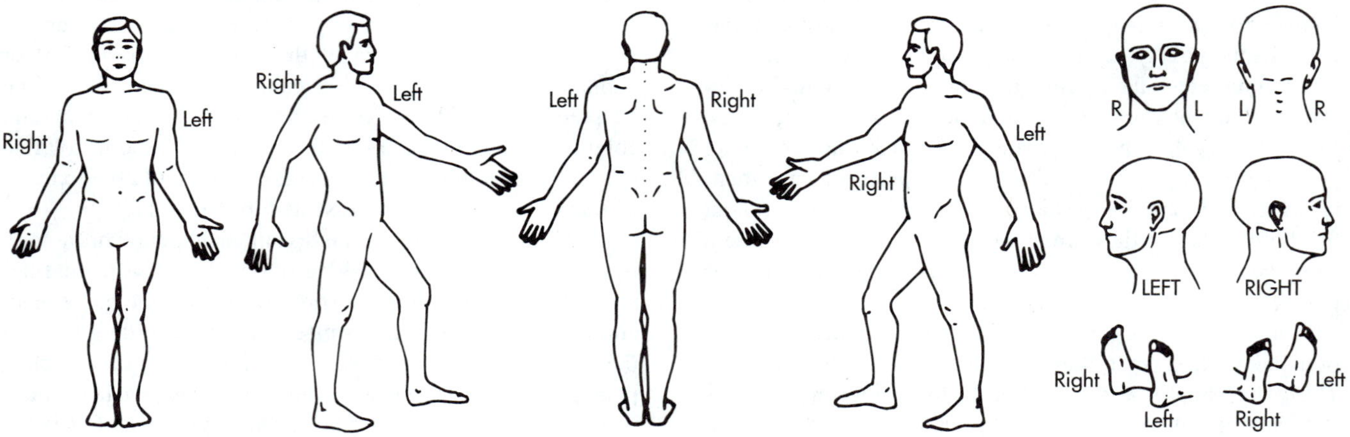

Right   Left   Right   Left   Left   Right   Left   Right   R   L   L   R
                                                                    LEFT   RIGHT
                                                           Right   Left
                                                                    Left   Right

II. INTENSITY: Patient rates the pain. Scale used _____

      Present: _____
      Worst pain gets: _____
      Best pain gets: _____
      Acceptable level of pain: _____

III. QUALITY: (Use patient's own words, e.g. prick, ache, burn, throb, pull, sharp) _____
   _____

IV. ONSET, DURATION VARIATIONS, RHYTHMS: _____
   _____

V. MANNER OF EXPRESSING PAIN: _____
   _____
   _____

VI. WHAT RELIEVES THE PAIN? _____
   _____
   _____

VII. WHAT CAUSES OR INCREASES THE PAIN? _____
   _____
   _____

VIII. EFFECTS OF PAIN: (Note decreased function, decreased quality of life.) _____
      Accompanying symptoms (e.g. nausea) _____
      Sleep _____
      Appetite _____
      Physical activity _____
      Relationship with others (e.g. irritability) _____
      Emotions (e.g. anger, suicidal, crying) _____
      Concentration _____
      Other _____

IX. OTHER COMMENTS: _____
   _____

X. PLAN: _____
   _____

Figure 9-1. Pain assessment. (From McCaffery M, Beebe A: *Pain: clinical manual for nursing practice,* St Louis, 1989, Mosby.)

Pain Distress Scales

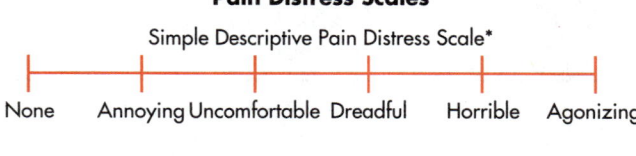

Simple Descriptive Pain Distress Scale*

None   Annoying Uncomfortable Dreadful   Horrible   Agonizing

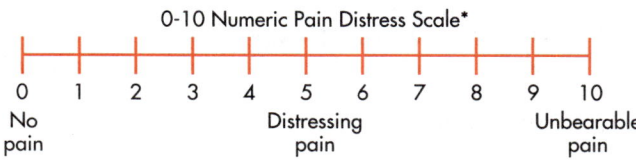

0-10 Numeric Pain Distress Scale*

0   1   2   3   4   5   6   7   8   9   10
No   Distressing   Unbearable
pain   pain   pain

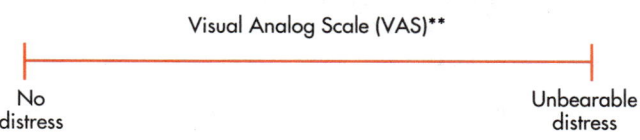

Visual Analog Scale (VAS)**

No   Unbearable
distress   distress

*If used as a graphic rating scale, a 10-cm baseline is recommended.
**A 10-cm baseline is recommended for VAS scales.

Figure 9-2. Example of pain distress scale. (From *Clinical practice guideline: acute pain management,* US Department of Health and Human Services, Public Health Service, Agency for Health Care Policy and Research, No. 92-0032.)

belonging, socialization, and self-esteem. The person who considers himself or herself strong and courageous may find it very humiliating to be forced to whimper or cry out with pain. What does the person want to be able to do? How does the person feel about himself or herself? Is the pain a mask for depression, of which one is unaware? Does the person feel useless, dependent, isolated? Has the pain changed interpersonal relationships? And last, can you, the nurse, help control the pain so that the individual can do what is most important to him or her?

The nurse may not be overtly aware of the influences that the patient's pain experience has on him or her as a participant and observer in the elder's care. If the elder patient is in control of the pain, it has a calming effect on the caregiver who observes and ministers. If the elder patient's pain is uncontrollable, it makes the caregiver agitated and irritated (Meinhart and McCaffery, 1983; Watt-Watson and Donovan, 1992), thus coloring the ability to accurately assess pain. Another impediment to accurate pain assessment is that the patient perceives pain as more severe than do the caregivers, namely, the physicians and nurses. Cultural expectations of the caregiver and preconceived gender expectations also affect the accuracy of assessment (Kosier et al, 1995; Vallerand, 1995).

Intervention

Approximately half the adults who undergo surgery continue to have pain after surgery as a result of the common

---

Box 9-11	**Immediate Help for Assessment**

Quick Assessment in Situations Where Patients are Unable to Tolerate Lengthy Questions

Time involved: Reading time, 5 minutes; implementation time, about 10 minutes.

Sample situation: Mr. M., 65 years old, with lung cancer and widespread metastasis is admitted to your floor. He is not able to concentrate long enough to answer many questions. He grimaces frequently and cries out saying "It hurts, please give me something." His wife states that he is not swallowing anything by mouth.

Possible solution: Assess pain with minimal number of questions in order to give initial analgesic safely.

Expected outcome: Patient states he is comfortable. Further pain assessment is completed at a later time so that a detailed plan of care may be implemented.

Tell the patient that you are going to work to get him comfortable as quickly as possible but that you must get some information first:

1. Point (on his body) to where the pain is. Mr. M. points to his lower back.
2. Is this the same location for the pain over the last several days?
   Mr. M. says that this is the same area that has bothered him over the last week, but it has gotten much worse since yesterday evening.

3. On a 0 to 10 scale (0 = no pain, 10 = worst pain), what number would you give your pain right now? Mr. M. becomes very agitated and yells "It is unbearable." This is a good enough answer under the circumstances.
4. What medication were you taking at home, and did it help the pain?
   Mrs. M. tells you that her husband was taking morphine 90 mg q4h with Motrin 800 mg q6h. He has not been able to swallow anything since late last night, so he has had nothing for pain since then. Prior to this, the medication was keeping the pain well controlled.

Due to Mr. M.'s condition, it was appropriate to ask only the most essential questions to initiate an analgesic regimen. The above four questions give you important baseline data and establish an initial narcotic dose.

Using a flow sheet, the immediate goal is to establish pain control quickly. Using Mr. M.'s words ask "Is the pain more bearable now?" Once Mr. M. is comfortable, additional questions from the initial pain assessment tool may be filled in, and a long-term plan of care may be reviewed with the patient and his wife.

From McCaffery M, Bebee A: *Pain: clinical manual of nursing practice,* St Louis, 1989, Mosby.

<table>
<tr><td>

Box 9-12

Content for Assessing Pain in the Elderly Patient

Pain description: Identify location, quality, intensity (present, worst, best), onset, duration, pattern of radiation or variation, manner of expressing pain, relationship to movement or position, time of occurrence, and related motor or sensory complaints.

Observations: Note vocalizations such as grunting or groaning and facial expressions including wrinkled forehead, tightly closed or widely opened eyes or mouth, or other distorted expressions. Observe body movements noting guarding, rocking, pulling legs into abdomen, increased hand/finger movements, inability to keep still, pacing behaviors, or other restrictive motions.

Alleviating or aggravating factors: Explore what intensifies or decreases the pain and what treatments, remedies, or activities relieve the pain.

Impact: Identify any changes in daily activities, gait, behaviors. Note onset of new behaviors such as confusion, irritability, increased activity; accompanying symptoms such as nausea, dizziness, sweating, fatigue; any changes in sleep, appetite, emotions, concentration, physical activity, relationships with others, social interactions, and common routines.

Social history: Explore functional status prior to onset of symptoms, marital status, family/community resource network, social and leisure activities, and environmental barriers to social activity.

From Herr KA, Mobily RR: Complexities of pain assessment in the elderly: clinical considerations, *J Gerontol Nurs* 17(4):12, 1991.

</td><td>

Box 9-13

Agency for Health Care Policy and Research Guidelines

1. A collaborative, interdisciplinary approach to pain control, including all members of the health care team, and input from the patient and the patient's family, when appropriate
2. An individualized proactive pain control plan developed preoperatively by patients and practitioners (since pain is easier to prevent than to bring under control, once it has begun)
3. Assessment and frequent reassessment of the patient's pain
4. Use of both drug and nondrug therapies to control and/or prevent pain
5. A formal institutional approach to management of acute pain, with clear lines of responsibility

From *Clinical practice guideline: acute pain management,* US Department of Health and Human Services, Public Health Service, Agency for Health Care Policy and Research, No. 920032.

</td></tr>
</table>

practice of PRN dosing of intramuscular opioids. Also the nurse often refrains from giving narcotics to the elderly due to the fear of patient complications, legal pressures, and misbeliefs about pain management. Needless suffering takes a toll physiologically and psychologically. These problems were addressed by the Agency for Health Care Policy and Research, Department of Health and Human Services, which after extensive research has established national guidelines, with intervention strategies, for the management of pain. These guidelines, published in 1992, should help health professionals improve the effectiveness of pain management for their patients. (See Box 9-13 for a brief summary of the guidelines.)

Pain can be minimized through gentle handling and touch. Use of pillows for support or body positioning, just sitting and holding the patient's hand, or allowing the individual to move at his or her own speed provides pain relief benefit.

Activity can be helpful in several ways. Gaumer (1974) indicates that the less active an individual, the less tolerable activity becomes. Anyone who becomes inactive will feel

more aches and pain than the active person. Distraction through the use of activity may help to change the behavior of the individual who uses pain to gain attention and sympathy (Box 9-8). It is important to identify activities that are compatible with the relief of anxiety. Use of analgesics in conjunction with activity may be necessary. The administration of a medication 20 to 30 minutes before a specific activity that elicits pain or giving an analgesic during activity to lessen or eliminate fear of discomfort experienced following activity can enhance greatly the individual's capacity for that activity. The nurse should learn the patient's body potential for coping with pain and work within those parameters.

The patient can be involved by keeping a weekly journal that includes an account of pain during the day; the times, type, and dose of medication taken; its effect; and the duration of its benefit. This type of information helps establish patterns that may be useful in improving pain management by adjusting activity, providing medications appropriately, and helping the patient feel useful and in control of some aspect of care. Patient-controlled analgesic devices (PCAs) have not been used as extensively with elders in the acute setting as they have with the other adult patients. This may be based on criteria that require the user of a PCA to be alert, mentally intact, and able to follow simple directions. In addition, elders with multisystem involvement are at high risk for respiratory and renal complications (Salerno and Willens, 1996). However, many elders meet the PCA criteria and still do not receive pain control with the PCA (Matteson et al, 1995). It is therefore important that elders receive ATC analgesia to alleviate pain.

The nurse's involvement in psychologic modulation of pain is in providing understanding and support for patients and learning and practicing hypnotic suggestion, biofeedback conditioning, TENS, and other psychologic practices that help patient relaxation and coping with pain. McCaffery (1979; Meinhart and McCaffery, 1983) suggests guidelines for individualizing pain control measures:

1. Use a variety of pain control measures.
2. Institute pain control measures before pain becomes severe.
3. Consider patients' ideas about what they feel is most effective in controlling pain when making the nursing care plan.
4. Consider patients' ability or willingness to participate in their pain control.
5. Listen to how patients describe the severity of pain. Physical signs and perceived severity are not predictably related.
6. Be aware that patients respond differently to different pain control measures. What is effective one day may not be effective the next day.
7. Encourage patients to use a pain control method more than one time. Repeated use may prove effective. A patient's bill of rights for pain appears in Box 9-14.

Whether the pain is brief or long standing, or the anticipated result of diagnostic procedures or surgery, a pain plan should be initiated. This should begin with a discussion between the nurse or physician and the patient of how much pain there might be and how long it might last, along with how will it be treated and what alternatives are available if the initial treatment does not adequately relieve the pain. In addition, for those who leave the hospital with pain or have chronic pain such as cancer, the plan should include the medications and when, how many, how often, and how to be taken; medications to be used if there are side effects; actions to ward off complications of medication therapy such as constipation, nausea, etc., any other pertinent instructions, and important numbers to call if necessary (Managing pain, 1996; *Focus on Geriatric Care and Rehabilitation,* 1996). Box 9-15 provides one type of pain control plan.

Evaluation

Evaluation or outcomes require reassessment of the patients'/clients' pain status. Physical indicators may include relaxation of skeletal muscles, which during pain were tense and rigid. The individual no longer assumes a constricted pain posture. Behavior may reflect an increased activity level and sense of self-worth and the ability to better concentrate, focus, and increase attention span. The individual is more able to rest, relax, and sleep. In fact, the individual may sleep for what might seem like excessively long periods, but this is a response to the exhaustion that pain imposes on the body. Verbal indicators reflect the patient/client referring to the decrease in pain or the absence of pain during conversation.

Chronic Pain. Nearly 90% of adults by the age of 50 have degenerative abnormalities of the lower spine. One of the most typical is thinning of the intervertebral disks, which

---

Box 9-14	**Pain Patient's Bill of Rights**

I have the right to:
- have my pain prevented or controlled adequately
- have my pain and pain medication history taken
- have my pain questions answered freely
- develop a pain plan with my doctor
- know the risks, benefits and side effects of treatment
- know what alternative pain treatments may be available
- sign a statement of informed consent before any treatment
- be believed when I say I have pain
- have my pain assessed on an individual basis
- have my pain assessed using the 0 = no pain, 10 = worst pain scale
- ask for changes in treatment if my pain persists
- receive compassionate and sympathetic care
- refuse treatment without prejudice from my doctor
- seek a second opinion or request a pain-care specialist
- be given my records on request
- include my family in decision making
- remind those who care for me that my pain management is part of my diagnostic, medical or surgical care

Modified from Batten M: Health: take charge of your pain, *Modern Maturity,* 38(1):80, 1995; Cowles J: *Pain relief,* New York, 1994, MasterMedia.

---

can eventually lead to arthritis and other painful conditions (*Low back pain,* 1989). Geriatric clients with benign chronic pain from musculoskeletal disorders have generally been treated pharmacologically without consideration of multidimensional, multidisciplinary rehabilitation programs that are frequently offered to younger patients. For some unknown reason many of these rehabilitation programs exclude individuals over 55 years of age. Middaugh et al (1988) debunked the bias that elderly patients do not benefit from such rehabilitation programs. The Middaugh study, using a group of young and old with chronic pain, showed that geriatric patients had as good if not better results than the younger group of patients. The study attributes some of the improvement that occurred to a high level of compliance, realistic expectations, and a lack of work-related obligations. Eland (1988) noted that studies indicate 60% of patients with chronic pain who were in a multidisciplinary program functioned better after 1 year of treatment. Sorkin et al (1990) stated that age should to be a significant factor in the offering of multidisciplinary treatment to patients with chronic pain.

Postherpetic Neuralgia (PHN). PHN (shingles) affects mostly those between the ages of 60 and 79. It has been estimated that about 50% of people who live to the age of 80 will have an attack of shingles (*Special Report on Aging,*

Box 9-15	**Pain Control Plan**

Pain Control Plan for _____

At home, I will take the following medications for pain control:

Medication	How to take	How many	How often	Comments
_____	_____	_____	_____	_____
_____	_____	_____	_____	_____
_____	_____	_____	_____	_____

Medicines that I may take to help side effects;

Side effect	Medicine	How to take	How many	How often	Comments
_____	_____	_____	_____	_____	_____
_____	_____	_____	_____	_____	_____
_____	_____	_____	_____	_____	_____

Constipation is a very common problem when taking opioid medication. When this happens, do the following:

_____ Increase fluid intake (8 to 10 glasses of fluid per day)
_____ Exercise regularly
_____ Increase fiber in diet (bran, fresh fruit, vegetables)
_____ Use a mild laxative, such as milk of magnesia, if no non-drug pain control methods
_____
_____

If you do not have a bowel movement in three days:
_____ Take _____ every day at _____ (time) with a full glass of water.
_____ Use a glycerine suppository every morning (this may help make a bowel movement less painful).

Additional instructions:
_____
_____

Important phone numbers:
Your doctor _____ Your nurse _____
Your pharmacy _____ Emergencies _____

Call your doctor or nurse immediately if your pain increases or if you have new pain. Also call your doctor early for a refill of pain medication. Do not let your medication get below 3 or four days' supply.

From Agency for Health Care Policy and Research: *Managing cancer pain,* consumer version, Clinical Practice Guide No 9, Washington, DC, 1994, Public Health Service, US Department of Health and Human Services.

1990). This may be due to the decrease in cellular immune response to the varicella zoster antigen, which is undetected in up to 30% previously immune healthy elders over 60. An attack of shingles can occur when there is reactivation of the varicella virus through immunosuppression, malignancy, trauma, surgery, or local radiation (Gilchrest, 1995). PHN is experienced because of irritation of the nerve roots that leave the spinal cord. The stinging, burning pain with or without an underlying sharp, jabbing sensation continues for weeks, months, and for some elderly indefinitely after the initial skin lesions have healed. Analgesics provide limited relief from the pain, although codeine is often prescribed.

More effective in providing relief is a combination of antiviral medications, steroids, aspirin, and topical anesthetics for pain. The U.S. Food and Drug Administration (FDA) has approved such prescription medications as Acyclovir and Famcyclovir, which shorten the duration of chronic shingle pain, and capsaicin (Zostrix) as an over-the-counter topical anesthetic (Reyes, 1994). The use of TENS and adjuvant therapy such as Despramine (which is considered one of the safe tricyclic drugs for use with the elderly) is effective (Portenoy, 1995; Watt-Watson and Donovan, 1992) (Box 9-16). Primary prevention of shingles (herpes zoster) and the subsequent PHN in the future may be attainable with widespread use of the varicella vaccine. When immunosuppressed individuals with herpes zoster eruptions are treated in the early eruption stage, it prevents or limits the dissemination of vesicles and herpetic pain.

Osteoarthritis. Osteoarthritis is one of the most common forms of joint disease with its prevalence increasing into the eighth decade. It is the leading cause of disability in persons 65 years of age and older (Ettinger, 1995). Joint pain and stiffness is initially intermittent and then can become constant. Pain is characterized by aching in the joints, surrounding muscles, and soft tissue, usually relieved by rest and exacerbated by activity. Such joints as the distal and proximal interphalangeal, cervical and lumbar spine, hips, knees, and toes are affected. Many older adults have other medical conditions in addition to osteoarthritis, which requires that the total picture be considered when the arthritic pain is treated. Generally treatment consists of anitinflammatory preparations such as aspirin; however, this is not recommended for elders because of the effect on the gastric mucosa. NSAIDs are also used, but they too can have an adverse effect on the gastrointestinal lining. Acetaminophen, while not as effective as antiinflammatory preparations, is preferred to salicylates. Effective pain relief can be achieved without the risk of gastric irritation or potential for gastric hemorrhage. Topical capsaicin may reduce osteoarthritis pain as well as PHN;

however, it is necessary to warn patients to wash their hands after application and to keep their hands away from their eyes. It is also important to tell patients to expect a strong sensation of burning. Nonpharmacologic pain management includes application of moist heat to relieve pain, spasm, and stiffness; orthotic devices such as braces and splints to support painful joints; weight reduction if the patient is overweight or obesity is a contributing factor; and occupational and physical therapy. Severe arthritis with unrelieved pain and extensive disability may require local anesthetics and corticosteroid injections into joints or epidural spaces for lumbar pain, or joint replacement for intractable pain.

Terminal Cancer Pain. Terminal cancer pain requires a thorough understanding of the dynamics of pain management. The nurse cannot be caught in the assumption that frequent use of analgesic drugs will create iatrogenic addiction; the real issue is adequate pain relief. Key to this relief is providing medication on time without the necessity of the patient asking for pain medication. Standard narcotic preparations or mixtures are effective. Present-day preparations contain morphine or methadone. Other ingredients such as mood elevators and antiemetics are added when necessary to control other symptoms produced by the disease and to temper the level of anxiety. Additionally, invasive anesthetics and neurosurgical or neurostimulating approaches may be used. Newer intraspinal pain relief approaches are used for pain relief below the midthorax. This requires persons with special expertise.

Pain management entails control of not only physical pain but also emotional, psychologic, and spiritual pain of the patient. The concept of the pain, anxiety, and anguish cycle mentioned earlier is crucial to successful management of pain in terminal cancer. Reduction or relief of anxiety can be achieved by allowing the individual some control over the pain situation. Self-medication is one method. Teaching the patient about his or her medication and allowing the patient to administer the medication and keep dosage records eliminate the fear that medication will not arrive on time and that the patient may have to suffer until someone arrives to provide relief. Obviously not all patients can administer their own medication, but the potential is there, and each situation must be assessed on an individual basis.

A flow sheet, kept by the patient or staff to rate pain on a scale of 0 to 10, provides the information to individually titrate the medication to the patient's pain need. Studies have shown that effective control of pain (attention to the psychologic, emotional, spiritual, and physical distress) in many instances has reduced the amount of medication needed.

The nurse need not look on pain with fear and trepidation. If assessment is correct and the patient listened to and handled gently and with care, anxiety can be controlled and interventions will prove more effective.

The following potential diagnoses must be considered as well as diagnoses unique to the particular individual:

Pain
Pain: chronic
Activity intolerance
Altered nutrition: Less than body requirements
Altered nutrition: More than body requirements
Anxiety
Constipation
Ineffective coping: individual
Fatigue
Fear
Hopelessness
Knowledge deficit
Impaired physical mobility

Powerlessness
Self-care deficit
    Bathing/hygiene
    Dressing/grooming
    Feeding
    Toileting
Low self-esteem
Sexual dysfunction
Sleep pattern disturbance
Impaired social interaction
Social isolation
Altered thought processes

NURSING PROCESS AND NURSING DIAGNOSIS
Chronic Pain

Etiology and Related Factors
Etiology
    Arthritis, postherpetic neuralgia, malignancies, low back pain, neuropathy of diabetes, peripheral vascular disease
Related Factors
    Persistent physical/psychologic disability
    Fear of reinjury
    Guarding movements
    Anorexia; weight gain
    Changes in sleep pattern
    Facial mask
    Altered ability to continue previous activity

Defining Characteristics
Verbal report of pain and/or observed pain over a 6-month period
Self-focusing
Social withdrawal
Impaired thought process
Depression

Knowledge
Response of older adults to pain
    Physiologic, cultural, social
    Pain theory and contributing factors
Assessment of pain
    Brief history
    Symptoms (defining characteristics)
    Nursing interventions to manage pain

Pharmacologic: drugs, interactions, how drugs affect pain management
Nonpharmacologic
    Relaxation/distraction
    Physical comfort measures
Client and family teaching on pain management
Community resources available to client and family

Clinical Judgments and Related Skills
Obtain history related to pain
Utilize standard pain assessment tools
Conduct brief assessment
    Observation of related behaviors
    Palpation of trigger points (as appropriate)
Administration of prescribed medications
Implementation of interventions to prevent or manage pain
        Client teaching
        Exercise/rest
        Distraction
        Positioning
        Heat/cold applications
        Behavior modification
        Biofeedback
        Family teaching and support

Evaluation
Pain has been eliminated or reduced to a level that client can accept and is functional.
Pain does not interfere with his/her physical, social, or psychological activities.

NEEDS ADDRESSED AND TASK STRENGTHS

Need to cope with acute and chronic discomfort; need to make own choices, express feelings and maintain self-worth (to meet need for basic survival, security, and self-esteem)

Assertive in seeking relief from pain
Ability to express feelings openly
Recognizing and discharging anger in acceptable ways
Accepting own personality changes when pain is present

KEY CONCEPTS

- The absence of pain does not necessarily imply comfort. Comfort is a state of ease and satisfaction of the bodily wants and freedom from pain and anxiety.
- Nurse's response to a client's pain is influenced by the degree of ability to imaginatively identify with another and how well the other is known. Nurses, like others, feel less concern for the stranger than for a loved one.
- Culture, ethnicity, family, and individual characteristics all influence one's tolerance and expressions of pain.
- Aged individuals with various degrees of cognitive impairment may demonstrate pain by increased levels of confusion, restlessness, or withdrawal.
- Though sometimes assumed, it has not been shown that pain sensitivity and perception decrease with age.
- Pain is what the elder says it is. The nursing goal is to assist in pain relief. Some pain medications are more appropriate for use with elders than others.
- Acute and chronic pain require different therapeutic approaches. Chronic pain predominates in the life of the aged.
- Various combinations of pharmacologic and nonpharmacologic pain control can be effective but must be individually designed with client decision making.
- Some elders may find autogenics helpful in pain control, though others may, depending upon personal background and expectations, find them totally ineffective.
- Giving a placebo (inert substance disguised as medication) "is never justified to determine the existence of pain" (McCaffery and Ritchey, 1992).
- Real placebo effects are a part of all successful pain management and incorporate the belief in efficacy by the client and caregiver and the acceptability of the substance or action.

▲ CASE STUDY

Katy was a 66-year-old diabetic and, following a stroke, her diabetes rapidly fulminated to uncontrollable fluctuations. Her blood sugar ranged from 20 mEq/ml to 800 mEq/ml. Some of this was due to erratic eating habits, almost no exercise, frequent urinary tract infections, and considerable stress related to her condition and her future. She bumped her toe while being assisted into her wheelchair after occupational therapy. In a few days the bruise had sloughed skin, and an open sore was evident. In spite of the use of local ointments and various dressings, the sore became necrotic and was debrided. Within a few weeks the debridement of necrotic tissue had removed half of her left great toe. She, who rarely complained, began to moan while she was sleeping and cry a lot during the day. She complained of a continuous burning sensation, and it felt as if her toe was "on fire." One day she threw her coffee cup across the room, simply unable to bear the discomfort without expressing her frustration and anger. Various pain medications were given by mouth on an incon-

sistent basis, but the relief she experienced was minimal. She began to beg to die. The nurses thought perhaps she was right—after all, her general condition was poor, and life held little satisfaction for her. Maybe she should be allowed to die.

Based upon the case study, develop a nursing care plan using the following procedure*:

List comments of client that provide *subjective data.*

List information that provides *objective data.*

From these data identify and state, using accepted format, two *nursing diagnoses* you determine are most significant to this client at this time. List two *client strengths* that you have identified from data.

Determine and state *outcome criteria* for each diagnosis. These must reflect some alleviation of the problem identified in the nursing diagnosis and must be stated in concrete and measurable terms.

Plan and state one or more *interventions* for each diagnosed problem. Provide specific documentation of source used to determine appropriate intervention. Plan at least one intervention that incorporates the client's existing strengths.

Evaluate success of intervention. Interventions must correlate directly with the stated outcome criteria in order to measure the outcome success.

STUDY QUESTIONS/ACTIVITIES

Discuss Katy's situation and her probable prognosis.

What could be done, based on the information you have, to improve Katy's condition?

Do you think Katy's focus on pain is realistic or an avoidance mechanism?

What do you think impedes the nurses' understanding of Katy's pain?

Do you believe elders feel the pain of a necrotic (dead tissue) toe in the same degree that you would feel pain if someone cut away half of your toe?

Discuss the reasons for sporadic pain medication and inattention to the patient's signals and requests.

Do you think nurses are concerned about addiction in cases like Katy's?

In what situations do you believe addiction to pain medications is a priority concern?

Discuss issues of power and control related to pain management.

RESEARCH QUESTIONS

How frequently is pain responsible for an elder's expressed desire to die?

---

*Students are advised to refer to their nursing diagnosis text and identify possible or potential problems.

Do pain perceptions generally diminish as one ages?

What type of chronic pain do elders find most intolerable?

How do elders describe the pain of arthritis?

Do elders really fear the physical pain that may accompany dying?

What nonchemical means of pain control do elders use most frequently?

What nonchemical means of pain control are effective, and in what circumstances do they provide pain relief?

What are the reliable ways of assessing pain in cognitively impaired elders?

How can pain and pain relief be evaluated in the cognitively impaired?

How effective is PCA use by elders?

For whom and under what circumstances should the various modalities of pain management be utilized?

RESOURCES

Organizations

American Chronic Pain Association
PO Box 850
Rocklin, CA 95677
(916) 632-0922

American Pain Society, National Chapter of the International Association for the Study of Pain
5700 Old Orchard Road
Skokie, IL 60077
(708) 966-5595

American Society of Pain Management Nurses
(404) 279-9022

International Association for the Study of Pain
For information on membership and the journal *Pain*
909 NE 43rd St
Room 306
Seattle, WA 98105
(206) 547-6409

National Chronic Pain Outreach Associations Inc.
4922 Hampden Lane
Bethesda, MD 20814
(301) 652-4948

National Headache Foundation
5252 N Western Avenue
Chicago, IL 60625
(312) 878-7715
(800) 843-2256
(800) 523-8858 (in Illinois)

Publications

Commission for Accreditation of Rehabilitation Facilities
101 N Wilmot Rd, Suite 500
Tucson, AZ 85711
(Lists 120 multidisciplinary pain clinics in the United States)

Acute Pain Management: Operative or Medical Procedures and Trauma—Clinical Practice Guideline, U.S. Department of Health and Human Services, Public Health Service, Agency for Health Care Policy and Research, AHCPR 92:0032.

Quick Reference Guide for Clinicians: Acute Pain Management in Adults—Operative Procedures, U.S. Department of Health and Human Services, Public Health Service, Agency for Health Care Policy and Research, AHCPR 92:0019.

REFERENCES

Acute pain management: Operative or medical procedures and trauma—clinical practice guideline, US Department of Health and Human Services, Public Health Service, Agency for Health Care Policy and Research, Washington, DC, 1992.

American Pain Society: *Principles of analgesic use in the treatment of acute and cancer pain,* ed 3, Skokie, Ill, 1992, American Pain Society.

Bates MS: *Biocultural dimensions of chronic pain,* 1996, Albany, State University of New York Press.

Boczkowski JA: Biofeedback training for the treatment of chronic pain in the elderly arthritic female, *Clin Gerontol* 2:39, 1984.

Chronic pain, *Harvard Medical School Health Letter* 16(2):6, 1992.

Davies P: Pharmacological management of pain in the elderly, *Analgesia* 7(1):4, April, 1996.

Chronic pain: medical essay, *Mayo Clinic Health Letter,* June 1, 1990.

Duff VG: Pain theories and their relevance to nursing practice, *Nurs Pract* 13:66, 1988.

Eland JM: Pain management and comfort, *J Gerontol Nurs* 14:10, 1988.

Eland JM: Minimizing pain associated with prekindergarten IM injections, *Issues Compr Pediatr Nurs* 5:361, 1981.

Ettinger HW: Joint and soft tissue disorders. In Abrams WB, Beers MH, Berkow R, editors: *The Merck manual of geriatrics,* ed 2, Whitehouse Station, NJ, 1995, Merck Research Laboratories.

Fakouri C, Jones P: Slow stroke back rub, *J Gerontol Nurs* 13:32, 1987.

Ferrell BA: Pain management in elderly people, *J Gerontol Soc* 39(1):64, 1991.

Ferrell BR, Ferrell BA: Easing the pain, *Geriatr Nurs* 11(5):175, 1990.

Ferrell BR, Ferrell BA: Pain in the elderly. In Watt-Watson JH, Donovan MI, editors: *Pain management: nursing perspective,* St Louis, 1992, Mosby.

Ferrell BR, McCaffery M, Rhiner M: Does the gender gap affect your pain control decisions? *Nursing* 92(8):48, 1992.

Fox AE: Confronting the use of placebos for pain, *Am J Nurs* 94(9):42, 1994.

Fulmer TT, Mion LC, Bottrell MM et al: Pain management protocol, *Geriatr Nurs* (17)5:222, 1996.

Gaumer WC: Psychological potentials of chronic pain, *J Psychiatr Nurs* 12:23, 1974.

Gilchrist BA: Skin changes and disorders. In Abrams WB, Beers MH, Berkow R, editors: *The Merck manual of geriatrics,* ed. 2, Whitehouse Station, NJ, 1995, Merck Research Laboratories.

Glickstein JK, editor: Managing chronic pain, *Focus Geriatr Care Rehab* 10(3):6, 1996.

Gordon DB, and Ward SE: Correcting patient misconceptions about pain, *Am J Nurs* 95(7):43, 1995.

Gray BB: Managed care policies affect nurses' ability to provide pain management, *Nurseweek* 9(3):1, 1996.

Griffin M: In the mind's eye, *Am J Nurs* 86:804, 1986.

Hamilton J: Comfort and the hospitalized chronically ill, *J Gerontol Nurs* 15(4):28, 1989.

Hamm BH, King V: A holistic approach to pain control with geriatric clients, *J Holistic Nurs* 11:32, 1984.

Hofland SL: Elder beliefs: blocks and pain management, *J Gerontol Nurs* 18(6):19, 1992.

Indeck W: Pain in geriatric patients, *Geriatrics* 32:43, 1977.

Jacox AK: Assessing pain, *Am J Nurs* 79:895, 1979.

Kastner M: Researching massage as real therapy, *Massage Ther J* 33(3):56, 1994.

Kosier B, Erb G, Blais K, Wilkinson JM: *Fundamentals of nursing: comfort and pain,* Addison-Wesley, Redwood City, Calif, 1995.

Kreiger D: Therapeutic touch: the imprimatur of nursing, *Am J Nurs* 75:784, 1975.

Krieger D: *The therapeutic touch: how to use your hands to help or heal,* New York, 1992, Prentice-Hall.

Low back pain: part I, *Harvard Medical School Health Letter* 15(1):5, 1989.

Mackey RB: Discover the healing power of therapeutic touch, *Am J Nurs* 95(4):27, 1995.

Managing pain: medical essay, *Mayo Clinic Health Letter,* supplement, pp 1–8, June 1996.

Marzinski LR: The tragedy of dementia: clinically assessing pain in the confused, nonverbal elderly, *J Gerontol Nurs* 17(6):25, 1991.

Matteson MA, Ruzicka S, Heye M, Bell M, Linton A: *Pain in cognitively impaired older adults,* 48th Annual Scientific Meeting, Gerontological Society of America, Los Angeles, Calif, October 1995.

McCaffery M: *Nursing management of the patient with pain,* Philadelphia, 1979, JB Lippincott Co.

McCaffery M, Beebe A: *Pain: clinical manual for nursing practice,* St Louis, 1989, Mosby.

McCaffery M, Ritchey KJ: Pain assessment: debunking the myths and misconceptions, *Nurseweek* 5(16):8, 1992.

Meek, SS: Effects of slow stroke back massage on relaxation in hospice clients, *Image J Nurs Sch* 25(1):17, 1993.

Meinhart N, McCaffery M: *Pain: a nursing approach to assessment and analysis.* East Norwalk, Conn, 1983, Appelton-Century-Crofts.

Melzack R: The McGill pain questionnaire: major properties and scoring method, *Pain* 1:277, 1975.

Melzack R, Wall PD: Pain mechanisms: a new theory, *Science* 150:971, 1965.

Middaugh SJ, Levin RB, Kee WG, Roberts FD: Chronic pain: its treatment in geriatric and younger patients, *Arch Phys Med Rehab* 69(12):1021, 1988.

National Institutes of Health: *Special report on aging,* Department of Health and Human Services, National Institutes of Health, Bethesda, Md, 1990.

Pain relief, *University of California Berkely Wellness Letter* 5(11):4, 1995.

Pearson BD: Pain control: an experiment with imagery, *Geriatr Nurs* 13:28, 1988.

Petrie A: In Bushman MS: *The roots of individuality—brain waves and perception,* an NIMH program report, Washington, DC, Oct 1975, US Department of Health, Education, and Welfare, Public Service, Alcohol, Drug Abuse and Mental Health Administration.

Portenoy RK: Pain. In Abrams WB, Beers MH, Berkow R, editors: *The Merck manual of geriatrics,* ed 2, Whitehouse Station, NJ, 1995, Merck Research Laboratories.

Preston TA: Placebo (letter), *Ann Intern Med* 97:781, 1982.

Reyes KW: Early treatment makes shingles easier to bear, *Modern Maturity* 36(6):79, Nov/Dec 1994.

Salerno E, Willens JS: *Pain management handbook,* St Louis, 1996, Mosby.

Sarvis CM: *Pain management in the elderly,* Sacramento, Calif, 1995, CME Resources.

Saxson SV, Etter MJ: *Physical changes and aging,* ed 3, 1994, New York, Tiresias Press.

Saxson SV: *Pain management techniques for older adults,* Springfield, Ill, 1991, Charles C Thomas.

Sengstaken EA, King SA: The problems of pain and its detection among geriatric nursing home residents, *J Am Geriatr Soc* 41:541, 1993.

Sorkin BA, Rudy TE, Hanlon RB et al: Chronic pain in old and young patients: differences appear less important than similarities, *J Gerontol* 45(2):64, 1990.

Spiro HM: The art and science of placebo, *Science Med* 3(2):6, April/May 1996.

Stewart ML: Measurement of clinical pain. In Jacox A, editor: *Pain: a source book for nurses and other health professionals,* Boston, 1977, Little Brown.

Templin MS et al: Placebos: how much do you know about them? *Nurs Life* 4:52, 1984.

Thomas BL: Elder care: pain management for the elderly—alternative interventions, part I, *AORN J* 52(6):1268, 1990.

Todd B: The placebo effect: real or imaginary, *Geriatr Nurs* 8:154, 1987.

Vallerand AH: Gender differences in pain, *Image J Nurs Sch* 27(3):235, 1995.

Watt-Watson JH, Donovan MI: *Pain management nursing perspective,* St Louis, 1992, Mosby.

Witt JR: Relieving chronic pain, *Nurse Pract* 9(1):36.

CHAPTER 10

Pharmacology and Drug Use

Patricia Hess, PhD, RN, GNP-CS and Samuel Lee, Pharm D

An elder speaks   *I think there's a pill or elixir for every human condition except aging, and, goodness knows, the search continues for that. With my luck, I expect it will come along sometime soon after I'm gone.*

Jerome, age 82

LEARNING OBJECTIVES   Upon completion of this chapter, the reader will be able to:

1. Describe the pharmacokinetic changes that occur in the aged.
2. Identify the altered effects of drugs on the aged.
3. Explain the effect of biorhythms on physiologic processes and the administration of medications.
4. Define chronopharmacology.
5. Discuss the information that the elderly should know about medication use.
6. Identify medications that may or may not be used by the aged.
7. Explain the factors that affect medication adherence.
8. Discuss the role that the health care professional has in assisting the aged with adherence to their medication regimen.
9. Develop a nursing plan to prevent drug toxicity.

DRUG USE

There has been a virtual explosion of new drugs in the past 15 years. Cardiovascular drugs including many beta-blockers, such as propranolol (Inderal); entirely new groups of calcium channel blockers such as nifedipine (Procardia); and angiotensin converting enzyme (ACE) inhibitors such as Captopril (Capoten) for hypertension have been introduced. New antiarrhythmic and anticholesterol medications have also appeared on the market. Digoxin FAB (Digibind) was the first drug available to treat digoxin toxicity, a life-threatening situation. A proliferation of nonsteroidal antiinflammatory drugs (NSAIDs) provided the beginning of greater relief for arthritic conditions. Additional support in the therapy of gastrointestinal ulcers was evidenced by the addition of the H_2 inhibitors, cimetidine (Tagamet), famotidine (Pepcid), ranitidine (Zantac), and nizatidine (Axid), and sucralfate (Carafate). Misoprostol (Cytotec) was specifically developed to counteract the gastrointestinal effects of

NSAIDs. By the end of the 1980s at least a dozen new antibiotics, penicillins, and cephalosporins were on the market as well as an expanded pneumococcal pneumonia vaccine. Less sedating and safer antihistamines such as terfenadine (Seldane), water-soluble radiologic contrast media, and many new rapid-acting psychotropic drugs, particularly for depression, appeared and were readily used.

New forms of old drugs have also come forth with increasing frequency: potassium supplements (Slow-K, Micro-K); digoxin transformed into capsule form (Lanoxicaps); and transdermal patches for nitroglyerin, scopolamine, and estrogen. Clonidine, fentanyl, nicotine, and Catopres are additional patches that have been added. The 1980s and early 1990s was also the time of recombinant DNA technology. Biosynthetic preparations such as human insulin (Humulin), a hepatitis B vaccine, and tissue plasminogen activator (TPA) appeared. Lastly, ibuprofen and calcium supplements initiated the conversion of prescription drugs to the nonprescription market (Todd, 1990). Many more prescription to over-the-counter (OTC) drugs continue to appear on the pharmacy and supermarket shelves.

During 1995 and 1996 additional cold and allergy medication (Tavist and Tavist-D), pain, arthritis, and antiinflammatory drugs (Aleve, Actron, Orudis KT), and H_2 inhibitors (Tagamet HB, Pepcid AC) have made the switch from prescription to OTC preparations. Still waiting for approval from the U.S. Food and Drug Administration are drugs with active ingredients of acyclovir, cholestyramine, and methocarbamol (Cameron, 1996).

While such advances in drug therapy are desirable, they bring with them concern about the effect of these new and improved drugs on the older person. Many nonspecialist physicians still do not realize older patients are vulnerable to drugs. Many new drugs differ only in subtle ways from older, less expensive therapeutic agents but have the potential for use by a relatively small group of patients. As new drugs are introduced, their advantages draw attention, and their potential side effects and other limitations or hazards are then obscured. At issue too is the tendency to think new is better, causing physicians to place older patients on newer, more expensive medications sometimes unnecessarily.

According to the World Health Organization (WHO), the world population of individuals 65 years of age in the year 2000 will be 600 million people. In the United States 16% of adults are over 60 years of age and take nearly 40% of the medications prescribed, the average being 4.5 drugs per person. A comparable number of elders in addition to their prescription drugs use between 40% and 50% of the OTC medications, with an average of 2 medications per person. Elders who reside in long-term care facilities take an average of 4 to 7 different medications (Hogstel, 1992). The trend of multiple drug use will continue as research produces more sophisticated therapies. A survey by the Pharmaceutical Manufacturers Association found 221 drugs at various stages of clinical development for 23 common diseases of the elderly (Stewart et al, 1991). The fast pace of drug research and development and the use of such drugs by elderly persons despite the lack of sufficient research with aged subjects requires an understanding of the changes in pharmacokinetics and pharmacodynamic effects in the aged. From a Maslovian perspective, drugs impinge on many levels of human needs. When used appropriately, drugs can enhance; when used inappropriately, they threaten all levels of the hierarchy of needs. At times, even when drugs are used appropriately, they may impinge on the elder's health. Figure 10-1 illustrates the possible negative influence drugs have on the hierarchy of needs.

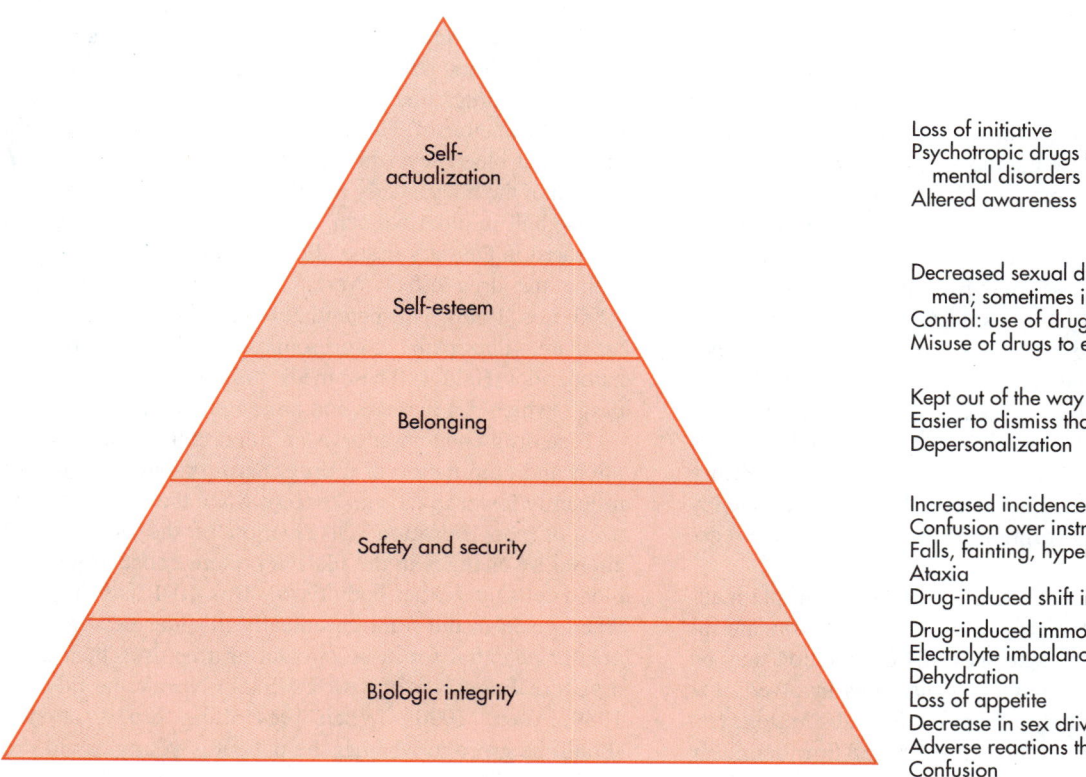

Figure 10-1. Possible negative influences of drugs on the hierarchy of needs.

PHARMACOKINETICS AND PHARMACODYNAMICS

Pharmacokinetics refers to those aspects of a drug involved in the distribution of the drug in the body from the point of administration through absorption, metabolism, and excretion (Vestal, 1985; Roberts and Tumer, 1988; DeMaagd, 1995). *Pharmacodynamics* refers to the processes involved in the interaction between a drug and the effector organ, ending in a response of the organ (Roberts and Tumer, 1988; DeMaagd, 1995).

Absorption

Absorption is the time required for a medication introduced into the body by oral, parenteral, or rectal route to enter the general circulation. Drug bioavailability, the amount of drug in the blood, depends on this (Cusack and Vestal, 1986; Demaagd,1995; Lee, 1996).

The small intestine is the organ in which maximum absorption occurs when medications are given by mouth. Parenteral routes of administration enter circulation either immediately by intravenous administration or at a steady rate through intramuscular injection. Drug absorption depends on two independent aspects of the process: the rate of absorption, which determines the time of onset, and the extent of absorption (the amount of drug that passes through the absorbing surface into the body). This differs from bioavailablity, which is the fraction of an administered drug that enters the systemic circulation.

In the aged there does not seem to be conclusive evidence that there is an appreciable change in the absorption process. Changes in gastrointestinal (GI) motility seem to be the one factor that might influence absorption, and that is only in the time it takes the medication to pass into the small intestine. This is significant because the increase or decrease in motility may enhance or interfere with the action of the drug. Delayed stomach emptying and delivery of the drug to the vast absorption surface of the small intestine may diminish or negate the effectiveness of short-lived drugs. Some enteric-coated medications, which are specifically meant to bypass stomach acidity, may be delayed so long that their action begins in the stomach and may produce undesirable effects such as gastric irritation or nausea. Increased motility of the small intestine lessens the drug contact time and diminishes the effect of the drug. Conversely, slowed intestinal motility can increase the contact time and increase drug efficiency because of prolonged absorption or can cause adverse reactions to occur.

Antispasmodic drugs, if taken as part of a multiple medication regimen, have the propensity to slow gastric and intestinal motility. In some instances this drug action may be useful, but when there are other medications involved, it is necessary to consider the problem of drug absorption. Impaired or slow mesenteric (splanchnic) blood flow definitely interferes with absorption. Sluggish blood flow lengthens the absorption time and increases the amount of drug absorbed. However, many authorities agree that the quality of the absorption process is unchanged even though it may be slowed (Cusack and Vestal, 1986; Demaagd, 1995; Lee, 1996). Diminished gastric pH in the aged will retard the action of acid-dependent drugs. Antacids or iron preparations affect the availability of some drugs for absorption by binding the drug with elements and forming compounds.

Distribution

Distribution or transport depends on the adequacy of the circulatory system. The largest portion of cardiac output and drug concentrations go to the heart, brain, kidneys, and liver, with lesser amounts directed to the muscles, bone, and fat (Cusack and Vestel, 1986; Lee, 1996). Altered cardiac output and sluggish circulation delay the arrival of medication at the target receptors and retard the release of a drug, or its by-products, from the body. In addition, distribution influences the amount of free and bound drug in the circulation system. This facet of distribution depends on the availability of plasma protein. In the younger adult adequate quantities of plasma albumin are present to bind with drugs. In the aged the amount of plasma albumin available for binding with drugs diminishes. This means that more free (unbound) active drug circulates in the aged person's blood and becomes a contributing factor in overdose and toxicity (Lee, 1996). The pharmacologic effect perceived originates from the free drug. Unbound, or free, drugs circulate and can be filtered through cell and organ membranes, excreted unchanged by the kidney, or metabolized to a less active inert form.

Changes in body composition during aging influence drug distribution. Total body water decreases, altering cellular distribution of drugs that are water soluble, such as cimetidine, digoxin, and ethanol. These drugs will be reflected in a higher than usual blood level in the elderly. Adipose tissue, or fat content of the body, nearly doubles in older men and increases by one half in older women. Highly lipid soluble drugs may be stored in the fatty tissue, thus extending and possibly elevating the drug effect (Vestal and Dawson, 1985; Vestal, 1990; Lee, 1996). This potentially occurs in such drugs as lorazepam, diazepam, chlorpromazine, phenobarbital, and haloperidol (Haldol). These medications can be stored in fatty tissue, which can increase and prolong their effect.

Free drug concentration is an important factor in distribution and elimination of a drug. Serum albumin is not significantly lower in the aged except when there is chronic illness or poor nutrition. Distribution of the drug may be altered by changes in the plasma protein concentration, red blood cells, and other body tissue. Box 10-1 lists drugs that when given to the frail, chronically ill older person have a greater potential for more circulating free drug than bound drug, creating a risk of toxicity (Santo-Novak and Edwards, 1989; Yuen, 1990). When prescribing drugs, attention should be given to whether the patient is young or old, frail or chronically ill, fat or lean, male or female. All these factors have a marked influence on drug action.

Metabolism

The microsomal enzyme system of the liver is the primary site of drug metabolism (biotransformation). Some studies using the drug antipyrine, which under normal circumstances should be totally metabolized by the liver, show a diminished metabolism in the aged (Cusack and Vestal, 1986; DeMaagd, 1995). Studies are conflicting in identifying universal age changes in the liver. The studies report differences in rates of metabolism, but there is consensus that there is a decreased blood flow to the liver whether from disease or normal aging or both. This results in decreased hepatic clearance (Lamy, 1990; Vestal, 1990); thus the half-life* of a drug increases as a result of diminished rate of metabolism in the aged.

The duration of drug action is determined by the metabolic rate. Slow metabolism suggests that the drug will remain in the body longer and produce a prolonged half-life. Sensitivity of the central nervous system alters receptor activity and produces greater receptor variation because of physiologic decline in autonomic nervous function, such as exaggerated or idiosyncratic reactions to hypotensive drugs or a hypothermic effect from phenothiazides.

A drug has specific affinity for receptor sites, which are designated areas inside or outside particular cells. When the drug reaches the receptor, it is translated into a chemical action that affects the body. This alteration at the receptor site is called pharmacodynamics.

Excretion

Under normal circumstances when a drug is taken by mouth, it is absorbed throughout the walls of the GI tract into the bloodstream, which facilitates distribution to various tissues of the body.

Degradation, breakdown of the drug into intermediate compounds, may occur with some drugs to produce a more excretable form. Elimination is primarily effected through the kidneys in urine; some, however, is eliminated through bile, the GI tract, feces, sweat, and saliva. Administration, supervision, evaluation, and education of the patient depend in part on this knowledge. Figure 10-2 illustrates the intricate relationship between physiologic age changes and pharmacokinetics/pharmacodynamics of drugs with the aged population. These interrelated processes are the basis for many of the positive and adverse responses of the aged to medications. Only a brief discussion of important issues will be presented here. Specific and more detailed information on the pharmacokinetics and pharmacodynamics of drugs can be found in numerous pharmacology textbooks.

Biologic half-life, the time required for half of the drug to be excreted, is affected by the degree of kidney function. Altered filtration and decreased plasma volume, which occur in dehydration, are common in the aged. These prolong

---

*Half-life (also called t½) is the time required for plasma concentration of a drug to be reduced by half.

and elevate blood levels of drugs. This can occur with penicillin. In some instances this situation can be beneficial, but with drugs such as streptomycin, toxic effects can overshadow the therapeutic value. Other drugs are ineffective in the presence of a low creatinine clearance.

Nurses need to be cognizant of kidney function in the aged, specifically the creatinine clearance (CrCl), which is a better index of renal function for the elderly than the serum creatinine. Accurate calculation of the creatinine clearance for men of normal weight is as follows:

$$CrCl = \frac{140 - Age\ (yr) \times Body\ weight\ (kg)}{72 \times Serum\ creatine}$$

Calculation for elderly women is obtained using the same formula and multiplying the answer (CrCl) by 0.85. A well elder usually has a creatinine clearance of 70 ml/min. Disease conditions may reduce this level of kidney function. When the creatinine clearance falls below 30 ml/min, the excretion of the drug eliminated by the kidney decreases, greatly increasing the risk of drug accumulation or if a nephrotoxic drug, a risk of renal damage (Lee, 1996).

Pharmacologic Chronobiology

Chronobiology is a developing science that may lead to more effective drug therapy. The best time to administer medications based on biorhythms of various physiologic processes is now being considered for therapeutic and toxic effects. With a new discipline or science, new terminology appears; Box 10-2 lists and defines chronobiologic terms.

Biorhythms exert a major impact on body processes involved in drug therapy. An awareness of biorhythmic influences on disease can have an effect on the care of the aged. For example, the aged individual with slow or altered physiologic processes of aging and/or disease may receive

---

Box 10-1 **Highly Protein-Bound Drugs**	
Aspirin	Haloperidol (Haldol)
Warfarin (Coumadin)	Thioridazine (Mellaril)
Phenytoin (Dilantin)	Nifedipine (Procardia)
Ibuprofen (Motrin)	Valproic Acid (Depakene)
Indomethacin (Indocin)	Verapamil (Calan, Isoptin)
Naproxen (Naprosyn)	Chlorothiazide (Diuril)
Phenylbutazone (Butazolidin)	Furosemide (Lasix)
Sulindac (Clinoril)	Hydrochlorothiazide (Hydrodiuril)
Chlorpropamide (Diabinese)	Diazepam (Valium)
Tolbutamide (Orinase)	Pentobarbital (Nembutal)
Chlorpromazine (Thorazine)	Secobarbital (Seconal)
	Chlordiazepoxide (Librium)

From Santo-Novak D, Edaeds RM: Rx: take caution with drugs for elders, *Geriatr Nurs* 10(2):72, 1989.

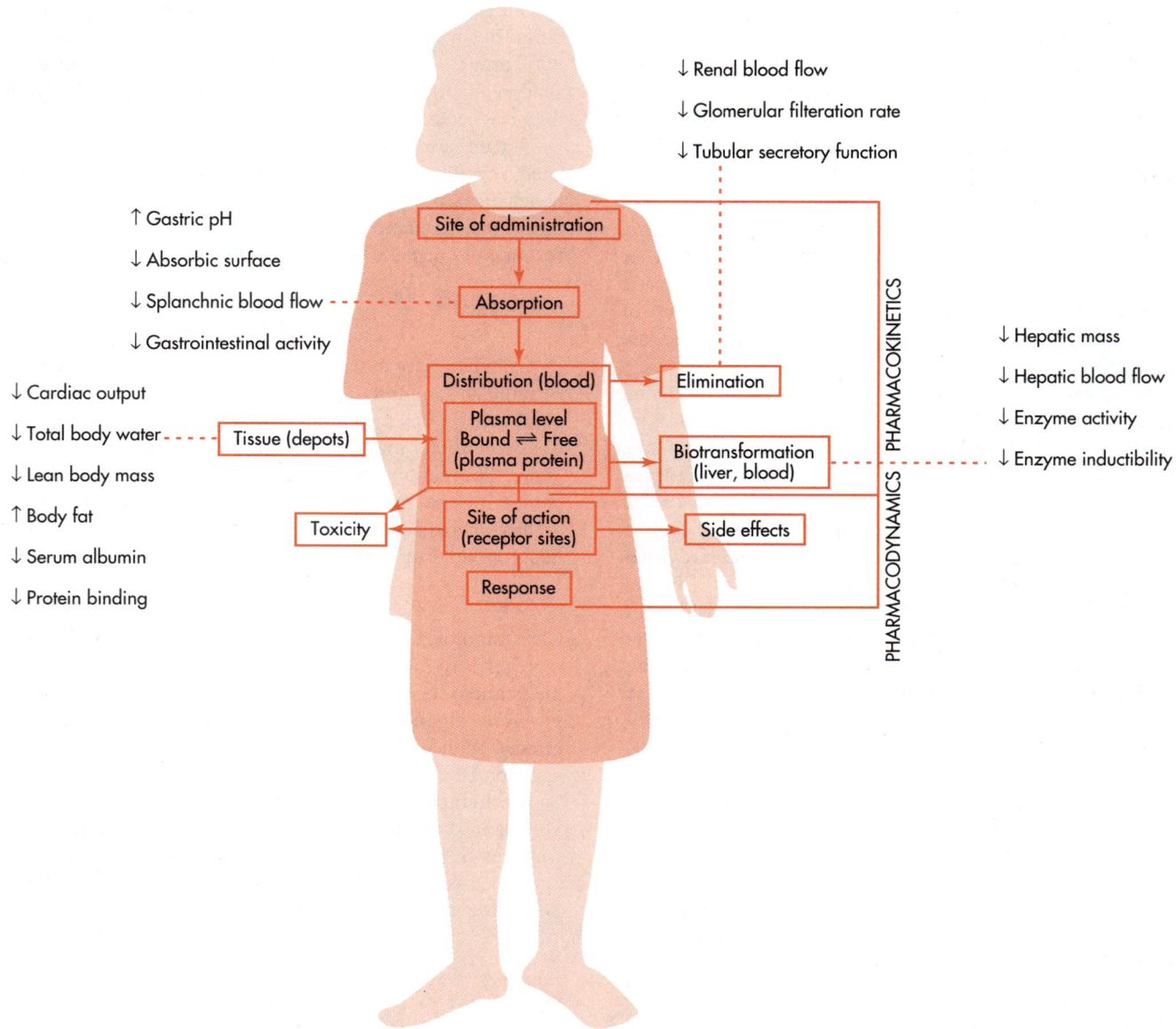

↓ Renal blood flow

↓ Glomerular filteration rate

↓ Tubular secretory function

↑ Gastric pH

↓ Absorbic surface

↓ Splanchnic blood flow

↓ Gastrointestinal activity

↓ Cardiac output

↓ Total body water

↓ Lean body mass

↑ Body fat

↓ Serum albumin

↓ Protein binding

↓ Hepatic mass

↓ Hepatic blood flow

↓ Enzyme activity

↓ Enzyme inductibility

Site of administration

Absorption

Distribution (blood)

Elimination

Plasma level
Bound ⇌ Free
(plasma protein)

Tissue (depots)

Biotransformation
(liver, blood)

Toxicity

Site of action
(receptor sites)

Side effects

Response

PHARMACOKINETICS

PHARMACODYNAMICS

Figure 10-2. Physiologic age changes and the pharmacokinetics and pharmacodynamics of drug use. (Data compiled from Lamy, 1982; Kane, Ouslander, Abrass, 1984; Vestal, 1985; Roberts, Tumer, 1988; Montatmat, Cusack, Vestal, 1989; and Bezon, 1991.)

a therapeutic or toxic effect from a medication because of the timing of the drug administration.

Pharmacokinetics and Pharmacodynamics. Our biorhythms strongly influence pharmacokinetics and pharmacodynamics. Absorption is dependent on gastric acid pH, emptying of the GI tract, and blood flow. All have been shown to have biorhythmic variations. Distribution of protein-bound drugs depends on albumin and glycoproteins produced by the liver. During the day, albumin levels are high, but they are low in the early morning hours. Drug metabolism also is influenced by biorhythmic activity. Oxidation, hydrolysis, de-

carboxylation, and demethylation by liver enzymes demonstrate rhythm variations. Renal elimination depends on kidney perfusion, glomerular filtration, and urine acidity. These also have shown variations in circadian rhythm. The brain, heart, and blood cells have also been found to have varied rhythmicity, resulting in a cyclic response for beta-blockers, calcium channel blockers, ACE inhibitors, nitrates, and other similar drugs. These are among the frequently prescribed drugs elders take for chronic cardiac conditions (Turkoski [in press]). Table 10-1 shows the rhythmic influence on diseases and physiologic processes.

Box 10-2	**Common Chronobiologic Terms**	
Chronobiology	The study of mechanisms of biological time structure	
Chronopharmacology	The study of interactions of biologic rhythms with medication	
Chronotherapeutics	Pharmacotherapy using drug delivery schedules or technologies based on biorhythms (predicted and/or individual)	
Chronothesy	Administration time differences in the effects of medications	
Chronotolerance	Rhythm-dependent changes in tolerance to medication	
Chronotoxicity	Adverse drug reactions as a function of biorhythms	
Circadian cycle	The approximately 24-hour biorhythms in living organisms	
Circamensual cycle	Biological rhythms with a frequency of about one month	
Circannual cycle	Biological rhythms with a frequency of one year $+/-3$ months	
Circaseptan cycle	Biological rhythms with a frequency of about a week	
Ultradian cycle	Biological rhythms with a frequency of more than 28 hours	
Oscillation	One cycle (Remains constant regardless of length of cycle)	
Infradian cycle	Biological rhythms of less than 20 hours	

From Turkoski BB: Medication timing for the elderly: the impact of biorhythms on effectiveness (in press).

Implications of Chronopharmacologic Therapy. The potential for decreasing the dose of medications and/or the frequency of administration for elders is the primary benefit of chronopharmacologic therapy. Both decreases may ultimately improve the therapeutic effect and decrease toxic effects for elders as well as the general population, and they may improve patient adherence to a medication regimen. In addition, chronotherapeutics may provide financial benefit to the patient by reducing the overall medication expense because fewer administrations are needed to achieve a therapeutic effect (Kresevic, 1996).

Nurse's Role. The nurse's role will be an important one. Nurses have a degree of discretion over drug administration. In the institutional setting it may occur as part of the nursing care plan; however, institutions still have rigid time schedules for medication administration. In the home care setting, there is a greater latitude to adjust medication time schedules and to explain to the patient why the medication is to be taken at a certain time (Kresevic, 1996).

The nurse needs to become a member of the therapeutics committee to help in an effort to make a change in medication administration timing. The nurse can also consult with the pharmacist. Lastly, the nurse can begin to bring research on chronotherapy to the attention of the physician and coworkers (Kresevic, 1996).

Instituting chronotherapy at an agency might begin with one classification of drugs, using chronopharmacologic standards from pharmacologic literature. When the staff has become comfortable with the chronotherapy of this one classification of drugs, additional medications should be added one by one on a regular basis (Kresevic,1996). Box 10-3 provides guidelines for application of chronotherapy.

Table 10-1	**Rhythmic Influences on Disease and Physiologic Processes**
Disease/Process	**Rhythmic Influence**
Allergic rhinitis	Symptoms worse in the morning
Arterial BP	Circadian surge—morning hours
Asthma	Greatest respiratory distress overnight (during sleeping)
	Symptoms peak in early morning (4:00-5:00)
Blood plasma	Plasma volume falls at night = hematocrit increases
Cancer	Tumor cells proliferate when normal cell miosis is low
Cardiac disease	Angina, myocardial infarction, thrombolytic stroke occur in the first 4 hours after waking (peak 9:00) (through 22:00)
	(Prinzmetal's angina—during sleep)
Catecholamines Fibrinolytic activity Platelet activation	Increase in early morning
Endogenous depression	May result from abnormality in circadian rhythm which affects cortisol levels, body temperature, sleep/wake cycle
Gastric system	Gastric acid secretion peaks every morning (2:00-4:00) circannual variability—incidence of gastric ulcers > winter
Osteroarthritis	Pain more severe in morning
Potassium excretion	Lowest in morning/highest in late afternoon
Rheumatoid arthritis	Pain more severe in late afternoon
Systemic insulin	Highest in afternoon

From Turkoski BB: Medication timing for the elderly: impact of biorhythms on effectiveness (in press).

Box 10-3	Applications of Chronopharmacology*	
Allergic rhinitis	H₁ receptor antagonists	Once daily/evening dose
Angina	Beta agonists/theophyllines	Once daily at night or ⅔ night, ⅓ morning
	Corticosteroids	Morning or ⅔ morning ⅓ late in day
	Respiratory treatment	Early evening
Duodenal ulcers	H₂ receptor antagonists	Once daily dose—evening
	Prophylactic	Once daily dose—morning
Edema	Furosemide	Once daily—morning
Hypertension	Infusion antihypertensives	
Ischemic activity	Long-acting beta blockers	Once daily at night
Osteoarthritis	NSAIDs	Once daily—morning
Platelet coagulation	Aspirin	Once daily—morning
	Plasminogen activators	Between noon and midnight
Rheumatoid arthritis	NSAIDs	Once daily—evening
Unstable diabetes mellitus	NPH Insulin	Bedtime dose

*General guidelines must be adjusted for individual clients.
From Turkoski BB: Medication timing for the elderly: the impact of biorhythms on effectiveness (in press).

Drugs designed to alter dose and frequency in accordance with biorhythms are already beginning to appear on the market. Among the first are antihypertensive drugs.

DRUG INTERACTIONS

Drug interactions are the result of two of more medications given simultaneously or in close sequence with an outcome response of drug synergism, which is rare, or more frequently drug potentiation or antagonism. Interactions may be precipitated by drug-drug, drug-nutrient, drug-disease, and social or psychological factors that influence drug response.

The interactions can occur within or outside the body. Many of the interactions are the result of pharmacokinetic activity. A variety of interactions occur. Within the body, absorption can be delayed by drugs exerting an anticholinergic effect. Tricyclic drugs (antidepressants) act in this manner to decrease GI motility and interfere with absorption of other drugs. Several drugs simultaneously compete to bind and occupy the binding sites needed by the other drug, creating a varied bioavailability of one or both of the drugs. Interaction may be blocked at the receptor site, preventing the drug from reaching the cells. Interference with enzyme activity may alter metabolism and cause drug deficiencies, or toxic and adverse responses may develop from altered tubular function. Outside the body, interactions can occur any time two medications are mixed before administration. An example of this is the improper preparation of more than one type of insulin for injection.

Table 10-2 illustrates outcomes of interactions that occur during absorption, distribution, metabolism, and excretion of some drugs. Table 10-3 indicates the manner of administration of drugs to reduce or prevent interactions.

Concern with the elderly's total response to drug therapy and its effect on the ability for activities of daily living and functional capacities such as vision, hearing, memory, and mobility is a substantial reason for a drug assessment of each aged person under the supervision of the nurse.

Adverse Reactions

Drug use and misuse are a combination of many factors and create a geriatric health problem, not exclusively the fault of the aged or their physicians. It is clear that as the person ages, altered biodegradability, nutritional and fluid status, inadequate assessment before prescribing (treating the symptoms rather than the underlying cause), polypharmacy, and compliance factors result in a three to four times higher rate of adverse drug reactions in the elderly than in the remainder of the population. At least 6 million elders are at risk for adverse drug reactions that will affect the development, adaptation, and social supports of the aged (Carruth and Boss, 1990; Wilcox et al, 1994). A study of 300 acute care hospital admissions showed that 16% were for adverse drug reactions. The total hospital cost for these reactions exceeds $200,000 (Col et al, 1990). Lamy (1986a, 1990) estimated that approximately 40% of the elderly in the community experienced adverse drug reactions, 80% of which occurred with well-known drugs given at usual dosages. Nolan and O'Malley (1989) estimated the number of geriatric admissions to the hospital due to adverse drug reactions to be 10%.

A study by Wilcox et al (1994) found 20 potentially inappropriate drugs prescribed for elders, including 3 controversial cardiovascular agents (propranolol, methyldopa, and reserpine). Among the most common drugs that produce adverse reactions are warfarin, digoxin, prednisone, diuretics, antihypertensives, insulin, aspirin, and antidepressants (Nolan and O'Malley, 1989; Hogstel, 1992; Lepkowsky,

Table 10-2	Pharmacokinetic Mechanisms of Drug-Drug Interactions

Mechanism	Example
Absorption from Gastrointestinal Tract	
1. Adsorption-drug gets "stuck on" to another substance	Charcoal, antacids, kaolin-pectin
2. Complexation or chelation—formation of insoluble, unabsorbable complex	Antacids, sucralfate, iron, calcium, tetracycline, quinolones, antibiotics, captopril, chloroquine
3. Resin binding	Cholestyramine, colestipol, warfarin, thiazide diuretics, thyroid hormones, digoxin
4. Altered intestinal flora	Broad spectrum antibiotics with digoxin
5. Change in gastrointestinal motility	Anticholinergics, opiates, aluminum hydroxide
6. Change in gastric pH	H_2 antagonists and ketoconazole
Alteration in Protein Binding	
Drugs that are highly protein bound (>80-90%) are affected	Warfarin, sulfa antibiotics, phenytoin, nonsteroidal anti-inflammatory agents (NSAIDs)
Alteration in Drug Metabolism	
1. Enzyme induction—increased metabolism of target drug results in lower drug levels	Enzyme inducers: Ethanol (chronic), barbiturates, carbamazepine (Tegretol), phenytoin (Dilantin), primidone (Mysoline), rifampin (Rifadin)
2. Enzyme inhibitors—reduce metabolism resulting in increased levels of target drugs	Enzyme inhibitors: allopurinol (Zyloprim), amiodarone (Cordarone), chloramphenicol, cimetidine (Tagamet), ciprofloxacin (Cipro), diltiazem (Cardizem), disulfiram (Antabuse), enoxacin (Penetrex), erythromycin, ethanol (acute), isoniazid (INH), ketoconazole (Nizoral), metronidazole (Flagyl), monoamine oxidase inhibitors (MOAI), omeprazole (Prilosec), phenylbutazone, quinidine, sulfonamides, trimethoprim (Trimpex), verapamil (Calan, Isoptin)
Alteration in Drug Excretion	
1. Reduced tubular secretion	Acidic drugs: cephalosporins, chlorpropamide (Diabinese), aspirin, indomethacin (Indocin), methotrexate, penicillins, probenecid (Benemid), thiazide diuretics Basic drugs: amiodarone (Cordarone), digoxin (Lanoxin), cimetidine (Tagamet), diltiazem (Cardizem), metformin (Glucophage), quinidine, quinine, ranitidine (Zantac)
2. Changes in urinary pH—affects acidic and basic drugs	

Developed by Samuel Lee, Pharm D, Clinical Pharmacy Supervisor, Veterans Administration Outpatient Department, Oakland, Calif.

1992; Wilcox et al, 1994). The most common reactions have been identified as sedation, lethargy, confusion, and falls (Palmieri, 1991; Hogstel, 1992).

Confusion perhaps is the most striking. The increase in confusion of a demented patient is often considered to be further decompensation due to the person's present illness and is treated by increasing the medication dose, when in fact the medication may have been causing the response. Confusion in any individual who previously has not been confused may be interpreted as a new symptom of some disease yet unidentified, and a new medication is inappropriately prescribed. In the classic work of Wolanin and Phillips (1981) drug intoxication and confusion are discussed in detail. Lethargy can also be misinterpreted as a symptom connected with cardiac, respiratory, or neurologic conditions rather than a medication response.

Polypharmacy (multiple medication use) with several psychoactive drugs exerting anticholinergic action is per-

haps the greatest precipitator of the adverse reaction: confusion. In addition, although the potential for an adverse drug reaction or interaction is only 6% when two drugs are taken, it rises to 50% when five drugs are ingested and to 100% when eight or more medications are taken together (Shaughnessy, 1992). Box 10-4 lists drugs that can lead to intellectual impairment, also cited by DeMaagd (1995). Box 10-5 presents the effects of systemic drugs on vision. Without going into detail, more than 200 medications interfere with or contribute to sexual dysfunction for adults of any age (Butler et al, 1994; Miller, 1995). The categories that are most responsible for this are cardiovascular drugs (antihypertensives and ACE inhibitors) and psychotropic drugs (antidepressants and phenothiazines).

Drug Toxicity

Drug toxicity is a condition that occurs when the amount of a drug in the body exceeds the amount necessary to bring

Table 10-3 | Proper Administration to Prevent Drug Interactions

Drug	Take with food, milk, meals	Do not take with milk or antacids	May impair nutrient and electrolyte uptake and use	Do not take with alcohol	Take on empty stomach
Alcohol			X		
Aminophylline and derivatives	X				
Ampicillin					X
Antihistamines					
Bisacodyl (Dulcolax)		X	X	X	
Chloral hydrate				X	
Chlorpropamide (Diabinese)				X	
Cholestyramine (Questran)			X		
Corticosteroids (oral)	X				
Folic acid inhibitors			X		
Ibuprofen (Motrin)	X				
Indomethacin (Indocin)	X				
Isoniazid (INH)			X		
Monoamine oxidase inhibitors				X	
Methotrexate			X		
Methylphenidate (Ritalin)				X	X
Metronidazole (Flagyl)	X			X	
Mineral oil			X		
Narcotics				X	
Neomycin			X		
Nitrofurantoin (Furadantin)	X				
Nitrofurantoin macrocrystals (Macrodantin)	X				
Penicillin (oral)					X
Phenytoin	X				
Tetracyclines		X			
Tolbutamide (Orinase)				X	

Data from Knoben JE, Anderson PO: *Handbook of clinical drug data,* ed 7, Hamilton, Ill, 1993, Drug Intelligence Publications.

Box 10-4 **Drugs with the Potential to Cause Intellectual Impairment**

Alcohol
Analgesics
Anticholinergics
Antidepressants
Antipsychotics
Antihistamines
Antiparkinsonian agents
Beta-blockers
Cimetidine
Digitalis
Diuretics
Hypnotics
Muscle relaxants
Sedatives
Sudden withdrawl of benzodiazapines

Data compiled from Nolan L, O'Malley K: Prescribing for the elderly: Part I, Sensitivity of the elderly to adverse drug reactions, *Am Geriatr Soc* 36(2):142, 1988; Lamy PP: Drug interactions and the elderly, *J Gerontol Nurs,* 12(2), 1986b; Lamy PP: Adverse drug effects, *Clin Geriatr Med* 6(2):1990.

about a therapeutic effect, exceeds the therapeutic level, or becomes a harmful agent in the body, producing adverse effects (Weitzel, 1991) (Box 10-6). A drug that has a cumula-tive effect has the potential for drug toxicity. Other drugs may produce drug toxicity under such circumstances as polypharmacy, slowed metabolism, altered excretion, dehydration, drug overdose due to self-medication errors, or excessive prescribed dosage. Table 10-4 presents specific drugs commonly prescribed for the elderly that may result in toxicity.

Drug toxicity is a major concern in the care of the elderly and should be regarded as a specific nursing diagnosis problem. Potential for drug toxicity appears as a subdiagnosis under the currently accepted NANDA diagnoses; it remains secondary in importance (Maas et al, 1991; Cox et al, 1993).

Nursing Interventions. The nurse is a key person in the prevention of drug toxicity and in the education of clients on the safe use and administration of medications. As part of an interdisciplinary approach, the nurse works with the physician, pharmacist, and dietitian to teach, monitor, and promote the actions necessary to prevent drugs from becoming toxic and to treat toxicity promptly should it occur.

Monitoring. The most effective way to prevent or minimize drug effects is by monitoring the client. The nurse's role includes knowledge of defining characteristics (signs and symptoms) indicative of toxicity and education of the elderly about drugs, dosage, and therapeutic and nontherapeutic indicators (Table 10-4).

Advocacy role. The nurse's advocacy role includes awareness of the elder's overall functioning in order to in-

---

Box 10-5   **Effects of Systemic Drugs on Vision**

Drug	Effect
Furosemide (Lasix)	Blurred vision, decreased tolerance to contact lenses, photophobia, allergic reactions to eyelids and conjunctivae
Propranolol (Inderal)	Transient blurred vision with diplopia, decreased accommodation
Dimetapp (antihistamine and anticholinergic effect)	Mydriasis (contraindicated in angle closure glaucoma), blurred vision, intolerance to contact lenses
Diazepam (Valium)	Allergic conjunctivitis
Digoxin (Lanoxin)	Diplopia, blurred vision, changes in color perception (warnings of toxicity)

Modified from Osis M: Drugs and vision, *Gerontion* 1(5):15, 1986.

Box 10-6   **General Physiologic System Characteristics of Drug Toxicity**

Cardiovascular
Arrhythmias
Tachycardias
Palpitations
Hypotension
Congestive heart failure
Hypertension
Bone marrow depression
　Leukopenia
　Thrombocytopenia
　Anemia
　Agranulocytosis

Central Nervous System
Confusion
Gait changes
Insomnia
Drowsiness
Blurred vision or visual changes
Slurred speech
Ototoxicity
Tremors
Irritability
Problems with temperature control
Anticholinergic effects
Seizures

Hepatic Changes
Jaundice
Clotting problems
Decreased liver function

Gastrointestinal
Anorexia
Nausea and vomiting
Diarrhea
GI bleeding
Pancreatitis

Renal
Electrolyte imbalance
Polyuria
Urinary retention
Fluid retention

Respiratory
Dyspnea
Asthmatic reactions

Skin
Rash
Urticaria
Pruritis
Photosensitivity

---

fluence the plan of treatment, clarify the treatment goals, and coordinate the activities of physicians and other clinicians to keep them focused on the goals of the client and family. For some drugs a periodic blood level determination may be wise to establish that the elder is remaining within the therapeutic parameters.

Drug holidays. Another intervention that may be used to decrease the potential of drug toxicity is a drug holiday, which is a planned omission of a specific drug or drugs for one or more days or weeks. Benefits of such an option were identified by Keenan (1983) in the institutional setting but might be extrapolated to elders in the community. The benefits of drug holidays include increased alertness of the individual, a decreased use of medications and subsequent reduction in overall medication cost, and easier scheduling of activities that can be restricted when certain medications are taken. For example, individuals who are on a diuretic might not be able to leave home until noon for fear there will not be a toilet accessible or that they cannot hold their urine long enough to find a toilet.

Though a drug holiday may be beneficial, questions arise regarding the length of time of a drug holiday. A variety of

| Table 10-4 | Toxic Characteristics of Specific Drugs Prescribed for the Elderly |

Drugs	Signs and symptoms

Benzodiazepines
    Diazepam (Valium)
    Flurazepam (Dalmane)
    Lorazepam (Ativan)
	Ataxia, restlessness, confusion, depression, anticholinergic effect

Cimetidine (Tagamet)	Confusion, depression
Digitalis	Confusion, headache, anorexia, vomiting, arrhythmias, blurred vision or visual changes (halos, frost on objects, color blindness) paresthesia
Furosemide (Lasix)	Electrolyte imbalance, hepatic changes, pancreatitis, leukopenia, thrombocytopenia
Gentamycin (Garamycin)	Ototoxicity (impaired hearing and/or balance), nephrotoxicity
L-dopa	Muscle and eye twitching, disorientation, asterixis, hallucinations, dyskinetic movements, grimacing, depression, delirium, ataxia
Lithium (Eskalith, Lithane)	Confusion, diarrhea, drowsiness, anorexia, slurred speech, tremors, blurred vision, unsteadiness, polyuria, seizures, muscle weakness
Methyldopa (Aldomet)	Hepatic changes, mental depression, fever, bradycardia, nightmares, tremors, edema

Nonsteroidal antiinflammatory agents (NSAIDs)
Ibuprofen (Advil, Motrin, Nuprin, Rufen)
    Indomethacin (Indocin)
    Fenoprofen (Nalfon)
	Photosensitivity, fluid retention, anemia, nephrotoxicity, visual changes

Phenylbutazone (Butazolidin)
    Piroxicam (Feldene)
    Sulindac (Clinoril)
    Tolmetin (Tolectin)
	Confusion plus all the above

Phenothiazide tranquilizers	Tachycardia, arrhythmias, dyspnea, hyperthermia, postural hypotension, restlessness, anticholinergic effects
Phenytoin (Dilantin)	Ataxia, slurred speech, confusion, nystagmus, diplopia, nausea, vomiting
Procainamide (Pronestyl, Procan, Promine)	Arrhythmias, depression, hypotension, SLE syndrome, dyspnea, skin rash, nausea, vomiting
Ranitidine (Zantac)	Liver dysfunction, blood dyscrasias

Sulfonylureas—1st generation
    Chlorpropamide (Diabinese)
    Tolbutamide (Orinase)
	Hypoglycemia, hepatic changes, CHF Bone marrow depression, jaundice

Theophylline (Theo-Dur, Elixophyllin, Slo-Bid)	Anorexia, nausea, vomiting, GI bleeding, tachycardia, arrhythmias, irritability, insomnia, seizures, muscle twitching
Tricyclic antidepressants Amitriptyline (Elavil, Endep, Amitril) Doxepin (Sinequan, Adapin) Imipramine (Tofranil)	Confusion, arrhythmias, seizures, agitation, tachycardia, jaundice, hallucinations, postural hypotension, anticholinergic effects

Data compiled from Skidmore-Roth L: *Nursing drug reference,* St Louis, 1992 Mosby; *Physician's desk reference,* Oradell, NJ, 1992, Medical Economics; Salzman C: Basic principles of psychotropic drug prescriptions for the elderly, *Hosp Comm Psychiatr* 33:133, 1982; Todd B: Identifying drug toxicity, *Geriatr Nurs* 4:231, 1985.

drugs taken by the elderly accumulate in body fat and take much longer to be depleted below therapeutic levels than other drugs. For those medications, a 1- or 2-day holiday may be ineffective. Perhaps rather than a drug holiday, reducing the number of medications prescribed and implementing a drug holiday in some situations would be more appropriate. Whatever the approach is, the nurse assumes the major intervention role.

PATTERNS OF DRUG USE

Individuals over the age of 65 are the largest users of prescription and OTC medications. It is estimated that people over the age of 60 constitute 16% of the population in the United States and take almost 40% of the prescribed medications (Hogstel, 1992). Although there is limited information about the number of OTC medications used by the aged, the number is thought to be as great or greater.

Darnell et al (1986) noted that 90% of the elderly took an average of three OTC drugs and five prescription drugs daily. DeMaagd (1995) cites the figure of at least two OTC drugs at any given time. The most commonly prescribed and used drugs are cardiovascular drugs, antiinfectives, antipsychotic drugs, antidepressants, and diuretics (Baum et al, 1986; Hogstel, 1992; DeMaagd, 1995). Analgesics, laxatives, and antacids are the most used OTC drugs, followed by cough products, acetaminophens, nonsteroidal topical preparations, milk of magnesia, Pepto-Bismol, eye washes, and vitamins (Hogstel,1992). Now with the conversion of prescription drugs to OTCs, additional use categories may appear (Miller, 1996).

Polypharmacy

The elderly often have multiple health problems or chronic conditions that are treated with multiple drugs. Because of this they are prone to excessive drug use. The polypharmacy that occurs is an attempt to treat several disorders simultaneously, creating high risks for interactions and adverse drug reactions. Polypharmacy stems from multichronicity, the prescribing methods of physicians, the beliefs and practices of the aged, and the ever-increasing practice of seeing more than one primary care provider, each of whom prescribes similar class drugs.

Self-Prescribing of Medications

Despite Medicare, the cost of medications continues to rise. Physician reimbursement for patient visits is low, and the number of physicians who will accept Medicare as total reimbursement continues to decrease markedly. So elders do not seek or get medical assistance because of the out-of-pocket cost or do not want to bother the physician unless they are very ill. They medicate themselves with former prescriptions, prescriptions borrowed from friends, or OTC drugs.

Symptoms experienced by the aged such as pain, constipation, insomnia, and indigestion are amenable to OTC self-treatment. Use of OTC drugs often enables elders to gain relief from symptoms less expensively than prescription drugs and to obtain sufficient comfort to continue their activities of daily living (Cameron, 1996).

Many OTC preparations have active ingredients that in large amounts would require a prescription; thus some drugs contain potentially dangerous substances. The elderly also use traditional medications such as folk medicine, herbs, and homeopathic remedies.

Today, with the frequent use of multiple concurrent medications, including prescribed and OTC drugs, the nurse needs to be aware of medications the aged person is taking and the possible interactions among them.

Over-the-Counter Medications

OTC preparations number over 300,000 products (SRx senior mini-class curriculum, 1988) and are increasing in number yearly as prescription drugs are released by the Food and Drug Administration to the OTC category. In the past few years over 600 prescription drugs have become available as OTC medications. While self-medication is an important part of our health care, the individual has the responsibility to be educated on the safe and wise use of these products. These products are just as much medications as those prescribed by physicians. OTC drugs are used by 75% of the aged to relieve symptoms of minor discomfort, illness, or injury and are stocked on supermarket, pharmacy, and drug emporium shelves. Undesirable effects can occur from these drugs as well as from prescription drugs.

Misuse of Drugs

Drug misuse is a problem for both the health profession and the elderly. Health, medical care, and personal habits of the aged foster the ingestion of a wide variety of drugs. The overwhelming majority of the aged have minimum supervision of their medications. Some of the misuse stems from the fact that physicians prescribe doses that have guidelines based on mature adults rather than the older adult. Normal age changes in the elderly create a difference in their ability to handle standard doses of drugs (refer to Figure 10-2).

Forms of misuse include overuse, underuse, erratic use, and contraindicated use. Most misuse is the result of inadequate physician training in geriatric pharmacology and inadequate assessment, as evidenced by treatment of a symptom rather than the cause of a symptom. An example of this is leg edema. This is generally associated with congestive heart failure, but in fact it may be just venous stasis from immobility. Prescribing a diuretic would be inappropriate, but if the assessment is inadequate, the likelihood of just such a prescription is highly probable, as is an incident of drug misuse. Nurses, too, have the responsibility to be knowledgeable about drugs and doses appropriate for elders and to question when a drug seems inappropriate.

Misuse of drugs by the aged may be deliberate. Personality response may be such that, under stress, oral intake may become either excessive or deficient, including over or underuse of drugs (prescribed or OTC). Misuse may also be the individual's means of asking for help. One cannot negate the self-destructive motive, the response to alienation or low social status. Drug misuse can also be a manifestation of certain psychopathologic states. Often, however, drug misuse by the aged is unintentional and based on inadequate knowledge; yet it is frequently judged as noncompliance regardless of the reason for misuse.

Noncompliance/Nonadherence

Investigators have individually defined compliance based on variations of criteria and have different interpretations of compliance or noncompliance.

Noncompliance is often considered deliberate misuse of medication. Seventy-five percent of elders intentionally do not adhere to their drug regimen by altering the dose either because it was ineffective or because of the uncomfortable side effects. Others stop the drug or drugs because they feel the medications are not needed anymore (Lamy, 1986a and 1986b) or because of the high cost of medications. The nurse and other health care personnel become exasperated and angry at the individual because of noncompliance with the established medical program or treatment plan. Factors that influence noncompliance appear in Box 10-7.

Nonadherence, while semantically the same as noncompliance, is a less harsh and accusatory term when addressing

Box 10-7	**Factors Affecting Medication Compliance**

Complexity of Drug Regimen

Number of drugs or doses
Duration of therapy
Convenience of refills
Ordering medication by mail or telephone leads to missed verbal directions, information, reinforcement, and mail delays in receipt of medication.
Failure to have prescription filled

Poor Drug Knowledge

Lack of knowledge about drug purpose, use, side effects, and possible interactions
Taking prescribed and OTC drugs without concern
Denial that certain OTC preparations such as vitamins and antacids are drugs

Physical Limitations

Vision or hearing impairments
Motion limitations
Inability to open medication container cap

Poor Patient–Health Professional Communications

Fragmentation of care through use of multiple healthcare providers
Dissatisfaction with care
Misunderstanding expected outcomes of medication
Lack of adequate directions for taking medication

Psychosocial Characteristics

Patient perception about drug efficacy
Social isolation

Data compiled from Delong MF: Caring for the elderly. Medication use and abuse, *NURSEweek* 8(8):8, 1995; Higbee MD: Consumer guidelines for using medications wisely, *Generations* 8(2):43, 1994; Spiers MV, Kutzik DM: *A multidimensional framework for understanding medication adherence: a prescription for rethinking,* Unpublished paper under review, 1995.

why elders do not follow a suggested or prescribed plan of treatment. In an attempt to help and do what they think is best for the patient, the nurse and other care providers tend to forget or ignore that *one cannot and will not comply with a prescription or treatment plan when there are incompatibilities that interfere with the practicalities of life or are distressful to the individual's well-being or when actual misinformation or disability prevents compliance.* For example, the aged individual cannot take medication three times a day with meals if he or she eats only two meals a day; the aged person may not continue to take a medication if it brings about lethargy and inability to participate in social activities. Nonadherence includes not only the person for whom the medication is prescribed but also the provider of care and the social support network (Spiers and Kutzik, 1993, 1995).

The aged person has been repeatedly blamed for noncompliance, but how can anyone comply if the directions are unclear or presented in a rapid-fire fashion in medical jargon? It is common to give discharge medication instructions when the person is leaving the hospital. It is also common to explain the treatment and give directions concerning medications when the patient is physically uncomfortable, to explain in English and not in the patient's primary language if other than English, or to explain in a noisy or busy place. It is no wonder that a problem of adherence occurs under such circumstances. One tends to forget that it takes longer for the aged to process information and that visual and hearing impairments and cultural or language barriers can interfere with adequate communication of important instructions.

Confusion about the frequency of taking medication and the identification of the medication to take are extremely common. Unintentional errors are made by the elderly because of too rapid or poor explanations, often given at times of high anxiety, fear, or physical distress. The elderly have been known to omit drugs by not purchasing them because of the expense or to alter the dosage in an attempt to stretch the medication over a longer period of time. When the person begins to feel better, drugs are sometimes stopped. Persons with little educational background and in economic difficulty are more likely not to adhere to therapies they do not understand or cannot afford, including medication. It should be noted that regardless of the setting, the elderly, whether experiencing failing sight (fewer than 15% of elders have 20/20 vision), hearing difficulties (by age 80, two thirds of the population have impaired hearing)(Shimp and Ascione, 1988), or memory lapses, can be educated if difficulties are compensated for rather than merely considered insurmountable hurdles.

A Multidimensional Framework. Spiers and Kutzik (1994) developed and revised (1995) a multidimensional framework for medication adherence that looks at the barriers to adherence by elders. The framework suggests that there is a simultaneous branching out between the three stages: intital instruction, regimen establishment, and self-management and the three levels: individual, provider-treatment, and social support network. The integration of the stages and levels provide a cogent approach to understanding the dynamics of elder adherence (Table 10-5).

In stage one of this framework, the individual must first comprehend and be committed to the treatment. The care provider must be able to communicate the information in a form(s) necessary to compensate for physical-sensory and cognitive changes so that the individual understands and is willing to follow the treatment plan.

The elder then can move to the second stage but must be able to carry what has been learned so that he or she can operationalize this information at this stage (obtain the medication, apply instructions, adjust to the regimen). The influence of the health professional is relatively strong in these two stages, with the social context having a less direct influ-

Table 10-5   A Multidimensional Framework for Medication Adherence

	Individual	Provider-Treatment	Social Support Network
Stage 1 Initial Instructions	Comprehension Committment to treatment	Communication effectiveness Number of providers	Community medical education Cultural beliefs
Stage 2 Regimen Establishment			
Attaining medications	Mobility Finances Beliefs (e.g., med sharing) Motivation	Medication cost Number of medications needed	Accessibility to pharmacies Financial aid
Application	Ability to reconstruct instructions Regimen strategy	Complexity of regimen Container design Label readability	Administration aid

Adjustment	Perception of effectiveness
	Self-manipulation of
	  dosage/regimen
		Rx manipulation
		Rx monitoring
			Level of emotional/functional
			  support

Stage 3 Self-Management			

Integration/reintegration	Emotional adjustment to long-
	  term medication
	  dependence
	Regimen routinization and
	  synthesis
	Response to challenges/
	  change
		Lifestyle change required by
		  regular medication taking
		Regimen changes
			Response to individual change
			Stability of support
			  network/living situation

Monitoring	Ability to self-monitor for
	  change
		Degree of comprehensive Rx
		  review
			Support network vigilance

From Spiers MV, Kutzik DM: *A multidimensional framework for understanding medication adherence in the elderly: prescription for rethinking,* Unpublished paper under review, 1995.

ence on the drug regimen. It is, however, affected by medical knowledge in the elder cultural/belief system.

Stage three is perhaps more strongly aligned with social network factors, mainly because of the constricting network elders have available to them. Success at this level depends on the number of persons in the elder's support network who are able to assist the elder, if necessary, with the integration and/or reintegration of the regimen and the monitoring of adherence. A similar approach to compliance by Conn et al (1995) also looks at the tasks necessary to manage medications, administration of medications, and evaluation of medication use.

Strategies for improving patient adherence in hospital settings require the caregiver to assess the patient's ability to open childproof caps (a request can be made for easily removable caps), to take prescribed medications (sufficient motor skills), and to read labels and accompanying instructions. The caregiver also needs to provide written legible directions and to teach and supervise self-administration of medications during the hospital stay.

In any setting the caregiver needs to be alert to assess the accuracy of comprehension of instructions and to reinforce the directions as needed. Placing the medications in view when giving directions to the client and using a variety of teaching aids, such as individualized teaching with demonstration and feedback or audiovisual aids, are helpful. It is

important to adjust teaching to those with hearing and visual deficits. If the individual has a hearing aid, make sure it is in place and working. If glasses are used, make certain they are on, the lenses are clean, and lighting is adequate. Individualized regimens that are consistent with the patient's routine and lifestyle provide better opportunities to facilitate compliance. Other methods to improve adherence include providing bold, large black-lettered information in the client's language and reading level, and when possible enlisting participation of a significant other.

Provision of memory aids such as a weekly calendar with pockets for medications indicating day, time, and date or a daily tear-off calendar remind the aged person to take daily medication. Larger calendars are helpful when multiple drugs must be taken; a check can be placed in the date square each time a medication is taken. Transparent envelopes or sandwich bags containing the medication can be affixed to the dated square. Each envelope or bag should state the name of the drug, dose, and times to be taken that day. In addition to a calendar, commercial drug caddies can be tried. These containers are available for single or multiple doses for a day, week, or month. Figure 10-3 shows some commercially available and homemade medication receptacles. Other methods include color coding the tops of the medication containers, circling the hours on a clock face affixed to the container, or setting an alarm clock to remind the elder when to take the medication. Today there are electronic pill containers that audibly let the person know when it is time to take his or her medication; however, they may be too expensive for some elder's limited resources. These methods can be of tremendous assistance to the aged person who is having difficulty managing medications.

Leirer et al (1991) showed that memory failures associated with nonadherence to medication regimens were of two general types: forgetting the way to correctly take medications and "prospective" recall failure (failure to remember to take medication at the correct times). This latter type of nonadherence was reported to increase with the number of different prescriptions taken. The research of Leirer et al (1991) showed that the use of voice mail that telephoned the elder each time a medication was to be taken to remind him or her of the type and amount of medication reduced nonadherence to as low as 2.1%. Studies prior to this time reduced nonadherence to only 10%. It was suggested that voice mail reminders could reduce nonadherence in three ways: (1) improve accuracy of the exact time elders remember to take their medication, (2) reduce the frequency of completely forgetting to take medication, and (3) reduce the frequency of self-overmedication.

For the individual who may not adhere because of low literacy, the use of matching colored dots on the drug container and a calendar or voice mail may be of value. Allow the individual to decide his or her own schedule and tailor it around his or her lifestyle. The use of cueing, that is, choosing daily events such as brushing teeth or dentures or watching a daily television program, is also useful in facilitating compliance by those individuals who have very limited literacy ability (Hussey, 1991).

One should not forget to ask if the individual has had any "bad reactions" (adverse drug reactions) to any drugs, what occurred, length of the reaction, and if it was necessary to see a physician if the drug was used after that time.

The caregiver will find that questions about medications the aged person ingests are perceived as very personal and almost as sensitive an issue as asking him or her to reveal a secret. It is important to be aware of this and ask questions in a nonthreatening, nonjudgmental manner. It is helpful to use open-ended questions, as well as some specific direct questions. For example, if you are trying to ascertain whether the patient has missed any doses of a medication, rather than asking how many times the doses were missed, it would be better or less threatening for the nurse to say, "It is quite common to forget to take your medication once in a while. How many times this month would you say you forgot to take your digoxin (or other specific drug)?" Many aged feel threatened by an authoritative manner and hesitate to reveal how they have been taking medications for fear that the caregiver will find fault and reprimand them. Taking medications has received most of the research in compliance; less investigation has been directed at elders' knowledge, that is managing medications. This is an important area that should be considered for further research.

Two issues still remain when one discusses or considers elders and adherence to medication regimens (or any therapy): (1) medication management is a complex activity that bears little resemblance to the simplistic notion of compliance (Conn et al, 1995) and (2) health professionals are frequently younger than their aged patients with little concept of how patients define their own quality of life or the quality of their therapy (Tobias, 1994). It is important then that the health professional listen to and start asking elders their perspective on their drug therapy in order to accomplish as smooth a regimen as is realistically feasible for the elder.

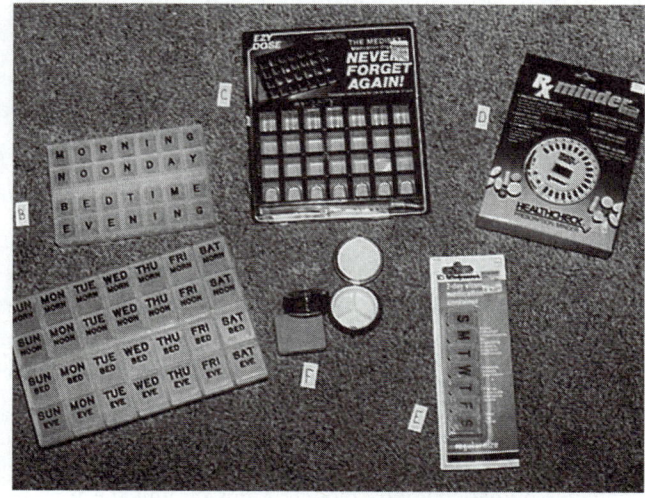 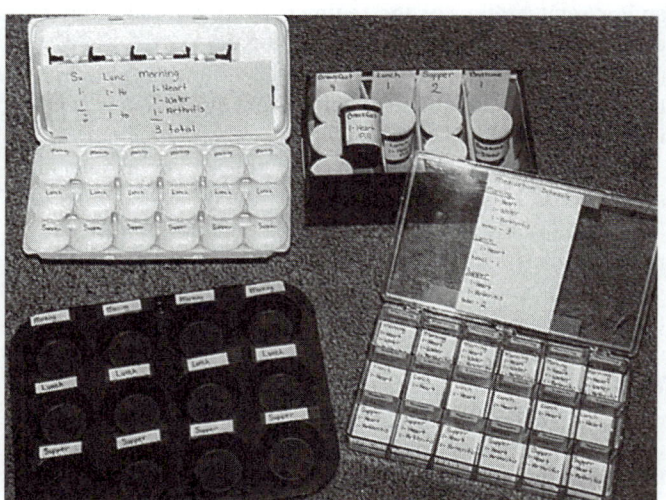

Figure 10-3. Medication reminder systems. **A,** Commercial. **B,** Homemade. (From Hahn K, Wietor G: Helpful tools for medication screening, *Geriatr Nurs* 13[3]:164, 1992.)

DRUG USE ASSESSMENT AND INTERVENTIONS

An adequate medication history should be the initial step in assisting the aged to achieve safe drug use so that information necessary to establish an individualized approach can be obtained. A comprehensive drug history should help maintain a therapeutic medication regimen, assist in identifying missing knowledge necessary to take medication correctly, eliminate unnecessary medications, and reduce the risk of adverse drug reactions.

Usually it is the role of the pharmacist to obtain a medication history. When there is no pharmacist, however, the nurse should be prepared to do so. One should start by asking, "What prescription medications are you taking?" A systematic way to gather information is to do a 24-hour medication history. If using the review of systems, the nurse may ask what medications are routinely used for headache, eye problems, ear problems, and endocrine problems (thyroid, insulin, etc.). Additional information about drug management can be gathered: as the medication is named, the individual is asked to describe the dose, frequency of administration, and purpose.

Open-ended questions such as "What do you take for headaches?" "What do you use for indigestion, or bowels?" should be asked. These provide information about motivation and beliefs concerning the taking of medications: current prescriptions and OTC preparations; current administration schedule; current medication status, the individual's knowledge about his or her medications; medication-related problems such as side effects or nonadherence; number of prescription drugs being taken; frequency of visits to the physician or primary care practitioner; level of sensory, memory, and physical disability; ability to pay for prescription medications; and the level of use of social drugs such as alcohol and caffeine (Ascione and Shimp, 1988; Ascione, 1994; Higbee, 1994). Information about "street" drugs (opiates, marijuana, and cocaine) should be discussed, and specifics of "back fence" drug use (drugs that are obtained from friends and relatives) should be identified. Use of vitamins and herbal preparations should also be noted. Many OTC preparations contain traces or lower doses of drugs that in higher dosage would require a prescription . These interact with other OTC or prescription drugs to reach toxic levels if an individual is taking several preparations that contain the same ingredients. Because many drugs take 2 to 4 weeks to be completely excreted, recently discontinued drugs as well as the reason for discontinuation may be significant.

When the aged person does not remember all that he or she is taking, ask that all medications be put in a paper bag and brought in for evaluation. Garner as much information as possible from the individual regarding amount, frequency, and reason for taking each drug. Figure 10-4 offers one form of a medication assessment tool.

Box 10-8 provides guidelines for subsequent visits.

Once the medication history is obtained, problem areas can be identified. Answers to the following questions should serve as a guide to definitive interventions.

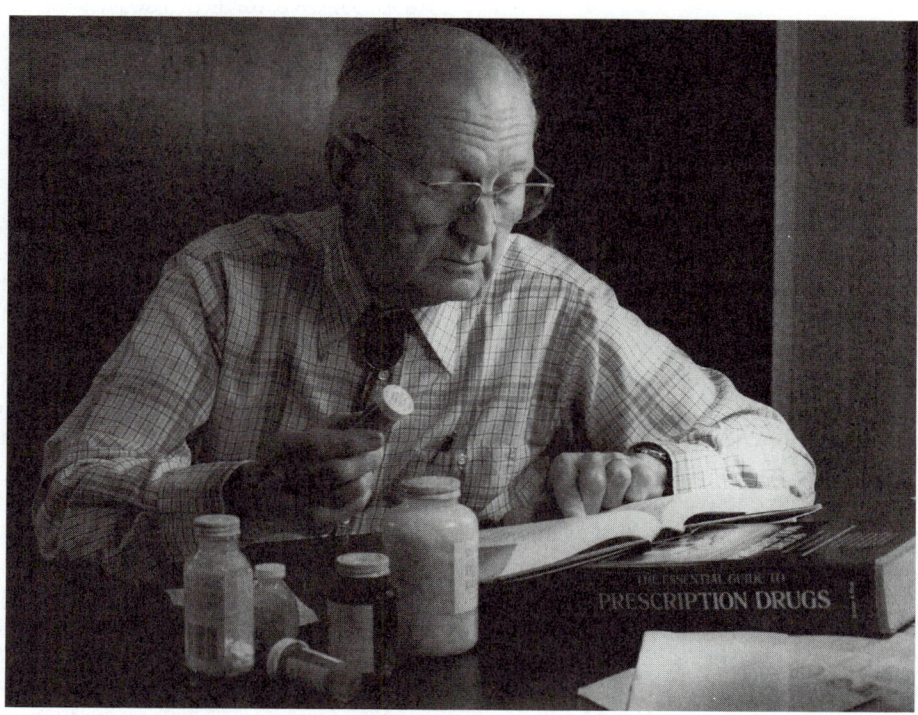

An elder prepares to take his medicine. (Courtesy Rod Schmall.)

General Considerations: What is the client/patient's:

1. Cognitive level _____
_____

2. Visual acuity and ability to read labels _____
_____

3. Hand/muscle coordination (to pour, uncap/cap bottle) _____

4. Ability to swallow without difficulty _____
_____

5. Level of ADLs: Independent [ ] needs help [ ] _____

6. Life-style patterns (alcohol, smoking, activity) _____

7. Beliefs and attitudes toward:
    Self _____
    Illness _____
    Treatments _____
    Prescribing physician or nurse _____

8. Living conditions: Alone [ ], with others [ ]
    Relationship with others _____
    _____

9. Ability to afford cost of medication _____
_____

SPECIFIC MEDICATION HISTORY:

10. Medications currently taking: (ALL prescribed by ALL
    physicians and nurses providing care)

    Prescribed: Over-the-counter
    _____   for pain _____
    _____   constipation _____
    _____   sleep _____
    _____   vitamins _____
    _____   health food products _____

11. Knowledge: (reason for taking drug) _____
    _____

    Times and frequency of self medication: _____
    _____
    _____

12. Are medications shared with: family [ ], friends [ ]
    If so who _____

13. ADR (adverse drug reaction(s)):
    Has experienced ADR(s) yes [ ]   no [ ]
    If yes, how was it handled _____
    _____
    _____

14. Incidence of overuse or underuse of medication:
    yes [ ]   no [ ]   Describe _____
    _____
    _____

15. Storage:
    How is medication stored _____
    Where stored _____
    Reason kept that way _____

16. Disposition of old drugs (how handled): _____
    _____

*If medications administered by spouse or other, the assessment should be done to ascertain caregiver's ability.

Figure 10-4. Medication assessment and history worksheet.

1. *Is the drug necessary?* Many elderly continue to take medication indefinitely or have had a large prescription that they did not want to waste, or the physician never told them to stop taking the drug. *Some aged are on drugs because of behavioral changes or symptoms that are the consequence of unrecognized toxicity from other medications.* Often the elderly do better without medication or may be able to follow a regimen when there are only one or two medications. The nurse should think about consolidating medications if there are medications with the same active chemicals that directly or indirectly accomplish the same end. For example, an individual who is on a hypnotic and a tricyclic medication can perhaps achieve better sleep with the tricyclic administered at bedtime since a side effect of the tricyclic is drowsiness. This would mean taking one medication instead of two and avoid other side effects such as hangover and daytime drowsiness.

2. *Does the drug have undesirable side effects?* The greatest lack of information by the aged is in the area of side effects. The nurse should know specific side effects before she cares for the person. Aged individuals should be alerted to the possible side effects of drugs they are receiving. The nurse should also tap as a resource the clinical pharmacist. Either with or without the assistance of the clinical pharmacist, when side effects exist, the nurse should assess what they are and if they interfere with the individual's ability to function fully. For example, sleeping pills trigger confusion, hallucinations, and excitation; excessive use of vitamin A can produce joint problems, headaches, blurred vision, night blindness, or loss of hair. All anticholinergic drugs, many of which are common to the pharmacopoeia of the aged, exacerbate some of the common problems of aging such as dry mouth, blurred vision, and anorexia. A helpful tip for nurses is to never allow

Modified from Higbee MD: Consumer guidelines for using medications wisely, *Generations* (2):43, 1994.

an elder to have lenses changed on glasses until medication routines are well established. Medication changes often produce temporary visual changes (Box 10-5). Another peculiarity of medication reaction among the aged is a tendency toward amnesic periods when taking benzodiazepines, especially Ativan. Haloperidol (Haldol), a psychotropic drug frequently used for behavioral control, is notorious for stimulating tardive dyskinesia in the aged (see Chapter 22). These few examples are meant to alert the nurse to observe carefully when instituting any new medication regimen; not all the possible adverse reactions will be found in textbooks. Geropharmacology is an area ripe for clinical research by nurses who are in the prime position to observe reactions over time.

3. *When more than one drug is involved, are interactions occurring?* If interactions are evident, are they detrimental? An account of OTC drugs should also be obtained to establish if these drugs have an independent or collective effect with prescription medications to produce interactions or interfere with the pharmacokinetics.

4. *Do the drugs induce malnutrition?* Many drugs leach vitamins and minerals from the body. The aged have a history of poor nutritional status and thus are more vulnerable to this problem. Table 10-6 is a limited chart showing which vitamins and minerals are affected by specific drugs. Depending on the degree of medication used, it might be helpful to the prescribing physician to pinpoint what vitamin and mineral supplements are necessary. See the appendices for a list of additional drugs that induce vitamin deficiencies.

LeSage and Stauffacher (1988) asked the following four questions to identify active or potential drug use or misuse: (1) What drug therapy or regimen is the older adult or caregiver actually following? (2) What is the older adult's or caregiver's knowledge base underlying decision making related to drug therapy? (3) Has the defined therapeutic outcome been achieved? (4) Does the person taking the drug have signs and symptoms that are commonly associated with adverse effects of drug therapy in older persons?

At the time of the drug assessment or anytime the client visits the physician or the hospital, clinic, or office, he or she should bring all prescribed medications. If this is not possible, the aged person should carry a current list of medications; Figure 10-5 illustrates a suggested format. It is a good idea for the nurse to initiate this if the aged person does not have a record of his or her drugs. The nurse should make a list for reference, for agency records and for the aged person to carry in a wallet or change purse.

Patient Education

The area in which nurses have the biggest impact on medication use is patient education. The elderly have problems understanding how and when medications should be taken. Language barriers, either because of poor vocabulary or because the aged person speaks a language other than English, have a direct bearing on the adequacy of explanations.

To minimize this kind of problem, the nurse should provide the patient with an adequate oral explanation supplemented by written instructions. Even with good directions, the elderly can become easily confused when more than one medication is involved. The suggestions for compliance that appear in Box 10-9 are directly applicable to patient education and address the noncompliance issues that appear in Box 10-7. The better informed the aged are about their medications, the better they will be able to respond to their prescribed regimen.

Ascione and Shimp (1988) discuss strategies for helping elders use medications safely. The strategies are of two types. One focus is on the dissemination of information about medications the elder is taking. The objectives are to provide the necessary knowledge so that the elder can take the medication appropriately, understand the reasons for taking the medication, minimize the harmful effects, and avoid practices that would aggravate the drug effect. These objectives can be accomplished by the use of oral instructions that match the language of the elder's level of understanding and that are delivered in a slow, deliberate, and paced manner. Written information provides reinforcement and can be in the form of graphics, information sheets, prescription labels, and booklets. One must be careful not to overload the individual with too much information or input at one time.

The second focus is on proper management of medications. This can be accomplished by reducing the number of medications and developing a schedule appropriate to or compatible with the individual's lifestyle. If one medication duplicates the action of another, consolidation of medications is appropriate (Mastrangelo, 1994).

It is important to remember that using one type of intervention on one occasion is insufficient to accomplish the goals of proper medication use or long-term compliance. A combination of interventions over an extended period of time has been shown to be the most effective approach (Haynes et al, 1987).

Table 10-6   Drugs That Contribute to Malnutrition by Their Pharmacokinetic or Pharmacodynamic Action on Vitamins and Minerals

Drug	Ascorbic acid	Folic acid	Niacin	Pantothenic acid	Pyridoxine	Riboflavin	Thiamine	Vitamin A	Vitamin B12	Vitamin D	Vitamin E	Vitamin K	Calcium	Iron	Magnesium	Potassium	Zinc
Adrenocorticosteroids	X	X			X			X		X			X			X	X
Alcohol	X	X	X		X	X	X	X	X	X				X	X	X	X
Antacids							X							X			
Anticonvulsants		X			X				X	X		X	X				
Barbiturates	X								X	X				X			
Chelating agents (penicillamine)																	X
Cholestyramine		X															
Cimetidine (H₂ blockers)									X								
Colestipol								X	X	X	X	X					
Cycloserine*					X												
Digitalis glycosides																	
Diuretics																	
Ethacrynic acid													X			X	X
Spironolactone						X	X						X				X
Thiazides						X	X						X		X	X	X
Triamterene		X															
Gentamicin																X	X
Hydralazine†					X												
Isoniazid†			X		X								X			X	X
Levodopa†					X								X			X	
Lithium	X	X															
Methotrexate		X											X			X	
Neomycin									X					X		X	
Penicillin	X																
Petrolatum liquid								X		X	X	X					
Phenolphthalein										X			X				
Potassium chloride									X								
Probenecid						X											
Salicylates	X	X										X			X	X	
Streptomycin				X													
Sulfonamides	X	X			X	X		X	X			X					
Tetracyclines	X	X				X	X					X	X	X	X		X
Vancomycin													X	X	X	X	
Warfarin												X					

Modified from Roe DA: *Diet and drug interactions*, New York, 1989, Van Nostrand Reinhold.

*Vitamin antagonist.

†Carbonate.

Medicines I Take

Name of Drug and What It's For	Color/Shape	Directions and Cautions	Times

Figure 10-5. Medicines I Take. (From *Using your medicines wisely: a guide for the elderly,* US Department of Health, Education and Welfare Public Health Service, Alcohol, Drug Abuse, and Mental Health Administration, PF1436 [1185], D317.)

Box 10-9 **Suggestions for Improving Medication Adherence Behavior**

Disseminate drug information
Audiovisual information
Individual or group instruction
Written instructions
   Information sheets, leaflets in bold
   Reasonably large print

Simplify the medication administration process
Clear prescription container labels
   Use lay terms ("twice a day" instead of BID)
Memory aids
   Calendars
   Day, week, month pill containers
   Voice mail reminders
Convenient medication refills
Easy-to-open medication containers
Reduce number of doses daily when possible
Reduce the number of medications when possible
Tailor medication regimen to lifestyle

Teach proper medication management skills
Medication administration and training program
Self-care instruction

Education of the aged in the safe use of drugs can be accomplished on an individual basis or in small groups. Pamphlets and booklets written in lay terms and in appropriate language should be available to the aged. If there are none that are appropriate, the nurse should be creative and develop a booklet or information sheet that will meet the drug information needs of the aged patient, taking into account sight and memory changes. Box 10-9 provides suggestions for better compliance with medication regimens.

Information is best presented in numbered line fashion rather than in paragraph form (Morrow et al, 1988). Written information should be in large boldface type. Audiovisual aids are available for health teaching, but if they are too expensive, the nurse should consider devising some. The elderly should be taught to exercise their right to question and know what they are taking, how it will affect them, and the alternatives open to them (Higbee,1994; Delong, 1995). The information elders need to know about their drugs and medication regimen and the specific interventions to be considered when teaching patients about medications appear in Boxes 10-10 and 10-11.

Dispensing Procedures

Containers and container labels are another problem area in which the nurse can be of assistance. Most childproof

---

Box 10-10 **What Elders Should Know about Their Medications and How to Take Them at Home**

- What is the name of each drug?
- What is the purpose of each drug?
- What is the dose per administration?
- What is the number of doses every day?
- What is the best time to take the medication?
- How should the medication be taken?
- Can the medication be taken with other drugs?
- Which medications can and cannot be taken together?
- Any special techniques, devises or procedures that are necessary to administer the medication?
- For how long should the medication be taken?
- What are the common side effects?
- If side effects occur: what to do, what changes in administration are necessary, when should the drug be stopped, when should the physician or pharmacist or both be called?
- What can be done at home to monitor for a therapeutic drug response?
- What should be done if a dose is missed?
- How many refills are allowed?
- How should the medication be stored?

- What are the nonprescription (OTC) preparations that should not be used with the present drug therapy?
- Take all medications prescribed unless the physician states otherwise.
- Stop taking the medication and report any new or unusual problems such as shortness of breath, nausea, diarrhea, vomiting, sleepiness, dizziness, weakness, skin rash, or fever.
- Never take medication prescribed for another person.
- Do not take any medication more than 1 year old or past the expiration date on the container.
- Store medications in a safe place, preferably the kitchen, rather than the bathroom, where moisture from bathing, especially showers, may affect the medicine.
- Do not keep medicines, especially sedatives and hypnotics, on the bedside stand, because when you are sleepy, you may forget that you have already taken the medication earlier.
- Do not place different medicines in the same container.
- Take a sufficient supply of all medicines in their individual containers when traveling away from home.
- Use a chart to keep track of medications.

---

containers are also "geriatric proof." For individuals who have arthritic hands or must open the container quickly, it is a frustrating, nearly impossible task. It is now possible for the aged person to ask that the medication be placed in a screw- or flip-top container. Nurses in the hospital, clinic, or physician's office who are responsible for ordering medications from the pharmacy should intercede and make such a request for the patient.

On most labels, much information is typed in a very small space. Not only are the patient's name and the directions for administration on the label but also the physician's name; prescription number; name, address, and phone number of the pharmacy; and at times, warning labels. So much in such a little space is difficult for the average adult to decode.

Current prescription labels should be reevaluated with geriatric patients in mind. Larger labels should be used to accommodate all information in readable form (and appropriate language), and to facilitate easier hand/muscle coordination. Color coding may be a way to help individuals with multiple medications keep the drugs and dosages correct. International signs and symbols exist that identify sport, travel assistance, and buildings for restrooms and other needs. Some kind of international coding should be developed for medication categories, which would appear on the bottles; for example, a red heart for heart preparations, perhaps purple for antihypertensive drugs, and other colors for other classifications may be effective. Since no standardized system of this nature currently exists, the

nurse may need to devise a color system for patients and a color key that would be kept with the medications to avoid confusion.

Braille labels for the blind and visually impaired are also available. The braille label, which is a clear piece of material affixed over the regular label, is embossed with the drug name, strength, and prescription numbers (*AARP News Bulletin,* Braille labels for drugs, 1983).

Computers are rapidly becoming entrenched in drug use review and monitoring safe drug usage. These increase information exchange between physicians and pharmacists in the surveillance of drug compatibilities. One of the first programs was begun in the Family Practice Clinic at the University of South Carolina Medical Center. Drug profiles of more than 6000 patients were stored in the computer system. When a new medication was prescribed for the patient, information was retrieved about the patient status (For example, Medicaid); interactional potential of the drug; educational information needed by the patient, including the prescription label data, patient history with dates of drug renewals, and a short sequence of characteristics of the drug and drugs other than the new prescription; and warnings about potential drug interactions with the new prescription and any other drug the patient was currently taking. Variations of this surveillance have become common, especially among large pharmacy chains.

Most medications are taken orally. Many of the tablets and capsules are difficult to swallow because of their size or because they stick to the buccal mucosa. Administration of

Box 10-11   Safe Use of Medicines by Older People

Most people, and especially the elderly, use medicines at some point during their lifetime. When used correctly, medicines can be of great value. They can help heal wounds, stop the spread of infections, bring on sleep, and ease pain, both physical and mental. But when used incorrectly, drugs have the ability to injure the patient or change the effects of other medicines being taken at the same time.

Drugs can be divided into two major groups; over-the-counter drugs (also called patent medicines), which can be bought without a doctor's prescription; and prescription drugs, which can be ordered only by a doctor and sold only by a pharmacist (druggist). Prescription drugs are usually more powerful and have more side effects than over-the-counter medicines.

People over 65 make up 11% of the American population, yet they take 25% of all prescription drugs sold in this country. One reason for this more frequent use of drugs by other people is that, as a group, they tend to have more long-term illnesses than younger people. Also, advancing age sometimes brings with it changes in physical abilities, eating habits and social contacts. The result of these changes—whether it is aching muscles, constipation from lack of certain foods, or depression after the loss of a relative or friend—may often lead an older person to seek medical help. Drug treatment may be suggested to help overcome many of these physical and emotional problems.

Safe drug use requires both a well-informed doctor and a well-informed patient. New information about drugs and about how they affect the older user is coming to light daily. For this reason, those taking drugs should occasionally review with a doctor their need for each medicine.

In general, drugs given to older people act differently than they do when given to young or middle-aged people. This is probably the result of the normal changes in body makeup that occur with age. For example, as the body grows older, the percent of water and lean tissue (mainly muscle) decreases, while the percent of fat tissue increases. These changes can affect the length of time a drug stays in the body, how a drug will act in the body, and the amount of drug absorbed by body tissues.

The kidneys and the liver are two important organs responsible for breaking down and removing most drugs from the body. With age, the kidneys and the liver often begin to function less efficiently, and thus drugs leave the body more slowly. This may account for the fact that older people tend to have more undesirable reactions to drugs than do younger people.

Because older people can often have a number of physical problems at the same time, it is very common for them to be taking many different drugs. Two or more medicines taken at the same time can sometimes react with each other and produce harmful effects. For this reason, it is important to tell each doctor you go to about other drugs you are taking. This will allow the doctor to prescribe the safest medicines for your situation.

By taking an active part in learning about the drugs you take and their possible side effects, you can help bring about safer and faster treatment results. Some basic rules for safe drug use are as follows:

1. Take exactly the amount of drug prescribed by your doctor and follow the dosage schedule as closely as possible.
2. Medicines do not produce the same effects in all people. For this reason, you should never take drugs prescribed for a friend or relative, even though your symptoms may be the same.
3. Always tell your doctor about past problems you had with drugs, and be sure to mention other drugs (including over-the-counter medicines) you are taking.
4. It may help to keep a daily record of the drugs you are taking, especially if your treatment schedule is complicated or you are taking more than one drug at a time.
5. If child-proof containers are hard for you to handle, ask your pharmacist for easy-to-open containers. Always be sure, however, that such containers are out of the reach of children.
6. Make sure that you understand the directions printed on the drug container and that the name of the medicine is clearly printed. This will help you to avoid taking the wrong medicine or following the wrong schedule. Ask your pharmacist to use large type on the label if you find the regular labels hard to read.
7. Throw out old medicines, since many drugs lose their effectiveness over time.
8. Ask your doctor about side effects that may occur, about special rules for storage, and about which foods or beverages, if any, to avoid.
9. Always call your doctor promptly if you notice unusual reactions.

From US Department of Health and Human Services, Public Health Service, National Institutes of Health. Rockville, Md, Fact sheet, *Safe use of medicines by older people,* 1990.

---

a drug in liquid form is sometimes preferable and allows flexibility; concentrations can be varied so that quantities of solution can be prepared and taken by the teaspoon, tablespoon, or ounce. For the aged person at home these are simply and commonly used measurements. When using liq-uid preparations, it is the nurse's responsibility to ascertain that the client is using an appropriate measure. *Crushing tablets or emptying the powder from capsules into fluid or food should not be done unless specified by the pharmaceutical company or approved by a pharmacist because it may interfere with the effectiveness of the drug or create problems in administration, as well as injure the mouth or GI tract.*

Enteric coatings are used to protect the stomach against irritating substances or to protect certain drugs from breakdown by the stomach acid. Some pharmaceutical companies coat the drug beads in extended-action capsules with different types of coatings to allow some of the medication to be released immediately and the remainder at predetermined intervals. Some tablets are made of an inert porous plastic matrix that is impregnated with the active drug. As the drug passes through the GI tract, it is slowly leached out and absorbed by the body, which is a timed-release effect. Coated beads, plastic matrix tablets, and layered tablets *should not be crushed,* since all the medication would be released at one time or inactivated by stomach acid. This is tantamount to administrating higher doses of medication than prescribed or none at all (Box 10-12). A particular noteworthy example is slow-release potassium tablets, which tend to be most frequently crushed and can lead to bowel wall injury, GI irritation, bleeding, obstruction, and perforation.

Placing capsules on the front of the tongue facilitates swallowing. Capsules are lighter than tablets and will float to the back of the buccal cavity when fluid is consumed, thus washing them back and, it is hoped, down. Tablets are pushed down the gullet with a surge of fluid imbibed.

Relatively new in drug administration is the transdermal patch, also called transdermal delivery system (TDDS) (Fischer and Clark, 1994). Although the medications of this type are limited (about 7 to 10), TDDS provides for a more constant rate of drug administration, eliminates concern for GI absorption variation, GI tolerance, and drug interaction. In addition, lower doses are needed and compliance is better due to the need for less frequent administration. It also provides for rapid drug therapy termination when necessary. Box 10-13 provides guidelines for the TDDS.

The drug regimen of nursing home patients consumes much of the time of professional nursing staff as they administer, record, and evaluate. Rover (1987) showed that two simple changes could reduce costs and release nurses to perform other functions. He recommended the following:

- Reduce the number of times per day a medication is given, considering its known pharmacokinetics.
- Reorganize the dose-interval schedule of the drugs making up the total drug regimen.

The nurse has enormous responsibility in the administration of medications to the elderly and in the education of the aged about drug use. Box 10-14 lists the specific responsibilities of the nurse in administering medications to older adults. A brief discussion of inhalers and medication associated with diabetes can be found in Chapter 8.

Outcomes

Reassessment of the elder will determine the outcomes of medication use. Observation of the aged client should be an ongoing process to determine if physical and/or mental changes have occurred, as well as whether the therapeutic goal or response has been achieved. Listen to the elderly when they describe how they feel or changes that they notice after they have begun a new medication, have had a dose adjustment, or even when they continue to take several medications. Periodically check blood levels of such drugs that have a cumulative effect or are enhanced or diminished by interaction with other medication such as coumadin, digitalis preparations, quinidine, theophylline, Dilantin, Tegretol, and various antibiotics.

Box 10-12	**Medications That Should Not Be Chewed or Crushed**

Type	**Rationale**
Enteric-coated tablets	Prevent destruction of drug in stomach
	Prevent irritation in stomach to achieve a prolonged action
Timed-release tablets	
Slow-release core	Give prolonged release
Mixed-release granules	Immediate and prolonged release
Multilayer tablets	One layer immediate dose; each layer released to maintain blood level of medication
Porous inert carriers	Slow release into gastric fluid
Soluble matrix	Wax matrix provides slow release into gastric fluid; prevents high concentration of drug in local area; prevents gastric upset

Box 10-13	**Guidelines for Transdermal Delivery Systems**

Proper Administration

- Know the proper place for administration (some require specific anatomic placement).
- Place on clean surface (if hairy, should be shaved).
- Press firmly for 10 seconds for secure contact (no wrinkles or raised edges).
- Wash hands after contact with patch.
- DO NOT cut patch in half to decrease dose (this can cause evaporation or spill out of medication, and decrease adherence to skin).

Site Rotation

- Do not reapply to same area for at least 7 days.

Rash Management

- Rash is most common side effect (occurs in about 50% of patients due to active ingredient or adhesive).
- Apply topical corticosteroid to site as a pretreatment or after patch is removed.

Proper Disposal

- Fold sticky edges together
- Dispose down toilet or in a closed garbage can to keep away from pets or children.

Modified from Fischer RG, Clark N: Skin contact: a clinical review of transdermal drug delivery systems, *Adv Nurs Pract* 2(10):15, 1994.

KEY CONCEPTS

- Individuals over 75 years old cannot be expected to react to any medication in the way they did when they were 25 years old.
- Any medication has side effects, and the therapeutic goal is to reduce the targeted symptom without undesirable side effects. Drug-drug and drug-food incompatibilities are an increasing problem of which nurses must be aware.
- Polypharmacy reactions are one of the most serious problems of elders today and are usually the first arena to investigate when untoward physiologic events occur.
- Drug misuse may be triggered by physician practices, individual self-medication, physiologic idiosyncrasies, altered biodegradability, nutritional and fluid states, and inadequate assessment prior to prescribing.
- Drug toxicity occurs when the amount of drug taken exceeds the amount necessary to bring about a therapeutic effect.
- Many drugs cause temporary cognitive impairment in older persons. These should be discontinued or if that is not possible the individual needs to be informed in order to forestall fears of Alzheimer's disease.
- Nurses must investigate drugs immediately if confusion is observed in an individual who is normally alert and aware.

Box 10-14	**Administration of Medications to Older People: Nursing Responsibilities**

Take a complete medication history, including the following:
    Past medications
    Present medications (prescription and OTC)
    Allergies of all kinds
    Patient's understanding of medications being taken (name, purpose, dose, method, times)

Space oral medications so that not more than one or two are taken at one time.

Have patient drink a little fluid *before* taking oral medications (to ease swallowing).

Encourage the patient to drink at least 5 to 6 ounces of fluid after taking medications (to assure that the medications have left the esophagus and are in the stomach and to speed absorption of the medication).

Do not routinely give analgesics for pain every 4 hours. Because of delayed absorption and distribution and the half-life of the medication, there may be an adverse cumulative effect.

If the patient has difficulty swallowing a large capsule or tablet, ask the physician to substitute a liquid medication if possible (cutting the tablet in half or crushing it and placing it in applesauce or fruit juice may distort the action of some medications, reduce the dose, or cause choking or aspiration of particles of medication or applesauce).

Teach alternatives to medications, such as the following:
    Proper diet instead of vitamins
    Exercise instead of laxatives
    Bedtime snacks instead of hypnotics
    Decrease in weight, salt, fats, stress, and smoking and increased exercise instead of hypertensive agents (if approved by the physician)

- Nonadherence of clients with medication regimens is a constant concern among health professionals. We recommend the nurse focus on possible reasons. One cannot and will not comply with a prescription or treatment plan when there are incompatibilities that interfere with the practicalities of life or are distressful to the individual's well-being or when actual misinformation or disability prevents compliance.
- An important aspect of medication administration is developing a reliable plan for dispensing the appropriate amounts and the correct time. Nurses may be most helpful is assisting the elder with such a plan.
- Chronopharmacology is a relatively new science that utilizes biorhythms of the body for the most effective medication therapy. It has the potential to decrease dose, frequency, and cost of a medication regimen and to improve adherence to drug therapy.

CASE STUDY

Rose was a 78-year-old lady who lived alone in a large city. She had been widowed for 10 years. Her children were grown and all quite successful. She was very proud of them because she and her husband had emigrated to the United States when the children were small and had worked very hard to establish and maintain a home. She had only a few years of primary education and still clung to many of her "old country" ways. She spoke a strange mixture of English and her mother tongue,

and her children were somewhat embarrassed by her. They thought she was somewhat of a hypochondiac because she constantly complained to them about various aches and pains, her knees that "gave out," her "sugar" and "water" problems, and her heart palpitations. She had been diagnosed with mild diabetes and congestive heart failure. She was a devout Catholic and attended mass each morning. Her treks to church events, the senior center at church, and to her various doctors (internist, orthopedic, cardiac, and ophthalmic specialists) constituted her social life. One day the recreation director at

▲ Nursing Diagnoses ▲▲▲

The following potential diagnoses must be considered as well as diagnoses unique to the particular individual:

NURSING PROCESS AND NURSING DIAGNOSIS
Risk for or Actual Poisoning: Drug Toxicity

Etiologies and Related Factors
Aging process of liver and renal function: metabolism or biotransformation of drugs excretion of drugs
Polypharmacy
Self-medication (OTC and Rx)
Inadequate or misunderstood instructions for prescribed medications

Defining Characteristics
Internal (individual) factors
  Reduced vision
  Cognitive or emotional difficulties
  Insufficient finances
External (environmental) factors
  Effects of polypharmacy
  Variables of drug administration
  Effects of drugs in the aging body

Knowledge
Therapeutic ranges of medication
  Pharmacokinetics
  Side effects
  Toxicity
Safe administration of drug
  Polypharmacy
  Medication/dietary interactions

Clinical Judgment and Related Skills
Administer drugs—all routes in institutional settings
  Plan and implement "drug holidays"
  Act as resource when use of "PRN" medication is being considered
  Plan and implement drug administration routines in home settings for aged individual or family to maintain
  Monitor for effectiveness, side effects and record
  Patient/family teaching
  Family/community teaching (health maintenance)

Evaluation
Medications correctly taken
Dosage prescribed is congruent with liver and kidney function
Clear instructions provided and evidence of client understanding demonstrated

NEEDS ADDRESSED AND TASK STRENGTHS

Need to cope with acute and chronic health disorders; need to make own choices (to meet need for basic survival, safety, and security)

Healthy skepticism
Inquisitive regarding effects of medications
Body awareness and monitoring ability
Follows directions but questions untoward effects

the senior center noticed her pulling a paper bag of medication bottles from her purse. She sat down to talk with Rose about them and soon realized that Rose had only a vague idea of what most of them were for and tended to take them whenever she felt she needed them.

Based upon the case study, develop a nursing care plan using the following procedure*:

List comments of client that provide *subjective data.*

List information that provides *objective data.*

From these data identify and state, using accepted format, two *nursing diagnoses* you determine are most significant to the client at this time. List two *client strengths* that you have identified from data.

Determine and state *outcome criteria* for each diagnosis. These must reflect some alleviation of the problem identified in the nursing diagnosis and must be stated in concrete and measurable terms.

Plan and state one or more *interventions* for each diagnosed problem. Provide specific documentation of source used to determine appropriate intervention. Plan at least one intervention that incorporates the client's existing strengths.

Evaluate success of intervention. Intervention must correlate directly with the stated outcome criteria in order to measure the outcome success.

STUDY QUESTIONS/ACTIVITIES

When you are given a prescription for medication, what do you ask about it?

How would you begin to help Rose if you were the recreation director at the senior center?

What factors about Rose's probable medication misuse would be most alarming to you?

What aspect of Rose's situation related to medications do you think are common among elders?

Do you think most elders seek adequate information about their medications before taking them?

Who should be responsible for teaching and monitoring medication use in Rose's case? In any case?

Is it possible to get sufficient drug information for ESL (English as a second language) persons? Where would you obtain it?

Is medication information provided that is geared to an individual who is barely functionally literate?

▲ ADDITIONAL CASE STUDIES FOR DISCUSSION

Ms. Snooze is a 65-year-old woman who has been falling asleep lately in the middle of her bridge games at her board

and care home. She has been her usual friendly, chatty self lately except for the frequent catnaps. Occasionally, she gets confused and forgets which card game she is playing (she keeps yelling "Fish"). She has begun asking someone else to shuffle the cards for her because she says her hands are weak. The only medication she takes is a small amount of Valium to help her sleep at night, so she knows the daytime sleeping, mild confusion, and weakened state are all part of growing old. She doesn't want to worry anyone by complaining.

What do you think about her attitude toward the changes taking place? What action would you consider taking with Ms. Snooze? Why?

Mr. Espinoza is a 75-year-old Hispanic man who has difficulty understanding English and is usually very nervous. He has a heart problem for which he takes digoxin and a diuretic to lower his blood pressure. Last week his doctor changed the doses of both medications. Mr. Espinoza has been complaining to you of feeling sick to his stomach, occasional vomiting, dizziness, and stumbling a lot. He stopped taking his medications today because he decided they were making him sick.

What do you think about his decision? What action would you consider taking with Mr. Espinoza? Why?

Ms. Jones is a 70-year-old retired school teacher who likes to drink a glass of wine with lunch and dinner to calm her nerves. She takes a narcotic pain medication, as needed, for her hip pain. Last month her doctor prescribed a mild sedative to help her sleep at night. She has been using an OTC cough syrup whenever she feels a cough coming on, which seems to be fairly often. Recently she has been more forgetful and sometimes can't remember where she lives. She continues to insist on a monthly doctor's appointment because she has great faith in modern medicine.

What do you think about the way she is handling her health care? What action would you consider taking with Ms. Jones?

RESEARCH QUESTIONS

Which elders tend to be given the most adequate information about their medications?

Who provides the most complete information about medications?

How many elders have access to sources for looking up their own medications?

What questions do elders ask before taking prescriptions?

---

*Students are advised to refer to their nursing diagnosis text and identify possible or potential problems.

What percentage of elders are not taking any prescribed drugs?

How many elders are aware of possible negative drug interactions?

What symptoms do elders recognize as possible drug reactions?

RESOURCES

Film and videos

The Medicated Generation
(Medication/elderly)
Addresses the special concerns of the elderly in medication management and the responsibilities of health professionals to support the elderly by communicating information and caring.

Publications

Using Your Medications Wisely: A Guide for the Elderly, National Institute on Drug Abuse. Available from Elder-Ed, PO Box 416, Kensington, MD 20795. Single copies free; multiple copies (lots of 100) purchased by writing The Superintendent of Documents, U.S. Government Printing Office, Washington, DC 20402.

Food and Drug Interactions (large size print). Originally published in the FDA Consumer Magazine. Send a postcard to FDA, HFE-88, 5600 Fishers Lane, Rockville, MD 20857.

National Institute on Aging, Age Pages Fact Sheet. For sale by Superintendent of Documents, U.S. Government Printing Office, Washington, DC 20402.

Drug Errors: Misleading Medication Labels Can Lead to a Fatal Mistake. To report drug errors or to confidentially or anonymously report a drug error, call (800) 23-ERROR. The hotline is sponsored by the Institute for Safe Medication Practice and the Federal U.S. Pharmacopeia, which sets standards for the FDA.

"Team Up and Talk About Prescriptions" *Prescription Medications and You: A Consumer Guide* (AHCPR Publication No. 96-0056, English; Spanish-language version available). For bulk copies (more than 10 copies), contact: NCPIE, 666 Eleventh Street NW, Suite 810, Washington, DC 20001-4542; (202)347-6711; Fax (202) 638-0773. (Cost = $25 per 50 copies.) Booklet also available on AHCPR's Web site by using Web browser, specifying URL http://www.ahcpr.gov/and click on "Consumer Health."

REFERENCES

Ascione FJ: Medication compliance in the elderly, *Generations* 18(2):28, 1994.

Ascione FJ, Shimp LA: Helping patients to reduce medication misuse and errors, *Generations* 2:52, 1988.

Bezon J: Approaching drug regimens with a therapeutic dose of suspicion, *Geriatr Nurs* 12(4):180, 1991.

Braille labels for drugs: *AARP Newsbulletin* 24(2):27, 1983.

Butler RN, Lewis MI, Hoffman E, Whitehead ED: Love and sex after 60: how physical changes affect intimate expression, *Geriatrics* 49(9):20, 1994.

Cameron KA: *Nonprescription medicines: new opportunities and responsibilities for self care,* Special Report 44, United Seniors Health Cooperative, Washington, DC, 1996.

Carruth AK, Boss BJ: More than they bargained for: adverse drug effects, *J Gerontol Nurs* 16(7):841, 1990.

Col N, Fanale JE; Kronholm P: The role of medication noncompliance and adverse drug reactions in hospitalization of the elderly, *Arch Intern Med* 150:1, 1990.

Conn VS, Taylor SG; Wienke JA: Managing medications: older adults and caregivers, *J Nurs Sci* 1(1-2):40, 1995.

Cox H, Hinz M, Luhno M et al. *Clinical applications of nursing diagnosis: adult, child, women's, psychiatric, gerontic and home health considerations,* Philadelphia, 1993, FA Davis.

Cusack BJ, Vestal RE: Clinical pharmacology: special considerations in the elderly. In Caulkins E, Davis PJ, Ford AB, editors: *The practice of geriatrics,* Philadelphia, 1986, WB Saunders.

Darnell JC, Murray MD, Martz BL et al: Medication use by ambulatory elderly: an in-home survey, *J Am Geriatr Soc* 34(1):1, 1986.

Delong MF: Caring for the elderly. 4. Medication use and abuse, *NURSEweek* 8(8):8, 1995 (second April issue).

DeMaadg G: High-risk drugs in the elderly population, *Geriatr Nurs* 16(5):198, 1995.

Fischer RG, Clark N: Skin contact: a clinical review of transdermal drug delivery systems, *Adv Nurs Pract* 2(10):15, 1994.

Haynes RB, Wang E, Gomez MD: A critical review of interventions to improve compliance with prescribed medications, *Patient Educ Counsel* 10:155, 1987.

Higbee MD: Consumer guidelines for using medications wisely, *Generations* 18(2):43, 1994.

Hogstel MO, editor: *Clinical manual of gerontological nursing,* St Louis, 1992, Mosby.

Hussey LC: Overcoming the clinical barriers of low literacy and medication noncompliance among the elderly, *J Gerontol Nurs* 17(3):27, 1991.

Kane RL, Ouslander JG, Abrass JB: *Essentials of clinical geriatrics,* New York, 1984, McGraw-Hill.

Keenan R: The benefits of a drug holiday, *Geriatr Nurs* 2:103, 1983.

Kutzik D, Spiers M: *Drug therapy adherence among the elderly: barriers to successful self management.* Paper presented at the Gerontological Society of America, San Francisco, Calif, November 21, 1993.

Lamy PP: Hazards of drug use in the elderly, *Postgrad Med* 76(1):50, 1982.

Lamy PP: Adverse drug reactions and the elderly: an update. In Ham RJ, editor: *Geriatric medicine annual,* Oradell, NJ, 1986a, Medical Economics.

Lamy PP: Drug reactions and the elderly, *J Gerontol Nurs* 12(2):36, 1986b.

Lamy PP: Adverse drug effects, *Clin Geriatr Med* 6(2):293, 1990.

Lee M: Drugs and the elderly: do you know the risks? *Am J Nurs* 96(7):24, 1996.

Leirer VO, Morrow DG, Tanke ED, Pariante GM: Elder's nonadherence: its assessment and medication reminding by voice mail, *Gerontologist* 31(4):514, 1991.

Lepkowski MI: General principles of drug therapy in the elderly. In Lantz J, editor: *Nursing care of the elderly,* San Diego, Calif, 1992, Western Schools.

LeSage J, Stauffacher MZ: Detection of medication misuse in the elders, *Generations* XII:32, 1988.

Maas M, Buckwalter KC, Hardy M: Nursing diagnoses and interventions for the elderly, Menlo Park, Calif, 1991, Addison-Wesley Nursing.

Mastrangelo R: Consolidating medications, *Adv Nurs Pract* 2(10):29, 1994.

Miller CA: Drug consult: medications and sexual functioning in older adults, *Geriatr Nurs* 16(2):94, 1995.

Miller CA: Drug consult: multiple choices in over-the-counter drugs, *Geriatr Nurs* 17(5) 1996.

Montatmat SC, Cusack BJ, Vestal RE: Management of drug therapy in the elderly, *N Engl J Med* 321(5):303, 1989.

Morrow D, Leier VO, Sheikh J: Adherence and medication instructions, *J Am Geriatr Soc* 36(12):1147, 1988.

Nolan L, O'Malley K: Adverse drug reactions in the elderly, *Br J Hosp Med* 41:446, 1989.

Palmieri DT: Cleaning up confusion: adverse effects of medication in the elderly, *J Gerontol Nurs* 17(10):32, 1991.

Roberts J, Tumer N: Pharmacodynamic basis for altered drug reaction in the elderly, *Clin Geriatr Med* 4(1):127, 1988.

Santo-Novak D, Edwards RM: Caution with drugs for the elderly, *Geriatr Nurs* 10(2):72, 1989.

Shaughnessy AF: Common drug interactions in the elderly, *Emerg Med* 24(21):21, 1992.

Shimp LA, Ascione FJ: Causes of medication misuse and error, *Generations* 12(2):17, 1988.

Spiers MV, Kutzik DM: *A multidimensional framework for understanding medication adherence in the elderly: a prescription for rethinking,* Paper under review, 1995.

SRx senior mini-class curriculum, SRx Regional Program, Medication Education for Seniors, 1988.

Stewart RB, Moore MT, May FE et al: Changing patterns of therapeutic agents in the elderly: a ten year overview, *Age Ageing* 20(30):182, 1991.

Tobias DE: Ensuring and documenting the quality of drug therapy in the elderly, *Generations* 18 (2):43, 1994.

Todd B: Prescription for the 90's, *Geriatr Nurs* 11(3):114, 1990.

Turkoski BB: Medication timing for the elderly: the impact of biorhythms on effectiveness, *Geriatr Nurs* 1997 (in press).

Vestal RE: Clinical pharmacology. In Andres R, Bierman LE, Hazzard WR, editors: *Principles of geriatric medicine,* New York, 1985, McGraw-Hill.

Vestal RE: Clinical pharmacology. In Hazzard W, Reuben R, Bierman E, Blass J, editors: *Principles of geriatric medicine and gerontology,* New York, 1990, McGraw-Hill.

Vestal RE, Dawson GW: Phamacology and aging. In Finch CE, Schneider EL, editors: *Handbook of the biology of aging,* New York, 1985, Van Nostrand Reinhold.

Weitzel EA: In Maas M, Buckwalter KC, Hardy M: *Nursing diagnoses and interventions for the elderly,* Redwood City, Calif, 1991, Addison-Wesley.

Wilcox SM, Himmelstein DU, Woolhandler S: Inappropriate drug prescribing for the community-dwelling elderly, *JAMA* 272(4):292, 1994.

Wolanin MO, Phillips LRF: *Confusion: prevention and care,* St Louis, 1981, Mosby.

Yuen GJ: Altered pharmacokinetics in the elderly, *Clin Geriatr Med* 6(2):257, 1990.

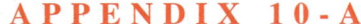

APPENDIX 10-A

Medications That Should and Should Not Be Used by Older Adults

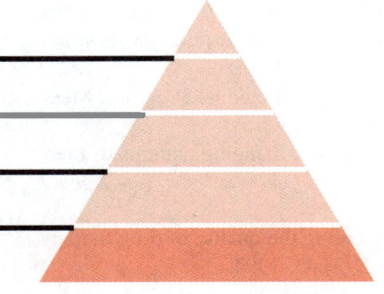

Category	Do not use	Limited use	Okay	Category	Do not use	Limited use	Okay
Cardiovascular	Aldomet	Capoten	Inderal	Pain and Anti-inflammatory	Bufferin		Advil
	Catapres	Diazide	Lopressor		Feldene		Aspirin
	Serpasil	Minipress	Tenormin		Darvocet		Ecotrin
	Persantine	Lasix	Lanoxin		Darvon		Empirin
	Cyclospasmol		Nitrobid		Demerol		Tylenol
	Pavabid		Coumadin		Talwin		Dilaudid
	Trental		K-Lor		Wygesic		Percodan
Tranquilizers and Hypnotics	Ativan	Serax					Vicodin
	Dalmane			Gastrointestinal	Mylanta	Antivert	Tagamet
	Halcion				Tigan	Compazine	Zantac
	Librium				Colace	Phenergan	Pepcid
	Nembutal				Dialose Plus	Reglan	Maalox
	Restoril				Doxidan	Milk of	Metamucil
	Valium					Magnesia	
	Xanax					Achromycin	
Antidepressants	Elavil			Antiinfectives			Bactrim
	Triavil						Gantrisin
Antipsychotics		Desyrel	Norpramine				Keflex
		Sinequan	Aventyl				Penicllin
		Tofranil	Pamelor				Septra
		Haldol	Lithium				Vibramycin
		Mellaril		Neurologic	Artane	Hydergine	Sinemet
		Navane			Cogentin		Dilantin
		Prolixin					Tegretol
		Stelazine		Nutritional	Vitamin E		Calcium
		Thorazine		Supplements			Feosol
							Fergon
							Niacin
							Vitamins
				Others	Norflex	Premarin	Synthroid

Compiled from Wolfe SM, Fugate L, Hulstrand EP et al: *Worst pills, best pills,* Washington, DC, 1988, Public Citizen Health Research Group; Lee, M: Drugs and the elderly: do you know the risks? *AJN* 96 (7):30, 1996.

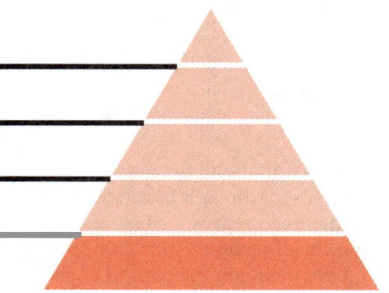

Special Drug Considerations for the Elderly

Drug	Special considerations
Analgesic Agents	
Acetaminophen (APAP) (Tylenol, Datril)	Acetaminophen is the preferred analgesic agent with noninflammatory pain and is as effective as propoxyphene and codeine. Chronic daily ingestion of more than 4 to 5 gm can lead to liver damage.
Aspirin (ASA)	Aspirin is the least expensive and is preferred over acetaminophen in inflammatory pain.
	It is as effective as propoxyphene and codeine.
	Gastrointestinal blood loss occurs in three fourths who take it and is of concern to patients with borderline anemia; concomitant liquid antacid minimizes. Antiplatelet effect may be of benefit in prevention of recurrent myocardial infarction and transient ischemic attack.
Propoxyphene and propoxyphene combinations (Darvocet-N 100 and Darvon compounds)	Single-ingredient propoxyphene is not as effective as aspirin or acetaminophen alone, but a combination is as effective as aspirin or acetaminophen. Confusional reactions are increased. Avoid long-term full-dose use.
Codeine and codeine combinations (Tylenol No. 1-4)	Codeine has equal potency with aspirin and acetaminophen. Combination has greater potency. Nausea, vomiting, and constipation are more common.
Pentazocine (Talwin)	Pentazocine is less effective than aspirin and is prone to causing confusional reactions.
Phenacetin	Never use phenacetin chronically, because both prescription and OTC medications will lead to analgesic nephropathy, especially in combination analgesics.
Meperidine (Demerol), morphine, hydromorphone (Dilaudid)	Use one-third to one-half usual adult dose, since much more potent. No side effect differences in equal analgesic doses, but incidence increases with age.
Antiinflammatory Analgesic Agents	
Phenylbutazone (Azolid, Butazolidin) and oxyphenbutazone (Tandearil)	Both have longer half-life and higher incidence of gastrointestinal upset and severe toxic reactions in older patients; therefore give with meals and/or liquid antacid to minimize gastrointestinal effect. These are not recommended in those over 60 years old by some authorities. Phenylbutazone and oxyphenylbutazone cause fluid retention, blood dyscrasias, and increased oral anticoagulant effect. Do not give full dose for more than 7 to 14 days.
Tolmetin (Tolectin), fenoprofen (Nalfon), sulindac (Clinoril), ibuprofen (Motrin), naproxen (Naprosyn)	All nonsteroidal antiinflammatory analgesics are less effective than aspirin in inflammatory disease but lower incidence of gastrointestinal side effects. These are much more expensive than aspirin.
Antidiabetic Agents	Weight reduction and dietary measures control up to 70% of maturity-onset diabetes. Oral agents may increase cardiovascular morbidity. Hypoglycemic signs of tremor, sweating, and tachycardia are not as readily discernible.
	Chlorpropamide (Diabenese) has an active metabolite and prolonged half-life.

Modified from Deverau MO, Andrus L, Scott C: *Elder care,* New York, 1981, Grune & Stratton.

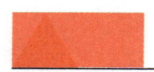

Drug	Special considerations
Cardiovascular Drugs	
Digitalis preparations	Digoxin (Lanoxin) is the preferred glycoside. Avoid digitoxin and digitalis leaf (long hepatic and renal half-lives). Although beneficial in low output failure and atrial fibrillation, digitalis preparations are successfully withdrawn in up to three fourths of patients. Subacute toxicity of anorexia with weight loss is more common than initial signs of gastrointestinal or cardiovascular effects. Baseline and follow-up electrocardiograms are essential. Dose is based on lean body weight and creatinine clearance with attention to electrolyte and thyroid status. One third to one half of patients are noncompliant.
Quinidine	Quinidine has higher serum levels if used concurrently with both drugs and digoxin. Half-life is prolonged. Cinchonism (gastrointestinal effects, light-headedness, tinnitus) occurrence is more common with low body weight. Decrease loading dose by one third in patients with
Propranolol (Inderal)	Toxic effects are more common, as is reduced beta-blocking responsiveness in older patients. Propranolol aggravates bronchospastic tendency in chronic obstructive pulmonary disease and can precipitate heart failure. Propranolol also affects diabetic control at higher doses, and there is increased tendency of "cold limb" effect in lower extremities in those with peripheral vascular or vasospastic diseases.
Nitroglycerin tablets (Nitrostat)	Nitrostat is the most stable form. Patient must sit down before sublingual dose placement. Beware of orthostatic effect of all vasodilators.
Nitroglycerin ointment (Nitrol)	Never rub into skin. Headache may be relieved with aspirin or acetaminophen.
Long-acting nitrates (isosorbide [Isordil, Sorbitrate] and pentaerythritol tetranitrate [Peritrate])	Long-acting nitrates are variably effective. Be careful about blood pressure-lowering effect.
Antihypertensive Agents	
Diuretics	All diuretics increase incontinence.
Thiazides (many; no significant difference; use hydrochloriazide generic)	Start with lowest possible dose. Patients must drink sufficient liquids. Watch volume, serum electrolyte, urate, and glucose effect.
Furosemide (Lasix)	Furosemide is most potent diuretic and should be held until thiazides no longer effective. It promotes calcium excretion and profoundly depletes sodium, potassium, and chloride. Cautious use of potassium supplements and salt substitutes is necessary because the elderly tend to have lower total body potassium with decreased muscle mass.
Spironolactone (Aldactone)	Spironolactone is a potassium-sparing diuretic often used in combination with thiazide (Aldactazide). Special caution is necessary if concurrent potassium supplement or salt substitute is used. Fatal hyperkalemia has been reported.
Triamterene (Dyrenium)	Triamterene is a potassium-sparing diuretic most often used in combination with thiazide
	(Dyazide) with similar precaution as spironolactone.
Sympatholytic Antihypertensive Agents	Beware of continued blood pressure below 120/70, orthostatic effects, impaired male sexual function, and drowsiness or sedation.
Methyldopa (Aldomet)	Reduce dosage when methyldopa is given in combination with thiazide (Aldoril). Sodium retention is seen when diuretic is not used. Daily dose at bedtime may take advantage of sedative effect, with therapeutic effect equivalent to multiple daily doses.
Propranolol (Inderal)	Propranolol is the only sympatholytic agent not requiring diuretic to prevent sodium retention. See cardiovascular section. If pulse is less than 50 to 60 beats per minute, drug is poorly tolerated.
Guanethidine (Ismelin)	Guanethidine is a profound sympatholytic agent with long second phase half-life. Use in small doses. Tricyclic antidepressants can interfere with antihypertensive effect.
Reserpine	Avoid giving reserpine to those with depression, sinusitis, peptic ulcer disease, and history of breast cancer.
Anticoagulant Agents	
Heparin	Heparin increases risk of bleeding with age, especially in women over 60 years old.

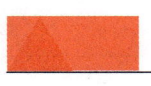

Drug	Special considerations
Anticoagulant Agents—cont'd	
Warfarin (Coumadin)	Warfarin increases risk of bleeding with age because of altered sensitivity with genetic, nutritional, and liver factors. Carefully evaluate use, and do serial prothrombin times. Beware of risk of hemorrhage, especially with possible hemorrhagic stroke, peptic ulcer disease, hiatal hernia, and diverticulosis or any bleeding diathesis. Concurrent aspirin usage is not possible except with heart valve prostheses.
Sedative-Hypnotics and Minor Tranquilizers	
Barbiturates (Butisol, Nembutal), phenobarbital, secobarbital (Seconal), amobarbital (Amytal)	With the exception of phenobarbital as an anticonvulsant, continued use of other barbiturates is irrational because of prolonged half-lives, paradoxic excitation in some, and tolerance and sleep pattern aberrations in all.
Benzodiazepines, chlordiazepoxide (Librium), diazepam (Valium), clorazepate (Tranxene), lorazepam (Ativan), oxazepam (Serax), and flurazepam (Dalmane)	Prolonged half-lives and cumulation of benzodiazepines have been reported with all except Ativan and Serax. Prolonged daily sedative (1 to 3 months) or hypnotic (7 to 14 days) use is not recommended because of depression of normal sleep pattern and resultant confusion, delirium, and psychologic changes. Serax is best choice because of short half-life. No hypnotic should be used nightly longer than 14 days; instead skip to every third night.
Chloral hydrate (Noctec)	Chloral hydrate is an excellent hypnotic in patients with no liver disease.
Antihistamines	
Diphenhydramine (Benadryl), hydroxyzine (Atarax, Visaril), phenylephrine (Dimetane), and chlorpheniramine (Chlor-Trimeton)	Antihistamines may be used for intercurrent use as needed for sedation and hypnotic effect. Beware of anticholinergic and tolerance effect with long-term use.
Nonbarbiturate Hypnotic Agents	
Ethinamate (Valmid), methaqualone (Quaalude), methyprylon (Noludar), glutethimide (Doriden), and ethchlorvynol (Placidyl)	None of these are recommended because of same types of problems as in barbiturates.
Major Tranquilizers—Antipsychotic Agents	
Phenothiazines, thioridazone (Mellaril), trifluoperazine hydrochloride (Stelazine), triflupromazine (Vesprin), and fluphenazine (Prolixin)	Use lowest possible dose and titrate approximately. Increased incidence of extrapyramidal symptoms in elderly. Postural (orthostatic) hypotension is a problem. Temperature control and tardive dyskinesia are more common with higher doses.
Butyrophenones (Haldol) and thioxanthene (Navane)	Highest incidence of extrapyramidal symptoms occur with these drugs. These are potent antipsychotic agents with low order of side effects and create episodes of amnesia and confusion.
Antidepressant Agents	Antidepressants are useful only in endogenous depression in up to one-half usual dosage.
Amitriptyline (Elavil), nortriptyline (Aventyl), imipramine (Tofranil), desipramine (Pertofrane), protriptyline (Vivactil), and doxepin (Sinequan)	These drugs can exacerbate tremors, psychosis, constipation, postural hypotension, benign prostatic hypertrophy, delayed micturition, and arrhythmias. Because of prolonged half-life, use caution in full-dose bedtime use, especially with Elavil and Tofranil.
Antiparkinsonian Agents	
Trihexyphenidyl (Artane), procyclidine (Kemadrin), benztropine (Cogentin), and diphenhydramine (Benadryl)	Prophylactic use with antipsychotic agents is generally not recommended. When extrapyramidal symptoms appear, 1 to 3 month use may be beneficial. Watch for constipation, tremors, and delirium resulting from prolonged use, especially with Cogentin.
Carbidopa-levodopa (Sinemet)	Carbidopa-levodopa is generally better tolerated than levodopa alone with less side effects (hypotension, syncope, anorexia, nausea, and emesis).

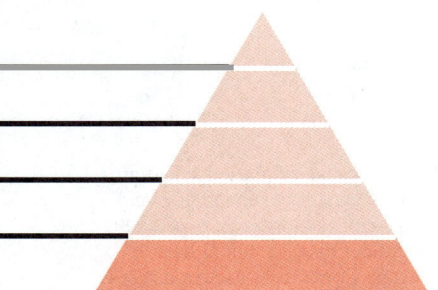

Side Effects of Drugs Used by the Elderly

Analgesic (mild)

ASA: Gastric irritant, allergic rhinitis, anticoagulant, uric acid precipitation

Analgesic (strong)

Depress CNS, circulation, and respiration; some cause constipation, sedation

Antacids

Decrease nutrient absorption; interfere with absorption of some other drugs; decrease stomach acidity; decrease calcium metabolism and absorption

Antiarrhythmics

Procainamide may cause agranulocytosis, fever, chills, and hypersensitivity; lidocaine needs careful monitoring in persons with impaired liver function; quinidine can cause tinnitus, nausea, and arrhythmias; idiosyncrasies are common; propranolol (beta-adrenergic blocker), use cautiously with the old

Antiarthritics

Phenylbutazone and oxyphenbutazone cause numerous side effects with high risk of severe or fatal toxic reactions; corticosteroids can cause gastrointestinal problems, depression, personality disturbance, irritability, and toxic psychoses

Anticholinergics

Blurred vision, dry mouth, urinary retention, intraocular pressure

Anticoagulants

Necessary to titrate to avoid internal bleeding; antibiotics and mineral oil decrease vitamin K production and thus potentiate anticoagulant effects

Anticonvulsants

Decreased folic acid activity, hypersensitivity, inhibit metabolism; primidone can cause anemia and visual hallucinations

Antidepressants

Imipramine, desipramine, amitryptyline, and nortriptyline all possess anticholinergic properties and must be used with caution in patients with glaucoma

Antihistamines

Drowsiness, blurred vision, and CNS depression, which is potentiated by alcohol

Antihypertensives

Thiazides and furosemide deplete potassium; triamterene or spironolactone may cause hyperkalemia; guanethidine and rauwolfia derivatives should be used together cautiously since they may cause excessive postural hypotension, bradycardia, and mental depression; hydralazine causes headaches, angina, and an arthritis-like syndrome

Antiinfectives

Hypersensitivity, gastrointestinal disturbance, pruritus, deafness, hepatic dysfunction, aplastic anemia; effects vary with the particular drug

Antiparkinsonians

Levodopa may cause nausea, hypotension, dyskinesia, agitation, restlessness and insomnia, cardiac and gastrointestinal effects; use with caution in patients with bronchial asthma or emphysema

Antipsychotics

In various degrees depending on the drug, all phenothiazines can cause photosensitivity, blood dyscrasias, agranulocytosis, and extrapyramidal effects (seen in 90% of patients after 10 weeks of therapy); haloperidol causes lethargy, decreased thirst and jaundice, dosage should be considerably reduced for geriatric patient; lithium carbonate has toxic level close to therapeutic; side effects are diarrhea, vomiting, tremors, sodium depletion, and muscular weakness; adequate salt and water intake is essential

Cough and cold preparations

OTC cough and cold preparations contain antihistamines and adrenergic decongestants; drugs with anticholinergic effects can contribute to a variety of drug interactions when taken with prescription drugs

Digitalis

Therapeutic and toxic levels close; frequent toxicity producing nausea, arrhythmias, hazy, yellow vision, and weight loss; potassium depletion sensitizes myocardium to digitalis and may also prolong toxicity, resulting in confusion and hallucinations

Diuretics

Thiazides can cause photosensitivity, pancreatitis, sodium and potassium depletion, and precipitate uric acid; ethacrynic acid can cause potassium depletion, vertigo, gastrointestinal problems, and hearing impairment; furosemide has similar side effects and may also alter color vision; spironolactone is potassium sparing but may cause hyperkalemia and drowsiness

Estrogens

Titrate dosage; use for 3 weeks with 1-week rest

Hypnotics

Barbiturates cause daytime drowsiness and hangover, aggravate cerebral anoxia, hypotension, delirium, and depress respiratory function, may cause decrease in REM sleep and rebound on withdrawal; chloral hydrate causes gastrointestinal irritation; dalmane may cause an arthritic-like allergic reaction

Hypoglycemics

Action altered by other drugs; avoid alcohol; oral preparations have numerous adverse side effects; some persons allergic to pork and/or beef insulin

Laxatives

Phenolphthalein may cause cardiac and respiratory distress in susceptible individuals

Psychotropics

Antianxiety drugs cause CNS depression and ataxia and may be habit forming with a definite withdrawal syndrome; benzodiazapines cause drowsiness, vivid dreams, ataxia, and convulsions on withdrawal; alcohol should be avoided

Vitamins

Ascorbic acids in dose of 1 g/day can cause diarrhea and precipitation of oxalic and uric acid crystals; vitamin D in large doses produces hypercalcemia, weakness, fatigue, headache, nausea, vomiting, and diarrhea

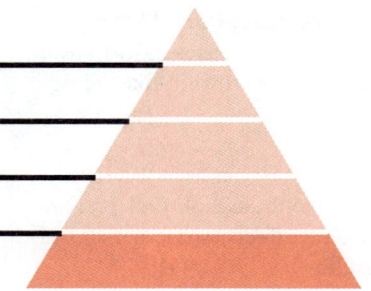

Drug-Induced Vitamin Deficiencies

Drug	Vitamin deficiencies
Aminopterin	Folic acid, vitamin B_{12}
Amitriptyline	Riboflavin
Aspirin	Folic acid, niacin, thiamin, vitamin C, vitamin K
Chloramphenicol	Riboflavin, vitamin B_6, vitamin B_{12}
Cholestyramine	Vitamin A, vitamin B_{12}, vitamin D, vitamin K
Cimetidine	Vitamin B_{12}
Colchicine	Folic acid, vitamin A, vitamin B_{12}
Coumadin	Vitamin K
Cycloserine	Folic acid, vitamin B_6, vitamin B_{12}
Digoxin	Thiamin
Erythromycin	Folic acid, vitamin B_{12}
Estrogen	Folic acid, riboflavin, thiamin, vitamin B_6, vitamin B_{12}, vitamin C
Ethotoin	Folic acid
5-Fluorouracil	Niacin
Glutethimide	Vitamin D
Indomethacin	Vitamin C
Mephenytoin	Folic acid
Methotrexate	Folic acid, vitamin B_{12}
Methyldopa	Folic acid, vitamin B_{12}
Neomycin	Folic acid, vitamin A, vitamin B_{12}, vitamin D, vitamin K
Nitrofuratoin	Folic acid
Phenelzine	Vitamin B_6
Phenformin	Folic acid, vitamin B_6, vitamin B_{12}
Phenobarbital	Folic acid, vitamin B_6, vitamin B_{12}, vitamin D
Phenolphthalein	Vitamin D
Phenothiazine	Vitamin B_{12}
Phenylutazone	Folic acid, niacin
Potassium chloride	Folic acid, vitamin B_{12}
Primidone	Folic acid, vitamin C, vitamin D
Probenecid	Riboflavin
Procarbazine	Vitamin B_{12}
Sulfasalazine	Folic acid
Sodium biocarbonate	Folic acid
Spironolactone	Vitamin A
Sulfonamides	Niacin, riboflavin, thiamine, vitamin B_6, vitamin C
Tetracycline	Folic acid, niacin, riboflavin, vitamin B_6, vitamin B_{12}
Thyroxine	Riboflavin, vitamin A
Triamterene	Folic acid, vitamin B_{12}
Trimethoprin	Folic acid
Vitamin E (megadose)	Vitamin K

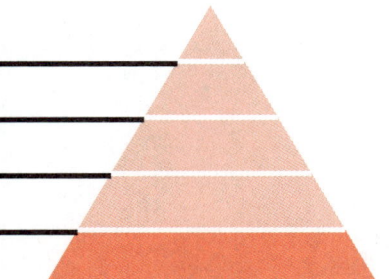

Examples of Mechanisms Causing Vitamin Deficiencies

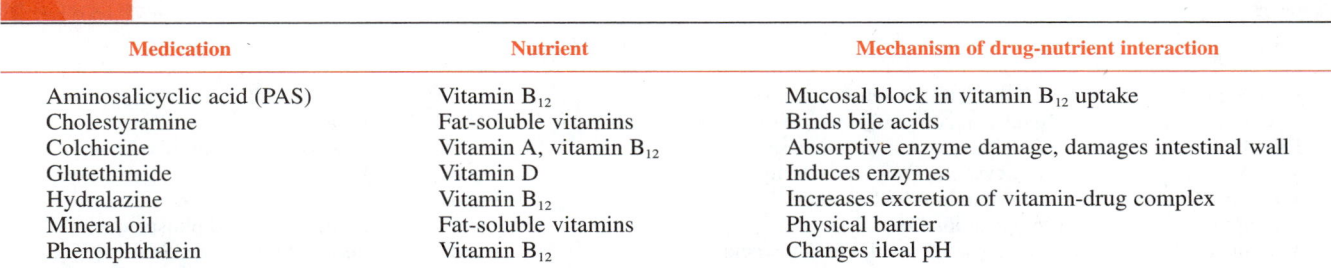

Medication	Nutrient	Mechanism of drug-nutrient interaction
Aminosalicyclic acid (PAS)	Vitamin B_{12}	Mucosal block in vitamin B_{12} uptake
Cholestyramine	Fat-soluble vitamins	Binds bile acids
Colchicine	Vitamin A, vitamin B_{12}	Absorptive enzyme damage, damages intestinal wall
Glutethimide	Vitamin D	Induces enzymes
Hydralazine	Vitamin B_{12}	Increases excretion of vitamin-drug complex
Mineral oil	Fat-soluble vitamins	Physical barrier
Phenolphthalein	Vitamin B_{12}	Changes ileal pH

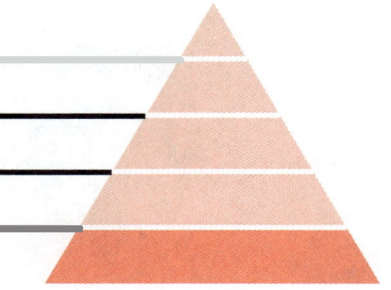

Screening Tests for Vitamin Deficiencies

Vitamin	Preferred laboratory test	Alternate tests
Folic acid	Red cell folate, histidine-load test	Plasma level
Niacin	N_1-methyl nicotinamide excretion	Urine niacin
Riboflavin	Erythrocyte glutatione reductase	Plasma level, urine riboflavin
Thiamin	Erythrocyte transketolase activity	Blood pyruvate
Vitamin A	Serum vitamin A and carotene	
Vitamin B_6	Tryptophan load test	Serum pyridoxal phosphate
Vitamin B_{12}	Serum B_{12}, urine methylmalonic acid	Serum thymidylate, Schilling's test
Vitamin C	Leukocyte ascorbic acid	Serum ascorbic acid
Vitamin D	Serum 25-hydroxycholecalciferol, serum alkaline phosphotase	Serum calcium and phosphorus
Vitamin E	Plasma level	
Vitamin K	Plasma level, prothrombin time	

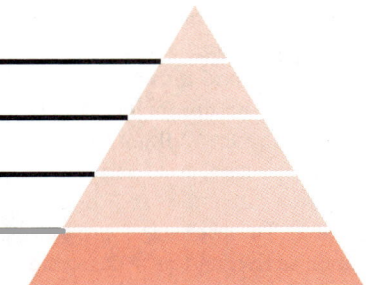

CHAPTER 11

Mobility

Students speculate

The thought of needing someone to help me shower and dress and transfer me from a chair to bed requires more acceptance than I have ever had to muster. I'm very good at making the best out of a bad situation, but somehow adapting to something like never walking again cannot be equated with a "bad situation." It is permanent, and it is the sacrifice of my precious independence. I was born on Independence Day! Thinking about these things overwhelms me with sadness.

Holiday, age 22

I feel like a trapped animal with the bars and straps they use when I'm in my bed and wheelchair, but they're worried about me falling, since I broke my arm the last time I slipped out of my wheelchair. I hate having to rely on people getting me around in my wheelchair, but it's necessary because of my arthritis.

Laura, age 30

Elders speak

I hate to have the family see me like this. You know, I was a military man. I took pride in the way I marched . . . or just stood at attention. I never imagined a time when I wouldn't be able to walk without assistance.

Jerry, age 78

Because of a CVA I have lost all sensation on my left side. That makes it difficult to walk. I use a cane and hold onto objects or persons. I am fortunate I have not lost any other sensory function.

Mary, over 70

The greatest challenges we have had are learning to adjust to increasing dependency, loss of physical strength, and lack of freedom to move about as we wish.

Leon and Alice, over 70

LEARNING OBJECTIVES

Upon completion of this chapter, the reader will be able to:

1. Describe age-related changes in bones, joints, and muscles that may predispose the individual to falls and accidents.
2. Discuss the effects of impaired mobility on general function and quality of life.
3. Discuss risk factors for impaired mobility.
4. Discuss factors that increase vulnerability to falls.
5. Describe the effects of restraints and alternative measures of protection.
6. Describe assessment measures to determine gait and walking stability.
7. Enumerate several measures to prevent falls and identify those at high risk.
8. Develop a nursing care plan appropriate to an elder at risk of falling.
9. Consider the impact of available transportation and driving in relation to independence.

Mobility is the capacity one has for movement within the personally available microcosm and macrocosm. In infancy moving about is the major mode of learning and interacting with the environment. In old age one moves more slowly and purposefully, sometimes with more forethought and caution. Throughout life, movement remains a significant means of personal contact, sensation, exploration, pleasure, and control. Movement is integral to the attainment of all levels of need as conceived by Maslow. Needs identified by elders (Wright and Aizenstein, 1993) include pride, maintaining dignity, social contacts, and activity. All of these are facilitated by mobility. Thus, in terms of Maslow's hierarchy and the needs identified by elders, maintaining mobility is an exceedingly important issue.

This chapter will focus on maintaining maximum mobility in health and in the presence of various disorders, the assessment of gait and mobility status, the effects of restraints and immobility, risk factors related to falls and preventive actions that nurses may take to reduce the risks, and aids and interventions that are useful when mobility is impaired. Also included are transportation and driving as essential aspects of environmental mobility.

Mobility and comparative degrees of agility are based upon muscle strength, flexibility, postural stability, vibratory sensation, cognition, and perceptions of stability (Roberts, 1988b). Aging produces changes in muscles and joints, particularly of the back and legs. Strength and flexibility of muscles decrease markedly and endurance to a somewhat lesser extent. Movements and range of motion become more limited. Normal wear and tear reduces the smooth coverings of joints. Movement is less fluid as one ages and joints change as regeneration of tissue slows and muscle wasting occurs. Some normal gait changes in late life include a narrower standing base, wider swaying when walking, the appearance of a "waddle," bowing of the legs, and less muscular control of the lower extremities. Steps are shorter and with a decreased stepping motion. These changes are less pronounced in those who remain active and at a desirable weight.

Inappropriate clothing may hinder mobility. Clothing that is fitted, back-closing, and knee-length is not comfortable for persons confined to wheelchairs, those with limited range of motion, or those who require catheters or prosthetic devices. Elders living alone have no one to help them button or zip the back of clothing. This can make dressing and undressing a time-consuming and frustrating experience. Adaptive fashions have been designed to facilitate easy or independent dressing and include features such as back and side openings, Velcro front openings, raglan sleeves, and cape-styled clothing. Slacks, with front flaps or extra room in back, or longer skirts are helpful. The fabric should be chosen for comfort, durability, attractiveness, and ease of laundering. Other items to facilitate moving about include wheelchair bags, catheter bags, and carefully chosen footwear (see Chapter 8).

Various degrees of immobility are often the temporary or permanent consequences of illness. On a broader scale, elders frequently have limited environmental mobility be-

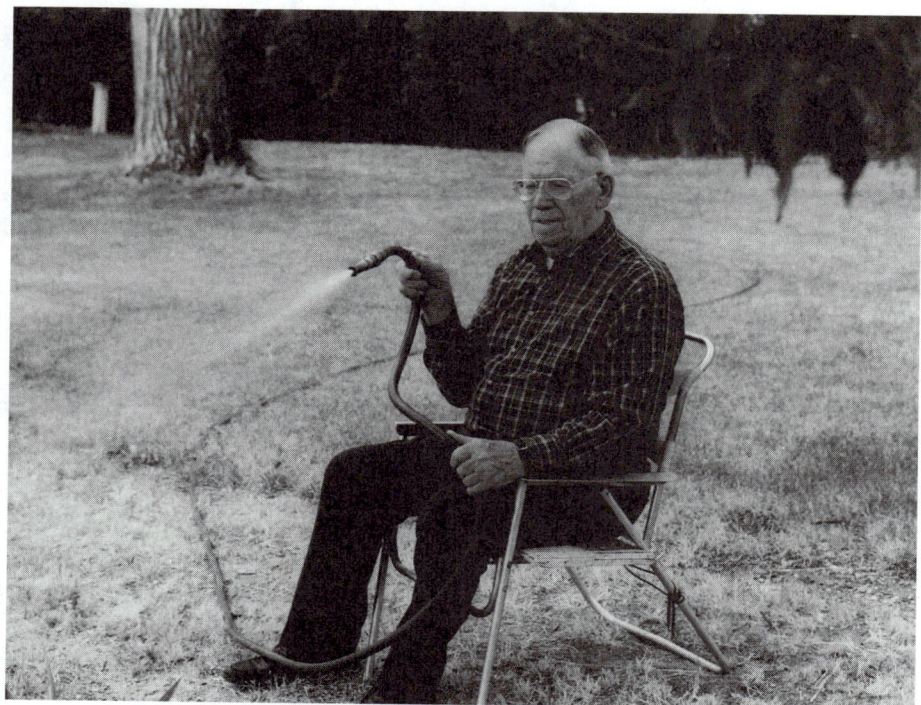

Adapting to impaired mobility. (Courtesy Rod Schmall.)

cause of lack of transportation or loss of driver's licence. On the most personal level, some elderly are immobilized by the fear of falling. In summary, many normal and abnormal changes affect the fluidity and comfort of movement and the capacity for involvement with surroundings. Limitations in mobility for whatever cause have serious consequences.

DISORDERS AFFECTING MOBILITY

Common conditions that accompany the normal changes of aging, as well as disorders that occur more frequently in the elderly, merit special attention. Such disorders or orthopedic impairments significantly impede the aged. Osteoporosis, gait disorders, Parkinson's disease, accidents, and fear of falling must be considered. Rheumatoid arthritis, osteoarthritis, and osteoporosis markedly affect movement and functional capacities. Mobility may be limited by paresthesias, hemiplegia, neuromotor disturbances, fractures, foot, knee, and hip problems, and illnesses that deplete one's energy. All of these conditions are likely to occur more frequently and have more devastating effects as one ages. More than one third (388 per thousand) of those over 65 years of age have some of these afflictions, with females significantly outnumbering males in this respect (U.S. Bureau of Census, 1995). Guralnik et al (1995) found various levels of difficulty among women in accomplishing mobility-related tasks. Table 11-1 shows the percentage of women having trouble with certain mobility-related tasks. The chronicity of these disorders is addressed in Chapter 8.

Osteopenia and Osteoporosis

Normally there is a gradual continual loss of cortical and trabecular bone in both men and women as they age. Osteopenia and osteoporosis are conditions in which a loss of bony tissue results in brittle bones that fracture easily. Osteopenia is defined as bone mineral density 1 to 2.5 standard deviations below that of the normal young adult female; osteoporosis is bone mineral loss that exceeds that amount. Fifty percent of women over age 50 have osteopenia; this increases to 57% for women 70 to 79 years old but decreases to 45% for women over 80 (Ezzati et al, 1994; Looker et al, 1995). This seems to indicate that those who survive beyond 80 may be generally of sturdier bone density (Figure 11-1). To determine the factors that contribute to osteopenia, Bauer (1993) evaluated a group of nearly 10,000 elderly community-residing women in Maryland, Minnesota, Oregon, and Pennsylvania. He found that greater bone mass was present in individuals with the associated variables listed in Box 11-1.

The dynamics of osteoporosis are complex, involving the interrelationship of dietary mineral metabolism, vitamin D, and hormone activity. The development of osteoporosis can be compared to a savings account (bone mass) with its assets (input of calcium for added bone density) and debits (the loss of calcium with the loss of bone density). As long as there is calcium intake in proportion to the other mechanisms, bone mass and density will be maintained and osteoporosis will not occur. When there is a deficiency of calcium, or a decrease in hormone levels that facilitate the absorption of calcium, there will be a greater loss of calcium than input. The result is less dense bone and the gradual development of osteoporotic manifestations. Gastrointestinal age-related changes and the inadequacy of dietary calcium of older adults are among the factors that leave elders prone to osteoporosis.

Toufexis (1994) reports genetic studies that indicate a gene that heightens the risk of osteoporosis by hampering the uptake of vitamin D. According to this research, the risk of osteoporosis depends heavily on whether one inherits the low–bone density (B) form or the high–bone density (b) form of this gene. Obviously a person who inherits the low-density gene from both parents (BB) would be at high risk. In the examination of 311 women they found that those with BB had serious fracture potential 18 years after menopause; those with Bb, four years later; and women with bb were not at the fracture threshold until 29 years after menopause. Compared with women at age 50 the incidence of osteoporosis increases exponentially with every decade of life. Vertebrae, wrists, and femoral neck bones lose the greatest proportion of trabecular tissue and are thus most fragile and likely to break with unusual pressure. It is estimated that osteoporosis affects 24 million people in the United States, including 50% of women over age 45 and 90% of women over 75 (Bourguet et al, 1991).

Bone Mass. Bone density is determined about 75% by heredity and 25% by environmental factors (Toufexis, 1994). Risk factors are well known and include being female, White or Asian, postmenopausal, nulliparous, small, lean, sedentary; having low calcium and vitamin D intake, high intake of nicotine, caffeine, alcohol, and phosphate; heredity; and advancing age. At this time there is equivocal evidence regarding alcohol intake and its effects on osteoporosis. A study utilizing data from the Framingham Heart Study found that moderate consumption of alcohol increased bone density in both men and women (Felson et al, 1995).

Osteoporosis can also result from prolonged steroid therapy and other medications such as thyroid, heparin, furosemide, tetracycline, anticonvulsants, and aluminum-containing antacids; endocrine disorders (notably Cushing's syndrome, parathyroidism, hyperthyroidism, premature menopause, and hyperadrenocorticism); gastrointestinal disorders such as malabsorption syndrome, peptic ulcer, lactase deficiency, and subtotal gastrectomy. Infection, injury, and synovitis may cause localized bone loss in affected areas.

Males with low levels of testosterone and hypogonadism have been found to be predisposed to osteoporosis and fractures. This suggests that osteoporosis prevention for older men may have been neglected because it has largely been considered a problem of postmenopausal women (Box 11-2).

Table 11-1   Percentage of Women Reporting Difficulty in Mobility-Related Tasks and Level of Difficulty Reported[a, b]

Task and level of difficulty	Total (N = 1002)	Age group			Disability level		
		65-74 (N = 388)	75-84 (N = 311)	85+ (N = 303)	Moderate[c] (N = 343)	ADL difficulty	
						Receives no help (N = 478)	Receives help (N = 181)
Stooping, crouching, or kneeling[d]	82.6	84.5	82.1	78.1	68.2	89.5	93.1
Level of difficulty[e, f]							
A little	10.3	11.7	9.8	7.5	14.4	8.4	7.1
Some	14.0	17.3	12.3	8.9	16.6	15.2	5.2
A lot	20.7	23.9	20.4	11.8	16.0	25.2	17.6
Unable to do	37.5	31.6	39.6	49.4	20.9	40.7	63.2
Doing heavy housework such as washing windows, walls, or floors[g]	81.6	80.4	82.8	82.0	77.1	79.7	96.4
Level of difficulty[e, f]							
A little	6.4	8.4	5.5	2.7	10.5	5.4	0.7
Some	9.2	11.5	8.5	4.0	11.0	10.1	2.7
A lot	11.1	15.6	8.5	4.6	15.7	10.4	3.5
Unable to do	54.8	44.6	60.3	70.1	39.9	53.7	89.0
Walking for a quarter of a mile, that is about 2 or 3 blocks[h]	74.4	69.7	76.5	82.4	66.0	75.4	89.0
Level of difficulty[e, f]							
A little	13.7	12.9	16.4	9.1	20.0	12.5	4.2
Some	14.8	14.8	16.3	11.1	17.5	13.9	11.8
A lot	19.1	20.7	19.6	13.3	17.2	22.6	13.6
Unable to do	26.3	21.0	24.3	47.4	11.2	25.9	58.8
Walking up 10 steps without resting[h]	51.9	49.3	53.3	55.3	37.2	53.5	77.6
Level of difficulty[e, f]							
A little	8.4	6.6	10.8	7.2	8.9	9.2	5.2
Some	15.0	17.4	13.7	11.7	14.8	15.4	14.3
A lot	15.1	16.6	13.8	14.4	9.4	17.1	21.4
Unable to do	13.2	8.8	15.1	21.5	4.1	11.6	36.7
Walking across a small room[d]	25.5	19.4	25.2	44.1	7.2	26.6	60.0
Level of difficulty[e, f]							
A little	4.4	2.5	4.4	9.8	3.0	5.1	5.3
Some	8.4	6.2	8.5	14.8	3.3	10.6	13.1
A lot	5.4	4.8	4.7	9.3	0.9	5.7	14.0
Unable to do	7.0	5.6	7.6	9.4	0.1	4.8	27.2

(Women's Health and Aging Study, screening and baseline interviews, 1992-1995)
From Guralnik JM et al: *The Women's Health and Aging Study: health and social characteristics of older women with disability,* NIH Pub No 95-4009, Bethesda, Md, 1995, National Institute on Aging.
[a]All variables have less than 2% missing data. Results are based on non-missing data.
[b]Descriptive statistics are based on weighted data.
[c]No ADL difficulty; disabled in two or more domains.
[d]The question is in the form "By yourself, that is, without help from another person or special equipment, do you have any difficulty . . . ?"
[e]How much difficulty do you have?
[f]The percents of participants reporting their levels of difficulty may not add up to the percent reporting difficulty due to (1) rounding (2) level of difficulty not reported.
[g]The screener question is the form "Because of a health or physical problem, do you have any difficulty . . . ?" The presence of the condition was confirmed in the baseline interview.
[h]The screener question is in the form "By yourself, that is, without help from another person or special equipment, do you have any difficulty . . . ?" The presence of the condition was confirmed in the baseline interview.

Assessment. Outward signs of osteoporosis are a loss of height, "dowager's hump," and fractures of vertebrae (Haskell, 1992) (Figure 11-2). Ideally it should be diagnosed by the use of a bone densitometer before becoming so grossly visible (Mastrangelo, 1994). Osteoporosis is termed a "silent thief" and seldom comes to anyone's attention un-til there is a fracture of the hip or vertebrae (Galsworthy and Wilson, 1996). Watts (1991) contends that primary physicians have the responsibility for identifying patients at risk and instituting appropriate preventive measures.

Measuring the rate of bone resorption is a sophisticated and complex procedure best accomplished by measuring the

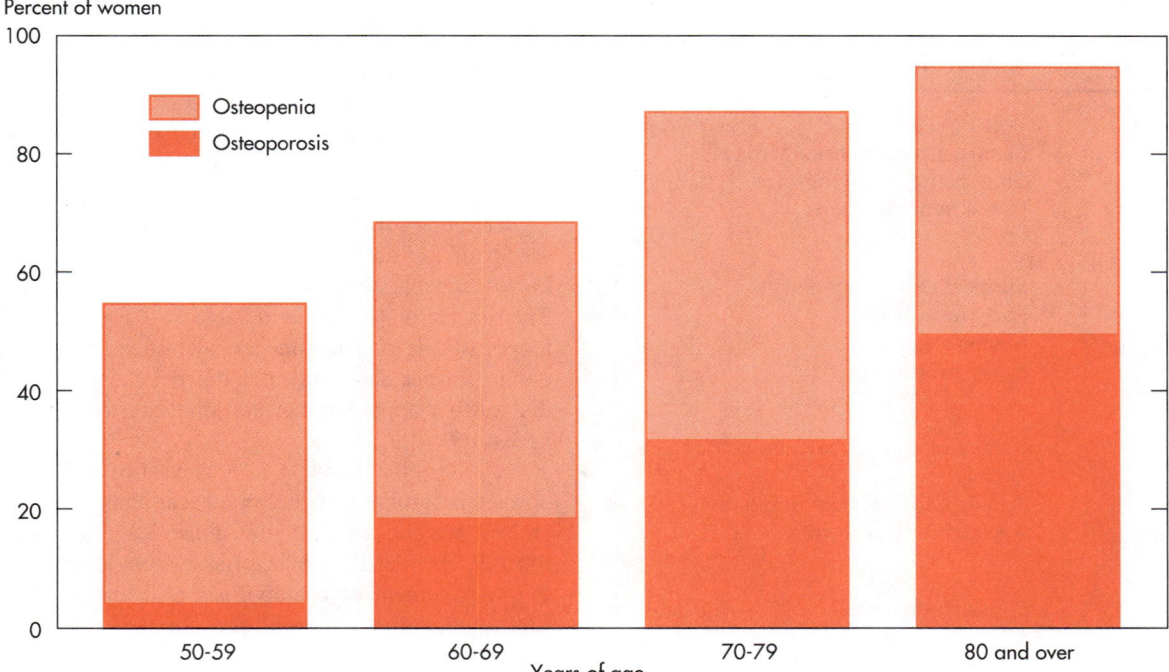

Notes: Osteopenia is defined as a bone mineral density 1 to 2.5 standard deviations below the mean of white, non-Hispanic women 20-29 years of age as measured in NHANES III (Phase I); osteoporosis is defined as a bone mineral density value of more than 2.5 standard deviations below the mean of young white, non-Hispanic women (WHO expert panel).

Figure 11-1. Prevalence of reduced hip bone density among women 50 years of age and over in the United States by age and severity, 1988-1991. (From Centers for Disease Control and Prevention, National Center for Health Statistics, National Health and Nutrition Examination Survey III [Phase I].)

urinary excretion of cross-linked peptides (Gertz et al, 1994). Standard x-ray examinations cannot reliably detect bone loss until the disease is advanced to at least 30% bone tissue loss. There is no simple, reliable, and risk-free diagnostic technique, although a recently approved blood test (Tandem-R Ostase) measures a blood marker known as ostase that gauges the rate of bone turnover (Mann, 1996). Preliminary trials of this method are encouraging. Presently, the most accurate technique is bone density measurement. This can be done through dual photon absorptiometry (DPA), quantitative computerized tomography (QCT), or dual-energy x-ray absorptiometry (DEXA) (Watts, 1991). Ultrasound examination of the patella is useful to identify women who have osteoporitic fractures. Although this procedure is less expensive and has considerably lower risk, it is revealing only for women with substantial bone loss. Most of the procedures are expensive and involve some degree of radiation exposure. Box 11-3 outlines several of these tests.

A major problem is the lack of attention to prevention or medical management of this common disorder (Lindsay, 1995). Bourguet et al (1991) found that only 10% of women seeing their family physician were assessed for risk of

---

Box 11-1 | **Variables Associated with Bone Mass in Aged Females**

Variables Listed in Descending Order of Association with Bone Mass Preservation
Estrogen use
Non–insulin dependent diabetes
Thiazide use
Increased weight
Greater muscle strength
Later age at menopause
Greater height

Variables Associated with Bone Mass Loss
Alcohol use
Decreased physical activity
Calcium deficiency
Pregnancies
History of breast-feeding
Parental nationality (European)
Hair color (blond, red)

Data from Bauer DC: Factors associated with appendicular bone mass in older women, *Ann Intern Med* 118:657, 1993.

Box 11-2	**Risk Assessment for Osteoporosis**	

Yes	No	**Heredity**
[ ]	[ ]	Family history of osteoporosis
[ ]	[ ]	Thin, petite, small muscled
[ ]	[ ]	Fair skin or thin skin

		Hormones
[ ]	[ ]	Surgical removal of ovaries
[ ]	[ ]	Early menopause
[ ]	[ ]	Menopausal
[ ]	[ ]	Never pregnant

		Calcium
[ ]	[ ]	Unsure of amount calcium getting daily
[ ]	[ ]	Avoids milk and dairy products
[ ]	[ ]	Avoided milk as a child

		Physical Activity
[ ]	[ ]	Physically inactive
[ ]	[ ]	Muscles weak and poorly toned
[ ]	[ ]	Seldom exercises

		Lifestyle
[ ]	[ ]	Drinks or smokes heavily
[ ]	[ ]	Taking medications
[ ]	[ ]	Diet contains a large amount of caffeine, salt, protein

Signs of Osteoporosis

(Height equals arm span, except for black people, whose arm span is generally greater than height) (Krames, 1985.)

[ ]	[ ]	Lost height
[ ]	[ ]	Upper back curves forward
[ ]	[ ]	Have fractured a wrist, spine, or hip or lost teeth lately

Living Safely with Osteoporosis

[ ]	[ ]	Wears high-heeled shoes
[ ]	[ ]	Does a lot of bending and lifting
[ ]	[ ]	Takes tranquilizers or drugs that cause drowsiness or dizziness
[ ]	[ ]	Safety hazards exist in home

TOTAL NUMBER OF RISK FACTORS

Modified from *Osteoporosis,* Daly City, Calif, 1986, Krames Communications.

osteoporosis and only 8% discussed risk factors with their physician, even though 19% received one or more interventions that would directly impact their osteoporosis risk. Even osteoporotic bone pain, a common and excruciating result of vertebral collapse, is often virtually ignored by professionals.

In assessing osteoporosis, the measure of disability is important. Helmes et al (1995) developed the Osteoporosis Functional Disability Questionnaire (OFDQ) to assess disability in persons with osteoporosis and back pain due to vertebral fractures. It appears to be a reliable instrument that correlates well with objective measures of spinal osteoporosis (see Appendix A).

Screening for risk factors of osteoporosis is an important aspect of the nurse's role. This requires that the nurse be knowledgeable about the risk factors and the disease itself. The risk factors are listed in Table 11-2 for types I and II osteoporosis. If risk factors are identified, the nurse should obtain further data and refer the person to a physician so that further appraisal can be done and treatment begun if necessary.

Living with Osteoporosis. Measures to prevent osteoporosis progression include physical activity, nutrition, exercise, weight bearing, adequate calcium intake, and lifestyle changes that reduce risk factors and are primary to the management of osteoporosis (Ali and Twibell, 1994). Education, fall prevention, and possibly estrogen replacement therapy (ERT) must be considered.

Physical activity plays an essential role in prevention of osteoporosis by maintaining bone mass. Weight-bearing activity such as brisk walking 20 minutes or more daily is excellent. It provides not only mechanical force, spine and long bone movement, but also sunlight exposure and vitamin D.

Exercise for those with osteoporosis provides increased muscle support of bones and improves flexibility and balance elements, which are extremely valuable in preventing fractures associated with the disease as well as maintaining general health. Postural exercises should be done to minimize the curvature and to maintain good posture. Physical activities such as dancing, walking, and swimming are very beneficial and a safe way for individuals with osteoporosis to remain active. An osteopathic physician or physical therapist is the best person from whom to seek an exercise program suited to individual condition and needs.

Muscle-building exercises help to maintain skeletal architecture by improving muscle strength and flexibility. Some evidence indicates muscle building also helps build bone (Osteoporosis Research, Education and Health promotion, 1990). Participation in a variety of exercises that include all parts of the body is important to prevent boredom and promote continued interest in maintaining a program. Research is underway into mechanical stress exercise applied to specific portions of the skeleton and the effect on bone strength in those sites. Ginsberg (1994) reports that weight training with professional trainers has helped develop muscle and bone strength in women who felt too fragile for such activity.

Lifestyle changes are necessary for those with osteoporosis, especially when there is evidence of eating and drinking patterns of excessive alcohol, protein, salt, and caffeine. Re-

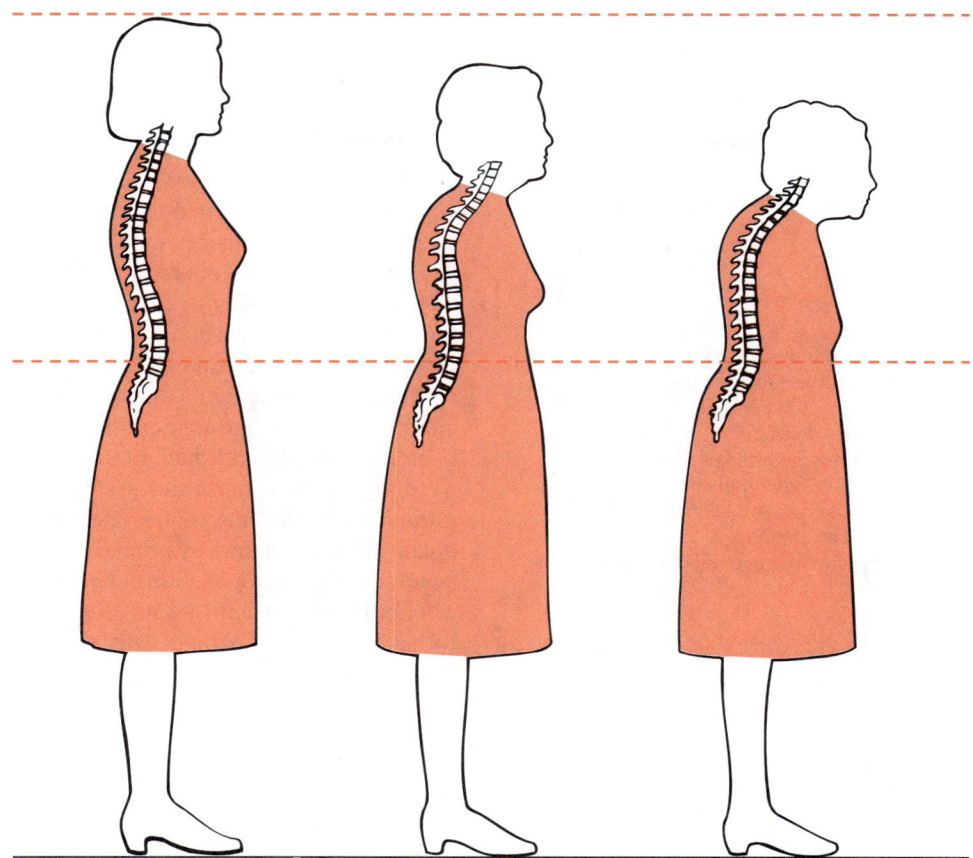

Figure 11-2. Osteoporosis spine alignment.

duction of cigarette smoking is another change that becomes necessary. All of these excesses cause bone to lose calcium.

Education/knowledge is perhaps the most important issue in prevention and treatment of osteoporosis. Knowledge about the sites most vulnerable to fracture through accidents, falls, back strain, and poor posture should be provided. Explanation should be given about changes in the upper spine that occur when vertebrae are weakened, and the pain that results from strain on the lower spine to compensate for balance and height changes due to alteration of the upper spine.

Personal safety should be addressed for those with osteoporosis to avoid falls. Shoes with good support should be worn. Handrails should be used and walking in poorly lighted areas should be avoided. Basic body mechanics such as not bending or lifting heavy objects should be learned. Use of step stools or chairs for reaching things in high places should be discouraged. Home safety should include good lighting, railings, and other aids as needed. Walkways should be kept free of obstacles; loose rugs and electrical cords should be arranged so that they do not cause falls.

Prevention and Treatment.   Actual prevention of osteoporosis must begin in the teen years. As women increasingly live into their 80s and 90s the treatment of osteoporosis is

---

Box 11-3	**Use and Value of Diagnostic Tests for Osteoporosis**

X-ray
Screening test; least sensitive

SPA (Single Photon Absorptometry)
Accurate; sensitive; safe; uses wrist to determine core bone; establishes severity of bone loss

DPA
Accurate; sensitive; safe; uses hips and spine; establishes severity of bone loss

QCT
Like CT or CAT scan, accurate; sensitive; safe; uses vertebrae; looks at cross-section of bone

Modified from Kaplan FS: Osteoporosis, *Clin Symp* 39(1):21, 1987.

becoming big business. In September 1994 the Pharmaceutical Research and Manufacturers Association of America reported that there were 23 different products in various stages of clinical trials by 16 pharmaceutical companies (NIAMS, 1996). Mundy (1995) notes that though we

Table 11-2   Risk Factors for Types I and II Osteoporosis

General factors	Specifics
Type I	
Genetic background	Predominantly white women
	Northwestern European
	Fair skin
Body characteristics	Small
	Slender
Activity level	Immobile
	Inactive
Diseases	Hyperparathyroidism
	Hyperthyroidism
	Cushing's syndrome
	Kidney disease
	Rheumatoid arthritis
	Advanced alcoholism
	Liver cirrhosis
	Diabetes mellitus
	Chronic obstructive pulmonary disease
Type II	
Drugs	Corticosteroids
	Isoniazid
	Tetracycline
	Some anticonvulsants
	Thyroid supplements
	Furosemide
	Heparin
Other	Gonadal hormone deficiencies
	Smoking

Compiled from Jennings J, Baylink D: Osteoporosis. In Calkins E, Davis PJ, Ford AB, editors: *The practice of geriatrics*, Philadelphia, 1986, WB Saunders; Miller G: Osteoporosis: is it inevitable?, *J Gerontol Nurs* 11:10, 1985; Spencer H et al: Disorders of the skeletal system. In Rossman I, editor: *Clinical geriatrics*, ed 3, Philadelphia, 1986, JB Lippincott.

presently have several effective drugs for osteoporosis, clinical trials show that even better ones are needed. At this time osteoporotic damage cannot be repaired, but prevention of the resorption of bone with various pharmaceuticals is an important goal.

Sodium fluoride has been thought to be useful in strengthening bone mass. Slow-release sodium fluoride and calcium citrate administered for 4 years has been shown to inhibit vertebral fractures (Pak et al, 1995); however, Sogaard et al (1995) found increasing reduction in bone strength and quality during long-term ingestion of sodium fluoride. Clearly, more study of sodium fluoride will be necessary.

The three pharmacologic treatments now available are by prescription only: hormone replacement therapy, calcitonin, and alendronate sodium (Fosamax). The standard treatment for osteoporosis has been estrogen (Prestwood et al, 1994) and calcium supplementation and recommendations for increased exercise and weight bearing. Long-term use of calcium supplementation, 5 years or more, reduces the lifetime fracture rate at all sites and by 50% at the hip (U.S. Department of Health and Human Services, 1995). However, the

public is becoming more cautious because the incidence of breast cancer has risen in tandem with the use of artificial hormones. Endometrial cancer is also a possibility when using unopposed estrogen. Estrogens must be used with special caution by individuals who have had thrombotic disorders and fibrocystic breast disease. Several longitudinal studies of women have demonstrated the efficacy of estrogen replacement therapy (ERT) in slowing the rate of bone resorption in women (National Osteoporosis Foundation, 1996).

Calcitonin was first discovered in 1962, but its physiologic role remains obscure. Its principal action is to inhibit osteoclastic bone resorption, which exerts a positive effect on bone mass. Rifat and colleagues (1992) found that calcitonin, a natural hormone produced by the parafollicular C cells of the thyroid, had an analgesic effect as well as bone regeneration capacities. Calcitonin may act as a neurotransmitter and may potentiate the body's endogenous opiate system and thereby relieve pain. This research could have significant implications. Recent developments with calcitonin-salmon indicate its effectiveness in nasal spray form, and there is strong evidence that it will decrease bone resorption and vertebral pain in the presence of osteoporosis (Rifat et al, 1992).

Therapeutic approaches for replacing lost bone, or restorative treatment, are still in the experimental stages, though the use of etidronate increased bone density among participants in an experimental study (Watts, 1991).

Recent pharmacologic research into the efficacy of alendronate sodium, an amino-biphosphonate, in the slowing of bone resorption is promising. Results of 2-year longtitudinal studies will soon be released. There is also some evidence that when given in combination with calcium, it restores some bone mass that has been lost (Merck, 1995). It is reported that side effects are mild and include abdominal and musculoskeletal pain, nausea, heartburn, and irritation of the esophagus.

One must be cautious, particularly with very old women, because long-range effects of none of these medications are known. Simple, effective, and risk-free diagnostic or treatment methods are not available at this time.

Nursing Interventions. Intervention, like prevention, should be directed toward educating clients about their medical regimen, assisting them in adapting to their disease, and preventing disease progression. Medical interventions of which the nurse should be knowledgeable include the various types of therapies used in the treatment of osteoporosis (Figure 11-3). Therapy includes the use of several drugs or combinations of drugs, some of which have not yet received Food and Drug Administration (FDA) approval. Estrogen replacement therapy for women who are in menopause or who have had surgical removal of their ovaries retards bone loss.

Nursing interventions for the individual with osteoporosis who is not hospitalized should focus on teaching and assisting the individual to maintain a positive approach toward

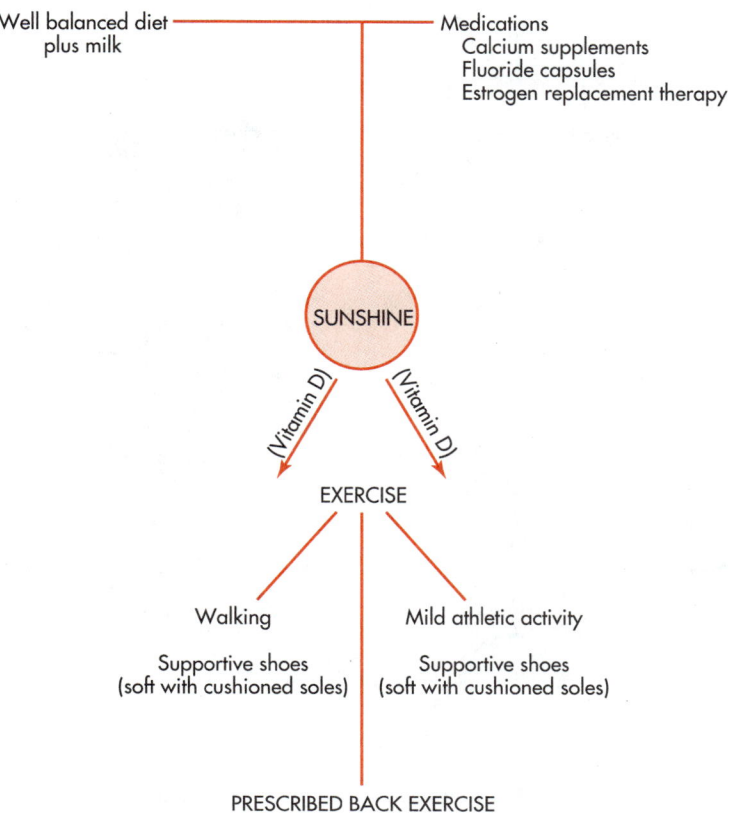

Well balanced diet
plus milk

Medications
   Calcium supplements
   Fluoride capsules
   Estrogen replacement therapy

SUNSHINE

(Vitamin D)   (Vitamin D)

EXERCISE

Walking

Supportive shoes
(soft with cushioned soles)

Mild athletic activity

Supportive shoes
(soft with cushioned soles)

PRESCRIBED BACK EXERCISE

Figure 11-3. Treatment of osteoporosis.

the disease and prevention of its progression or complications. Interventions include the following:

1. Teaching about nutritionally balanced calcium-rich diets including milk, or milk substitutes for those who are lactose intolerant (see the discussion of nutrition in Chapter 6)
2. Teaching the client to take 1500 mg calcium daily through diet and/or calcium supplements
3. Teaching about the factors that inhibit calcium absorption, such as excess protein or salt, and excretion enhancers, such as caffeine, excess fiber, phosphorus in meats, sodas and preserved foods, and the influence of the body's response to stress (decreased calcium absorption and increased excretion of calcium in the urine)
4. Discussing the pros and cons of ERT
5. Ensuring understanding of medication and adjunct regimen
6. Encouraging women to maintain a daily schedule or alternate-day schedule of weight-bearing exercises such as walking, low-impact aerobics, workout machines, swimming, or a combination of activities

Much remains to be done in preventing osteoporosis. Young women must be taught preventive measures in order to forstall the development of osteoporosis and reduce the enormous cost of osteoporotic fractures and the painful disability and discomfort to the individual.

Degenerative Joint Diseases

Degenerative arthritic and rheumatic disorders are the most common of the afflictions that disable elders. It is estimated there are 120 types of these problems that arise from various combinations of overuse, obesity, enzyme imbalances, and infections. They affect up to 37 million individuals in the United States, young as well as old (Dalton, 1995), and include disorders of joints and connective tissue throughout the body. These disorders create pain, depression, immobility, and functional and self-concept disturbances. Arthritis, though the most prevalent disorder of aging, is by no means equally distributed throughout the elderly population by age, gender, or geography. At age 65 more than 373 per thousand of these are men and 533 per thousand are women (U.S. Bureau of the Census, 1995). Those states with the most cases can be seen in Figure 11-4. Thirty eight percent of those over 65 years of age have limitation of activity; this figure increases to 44% by age 75 (U.S. Department of Health and Human Services, 1995).

Osteoarthritis. Osteoarthritis (OA), a "wear and tear" noninflammatory joint disorder that affects at least 16 million Americans, is characterized by the deterioration of articular

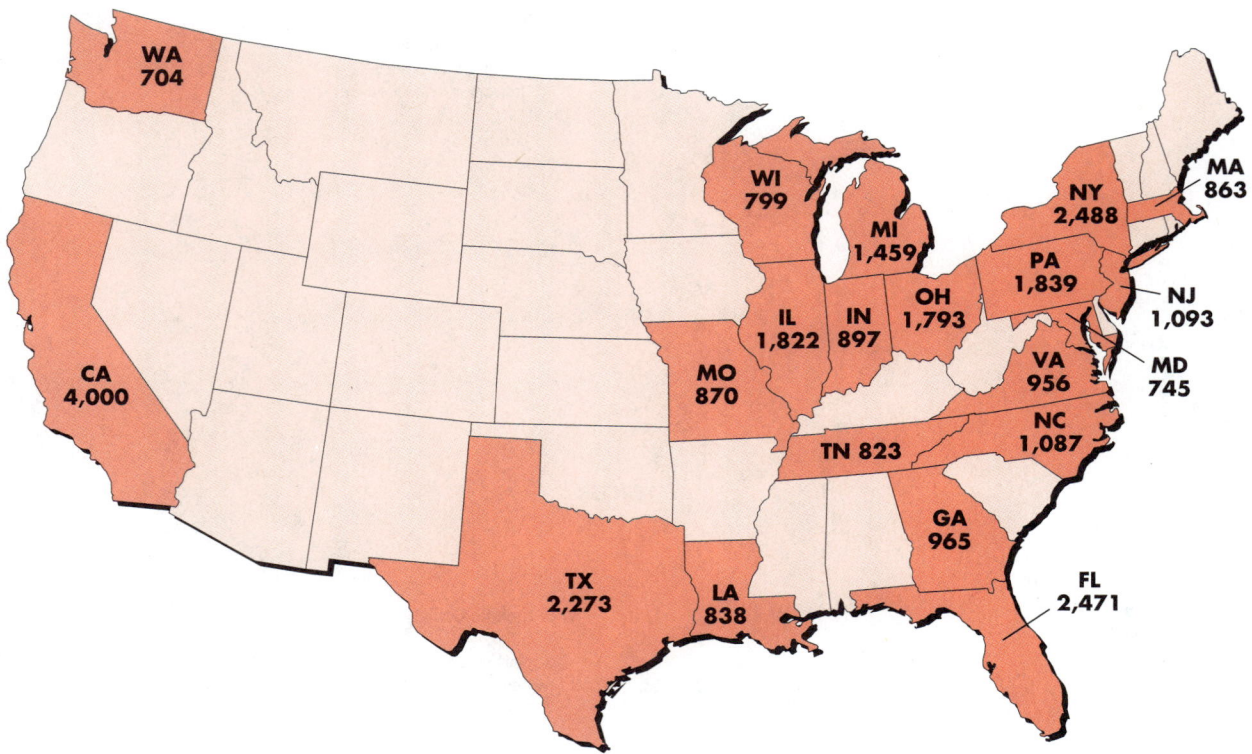

Figure 11-4. Cases of self-reported arthritis and activity limitation attributable to arthritis—United States, 1990 (in thousands). (From US Department of Health and Human Services, *Research News,* Bethesda, Md.)

cartilage, which continues to slowly progress. It is the most common of the arthritic disorders, and 90% of elders show some evidence of these changes on x-ray examination, though they are not necessarily aware of arthritic changes. Elderly persons with OA experience joint deterioration more often than younger persons because joint protective mechanisms such as neuromuscular response and muscle conditioning are impaired in elders (Felson, 1993). Excess weight exacerbates the problems. Many find movement restricted and joints hypertrophied, stiff, and painful. Discomfort tends to be worse in the morning after a night of inactivity, after excessive use, and when there is change in the weather. Major areas affected are hands, knees, hips, lumbar spine, and cervical spine. One may hear a grinding or grating sound, particularly in the neck, when moving. This crepitation is an indication of the deterioration of the synovial covering of the joint (Figure 11-5).

About 85% of people over 70 years of age have varying degrees of neck pain due to OA (Mayo Foundation for Medical Education and Research, 1994). OA of the knee occurs in about 10% of individuals over age 65 and accounts for considerable pain, disability, and costly care. Most total knee replacements are done because of OA (Galanos, 1992). OA of the hip is the most prevalent form of arthritis in the United States. Persons with OA of the hip experience pain, localized to the groin and anterior or lateral thigh, morning stiffness, and gel phenomenon (feeling that the joint is frozen in one position) (Hochberg et al, 1995). While not as frequent, OA of the hand may be particularly troublesome because so much of our daily life depends upon object manipulation. Characteristically, it limits movement at the base of the thumb and the end joints of the fingers (Johns Hopkins Medical Letter, 1993).

Assessment. Various assessment tools have been devised to measure joint movement limitations. Grip and the pinch gauge measure strength. Range of motion (ROM) and pain in hands and fingers demonstrate movement limitations. Overhead lift of weight and shoulder rotation test strength and ROM of shoulder. Knee extensor and hip flexion measure ROM, strength, and discomfort (Guralnik et al, 1995).

Interventions. The goals of intervention and management of OA are to control pain, to minimize disability, and to educate the client (Hochberg et al, 1995). It is clear that obesity aggravates the symptoms of OA of the knee. Therefore the first positive action an individual might take is weight reduction. Cowan and Galanos (1992) describe a supervised fitness walking regimen for OA of the knees designed to maintain mobility and functional status. They found that when carefully supervised, walking for short periods was successful in reducing pain and increasing walking capacity. There is still disagreement in the literature about the wisdom of walking any more than necessary with an osteoarthritic knee. The value of walking, if these findings can be replicated, may be in morale and weight control as well as weight bearing and movement. Figure 11-6 illus-

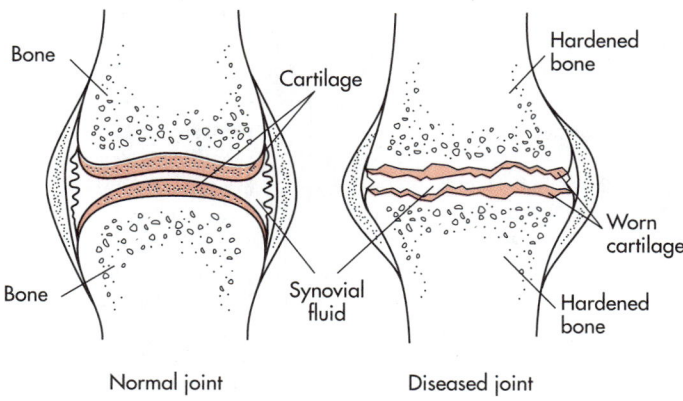

Figure 11-5. Normal joint and diseased joint.

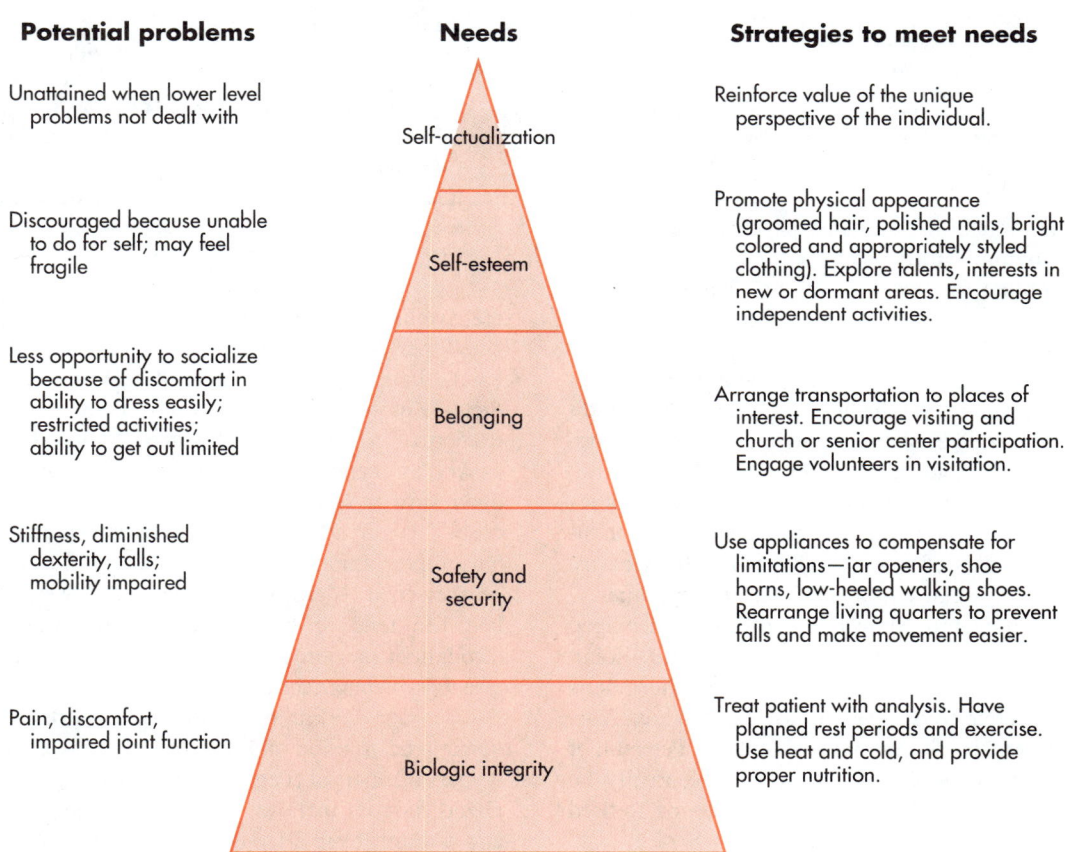

Potential problems	Needs	Strategies to meet needs
Unattained when lower level problems not dealt with	Self-actualization	Reinforce value of the unique perspective of the individual.
Discouraged because unable to do for self; may feel fragile	Self-esteem	Promote physical appearance (groomed hair, polished nails, bright colored and appropriately styled clothing). Explore talents, interests in new or dormant areas. Encourage independent activities.
Less opportunity to socialize because of discomfort in ability to dress easily; restricted activities; ability to get out limited	Belonging	Arrange transportation to places of interest. Encourage visiting and church or senior center participation. Engage volunteers in visitation.
Stiffness, diminished dexterity, falls; mobility impaired	Safety and security	Use appliances to compensate for limitations—jar openers, shoe horns, low-heeled walking shoes. Rearrange living quarters to prevent falls and make movement easier.
Pain, discomfort, impaired joint function	Biologic integrity	Treat patient with analysis. Have planned rest periods and exercise. Use heat and cold, and provide proper nutrition.

Figure 11-6. Osteoarthritis wellness perspective.

trates management of OA from a wellness perspective. Medical management guidelines can be seen in Table 11-3.

Particular guidelines for the best ways to relieve OA of the hand can be seen in Box 11-4.

General principles for all types of OA are intermittent rest periods interspersed with periods of mild activity; cold applications to ease pain and warmth to relax muscles (applications not to exceed 20 minutes for each); in some cases immobilization with braces when pain is aggravated by movement; and NSAIDs judiciously used and never on an empty stomach (Mayo, 1994). Arthroscopy, or surgery through a thin telescope inserted directly into the joint, is sometimes helpful but is not suitable for everyone.

Surgical total joint arthroplasty (replacement of hips and knees) brings relief from pain and functional limitations. Consideration must be given to the potential for

Table 11-3   Medial Management of Patients with Osteoarthritis of the Hip*

Nonpharmacologic therapy

Patient education
  Self-management programs (e.g., Arthritis Self-Help Course)
Health professional social support via telephone contact
Weight loss (if overweight)
Physical therapy
  Range of motion exercises
  Strengthening exercises
  Assistive devices for ambulation
Occupational therapy
  Joint protection and energy conservation
  Assistive devices for ADLs and IADLs
Aerobic aquatic exercise programs

Pharmacologic therapy

Non-opioid analgesics (e.g., acetaminophen)
Nonsteroidal antiinflammatory drugs
Opioid analgesics (e.g., propoxyphene, codeine, oxycodone)

From Hochberg MC et al: Guidelines for the medical management of osteoarthritis. I. Osteoarthritis of the hip, *Arthritis Rheum* 38:1535, 1995.
*ADLs = activities of daily living; IADLs = instrumental ADLs.

Box 11-4   Activities for Management of Arthritis of the Hands

Start exercising slowly with no more than 4 or 5 repetitions 1 or 2 times daily.
Consider consultation with an occupational therapist for individually designed exercises.
Use one hand to gently massage the other from knuckle joints to fingertips and then reverse the process; then do the same with the other hand.
Stretch wrist in circular motion then bend backward as far as possible without discomfort.
Stretch muscles and ligaments in forearm by resting arm with palm down and rotating lower arm until palm faces upward.
Avoid overuse of any set of muscles.
Avoid repetitious movements.
Lift objects with both hands.
Press on plunger type spray bottles with both hands.
Rise from armchair by pushing down on both palms (do not push with knuckle pressure).
Hold a coffee mug with both hands wrapped around the mug.

Modified from The best ways to relieve osteoarthritis of the hand, *Johns Hopkins Medical Letter* 5(8):3, 1993.

wound healing, rehabilitation, and psychosocial factors. Changes in synovium, cartilage, and soft tissues must be assessed before opting for surgical options such as synovectomy, arthroplasty, arthrodesis, bone grafting, and others. (See glossary at end of text for definitions of terms.) Outcomes depend on the timing of surgery, the number of procedures that the surgeon and the hospital have to their credit and the patient's medical status, perioperative and postoperative management, and rehabilitation (Hochberg et al, 1995). Nearly twice as many females as males have joint replacements, and over 60% of all joint replacements are in individuals over 65 years of age (U.S. Bureau of the Census, 1995). Swedish physicians have devised an experimental cartilage-regeneration procedure that can replace damaged cartilage by harvesting healthy cartilage from the joint, growing the healthy cells in a culture serum, and then suturing this new protective covering over the damaged area. This has been used to repair injuries and tears, but Dr. Peterson of the University of Goteberg believes it will eventually be applicable to all joints (American Association of Retired Persons, 1995).

Rheumatoid Arthritis. Rheumatoid arthritis (RA) is thought to be one of the autoimmune disorders that involve both environmental and genetic factors (Davis, 1995). It may occur at any age, but it tends to become more frequent in individuals, particularly women, after age 60. In contrast to OA, where the synovial covering of a joint is worn away, in RA the affected synovium becomes massively hypertrophic and edematous with projections of synovial tissue protruding into the joint cavity (Davis, 1995). This is thought to be possibly due to a smoldering infection stimulated by an unknown antigen. Generally it begins with bilat-

eral swelling and inflammation of the synovial membrane of small, peripheral joints, particularly wrist, knee, ankle, and hand, though it affects large joints as well. It is unpredictable in its course and may have periods of remission and exacerbation that seem influenced by psychosocial factors as well as changes in synovia. The course usually continues downward in spite of periods of remission. Ten years after onset 50% of afflicted individuals are unable to work and have other limitations in function, and life expectancy may be shortened (Marino and McDonald, 1991). Symptoms in late life tend to be acutely uncomfortable and spread throughout the joints of the body. Sometimes the disorder affects systems other than joints.

Assessment. Early diagnosis is important because irreversible destruction of affected joints may occur within 1 to 2 years after onset (Paget, 1995). Early signs include generalized fatigue, malaise, stiffness with swelling, erythema, and warmth over affected joints. Weight loss is common. Usually joint involvement is symmetrical rather than asymmetrical as in osteoarthritis. Elevated rheumatoid arthritis factor (RF) and erythrocyte sedimentation rate (ESR) are most suggestive of rheumatoid arthritis.

Interventions. Prostaglandins play a primary role in both the onset and relief of the inflammation of arthritis, and the balancing of prostaglandins is the key to controlling inflammation (Dalton, 1995). Excess prostaglandins and other metabolic byproducts can be inactivated and flushed from the body by increased dietary fiber and sufficient fluid intake; lacking these, arthritis may either be induced or aggravated. Dalton (1995) makes a strong case for dietary supplementation with fiber and increasing fluid intake as well as nutritional supplements. She also suggests that individuals monitor their reactions to other dietary substances, particularly the foods that are categorized as "nightshades" (tomatoes, peppers, potatoes, and eggplants). In some people these will exacerbate symptoms and should be eliminated from the diet (Dalton, 1995).

The client needs psychologic support, rest, analgesics, and antiinflammatory medications (both NSAIDs and corticosteroids). Flexion contractures of the involved joints are common, resulting in limitation of movement and pain. Pain in all stages of arthritis is a serious consideration. See Chapter 9 for suggestions regarding pain management.

Most recent philosophy tends toward vigorous treatment of RA with disease-modifying antirheumatic drugs (DMARDs) and use of NSAIDs as adjunctive rather than primary modes of pain management. Nurses must advocate for clients because they may not be aware of the importance of rapid and aggressive treatment. The Arthritis, Rheumatism, and Aging Medical Information System (ARAMIS) data banks have clearly shown the following: (1) RA is not a benign, self-limiting disease but one that increases morbidity and mortality; (2) NSAIDs are not benign but create serious gastrointestinal disorders and hemorrhage, and though they may relieve pain, they have no effect on the progression of the disease; and (3) even though DMARDs are more toxic than NSAIDs, the disability and pain were significantly reduced (Fries) (Table 11-4 and Figure 11-7).

J. Bruce Smith published a study in the February 1996 issue of *Journal of Rheumatology* reporting that a vaccine that imitates the effects of pregnancy on a woman's immune system is being studied as a possible treatment for RA based upon the observation that pregnancy triggers a remission of the disease in about 70% of cases (Smith, 1996). Eleven women, none of them over the age of 55, were given the vaccine with 75% success. Large-scale clinical studies are now in progress (NURSEweek, 1996).

Additional studies from the Netherlands have shown an antigen-driven expansion of T lymphocytes in the inflamed joints. Attenuated nonspecific T-cell lines were used as a vaccine with some evidence for a modulated T-cell reactivity in vivo and in vitro. Breedveld et al (1995) suggest that further studies focus on the effect of vaccination using vaccines prepared from disease-inducing cells. The importance of this for nurses is to encourage patients that progress is being made in understanding the disorder. Until now the outlook was grim.

Because of the unknown causes and unpredictable but persistent nature of arthritis, people often fall prey to worthless cure tactics. However, some may be effective because they act as placebos. Self-help and support groups are useful, but the individual often must simply learn to live with a certain degree of constant discomfort. Lorig et al (1985)

Table 11-4 Comparative Toxicity of DMARDs and NSAIDs

Rank	DMARD	Toxicity index	NSAID	Toxicity index
1			Salsalate	1.28
2	Hydroxychloroquine	1.38		
3			Ibuprofen	1.94
4			Naproxen	2.17
5			Sulindac	2.24
6	Intramuscular gold	2.27		
7			Piroxicam	2.52
8			Fenoprofen	2.95
9	Penicillamine	3.38		
10			Ketoprofen	3.45
11	Methotrexate	3.82		
12			Meclofenamate	3.86
13	Azathioprine	3.92		
14			Tolmetin	3.96
15			Indomethacin	3.99
16	Auranofin	5.25		

From Fries JF et al, 1993
From Fries JF: A new treatment approach: DMARD-based sequential therapy. In *Diagnosis and treatment of rheumatoid arthritis,* Laguna Niguel, Calif, 1995, The Institute for Medical Studies, HP Publishing Co.

found that patients with osteoarthritis and/or rheumatoid arthritis were helped by a self-management program that relied largely on the efficacy of six 2-hour sessions in a self-help group for arthritics. In a 4-year follow-up it was found that knowledge of the disorder had increased and pain had decreased even though the physical disability had progressed. Though this is an old study, it would seem to indicate that feelings of self-efficacy, induced by increased knowledge and feelings of control, may have very positive outcomes even in the presence of increasing debilitation. Replication of these data are needed.

Management of arthritis through providing classes in specially designed exercises, relaxation, and pain management techniques have been useful. (Box 11-5 lists management goals.) Participants are also given general information about their disease and taught to use medication wisely. These classes have shown that arthritics can take control of their situation and increase functional independence with a minimum amount of discomfort. Based on the success of this effort the National Arthritis Foundation is now offering similar courses throughout the United States. Many medical centers and senior care centers now have arthritis clinics, and these should be sought for a thorough evaluation and individualized treatment program. At present, arthritis cannot be prevented or cured.

Geriatric Shoulder Pain. Shoulder pain in the geriatric patient is commonly seen by primary physicians. Often it is dismissed as rather inconsequential, because it does not inhibit general mobility, tends to persist for long periods, and is difficult to assess properly (Glockner, 1995). Proper evaluation requires an understanding of patient anatomy, a thorough physical examination, and a knowledge of common shoulder disorders that occur in the aged population (Vecchio et al, 1995). Because it is seldom seen as serious by the client or the physician, the nurse may be the one to observe the limitations imposed by a shoulder disorder.

The most demonstrable effects of a shoulder disorder are impairment of personal care, inability to accomplish some household tasks, and pain on movement (Vecchio et al, 1995). Often the pain interferes with sleep, and the client has difficulty moving the arm to eat if the pain is in the dominant side. One man suffered intense pain for a period of 6 months, but because the physicians attending him paid little attention, he felt he was doomed to this for the remainder of his life. Medications did not seem to help, and in addition most of the activities he enjoyed required the use of his right arm, which he could not extend or rotate externally. He held his arm as if he were hemiplegic. With aggressive examination and diagnosis it was determined he had a rotator cuff

separation. Intensive therapy, prescribed exercises, and medication finally alleviated the problem.

Shoulder pain may be a result of inflammatory disorders, degenerative problems, fractures or contusions, shoulder separation involving the clavicle, impingement syndrome involving the rotator cuff, or biceps tendinitis or referred pain from other areas (Glockener, 1995).

Assessment. The shoulder comprises four separate articulations: the glenohumeral, acromioclavicular, sternoclavicular, and scapulothoracic. The combined motion of these joints provides the wide range of motion possible in the shoulder. The shoulder has a more extensive range of motion than any other joint. To effectively use this wide range of motion the soft tissues of the shoulder must provide the necessary stability.

During assessment, the onset, nature, location, and duration of pain and its relationship to daily activities should be determined. Pain patterns can provide important diagnostic

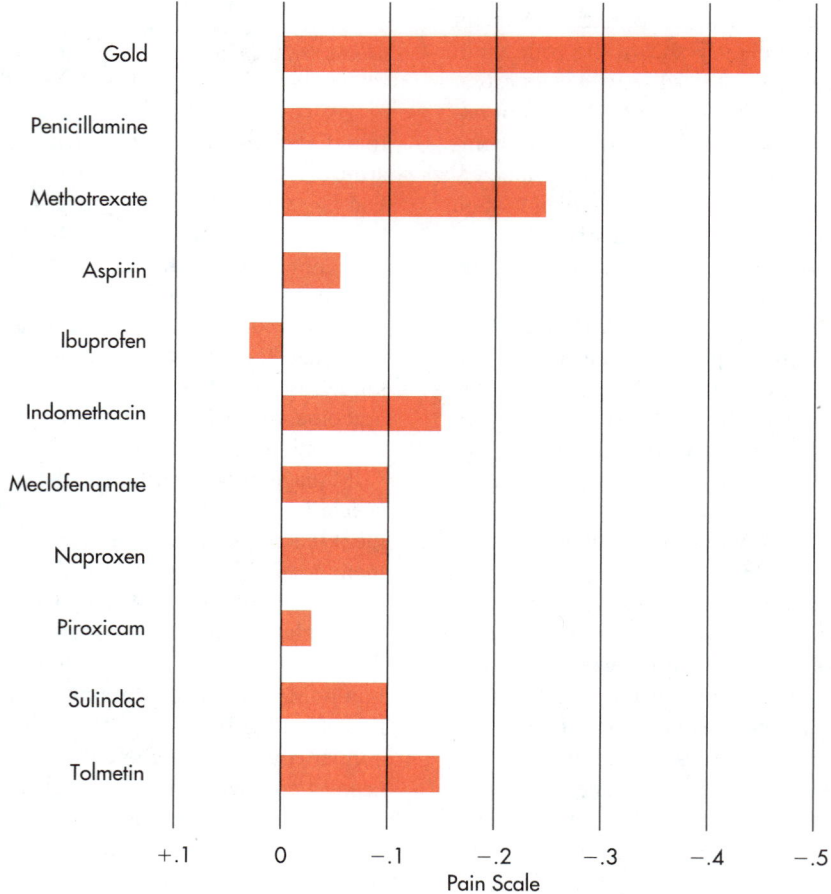

Figure 11-7. Average pain levels at baseline and 9 months after initiation of therapy in an early study of ARAMIS data were substantially improved by DMARDs (gold, penicillamine, or methotrexate), compared with no, insignificant, or only modest changes with NSAIDs. (From Fries JF: A new treatment approach: DMARD-based sequential therapy. In *Diagnosis and treatment of rheumatoid arthritis: a special report for primary care physicians,* The Institute for Medical Studies, Laguna Niguel, Calif, 1995, HP Publishing Co.)

clues. Pain that increases with activity suggests tendon impingement or degenerative arthritis. Pain with numbness and tingling may indicate cervical radiculopathy. Pain that occurs most severely at night is often seen with rotator cuff tears.

Chronic rotator cuff tears are most commonly seen in elderly patients. They represent the cumulative effects of many years of wear as the rotator cuff tendons glide under the acromion. Repetitive overhead motion impinges the undersurface of the acromion (Zuckerman and Shapiro, 1997). Range of motion of the shoulder should be tested with the patient sitting, and roentgenographic examination should include two views taken at 90 degrees to each other. When these are not done, the assessment will be incomplete. The drop-arm test may be helpful in diagnosing a rotator cuff tear. While sitting, the patient is asked to slowly lower the arm. Inability to do so indicates a rotator cuff tear.

Interventions. Antiinflammatory medications and injected steroids may provide relief. When pain persists for more than 2 months, surgical treatment may be indicated. Shoulder replacement has been shown to provide excellent pain relief in 90% to 95% of persons undergoing the surgical procedure, but shoulder replacement has been reserved for patients in severe pain unalleviated by other methods. Surgical intervention for older patients is not to be discouraged. Hattrup (1995) reports that in those over 65 years of age, 77% had excellent results.

The nursing role in dealing with persons who have intractable shoulder pain is to encourage them to emphasize to the physician the need for a thorough examination and to keep an extensive log of the patterns of pain, intensity, frequency, and specific positions that cause the most pain. Often the nurse must act as patient advocate to encourage surgery if pain resolution has not occurred within 6 to 8 weeks (Glockner, 1995).

Gait Disorders

Gait disorders make one vulnerable to tripping and falling. In addition, they impede activity and increase anxiety in the elder who is aware of instability in gait. More than 2.5 million individuals over 65 years of age in the United States need assistance to walk; almost 1% of the total population. Given the magnitude of this problem, routine examination of the elderly should include gait and postural assessment (Box 11-6). Normal gait involves the vestibular system of balance, proprioception (sensitivity to body in motion), neurophysiologic integrity, and vision.

A mnemonic device for remembering etiology of gait disorders is CANE (cardiovascular, arthritic, neurosensory, and etiology unknown). Arthritis of hip, knee, or foot is the most common cause of instability. Arthritis of the knee may

---

Box 11-5   Goals of Nursing Management and Interventions in Arthritis

Goals
Pain management and promotion of comfort
Exercises and rest interspersed
Psychologic support
Reduction of swelling and inflammation
Prevention of deformity
Promotion of optimal life-style

Suggested Interventions
Provide realistic information
Teach client self-care to promote comfort
Assist client to modify life-style appropriately
Prescribed exercises for muscle maintenance
Participation in weight reduction program if necessary
Balance rest and activity
Teach relaxation and stress reduction
Teach to avoid bending painful joints, splint when inflamed
Teach to maintain body alignment when standing, sitting, and lying down

Summarized from Heckheimer EF: *Health promotion of the elderly in the community,* Philadelphia, 1989, WB Saunders.

Box 11-6   Gait Disorders

Ataxia
Wide-based gait with frequent side-stepping

Normal Pressure Hydrocephalus
Step height reduced, shuffling gait as if feet stuck to floor; short steps, unsteady speed, and ataxia

Parkinson's Disease
Stooped posture, short rapid shuffling gait, uncontrollable propulsion or retropulsion; "freeze" walk when feet abruptly halt while body continues to move forward

Spondylotic Cervical Myelopathy
Spastic, shuffling gait, deep tendon reflexes below level of compression increase muscle tone; sometimes nonspecific, e.g., "clumsy feet," "legs gave way"

Senile Gait
Associated with stooped posture, hip and knee flexion, diminished arm swing, stiffness in turning, broad-based, small steps with poor gait intention

Hemiplegia
Poor arm and leg swing, affected limb does not bend at knee; ankle fixed and inverted as leg swings in wide circle; foot tends to drag

Osteomalacia
Ill-defined skeletal pain, pain on weight bearing, unstable waddling gait

result in ligamentous weakness and instability, causing legs to give way or collapse. Muscle weakness is often experienced in hyperthyroidism and hypothyroidism, hypokalemia, hyperparathyroidism, osteomalacia, hypophosphatemia, and in some cases is brought on by various drug therapies. Diabetes, alcoholism, and vitamin B deficiencies may cause neurologic damage and resultant gait problems. Vestibular dysfunction causes unsteadiness in walking and listing to one side or the other when eyes are closed. The individual cannot focus well on a fixed target while moving or on a moving object while standing still. Elderly diabetics and individuals on certain medications may experience dizziness, unsteadiness, and lightheadedness. Postural instability increases and is exacerbated by some medications. Extrapyramidal symptoms produce a shuffling gait in some individuals taking psychotropic medications (see Chapter 23) and in those who have a propensity toward Parkinson's disorder. Postural reflex impairment occurs with aging, and

postural sway, forward and backward, can be observed when an individual stands still. A cane or supportive device may be essential to provide a sense of security.

Assessment. Neurologic damage is best determined by the positive Romberg sign and impaired vibratory sense in the legs (Catanasos and Israel, 1991). Spontaneous lateral postural sway is a predictor of fall risk (Maki et al, 1994). Gait speed and agility have been found to correlate well with functional level (Potter et al, 1995). A senile balance and gait disorder is thought to be an aspect of advanced age, but as yet this remains poorly defined. Marked gait disorders are not normally a visible consequence of aging alone but are more likely indicative of an underlying pathologic condition.

Investigation of gait disorders in the elderly is a very complex issue and, even though nurses will not be responsible for these diagnostic activities, it is important that they recognize and advocate for proper and thorough assessment and diagnosis. Nurses are the most likely providers to observe

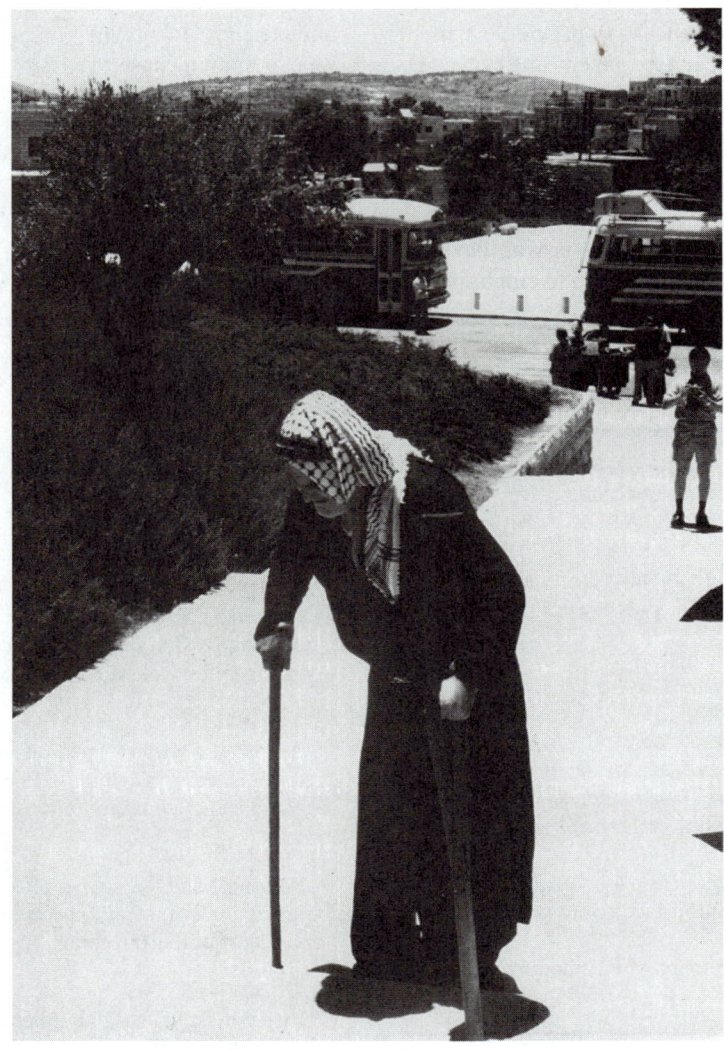

Stabilizing gait. (Courtesy Patricia Hess.)

gait disturbances and make initial descriptive assessments. Using the appropriate terminology will assist other professionals in investigation of the problem.

A guide nurses can use for gait and balance assessment is provided in Box 11-7. The Tinetti Balance and Gait Evaluation is most precise and has been tested for validity and reliability (Tinetti, 1986) (Figure 11-8).

In most gait disturbances, nervousness or anxiety aggravates the condition. Nurses may assist by gently holding the arm on the unaffected side and supporting the client's efforts.

Interventions. Often well-fitting shoes, canes, leg braces, pain relief, handrails, or walkers may improve mobility status. The nurse is responsible for initial assessment of gait disturbance and gaining appropriate professional evaluation for gait training and prostheses. Rehabilitative teams are usually responsible for teaching patients, but nurses must understand concepts and specific methods because they will assist the patient to carry out correct procedures on a daily basis. Gait disorders may be the prelude to increasing loss of mobility. Gait involves a complex set of simultaneous movements (Cunha, 1988). A complete analysis of gait patterns and characteristics requires special equipment and expertise, but simple gait observation by nurses can yield valuable information regarding a client.

Parkinson's Disease

Parkinson's disease (PD) affects over 1 million people in the United States and is the most predominant neurologic disease of elderly persons. In addition, many elders develop parkinsonian reactions in response to psychotropic drugs. Parkinson's disease (PD) is a slowly progressive disease of the basal ganglia of the nervous system that leads to difficulty with movement. Early signs are mild tremor of the hands and feet, generalized slowing of movement, rigidity, loss of motor skills and facial expression, and characteristically small handwriting. There is also a tendency toward stooped posture, shuffling gait, and keeping the arms fixed at the side when walking (Parkinson's Disease Foundation, 1996). Some individuals with PD have a festinating gait in which steps become smaller and smaller and faster and faster. Invisible symptoms, including erosion of recent memory, depression, hallucinations, low backache due to poor posture, mild vision loss, cramps, and burning sensations of thighs and legs, become very troublesome. Athough tremor, rigidity, and slowness of movement are the characteristic triad of symptoms, other problems that occur quite frequently include freezing (sudden difficulty in walking or turning around), dementia, excessive perspiration, oily skin, and feeling hot or cold. Box 11-8 lists symptoms of PD. PD occurs with increasing frequency as individuals age. In persons over 80 years old about 1 in 100 will experience some degree of PD. Men are more commonly affected than women. There is uncertainty about cause and predictability of symptoms. Risk factors are not clear, but preliminary investigation suggests that environmental toxins may be a factor, and there is a correlation between increased incidence of dementia and PD in late life (Marder, 1992). Eighteen PD centers across the nation and in Canada are investigating the manifestations and management of the disorder.

Essential tremor is somewhat similar in appearance to PD and is said to be the most prevalent movement disorder,

Box 11-7	**Gait Description and Assessment**
Pain in back and lower limbs	Antalgic gait; short steps flexed toward affected side
Contracture or ankylosis	Short-leg gait; wide outward swing of affected side, unaffected knee flexed and body bent forward
Foot deformities	Loss of spring and rhythm in step, toes inward or outward bilaterally or unilaterally
Footdrop	Foot slap heard due to knee raised higher than usual
Gluteus medius weakness	Waddle gait; drop and lag in swing phase of unaffected side, seen in osteomalacia and senile gait in women
Stroke	Wide, open, flinging foot on affected side, uncoordinated
Cerebroarteriosclerosis	Bilateral involvement manifested by extremely short steps
Parkinsonism	Festinating gait; short, hurried, often on tiptoe, or rigid, tremorous, slow, tends toward retropulsion, mincing
Etat lacunaire	Similar to Parkinson's gait, irregular footsteps
Dementia	Slow, shuffling, apraxic, short steps
Peripheral neuropathy	Difficulty lifting feet, stumbles easily
Subdural hematoma	Ataxic, prominent feature is gait disturbance
Cerebellar ataxia	Staggering, unsteady, irregular, wide-based gait, inappropriate foot placement
Vitamin B_{12} deficiency	Paresthesias, unsteadiness, foot dragging
Endocrine disorders	Gait ataxia, particularly with hypothyroidism
Medications	Ataxia, Parkinsonian gait, imbalance

Tinetti Balance and Gait Evaluation

Balance
Instructions: Subject is seated in a hard, armless chair. The following maneuvers are tested:

1. Sitting balance
   0 = Leans or slides in chair
   1 = Steady, safe
2. Arise
   0 = Unable without help
   1 = Able but uses arm to help
   2 = Able without use of arms
3. Attempts to arise
   0 = Unable without help
   1 = Able, but requires more than one attempt
   2 = Able to arise with one attempt
4. Immediate standing balance (first 5 seconds)
   0 = Unsteady (staggers, moves feet, marked trunk sway)
   1 = Steady but uses walker/cane or grabs other object for support
   2 = Steady without walker or cane or other support
5. Standing balance
   0 = Unsteady
   1 = Steady, but wide stance (medial heels > than 4" apart) or uses cane/walker or other support
   2 = Narrow stance without support
6. Nudge (subject at maximum position with feet as close together as possible. Examiner pushes lightly on subject's sternum with palm of hand 3 times.)
   0 = Begins to fall
   1 = Staggers, grabs, but catches self
   2 = Steady
7. Eyes closed (at maximum position #6)
   0 = Unsteady
   1 = Steady
8. Turn 360°
   0 = Discontinuous steps
   1 = Continuous steps
   0 = Unsteady (grabs, staggers)
   1 = Steady
9. Sit down
   0 = Unsafe (misjudged distance; falls into chair)
   1 = Uses arms or not a smooth motion
   2 = Safe, smooth motion

_____ **/16**   BALANCE SCORE

Figure 11-8. Tinetti Balance and Gait Evaluation. (From Brady R et al: Geriatric falls: prevention strategies for the staff, *J Gerontol Nurs* 19(9):26, 1993.) (Reprinted with permission, Mary Tinetti, M.D.)

Tinetti Balance and Gait Evaluation

Gait

Instructions: Subject stands with examiner. Walks down hallway or across room, first at his/her usual pace, then back at a "rapid but safe" pace (using usual walking aid such as cane/walker).

10. Initiation of gait (immediately after told 'go')
    0 = Any hesitancy or multiple attempts to start
    1 = No hesitancy
11. Step length and height (right foot swing)
    0 = Does not pass L. stance foot with step
    1 = Passes L. stance foot
    0 = R. foot does not clear floor completely with step
    1 = R. foot completely clears floor
12. Step length and height (left foot swing)
    0 = Does not pass R. stance foot with step
    1 = Passes R. stance foot
    0 = L. foot does not clear floor completely with step
    1 = L. foot completely clears floor
13. Step symmetry
    0 = R. and L. step length not equal (estimate)
    1 = R. and L. step length appear equal
14. Step continuity
    0 = Stopping or discontinuity between steps
    1 = Steps appear continuous
15. Path (estimated in relation to floor tiles, 12" wide. Observe excursion of one foot over about 10 feet of course.)
    0 = Marked deviation
    1 = Mild/moderate deviation or uses a walking aid
    2 = Straight without walking aid
16. Trunk
    0 = Marked sway or uses walking aid
    1 = No sway but flexion of knees or back or spreads arms out while walking
    2 = No sway, no flexion, no use of arms and no walking aid
17. Walk stance
    0 = Heels apart
    1 = Heels almost touching while walking

_____ **/12**   GAIT SCORE

_____ **/28**   TOTAL MOBILITY SCORE (BALANCE AND GAIT)

Figure 11-8, cont'd. For legend see opposite page.

peaking in the sixth decade of life. It primarily affects the hands and the head and may significantly impair communication and activities requiring fine motor control as well as impact psychosocial adjustment. The disorder may become apparent in young adulthood and will grow progressively worse as one ages (Lundervold and Poppen, 1995). Etiology and management are poorly understood, though tremor-lytic medications and alcohol are helpful in most cases. See resources at the end of the chapter for further information.

Management. Typically, individuals are maintained on a combination of carbidopa and levodopa (Sinemet), which often loses effectiveness as the amino acid L-dopa competes with other amino acids for absorption at both the intestinal wall and the blood-brain barrier. Restricting dietary protein is sometimes effective. Recently the experimental drug lazabemide (RO 19-6327) has been used in clinical trials. The Parkinson's Disease Foundation (1996) warns that patients with PD must be maintained on their medication even during acute illness because some persons deprived of their antiparkinsonian medication have died. See Chapter 23 for discussion of parkinsonian movement disorders as a result of psychoactive medication use and for the AIMS evaluation tool.

Because of the slow progression of the disease and the disability that accompanies it, individuals experience a change in role, activities, and social participation. The reflected appraisal from others of incapacity may exacerbate feelings of inadequacy. The expressionless face, slowed movement, and soft, monotone speech may give the impression of apathy, depression, and disinterest. Tremors may produce embarrassing moments. A sensitive nurse is aware that the visible symptoms produce an undesired facade that may hide an alert and responsive individual who wishes to interact and generate interest. Persons with PD experience great functional problems in mobility, communication, and home management (Longstreth et al, 1992). Two commonly identified problems are trouble with writing or typing and decreased sexual activity. Lipe et al (1990) found in a comparison between men with PD and those with arthritis that in both disorders more than 80% experienced decreased sexual function. Another problem, studied by Madeley et al (1990), was that of marked impairment in driving skills in severe cases of PD. In many patients with PD the medication regimen may create illusions or hallucinations. Meco et al (1990) found that these were more common in individuals with cognitive impairment. A problem of lesser frequency but very distressing is dystonic cramps, particularly those that result in curling and twisting of the toes and the feet. Surgery does not correct this problem. A neurologic consultation is advised.

Topp (1987) suggests the following ways of coping with some of the symptoms that disturb the client with PD:

1. Movement of the limbs decreases the tremors; when walking, one should swing the arms.
2. Holding an object helps control the tremors; individuals should hold something in their hands when sitting quietly.
3. Contractures and deformities are avoided if the individual walks as much as possible and avoids remaining still for long periods; range of motion and balancing exercises need to be prescribed by a physical therapist and practiced faithfully. Van Oteghen (1987) has prescribed particular exercises found helpful with her father.
4. Skin must be kept dry and clean and oil-free lotion applied every few hours to avoid seborrhea and skin breakdown; air mattresses and sheepskins are advisable for beds.
5. Constipation may be avoided by high fluid intake and a high-residue diet.

6. Speaking and reading aloud should be encouraged to enhance communication; sometimes speech therapy is warranted.
7. Depression and low self-esteem may be partially countered by direct discussion of feelings about changes in self-image, sexuality, and functional ability.
8. Support system encouragement and information about the disease are essential if the family is to cope with the slow responses, clumsiness, and poor communication of the afflicted individual.
9. Self-help groups are often helpful, because the members solve their problems collectively.

The Sickness Impact Profile (SIP) is a useful tool that can be used by nurses to determine problems most troublesome from the client's perspective (Table 11-5).

Interventions to Manage Gait and Balance Disorders

A thorough physical and medication review is essential to identify, describe, and assess causes of gait and balance disorders. The physical examination must include vision, blood pressure, range of motion, muscle strength, balance, posture, podiatric examination, and neurologic and cognitive assessment.

Buchner and Wagner (1992) found that exercise often produced improvements in gait and balance. In addition, Lord et al (1996) found that older persons actively engaged in exercise develop strength in lower limbs, faster walking pace, longer strides, and improved ankle dorsiflexion strength. Exercise can also benefit individuals with arthritis, increase bone density in osteopenia, and enhance cognitive function. Specific gait training as individually prescribed by a physical therapist was found effective in reducing falls in individuals who were fall-prone (Galindo-Ciocon et al, 1995).

The interventional issue is not only to "educate" the individual but also to identify ways to motivate the elderly to routinely exercise in a manner designed to facilitate health. Exercises to improve flexibility and muscle tone while lying, sitting, standing, and walking are included in Chapter 3. We must remember that the very problems exercise may impact are the ones that may cause the individual to avoid participation: lack of strength, fear of falling, and lethargy. Creating security and confidence in movement includes encouraging the elder to employ the following strategies:

1. Participating in home exercise programs
2. Wearing carefully fitted shoes that are low-heeled and rubber-soled
3. Walking with a companion on smooth ground as a form of exercise and muscle strengthening
4. Asking bystanders for help in navigating high curbs or other hazards to walking
5. Participating in gait training
6. Remembering good posture
7. Evaluating and modifying home hazards

Care of the Feet. Care of the feet is an important aspect of comfort, stable gait, and mobility and one that is often neglected. Some aged persons in the hospital have been unable to walk comfortably, or at all, due to neglect of corns, bunions, and overgrown nails. Other causes of problems may be traced to loss of fat cushioning and resilience with aging, ill-fitting shoes, poor arch support, excessively repetitious weight-bearing activities, obesity, uneven distribution of weight on foot (Mayo Foundation for Medical Education and Research, 1996b). As many as 35% of persons living at home may have significant foot disability that goes untended. The following are common disorders:

1. Arthritic foot disorders resulting from rheumatoid arthritis, osteoarthritis, and gout
2. Atrophy of the plantar pad that leads to loss of shock absorption and metatarsalgia with increased difficulty in walking
3. Onychogryphosis, or overgrown, clawlike toenails that cause walking pain, immobility, and falls
4. Corns that cause pain and may reduce mobility
5. Hallux valgus that may cause little difficulty unless ulceration or bursitis sets in
6. Foot surgery, which may give rise to severe walking difficulty for several months (Cunha, 1988).

Appropriate care of the feet has been discussed earlier in Chapter 7.

FALLS—CAUSES AND CONSEQUENCES

Falling is one of the most serious and frequent problems associated with the aging process. Falls are a symptom of a problem, though they become the focus of the problem when they occur. Because falls may indicate neurologic, sensory, cognitive, medication, or musculoskeletal problems, it is important for nurses to evaluate each older client's biopsychosocial vulnerability to falling (Table 11-6). Intrinsic changes in the capacities of the aged (see Chapter 15 for discussion of frailty), disease processes, psychologic and extrinsic factors (see Chapter 13 for discussion of environmental hazards) all contribute to a greater vulnerability to falls as one ages.

The National Institute on Aging (NIA) (1990) estimates that each year one third of all persons age 65 and older who live at home fall, and about half of those fall repeatedly. Falls and the consequent broken hips cause 40% of nursing home admissions annually, according to the NIA. Up to 20% of hospitalized patients and 45% of those in long-term care facilities will fall. Fall-related mortality increases with advanced age and more than doubles with each decade of life (Tideiksaar, 1990). The problem is particularly prevalent in the very old and is the leading cause of accidental death in men and women over 85.

Factors Contributing to Falls

Falls are generally classified as extrinsic (related to environment), intrinsic (related to host factors), or iatrogenic

Table 11-5   Items in the SIP Endorsed by a Third or More of Patients with Parkinson's Disease*

SIP category	SIP item	Percent (no.) of PD patients endorsing item	Percent (no.) of controls endorsing item
Ambulation	I walk more slowly.	59 (26)	30 (13)
Body care and movement	I move my hands or fingers with some limitation or difficulty.	39 (17)	11 (5)
	I dress myself, but do so very slowly.	46 (20)	9 (4)
Mobility	I stay home most of the time.	50 (22)	7 (3)
Emotional behavior	I act nervous or restless.	43 (20)	30 (13)
Social interaction	I am going out less to visit people.	50 (22)	14 (6)
	I am doing fewer social activities with groups of people.	50 (22)	27 (12)
	My sexual activity is decreased.	61 (27)	16 (7)
Alertness behavior	I have more minor accidents, drop things, trip and fall, bump into things.	46 (20)	14 (6)
	I forget a lot, for example, things that happened recently, where I put things, appointments.	36 (16)	25 (11)
Communication	I am having trouble writing or typing.	75 (33)	14 (6)
	I often lose control of my voice when I talk, for example, my voice gets louder or softer, trembles, changes unexpectedly.	41 (18)	2 (1)
	I do not speak clearly when I am under stress.	52 (23)	5 (2)
Sleep and rest	I sit during much of the day.	41 (18)	27 (12)
	I lie down more often during the day in order to rest.	34 (15)	16 (7)
	I sleep less at night, for example, wake up too early, don't fall asleep for a long time, awaken frequently.	46 (20)	25 (11)
Home management	I do work around the house only for short periods of time or rest often.	41 (26)	23 (10)
	I am doing *less* of the regular daily work around the house than I would usually do.	59 (26)	25 (11)
	I am not doing *any* of the maintenance or repair work that I would usually do in my home or yard.	39 (17)	11 (5)
	I have difficulty doing handwork, for example, turning faucets, using kitchen gadgets, sewing, carpentry.	39 (17)	9 (4)
	I am not doing heavy work around the house.	48 (21)	23 (10)
Recreation and pastimes	I do my hobbies and recreation for shorter periods of time.	43 (19)	18 (8)
	I am going out for entertainment less often.	43 (19)	32 (14)
	I am cutting down on *some* of my usual physical recreation or activities.	46 (20)	30 (13)

*Patients are instructed to endorse those items that apply to themselves and are related to their health.

(related to treatment factors) (Commodore, 1995). Shepherd et al (1992) studied falls in 431 patients seen in family practice and found that after age 65 individuals fell most frequently due to external reasons, however, with increasing age, internal and locomotor reasons became increasingly prevalent. Fall risk factors that increase proportionally as one ages are disturbances in visual acuity, postural hypotension, and cardiac arrhythmias (Shepherd et al, 1992; Maki et al, 1994; Lipsitz, 1995). Decline in depth perception, proprioception, vibratory sense, and normotensive response to postural changes are important factors, though the majority of falls occur in individuals with multiple medical problems (Tideiksaar, 1990).

Lipsitz and colleagues (1991) evaluated 126 individuals (mean age, 87 years) in long-term care facilities to determine the most prevalent causes of falling. They found stroke, parkinsonism, blindness, drug-related hypotension, and arthritis were most predominant. Those who fell were more often women, were more functionally impaired, and took more medications than those who did not fall. They

Table 11-6	Fall Factors	
Psychogenic	**Physiologic**	**Environmental**

Dementia
  Alterations in gait and vitamin B$_{12}$ level; poor evaluation of ability and environment
Depression
  Disinterest in surroundings, no concern for safety, subliminal suicide
Fear/anxiety
  Distraction, scattered perceptions
	Neurologic
	  Dementias
	  Somnolence
	  Normal pressure hydrocephalus
	  Neurosensory and visual deficits: loss of proprioception; peripheral neuropathy; vestibular dysfunction; dizziness; vertigo; syncope; seizures, brain tumors, or lesions; Parkinson's disease; cervical spondylosis
	Cardiovascular disorders
	  Cerebrovascular insufficiency, strokes and TIAs, carotid sinus syncope, vertebral artery insufficiency
	  Arrhythmias: Stokes-Adams
	  Valvulopathies
	  Congestive heart failure
	Hypotension: postural hypotension, postprandial drop in blood pressure, medication induced, male micturation when urethral obstruction present, hypovolemia (dehydration, hemorrhage), impaired venous return (venous pooling, valsalva), impaired vasoconstriction (autonomic disorders, vasovagal)
	Metabolic disorders: anemia, hypoxia, hypoglycemia, hyperventilation
	Debilitating disease: cancer, pulmonary disease, immunosuppressant disorder
		Slippery floor: urine or fluid on the floor, loose throw rugs
		Uneven and obstructed walking surfaces: electrical cords, furniture, pets, children, uneven door steps or stair risers, loose boards, cracked sidewalks
		Inadequate visual supports: glaring; low wattage bulbs; lack of night-lights for bathroom, stairs, and halls; poor marking of steps and other hazards
		Inadequate construction: absence of railing, lack of grab bars on shower or tub, poorly designed stairs and walkways

tended to have more difficulty rising from a chair or turning 360 degrees, had impaired positional sense, and had a higher prevalence of antidepressant use. These few variables accounted for three quarters of the ambulatory elderly with recurrent falls in that study group.

Vision Problems. Sudden unexpected visual problems become major fall risks; visual changes may be transient, a symptom of other problems such as hypotension, cardiac arrhythmia, temporal arteritis, or vertebrobasilar artery insufficiency. Additionally, new glasses or recent cataract surgery may be impediments. The more gradual and progressive visual changes become serious fall risks when they interfere with depth vision.

Balance Problems. Vertigo and dizziness are the result of dysfunction in balance control systems and vestibular apparatus. Benign positional vertigo is the most common form experienced by the elderly. Ear infection or head trauma are common precipitants. Labyrinthitis is an infectious or toxic process that results in dizziness and gait ataxia. Drug toxicity causes tinnitus and hearing loss, which may become permanent. Treatment of the infection, discontinuation of the drug, or removal of cerumen impaction often resolves the problem. Disequilibrium may arise from many disorders including Parkinson's disease, Alzheimer's disease, peripheral neuropathy caused by pernicious anemia, alcoholism, or diabetes. Patients experience unsteadiness and a tendency to fall. They often need an assistive device for walking and a medication evaluation (Tideiksaar, 1990). Contributing factors are summarized in Box 11-9.

Interruption of Cerebral Oxygenation. Transient ischemic attacks (TIAs) affect the perfusion of the brain and cause intermittent dizziness. It is estimated that up to 25% of falls are due to drop attacks associated with TIAs. The individual may not have a loss of consciousness but will feel as if the legs gave way. Patients subject to these attacks should wear cervical collars to prevent backward flexion of the head.

Syncope, or a brief loss of consciousness due to cerebral ischemia, has many causes. Vasodepressor syncope typically occurs during emotional upset, injury, excessive fatigue, or during prolonged standing in a warm environment. Orthostatic syncope is a compensatory response to rapid rising to a standing position when depletion of body fluids or medications interfere with rapid venous return and dynamic homeostatic responses. Postprandial reductions in blood pressure may also occur sufficiently to produce syncope. Hypoglycemia is usually only syncopal in the diabetic and then usually 3 to 5 hours after a meal.

About 15% to 20% of noninstitutionalized elders are susceptible to orthostatic hypotension. Paradoxically, age-related elevations in blood pressure increase the risk of hypotension (Lipsitz, 1995). Baroreflex responses mediate both hypertension and hypotension, and in old age the efficiency of this function progressively declines, thus the aged are more vulnerable to episodes of cerebral ischemia with rapid changes of posture.

<table>
<tr><td colspan="2">

Box 11-9   **Fall Risk Factors for Elders**
</td></tr>
<tr><td>

Conditions

Female or single (incidence increases with age)
Sedative and alcohol use, psychoactive medications
Previous falls, unsteadiness, dizziness
Acute and recent illness
Pathologic conditions, drop attacks
Cognitive impairment, disorientation
Disability of lower extremities
Abnormalities of balance and gait
Foot problems
Depression, anxiety
Decreased vision or hearing
Fear of falling
Terminal drop (dies in following year to 2 years)
Skeletal and neuromuscular changes that predispose to
    weakness and postural imbalance
Acute and severe chronic illness, debilitation
Functional limitations in self-care activities
Women (75 years and older)
Multiple disorders and medications
Wheelchair-bound
Sensory deficits
Impaired locomotion
Predisposing physiologic and psychologic conditions
Preoccupation with stressors
Anxiety related to previous falls
Confusion, dementia
</td><td>

Situations

Urinary urgency, particularly nocturia
Environmental hazards
Recent relocation
Assistive devices needed for walking
Inadequate or missing safety rails, particularly in bathroom
Poorly designed or unstable furniture
Low stools
High chairs and beds
Floor surfaces
Glossy, highly waxed floors
Wet, greasy, icy surfaces
Inadequate lighting
General clutter
Pets that inadvertently trip an individual
Electrical cords
Loose or uneven stair treads
A detailed discussion of these can be found in Chapter 13.
</td></tr>
</table>

Data from Tinetti et al (1988); Craven and Bruno, 1986; Kaufmann (1985); Barbieri, 1983; and Fife et al, 1984.

Carotid sinus syncope occurs frequently in older people who have sinus node disease. This hypersensitivity to pressure or mechanical obstruction makes the individual vulnerable to syncope when applying pressure to carotid in shaving, turning head sharply to one side, or wearing tight collars. Drugs such as propranolol and digitalis may produce carotid hypersensitivity (Tideiksaar, 1990).

Unusual and rarely mentioned is micturation syncope, which occurs immediately following voiding in some elderly males with bladder outlet obstructions (often prostatic hypertrophy). The loss of consciousness is due to vagal bradycardia. These individuals should sit during urination.

Cardiac arrhythmias are a common cause of syncope, particularly supraventricular tachycardias. Heart monitoring for 24 to 48 hours is often necessary to reveal these bradyarrhythmias or tachyarrhythmias.

Fatigue Factors.   Postural training for individuals has many advantageous benefits. Few individuals realize that fatigue may result or be more pronounced due to poor posture. In addition, poor posture contributes to the incidence of falls. Physiotherapists should be engaged to teach nurses and clients correct postural habits.

Fear of Falling.   Fear of falling may actually be a more pervasive problem than falling, and the fear that becomes obsessional can become detrimental and limiting. Fear can result in avoidance phobias that continually and gradually restrict the environment until one is confined to bed. In addition, Gray-Miceli (1995) notes that the fear of falling is an important predictor of general functional decline.

Mr. Chang was a sprightly 83-year-old widower, the son of an immigrant laundry worker. He had lived in San Francisco's Chinatown all his life. He hurried about in the crowded area and bartered with the market vendors for his fresh vegetables and other needs. He tripped and fell one day for no known reason and suffered shoulder contusions and a mild concussion. After an examination and thorough radiographic studies, he was released from the emergency room with the physician's warning, "Be careful, you are an old man." Gradually Mr. Chang began to believe this and slowed his pace, carefully watching the ground to see that there was nothing to trip him. He began to shuffle rather than walk. All of this was so gradual that it was a year before his family realized he was not leaving his room very often. In deference and respect they did not interfere until during a surprise visit they discovered he had no food in his flat, dirty clothes were heaped about, and it appeared he rarely left his bed. He had obeyed the physician.

Tinetti (1989) studied 300 community-residing people over the age of 65 to determine their fall propensity and frequency. A quarter of the people who fell restricted their activities following the fall. The fear of falling became a psychosocial impediment. This study identifies risk factors and interventions that minimize the risk of falling. Similarly, studies by Walker and Howland (1991) showed almost one half of a group of 115 community-residing elders limited their activities for fear of falling, and 30% had fallen within the previous year. In both studies fear of falling became a major life impediment and rated a greater concern than fears of robbery or financial difficulties.

Tinetti et al (1990) developed a Falls Efficacy Scale (FES), an instrument to measure fear of falling based on self-perceived ability to avoid falls during normal nonhazardous activities of daily living. It was found that anxiety, depression, and slowed walking pace were correlates of the fear of falling. The FES proved useful in predicting functional decline based on limitations induced by fear. Health care providers felt that getting dressed, getting on and off the toilet, preparing meals, and taking baths or showers were the most demanding activities. Elderly individuals named activities they most avoided because of fear of falling as reaching into cabinets or closets, taking a bath or shower, walking around the house, and getting in and out of bed. These data may be useful because home health nurses may assess these particular activities and suggest ways the individual can alter activities and feel more secure.

Maki et al (1991) studied 100 ambulatory, community-residing elders to determine correlations between fear of falling and actual falls. Their previous studies showed that individuals tend to stiffen their posture when afraid of falling and that this actually induces more falls. In this replication study they found that postural changes could not unequivocally be attributed to fear of falling, and therefore the current trend to measure postural sway and one leg stance as evidence of fall potential should be interpreted carefully when used with apprehensive individuals.

Drop Attacks. When an elderly person falls "just because my leg went out from under me," we often call these drop attacks. These falls cause hip trochanter cracks or femur fractures, sometimes both. This is thought to be due to osteoporotic bone erosion that accompanies old age and in some women with a high-risk profile (Watts, 1991), reaches pathologic proportions. When osteoporosis of this magnitude occurs, the bone can no longer bear the weight of the individual in walking. It is sometimes difficult to determine whether the fall creates the fracture or the fracture creates the fall. It is of little consequence which precedes the other. In fact, numerous conditions may precipitate a drop attack. Zeiler and Zeitlhofer (1988) found that many neurologic disorders may lead to snycope and/or drop attacks. Seizures, sleep and arousal disorders, vagotonic and several other central autonomic disorders are sometimes culprits; even psychogenic seizures must be considered. Cerebrovascular disorders account for a high incidence, and some metabolic disorders, such as hypophosphatemia, may cause muscle weakness and periodic paralysis (Delage and Lebel, 1990). Regardless of cause, the end result is often immobility, restrictions in movement, institutional living, and all of the physical ailments that tend to follow immobility, especially in the very old and frail elders (Box 11-10).

In summary, numerous situations and conditions make old people susceptible to falls:
- Transient ischemic attacks with vertigo, syncope, or stroke
- Muscle weakness
- Interference with the sense of balance
- Poor eyesight and faulty evaluation of spatial relationships, often resulting from neural deficiencies
- Urinary frequency and urgency leading to unsafe maneuvering at toileting
- Unsteady gait because of pain, fatigue, arthritic changes, or osteoporosis
- Improper footwear or podiatric difficulties
- Improper clothing such as long nightclothes or robes
- Improper use of wheelchairs and walkers, especially on transfer
- Mental confusion and faulty judgment
- Incontinence and dribbling of urine

Assessment. Patients who fall present a complex diagnostic challenge to physicians and nurses. It is helpful to classify a fall in order to better understand the origins as well as the management. Gray-Miceli (1995) provides a specific classification of falls that is useful. *Premonitory* falls are those that are secondary to a medical problem, multifactorial in nature, and preceded by a symptom. These are subject to treatment. *Prodromal* falls are those that precede and predict the onset of disease. *Extrinsic* falls are related to environmental factors. The fall may be accidental or intentional. *Isolated* falls are those rare occurrences that might be considered "freak" accidents. *Cluster* falls describe a situation in which an individual falls frequently at a particular time or place (Gray-Miceli, 1995) (Box 11-11).

Chipman (1990) recommends that any patient with an unexplained fall should have postural pulses and blood pressures taken, a rectal examination for stool guaiac, and a hematocrit level. Nursing observations may be essential to establishing an accurate diagnosis. The nurse may be the only professional who has been in the home and seen the elder function in a familiar setting; the nurse may be the one who has knowledge of the elder's usual lifestyle and needs; the nurse is the one most likely to view the elder holistically and to advocate for protection from unnecessary diagnostic testing.

Functional reach is thought to demonstrate the degree of risk among elderly men for recurrent falls (Duncan et al, 1992). Those individuals who are able to reach forward from 6 to 10 inches beyond arms' length have only one fourth the fall risk of those who could reach lesser amounts.

Box 11-12 provides assessment information.

Interventions. Environmental factors (extrinisic) need modification for safety as enumerated in Chapter 13. Psychosocial intrinsic factors such as confidence and feelings of self-efficacy are seen to reduce the fear of falling (Tinetti et al, 1994). Proprioception and visual acuity contribute markedly to dynamic balance. Therefore any interventions that enhance sensory function and spatial awareness will reduce falls. The aged can adapt quite well to changes in the environment and reduced sensory input if gradually occurring, though the very old do not (Judge et al, 1995). All aged persons should be cautioned against sudden rising from sitting or supine positions, particularly after eating.

As a general principle, any action that increases the individual's confidence and ability to relax is likely to decrease the propensity toward falls.

Actions to increase patient safety include the following:

1. Individualize care planning in terms of patient's level of disorientation.
2. Consistently make efforts to reduce anxiety and uncertainty in new residents. Fear and agitation create clumsiness at any age.
3. Early case finding of the accident-prone individual and concerted efforts by the entire team to minimize unsafe activities and behavior are essential.
4. Review of medications, especially tranquilizers, as to need, dosage, and side effects must be continuous.
5. Adequate staffing, especially at the most dangerous hours, is important.
6. A safe environment, especially for all ambulatory residents, must be maintained.
7. Attempt to deal with confused and agitated individuals through reality therapy, behavior modification, and tender loving care.
8. Residents should be taught the safe use of wheelchairs and walkers.
9. The ambulatory resident should be observed for signs of weakness or fatigue and be assisted as necessary.
10. Continue to gather further information to initiate a program of accident prevention.

The consequences of falls are more serious for old people, and the mortality for various types of accidents rises dramatically. To prevent accidents assess mobility impairments and individual strengths (Box 11-13).

Walker and Howland (1991) found assertiveness training and education regarding hazards reduced fears of falling. Other suggestions include encouraging the elder to be matter of fact about using a cane or walker to help maintain balance and advising not to hurry to answer phones or doorbells. Haste can be dangerous. Gait training, postural reminders, evaluation of home hazards, and modification of environment have all been effective in reducing fall rates.

Box 11-10   Types of Falls

1. Slips and trips: The patient may falsely attribute the fall to these causes when in reality it is due to a physical deficit.
2. Falls while attempting a difficult maneuver (such as climbing over a bed rail).
3. Syncope: The loss of consciousness immediately precedes the fall, and may, itself, be preceded by a brief interval of giddiness or unsteadiness.
4. Seizure: The loss of consciousness accompanies the fall. It may be preceded by an aura. It may or may not be accompanied by clonic movements and incontinence.
5. Drop attack: Sudden loss of muscular tone without loss of consciousness.
6. Vertigo: The patient experiences true dizziness (the room seems to spin) and falls to one side or the other.
7. Sliding off furniture: Due to weakness or somnolence.

From Wieman H, Calkins E: Falls. In Calkins E et al, editors: *The practice of geriatrics,* Philadelphia, 1986, WB Saunders.

(See Chapter 13 for suggestions regarding safety in the home). Correcting environmental hazards and modifying gait problems by increasing lower extremity truncal strength reduced the risk of falling (Shepherd et al, 1992). Box 11-9 lists fall risk factors for elders in an institution and in the community.

With training and increased awareness comes a sense of competence and confidence that may obviate the fear of falling. The National Institute on Aging (1996) reports two studies under their aegis that improved balance of elders and decreased fear of falling. One showed a 47.5% reduced risk of falling after 15 weeks of tai chi training (Wolf, 1996) and the second a 25% to 50% improvement in balance after 3 months of balance and strength training (Wolfson, 1996).

Risk of Falling

Acute illness is associated with functional impairments that tend to increase the risk of falling. Confusion, generalized weakness, postural instability, and foreign environment are major contributors to falling when hospitalized. Loss of proprioception in the legs due to disuse is also an important factor. Bed rest, understaffing, serious illness, and rapid hospital discharge have contributed to an unknown number of falls. There is an increased vulnerability if the individual has a history of falls, is receiving intravenous therapy, has impaired mental status, and needs assistive devices to walk.

Fractures

Osteoporosis of the hip increases with each decade of women's lives, particularly after menopause. This is an im-

Box 11-11   Fall Typology and Common Etiologies

Multifactorial Falls

- Visual loss from macular degeneration, cataracts, hemianopsia, retinal artery/vein occlusion, temporal arteritis
- Hearing loss from sensorineural factors or conductive reasons, neuromas
- Orthostatic hypotension linked to aging, volume depletion, medications or diseases such as diabetes mellitus, Parkinson's disease
- Peripheral neuropathies of lower extremities from B_{12} deficiency, diabetes mellitus, spinal lesions/tumors, cervical arthritis
- Lower extremity weakness from degenerative joint disease, hypothyroidism, hyperthyroidism, electrolyte imbalances, CVA, polymyalgia rheumatica
- Poor balance from cerebrovascular accidents, Parkinson's disease, parkinsonism (related to medications, cerebrovascular dementia)
- Gait abnormalities from dementia (apraxic gait), Parkinson's disease, normal pressure hydrocephalus, B_{12} deficiency, posterior column diseases

Premonitory Falls

- Seizure-associated with post-ictal state, loss of urine control from previous head trauma, stroke or de novo Alzheimer's disease
- CVA associated with sudden extremity weakness, speech or visual change
- Cardiac arrhythymia associated with palpitations or shortness of breath from sick sinus syndrome, sinus bradycardia or tachycardia, junctional rhythms or blocks, or uncontrolled atrial fibrillation
- Orthostatic hypotension associated with lightheadedness and positional changes, caused by diuretic or other factors
- Vertigo associated with dizziness caused by labyrinthitis, vertebrobasilar insufficiency
- Syncope caused by sudden blood loss, vasovagal, post-micturation, hypersensitive carotids, carotid stenosis or neurological etiology

Prodromal Falls

- Congestive heart failure
- Infections such as cholelithiasis
- Functional decline with impairment in mobility, daily living

Extrinsic Falls

- Improper shoewear (poor soles, poor fit)
- Loose or frayed carpeting
- Poor lighting
- Cluttered environments with obstacles
- Sidewalk edging that is difficult to see
- Tripping over cords, walkers (in patients with dementia)
- Slips on floor (from spills, slippery substances)
- Sitting/leaning on moving object (unlocked bed or wheelchair)
- Glare on floor, causing temporary vision impairment
- Steps in poor condition
- Lack of grab rails or devices to lean on
- Missing a step (while descending)

From Gray-Miceli D: Evaluation and treatment of falls, *ADVANCE for Nurse Pract* 3(11):29, 1995.

portant cause of hip fractures in older women (Wolinsky and Fitzgerald, 1994). Decreased bone mass density puts one at high risk of future hip fracture. The treatment of hip fracture has been estimated to cost from $10 to $20 billion annually (Lindsay, 1995). Each year approximately 1.5 million aged experience fractures: one third of these are vertebral, one sixth are hip fractures, 200,000 are wrist fractures, and the remaining 300,000 of various other types (Moran, 1996). While the economic cost is enormous, it is impossible to estimate the human cost in terms impaired function.

Lukens (1986) studied recovery from hip fracture and found that emotional status and degree of social isolation are factors that affect speed and quality of recovery. Active and alert elderly clients are more likely to achieve complete recovery. Age and preoperative health status affect postfracture ambulation. Those over 70 years of age with previous disabilities are most likely to experience increased disability following fracture. Stable emotional states, mental clarity, and frequent activity outside the home before fracture portend a good return to prefracture function. A younger age

Box 11-12	Assessment of Fall Risk

Obtain history of previous falls and precipitants

Evaluate for orthostatic hypotension (increases with age)

Evaluate visual acuity: peripheral, depth, and color vision

Determine presence of arrhythmias

Massage carotid bulb for carotid sinus sensitivity

Rotation of neck to assess vertebrobasilar artery involvement

Observe movements and evaluate muscle strength and balance:
  Test functional reach (Duncan et al, 1992)
  Rising from chair
  Performing deep knee bend
  Walking 10 feet in a straight line, turning full circle
  Climbing and descending stairs
  Romberg test for increased sway
  Standing on tiptoes and reaching upward
  Bending down to pick up object from floor
  Raising feet while walking; tandem walking

Check feet for abnormalities that affect gait

Evaluate mental status and medication regimen, particularly note psychoactive drugs

Observe ease of routine daily mobility maneuvers

All of these evaluations must be carried out with sufficient support and encouragement to avoid activities threatening to the individual's sense of security or that are potentially dangerous

Data complied from Tideiksaar R: Falls in the elderly: etiology and prevention. In Bosker G, Schwartz G, Jones J et al, editors: *Geriatric emergency medicine,* St Louis, 1990, Mosby; Tinetti M, Speechley M, Ginter S: Risk factors for falls among elderly persons living in the community, *N Engl J Med* 319(26):1701, 1988.

Box 11-13	Actions to Prevent Falls

Regular testing for vision and hearing; aids if needed; keep glasses clean and ears free of cerumen and infection.

Seek evaluation and modification of medications (e.g., diuretics, nitrates, hypnotics, antidepressants, antianxiety agents, antihypertensives, and hypoglycemics) that affect balance, coordination, and cardiovascular sufficiency

Limit alcohol intake

Rise slowly from bed or chair to avoid sudden drop in blood pressure, avoid sudden changes in position

When outdoors watch for wet or slippery surfaces; use extra care getting into and out of vehicles, negotiating curbs and crowds

Ask for assistance when needed

Reduce hazards in home

Stay physically and socially active, increase activities gradually

Wear appropriate footwear, avoid high heels and slippery soles

Use assistive devices for ambulation

Consult with physician if feeling unsteady or ill

Data compiled from Tideiksaar R: Falls in the elderly: etiology and prevention. In Bosker G, Schwartz G, Jones J et al, editors: *Geriatric emergency medicine,* St Louis, 1990, Mosby; Tinetti M, Richman D, Powell L: Falls efficacy as a measure of fear of falling, *J Gerontol* 45(6):239, 1990.

was the most significant factor in return to prior function. The number and quality of social supports significantly impact recovery. Physical and mental resources, sociocultural factors, and availability of support systems markedly influence recovery potential (Lukens, 1986). Prerequisites to discharge with the expectation of complete recovery include the ability to maintain (1) balance, (2) motor coordination, (3) stamina, and (4) walking and ADLs within 2 weeks after surgery.

A client's attitude toward recovery during the period of hospitalization does not necessarily indicate capacity for return to function. Thus this should not influence the degree of effort or amount of encouragement given toward recovery. In fact, there was some indication that those with high expectations needed extra support, since their recovery might be slower than anticipated (Lukens, 1986).

Maximum recovery for the client entails intensive and consistent physical therapy and muscle building and range-of-motion exercises, regaining strength, participating in decision making regarding care, maintaining social contacts, fostering feelings of self-worth, as well as tolerating some dependency in the recovery period. Prefracture level of activity provides a baseline for the formation of appropriate goals. When progress is slow, small signs of progress must be discussed with the individual and frequent encouragement given. Resources should be mobilized for return to the home environment, which is psychologically preferable to convalescence in an extended care facility. Emphasis on the activities the individual desires and is capable of achieving is essential. Given the strong relationship of social supports to recovery (Cummings et al, 1988), nurses should assist the individual in maintaining existing support systems.

Fractures are a common result of osteoporosis that lead to many residual chronic problems and various degrees of impaired mobility if the fracture is not well managed after hospitalization. Because these are such common accidents among the old, an example is included to demonstrate the need for continuing, coordinated, and well-managed services in the home if full return to prior status is to be obtained (see case study on p. 429). Recovery from hip fracture demands appropriate education to prevent residual problems or dislocation. The suggestions from *Focus on Geriatric Care and Rehabilitation* (1992) may be given to individuals recovering from hip surgery:

Do not do the following:
1. Turn toes in
2. Bend over too far
3. Cross legs when sitting
4. Lie on side in bed without a pillow between legs
5. Lean forward in bed
6. Forward flex when sitting up or down on a chair or toilet that is too low
7. Keep operated leg planted when turning
8. Have foot rest too high on wheelchair or chair
9. Cross foot of operated hip over the other leg

Falls and fractures often produce periods of immobility. The complications of immobility include the following:

Dehydration
Bronchial pneumonia
Contractures
Constipation
Pressure sores
Hypothermia
Iatrogenic complications
Disability
Institutionalization
Loss of independence
Isolation and depression

Repeated falls are a major precipitant to long-term care admission, and even in a protected setting 25% of these persons continue to fall.

Prevention of Falls

Prevention of falls requires education of the individual in all aspects of environmental hazards and the awareness that falling may be an indication of other underlying problems. Box 11-13 lists actions that help prevent falls. In addition, each facility needs a well-developed falls prevention protocol (Brady et al, 1993) (Figure 11-9).

Management of Falls

Falls, while devastating events, do not ordinarily present an immediate life threat. Chipman (1990) therefore suggests that the physician's approach to the patient should be gentle and unhurried, making sure the patient has heard and understood what is happening. The hospital experience should afford comfort, dignity, and sympathy. Initial considerations are evaluation for head, cervical spine, and torso injuries. Most common are Colles' fracture of the wrist, fracture of the humerus (often accompanied by dislocation of the shoulder), and femoral fractures with a tendency toward intertrochanteric and subtrochanteric fractures.

Prevention of hip fractures can be accomplished in many cases by the wearing of padded undergarments that protect the hips. Several types of these are under investigation and

have proved effective in reducing hip fracture in those prone to falls (University of California, San Francisco, 1995; Chipman, 1996).

Functional Restoration

Kaufmann (1988) states, "Promoting functional restoration and maintenance is more beneficial to the elderly patient than applying restraints to prevent the risk of injury." She suggests the following considerations that have proved beneficial in reducing falls and increasing self-esteem among the fall-prone elderly.

1. Immediately upon admission conduct a fall assessment risk analysis and, if necessary, institute a fall prevention program.
2. Analyze the effectiveness of each intervention in the fall prevention program. Determine whether the interventions are primarily for the protection of the patient or the institution.
3. Institute a written policy regarding the management of the fall-prone client. Discuss the policy regarding the use of restraints with the family, client, doctor, and nursing staff. Document the conversation regarding the wishes of the family and the client. This must be signed by the family and the client.
4. Purchase beds that are as low to the floor as possible; possibly invent beds that are safe.
5. Increase muscle strength through carefully designed exercise programs.
6. Recognize and reduce fatigue factors.
7. Teach walking exercises in which the client learns to lift up the feet rather than shuffling them.
8. Provide appropriate shoes and slippers that have nonskid soles and broad heels of a height comfortable to the individual.

Prerequisite to a fall prevention program is a thorough assessment of persons who have fallen, including a detailed history and physical examination and assessment of risk of falling (Figures 11-10 and 11-11).

RESTRAINTS

Restraints have been used historically for the "protection" of the client and for security of the client and the staff.

Physical Restraints

Stilwell's (1988) definition of physical restraints was developed as a part of her investigations as an expert witness and remains the clearest and most inclusive:

Physical restraints are devices, material and equipment which: (1) are attached to or are adjacent to the patient's body; (2) prevent free bodily movement to a position of choice (standing, walking, lying, turning, sitting); and (3) cannot be controlled or easily removed by the patient. Temporary immobilization of a part of the body for the purpose of treatment, such as casts, splints and arm boards, is not included in this definition.

Falls Prevention Protocol

Initiated	Discontinued
Date: _____	Date: _____
Time: _____	Time: _____
RN: _____	RN: _____

PURPOSE

To outline nursing responsibilities and management for a patient at risk for falling.

LEVEL

Independent (requires nursing order only).

SUPPORTIVE DATA

A fall is defined as an uncontrolled and undirected occurrence in which the patient comes to rest on the floor. All patients are at risk for falls by virtue of hospitalization and treatment. Two levels for falls are identified. As the levels progress, the potential for falls becomes greater.

NURSING INTERVENTIONS

Assessment

1. Perform admission assessment and every 8 hours in the following areas: cognitive, sensory, and mobility.
2. Assess degree of risk for falling according to the following criteria:
   Level 1 patients: Demonstrate no cognitive, sensory, or mobility deficits.
   Level 2 patients: Demonstrate a deficit in one or more areas: cognitive, sensory, or mobility (i.e., untreated visual impairment, impaired judgment, unsteady gait, disorientation); and/or a previous history of falls.

Intervention

3. If patient is assessed as Level 1:
   Ensure the call bell is in reach.
   Lower the bed.
   Lock the wheels of beds and wheelchairs, as appropriate.
4. If patient is assessed as Level 2:
   Address potential for injury through standard care plan or other related nursing care plans.
   Alert all caregivers and staff of the patient's potential for falling by:
      Replacing patient's identification band with yellow ident-a-band.
      Placing yellow signs indicating implementation of the falls program over the patient's bed and outside the patient's room.
      Assess cognitive, sensory, and mobility deficits every shift.
   Every 4 hours as necessary:
      a) Implement Level 1 interventions.
      b) Ensure the side rails are up.
      c) Reinforce calling for assistance.
      d) Offer assistance for toileting.
      e) Offer fluids and nutrition.
      f) Offer transfer assistance.

Reportable conditions

5. Any patient falls.
6. Any significant changes in cognitive, sensory, or mobility conditions.

Patient/significant other instruction

7. Orient to and reinforce falls program.

Documentation

8. Record initiation of falls prevention protocol on progress note in the medical record.
9. Record changes in assessment findings in the medical record.
10. Initiate or discontinue the intervention levels based on ongoing patient assessment.

Note. Adapted from Dallaire, L.B. Reducing patient falls. Nursing 89 1989; 19(5):78-79; and Hendrich, A.L. An effective unit-based fall prevention program. Journal of Nursing Quality Assurance 1988; 3(1):28-36.

Figure 11-9. Falls prevention protocol. (From Brady R et al: Geriatric falls: prevention strategies for the staff, *J Gerontol Nurs* 19(9):26, 1993.)

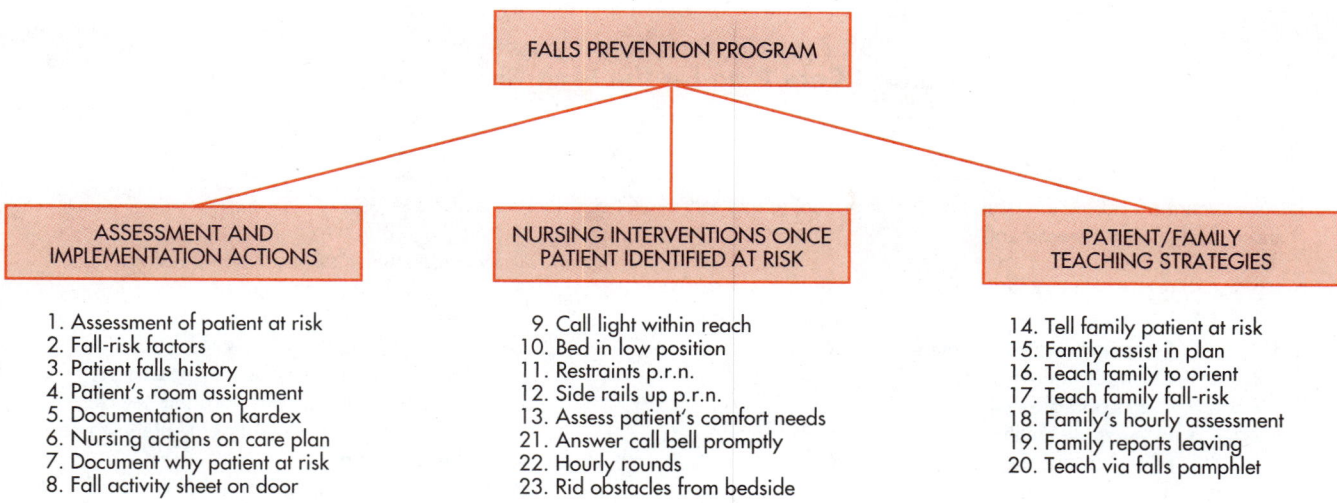

Figure 11-10. A schematic representation of the nursing measures in each major section of the patient falls prevention program. *Note:* The numbering of the interventions in this figure parallels the numbering of the nursing interventions in Part A of the study instrument. (From Kaufmann M: *A patient falls prevention program—do nurses perceive it to be an effective intervention,* unpublished master's thesis, Case Western Reserve University, Cleveland, Ohio, 1985.)

The problems of restraint usage were first brought to the forefront of nursing attention by a request from Doris Schwartz, one of the pioneer gerontic nurses, for information from practicing nurses regarding their observations and concerns about restraint usage. In the intervening time, and largely through efforts of her friends and herself, the use of restraints has been drastically reduced (Evans and Strumf, 1989).

Studies (Tinetti, 1989; Tinetti et al, 1990, 1991, 1992) have shown that mechanical restraints were associated with serious injuries, such as higher mortality, injurious falls, longer hospital stays, nosocomial infections, incontinence, immobility and contractures, and decubitus ulcers (pressure sores).

Characteristics of those who were restrained: older, disoriented, dependent for help with dressing, unsteady, disruptive, agitated, and wanderers. Those who were restrained most frequently seemed to have higher levels of need and interactional desires. When unrestrained, they used fewer antidepressants and participated to a greater extent in social activities. It may be that the quiet, noninvolved, nondemanding patients are simply restrained less frequently. The difference in personality types and activity levels is an area needing further nursing research. Factors that increase the likelihood of restraint application are cognitive impairment, severe limitation in activities of daily living (ADLs), depression, wandering (Burton et al, 1992), and dementias.

Miles and Irvine (1992) investigated 122 deaths caused by vest and strap restraints and found most occurred in nursing homes among women over 70 who suffered various degrees of dementia and had major, involuntary escape-directed movements. These findings reinforced the need for safe systems of surveillance (see resources at the end of the chapter).

Within the last decade and in compliance with the Omnibus Reconciliation Act (OBRA) of 1987 requirements, there has been a concerted effort to reduce the use of restraints in long-term care settings. Whereas physical restraints were the first consideration in preventing falls, they have now been largely replaced by methods of reducing the agitation that precipitates falls and the interference with treatments (Bryant and Fernald, 1996). Fear of litigation was often the impetus for restraints. Now, family members and the client are engaged in discussions regarding legalities and problem solving to avoid the use of restraints. In acute care settings more than 90% of nurses are not aware of OBRA requirements and tend to use restraints to prevent the patient from detaching invasive devices (Bryant and Fernald, 1996).

Rather than augmenting patient care, restraints often increase agitation and attempts to free oneself from uncomfortable catheters, tubes, and lines. Strumpf and Evans (1988), leaders in the move to untie the elderly, found that restrained elders responded with anger, fear, humiliation, demoralization, discomfort, and resignation. Even though physical restraints are used to prevent falls, patients who are restrained are more likely to be injured than those who are not. Reports of deaths as a result of restraints (Katz et al, 1981; DiMaio et al, 1986) emphasized the fact that restraints were not safe.

Many nurses feel that the use of restraints is directly related to a lack of sufficient personnel, and they must be used to prevent falls, injuries, and wandering. However, with the restrictions on restraint usage dictated by OBRA the reliance on them has been markedly reduced, and other safety measures have proved more effective. Most nurses still feel

---

St. Francis Memorial Hospital
Standard Care Plan for the High-Risk Patient

Objectives	Nursing Actions

1. Assessment on admission of the high-risk patient (circle for individual patient assessment).
 	
0 1 2 3 4 5 Unsteady on feet
0 1 2 3 4 5 Poor eyesight (if corrected with glasses rate 0)
       15 Confused and disoriented
0 1 2 3 4 5 Changes in environment
0 1 2 3 4 5 Drugs and alcohol
0 1 2 3 4 5 Physical disabilities
0 1 2 3 4 5 Footwear unsafe
0 1 2 3 4 5 Multiple diagnoses
0 1 2 3 4 5 Language barrier
0 1 2 3 4 5 Neurological problems
0 1 2 3 4 5 Postoperative condition
0 1 2 3 4 5 Attitude
       15 Patient has fallen previously
 	
Add points. If total is 15 or more, continue with plan of care and nursing actions.
	Check nursing actions taken.
	
	a. _____ Assign near nurses station when possible
	b. _____ During nursing interview
	      _____ Ask if patient has fallen
	      _____ Flag on care plan (use color sticker)
	      _____ Recommend safety belt if necessary
	      _____ If family present consider their use during hospitalization—question if sitters would be necessary
	      _____ Continually assess and update record

2. Patient and family education	a. _____ If appropriate, inform the patient and family of the risk of falling b. _____ Repeatedly reinforce this concern to patient c. _____ Involve family members as much as possible
3. Prepare safe environment	a. _____ Special poster in room b. _____ Side rails up c. _____ Bed in low position (brakes working) d. _____ Unnecessary furniture removed e. _____ Call light within easy reach and working f. _____ Night light working g. _____ Footwear checked h. _____ Color sticker on patient's door
4. Maintaining a safe environment	a. _____ Close door (reduce noise level) b. _____ Check patient frequently/talk with patient when awake c. _____ Be alert for equipment maintenance (carpet, floors, lights)
5. Assessing pharmacologic effects	a. _____ Be aware of all medications the patient is receiving, particularly hypnotics b. _____ At night when giving hypnotics, be especially aware of side effects in elderly or postoperative patients c. _____ Note if laxatives are given at night d. _____ Note if diuretics are given

Documentation in nurses' notes should reflect all nursing actions taken.

Figure 11-11. Care plan for the prevention of patient falls developed by the nursing quality assurance and education departments and included in each patient record. A score of 15 on Part 1 places the patient in the high-risk category. Nursing actions are also delineated. (From the Joint Commission on Accreditation of Healthcare Organizations, Chicago, 1989.)

they have been inadequately educated about the use of restraints (Bryant and Fernald, 1996).

Electronic devices are available to alert nurses when an individual is attempting to get out of bed; these are becoming much more frequently used as human rights are more rigidly enforced (see resources at the end of the chapter). Nursing skills are often needed far more than restraints or electronic devices. Communication and creative planning can reduce the anxiety and agitation in the client (Werner et al, 1994). Questions the nurse needs to address include What is frightening the patient? Is there anything in the environment that is familiar to provide security for the client? Is the client cognitively impaired? Is the client isolated, or can contact with the environment be more constant? Information given in measured quantities and frequent brief interactions may reduce the anxiety and agitation to manageable levels.

Some alternatives to restraint use are enumerated in Table 11-7. The methods are limited only by the creativity of the nurse. When the safety and agitation of the client cannot be managed with any known methods, it is the nurse's obligation to insist that the family or facility engage a sitter or companion for the individual.

Just a few years ago, the quality of nursing care and specific requirements for facilitating individual mobility of the aged in long-term care was a concern mainly of a few enlightened nurses and administrators. Now OBRA, the National League for Nursing, and the Joint Commission on Accreditation of Health Care Organizations all have specific

requirements by which outcome criteria and goal achievement can be measured. No longer can facilities be casual about the requirements of OBRA and the accrediting bodies. There has been a proliferation of materials related to the development of measurable outcomes. All long-term care facilities must comply with statements from the *Federal Register* (V56187) that relate to restraints and abuse in order to receive Medicare licensure (Box 11-14).

Environmental Restraints

Intentional environmental impediments may be effective in limiting movement and in some cases may avoid the more devastating alternative of applying physical restraints. Doors may be locked, chairs may be difficult to rise from. These effectively limit individual movement.

In institutions it is sometimes deemed easier to encourage the use of a wheelchair or geri-chair than to modify the environment to increase safety and reduce hazards. Hiding an individual's clothing to prevent venturing away or wandering aimlessly is an infringement on personal rights and is often an unsuccessful deterrent. Recognizing the impact on self-esteem when one is discouraged from the use of maximum capacities should alert the caregiver to provide the aged with more opportunities for independence. If the individual decides to conserve energy by using a wheelchair, it must be a personal decision rather than one imposed for the convenience of others. Attending to individual desire and capacity is a message of affirmation to one who may feel an impending loss of independence in many spheres.

Environmental barriers often discourage ambulation among persons in various settings. In the outer environment steps and curbs may be too high. Buses, subway trains, elevators, revolving doors, and escalators may move too rapidly for the slow-moving elderly person to enter and exit comfortably. Thus the individual may find the interactional

Table 11-7	Alternatives to Restraint Use		
Type of Method Used		**Chronic**	**Acute**
Pain relief		34%	54%
Other comfort measures, i.e., repositioning		69%	71%
Reality orientation		62%	86%
Pet therapy		3%	0%
Music therapy		36%	14%
Therapeutic touch		31%	11%
Reminiscence		24%	3%
Behavior modification		66%	26%
Companionship		55%	60%
Crafts		21%	6%
Active listening		34%	26%
Clear pathways		31%	11%
Increased lighting		21%	43%
Placement of patient near nursing station		86%	80%
Beds lower to floor		21%	43%
Accessible call light		66%	29%
Regular routine		52%	31%
Defusing agitated behavior		66%	29%
Diversional activities		62%	46%
1-1 supervision		69%	69%
Other		14%	0%

From Bryant H, Fernald L: Nursing Knowledge and use of restraint alternatives: acute and chronic care, *Geriatr Nurs* 18(2):57, 1997.

Box 11-14   Statements on Use of Restraints and Abuse

The resident has the right to be free from any physical or chemical restraints imposed for purposes of discipline or convenience, and not required to treat the resident's medical symptoms. The resident has the right to be free from verbal, sexual, physical, and mental abuse, corporal punishment, and involuntary seclusion.

The facility must develop and implement written policies and procedures that prohibit mistreatment, neglect, and abuse of residents.

The facility must ensure that the resident environment remains as free of accidental hazards as is possible; and that each resident receives adequate supervision and assistance devices to prevent accidents.

From *Federal Register* (V56187), Sept 26, 1991, p. 48825.

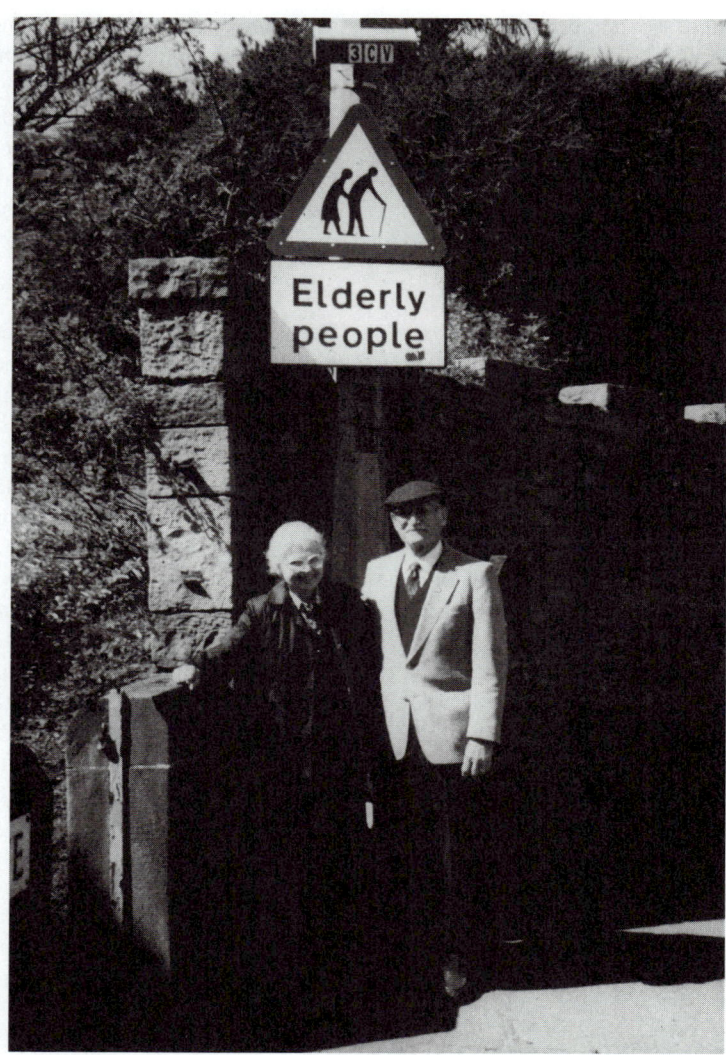

Crossing safely. (Courtesy Patricia Hess.)

world gradually shrinking because of factors that are unintentional. Fortunately, in the last 2 decades there has been a concerted effort by government to encourage the elimination of environmental barriers for the disabled, and this has had a beneficial effect on the elderly as they negotiate the environment.

Wanderers. Wandering is one of the most difficult management problems encountered in institutional settings. Each year some residents wander away from a facility and are later found injured or dead. Media attention and litigation may suggest that staff has been lax in allowing this to happen. Some elders are obsessed with the thought of leaving a facility.

Ambulation, in and of itself, is necessary, and sufficient opportunities to do so in areas that are not hazardous are necessary in institutional settings. Individuals whose lifestyle has included great amounts of ambulation are particularly in need of opportunities to continue this behavior. The

rate or amount of ambulation may seem excessive, but if it is not inherently dangerous, it should be allowed without interference. The pattern and route of ambulation as well as the point at which it terminates are significant. There are many possible patterns and causes for wandering behavior. Some of the most predominant include the following:

- Akathisia-induced ambulation, which is usually a result of long-term use of neuroleptics and is associated with other signs of akathisia, such as inability to sit still, repetitive movements, and other extrapyramidal symptoms. Antiparkinsonian medication may reduce motor restlessness. Usually these persons will not do anything dangerous if made aware of the hazards.
- Self-stimulatory behavior that takes the form of ambulation. This is often seen in advanced dementia and is associated with other stereotyped actions, such as furniture rubbing, hand clapping, and repetitive

vocalizations. Little has been done to deal effectively with stereotypy—the persistent, inappropriate mechanical repetition of actions or verbalizations. These may be a form of self-stimulation in the absence of stimulation that is more meaningful. Providing other forms of stimulation such as paper, cloth, or stuffed toys to manipulate may reduce the meaningless repetitive behavior. Continuous self-stimulation may indicate a lack of external sensory stimulation in the environment.

- Modeling, which occurs when a severely demented client shadows an ambulator and will follow him or her everywhere. Engagement in other activities has proved useful to deter the shadowing.
- Exit-seeking behavior, most often exhibited in recently admitted patients on locked wards. The behavior is accompanied by statements reflecting a desire to go home. Distracting activities may be temporarily useful. Exit-seeking behavior is highly motivated and may persist until the individual finds some gratifications in the present environment that reduce the desire to leave. It may be useful to bring some significant items from the home to help the individual feel more comfortable in the unfamiliar setting. It is important for the nurse to determine how actively the individual was involved in the decision to move to the institution and whether there was adequate orientation to the move.

The first two of these are secondary forms of wandering that are not motivated by the primary desire to move about and are, in fact, evidence of neurologic or cognitive disorders. The interruption of these behaviors may cause more distress for the client and is usually not necessary. When any behavior is negated or discouraged, it is important to provide something to take its place. It is most productive to modify the environment so that the wandering is not likely to be hazardous.

In one facility it was noted that Harvey always tended to walk out of his room and turn right, toward the exit. By recognizing this pattern and changing his room so that a right turn led him to the lounge area, his tendency to wander outside was abated. Past patterns undoubtedly had something to do with his penchant to make a right turn whenever leaving his room. We might assume that in his home the kitchen was to the right of his bedroom. Alert staff were able to realize his pattern and intervene effectively.

Stimulus for wandering arises from many internal and external sources. Agenda behaviors were identified and studied by Rader et al (1985). They found that many wanderers had a specific pattern that gave clues as to their needs. When the need was met, the wandering abated. Three psychosocial factors are correlated with types of wandering: previous work roles, lifelong patterns of coping with stress, and the search for security. Attention to the wanderer's nonverbal behavior, past coping strategies, and present mood are essential. Before attempting to manage wandering be-

havior, you need answers to the following questions:

What is being sought?

When does the behavior most frequently occur?

What would be done if the person were 20 years old instead of 80?

Is the present setting too restrictive?

How dangerous is the wandering?

What psychologic need or energy process causes the wandering?

Discussion of these questions with caregivers and the wanderer may help arrive at intervention that will diminish the need to search. The following interventions may be helpful:

- Care plans that included past coping styles and work orientation
- Memory training group sessions for wanderers
- Assistance to residents in building cognitive maps
- Interesting activity programs to meet varied needs
- Interpersonal contact with significant people
- Availability of items to meet basic needs (for example, food, drinks, blanket)
- Activities that dissipate energy
- Continuity of personnel
- Group relationships and meetings to establish feelings of connection
- Established territory and cognitive maps
- Music, exercise groups, and dances to provide opportunities to move in an integrated manner
- Massage to reduce generalized tension
- Imagery exercises to take mental trips to places one enjoyed
- Nature walks outside the facility to provide relief from the institutional setting
- Visits to places of importance such as work sites and homes

Most important, on admission the patient and family should discuss the hazards of wandering versus the hazards of confinement and make a deliberate decision about when and if an individual should be restricted. Electronic ankle bracelets embedded in plastic, for comfort and ease of bathing, can be put on individuals who have been identified as "wanderers." These will activate alarms that are installed at exits. A lighted panel alerts staff to the exit one has crossed. This system allows others to enter and leave the facility at will and eliminates the need for locked exits. There are other electronic tracking devices that are being used to follow the wanderings of some individuals.

A particularly appealing method of dealing with the wandering patient is to form a buddy system with an individual who is willing and able to provide companionship for varying periods and can account for the patient's presence. This might increase the socialization of each, protect the wanderer, and enhance the ego of the "buddy." The "buddy" must not be coerced into such an arrangement. Sometimes they have formed spontaneously.

We have found no better guidelines than those proposed by Rader et al (1985) to manage an individual who is trying to leave a protected setting. Following this plan reinforces the nurse's interest in the patient's feelings and needs and may relieve distress. It seems that tone of voice and eye contact may provide sufficient focus, somewhat like a radar beam, that keeps an individual on course. Perhaps the personal attention filled the empty restlessness that activated the wanderer.

A wanderer's lounge was developed in a nursing home in Long Beach to provide beneficial activities for confused residents and respite for staff and the more alert residents who were annoyed by the intrusions of the wanderers. The lounge was made safe, and everything in it could be touched by the residents. Each day just before 3 PM, the time when these residents seemed to become the most confused and agitated, a small group of 15 to 20 residents is taken to the designated area. The group members are introduced to each other daily and involved in simple exercises and activities. Refreshments are served. The program employs music, exercise, sensory stimulation, nourishment, and dancing each day. Activities vary from day to day and may include entertainers, poetry readings, sing-alongs, cosmetic sessions, and reminiscing. The program lasts for about 1 1/2 hours.

An activity coordinator, a nursing assistant, and a registered nurse are involved in designing and administering the activities. The nurse evaluates the individual's ability and status during the program, the nursing assistant attends to individual problems such as aggression, and the activity director guides and leads the exercises. Staff members maintain positive attitudes and are not allowed to say "no." Residents are allowed to wander about during the planned activities and to do anything they wish that is not harmful to themselves or others. The observed benefits of this program have been increasing communication among the group members, fewer aggressive episodes, ability to eat finger foods without assistance, and improved nighttime sleep (McGrowder-Lin and Bhatt, 1988).

Holmberg (1996) reported the success of an "evening walker's" group in reducing aimless wandering in a group of persons who had various degrees of dementia but were physically quite active. Conducted in the early evening by volunteers, 8 to 10 individuals would be assembled each evening just after dinner for a planned walk. The volunteers were given information about past interests of individual group members and used this knowledge to keep a conversation going during the walk. Those who participated in the walks seemed calmer afterward and tended to sleep well.

Nursing home residents who participated in a 3-week walking regimen outside the nursing home reported they felt significantly less fatigued. It was suggested that regular outdoor walking programs be instituted as a standard intervention for all nursing home residents who are ambulatory, even if canes and walkers are necessary. In urban settings where traffic and crime may present special problems, internal courtyards may be created or special routes selected for ele-

ments of safety. It might also be possible to transport groups to more pleasant settings for walking. Staff accompaniment is usually necessary for the walking group, but in certain cases individuals may be encouraged to walk in pairs or small groups without staff accompaniment. Visitors can also be encouraged to take residents for walks outside a facility.

Reducing environmental hazards, keeping an individual moving about to increase endurance and function, and identifying persons most at risk of falling are methods that may be used to avoid accidents and falls and maintain mobility. Thoughtful, clear communication, creative planning, and nursing skills can obviate the need for restraints. Nurses in many settings are working together to solve the problems inherent in restraint use but there is still much to be done.

MOBILITY AIDS
Assistive Devices

In ancient times the cane or staff was a symbol of authority. The caduceus is the one with which we are most familiar; the symbol of the Greek god Hermes and the Roman god Mercury. It conveys the authority and distinction of Caducifer's staff with the sacred serpents of wisdom entwined on it and is the emblem of the U.S. Army Medical Corps (Donahue, 1985). In Victorian times a walking stick was essential to a gentleman's attire. Canes and walkers are now designed to be functional.

Catherine had a lovely gnarled, hand-carved, and highly polished wooden walking stick. It was an assistive device, but because of its beauty it was much more. It represented her defense, her power, and her distinctive personality. It provided her security and independence.

Arthritic hips and knees cause considerable pain. To relieve the pressure, the use of a cane on the uninvolved side is helpful. When both sides are involved, a walker may relieve the pressure equilaterally. Many devices are available that are designed for very specific benefits (Figure 11-12).

When helping someone select a walking assistance device, begin with correct shoes. In 1993 it was estimated that sales of walking devices, excluding special shoes, totaled $177 million. Marketers are always ready to sell. If you think your client could benefit by an assistive device, consult specialists and/or rehabilitation therapists. Physicians who are not specialists in orthopedic or physical medicine are not likely to be much help. Assist your client in obtaining a written prescription from the appropriate therapist because Medicare may cover up to 80% of the cost of the device if this is done; other insurance coverage is variable.

When the correct device is obtained, then the client will need assistance in learning to use it correctly. This, again, should be taught by specialists in physical therapy. In general, the following principles should be observed:
- Move the assistance device first, then the weaker leg, and finally the stronger leg.
- Always wear low-heeled, nonskid shoes.

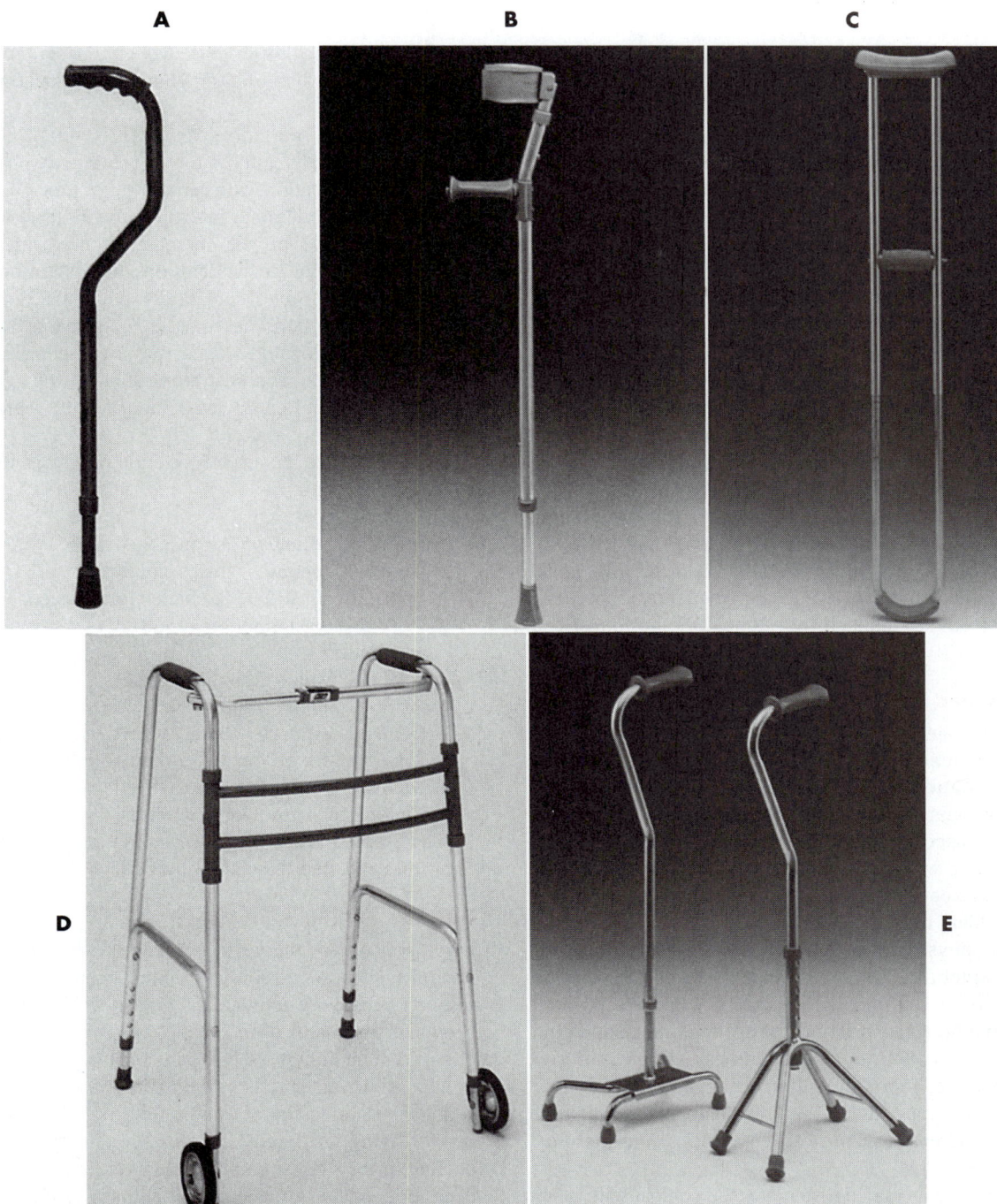

Figure 11-12. Assistive devices. **A,** Standard ortho cane with swan neck. **B,** A forearm crutch stabilizes your elbow while you walk. **C,** New "rolling crutch" provides smoother contact with the ground. **D,** Walker with front wheels allows constant contact with the ground. **E,** Quad cane offers more support than a single-stem walker. (Courtesy Lumex, Inc, New York.)

- When using a cane on stairs, step up with stronger leg and down with the weaker leg. Use the cane as support when lifting the weaker leg. Bring the cane up to the step just reached before climbing another step. When descending, place cane on next step down, move disabled leg down, followed by good leg.

- When using a walker, stand upright and lift walker with both hands.
- Place all of its legs down at a comfortable distance. Step toward it with the weaker leg and then bring the stronger leg forward. Don't climb stairs with a walker.
- Every assistive device must be adjusted to individual height; top of cane should align with crease of wrist.

- Choose a size and shape of cane handle that fits comfortably in the palm; like a tight shoe, it will be a constant irritant if it is not properly fitted.
- Cane tips are most secure when they are flat at the bottom and have a series of rings. Replace frequently because they wear out and a worn tip is insecure.

Wheelchairs.

Winifred glides about the center in her motorized chair, forward and back, negotiating sharp turns, and all the time sitting straight, appearing totally at ease and quite regal. There is no hint of impairment in her bearing.

We have come a long way with assistive devices, but due to maldistribution and sparse budgets there are still places in which the old wooden wheelchairs can be found in use.

Wheelchairs are a necessary adjunct at some level of immobility. These can be used in a healthful way and without demeaning the individual. The various types of motorized chairs can be handled with ease and do not leave the impression of an individual encased in metal trappings. Some are quite attractive. There are frequently opportunities to buy them secondhand from those who no longer can use them.

Transportation

Even though one is physically able to move about there may be many hindrances to full use of public space. Available transportation is a critical link in the ability of the elderly to remain independent and functional. The lack of accessible transportation may contribute to other problems, such as social withdrawal, poor nutrition, or neglect of health care. Even when municipal transportation service is available, elders may not use it. Urban buses and subways not only are physically hazardous but are often dangerous. A "crisis in mobility" exists for many aged people because of the lack of an automobile, an inability to drive, limited access to public transportation, health factors, geographic location, and economic considerations. Older minority people experience more difficulty getting around than older whites and rural more than urban residents. Add to that being female (increased poverty levels), and severe mobility problems exist.

Aged individuals may desire increased contact with other people, particularly relatives; however, even more crucial is the need to reach medical services, shopping areas, and service agencies. If mobility is hampered, both security and the sense of belonging to the mainstream of society may be blocked. The emphasis on a "barrier-free" (structurally revised) transportation system and reduced fares has been helpful to many aged, but some cannot avail themselves of public transportation because of physical disability or residence in a high-crime area. County, state, or federally subsidized transportation is being provided in certain areas to assist aged people in reaching social services, nutrition sites, health services, emergency care, medical care, recreational

centers, mental health services, day-care programs, physical and vocational rehabilitation, continuing education, and library services.

Although transportation can often be found for special needs, it is virtually impossible to locate transportation for pleasure or recreation. Nurses working with the aged find themselves in a dilemma. Interest and concern may suggest that we, acting as private citizens, provide transportation. Aside from liability considerations, this solution presents other problems. Small cars rarely have space for wheelchairs; access to buildings must be checked before an outing; and institutionalized aged may need permission from families as well as administration. Finally, the aged should not need to depend on the available time of a few people of good will and compassion.

Some effective local transportation programs include the following services:

- Reduced fares
- Informal, volunteer drivers
- Demand-response transit vehicles
- Specially constructed vehicles for handicapped
- Door-to-door minibuses requiring advance reservations
- Use of subsidized taxicab services
- Radio-equipped response vehicles
- Demand-response vehicles with a large pool of volunteer drivers (many of them aged)
- Dial-a-ride
- Charter bus trips to special events

The greatest problems in transportation still exist among the rural aged, and this deficit needs increased attention.

Automobiles and Older People

Driving is one of the instrumental activities of daily living for most elders because it is essential to obtaining necessary resources for those individuals who live in rural and suburban areas. Assessments of functional capacities often neglect this important activity. We should evaluate whether an individual can drive, feels safe driving, and has a driver's license.

Changes in vision, reaction time, and physical agility make driving hazardous for some elders. Typically, elders decline in their driving ability around age 75, and dramatic decline is evident by age 85. Kline et al (1992) found that most problems experienced by older drivers involved the following: unexpected vehicles, moving too slowly for the flow of traffic, problems reading road signs, and seeing the roadway clearly enough. Problems that tend to precede driving cessation include neurologic disease, advanced age, cataracts, reduced functional capacities and strength, and lower income (Marottoli et al, 1993).

Peripheral vision is critical to driving because 98% of visual information that a driver receives comes through the periphery and those with poor peripheral vision in both eyes have accident rates twice as high as those with normal vision. In aging the development of arcus senilis, decrease in pupil diameter, eyelid ptosis, cataracts, and decreases in retinal vessel oxygenation all mitigate against good peripheral vision (Fox, 1989).

Kumar et al (1991) discuss perceptual dysfunction related to hemiplegia and automobile driving. These are individual and environmental issues that are addressed in Chapter 12 in relation to the importance of an integration of perceptual abilities, including speed of reaction.

Unfortunately, when judgment is impaired, an individual may believe and insist that he or she retains the capacities for safe driving even though objective assessment shows this is not true. Giving up the mobility and independence afforded by driving one's own car has many psychologic ramifications as well as inconveniences.

When Albert had an unexplained seizure, his doctor told him he could no longer drive. He had been an auto addict all of his adult life and found his major pleasures behind the wheel of the new car that he would buy each year. As a young man having an auto was a major status symbol because few teenagers owned a car in 1935. Driving was much more than a means of transportation for him.

At this time it is often the physician who determines when an individual should no longer drive. In some states physicians are liable if they have allowed an individual to continue driving when it is dangerous. However, there are systematic and comprehensive performance-based road tests that can identify older drivers who are hazardous on the road (Odenheimer et al, 1994). To augment the necessity of such objective performance, Kapust and Weintraub (1992) found that patients with the same level of mild to moderate dementia performed quite differently on actual road tests. Some were deemed safe to drive. Therefore they recommend a road competency test be given before making a determination of such importance to an individual as the revoking of a driver's license. A self-test of driving adequacy has been devised (Mayo Foundation for Medical Education and Research, 1996a) that might be used as a gross assessment tool by health care providers to determine driving adequacy (Box 11-15).

To the 10 million people over 65 years of age who drive automobiles, freedom and independence are equated with keeping a "clean" driving record and their driver's license. Some avoid freeways and take circuitous routes to reach their destination. Their concerns are realistic. Accidents involving the elderly increase insurance rates and are twice as likely to be fatal as compared to younger drivers. These considerations tend to make them overly cautious, which is often very dangerous.

Most states require special testing before reissuing licenses to those over 70 years old. Some people have limited licences that restrict driving to specific areas and distances. Good insurance coverage is imperative and can be obtained through the American Association of Retired Persons (AARP). AARP also provides a course, "55 Alive/Mature Driving," that is helpful and in some cases will qualify one for lower insurance rates.

The older person, if continuing to drive, should be advised to do the following: plan the route beforehand; bring someone to act as navigator when possible; allow plenty of room between cars; avoid night driving; wear hearing aids and glasses to augment sensory awareness; avoid driving under the influence of medications or alcohol; avoid driving in fog, heavy rain, snow, and ice; plan relief periods or drivers for long distances; and keep car in good repair. These tips are particularly critical for older drivers.

Von Mering et al (1994) state that the basic issues of personal autonomy, safety, quality of life, and lack of realistic transportation alternatives for elders dictate the need to find ways to keep older drivers safe on the road and to allow them to remain on the road longer.

In summary, the capacity to move about, on two legs, horses, and wheeled vehicles has been portrayed from the earliest recorded time. The nurse can be significant in facilitating this most fundamental human need, to assist our clients to move as far as their reach extends and as far as our imagination will allow.

Box 11-15   Driving Skills Quiz

If you answer yes to one or more of the following questions, you may want to limit your driving or take steps to improve a problem.

If you answer yes to most of the questions, it may be time to consider letting someone else do your driving for you.

The quiz is based in part on an American Association of Retired Persons publication.

- Does driving make you feel nervous or physically exhausted?
- Do you have difficulty seeing pedestrians, signs and vehicles?
- Do cars frequently seem to appear from nowhere?
- At night, does the glare from oncoming headlights temporarily "blind" you?
- Do you find intersections confusing?
- Are you finding it harder to judge the distance between cars?
- Do you have difficulty coordinating your hand and foot movements?
- Are you slower than you used to be in reacting to dangerous situations?
- Do you sometimes get lost in familiar neighborhoods?
- Do other drivers often honk at you?
- Have you had an increased number of traffic violations, accidents or near-accidents in the past year?

From Mayo Foundation for Medical Education and Research: Driving: how safe are you behind the wheel? *Mayo Clinic Health Letter* 14(7):7, 1996.

Nursing Diagnoses

Activity intolerance
   Gait disorder
   Depression
   Fear of falling
   Sensory/perceptual changes
   Generalized muscle weakness
   Pharmacotherapeutics
   Dyspnea
   Report of fatigue
Impaired physical mobility
   Prolonged bed rest
   Limited range of motion
   Decreased muscle mass, control and/or strength
   Sensory/perceptual impairments
   Severe depression, apathy
   Muscular incoordination
   Cardiovascular and/or respiratory problems
Ineffective management of therapeutic regimen

Risk for caregiver role strain
Anxiety
Fear
Body image disturbance
Cardiac output decreased
Risk for disuse syndrome
Altered health maintenance
Impaired home maintenance management
Risk for injury
Risk for impaired skin integrity
Pain
Fluid volume deficit/excess
Diversional activity deficit
Powerlessness
Sensory/perceptual alterations
Sleep pattern disturbance
Social isolation
Altered thought processes

NURSING PROCESS AND NURSING DIAGNOSIS
Impaired Physical Mobility

Etiologies and Related Factors
Medications
Pain
Neurologic impairment
Sensory impairment
Musculoskeletal impairment
Trauma
Surgery
Systemic and debilitating diseases
Bed-bound
Malnutrition

Defining Characteristics
Activity intolerance: decreased muscle
   strength/endurance
Pain with movement
Prolonged bed rest
Inability to move purposefully in environment
Limited range of motion
Impaired coordination
Presence of prosthetic/adaptive devices
Restraints
Altered body perception

Knowledge
Normal anatomic and functional age changes
Range-of-motion and transfer techniques, positioning
Impact of medications
Physical assessment skills
Activities of daily living assessment skills
Counseling skills
Therapeutic communication
Coping strategies

Collaboration skills with other disciplines
Pain control
Principles of rehabilitation
Common prosthetic/adaptive devices
Interventions for various immobilizing conditions
Hazards of immobility
Community resources

Clinical Judgment and Related Skills
Obtain a client history or history through caregiver(s),
   including nutritional and medication history
Perform a physical assessment with attention to
   neurologic and musculoskeletal systems
Perform range of motion
Assess activities of daily living; ability to transfer, stand, etc.
Develop an exercise program compatible with established
   prescription plan by physical therapist or physiatrist
Promote and encourage self-care
Teach client/caregiver/family needed skills to improve or
   maintain mobility; the use of prosthetic/adaptive
   devices/equipment
Implement pain control measures as appropriate
Design, implement, and evaluate a plan of care for
   client/family/caregiver that maintains or improves
   client mobility
Refer to community support groups, home care services,
   or other appropriate agencies

Evaluation
Contributing factors are reduced or eliminated
Adaptive devices are used successfully
Increased independence/mobility evident
Further decline is prevented

KEY CONCEPTS

- Mobility provides opportunities for exercise, exploration, and pleasure and is the crux of maintaining independence.
- Changes in bones, muscles, and ligaments affect one's balance and gait as they age and increase instability.
- Ease of mobility is thought to be the most visible measure of one's overall health and survival capacity.
- Muscle weakness must be investigated because it is often a result of reversible problems such as endocrine imbalances, particularly hypothyroidism, or medication reactions.
- Gait disorders are often the obvious indexes of systemic problems and should be investigated thoroughly.
- A thorough nursing assessment must include descriptions of gait and mobility patterns.
- Prevention of falls is one of the most important proactive considerations to preserve health and function for the elderly.
- Each institutionalized individual should be assessed for fall risk factor to which they are exposed or inclined.
- Paradoxically, fear of falling and extreme caution actually increase falling propensity in the elderly.
- Physical restraints are to be used only under very specific conditions, with a doctor's order and for a very limited time until a better solution can be found. They are not appropriate for "safety" and are not allowed under OBRA guidelines except in very specific situations.
- Elders who continue to drive may be tested more frequently and may be given restricted licenses.
- Transportation for the elderly is critical to their physical, psychologic, and social health.

▲ CASE STUDY

Osteoporosis

Midge was a tiny lady; she was 5 feet tall, weighed 100 pounds, and was 75 years old. She had retired from a position as director of the water department in a major U.S. city. She had been active politically and involved in numerous causes and campaigns. In short, she was a dynamo, often working 12 to 14 hours a day and so intensely involved she would forget to eat. During her menopausal years she blithely ignored the whole process and was only slightly aware of vasomotor instability (hot flashes). When her friends argued the pros and cons of estrogen therapy, she postulated that it was unnatural and she was not interested. And when discussing nutrition, she said, "Milk!! You must be kidding—my diet is cigarettes and coffee." When she fell from a stool and braced herself with her right hand, her wrist swelled terribly but was not extremely painful. The bruise extended over the palm of her hand and up her forearm. After several days the pain increased and she went to see a doctor, a member of a preferred providers organization (PPO) of physicians to which she had belonged through her employment. She was very surprised to find that her wrist was broken. She had always climbed about and done whatever she wished with little concern for safety. When the physician casted her wrist, he told her she might have osteoporosis. She usually gave little thought to her physical status, but she began to worry about her bones.

She knew that she could manage whatever came along, as she always had, but she wanted to know exactly what her future might hold in relation to osteoporosis and the possibility of broken bones. In order to reassure herself regarding the integrity of her bone structure she called the PPO to schedule an evaluation. You are the clinical nurse specialist she will see initially to determine her need for follow-up.

Based upon the case study, develop a nursing care plan using the following procedure*:

List comments of client that provide *subjective data*.

List information that provides *objective data*.

From these data identify and state, using accepted format, two *nursing diagnoses* you determine are most significant to this client at this time. List two *client strengths* that you have identified from data.

Determine and state *outcome criteria* for each diagnosis. These must reflect some alleviation of the problem identified in the nursing diagnosis and must be stated in concrete and measurable terms.

Plan and state one or more *interventions* for each diagnosed problem. Provide specific documentation of source used to determine appropriate intervention. Plan at least one intervention that incorporates the client's existing strengths.

Evaluate success of intervention. Interventions must correlate directly with the stated outcome criteria in order to measure the outcome success.

STUDY QUESTIONS/ACTIVITIES

What characteristics put one at risk of osteoporosis?

How would you evaluate Midge regarding risk of developing osteoporosis?

---

*Students are advised to refer to their nursing diagnosis text and identify possible or potential problems.

Discuss lifestyle changes that you would suggest to Midge.

What do you imagine her internist will do to determine her propensity for osteoporosis?

What ideally should have been done for Midge or what should she have done for herself?

RESEARCH QUESTIONS

Compare the accuracy and expense of the various methods of measuring bone density.

What remedial measures have produced the best results in slowing or stopping bone deterioration?

What is the earliest age at which it is possible to detect bone resorption and to predict osteoporosis?

Has the incidence of osteoporosis decreased in particular geographic areas where fluorides have been added to drinking water?

Does the condition of dentition have any correlation with the condition of skeletal bones?

▲ CASE STUDY

Rheumatoid Arthritis

Shirley was a very devout Southern Baptist black lady who developed rheumatoid arthritis in her midfifties. She had learned to manage the pain fairly well, but as she neared 70 years old, the combination of rheumatoid arthritis and the "wear and tear" of osteoarthritis had created deformities and pain that restricted her movement considerably. She could no longer move her arms in positions above her chest, and her shoulders felt stiff. She found it difficult to twist jar lids and to open containers. It was particularly difficult to climb the stairs to her bedroom. Sometimes a soak in a hot tub, or a heating pad, or ice packs would bring relief. She often prayed for relief and usually felt better afterward. For a while she participated in a research program using dimethyl sulfoxide (DMSO). She tried to keep active by walking her dog every morning, but she was becoming discouraged and said, "It upsets me that I never know whether I'm going to have a good day or a bad day." She sometimes found herself tempted to try some of the "miracle cures" that she knew were probably fraudulent but seemed to offer some hope.

Based upon the case study, develop a nursing care plan using the following procedure*:

List comments of client that provide *subjective data.*

List information that provides *objective data.*

From these data identify and state, using accepted format, two *nursing diagnoses* you determine are most signifi-

cant to this client at this time. List two *client strengths* that you have identified from data.

Determine and state *outcome criteria* for each diagnosis. These must reflect some alleviation of the problem identified in the nursing diagnosis and must be stated in concrete and measurable terms.

Plan and state one or more *interventions* for each diagnosed problem. Provide specific documentation of source used to determine appropriate intervention. Plan at least one intervention that incorporates the client's existing strengths.

Evaluate success of intervention. Interventions must correlate directly with the stated outcome criteria in order to measure the outcome success.

STUDY QUESTIONS/ACTIVITIES

Describe the differences between rheumatoid arthritis and osteoarthritis.

Discuss Shirley's lifestyle and beliefs as they may affect her arthritis.

What are some of the modifications in her activities that might be useful?

How would you incorporate her beliefs into a care plan?

Discuss the meanings and the thoughts triggered by the students' and elders' viewpoints expressed at the beginning of the chapter. How do these vary from your own experience?

RESEARCH QUESTIONS

What factors predispose one to osteoarthritic changes?

What types of alternative comfort measures are actually sought and used by sufferers of arthritis?

What do elders say reduces the discomfort of arthritis?

What aspects of arthritis cause most distress for elders?

What do demographic comparisons reveal about the geographic, gender, and age distribution of arthritis?

What is the potential for use of vaccines to prevent rheumatoid arthritis?

FURTHER STUDY QUESTIONS/ACTIVITIES

List all of the risk factors in your home that may contribute to falls.

Discuss psychosocial and physiologic issues that impact mobility.

List five hazards of immobility in old age and discuss the effects on an elder's health and function.

Spend 30 minutes in a shopping mall observing older individuals and identify as many types of gait disorders and mobility assistive devices as possible.

Enumerate and discuss the reasons that falls increase in frequency as one ages.

What are some of the practical tips you would give an elder to prevent falls?

---

*Students are advised to refer to their nursing diagnosis text and identify possible or potential problems.

Discuss concerns you have about falling now. What do you think your concerns will be when you are 80 years old?

Discuss the reasons why restraints may be necessary to apply when you are caring for an aged person who is confused, hospitalized, has a foley catheter, and is receiving an intravenous infusion.

Discuss the reasons you would avoid applying restraints.

Identify several alternatives to restraint use.

Work with a partner and take turns restraining each other in a chair with soft restraints. Leave the restrained individual alone for 20 minutes, and after both have experienced this discuss your thoughts and feelings.

What are some of the ways that older individuals could be assisted to drive safely? What criteria would you use to deny an individual a driver's license?

FURTHER RESEARCH QUESTIONS

What types of gait disorders trigger falls and in what situations?

What activities/exercises are most useful in maintaining mobility in the aged?

What are the psychologic reactions of elders to the use of assistive devices for ambulation?

What factors in the institutional environment induce immobility?

What factors outside home and institution (in the community) are most hazardous for the mobility of elders? Where do the most falls occur?

How does a new environment affect mobility? Is there a higher incidence of falls in the first few weeks of adaptation to a new environment as compared to later?

How does obesity affect agility and mobility?

Does obesity predispose one to falling?

How often and in what circumstances are falls precipitated by the distractions or actions of another individual?

How effective are hip pads in reducing fractures?

RESOURCES

American Academy of Orthopedic Surgeons
6300 North River Road
Rosemont, Illinois 60018
Publishes numerous patient education booklets, available free for distribution to clients, on topics such as arthritis, joint replacement, low back pain, and fractures.

Patient Alarms*

Pressure-sensitive alarms usually include a monitor or control unit and some type of pressure-sensitive pad or strip that is positioned un-

*This section was compiled to provide both an overview of the types of alarms currently available and contact information for further inquiries regarding the products. This listing is not meant to imply an endorsement of the products' safety or effectiveness and is not exhaustive.

der the patient. As the pressure is released or varied, the alarm sounds. Units can sound at bedside and/or the nurses' station through the nurse call system. Various adjustments can be made by nurses to tailor these systems to the patient's needs, including alarm time delay, mute settings, or weight sensitivity. Portable units use disposable sensor pads; however, permanently installed units are also available.

For more information on pressure-sensitive alarms, contact:

Bed-Check Corporation PO Box 170 Tulsa, OK 74101	Alarm: Phone:	Bed-Check and Chair-Check (800) 523-7956
Hill-Rom 1069 State Route 46E Batesville, IN 47006	Alarm: Phone:	Bed Exit System (800) 445-3730
Posey Company 5635 Peck Road Arcadia, CA 91006-0020	Alarm: Phone:	Posey Sitter (800) 447-6739
RF Technologies, Inc. 3125 N 126th Street Brookfield, WI 53005	Alarm: Phone:	Code Alert Bed/ Chair Alarm (800) 669-9946
Stryker Medical 6300 Sprinkle Road Kalamazoo, MI 49001-9799	Alarm: Phone:	Bed Exit Alarm (800) 669-4968
Tactilitics, Inc. 5595 Arapahoe Road Boulder, CO 80303	Alarm: Phone:	RN+ Systems (800) 866-4544
Tapeswitch Corporation 100 Schmitt Boulevard Farmingdale, NY 11735	Alarm: Phone:	Nurse Alert (516) 694-6312

Magnetized sensor alarms sound when a magnet is disconnected from the control unit as the patient moves beyond the range of the connecting line. The connecting line is secured to the patient's clothing, to the bed linens, or even across a door. When the line is extended beyond its length, the magnet is disconnected from the control unit and the alarm rings. Units are portable, and the length of the connecting line can be adjusted to meet the patient's individual needs for monitoring. For more information contact:

Alert Care, Inc. 591 Redwood Hwy. Suite 2125 Mill Valley, CA 94940	Alarm: Phone:	Tether Alarm (800) 826-7444
Posey Company 5635 Peck Road Arcadia, CA 91006-0020	Alarm: Phone:	Posey Personal Alarm (800) 447-6739
Wander Guard, Inc. PO Box 80238 Lincoln, NE 68501-0238	Alarm: Phone:	TABS Mobility Monitors (800) 824-2996

Patient-worn movement detectors are positioned on the patient's leg (worn above the knee) so that movement to a near-vertical position is detected. The alarm sounds from the control unit on the patient device. The control units are attached to the patient-worn device, which is patient specific and can be laundered.

Ambularm emits an intermittent sound when the patient swings a leg over the edge of the bed.

For more information on patient-worn movement detectors, contact:

Alert Care, Inc.   Alarm: Ambularm
591 Redwood Hwy.
Suite 2125
Mill Valley, CA 94940   Phone: (800) 826-7444

Films and Videos

Everyone wins! Quality Care without Restraints, a comprehensive multipart training program that offers practical and creative strategies for providing long-term care without the use of restraints. Given the National Media OWL Award. Available from Independent Production Fund and Toby Levine Communications, New York, New York.

Preventing Falls in the Geriatric Patient discusses common causes of falls, assessment of patients at risk, and nonrestrictive interventions. Available from Geriatric Video Productions, PO Box 1757, Shavertown, PA 18708-0757, (800) 621-9181.

Restraints, the Difficult Decision. Diehl P. Westport, Jacoby/Storm Productions, Inc., JB Lippincott Company 1986. A series of five videotapes related to the appropriate use of restraints: the safety, legal, social, and emotional issues are presented in a usable and practical manner.

The following are available from Video Press, University of Maryland at Baltimore, School of Medicine, Suite 133, 100 Penn Street, Baltimore, MD 21201, (800) 328-7450 or (410) 328-5497, fax: (410) 328-8471.

A Choice among Risks: Physical Restraints Rejected, A. Herb, Montefiore Medical Center, Bronx, NY (30 minutes). This video examines the use of physical restraints, including the restraint experience as described by two residents and the dilemmas articulated by caregivers.

Assessment of the Geriatric Patient with a Total Hip Replacement, Rick Violand, Violand and McNerney, 31 minutes, (purchase, $200; rental, $100). The patient in this video program presents a wide range of problems in addition to osteonecrosis of the femoral heads. Four weeks prior to the videotaping, the patient underwent surgery for a total hip replacement. Assessment begins in observing the patient perform activities of daily living. Assessment considerations include the right and left lower extremity, upper extremity strength, incision site, range of motion and leg length, sitting balance and ability to transfer, gait characteristics, and stair climbing. In conclusion, an overview of assessment findings is presented and treatment goals are defined.

Reducing Restraints through Individualized Care, Lois K. Evans, Neville E. Strumpf, and Joanne E. Patterson, Lecture, 24 minutes (purchase, $300; rental, $100). Physical restraints are often used with three groups of institutionalized frail elders: those at risk of falling, those who are noncompliant with medical treatment, and those with disruptive behaviors. Yet restraints are rarely the most appropriate management and frequently result in poor outcomes. This video program briefly describes the problem of physical restraints from a historical perspective and examines the outcomes for residents and staff when restraint use is routine.

Organizations

55 Alive/Mature Driving
AARP
601 East Street NW
Washington, DC 20049

American College of Rheumatology
60 Executive Park South, Suite 150
Atlanta, GA 30329
(404) 633-3777; fax: (404) 633-1870.

Arthritis Foundation
1314 Spring Street
Atlanta, GA 30309

Arthritis Information Clearing House
PO Box 9782
Arlington, VA 22209
(703) 558-8250

National Osteoporosis Foundation
1150 17th Street, NW, Suite 500
Washington, DC 20036 (202) 223-2226,
fax: (202) 223-2237

Older Women's League (OWL)
666 11th Street, NW, Suite 700
Washington, DC 20001

Parkinson's Disease Foundation
Columbia-Presbyterian Medical Center
650 West 168th Street
New York, NY 10032
(800) 457-6676 or (212) 923-4700

Rigid Systems, Inc
Shelter Point Business Center
591 Redwood Highway, Suite 5285
Mill Valley, CA 94941
(415) 381-9009

REFERENCES

Ali N, Twibell R: Barriers to osteoporosis prevention in perimenopausal and elderly women, *Geriatr Nurs* 15(4):201, 1994.

Medicare and medicaid: requirements for long term care facilities and nurse aide training and competency evaluation programs—final rules, Health Care Financing Administration, Department of Health and Human Services Federal Register 56(187):48825, 1991.

American Association of Retired Persons: New cartilage for old, *Modern Maturity* 38(5):22, 1995.

Barbieri EB: Patient falls are not patient accidents, *J Gerontol Nurs* 9(3):171, 1983.

Bauer DC: Factors associated with appendicular bone mass in older women, *Ann Intern Med* 118:657, 1993.

Bourguet C, Hamrick G, Gilchrist V: The prevalence of osteoporosis risk factors and physician intervention, *J Fam Pract* 323:265, 1991.

Brady R, Chester F, Pierce L: Geriatric falls: prevention strategies for the staff, *J Gerontol Nurs* 19(9):26, 1993.

Breedveld F, Struyk L, van Laar J, Miltenburg A, de Vries R, van den Elsen P: Therapeutic regulation of T cells in rheumatoid arthritis, *Immunol Rev* 144:5, 1995.

Bryant H, Fernald L: Nursing knowledge and use of restraint alternatives: acute and chronic care, *Geriatr Nurs* 18(2):57, 1997.

Buchner D, Wagner E: Preventing frail health, *Clin Geriatr Med* 8(1):1, 1992.

Burton L, German P, Rovner B et al: Mental illness and the use of restraints in nursing homes, *Gerontologist* 32(2):164, 1992.

Catanasos G, Israel R: Gait disorders in the elderly, *Hosp Pract* 26(12):67, 1991.

Chipman A: Airbag for hip protects elderly, *San Francisco Examiner,* p. B1, April 8, 1996.

Chipman C: Evaluation of falls and their traumatic consequences. In Bosker G, Schwartz G, Jones J et al, editors: *Geriatric emergency medicine,* St Louis, 1990, Mosby.

Commodore D: Falls in the elderly population: a look at incidence, risks, healthcare costs, and preventive strategies, *Rehab Nurs* 20(2):84, 1995.

Cowan K, Galanos AN: Fitness walking for osteoarthritis of the knee, *Geriatr Med Curr* 13(2):7, 1992.

Craven R, Bruno P: Teach the elderly to prevent falls, *J Gerontol Nurs* 12(8):27, 1986.

Cummings S, Phillips S, Wheat M et al: Recovery of function after hip fracture: the role of social supports, *J Am Geriatr Soc* 36(9):801, 1988.

Cunha U: Differential diagnosis of gait disorders in the elderly, *Geriatrics* 43(8):33, 1988.

Dalton C: Complementary therapies in arthritis treatment, *Advance for Nurse Practitioners* 3(11):33, 1995.

Davis J: Disease mechanisms and therapeutic options. In *Diagnosis and treatment of rheumatoid arthritis: a special report for primary care physicians,* The Institute for Medical Studies, Inc, Laguna Niguel, Calif, 1995, HP Publishing Co.

Delage R, Lebel M: Potential role of acute hypophosphatemia during hypokalemic periodic paralysis attack, *Med Hypoth* 32(4):273, 1990.

DiMaio V, Dana E, Bux R: Deaths caused by restraint vests, *JAMA* 255(7):610, 1986.

Donahue M: *Nursing: the finest art,* St Louis, 1985, Mosby.

Duncan P, Studenski S, Chandler J et al: Functional reach: Predictive validity in a sample of elderly male veterans, *J Gerontol* 47(3):93, 1992.

Evans L, Strumpf N: Tying down the elderly: a review of literature on physical restraint, *J Am Geriatr Soc* 37:65, 1989.

Ezzati TM, Massey Jt, Waksberg J: Plan and operation of the Third National Health and Nutrition Examination Survey, 1988-1995, National Center for Health Statistics, *Vital Health Stat* 1(32): 48825, 1994.

Federal Register (V56187), p. 48825, Sept 26, 1991.

Felson D: The course of osteoarthritis and factors that affect it, *Rheum Dis Clin North Am* 19(3):607, 1993.

Felson D, Zhang y, Hannan M, Kannel W, Kiel D: Alcohol intake and bone mineral density in elderly men and women: the Framingham study, *Am J Epidemiol* 145(5):495, 1995.

Fife D, Solomon P, Stanton M: A risk/falls program: code orange for success, *Nurs Manage* 15(11):50, 1984.

Focus on geriatric care and rehabilitation (brochure), Gaithersburg, Md, 1992, Aspen.

Fox M: Elderly drivers' perceptions of their driving abilities compared to their functional visual perception skills and their actual driving performance. In E Taira, editor: *Assessing the driving ability of the elderly.* Binghamton, NY, 1989, Haworth Press.

Fries J: A new treatment approach: DMARD-based sequential therapy. In *Diagnosis and treatment of rheumatoid arthritis: a special report for primary care physicians,* The Institute for Medical Studies, Laguna Niguel, Calif, 1995, HP Publishing Co.

Galanos AN: Effect of obesity on symptomatic knee osteoarthritis, *Geriatr Med Curr* 13(2):6, 1992.

Galindo-Ciocon D, Ciocon J, Galindo D: Gait training and falls in the elderly, *J Gerontol Nurs* 21(6):10, 1995.

Galsworthy TD, Wilson PL: Osteoporosis: it steals more than bone, *Am J Nurs* 96(6):27, 1996.

Gertz BJ, Shao P, Hanson DA et al: Monitoring bone resorption in early postmenopausal women by an immunoassay for cross-linked collagen peptides in urine, *J Bone Miner Res* 9(2):135, 1994.

Ginsburg M: Weights strengthen older women's bones, *San Francisco Examiner,* 171, p. A1, 1994.

Glockner SM: Shoulder pain: a diagnostic dilemma, *Am Fam Physician* 51(7):1677, 1995.

Gray-Miceli D: Evaluation and treatment of falls, *Advance for Nurse Practitioners* 3(11):29, 1995.

Guralnik JM, Fried LP, Simonsick EM, Kasper JD, Lafferty ME: *The women's Health and Aging Study: health and social characteristics of older women with disability,* Bethesda, Md, 1995, National Institute on Aging, NIH Pub No 95-4009.

Haskell W: Fracture intervention trial, Stanford Center for Research in Disease Prevention, Musculoskeletal Research Laboratory, Stanford University Medical Center, 1992, Palo Alto, Calif.

Hattrup SJ: Rotator cuff repair: relevance of patient age, *J Shoulder and Elbow Surgery* 4(2):95-100, 1995.

Helmes E, Hodsman A, Lazowski D et al: A questionnaire to evaluate disability in osteoporotic patients with vertebral compression fractures, *J Gerontol* 50A(2):M91, 1995.

Hochberg M, Altman R, Brandt K et al: Guidelines for the medical management of osteoarthritis, *Arthritis Rheum* 38(11):1535, 1995.

Hofland S, Powers J: Sexual dysfunction in the menopausal female: hormonal causes and management, *Geriatr Nurs* 17(4):161, 1996.

Holmberg S: A walking program for wanderers: volunteer training and development of an evening walker's group, *Geriatr Nurs* 18(3):120, 1997.

Judge J, King M, Whipple R, Clive J, Wolfson L: Dynamic balance in older persons: effects of reduced visual and proprioceptive input, *J of Gerontol* 50A(5):M263, 1995.

Kapust LR, Weintraub S: To drive or not to drive: preliminary results from road testing of patients with dementia, *J Geriatr Psych Neurol* 5(4):210, 1992.

Katz L, Weber F, Dodge P: Patient restraint and safety vests: minimizing the hazards, *Dimensions of Health Service* 58:10, 1981.

Kaufmann M: *Falls and the consequences,* Lecture, Frances Payne Bolton School of Nursing, Cleveland, November 9, 1988. Case Western Reserve University.

Kessenich C: Osteoporosis in aged men, *Geriatr Nurs* 17(4): 171, 1996.

Kline DW, Kline TJG, Fozard JL et al: Vision, aging, and driving: the problems of older drivers, *J Gerontol* 47(1):P27, 1992.

Kumar R, Powell B, Tani N et al: Perceptual dysfunction in hemiplegia and automobile driving, *Gerontologist* 31:807, 1991.

Lindsay R: The burden of osteoporosis: cost, *Am J Med* 98:9S, 1995.

Lipe H, Longstreth WT Jr, Bird TD et al: Sexual function in married men with Parkinson's disease compared to married men with arthritis, *Neurology* 40:1347, 1990.

Lipsitz L: Hypotension. In Abrams WB, Beers MH, Berkow R, editors: *Merck Manual of Geriatrics,* ed 2, 1995, Whitehouse Station, NJ, Merck Research Laboratories.

Lipsitz L, Jonsson P, Kelley M, Koestner J: Causes and correlates of recurrent falls in ambulatory frail elderly, *J Gerontol* 46(4):114, 1991.

Longstreth WT, Nelson L, Line M et al: Utility of the sickness impact profile in Parkinson's disease, *J Geriatr Psych Neurol* 5:142, 1992.

Looker AC, Johnston cc, Wahner HW, et al: Prevalence of low femoral bone density in older US women from NHANES III, *J Bone Miner Res* 10:796, 1995.

Lord S, Lloyd D, Nirui M, Raymond J, Williams P, Stewart R: The effect of exercise on gait patterns in older women: a raondomized controlled trial, *J of Gerontol* 51A(2):M64, 1996.

Lorig K, Lubeck D, Kraines RG et al: Outcomes of self-help education for patients with arthritis, *Arthritis Rheum* 28:680, 1985.

Lukens L: Six months after hip fracture, *Geriatr Nurs* 7(4):202, 1986.

Lundervold D, Poppen R: Biobehavioral rehabilitation for older adults with essential tremor, *Gerontologist* 35(4):556, 1995.

Madeley P, Hulley JL, Wildgust H et al: Parkinson's disease and driving ability, *J Neurosurg Psych* 53:580, 1990.

Maki B, Holliday P, Topper A: Fear of falling and postural performance in the elderly, *J Gerontol* 46(4):123, 1991.

Maki B, Holliday P, Topper A: A prospective study of postural balance and risk of falling in an ambulatory and independent elderly population. 49(2):M72, 1994.

Mann D: New blood test quickly assesses bone health, *Medical Tribune News Service,* Oct 24, 1996.

Marder K: Epidemiology of PD in Northern Manhattan, *Parkinson's Disease Foundation Newsletter,* Columbia-Presbyterian Medical Center, New York, NY, Summer, 1992.

Marino C, McDonald E: Differential diagnosis of rheumatoid arthritis. *Arthritis* 90:237, 1991.

Marottoli R, Otsfeld A, Merrill S, Perlman G, Foley D, Cooney L: Driving cessation and changes in mileage driven among elderly individuals, *J of Gerontol* 48(5):S255, 1993.

Mastrangelo R: The silent disease: diagnosing and treating osteoporosis, *Advance for Nurse Practitioners* 2(4):23, 1994.

Mayo Foundation for Medical Education and Research: Neck pain, *Mayo Clinic Health Letter* 12(10):4, 1994.

Mayo Foundation for Medical Education and Research: Driving: how safe are you behind the wheel? *Mayo Clinic Health Letter,* 14(7):7, 1996a.

Mayo Foundation for Medical Education and Research: Heel pain, *Mayo Clinic Health Letter,* 14(7):1, 1996b.

McGrowder-Lin R, Bhatt A: A wanderer's lounge program for nursing home residents with Alzheimer's disease, *Gerontologist* 28(5):607, 1988.

Meco G, Bonifati V, Cusimano G et al: Hallucinations in Parkinson disease: neuropsychological study, *Italian J Neurol Sci* 11:373, 1990.

Merck & Co, Inc: FDA clears Merck's Fosamax as first nonhormonal drug to treat osteoporosis in women after menopause, *Merck Media Alert,* Oct 2, 1995, West Point, Pa.

Miles SH, Irvine P: Deaths caused by physical restraints, *Gerontologist* 32:762, 1992.

Moran G: Osteoporosis fact sheet, Bone Matters Tour, May 1996, Sandoz Pharmaceuticals, NJ, (201) 503-5567.

Mundy GR: No bones about fluoride, *National Medicine* 1(11):1130, 1995.

National Institute on Aging: *Special report on aging,* US Department of Health and Human Services, Bethesda, Md, 1990, Public Health Service.

National Institute on Aging: *Tai Chi for older people reduces falls, may help maintain strength,* National Institute on Aging, news release, May 2, 1996.

National Osteoporosis Foundation: *Osteoporosis facts, Legislation Issue Brief,* Washington, DC, Feb 1996, National Osteoporosis Foundation.

NURSEweek Newsbriefs: Researchers hope new vaccine helps treat rheumatoid arthritis, *NURSEweek* 9(5):23, 1996.

Odenheimer G, Beaudet M, Jette A, Albert M, Grande L, Minaker K: Performance based driving evaluation of the elderly driver: safety, reliability and validity, *J Gerontol* 49(4):M153, 1994.

Osteoporosis research, education and health promotion: US Department of Health and Human Services, National Institutes of Health, Part I, Bethesda, Md, 1990, Public Health Service.

Paget S: Diagnostic guidelines. In *Diagnosis and treatment of rheumatoid arthritis: a special report for primary care physicians,* The Institute for Medical Studies. Laguna Niguel, Calif, 1995, HP Publishing Co.

Pak CY, Sakhaee K, Adams-Huet B, Piziak V, Peterson RD, Poindexter JR: Treatment of postmenopausal osteoporosis with slow-release sodium fluoride, *Ann Intern Med* 123(6):401, 1995.

Parkinson's Disease Foundation Newsletter: *About Parkinson's disease,* Parkinson's Disease Foundation, Columbia-Presbyterian Medical Center, New York, NY, Summer 1996.

Potter J, Evans A, Duncan G: Gait speed and activities of daily living function in geriatric patients, *Arch Phys Med Rehabil* 76(11):997, 1995.

Prestwood KM, Pilbeam CC, Burleson JA et al: The short term effects of conjugated estrogen on bone turnover in older women, *J Clin Endocrinol Metab* 79(2):366, 1994.

Rader J, Doan J, Schwab M: How to decrease wandering, a form of agenda behavior, *Geriatr Nurs* 6:196, 1985.

Rifat S, Kiningham R, Peggs J: Calcitonin in the treatment of osteoporotic bone pain, *J Fam Pract* 35(1):93, 1992.

Roberts B: Risk of falling among persons discharged from intensive care, Unpublished manuscript, Cleveland, 1988, Case Western Reserve University.

Shepherd J, Lutz L, Miller R, Main D: Patients presenting to family physicians after a fall: a report from the ambulatory sentinel practice network, *J Fam Pract* 35(1):43, 1992.

Sogaard CH, Mosekilde L, Richards A: Loss of trabecular bone strength and bone quality after 5 years of fluoride therapy for osteoporosis, *Ugeskr Laeger* 157(14):2004, 1995.

Stilwell E: Use of physical restraints on older adults, *J Gerontol Nurs* 14:42, 1988.

Strumpf NE, Evans LK: Physical restraint of the hospitalized elderly: perceptions of patients and nurses, *Nurs Res* 37(3):132, 1988.

The best ways to relieve osteoarthritis of the hand, *Johns Hopkins Medical Letter* 5(8):3, 1993.

Tideiksaar R: Falls in the elderly: etiology and prevention. In Bosker G, Schwartz G, Jones J, Sequeira M, editors: *Geriatric emergency medicine,* St Louis, 1990, Mosby.

Tinetti M: Performance oriented assessment of mobility problems in elderly patients, *J Am Geriatr Soc* 34:199, 1986.

Tinetti M: Instability and falling in elderly patients, *Semin Neurol* 9(1):39, 1989.

Tinetti M, Ginter S: The nursing home life-space diameter: a measure of extent and frequency of mobility among nursing home residents, *J Am Geriatr Soc* 38(12):1311, 1990.

Tinetti M, Liu W, Ginter S: Mechanical restraint use and fall related injuries among residents of SNFs, *Ann Intern Med* 116(5):369, 1992.

Tinetti M, Liu W, Marottoli R et al: Mechanical restraint use among residents of skilled nursing facilities: prevalence, patterns, and predictors, *JAMA* 265(4):468, 1991.

Tinetti M, Mendes de Leon C, Doucette J, Baker D: Fear of falling and fall-related efficacy in relationship to functioning among community-living elders, *J Gerontol* 49(3):M140, 1994.

Tinetti M, Richman D, Powell L: Falls efficacy as a measure of fear of falling, *J Gerontol* 45(6):239, 1990.

Tinetti M, Speechley M, Ginter S: Risk factors for falls among elderly persons living in the community, *N Engl J Med* 319(26):1701, 1988.

Topp B: Toward a better understanding of Parkinson's disease, *Geriatr Nurs* 8(4):180, 1987.

Toufexis A: Why the bones break, *Time* 143(5):97, Jan 31, 1994.

US Bureau of the Census: *Statistical abstract of the United States: 1995,* ed 115, Washington, DC, 1995.

US Department of Health and Human Services: *Research News,* Bethesda, Md, 1995, National Institute of Arthritis and Musculoskeletal and Skin Diseases (NIAMS), National Institutes of Health News Release.

US Department of Health and Human Services: *Health United States 1995*, National Center for Health Statistics, Hyattsville, Md, 1996, US Government Printing Office, Washington, DC, DHHS Pub No (PHS) 96-1232.

University of California, San Francisco: A hip pad to prevent injuries during a fall, *To Our Neighbors* 20(4):1, 1995.

Vecchio PC, Kavanagh RT, Hazelman BL, King RH: Community survey of shoulder disorders in the elderly to assess the natural history and effects of treatment, *Ann Rheum Dis* 54(2):152, 1995.

Von Mering O, Donnelly M, Kaplan H: Driving smart: a quality of life issue for elders, *Aging Today* 15(5):12, 1994.

Walker J, Howland J: Falls and fear of falling among elderly people living in the community: occupational therapy interventions, *Am J Occupa Ther* 45(2):119, 1991.

Watts N: Prevention of osteoporosis: The role of primary physicians, *J Fam Pract* 32(3):261, 1991.

Werner P, Koroknay V, Braun J, Cohen-Mansfield J: Individualized care alternatives used in the process of removing physical restraints in the nursing homes, *J Am Geriatr Soc* 42:321, 1994.

Wolf SO: Reducing frailty and falls in older persons: investigation of Tai Chi and computerized balance training, *J Am Geriatr Soc* 44(5):489, 1996.

Wolfson L, Whipple R, Amerman P et al: Gait and balance in the elderly: two functional capacities that link sensory and motor ability to falls, *Clin Geriatr Med* 1:649, 1985.

Wolinsky F, Fitzgerald J: The risk of hip fracture among noninstititutionalized older adults, *J of Gerontol* 49(4):S165, 1994.

Wright B, Aizenstein S: Behavioral diagnoses of an elderly nursing home population: how a multi-disciplinary team named behaviors, *Geriatr Nurs* 14(1):30, 1993.

Zeiler K, Zeitlhofer J: Syncopal consciousness disorders and drop attacks from a neurological viewpoint, *Wien Klini Wochenschr* 100(4):93, 1988.

Zuckerman J, Shapiro I: Geriatric shoulder pain: common causes and their management, *Geriatrics* 42(9):43, 1987.

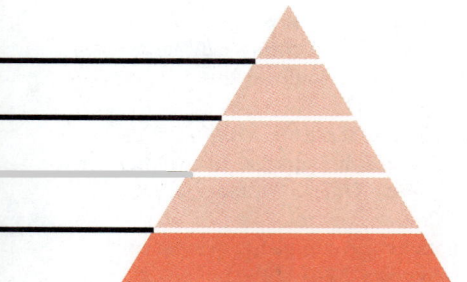

Osteoporosis Functional Disability Questionnaire

The osteoporosis functional disability questionnaire was developed as a specific instrument to measure disability in several domains: feelings of adequacy, comfort, mood, activities of daily living, instrumental activities of daily living, and social activities. Self-evaluation of impairment (on a Likert scale 1-5 indicating frequency and/or severity of problems) provides information for designing and planning self-care and supportive activities.

Motivation and need for participation in therapeutic regimens and exercise programs is evaluated by the following indications:

Please indicate in degrees of 1 (good) to 5 (poor) your estimation of your general health aside from your osteoporosis _____

Please indicate in degrees of 1 (no difficulty) to 5 (very difficult) any problems meeting your financial commitments in the following areas.

Housing _____
Food _____
Personal expenses _____
Transportation _____
Medical expenses _____
Other _____

Please indicate in degrees of 1 (least) through 5 (most) items below that are of most concern related to your osteoporosis.

Pain _____
General health _____
Appearance _____
Interferes with social activities _____
Interferes with work _____
Other _____

Mark in degrees of 1 (least) through 5 (most) the organizations or groups of importance to you that you are hindered from enjoying because of your osteoporosis.

Church _____
Job related _____
Recreational _____
Fraternal _____
Civic/political _____
Other _____

Indicate by numbers 1 (least) through 5 (most) the intensity/frequency of feelings you have experienced in the past week.

I was bothered by things that usually don't bother me. _____
I did not feel like eating; my appetite was poor. _____
I was unable to shake off the blues even with help from family and friends. _____
I felt I was just as well off as other people. _____
I had trouble keeping my mind on what I was doing. _____
I felt depressed. _____
I felt as if everything I did was an effort. _____
I felt hopeful about the future. _____
I thought my life had been a failure. _____
I felt fearful. _____
My sleep was restless. _____
I was happy. _____
I talked less than usual. _____
I felt lonely. _____
People were unfriendly. _____
I enjoyed life. _____
I had crying spells. _____
I felt sad. _____
I felt that people disliked me. _____
I could not get going. _____

Indicate by numbers 1 (unable) through 5 (independent) your ability to accomplish the following activities without assistance.

Get in and out of bed _____
Use the toilet _____
Bathe yourself _____
Dress yourself _____
Put on your shoes _____
Cut your toenails _____
Prepare light meals _____
Prepare meals for family or entertainment _____

Wash the dishes _____

Do laundry _____

Do light housework _____

Do your vacuuming _____

Do heavy housework _____

Go shopping _____

Go on social outings _____

Walk around your house _____

Climb stairs _____

Walk down stairs _____

Hold a book to read _____

Walk outdoors for over 15 minutes _____

Board a bus _____

Drive an automobile _____

Do gardening _____

Bend down _____

Reach overhead _____

Sit down and get out of chair _____

Ideally, this self-evaluation tool should be used before and after program interventions.

Modified from Helmes E, Hodsman A, Lazowski D, Bhardwaj A, Crilly R, Nichol P, Drost D, Vanderburgh L, Pederson L: A questionnaire to evaluate disabiilty in osteoporotic patients with vertebral compression fractures, *J Gerontol* 50A(2):M91-M98, 1995.

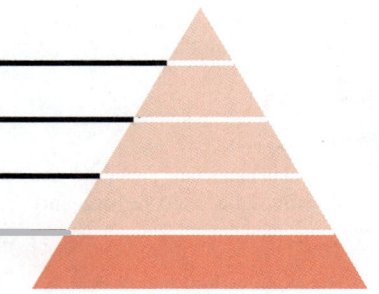

CHAPTER 12

Maximizing Sensory Function

A student learns   ***During the years I worked as a food server I grew accustomed to waiting on older people. They can't always read the menu, they complain that the lighting in the restaurant is too low, they like their dinner experience to be slower, they can't find their silver when they need it, the soup is never hot enough and the cup of coffee is never full enough. They would yell at me because they could not hear me. It used to make me mad, but now I understand they are just real people experiencing growing old. Yes, they may have problems like losing some of their senses and other physical changes, but in actuality they are the same as me.***

Debbie, age 27

Elders speak   ***You know how much Erma loves her soup for lunch. The other day she said that the soup here isn't good anymore. I think it is because her taster isn't good anymore. You know, we have had the same cook in this center for 25 years.***

Laura, age 80

One of the great frustrations is the matter of eyesight. One can get used to large print and hope for black letters on white paper but why do modern publishers seem to prefer the shiny, slick off-white paper and pale ink in miniscule print? And, my new prescription glasses have not restored my ability to cut my own toenails without danger of wounding myself. I find myself wishing for some treatment for incipient cataracts. Please researchers, let's get rid of this scourge of the elderly.

Lyn, age 85

LEARNING OBJECTIVES   Upon completion of this chapter, the reader will be able to:

1. Identify several sensory changes accompanying aging that alter the perceived world of the aged.
2. Explain changes in the aging system that impair sensation.
3. Relate sensory changes to perceptual and environmental insecurity and behavioral disturbances.
4. Discuss the use of various accoutrements that assist the aged with sensory deficits and how they are best used.
5. Describe several conditions that affect sensory function and awareness.
6. Identify several interventions that enhance sensory function and perceptual integration.
7. Develop a nursing care plan appropriate to the care of an elder experiencing a sensory deficit.

THE SENSORY APPARATUS

Huxley (1954) wrote an interesting monograph formulating a paradoxic theory of sensory function. He believed sensory apparatus was meant to filter out the impinging universe. This is in contrast to the common view that sensory organs are our windows on the world. Huxley believed our senses protect us from the overwhelming bombardment of environmental messages that are not necessary for human function. He thought our senses are filters rather than feelers. They filter out the extraneous messages and let in only those that increase our adaptability. The senses seem to put boundaries and order into our lives, and when they are understimulated or overloaded, the structure weakens and unconscious processes break through. (See later in the chapter and chapter 21 for further discussion of perceptual disorganization.)

Appreciation of Sensory Changes

With old age, all senses gradually lose their acuity (see Chapter 4). Although the normal changes of age do not result in any abrupt awareness of sensory loss, the accumulated atrophy of sensory receptors in the eye, ear, nose, buccal cavity, and peripheral afferent nerves substantially reduce the vividness of environmental impressions. Events no longer alert the nervous system with such clarity as in youth. Habituation to certain sensations may also diminish their impact. When the senses are impaired, the sense of self is altered.

The natural gradual loss of sensory functioning with old age may be pragmatically sound. It lends some credence to the disengagement theory. With age the filters atrophy and the perceptible universe shrinks. This may be a mechanism of gradual withdrawal from the experienced universe. Is it less traumatic to gradually disengage from the impressions of life than to abruptly cease to exist? Perhaps we should consider the possibility of sensory disengagement as well as social disengagement. A world that is not so bright and vivid as that of the child's may not be so hard to leave. Perhaps the muting of sensory detail is an aspect of the development of wisdom. The elder is less distracted from the larger sense and meanings.

The issues of concern to nurses are devising methods to keep the organismic senses functional enough to negotiate the environment effectively: to enjoy the beauty and respond to the pain. Both joy and pain are meaningful; pain perception signals danger but also can be ambivalently mixed with pleasure. Pain and pleasure are often intertwined; both are part of living and experiencing. We must dull excruciating pain but avoid dulling awareness with medications and mechanistic limitations that effectively reduce one's appreciation of pleasure and sorrow.

The caregiver's job is to keep the environment within reach; to supplement sensory loss with additional pleasures to the remaining senses; to provide touching and stroking, color and variety; to refrain from pushing and shoving the elements in haste and irreverence. The sensory environment is to be revered and cultivated. Therein lie many problems. Old age subjects one to decreased appreciation of the environment through drugs, machines, treatments, paresthesias, presbyopia, presbycusis, agnosia, etc. Life may be more cautiously sampled. Stored experiences often come to the rescue, and old people remember things they can no longer perceive.

When describing the capacities and changes in the various sensory apparatus, we must understand that they all work in consensus. Situations are experienced through sight, sound, smell, and touch simultaneously (Sacks, 1989). The senses are tightly interwoven in forming the perceptual base of our world. Possibly the "sixth sense" (intuition, or the power of perception that goes beyond that of the five senses) is really the consensus of all the senses in an acutely aware individual. In some cases a disorder of one of the senses may stimulate the others in a compensatory manner. No one has studied this in the aged, but anecdotally some elders have experienced and escribed enhancement of the sense of hearing when sight was poor or vice versa.

Age-related declines are variable and cannot be generalized to all sensory systems (Meeuwsen et al, 1992). Personal hardiness and an environment that conveys order and meaning contribute in ways yet unidentified to good perceptual processing and high level functioning. It is not uncommon that elders are thought to be cognitively impaired when, in fact, attention to enhanced sensory function through an adapted environment and well-fitted accoutrements reveal much higher functional levels. General perceptual organization and efficiency are modified by health status, frailty of aging, illness, medications, fatigue, and stress and anxiety (see chapters 10, 15, 19, 21 and 23).

Through stroke studies it has become evident that the degree of tactile acuity is highly predictive of levels of perceptual integrity and can be predictive of functional recovery (Barer, 1990). Though this has not been studied sufficiently, we would expect the sensitivity to touch to be useful in assessment of sensory integrity. Further discussion of the importance of touch can be found in chapter 16.

In this chapter we focus on the major sensory organs, the normal age-related alterations as well as the most commonly experienced problems. How these affect the individual and his or her ability to successfully negotiate the environment is the nurse's concern. The task is to augment sensory experience when senses are diminished and to help design a colorful, rewarding environment that fits the needs and abilities of the individual (Table 12-1).

Alteration in Sensory Experience

The normal gradual diminution of the senses during the aging process is usually well accommodated by experience. When the experience remains within the boundaries of constancy and familiarity, normal sensory loss is not detrimental to function. It may in fact be desirable. An old person, because of lowered energy and concentration, may be more

Table 12-1   Age-Related Sensory Changes, Outcomes, and Prevention, Health Promotion, and Maintenance Approaches

Age-related changes	Outcomes	Health prevention, promotion, and maintenance
Vision		
Lid elasticity diminishes	Pouches under the eyes	Use isotonic eye drops as needed
Loss of orbital fat	Excessive dryness of eyes	
Decreased tears		
Arcus senilis becomes visible		
Sclera yellows and becomes less elastic		
Yellowing and increased opacity of cornea	Lack of corneal luster	
Increased sclerosis and ridgidity of the iris		
Decrease in convergency ability	Presbyopia	Have eyes examined at least once a year
Decline in light accommodation response	Lessened acuity	Use magnifying glass and high intensity light to read
Diminished pupilary size	Decline in depth perception	Increase light to prevent falls
Atrophy of ciliary muscle	Diminished recovery from glare	Clip on sunglasses, visors, sun hat, nonglare coating on prescription glasses/sunglasses
Night vision diminishes	Night blindness	Don't drive at night
		Keep night-light in bathroom and hallway
		Paint first and last step of staircase and edge of each step between with a bright color
Yellowing of lens	Diminished color perception (blues and greens)	
Lens opacity	Cataracts	Surgical removal of lens
Increased intraocular pressure	Rainbows around lights	Have a yearly eye examination including tonometer testing
Shrinkage of gelatinous substance in the vitreous	Altered peripheral vision	
Vitreous floaters appear		
Ability to gaze upward decreases		
Thinning and sclerosis of retinal blood vessels		
Atrophy of photoreceptor cells		
Degeneration of neurons in visual cortex		
Hearing		
Thinner, drier skin of external ear		
Longer and thicker hair in external ear canal		
Narrowing of auditory opening		
Increased cerumen		Check ears for wax or infection
Thickened and less resilient tympanic membrane		
Decreased flexibility of basilar membrane	Difficulty hearing high-frequency sounds (presbycusis)	Formal hearing test
Ossicular calcification		
Diminished neuron, endolymph, hair cells and blood supply to inner ear and auditory nerve	Gradual loss of sound	Consultation for proper hearing and speaking tone-shouting distorted
Degeneration of spiral ganglion and arterial blood vessels		
Weakness and stiffness of muscles and ligaments		
Smell		
Decreased olfactory cells	Decreased appetite	Encourage social dining
	Decreased protection from noxious odors and tainted food	
Taste		
Possible decrease in size and number of taste buds	Poor nutrition	Nutritional supplementation. Use of stronger flavors

vulnerable to sensory overload than to sensory deprivation. We are all subject to alterations in our sensory experience, and with increasing age it is likely that these circumstances will occur more frequently and perhaps be more devastating. They occur in the following ways:

A. Environmental alterations
   1. Protective isolation
   2. Experimental isolation
   3. Environmental overload: size, frequency, intensity
   4. Noxious agents: noise, glare, temperature
B. Organic alterations
   1. Pain and illness (for example, ability to smell and taste altered by a cold)
   2. Receptor changes of biologic origin
   3. Receptor changes of chemical origin
C. Perceptual alterations
   1. Selective inattention
   2. Habituation
   3. Expectations derived from past experience
   4. Conflicts and psychologic defenses

Alterations in sensory input may contribute to increased anxiety in the aged population. Caregivers of the aged are concerned about manipulating stimuli and enhancing sensory apparatus to induce an optimum functional level of perceptual adequacy. When the senses are grossly underloaded or overloaded, perception and reactions are distorted. The world becomes an alien, confusing place. Fear and anxiety increase, or one withdraws into a fabricated world that provides security. Altered sensory experience will affect one's view of self and one's ability to relate to others (Figure 12-1). Isolation and loneliness may be the result (see Chapter 18). Emotional responses to altered sensory input include boredom, diminished concentration, incoherent thoughts, anxiety, fear, depression, lability of affect, and even hallucinations. Clear and sometimes repetitive data about the environment must be given when perceptions are impaired. Manipulating the environment to reduce demands and enhance sensory function should decrease these symptoms, although studies show that signs may persist for several days. Significant research on elders' varied adaptations to sensory losses is limited. The assumption of increasing loss of acuity of all senses and the importance of well-designed and well-fitted accoutrements comprise the bulk of attention given to the topic. Adequate input is essential to continued cognitive development.

Sensory Deprivation. There are at least three types of sensory deprivation: (1) reduced sensory capacities, (2) elimination of patterns and meaning from input, and (3) restrictive, monotonous environments. Prisoners, astronauts, and solitary explorers have made the public aware of the effects of isolation from ordinary environmental stimulation. Psychologic and physiologic effects of such situations have been reported through personal accounts and from studies of artificial situations constructed for the express purpose of studying sensory deprivation. None of the natural or laboratory experiences demonstrated the particular significance of age variables. It has been more or less assumed that aged people who are isolated from adequate stimuli by failing sensory organs or reduced environmental variation react with the same symptoms as younger adults. Certain effects thought to be "confusion" or "old age" may arise from sensory deprivation. Box 12-1 summarizes some effects of sensory deprivation. Any situation lacking varied environmental stimuli deprives the senses of adequate material for perceptual integrity.

Common contributors to sensory deprivation in the elderly are altered sensory capacities and restrictive environments. Problems such as poor vision, decreased energy, poor hearing, extended periods in a supine position, debilitating illness and chronic disorders, few pleasant sounds, and limited meaningful contact with others often result in disorientation. Late afternoon may aggravate the deprivation if daylight is diminished and there is inadequate indoor lighting. Simple nursing actions will alleviate this barren existence. Open drapes and the window a crack; sights, sounds, and smells of outdoors and life can be enjoyable and reassuring. Turn on lights; raise the head of the bed or assist person to a chair bolstered comfortably with pillows; bring a flower to the room; sit down; speak, touch, and listen to the client's feelings and perceptions. Discuss the isolated person's interests; radio, television, computers, books, puzzles, and handicrafts may all amuse the solitary person. It is essential to plan with them, not for them. When these efforts fail, it is because of inadequate assessment. If the individual is concerned about more fundamental issues such as maintaining biologic integrity, comfortable and nondemanding surroundings will be a priority.

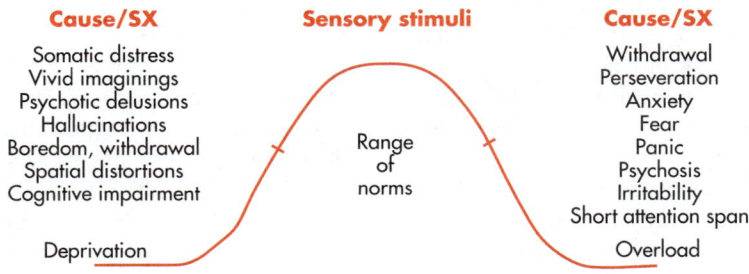

Figure 12-1. Reaction to sensory and environmental alterations. (Illustration by Joseph Pierre.)

Effects of Sensory Deprivation

- Sensory deprivation tends to amplify existing personality traits. Vernon and Makowsky (1961) believe sensory deprivation generates a great need for socialization and physical stimulation.
- Perceptual disorganization occurs in visual/motor coordination, color perception, apparent movement, tactile accuracy, ability to perceive size and shape, and spatial and time judgment. Sensory deprivation brings about temporary loss in color perception, motor coordination, and weight loss.
- Affectual changes include boredom, restlessness, irritability, anxiety, and panic.
- Sensory deprivation alters mechanisms of attention, consciousness, and reality testing, resulting in general disorganization of brain function similar to that produced by anoxia.
- Marked changes of behavior occur, such as inability to think and solve problems, affectual disturbance, perceptual distortions, hallucinations and delusions, vivid imagination, poor task performance, increased anxiety and aggression, somatic complaints, temporal and spatial disorientation, emotional lability, and confusion of sleeping and waking states.
- Monotony produces a disruption of the capacity to learn and the ability to think. In the absence of varied stimulation, brain function becomes less efficient; an electroencephalogram shows slowed alpha waves maintained by constant sensory flux.
- Illness often increases the perceptual confusion, particularly among the aged, although studies show that adults of all ages experience distortion and depersonalization when environmental stimuli are bland.

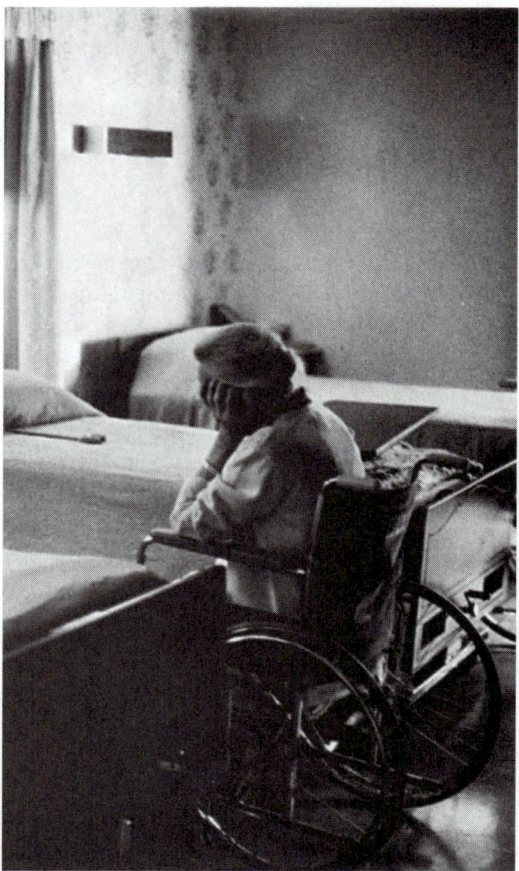

Sensory deprivation. (Courtesy Patricia Hess.)

When the ambiance is one of monotony, even a small stimulus may trigger a strong response. Knowing this makes it easier to understand the overreactions displayed when a routine is interrupted. One lady became extremely upset when a large sign was hung above her bed; another refused to return to her room after it had been rearranged. People are more sensitive to changes of any sort when there are so few and they feel deprived of control. Following sensory deprivation, there is a good response to gradual environmental enrichment. Rapid increases may produce emotional outbursts. The benefits of orderly, gradual environmental enrichment geared to individual personality and interests are yet to be thoroughly studied.

Meanings and patterns that throughout life have formed the basis of percepts, and on a preconscious level have sorted data in ways meaningful to the individual, may be shattered in crises, unnatural events, and catastrophes. The senses are no longer reliable. An example that illustrates this point occurred for me during an earthquake. It seemed to me I was experiencing vertigo because my perceptual filter did not recognize the source of the movement.

Sensory Overload. Neuroexcitability and secretion of stimulating neurotransmitters decrease as one ages. Over-arousal is most often from abrupt, unexpected environmental change such as accident or hospitalization. These are situations of sensory overload precipitated by actual or perceived environmental demands. Emergency reactions sustained for long periods exhaust the organism's physiologic adaptive mechanisms (Selye, 1956). An individual with marginal adaptation and cognitive decrements is particularly vulnerable. Sensory overload is a very individual matter, often related to cognitive capacity. It can be recognized by certain symptoms: thoughts may race, and attention scatters in many directions. People find it difficult to sit still. Aberrant thoughts or actions may occur. Evidences of anxiety are present. The amount of stimuli necessary for healthy function varies with each individual; relevance and familiarity of stimuli may be more important than amount. Biorhythms are another important consideration. Individuals may be more subject to environmental overload at one time than another. Sensations are generally most acute in the late afternoon when cortisol levels are highest, although effects on the aged have not been established.

Chapters 13 and 19 discuss reactions to multiple, rapid environmental changes and the concomitant vulnerability to increased physical illness. Sensory overload cannot always be avoided, but when one is extremely stressed and bombarded with adaptive demands, time must be arranged for peacefulness and frequent rest periods. It is often helpful to sit quietly with the person, saying very little, or engage him or her in a nondemanding repetitive activity that will help focus attention on something that provides security and reduces stress. Walking can be beneficial.

One must be cautious in arbitrarily attributing anxiety, agitation, mood swings, or disorientation to sensory overload. One man was intermittently disoriented for several days following hip surgery. A nursing assistant reported his disorientation and anxiety and concluded he was suffering sensory overload. She therefore wanted to keep the lights dim, reduce noise, move the patient to a private room, and advise others to disturb him as little as possible. Although these interventions would be useful in one experiencing overload, it would further reduce this man's ability to remain in touch with his surroundings. It is likely he was reacting to medications, tenuous physiologic balance, dehydration, infection, and the stress of translocation and major surgery. It is best to have a consistent attendant with him to reassure him repeatedly that this is a reaction to surgery and to interpret sounds, actions, and items that are in his present environment.

TASTE AND SMELL

Age-related losses of smell and fine taste normally begin in the sixth decade and are accelerated by cigarette smoking. Four basic tastes have been identified (sweet, sour, salty, and bitter), conveyed by approximately 9000 taste buds. Scientists believe there are more yet to be identified and an unknown number of basic and subtle odors. The senses of taste and smell (chemosenses) are intertwined and can when acute provide great pleasure as well as protection from harm. Fine taste, such as the subtle differences between turkey and chicken, is an olfactory function; crude taste such as sweet and sour is dependent on the taste buds. It is thought that there is about a 40% decrement in smell (hyposmia) and taste (hypogeusia) in old age (Wilson, 1995). Subtle changes occur during the aging process, but these are not sufficiently well documented to consistently verify their existence and normally do not interfere with one's pleasure or safety.

Overall, enjoyment of taste is really the totality of the experience of temperature, texture, smell, appearance, and flavors. In fact, some believe the trigeminal nerve endings that lie close to the surface of the lips and nose contribute a great deal to the sensations of eating. People who have lost some of the sense of smell or taste may still identify many foods

through the stimulation of the trigeminal nerve endings (Taste and Smell, 1991). It therefore becomes quite difficult to determine the significance of any one sensory response. Significant, rapid, and noticeable changes in smell and/or taste may be the result of medication, disease or, in rare situations, hallucination. Gustatory and olfactory hallucinations are danger signals of brain lesions and should be immediately suspect.

Olfaction

One of two persons over 65 has lost some sense of smell. A study of 85 males and 76 females, part of the Baltimore Longitudinal Study of Aging, demonstrated the progressive deterioration of the sense of smell with age, though women lose less odor discrimination than men (Ship et al, 1996). Most, however, lose some olfactory discriminatory capacity, resulting in a lowered capacity for enjoyment of scents and fragrances and a stronger reliance on texture and visual cues. The National Institute on Aging (1990b) reports research that has found age takes a greater toll on olfaction than on taste. Smell losses outnumber taste problems three to one.

A decreased sensitivity to odors may be dangerous for the older person, such as when one may fail to detect the odor of leaking gas, a smoldering cigarette, or tainted food. The loss of smell may also present social problems. We all experience habituation to, and unawareness of, our own body odor. Some elders are unaware that the odor of urine accompanies them even though they only have slight leakage. This particular sensory reduction can be an alienating factor unless attended to.

Three causes can explain 60% of the problems with loss of smell. These include nasal sinus disease that results in obstruction of passages, thereby interfering with odors reaching the smell receptors, and repeated injury to olfactory receptors through viral infections (Figure 12-2). The third and least common reason for the aged to lose the sense of smell is head trauma that results in bleeding into the nasal mucous membrane. The older one is the more likely that a viral infection will result in permanent changes to the sense of smell. Abrupt loss of the sense of smell may occur after a viral nasal infection, though usually that will need immediate attention as it may signal a serious disorder (Wilson, 1995).

Recent research from the National Geographic Smell Survey found that exposure to medications and environmental agents affect chemosensation, especially in men and particularly those who have worked in factories. The accumulation of noxious agents over time results in an impaired sense of smell (Corwin et al, 1995). Olfactory dysfunction is among the first signs of Parkinson's disease and may in fact be a preclinical indication of the disease (Doty et al, 1995).

Olfactory nerve cells are thought to be the only sensory nerves capable of regeneration (Figure 12-3); however, if the sense of smell has been absent for 6 months or more it is unlikely that it will return (Taste and Smell, 1991) (Box 12-2). There has been some indication that zinc sulfate tablets may be helpful, but this is as yet unproved (Wilson, 1995).

Assessment. A reliable and easy odor recognition tool is the University of Pennsylvania Smell Identification Test; a prepackaged scratch-and-sniff test that can be done with ease in any setting. Dysosmia (the sensation of unpleasant smell) may be individually idiosyncratic. For example, one lady found a particular incense nauseating, others are repelled by certain perfumes. Duffy et al (1995) measured the nutritional risk associated with olfactory dysfunction among a large group of older women. They found the subjects had less interest in food, a higher intake of sweets, less appreciation of pungent tastes, lower intake of low-fat milk products, and a nutrient intake profile that put them at higher risk for cardiac disease. They suggest that practitioners pay special attention to nutritional counseling for women with olfactory dysfunction. Their study was only of women, but we feel certain it is equally important for men.

Taste

Taste acuity is at least two thirds dependent on the olfactory sense. However, it is not only taste but also the sensual aspects of food that are enjoyable. The pleasure of eating comes more from masticating than from the taste buds or the hunger center in the lateral hypothalamus. This knowledge can be important in preparing food for older people.

Taste buds that seem most affected by aging are those for sweet and salty at the tip of the tongue. These supposedly are exposed to more contact and thus may deteriorate slightly. This theory is based on the knowledge that taste buds begin to atrophy in midlife, for some as early as age 40, and the observation that many elders tend to salt and sweeten their foods more than when they were younger. Bitterness, located at the very back of the tongue, seems to remain a strong sensation at all ages.

Individuals have varied levels of taste sensitivity that seem predetermined by genetics and constitution, as well as age variations. Comparatively little interest has been demonstrated in studying these differences. Many denture wearers say they lose some of their satisfaction in food, possibly because texture is such a very important element in food enjoyment. The sensory pleasure of food combined with the symbolic nurturance inherent in eating and feeling satiated are important ways one maintains a sense of security. Indeed, when feeling insecure, many people begin to eat com-

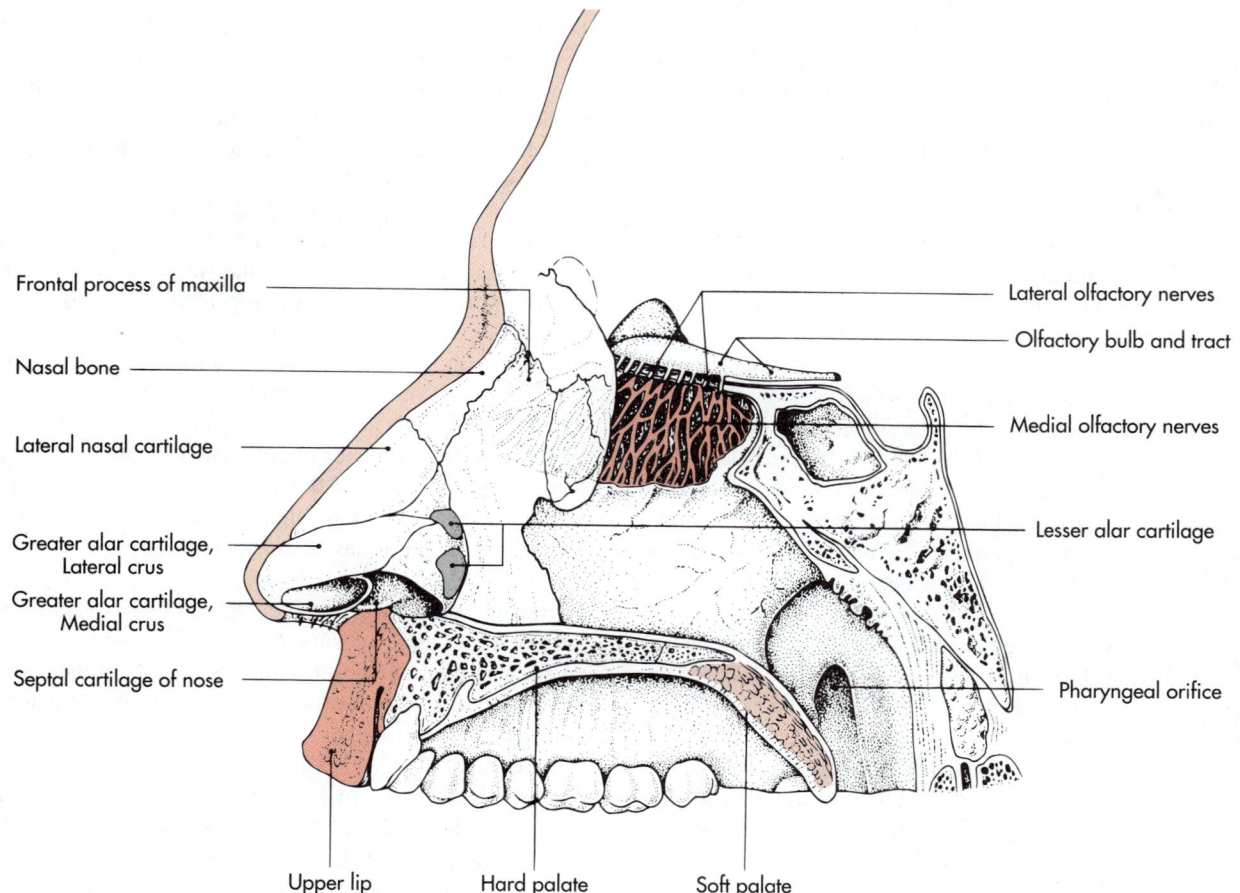

Figure 12-2. Key structures of the nose. (From Knapp MT: A rose is still a rose: how does losing the sense of smell affect an elder's life? *Geriatr Nurs* 10(6):290, 1989.)

pulsively. Difficulties measuring flavor appreciation come from individual variables such as smoking, olfactory sensitivity, attitude toward food and eating, and the presence of moistening secretions. There are also aberrations in flavor sensations caused by certain medications.

Assessment. Detailed and meaningful gustatory evaluations are difficult to administer. Wilson (1995) suggests asking clients if they taste salt when added to soup, sugar when added to tea, sourness of lemon juice, and bitterness of coffee. Individuals complaining of dysgeusia (unpleasant taste in mouth) should be evaluated for dental disease and dental hygiene, medication side effects, head trauma, upper respiratory disease, and first, seventh, ninth and tenth cranial nerve integrity. If these screening procedures are inadequate, the individual may need to be referred to a chemosensory center for intensive testing (Wilson, 1995).

There are no known therapies for primary gustatory dysfunction. If all secondary causes have been eliminated, the most useful approach to the client is simply being concerned and supportive. Help the person experiment with various herbs and flavors and identify foods that are most enjoyable. Encourage smokers to refrain from smoking. Do not burden them with a bland, soft, or liquid diet unless it is absolutely essential. They may enjoy the sensations of the food and chewing even if their taste for flavors is not acute.

VISION

Visual acuity and accommodation normally, as mentioned in Chapter 4, decrease with age. These changes, particularly presbyopia, begin making themselves felt in the mid-40s for many people. They are not usually great problems but mainly an inconvenience. Although major aging of the eye

(presbyopia) occurs between 45 and 55 years of age, 80% of the aged have fair to adequate vision past 90 years of age. According to the *Statistical Abstract of the United States* (U.S. Bureau of the Census, 1995), there are over 9 million people in the United States with visual impairments. At ages 75 and beyond 154/1000 males and 133/1000 females have

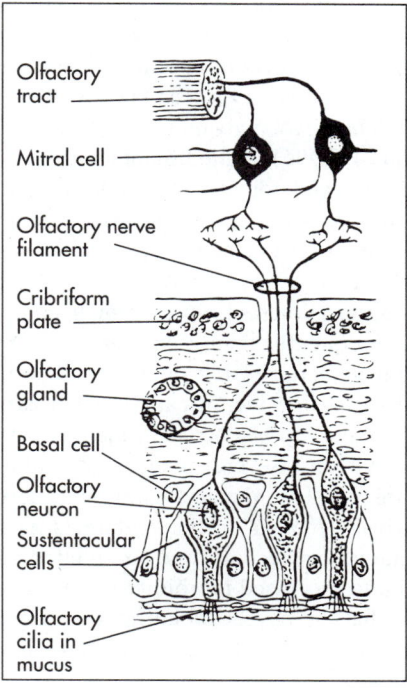

Figure 12-3. Scheme of cell and fiber arrangement in olfactory epithelium. (From Mosby's *Medical, nursing, and allied health dictionary,* ed 2, St Louis, 1986, Mosby.)

Box 12-2	**Assessing the Nose**

- Visually inspect the nose. Note any asymmetry that could interfere with breathing or smell. Expect that the nose will be relatively long and broad because of the ongoing formation of cartilage through the years. Examine the color and texture of the surface of the nose. Diffuse redness, papules, pustules, and dilated venules can signal excess alcohol intake.
- Palpate the nose. Feel for raised bumps along the frontal bone at the base and hard nodes in the cartilage. Note any frontal bone depression suggesting nose fracture in the past.
- With an otoscope, look inside the vestibule of each nare. With age, nasal hair becomes coarser and thicker. Inspect the base of the hairs for signs of irritation or infection caused by clipping the hairs too close. Examine the nasal mucosa: Is it moist and intact? or dry and broken? With age, the mucosa becomes fragile and easily broken. A

smooth, shiny membrane with engorged turbinates is a sign of vasomotor rhinitis. Check the arterier septum and note whether it appears straight or deviates to the left or right of the columella separating the nares. At least a mild degree of septal deviation is common in adults.
- Occlude each nostril, one at a time, and ask the person to close his mouth and breathe through the open nostril. Note whether both nostrils are patent.
- Test olfactory nerve function by asking the person to identify various smells: Nerve fibers in the olfactory bulb decline at a rate of about 1% per year, which may account for a decreased ability to recognize or distinguish smells with age.
- Palpate the paranasal sinuses to detect swelling or any sign of tenderness that may indicate sinusitis or postnasal drip.

From Knapp MT: A rose is still a rose: how does losing the sense of smell affect an elder's life? *Geriatr Nurs* 10(6):290, 1989.

visual impairments. Many of these have "low vision." Low vision is that which cannot be corrected by ordinary lenses, medical treatment, or surgery (Stuen, 1996). Records of 261 patients (mean age 73.5 years) attending a low vision clinic showed various problems. The causes of visual impairment were macular degeneration (38.9%), diabetic retinopathy (16.1%), glaucoma (8.4%), and cataract (7.4%). Low vision aids were prescribed for 80% of the clients, and 77% of those were found, in a 1-year follow-up, to use them regularly (van Rens et al, 1991). It seems evident that much can be done to improve vision for the majority of elders and that compliance is high when vision is affected.

Rovner et al (1996) studied community-residing elders with low vision and found symptoms of depression and excess disability prevalent. About 3 million of those with low vision are so seriously impaired that they are unable to read (Schneider, 1996). Approximately 2% of the aged are totally blind (Stuen, 1996). Women completely lose vision more frequently than men, and in both sexes it is common to have better vision in one eye than in the other. It is probable that the identification and treatment of depression is frequently neglected in the care of those with low or no vision. Severe nuclear sclerotic cataracts, cataract surgery, and visual impairment correlate with poorer survival, whereas cortical cataracts, posterior subcapsular cataracts, glaucoma, and age-related maculopathy are unrelated to increased morbidity (Klein et al, 1995). It seems clear that the psychosocial ramifications of various kinds of visual impairment are, at this time, poorly understood and treated.

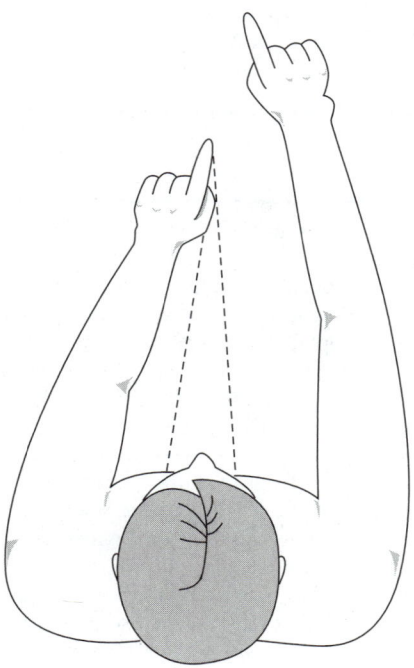

Figure 12-4. Eye muscle exercise.

There are several ophthalmologic changes that occur with aging that are not serious but may cause discomfort or alarm in the elder experiencing them. Headache accompanied by eye muscle pain can be caused by the tendency with aging for a gradual decrease in the tone of the medial rectus muscle, which turns the eye inward while focusing on close objects. This then creates *exophoria* (slight towing outward of the eye) and may result in headache when doing close work for an extended period. Headaches associated with this condition can be remedied by taking more rest breaks during close-range work, advising the patient to do close work early in the day, and engaging in eye muscle exercises 3 times daily for 5 minutes each session (Figure 12-4). Symptomatic relief is usually achieved in 4 to 6 weeks.

Decrease in pupil size, which hinders light from reaching the retina, is a major factor in visual changes of aging. Small objects cannot be seen at a distance. Adaptation to darkness is also deficient in old age with depletion of rhodopsin restitution in the retina.

Night vision decreases and may become a great source of insecurity to those aged who must drive at night. In addition, individuals who have surgical radial keratotomy to correct nearsightedness may develop impaired night vision related to scarring (Radial keratotomy, 1995). Many limit themselves to daytime driving. Many safety factors are obviously attached to visual adequacy, although people with limitations often adapt remarkably well.

Vitreous floaters and occasional lightning flashes in the visual field may be alarming. As the vitreous undergoes liquefaction with eye movements the vitreous attachment is placed under intermittent tension. This creates a mechanical stimulation of the peripheral retina that causes vertically oriented flashing lights unilaterally. In addition, other lines, spots, clusters of dots, and webs may move slowly across the visual field. Though none of these conditions are serious, explanation and client reassurance are essential because the threat of blindness is one of the most devastating thoughts one can entertain. These ever-present, manifest changes are constant reminders of one's aging process.

Some visual distortions that require immediate attention and may signal retinal detachment include any change that persists and is accompanied by a decrease in the visual field, a shower of opacities accompanied by flashing lights in the peripheral visual fields, or a feeling of a "veil over the eye."

Presbyopia

Accommodation, or the ability to focus on objects at various distances, decreases from 5 years of age onward, and by the mid-40s most people become aware of the need to hold objects farther away to properly focus their gaze. This change is presbyopia. For most individuals the reading lens must be increased in strength every 2 or 3 years between the ages of 45 and 65. For the farsighted (hyperopic) the presbyopia tends to occur earlier than for the nearsighted (myopic). As lens opacity increases some refractive power increases at the same time accommodation, or lens resilience, decreases. The result is a temporary shift toward myopia and improved close vision. Thus some individuals at 60 or 70 years of age develop "second sight" in which they can again read without glasses (Kupfer, 1995a). Increasingly, ophthalmologic journals are reporting the use of contact lenses to correct presbyopia with varying degrees of acceptance and success (Back et al, 1989; Collins et al, 1989; Stein, 1991).

Glaucoma

Glaucoma is a chronic, progressive, degenerative disease involving increased intraocular pressure, usually bilaterally, that can lead to permanent damage of the optic nerve. Open-angle glaucoma accounts for about 80% of the cases and is asymptomatic until very late in the disease, when there is a noticeable loss in visual fields (Kupfer, 1995). Age is the single most important predictor of glaucoma, and it is the most common cause of blindness in Americans over the age of 65. Aged females are afflicted twice as frequently as aged males (Schappert, 1995). Blacks develop glaucoma at younger ages and with more frequency than Whites. Orientals, particularly the Chinese, are prone to develop glaucoma. Other risk factors have been identified and can be seen in Box 12-3. Many drugs that are given to elders, with little or no thought to the ramifications, will exacerbate glaucoma. Drugs with anticholinergic properties or those that cause pupil dilation are particularly dangerous for patients predisposed to angle-closure glaucoma (Table 12-2).

Though the etiology is variable and often unknown, the problem occurs when the natural fluids of the eye are blocked by ciliary muscle rigidity and the buildup of pressure, which damages the optic nerve (Figure 12-5). An acute attack of angle-closure glaucoma is characterized by a rapid rise in intraocular pressure (IOP) accompanied by redness and pain in and around the eye, severe headache, nausea and vomiting, and blurring of vision. Usually medication can control glaucoma, but when surgery is necessary it is only successful if scar tissue does not later obstruct the drainage channel. The National Eye Institute has reported the increased success of surgery for glaucoma when followed by injections of the antimetabolite drug, 5-fluorouracil (National Institute on Aging, 1990c).

Glaucoma screening is frequently the responsibility of the primary care nurse or nurse practitioner. Ralston et al (1992) developed a simple noncontact method of tonometry that can be used to identify 90% of patients with IOPs greater than 22 mm Hg. The handheld, air-puff, noncontact tonometer has been in use for measurement of IOP since 1972. A direct jet of air that exceeds the pressure of the IOP is directed at the cornea of the patient. Ordinarily, a tonometry reading of 10 to 20 is considered acceptable, although there are many complicating factors. Persons with measurements of pressure over 21 mm Hg are "ocular hypertensives" and may not yet need treatment but will need visual field testing at 6-month intervals (Kupfer, 1995b).

About one sixth of patients with diagnosed glaucoma do not have IOPs above those considered normal. These persons are categorized as having "normal tension glaucoma." While tonometry alone is clearly not sufficient to diagnose glaucoma, that in conjunction with ophthalmoscopic visualization of the optic disc is within the purview of primary care nurses and will determine the need for referral to an ophthalmologist. Presently many elders may have undiagnosed glaucoma that has not been screened or evaluated. The "silent thief" will steal vision with no forewarning. It is recommended that individuals with any of the risk factors identified should be evaluated annually and those with medication-controlled glaucoma should be examined at least every 6 months (Kupfer, 1995a).

Cataracts

Another prevalent disorder among the aged is the development of cataracts caused by oxidative damage to lens protein and the deposit of lipofuscin in the ocular lens. When lens opacity reduces visual acuity to 20/30 or less in the central axis of vision, it is considered a cataract. Cataracts are categorized according to their location within the lens. They are virtually universal in the very old but may be only minimally visible, particularly in individuals with pale irises. Cataracts are recognized by the clouding of the ordinarily clear ocular lens. They are normal in the aging process but may be worsened by diabetes, hypertension, kidney disease, and injuries or exposure to toxic situations. The cardinal sign of cataracts is the appearance of halos around objects as light is diffused. Other common symptoms include blurring, seeing double moons, decreased perception of light and color, and sensitivity to glare. The hallmark of cataracts is painless, progressive loss of vision (Kupfer, 1995b). Cataracts are the second leading cause of blindness in the United States. Eighteen percent of people between 65 and 74 years of age have cataracts, and 46% of those aged 75 to 84 years have

---

> **Box 12-3**   **Risk Factors for Glaucoma**
>
> - Elevated IOP ($\geq$22 mm Hg)
> - Age >50 years
> - Black race
> - Family history
> - Associated conditions
>   Diabetes mellitus—strongest association with
>   glaucoma
>   Thyroid disease
>   Nearsightedness
>   Hypertension
>   Cardiovascular disease
>
> From Ralston ME, Choplin NT, Hollenbach KA et al: Glaucoma screening in primary care: the role of noncontact tonometry, *J Fam Pract* 34(1):73, 1992. Reprinted by permission of Appleton and Lange.

Table 12-2   Drugs Commonly Prescribed for Elders That Are Contraindicated or Must be Used with Caution in the Presence of Glaucoma or Prodromal Signs of Glaucoma

Generic name	Trade name*	Generic name	Trade name*
Aminophylline or theophylline with ethylenediamine	Aminophyllin Corophyllin	Lorazepam Loxapine succinate	Ativan Daxolin
Amitriptyline hydrochloride*	Amitril		Loxitane
	Elavil	Mesoridazine	Serentil
Amyl nitrate*		Methamphetamine hydrochloride	Desoxyn
Atropine*			
Benztropine mesylate*	Cogentin	Nitroglycerin	Nitrostat
Biperiden hydrochloride*	Akineton	Nortriptyline hydrochloride*	Aventyl
Carbamazepine	Tegretol		
Chlorpheniramine maleate	Chlor-Trimeton preparations	Orphenadrine citrate	Norflex
		Papaverine	Pavabid
Chlorphenoxamine hydrochloride	Phenoxene	Pentaerythritol tetranitrate	Peritrate
Chlorpromazine*	Thorazine	Perphenazine	Phenazine
Chlorprothixene	Taractan		Trilafon
Clorazepate dipotassium	Tranxene	Phenylephrine hydrochloride	Neo-Synephrine
Clonazepam	Clonopin		Tear-Efrin
Cyclobenzaprine hydrochloride	Flexeril	Prochlorperazine	Compazine
Cyproheptadine hydrochloride	Periactin		Stemetil
Desipramine hydrochloride*	Norpramin	Promazine hydrochloride	Sparine
	Pertofrane	Promethazine hydrochloride*	Phenergan
Diazepam*	Valium	Protokylol hydrochloride	Ventaire
Dimenhydrinate	Dramamine	Protriptyline hydrochloride	Vivactil
Diphenhydramine hydrochloride*	Benadryl	Pseudoephedrine hydrochloride*	Sudafed
Doxepin hydrochloride*	Adapin	Succinylcholine chloride	Anectine
	Sinequan	Tetrahydrozoline hydrochloride	Murine
Ephedrine sulfate	Efedron		Visine
Epinephrine	Bronkaid mist	Theophylline*	Aerophylline
	Primatene mist		Theo-Dur
Fluphenazine hydrochloride*	Prolixin	Thioridazine hydrochloride	Mellaril
Glutethimide	Doriden	Thiothixene hydrochloride	Navane
Glycopyrrolate*	Robinul	Trifluoperazine hydrochloride	Stelazine
Haloperidol*	Haldol	Trihexyphenidyl*	Artane
Hydrocodone bitartrate	Hycodan	Trimeprazine tartrate	Panectyl
Imipramine hydrochloride*	Antipres	Tripelennamine hydrochloride	Pyribenzamine
	Impril	Triprolidine hydrochloride	Actidil
	Tofranil	Tropicamide	Mydriacyl
Isopropamide iodide	Darbid	Xylometazoline hydrochloride	Neo-Synephrine II
Isosorbide dinitrate	Isordil	Zinc sulfate	Op-Thal-Zin
Levodopa*	Bendopa Dopar Levopa		

*Multiple trade names not listed.

cataracts that impair their daily activities and ability to live independently (Bass et al, 1995).

There was a time when cataracts were allowed to "ripen" before surgery was undertaken, and in those cases many elders became virtually blind prior to cataract removal. Some stories still remain of individuals who were blind until their cataracts were removed, some not even aware that cataracts were the problem. Now aged individuals are considered for surgery whenever the visual disturbance becomes an impediment in the individual's daily life. However, recent Medicare policies restrict payment for surgery to those unable to function normally without the surgery or those whose problem cannot be corrected with eyeglasses. These restrictions have been put in place because of the enormous number of individuals having cataract surgery: 2 million individuals in 1994 at a cost of nearly $1.5 billion (U.S. Department of Health and Human Services, 1995b).

Most often cataract surgery involves removing the entire lens capsule and replacing it with an artificial lens. At present these are often slipped into place without the need for suturing. When necessary, cataract surgery has the potential to improve not only sight but quality of life as well. Tielsch et al (1995) report a study of 772 patients undergoing first-eye cataract surgery that showed 61% achieved or surpassed

Sight

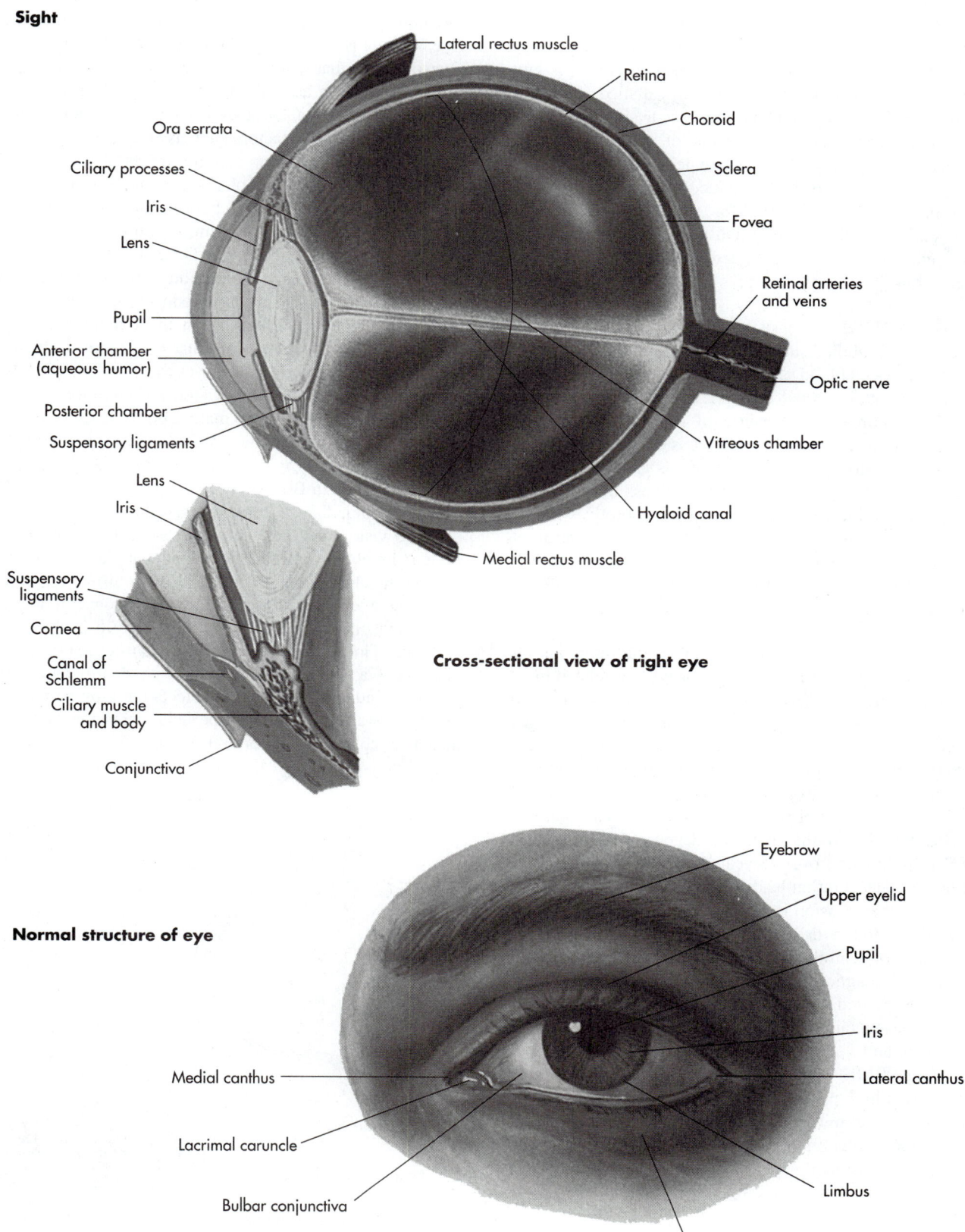

Cross-sectional view of right eye

Normal structure of eye

Figure 12-5. Cross-sectional view of right eye. (From Mosby's medical, nursing, and allied health dictionary, ed 2, St Louis, 1986, Mosby.)

their expected level of postoperative functioning. The rate of satisfaction for those who had surgery in both eyes was significantly higher (Javitt et al, 1995). The group over 75 with coexisting visual problems were less satisfied. Unfortunately, glaucoma and cataracts often occur simultaneously, which complicates the management of each. Individuals who have had cataract surgery are less likely to be surgically treated effectively for glaucoma. The nursing role is to prepare the individual for significant changes in vision and adaptation to light and to be sure they have received adequate counseling regarding realistic postsurgical expectations.

Diabetic Retinopathy

Some visual disabilities are acquired through the deleterious effects of elevated blood sugar due to diabetes, which creates microaneurysms in retinal capillaries. These are the source of diabetic retinopathy. Because of vascular and cellular changes accompanying diabetes, there is often rapid worsening of other vision pathologic conditions as well. Diabetic retinopathy accounts for 7% of the blindness in the United States, and the incidence curves upward abruptly with increasing age (Kupfer, 1995b). Constant, strict control of blood sugar and photocoagulation laser treatments can halt progress of the disease (National Institute of Aging, 1995).

Macular Degeneration

The macula is the central visual point of the retina and as such is the source of central visual clarity. Age-related macular degeneration (ARMD) results from systemic changes in circulation, accumulation of cellular waste products, tissue atrophy, and growth of abnormal blood vessels in the choroid layer beneath the retina. It is the most common visual impairment of individuals over 50. It leads to permanent visual deficits but not blindness (Figure 12-6). The National Eye Institute found that macular degeneration occurs in 36.8% of individuals over 75 years of age (Eastman, 1996).

Macular degeneration leads to loss of central visual acuity, but peripheral vision is not affected. The etiology is unknown. Early in the disease an Amsler grid is used to determine clarity of central vision (Figure 12-7). A perception of wavy lines is diagnostic of beginning macular degeneration and can be halted by laser treatment if diagnosed early (Macular degeneration, 1990).

Virtanen and Laatikainen (1991) found that 91% of patients with ARMD were able to read newsprint with simple magnifiers or high-powered (5X to 9X) reading glasses. Antioxidants, thalidomide, blocking ultraviolet light rays, and laser photocoagulation are some of the treatments that are being used. Transplanting healthy retinal cells to replace degenerating ones is under investigation (Eastman, 1996).

Assessment of Vision

Although low vision is defined in terms of visual acuity and visual field, these parameters are insufficient to understand individual treatment and rehabilitation needs. The National Eye Institute is developing a comprehensive Visual Function Questionnaire that will be used to assess levels of functional impairments such as mobility, near vision, ability to read, drive, work, and manage independent living and the influence of psychosocial factors such as stress, frustration, isolation, loss of privacy and existing levels of social support (Kupfer, 1995a). For example, nearly one fourth of nursing home residents were found to have vision impairment. Even considering numerous other chronic impairments, low vision was a most significant predictor of functional dependency (Horowitz, 1994). In addition, it has been found that increased visual cues and aids reduced agitation and improved function of individuals with Alzheimer's disease (Koss, 1995). It seems evident that the complex effects of low vision on function are not yet fully understood. However, various problems with vision are common in aging, and nurses are most likely to make a preliminary assessment prior to referral for further evaluation. Certain signs and symptoms of visual problems that should alert the nurse to action are noted in Box 12-4.

The Snellen chart is commonly used by nurses to test for distance vision. Testing the aged should be done in good light and with the bulb shielded to prevent glare. If the 20/40 line on the chart cannot be read, looking through a pinhole in a piece of cardboard should improve vision. If it does improve, that indicates a need for a change in eyeglass prescription. Gross visual field deficits can be determined by displaying a wide arc with outstretched arm and noting when the individual no longer detects the moving finger of the nurse's arm. These are superficial assessments and not meant to replace more thorough examination by specialists.

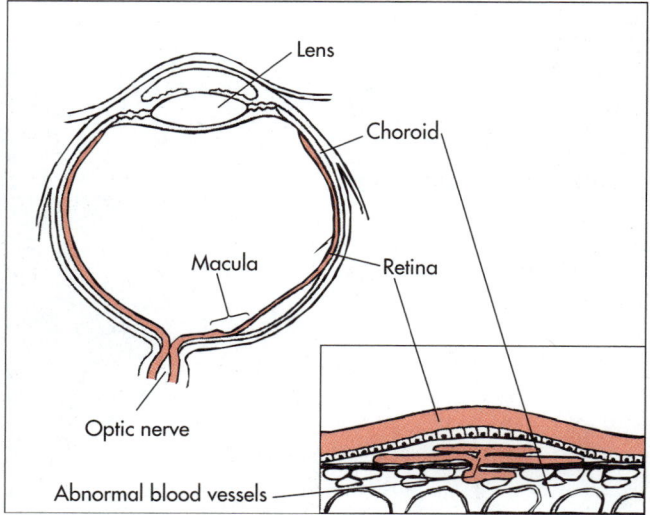

Figure 12-6. Age-related macular degeneration (ARMD) results if abnormal blood vessels grow in the choroid layer beneath the retina or if any part of the retina fails to receive proper nutrients. (From Macular degeneration, *Mayo Clinic Health Letter* 8[9]:5, 1990.)

Observation of the retina and optic nerve disc reveals important systemic, circulatory, and vision information, but pupillary constriction and clouding of the vitreous and lens often hamper the eyeground ophthalmologic examination of an older person. Also, one must be cautious because pupil dilation with phenylephrine for the purposes of examination may precipitate an acute attack for those predisposed to angle-closure glaucoma.

Other methods of assessment such as infrared scanning of the retina and the laser scanning ophthalmoscope (SLO) are providing safer and more sophisticated data. The SLO generates digital imaging computerized projections that measure specific visual changes corresponding to retinal damage of various degrees and types (O'Connell, 1995). Advanced equipment such as the retinal scanner will be-

come commonplace in providing computer-generated exact replicas of the pattern of blood vessels in the retina. It has even been suggested that the uniqueness of each individual's retinal capillary patterns may generate an identification even more reliable than a fingerprint (Look me in the eye, 1990).

Caring for the Elder with Visual Impairment

General principles in caring for the elder with visual impairment include the following: use warm incandescent lighting, control glare by using shades and blinds, suggest yellow or amber lenses to decrease glare, suggest sunglasses that block all ultraviolet light, select colors with good contrast and intensity, recommend reading materials that have large, dark, evenly spaced printing (Stuen, 1996).

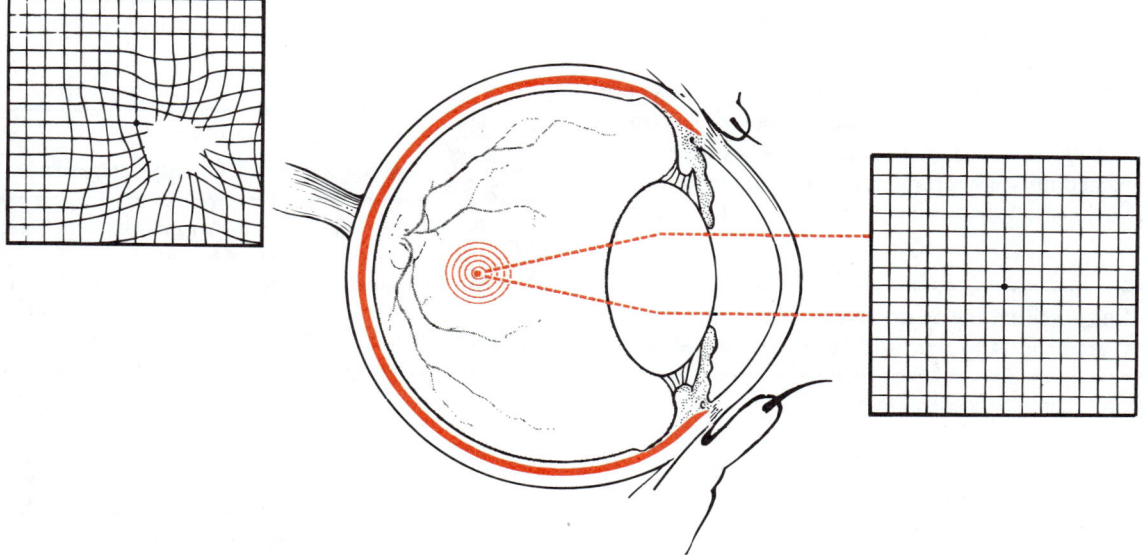

Figure 12-7. Macular degeneration: distortion of center vision; normal peripheral vision. (Illustration by Harriet R. Greenfield, Newton, Mass.)

Box 12-4	**Signs and Behaviors That May Indicate Vision Problems**

Client May Report
- Pain in eyes
- Difficulty seeing in darkened area
- Double vision/distorted vision

Staff May Notice
- Getting lost
- Bumping into objects
- Straining to read or no reading
- Stumbling/falling
- Spilling food on clothing
- Social withdrawal

- Migraine headaches coupled with blurred vision
- Flashes of light
- Halos surrounding lights

- Less eye contact
- Placid facial expression
- TV viewing at close range
- Decreased sense of balance
- Mismatched clothes

Modified from McNeely E, Griffin-Shirley N, Hubbard A: Diminished vision in nursing homes, *Geriatr Nurs* 13(6):332, 1992.

Environmental Lighting. The pupil of the aged eye admits less light to the retina. This is a normal condition known as senile miosis. A simple and effective intervention for the visually impaired is often neglected: increased environmental lighting (Kolanowski, 1992). Behavioral responses to light fall within three variables: intensity, spectral power distribution (color), and temporal pattern of exposure (Kolanowski, 1992).

In the process of aging the intensity of illumination needs to be three times as powerful to produce the same visual capacity. Intensity must be tempered by appropriate diffusion to avoid glare. Sensitivity to glare increases markedly in the aged due to clouding of the lens and vitreous that results in scattering of light as it passes through the lens. This is particularly noticed in night driving or in low levels of illumination when the pupil is slightly dilated (Kupfer, 1995b). This may cause eyestrain, fatigue, tension, and actual pain. Individuals are advised to avoid night driving and looking directly at oncoming headlights.

Fluorescent lighting has been shown to have adverse effects on behavior because it contributes to sensory overload (Wolanin and Phillips, 1981). The quality of artificial light becomes exceedingly important for the aged, particularly those who are institutionalized, because they often spend a great deal of their time indoors. Although we often think of light in terms of visualization only, it is also significant in several other respects. The characteristic color of a particular light source is another issue of concern. This "spectral power" is the radiant power emitted at each wavelength over the visible electromagnetic spectrum (Kolanowski, 1992). Some fluorescent lights filter out the red (longer wavelengths), and others filter out the blue (shorter wavelengths). Kolanowski found that a significant number of elders preferred broad-spectrum fluorescent lighting that simulates natural sunlight. There is some evidence that these types of lighting also produce calmness and relaxation.

Contrasting Colors. Color contrasts are used to facilitate location of items. Sharply contrasting colors assist the partially sighted. For instance, a bright towel is much easier to locate than a white towel hanging on a beige wall. Boxes 12-5 and 12-6 provide further ideas regarding caring for the visually impaired elder. Most visually impaired people have

---

Box 12-5   Suggestions for Communicating with and Caring for the Visually Impaired Patient

1. Always identify yourself clearly.
2. Always make it clear when you are leaving the room.
3. Make sure you have the resident's attention before you start to talk.
4. Try to minimize the number of distractions.
5. Whenever possible, choose bright clothes with bold contrasts.
6. Check to see that the best possible lighting is available.
7. Assess your position in relation to the resident. One eye or ear may be better than the other.
8. Try not to move items in resident's room.
9. Staff members should try to narrate their actions.
10. Try to keep resident between you and the window, or you will appear as a dark shadow.
11. Use some means to identify residents who are known to be visually impaired.
12. Use the analogy of clock hands to help locate objects.
13. Keep color and texture in mind when buying clothes.
14. BE CAREFUL ABOUT LABELING A RESIDENT AS CONFUSED. He or she may be making mistakes due to poor vision!

From McNeely E, Griffin-Shirley N, Hubbard A: Diminished vision in nursing homes, *Geriatr Nurs* 13(6):332, 1992.

Box 12-6   Caring for the Visually Impaired

- Remember there are many degrees of blindness; allow as much independence as possible.
- Speak normally but not from a distance; do not raise or lower voice, and continue to use gestures if that is natural to your communication. Do not alter your vocabulary; words such as "see" and "blind" are parts of normal speech. When others are present, address the blind person by prefacing remarks with his or her name or a light touch on the arm.
- When entering the presence of a blind person, speak promptly, identifying yourself and others with you. State when you are leaving to make the person aware of your departure.
- Speak descriptively of your surroundings to familiarize the blind person. State the position of people who are in the room.
- Do not change room arrangement without explanation.
- Speak before handing blind person an object. Describe positions of food on plate in relation to clock position (e.g., 3 o'clock, 6 o'clock).
- When walking with a blind person, offer your arm. Pause before stairs or curbs; mention them. In seating, place the person's hand on the back of the chair. Let him or her know position in relation to objects.
- Blind people like to know the beauty that surrounds them. Describe flowers, scenery, colors, and textures. People who have been blind since birth cannot conceive of color, but it adds to their appreciation to hear full descriptions. Older people most frequently have been sighted and can enjoy memories of beauty stimulated by descriptive conversation.

enough residual vision to use their eyesight with proper aids or training to read, write, and move around safely. Unfortunately, many older persons with serious visual impairments consider themselves blind and are usually treated as if they are. Adequate training in using residual vision can prevent partially sighted older persons from falling into unnecessarily dependent lifestyles.

Low-Vision Devices. Technology advances in the last decade have produced some low-vision devices that may be used successfully in the care of the visually impaired elder. An array of assistive devices are now available for these individuals, such as Microspiral Galilean Telescopes, Telephoto Microscopes, Clear Image Lens, Behind the Lens Telescopes, and the Low Vision Enhancement System. This last device uses tiny cameras to place an enlarged image on a video screen in front of the eyes. This is worn as a headset and can be used for distance viewing as well as reading (O'Connell, 1995). Persons with reduced visual acuity should be encouraged to consider some of these sophisticated aids because severe visual deficits may result in mobility restrictions, as well as creating cognitive, sensory, and behavioral disturbances.

Magnifying lenses are available in many forms in addition to those commonly found in spectacle frames (Figure 12-8). These can be recommended in relation to the use for which they are desired. The most complex of the low-vision devices are telescopes that can be focused at various distances, thus increasing the number of tasks that can be performed. In addition, closed-circuit television magnifying units are available that can enlarge written characters up to 45 times. Although these are currently expensive, the prices are rapidly dropping as they become more commonly available.

Another method of magnification is through the use of a standard copying machine that has magnifying capabilities. One need not buy one of these but only make use of those available to the public. By repeatedly magnifying printed words or images, even small print can be made as large as desired.

Eyeglasses, once heavy and bulky, are now cosmetically appealing. Many also incorporate prismatic lenses that expand the visual field. Sunglasses are designed to filter out ultraviolet rays that may be harmful to sensitive retinas. Some eyeglasses adjust to light source and become darker in the sun. Magnifiers have been redesigned for ease of changing batteries and bulbs, positioning and grasping. Telescopic lens eyeglasses are smaller, easier to focus, and have a greater range (Figure 12-9). It is now possible to electronically magnify video- and computer-generated text. Some software converts text into artificial voice output. All of these resources must be considered when attempting to help the visually impaired elder achieve the visual activities that are important to his or her quality of life (Silverstone, 1988). Because individual needs are unique, it is recommended that prior to investing in any of these vision aids, the client be advised to consult with a low-vision center or low-vision specialist. Information regarding these is provided in the resources at the end of the chapter.

Orientation Strategies for the Nonsighted

Methods to assist those individuals with total lack of sight are not generally included in nursing curricula. Methods in common use include the following: (1) the clock method, in which the individual is simply told where the food or item is as if it were on a clock face; (2) the sighted guide, in which a companion guides the visually impaired and enables safe mobility, (3) the cane sweep, which encounters obstacles, (4) varied textured surfaces, (5) sound signals, for example, at street crossings; and (6) seeing-eye dogs.

A Sighted Guide. Ask the blind person if he or she would like a "sighted guide." A strong element of dependency and trust is necessary in this method, and many people

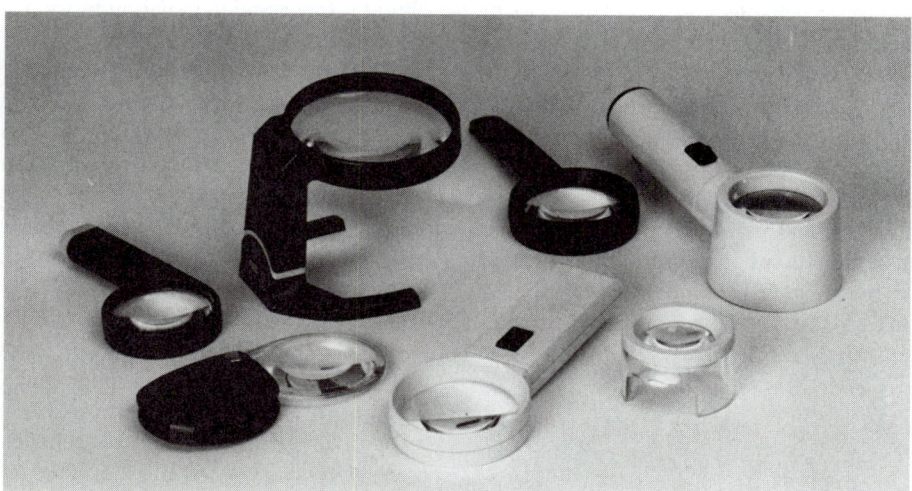

Figure 12-8. Hand and stand magnifiers. (From *Focus Geriatr Care Rehab,* Vol 10, #1, May, 1996.)

would rather manage on their own. Initially, as a person is adjusting to blindness, it can be helpful. If assistance is accepted, offer your elbow or arm. Instruct the person to grasp your arm just above the elbow. If necessary, physically assist person by guiding his or her hand to your arm or elbow.

Go one half step ahead and slightly to the side of the blind person. The shoulder of the person should be directly behind your shoulder. If the person is frail, place the hand on your forearm. With this modified grasp, the person will be positioned laterally to your body.

Relax and walk at a comfortable pace. Tell the person when approaching doorways or a narrow space.

Cane Sweep. White canes, sometimes called "long canes," are used by about 109,000 persons in the United states to alert others to their presence as a nonsighted person, as well as to signal the blind person to obstacles in the space ahead (American Foundation for the Blind, 1996). However, an architectural design that includes slanted beams and inverted pyramidal designs can be deceiving. In the early 1970s there were numerous college students who were blind as a result of being exposed at birth to concentrated oxygen in isolettes. One brought to my attention the difficulty he had negotiating the student center with a cane. It was designed with large angled concrete beams from floor to ceiling, and when the path at cane level seemed clear, the beam would surely present a hazard at the level of his head.

Sound Signals. In some U.S. cities and most European and Japanese cities intermittent sound signals alert the nonsighted when it is safe to cross the street—a simple solution, surprisingly not common in the United States. As nurses become more involved in political activist groups, this would be an area on which to focus county and state lawmakers' attention.

Varied Textures. Those elders who have been blind for quite some time have developed hypersensitivity to textural variations. This sensitivity can be incorporated into the environment in numerous ways to assist the blind person (see the resources at the end of the chapter).

Guide Dogs. There are 14 guide dog schools in the United States, and about 10,000 persons use dog guides to assist them in mobility. Trained guide dogs are matched to individuals' needs and personalities, and those elders who have guide dogs have had several during the course of their adult years (Schneider, 1996). Each dog becomes a companion, as well as a guide, and the elder grieves upon its demise, though no specific studies regarding this could be found. Some altruistic nurses have become involved in raising and training guide dogs. See the resources for additional information regarding this.

HEARING AND HEARING IMPAIRMENT IN THE AGED

Oliver Sacks, author of the well-known film story *Awakenings,* wrote *Seeing Voices* (1989) to elucidate "a journey into the world of the deaf." Sacks presents a view that blindness

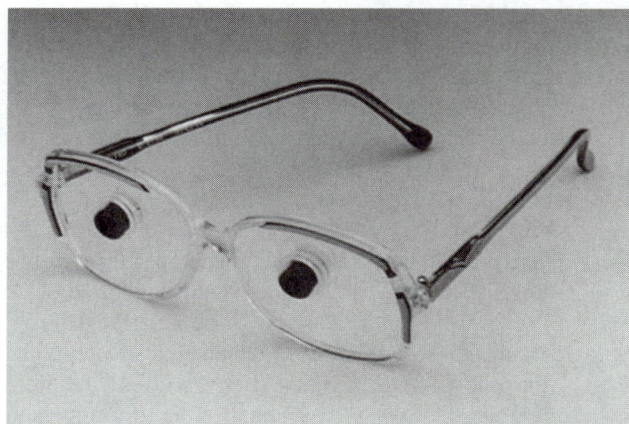

Figure 12-9. Keplerian telescopic lenses. (Courtesy The Lighthouse Inc, New York.)

may in fact be less serious than loss of hearing because of the interference with communication with others and the interactional input that is so necessary to stimulate and validate. One old man said a great annoyance of hearing loss is in the subtle aspects of living with a partner who also most probably has a hearing loss as well . "You must often repeat what you say, and in lovemaking, whispering sweet words becomes a gesture for yourself alone." Perhaps Helen Keller was most profound in her expression: "Never to see the face of a loved one nor witness a summer sunset is indeed a handicap. But I can touch a face and feel the warmth of the sun. But to be deprived of hearing the song of the first spring robin and the laughter of children provides me with a long and dreadful sadness" (Keller, 1902).

For those deafened in later life after hearing was well established the world may remain full of "phantasmal," or imagined sounds. This is a unique type of imagined sound in which visual experience (movement and speech) is rapidly and unconsciously translated into an auditory correlate. It is thought that special visual-auditory neurologic connections are established (Sacks, 1989).

Today in the United States there are more than 24 million people with impaired hearing (U.S. Bureau of the Census, 1995). It is estimated that 50% of persons over age 65 have a hearing problem; the occurrence is as much as 90% among the institutionalized aged. Reasons for this are not clear because hearing impairment is not ordinarily a trigger to institutionalization. As a review, we have included the anatomy of the ear in Figure 12-10.

Presbycusis

Changes in the middle and inner ear make many elders intolerant of loud noises and incapable of distinguishing between some of the sibilant consonants. The condition progressively worsens with age. The influence of genetics, noise exposure, cardiovascular status, central processing capacity, systemic disease, smoking, diet, personality, and stress have all been implicated to varying degrees in the eti-

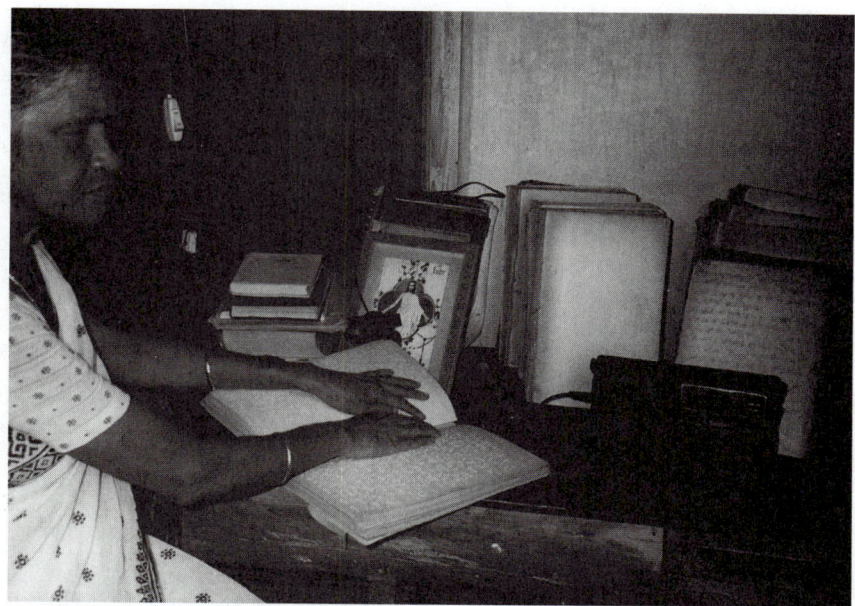

Congenital blindness. (Courtesy Priscilla Ebersole.)

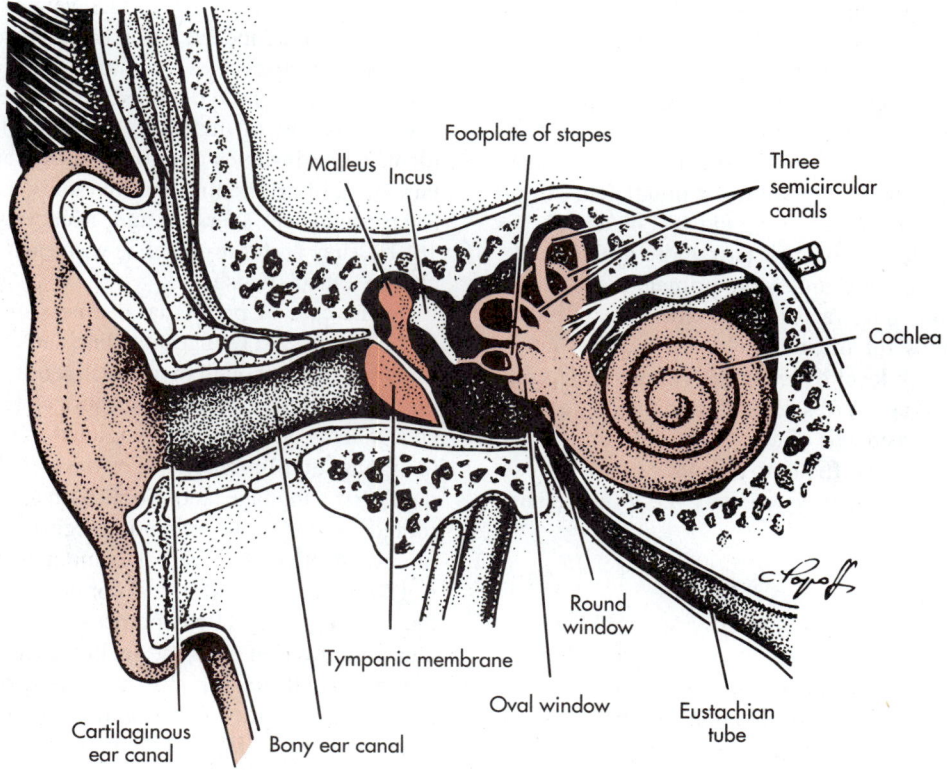

Figure 12-10. External auditory canal, middle ear, and inner ear. (From Malasanos L, Barkauskas V, Stoltenberg-Allen K: *Health assessment,* ed 4, St. Louis, 1991, Mosby.)

ology of impaired hearing (National Institute on Aging, 1990a). The common problem of cerumen in the ear canal is a frequent and treatable cause of conductive hearing loss. There is even some suspicion that hyperlipoproteinemia may be related to presbycusis (Ray, 1991).

Presbycusis is primarily an affliction of individuals over 50 but is not a universal change and though age-related may really be more reflective of environmental conditions and lifestyle than of age. Ritter (1991) reported on National Institute of Aging research being conducted by Pearson, who found that men are losing their hearing at younger ages each generation and that men over 30 are losing hearing twice as fast as women 80 years old and older.

Across the life span there are one quarter more males than females with hearing impairment. According to the *Statistical Abstract of the United States* (U.S. Bureau of the Census, 1995), about 27% of individuals between 45 and 64 years old are using some type of hearing augmentation device. This percentage rises to 41% for those 65 to 74 and 39.7% for individuals over 75 years old. There may be many others that have not been tested and/or whose hearing impairment has not been recognized or documented. Interestingly, although the legally blind have always received categorical aid, the hearing impaired have not. The reasoning behind this is unknown.

Impaired hearing increases isolation and suspicion that sometimes progress to paranoia. Feeling cut off from others, a deaf individual may act angry even when someone attempts to break through the barrier to sound (Chen H-L, 1994). There is normally a loss of speech, tone, and directional discrimination. Older persons are often unaware of hearing loss because of the gradual manner in which it usually develops. Some people are aware of a hearing loss and are disturbed by misperceptions and distortions, often imagining derogatory remarks said about them. However, knowing that one has a hearing loss is not sufficient. Testing must be done to determine the nature of the loss, how much it interferes with communication, whether it is treatable (as may be the case with metabolic alterations or middle ear structural changes), and whether a hearing aid will be useful.

Elderly persons with presbycusis have more difficulty filtering out background noise unless the primary signal is 10 times louder than the noise factor (von Wedel et al, 1990a). This has implications for institutional noise factors, intercoms and general high level of extraneous sounds. Hearing loss after 65 years of age varies according to the degree and type of loss being considered (Table 12-3). Certain sounds and words are much more difficult to hear than others. Those less than 40 decibels and of frequencies over 1000 are particularly difficult.

Prelingual Deafness

Prelingual deafness in the aged is rarely addressed because it is assumed that individuals deaf since childhood have learned early on to communicate through the use of sign language. Until 50 years ago it was common for deaf children to be placed in a state school for the deaf to develop within a culture of their own; therefore many elders with prelingual deafness will have had an entirely different childhood than those with hearing and have memories of knowing they were considered "deaf and dumb." The remnants of these early unfortunate discriminations are still embedded in the culture: deaf people are often treated as if they are mentally impaired. Of course, elders understand that "dumb," as then used, simply described the incapacity for intelligible

| Table 12-3 | Common Causes of Bilateral Symmetric Sensorineural Hearing Loss in the Aged |

Disorder	Characteristics
Hypothyroidism	Slowly progressive sensorineural and conductive hearing loss; affects all frequencies equally
Ototoxic drugs	Hearing loss with or without vestibular dysfunction, following treatment with known ototoxic drugs
Noise-induced hearing loss	History of prolonged exposure to loud continuous noise or brief exposures to loud impulse noise
Presbycusis	Gradual, progressive loss of hearing after 20 years; affects reception of high-frequency sounds

Hearing loss from any of these disorders may be improved with hearing aids; in cases of profound sensorineural hearing loss cochlear implant may be considered.

Adapted from Anderson R, Meyerhoff W. In Calkins E, Davis P, Ford M, editors: *The practice of geriatrics,* Philadelphia, 1986, WB Saunders.

speech—another misnomer. The prelingual deaf often learn audible speech very well. In the event of later institutionalization they may indeed find it easier to adapt to a collective lifestyle reminiscent of childhood experiences. No studies concerning this could be found. Those individuals who have been deaf most of their lives are said to share a collective identity that involves their own values, appreciation of certain types of art, drama, and literature, as well as American Sign Language (Vernon and Makowsky, 1961; Schein, 1991). They prefer to socialize with each other and typically choose a deaf spouse.

In the case of prelingual deafness of an elder, Andrews and Wilson (1991) suggest reading and writing skills may be impaired. Even though their intelligence is normal, they may not have had the common educational opportunities of their cohort. This is thought to be related to the early orientation to signing and lip reading. For these individuals, signing is their first language and English their second. Signing is rooted in iconic and mimetic origins and as such may be more evocative than verbal communication (Sacks, 1989, p. 120*). Subtleties of verbal communication may be lost to them, though they often compensate and become extremely alert to nonverbal cues and feelings. At times a certified interpreter, well enmeshed in the world of the deaf, will be needed. For additional information in this regard the reader might contact Gallaudett University (see resources at the end of the chapter).

Andrews and Wilson (1991) list a number of common myths and assumptions about the deaf that are worth repeating for emphasis (Box 12-7). It is often incorrectly assumed that an elder can read lips; more likely it is body language

*Individuals desiring sophisticated and in-depth discussions of hearing impairment are referred to Oliver Sacks's book, *Seeing Voices,* Berkeley, Calif, 1989, University of California Press.

Myths and Assumptions about the Deaf

The deaf elderly should be treated like children.
Congenital deafness is a form of mental retardation.
Deaf people can understand speech through lip reading.
Deaf people can read and write English.
Smiling and head nodding indicate agreement or comprehension.
A hearing aid and talking louder help the deaf person to hear better.
Anger, stubbornness, and uncooperative behavior mean the deaf person is becoming senile.
Consistency of personnel is no more important for the deaf than anyone else.

Protocol for Cerumen Removal

Box 12-8

Assess for ear pain, traumas, abnormalities, drainage, surgeries, or perforations. These or any other unusual findings should be referred to an otolaryngologist.
When aural exam reveals cerumen impaction with no other abnormalities the nurse may irrigate for cerumen removal using the following techniques:

- Carefully clip and remove hairs in ear canal
- Instill a softening agent, such as slightly warm mineral oil, 0.5 to 1 ml twice daily for several days until wax becomes softened
- Protect clothing and linens from drainage of oil or wax by small cotton ball placed in each external ear canal
- When irrigating the ear use hand held bulb syringe, a 2 to 4 ounce plastic syringe or Water Pik with emesis basin under ear to catch drainage; tip head to side being drained
- Use solution of 3 ounces 3% hydrogen peroxide in quart of water warmed to 98 to 100 degrees; if client is sensitive to hydrogen peroxide use sterile normal saline
- Place towels around neck, empty emesis basin frequently, observing for residue from ear; keep client dry and comfortable; do not inject air into client's ear or use high pressure when injecting fluid
- If the cerumen is not successfully washed out begin the process again of instilling a softening agent for several days

Adapted from Webber-Jones J: Doomed to deafness. *Am J Nurs* 92(11):37, 1992.

and the context of a situation that clues an elder to words being said. In addition, it seems common to overlook the fact that vision may also be fading, thus impinging on lip-reading ability. Perhaps it is the desire of nursing personnel to believe that lip reading is common rather than face the fact that communication can be extremely difficult for some elders. Some elders become dependent on vision for understanding speech at the same time their vision is becoming compromised (Thorn and Thorn, 1989). Nurses will need to seek resources appropriate to augment vision to the greatest degree possible in these unfortunate individuals.

Cerumen Impaction

Cerumen impaction is the most common and easily corrected of all interferences in the hearing of the aged. The reduction in the number of cerumen-producing glands and activity of the glands results in a tendency toward cerumen impactions in the aged. This can be removed and must be before accurate audiometry can be done. A protocol for removal can be seen in Box 12-8.

Long-standing impactions become hard, dry, and dark brown in color. Many elderly admit to using foreign objects to clean their ears. Some have perforated the tympanic membrane in the process and thus suffered severe hearing loss in the injured ear. Individuals at particular risk of impaction are those old men with large amounts of ear canal tragi (hairs in the ear) that tend to become entangled with the cerumen, which prevents dislodgment.

A student was examining Ed's ear with the aid of an otoscope and was having great difficulty visualizing anything. In the process she dislodged a hard ball of cerumen that became lodged even farther in the ear. In panic he yelled that she had deafened him. He was immediately taken to his physician, who removed the wax with the aid of an aural speculum and a cerumen spoon. Then Ed was all smiles, saying he hadn't heard so well in years.

Others who may develop excessive cerumen are those who habitually wear hearing aids, those with benign growths that narrow the external ear canal, and those who have a predilection to cerumen accumulation. Box 12-8 contains suggestions for wax removal.

Irrigation is contraindicated if the tympanic membrane has been perforated because it may induce an infection. Cautions are also necessary for those with especially sticky cerumen, which can damage the mechanism of a hearing aid and involve costly repairs. The factory cost for placing a wax guard is approximately $100; however, adhesive covers and wire baskets are available for less than $10.

Tinnitus

Tinnitus (ringing, buzzing, hissing, whistling or swishing sounds arising in the ear) is a condition that afflicts many aged and can interfere with hearing as well as become very irritating (see Chapter 4). It is estimated that nearly 50 million adults in the United States are afflicted, 12 million severely enough to seek medical help (American Tinnitus Association, 1996). The incidence of tinnitus peaks between ages 65 and 74 and then seems to decrease in males. About 11% of that cohort of older persons experience tinnitus, more males than females in that age group. After age 75 females experience tinnitus far more frequently than males (U.S. Bureau of the Census, 1995).

Tinnitus can be caused by loud noises, excessive cerumen or auditory canal obstruction, disorders of the cervical vertebrae or the temporomandibular joint, allergies, underactive thyroid, cardiovascular disease, tumors, conductive hearing loss, anxiety, depression, degeneration of bones in the middle ear, infections, or trauma to the head or ear. In addition, more than 200 prescription and nonprescription drugs list tinnitus as a potential side effect, aspirin being the most common. (American Tinnitus Association, 1996; Gulya, 1995). Tinnitus has a significant impact on daily life even in those with normal or very mildly impaired hearing. It is exacerbated by noise and increases in severity over time in many elders.

Assessment. Tinnitus may be described as pulsatile, matching the beating of the heart, or nonpulsatile; unilateral, asymmetric, or symmetric. Tinnitus may be subjective (audible only to the person) or objective (audible to the examiner). Subjective tinnitus is more common. Objective tinnitus is rare and is frequently due to a vascular or neuromuscular condition (Ciocon et al, 1995). The mechanisms of tinnitus are unknown but have been thought to be like crosstalk on telephone wires, or phantom limb pain, or transmission of vascular sounds such as bruits, and are sometimes hallucinatory.

Mabel, 80 years old, was complaining of sounds in her ears that would not go away. A complete physical examination, aural examination, and audiometric testing were prescribed. At the completion of testing the audiometrist asked Mabel to describe the sounds.

Mabel began singing, "I'll Be Loving You Always." Perhaps the first question should have been, "Describe the sounds you hear that won't go away."

Newman et al (1995) have devised a Tinnitus Handicap Questionnaire that is a self-report measure of the physical, emotional, and social consequences of tinnitus. It can also be used to remeasure the changes an individual experiences after treatment. However, in spite of intensive testing, questioning, and treatment, some sufferers of tinnitus can never discover the cause and may find little relief. In other cases the problem may quite arbitrarily disappear.

Nursing Management. Therapeutic modes of treating tinnitus include transtympanal electrostimulation, iontophoresis, biofeedback, tinnitus masking with alternative sound production, dental treatment, cochlear implants, and hearing aids (American Tinnitus Association, 1996). Interestingly, the benefits of a hearing aid prove helpful to some, but for others hearing aids increase the problem. In one study about 3% of patients were helped by tinnitus maskers and only 1% by the other methods tried (von Wedel et al, 1990b). Some have found hypnosis, acupuncture, chiropractic, naturopathic, allergy, and drug treatment effective. Lidocaine is helpful to a large number of persons but impractical due to the necessity of intravenous administration and the brevity of relief. Researchers are attempting to identify drugs that can be effective without serious side effects.

Nursing actions include discussions with the client regarding times when the noises are most irritating; perhaps suggest a diary in order to identify patterns. There is some

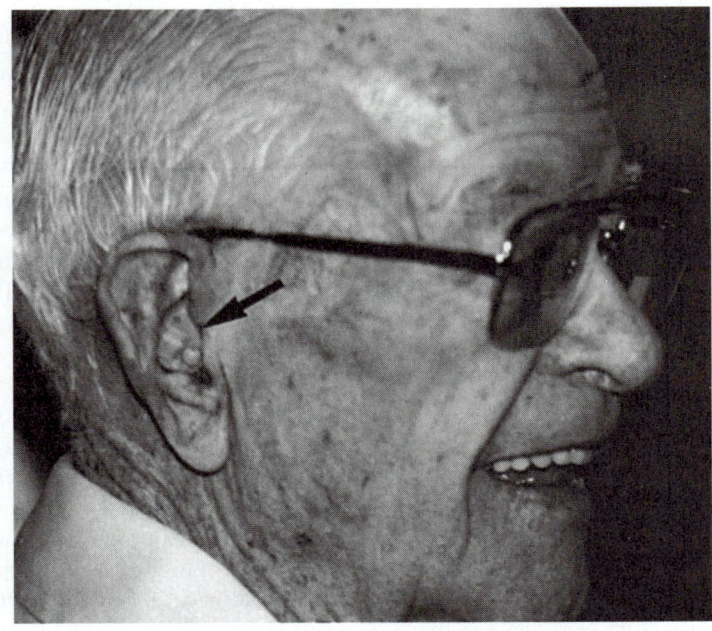

Sensory augmentation of vision and hearing. (From Castillo HM: *The nurse assistant in long-term care: a rehabilitative approach,* St Louis, 1992, Mosby.)

evidence that caffeine, alcohol, cigarettes, stress, and fatigue may exacerbate the problem (Gulya, 1995). Assess medications for possible contribution to the problem. Discuss lifestyle changes and alternative methods that some have found effective. Also, refer clients to the American Tinnitus Association for research updates, education, and support groups (see the resources at the end of the chapter).

The Hospitalized Hearing-Impaired Person

Andrews and Wilson (1991) suggest the following aids to assist the hospitalized hearing-impaired person:

- Note on the intercom button and the patient's chart that the patient is deaf.
- Note the most effective way to communicate with the patient.
- Never restrict movement in the arms of deaf patients who use sign language as the primary means of communication.
- Use charts, pictures, or models to explain medications and procedures.
- Adequate lighting is essential.
- If the patient has a hearing aid, encourage its use.
- Determine a means of readily identifying the hearing impaired.
- Obtain a certified sign language interpreter for obtaining consent for any procedure. It is essential that the patient understand possible risks and outcomes.

Assessment of Those with Impaired Hearing. Assessment of a hearing disability may be done in a superficial manner by almost any observant health care professional. However, the responsibility for the initial identification of hearing problems usually falls upon the nurses, and therefore rapid, reliable, effective screening methods must be available to them. To this end, the effectiveness of a hearing screening protocol was evaluated by O'Rourke et al (1993). The screening included use of the Hearing Handicap Inventory for the Elderly—Screening (HHIE-S), visual inspection of the ear, pure-tone screening, and the client's history, which can begin with these questions:

1. In the past 3 months, have you had discharge from your ears?
2. In the past 3 months, have you experienced dizziness (not related to sudden changes in position)?
3. In the past 3 months, have you had pain in your ears?
4. In the past 3 months, have you noticed a sudden or rapid change in your hearing?
5. Have you ever experienced tinnitus, vertigo, sudden or gradual loss of hearing?
6. How much does this problem interfere with your communications?
7. In which situations do you have difficulty hearing?
8. In the past have you experienced ear infections, surgery, treatment, or hearing aid use?
9. Is there a family history of hearing loss?
10. What drugs have you used or are now using? (Note particularly toxic levels of streptomycin, Mycifradin [neomycin], or aspirin.)

It is important that nurses become aware of these considerations. The client's history and visual inspection require little time to administer and effectively identify subjects who need medical referral. Hearing handicap scales vary in their predictive accuracy.

Pure-tone screening is highly reliable but is sometimes difficult to administer to elders. Each elder is entitled to a complete and thorough audiometric exam if there is any doubt about adequate hearing capacity. Early detection of hearing loss often depends on a nurse's observational assessment. The following are useful initial screening observations:

- Does the person often seem inattentive to others?
- Does the person respond with inappropriate anger or irritation when spoken to?
- Does the person believe people are talking about him or her?
- Does he or she lack a movement response to sounds in the environment?
- Does the person have difficulty following clear directions?
- Is he or she withdrawn and alone much of the time?
- Does the person frequently ask to have something repeated?
- Does he or she tend to turn one ear toward a speaker?
- Does the person have a monotonous or unusual voice quality?
- Is speech unusually loud or **soft**?

Before concluding that any of these **signs are** evidence of "senility" or other aberrant behaviors, consider the possibility of a hearing problem. When there is any **doubt**, referral should be made to an otologist or otolaryngologist to identify possible medical conditions and then to an audiologist or a speech-hearing clinic for an audiologic evaluation before contacting a hearing aid representative.

Nurses are reminded that the best judge of adequate hearing capacity will come from the aged individual's own evaluation (Figure 12-11). Clark et al (1991) found high levels of accuracy of self-reported hearing loss among old women if it hampered their daily life. However, older persons are often unaware of mild to moderate hearing loss because of the gradual manner in which it usually develops. Jupiter (1989) reports a community hearing screening program for the elderly. Over 800 individuals from 20 senior centers participated. Sixty-six percent failed the pure tone test. The majority of the respondents indicated that they did not feel handicapped by a hearing deficit and were not interested in obtaining a hearing aid. It seems that wearing hearing aids is problematic in the minds of many, whether because of cost or inconvenience, and unless hearing loss significantly impairs life quality, it may be ignored.

Hearing Evaluation. Few elders have had audiometric testing though nearly half of elders over 75 years old have hearing impairment (458 per 1000 males, 360 per 1000 females) (U.S. Bureau of the Census, 1995). Nursing service can and should provide initial assessment by investing in a tuning fork, an otoscope, and an audioscope and learning to use them appropriately. An otoscope allows visualization of the ear and discovery of perforated eardrums and cerumen impaction.

A tuning fork placed on an individual's forehead will determine the presence of unilateral conductive hearing loss. This is a nonspecific test and does not measure bilateral

---

Hearing Handicap Scale

Rating:

Always—1 or 2
Frequently—3 or 4
Never—5

Scoring:

Raw score − 29 × 1.25 = %

Scores:

No handicap	0% to 20%
Mild hearing handicap	21% to 40%
Moderate hearing handicap	41% to 70%
Severe hearing handicap	71% to 100%

	Score
1. At 2 to 4 m from radio or television, do you understand speech?	
2. Can you converse on telephone easily?	
3. Can you carry on conversation comfortably when in a noisy place?	
4. Can you understand speech when in a noisy bus, on an airplane, at a movie, on the street corner?	
5. Can you understand a person when seated beside him and you cannot see his face?	
6. Can you understand speech if someone is talking to you while chewing crunchy foods?	
7. Can you understand a whisper when you cannot see a person's face?	
8. Can you carry on conversation across a room when someone speaks in normal tone of voice?	
9. Can you understand women when they talk?	
10. Can you carry on conversation outdoors when it is reasonably quiet?	
11. When in a meeting or a large dinner would you know what speaker said if lips were not moving?	
12. Can you follow conversation at a large dinner or in a small group?	
13. When seated under balcony of a theater or auditorium, can you hear what is going on?	
14. When in church, lodge meeting, or lecture hall, can you hear if speaker does not use a microphone?	
15. Can you hear telephone ring when it is located in another room?	
16. Can you hear warning signals such as automobile horns, railway crossing bells, or emergency vehicle sirens?	
17. Can you carry on conversation in car with windows open?	
18. Can you carry on conversation in car with windows closed?	
19. Can you hear when someone calls from another room?	
20. Can you understand when someone speaks to you from another room?	
21. Can you carry on conversation with someone who speaks quietly?	
22. When you ask for directions, do you understand what is said?	
23. When you are introduced, do you understand the name the first time it is spoken?	
24. Can you hear adequately when conversing with more than one person?	
25. When seated in the front of an auditorium, can you understand most of what is being said?	
26. Can you carry on everyday conversations with family members without difficulty?	
27. When seated in the rear of an auditorium, can you understand most of what is said?	
28. When in a large formal gathering, can you hear what is said if speaker uses a microphone?	
29. Can you hear night sounds, such as dogs barking, distant trains, bells, trucks passing, etc.?	

Figure 12-11. Hearing Handicap Scale. (Modified from High WS et al: *J Speech Disord* 29:215, 1964.)

hearing loss. The audioscope can then be used, following the instructions in Figure 12-12, to determine the frequency range of hearing. Human speech is usually heard below the 2000 to 3000 Hz range. Those who have used the audioscope find it a highly valid screening instrument. Although it should not be used exclusively for determining etiology and degree of hearing loss, it is a simple, fast, and accurate method of screening for hearing loss. Assessment of hearing disorders is done with audiometric and nonaudiometric testing tools. Assessment of structural changes and gross evidence of hearing loss is part of a physical examination. Audiometry is needed for more precise information.

Because many elders are very sensitive about admitting losses, they may be reluctant to share such information. It can best be obtained by first establishing rapport with the elderly person and then proceeding to open interviewing with a comment such as, "Many people have difficulty hearing in certain situations. Have you experienced any difficulty?" "Describe these for me." If friends and relatives have insisted the older person needs hearing evaluation, he or she may be doubly resistant.

Interventions for Those with Impaired Hearing.
Physical examination, interview, self-assessment, relative or friend assessment, and audiometric findings are all nec-

essary to arrive at a meaningful recommendation for the hearing-impaired aged person. Counseling includes specific information regarding the problem, encouragement that sensorineural loss (nerve deafness) can often be partially counteracted by a hearing aid, assistance in the adjustment phase of wearing a hearing aid, and work with family members to improve their communication techniques.

Hearing aids. Many factors may influence an individual who refuses to wear a hearing aid. If the person has been taught to use an aid gradually and correctly and yet does not do so, the nurse should attempt to discover the reasons: the appearance of having an infirmity, the difficulty manipulating a small object, lack of energy, uncomfortable fit, forgetfulness, anger expressed through passive resistance, cost, or simply self-neglect. In this era of highly sophisticated, personalized and computerized hearing aids, almost anyone can find some hearing enhancement that is acceptable to them. Hearing aids have changed dramatically in recent years, but many individuals, having tried one several years ago, have decided against using them.

A hearing aid is a personal amplifying system that includes a microphone, an amplifier, and a loudspeaker. The appearance and effectiveness of hearing aids have greatly improved in recent years. Hearing aids have been miniaturized,

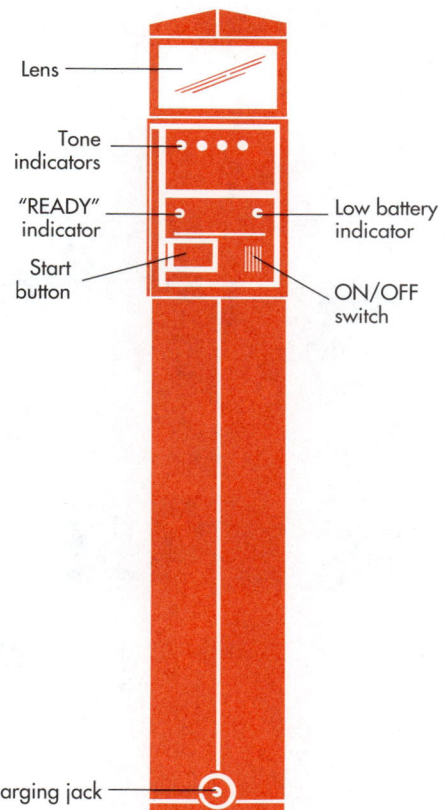

Lens

Tone indicators

"READY" indicator

Low battery indicator

Start button

ON/OFF switch

Charging jack

1. Turn on the instrument by sliding the ON/OFF switch up.

2. Inform the client that he/she will hear some faint tones and ask the client to raise the index finger each time the sound is heard.

3. Gently pull the ear canal up and back and then carefully insert the audioscope into the ear canal using the largest ear speculum that can be comfortably inserted into the ear canal.

4. The tip is positioned so that the tympanic membrane is visualized.

5. Depress the start button.

6. The tone indicators illuminate sequentially (with a red light) as each tone is presented to the client for 1.5 seconds.

7. Repeat the same procedure in the opposite ear.

NOTE: Occluding the opposite eardrum does not appear to influence the accuracy of the test results.

Figure 12-12. The audioscope. (From Campbell S: The audioscope: a valuable hearing assessment tool, *J Gerontol Nurs* 12(12):28, 1986.)

but the small size may present difficulties for the aged with visual deficits, loss of sensation, or arthritic hands. A recent advance has been the introduction of a remote control device that contains an on/off switch and volume device. There are approximately 50 different manufacturers of hearing aids, and thus the informed consumer has a broad selection from which to choose.

The law requires that audiologic testing be preceded by an examination by a physician to rule out ear, nose, and throat (ENT) disorders. Many ENT specialists have an audiologist and audiologic testing available in the office. Audiologists may favor certain models, and it is wise for a client to shop around for fit and sound regardless of what the physician and audiologist recommend. The investment in a good hearing aid is considerable, and a good fit is crucial.

Styles. There are numerous hearing aids and assistive devices to improve hearing (Figure 12-13).

The "behind-the-ear aid," which looks like a shrimp and fits around behind the ear, is less commonly used now than the "in-the-ear aid," which is small and fits in the concha of the ear. There is also a larger one that is custom made to fit the entire external auricular cavity (Silverstein et al, 1992). Today the entire system can fit easily in the ear canal.

Whereas these analog hearing aids are designed to be worn at all times, there are other devices designed to solve specific problems (Wylde, 1988). For instance, some products are designed to overcome the effect of noise and distance. These transform sound waves to a different energy spectrum such as infrared or electromagnetic waves that are then transmitted from the microphone to the receiver. These are designed to deliver a clear signal directly in the person's ear.

Digitally programmed hearing aids are becoming available that have more than a million different settings from which to select. These are matched to the individual's hearing loss.

In the past 5 years a miniaturized computer with a memory chip has been integrated into a hearing aid that eliminates many of the major problems with aids, such as adjustment levels, background noise, and whistling. These aids automatically electronically separate incoming sound without the need to adjust the volume (Resound, 1996).

With the rapidly developing technology it behooves the hearing-impaired individual to be thoroughly evaluated in an audiologic center that is not marketing specific hearing aids. Many hospitals and health centers have such services and may have dozens of models an individual can try until one is

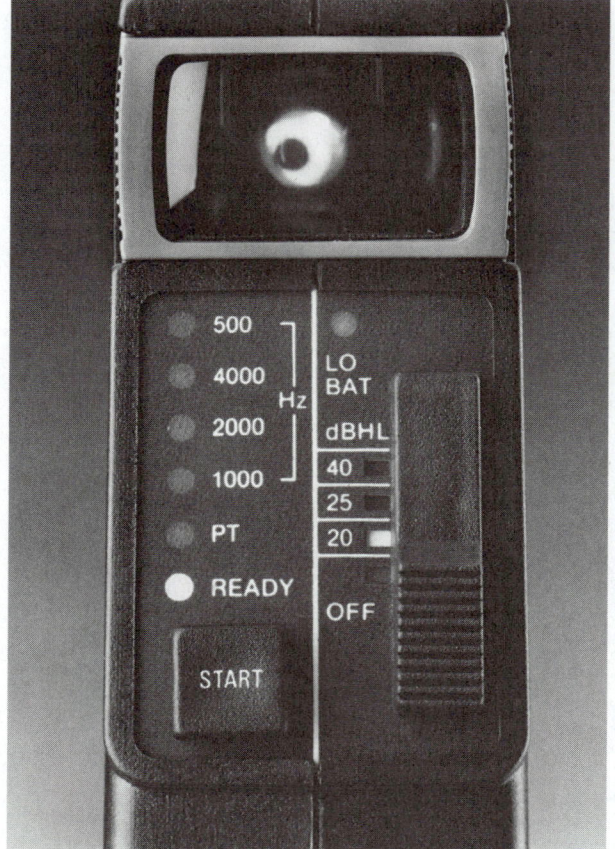
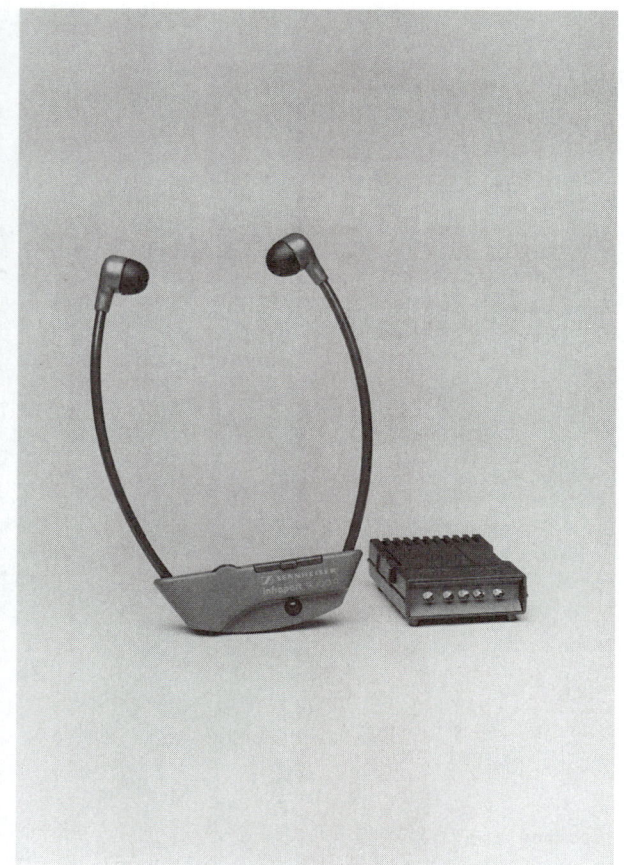

Figure 12-13. **A,** Audioscope. **B,** DirectEar (personal listening system). (**A,** Courtesy Welch Allyn, Inc., Skaneateles Falls, New York; **B,** courtesy Sennheiser, Old Lyme, Conn.)

found that is most suitable. Wylde gives the following guidelines for anyone who is thinking of purchasing a hearing aid:

- Have a complete hearing evaluation by a qualified audiologist.
- "Nerve deafness" is no longer a reason for not seeking a timely evaluation.
- Hearing aids of whatever type will require individual motivation to adapt and adjust to the aid.

Suggestions for using and caring for a hearing aid are given in Table 12-4. At least a 30-day trial should be given before purchasing a hearing aid. If problems occur during that time, return to the audiologist for assistance. Recent federal regulations have influenced hearing aid manufacturers toward more careful marketing and fitting procedures.

Currently before a hearing aid can be purchased, medical clearance of a signed waiver from a physician is mandatory, stating that none of the following conditions exist:

1. Visible congenital or traumatic deformity of the ear
2. Active drainage from the ear in the last 90 days
3. Sudden or progressive hearing loss within the last 90 days
4. Acute or chronic dizziness
5. Unilateral sudden hearing loss within the last 90 days
6. Visible evidence of significant cerumen accumulation or a foreign body in the ear canal
7. Pain or discomfort in the ear
8. Audiometric air-bone gap equal to or greater than 15 dB

Nurses can on physical examination detect the first seven of these conditions and advise clients to seek further counseling from an otolaryngologist. They must also advise clients that charges for hearing aids or routine hearing loss examinations are not paid for by Medicare (Health Care Financing Administration, 1995). There are nine standard Medigap insurance plans, and among them only two, Plan E and Plan J Medigap insurance policies, reimburse for some preventive health services. Plan E states "The preventive medical care benefit pays up to $120 per year for physical exams, serum cholesterol screening, hearing test, diabetes screening, and thyroid function test" (Health Care Financing Administration, 1995). Neither Medicare nor insurance covers any of the cost of hearing aids.

The sound booster hearing accessory. There are now sound amplifiers on the market that fit in a pocket and are inexpensive walkabout-style hearing boosters. They appear to be like a common Walkman. These are particularly useful for individuals with conductive hearing loss and in situations where background noise is inevitable. The amplifying microphone can be attached to the TV, telephone, or clipped on a friend's collar. In situations where a primary sound source is desirable, these devices are ideal. Headsets with small or large earphones are available. Thus hearing aids are not necessary but amplification of desired sounds is available (Figure 12-13*B*).

Cochlear implants. In the 1980s cochlear implants became available to profoundly deaf individuals with sensorineural hearing loss. These have been refined considerably since then and are most successful for those elders who have not been deaf for long and have a strong desire to hear (Cochlear implants, 1991). Unlike hearing aids that amplify noises, the cochlear implant converts sound waves into electrical impulses and transmits them to the inner ear. A cochlear implant is surgically implanted in the mastoid bone behind the ear and electrically stimulates the primary hearing organ, the cochlea, setting the cilia in motion and transmitting impulses along the auditory nerve to the brain's hearing center (Figure 12-14). Although these are not yet in

---

Table 12-4   The Care and Use of Hearing Aids

Hearing aid use	Care of the hearing aid
• Initially, wear aid 15 to 20 minutes daily. • Gradually increase time until 10 to 12 hours. • Hearing aid will initially make client uneasy. • Insert aid with canal portion pointing into ear, press and twist until snug. • Turn aid slowly to $^1/_3$ or $^1/_2$ volume. • A whistling sound indicates incorrect ear mold insertion. • Adjust volume to a level comfortable for talking at a distance of 1 yard. • Do not wear aid under heat lamps or hair dryer or in very wet, cold weather. • Do not wear aid while bathing or perspiring heavily. • Concentrate on conversation, request repeat if necessary. • Sit close to speaker in noisy situations. • Continue to be observant of nonverbal cues. • Be patient with self and realize the process of adaptation is difficult but ultimately will be rewarding.	• Insert battery when hearing aid is turned off. • Store hearing aid in a dry, safe place. • Remove or disconnect battery when not in use. • Batteries last 1 week with daily wearing 10 to 12 hours. • Clean cerumen from tip weekly with the pipe cleaner. • Common problems include switch turned off, clogged ear mold, dislodged battery, twisted tubing between ear mold and aid. • Ear molds need replacement every 2 or 3 years. • Check ear molds for rough spots that will irritate ear. • Avoid exposing aid to excess heat or cold. • Clean batteries occasionally to remove corrosion; use a sharpened pencil eraser and gently scrape.

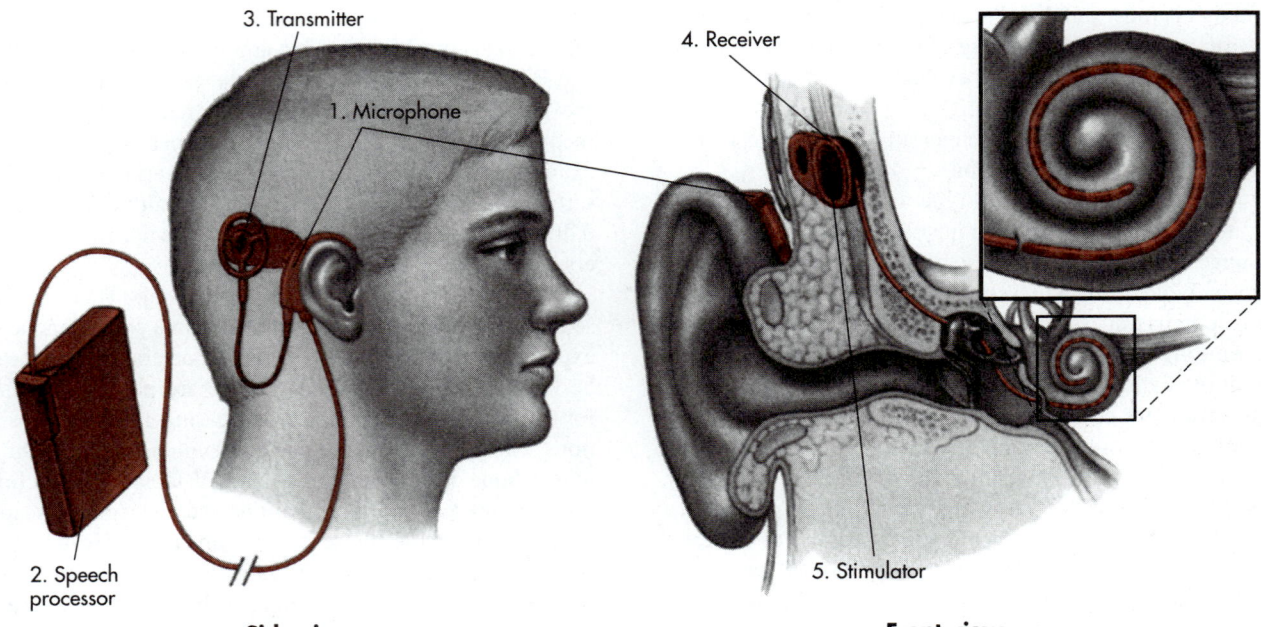

3. Transmitter

1. Microphone

4. Receiver

2. Speech processor

5. Stimulator

Side view   **Front view**

Figure 12-14. How cochlear implants work: A microphone (*1*) picks up sound. The sound travels through a thin cable to a speech processor (*2*). The processor can be worn on a belt or in a pocket. The processor converts the signal into an electrical code and send the code back up the cable to a transmitter (*3*) fastened to the head. The transmitter sends the code through the skin to a receiver-stimulator (*4* and *5*) implanted in bone directly beneath the transmitter. The stimulator sends the code down a tiny bundle of wires threaded directly into the cochlea (snail-shaped primary hearing organ). Nerve fibers are activated by electrode bands on this bundle of wires. The auditory nerve carries the signal to the brain, which interprets the signal. (From Cochlear implants, *Mayo Clinic Health Letter* 9[11]:4, 1991.)

common use, they offer hope to some and are harbingers of even more effective refinements that can be expected in electronic hearing devices.

In 1995, the Food and Drug Administration (FDA) issued guidelines for selecting individuals considered appropriate for cochlear implants. The National Institutes of Health (NIH) finds them most effective in those who receive the implant soon after the hearing loss. The NIH recommends use of the hearing device in adults who are not totally deaf but are not helped sufficiently by hearing aids (Newsline, 1995). The implant carries some risk because the surgery destroys any residual hearing that remains. Therefore cochlear implant users can never revert back to using a hearing aid.

Adaptive devices. Many devices have been developed to assist the hard of hearing. These include alarm clocks that shake the bed or activate a flashing light; television and telephone amplifiers; and sound lamps that respond with light to sounds such as doorbells, babies crying, telephones, or other noises. These can be purchased from hearing aid dealers, telephone companies, electronic and appliance shops, or by writing.

Any facility that receives financial aid from Medicare is required by the Americans with Disabilities Act to provide

equal access to public accommodations. Such facilities are required to have sign language interpreters, telecommunication devices (TDDs), flashing alarm systems, and telecaptioning devices on TVs for the deaf. Unfortunately, these are seldom seen.

When the nurse is considering the basis for making a nursing diagnosis of sensory/perceptual disorder due to impaired hearing, Janken and Cullinan (1990) suggest a redefinition of significant variables. In a study of acutely ill geriatric patients they found that psychosocial dysfunction is not a significant indication of sensory/perceptual alterations due to hearing impairment but must be considered in conjunction with other variables such as levels of depression, cognitive function, social contacts, self-reported hearing ability, and overall health status.

Extensive nursing care plans related to presbycusis can be found in many recent clinical manuals. We suggest that these plans, such as the ones provided by Hogstel (1992), be reviewed for routine management but carefully and thoughtfully modified in relation to the patient's unique needs.

Some very innovative people have developed ideas and products to enrich the lives of the hearing impaired. One group has recorded music especially for the profoundly hearing impaired that is focused only in the low-frequency cycles that are most easily heard (see the resources at the end of the chapter).

Another program that is gaining recognition is Hearing Dogs for the Deaf. There are 17 locations in the United States that train hearing dogs for the deaf. In some locations the Society for the Prevention of Cruelty to Animals (SPCA) trains "shelter dogs," some dogs are especially bred and raised to be hearing dogs, and in some locations the individual's own dog is trained appropriately. Hearing dogs serve to warn the hearing impaired of impending danger, audible signals, phones, fire and smoke alarms, emergencies, and intruders. While there are other, electronic means of dealing with many of these problems, the hearing impaired most consistently comment on the alleviation of the sense of isolation that so often accompanies hearing impairment. With a hearing dog companion, elders express renewed courage, confidence, and freedom (Hearing Dog Program brochure, see the resources at the end of the chapter).

Self-help groups. In a small group discussion I conducted with elders, a portable microphone was brought in and tried by all the participants. After a few moments of play they put it on the table and never used it again during the group. But there was a noticeable difference in how they addressed each other and the level of feedback that was given. They reminded each other when the speaker was mumbling, speaking into his or her own lap, covering the mouth, or could not be heard. The auditory consciousness of the group had been raised by a few moments of discussion at the beginning. In years of conducting groups, this was the first time a real discussion of hearing helps preceded the group. Perhaps it was my consciousness that was raised more than that of anyone else in the group.

In old age, when people have transcended work and have more time to communicate for pleasure, they often develop hindrances to the communication process. When interactions are thwarted by sensory disturbances and motor disabilities, isolation and withdrawal soon follow. However, some people are able to transcend the limitations amazingly well. One very deaf old lady remained responsive and warm, often carrying the conversation by sharing her life experiences and observations. The conversation was one sided but enjoyable to those who listened. She was very aware of verbal and nonverbal cues, which encouraged her to continue or to cease sharing.

Health care professionals may need to focus on ability rather than disability and not assume a deaf person does not wish or is not able to talk. The ability to communicate verbally is gratifying to most persons. One aged man said he missed hearing conversations around him almost as much as the ability to comfortably converse. Listening and talking can be comforting, enlightening, and reassuring, particularly for those who may have been surrounded by conversation for most of their lives. For discussion of other problems of communication see chapter 18.

This small group of elders enumerated a few simple suggestions that make a significant difference in their ability to hear:

- Speakers need to keep hands away from mouth and project voice by controlled diaphragmatic breathing.
- Facial and hand expressions used liberally facilitate understanding.
- Careful articulation and moderate speed of speech are helpful.
- Some languages and some cultural levels of verbal expressiveness facilitate understanding more than others; for example, rapid, romance languages are more difficult to understand and stolid or stoic individuals are more difficult to understand.
- If one has a hearing deficit, wear two hearing aids; in most cases there is a "better ear," but both should be augmented for best results. Hearing is a binary process and is most effective when both ears are functioning at the maximum. Cost and convenience are factors that hamper many elders from following through on this.
- Face the individual and stand or sit on the same level.
- Gain the individual's attention before beginning to speak.
- Avoid conversations in which the speaker's face is in glare or darkness.
- Avoid speaking from another room or while walking away.
- Enunciate carefully and speak in normal cadence.
- Avoid eating, chewing, or smoking while speaking.
- Realize that the listener will hear less well if ill or fatigued.
- Pause between sentences or phrases to confirm understanding.
- When changing topics, preface the change by stating the topic.
- Provide visual cues to locate noise direction, since there appears to be an age-related deficit in picking up directional cues.
- Restate with different words when you are not understood.
- If paranoia has developed, the individual may not respond well to touch. A handshake is a benign gesture and will signal acceptance or rejection of your efforts to communicate.
- Reduce background noise such as radio or television.

Their mutual problem-solving efforts not only afforded an opportunity for shared concerns but resulted in practical ideas helpful to individuals and their caregivers.

PERCEPTUAL ORGANIZATION

Perception arises from the integration of sensory signals into percepts that give meaning to raw data. Perception depends on sensations and experience. An old person has a wealth of experience to draw from when interpreting data, but at times the sensation is incomplete or experience distorts the present reality. When this happens, we may label the person "confused." Confusion is a term frequently misplaced. It often refers to the nurse as much as the client. When nurses are confused, they need more data. When clients are confused, nurses need to find out the specific source and limits of their data. Confusion and disorientation are sometimes used synonymously, although "confusion" is a catchall diagnosis of unexplained symptoms, and disorientation can be very specific. For thorough understanding we recommend Wolanin and Phillips, *Confusion: Prevention and Care* (1981). It is the classic work on this subject. Disorientation and illusions most frequently have an organic base. Hallucinations may be organic or functional in origin. Further consideration of these concepts can be found in chapters 21 and 22.

Disorientation

Thoreau (1946, p. 285) said, "If a man does not keep pace with his companions, perhaps it is because he hears a different drummer." When people are disoriented, they are listening to a different drummer in another time or place, but the beat is uneven and the impulses disquieting. Following their inner drummer brings insecurity and uncertainty. Sensory impressions are confusing and disconnected rather than intermingling in the subtle manner necessary for integration and accurate perception.

Perception of Time. The first level of disorientation to emerge is often related to timing of events. Being unclear about time measurement puts one out of step with the world at large and subject to an altered sense of linear time. Time orientation is evidence of a personal organization and structure and is somewhat more subjective in the old than in the young. It is the first level of individual awareness to be distorted by stressful circumstances, monotonous environments, or altered awareness. Illness, loss, and crises are frequently accompanied by an expanded, contracted, or muted sense of time passage. Keeping track of time requires attention, devices, and interest; all of these are easily diverted by biologic, psychologic, and sociologic disruption. When stress is severe enough, personal time may remain out of synchronization with the world of clocks and dates or become totally submerged. Widows often move in slow motion for several weeks after the spouse's death. People in these major crises are preoccupied and experience sensory distortion. This kind of reaction has important implications for caregivers. When the world is perceived as threatening and chaotic, we must attempt to move slowly and patiently to restore order. Reassure the client that altered time perception is not abnormal.

The elderly in monotonous environments who lack contrasting events and experiences that mark progression in most peoples' lives eventually lose interest and pay little attention to the flow of time. Organic impairment most often produces disorientation toward recent events such as

whether the last meal was lunch or breakfast. It is difficult for the individual with physiologic disturbance in cerebral function to focus attention or to remember events.

In these situations our interventions are aimed toward capturing the elderly person's attention by direct, personalized communication and through provision of cues in the form of cards, name tags, calendars, clocks, reality boards, and schedules. Daily living patterns should remain as constant as possible. Meaningful stimulating events introduced into a consistent supportive atmosphere may produce improved client affect and function.

Some clients will be experiencing time disorientation of multiple origins: organic impairment, personal crises and loss, and colorless and boring environment. These are the clients whose time sense is likely to be most profoundly impaired.

Perception of Place. The second level of orientation is interrupted when a person is uncertain of territory. Chapter 13 discusses several kinds of territories as they influence the security of an individual. At this time we will explore the internal perception of placement. Distortion of perception relating to one's place usually occurs following translocation. It seems as if one's subconscious lends itself toward establishing security. An individual will perceive characteristics in the environment that relate to previous life experiences; for example, "Did you hear that ringing? It must be the trolley going by," or "What kind of hotel is this? I can't find the bar." Misconceptions of the environment are intensified by poor lighting, intercoms, and room transfers.

Frequently an individual is disoriented toward time and place; most often the aged slip into the security of the familiar past; for example, "I heard the clattering pans and thought Mother would call me for breakfast any minute." The nurse who responds with, "Mr. Jones, this is a hospital and it will soon be lunchtime," is listening and assessing on a most superficial level. It would be far more useful to sit with the client for a few moments, ask about his remembrance of breakfast when he was a child, note the strange noises that disturb one's rest in the hospital, and ask if the client may have been dreaming about a time that was more comfortable and secure.

The nurse will recognize themes of dependence, fears, unfamiliar expectations, and pain. All these commonly expected reactions to illness and hospitalization may be exacerbated by medications, lying in bed (alters perceptions), and slipping from waking to dozing state and states of hypnagogic and hypnopompic reverie. If the client consistently insists he is not in the place he should be or repeatedly calls for someone who is not there, interventions aimed toward increasing security and orientation may be helpful.

1. Gear activity to client level and reduce or increase stimulation toward a more normal range because either extreme will increase psychologic stress and the need to hold onto delusion.

2. See client frequently, introduce self each time, and explain what you would like to do.
3. Obtain some objects that provide comfort or familiarity; for example, pictures or sentimental objects. If the client has no family, find out comfort routines; for example, a glass of warm water with lemon before breakfast, a spread carefully folded on the foot of the bed, or a particular brand of toothpaste or denture cleanser on the nightstand. In long-term care situations it is imperative to alter the environment toward personalization.

Perception of Person. The third level of disorientation is to person and often is closely tied to confusion about one's whereabouts. A patient who believes he or she is at home may expect a family member to enter the room. Quite often health care personnel resemble a significant person in one's past and are believed to be that person. Sometimes it is not disorientation but rather longing that precipitates identity confusion. One aged man wandered the halls of a nursing home calling his wife's name toward the backs of departing female patients. This phenomenon is not limited to the old. Younger people also sometimes imagine they see a dead loved one (Parkes, 1972).

Disorientation regarding one's identity is the most profound insecurity. Even stuporous patients will usually give some response to their own name. Standing very close to a comatose patient, holding the hand firmly but gently, and calling the patient by name close to his or her ear may bring a flicker of recognition.

Disorientation Resulting from Traumatic Treatments. It is common to encounter patients who have transient periods of disorientation related to abrupt or massive interference with body integrity. Cardiac surgery can be a precipitant of disorientation and hallucinatory experiences. Cataract surgery in the past was considered a threat to orientation due to sensory deprivation resulting from eye patches and the general stress of hospitalization, medications, and surgery. With the rapidity of same-day surgery and home recovery this problem is now seldom seen.

Illusions

Illusions are visual misinterpretations of the environment. They are often concomitant with disorientation and may arise from similar sources. A classic example of an illusion seen by one aged lady was her perception of a huge spider on the wall; actually it was an oxygen outlet. The clouding of her sensorium by anoxia made her particularly vulnerable to illusions. In this case her familiarity with spiders and her unfamiliarity with oxygen outlets may have influenced her interpretation of the visual stimuli. Illusions seem to function as a connection with a more familiar environment. However, people within their own homes are not immune to illusions. In some cases illusions are definitely frightening, such as those in which a person imagines the call bell cord to be a snake or a shadow in the corner to be an intruder.

Nurses need to repeatedly explain the source of the illusion and reassure the patient regarding the temporary nature of the misperception.

Perceptual Integration through Movement

We often neglect the critical importance of movement and balance in sensory coordination and perceptual integration. Proprioception has been considered in Chapter 11 in the discussion of mobility. It will suffice to say here that bodily movement is significant to overall adaptation, satisfaction, and environmental interpretation. Vestibular stimulation and tactile stimulation occur as our bodies move in space and give us clear signals about our relationship to objects around us.

A significant amount of vestibular stimulation, information, and sensual gratification come about through touching. Touch intensifies bonding and defines boundaries of self. Those who have visual and hearing impairment often compensate by cultivating the sense of touch to a high degree. For a more thorough discussion of the significance of touch see Chapter 16, which deals with sensuality and sexuality.

Movement gives us an integrated awareness of self and our communication with the surroundings (King, 1974). Perception is influenced by our movement patterns. When movement is limited, there are changes in how one interprets the environment: surroundings seem different, perspectives shift, things seem larger, smaller, flatter, or out of shape. Bedridden people begin to lose perception. Old and young people are more prone to hallucinatory experiences when mobility is restricted. Recent progress in discontinuing the use of restraints is partially due to growing awareness of the devastating effects they have on sensory integration.

In old age certain changes occur in total body awareness (proprioception) that affect one's sensorium. Reaction time increases and movement decreases steadily after 20 years of age. Psychomotor slowing seems to be related to four central nervous system processing factors: (1) functional neuron loss reduces signal strength and processing capacity, (2) an increase in random neural activity creates "noise" interference in processing, (3) reconstitution after neural activity takes longer, and (4) arousal levels are diminished. Some people find natural ways to stimulate vestibular function and movement integration. Perhaps old people rock frequently in response to a subliminal need for body movement.

Movement and vestibular and tactile stimulation may need to be adapted to the needs of the elderly. When a patient has been bedridden for some time, it is important for the nurse to alert the patient to unfamiliar environmental sensations and support the patient as he or she regains upright bearings. The patient is in fact seeking navigational bearings to reorient himself or herself, just as a sailor develops sea legs and must adapt to the feel of the land again. An old person is particularly vulnerable to this disorientation because the sensory/spatial body systems do not reintegrate as quickly as in youth. Both physical and psychologic support is necessary as older persons regain strength and movement.

Perception, feeling, and ideation may not be an end in themselves but are instead the instruments of wise, efficient, and smooth action. Interference with muscular expression may be fundamental to personality disorganization. The brain connects perceptions to the deep centers of the cerebellum where specific sets of intricate actions express satisfaction through energy discharge. We do know that people gain security when they can effectively move about in the environment and feel the effects of their actions and influence on the surroundings.

Nursing to Integrate Sensory Stimuli

Throughout this chapter we have examined the aged person's communication with the environment through the senses and perceptual organizational processes. These factors are fundamental to the maintenance of safety and security. When in disorder, these limitations hinder one's ability to obtain what is needed from the environment. Many of the aged rely on devices to assist them in this process. Those most frequently used to facilitate environmental contact are hearing aids, spectacles, wheelchairs, dentures, canes, and crutches. The nurse's presence in the environment provides a lighthouse to those running aground in their perceptual storms. The intricacies of interpersonal communication will be explored more fully in the discussion of belonging (see Chapter 17) and the obstacles to overcome (see Chapter 18). Here our goal has been to increase the nurse's understanding of how one may assist an aged person to effectively negotiate and make meaning of the personal environment, using all capacities to an optimum level.

KEY CONCEPTS

- The sensory apparatus all lose some degree of acuity in the aging process; hearing is the most prevalent loss.
- The importance of cerumen removal is frequently overlooked and often greatly improves hearing.
- Those with hearing impairment often find it difficult to adapt to hearing aids. If they have not recently been to a certified audiologist they should do so. Many improvements have recently been made, and a proper assessment is essential in order to an obtain a recommendation for the most appropriate hearing aid.
- The loss of vision is greatly feared by many elders, though vision impairment is only one third as common as hearing loss, and total loss of vision is rare and due to pathologic processes rather than aging per se.
- When working with the visual impairment, announcing your presence and vivid, detailed descriptions of surroundings are usually greatly appreciated.

- Some believe that "sundowners'" confusion is magnified by sensory impairment and that all experiences of confusion and illusion are magnified by sensory losses.
- Many stimuli in the environment are not perceived within the narrow parameters of the human sensory equipment. Therefore we may sometimes "sense" things that are not clearly discerned by the senses. Some of these may be labled intuition, paranormal or extrasensory perception. These would be an area of fruitful investigation with the aged.
- Environments and environmental changes have major effects on the sensory input available to elders.
- Environmental sensory deprivation may have seriously disorienting consequences for the elderly.
- Sensory overload when individuals are physically depleted by illness may cause behavioral disturbances and great anxiety. Maintaining a quiet and peaceful environment allows for the use of healing energies toward recovery.

▲ CASE STUDY

Harriet was a 67-year-old high school nurse/consultant. She had retired from the Army Nurse Corps with an officer's rank after having served 20 years, much of it in the Korean conflict with heavy exposure to shelling in the early part of her career. She became aware of hearing loss at about age 40, and by age 50 it had became severe. While in the service she had considerable assistance from noncommissioned personnel and functioned very well. When she entered civilian life, it became more difficult for her to manage, but she was unwilling to admit to others her major hearing deficit. During those years she simply attempted to cover it as much as possible, and some of her co-workers felt she was rather obtuse—others suspected her deafness. When she took the position with the school district, she was involved with three high schools, numerous faculty, and students, and interpersonal communication was a major aspect of her position. When she was evaluated at the end of the first year, it was pointed out that feedback indicated she was inattentive. She did then admit her hearing problem and was advised to get hearing aids. She said, "I've known several people over the years that have hearing aids, and none of them were really satisfied with them. I guess that is why I have not gotten them before now." She complied but, after a few weeks, rarely wore them. The personnel officer of the school board, after hearing several more complaints of inappropriate communication, told her she must wear the hearing aids if she wished to continue in her position. Harriet knew that hearing aids were essential, not only for communication but she had almost been hit by a car while walking because she simply didn't hear it coming. Yet she didn't want to go back to the audiology clinic, because they didn't seem to know what they were doing, and each time she saw someone they gave

Nursing Diagnoses

The following potential diagnoses must be considered as well as diagnoses unique to the particular individual:

Risk for impaired communication related to hearing deficits

Risk for ineffective individual coping related to misinterpretation of environment

Grieving related to loss of sensory acuity

Personal identity disturbance related to waning ability to cope

Self-care deficit related to visual impairment

Sensory, perceptual alteration related to impaired hearing, visual, auditory, kinesthetic, gustatory, tactile, olfactory hallucinations, delusions

Impaired social interaction related to disturbances in perception:

Anxiety

Diversional activity deficit

Fear

Injury, risk for

Knowledge deficit

Personal identity disturbance

Protection, altered

Thought processes/altered

NURSING PROCESS AND NURSING DIAGNOSIS
Alteration in Sensory Perception: Hearing

Etiologies and Related Factors

Normal auditory age changes

Uncompensated deficits

Impaired communication

Environmental factors

Defining Characteristics

Inability to identify whispered sounds or normal voiced words

Repeatedly asks for words to be repeated

Cups hand behind ear

Talks too softly or too loudly

Withdrawal from activities

Decreased socialization

Knowledge

Older adult's response to alterations in hearing (physical, psychologic, emotional, cultural/social)

Normal anatomic and functional age changes

Auditory (and as necessary visual) assessment and screening

Types, advantages, disadvantages, and cost of assistive devices

Techniques for assisting hearing impaired

Cerumen removal

Pharmacologic impact

Community resources and referral options

Clinical Judgment and Related Skills

Obtain auditory history: environmental, medications, childhood diseases, allergies, trauma

Inspection of external ear and tympanic membrane

Inspection with otoscope

Conduct a hearing assessment with tuning fork, ticking watch, verbal cues, pure tone testing with audioscope

Evaluation of medications and interactions that affect hearing deficit

Referral to appropriate resources

Teach ear care, safety precautions relative to deficit

Design, implement, and evaluate a plan of care for client/family to facilitate more effective communication between client and others

Evaluation

Communicates appropriately with others

Resumes social activities

If hearing aid is recommended: wears hearing aid

States is satisfied with hearing aid

States life satisfaction better

NEEDS ADDRESSED AND TASK STRENGTHS

Need for sensory stimulation and social interaction (to meet need for safety, belonging, and self-esteem)

Assertive in obtaining services and assistive devices

Seeks and accepts augmentation for sensory decline

Uses accoutrements when personally desirable

Recognizes energy demands of adaptation to sensory change

her different information. She had tried three different types of aids that seemed of little help. She had lost confidence in her ear, nose, and throat specialist because he had been unable to help her resolve the ringing in her ears. Now her school district had contracted with an HMO for health care, and she wasn't even sure whom she should see.

Based upon the case study, develop a nursing care plan using the following procedure:*

List comments of client that provides *subjective data.*

List information that provides *objective data.*

From these data identify and state, using accepted format, two *nursing diagnoses* you determine are most significant to this client at this time. List two *client strengths* that you have identified from data.

Determine and state *outcome criteria* for each diagnosis. These must reflect some alleviation of the problem identified in the nursing diagnosis and must be stated in concrete and measurable terms.

Plan and state one or more *interventions* for each diagnosed problem. Provide specific documentation of source used to determine appropriate intervention. Plan at least one intervention that incorporates the client's existing strengths.

Evaluate success of intervention. Interventions must correlate directly with the stated outcome criteria in order to measure the outcome success.

STUDY QUESTIONS/ACTIVITIES

What are some of the possible reasons Harriet suffered severe hearing loss at so young an age?

Discuss the stigma of hearing loss and hearing aids.

Obtain a "hearing aid loaner." Instruct students to wear it for several hours and report their reactions in writing. List difficulties experienced.

How would you advise Harriet if you were her nurse/friend?

Discuss the various kinds of hearing aids and how they differ.

Discuss reasons why Harriet may have discontinued wearing her hearing aids.

What might you suggest that would be helpful in adapting to the wearing of a hearing aid?

What are some of the options you would discuss with Harriet?

Which of the various sensory/perceptual changes of aging would you find most difficult to cope with?

Discuss the meanings and the thoughts triggered by the student's and elders' viewpoints expressed at the beginning of the chapter. How do these vary from your own experience?

*Students are advised to refer to their nursing diagnosis text and identify possible or potential problems.

RESEARCH QUESTIONS

How frequently is cost a factor that prohibits elders from the use of eyeglasses or hearing aids?

Do participation in sensory loss simulated experiences change a provider's attitudes towards these losses in the aged?

What environmental hazards are most detrimental to hearing?

What percentage of older individuals are troubled by ringing or other internally generated sounds?

What methods are most effective for reducing the interference of tinnitus?

Which sensory losses are elders most aware of experiencing?

Do aged individuals who grew up in urban/industrial cities experience sensory losses earlier in their life span than those individuals from a more pastoral environment?

Are there distinct cohort differences in the types and degrees of sensory loss older individuals experience?

How many elders are aware of the specific sensory/perceptual changes that occur with the use of certain medications?

What assistance is most commonly sought for hearing impairment and/or tinnitus, and is satisfaction obtained?

RESOURCES FOR THE HEARING IMPAIRED

AARP Resource List for the Deaf and Hearing Impaired (D14925), AARP Fulfillment (EE0569), PO Box 22796, Long Beach, CA 90801-5796.

Self Help for the Hard of Hearing (SHHH) offers *Resources for Hearing Impaired Adults,* 7910 Woodmont Ave., Suite 1200, Bethesda, MD 20814.

Organizations

Alexander Graham Bell Association for the Deaf, Inc.
3417 Volta Place, NW
Washington, DC 20007-2778
(202) 337-5220

American Academy of Audiology
1735 North Lynn Street, Suite 950
Arlington, VA 22209
(800) 222-2336

American Speech-Language-Hearing Association
10801 Rockville Pike
Rockville, MD 20852
(800) 638-8255

Better Hearing Institute
PO Box 1840
Washington, DC 20013
(800) 327-9355

Johns Hopkins Center for Hearing and Balance
Baltimore, MD 21205
(410) 955-1078

National Captioning Institute, Inc.
5203 Leesburg Pike
Falls Church, VA 22041
(800) 533-WORD

National Information Center on Deafness
Gallaudet University
800 Florida Avenue, NE
Washington, DC 20002
(202) 651-5051

Self Help for Hard of Hearing People
7910 Woodmont Avenue, Suite 1200
Bethesda, MD 20814
(301) 657-2248

Publications

Coping with hearing loss: a guide for adults and their families, by Rezen and Hausman, Barricade Books, 1993.

Missing words: the family handbook on adult hearing loss, by Thomsett and Nickerson, Gallaudet University Press, 1993.

Living well with hearing loss: a guide for the hearing-impaired and their families, Huning, Wiley 1992.

RESOURCES FOR THE HEARING IMPAIRED ELDERLY

Product Sources for Hearing Loss

COMTEK, 1748 West, 12600 South, Riverton, UT 84095; (801) 254-9263. Personal FM systems.

Gentex Corporation, 10985 Chicago Drive, Zeeland, MI 49464; (616) 392-7195. Portable smoke detector, Lite-alert smoke alarm.

NFSS, 8120 Fenton Street, Silver Spring, MD 20910; (301) 589-6671. Alarm and alerting devices, telephones, smoke alarms, alarm clocks.

Resound Corporation, 220 Saginaw Drive, Seaporte Center, Redwood City,CA 94063; (800) 582-HEAR. Electronically separates incoming sound, no need to adjust volume.

Special Instruments Department, Telex Communications, Inc, 9600 Aldrich Avenue, South, Minneapolis, MN 55420; (800) 328-8212. Personal FM systems.

Williams Sound Corporation, 5929 Baker Road, Minnetonka, MN 55345-5997; (800) 328-6190. Assistive listening devices, personal FM systems, loop systems, telephone amplifiers.

Audio-EX2 Sound Booster, #ASM702, $169, produced by Sony Corporation.

Music For All To Hear, Inc, PO Box 6347, Evanston, IL 60204; (708) 475-6336. Music recorded in the HZ range frequency accessible to those with moderate to severe hearing loss. It has been arranged and acoustically prepared especially for the hard of hearing.

For hearing aid information, look in the Yellow Pages under "Audiologists," "Hearing Aids," or "Speech and Hearing Services."

Organizations

American Association of the Deaf-Blind
814 Thayer Avenue, Room 300
Silver Spring, MD 20910.

American Tinnitus Association
PO Box 5
Portland, OR 97207-0005
(503) 248-9985; fax (503) 248-0024

Association for Macular Diseases
210 E 64th Street
New York, NY 10012

Association for Late-Deafened Adults
PO Box 641763
Chicago, IL 60664-1763

National Association for Speech and Hearing Action
10801 Rockville Pike
Rockville, MD 20852
(800) 638-8255

Better Vision Institute
1800 N Kent Street, Suite 904
Rosalyn, VA 22209

Deafness Research Foundation
9 E. 38th Street, 7th Floor
New York, NY 10016

National Eye Research Foundation
910 Skokie Boulevard #207A
Northbrook, IL 60062

Self Help for Hard of Hearing People, Inc. (SHHH)
4848 Battery Lane, Suite 100
Bethesda, MD 20814
(301) 657-2248

American Foundation for the Blind:
"What Are Older Friends For?"
Self-Help Groups for Older Persons with Sensory Loss
The U.S.E. Program
15 West 16th Street
New York, NY 10011
(212) 620-2000

The Hearing Dog Program
San Francisco SPCA
2500 16th Street
San Francisco, CA 94103
(415) 554-3020 Voice, (415) 554-3022 TDD

Publications

Booklets and pamphlets on hearing loss and hearing rehabilitation are available from The Volta Bureau, 3417 Volta Place, NW, Washington, DC 20007.

In addition, telephone amplifiers, loud door buzzers, and radio and television earphone attachments are available from local companies.

For nursing care plans related to presbycusis refer to Hogstel M: *Clinical manual of gerontological nursing,* St Louis, 1992, Mosby.

RESOURCES FOR THE VISUALLY IMPAIRED ELDERLY

U.S. Library of Congress

The National Library Service for the Blind and Physically Handicapped, a service of the Library of Congress, cooperatively with selected American libraries, operates a national library program for the visually and physically handicapped. Any resident unable to turn pages or to see print clearly and comfortably for a reasonable length of time without special devices, other than regular eyeglasses, is eligible for the program. Braille books and magazines, recorded disks, cassette tapes, and music instruction scores are available. Talking Book machines and cassette players are lent free to eligible persons. (Available from Division of the Blind and Physically Handicapped, Library of Congress, Washington, DC 10542,: [202] 882-5500, [800] 453-4923.)

American Foundation for the Blind Resource Materials

Catalog of Publications (free). A listing of approximately 200 publications concerning the blind.

Directory of Agencies Serving the Visually Handicapped in the U.S.A.

What Do You Do When You See A Blind Person? (free). The do's and don'ts of how to be more helpful and comfortable with the blind. Also available in film (13 1/2 minutes, 16 mm, color). (Cost: on loan, $12 per screening.)

Step-by-Step Guide to Personal Management for Blind Persons. (Cost: $3.50.)

Introduction to Working with the Aging Person Who Is Visually Handicapped. Basic information and education on special needs of the aging blind for those working with the elderly and blind. (Cost: $3.00.)

How to Integrate Aging Persons Who Are Visually Handicapped Into Community Senior Programs. Report of a 1-year study in five New York cities to develop effective methods to integrate older blind persons into senior centers. (Cost: single copy free, additional copies $1.75.)

All the preceding are available from American Foundation for the Blind, 11 Penn Plaza, Suite 300, New York, NY 10001; (212) 502-7600, fax (212) 502-7773.

Other Resources

Aids and Appliances for the Blind and Visually Impaired, ed 22, 1976-1977. A catalog of items for the blind person. Published by American Printing House for the Blind, 1839 Frankfort Avenue, PO Box 6085, Louisville, KY 40206. (Cost: printed copy free; braille edition $6.00.)

Standard First Aid and Personal Safety. 1973, catalog number 6-2250; in braille. Published by American Printing House for the Blind, 1839 Frankfort Avenue, PO Box 6085, Louisville, KY 40206. Three volumes. (Cost: $12.60.)

The Jewish Guild for the Blind, 15 West 65th Street, New York, NY 10023. Curriculum and videotape for training staff in the care of the visually impaired. Pennsylvania College of Optometry, Institute for the Visually Impaired, 1200 W Godfrey Avenue, Philadelphia, PA 19141.

The Lions World Services for the Blind, PO Box 4055, Little Rock, AR 72214-4055; (501) 664-7100, fax (501) 664-2743.

Aids that can assist the blind or visually impaired may be obtained from the American Foundation for the Blind. These are some of the many products offered:
  Open-faced wristwatches, clocks, and timers
  Kitchen appliances designed for use by touch
  Bathroom scale with raised numerals
  A large taxi button
  LowVision large-figure playing cards, puzzles, and games, including Braille scrabble and raised-numeral bingo

Braille calculator
Speaking calculator
Braille writers
Magnifying glasses
Carpenter's tools with Braille or raised markings
Syringes, needle guide caps

American National Red Cross Publications

Loss of Sight (ARC 1275). Information for families and friends of veterans, applicable to others.

Self-Help Groups for the Visually Impaired

Self-Help/Mutual Aid Support Groups for Visually Impaired Older People: A Guide and Directory is available for $10.00 by telephoning (800) 334-5497 or by writing the Lighthouse National Center for Vision and Aging.

Low Vision Devices, 800 Second Avenue, New York, NY 10017.

A catalog of low-vision products is also available by calling (800) 453-4923. Some of the 250 items included in the catalog are watches (large numerals and Braille), clocks and calculators, cassette players and recorders, lighting devices, games and toys, large print books and writing supplies, and numerous other products to enhance vision.

Organizations for the Visually Impaired

American Foundation for the Blind
11 Penn Plaza, Suite 300
New York, NY 10001
(800) 232-5463; TDD (212) 502-7662.

Association for Macular Diseases, Inc.
210 E 64th Street
New York, NY 10021
For information send business size self-addressed stamped envelope (SASE).

The Center for the Partially Sighted
720 Wilshire Boulevard, Suite 200
Santa Monica, CA 90401-1713
(800) 481-3937

Foundation Fighting Blindness
Local affiliates nationwide
(800) 683-5555, TDD (800) 683-5551
Free Amsler grid, pamphlets, information, support networks, and/or referrals for people with retinal degenerative disease.

Glaucoma Research Foundation
490 Post Street, Suite 830
San Francisco, CA 94102-1409
(800) 826-6693
Material on glaucoma, newsletter, eye donor and phone support networks.

The Lighthouse, Inc.
111 E 59th Street
New York, NY 10022
(800) 334-5497
Send SASE with 64 cents postage for low-vision information.

The Lions World Services for the Blind
PO Box 4055, Little Rock, AR 72214-4055
(501) 664-7100

National Association for Visually Handicapped
22 W 21st Street
New York, NY 10010
(212) 889-3141

National Eye Institute
National Institutes of Health
2020 Vision Place
Bethesda, MD 20892-3655

New York Association for the Blind
111 East 59th Street
New York, NY 10022
(800) 334-5497 or (212) 355-2200

Kit for Simulation of Sensory Loss

Vicki Schmall (Schmall V: Create a tool kit that simulates sensory losses, *Aging Connection* 4(4):7, 1988) suggests these ideas for a kit to simulate sensory loss.

Touch: Wear surgical or latex gloves; apply water soluble glue to fingertips and let it dry.

Taste: Provide bland, salt-free foods, crackers, unsweetened Kool-aid, weak lemonade, and pureed food.

Smell: Place nose plugs or cotton in the nostrils. Blindfold individuals and ask them to identify fragrances, extracts, or spices; try to identify differences in taste of potato, turnip, onion, and apple.

Vision: Obtain spectacles from thrift store; cover with yellow cellophane or plastic wrap. Cover sides of spectacles with black paper to simulate loss of peripheral vision. Simulate central vision loss by covering middle of spectacle lens, and simulate total blindness by night shades.

Hearing: Use industrial earplugs, swimmer earplugs, earmuffs, headphones, or cotton in ears for varying degrees of hearing loss. The Institute of Gerontology at University of Michigan, Ann Arbor, produced a useful tape, *Challenging Listening Situations for Older People,* that can be used to check hearing.

Give the student some ordinary situations to complete such as threading a needle, peeling an apple, making a phone call, or eating soup with the various sensory loss simulations.

REFERENCES

American Foundation for the Blind: *Fact sheet: guide dogs for the blind,* New York, 1996, American Foundation for the Blind.

American Tinnitus Association: *Information about tinnitus,* Portland, Ore, 1996, American Tinnitus Association.

Andrews JF, Wilson HF: The deaf adult in the nursing home, *Geriatr Nurs* 12(6):279, 1991.

Back AP, Holden BA, Hine NA: Correction of presbyopia with contact lenses—comparative success rates with 3 systems, *Optom Vis Sci* 66(8):518, 1989.

Barer D: The influence of visual and tactile inattention on predictions of recovery from acute stroke, *Q J Med* 74:273, 1990.

Bass E, Steinberg E, Luthra R: Do ophthalmologists, anesthesiologists, and internists agree about preoperative testing in healthy patients undergoing cataract surgery? *Arch Ophthalmol* 113:1248, 1995.

Campbell S: The audioscope: a valuable hearing assessment tool, *J Gerontol Nurs* 12(12):28, 1986.

Chen H-L: Relation of hearing loss, loneliness, and self-esteem, *J Gerontol Nurs* 20(6):22,1994.

Ciocon J, Amede F, Lechtenberg C, Astor F: Tinnitus: a stepwise workup to quiet the noise within, *Geriatrics* 50(3):16, 1995.

Clark K, Sowers MF, Wallace RB et al: The accuracy of self-reported hearing loss in women aged 60-85 years, *Am J Epidemiol* 134(7):704, 1991.

Cochlear implants: Technological advances offer new worlds of sound, *Mayo Clinic Health Letter* 9(11):4, 1991.

Collins MJ, Brown B, Verney SJ et al: Peripheral visual acuity with monovision and other contact lens corrections for presbyopia, *Optom Vis Sci* 66(6):370, 1989.

Corwin J, Loury M, Gilbert AN: Workplace, age, and sex as mediators of olfactory function: data from the National Geographic smell survey, *J Gerontol* 50B(4):P179,1995.

Doty R, Bromley S, Stern M: Olfactory testing as an aid in the diagnosis of Parkinson's disease: development of optimal discrimination criteria, *Neurodegeneration* 4(1):93, 1995.

Duffy V, Backstrand J, Ferris A: Olfactory dysfunction and related nutritional risk in free-living, elderly women, *J Am Diet Assoc* 95(8):879, 1995.

Eastman P: When the light fades . . . macular degeneration in the spotlight, *AARP Bulletin* 37(7):2, 1996.

Gulya AL: Ear disorders. In Abrams WB, Beers MH, Berkow R, editors: *Merck manual of geriatrics,* ed 2, Whitehouse Station, NJ, 1995, Merck Research Laboratories.

Health Care Financing Administration: *1995 guide to health insurance for people with Medicare,* Washington, DC, 1995, US Government Printing Office.

Hogstel MO: *Clinical manual of geriatric nursing,* St Louis, 1991, Mosby.

Horowitz A. Vision impairment and functional disability among nursing home residents, *Gerontologist* 34(3):316, 1994.

Huxley A: *The doors of perception/heaven and hell,* New York, 1954, Harper & Row, Publishers, Inc.

Janken JK, Cullinan CL: Auditory sensory/perceptual alteration: suggested revision of defining characteristics, *Nurs Diag* 1(4):147, 1990.

Javitt J, Steinberg E, Sharkey P: Cataract surgery in one eye or both? *Ophthalmology* 102(11):1583, 1995.

Jupiter T: A community hearing screening program for the elderly, *Hearing J* 42(1):14, 1989.

Keller H: *The story of my life,* Garden City, NY, 1902, Doubleday.

King LJ: A sensory-integrative approach to schizophrenia, *Am J Occup Ther* 28(9):529, 1974.

Klein R, Klein B, Moss S: Age related eye disease and survival: the Beaver Dam eye study, *Arch Ophthalmol* 113(3):333, 1995.

Kolanowski AM: The clinical importance of environmental lighting to the elderly, *J Gerontol Nurs* 18(1):10, 1992.

Koss E: Increasing visual cues to reduce agitation in patients with Alzheimer's disease, *Research Reports on Aging* 2(2):4,1995.

Kupfer C: Measuring quality of life in low vision patients, *Aging and Vision News* 7(2):5, 1995a.

Kupfer C: Ophthalmologic disorders. In Abrams WB, Beers MH, Berkow R, editors: *Merck manual of geriatrics,* ed 2, Whitehouse Station, NJ, 1995. Merck Research Laboratories.

Lee MH, Itoh M: General concepts of geriatric rehabilitation. In Abrams WB, Berkow R, editors: *Merck manual of geriatrics,* Rahway, NJ, 1990, Merck Sharp & Dohme Research Laboratories.

Lighthouse, Inc: Educating professionals about low vision, *Aging and Vision News* 7(2):3,1995.

Lighthouse, Inc: Current and future treatments for macular degeneration, *Aging and Vision News* 8(1):1, 1996.

Lighthouse, Inc: Glaucoma: new concepts, new treatments, *Aging and Vision News* 8(1):4,1996.

Lighthouse, Inc: Preventing diabetic vision loss, *Aging and Vision News* 8(1):6,1996.

Look me in the eye, *Discover* 11(2):8, 1990.

Lynch MP, Steffens ML: Effects of aging on processing of novel musical structure, *J Gerontol* 49(4):165,1994.

Mangione E, Orav J, Lawrence M: Prediction of visual function after cataract surgery, *Arch Ophthalmol* 111:1305, 1995.

McNeely E, Griffin-Shirley N, Hubbard A: Diminished vision in nursing homes, *Geriatr Nurs* 13(6):332, 1992.

Meeuwsen HJ, Tesi JM, Goggin NL: Psychophysics of arm movements and human aging, *Res Q Exer Sport,* 63(1):19, 1992.

National Institute on Aging: *Hearing problems common in older people studied,* National Institute on Deafness and Other Communication Disorders, Baltimore, Md, 1990a, National Institutes of Health, US Department of Health and Human Services.

National Institute on Aging: Relationship of age and smell explored. In *Special report on aging,* Baltimore, 1990b, National Institutes of Health.

National Institute on Aging: *Scientists study treatment for glaucoma,* National Eye Institute, Baltimore, Md, 1990c, National Institutes of Health.

National Institute on Aging: *Diabetic retinopathy and blood sugar management,* 1995, Bethesda. Md, National Institutes of Health.

Newman C, Wharton J, Jacobson G: Retest stability of the tinnitus handicap questionnaire, *Ann Otol Rhinol Laryngol* 104(9 part1):718, 1995.

Newsline: FDA considers expanded use for cochlear implant, *NURSEweek* 8(11):30, 1995.

O'Connell WF: Low vision—new developments and future directions, *Aging and Vision News* 7(2):3, 1995.

O'Rourke CM, Britten CF, Krien TL: Effectiveness of a hearing screening protocol for the elderly, *Geriatr Nurs* 14(2):66, 1993.

Parkes C: *Bereavement: studies of grief in adult life,* New York, 1972, International Universities Press, Inc.

Radial keratotomy, *Mayo Clinic Health Letter* 13(4):4, 1995.

Ralston ME, Choplin NT, Hollenbach KA et al: Glaucoma screening in primary care: the role of noncontact tonometry, *J Fam Pract* 34(1):73, 1992.

Ray J: Is there a relationship between presbycusis and hyperlipoproteinemia: a literature review, *J Otolaryngol* 20(5):336, 1991.

Resound Corporation, 220 Saginaw Drive, Seaporte Center, Redwood City, Calif, 94063.

Ritter M: Study suggests men losing hearing earlier, *Erie Daily Times,* Nov 26, 1991.

Rovner B, Zisselman P, Schmuley-Dulitzki Y: Depression and disability in older people with impaired vision: a follow up study, *J Am Geriatr Soc* 44(2):181, 1996.

Sacks O: *Seeing voices: a journey into the world of the deaf,* Berkeley, 1989, University of California Press.

Sandler RL: Glaucoma, *Am J Nurs* 95(3):34,1995.

Schappert SM: Office visits for glaucoma: United States, 1991-1992, *Advance data from vital and health statistics,* No 262, Hyattsville, Md, 1995, National Center for Health Statistics.

Schein JD: The deaf community in the twenty-first century. In Garretson M, editor: *Perspectives on deafness: a deaf American monograph,* 41:131, 1991.

Schmidt E: Personal communication, American Foundation for the Blind, July 16, 1996.

Schneider E: *Demographics update: blind persons who use guide dogs,* New York, 1996, American Foundation for the Blind.

Selye H: *The stress of life,* New York, 1956, McGraw-Hill.

Ship JA, Pearson JD, Cruise LJ, Brant LJ, Metter EJ: Longitudinal changes in smell identification, *J of Gerontol* 51A(2):M86,1996.

Silverstein H, Wolfson RJ, Rosenberg S: Diagnosis and management of hearing loss, *Clin Symp* 44(3):2,1992.

Silverstone B: Technology and low-vision aids, *Aging Connection,* 4(4):5, 1988.

Stein HA: Contact lenses in the management of presbyopia, *Int Ophthalmol Clin* 31(2):61, 1991.

Stuen C: Vision care and rehabilitation, *Focus on Geriatric Care and Rehabilitation* 10(1):1,1996.

Taste and smell, *Mayo Clinic Health Letter* 9(10):1, 1991.

Thoreau HD: *Walden XVIII,* Conclusion, New York, 1946, Dodd, Mead & Co.

Thorn F, Thorn S: Speechreading with reduced vision: a problem of aging, *J Optical Soc Am* 6(4):491, 1989.

Tielsch J, Steinberg E, Cassard S: Preoperative functional expectations and postoperative outcomes among patients undergoing first eye cataract surgery, *Arch Ophthalmol* 113:1312, 1995.

US Bureau of the Census: *Statistical Abstract of the United States: 1995,* Washington, DC, 1995, Superintendent of Documents, US Government Printing Office.

US Department of Health and Human Services: *HCFA announces toll-free Medicare hotline for hearing and speech impaired,* HHS News press release, Sept 14, 1995a.

US Department of Health and Human Services: *Medicare policy proposed for eye surgery,* HHS News press release, Oct 5, 1995b.

US Department of Health and Human Services: *Healthy people 2000: midcourse review and 1995 objectives,* Washington, DC, 1995c, National Institutes of Health.

van Rens GH, Chmielowski RJ, Lemmens WA: Results obtained with low vision aids: a retrospective study, *Doc Ophthalmol* 78(3-4):205, 1991.

Vernon M, Makowsky B: Deafness and minority group dynamics, *Deaf American* 21:3, 1961.

Virtanen P, Laatikainen L: Primary success with low vision aids in age-related macular degeneration, *Acta Ophthalmol* 69(4):484, 1991.

von Wedel H, von Wedel UC, Streppel M: Selective hearing in the aged with regard to speech perception in quiet and in noise, *Acta Otolaryngol* 476(Suppl):131, 1990a.

von Wedel H, von Wedel UC, Zorowka P: Tinnitus diagnosis and therapy in the aged, *Acta Otolaryngol* 476(Suppl):195, 1990b.

Wilson WR: Nose and throat disorders. In Abrams WB, Beers MH, Berkow R, editors: *Merck manual of geriatrics,* ed 2, Whitehouse Station, NJ, 1995, Merck Research Laboratories.

Wolanin MO, Phillips LRF: *Confusion: prevention and care,* St Louis, 1981, Mosby.

Wylde M: Technologies help compensate for hearing loss, *Aging Connection* 4(4):6, 1988.

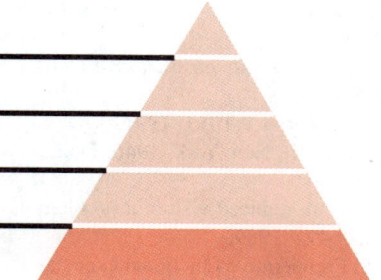

CHAPTER 13

Environmental Safety and Security

A student learns **I think the public should become more educated about what it is really like to live in a facility day after day. My anticipated hope behind doing this would be a shift in the health care system to place a greater emphasis on home health care. I think it is true to say that if family members were offered more help in all areas, that is, physically, emotionally and monetarily, there would be a greater proportion of older adults living out their last years with family members versus institutionalized care.**

Dena, age 28

An elder speaks **How to choose, what to choose, when to choose? Gradually I am confronted with the need to plan for an unknown future. Where will I be safe? Where will I have the services and the help I need? With no children to rely upon I must select living quarters and arrangements for my physical care over the long haul. My mother lived with me in her later years, and we were both unhappy about it.**

Lyn, age 69

LEARNING OBJECTIVES Upon completion of this chapter, the reader will be able to:

1. Identify numerous factors in the microenvironment and macroenvironment that ideally contribute to the safety and security of the aged.
2. Relate strategies for protecting the aged person from injury and accident in the home and in the community.
3. Compare the major features, advantages, and disadvantages of several housing situations available to the aged.
4. Specify symptoms indicative of hypothermia and hyperthermia and enumerate interventions both proactive and therapeutic.
5. Explain the significance of personal space and environmental demands on adaptation in late life.
6. Discuss changes in environment and the effects on individual function.

PERSONAL SPACE

The environment includes one's personally significant space and extends to the outermost boundaries of potential life space. These spaces are geographically and perceptually defined and subject to enlargement, constriction, and energy exchanges. Although one's personally significant geographic space may be limited to a 5- by 10-foot cubicle, perceptual life space is limited only to the creativity and capacity of the individual. In this chapter we consider older individuals and their personal and geographic life space. Chapters 8, 9, 11, 18, 21, 22, 25, 26 and 27 all present other elements of life space.

As you immerse yourself in the text, it will become apparent that one's perceptions of possibilities and one's cognitive capacities greatly influence life space and satisfaction regardless of where one resides. However, it is incumbent on nurses to assist the individual to maximize comfort and safety in geographic space. In this chapter we will address the specifics that are considered in doing so. Figure 13-1 addresses the basic environmental supports elders require to function maximally at each level of need. We will also address select environmental hazards that are particularly dangerous to the vulnerable elderly.

Personal space embodies two main concepts: privacy and periphery. Each person needs an inviolable space for solitude, intimacy, anonymity, and centering oneself. The amount of time needed and the boundaries of this private space are individually variable. Likewise, one needs personalized boundaries, which define one's limits of control and energize one to seek the periphery for stimulation. An aged person with no opportunity for privacy may cease to care about the activities on the perimeter. This person will usually erect psychologic walls for self-protection from personal invasion and will no longer care about seeking enlargement in life space. Problems such as sensory overload (related to loss of environmental control), medication haze, isolation from significant persons, pain, and biologic disorders all affect one's sense of personal space. These are all discussed in various other chapters. Insufficient personal space and lack of privacy seem to cause stress and anxiety. Aged people characteristically maintain a sense of personal space by clutter and environmental props (significant personal items). A thoughtful nurse will respect these territorial boundaries, will not move into private space or thought too rapidly, and will bring together health and illness behavioral needs to establish a secure place.

Suggestions and nursing interventions throughout this chapter are designed to restore pattern and order and environmental predictability: a sense of safety and security.

There are several areas of concern to gerontic nurses interested in maximizing the environmental satisfaction of elders:

- Housing
- Migration patterns
- Weather
- Relocation stress
- Institutionalization
- Environmental safety and convenience

All of these will be considered in this chapter in terms of maintaining personal space and life space in a safe and satisfactory manner.

COMMUNITY

Community means different things to different people. It is defined as a social group of any size whose members reside in a specific locality, share government, and have a common cultural and historic heritage. An alternative definition is that of any group sharing common characteristics or interests. In a sense the aged form a community within other communities. Certain communities of the aged such as senior communities may be readily identified. "Community" as applied to the aged often takes on the connotation of

available resources, and for many this is the limit of their contact with the community.

Senior Center Linkages to the Community

The growth and development of senior centers as service centers for the community-residing elderly were given impetus by the Older Americans Act of 1975. Title III of this act directed development of comprehensive and coordinated services to address the needs of the aged. In 1978 the act was amended to declare senior centers as appropriate and desirable service delivery focal points. There is considerable concern that the senior centers are unable to serve as focal points for the coordination of resources needed by many seniors. Location, availability of transportation, budget, and staff expertise are all critical to the quality and range of services provided. The senior center's role in serving the "at-risk" elderly is even more dubious. Senior centers often serve a segment of the aged population who are likely to cope well with or without the senior center, although life enrichment is certainly a part of that which is best accomplished.

Rural Communities

Nearly half of America's elders live in nonmetropolitan areas. Within the past 10 years twice as many elderly people have moved from urban to rural areas as have moved from rural to urban areas, and this trend is growing. It is generally attributed to the desire to avoid urban crowds, crime, and high costs in the cities and to seek the neighborliness, the tranquility, and the lower costs in rural areas. However, every problem encountered by their urban counterparts is

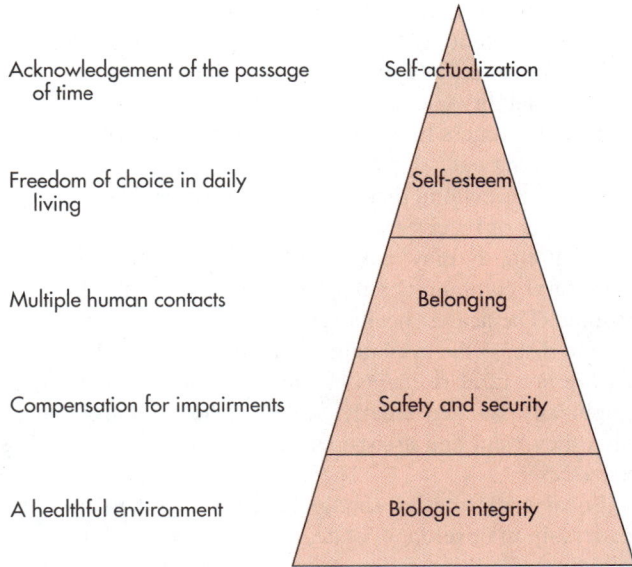

Figure 13-1. Environmental needs of older Americans. (Modified from Herreth J, Orr P, Jones B: *Environmental needs of older Americans,* Atlanta, 1984, The Exchange.)

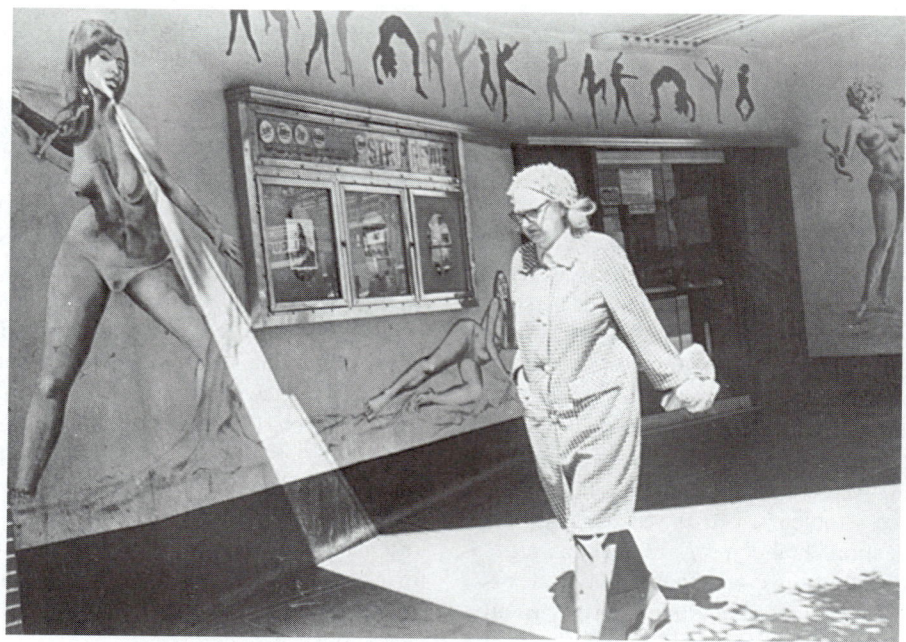

Life space.

likely to be compounded by distance in rural sites. Transportation and health care may be hindrances to rural living, yet rural elders are more likely to describe themselves as satisfied with their situation. Although rural people may have fewer agency supports, they often have strong social supports sustained through family, church, and neighbors. The mutually supportive relationships among older rural dwellers may sustain elders in the following ways:

- Motivation to help whether from altruism, reciprocity, or moral responsibility
- Commonality of experience in which the participants share central life interests and problems
- Availability
- Attentiveness to potential need and voluntary reaching out
- Role reversal in that each would assume the role of helper or receiver whenever the need occurred.

Rural elderly may lack access to medical attention. Remote rural communities may have no physician, clinic, or hospital. The nearest health service may be miles away. It is wise to discuss the availability of medical care. Policy makers are not rural residents. To meet the needs of the geographically isolated elderly, we must find out from them what they want and assist them in identifying and seeking resources.

Local communities should be encouraged to take the leadership to develop, operate, and monitor programs with minimum direction from state and federal governments. Federal regulations, frequently developed around urban models, may be inappropriate if not impossible to implement in rural areas. When assessing the need for services

in a rural area, one must evaluate formal and informal systems. This is only possible with a real understanding of the community and its inhabitants. Medical, podiatric, and dental services, legal aid, adult protective services, visiting nurses services, services for the blind and deaf, extended care facilities, acute and emergency health and psychiatric care, and senior centers may best be provided formally.

Services may be more acceptable if met through churches and neighbors in the community. In many rural communities, churches occupy a central role. As holistic health care providers, we must be flexible enough to evaluate services according to the modes most acceptable to clients from their unique community perspective.

The very remote rural elderly present special problems. In a Colorado mountain area older, isolated persons are given a red flag and a white flag. When all is well, the white flag flies, and when assistance is needed, a red flag flies. The Bureau of Land Management monitors the area with helicopters. With recent updates in the capacities of cellular phones this would seem unnecessary, yet many elders are not able or willing to deal with the cost and unpredictability of cellular phones.

Finally, it must be recognized that many elders maintain their rural life style by choice and may be the last remnants of the idealized rugged individualists so characteristic of an earlier era. Self-reliance and individual responsibility may be more highly valued than the services state or government might offer. Stoller (1993) notes this may be the price of maintaining pride. Vrabec (1995) suggests key members of the community may be cultivated as proponents in establishing nurse-managed clinics that use local, respected residents as ancillary or primary providers to the greatest extent possible.

NEIGHBORHOOD

The idea of neighborhood is a smaller concept than community and is more attuned to the convenience and friendliness of daily contacts. It usually includes the corner grocery, paper stand, mail carrier, small cafes, barbershops, and, it is hoped, the clinic one uses. Nine blocks roughly corresponds to the size of a neighborhood. Low morale and isolation are inversely correlated with one's sense of "neighborhood." The neighborhood seems to be a most important environmental unit for the elderly. The character of a neighborhood may be an important source of satisfaction or alienation. Many older people who once belonged in their neighborhood have been left behind by migration to the suburbs and find themselves in a neighborhood that has evolved into an alien and often frightening place. A significant contributor to fear of crime among the elderly is the socioeconomic deterioration of the neighborhood.

Crimes Against the Elderly

Crime is of particular concern to many older persons. Crimes against their person or property are magnified because of their sense of vulnerability (Garcia and Luck, 1987). Fear of victimization has been studied and identified frequently as more predominant in the aged than in younger people. Studies have yielded somewhat different conclusions but generally upheld the basic assumption. Ferraro and LaGrange (1992) challenge these findings using an alternative strategy for measuring fear of crime and found that younger persons are more likely than the old to be afraid of most types of crime.

In many communities special programs such as escort services, victim counseling, and safety information have been initiated. The American Association of Retired Persons (Leach, 1996) conducted a national search to identify programs in crime prevention that have proved effective. One of the model programs is in Broomfield, Colorado, where a specially assigned police officer presents crime education at senior and community centers within the city, as well as advising individual isolated elders on ways to reduce vulnerability to crime. Another program in Chicago, dubbed SHARE, involves low-rent housing occupants who act as representatives of their units to work directly with police to improve building safety. In Dana Point, California, older persons are recruited as volunteers to work with police. They are issued special uniforms and work in canvasing their neighborhoods performing vacation and neighborhood checks, serve to control crowds and traffic at special neighborhood events, and perform foot patrols in business and shopping areas. Several other creative methods of involving elders and the police in cooperative programs to reduce

crime are reported in the AARP (Leach, 1996) publication (see resources at end of chapter). Nurses need to learn about programs in crime protection, prevention, assistance, and how to obtain legal redress.

Street Crime. Surveys indicate that the elderly are no more likely to suffer physical injury or financial loss from crime than other age groups, although this has been a common assumption. Although crime is no more frequent or severe against the aged, the disturbance and consequences are often more devastating. For instance, an attack resulting in a fall and broken leg may end in death for an old person but only a few weeks of limited activity for a young adult. A purse snatching and the loss of $100 may mean 2 months' food to a poor elderly citizen. Location and income often are far more significant than age in predicting crime rate. In fact, with age as the variable, the elderly are the least likely to be victims of crime. However, there is still much national attention paid to crimes against the elderly because of the recognized serious consequences.

One effort to reduce street muggings of the elderly involved an ex-Marine in his mid-50s who impersonated an old man. Using makeup, he grayed his hair, mottled his skin, drew facial lines, wore an orthopedic shoe to mimic a limp, and used a cane. In league with the police he worked a slum area to identify and arrest attackers. He was mugged 256 times and nearly fatally stabbed but has cleared that area of criminals who attack the vulnerable elderly. Although this is an extreme and well-planned measure to reduce street crime, it demonstrates that something can be done (Steinberg, 1994).

Federal programs through the Law Enforcement Assistance Administration sometimes assist those aged who have been victims of crime. In most communities the Office of Community Victim Assistance offers both crime prevention and victim assistance. In addition, the National Crime Prevention Council can assist in establishing appropriate programs (see resources at the end of the chapter). For specific community programs contact the mayor's office of aging in the community.

Fraud: "White-Collar Crime." Muggings and robbery involving the elderly are frequently brought to public attention, but a larger, less socially visible problem is the numerous fraudulent schemes victimizing the aged daily. Medical quackery, door-to-door salespersons, unreliable repair people, and unethical businesspersons are among those who prey on the elderly. Aged widows are particularly vulnerable if they have always relied on their husbands to manage household affairs. Grief and inexperience in making business decisions combine to create many problems stemming from naivete and poor judgment. One aged lady sold a valuable plot of land to a neighbor for $2000 because he was "such a nice young man." Another had a complicated heating/cooling system installed that was expensive and tripled her fuel bill.

Although nurses are not often in a position to assist in such decisions, they can alert aged people to specific schemes through community education programs. Isolated elderly may be inaccessible but can often be warned against hasty decisions made with inadequate background information. This can be accomplished through spot announcements on public television. Most aged people are more cautious about unnecessary expenditures than when younger but during crisis or illness may search for quick relief. The old caveat "buyer beware" is still important advice.

Recently elderly persons have been victims of fraudulent tax payment schemes such as (1) contacting new widows or widowers to arrange payment of deceased's "back taxes" and (2) bogus Internal Revenue Service (IRS) agents contacting the person for a tax audit meeting in an attempt to extort money. If unsure of the agent's credentials, call nearest IRS office for confirmation.

Most recently, medical fraud has become a national concern. Supplies and equipment brought into the home by various suppliers have been grossly overpriced, and at times there are charges for items not supplied. The Health Care Financing Administration (HCFA) has established offices to inform Medicare and Medicaid beneficiaries of ways to decrease these practices. The expectation is that reduction of the expense of these enormous abuses will ultimately preserve the integrity of the Medicare and Medicaid systems (U.S. Department of Health and Human Services, 1995).

Crime Prevention. Crime prevention programs for the elderly have been established through the Law Enforcement Assistance Administration, the Community Services Administration, and the Department of Housing and Urban Development. These projects have shown the effectiveness of neighborhood crime prevention networks, public education in self-protective measures, avoidance of fraudulent schemes, community safety inspection programs, security advice in homes, and civic and organizational assistance in obtaining security devices and escort services. In some instances, elderly volunteer peer counselors provide support and counseling to elderly victims of crime and violence. Working individually or in teams, these volunteers receive referrals from law enforcement agencies and work with elderly victims to reduce the financial, physical, and emotional traumas of victimization (Burke, 1983).

Crime prevention programs should increase security conscious behaviors that will decrease vulnerability to criminal victimization. Positive aspects of security consciousness should be emphasized. Nurses can be instrumental in reducing fear of crime, and assisting elders in exploring ways they may protect themselves and feel more secure. The following information is useful:

- Purse and wallet snatchers are usually not interested in injuring anyone. People can be advised to carry little money and personal items in a wallet or purse; house keys, larger amounts of money, and credit cards should be kept in an inside pocket of clothing.

Women may need to sew a special pocket inside a coat or jacket. When accosted, hand over purse or wallet readily.
- Some older persons travel about in groups of three and feel quite secure.
- Some people wear a small police whistle around their necks.
- A cane or an umbrella can be a deceptive weapon of defense.
- The Social Security payment is a prime target of muggers, and the elderly should be encouraged to have their checks mailed directly to their banks.
- News media sometimes alert people to fraud and protective actions.
- Whenever someone wants to gain entrance to their home by showing identification, elders should phone the agency involved to verify the authenticity of the identification.
- Increased police surveillance of areas frequented by the elderly, self-defense courses, and availability of youth escort services have all been helpful. See Box 13-1 for other suggestions.

Accidents and Injury

Falls, driving accidents, and thermal injury account for many hospitalizations of persons over 60 years old. The overall mortality in these persons is near 20%. Those who survive may not return to their previous level of independence. Surprisingly, health status before injury has little to do with survival rate after accident. The explanation seems to indicate that prior health status may not provide a true index of functional capacity (see Chapter 11 for further discussion of falls).

In the United States the overall accidental death rate is 34 per 100,000 population and has been consistently dropping in all causes since 1970 with one exception. There are now more than twice as many deaths from accidental poisoning by drugs and medicines. Individuals over 75 are particularly subject to falls, suffocation, and motor vehicle accidents. Falls create the most accidental fatalities, and the majority of these occur in the home (Box 13-2). The second highest cause of accidental deaths of individuals over 80 is motor vehicle accidents. The incidence of these deaths has gradually increased since 1980, while in all other age categories the incidence of vehicular accident deaths has decreased significantly (U.S. Bureau of the Census, 1995) (Table 13-1).

A common assumption is that the environment is hazardous to the aged. We must keep in mind that old people have considerable experience negotiating their environment and have survived many dangerous situations. They are usually more aware of potential dangers and exert more caution than younger people. In fact, excessive caution may create some of the accidents. Others are a result of illness or sensory impairment (see Chapter 12). In those cases it is the microenvironment that is a problem. The following conditions increase susceptibility of the old to accidents:

- Transient ischemic attacks with vertigo, syncope, or stroke
- Muscle weakness
- Interference with the sense of balance
- Poor eyesight and faulty evaluation of spatial relationships, often resulting from neural deficiencies
- Urinary frequency and urgency leading to unsafe maneuvering at toileting
- Unsteady gait because of pain, fatigue, arthritic changes, or osteoporosis
- Orthostatic hypotension, usually due to medications
- Improper footwear or podiatric difficulties
- Improper clothing such as long nightclothes or robes

Box 13-1

Crime Reduction Suggestions

- Do not wear flashy jewelry in public places or carry deadly weapons.
- Identify police and security personnel that are available in high-risk areas.
- Institute informal surveillance agreements by tenants to increase security.
- Receive a home security check by police and follow through on their security suggestions.
- Attend a crime prevention program.
- Keep doors locked, install deadbolt locks, and choose locks that you can easily manipulate. If key is lost, or if you move, have locks replaced. Don't attach ID tag to key ring.
- Use peephole (install one if necessary). Confirm authenticity of a service person's ID by calling that service agency before opening the door. Never open doors to strangers or let them know you're alone.
- Lock windows. Get fire department–approved grates put on ground floor/fire escape windows. Keep all hidden entries locked (garage, basement, roof, etc.) Draw curtains and blinds at night.
- Protect valuables:
  Keep money, securities in a bank.
  Have Social Security pension check deposited directly to your account.
  Mark all valuables with Social Security number, record serial numbers.
- Beware of phone tricks.
  Hang up on (and report) nuisance callers.
  Don't give any information to strangers over phone.
- Consider a pet. A dog—even a small one—can provide excellent protection and good company if you're willing to care for one.
- Organize a buddy system.
  Neighbors can watch out for each other, go to basement/laundry room together, etc.

- Improper use of wheelchairs and walkers, especially on transfer
- Mental confusion and faulty judgment
- Mental depression, with suicidal tendencies
- Hostility and anger at confinement with attempts to gain attention.

Many of these conditions occur more frequently as one ages and are discussed elsewhere in the text.

Nurses often work with aged people who are in an unfamiliar environment with increased potential for accidents. It is incumbent on us to reduce hazards (see Chapter 11 for additional discussion). Although healthy old people in a familiar environment may be somewhat more accident prone than younger people, the consequences of accidents are usually more serious. The mortality for various types of accidents rises dramatically among older people. Checklists of home safety can be seen in appendixes B and C at the end of this chapter.

Injury Prevention in the Home. In general, the most dangerous rooms for elders are the bedroom and the bathroom. Injuries, other than falls, include burns, suffocation, poisoning, scalding, electrical shock, and drowning. The kitchen is the source of many nonfatal injuries such as cuts, burns, and falls. Parsons and Levy (1987) developed a home safety assessment tool that can assist in identifying risk factors for elderly clients in the home. The assessment is of the individual rather than the environment itself. Major factors are altered thought processes, sensory-perceptual alteration, and impaired home maintenance management. In addition, they suggest areas of environmental assessment.

Tynan and Cardea (1987) report the implementation by a long-term care staff of a program to reduce accidents in the home. Letters were sent to all agencies in Tucson that provided service to elders. In addition, a publicity campaign in newspapers and television was launched. Free home assessments were made for the 125 elderly participants in the project. These included recommendations for environmental changes, education in drug use, and referrals for assistance

---

Box 13-2

Assessment of Potential Risks for Accidents in the Home

- Activities of daily living (level of function)
- Cognition, emotional state (memory, depression)
- Clinical findings (health history)
- Incontinence
- Drugs (complete inventory)
- Eyes, ears, environment (sensory deficits)
- Neurologic deficits (gait, balance)
- Travel history (driving ability)
- Social history (alcohol, drug)

From Escher JE et al: *Geriatrics* 44:54, 1989. Copyright by Advanstar Communications, Inc. Advanstar Communications retains all right to this article.

Table 13-1	Death Rates from Accidents and Violence: 1990 to 1992

[**Rates are per 100,000 population.** Excludes deaths of nonresidents of the United States. Beginning 1980, deaths classified according to the ninth revision of the *International Classification of Diseases*. For earlier years, classified according to the revisions in use at the time.]

	White						Black					
	Male			Female			Male			Female		
Cause of Death and Age	1990	1991	1992	1990	1991	1992	1990	1991	1992	1990	1991	1992
Total*	81.2	78.7	76.2	32.1	31.5	30.4	142.0	143.9	134.5	38.6	38.4	36.7
Motor vehicle accidents .	26.1	24.4	22.4	11.4	10.8	10.2	28.1	25.6	24.0	9.4	8.7	8.8
All other accidents	23.6	23.3	23.4	12.4	12.6	12.4	32.7	34.2	30.9	13.4	13.5	12.7
Suicide	22.0	21.7	21.2	5.3	5.2	5.1	12.0	12.1	12.0	2.3	1.9	2.0
Homicide	9.0	9.3	9.1	2.8	3.0	2.8	69.2	72.0	67.5	13.5	14.2	13.1
15 to 24 years old	107.3	104.2	97.4	30.5	31.2	28.4	208.0	231.9	222.2	34.9	37.0	34.9
25 to 34 years old	97.4	94.2	90.4	26.0	24.7	23.6	218.1	213.8	193.6	48.1	47.7	46.1
35 to 44 years old	82.3	78.5	80.3	24.4	23.5	23.5	176.6	171.8	159.8	38.5	40.0	38.9
45 to 54 years old	73.5	72.9	69.8	25.3	25.2	24.2	138.5	132.4	132.9	30.7	33.1	29.5
55 to 64 years old	79.5	75.6	73.0	29.4	26.6	25.7	129.9	124.7	118.7	36.1	32.5	31.8
65 years old and over . . .	150.7	147.4	145.4	80.1	79.6	78.6	175.5	182.2	165.7	81.6	78.6	72.6
65 to 74 years old . . .	99.7	94.8	94.0	40.5	39.0	38.7	141.8	142.6	130.8	50.4	48.1	43.9
75 to 84 years old . . .	195.7	190.5	186.2	89.4	87.1	83.9	206.1	213.5	201.4	95.8	89.7	89.5
85 years old and over .	428.3	433.3	421.4	232.4	234.8	234.2	359.1	373.9	340.0	213.0	209.8	178.4

From U.S. Bureau of the Census: *Statistical abstract of the United States: 1995,* ed 115, Washington, DC, 1995.
*Includes persons under 15 years old, not shown separately.

when needed. More than 50% of participants needed environmental alterations, and 28% were given drug and health care recommendations. Approximately 20% were encouraged to use state or federal programs for which they were eligible but had not accessed, and 10% were advised to obtain home health care. Increased social activity and emotional support were also recommended in a number of cases. The means of financing the institutionally based staff time was not reported, but the cost of $50,000 for preventive care undoubtedly saved far more than would have been spent in the health care system had it not been provided. Additionally, the link between long-term care providers and the community has great potential for serving rural and urban elders.

Environmental Hazards

The aged are more susceptible than younger people to the impact of environmental variations, including pollutants, pesticides, impure water supplies, and climatic and altitudinal environmental extremes. In this text we will not focus on man-made environmental hazards but only on climate and altitude as it affects the aged and particularly the frail aged. When people briefly visit areas of high altitude, they may become hypotensive or develop cardiac symptoms. They should be advised to rise to a standing position slowly and to reduce their activity level to a point of comfort. They may need additional rest periods. High altitudes and air travel may precipitate aural discomfort or disequilibrium as a result of changes in atmospheric pressure. Nurses are often able to provide anticipatory guidance in general and specific ways. It is helpful to let people know that any major envi-

ronmental change is likely to be stressful, but specific discomforts should not be ignored. When an older person experiences a specific, intermittent uncomfortable reaction or one sustained over several hours, he or she should seek medical attention. Too often a real problem is dismissed as just another symptom of old age.

Thermal Stress. It is generally well known that the ability to respond to thermal stress (the ability to feel and adapt to extremes of heat or cold) is impaired in the aged. It takes an aged individual nearly twice the time of a younger person to return to core body temperature following exposure to extreme heat or cold. These effects become evident after 70 years of age and increase progressively thereafter.

Excessive deaths of the elderly during heat waves and cold spells are well documented and are usually preventable. During a 7-year period 5,403 deaths among people 60 years or older were attributed to excessive heat or cold. The percentage due to cold remains relatively constant each year, but the number dying from heat prostration varies considerably depending upon the heat waves of a given year (Macey and Schneider, 1993). Many older persons feel they cannot afford the cost of air conditioning or additional heat even when they are uncomfortable with extreme temperatures.

Minority, rural, and inner city elderly are most likely to die from temperature-related causes. Interestingly, it is found that there is a gender bias in thermal stress: more females die of excessive heat and more males from excessive cold (Macey and Schneider, 1993).

Heat. Heat-related illnesses (hyperthermia) are classified as medical emergencies. There are numerous deaths an-

Table 13-2	Hyperthermia		
Illness	**Causes**	**Symptoms**	**Treatment**
Heat stroke	Breakdown of body's cooling system	Hot, dry skin, high temperature (106°), rapid pulse, nausea, hypotension, headache, dizziness, syncope	Move patient to shade, wrap in wet sheet, call for emergency equipment, give fluids
Heat exhaustion	Loss of fluid and sodium, often follows heavy exertion and precedes heat stroke	Fatigue, giddiness, elevated temperature, muscle cramps, delirium, skin cold and clammy	Lie down away from source of heat, keep feet elevated, give patient cold fluids with 1 tsp salt per liter added, wrap in cold, wet towels
Heat syncope	Sudden exertion or sudden exposure to unusual heat	Dizziness, lower than usual blood pressure, slowed pulse, sudden fainting, cool and sweaty skin	Get out of the sun, put head between knees, and drink fluids

nually from hyperthermia, and these could be almost entirely prevented with education and caution. Perspiration, blood vessel dilation, and thirst are the mechanisms that lower body temperature. Older people are not as sensitive to thirst and as the ability to perspire declines, peripheral capillary dilation burdens the heart. In addition, humid climates slow evaporation from the skin and interfere with the effectiveness of perspiration as a cooling mechanism. Particularly during the night, when metabolic and cardiac activity is slowed, it is imperative that arrangements are made to cool the ambient air (Sweet, 1995). Due to all these factors, elders with cardiovascular disease, diabetes, peripheral vascular disease, and those on certain medications (anticholinergics, antihistamines, diuretics, beta-blockers, antidepressants and antiparkinsonian drugs) are at risk of hyperthermia (Texas Heart Institute, 1992).

There are three distinct types of hyperthermic emergency: heat stroke, heat exhaustion, and heat syncope. See Table 13-2 for distinguishing characteristics. Interventions to prevent hyperthermia when Fahrenheit temperature exceeds 90 degrees include the following:

- Drink 2 to 3 L of fluid daily.
- Avoid exertion, especially during the heat of the day.
- Acclimate gradually over 2 or 3 weeks to hot climates.
- Alternate periods in heat with cooling periods.
- Stay in air-conditioned places or use fans when possible.
- Wear a hat and loose clothing of natural fibers if outside; remove clothing if indoors.
- Take tepid tub bath or shower.
- Use cold wet towels or dampen clothing in extreme heat.
- Avoid heavy, hot foods.
- Ask your physician or pharmacist if any of your medications put you at risk of hyperthermia.
- Fan self.
- Avoid alcohol.
- The simplest and most essential steps to avoid hyperthermia are liberal intake of fluids, rest, and cool surroundings.

Communities subject to summer heat waves can take steps to provide heat relief. Philadelphia instituted an Emergency Cooling Project in 1995 in response to record summer temperatures. The project included grants to residents toward purchase of a fan or air conditioner and a telephone HEATLINE providing emergency assistance, information, and referrals to elders at risk. Specially trained volunteers worked the phone lines on hot days. A supervisor and city health department nurse were on site. The nurse reviewed callers' cases and was authorized to dispatch a health department mobile team for elders needing assistance (Mudd, 1995). This project provides a model for other communities and nurses to replicate.

Cold. Hypothermia, or fatally low body temperature, kills an estimated 25,000 elderly persons each year, but most elderly and most professionals know little about the condition (Wollner and Collins, 1992). The prevalence of deaths from exposure and cold has parallelled the increase in energy costs, although the full extent of the problem in the United States is unknown. The elderly are especially vulnerable to hypothermia for numerous reasons, as seen in Box 13-3.

Unfortunately, a dulling of awareness accompanies hypothermia, and persons experiencing it rarely seek assistance. For the very old and frail, environmental temperatures below 65° F (18° C) may cause a serious drop in core body temperature to 95° F (35° C) or less. Median oral temperature of elderly persons is 96.8° F (36° C). Factors that increase the risk of hypothermia are numerous, as shown in Box 13-3. The factors associated with low body temperature in the elderly are summarized in Box 13-4.

Nurses are responsible for keeping frail elders warm for comfort as well as prevention of problems. Recognition of the clinical signs and the severity of hypothermia is the first nursing responsibility because it frequently goes unrecognized (Table 13-3).

Specific interventions to prevent hypothermic reactions are shown in Box 13-5.

Because much of nursing care has moved into the home, it is imperative to assess the available warmth in the environment, demonstrate how to prevent heat loss and maintain

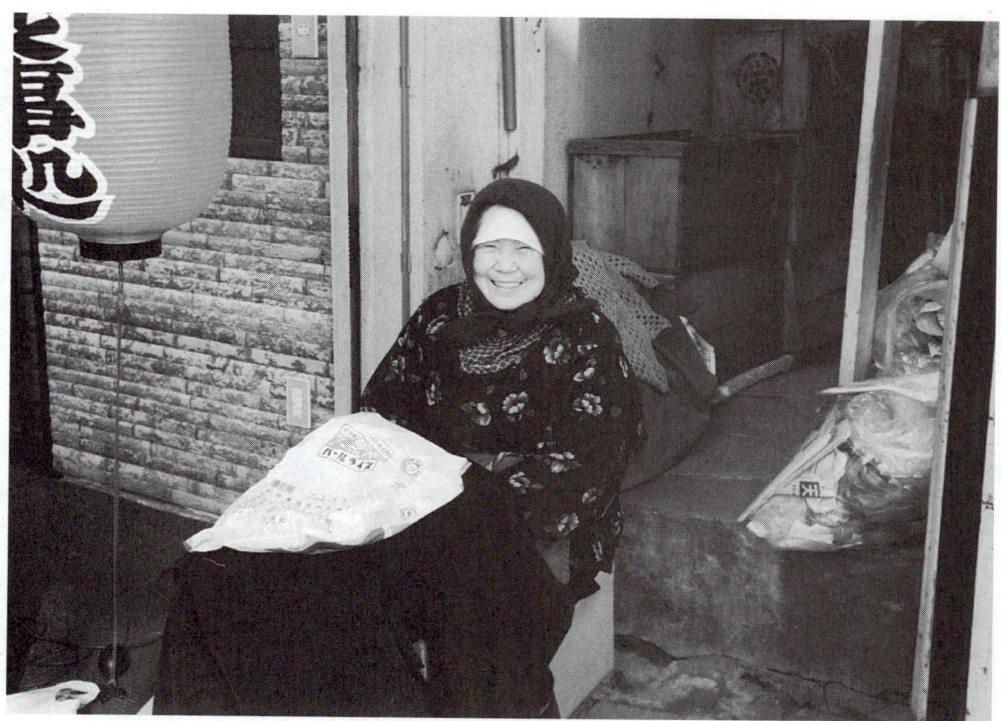

Keeping warm. (Courtesy Priscilla Ebersole.)

core body temperature, and give clients information about the energy assistance that is available in most communities for those on limited incomes.

Fire. There are probably both conscious and subconscious realities in an old person's fear of and respect for fire. Fire symbolizes purification, productivity, punishment, and vigilance, all of which may be subconscious issues of aging. Most of the literature reviewed relates to fire in nursing homes, possibly because the residents of any congregate setting are vulnerable to fire, particularly the frail, immobilized elderly. However, many independent elderly fear fire. They may reside in dilapidated wooden buildings, walk-up tenements, downtown hotels, or other settings where they are at the mercy of others' careless behavior. Of course, residents of free-standing dwellings are also victims of fire. Even though one survives a fire, the loss of treasured belongings can be devastating.

The mortality of those 65 years and over because of fire is more than twice that of any other age group except children 1 through 4 years old. Interestingly, old men are twice as likely to die by fires as old women. This might be related to their greater tendency to smoke and consume alcohol. Most fires occur in the home, and more people die by smoke inhalation than by flame. Noxious fumes produced by burning plastic substances are particularly deadly to aged people with decreased vital capacity or respiratory disorders, who succumb to smoke inhalation quickly. For protective measures to prevent fire and burns in the home, see Box 13-6.

Suggestions advanced to promote a fire-safe institutional environment include use of noncombustible building materials, sprinkler systems, smoke detectors, closed air spaces, written fire procedures, and assessment of environment by fire prevention officials. Flame-retardant fabrics have been recommended by some, but there are those that exude noxious gasses in the presence of fire. We would caution against their general use. Nurses are in a position to ensure personnel familiarity with fire safety procedures and evacuation protocol and also to report or remove any potential fire hazards. Protocol should address these issues:

1. Predetermined staff members should be given specific duties and posts.
2. Notification of fire department and personnel should be clearly described.
3. Management of exit maneuvers should be assigned and specifically described.

The following are practical suggestions of use to nurses personally and to educate patients in home safety:

1. When you smell smoke, see flames, or hear the sound of fire, evacuate everyone in the house before doing anything else.
2. Use normal exits unless blocked by smoke or flame. Do not use elevators.
3. Stay near the floor because gases and smoke collect near the ceiling.
4. In a high-rise apartment remain in room with doors and hall vents closed unless smoke is in your

Box 13-3	**Factors that Increase the Risk of Hypothermia in the Elderly**

Thermoregulatory Impairment

Failure to vasoconstrict promptly or strongly on exposure to cold.

Failure to sense cold.

Failure to respond behaviorally to protect oneself against cold.

Diminished or absent shivering to generate heat.

Failure of metabolic rate to rise in response to cold.

Conditions that Decrease Heat Production

Hypothyroidism, hypopituitarism, hypoglycemia, anemia, malnutrition, starvation.

Immobility/decreased activity (e.g., stroke, paralysis, parkinsonism, dementia, arthritis, fractured hip, coma).

Diabetic ketoacidosis.

Conditions That Increase Heat Loss

Open wounds, generalized inflammatory skin conditions, burns.

Conditions That Impair Central or Peripheral Control of Thermoregulation

Stroke, brain tumor, Wernicke's encephalopathy, subarachnoid hemorrhage.

Uremia, neuropathy (e.g., diabetes, alcoholism).

Acute illnesses (e.g., pneumonia, sepsis, MI, CHF, pulmonary embolism, pancreatitis).

Drugs that Interfere with Thermoregulation

Tranquilizers (e.g., phenothiazines).

Sedative/hypnotics (e.g., barbiturates, benzodiazepines).

Antidepressants (e.g., tricyclics).

Vasoactive drugs (e.g., vasodilators).

Alcohol (causes superficial vasodilation; may interfere with carbohydrate metabolism and judgment).

Other: methyldopa, lithium, morphine.

From Worfolk JB: Keep frail elders warm, *Geriatr Nurs* 18(1):7, 1997.

Box 13-4	**Factors Associated with Low Body Temperature in the Elderly**

Aging

Increases risk of thermoregulatory dysfunction.

Increases risk of acute and chronic conditions that predispose to hypothermia.

Low Environmental Temperature

Risk of hypothermia increased below 65° F.

Thinness/Malnutrition

Very thin people have less thermal insulation, higher surface area-to-volume ratios

Prolonged malnutrition can decrease the metabolic rate by 20-30%.

Poverty

Increases risk of thinness/malnutrition, inadequate clothing, low environmental temperature secondary to poor housing conditions and inadequate heat.

Living Alone

Associated with poverty, delayed detection of hypothermia, delayed rescue if person falls.

Nocturia/Night Rising

Associated with falls; if rescue delayed and person lies immobilized for a long time, hypothermia may develop as heat is conducted away from the body to the cold floor.

Orthostatic Hypotension

An indicator of autonomic nervous system impairment; dizziness and postural instability are associated with falls.

From Worfolk JB: Keep frail elders warm, *Geriatr Nurs* 18(1):7, 1997.

apartment. Open or break a window to obtain fresh air.

5. Define and discuss evacuation plans with other residents of setting.

6. Home fire alarm systems and smoke detectors should have a label indicating Underwriters' Laboratories approval. Smoke detectors should be installed outside of each sleeping area, at the top of the basement stairs, in the bedroom of smokers, and in all other rooms more than 4.5 m from a smoke detector.

7. If clothing catches fire, lie down, and roll over and over; do not run. If someone else's clothing is burning, smother the flames with the handiest item: rug, coat, blanket, drapes, etc.

Some common fire hazards in the home are (1) flammable liquids (gasoline, acetone, lacquer thinner), (2) combustible liquids (lighter fluid, kerosene, turpentine), (3) gas leaks, (4) rubbish and trash stored near stove, water heater, or furnace, (5) Christmas trees and tree lights that are frayed or poorly insulated, (6) smoking in bed or discarding burning cigarettes, and (7) overloaded or worn electric systems.

Promoting Home Safety

Community health nurses are in frequent contact with the actual living conditions of the aged. Our responsibility to survey the safety of their environment is obligatory. Although poverty may greatly affect one's ability to keep all things in good repair, it is the responsibility of a community nurse to alert individuals to unsafe situations. One nurse attached red stickers (such as purchased in a stationery store) to dangerous areas. Yellow stickers could be used to indicate

Table 13-3	Clinical Presentation of Hypothermia: Stages and Assessment Findings

Mild (89.6-95° F)	Moderate (82.4-89.6° F)	Severe (82.4° F and below)
Cold skin; pallor	Very cold skin; increasing pallor	Extremely cold skin; extreme pallor, blue blotches, cyanosis
May not complain of cold	Puffy face; generalized edema	Deathlike appearance
Slurred speech	No complaints of cold	Muscle rigidity; may become flaccid below 80° F
Intense shivering (elderly may not shiver)	Speech difficult	Comatose; unresponsive to stimuli
Incoordination; slow gait; may stumble and fall	Shivering stops; muscle rigidity develops	Areflexia; pupils fixed and dilated
Confusion, disorientation	Slowed reflexes; poorly reactive pupils	Apnea
Apathy or irritability, may be combative; (elderly may sit immobile in a chair)	Stupor; semicomatose	No detectable pulse; ventricular fibrillation
Increased BP, HR	Bradycardia, hypopnea	
	Atrial and ventricular arrhythmias (atrial common in the elderly)	
	Polyuria or oliguria	
	Dehydration; signs of shock	

From Worfolk JB: Keep frail elders warm, *Geriatr Nurs* 18(1):7, 1997.

Box 13-5	Nursing Interventions to Prevent Cold Discomfort and the Development of Accidental Hypothermia in Frail Elders

Desired outcomes: Hands and limbs warm; body relaxed, not curled; body temperature >97° F; no shivering; no complaints of cold.

Interventions

Maintain a comfortably warm ambient temperature no lower than 65° F. Many frail elders will require much higher temperatures.

Provide generous quantities of clothing and bedcovers. Layer clothing and bedcovers for best insulation. Be careful *not* to judge your patient's needs by how *you* feel working in a warm environment.

Limit time patients sit by cold windows to short periods in which they are warmly dressed

Provide a headcovering whenever possible—in bed, out of bed, and particularly out-of-doors.

Cover patients well during bathing. The standard—a light bath blanket over a naked body—is not enough protection for frail elders.

Cover naked patients with heavy blankets for transfer to and from showers; dry quickly and thoroughly before leaving shower room; cover head with a dry towel or hood while wet.

Dry wet hair quickly with warm air from an electric dryer. *Never* allow the hair of frail elders to air dry.

Use absorbent pads for incontinent patients rather than allow urine to wet large areas of clothing, sheets, and bedcovers. Avoid skin problems by changing pads frequently, washing the skin well, and applying a protective cream.

Provide as much exercise as possible to generate heat from muscle activity.

Provide hot, high protein meals and bedtime snacks to add heat and sustain heat production throughout the day and as far into the night as possible.

From Worfolk JB: Keep frail elders warm, *Geriatr Nurs* 18(1):7, 1997.

the need for caution. For example, red tape indicates when kitchen stove burners or oven present hazards; yellow tape is placed on risers of steps or jutting corners of objects in the environment. Nurses alert to dangers will find many innovative ways to assist the client in making the environment safe (see appendixes).

Relocation

Recognizing the strong instinctual nature of territorial needs, it is not surprising that much attention has been given to the crisis of relocation. Relocation as defined in the Springer *Encyclopedia of Aging* (Maddox, 1995) includes relocation, migration, and residential mobility. Regardless of the type of move and its desirability or undesirability,

some degree of stress will be experienced (box 13-7). With each move one must begin to claim personal space by in some way placing the stamp of individuality upon an area if the adaptation is to be satisfying. Since the elderly are particularly likely to move or be moved, the subject of relocation is significant.

Migration. Elders generally migrate for the following reasons: health, affiliation, economic security, comfort, maintaining functional independence, and getting on with life after a family crisis. Disability and health were not as strong motives as is commonly thought. However, the very old most often migrate or move for reasons of health, affiliation, economic security and comfort (DeJong et al, 1995). Although levels of elder migration are much lower than for

Box 13-6	**Measures to Prevent Fire and Burns**

Do not smoke in bed or when sleepy.

When cooking, do not wear loose-fitting clothing (bathrobes, nightgowns, pajamas).

Set thermostats for water heater or faucets so that the water does not become too hot.

Install a portable hand fire extinguisher in the kitchen.

Keep access to outside door(s) unobstructed.

Identify emergency exits in public buildings.

If you consider entering a boarding or foster home, check to see that it has smoke detectors, a sprinkler system, and fire extinguishers.

Wear clothing that is nonflammable or treated with a permanent flame-retardant finish. Fabrics of animal hair, wool, or silk are less flammable.

Use several electrical outlets to avoid overloading.

From Age Page, *Bulletin of National Institute on Aging,* 1980.

the population as a whole, a few states are disproportionately impacted. Many elders voluntarily migrate on a seasonal basis. These persons are relatively affluent and maintain residences in two states. They migrate as the weather dictates, often from northeast to southeast or southwest. These have been given considerable attention in the literature and the media and by market analysts and real estate promoters.

Another group that continually shifts the balance of the aged population in any state and has received little attention is the "new elderly births" (those that become of age to enter the ranks of those classified as old). These new elderly may migrate to other states, or countries, where retirement dollars have more purchasing power. Thus the aged population in any state is continually shifting, and those "newborn" elderly who sought educational and job opportunities in pre-elderly years may now seek to retire in places with entirely different demographic characteristics. Frey (1995) contends that these elderly births have a greater impact on the demographic composition of a state than any of the migrants or immigrants. States particularly experiencing these "in-migrant elderly newborns" as contributing to an increase in good demographics (high education, lower poverty levels, and husband-wife couples) are Maryland, Virginia, Georgia, Colorado and Texas. Recent shifts in retirees' desires is reflected in the largest increases of in-migrants going to Nevada and Alabama. The sites are selected based on cost, climate, housing, safety, services, and leisure activities (American Association of Homes and Services for the Aging, 1995b).

A group we know little about are those aged people who migrate from one willing (or unwilling) relative to another and often evidence considerable satisfaction with this lifestyle. This is probably most satisfactory if one has a large family who willingly support this migratory pattern. People who move about in this fashion are usually highly functional.

A diminishing kind of migratory activity among the aged is that of aging veterans who move from one hospital to another and are quite expert at planning their itinerary to include hospitals with certain advantageous features. This type of activity has become less frequent as the Veterans Hospital Administration resources are becoming less available and criteria for admission more stringent.

Immigration. Since immigration laws now permit the entry of family members, including elderly parents of current naturalized U.S. citizens, increasingly large streams of elderly immigrants from the Pacific Rim and Latin America are joining their children who reside in the United States. In Hawaii, California, Florida, and New York these immigrants account for 1% of the elderly population. Immigration of elders to the United States to join children is becoming quite common. This type of relocation is particularly difficult because it involves adaptation to a foreign culture, language, weather, and living situation. This is especially challenging to home care providers and requires that the nurse recognize the grief entailed in such major loss. Cultural considerations will be discussed more fully in Chapter 24.

Many studies on the effects of relocation on the individual have been published, but there are few studies of the effects on certain states of massive migrations. What are such states doing to respond to the large influx of aged people, many of them over 75 years old and in need of multiple support services? States within the migratory patterns of the aged will need intensive planning to meet the needs of their residents, young and old. Elders should be advised to investigate service availability before moving.

Moving. Pertinent to the adjustment of elders to long distance moves are the following:

- Maintenance of continuity and affective congruence essential to satisfactory adjustment
- Physical and social resources
- Control of events and situations relative to satisfaction
- A sense of cultural and social belonging
- Threads of lifestyle consistency before and after relocation
- A sense of meaning and purpose in the new location

The decision of the elderly to move or not depends on several factors: (1) retirement benefits, (2) available benefits in another state, (3) social and economic conditions where they are, and (4) level of economic independence. When considering retirement relocation, such factors as low taxes, fuel, living costs, and the availability of modestly priced housing and medical services should receive serious consideration. Other factors affecting desirability are potential for employment, the ratio of retirees to working-age population, weather conditions, and utility rates.

Florida and Arizona, two popular retirement areas, were not rated highly in some of these aspects because of an

---

Box 13-7 **Relocation Stress Syndrome**

Relocation stress syndrome is a physiologic and/or psychosocial disturbance as a result of transfer from one environment to another.

Defining Characteristics

Major

Change in environment or location
Anxiety
Apprehension
Increased confusion (elderly)
Depression
Loneliness

Minor

Verbalization of unwillingness to relocate
Sleep disturbance
Change in eating habits
Dependency
Gastrointestinal disturbances
Increased verbalization of needs
Insecurity
Lack of trust
Restlessness
Sad affect
Unfavorable comparison of posttransfer/pretransfer staff
Verbalization of being concerned/upset about transfer
Vigilance
Weight change
Withdrawal

Related Factors

Past, concurrent, and recent losses
Losses involved with the decision to move
Feeling of powerlessness

Lack of adequate support system
Little or no preparation for the impending move
Moderate to high degree of environmental change
History and types of previous transfers
Impaired psychosocial health status
Decreased physical health status

Sample Diagnostic Statement

Relocation Stress Syndrome related to admission to long-term care setting as evidenced by anxiety, insecurity, and disorientation.

Expected outcomes include

1. The resident will socialize with family members, staff, and/or other residents.
2. Preadmission weight, appetite, and sleep patterns will remain stable. If previous patterns were dysfunctional, more appropriate health patterns will develop.
3. The resident will verbalize feelings, expectations, and disappointments openly with members of the staff and/or family.
4. Inappropriate behaviors, i.e., "acting out," refusing to take medicines, will not occur.

Expected short-term goals include

1. The resident will become independent in moving to and from areas within the facility during the next 3 months.
2. The resident will react in a positive manner to staff effort to assist in adjusting to nursing home placement in next 3 months.

---

already overabundant retiree population and high unemployment levels. California has lost favor because of excessive taxes and the difficulty in finding moderately priced housing.

Extended family availability is not the most salient factor in decisions of the elderly to move or not to move, but when illness or loss occurs, it is not uncommon for distant family to become adamant about moving the aged person near them. It is a poor idea to move one who is already stressed, but at times there seem to be few options. Social supports are the key variable in helping individuals to adapt successfully in a particular environment.

Nurses may help older people considering moves to articulate their reasons for moving, to realistically appraise the potential benefits and liabilities of the new situation and what supports they will need and expect, and to consider all their options. If at all possible, the aged person should test the new situation with a visit of a few months before making an irrevocable decision to migrate. A brief visit will not give sufficient data on which to base a decision to move. Perhaps a brief change of scene is all the individual really wants anyway.

The single most crucial factor in adjustment to relocation seems to be the element of perceived control. The implications for nurses and families lie in their responsibility to the aged to make them aware of options and to enhance their sense of autonomy in new situations by providing advance inspection of and thorough orientation to any new setting.

Mrs. L went to live with her son in another state soon after her husband died. It seemed ideal. The move was difficult in many ways but was compensated by the opportunity of being with her son. She knew that at 85 years old she would soon need help, though at present she managed all the activities of daily living very well. She was so relieved that this son whom she adored was eager to have her move in. His wife was not as eager; however, she was agreeable and adjusted to the changes necessary. Unfortunately, Mrs. L's son had a massive heart attack 3 months after she moved in. She had just become settled in, and it had never oc-

Relocation Stress Syndrome—cont'd

3. The resident will express his or her thoughts on his or her concerns about placement when encouraged to do so during individual contacts in the next 3 months.
4. During the next 3 months, the resident will not develop physical and/or psychosocial disturbances indicative of translocation syndrome as a result of the change in living environment.

Expected long-term goals include

1. The resident will verbalize acceptance of nursing home placement within the next 6 months.
2. The resident will indicate acceptance of nursing home placement through positive body language within the next 6 months.

Specific nursing interventions include

1. Identify previous coping patterns during admission assessment. Clearly document these and share the information with other staff members.
2. Include the resident in assessing problems and developing the care plan on admission.
3. Adjust for limitations in sensory-perceptual disturbances when planning care for residents. Visual disturbances need special intervention to assist residents in finding their way around.
4. Staff members will introduce themselves when entering the resident's room, indicating the nature of their relationship with the resident. Example: "Hello, Mr. Smith. My name is Nancy. I'll be your nurse attendant today, helping you with your meals and your bath."

5. Each staff member providing care for the resident should make it a point to spend at least 5 minutes each day with new admissions to "just visit."
6. Allow the resident as many opportunities to make independent choices as much as possible.
7. Identify previous routines for ADLs. Try to maintain as much continuity with the resident's previous schedule as possible. Example: If he has taken a bath before bed all of his life, adjust his schedule to continue that practice.
8. Familiarize the resident with unit schedules.
9. Encourage family participation through frequent visits, phone calls, activity sessions. Be sure to let them know schedules.
10. Establish familiar landmarks for resident when leaving his or her room so that he or she can recognize areas more quickly.
11. Encourage family members to bring familiar belongings from home for the resident's room decorations.
12. Provide reorientation cues frequently. Example: "You are in the dining room. Your room is down the hall three doors just past the window."
13. Encourage the resident to talk about expectations, anger, and/or disappointments and the recent life changes that he or she has experienced.
14. Review medication list with physician to verify the need for medications that might promote disorientation.
15. Provide for constructive activities. Initiate activity therapy consultation.

curred to her that her son, at 65 years old, might not outlive her. The two widows were too enmeshed in their own adjustments to give their energies to developing a relationship. Soon Mrs. L decided she would move to the state where her daughter lived, even though they had never gotten along particularly well. The daughter agreed it would be wise if she were near family members. After a short time at her daughter's they mutually decided it would be best if Mrs L moved to a nearby retirement center. The moves and attendant losses took their toll on her vitality; Mrs L was soon moved to an assisted living center and seemed to have lost her will to live.

The first issue to address in any move is whether it is necessary and whether it will provide the least restrictive lifestyle appropriate for the individual. Questions that must be asked to assess the impact on the individual after a move include the following:

Are significant persons as accessible in the new location as they were before the move?

Is the individual developing new and reciprocal relationships in the new setting?

Is the individual functioning as well, better, or not as well in the new location? This determination cannot be made immediately but must be assessed at least 6 weeks after the move.

Was the individual given options before the move?

Was the individual given the opportunity to assess the new environment before making a decision to move?

Has the individual been able to move important items of furniture and memorabilia to the new setting?

Has a particular individual who is familiar with the environment been available to assist with orientation?

Was the decision to move made hastily or with inadequate information?

Does the new situation provide adequately for basic needs (food, shelter, physical maintenance)?

Are individual idiosyncratic needs recognized, and is there the opportunity to actualize them?

Does the new situation decrease the possibility of privacy and autonomy?

Is the new living situation an improvement over the previous situation, similar, or worse?

King et al (1987) found many factors that contributed to positive readjustment in relocation. In addition to high self-esteem and perceived good health they identified mood stability, few worries, and available confidantes as important. To make a cursory determination of these factors a nurse might ask the following questions (modified from King et al, 1987):

- Do you have a confidante who will be available to you?
- Do you tend to worry a lot or very little?
- In general, how do you rate your feelings about yourself?
- How would you rate your health on a scale from very good to very poor?
- Do you prefer being alone or in groups?
- Do you expect the move to be easy or difficult for you?

The four types of relocation must be looked at individually because they are increasingly stressful:

- Residential, in which the individual moves from one home to another
- Residential/institutional, involving the transfer from home to institution and vice versa
- Interinstitutional, in which the individual is transferred from one institution to another
- Intrainstitutional, in which the individual is transferred from one room to another, often involving different levels of care and dependency

Residence-to-Residence Relocation. Forced residential relocation is generally thought to have negative consequences, yet Dimond et al (1987) studied a group of noninstitutionalized elders forced by industrial expansion into residential relocation and were able to identify those persons at risk of such consequences. The family home can be a stabilizing force for widows in coping with the grief of bereavement, yet they are most vulnerable to being moved when they lack the energy to resist the good intentions of their children. Some are forced by circumstances to do so. Nurses can be instrumental in encouraging the delay of relocation if possible and assessing the relocation risk (Table 13-4).

Residential-to-Institutional Relocation. In 1994 1.6 million persons over 65 years lived in nursing homes. This amounts to 42 persons for every thousand elders in the United States (US Department of Health and Human Services, 1995). Although, slightly over 5% of the aged population overall are in nursing homes at any given time, the

---

Table 13-4   Assessment of Relocation Risk, Nursing Interventions, and Continuum of Care

	Low risk	Moderate risk	High risk
Patient characteristics	High self-esteem Confidante available No worries Low alienation Stable mood Perceived health good Old-old	Moderate self-esteem Confidante Some worries Some alienation Mood fluctuations Perceived health fair Younger-old	Low self-esteem No confidante Many worries High alienation Depressed Perceived health poor Younger-old
Nursing interventions	Provide information and support as needed Not likely to come to the attention of health care providers	Identify needs for information and support Provide empathy for losses Teach problem-solving skills Assist with management as needed Attend to health needs and provide intervention	Identify needs for ongoing support Identify those at risk of suicide Actively assist in problem-solving and obtain assistance from social support services Involve the client in a network of effective professional helpers Assist the client to maintain contacts with friends, if needed Attend to potential decline in health Coordinate medical and nursing care for actual declines in health
Continuum of care	Concern Listening Information	Empathy Information Assist problem-solving Empathy and relabeling	Support services Skills building and problem-solving Referral for individual psychologic assessment and therapy

From Dimond M, McCance K, King K: Forced residential relocation: its impact on the well-being of older adults, *West J Nurs Res* 9(4):445, 1987.

vulnerability of those over 80 increases the likelihood of their residing in a nursing home to nearly 25% (American Association of Retired Persons, 1996). Nursing home utilization varies substantially from state to state, with Hawaii and Nevada having the least and Iowa and South Dakota the greatest number in nursing homes (U.S. Department of Health and Human Services, 1995).

Translocation confusion is a predictable result of abrupt moves to an environment that is vastly different than the one usually occupied. It is often a symptom of anxiety and uncertainty. Many times drugs and treatments contribute to the confusion. An abrupt and poorly prepared transfer actually increases illness and disorientation. An individual who has functioned quite well prior to a major move may show previously unrecognized signs of dementia when in an unfamiliar environment. An accurate assessment of mental status before the move must be obtained from family or significant others. If this is not possible, it must be temporarily assumed that the confusion is a transient response. An elder who has been transferred to an institution from a residence in which considerable autonomy was possible may react more intensely than one where the disjuncture in lifestyle has not been so severe. Some, of course, move to a much more comfortable and supportive situation and adapt well.

To avoid some of the translocation confusion the individual must have some control over the environment, prior preparation regarding new situations, and maintenance of familiar situations to the greatest degree possible (Petrou and Obenchain, 1987). Some familiar and some treasured items must also accompany the transfer. Table 13-1 shows the specific needs met in a sufficient environment. Family members will need considerable support when an elder is moved into an institution. No matter the circumstances, the family invariably feels they have in some way failed the elder. These issues are discussed in more depth in Chapter 17.

Interinstitutional Relocation. Serious consideration has been given to the deleterious effects of relocation, to the extent that a nursing diagnosis related to relocation stress has been adopted by the North American Nursing Diagnosis Association (NANDA). In one study, measuring the impact of relocating individuals from an old institution to a newer one with the same level of institutional care, it was found that prior preparation, anticipation, and involvement in the process made for a smoother, less stressful move (Grant, et al, 1992). Profiles of residents' physical, social, and emotional needs as well as careful inventories of personal possessions and specific needs contribute to more comfortable relocation. Nurses' concerns are on assessing the impact of relocation and the determination of methods to mitigate any negative reactions. The growing numbers of persons who will spend some of their later years in institutions have made this an urgent issue.

Cognitive maps. The preceding discussion of territorial needs, major moves, and relocation adaptation leads to spec-

ulation regarding the process by which one reorganizes spatial relationships. Territory is only as meaningful and available as it is cognitively perceived to be. Cognitive maps, originally conceptualized by Tolman (1948), have come to mean one's perceptual image of one's environment. The implication is that one's state of security depends greatly on perceived environmental order or disorder and how it is visualized. People in unfamiliar settings often need assistance developing cognitive maps. Some of the following suggestions may be useful:

1. Maps of building and surroundings need to be displayed in centrally accessible areas.
2. Individuals feel more secure with directional orientations (north, south, east, west). These should be given.
3. Location of important services must be emphasized.
4. A person familiar with the environment can be asked to orient a newcomer.
5. Discussion of visual points of reference may assist (for example, "Did you notice the large red painting?").
6. Important reference points or services should not be arbitrarily moved without prior preparation. In a public building one women's restroom was temporarily assigned to men. Several women automatically wandered in and left looking rather bewildered.
7. Preparation should be made before relocation of a familiar item or service.
8. Orientation to new surroundings should be delayed until persons have become settled in their individual space. Give time for them to establish some security and reduce anxiety. Poorly timed orientation tours are of little help.
9. Recap and ask for questions at the end of the tour.
10. In a large facility or neighborhood, orientation sessions should be spread out over several days.

Preventing Relocation Stress. See summary of relocation stress syndrome and nursing actions in Box 13-7.

THE CONTINUUM OF HOUSING OPTIONS FOR THE ELDERLY

There are currently approximately 32 million people over 65 years old in the United States living in numerous types of independent, partially dependent, and fully dependent situations. This portion of the chapter examines the options available to the aged along the continuum of housing, from those who are fully independent to those requiring long-term sheltered care (Figure 13-2). Questions are being posed as to the effects of managed care on the continuum of housing options for the elderly (American Association of Homes and Services for the Aging, 1996). As Medicare HMOs continue to expand, managed care providers will find it necessary to establish more networks with housing providers because

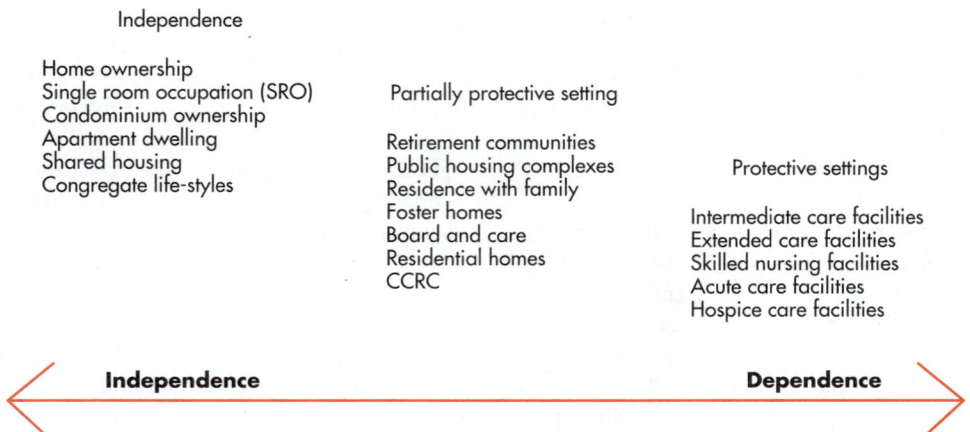

Figure 13-2. Continuum of housing security.

the living site of elders will ultimately also be the site where most economical and preventive health services will be dispensed.

Independent Residences

Almost 21 million households are headed by elders. Of these, 78% are owners and 22% renters. Over 80% of the owners have homes free of mortagage, but many of the homes (57%) were built 40 or more years ago and are badly in need of repair (American Association of Retired Persons, 1996). Home ownership rates among the aged are highest in Utah, Idaho, and West Virginia and lowest in New York, Washington, DC, and Rhode Island (American Association of Retired Persons, 1995). Depending upon the states where they reside, some elders may literally be taxed out of their homes. It is estimated that 1.5 million elderly homeowners have incomes below the poverty level, and 700,000 desperately need housing assistance (American Association of Homes and Services for the Aging, 1992). Three quarters of heads of household own their own homes, and 80% are mortgage free. Homeowners over 75 years of age occupy the highest percentage of substandard housing and often spend 30% to 50% of their total income on utilities. The elderly reside disproportionally in older and more dilapidated housing, which tends to be even worse among rural dwellers. Older persons increasingly identify housing as a major concern. Almost half of all older women living alone spend 50% or more of their income on rent. In addition, many areas have no rent control, and these women are constantly anxious about increasing rents. In the states of California, Nevada, and Florida excessive housing costs are a serious problem for more 60% of elderly renters (American Association of Retired Persons, 1995).

At present many states are designing property tax structures that allow aged residents to remain in their homes by deferring taxes until their death and estate settlement, at which time the taxes will be deducted from the sale of the property. Another option is to borrow money against home equity (reverse equity payment), thereby giving aged people an opportunity to remain in their home and enjoy financial ease (see Chapter 14).

Remaining at Home. "Home" provides basic shelter, is a place to establish security, and is the place where one "belongs." It should provide the highest possible level of independence, function, and comfort. Most people have found basic shelter, but security within that shelter may be minimal. When planning housing for the elderly, the major task is to help the older person stay where he or she wants to be with appropriate support. The Program for All inclusive Care of the Elderly (PACE) in several sites nationwide provides models for keeping individuals in their own homes with sufficient supports.

The living arrangements of the aged are shown in Figure 13-3. More and more, however, for the aged the hospital has been brought to the home in the equipment needed for high-tech care. Some refer to this as the "hypermedicalization" of the home (Arras and Dubler, 1994). The nurse must adapt to the space of the client and forgo the traditional security of our professional home and institutional care. Even more difficult, the client and family requiring high-tech home care must forgo the security of the hospital and take on responsibilities that they may not feel capable of or willing to manage. Although we may find our own adaptation to the client's home and personal space provokes some anxiety, we will also experience some of the patient's anxiety regarding invasion of the home. Arras and Dubler (1994) suggest that patients and their families be informed of the benefits and the burdens of such care and the alternatives. For some people high-tech home care may not be a reasonable expectation or one that they can accept. Clients in the home need the following:

1. Acknowledgment that the nurse is intruding into the client's domain
2. Assistance in arranging medical equipment comfortably and instruction in safety issues

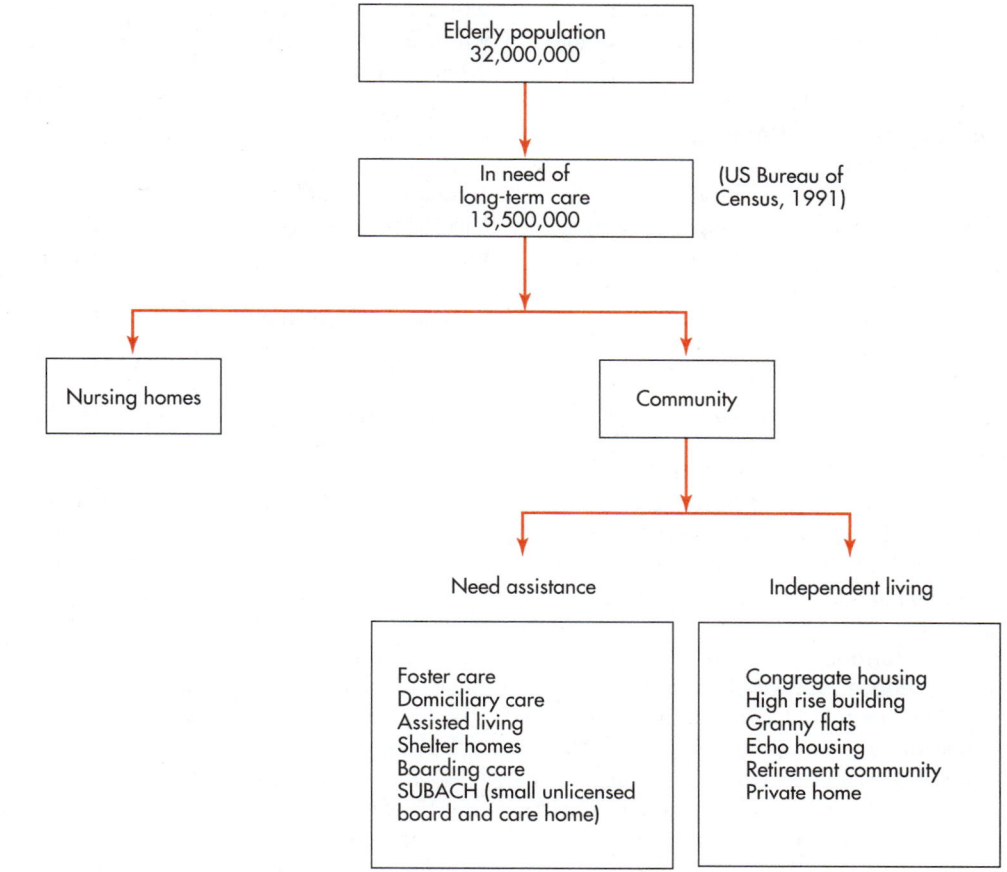

Figure 13-3. Living arrangements of the elderly. (By Kevan H. Namazi, Director of Research, Corinne Dolan Center for the Study of Alzheimer's Disease, Case Western Reserve University, Cleveland, 1988.)

3. Explanations of rationale and demonstrations of appropriate disposal of potentially contaminated or toxic materials

4. Acknowledgment that home care brings intrusions into the client's surroundings and assistance with lifestyle modification to produce the most acceptable ambiance

5. Information about alternatives that may be more feasible for the client than those typically recommended

6. Discussion of any modifications needed to ensure safety

7. Ready access to assistance when needed and emergency responses for necessary services

Home modifications. Minor repairs may present a major problem for elderly homeowners. Those who do not have the strength or skills to make needed repairs often rely on friends and relatives, but many elders have no one to assist them. Some communities have organized a home repair service particularly for the low-income elderly and disabled. Home maintenance service can be managed by retired workers with special skills, and the work can be done by youths who need jobs. The retirees can teach badly needed job skills to youths while providing an inexpensive service to elders in the home. No programs are available across the country; it is therefore suggested that resources might be allotted through Housing and Urban Development (HUD) or by creating a national home modification program modeled after the demonstration program of the 1980s that was funded through HUD (Pynoos, 1992). Until it is recognized that adequate living situations actually promote health and reduce illness costs it is unlikely that this will be done.

Elders who have planned ahead and have adequate resources often modify their home or buy a more convenient home long before they become frail. Some of the features they seek are no stairs, roomy bathrooms with grab bars strategically placed, closets and shelves that are easily accessible without reaching, security systems, lights that may be dimmed at night, and other convenience features. Architectural design and remodeling for the individual owner and institutions has become a thriving business.

Basic services that may keep old people in their homes longer than would otherwise be feasible include: (1) home health maintenance, (2) rehabilitation and medical services when necessary, (3) home household help, (4) mobile meals, (5) transportation services, and (6) counseling, crisis intervention, and advocacy (case management).

Housed with Families: Multigenerational Residences. The factors most likely to predict shared housing among adult children and dependent elders are widowhood, a small support network, and low economic status. However, strong cultural influences predict the frequency of multigenerational residences. Among Asians and South Americans it is often an expectation, though increasing industrialization in any country changes these traditional patterns. Clarke and Neidert (1992) found that older persons with Central, Eastern, or Southern European roots were more likely to live with relatives than those individuals from Northwestern Europe. There are many possible cultural explanations. The important issue is for social policy and supports to support the choice of the individual and the family; often this is not the case.

The "Granny Flat" Solution. Almost two decades ago the "granny flat" was developed in Australia as a model for providing independent housing for elders by construction of prefabricated small housing units on family property. This allowed families to be close enough to be of assistance if needed but remain separate. These were practical and economical, and their production has continually expanded in Australia. Private contractors have been more productive than government administration in making these flats available (Lazarowich, 1990). In the United States there has been little indication of this model being used, though existing "mother-in-law" cottages and apartments have served a similar purpose for many families. An additional model that has great popularity in certain areas is the use of mobile homes. These, may in fact, be mobile and moved onto family property or may in reality be quite immobile and set in established mobile home parks that cater to older people and their needs.

Gated Communities. Gated communities are designed for affluent individuals who wish seclusion, protection, maintenance, and high security. These communities tend to be designed for and to cater to older individuals. They often have golf courses, health clinics, entertainment centers, restaurants, gymnasiums, tennis courts, clubhouses, pools, transportation, and convenient services within the compound. One such, characteristic of many, is described thus: ". . . facilities resemble that of a small city. One member of each household must be 55 years of age or older. The resident mix includes currently active and retired professionals. Housing options vary from single family dwellings to single or multi-story condominiums and co-operatives. Health and medical facilities, commercial and retail centers and houses of worship are nearby." (Leisure World, 1996) These communities are flourishing throughout the United States and

will undoubtedly increase because the numerous young-old who can afford them value the advantages they offer. The disadvantages are apparent when one becomes old and frail and must hire from outside any live-in assistance that may be necessary.

In some ways these are similar to upscale life-care communities, and nurses need to be aware of the differences. Providing health services is not part of the entitlements in these leisure communities as they are in life-care communities.

Senior Retirement Communities. Communities designed for elders are proliferating. There are numerous combinations of cottages, apartments, activities, optional services, meals in the home, cafeterias, restaurants, housekeeping, golf, tennis, security, and emergency services and clinics. Some have sections designed especially for assisted living. These are all designed to make independent living feasible with the least effort on the part of the elder. They are usually expensive, and services are purchased outright. The various names for such communities include "retirement community," "independent living centers," and "life care." Considerations important to a client who is contemplating entering one of these communities include the following:

- Plan far ahead and anticipate needs. Good facilities have long waiting lists.
- Meals, activities, health care, and housekeeping must be readily available and affordable if desired or needed.
- Examine the compatibility of the residents; look for evidence of interaction and involvement in activities and committees.
- Study the effectiveness of the staff from administrator to maintenance personnel.
- Determine the community's compliance with standards, by licenses, certificates, or other evidence.
- Inquire about the availability of financial statements and marketing projections.
- Contracts should include fixed increases over time or amounts directly related to the inflation index; costs and limits of nursing care should be clearly stated. What amount of the fee is refundable if the client dies or moves?
- Does the resident have a voice in management?
- If a complex is not yet in operation, request a financial incentive before signing up, and put up only a nominal, fully refundable deposit before operation begins.

Continuing Care Retirement Communities. There are more than 1000 nonprofit continuing care retirement communities (CCRCs) across the country and many that are corporate-for-profit. This mode of service to the aged has chiefly emerged since 1974, though some church-affiliated CCRCs have been in existence for nearly 100 years. These are sometimes called life care communities because that is precisely what they guarantee. CCRCs are flourishing.

These are designed only for the middle class or wealthy elder. There is a large ($50,000 to $500,000) one-time entrance fee and monthly payments of $800 to $3000 thereafter. There are several basic combinations of service, but the commonality is of lifelong care. The communities usually contract with a nearby hospital for acute care, but aside from that they are equipped to provide whatever level of assistance and health care is needed by the elder resident. Dining rooms and meals are often exquisite. Residents are predominantly females in their 80s who entered the community in their late 70s. They are often very involved in the community activities and find this a pleasant life. Resident satisfaction is a major thrust of these communities, and they focus on such things as excellent food and service, comfort, convenience, security, intellectual and artistic pursuits, and socialization.

Increasingly, dynamic and financially secure older women are taking the initiative to move into life-care communities while they are active and in good health. They often select them because of the security and the stimulation. The decision to enter a life-care facility is often made in response to a growing awareness of the eventual need for more assistance and support. It is also stimulated by observing friends who suddenly lose the capacity for independent living and are abruptly relocated without sufficient time to select a situation to their liking. Hartwigsen (1987) termed these "vicarious crises."

In making the decision to move to a life-care facility, the elder should explore several of them. Selection of the CCRC that best meets the individual's needs and preserves much of the past way of life is important.

Federally Assisted Housing. There are several federally subsidized rental options, and nearly 40% of poor elderly renters are benefiting from one of these options (U.S. Government General Accounting Office, 1992). The largest number of elderly are assisted through HUD-subsidized rental housing. These are not specific to the aged, but nearly 45% of the units are occupied by elders. Section 202 approved the construction of low-rent housing units especially for elders. These units also have provisions for health, recreation, and transportation. More than 91% of these apartment units have waiting lists of eight or more applicants for each vacancy as it occurs. Under Section 8 of the Housing Act of 1983, tenants locate their own unit. Usually, the tenant will pay 30% of his or her adjusted gross income toward the rent, and HUD can assist by supplementary vouchers from 30% to 120% of the tenant's contribution in order to meet the fair market value of the rental.

These federal housing assistance programs have been a boon to poor elders, but many who need assistance are not being served. Over 600,000 units of public housing in the United States are occupied by the elderly; half of these have been specifically designated and some specially designed for them. Public housing for the elderly is predominantly occupied by white women living alone.

In a study of 333 elders on waiting lists for public housing it was found that applicants had waited on average more than 2 years and 15% for 4 years or more to obtain assistance or placement. Over half were poor, living in unsafe dwellings lacking sufficient heat and functional plumbing and paying more than 60% of their income for housing. They applied for government assistance hoping to reduce housing expenditures and hazardous living conditions (Pynoos et al, 1995). Eighty three percent of rental applicants for federal housing assistance experienced excessive housing costs (Figure 13-4) (American Association of Retired Persons, 1995).

People in public housing are generally in need of many services, although most sponsored housing projects have not provided space or personnel for those needs. Projects are often built in inconvenient and undesirable neighborhoods. An ideal public housing complex for low-income aged residents will provide modern facilities, security, accessible services, privacy, and some entertainment and activities. An important consideration in planning low-cost housing units for the elderly is the potential for evolution of services. Residents rarely move out, and as they age their ability and independence are likely to decrease. Retirement communities often solve this dilemma by building semidependent units. For those less affluent people currently in subsidized public housing, the only alternatives may be residential care facilities or nursing homes.

Group Residences

There are many housing options available before one must consider institutionalization (Table 13-5). Facilities for elders who cannot live independently but do not need nursing home care include adult foster-care homes, senior-assisted housing, group-assisted living, domiciliary care, congregate care, supportive housing, continuing care, life care, residential care, board and care, and personal care facilities. These are collectively classed as "assisted living" situations.

Certain fair housing laws have been enacted to protect the rights of frail older persons in group residences (Edelstein, 1995) that are under state and federal jurisdiction. These are primarily focused on antidiscrimination, access accommodations, and health and safety concerns. These are all important in maintaining independence, control, and quality of life.

The number of individuals in a group residence and the variety and quality of services vary considerably. They may be under local, state, or federal jurisdiction or privately owned and operated. Some accept only private pay, and some are partially or fully subsidized. It would be virtually impossible to define each of these in terms of opportunities, quality, and limitations, but nurses will be asked about them. Elders and their families should be advised to ask about and carefully consider the following:

What services are offered?
What is the out-of-pocket cost?

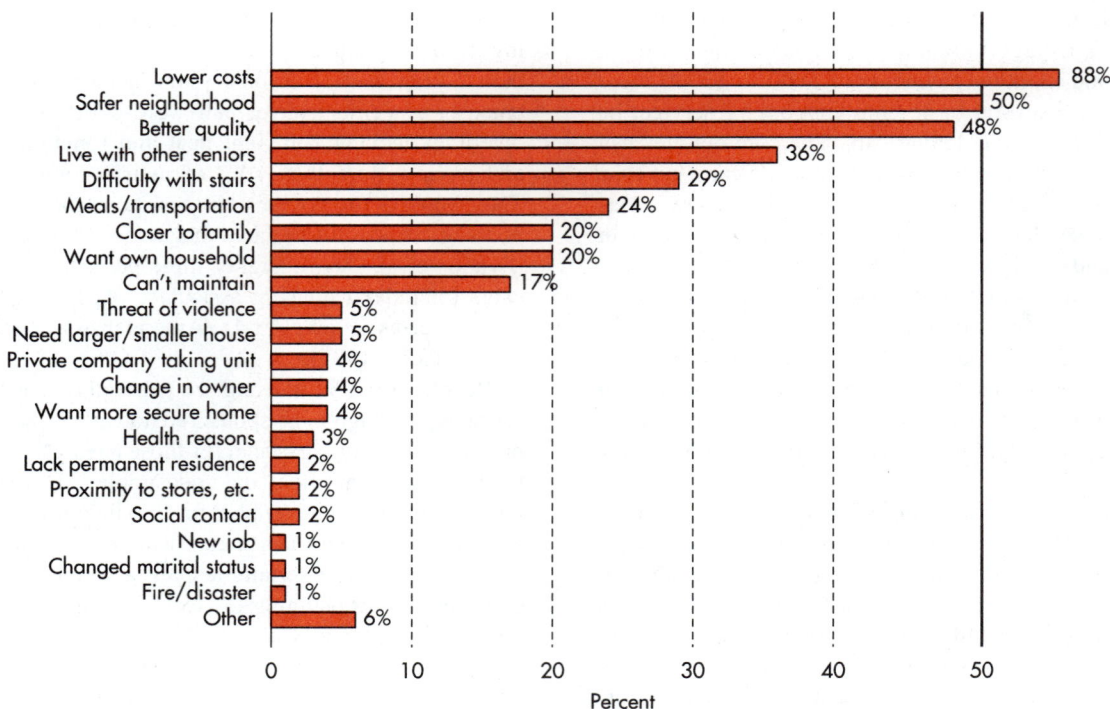

Figure 13-4. Reasons for seeking federal housing. (From Pynoos J, Reynolds SL, Salend E, Rahman A: *Waiting for federally assisted housing: a study of the needs and experiences of older applicants,* 1995, American Association of Retired Persons, 601 E. Street NW, Washington, D.C. Reprinted with permission.)

What levels of assistance are available?

What safety factors are in place?

Are individual preferences respected?

What range of physical and cognitive impairments can be accomodated?

What are the security measures?

What agencies, if any, are responsible for monitoring quality?

What are the special features designed for the frail or disabled?

What is the process for reporting abuse, neglect, or exploitation?

Shared Housing. Since so many elderly own their homes, house sharing has been proposed as a feasible way to keep one's home. Older people often live in houses geared to family life, purchased in their young adult years. It is estimated that half the space is underused. Sharing a house can be easily implemented by locating, screening, and matching older people looking for houses to share with those who have them. The National Shared Housing Resource Center (NSHRC) has established 350 subgroups nationally to assist individuals interested in home-sharing. Those who have done so report feeling safer and less lonely. Home-sharing studies need to focus on the effects on well-being, finances, health, social life, and daily satisfaction. Most successful are

the intergenerational model, in which an elder with a home locates a younger person to share the home (Bergman, 1994). In each situation the individuals must consider the following:

• Should both men and women live together?

• Should the house include aged peers only or people of all ages?

• Should there be equal or reciprocal exchange?

• Should the house provide temporary or permanent residence?

• Should residents sign an agreement form?

• Will residents respect privacy?

• What is the motivation for moving into a shared house: financial need, companionship, or services/assistance?

Shared housing as a method of providing for the needs of several frail elderly in one renovated home has been used with varying degrees of success, but little has been done to explore the impact on the private housing market, the implications of sharing among aged citizens in general, and the intergenerational possibilities of this type of shared housing. The major reason this has not been developed and used to its fullest extent probably has to do with zoning laws in residential areas and other obstacles in public policies. Shared housing policy problems include the role of local planning

Table 13-5   Advantages and Disadvantages of Selected Alternative Housing Options

Options	Advantages	Disadvantages
Board and care homes	Homelike; economical	Not licensed in some states or concerned with standards; owner/operators often lack training; little planned social activities
Congregate housing	Provides basic support services that can extend independent living; reduces social isolation	Tendency to promote dependency; expensive for most elderly without subsidy
Elder cottages—"granny flats"	Facilitate older persons receiving support from younger family members	Concerns about housing and building code violations
Home equity conversion	Converts lifetime investment into usable income; can be used to finance housing expenses, i.e., make necessary repairs, utilities, taxes	Reluctance by homeowner to utilize due to lack of information, concern for lien on property, and/or impact on estate for heirs
Life-care facilities	Offer prepaid health care; wide range of social activities with health and support systems	Too expensive for many elderly; no guarantees that monthly payment will not rise
Shared housing	More extensive use of existing housing; program inexpensive to operate	Problems with selection of individual to share home; amount of privacy reduced; city zoning ordinances may prohibit

Modified from Mutschler PM: Where elders live, *Generations* 16(2):7, 1992.

and zoning regulatory bodies in making changes that will allow more unrelated individuals to live together (Tassy, 1995). Problems might arise from long-standing patterns of living, privacy, and interpersonal needs. Modifications to units that would maximize privacy may be cost prohibitive. However, small groups of elderly living under the same roof are a growing trend. The following are characteristic of successful group homes:

- They usually have a nonprofit sponsor.
- Services include housekeeping, cooking, maintenance, and social services.
- Spontaneity and interaction are encouraged but not forced.

Foster Care. Adult foster care is meant to provide assistive care in a homelike setting that will enhance function, and quality of life and allow the elder to remain in a community-based setting. This foster care is different from other residential care settings in both the size of the homes and the family-oriented care setting (Folkemer et al, 1996). The operational definition of adult foster care is as follows: adult foster care offers a community-based living arrangement to adults who are unable to live independently because of physical or mental impairment or disabilities and are in need of supervision or personal care.

Homes providing adult foster care offer 24-hour supervision, protection, and personal care in addition to room and board. They may also provide additional services. Adult foster care serves a designated, small number of individuals (generally from one to six) in a homelike and family-like environment where one of the primary caregivers often resides in the home (Folkemer et al, 1996). A survey of states having adult foster care programs indicated 26 states have programs consistent with the federal guidelines. Eight states have no such program, and 16 states did not respond to the questionnaire (Table 13-6).

A growing number of homes are under corporate ownership, and in these situations the homelike atmosphere tends to be lost. However, with state regulated outcome-oriented quality assurance strategies focused on achieving maximum function, autonomy, and social integration, adult foster care may fill a real need.

Some communities have organized foster care programs in which foster families are supervised in the adoption and care of one or two disabled geriatric clients. Braun and King (1989) report such a program in Honolulu, modeled after similar programs in Boston and Baltimore. These are all part of community care programs affiliated with hospitals. The Queen's Medical Center (Honolulu) developed the program as an additional discharge option for long-term care patients. The foster patients are eligible for nursing home placement but need more care than can be provided in a residential setting. The hospital's social work department manages and monitors the program. A home care team makes visits as needed or required. Case managers visit monthly and at other times when needed. Applicant families are thoroughly screened, and a home assessment is made. A training program prepares them for the experience. Foster families provide personal care, homemaking, transportation, and other services as needed. They are reimbursed by Medicaid. Costs and outcomes of such care are favorable in comparison to institutional settings. When families and elders are carefully matched, the elder is nurtured and cared for as if a member of the family.

Although this model has unlimited potential, it has not been developed to full advantage. Families already caring for an elderly member might find it advantageous both socially and economically to adopt one or two other elders. Problems could be expected if families were not appropriately screened or the care needs of the elder were too demanding.

| Table 13-6 | Adult Foster Care Program Names, Number of Homes, Number of Residents, and Use by the Elderly by State | | | |

State	Name of Program	# Homes	# Residents	% Older Population
Alabama	Adult Foster Care	n/a	3,402	n/a
Arizona	Adult Foster Care	231	511	80%
Colorado	Adult Foster Care	71	427	24%
Delaware	Family Care Rest Home Program	n/a	319 beds	65%
Florida	Adult Family Care Homes	570	900	95%
Hawaii	Adult Residential Care Home-Type I	494	2,620*	95%
Idaho	Adult Foster Care Home	n/a[b]	n/a	n/a
Iowa	Family-Life Home Program	n/a	41	n/a
Kentucky	Family Care Homes	n/a	450	66%
Maryland	The CARE Program or Project Home	450	745	32%
Massachusetts	Family Adult Foster Care (AFC)	n/a	800[c]	70%
Michigan	Adult Foster Care Homes	1,550	n/a	n/a
Minnesota	Adult Foster Care (Homes Plus)	2,160	4,354	20%
Montana	Adult Foster Family Care	128	380	40%
Nebraska	Adult Family Home	132	265	38%
Nevada	Residential Facilities for Groups	300	1,200	70%
New York	Family-Type Homes for Adults	776	1,414	60%
North Carolina	Family Care Homes	698	3,799	73%
Ohio	Adult Family Homes	512[d]	4,120 (across)	50% (across both
	Certified Foster Home	75	both categories)	categories)
Oregon	Adult Foster Care	2,242 commercial homes	9,396 in commer-	70%[e]
		1,500 relative homes	cial homes	75%
Pennsylvania	Domiciliary Care Services for Adults	969	2,054	27%
Texas	Adult Foster Care Program (AFC)	282	n/a	n/a
	Nursing Facility Waiver Adult Foster Care (NFW)	26		
Virginia	Adult Foster/Family Care Program	180	191	n/a
Washington	Adult Family Home	1,334	5,797	65%
West Virginia	Adult Family Care	324	597	n/a
Wisconsin	Adult Family Homes	1,700	n/a	n/a

From Folkemer D et al: *Adult foster care for the elderly: a review of state regulatory and funding strategies,* 1996, American Association of Retired Persons, 601 E. Street NW, Washington, DC. Reprinted with permission.
[a]Count includes some residents from a limited number of larger residential homes. [b]All records kept at regional level. [c]Count includes residents of group foster care. [d]Count includes some group homes that are also called adult family homes. [e]Seventy percent of publicly funded residents are older. No data are collected on private pay residents, but they are primarily older.

Board and Care. Board and care are usually provided in small homes serving six to eight residents. They serve individuals who are not in need of the professional nursing care provided in nursing homes but need considerable personal care and assistance. This care is often funded by Medicaid. They vary from foster care in that the simulation or reality of a family setting is not the focus of the setting, though the distinction between foster care and board and care is in individual circumstances not at all clear at times. In addition, foster care programs usually provide guidelines and education for the participants, but this is often not the case with board and care operators. Most caregivers of the aged in board and care settings have not been recruited by agencies but rather have taken this function on their own initiative or at the suggestion of friends or relatives. It is not uncommon that they rent a small house, row house, or a flat and maintain it as a business. Although their intentions may be humanitarian, they often need training in the special needs of the elderly.

The National Association of Residential Care Homes is an organization of board and care operators that is growing in strength and brings professionalism to its members. Board and care regulation and licensing is within the domain of the respective state. It is generally agreed that licensing and provider education should be increased, but few funds are budgeted for the monitoring and improvement of these small facilities. Where these are poorly funded, there is less incentive among operators to meet quality standards. Board and care operators cannot provide the quality of care desirable unless there is both financial incentive and continuing supportive resources available to assist them (Reschovsky and Ruchlin, 1993).

Assisted Living. Assisted living is emerging as the option of choice for elders who can no longer remain in their own homes but do not need nursing home care (American Association of Homes and Services for the Aged, 1995a). Although some states have developed regulations, there are as yet no federally defined standards. In the absence of such

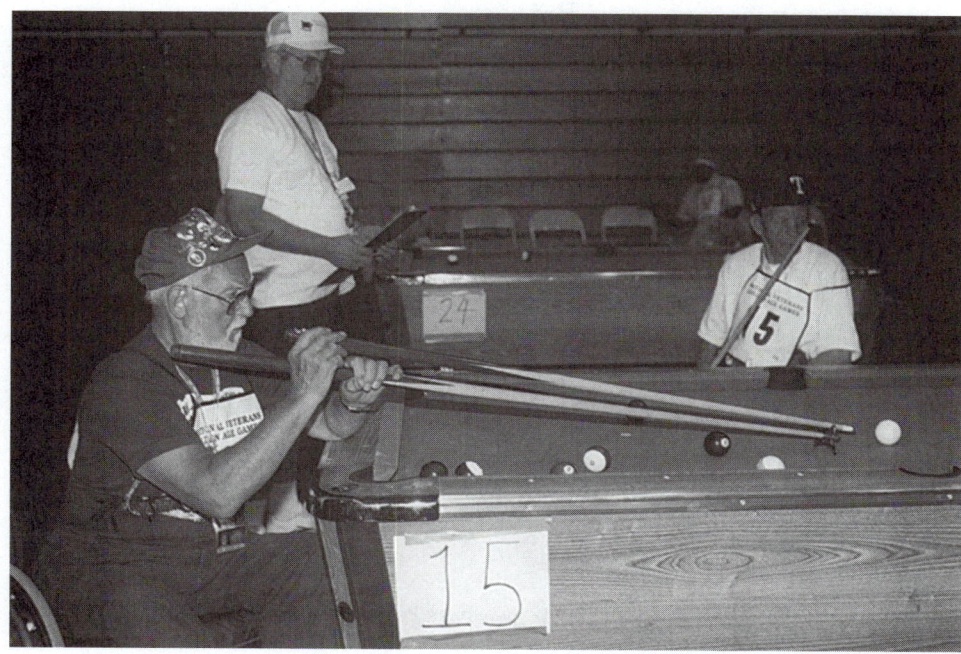

Enjoying life space. (Courtesy National Veterans Golden Age Games, Department of Veterans Affairs.)

standards the American Association of Homes and Services for the Aged has taken on the challenge of developing prototypes that will provide models for sponsors and developers of such facilities (American Association of Homes and Services for the Aged,1995a). Assisted Living Facilities (ALFs) are usually small (average size of 25 residents) congregate living sites that provide help with activities of daily living (ADLs). Nationwide there are 1.5 million residents in ALFs. These facilities may also be designated "personal care." The distinction between these and residential care is often blurred, though residential care most often is limited to independent apartments with meals available, housekeeping, and emergency response systems on site to assist with problems. There are no reimbursement mechanisms for these settings. The costs are borne entirely by the residents.

Subacute care and rehabilitation units.   The route taken by many elders has been changed in the current health care system. It is often from a few days in an acute hospital to either a rehabilitation hospital for specific therapies expected to increase the elder's function or to a subacute unit that functions much like general medical/surgical hospital units of the past, though most often they are located in nursing homes. These stays are likely to be short but constitute one or two more moves an elder must make in the course of an illness. Too frequently the elder is sent directly home from an acute illness episode. While theoretically this seems the most humane, it often is downright dangerous. Family members may not be willing or able to give the sophisticated care needed for the elder's maximum recuperation. Nurses must

advocate for appropriate levels of care and object to pushing people through a system based entirely on economics.

At the present time a 3-day hospitalization is required by Medicare prior to a move into a nursing home. The American Health Care Association and other organizations have been trying for some time to have this ruling rescinded. In fact, if the 3 days are used for a thorough work-up, it is advantageous because it will facilitate the most appropriate assessment and placement of the elder.

Nursing Homes.   Nursing homes provide round-the-clock care for those needing subacute, chronic, and rehabilitative nursing care (see chapters 8 and 14 for further discussion of nontraditional nursing home care). They range from 10 to over 1000 beds, with a national average of 106. Though called nursing homes, they resemble hospitals far more than homes, and private rooms are at a premium. Because of rapid changes in the industry and the intensity of care provided, it is difficult to estimate the numbers nationally, though the estimate is over 33,000. About 17,000 of these are traditional nursing homes that indeed are home for 1.5 million elders, 75% of whom are women (American Health Care Association, 1996). This figure excludes hospital-based nursing home units, which at present number are emerging with great rapidity (U.S. Bureau of the Census, 1995).

Costs vary significantly with the location but average $38,000 annually for basic nursing home care. Fees are usually obtained through a combination of Medicare (5%), Medicaid (45%), out-of-pocket (45%), and insurance (1%)

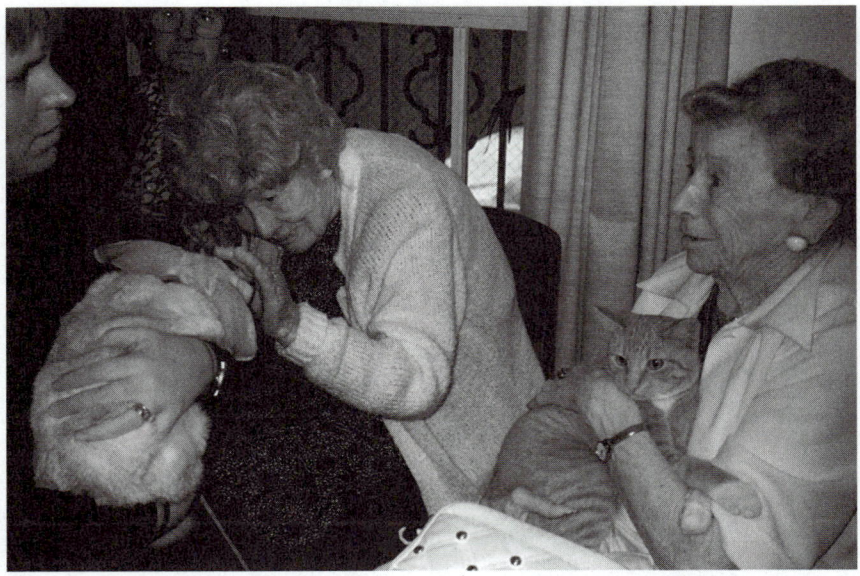

Pets in nursing home. (Courtesy Priscilla Ebersole.)

payments. Federal and state regulations have become more onerous and time consuming than the care. OBRA (Omnibus Budget Reconciliation Act) 1987 and the frequent revisions and updates are designed to impact the actual quality of resident care, and the system is beginning to show results in this respect and in observation of resident rights and privileges. OBRA laws require that nursing homes must do the following:

- Increase their nursing and social work staff
- Train nurses' aides
- Institute activities programs
- Set standards for nursing home administrators
- Expect increased financial sanctions for noncompliance with regulations
- Guarantee the right to one's own physician
- Guarantee freedom from drug or physical restraint for convenience or discipline
- Guarantee resident participation in care and treatment decisions
- Guarantee resident privacy
- Investigate the background of individuals applying for work in long-term care facilities.

With the inroads of managed care, block grants, and the shift of responsibility to the states, there is great concern that some of these hard-won gains may be diminished.

Even with the safeguards of OBRA legislation there is much more to be done to support life quality. With institutionalization, individuals are in an environment where the usual noises of life, odors, shifting temperatures and wind patterns, vegetation, and natural diurnal light variations are altered. These changes affect individuals in as yet unknown ways. Elders in restricted living situations and those who are housebound or institutionalized suffer a type of deprivation

that is not understood, but we sense that the quality of life is somehow diminished. Disorientation may ensue because natural and man-made cues are often missing. Most of the man-made cues are inexpensive enough to ensure general availability, yet situations still exist where clocks, calendars, location of important events, facility maps, and individual room identification are missing. Friedman and Ryan (1986) conclude that "many of the problem behaviors observed in the nursing home setting can be viewed as attempts on the part of the elderly resident to actively reestablish a sense of control, dignity, and self-worth in the face of an ecological crisis" (p. 268). One lady said, "I believe being able to watch that garden from my room has played a major part in my getting better" (Williams, 1990, p. 27). In all situations where the elder is at the mercy of an unnatural environment, thought must be given to the artificial aspects of the surroundings.

Williams (1990) believes exposure to nature is important to personal growth and self-expression. In the future, we hope considerations of the environmental needs of the aged may result in a more balanced view of natural and synthetic environments.

Intrainstitutional relocation. Studies do not agree regarding the effects of intrainstitutional relocation. Some find an increase in mortality, and others find no change. In some cases the move undoubtedly has positive outcomes. However, Mirotznik and Lombardi (1995) found that older persons had more deleterious health effects following a room change than did younger persons. As in most situations, the degree of familiarity, control, and desire will directly affect the adaptation of the individual regardless of age.

Effects of relocation on the mentally frail. Familiarity with the environment is even more important in the care and

<table>
<tr><td>

Box 13-8   **Environmental Cueing**

Physical Cues

Mealtime may be signaled by a chime and food-scented air fresheners.

Bedtime may be signaled by dimmed lights, lowered noise level, and sounds of ocean waves.

Redundant cueing of physical space by room with name, number, color, and photograph.

Social Cues

24-hour reality orientation.

Clear information, with demonstration before activities or expectation of behavior by patient.

Use of idioms from individual's previous life experience.

Physical Stability

Reduce range of environment but increase access to anything within that environment.

When change is necessary, introduce one change at a time to allow incorporation to the greatest extent possible.

Multipurpose rooms produce confusion.

Social Stability

Continuity of personal contacts, numbers limited but frequency expanded.

Predictable daily routines; activities may differ but place and time remain the same.

Complexity of cues may need to be reduced even further as the patient's condition declines.

</td></tr>
</table>

function of mentally frail elders. When objects and persons in the environment are familiar, less integrative capacity is needed in order to cope effectively. In unfamiliar places disorientation and catastrophic reactions may occur. Cues in the environment are fundamental to designing interventions to modify such behaviors (Box 13-8).

An environment rich in physical and social cues most helpful to the demented person will label locations and activities with color and pictures or simple words. Verbal instructions will be congruent, augmented by hand motion or demonstration. Smiling, touching, and direct eye contact provide assurance of interest. Personalization of individual space is also important for orientation as well as security. For stability and security, cues should remain constant and predictable. Changes in room assignment, staff, furniture arrangement, and interior decoration all elicit confusion. Intercoms, buzzers, continuous music, and excessive light at night are additional distractors.

Throughout the long-term care industry numerous facilities have established special care units (SCUs). Nurses must be involved in the design of these units and carefully assess the adaptational cues.

Roberts and Algase (1988) give some specific suggestions to enhance physical and social cues and physical and social stability in the environment of the individual with dementia (Box 13-8). The authors note that these suggestions are based on anecdotal information and suggest any of these items as subjects of further nursing research.

Evergreen Retirement Community in Oshkosh, Wisconsin, has developed a "home" unit in which the design and activities mimic those of a home and family setting (Green, 1994). Eight resident rooms surround the "farm kitchen," where all activities and meals take place. The results are a close-knit, interactive group of residents and staff. Informality and interaction are stressed. This approach has resulted in greater interest and involvement of families of those residents as well.

When structural changes are not possible, Schafer (1985) suggests ways to modify the environment to more nearly resemble the patient's previous living situation:

1. Individualize care.
2. Learn who the patient was.
3. Recognize strengths.
4. Foster sense of control.
5. Provide environmental cues for orientation.
6. Maintain patient's home schedule.
7. Adapt schedule of diagnostic procedures to patient's needs.
8. Communicate.
9. Time the giving of information.
10. Maintain consistency in staff-patient interactions.
11. Maintain ADLs using patient's coping resources and social supports.

All of these suggestions require rethinking methods of providing care.

Individualized care might begin with a psychosocial admission assessment that would include data about the client's preferences, home schedules, strengths, and ability to accomplish ADLs before admission to the facility. The Minimum Data Set (MDS 2.0) now required by OBRA has made great progress toward individualized care plans. Ideally the staff who will work up the MDS 2.0 will also obtain a life history of significant roles, events, and activities that have given the individual his or her sense of identity.

Suggestions about ways that family and community members may enhance nursing home life:

1. Donate clothing, supplies, fruit, flowers, art objects, books, televisions, and pianos to nursing homes.
2. Offer positive feedback to the overworked, underpaid personnel.
3. Volunteer your services or special talents.
4. Adopt a grandparent and include in family outings and holidays.
5. Assist children in getting acquainted with individuals in nursing homes. The aged enjoy this immensely, and the children may learn more about the aged than we know.

6. Give input to the director of nursing regarding beneficial services available in the community.
7. Develop forums (schools, city council meetings, religious organizations) for the aged to express their community needs.
8. Educate children to effectively interact with the aged.
9. Provide group meetings for families with aged members to share problems and solutions and to vent their feelings about their situations.
10. Form support groups and network for counseling older adults in institutional settings to adapt to and work on life issues: grieving, stresses, living situations, etc.

Making a home. Fifteen factors have been identified in rank order as contributing to satisfaction in a nursing home (Figure 13-5) (Kane et al, 1986) and improving morale among patients. Other studies reinforce the importance of personal possessions in the milieu of the institutionalized elderly; suggested possessions may include pictures, paintings, photographs, bureaus, bookcases, bedspreads, quilts, lamps, and any item of special significance to the elderly.

Responsibility. Many persons believe the difference between housing and a home is measured by responsibility and caring. In nursing homes, residents who have responsibility for the care of a bird, a fish, or a plant remain more active and spontaneous than the residents who have nothing to care for. Behaviors reinforcing dependence are frequently noted among nursing home residents. When looking at the inter-

action patterns between elderly residents and their social partners, often the more dependent resident gains more attention from social partners. From these data we might conclude that many residents demonstrate a strong need to care for someone who seems to need them. Studies have previously identified the therapeutic effects of plants in rooms with the elderly in nursing homes. A study was done by Roush and Banzinger (1982) of the implications and importance of bird feeders outside residents' windows to establish responsibility for the wild birds. It was found that life satisfaction, perceived control, happiness, and activity were significantly improved for those residents. Nurses also rated these individuals as being more active, happy, alert, and sociable.

Pets. Much has been reported about companion therapy with animals, and it has been empirically accepted that they increase morale and provide emotional satisfaction to many elderly people. Instances when pets may be especially helpful to the elderly are in the presence of (1) chronic disability or illness, (2) depression, (3) a previous relationship with pets, (4) role reversal, (5) negative dependency, (6) loneliness and isolation, (7) helplessness, (8) low self-esteem, (9) hopelessness, and (10) absence of humor. A pet can often expand the sociability of aged residents, decrease their sense of regimentation, give them some purpose, help them to feel needed and loved, and provide tactile comfort. Rosenkoetter (1992) reported an increase in communication among nursing home residents as they talked about Brutus in anticipation of and after his weekly visits.

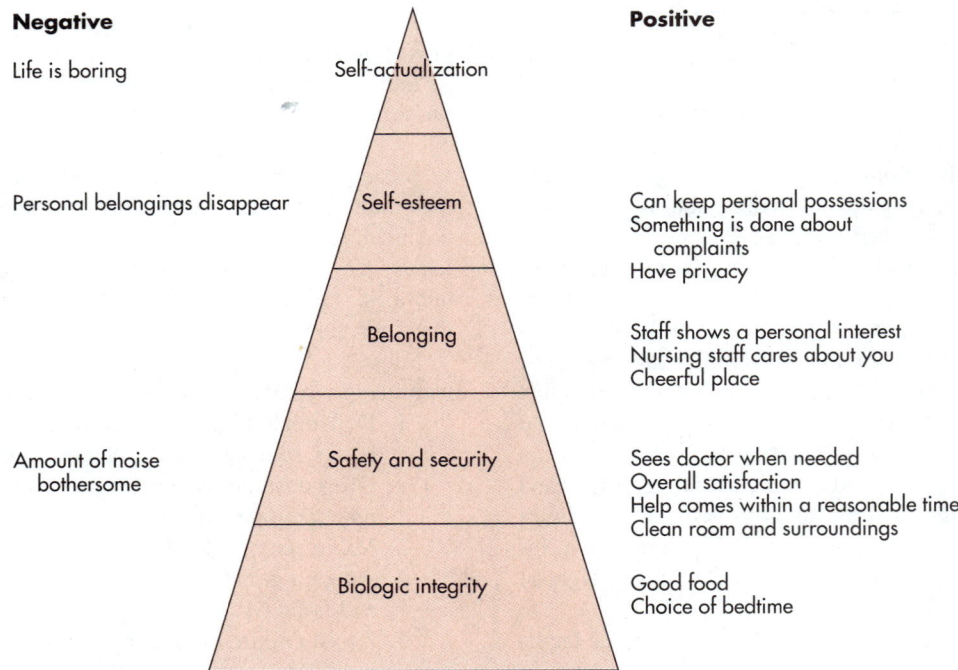

Figure 13-5. Satisfaction factors reported by nursing home patients. (Developed from Kane R, Bell R, Riegler S: Value preferences for nursing home outcomes, *Gerontologist* 26[3]:303, 1986.)

The California Veterinary Medical Association Guidelines suggest it is important to survey staff and resident preferences regarding pets in nursing homes. In assessing nursing home characteristics, physical space and social space are important, and certain rules and regulations regarding the pets need to be established. If it is not deemed suitable to have a pet continuously in a given facility, there are volunteer programs that provide animals for a short period.

Common sense considerations when including an animal in the facility or when visiting are that the animal must be clean and healthy and have required immunizations, the animal should be on leash or in an appropriate cage, the animal should be kept out of food preparation areas, people allergic to animals in the nursing home should be warned of their presence, and any scratches or injuries that result from animals must be reported (Bustad and Hines, 1983).

Nature hikes for nursing home residents. Morganett (1987), a park naturalist, suggests nature hikes for nursing home residents as a means of heightening awareness and increasing quality of life. Hikers are encouraged to use all their senses to experience nature: tasting wild berries; listening to birds, frogs, and crickets; seeing different colors of soil and sand; touching flower petals and leaves; and smelling flowers and plants. If hiking is too difficult, some of these items can be brought to the nursing home for demonstrations. Before beginning such a program, she gives some directions: (1) do not contact poisonous plants; (2) do not pick things in state and national parks since this is illegal; and (3) treat animals gently and set them free immediately after any demonstration.

She suggests careful planning and assembling of materials before departure. An insect box and a magnifying glass are not necessary but will be useful. You may wish to augment the walk with large pictures of birds and recorded bird calls. Berries can be brought back and made into jam. Wild flowers may be placed in pots in the facility. She gives abundant information about special characteristics of plants, animals, and birds. For the neophyte it would be useful to obtain assistance from the park service. Nature hikes can be adapted to many settings in addition to parks.

Plush animals. Another unlikely, and somewhat controversial, means of individualizing the environment is to provide plush animals for residents. The critical issue in doing so is to view it as a comfort rather than as a childish condescension. Francis and Baly (1986) found that if the animals were self-selected and made available but not recommended the results were positive. Residents who chose plush animals often became quite attached to them, named them, and commented on how they enjoyed them. It was also observed that having a plush animal promoted interpersonal interaction, provided comfort, and improved interest in social activities. Although all these things are useful, it is well to remember Wolanin's comment: "In the absence of a comforting human interaction a plush animal may provide some small measure of comfort."

Libraries. Almost all facilities have a library of some sort that is hardly ever noticed. Reading and discussion groups have been implemented in some settings successfully. We might find residents more interested in reading if there was a monthly trip to the community library for those who are able and a list of reading materials desired by those who are unable to obtain them. Readings of great books and poetry might become a focus for discussion of philosophy. Bond and Miller (1987) instituted regular reading groups and the building of a library in a long-term care facility and found residents quite interested. Magnifying lights and current news should always be available. A library keeps one in touch with great ideas and expands one's sights beyond the surrounding walls to the larger community of mankind.

Art. Art activities help an elder remain in touch with the creative self, the outside world, and provide expressions of control and self-disclosure (Sterritt and Pokorny, 1994). O'Connor (1987) has devised a method of enriching the environment of bed-bound patients by use of art placed on the ceiling. She has dubbed this "ceiling therapy." Such creative efforts to enhance surroundings for immobilized patients are encouraged.

The following are suggested ways to promote a sense of personal security for clients in institutions:

1. Patients' rooms need a "Please do not disturb" sign that can be hung on the door when the patient chooses.
2. Transfer patients from one room to another infrequently or not at all.
3. Include objects of personal significance in the environment.
4. Respect the arrangement of the patients' space; do not move things without permission.
5. Prepare people for intrusive procedures, even though routine to personnel, and verbally assure them you are aware of intruding into their space. Respect patients' dignity and modesty. Do not leave body exposed.
6. Ask whether patient wants door open or shut and curtains closed or open.
7. Avoid direct eye contact during care of intimate body areas.
8. Be alert to cues. Touching may increase or decrease anxiety.
9. Communicate territorial preferences of patient to other health care team members.
10. Confer with patients regarding arrangement of public space.
11. Give choices as much as possible, which in turn will give you territorial clues about patients' desires.

Innovative Environmental Design

Teams of environmental consultants across the nation have begun to take note of the special design needs of congregate living facilities. The owners/investors of such facilities welcome their input for several reasons: a well-designed facility will be more effectively operated, services and care will be more easily provided, appearance is important in marketing, and good design may avert accidents and incidents. Residents will also negotiate the environment more easily and have fewer restrictions; restlessness and confusion will be reduced and quality of life improved (Hiatt, 1988).

Environment is more than a backdrop; it is integral to care. Environment can enhance the abilities of older adults and provide a heightened sense of autonomy for both residents and staff. We have seen the redesign of obstetric units to birthing centers. It is not impossible to design appropriate living centers for the aged in institutions (Noell, 1996).

Whereas in the past architects might dictate design, it is now more common for the design to be a result of interdisciplinary input. The innovative architect listens, reads, tours facilities, and works from the start with functional needs and cost in mind. Hiatt (1988) says there is still a great need to look to the future and what care should be, how staff should work, and what will contribute more to the quality of life. At present there are numerous "special care units" designed for persons suffering dementia, but they vary greatly in the efficiency and effectiveness of the design.

Crawford (1988) states, "Designing a long term care facility is like designing a small town." People with diverse needs and tastes are to be considered. Designers must also be very sensitive to the processes of aging. There is a challenge to designing a setting that keeps everyone operating at peak independence as long as possible. For example, in one progressive facility alternative routes from one place to another were built. One could cross an arched foot bridge if able to climb, but if not the person could take the other route, which was flat but somewhat longer. Both provided an equal amount of exercise.

Hiatt (1988) reports great progress toward the development of enhancing environments in long-term care facilities. Such factors as spatial relationships, acoustics, lighting, and furnishings are major considerations in designing environments that are functionally durable yet aesthetic and comfortable. The impetus for this new wave of interest in design is economic. Success in the design of long-term facilities is based on how long the building will be useful and how marketable it will be over time (Crawford, 1988). It must accommodate to the residents' changing needs over time as well. In life-care centers this is particularly essential, and many have been unable to remain operational because they were not designed to respond to the changing needs of the client population when the majority of them have become old and frail. Flexibility in planning the life-care center can accommodate to the needs of the young-old and the old-old. For instance, residential-oriented planning sessions will help identify options that are available (Crawford, 1988). Some elders wish to be near children, and others do not. A solution for one center was to build a freestanding day-care center on the grounds of the facility but far enough away not to annoy residents who did not wish contact with children.

Creating interiors for a changing clientele is an additional challenge for the designers of long-term care settings and perhaps the most significant from a nursing perspective. In Tucson, La Posada nursing home administration responded to the needs of their residents by creating specially designed light fixtures with a silk-screened cultural symbol (God's eye) on each, and the same symbol was used on the padded designer headboards. These small touches reduced the institutional appearance and were practical and money-saving modifications. The light fixture was designed to emit a softer, more diffuse light that reduced glare considerably, and the padded designer headboards of vinyl resisted staining and provided a soft contact for the individual who moves too far up toward the head of the bed (Smith and Karras, 1988).

Facilities that are well designed are most likely to operate more efficiently. Benefits are reaped by employees who find their work easier to organize and more satisfying. Most importantly, from a nursing perspective, better layout, facility organization, technology, and furnishings may reduce the need for restraints while preserving the security of the patient. Other benefits that have been observed include (1) more normalized patient responses and reduction of excess disabilities and (2) the transformation of nursing to habilitative nursing since the nurse has more time to work with the patient because less time is needed to accomplish the task-oriented activities. Well-designed facilities provide access to porches and protected gardens; freedom is maximized. It is being recognized that environment is a vital aspect of care (Hiatt, 1988).

Monitoring environmental safety is a significant proactive nursing commitment and one of the least expensive and most straightforward means of prevention. When it is possible, make home assessments and modifications that are most effective. At times one must be very creative in matching safety needs with comfortable rituals to arrive at an environmental alteration that is both comfortable and safe. For example, Drysdale (1988) surveyed the accident precipitants in a large number of elders admitted to an acute rehabilitation facility following hip fractures. The three most common causes of accidents were (1) being tripped by a pet, (2) tripping over an electrical cord, and (3) falling down stairs. Quite obviously a nurse would not suggest removing a pet from an elder's home. One might, however, suggest tying a bell to the pet's collar to alert the individual of the animal's presence. An elder with hearing impairment might be given information regarding the problem and a mnemonic device as a reminder to be aware of the pet.

Environmental design may also present hazards that are highly valued and thus may be considered worth the inconvenience. An example of this is observed in Margaret Wagner House in Cleveland. Margaret Wagner House is the long-term care center of the Benjamin Rose Institute and was a participant in the Teaching Nursing Home Project sponsored by the Robert Wood Johnson Foundation. This is a model facility and highly regarded nationally for the standards of care maintained. On the first floor the long polished hall of white tile is boldly contrasted with black tile squares placed intermittently down the center of the hall. Staff introduced to the resident council the idea of having it changed, and the residents vetoed it because they felt the hall was attractive and lent a palatial feeling to the facility.

Liu (1988) suggests that Chinese elders are even more prone to falls when living in their traditional homes than when institutionalized. Each room has a sill separating it that is several inches high, thus requiring the elder to step up and over it each time he or she enters or leaves a room. The Chinese also like beds that are high above the floor. These environmental design issues may be traditionally important to them and emotionally more significant than the hazards they present. This is a fertile field for cross-cultural and interdisciplinary research involving schools of nursing, environmental design, and architecture.

Those who design housing especially for the elderly would be most successful in providing satisfactory arrangements if they consulted the elderly first and then built prototypes to be tested by the aged. There are now several organizations devoted to designed living environments for elders. Two of the most well known are the Society for the Advancement of Gerontological Environment, based in Huntington Woods, Michigan, and the Center of Design for an Ageing Society, in Portland, Oregon (Noell, 1996).

The following are some special considerations:
Easily activated emergency and security systems
Phones by beds
Sufficient storage space
Convenient places to obtain meals
Mail drops conveniently placed
Window arrangements that allow for privacy and natural outdoor views
A place to grow things

In summary, personal territories and life space are the fabric of human existence. How people cluster together, where they establish their roots and personally define the limits of their range influence all other aspects of adaptation. When one reaches old age, environmental response is strongly rooted in experience and the emotional impact of certain houses, areas, and events connecting them. When relocation is essential, the environment should be matched as carefully as possible to previous desirable aspects. Most positive outcomes are seen when the individual has a sense of control and transitional supports. We will be much more effective in dealing with environmental issues if we remember the strong instinctive nature of territorial occupancy.

KEY CONCEPTS

- A familiar and comfortable environment allows an elder to function at his or her highest capacity.

- Relocation has variable effects depending upon individual personality, health, cognitive capacities, self-esteem, and preferred lifestyle.

- Environmental cues such as wall maps, clear directive lables, calendars, and clocks will assist individuals to adjust to a new setting and remain oriented.

- Noise pollution and abysmal lighting are seldom given sufficient attention in institutional living.

- Those individuals residing in long-term care institutions need regularly scheduled opportunities to go outside and participate in natural environments; gardens, lakes, and natural beauty are restorative.

- Quiet, private places for reflection, contemplation, or intimacy should be available to those individuals living in congregate settings.

- Wanderers are vulnerable to injury. The nursing function is to assess the stimulus for wandering and make attempts to meet the inherent need in the best way possible. Restraints are **never** a solution to wandering.

- Maladaptive behaviors are a result of environmental pressures beyond an individual's adaptive capacity (Lawton and Nahemow). Environmental competence results when individuals and environment in adaptive balance. This balance may require lifestyle modifications of the individual and of the environment and may be a time-consuming process.

- An environmental safety check and client education to prevent crime may prevent many problems and is a nursing responsibility when working with individuals and families in the community.

▲ CASE STUDY

Celeste was the 88-year-old grande dame of her neighborhood and local temple. Even the rabbi seemed cowed in her presence. She had great dignity and pride but was a warm and caring friend. She exuded independence and strength. Throughout her adult years she held a managerial position in a small hotel. With work and family she had little time to pursue the arts or recreational activities. Most of her interests and activities were focused on family and temple. There is little question she had been the matriarch of her family. Though some thought Celeste domineering, her husband, a rather quiet and scholarly man, had been content. Her husband, after numerous bouts of illness and hospitalization, died. She managed very well through all of his illnesses and with the support of neighborhood, temple, and close friends seemed to be adapting to his loss. However, in the grief over the loss of her husband she felt the need to have her daughters close. Both lived at considerable distance and were highly involved in their own communities and professional lives. Celeste began insisting they spend more time with her. They began to feel guilty and distressed because it was

Nursing Diagnoses

The following potential diagnoses must be considered as well as diagnoses unique to the particular individual:
Fear
Home maintenance management, impaired
Hyperthermia
Hypothermia
Injury, risk for

Knowledge deficit
Protection, altered
Role performance/altered
Sleep pattern disturbance
Social isolation
Relocation stress syndrome

NURSING PROCESS AND NURSING DIAGNOSIS
Hypothermia

Etiologies and Related Factors
Age related changes
Exposure to a cool or cold environment
Inappropriate clothing for climate
Illness or trauma
Alcohol consumption
Evaporation from skin in cool environment
Inactivity
Inadequate shelter/substandard housing
Lives alone
Extremes in weight
Immediate postoperative period
Inactivity
Medications that cause vasodilitation
Inability or decreased ability to shiver
Damaged hypothalamus

Defining Characteristics
Reduced body temperature below normal
Cool skin
Slow capillary refill
Cyanotic nail beds
Tachycardia
Hypertension
Mental confusion
Shivering
Drowsiness
Decreased pulse and respiratory rate

Knowledge
Normal integument age changes
Medications that interfere with maintenance of temperature
Physiologic conditions that interfere with or damage body defenses against cold
Risk factors
Signs and symptoms of hypothermia
Interventions to prevent and treat hypothermia
Community resources: financial; utility company programs

Clinical Judgment and Related Skills
Assess for risk factors
Monitor body temperature
Reduce or eliminate causative or contributing factors
Health teaching (client/family/community) risks, early signs and symptoms, proper clothing to wear, resources for assistance
Make referrals
Design, implement, and evaluate a plan of care for a client to prevent or treat hypothermia

Evaluation
Normal body temperature
Appropriate clothing worn
Environmental temperature appropriate
Client has taken preventive measures for hypothermia
Client states signs and symptoms of hypothermia

NEEDS ADDRESSED AND TASK STRENGTHS

Need for privacy, activity, and social interaction; to make own choices (to provide for safety, belonging, and self-esteem)
Awareness of environmental impact on function

Modifies environment for ease of function
Identifies own environmental preferences
Recognizes need for private time and space
Personalizes environment

not possible for them to drop everything and be with her when she felt lonely. The daughters convinced her to move near them, and in her loneliness she agreed. They leased a large apartment in a lovely complex and with assistance of friends and relatives managed to get her and most of her prized possessions moved in. Celeste soon began pleading to "go back home." The daughters recognized the relocation stress and visited as frequently as possible. They encouraged her to go to temple or a senior center, but she resisted getting to know new people. "I miss my friends. At my age it is just too much trouble to get to know new people. I want those I have known all my life." Soon she began insisting she needed a larger apartment and suggested perhaps one of the daughters could live with her. Knowing her need to "be in charge," the daughters both resisted this idea. It became apparent after several months that the relocation stress was not subsiding but was beginning to impair Celeste's function. She began neglecting her laundry and seldom picking up her mail. She was moved into an apartment closer to the center of the complex. She seemed somewhat more content for a few weeks though she seldom left her apartment and never participated in any activities in the center or the temple. One day her daughter came to visit and found four bags of garbage in the kitchen of her mother's apartment. She was horrified because her mother had always been so fastidious. When she mentioned it, her mother said, "I can't go out. I'm afraid."

Based upon the case study, develop a nursing care plan using the following procedure*:

List comments of client that provide *subjective data.*

List information that provides *objective data.*

From these data identify and state, using accepted format, two *nursing diagnoses* you determine are most significant to this client at this time. List two *client strengths* that you have identified from data.

Determine and state *outcome criteria* for each diagnosis. These must reflect some alleviation of the problem identified in the nursing diagnosis and must be stated in concrete and measurable terms.

Plan and state one or more *interventions* for each diagnosed problem.

Provide specific documentation of source used to determine appropriate intervention. Plan at least one intervention that incorporates the client's existing strengths.

Evaluate success of intervention. Interventions must correlate directly with the stated outcome criteria in order to measure the outcome success.

*Students are advised to refer to their nursing diagnosis text and identify possible or potential problems.

STUDY QUESTIONS/ACTIVITIES

Discuss housing options that might be suitable for individuals like Celeste.

What aspects of her environment do you believe she has the power to change?

Locate low cost housing in your area and assess for convenience and safety.

Is purse snatching and mugging of elders commonplace in your city?

What resources are available to prevent or assist those who may be vulnerable to attack?

Discuss how you would assist your parents in making a decision regarding a change in living situations as they become increasingly disabled and unable to care for themselves.

List several aspects of your environment that are important to you and discuss their particular significance.

Discuss relocation stress and the significance it has to aged individuals.

Discuss housing options that would be most suitable and feasible for you if you were unable to get around without the assistance of a walker.

Discuss the meanings and the thoughts triggered by the student's and elder's viewpoints expressed at the beginning of the chapter. How do these vary from your own experience?

RESEARCH QUESTIONS

What are the differences in crime victimization of the elderly in the inner city as compared to suburbs and rural areas?

What criminal activities are of most concern to the aged?

What percentage of major cities or states have crime victimization programs in place?

What are the environmental safety factors most frequently neglected by the aged?

What are the home safety factors most frequently causing trouble for the aged?

What have proved to be the most effective crime stoppers in relation to protecting the aged from victimization?

What is the geographic distribution and incidence of hypothermia and hyperthermia in the United States?

What changes in behavior occur when institutionalized elders are routinely taken outdoors for exposure to nature?

What services or lack of services contributes to the increased morbidity of nursing home patients in the first 2 years of institutionalization?

What are the outcomes of various services in institutions?

RESOURCES

Films and Videos

Training series "Injury Prevention for the Elderly" includes falls, burns, abuse, hypothermia and hyperthermia. Aspen

Publishers, Inc, 200 Orchard Ridge Drive, Gaithersburg, MD 20878; (800) 638-8437, fax (301) 417-7650.

Closer from Home, L. Bloise, Terra Nova Films, Chicago, IL (38 minutes). This videotape depicts an elderly man who becomes homeless when he loses his apartment and cannot move into a new one until his Social Security check arrives.

Miss Nora's Store (Rural Elderly) (28 min). Captures the beauty and hardship of rural life for elderly Americans. This documentary presents life experiences of individuals 65 to 97 years of age who personify the strength of character, desire for independence, and treasury of memories inherent in many elderly rural Americans. The program also reveals the geographical, psychosocial, and cultural barriers that may prevent access to necessary health and social services. Highly recommended for preservice training of all health professionals to encourage practice in rural areas and to provide an understanding of the special needs of elderly individuals living in rural communities. From Video Press, University of Maryland at Baltimore, School of Medicine, Suite 133, 100 Penn Street, Baltimore, MD 21201; (800) 328-7450 or (410) 328-5497; fax (410) 328-8471.

Organizations

HUD USER, PO Box 6091, Rockville MD 20850; (800) 245-2691, (301) 251-5154. Assistance in obtaining low-cost housing.

Lifeline Systems, Inc, One Arsenal Marketplace, Watertown, MA 02171; (617) 923-4141. Provides a personal emergency response system to a signal from an individual wearing a transmitter.

National Center for Home Equity Conversion, 110 East Main Street, Room 601, Madison, WI 53703; (608) 256-2111. Information regarding obtaining home equity loans.

National Environmental Health Association, 720 s Colorado Boulevard, Suite 970, South Tower, Denver, CO 80222. For professionals working with environmental disorders.

Golden Age Passports may be obtained from the National Park Service, Washington, DC 20242 (209) 252-2548, or from regional park offices. These passports provide free entry at all federal recreational sites for individuals over 62 years of age.

Secure Care Systems, Inc, PO Box 1180, Portland, ME 04104. Provides individual electronic monitoring of patients who may wander from premises.

U.S. Consumer Products Safety Commission, Washington, DC 20207; (800) 638-2772. Regulates products used in and around the home. Free home safety publications are available.

Many states have programs designed to assist victims of crime. To learn more about such resources in your area, write to the National Organization for Victim Assistance, 1757 Park Road, NW, Washington, DC 20010.

The Food and Drug Administration can advise you on quack products and devices. Write to FDA, Bureau of Medical Devices, Consumer and Regulatory Affairs Branch (HFK-131), 8757 Georgia Avenue, Silver Spring, MD 20910.

The Crime and Prevention Coalition (Box 6700, Rockville, MD 20850) can send you the free brochure *Senior Citizens against Crime,* published by the U.S. Department of Justice. The Council of Better Business Bureaus has published a pamphlet entitled *Consumer Problems of the Elderly.* Single copies can be obtained by sending a self-addressed stamped envelope to the Council of Better Business Bureaus, 1515 Wilson Boulevard, Arlington, VA 22209.

The National Crime Prevention Council, 733 15th Street, NW, Washington, DC, 20006, (202) 393-7141.

For more information about crime prevention for older people, contact the American Association of Retired Persons, Criminal Justice Services, 1909 K Street, NW, Washington, DC 20049. Also, your local police or sheriff's office may have a crime prevention unit to provide assistance in your area.

Publications

Booklets

Making Your Community Livable: Programs That Work, Public Policy Institute, American Association of Retired Persons (AARP), 601 E Street, NW, Washington, DC 20049. Available free. Describes programs in crime prevention, home repair and modification, and transportation that have proved effective in helping older people live independently in their homes.

Too Good to Be True: A Consumer Guide to Fraud. Deals with numerous categories of fraud and supplies agency addresses and phone numbers to contact for assistance in each type of fraud. Booklet available free from Consumer Information Center, Pueblo, CO 81009.

Telephone California Association of Health Facilities (916) 445-2070 for copies of *Your Rights as a Resident in a Nursing Home* (in English, Spanish, Chinese and Tagalog), *Residents' Rights* (17 different fact sheets), and *Consumer Guide: Special Care Programs for Persons with Alzheimer's Disease or Other Dementias.*

Telephone Shelly Jenkins at the California Healthcare Association at (916) 443-7401 or the California Medical Association at (415) 541-0900 for copies of *HCFA's Guide to Choosing a Nursing Home* and *Durable Power of Attorney for Health Care* (forms in English and Spanish).

Telephone the Medicare Rights Center at (212) 869-3850 for copies of *Medicare Appeals and Grievances: Strategies for System Simplification and Informed Decisionmaking.* Written for assistance in cases of denial of coverage, this 48-page booklet explains the difference between Medicare fee for service and Medicare risk programs. First copy free.

The Pacific Center for Health Policy and Ethics publishes *Your Rights to Make Decisions about Medical Treatment,* which healthcare providers are required to issue to patients or residents upon admission. For copies of this brochure, telephone (213) 740-2541.

Directories of retirement housing

The American Association of Retired Persons publishes a "Better Retirement" series that includes two booklets on the subject of retirement housing: *Your Retirement Housing Guide* and *Your Retirement Home Repair Guide.* These booklets offer useful suggestions that will help in making decisions regarding housing in the retirement years. Individual copies of these booklets are free on request from the American Association of Retired Persons, 1909 K Street, NW, Washington, DC 20006.

Listed below are several directories that provide information on retirement housing and facilities. Most of these should be available in local libraries or bookstores or can be ordered directly from the publisher.

Musson N: *The National Directory of Retirement Residences: Best Places to Live When You Retire,* Frederick Fell, Inc, 386 Park Ave South, New York, NY 10016. (Cost: $9.95.) This book contains brief, concise descriptions of 1000 retirement residences, including villages or single dwellings, groups of apartments, group residences, and multitype facilities built or modernized since 1950. A short description of climatic and geographic conditions for each state is included. The listings include type of facility, number of units, fees, type of sponsorship, special features and services on the premises, type of locale, and proximity to needed facilities. The directory also includes detailed introductory chapters offering guidance in choosing a retirement residence and financial, legal, and health needs in retirement, and gives points on selling a house and surplus belongings when moving to a retirement home.

Woodall's Retirement and Resort Communities Directory, Woodall Publishing Co, 500 Hyacinth Place, Highland Park, IL 60036 (published annually). (Cost $5.95.) This directory is a complete guide to retirement and leisure living. It lists thousands of housing opportunities including apartments, condominiums, mobile home and recreational vehicle parks, and single family developments. Features illustrated listings or floor plans of specific homes available. Includes thoroughly researched facts about climate, cost of living, recreation, and medical care available. More than 400 retirement regions to choose from throughout the country, plus special features written to help determine which housing facility or lifestyle suits the reader best.

Your Home . . . and Your Retirement, Retirement Living, 150 East 58th Street, New York, NY 10022. (Cost: $1.25.) This is a general survey that provides an outline of the types of retirement housing available and surveys the cost of living, availability of housing, and climate conditions by state.

REFERENCES

American Association of Homes and Services for the Aging: *Fact Sheet,* Washington DC, 1992, American Association of Homes and Services for the Aging (AAHSA).

American Association of Homes and Services for the Aging: AAHSA creates subsidiary for assisted living, *Provider News* 10(3):1, 1995a.

American Association of Homes and Services for the Aging: Trends and issues, *Currents* 10(9):4, 1995b.

American Association of Homes and Services for the Aging: Managed care: LTC funding likely to affect senior housing, *Currents* 11(1):3, 1996.

American Association of Retired Persons: *Expanding housing choices for older people,* AARP WHCoA Mini-conference, Jan 26, Conference Papers and Recommendations.

American Association of Retired Persons: *Experience of older applicants waiting for federal assisted housing,* Public Policy Institute, Washington DC, AARP, FS #43:1-2, 1995.

American Health Care Association: *AHCA applauds senate passage of long term care insurance provisions,* press release April 19, 1996, American Health Care Association, Washington, DC.

Arras JD, Dubler NN: Bringing the hospital home: ethical and social implications of high-tech home care, *Hastings Center Report* 24(5):Suppl 19,1994.

Bergman G: Shared housing—not only for the rent, *Aging Today* 15(1):1, 1994.

Bond C, Miller M: Reading: the ageless activity, *Geriatr Nurs* 8(4):192, 1987.

Braun K, King R: Assuring quality in foster care, *Generations* 13(1):48, 1989.

Burke MJ: Operation victim support: elderly peer counseling project, *Gerontologist* 23:275 (special issue), 1983 (abstract).

Bustad LK, Hines LM: *Placement of animals with the elderly: benefits and strategies,* Moraga, Calif, 1983, California Veterinary Medical Association.

Chardon, Ohio, 1988, Corinne Dolan Alzheimer Center.

Clarke CJ, Neidert LJ: Living arrangements of the elderly: an examination of differences according to ancestry and generation, *Gerontologist* 32(6):796, 1992.

Crawford R: Plan with flexibility as the top priority, *Provider* 14(9):17, 1988.

DeJong GF, Wilmoth JM, Angel JL, Cornwell GT: Motives and the geographic mobility of very old Americans, *J Gerontol SS*50B(6):S395, 1995.

Dimond M, McCance K, King K: Forced residential relocation: its impact on the well-being of older adults, *West J Nurs Res* 9(4):445, 1987.

Drysdale A: Personal communication, 1988.

Edelstein S: *Fair Housing laws for group residences for frail older persons,* Washington, DC, 1995, American Association of Retired Persons.

Ferraro KF, LaGrange RL: Are older people most afraid of crime? Reconsidering age differences in fear of victimization, *J Gerontol* 47(5):S233, 1992.

Folkemer D, Jensen A, Lipson L, Stauffer M, Fox-Grage W: *Adult foster care for the elderly: a review of state regulatory and funding strategies,* Washington, DC, 1996, American Association of Retired Persons.

Francis G, Baly A: Plush animals, *Geriatr Nurs* 7(3):140, 1986.

Frey WH: Elderly demographic profiles of US states: impacts of "new elderly births," migration, and immigration, *Gerontologist* 35(6):761, 1995.

Friedman S, Ryan LS: A systems perspective on problematic behaviors in nursing homes, *Family Therapy* 8(3):265, 1986.

Garcia E, Luck R: Crime and the older adult, *Aging Network* 3(12):4, 1987.

Grant PR, Skinkle RR, Lipps G: The impact of interinstitutional relocation on nursing home residents requiring a high level of care, *Gerontologist* 32(2):834, 1992.

Green DA: A resident-centered model for nursing home design, *Aging Today* 15(2):15,1994.

Hartwigsen G: Older widows and the transference of home, *Intl J Aging Human Develop* 25(2):195, 1987.

Hiatt L: Does innovative design exist? *Provider* 9:12, 1988.

Kane R, Bell R, Riegler S: Value preferences for nursing home outcomes, *Gerontologist* 26(3)303, 1986.

King K, Dimond M, McCance K: Coping with relocation, *Geriatr Nurs* 8(5):258, 1987.

Lazarowich NM: A review of the Victoria, Australia granny flat program, *Generations* 30(2):171, 1990.

Leach D: *Making your community livable: programs that work,* AARP Public Policy Institute, 1996, Washington, DC.

Leisure World Laguna Hills, press release, May 1996, 23522 Paseo de Valenica, Laguna Hills, CA 92653, (800) 711-9273.

Liu H: Personal communication, 1988.

Macey SM, Schneider DF: Deaths from excessive heat and excessive cold among the elderly, *Gerontologist* 33(4):497, 1993.

Maddox G: *Encyclopedia of aging,* New York, 1995, Springer.

Mirotznik J, Lombardi TG: The impact of intrainstitutional relocation on morbidity in an acute care setting. *Gerontologist* 35(2):217-224, 1995.

Morganett B: Nature hikes for nursing home residents, *Geriatr Nurs* 8(4):178, 1987.

Mudd K: *Philadelphia leads nation in efforts to provide heat relief,* news release, Philadelphia Corporation for Aging, Philadelphia, Oct 13, 1995.

Namazi K: *Summary of environmental design issues,* Unpublished manuscript.

Noell E: Design in nursing homes: environment as a silent partner in caregiving, *Generations* 19(4):14,1996.

O'Connor C: Psychosocial aspects of care with elderly veterans by a gerontological clinical specialist in a US Veterans Administration Hospital. *Proceedings of the Third Congress of the International Psychogeriatric Association* 3:111, Chicago, 1987, (abstract).

Omnibus Budget Reconciliation Acts (OBRA) of 1987 (Public law #100-203): amendments 1990, 1991, 1992, 1993, 1994, Rockville, Md), Health Care Financing Administration, US Department of Health and Human Services.

Parsons M, Levy J: Nursing process in injury prevention, *J Gerontol Nurs* 13(7):36, 1987.

Petrou M, Obenchain J: Reducing incidents of illness post transfer, *Geriatr Nurs* 8(5):264, 1987.

Pynoos J: Strategies for home modification and repair, *Generations* 16(2):21, 1992.

Pynoos J, Reynolds SL, Salend E, Rahman A: *Waiting for federally assisted housing: a study of the needs and experiences of older applicants,* Reprint 9506, Washington, DC 1995, American Association of Retired Persons.

Reschovsky JD, Ruchlin HS: Quality of board and care homes serving low-income elderly: structural and public policy correlates, *J App Gerontol* 12(2):225, 1993.

Roberts B, Algase D: Victims of Alzheimer's disease and the environment, *Nurs Clin North Am* 23(1):83, 1988.

Rosenkoetter MM: Brutus is making rounds, *Geriatr Nurs* 12(6):277,1992.

Roush S, Banziger G: *Nursing homes for the birds: a control-relevant intervention with bird feeders.* Paper presented at the meeting of the Gerontological Society of America, Boston, Nov 21, 1982.

Schafer S: Modifying the environment, *Geriatr Nurs* 6:127, 1985.

Smith D, Karras T: Creating interiors for a changing clientele, *Provider* 14(9):20, 1988.

Steinberg D: Fearful elders can learn alot from an ex-rat, *San Francisco Examiner,* Section C-7, Feb 19, 1994.

Sterritt PF, Pokorny ME: Art activities for patients with Alzheimer's and related disorders, *Geriatr Nurs* 15(3):155, 1994.

Stoller EP: The price of pride, *Aging Today* 14(5):7,1993.

Sweet H: Can't take the heat, *Remedy* 11(4):31, 1995.

Tassy E: Senior home elicits community contention, *Baltimore Sun,* p 1B, Sept 2, 1995.

Texas Heart Institute: Coping with the heat, *Vision,* p 2, Summer, Houston, 1992.

Tolman EC: Cognitive maps in rats and men, *Psychol Rev* 55:189, 1948.

Tynan C, Cardea J: Home health hazard assessment, *J Gerontol Nurs* 13(10):25, 1987.

US Bureau of the Census: *Statistical abstract of the United States: 1995,* ed 115, Washington, DC, 1995.

US Department of Health and Human Services: *HCFA opens first health care fraud satellite office,* Health Care Financing Administration Press Office, Sept 5, 1995.

US Government General Accounting Office: *Elderly Americans: health, housing and nutrition gaps between the poor and nonpoor,* Gaithersburg, Md, 1992, GAO.

Vrabec NJ: Implications of US health care reform for the rural elderly, *Nurs Outlook* 43(6):260, 1995.

Williams CC: Long term care and the human spirit, *Generations* 14(4):25, 1990.

Wollner L, Collins KJ: Disorders of the autonomic nervous system. In Brocklehurst JC, Tallis RC, Fillit HM, eds. *Textbook of geriatric medicine and gerontology,* ed 4, Edinburgh, 1992, Churchill Livingstone, pp 399–403.

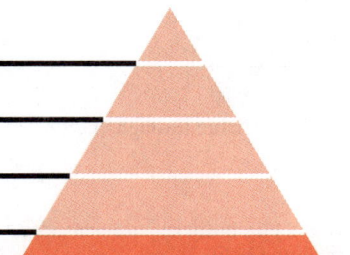

Home Care: A Checklist for Assessment of the Physical Setting and Tasks of Home Care

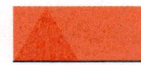

Housing (Satisfactory Physical Setting for Care)

Comfort, cleanliness, spaciousness
Safety and comfort of the neighborhood
Access for patient, family, friends
Consider housing assistance programs (e.g., mortgage
   maintenance and rental supports)
Consider special housing (for independence or assisted living)
   Handicapped housing
   Senior citizen housing
   Foster homes

Room

Where will patient be? Consider rearranging rooms.
Where will others sleep and carry on their lives?

Bed (Rent, Buy, or Borrow Bed for Special Needs)

Elevated, adjustable (mechanical or electrical adjustments)
Side rails, trapeze
Mattress (foam, air, water, or regular)
Bedding (e.g., sheepskin, plastic sheets, underpads)
   Changing bedding
   Moving, turning
   Washing
   Special skin care (preventing and treating decubitus ulcers)

Mobility

Transfer techniques (e.g., lifting, mechanical devices)
Special chairs, couches
Assistance in ambulation (e.g., canes, walkers, wheelchairs, rails,
   ramps, bars)
Check for safety hazards (e.g., loose rugs, obstructions)
Exercise (active and passive), physical therapy

Dressing

"Bedclothes" and normal clothes
Laundry

Grooming

Hair and nails
Makeup

Bathing

Aids (e.g., flexible shower heads, long-handled brushes, adhesive
   strips to prevent slipping, safety bars)

Bowel and Bladder Function

Continent
   Use of bedpan, urinal, bedside commode, elevated toilet seat
   Access to the bathroom
   Bowel regimens, suppositories
Incontinent
   Underpads, plastic sheets, towels, hampers, diaper service
   External or indwelling urinary catheter
   Drainage systems and their management

Feeding

Shopping or ordering food; Meals-on-Wheels
Preparation
   Soft and liquid diets
   Tube feedings
   Assistance in eating
   Bedside fluids, snacks
   Special utensils, straws
Alcohol
Food stamps and other nutritional support programs

Medication

Purchase and delivery
Storage and safety
Refilling
Monitoring
Recording
Adjusting
Self-administered versus given by family member
Aid in swallowing (e.g., mashing pills, mixing with food, liquid
   preparations)
Suppositories
Topical treatments
Injections

Supplies and Equipment

Purchasing, borrowing, or renting
Delivery
Storage and safety
Proper use of gloves, syringes, needles, sterile dressings,
   solutions
Catheter equipment
Oxygen, suction equipment
Intravenous therapy, hyperalimentation
Dialysis

From Tideiksaar R: Ritter Department of Geriatrics and Adult Development, New York, 1983, The Mount Sinai Medical Center.

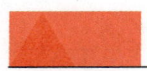

Attending

Professional "skilled" help versus "unskilled" help
    Visiting nurses
    Physical therapy, speech therapy, occupational therapy
    Home health aides
    Homemakers, chore services
    Companions and volunteer services
Training nonprofessional helpers (e.g., to change dressing, give injections, monitor vital signs)
Constant versus intermittent availability of help
Regular, anticipated chores (e.g., dressing changes, meals, skin care, medications) versus intermittent needs (e.g, snacks, "as needed" medications, some transfers)
Night call
Methods for calling for help (e.g., phones, buzzers, bells, intercoms)
What to do when questions arise? Caretakers absent? Emergencies?

Diversions, Entertainment, Recreation

Hobbies, books, television, radio, tapes, records
Personally important objects (e.g., photographs, paintings, gifts, souvenirs, and mementos)
Family access and visitors
Excursions

Pastoral Care

Awareness of services and resources available through church affiliation

Legal Aid

Knowledge of the availability of and eligibility requirements for services and the process of obtaining help

Financial Aid

Knowledge of the availability of and eligibility requirements for services and the process of obtaining help
Hospital-based and community-based social service agencies
Sources
    Third-party health insurance (e.g., Blue Cross/Blue Shield, Medicare, Medicaid, and other private insurers)
    Social Security, general relief
    Area agency on aging
    United Way and other community charities
    Special funds (e.g., American Cancer Society, local and national philanthropic organizations, hospital funds)

Out of Home Help

Senior citizens' center for meals, recreation
Day care
Respite care
Rehabilitation services
Transportation

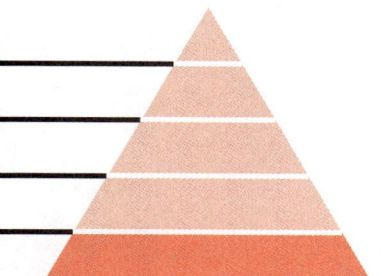

Home Assessment Checklist

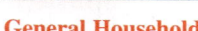

General Household

1. Is there good lighting available, especially around stairwells?
2. Are there handrails (which can be easily grasped) on both sides of the staircases, designed to indicate when top and bottom steps have been reached?
3. Are top and bottom steps painted in easily seen colors? Are nonskid treads used?
4. Are the edges of rugs tacked down? (Suggest the use of wall-to-wall carpeting.)
5. Is a telephone present? Does the telephone have a dial that is easily readable? Are emergency numbers written in large print and kept near the telephone?
6. Are electrical cords, footstools, and other low-lying objects kept out of walkways?
7. Are electrical cords in good condition?
8. Is furniture arranged to allow for free movement in heavily traveled areas?
9. Is furniture sturdy enough to give support?
10. Is furniture designed to accommodate easy transfers on and off?
11. Is the temperature of the home within a comfortable range?
12. If fireplaces or other heating devices are present, do they have protective screens?
13. Are smoke detectors present (especially in the kitchen and bedroom)?
14. Are rapidly closing doors eliminated?
15. Are there alternative exits from the house?
16. Are basements and attics easy to get to, well lighted, and well ventilated?
17. Are slippers and shoes in good repair? Do they fit properly and have nonskid soles?

Kitchen

18. Are there loose extension cords, small sliding rugs, slippery linoleum tiles present? (Suggest the use of rubber-backed, nonskid rugs and nonskid floor wax.)
19. Is the cooking stove gas or electric?
20. Are there large easily readable dials present on the stove or other appliances, with the "on" and "off" positions clearly marked?
21. Are refrigerators in good working order? Are refrigerators placed on 18-inch platforms to avoid bending over?
22. Are spaces for food storage adequate? Are shelves at eye level and easily reachable?
23. Is a sturdy stepladder present for reaching?
24. Are electrical circuits overloaded with too many appliances?
25. Are electrical appliances disconnected when not in use?

26. Are sharp objects (such as carving knives) kept in special holders?
27. Are cleaning fluids, polishes, bleaches, detergents, and all positions stored separately and clearly marked?
28. Are kitchen chairs sturdy, with arm rests with high backs?
29. Is stove free from flammable objects?
30. Are pot holders available for removing pots and pans from the stove?
31. Is baking soda available in case of fire?

Bathroom

32. Are there grab bars in the bath, in the shower, and around the toilet?
33. Are toilet seats high enough to get on and off of without difficulty?
34. Can the bathroom door be easily closed to ensure privacy (Avoid locks.)
35. Are bathroom doorways wide enough for easy wheelchair and walker access?
36. Are there nonskid rubber mats in the bath, in the shower, and on the floor?
37. Is there good lighting in the area of the medicine cabinet?
38. Are internal and external medications stored separately? And safely (especially important with young grandchildren present in the house)?
39. Do medication containers have childproof tops? Are they labeled in large print? Is a magnifying glass present for reading medication instructions?
40. Have all outdated medications been discarded?
41. Do you notice any medications (both prescription and over-the-counter) that could cause adverse side effects or drug-drug interactions that the patient is unaware of?
42. Can the water temperature be easily regulated?
43. Are electrical cords, outlets, and appliances a safe distance from the tub?
44. Are razor blades kept in a safe place?
45. Is a first aid kit available?

Bedroom

46. Is there adequate lighting from the bedside to the bathroom?
47. Are lights easily accessible? (If not, suggest keeping a flashlight by the bedside or using a flashlight for entry into dark rooms if light switch is not within easy reach.)
48. Are beds in good repair?
49. Are beds at the proper height to allow for easy transfer on and off without difficulty?
50. Do bedroom rugs have nonskid rubber backings?

From Tideiksaar R: Ritter Department of Geriatrics and Adult Development, New York, 1983, The Mount Sinai Medical Center.

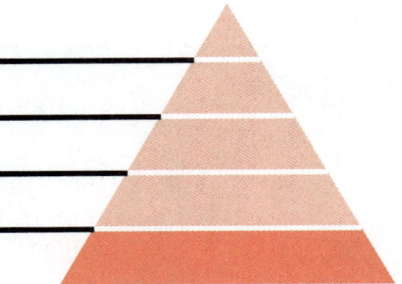

Guidelines for Home Safety Assessment

	Okay (y/n)	Plan to improve
Basic Structure		
Intact roof		
Solid floors and stairs		
Functioning toilet (or outhouse)		
Source of fresh water		
Wheelchair ramp		
Temperature Control		
Fan/air conditioner		
Proper use of heating pads		
Proper hot water heater temperature		
Adequate heat/insulation		
Nutrition		
Kitchen condition/food storage		
Evidence of alcohol use		
Pests		
Fire Prevention and Response		
Use of kerosene heaters		
Use of open gas burners on stove for heat		
Smoking in bed		
Use of oxygen		
Dangerous electrical wiring		
Smoke alarms		
Exit plans in case of fire		
Self-Injury/Violence Prevention		
Locks		
Method of calling for help		
Proximity of neighbors		
Surrounding criminal activity		
Emergency phone numbers by telephone		
Loaded guns/knives		
Household toxins		
Water/bathtub		
Power tools		
Medication Management		
Duplicate medicines, outdated drugs, pill box		
Correct labeling		
Storage safety, accessibility, refrigeration		
Caregiver familiarity		
Wandering Control (for confused patients)		
Doortap latches, special locks		
Fenced yards with hidden latches		
Identification bracelets		
Electronic wandering alarms		

Use for:
___ client
X clinician

Client's signature _____

Clinician's signature _____

RESIDENCE _____

Date _____

Adapted from Yoshikawa TAT, Cobbs EL, Brummel-Smith K: *Ambulatory geriatric care,* St Louis, 1993, Mosby, p 162.

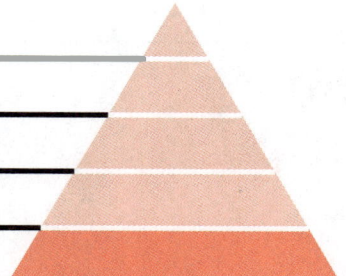

Community Assessment Guide

Overall Features

Climate
Location
Topography
Roadways
Open space

Distribution of building
Noise level
Economic state
Community planning

Population Characteristics

Overall age, sex, ethnic distribution
Proportion of elderly in population

Ethnic/socioeconomic characteristics of elderly
Intergenerational relations

Service Facilities

Shopping/basic service

Food, drug, clothing stores
Dry cleaners
Shoe repair
Restaurants
Banks
Post office

Educational

Public library
Adult education programs

Transportation

Private cars
Taxis
Subways and/or buses

Health care

Ambulance service
Clinics
Hospitals
Physicians
Dentists
Home care services
Pharmacists
Folk healers

Social/recreational

Places of worship
Outdoor parks
Indoor facilities:
   The "Y"
   Cinemas
   Bowling
   Private clubs

Social services

Social Security office
Welfare office
Senior citizens' programs:
   Senior centers, clubs, nutrition programs, outreach services

Environmental/Safety Conditions

Pavements/curbs
Crosswalks
Street lighting
Air quality

Sanitation services
Unleashed animals
Police department (crime rate)
Fire department (fire, arson rate)

From Rauckhorst LM et al: *J Gerontol Nurs* 6:321, 1980.

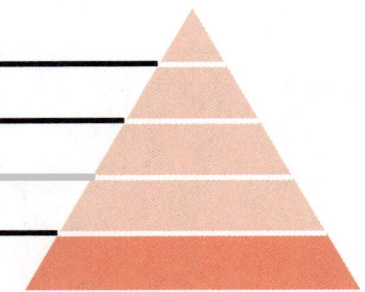

CHAPTER 14

Health Care, Economic, and Legal Concerns of the Aged

A student learns

A myth I had about the aged was that most elderly people were financially well off. The realization that many live on a fixed income and sometimes lack the family support that would help cover their needs has become clear to me. Inflation and health care costs have made it so that many elders are unable to keep up with the financial demands of their aged lifestyle.

Laura, age 36

Elders speak

I remember how my grandmother talked of the hard times when she was old, during the depression. There was no economic assistance or health care for the poor. Times have changed. I have enough money now and good health care, but I'm afraid I may outlive both.

Rachel, age 76

In these days of inflated values for desirable items such as housing, clothing, food, and medical care, the plight of the elderly is particularly acute. Everything costs more, but our incomes are reduced; our assets are facing a constant attack, and as they are diminished our incomes are further reduced. Even in a guaranteed existence such as I enjoy here at the Meadows, there is a constant reminder that there will be less and less money available as, with improved care and increased longevity, I try to maintain adequate funds for my own care. This, I think, is my greatest worry—and if I, cosseted as I am in my present circumstances, find little solace in my good fortune, what about all the others who have not been so lucky?

Lyn, age 85

The most pressing problems of our era are the increasing number of elders dependent upon care and the cost of this care to patient and family.

Leon and Alice, over 70

LEARNING OBJECTIVES

Upon completion of this chapter, the reader will be able to:

1. Identify several economic factors that influence the lives of the elderly.
2. Discuss income and expenditures of the aged and the multiple sources of these.
3. Relate economic dilemmas of old and young.
4. Explain fundamentals of Medicare and Medicaid sufficiently to assist elders in obtaining more specific information.
5. Specify and explain legal issues of concern to the aged.
6. Describe the role of the nurse-advocate in relation to legal, health, and economic issues of concern to the aged.

This chapter is designed to inform and update students and practitioners on the current economic, legal, and health policies that one must comprehend in order to provide appropriate guidance and resource information to elders within our care or under our jurisdiction. As almost everyone is aware, our service systems to elders and others are in a state of chaos, and thus it is difficult to present information that will be accurate and currently useful even a year from now. Predictions aside, we do know that states and large corporations are increasingly in control of the directions of health and entitlements for the aged. Individuals must, more than ever before, have knowledge of the options available to them and the resources and advocates they can trust.

Nurses are increasingly in the front lines as primary care providers and gatekeepers to care. Advanced practice nurses are being given more responsibility in triage and management of the common disorders that accompany the aging process. We recognize the chaos and complexity of health care and the sophistication necessary to survive economically and legally in the present era. We are aware that many of the concepts that underlie decisions nurses are making with clients on a daily basis are very advanced and becoming increasingly intricate. These are not arenas in which even the experts agree, but we will present them as cogently as possible for the background of students and practitioners with the full knowledge that neither we nor our readers can fully comprehend the massive changes occurring. The movement in general is toward increasing client and family responsibility for their own welfare, the development of numerous methods to provide care outside of institutions, and moving away from the private provider model. Many of these issues are dealt with in more depth in other chapters,

but this chapter is designed to summarize important information that the reader may need in planning care.

THE ECONOMIC FACTS OF AGING

More people are living into advanced old age and requiring more legal, social, medical, and economic supports. There are now nearly 34 million persons over 65 years of age, and because births and deaths annually have gradually decreased since 1990, the median age of the United States population has risen to 34 years. This is a 6-year gain since 1970. Currently 33% of the population are not in the labor force, which means that the support/dependency ratio is 2:1. Individuals 75 years of age and over have increased by 30% since 1981 (U.S. Bureau of Census, 1995). In a decade the largest population group, the baby boomers, will begin to need supports and services in their aging process. These trends lead to increasing concerns about the future of the aged.

Economic Status of the Aged

The income distribution of individuals working full time and the comparison with elders can be seen in Table 14-1. However, most elders do not work full time. In 1995 one in every 13 elders had an income of less than $5000, and only 12% had incomes over $30,000 annually (American Association of Retired Persons, 1996). However, net worth, calculated by assets minus liabilities, reflects a median of $86,300, accounted for mainly by homes and real goods. The national average is only $37,600 while the net worth for 17% of elders is well over $250,000 (American Association of Retired Persons, 1996). Sources of income are noted in Table 14-2.

Assets and Income. Household net worth includes ownership of stocks, bonds, savings, homes, other real estate,

Table 14-1   Median Income of Year-Round Full-Time Workers with Income: 1980 to 1993

[Age as of March of following year. Prior to 1990, earnings are for civilian workers only.]

Item	Female					Male				
	1980	**1990**	**1991**	**1992**	**1993**	**1980**	**1990**	**1991**	**1992**	**1993**
Total with income	**$11,591**	**$20,591**	**$21,245**	**$22,093**	**$22,469**	**$19,173**	**$28,979**	**$30,332**	**$30,832**	**$31,077**
15 to 19 years old	6,779	*13,944	*14,242	*14,662	*15,227	7,753	*15,462	*15,307	[1]15,658	[1]15,948
20 to 24 years old	9,407	(NA)	(NA)	(NA)	(NA)	12,109	(NA)	(NA)	(NA)	(NA)
25 to 34 years old	12,190	20,184	21,022	21,941	21,949	17,724	25,355	26,100	26,410	26,087
35 to 44 years old	12,239	22,505	23,385	24,125	25,282	21,777	32,607	33,588	34,714	35,233
45 to 54 years old	12,116	21,938	22,630	24,489	24,412	22,323	35,732	37,198	37,926	39,685
55 to 64 years old	11,931	20,755	21,325	22,581	22,587	21,053	33,169	35,720	35,537	35,736
65 years old and over ..	12,342	22,957	21,780	21,556	24,875	17,307	35,520	34,473	35,341	37,085
White	11,703	20,839	21,555	22,349	22,979	19,720	30,081	30,953	31,565	31,832
Black	10,915	18,544	19,134	20,258	20,315	13,875	21,481	22,628	22,991	23,566
Hispanic†	9,887	16,181	16,548	17,674	17,112	13,790	19,358	20,027	19,855	20,423

From US Bureau of the Census: *Statistical Abstract of the United States: 1995,* ed 115, Washington, DC, 1995.
NA, Not available. *15 to 24 years old. [1]Persons of Hispanic origin may be of any race.
Source U.S. Bureau of the Census. *Current Population Reports,* P60-188, and earlier reports, and unpublished data.

Table 14-2   Income Sources in the Survey of Income and Program Participation (SIPP) Database

Income variables	SIPP income sources included
Social Security	Social Security
Pensions	Railroad retirement
	Veterans compensations or pensions
	Pension from company or union
	Federal civil service or other federal civilian employee pensions
	Military retirement pensions
	State government pensions
	Local government pensions
	Other payments for retirement, disability or survivor lump sum payments
Gifts	Income assistance from a charitable group
	Money from relatives or friends
Earnings	Incidental or casual earnings
	Wage income (nonfarm self-employment income, farm self-employment income)
Asset income	Regular/passbook savings accounts in bank; savings and loan or credit union; money market deposit accounts; certificate of deposit or other savings certificates; NOW, super NOW or other interest-earning checking account; money market funds; U.S. government securities; municipal or corporate bonds; other interest-earning assets; stocks or mutual fund shares; income from rental property; mortgages held; royalties and other financial investments
Unemployment compensation	State unemployment compensation
	Supplemental unemployment benefits
	Other unemployment compensation
	Workers compensation
	Employer or union temporary sickness policy
Insurance/Estate	Payments from a sickness, accident, or disability insurance policy purchased on own
	Income from paid-up life insurance policies or annuities
	Estates and trusts
	Income from roomers or boarders
Other support	State SSI; black lung; state temporary disability benefits; Indian, Cuban or refugee assistance; national guard or reserve forces retirement
	AFDC, ADC
	Foster child care payments
	Other welfare
	WIC
	Child support payments
	Alimony payments
	Other cash income not included elsewhere
	National guard or reserve pay

From Dodge HH: Movements out of poverty among elderly widows, *J Gerontol: Social Sciences* 50B(4):S240, 1995.

and vehicles. Those 65 years and over average $73,471 of assets, which is more than all other age groups with the exception of householders 55 to 64 years, who have the largest net worth, averaging $80,032. Median income for those over 65 years is $17,751, a precipitous drop from ages 55 to 64, when the median income is $33,474. At present the highest median income, $46,207, is achieved between the ages of 45 and 54 (U.S. Bureau of the Census, 1995). The median annual income of persons in 1994 who were over 65 was $15,250 for males and $8,950 for females; the mean monthly overall income for those over 65 years old was $1,329. This has more than doubled since 1989 (U.S. Bureau of Census, 1995).

Social Security provides 40% of the income of older couples and individuals (average monthly Social Security benefits are $720); assets are the source of 21%, earnings 17%, and public and private pensions 19%. Other sources provide

3% of elders' income. Even though Social Security tends to be an equalizing factor in the income of old people, private pensions, savings, and other important retirement income vary greatly and are often education-dependent. In fact, average annual income for individuals with graduate degrees is more than twice that of those persons with only high school or less (U.S. Bureau of the Census, 1995). Old people with high levels of education usually experience economic well-being. This certainly has implications for the upcoming generation of elders who have to a large extent had at least some college education.

Home ownership as an asset.   Nearly 7.5% of the elderly are homeowners, 80% of whom have paid their mortgages. Often a home that has increased immensely in value is the major asset of an elder. Taxes and maintenance costs have likewise risen. If monthly income is low, a deprived state of existence may be chosen over selling one's home. If one does choose to sell, a once-in-a-lifetime exemption from the capital gains tax is allowed, up to $125,000 profit from the sale of a personal residence. This means that a person (over 55 years old) who wants to sell and move to a small apartment will be able to use much of the profit from the sale of his or her home for living expenses rather than paying a large part of it in taxes.

If one does not wish to sell the home and cannot afford the upkeep, a reverse annuity mortgage (RAM) plan may be a reasonable solution. This is designed to allow the use of home equity without forcing the elderly to move. The RAM can be used by a homeowner who owns the home completely to generate monthly payments for a period of 3 to 12 years to a total of 80% of the home value. The owner retains title to the property, and the monthly payments do not interfere with eligibility for other senior benefits. However, when the term is up, the loan must be repaid with interest. This type of RAM loan is really designed for people with short-term financial needs.

The reverse shared appreciation mortgage (RSAM) is also available in many states. It allows the homeowner to occupy the home for life, and the lender receives a portion of the home's appreciation on the death of the owner and the sale of the home. The monthly check is in direct proportion to the current value of the home and the percentage of appreciation assigned to the loan agency.

In 1989 the Federal Housing Authority (FHA) entered the home conversion market with four different plans. Briefly, the four plans are as follows: (1) a line of credit established based on the borrower's age and the value of the home; (2) a tenure loan that offers lifetime payments not based on shared appreciation; (3) a fixed rate, shared appreciation tenure mortgage based on life expectancy of the younger spouse and a cap of 25% appreciation contribution to the lender; and (4) a monthly payment similar to the RAM loan but that need not be repaid until the homeowner dies, sells the home, or moves (McGurk, 1989). To qualify for an FHA home equity conversion one must be at least 62 years old, fully own and live in the home, and receive independent financial counseling from a disinterested party. For additional information one may contact the FHA or the American Association of Retired Persons (AARP). Banks have various methods and policies regarding reverse mortgages, and interested individuals need to contact several before making a decision.

Poverty. About 3.7 million elders live below the poverty level (12.2%). Females living alone are among the poorest. Seven percent of the elderly are "near poor," with incomes below 125% of the poverty level (American Association of Retired Persons, 1996) (Table 14-3). Sadly, the percentage of individuals living in poverty has gradually increased in the United States since 1978, when it reached a 30-year low of 11.4%. It now stands at 16%. Ten percent of whites and 28% of blacks over 65 years old are below the 1996 poverty threshold of $7,740 annual income (Table 14-4 has a more extensive breakdown of poverty guidelines).

Although the number of white elders living in poverty has gradually decreased, the number of children and ethnic elders in poverty continues to grow. Categorically, persons over 65 years of age who suffer the worst poverty are elderly black* women. Regionally, Hispanics in the Northeast and blacks in the Midwest are the poorest, contrary to the popular assumption that blacks are poorest in the South (Table 14-3). The most unfortunate are children under age 18 (22.7% in poverty) and particularly black children (46.1%) (U.S. Bureau of the Census, 1995). Frequently, in the poorest families the Social Security benefits of the elderly widow residing with the family sustain them economically and contribute to the survival of the group (Waehrer and Crystal, 1995).

Poverty rates among very old women living alone have remained high in the last 3 decades. Women living with a spouse or family have far lower rates of poverty. It is thought that the high poverty rates are caused not only by income differences between cohorts of women but also by their increasing longevity and propensity to live alone; at present, 40.2% of those females over 65 years of age live alone (U.S. Bureau of the Census, 1995). Nurses must be alert to the fact that very old women who have been living alone may suffer the results of lengthy economic deprivation. Health care may be delayed until an emergency occurs, and nutrition may be inadequate. Neglect of health care is only a part of the picture; only half receive any kind of means-tested assistance. Often they are unaware that they qualify. The older one becomes, especially if female, the more likely she or he is to sink deeper into poverty.

Social Security and SSI. Our Social Security plan was developed during the height of the Great Depression, when poverty and unrest were rampant in the United States. It was designed as an insurance trust fund with benefits based upon a retired worker's contributions. It was meant to provide minimal sustenance for those over 64 years of age at a time when the average life expectancy did not extend very far beyond that. Over the years the purposes of the Social Security Trust Fund have been expanded to provide old age and survivors insurance, disability income, and partial subsidies of hospital insurance for Medicare Part A and supplementary medical insurance for Medicare Part B. The principal goal of Social Security is to provide economic protections, through payroll contributions, for the retired, disabled, and bereaved. There is a $60 billion surplus now in the fund (Quinn, 1996).

In 1995 Social Security was established for the first time as a separate agency apart from the umbrella of the United States Department of Health and Human Services. Shirley Chater, a nurse, was appointed as its head. This seperation ensures that trust funds for Social Security will remain in that trust rather than being used for other purposes. At

---

*Statistical tables issued by the U.S. Bureau of the Census use the category "blacks," not African-Americans.

Table 14-3   Persons below Poverty Level, by Selected Characteristics: 1993

[Persons as of **March 1994.** Based on Current Population Survey.]

Age and region	Number below poverty level (1,000)				Percent below poverty level			
	All races*	White	Black	Hispanic†	All races*	White	Black	Hispanic†
Total	39,265	26,226	10,877	8,126	15.1	12.2	33.1	30.6
Under 18 years old	15,727	9,752	5,125	3,873	22.7	17.8	46.1	40.9
18 to 24 years old	4,854	3,274	1,264	1,047	19.1	16.0	34.4	31.0
25 to 34 years old	5,804	3,885	1,556	1,279	13.8	11.3	28.4	25.4
35 to 44 years old	4,415	3,001	1,156	879	10.6	8.7	23.0	23.8
45 to 54 years old	2,522	1,776	586	446	8.5	7.0	19.2	20.2
55 to 59 years old	1,057	742	254	154	9.9	8.0	23.6	20.6
60 to 64 years old	1,129	857	233	151	11.3	9.7	24.4	24.4
65 years old and over ...	3,755	2,939	702	297	12.2	10.7	28.0	21.4
Northeast	6,839	4,817	1,744	1,527	13.3	11.0	31.2	37.3
Midwest	8,172	5,454	2,413	476	13.4	10.3	35.9	26.5
South	15,375	8,876	6,063	2,349	17.1	12.8	33.6	28.0
West	8,879	7,080	658	3,774	15.6	14.6	25.9	30.7

From US Bureau of the Census: *Statistical Abstract of the United States: 1995,* ed 115, Washington, DC, 1995.
*Includes other races not shown separately. †Persons of Hispanic origin may be of any race.
Source U.S. Bureau of the Census, *Current Population Reports,* P60-188, and unpublished data.

present there are numerous plans proposed to ensure the long-range integrity of the system as the cohort of the baby boomers will soon reach the age to be drawing benefits. Social Security reform options include reducing or eliminating cost-of-living increases (COLA), removing or adjusting the taxable ceiling, increasing the payroll tax, allowing individuals to invest a portion of their assets in private market funds for later Social Security benefits, computing benefits over 38 rather than 35 years, taxing benefits like private pensions, and gradually increasing the eligible retirement age (Kingson, 1995; Quinn, 1996). The resolution will probably include elements of several of these proposals.

Although Social Security benefits are entitlements and not categorical aids, there is a factor of means assessment and certain inequities exist, particularly for women. The average monthly benefit in 1996 was $720 for a retired worker. Persons with low lifetime incomes receive more proportionately than those with higher incomes. Widows' benefits range from 71½% to 100% of the deceased husband's benefit, depending on age and disability. In addition, calculations of benefits are based on a formula applied to the previous 35 years of work. Clearly, housewives who entered the workforce after children were raised will be penalized for numerous zero wage years in the calculation formula.

In 1994, 26.4 million retired workers and 10 million other adults and children received Old Age Survivors Insurance (OASI) benefits totaling $279.1 billion. Wives who have worked may receive their own benefits or 50% of the amount their husbands receive, whichever is the greater sum. If they opt for the second choice, their own benefits are forfeited. A widow over 60 years old may collect her husband's benefits, prorated according to how long he collected them, or 100% of his benefits if he dies before retirement age. If she has been receiving her own benefits, she may continue receiving them if they are larger than the widow's benefits would be. On remarriage there are three choices: (1) to continue her own benefits, (2) to receive benefits based on those of her dead husband, or (3) to receive benefits based on those of her new husband. Benefit reduction rules applying to the newly married over 60 years of age have been eliminated. Divorcees over 62 years of age are allowed to collect Social Security based on their former husband's earnings if they were married for at least 10 years (U.S. Department of Health and Human Services, 1994).

Those individuals age 65 through 69 who attempt to supplement their Social Security income by working must be aware that of every $3 earned over $11,520 annually (1996 figure), $1 will be deducted from Social Security benefits. For those individuals under 65 years old it is $1 of every $2 earned. However, after age 70 individuals may earn as much as they wish with no deduction from Social Security benefits. Because the government wishes to encourage individuals to continue working and apply later for Social Security benefits, there will be gradual increases in exempt earnings. By 2002 the exclusion will be raised to $30,000 (American Nurses' Association, 1996). It is required that annual income reports be sent to the Social Security Administration to verify earnings and the accuracy of benefit calculations.

An aged person who is dissatisfied with rulings from the Social Security Administration may challenge benefit allotments by contacting the Bureau of Hearings and Appeals of the Social Security Administration. This must be done within 60 days after receiving notice of a decision. Information about this procedure can be obtained from the local Social

	Poverty guideline		
Size of family unit	**48 contiguous states and the District of Columbia***	**Alaska**	**Hawaii**
1	$7,740	$9,660	$8,910
2	10,360	12,940	11,920
3	12,980	16,220	14,930
4	15,600	19,500	17,940
5	18,220	22,780	20,950
6	20,840	26,060	23,960
7	23,460	29,340	26,970
8	26,080	32,620	29,980

Table 14-4   1996 Poverty Guidelines

Modified from *Federal Register* 61(43) p. 8286, Mar 4, 1996.
*For family units with more than 8 members, add $2.620 for each additional member. (The same increment applies to smaller family sizes also, as can be seen in the figures above.)

Security office listed in United States Government section of the phone book. Unusual amounts received should be reported; when an error is discovered, the Social Security office will deduct it from future payments or ask that it be returned.

Supplemental Security Income (SSI). This income is provided through the Social Security Trust Fund for the blind, aged, or disabled with inadequate resources. The average monthly benefit was $642 in 1993, and in addition, these individuals are covered by Medicare regardless of age. Aged people may qualify for SSI in addition to or in lieu of Social Security benefits. Eligibility varies from one state to another, as do allowances and retention of personal assets. Individuals should be encouraged to contact their local Social Security office if they believe it is possible they qualify.

Social Security and SSI may be inadequate, but they are reliable. One is assured of a certain amount of money each month. There is security in that. Social Security and SSI checks arrive quite dependably on the third day of each month. This can be a cause of insecurity as well. Aged people often proceed to the bank immediately after their check arrives. In any large urban area a number of checks are stolen from mailboxes or from the recipients on their way to or from the bank. To avoid this some have their checks mailed to the bank and deposited directly into their accounts. This is a wise idea because it saves time and is much safer. Those who wish to follow this plan should contact their bank, savings and loan, or credit union and ask for a direct deposit form (SF-1199) to authorize direct deposits.

Persons who do not use direct deposit should be advised to endorse checks only at the teller's window in the bank. The treasury department can issue substitute federal benefit checks to replace lost, stolen, or destroyed checks without generally requiring statements of indemnity. This regulation affects checks issued under the Social Security, SSI, and Aid to Families with Dependent Children programs. A statement of indemnity will be required only if the check exceeds $1000 or there is reason to suspect fraud.

Social Security has functioned well for the purpose it was intended and is currently reported to be financially sound. Aged persons are advised to contact their Social Security office (listed in the telephone directory under U.S. Government, Department of Health and Human Services) at least 1 year before they plan to retire, since benefits will not be processed immediately or automatically.

Private Pension Plans. Forty-eight percent of working women and 54% of working men in the age bracket from 45 to 64 years have pension plan coverage (U.S. Bureau of the Census, 1995). These figures have diminished slightly in the last 5 years, perhaps because of downsizing in many corporations. However, recent passage of legislation to ensure portability of retirement packages and health coverage will increase the potential for retaining these important benefits. Problems occur when Social Security and pensions are linked together and when direct Social Security benefits are offset in the private pension formula. In these plans the pension benefit paid by the private employer is directly reduced by some percentage of the Social Security benefits received. Business people are therefore concerned that Social Security reductions will increase private pension costs and that the private pension benefits will be expected to mitigate against the effects of Social Security reductions. Additional discussion can be found in Chapter 20.

Private pensions do not necessarily increase if one works after 65 years of age. The 1974 Employment Retirement Income Security Act (ERISA) exempts employers from crediting time worked after 65 years of age. ERISA, despite some deficiencies, made it possible for the future aged to have some confidence in their pension plans; however, many of the present aged are suffering the results of pension system abuse such as the following:

1. Underfunding: company controls system in which vested liabilities exceed pension plan assets.
2. Minimum age of retirement: employee may be forced to quit before the time and forfeit all retirement benefits.

3. Portability: transferring from one location to another within a company or to another company may threaten pension benefits already earned.
4. Overfunding: companies accumulate much more money than accrued vested benefits.
5. Corporation mergers: company downsizes to increase corporate profit returns, or there are insufficient benefit transfers.

In all these cases the employee may be taken advantage of and legal action accomplishes little; often the particular company is bankrupt or no longer in existence. Pension plans have been under investigation and legislative reform since ERISA established an office of Employee Benefits Security under the aegis of the U.S. Department of Labor. Many private pension plans were not reliable. Factors such as company instability, poor investment of pension funds, job layoffs, and mismanagement of programs resulted in no pensions for many workers who had contributed throughout their working years. Though these abuses will not continue, there are present retirees suffering from them.

Harvey was a lumber company manager for one of the nationally known companies in the Northwest. He had worked his way up through the ranks by his knowledge of mill management. His expertise was troubleshooting; he could bring a faltering mill operation back into full production and produce a profit. When the lumber industry began to falter in the 1980s, he was transferred within the company to a mill that was soon sold. He was then given a 30-day option to retire and accept severance pay or stay with the new company. The legal machinations of the powerful company had not given him a clear idea of what was transpiring. It soon became evident to him he was to forfeit his pension benefits of 20 years and that had been the intent of the company when they abruptly transferred him. Harvey and several other midlevel executives in similar situations within various companies have been in litigation for several years. Many similar cases are now in the courts.

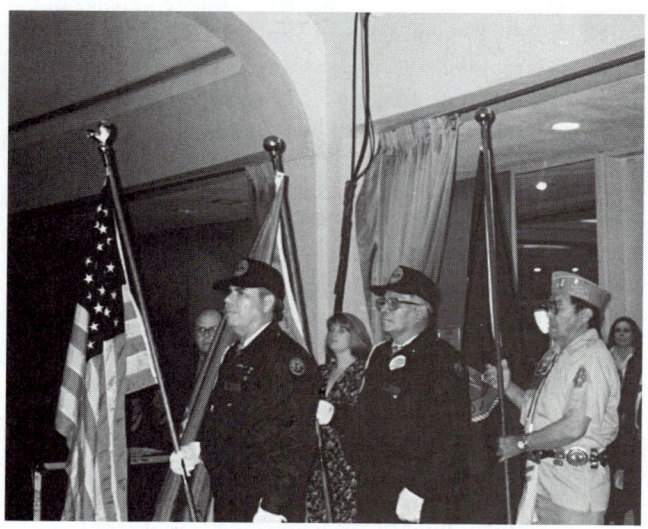

Recognizing veterans. (Courtesy Priscilla Ebersole.)

Women and pensions. The Economic Equity Act, a package of bills aimed at reducing pension discrimination against women, is a beginning but does not address the biggest factors that often keep women from having adequate retirement incomes. The pension legislation contained in the Employment Equity Act has resulted in nondiscrimination clauses being instituted by several major pension benefit purveyors. Of course, they never intended to discriminate against women, but because women lived longer, it seemed reasonable to calculate benefit actuarial tables on expected life span.

Another problem is that pension participants often must choose whether or not to elect survivor benefits for the spouse. The monthly benefit will be reduced considerably if they choose survivor benefits. Many widows do not find out about their lack of pension rights until after the funeral of their spouse. Mary and Bill were an exception. They discussed this issue thoroughly, and because both were healthy and planning an early retirement, they decided to select the greater pension retirement option. Unfortunately, Bill unexpectedly died of a massive heart attack, and Mary received none of his pension benefits. The choice they made had seemed the best at the time, but it made a difficult future for Mary, who at 49 years old could look forward to a future of low-paying jobs with minimal benefits until she could retire at 62 by drawing upon her husband's Social Security benefits or her own, whichever was the larger.

Veterans' Benefits. Pensions and compensation for the veterans of our wars has become a major fiscal responsibility, totaling $16.3 billion in 1994. Although the costs of benefits to our aged veterans are an obligation that most of society fully accepts, the increasing costs of providing adequately for veterans' old age, pensions, and health care are becoming grave concerns. Nearly 8 million World War II veterans and 1.5 million Korean War veterans are now over 65 years old. However, the number of World War II veterans receiving compensation for disabilities (731,000) is only slightly higher than the number with disabilities (694,000) from the Vietnam War (U.S. Bureau of the Census, 1995).

Multiple Pensions. In annual income, many elders are faring very well with Social Security, veterans' pensions, and private pensions. These have been dubbed "double dippers" because they dip twice from the public trough. The "dippies," a term attributed by Neal Cutler (1992) to Richard Rose of Scotland, are the two-earner couples with double benefits and double pensions. An example would be that of a husband and wife, who both retired at 62 years of age, both with veterans' pensions, both receiving Social Security benefits, and both having state or federal pensions from 20 years of civil service work following their 20 years in the United States military service. In addition, they have access to veterans' medical benefits and state-sponsored HMO benefits. Many question whether our system can afford to maintain people in such relative comfort for a possible 20 or 30 years of retirement from the workforce. Most serious are the projections for the future as the baby boom generation enters fully into the entitlement programs in about the year 2020. These situations are being scrutinized carefully given the present budget constraints, national expenditures, and national debt.

Tax-Deferred Funds. Individuals are increasingly setting aside current income in deferred tax accounts to reduce present taxable income and save for the retirement years. More than 40% of persons employed for pay between the ages of 55 and 59 years old (peak earning years for most) are using this method of planning for retirement income. Although this method has gained popularity, there are some risks: inflation will reduce the purchasing power of the money when it is withdrawn, accounts may be as vulnerable to mismanagement and misappropriation as pension funds, the tax base when the individual withdraws funds and pays the deferred tax may be considerably higher than it is now, and there are restrictions and penalties on withdrawing funds before age 59½.

Goods and Services

Senior centers, nutrition sites, senior discounts on numerous goods and services, surplus foods, food stamps, homemakers, and family caregiving are a few of the items that increase the buying power of the elderly. However, throughout the United States there are great discrepancies in the costs of goods and services in relation to income. Fixed incomes that have no adjustment for geographic location put some people in jeopardy. One person may live in abject poverty in a central city hotel, while another may manage nicely on the same income in a "mother-in-law" apartment located in the Midwest. The overall average annual expenditures can be seen in Table 14-5. Housing, fuel, and health care are the major expenditures of the aged and of others as well.

Business is sensitive to market trends. It creates products and advertising aimed at the population most likely to spend money. Marketing departments of many companies are increasingly responding to the affluence and militancy of the over-65 segment of the nation and the purchasing behaviors of aged consumers. When designing packages for older consumers such elements as size, typeface, design layout, color-ground relationships, and ease of opening may be important in making decisions. Many elders find the packaging of foods extremely frustrating, since they can be difficult and sometimes impossible to open. Labels with nutritional information that can be easily read and understood will assist older shoppers to choose foods wisely. Elderly shoppers who are alert and cost conscious may find shopping a source of pleasure and recreation when their particular needs are taken into consideration.

Changes in Expenditure Patterns of Retirees. The last two decades show significant increases in health care and leisure expenditures but less for food, apparel, and charitable contributions (Nieswiadomy and Rubin, 1995). Expenditures and average income of all consumers over 65 is notable because over one third of income is spent on housing. At age 75 the total annual average expenditures exceeds income before taxes (U.S. Bureau of the Census, 1995). Although the median income of those over 65 years of age is $17,751, the average annual expenditures are $21,322. Quite obviously, many retirees are drawing upon assets and undoubtedly hoping these will outlive them. The out-of-pocket health expenditures for retirees and nonretirees are equitable when considering costs of insurance premiums and medical goods and services (Rubin et al, 1995).

Economics are extremely complex, and even the experts often disagree. Our point in discussing them is to orient nurses to some of the issues elders face and to increase awareness in a general sense to the numerous factors that contribute to an economically comfortable old age. Nursing functions in respect to the budgets of elders might include discussion and provision of access to resource materials for those who wish to have guidance. The Area Agency on Aging and most senior centers have resource guides to discounts for various goods and services to the aged. It is also useful for the nurse to have a general understanding of the goods and services aged clients use. Most important is a discussion with the client of their priorities when spending. One old gentleman on a limited budget was willing to forgo many small luxuries in order to buy a season ticket to the opera. Another elder spent a much larger portion of her monthly income than the recommended 40% in order to live in an exclusive high-rise apartment. These individuals choices contributed to their quality of life and must be respected even though not fitting a typical profile.

Intergenerational Equity

Concern over the public and private cost of providing a reasonable subsistence compatible with health and decency for increasing numbers of elderly persons within our society has generated much discussion about the impact on the working population and on youth. The dependency ratio in a society is based on the demographics of age and work; however, there are other factors to consider. Projections for the future dependency ratio are unreliable because several elements may affect them drastically: the elevated retirement age policies enacted in 1977 may induce many older persons to work longer, and, on the other hand, if a great number of people decide to retire early, the dependency ratio could double. Conflict between the generations in the midst of tight budgets and a large federal deficit has received attention in the media. Some believe the aged are receiving more than their share of the economic pie at the expense of younger persons. It is too easy to be misled by this approach and believe that the solution lies in taking from one group and giving to another.

In reality, the ratio of children under 18 years of age to the number of working adults is continually decreasing. The

Table 14-5   Average Annual Expenditures of All Consumer Units, by Race and Age of Householder: 1993

[In dollars. Based on Consumer Expenditure Survey. Data are averages for the noninstitutional population. Expenditures reported here are out-of-pocket]

Item	All consumer units	White and other	Black	Age Under 25 yrs	25 to 34 yrs	35 to 44 yrs	45 to 54 yrs	55 to 64 yrs	65 yrs and over
Expenditures, Total	**30,692**	**31,967**	**20,684**	**17,468**	**28,594**	**37,429**	**41,020**	**32,973**	**21,322**
Food..........................	4,399	4,517	3,399	2,631	4,170	5,360	5,485	4,638	3,245
Food at home	2,735	2,772	2,421	1,339	2,519	3,336	3,212	2,897	2,344
Cereals and bakery products	434	444	348	206	392	544	522	434	375
Cereals and cereal products	160	161	151	86	153	206	200	143	127
Bakery products	274	283	196	119	239	338	322	292	248
Meats, poultry, fish, and eggs	734	720	862	337	636	892	876	844	629
Beef	234	234	238	110	209	287	273	278	190
Pork	154	148	200	66	130	185	178	180	142
Other meats	98	97	101	41	84	116	120	120	81
Poultry	131	127	169	61	114	166	163	135	110
Fish and seafood	87	84	118	42	70	104	109	99	79
Eggs	30	29	35	16	29	34	34	32	28
Dairy products	295	307	193	141	283	368	333	304	251
Fresh milk and cream	128	132	93	65	125	164	139	127	107
Other dairy products	167	175	100	77	158	204	194	177	144
Fruits and vegetables	444	450	387	186	387	509	518	470	451
Fresh fruits	137	140	108	46	110	158	165	151	146
Fresh vegetables	132	135	107	52	113	150	159	143	134
Processed fruits	96	97	86	49	93	109	105	92	96
Processed vegetables	79	78	86	40	71	92	89	84	75
Other food at home	827	850	631	469	821	1,023	962	845	639
Nonalcoholic beverages	225	230	181	126	203	288	281	228	169
Food away from home	1,664	1,746	978	1,293	1,651	2,024	2,273	1,741	901
Alcoholic beverages	268	288	98	304	307	324	293	250	148
Housing	9,636	9,928	7,341	5,297	9,683	12,005	12,027	9,683	6,908
Shelter	5,415	5,585	4,106	3,297	5,794	7,002	6,744	5,017	3,440
Owned dwellings	3,331	3,559	1,585	424	2,719	4,804	4,803	3,583	2,197
Mortgage interest and charges	1,878	2,001	936	300	1,900	3,301	2,818	1,633	417
Property taxes	825	886	359	73	471	912	1,204	1,115	883
Maintenance, repair, insurance, other	628	672	290	50	348	592	782	835	896
Rented dwellings	1,714	1,625	2,395	2,678	2,857	1,817	1,297	929	966
Other lodging	370	402	126	196	219	380	643	505	278
Utilities, fuels and public services	2,112	2,121	2,048	1,082	1,886	2,351	2,580	2,425	1,920
Natural gas	279	274	318	110	223	295	329	342	302
Electricity	836	845	769	389	727	947	1,046	963	754
Fuel oil and other fuels	99	106	46	13	69	97	118	118	133
Telephone	658	650	719	512	687	734	782	707	484
Water and other public services	241	247	196	58	180	277	304	295	247

From US Bureau of the Census: *Statistical Abstract of the United States: 1995,* ed 115, Washington, DC, 1995.
Source U.S. Bureau of Labor Statistics, *Consumer Expenditures in 1993;* and unpublished data.

poverty rate for children is higher than for the aged, but we must remember that the aged are not taking resources from the children. Children are poor because of the increasing number of female-headed households, increasing number of adolescent pregnancies, fluctuating levels of unemployment, variations in economic conditions, cuts in essential federal programs for children and needy families, and the continuing imbalance in female wages as compared to those of males.

Bengtson (1992) adds the confounding factor of the transfer of an estimated $7 trillion of assets to the middle aged on the deaths of their parents (the present generation of elders) to the equation of dependency. This complicates the predictions and tends to balance the picture of generational inequity that seems to appear when examining only Social Security and taxes. Numerous policy changes are being proposed in response to the realistic concerns of the baby boomers as they begin to seriously approach old age. Pitting the young against the old is a divisive tactic, often meant to obscure the real issues. Fundamental changes in national priorities are necessary.

Item	All consumer units	White and other	Black	Age					
				Under 25 yrs	25 to 34 yrs	35 to 44 yrs	45 to 54 yrs	55 to 64 yrs	65 yrs and over
Expenditures, Total, cont'd									
Household operations	469	496	256	156	514	671	408	377	433
Personal services	228	238	148	113	402	408	106	85	100
Other household expenses	241	258	109	43	112	263	302	292	333
Housekeeping supplies	410	427	263	161	356	458	537	424	396
Household furnishings and equipment ...	1,230	1,299	667	600	1,133	1,524	1,758	1,439	718
Household textiles	102	107	66	21	67	126	160	106	94
Furniture	317	325	257	224	368	402	426	302	144
Floor coverings	87	94	34	14	69	91	140	163	40
Major appliances	143	150	88	73	112	171	174	191	118
Small appliances, misc. housewares ...	87	93	40	43	71	114	103	107	68
Miscellaneous household equipment ...	493	530	182	225	445	620	755	570	254
Apparel and services	1,676	1,681	1,638	1,198	1,752	2,071	2,200	1,695	937
Men and boys	426	437	334	274	457	574	551	410	203
Women and girls	658	658	662	332	566	828	883	749	456
Children under 2 years old	79	77	103	104	166	78	61	47	20
Footwear	249	244	292	248	257	289	327	236	142
Other apparel products and services ...	264	266	247	241	307	302	377	253	116
Transportation	5,453	5,759	3,092	3,948	5,099	6,651	7,479	6,340	3,081
Vehicle purchases (net outlay)	2,319	2,493	981	2,139	2,146	2,847	3,104	2,833	1,137
Cars and trucks, new	1,216	1,328	349	1,077	1,023	1,427	1,752	1,665	577
Cars and trucks, used	1,079	1,137	631	1,053	1,069	1,388	1,329	1,151	560
Gasoline and motor oil	977	1,017	666	652	960	1,199	1,299	1,069	589
Other vehicle expenses	1,843	1,932	1,154	1,008	1,711	2,272	2,622	2,032	1,129
Vehicle finance charges	244	254	172	154	282	331	345	256	72
Maintenance and repair	620	649	396	368	560	781	833	685	404
Vehicle insurance	678	711	422	364	598	767	964	773	500
Rent, lease, licenses, other	301	319	164	123	270	393	480	318	153
Public transportation	314	317	291	148	282	333	453	406	225
Health care	1,776	1,890	894	349	1,128	1,673	1,817	2,176	2,733
Entertainment	1,626	1,734	772	910	1,511	2,094	2,490	1,527	918
Personal care products and services	385	393	310	228	358	455	478	384	323
Reading	166	177	83	72	137	191	212	197	150
Education	455	475	305	907	270	438	1,114	209	107
Tobacco products and smoking supplies ..	268	277	198	202	280	324	345	316	141
Miscellaneous	715	751	434	266	646	898	893	921	503
Cash contributions	961	1,029	436	95	465	811	1,473	1,301	1,292
Personal insurance and pensions	2,908	3,067	1,685	1,061	2,787	4,133	4,716	3,336	837
Life and other personal insurance	399	414	284	56	229	431	717	579	302
Pensions and Social Security	2,509	2,653	1,401	1,006	2,558	3,702	3,999	2,757	535
Personal Taxes	**2,978**	**3,173**	**1,413**	**873**	**2,701**	**4,127**	**5,138**	**3,318**	**1,110**

HEALTH CARE

The most important issues on the political scene according to a Kaiser/Harvard survey of voters were health care (33%), crime (29%), and taxes (23%) (American Association of Homes and Services for the Aging, 1996). National health expenditures reached $949.4 billion in 1994 (U.S. Department of Health and Human Services, 1996). Private consumer outlay for health care has risen from $41.8 billion in 1970 to $484.3 billion in 1993, of which $296.1 billion was paid in insurance premiums (U.S. Health Care Financing Administration, 1995). Health care respresents 13.9% of the gross domestic product (GDP) and an average of $3,510 per capita (U.S. Department of Health and Human Services, 1995) (Figures 14-2 and 14-3).

This enormous rise in health care costs has occurred while more than 40 million of our citizens have no health care available to them. However, the annual percentage increase in health care costs has been halved, from 15% in 1980 to 7.8% in 1993. From 1980 to 1994 the out-of-pocket expenditures for health care declined 2% for hospital care,

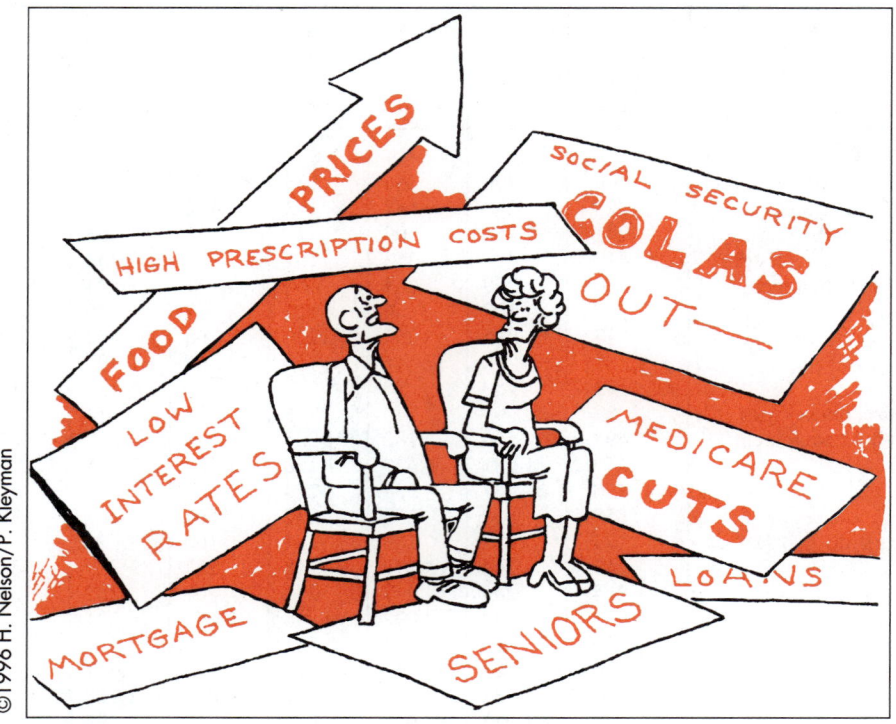

©1996 H. Nelson/P. Kleyman

"I wish we could afford to be greedy geezers."

Figure 14-1. Greedy geezers. (From *Aging today* 17[4], p. 3, July/Aug 1996.)

5% for nursing home care, and 13% for physician services. In 1983 7% of Medicare beneficiaries were enrolled in HMOs, and by 1995 this had increased to 18% (U.S. Department of Health and Human Services, 1996). This percentage is rapidly rising.

Health care heads the list of economic considerations in old age. It is the one item that judicious planning and careful consideration can do little to control. Admittedly, lifestyle changes and self-care have become popular ideas and can improve health status over time, but, realistically, most elders have accrued the dividends from decades of healthy or unhealthy habits and now are the main consumers of health care.

The chaos of the health care system and the insistent pressure to fit everyone into the mold of managed care has greatly altered the care of the aged. The 8-minute average visit, the gold standard of managed care, hardly allows time for writing the six prescriptions that are the average for elders. Some elders have steadfastly refused to be coerced into these capitated models and remain loyal to the private health care providers outside HMOs (Archer, 1996). However, serious problems are occurring for these traditional Medicare recipients. Most care is now provided on an outpatient basis. Medicare Part B ostensibly covers 80% of care after the first $100 deductible each year. Hospitals providing same-day service frequently charge much more than the Medicare-approved reimbursement amount; the client pays the difference, which sometimes amounts to as much as 50% of the

charges. Secretary of Health and Human Sevices Donna Shalala says the client's copayment will likely rise to 70% by the year 2000. Congress says it cannot limit what hospitals charge for outpatient services, but they definitely limit how much Medicare will pay (San Francisco Examiner, 1996).

Health care in the United States has been under scrutiny for all the years since it was realized that Medicare had no brakes (Figure 14-4). In 1955, before Medicare, there were nearly 7000 hospitals in the United States, and the occupancy rate was 85%. These figures have consistently dropped each year since, though the population of the United States has increased enormously. Now there are less than 6400 hospitals, and the occupancy rate is about 66% (U.S. Bureau of the Census, 1995).

Overall, Medicare paid slightly less than half the health care expenses for elderly persons. Most Medicare beneficiaries supplement their Medicare coverage with privately purchased Medigap policies.

Average per capita personal health care costs are difficult to estimate since they are not inclusive. For example, the Department of Health and Human Services statistics exclude the cost of nonprescription drugs, nursing home care, and health insurance premiums. No figures include the cost of transportation for medical care. From various reports it appears annual health care expenditures of the aged are about $3000, or two and one-half times the national average. About 37% of personal health care costs are out-of-pocket.

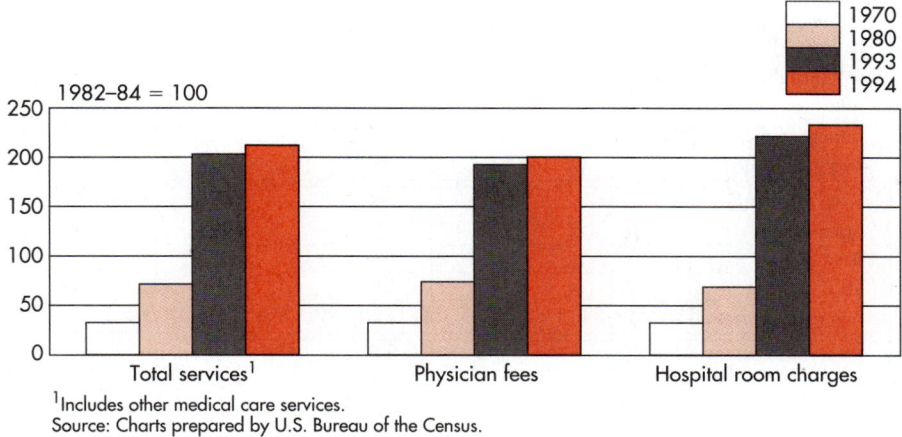

Figure 14-2. Consumer price indexes—medical services: 1970 to 1994. (From *Statistical Abstract, 1995.*)

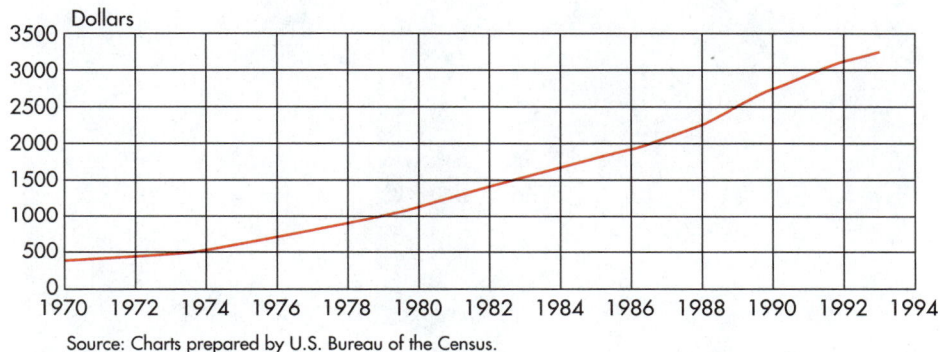

Figure 14-3. Personal health care expenditures per capita: 1970 to 1993. (From *Statistical Abstract, 1995.*)

Almost 30% of the total personal health care expenditures are made by the aged, although they comprise only 12.6% of the population. Those over 75 years of age have spent an average of 15.7% of their annual budget on health care during the years 1985-1993 (U.S. Bureau of the Census, 1995). Costs have increased an average of 10% annually in those years. Hospital charges and physicians' fees have tripled in that time, and home health charges have increased 1000%. In 1993 49.6% of hospital charges for individuals over 65 were reimbursed, a drop from 70% in 1980 (U.S. Bureau of the Census, 1995). The fastest growing expenditures today are for home health and skilled nursing care. In general, health care costs have not risen as sharply in recent years; beneficiaries are paying a larger share, and 40 million citizens are uninsured.

Medicare and Medicaid

In 1965 the Social Security Act was amended to provide Medicare (Title XVIII) and Medicaid (Title XIX). Medicare was meant to provide medical care to the elderly regardless

of their financial situation. Medicaid was designed to defray expenses for those who could not meet the cost of Medicare contributions or who exhausted their Medicare benefits. Medicaid, however, was left to individual state's discretion; therefore it varies in coverage nationwide. Almost all aged persons receive either Medicare or Medicaid benefits.

Medicare is a major payer in the U.S. health care system, accounting for 28% of all hospital and 20% of all physician payments. It also covers 45% of health care spending for the elderly overall (National Academy on Aging, 1995). Five percent of Medicare beneficiaries incur 50% of the costs, and 10% incur 70% of the costs (Rini, 1996). The greatest inadequacies in Medicare are for the most common needs of the aged: hearing aids, eyeglasses, medications, and long-term care. Comparisons of Medicare and Medicaid are shown in Table 14-6.

Medicare. Medicare was instituted as a federally administered universal health insurance program for people over 65 years of age and disabled people under 65 years of age. Medicare has two parts: Part A is designed as hospital

Payments* ($bil)	1967	1975	1985	1995**	2005**
HI (Part A)	3.0	10.5	42.3	110.2	240.0
SMI (Part B)	1.3	4.0	21.6	64.0	209.3
Total	4.2	14.5	63.8	174.2	449.3
Total as % GDP	0.52	0.92	1.58	2.45	3.70
Avg growth/year: 1967-75: 17%; 1975-85: 16%; 1985-95: 11%; 1995-2005: 10%					

Enrollment (mil)	1967	1975	1985	1995*	2005*
Aged	19.5	22.8	28.2	33.3	35.3
Disabled	—	2.2	2.9	3.9	6.8
Total	19.5	25.0	31.1	36.2	42.1
Avg growth/year: 1967-75: 3%; 1975-1985: 2%; 1985-1995: 2%; 1995-2005: 2%					

$ per enrollee	217	583	2,055	4,818	10,677
Adj for CPI	217	362	638	1,066	1,645

*Not including administrative costs. **Projected.

Figure 14-4. Medicare growth. (*Facts on Medicare and supplementary insurance,* National Academy on Aging, A Policy Institute of the Gerontological Society of America, October, 1995.)

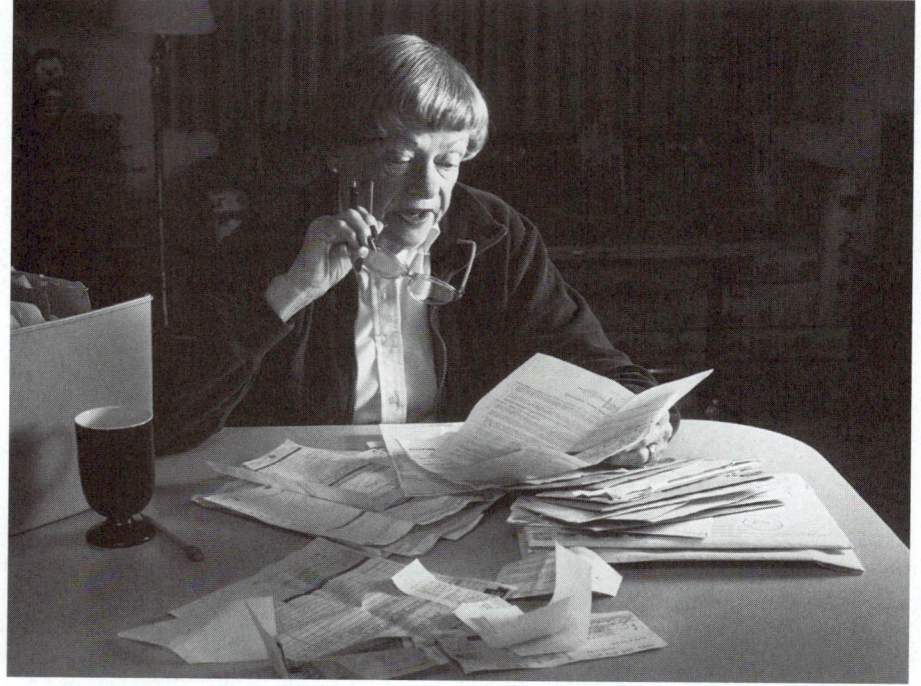

Filling out forms. (Courtesy Rod Schmall.)

insurance, and Part B covers physician and certain outpatient service fees. As of January 1996, Medicare Part B Supplementary Medical Insurance monthly premiums were $42.50 monthly, and Part A, Hospital Insurance, is financed through a dedicated payroll tax on current workers and partially financed by current beneficiaries (Rini, 1996). Hospitalization requires a $736 deductible payment and step increases in copayments after the sixty-first day of hospitalization (Legal Eye Newsletter, 1995).

Most people do not pay monthly premiums directly for Parts A and B because premiums are deducted from the monthly Social Security check. If one is covered by both Parts A and B, there are still many exceptions. Each year all Social Security recipients receive a booklet explaining the many exclusions and complexities in the Medicare reimbursement system. It is very difficult for the average person to determine what he or she will be reimbursed, since there are many confusing and ambiguous statements. Because of gaps in Medicare coverage, prescription drugs, adaptive devices, preventive care, and long-term care are generally not reimbursable.

Claims are handled through specific major insurance companies in each state, which are called carriers. Some of

Table 14-6   Comparisons of Medicare and Medicaid

Health care benefit	Medicare	Medicaid
Hospitalization	Beneficiary pays Part A deductible $736 (1996); Medicare coves almost all hospital expenses for 1st 60 days; Medicare then pays all covered costs but $184/day for days 61-90, and $368 per day for days 91-150; Medicare pays nothing after 150 days.	For low-income persons who are aged, blind, disabled (or members of families with children), inpatient hospital services covered.
SNF Care	Medicare pays all SNF care for first 20 days if beneficiary has been hospitalized for at least 3 days prior to the SNF care; from day 21-100, Medicare pays all but $92/day; after 100 days, Medicare pays nothing.	Covered.
Home Health Care	Medicare covers home health care on part-time or intermittent basis if beneficiaries homebound, in need of skilled nursing care or PT/ST; services must be ordered and regularly reviewed by a physician. Medicare pays 80% of approved amount for durable medical equipment and supplies.	Covered.
Hospice Care	Medicare covers up to 210 days of hospice care for a terminal illness; additional coverage is available if necessary.	Individual states may elect to cover.
Blood	Medicare pays 80% of approved amount (after $100 deductible and starting with 4th pint).	Covered.
Medical Expenses	Beneficiary must meet an annual $100 deductible; then Medicare Part B pays 80% of an amount based on a government fee schedule for physician services. Monthly premiums $42.50	Physician services covered.
Clinical Laboratory Services	Medicare pays 100% of approved amount.	Laboratory and x-ray services covered.
Outpatient Hospital Services	Unlimited if medically necessary; beneficiary pays 20% of billed amount after $100 annual deductible.	Covered.
Services of Special Practitioners	Medicare Part B helps pay for covered services from certain specially qualified practitioners who are not physicians: certified nurse anesthetist, certified nurse midwife, clinical psychologist, clinical social worker, physician assistant, nurse practitioner and clinical nurse specialist in collaboration with a physician.	Nurse practitioner services covered; individual states may elect to cover services of other special practitioners.
Prescription Drugs	Medicare pays only for prescription drugs administered in hospital and in limited outpatient situations. Medicare does not cover most outpatient prescription drugs, but does help pay for: antigens, epoetin alfa, hemophilia clotting factors, immunosuppressive drugs, certain oral cancer drugs.	Individual states may elect to cover prescribed drugs.
Ambulance Service	Medicare Part B helps pay only if transportation in any other vehicle would endanger health, but only to hospital or SNF.	Individual states may elect to cover transportation services.
Outpatient Mental Health	Outpatient mental health treatment limitation—once annual deductible met, Medicare Part B pays only 50% of approved amount.	Individual states may elect to cover.
Inpatient Psychiatric Care	Part A helps pay for no more than 190 days of inpatient psychiatric hospital care (lifetime limit); however, psychiatric care in general hospitals is not subject to this 190-day limit.	Individual states may elect to cover.
Preventive Health Care: Mammography Screenings	Medicare Part B helps pay if provided by a Medicare-approved supplier; every 24 months for a screening mammogram; as needed for diagnosis.	Individual states may elect to cover preventive services.
Pap Smear	Medicare Part B helps pay once every 3 years for Pap smears; helps pay more frequently for certain women at high risk and for diagnostic Pap smears when symptoms present.	Individual states may elect to cover.

From Melillo KD: Medicare and Medicaid: similarities and differences, *J Gerontol Nurs* 22(7):12, 1996.
Source Information from this chart is compiled from the reference list and personal communication with the *Medicare Hotline,* 1-800-638-6833 (February, 1996).   *Continued*

Table 14-6	Comparisons of Medicare and Medicaid—cont'd	
Health care benefit	**Medicare**	**Medicaid**
Immunizations: Pneumococcal pneumonia, Influenza, Hepatitis B	Medicare Part B pays full approved charges for flu and pneumonia vaccines and their administration; neither the $100 annual deductible nor the 20% coinsurance applies; Medicare Part B helps pay for hepatitis B vaccine administered to those considered to be at high or intermediate risk of contracting the disease.	Individual states may elect to cover.
Dental Surgery	Medicare Part A may pay for inpatient hospital stay if hospitalization required because of the severity of a dental procedure.	Medical and surgical services furnished by a dentist are covered.
Routine Dental Services & Dentures	Not covered by Part B, unless a medical problem is more extensive than the teeth or supporting structures.	Individual states may elect to cover.
Services of: Chiropractor	Medicare helps pay for only one kind of treatment furnished by a licensed chiropractor: manual manipulation of the spine to correct a subluxation that is demonstrated by x-ray.	Individual states may elect to cover.
Podiatrist	Medicare helps pay for services to tx injuries and DZs of the foot (ingrown toenails, hammer toe, bunion deformities, heel spurs)	Individual states may elect to cover.
Optometrist	Medicare helps pay for Medicare-covered vision care and cataract glasses/lens after cataract surgery	Individual states may elect to cover.
Vision Exams and Glasses	Not covered by Part B if exam for prescription or fitting eyeglasses	Individual states may elect to cover.
Routine Foot Care	Not covered (cutting or removal of corns or calluses, trimming of nails) unless being treated for DM or PVD.	Individual states may elect to cover.
Hearing Tests and Hearing Aids	Not covered if ear examination is to prescribe or fit hearing aid	Individual states may elect to cover services for persons with hearing disorders.
Long-Term Nursing Home	Medicare Part A helps pay for a maximum of 100 days in each benefit period for SNF care only.	Nursing facility services are covered.
Custodial Care in Nursing Home	Medicare does not pay when care is primarily for the purpose of helping the patient with daily living or meeting personal needs and could be provided safely by people without professional skills or training.	Nursing facility services are covered.
Homemaker Services	Not covered, although homemaker aids may be furnished by a home health agency to a homebound beneficiary if part of a formal plan of treatment.	Home health services are covered; individual states may elect to cover personal care services.
Private Duty Nursing	Not covered.	Individual states may elect to cover.
Routine CPE	Most routine physical examinations and tests related to such exams not covered by Part B.	Individual states may elect to cover screening and preventive services.

these carriers have recently opted out in favor of managed care programs (California Association of Health Facilities, 1996). Copayments, deductibles, and premiums change each year and are burdensome to the poor elderly. Only about one in four of the poor elderly can afford the supplemental insurance necessary to partially cover these gaps and, in spite of their poverty, only one in three obtain Medicaid assistance. Poor elders spend nearly 20% of their total income on out-of-pocket health care expenses (U.S. Government General Accounting Office, 1992). Details about Medicare coverage can be obtained by requesting the *Medicare Handbook* from the Consumer Information Center, Department 59, Pueblo, CO 81009 or from the local Social Security office.

In spite of diagnosis related groups (DRGs), attempts to control physicians' fees, and rampant claims reductions and denials, the cost of the federal Medicare program increased from $109 billion in 1990 to $178 billion in 1995. The Health Care Financing Administration (HCFA) estimated a $345 billion budget in 2002, making it the twelfth largest government budget of any kind in the world (USHCFA, 1995). Schwartz reports that in 1991 20% of Medicare claims were denied outright, and 75% had reduced payment.

An issue that needs to be addressed is the conflict of interest inherent in the Medigap insurance carrier serving as the Medicare fiscal intermediary, as well as the underwriter of the Medigap policy. Some people do not realize that if Medicare payment is delayed or denied the Medigap policy is not obligated to pay either. Medicare has undergone many changes and will continue to do so until we arrive at a realistic and affordable system of providing and financing care.

Clearly some very significant changes are occuring in the Medicare system, though it has been a political football for various pressure groups and will undoubtedly continue to be one (Box 14-1). Suggestions for maintaining the viability of

> **Box 14-1** **Medicare-Related Activities of the Past Decade**
>
> **1981** The Omnibus Budget Reconciliation Act (OBRA) created block grants for some health programs and imposed cutbacks on Medicare benefits.
>
> **1982** The Medicare budget was further cut with the Tax Equity and Fiscal Responsibility Act (TEFRA). This act called for the development of a prospective payment system for Medicare's hospital reimbursements. During the following year, diagnosis-related groups (DRGS) were enacted.
>
> **1983** Hospice services became covered through TEFRA, but a limited number of hospice agencies are certified because the regulations are very strict (e.g., having to provide inpatient care if necessary) and many agencies cannot afford to provide the service. Employers were mandated to offer employees age 65 and older the same health insurance they offer younger employees.
>
> **1984** Congress put a temporary freeze on the Medicare fee reimbursement scale for physicians.
>
> **1986** Employers were mandated to continue health insurance benefits for dismissed employees. That created the potential for discrimination against the hiring of older workers.
>
> **1987** OBRA amendments called for major changes in Medicare provider certification for long-term care facilities. Residents' rights, timely assessments, and mandatory personnel training were some of the major changes.
>
> **1988** Congress enacted a Medicare Catastrophic Coverage Act that protected the elderly from financial ruin. This enactment was considered the most significant expansion of Medicare since the program was created and included prescription coverage and limitations on spousal spend-down.
>
> **1989** The Medicare Catastrophic Coverage Act was repealed. There were conceptual flaws in the Act. One flaw was that the coverage and cost were limited to one group, Medicare beneficiaries, rather than spread across all age groups. There was only minimal coverage for long-term care settings, such as home care and nursing homes.
>
> **1990** The Bipartisan Pepper Commission on Comprehensive Health Care was created. Commission members proposed a solution to the problem of the elderly, the disabled, and all uninsured people's health needs. The plan combined public and private funding and included long-term care reform. Government or social insurance would keep community-based care available and affordable, and nursing home users would be protected against impoverishments. These recommendations did not include specific cost-containment measures.
>
> **1993** National health care proposals resurface again (as in the Johnson era). In addition to the Pepper Commission's proposal, Congressman John J. Rhodes put forward The Incentives Act, and nursing leaders developed an Agenda for Health Care Reform. Both of these proposals addressed long-term care issues, including an emphasis on home and community-based care rather than acute care.
>
> **1995** The Health Care Financing Administration regulates fees for providers, investigated fraud, allowed numerous capitated care plans, and considered benefit reductions.

Adapted from Gale BJ, Steffl BM: The long-term care dilemma: what nurses need to know about medicare, *Nursing Health Care* 13(1), 1992.

the Medicare system include providing vouchers for care, raising the eligibility age limit while creating more relaxed standards for disability qualification above a certain age, and removing age criteria from Medicare entirely while instituting some forms of means testing (Moon, 1995). Moon suggests that changes in Medicare's benefit package would make the most sense if the program were targeted toward those aged 75 and older. However, while all these changes are contemplated, a large mass of Medicare participants are already enrolled in managed care programs. It is imperative nurses know the differences in these programs because they are rapidly proliferating.

Several variations of HMOs are available to Medicare beneficiaries:

Medicare risk HMOs. These are the most popular and least expensive for breadth of health care services. These plans are required by HCFA to provide all of the services ordinarily available through Medicare with the exception of hospice services. Access to physicians and hospitals is limited to the HMO provider network unless a feature called point of service (POS) is included. In those cases beneficiaries may see a physician of their choice but usually will pay more for that option. The word "risk" refers to the financial risk assumed by the provider when costs exceed per capita reimbursement.

Medicare cost HMOs. These are more costly to beneficiaries and companies than risk HMOs because the reimbursement through HCFA is for actual Medicare-approved costs of care, retrospectively. These HMOs are less frequently available through employee health plans because they are more costly than capitated plans.

Medicare eligible preferred provider organizations. These include a very large network of doctors and other providers for beneficiaries to choose from and also offer, for additional cost, the choice of physicians outside the plan (United Seniors Health Cooperative, 1996).

Fundamentals of Medicare that every nurse and elder should be aware of are found in Box 14-2.

Medicaid. Medicaid provides health care insurance to more than 34 million low-income Americans, more than half of whom are poor children. (Twentieth Century Fund, 1995). In contrast to Medicare, Medicaid provides an array of preventive services as well as medical services: eye care, dental care, prescription drugs, physical therapy, hospice care, and rehabilitation services with no out-of-pocket fees, premiums, co-payments, exclusions, or deductibles.

In 1994 7.8 million Medicaid beneficiaries were enrolled in managed care programs, most of whom were poor families. There are questions about whether managed care is suitable for Medicaid recipients because the profit margins for their care would be slimmer than for those of other enrollees. They might be given short shrift, as they were in Florida for a period of time.

Though Medicaid constitutes only 6% of federal budget outlays, concerns about escalating costs have generated plans to move the majority of responsibility to states in the form of federal block grants as opposed to the present method of cost splitting between states and the federal government.

Medicaid is the health care financing program that complements Medicare and at present provides assistance to more than 1 in 10 Americans age 65 and older; the great majority of these are in long-term care situations. Two thirds of all Americans in nursing homes receive assistance from Medicaid. An elderly Medicaid eligible residing in a nursing home costs an average of $38,000 annually. Because home care is generally less expensive and more desirable, all states have received federal waivers allowing them to pay for home and community care for elderly beneficiaries who otherwise would end up in nurisng homes. Nearly 4 million low-income elderly people receive Medicaid assistance, accounting for over one quarter of total Medicaid expenditures (Lyons et al, 1996). Medicaid expenditures averaged nearly $10,000 per elderly beneficiary in 1993 and barely over

---

Box 14-2	**Fundamentals of Medicare**

Medicare Part A

Medicare Part A is designed primarily to partially cover the costs of inpatient hospital care and other specialized care as listed below:

- Acute hospitalization coverage includes costs of semiprivate rooms, meals, nursing services, operating and recovery room, intensive care, drugs, laboratory and radiology fees, blood products, and other necessary medical services and supplies. Certain deductibles must be paid by the patient. These vary each year and increase incrementally as patients are hospitalized beyond 60 days. Most individuals meet these expenses through Medigap policies or HMO membership. Further discussion of these is found later in the chapter in relation to managed care and its development.
- Skilled nursing facility care is covered by Medicare for a maximum of 100 days and then only if the individual has been hospitalized in acute care for a minimum of 3 days within the prior 30 days and only if deemed medically necessary. With the emergence of subacute care in skilled nursing facilities, these rules are likely to change, particularly the requirement for 3-day hospitalization prior to nursing home admission. The patients pay a deductible for each day after 20 days.
- Home health care may be covered by Medicare on an intermittent and/or part-time basis for skilled nursing care, physical therapy, and rehabilitative services; however, chronic disorders requiring custodial care, such as Alzheimer's disease, must be paid out-of-pocket by the patient or caregiver. Cost of care is covered as long as individuals meet Medicare requirements; Medicare pays 80% of the approved amount for durable equipment.
- Hospice care is provided for terminally ill persons expected to live less than 6 months who elect to forgo traditional medical treatment for the terminal illness. Medicare pays for all but limited costs for outpatient drugs and inpatient respite care (U.S. Health Care Financing Administration, 1996).
- Psychiatric care is limited to 190 days of care in a lifetime; partial payment and other limitations apply.

Medicare Part B

Medicare Part B is designed to pick up where Part A leaves off. It pays partially for a wide range of medical services, supplies, and doctor bills:

- Doctor's services, supplies and diagnostic tests, physical and speech therapy, durable medical equipment and other services are included for unlimited periods, deductibles are applied.
- Clinical laboratory services are fully covered if deemed medically necessary.
- Outpatient hospital treatment, blood, and ambulatory surgical services have deductibles of $100 each and patient payment of 20% of charges (Health Care Financing Administration, 1996).

Booklets explaining the details of Medicare are provided annually to all beneficiaries.

$1000 per child. Nearly three quarters of Medicaid spending on the elderly goes to long-term care. Medicaid spent more than $25 billion for long-term care provided in nursing homes during 1993 (U.S. Bureau of the Census, 1995).

Problems with Medicaid that need to be resolved are disproportionately large outlays for elders in nursing homes, dramatic increases in the population over age 85 needing an array of Medicaid services on a continuing basis, and federal legislation requiring costly care in nursing homes (Figure 14-5). In addition, Medicaid eligibility requirements are complicated and cumbersome (Box 14-3).

Nursing home care and Medicaid. Medicare was designed to ensure a basic hospital benefits package, which was well defined. There has been no similar national consensus for a defined package of long-term care and social services. These have been developed at state discretion under the federal guidelines of Title XIX (Medicaid) of the Social Security Act. Long-term care and social services programs are administered locally, and therefore the scope of services, extent of funding by county, state, and federal governments, and eligibility requirements differ from community to community. The result is a maze of services that may be duplicative, of variable quality, and of uncertain durability.

Medicaid and the Veterans Administration are the chief fiduciary agents of long-term institutional care. Medicare reimbursement for nursing home care applies only to a few pa-

tients and then it is of short duration. However, the impact of DRGs of disorders has changed this because many patients requiring subacute care are not placed in nursing homes. Placement is becoming increasingly difficult since some facilities are unable to provide the services required

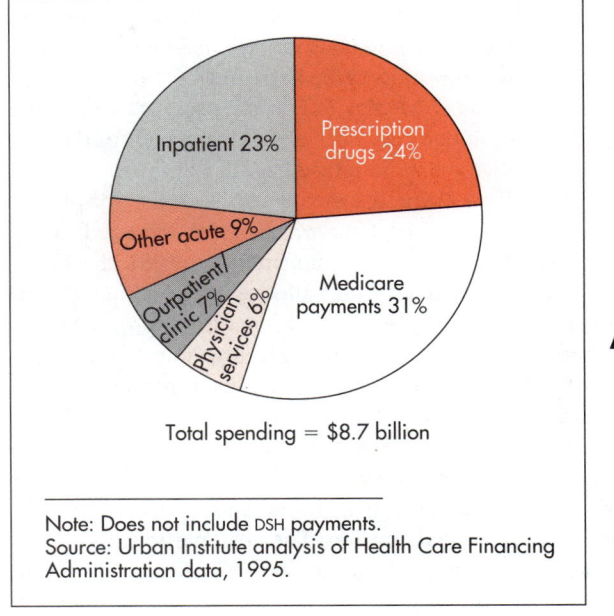

Total spending = $8.7 billion

Note: Does not include DSH payments.
Source: Urban Institute analysis of Health Care Financing Administration data, 1995.

A

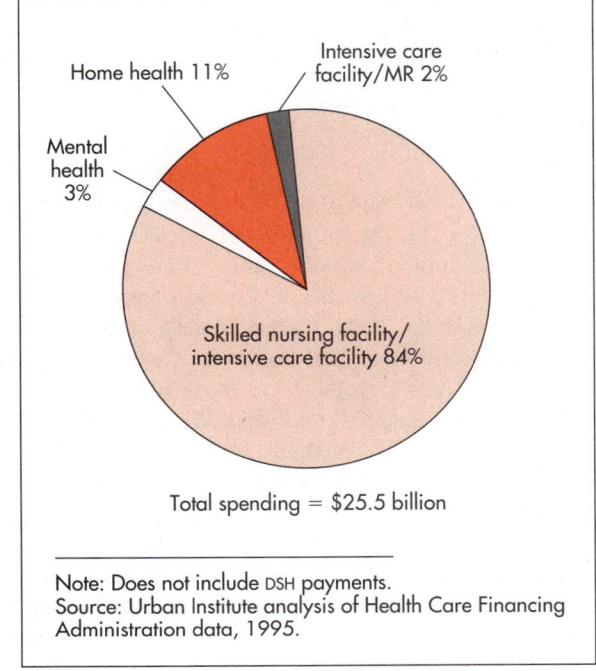

Total spending = $25.5 billion

Note: Does not include DSH payments.
Source: Urban Institute analysis of Health Care Financing Administration data, 1995.

B

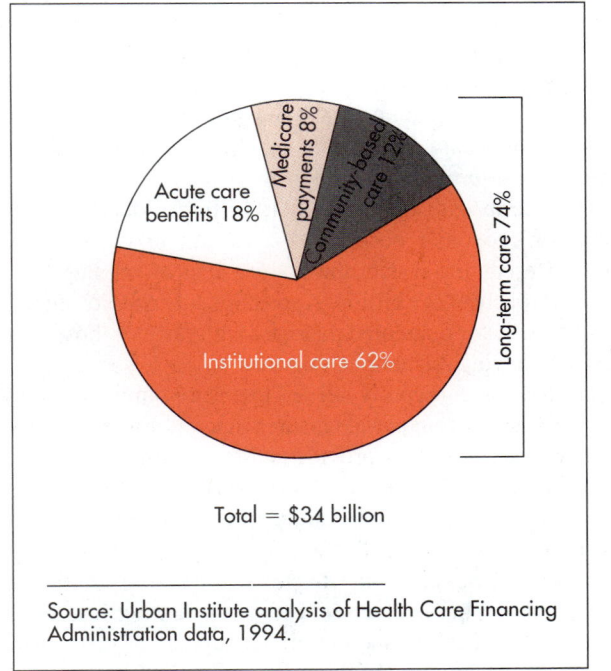

Total = $34 billion

Source: Urban Institute analysis of Health Care Financing Administration data, 1994.

C

Figure 14-5. **A,** Medicaid acute care spending for the elderly to supplement Medicare, 1993. **B,** Long-term care Medicaid expenditures for the elderly, by type of service, 1993. **C,** Medicaid expenditures for the elderly, 1993. (From Lyons B, Rowland D, Hanson K: Another look at medicine, *Generations* 20[2]:24, Summer 1996.)

for certification and others do not want clients who have the time limitations and restrictions imposed by Medicare. Medicaid is primarily the payer of long-term care. Nearly half of the nursing home costs are borne by Medicaid (46%), 2% by Medicare, 2% by private insurance, and the remaining 50% by individuals and their families.

Problems that confront patients and their families are the imposition of additional fees for specific services such as incontinent care and various private payment contractual arrangements they must agree to before a facility will accept a patient receiving Medicaid. Facilities seek patients requiring the least skilled care or those who can pay for their own care. The others may be refused admission.

Nurses have borne the major responsibility for planning and implementing the long-term care of the aged. Recognition of this is becoming apparent: in 1981 the Federal Omnibus Reconciliation Act allowed geriatric nurse practitioners to recertify Medicaid patients for appropriate levels of care, and in several states geriatric nurse practitioners may be directly reimbursed by Medicaid for specific types of care.

Costs of Nursing Home Care.   Most persons (estimates of up to 56%) now 50 years of age or older will need nursing home care at some time for themselves or a parent. It is an issue of national concern. The cost, particularly, is often devastating to spouses and families. Placement in a nursing home reminds one economically of the funeral home: one does not quibble about price but seeks the best. The need to seek the most desirable situation and status for a loved one is an inherent aspect of demonstrating caring and concern. Families and spouses, unless the individual qualifies for Medicaid, spend from $25,000 to $60,000 per year for nursing home care for a spouse or parent. A nest egg of $100,000 may be entirely consumed in 4 years or less by payment for nursing home care. Because of this, many people have considered long-term care (LTC) insurance.

Long-term care of the aged is in transition chiefly because of economic necessity. According to the Congressional Research Service, the annual cost of nursing home care approaches $33 billion. Approximately 58% of nursing home cost is for demented patients, with 50% of those diagnosed as having Alzheimer's disease.

Legislation is urgently needed to ensure families of some reimbursement from private insurers and public funds for the necessary services they provide and for diagnoses, day care, respite care, home care, and transportation (Figure 14-6). If such services were more readily available, families might avoid costly institutionalization in many cases (see further discussion of caregivers in Chapter 17). The best solutions to costly nursing home care seem to be preventing institutionalization by financial and emotional support of the primary caregivers of the aged in the community, shifting the medical model of reimbursement to a functional base, providing national health insurance for long-term care, and increasing use of HMOs and nurses as primary case managers.

Box 14-3	Verification Documents for Medicaid Eligibility

To determine eligibility, an applicant is generally required to provide the following information when meeting with case workers.
1. Social Security cards for all household members
2. Multiple pay stubs or earnings statement from employer
3. Proof of income from rental property
4. Verification letters from Social Security, Supplemental Security Income, Department of Veterans Affairs, unemployment compensation, or workers compensation
5. Proof of support or alimony payments
6. Bank statements, checking accounts, savings accounts, credit union records, stocks, and bonds
7. Rent or mortgage payment receipts
8. Utility receipts
9. Proof of citizenship or alien status
10. Verification of age of children
11. Proof of the absence of disability of a parent
12. Verification of address
13. Collateral verification of family composition and address
14. Tag receipt or title of all motor vehicles
15. Tax notice on real estate
16. All life and health insurance policy and insurance identification cards
17. Written statement of child care expenses
18. Written statements from anyone making a contribution (cash or vendor payments)
19. If pregnant, written statement verifying pregnancy

Data from Shuptrine S: Reforming Medicaid eligibility rules, *The Safety Net,* p. 5, Summer 1991.

Long-term care insurance.   Long-term care insurance (LTCI) to defray the cost of nursing home care and, in some policies, also home care is becoming more affordable and reliable (Figure 14-7). As of 1994, private insurers had sold 3.4 million policies. Most of these were purchased directly by individuals (International Longevity Center, 1995). The triggers for benefit payments are more likely to be functional losses than medical conditions. With the shift in venue and health care delivery methods, traditional LTCI designed around a flat-fee daily reimbursement rate for nursing home care and home care must change to reflect the newer alternatives. McSweeney (1995) found that some LTCI policies are already responding with reimbursement for a richer set of alternatives, particularly noninstitutional options. In August 1996 the U.S. Congress passed S.1658 (the Health Insurance Reform Act of 1996), which has a number of features related to insurance portability. It also provides incentives for individuals to finance their own LTCI (Newsview, 1996).

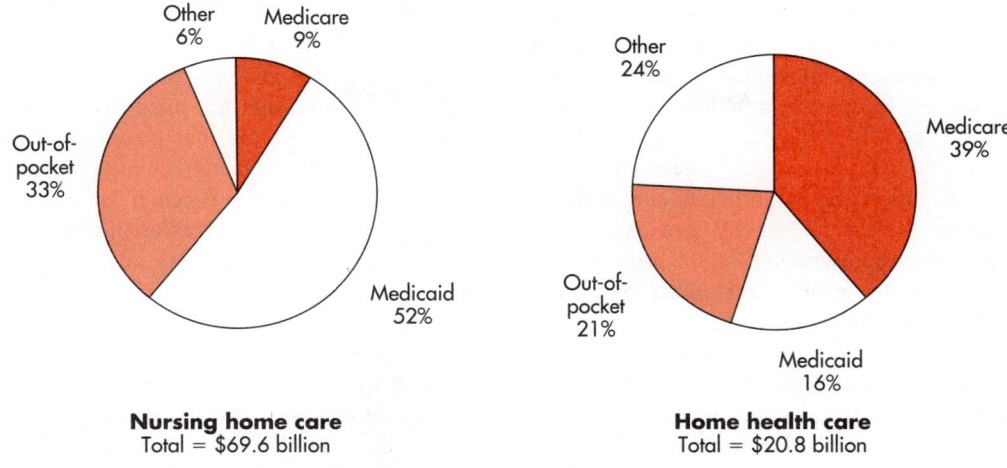

Source: Kaiser Commission on the Future of Medicaid, 1995

Figure 14-6. Sources of long-term care funding, 1993. (From Kaiser Commission on the Future of Medicaid, 1995, *The Public Policy and Aging Report* 6[6]:4, 1995.)

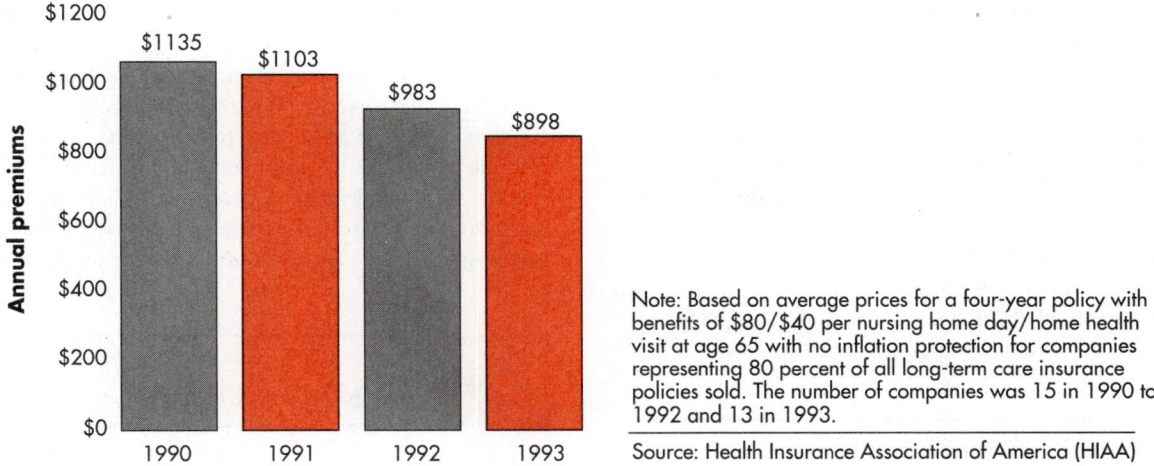

Note: Based on average prices for a four-year policy with benefits of $80/$40 per nursing home day/home health visit at age 65 with no inflation protection for companies representing 80 percent of all long-term care insurance policies sold. The number of companies was 15 in 1990 to 1992 and 13 in 1993.

Source: Health Insurance Association of America (HIAA)

Figure 14-7. Declining long-term care insurance premiums. (From Health Insurance Association of America [HIAA]: Trends and issues, *Currents* 11[7]:10, 1996.)

Many plans are being marketed at present. Even the American Nurses' Association (ANA) has a plan available to ANA members, underwritten by American Express. The purchaser of LTCI must be especially prudent and consider all the exclusions most thoughtfully before enrolling. There are particular concerns related to Alzheimer's disease because many policies exclude these individuals from home benefits and include very limited institutional benefits. Some information sources can be found at the end of this chapter. An extensive report of the status and ratings of nursing home insurance appeared in the May 1988 edition of *Consumer Reports* (Who can afford a nursing home?, 1988). The infant industry has grown considerably since that time, but the guidelines for policy selection remain valid (Box 14-4). It is important to review all the benefits and restrictions before advising consumers to purchase a policy, since this burgeoning aspect of the industry is still poorly understood by the insurance agents. The best LTCI packages are those negotiated by a large employer or state organization or association.

Consumer reports of the particular insurance company and its reliability will be important as well as understanding that the older one is when applying for the policy, the higher the rates will be. When purchasing as an individual, a 55 year old can buy a policy for $600 + per year, whereas a person 75 years of age must pay more than $3000. Rates are considerably better when purchasing LTCI through a group policy. California state employees can purchase a good

LTCI policy for $100 per month at age 65. Minimal policies cost significantly less. Currently Congress is considering two bills that would encourage individuals to purchase LTCI and would provide tax incentives for doing so (CalPERS, 1996).

Managed care and long-term care. These are coming under scrutiny by providers and major health care organizations, such as the American Health Care Association (AHCA), as the major representative of for-profit nursing home care providers. In life-care organizations, model programs such as On Lok/PACE (Program for All inclusive Care of the Elderly), social health maintenance organizations (SHMOs), the Arizona Long-Term Care System, and the Oregon Health Care system, there is mounting evidence that this can be done successfully. However, there is concern that long-term care providers would be shortchanged in fiscal resources (Wiener, 1996). In fact, considerable protest and congressional testimony have already been mounted regarding the differential in reimbursement for similar conditions in the acute care setting and in subacute long-term care (Bailis, 1996).

Stone and Reublinger (1995) enumerate some of the dramatic changes that have taken place in long-term care. Formerly considered an insignificant part of health care, it is now seen as a cost-saving method of providing subacute care through hospice care; home health care; social, medical, and rehabilitative day care; and assisted living and congregate care. The nursing home is being transformed into a center for the coordination of the continuum of care as the hospital is being redefined as a surgical, emergency, and intensive care center. These changes will require many attitudinal and personnel shifts because many health professionals remain in the outdated mode of health care delivery.

Health Maintenance Organizations and Managed Care

Health maintenance organizations (HMOs) and managed care are terms that are used interchangeably to indicate health care systems that provide various services for a set monthly fee. These fees may be paid by an employer, agency, individual subscriber, or any combination. These organizations have a vested interest in maintaining the health of their subscribers and keeping costs of care as low as possible. There are some excellent plans and some that are notoriously bad. Questions that should be considered prior to enrolling in any are enumerated in Box 14-5.

Good managed care has demonstrated its potential to reduce the overall cost of health care for consumers and the government (National Policy and Resource Center on Women and Aging, 1995). The premise of Medicare managed care is that better outcomes will result from systems of care that integrate professionals in responsive teams, widely use subacute care, and provide incentives to reduce the reliance on institutional acute care (Rosenfeld, 1996). Yet, while these positive claims are being made, Rovner (1996) says, "One thing experts do agree on is that in its current form, Medicare's managed-care program has cost more to date than it has saved." "Whether or not managed care is ultimately good for Medicare, most experts agree that it can provide as good . . . and in some cases better . . . care than fee for service." Managed care systems are most effective for individuals enrolled over a long period of time who use ongoing primary care and preventive strategies to maintain

---

Box 14-4 | **Benefits Included in a Good Long-Term Care Policy**

- Daily benefit of $100
- Waiting period of not over 20 days
- Maximum benefit for one stay of at least 4 years
- Unlimited maximum benefit for all stays
- Payment for skilled nursing facility (SNF), intermediate care facility (ICF), or custodial care
- Partial payment for subacute care not covered by Medicare
- Coverage should begin within 20 days of a hospital stay of 3 days
- Home care benefits should be paid without requiring a hospital stay or previous nursing home care
- Waiver of premium when hospitalized
- Guaranteed renewability for life
- Specific coverage of Alzheimer's disease
- Constant premium level for life

Box 14-5 | **Managed Care Checklist**

If you now have a doctor, is he or she affiliated with a plan you can join?

Can you easily switch doctors in the plan if you are dissatisfied?

What is the quality of care rating (see resources at end of chapter)?

Can you switch plans without undue difficulty if you are dissatisfied?

Are the various services conveniently located?

Is advice and care readily available on evenings and weekends?

How accessible are mental health services within the plan?

Does the plan supply information in your primary language?

Where and how can you obtain health services if you are traveling?

Does the plan cover alternative therapies such as acupuncture, chiropractic, and homeopathy?

health and avoid high-cost emergency services and intensive treatment (Twentieth Century Fund, 1995).

Managed care and HMOs have captured the health care market with remarkable growth in the past 3 years. From 1993 until 1996 enrollment increased from 1,624,000 to 3,465,916, and Medicare risk contracts approved by HCFA more than doubled (Fox and Fama, 1996) (Figure 14-8). The managed care models vary considerably in qualtiy, and this is being extensively evaluated. All are based on a per-capita asset accrual to sustain individuals in as healthy a manner as possible. Most of these organizations are guided by waivers to states that have been granted by the HCFA to reduce Medicare expenditures and move the locus of control from the federal bureaucracy to that of the states. Many of the managed care groups control costs by retraining professionals and lay persons for specific roles that supplement or replace the services of more costly personnel.

Have all these changes been advantageous for the aged participants? It is not yet known because there are many variables within each managed care plan. However, HMOs that have been granted Medicare per-capita waivers cannot refuse applicants based upon preexisting health conditions, and the supplemental services offered may save the participant a considerable amount in medications, assistive devices, and professional consultation charges. The negative

aspects of HMOs/managed care are the access barriers to specialists and high-tech procedures and treatments. Some HMOs provide extensive health education services, support groups, and telephone support services to the homebound. Information and improvements that are needed in the system are summarized in Box 14-6.

Core concepts behind managed care systems can be seen in Box 14-7.

Each month more and more companies and hospitals form conglomerates to provide managed care under the Medicare waiver risk benefit plan. Kaiser Foundation has been the leader and time-tested provider in this realm and continues to be the most reliable based upon its history. However, it is becoming a highly competitive market, and each provider-group will ultimately survive based on the quality and accessibility of the care given to consumers. Consumers are becoming well informed and wise purchasers. An example of a common type of news release shows the type of marketing we can expect:

Access Health Announces Million Member Contract with Blue Cross Blue Shield of Florida:

Members can receive information 24 hours a day, seven days a week via the telephone, the Internet, fax, printed materials or cable TV. Registered nurse counselors are available anytime of the day or night to answer questions and provide other health related

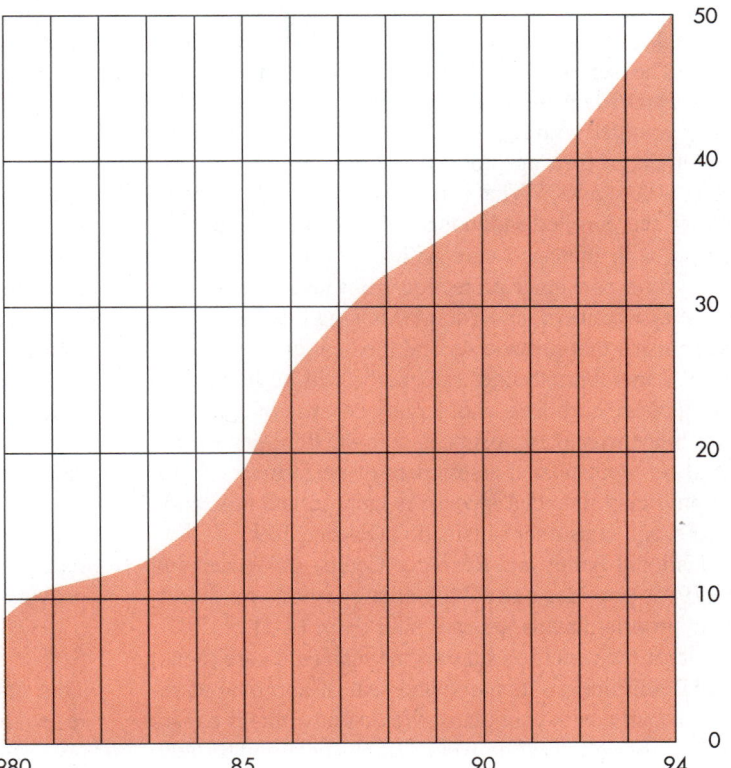

Note: "Health Maintenance Organizations (HMOs)" include Individual Practice Arrangements (IPAs), networks, group, staff, and mixed-model HMOs.

Source: Group Health Association of America. *Patterns in HMO Enrollment.* Washington, DC: Group Health Association of America, 1994. Table 2, p. 7.

Figure 14-8. Growth in the number of Americans receiving their care in HMOs, 1980-1994 (in millions). (From The Robert Wood Johnson Foundation: *Annual Report,* 1994.)

assistance as necessary . . . Under the terms of the agreement, Blue Cross and Blue Shield of Florida and Health Options, Inc., the company's HMO, will initially offer Personal Health Advisor to 220,000 Medicare Supplement customers and 155,000 of its commercial managed customers in Florida's northeast region as of Oct. 1, 1996. (Access Health, 1996, p. 1.)

There has been considerable negative reaction to this by the media, health professionals, and somewhat less so by the public. Both HMOs and managed care categories of care provision range from excellent to abominable, and all are based on a capitated per diem reimbursement mechanism; the healthier and less costly the interventions, the greater the profit.

In 1996 HCFA paid monthly rates of $313.55 to $760.66 per person enrolled in Medicare HMOs (U.S. Health Care Financing Administration, HCF, 1998). As the fiscal solvency of the Medicare program becomes more tenuous, means of sustaining quality care at an affordable cost for the elderly are an ever-growing concern. Medicare has contracted with several HMOs to provide comprehensive services for the elderly, financed by Medicare premiums. These are complete health care systems with highly trained physicians and nurses working out of a single, completely equipped medical center. HMOs differ from other medical services in that they emphasize preventive medicine, comprehensive care, and periodic physical examinations, and they cover more services than are ordinarily covered under Medicare. There is a minimum monthly charge to the participant and a service fee for each visit and for each prescription. The senior citizens who currently tend to subscribe to HMO/Medicare programs tend to be those who are relatively younger with higher educational and income levels than others in their age cohort.

Rother (1996) asks, "What is the best way to safeguard the interests of the enrolled individual?" He suggests consumer satisfaction with managed care will be a generational phenomenon: now, consumer protection from insufficient attention is a major concern, and good HMOs will develop internal mechanisms that provide second medical opinions at the request of a member; second, safeguards will be in place to protect Medicare enrollees who, largely because of age, form a pool of higher risk participants; and, in the third generation, there will be sophisticated assessment of performance in regard to physician financial incentives, appropriate utilization of services, and consumer satisfaction (Rother, 1996).

The National Policy and Resource Center on Women and Aging (1995) provides a checklist of suggestions for selecting the appropriate managed care plan (Box 14-5).

In spite of the unsettled state of the managed care industry, AARP will license its name and seal of approval to selected managed health care plans. We do know this is a massive change in health care delivery that has occurred through corporate insistence while Congress has bandied about numerous ideas and made no clear decisions. Above all, in this present system beneficiaries must be aggressive in demanding the care they need (Figure 14-9). There are several indi-

Box 14-6	**Managed Care Improvements Needed**

- Better monitoring by HCFA of the impact of Medicare risk programs is needed.
- Consumers need more and better information about the quality of various plans.
- Medicare beneficiaries need to understand limitations of access to providers outside the plan.
- Providers need to make the range of services and limitations clear to the participants.

cations that consumers will soon have considerably better information at their disposal in order to make informed choices. A decision by the California Supreme Court (San Francisco Chronicle, 1996) ruled that the state's medical licensing agency can obtain personnel files and other documents, previously held confidential, that report physician incompetence or misconduct. In addition to less patronage protection of physicians by physicians and hospitals, we are seeing frequent reports of quality of care evaluation by consumers of managed care (Table 14-7).

We believe this signals important and positive changes in the delivery and accountability of health care providers and systems even though at present they still swing chaotically from one extreme to another.

Case Managed Care

To provide more comprehensive, individualized, and economic care, case management and managed care have emerged as solutions to the cost and fragmentation now experienced by elders. Managed care simply means care is guided by economic concerns, and case management implies an individual provider who functions as a primary care agent concerned about both cost and quality of services. Many variations of these mechanisms exist throughout acute and long-term care. Elders must have an advocate or individual who can provide answers based on a comprehensive view of their situation. Problems arise chiefly because the case manager may have a title but insufficient authority and flexibility allowed in which to actually manage the case for the best client outcome. More often at this time we hear of restrictions dictated by the economic interests of agencies providing care.

The Veterans Health Care System

This system has long held a leadership position in geriatric research, medical care and extended care. In fact, a great deal of the research that has guided gerontologists in earlier years was generated through the veterans health system as were innovations in care. In addition, the vast majority of geriatric fellowships have been provided through the Department of Veterans Affairs (VA) hospitals. The VA system

---

**Box
14-7**   **The Seven Cs of Managed Care: The Core Concepts behind Managed Care Systems**

COMMON FEATURES: Managed Care Systems aim to be:

1. CONSOLIDATED in auspice and funding, so there is one-stop shopping
2. COMPREHENSIVE, offering services across the continuum
3. CONTINUOUS, following people from acute to long-term care
4. COORDINATED, with more integration of services and information
5. CONTROLLED, with authority over providers, services, and costs
6. COST-CONSCIOUS, and aim to be cost-competitive or capitated
7. COMMUNITY-BASED, emphasizing noninstitutional approaches

These systems are also becoming more and more CONSUMER-ORIENTED.

DIFFERENCES BETWEEN VARIOUS TYPES OF MANAGED CARE SYSTEMS:

Managed Care Systems differ from one another in:

1. The RANGE OF SERVICES they provide (acute vs. long-term care; medical vs. health vs. social support services; whether or not housing is included)
2. The POPULATION targeted for recruitment, or eligible for enrollment
3. The extent to which they assume COMPLETE and LONG-TERM RESPONSIBILITY for their enrollees
4. The TYPES OF FUNDING used to support services
5. The MODEL used to bring together services and providers
6. The MECHANISMS used FOR CONTROLLING COSTS
7. The SOPHISTICATION OF their systems for INFORMATION MANAGEMENT and SERVICE COORDINATION

The above differences result in a CONTINUUM OF MANAGED CARE SYSTEMS

| basic health——augmented health——chronic care——long-term care |
| HMOs   S/HMOs   CCRCs   CCODAs |

From Laura Reif, RN, PhD, School of Nursing, University of California, San Francisco, 1994.

---

has been a forerunner of the various continuum-care providers in place at present as early on they provided VA-run nursing homes, home care and community-based programs, respite care, blindness rehabilitation, mental health, and numerous other services in addition to acute medical/surgical provisions. There is now concern that federal budgetary restrictions will virtually annihilate this system that has for several decades led the way in the continuum of health care (Custis and Fuller, 1996).

Subacute Care

The development of subacute units has become a massive move by the larger nursing home chains and hospitals to meet the needs of the aged who are discharged "quick and sick." The AHCA and the Joint Commission on Accreditation of Health Care Organizations (JCAHO) provide the following definition of subacute care:

Subacute care is comprehensive inpatient care designed for someone who has an acute illness, injury, or exacerbation of a disease process. It is goal-oriented treatment rendered immediately after, or instead of, acute hospitalization to treat one or more specific active complex medical conditions or to administer one or more technically complex treatments, in the context of a person's underlying long-term conditions and overall situation.

The definition goes on to explain in more detail all of these factors and is reproduced in Box 14-8. Copies are available from JCAHO.

As hospitals eject patients with ever greater rapidity, nursing homes are increasingly taking on the form and functions of the traditional medical unit in a general hospital, under the category of providing subacute care. Subacute care is more intensive than traditional nursing facility care and several times more costly, but it is far less costly than similar care in an acute care hospital.

Guidelines have been established for these subacute units for accreditation standards and physician responsibilities. These are, in large part, in response to the necessary upgrading of many long-term care facilities in which staffing, equipment, and structures were not adapted to the level of care needed by some of the patients admitted directly from acute care hospitals. The American Medical Association (AMA) established guidelines in 1995 that are especially important in assuring prompt and adequate care because typically long-term care has been the stepchild of physicians. Now, physicians are required to be responsible for patient care 24 hours a day, 7 days a week. The patient is to remain under the primary coordinating care of the admitting physician rather than being transferred to a house physician.

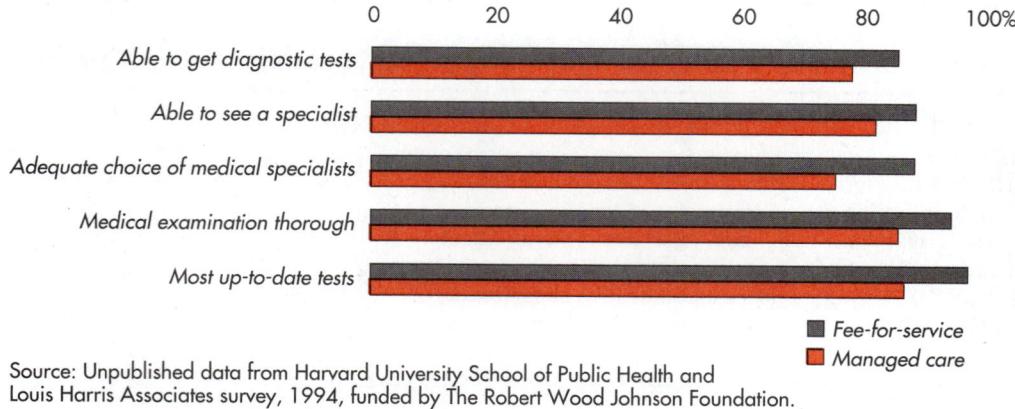

Source: Unpublished data from Harvard University School of Public Health and Louis Harris Associates survey, 1994, funded by The Robert Wood Johnson Foundation.

Figure 14-9. Americans' experience with health care. (From The Robert Wood Johnson Foundation: *Annual Report,* 1994.)

Table 14-7	Member Recommendation Survey Basic Plan Results Only

Plan name	Percent of those likely to recommend*
Aetna Health Plans	86%
Blue Shield HMO	82%
CAHP	100%
CCPOA	51%
CIGNA	89%
CPFA	73%
FHP/TakeCare (merged)	88%
Foundation Health	80%
Health Net	93%
Health Plan of the Redwoods	87%
Kaiser North	93%
Kaiser South	95%
Lifeguard	94%
Maxicare	94%
National HMO	86%
OMNI Healthcare	89%
PacifiCare	88%
PERSCare	93%
PERS Choice	88%
PORAC	97%

From Open Enrollment Materials, 1998 Health plan/quality report, CalPERS.
*NOTE: Represents the percentage of respondents who would recommend their plan to someone else.

Other features of the guidelines include assurance that education and skills of staff are sufficient to provide the necessary care, peer evaluation will monitor quality of care, a comprehensive patient assessment and plan of care will be in place within 24 hours of admission, and there will be a minimum of once weekly visits and progress notes for each visit (American Medical Association, 1995).

A present concern in the long-term care provider industry is the need to institute staff development programs that include skills and procedures traditionally limited to the acute care setting. Nurses who have devoted their careers to providing the real "nursing home" care so essential to long-term residents fear that it will be lost as the industry gears up to provide hospital care.

The HCFA ruling that acute hospitalization for 3 days must precede admission to a nursing home is problematic and may be eliminated if the subacute care providers' testimony is incorporated into policy (Bailis, 1996). This policy is estimated to generate unnecessary costs of from $2700 to $4000 per patient. Bailis, representing the membership of the AHCA, contends that equity in the acute care and subacute care payment systems could save Medicare between 7.5 and 9 billion dollars annually. A HCFA estimate released in 1995 found that hospital-based SNF care cost, on average, $150 more per day than similar care in a free-standing SNF. Hospital-based SNFs and subacute care units are proliferating 6 times more rapidly than the free-standing SNFs and subacute care units (Bailis, 1996). Given the number of empty hospital beds, this trend is likely to increase. However, with a potential market of $20 billion, major providers of long-term care, such as Beverly Enterprises, Hillhaven Corporation, and Manor Health Care, are moving rapidly into the provision of subacute care (Hicks and Miner, 1993).

Home Care

An array of public and privately financed services has developed across the United States to support the desire of impaired elders to live out their lives in the comfort and independence of their own homes. Ideally, the services provide a

Subacute care is comprehensive inpatient care designed for someone who has an acute illness, injury, or exacerbation of a disease process. It is goal-oriented treatment rendered immediately after, or instead of, acute hospitalization to treat one or more specific active complex medical conditions or to administer one or more technically complex treatments, in the context of a person's underlying long-term conditions and overall situation.

Generally, the individual's condition is such that the care does not depend heavily on high-technology monitoring or complex diagnostic procedures. Subacute care requires the coordinated services of an interdisciplinary team including physicians, nurses, and other relevant professional disciplines, who are trained and knowledgeable to assess and manage these specific conditions and perform the necessary procedures. Subacute care is given as part of a specifically defined program, regardless of the site.

Subacute care is generally more intensive than traditional nursing facility care and less than acute care. It requires frequent (daily to weekly) recurrent patient assessment and review of the clinical course and treatment plan for a limited (several days to several months) time period, until the condition is stabilized or a predetermined treatment course is completed.

From American Health Care Association, 1201 L Street, NW, Washington, DC.

combination of health care, day-care supervision, housekeeping, counseling, meal deliveries, transportation, visits from friendly companions, home repairs, and other services as needed. The cost of such services has been the subject of much debate, and thus all services are often not available to those who need them. The government fears that many individuals would emerge to claim services if they were publicly financed. Demonstration projects have shown varying costs and do not necessarily reflect cost savings when compared with nursing home placement. Freedom and commitment to quality of life are valued principles of American life but have yet to be fully supported economically.

It is estimated that 10% to 20% of persons in nursing homes could have remained in their own homes if some of these services had been available to them. In many cases a wide range of services is available to those who can afford them, but persons may be unaware of what is needed or where it can be obtained. In these situations, case managers may help individuals identify their specific needs and find the appropriate services. Case managers may be found through city and county referral services or private agencies that provide case management on a fee-for-service basis.

Community services such as home health care may be funded under Medicare and Medicaid (Title XVIII and XIX, Social Security Act), the Social Services Amendment (Title XX, Social Security Act), the Older Americans Act (Title III), and by the Department of Veterans Affairs. Provision of and reimbursement for community services focus on the individual and often do not support the family in its efforts to care for the functionally dependent older person in the home. The net effect restricts the provider's capacity to develop or manage a comprehensive treatment plan. In the past few years home health care has expanded enormously. Numerous demonstration projects and Medicare waivers have provided policy makers with a more accurate picture of the potential quality and cost issues addressed by comprehensive home care.

Home care can be a desirable alternative to institutional care if caregivers, nurses, family, social workers, physicians, homemakers, and home health aides are available when needed. However, these ideal conditions may not exist, and if available, there are strict Medicare limits. Some aged people manage to remain in their homes with few services and minimal assistance. Conditions may be less than desirable from professional standards but by the standards of the individuals are much more acceptable than institutionalization.

Total expenditures for home health care have increased enormously as more people are finding it possible to remain at home and as costs, particularly of durable goods, have increased exponentially. In 1980 national expenditures for home care were $1.9 billion; in 1993 costs were $20.8 billion (U.S. Bureau of the Census, 1995). Of this, about one third were out-of-pocket expenditures ($2.6 billion). The cost is continuing to rise. Earlier it was estimated to reach $19.8 billion by the year 2020, but clearly that was a gross underestimation. Considering that many hidden costs and most of the actual care are provided by family members, the real cost of care in the home cannot be compared with that of other venues.

There is much debate about the cost effectiveness of home care, yet reliance on home health care has grown out of necessity because of the rapid discharge of hospitalized patients.

Home care reimbursement has been abused to some extent because it has not been under the restrictions of hospitals and nursing homes in terms of prospective reimbursement. From personal experience we learned that some home health agencies charge Medicare for visits that have not been made. Stories of outrageous charges for medical equipment are commonplace. However, there is now a concerted effort to curb fraudulent claims and excessive charges. In 1997 the HCFA plans for prospective reimbursement should reduce the costs of home care considerably.

Interestingly, supermarkets of home care supplies and medical equipment designed to provide individual and personalized service directly to consumers are appearing nationwide and drawing crowds of careful shoppers (Chriss, 1996). These retailers often have professionals available to advise, instruct, and answer questions. In one such outlet most of the employees are registered nurses or licensed vocational nurses and have special training in the use of medical equipment. In some situations, follow-up home assessments are made to ensure client satisfaction and proper usage. This is reassuring evidence of the growing trend for clients to take charge of their own care. Nurses are case managers and primary care coordinators in the home, and at present, home health care is the most important issue at stake in the care of the aged. We expect nurses will continue to occupy a pivotal role in home care as client advocates as we carefully evaluate quality, outcomes, costs, and cost savings (see discussion of nursing role in Chapter 28).

Where Is Health Care Headed?

An entire issue of *Generations*, the journal of the American Society on Aging, was devoted to examining the future direction of health care of the aged (American Society of Aging, 1996). None of the comprehensive health care plans introduced in 1993 came to pass. Yet, polls show that from 1984 until 1994 from 75% to 85% of the American public were satisfied with the medical care available to them (Zis et al, 1996). In 1994 and 1995 it appeared that Medicare and Medicaid were increasingly vulnerable to political manipulations. When Medicare was put into effect more than 30 years ago, it was expected that it was a major step toward universal national health insurance (Ball, 1996). Now this seems at least a decade away. In 1996, there were 4.5 million Medicare beneficiaries, and 10% of these were enrolled in managed care plans. Participants in these plans increased 16% from 1994. The greatest number of members are from California. In Orange County, California, fully 50% of Medicare-eligible residents are enrolled in managed care risk contracts. The competitive managed care marketplace seems to be in control of health care direction for the foreseeable future.

LEGAL ISSUES OF THE ELDERLY

Old people may need legal assistance to wade through the complex, ever-changing laws that affect (1) taxation, (2) wills and estate planning, (3) appeals to Social Security and Medicare, (4) conservatorships and guardianships, (5) property management and sales, (6) contracts, (7) housing disputes, (8) pensions, and (9) the right to work. Other legal considerations in late life include advance directives regarding health care (discussed in Chapter 26), provisions for temporary or long-term inability to manage personal affairs, and avoiding contractual arrangements in which the elder will be at a disadvantage. More specifically, there may be concerns about property division among heirs, life being sustained by artificial means, mental incompetence, func-

tional disabilities, fraud, appropriate insurance coverage, property management, familial obligations, funeral plans, organ donation, retirement, veterans and Social Security benefits, and late marriage. All of these issues are ones in which legalities are important and must be considered (Heckheimer, 1989).

Some elders delegate power of attorney to another individual who then has power to act in the elder's behalf and make decisions regarding assets and legal affairs. This can be for a specified period of time or indefinitely. Normally, a power of attorney is revoked if the maker becomes incompetent; however, a durable power of attorney, specifically stated to be such, continues in effect during incompetence. Guardianships and conservatorships are another method by which an individual's powers of decision making are given over to a named representative of the client appointed by the court. These are used in cases where the court judges an individual to be in need of protective services. (See Chapter 15 for further discussion of these issues.) The durable power of attorney for health care deals with issues of care management and is discussed fully in Chapter 26.

Legal Aid

Because of the complexity and changing nature of statutory, regulatory, and decisional law, the elderly may need counseling or legal services to protect their rights, assets, and eligibility for various services. Information about legal aid to the elderly may be obtained by looking in the Yellow Pages under "Attorneys, elder law." The federal Office of Economic Opportunity's (OEO's) legal services division and the move toward case management as a part of law school education have increased the availability of legal services to the indigent, but this has not produced a dramatic change in the availability of services to the elderly.

There are over 780,000 lawyers in the United States at present. About 5% of these are retired or inactive (U.S. Bureau of the Census, 1995). An active recruitment of their services for the assistance of the elderly would benefit both clients and lawyers. However, pro bono or carefully regulated fees for service would be essential.

Currently, many senior newsletters and magazines provide a monthly legal advice column. Legal aid to the aged is available in many communities under county health and welfare services. It is often provided by paralegal aides or law students. Most county bar associations also have provisions for brief consultations at a nominal fee. Senior centers provide information and legal assistance, and the local phone book lists legal offices and organizations that can advise seniors about their rights and obligations. Additional discussion of legalities particular to nurses working with the aged can be found in Chapter 28.

Testimonial and Contractual Capacity. Testimonial capacity involves an individual's capacity to testify in court. An issue may arise as to an aged person's ability to accurately recollect significant data. Some criminal suits for homicides and assaults in institutions have been dropped when the only witnesses were elderly. Because of the long delay before a case reaches the courts, an elderly witness may no longer be a reliable informant or, perhaps, may not be alive. Testamentary capacity regarding wills, marriages, and other contracts may be questioned in cases that involve elders.

Capacity to contract involves the ability to know the nature and effect of the transaction. Generally speaking, courts are loath to invalidate a marriage, although family members may be especially concerned when an elderly parent marries someone they suspect is a "fortune hunter." Divorce is rarely a problem area legally, since most states permit a no-fault divorce, and many elders in late marriages have established prenuptial exclusions and agreements.

Wills are frequently disputed; thus many lawyers request a psychiatric examination concurrent with the making of a will by a very old person. Because the law recognizes the existence of "lucid intervals" in which an otherwise impaired person may be capable of effectuating a will, it is wise for the psychiatrist and the lawyer to obtain some longitudinal data. If the will is contested, the psychiatric evaluation will be used in court and will not remain confidential.

Codicils, or subsequent additions to the will, are also often contested if they benefit one relative over another. "Undue influence" may be charged legally when a person has testamentary capacity but is so impaired that he or she is subject to manipulation. However, many families simply wrangle among themselves without taking legal action but with the result of breaches in family relationships and wounds that do not heal.

Currently there is a trend for elders to establish living trusts in order to avoid the time-consuming process and cost of probate court. However, when families are not altogether in harmony, a living trust can cause significant problems because the named executor or executors have full control of decisions regarding these estates.

Gerald had amassed a fair-sized fortune through real estate investments and astute management of his money. Though he had made a will during midlife, in later life he began to consider the costs of probate and the lengthy time his estate would be tied up in court proceedings. He rescinded his will and set up a Living Trust with his present, but second, wife as executrix. Though he intended the estate to be divided among his second wife and the three children of his first marriage, this did not happen. He died unexpectedly at age 63 in an auto accident, and the suit against his estate consumed a significant portion of his fortune. His children fought for the remainder of his estate, contending he had been incompetent and unduly influenced by his wife when he rescinded the original will. This situation is yet unresolved 4 years after his death.

Consent for Treatment. Consent for medical treatment is traditionally the prerogative of the adult individual of sound mind. The exceptions to this rule are determined by law, regulatory policy, and judicial decision. Usually the patient's wishes prevail if judged competent. When the patient is incompetent, a variety of factors will be considered. Even with the most careful presentation of data, judges frequently decide these matters based on the individual case rather than any overriding principle (Gilfix, 1987).

Involuntary hospitalization is governed by two principles: Is the person dangerous to self, or is the person dangerous to others? In some states this concept includes inability to meet one's own survival needs. Some jurisdictions maintain it is the responsibility of government to take care of those unable to care for themselves. Many abuses have occurred in applying these principles to the involuntary hospitalization of the aged. The U.S. Supreme Court has stated that involuntary hospitalizations should be permitted only when "clear and convincing evidence" is present (*Addington v. Texas*). The most useful stance is to seek the "most beneficial alternative" as an essential element of the "least restrictive choice." Placement in a setting where adequate care is not provided makes these phrases mere euphemisms. Missouri specifically excludes disorders such as senility, when not of an active psychotic nature, as a basis for involuntary hospitalization. Further discussion of legal issues in geriatric psychiatric can be found in Chapter 21.

Consent for Research. Consent for research leads to another set of issues regarding consent, particularly since Alzheimer's disease is one of researchers' major interests in the geriatric patient. Ideally, a living will or advance directive for health care would designate the willingness of an individual to participate in research, but realistically this is rarely the case. Patients with a diagnosis of senile dementia or psychosis may be incompetent in some respects but not in all (Sansone and Schmitt, 1996). Specific alterations of the consent process to obtain the patient's consent are suggested:

1. Make the material more readable.
2. Tailor the information to the needs of the patient.
3. Allow patients to review the material for a longer time than usual before determining competence to consent.
4. Use teaching, review, and testing regarding the patient's ability to understand material.
5. Develop rapport with the patient and encourage questions.
6. Involve the patient's family in the consent process. They may use language more familiar to the patient and make the material more understandable to the patient.

Over a decade ago, the National Institute on Aging (NIA) established a task force to design a set of guidelines that might be helpful in the review of research protocols concerning senile dementia of the Alzheimer's type (SDAT). When these were established, Melnick et al (1984) specifically addressed the fifth guideline, the determination of a subject's capacity for understanding a specific protocol. These authors state that consent should not be based on overall competency because an individual may retain the capacity to consent but lack the capacity to manage his or her affairs in other respects. This has been confirmed in studies by Sansone and Schmitt (1996). (See Chapter 28 for additional discussion of nursing research.)

Rights of Patients

Patients' rights in institutions of all types are mandated by federal and state laws and the Constitution, as are the rights of the general population. Legal rights vary according to the setting and individual competency. Rights in institutions are to be posted in a place visible to all and are to be reviewed with the individual soon after admission to a facility. In some settings, because of the difficulty of enforcement, rights are often not respected or protected.

Nursing responsibilities are (1) to ensure that the patient has seen, read, and/or understands the rights, (2) to document explicitly when and why any rights may be temporarily suspended, (3) to observe and record observations attesting to the individual's ability or inability to manage daily affairs; and (4) to be sure the patient's status is reviewed at appropriate time intervals (these vary from one state to another) and that he or she obtains legal assistance in presenting his or her defense. The rights of patients are enforced largely because of the integrity of nurses and our willingness to act as patient advocates.

Ombudsman

Advocacy organizations for nursing home residents began flourishing between 1975 and 1979. The various activities they are engaged in include complaint resolution, confrontation and/or negotiation with nursing homes, community education, legal intervention, and legislative reform. *Ombudsman* as the term is used today most commonly denotes the nursing home advocate prepared to deal squarely but sensitively with the realities of a nursing home resident's life. An ombudsman must view the resident's problem as impartially as possible and act as advocate but not in an adversarial role with the nursing home administration.

In addition to acting as advocate, the ombudsman often locates appropriate resources and links residents to them, trains friendly visitors, provides a clearinghouse for problems or complaints, gives legislative updates, and provides assistance in conducting family councils and resident councils. The ombudsman must also assist families in transferring or discharging patients from a nursing home to another setting. The ombudsman is concerned about maintaining good relationships with nursing home personnel. Ways that a nursing home can ensure a more collaborative relationship with the ombudsman are summarized in Box 14-9.

The long-term care ombudsman program is mandated by the Older Americans Act (OAA). Each state must have an Office of the State Ombudsman to which all substate programs report. Models may vary to reflect the needs and conditions within the state. Nursing home and board and care residents must have direct and immediate access to an ombudsman when needed for protection and advocacy. Netting et al (1992) studied and reported the type of complaints registered nationwide through state agency offices in 1990. The largest number (38,100) were about care issues such as abuse, neglect, poor care, poorly trained staff, and poorly dressed patients. The second largest area of complaint was against administration for understaffing, inadequate laundry procedures, roommate conflicts, and other items (21,500). The third area of complaint was for denial of rights, violation of privacy, and lack of grievance procedures (18,700). Given these patient concerns, it is clear that professional nurses must remain alert to their advocacy role in institutions. Nurses need to be aware of the procedure for filing a complaint against a nursing home. Some may wish to do so and will need the support of the legal system and other nurses in the advocacy of humane care for clients.

1. A complaint about practices, procedures, physical conditions, or quality of care in a nursing home is initially a request to the state health department to inspect a particular home and determine if a violation exists. Any person may file such a request simply by writing a letter. The letter should specifically detail the incidents of concern. However, even vague complaints such as lack of attention will be investigated. Numbers to call can be found in the telephone book.
2. Copies of licensing surveys are available to the public through the facilities licensing section of each state. They will show the violations that have been noted.
3. Copies of regulations are available through the state publications office. These will provide a basis for measuring violations.

ADVOCACY FOR THE AGED

Advocacy is representing the interest of others by acting in their behalf or by attempting to influence the formulation of administrative, institutional, and legislative policies that affect them. Instruments of advocacy include protest, disruption, representation, demonstration, and argument appropriate to the protection of rights, entitlements, and privileges of specifiable persons. Advocates may or may not be legal representatives of the individual. Nurses are advocates of the people they serve and may employ legal representatives to assist in defending their position. No nurse can be entirely exempt from the role of advocate. We have the opportunity and the obligation to plead the cause of our aged clients.

There are three levels of advocacy based in ethical positions:

1. Justice affords equal opportunities and protection to all persons within the framework of formal and informal institutions and practices.
2. Corrective justice involves the selective consideration of the needs of deprived groups and the institution of different provisions for them in light of their present condition and past deprivations.
3. Distributive justice makes adequate provision for inequalities between the parties to a transaction.

Box 14-9	**Working Effectively with an Ombudsman**

1. The administrator should become acquainted with the ombudsman.
2. The administrator should introduce the ombudsman to the entire staff.
3. The ombudsman should be invited to the facility on a routine basis and on special occasions to become a part of the facility resource rather than an adversary.
4. The ombudsman and administrator should share perceptions and facts openly with each other while maintaining confidentiality.
5. The administrator should discuss some of his or her concerns and legislative issues that need attention.
6. The administrator should inform the residents' council that an ombudsman is available.
7. The administrator should likewise inform the family council about the ombudsman.

Box 14-10	**Principles of Advocacy**

1. Gather as much specific data as possible to make your case.
2. Be informed regarding pros and cons of the issue.
3. Know the policies that will influence decisions in the case.
4. Involve others who will support or augment your case.
5. Work with those who have power to make relevant decisions.
6. Make a clear decision regarding risks you are willing to take to win your case.
7. Inform and involve client groups who will benefit from your position in the case.
8. If the client is at risk, be sure he or she is aware of the risk.
9. Take an offensive rather than a defensive position.
10. Be calm and clear when presenting your case.
11. Emphasize positive aspects of the case.
12. Be tolerant of opposing viewpoints.
13. Consider alternatives to your position that would be acceptable.

Equal opportunities and provisions are not always sufficient for persons in groups or deprived circumstances. Services and policies may be administered fairly, but if one is hampered by language, distance, or comprehension in obtaining a service, it is not fairly distributed.

The second and third definitions are especially applicable to the aged. Our potential clients, who are unaware of services or unable to obtain them, must become a concern of nurses if we are to correct the unequal distribution of the goods and benefits in our nation. Additional discussion of ethics and advocacy can be found in Chapter 28.

Principles of advocacy useful in formulating and presenting a case are summarized in Box 14-10.

National Issues in Advocacy

- Tax counseling for the elderly should be readily available to cut through the morass of calculations that make it no longer possible for ordinary citizens to file their own tax statements.
- The Social Security Trust Fund is now managed separately, but there remains concern that funds may be diverted for uses other than paying benefits and administering the agency.
- Provision for adequately financing long-term care in home and institutions and with improved quality assurance is desperately needed.
- Cash assistance and in-kind support of all individuals living below the poverty level is a concern of all nurses who recognize the relationship of health and wealth.
- Removal of covert and overt barriers to participation in the labor force remains a significant issue in spite of federal regulations against such discrimination.

- Housing and energy assistance programs are critical to survival for many aged.
- Consumer protection against fraud and enforcement of personal and legal rights must be a constant concern.
- Increased attention must be given to the financial abuses of elders that are perpetrated by some guardians and conservators.

Gerontic nurses share a responsibility to the young and the old, individually and collectively. Future possibilities will depend on more equal distribution of resources and protection of rights. We are aware of the remnants of our "child within," but are we as cognizant of the present structuring of our "elder within"? Our children must be adequately supported and treasured as youth in order to move forward through each developmental stage and reach a satisfying old age. Let us mobilize our strength to enrich the experience of growing and aging for our elders, our own present and future, and that of our children.

KEY CONCEPTS

- Aged individuals range from the poorest to the richest in our nation with very old black widows being the poorest segment of the population.
- There is rising concern among the baby boomers regarding the viability of the Social Security and Medicare systems because the predictions, for the most part, have been ominous.

Nursing Diagnoses

The following potential diagnoses must be considered as well as diagnoses unique to the particular individual:
Anxiety
Conflict/decisional
Denial/ineffective
Fear
Health maintenance/altered
Knowledge deficit
Powerlessness
Protection/altered

NURSING PROCESS AND NURSING DIAGNOSIS
Powerlessness

Etiologies and Related Factors
Personal characteristics
Institutionalization
Physical and mental changes
Loss of autonomy

Defining Characteristics
No directives regarding emergencies, trusted persons for decision making, preferences for where/when to die, organ donation, funeral arrangements
Lack of social contacts
Incongruence between what is stated and what is documented
Change in responsibility patterns
Change in others' perception of client
Family questions client competency
Institutionalization imminent
Lack of knowledge

Knowledge
Legal directives and options
Communication skills
Normal age changes
Chronic disease conditions
Teaching skills
Community resources

Clinical Judgment and Related Skills
Respect premise that client "knows best"
Show respect
Bolster self-worth
Collaborate with client
Provide information on request
Give comprehensive information that covers essential points
Encourage documentation of wishes
Teach client about various directives, advantages and disadvantages of each
Assist client with completion of document(s)
Document client's wishes

Evaluation
Client statements and documents are congruent
Completes an advance directive

NEEDS ADDRESSED AND TASK STRENGTHS

Need to make own choices; need for protection from uninformed judgment; need to maintain dignity (to assure safety, security, and self-esteem)

Plans for various contingencies that may occur
Seeks professional guidance when needed
Develops awareness of resources to obtain service
Seeks knowledge of rights and privileges

- Social Security and Supplemental Security Income, while not adequate of themselves, provide an economic safety net for most elders in the United States.
- Pensions, veterans benefits, and investments form part of the economic base for most elderly white males, but ethnic minorities and women fare less well, though the gender gap is slowly closing.

- The burden of medical expenses for the aged is shifting because almost half of Medicare beneficiaries are now subscribers of an HMO or managed care provider. The healthier aged are quite satisfied with the system, though the ill aged often feel they are not getting the expert attention they need or sufficient time with providers to properly address their complex problems.

- Nursing home care consumes the largest share of the Medicaid budget, and the provision of long-term care insurance is an ongoing concern of both young and old. It is costly and at present few individuals have long-term care policies.
- Legal and ethical protection of aged research subjects is a significant concern of gerontologists and nurses. The legal parameters are especially unclear for elders with various degrees of dementia.
- There are several groups that advocate for the aged and particularly for those in nursing homes.
- A major nursing responsibility is to advocate for the aged who lack family or capacity to represent their own best interests.
- Ethical and legal issues concerning active euthanasia are increasingly significant as they receive more media attention.

▲ CASE STUDY

Mr and Mrs J, age 62, and 60, respectively, have been married for 35 years. Mr J was a midlevel executive with a flourishing company. With company stock options and an attractive pension plan their future looked bright. They owned their home, a split-level, four-bedroom house in a lovely suburban community located on the bay. Their small cabin cruiser gave them a great deal of pleasure and they also frequently took commercial cruises. Their lifestyle was geared to their uppermiddle class income as were their friends. When Mr J was 58 years old, the company was sold to a multinational corporation based outside the United States, and Mr J no longer had a position with the new company. The stock dropped in price, the pension plan was inadequate if drawn upon early, and there was a penalty for drawing upon tax-deferred funds prior to age 59½. It appears the pension funds were poorly invested and may not bring the expected returns. Though their health is presently good, they are concerned about the future of Medicare, managed care, and whether to buy long-term care insurance. Mrs J had never worked outside the home and had no salable skills. What they had thought to be a very comfortable retirement became one of serious concern. They had saved a considerable amount in their middle years, but it was soon depleted as it was used for general expenses. Now Mr J has begun to draw upon his Social Security at a reduced benefit rate, and Mrs J is collecting Social Security based on her husband's benefits. Combined, their retirement income is about $2800 per month. This is insufficient to maintain the style of living to which they are accustomed. They are able to get by, but their income will not be adequate for maintaining and repairing their 35-year-old house, maintaining their boat, or their present social life. In addition, taxes keep going up as property values continue to rise. Mrs J says, "We really don't know what to do to ensure that we will have sufficient income for our needs 20 years from now. I'm really frightened about our future."

▲ CASE STUDY

Jake had retired after 20 years as a sergeant in the U.S. Army. For several years he did odd jobs, often as a mechanic in a nonunion shop or helping friends with home and mechanical repairs. He simply never found his niche after leaving the service. Some thought his war experiences had created serious psychologic problems for him. His wife, a successful nursing faculty person, had a good retirement plan. When his wife realized she was dying of cancer, she selected spousal survivor benefits in her retirement and insurance policies. After her death, Jake was financially secure though grief stricken because he had depended on his wife's practical and emotional support. Two years later Jake met Jane and soon realized he wished to marry her but found that his spousal retirement and Social Security benefits would be terminated if he married. Jake contacted a friend of his deceased wife to discuss his feelings and thoughts with her. He said, "I will not be content unless I marry Jane, but without the benefits I now receive I won't be able to manage. I wonder what I should do?"

Based upon one of the case studies, develop a nursing care plan using the following procedure*:

List comments of client that provide *subjective data.*

List information that provides *objective data.*

From these data identify and state, using accepted format, two *nursing diagnoses* you determine are most significant to this client at this time. List two *client strengths* that you have identified from data.

Determine and state *outcome criteria* for each diagnosis. These must reflect some alleviation of the problem identified in the nursing diagnosis and must be stated in concrete and measurable terms.

Plan and state one or more *interventions* for each diagnosed problem. Provide specific documentation of source used to determine appropriate intervention. Plan at least one intervention that incorporates the client's existing strengths.

Evaluate success of intervention. Interventions must correlate directly with the stated outcome criteria in order to measure the outcome success.

STUDY QUESTIONS/ACTIVITIES

What would be the focus of your first interaction with Mr and Mrs J?

---

*Students are advised to refer to their nursing diagnosis text and identify possible or potential problems.

Discuss various options that may provide them more economic security. Compare the benefits they might obtain from a reverse annuity mortgage with the benefits of selling the home and entering a life-care community. Discuss the pros and cons. How would you initiate such a discussion?

Discuss the limitations of Medicare and the out-of-pocket costs elders experience.

How common is a situation such as the Js'?

What major economic and legal issues are a concern of yours as you contemplate your old age?

Discuss the pros and cons of managed health care.

Do you believe it is acceptable to spend the great majority of our health dollars on the very old when several million children have no health care?

Is age a valid criterion for denial of certain medical services?

Discuss the meanings and the thoughts triggered by the student's and elders' viewpoints expressed at the beginning of the chapter. How do these vary from your own experience?

Discuss Social Security with an older relative and its effectiveness for him or her.

Consider Jake's dilemma and propose various solutions, remembering his personal history and cohort.

How have your parents expenditure patterns changed as they age?

What do you believe the "baby boomers" should do about their future economic situation and health care?

RESEARCH QUESTIONS

What do elders find most helpful about Medicare? Least helpful?

How would elders like to see Medicare changed?

What are elders' thoughts and attitudes about managed care?

Whom do elders most frequently contact when they need legal and economic advice?

How many elders feel secure about their economic future?

What are the current average out-of-pocket costs for elder health care?

How do elders feel about the rationing of health care based on age and/or survivability?

Are the poverty-inducing effects of widowhood and retirement different in specific ways in various ethnic groups?

What are the prevalent attitudes of the aged persons with whom you are acquainted regarding their economic future?

RESOURCES

Your Medicare Handbook, Health Care Financing Administration, U.S. Government Printing Office, U.S. Department of Health and Human Services, 7500 Security Blvd, Balti-

more, MD 21244-1850. The handbook is updated and issued each year to Medicare eligibles and may also be requested by other interested persons.

Social Security Retirement and Survivors Benefits booklet is available from all Social Security offices listed in the telephone book or by calling 1-800-772-1213.

Self-Help for Public Benefits, brochure prepared by Legal Counsel for the Elderly/AARP, PO Box 96474, Washington, DC 20090-6474.

Organizations

The American Bar Association
Commission on Legal Problems of the Elderly
1800 M Street NW
Washington, DC 20036
(202) 331-2297

Gray Panthers Project Fund
311 S Juniper St, Suite 601
Philadelphia, PA 19107

Advocates Senior Alert Process (ASAP)
134 G Street NW
Washington, DC 20005

National Center for Home Equity Conversion (NCHEC)
110 East Main, Room 1010,
Madison, WI 53703

Leo Baldwin
Consumer Housing Information Service
American Association of Retired Persons
1909 K Street NW
Washington, DC 20009

Publications

Long-Term Care Insurance
Shoppers Guide to Long-Term Care Insurance
National Association of Insurance Commissioners
(Call your state insurance commissioner and request copy)

HIAA's Consumer's Guide to Long-Term Care Insurance
(call 1-800-942-4242)

Take Charge of Your Money. A manual on how to manage your financial resources during retirement published by AARP that helps you establish goals, handle risk, and identify assets you did not know you had (or that are not working as hard as they should). For a free copy, send a postcard to Take Charge of Your Money, AARP Fulfillment, PO Box 2240, Long Beach, CA 90801.

15 Money Blunders. This booklet put out by Aetna Life Insurance helps persons to avoid the most common money-managing mistakes. It outlines some of the errors people make when budgeting, buying insurance, doing their taxes, etc. For a free copy, write to 15 Money Blunders, DA23, Aetna Life & Casualty, 151 Farmington Avenue, Hartford CN 06156.

Medicare

Guide to Health Insurance for People with Medicare. The free 30-page booklet, which is available from state insurance departments, is circulated by many Medigap insurance agencies (most state laws require insurers to offer clients the information contained in the booklet) or can be ordered from HCFA Publications, 6325 Security Blvd, Baltimore, MD 21207.

National Committee to Preserve Social Security and Medicare. Provides information, resources, addresses, and guidance for seniors to make services more readily available. 2000 K Street NW, Suite 800, Washington, DC 20006 (202) 822-9459.

Legal matters

It is advisable to consult a lawyer before setting up power of attorney, durable power of attorney, joint accounts, trusts, or guardianships. Be sure to ask for the cost of a legal consultation before you visit a lawyer. Most libraries have legal directories, or you can contact the American Bar Association, Lawyer Referral and Information Service, 750 North Lake Shore Drive, Chicago, IL 60611 (312/988-5760) and ask for help in locating a lawyer.

Free legal and financial services are often available to help older people and their families. For assistance, you can call or write the following organizations to be referred to your local, area, or state Agency on Aging:

National Senior Citizens Law Center
1052 W 6th Street, Suite 700
Los Angeles, CA 90017

National Association of Area Agencies on Aging
600 Maryland Avenue SW, Suite 208
Washington, DC 20024
(202) 484-7520

National Association of State Units on Aging
2033 K Street NW, Suite 304
Washington, DC 20006
(202) 785-0707

Legal Eye Newsletter for the Nursing Profession
8500 Fremont Avenue N, Suite 103
Seattle, WA 98103

Nolo Press Self-Help Law Books
Berkeley, CA
(510) 549-1976

Complaints against health care service plans in California can be filed with the Department of Corporations (DOC), (800) 400-0815. This should be done only after first contacting the health plan's grievance representative and attempting a resolution.

Consumers' Guide to Health Plans is a publication that has rated HMOs across the nation as excellent, very good, good, fair, or poor. This guide also gives information on keeping costs down and getting the best care when enrolled in a plan. Contact Health Plan Guide, 733 15th Street NW, Suite 821, Washington, DC 20005. (Cost, $12 including postage.)

Consumers' Guide to Health Plans, a similar publication, available from Center for the Study of Services, 1995; (202) 347-7283 or (510) 397-8305 or (800) 475-7283.

To obtain the free *Status List of the National Committee for Quality Assurance,* call (202) 955-3515.

1996 Accreditation Manual for Home Care, available from the Joint Commision of Health Care Organizations (JCHCO), One Renaissance Blvd, Oakbrook Terrace, IL 60181, (708) 916-5800.

REFERENCES

Access Health: Access Health announces million member contract with Blue Cross Blue Shield of Florida, *Access Health* news release # 35321723-013-86-0018, Sept. 13, 1996.

American Association of Homes and Services for the Aging: Most important issues in deciding 1994 US house vote, *Currents* 11(8):4, 1996.

American Association of Retired Persons: *A profile of older Americans: 1995,* AARP PF3049 (1295), Washington, DC, 1996, The Association.

American Medical Association: *AMA guidelines for physician responsibilities in subacute care,* Washington, DC, 1995, AMA Board of Trustees.

American Nurses' Association: Bill approved to raise debt limit includes line item veto and Social Security earnings limit, *Capital Update* 14(6):3, 1996.

American Society on Aging: Where is healthcare headed? *Generations* 20(2), entire issue, Summer 1996.

Archer D: Medicare HMOs sound good, but consumers have questions. In United Seniors Health Cooperative: More or less cost/more or less choice in today's health care, *United Seniors Health Report,* p. 1, summer 1996, Special Edition, United Seniors Health Cooperative, Washington, DC.

Bailis S: *Post acute care and prospective payment systems.* Testimony before the subcommittee on health of the House Committee on Ways and Means, July 23, 1996, Washington, DC, on behalf of the American Health Care Association.

Ball R: Medicare's roots: what Medicare's architects had in mind, *Generations* 20(2):13, Summer 1996.

Bengtson VL: Generational accounting doesn't add up, *Aging Today* 13(6):10, 1992.

California Association of Health Facilities: Fiscal intermediary to quit, *CAHF Long-Term Care News* 15(21):3, August 2, 1996.

CalPERS: Making your health plan decision, *Perspective, a California Public Employees' Retirement System Newsletter,* p. 1, Fall 1996.

Chriss L: Retailers cash in on home health market, *Nurseweek* 9(17):1, 1996.

Custis D, Fuller R: The VA will be there: the future of veterans' health care, *Generations* 20(2):71, summer 1996.

Cutler NE: Middle aging and the complexity of financial decisions, *DVMAGEC NEWS (Delaware Valley Mid-Atlantic Geriatric Education Center)* 6(3):3, 1992.

Fox P, Fama T: Managed care and the elderly: performance and potential, *Generations* 20(2):31, Summer 1996.

Gale BJ, Steffl BM: The long-term care dilemma, *Nursing Health Care* 13(1):34, 1992.

Gilfix M: Legal planning is essential for Alzheimer's victims, *Senior Spectrum* 6(12):5, 1987.

Heckheimer EF: *Health promotion of the elderly in the community,* Philadelphia: 1989, WB Saunders.

Hicks W, Miner K: The post-acute spectrum of care, *Cowen Industry Strategies* p. 4, May 19, 1993.

International Longevity Center: United States long-term care insurance: status report, *Longevity News* 3:4, 1995.

Kingson E: *A broader policy discussion is needed to plan for the aging of the baby boom cohorts and those who follow.* Paper presented at the 42nd Annual Meeting of the American Society on Aging, Anaheim, Calif, March 16, 1995.

Lyons B, Rowland D, Hanson K: Another look at Medicaid, *Generations* 20(2):24, Summer 1996.

McGurk M: Home equity conversion: could it be for you? *Senior Spectrum* 8(3):6, 1989.

McSweeney M: Long-term care insurance and alternatives: a comparison of employer and individual policy markets. *Health Care Finance* 22(1):72, 1995.

Medicare: 1996 deductibles, coinsurance, premiums, *Legal Eye Newsletter for the Nursing Profession* 4(3): 3, 1995.

Medicare patients footing big part of outpatient bills, *San Francisco Examiner,* p. A8, July 1, 1996.

Melnick V, Dubler N, Weisbard A: Clinical research in senile dementia of the Alzheimer type: suggested guidelines addressing the ethical and legal issues, *J Am Geriatr Soc* 32(7):531, 1984.

Moon M: Medicare: an appropriate age-related program? *Generations* 19(3):50, 1995.

National Academy on Aging: Medicare: hospital insurance and supplementary medical insurance, *Gerontology News,* p. 10, Oct 1995.

National Policy and Resource Center on Women and Aging: What do you know about managed care? *The Women and Aging Letter* 1(1):1, 1995.

Netting FE, Paton RN, Huber R: The long-term care ombudsman program: what does the complaint reporting system tell us? *Gerontologist* 32(6):843, 1992.

Nieswiadomy M, Rubin R: Change in expenditure patterns of retirees: 1972-1973 and 1986-1987, *J Gerontol* 50B(5):S274, 1995.

Quinn J: Entitlements and the federal budget: a summary, *Gerontology News* 23(8):4 pp. insert between pp. 4 and 5, Aug 1996.

Rini A: Elderlaw for nurses, *New Horizons* 5(25):2, 1996.

Rosenfeld A: Managed care for the elderly: what's the problem, where's the problem? *The Public Policy and Aging Report* 7(2):1, 1996.

Rother J: Consumer protection in managed care: a third-generation approach, *Generations* 20(2):42, 1996.

Rovner J: Moving to managed care: whole new game in the works for Medicare beneficiaries, *AARP Bulletin* 36(7):2, 1996.

Rubin R, Koelln K, Speas R: Out-of-pocket health expenditures by elderly households: change over the 1980s, *J Gerontol* 50B(5):S291, 1995.

Ruling a blow to some doctors, *San Francisco Chronicle,* p. A23, Oct 4, 1996.

Sansone, Schmitt: *Elderly with dementia can decide own treatment at end of their lives.* Unpublished study conducted at Frances Schervier Home and Hospital in the Bronx, New York, under the auspices of the Bureau of Long Term Care Services of the New York State Department of Health, news release, April 17, 1996.

Schwartz R: Heartless Medicare claims denials, *Contemporary Long Term Care* 15(11):24, 1992.

Stone D, Reublinger V: Long-term care reimbursement issues, *Clin Geriatr Med* 11(3):517, 1995.

Twentieth Century Fund: *Medicaid reform: a twentieth century fund guide to the issues,* New York, 1995, Twentieth Century Fund Press.

United Seniors Health Cooperative: More or less cost/more or less choice in today's health care, *United Seniors Health Report,* p. 1, summer 1996, special edition, United Seniors Health Cooperative, Washington, DC.

US Bureau of the Census: *Statistical Abstract of the United States: 1995,* ed 115, Washington, DC.

US Department of Health and Human Services: *Social Security: what every woman should know,* Social Security Administration, SSA Publication No. 05-10127, September 1994.

US Department of Health and Human Services: *Health United States: 1995,* Centers for Disease Control and Prevention, National Center for Health Statistics, Data Dissemination Branch, Hyattsville, Md, 1996, DHHS Pub No (PHS) 96-1232.

US Department of Health and Human Services: *The Medicare handbook,* Baltimore, 1996, Health Care Financing Administration.

US Government General Accounting Office: *Elderly Americans: health, housing and nutrition gaps between the poor and nonpoor,* Gaithersburg, Md, 1992, GAO.

US Health Care Financing Administration: *Health care financing review,* Washington, DC, Summer, 1996, US Government Printing Office.

US Health Care Financing Administration: *Your Medicare Handbook: 1996,* Baltimore, Md, 1996, US Government Printing Office, Pub No HCFA-10050.

Waehrer K, Crystal S: The impact of coresidence on economic well-being of elderly widows, *J Gerontol* 50B(4):S250, 1995.

Who can afford a nursing home? *Consumer Reports* 53(5):308, 1988.

Wiener J: Managed care and long-term care: the integration of financing and services, *Generations* 20(2):47, 1996.

Zis M, Jacobs L, Shapiro R: The elusive common ground: the politics of public opinion and healthcare reform, *Generations* 20(2):7, 1996.

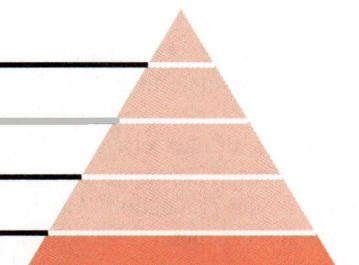

CHAPTER 15

Frailty, Vulnerability, and Neglect*

A student speculates

I imagine myself at 90; I have been living in a convalescent hospital for 6 years. Most of my friends have passed on, and it's very lonely here. I'm frustrated because I can't remember all my grandchildren's names, but I can still remember what happened on my wedding day. I also get confused as to where I am and who is visiting me.

Laura, age 36

Elders speak

I'm absolutely fine, but my legs feel as if they have lead weights tied to them. It is so hard to get around, and it takes all my energy. Sometimes I'm just too tired to concentrate. It's harder each day to do the things I must.

Ernie, age 84

A real concern of mine is that I will become incapacitated and hang on too long.

Alice, over 70

LEARNING OBJECTIVES

Upon completion of this chapter, the reader will be able to:

1. Identify several characteristics of the oldest-old.
2. Compare attributes of the frail old and the hardy old.
3. Specify problems that are characteristic of the frail and vulnerable old.
4. Enumerate important considerations in caring for the frail old.
5. Develop a nursing care plan addressing comprehensive needs of a frail elder.
6. Explain the fundamental concept of hardiness and apply it to understanding elder persons.
7. Relate essential aspects of conservatorships and guardianships and nursing responsibilities in relation to these.
8. Explain several of the dynamics of elder abuse.
9. Describe several situations that may trigger elder abuse.
10. Discuss the nurse's responsibility in regard to assessing, intervening, and reporting in cases of suspected elder abuse.

THE OLDEST-OLD

In 1995 it was estimated that 3.3 million individuals in the United States are over 85 years old (Zusman, 1995). These oldest-old, from age 85 to 123, range across the entire con-

tinuum of functional, emotional, and spiritual capacities from the totally dependent and oblivious to those who are hardy with startlingly predominant personality characteristics.

James was an example of the latter. A small, vigorous man at 103 years old, he had been a small-hotel owner in San Francisco in the days when an energetic and independent businessman could become very successful. He carried many of his skills and much of his energy into old age and could continually be seen organizing

*Our thanks to Mary Joy Quinn, Director of Probate Court Services, San Francisco Superior Court, City and County of San Francisco, who has contributed substantially to the accuracy and content of this chapter and whose contribution is essential to the substantive aspects of this chapter.

the retirement center in which he resided, much to the dismay of the administrator and, occasionally, the corporate directors. Even so, James was vulnerable to disturbances in his routines, infections, and any number of potential problems that could disturb his delicately balanced system of survival. He was balanced on a highly stretched and narrow tightrope of physiologic function. Any disturbance that created slackness in that tightrope would bode disaster for James. The last time we saw James, at his birthday celebration, he appeared rather dazed though charming and sociable. He had contracted an upper respiratory infection, possibly from communal exposure so common among residents of congregate living sites, and quickly developed pneumonia. Two months later he was dead. James was one of the fortunate of the frail and vulnerable. He demonstrated the concept of compressed morbidity (Fries, 1993; 1995), remaining hardy and functional until a very short time before death.

The concept of compressed morbidity, introduced by Fries in 1980, is of continuing interest in gerontology. Essentially the hypothesis envisions a reduction of extended morbidity and health care costs, now concentrated in the very old, and an extension of healthy aging, thus shortening the period of morbidity prior to death (Fries, 1993).

There are now many elders, not so fortunate as James, who have extended periods of impaired function, physically, socially, and mentally. The most important issue in facilitating shortened morbidity is to be aware of the vulnerability of the very old, even when they appear competent in all ways. They are not only vulnerable to physiologic disturbance but socially vulnerable to various abuses, mentally vulnerable to stressors, and spiritually vulnerable to deprivation of altruistic opportunities. Recognition of this vulnerability and proactive interventions are the key to longer periods of healthy survival and shorter periods of disability before death.

Characteristics of the Oldest-Old

From 1970 until 1994 the population over 85 years of age increased from 1,408,000 to 3,522,000, more than doubling in 25 years and now comprising 1.4% of the entire population of the United States (U.S. Bureau of the Census, 1995). It is common knowledge that this group is proportionately the most rapidly growing group of the population. Among the oldest-old, women vastly outnumber men (Table 15-1).

The oldest of the old are little known or understood other than in relation to their degrees of dependency. The element they all share is the recognition that they are old, although many still feel that the essence of self is not old . . . only the outer trappings. The major traumas of life, such as widowhood and retirement, are long since past for many of these elders. They have survived all the significant life transitions and are in various ways dealing with their own dependency and impending death. Others with whom they have been close have doubtless provided models for these events. These are the survivors; those who have learned most about life. Some gerontologists have termed this "the fifth age": the time when the dominant theme of life is self-determination versus dependence (Maddox, 1995).

Although many of the oldest-old live alone or with family, 23% are institutionalized. In addition to great numbers in nursing homes, many must rely on others for various types of assistance. The key concern of these very old is remaining in charge of their own lives. Fifty-five percent are managing to do so. With limited economic resources, few community supports, and nonaffordable housing they yet remain able to negotiate this complex society, if not to their satisfaction at least to maintain autonomy. Studies by Tsuji

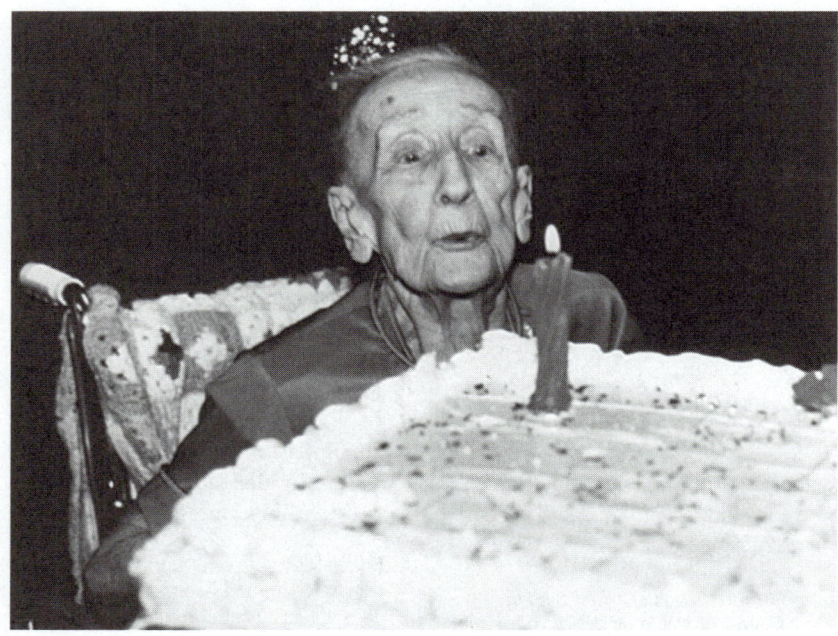

Hardy at 100. (Courtesy Mary Jane Prout, American Society on Aging.)

et al (1995) indicate that elders are vulnerable to institutionalization when they lose control of behavior or bodily functions or when their needs interfere greatly with those of the caregivers. Obviously, more attention needs to be given to the needs of care providers who are critical to sustaining the very old. Maintaining a social support network of interdependent caring and exchange is often the critical factor. Prevention of abuse and neglect is directly related to the availability of resources and respite from the burden of care. Discussion of caregivers can be found in Chapter 17.

Ethnic Minorities and the Oldest-Old

Among the oldest-old, minority populations form a small group (Table 15-2). They may be a very select group of survivors, having overcome the effects of poorer education, poverty, and discrimination. Few are institutionalized. Often they are living in their own homes with extended family members who assist them or in a home with "family" to whom they are not biologically related. Most of the minority persons of great old age have been severely disadvantaged and have learned to cope with a lifetime of stress and poverty. These patterns will undoubtedly change in the coming decades as more opportunities have been available to the minority groups in their young adult years.

The group of very old Hispanics is increasing rapidly, and although few in number, they are concentrated in: New York, Illinois, Florida, Texas, and California, with the majority in Texas and California (U.S. Bureau of the Census, 1995).

Twenty one percent of those over 65 years old live below the poverty level as do 28% of black elders. Though an age category is not readily available, 15% of Asians and 27% of American Indians are below the poverty level, and if the pattern is similar to other elderly groups, the poverty level gradually increases every year after age 65. These very old survivors of discrimination and disadvantage merit serious study. Risk taking and abusive behaviors in minority communities that include substance abuse, high-risk sex, accidents, and violence have destructive effects on the elders who manage to maintain residence in those communities (Castro et al, 1995). In addition, these problems in their youth have residual effects that may mar old age for those who manage to survive. Poverty and ill health are often addressed as problems of the ethnic aged, but the psychologic ramifications of a lifetime of exclusion, danger, and fear have scarcely been addressed at all. Frequency of abusive situations is unknown. Additional discussion of old age and ethnicity can be found in Chapter 24.

Frailty

Frailty is the term commonly used to indicate that an aged person is tenuously able to carry out important practical and social activities of daily living, though conceptualization of "frailty" is poor at best (Brown et al, 1995). Buchner and Wagner (1992, p. 1) describe frailty as follows:

A state of reduced physiologic reserve associated with increased susceptibility to disability. Reduced physiologic capacity in neurologic control, mechanical performance, and energy metabolism are

---

Table 15-1   Resident Population, by Age and Sex: 1970 to 1994

[In thousands, except as indicated. **1970, 1980,** and **1990** data are enumerated population as of **April 1;** data for **other years** are estimated population as of **July 1.** Excludes Armed Forces overseas.]

Year and sex	55-59 years	60-64 years	65-74 years	75-84 years	85 years and over	5-13 years	14-17 years	18-24 years	Median age (yr)
1991, total . . .	10,423	10,584	18,275	10,311	3,179	32,496	13,419	26,341	33.1
1992, total . . .	10,485	10,444	18,451	10,527	3,294	33,008	13,653	25,939	33.4
1993, total . . .	10,680	10,242	18,640	10,720	3,413	33,491	13,928	25,661	33.7
1994, total . . .	**10,936**	**10,082**	**18,712**	**10,925**	**3,522**	**33,863**	**14,428**	**25,263**	**34.0**
Male	5,244	4,740	8,290	4,206	980	17,339	7,412	12,856	32.9
Female	5,692	5,342	10,422	6,719	2,542	16,524	7,016	12,407	35.2
Percent:									
1970	4.9	4.2	6.1	3.0	0.7	18.0	7.8	11.7	(X)
1980	5.1	4.5	6.9	3.4	1.0	13.8	7.2	13.3	(X)
1990*	4.2	4.3	7.3	4.0	1.2	12.8	5.4	10.8	(X)
1994	**4.2**	**3.9**	**7.2**	**4.2**	**1.4**	**13.0**	**5.5**	**9.7**	**(X)**
Male	4.1	3.7	6.5	3.3	0.8	13.6	5.8	10.1	(X)
Female . .	4.3	4.0	7.8	5.0	1.9	12.4	5.3	9.3	(X)

From U.S. Bureau of the Census: *Statistical abstract of the United States: 1995,* ed 115, 1995.
*X, Not applicable.
*The data shown have been modified from the official 1990 census counts. The April 1, 1990, census count (248,718,291) includes count resolution corrections processed through March 1994 and does not include adjustments for census coverage errors.
Source U.S. Bureau of the Census, *Current Population Reports,* P25-917 and P25-1095; and Population Paper Listing 21.

Table 15-2   Resident Population, by Race, Hispanic Origin, and Single Years of Age: 1994

[In thousands]

Age	Total	Race				Hispanic origin*	Not of Hispanic origin			
		White	Black	American Indian, Eskimo, Aleut	Asian, Pacific Islander		White	Black	American Indian, Eskimo, Aleut	Asian, Pacific Islander
45-49 yrs. old	16,679	14,249	1,740	120	571	1,230	13,130	1,669	107	544
45 yrs. old	3,659	3,096	407	26	130	278	2,844	391	23	124
46 yrs. old	3,550	3,036	369	25	120	259	2,800	354	22	114
47 yrs. old	3,843	3,322	375	26	120	258	3,088	360	23	115
48 yrs old	2,652	2,269	267	20	96	213	2,074	255	18	92
49 yrs. old	2,974	2,525	322	22	105	222	2,323	309	20	100
50-54 yrs. old	13,191	11,355	1,340	91	406	913	10,522	1,287	82	387
50 yrs. old	2,890	2,483	293	21	93	204	2,298	282	19	88
51 yrs. old	2,931	2,549	278	19	85	195	2,371	267	17	81
52 yrs. old	2,549	2,191	263	18	78	174	2,032	253	16	74
53 yrs. old	2,440	2,099	250	17	75	172	1,941	240	15	72
54 yrs. old	2,381	2,033	256	17	76	167	1,880	246	15	72
55-59 yrs. old	10,936	9,436	1,110	71	318	738	8,760	1,069	64	304
55 yrs. old	2,283	1,950	246	16	71	157	1,808	237	14	67
56 yrs. old	2,281	1,966	234	15	66	154	1,825	226	13	63
57 yrs. old	2,178	1,876	224	14	64	147	1,742	215	13	62
58 yrs. old	2,021	1,758	195	12	56	137	1,632	187	11	54
59 yrs. old	2,173	1,886	212	14	61	144	1,754	204	13	59
60-64 yrs. old	10,082	8,773	984	57	268	616	8,208	950	51	257
60 yrs. old	1,981	1,714	198	12	56	128	1,597	191	11	54
61 yrs. old	1,953	1,693	194	12	54	123	1,581	187	11	52
62 yrs. old	1,965	1,705	196	11	53	118	1,597	189	10	50
63 yrs. old	2,065	1,810	192	11	52	125	1,695	185	10	50
64 yrs. old	2,118	1,850	204	11	54	123	1,737	197	10	51
65-69 yrs. old	9,970	8,792	906	47	226	521	8,312	878	42	217
65 yrs. old	2,059	1,796	202	10	50	116	1,689	196	9	48
66 yrs. old	2,071	1,822	193	10	47	111	1,720	187	9	45
67 yrs. old	2,003	1,765	184	9	45	103	1,670	179	8	43
68 yrs. old	1,897	1,678	168	9	43	96	1,589	163	8	41
69 yrs. old	1,940	1,730	159	9	42	94	1,643	155	8	40
70-74 yrs. old	8,741	7,840	694	36	171	383	7,485	676	33	164
70 yrs. old	1,875	1,674	153	8	40	88	1,592	149	8	38
71 yrs. old	1,801	1,611	146	8	37	83	1,534	142	7	36
72 yrs. old	1,811	1,630	138	8	35	77	1,558	135	7	34
73 yrs. old	1,695	1,527	130	7	31	71	1,461	127	6	30
74 yrs. old	1,559	1,398	127	6	28	63	1,340	123	5	27
75-79 yrs. old	6,574	5,949	499	24	102	243	5,724	487	23	98
75 yrs. old	1,473	1,326	117	6	24	56	1,274	114	5	23
76 yrs. old	1,369	1,243	101	5	21	51	1,196	98	5	20
77 yrs. old	1,294	1,173	96	5	20	47	1,130	94	4	19
78 yrs. old	1,254	1,139	92	5	19	46	1,097	90	4	18
79 yrs. old	1,184	1,068	94	4	18	44	1,028	91	4	17
80-84 yrs. old	4,351	3,962	316	16	57	162	3,810	309	15	54
80 yrs. old	1,048	953	77	4	14	39	917	75	4	14
81 yrs. old	966	878	72	4	12	36	844	70	3	12
82 yrs. old	855	783	58	3	11	32	753	57	3	10
83 yrs. old	784	716	55	3	10	30	688	54	3	10
84 yrs. old	699	633	54	3	9	25	609	53	2	9
85-89 yrs. old	2,274	2,083	161	8	22	80	2,008	158	8	21
90-94 yrs. old	948	859	77	4	8	32	828	76	4	8
95-99 yrs. old	249	225	20	1	3	8	218	20	1	3
100 yrs. old and over . . .	50	42	7	—	1	2	40	7	—	1
Median age (yr.)	34.0	35.0	29.0	26.7	30.4	26.1	33.2	291	27.2	30.7

From U.S. Bureau of the Census: *Statistical abstract of the United States: 1995*, ed 115, 1995.
— Represents or rounds to zero. *Persons of Hispanic origin may be of any race.
Source U.S. Bureau of the Census, unpublished data.

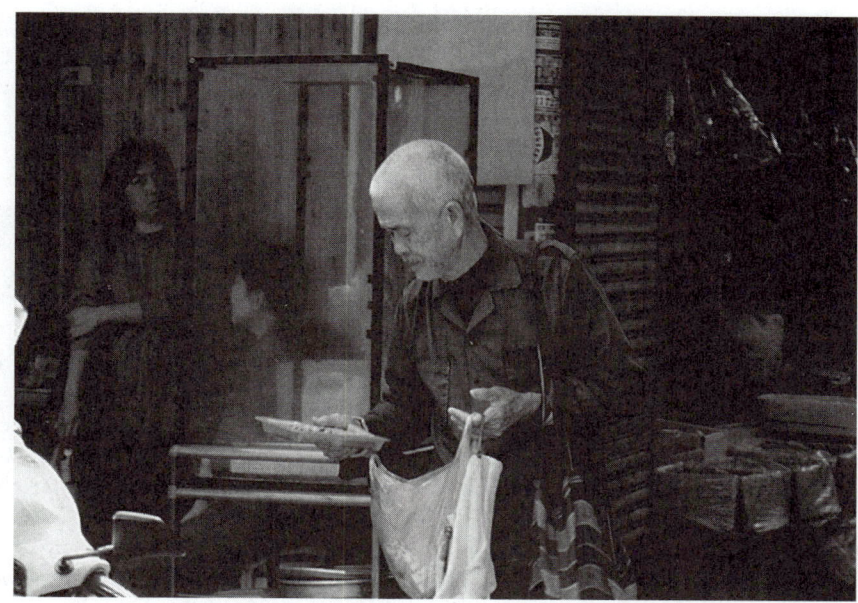

An elder in his ethnic enclave. (Courtesy Priscilla Ebersole.)

the major components of frailty. Although disease is an important cause of frailty, there is sufficient epidemiologic and experimental evidence to conclude that frailty is also due to the additive effects of low-grade physiologic loss resulting from a sedentary life style and more rapid loss due to acute insults (illness, injuries, major life events) that result in periods of limited activity and bed rest. The pathogenesis of frailty involves a complicated interaction of factors that block recovery from rapid physiologic loss. To some extent, frailty is preventable. Approaches to prevention include (1) the periodic monitoring of key physiologic indicators of frailty, (2) the prevention of physiologic loss and acute and subacute episodes of physiologic loss, (3) the prediction of episodes of physiologic loss and the reduction of frailty prior to the loss, and (4) the removal of obstacles to recovery once physiologic loss has occurred.

Anderson and Johnson (1996) say, "In any practice that includes elderly patients, you'll find frail, older individuals teetering on the edge of decline." Further they find that 46% of community-dwelling elders over age 85 are frail, meaning they have significant functional loss in the neurologic, musculoskeletal, and energy metabolism domains. They are at risk of a rapid downhill spiral when any acute insult, physiologic or psychologic, is added to the existing chronic, low-grade physiologic losses and changes of aging. They are much less likely to return to their previous functional baseline after any acute episode.

Individuals may be mentally or physically frail or both. Jones (1990) found that frailty was evidenced by increased susceptibility to disease and accident, diminished physiologic function, and compromised host-defense mechanisms. Often the frail and vulnerable are seen when they are incontinent, demented, or immobilized. These vulnerable individuals frequently develop urinary tract infections, skin infections and wounds, pneumonias, and gastroenteritis (Tennstedt and McKinlay, 1994).

Mental frailty will be addressed more fully in Chapter 22 but needs to be mentioned here because it is often the first evident sign of physical frailty. Mental frailty can be conceptualized as the narrowing of the sense of self as the trappings of identity are eroded by loss, changing appearance and insufficient physiologic reserve to support the lifestyle that has formed one's persona. Wolanin (1996) conceptualizes mental frailty as the increasing difficulty in the later years of maintaining the "continuity of self" that characterizes one's identity and capacity for personal integration.

We believe frailty of the very old is conveyed by words such as fragile, delicate, brittle, tender, easily disturbed, and confused.

Angie, at 92 years old, is frail. She is "independent" in her small apartment and requires no assistance in activities of daily living (ADLs). She stands straight, expresses herself well, and conveys a sense of power and dignity. Even though her apartment is air-conditioned, an unexpected spell of very hot weather disturbed her peace of mind and feelings of security. She didn't go out of the apartment to empty garbage or pick up mail; her appetite failed completely. Within a week she was marginally functional. By contrast, Madge, at 89 years old, lives in the same apartment complex and functions in much the same manner as Angie, but she has pronounced familial tremor, shuffles when she walks, is bent over with osteoporosis, and has joints deformed by arthritis. She is frail in a different way than Angie, but both are vulnerable.

These examples point to the fact that very old persons cannot be judged by external appearance. They are often less vulnerable than they physically appear to be, and many are more vulnerable. The point is, we are prone to judge by outward appearance, and this gives little information about the capacities or the reserve of an individual.

The Frail Elderly Functional Assessment Questionnaire (FEFA) seems to be a reliable instrument in assessing the functional ability of frail elders (Gloth et al, 1995), but even the most comprehensive geriatric assessment instruments fail to evaluate an elder's degree of vulnerability. Siu et al (1996) state that further efforts are needed to develop and to evaluate realistic approaches to comprehensive geriatric assessment. At present, none seem sufficient to give prognostic data, though Shats et al (1995) have found that elders who survive beyond the dangerous decade (70-79 years of age) seem to stabilize and perhaps show functional improvement. This concept is being seriously considered and studied.

These findings are, of course, complicated by the fact that many individuals who would have died of various disorders have been kept alive through sophisticated medical technology. Therefore, among the very old we find two distinct groups: those hardy souls genetically meant to endure for a century and the extremely frail who have walked the tightrope between survival and death for several decades. In general, those who are most frail present with atypical symptoms, most usually delerium, regardless of the disorder or problem and will have significiantly poorer responses to hospitalization (Jarrett et al, 1995). Siu et al (1993) found that self-reports regarding capacities and abilities are, for the most part, valid. The significance for nursing is that in general clients are the best judges of what they are and are not able to do comfortably.

Growth hormone is under investigation as a possible factor in preventing frailty. Normally, growth hormone diminishes during aging. A National Institute on Aging (NIA) study is aimed at determining whether administration of growth hormones on an ongoing basis will keep people strong and fit and in essense delay morbidity. In a small study it was shown that administration of growth hormone increased strength, muscle mass, and skin integrity in healthy men over 65 years of age. This larger NIA study is aimed at increasing healthy aging and reducing frailty.

Hardiness

Hardiness, a concept at the opposite end of the continuum from frailty, is important in the assessment of the adaptation and survival of the very old. Hardiness is defined as a personality style characterized by three elements: feelings of control, deep commitment to something or someone, and enjoyment of challenge (Pappas, 1995). The concept is based in the existential belief that stressors provide the impetus for making choices and taking responsibility for actions (Kobasa, 1979). Challenge is perceived as normal and beneficial, and these personality characteristics function as a resource in the face of adversity (Kobasa et al, 1982).

Hardiness is increasingly popular as a research variable used to explain survival capacity of the frail and vulnerable. Investigators have for almost two decades investigated the concept of hardiness as it relates to survival and coping among the oldest-old with chronic illness and multiple stressors (Bowsker and Keep, 1995).

Though we may experience an overwhelming need to assist, it is our professional obligation to ask, "What kind of help will make it possible for you to do the things that are important to you?" There are risks for professionals and for clients, but few actions are risk-free. Clark (1995) contends that professionals are becoming more cognizant that the patient must define the means and ends of care and that the restructuring of health care around the uniqueness of the individual has been a distinct shift in medical practice. The emphasis on basic values and meanings in each health care encounter must fit in relation to the individuals' life goals.

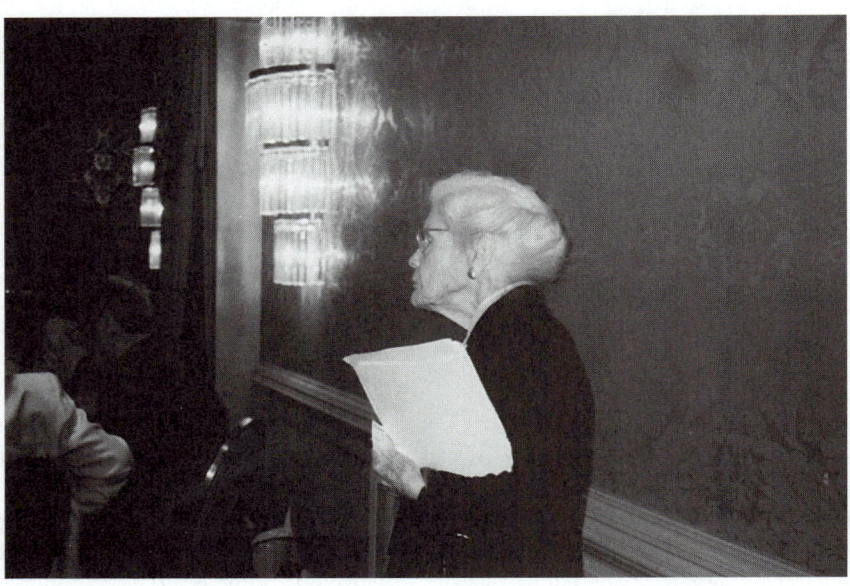

Frail but powerful. (Courtesy Priscilla Ebersole.)

This, when genuinely activated, is fundamental to hardiness at any age. The relinquishment of professional control to the individual activates the person's inherent power, accountability, and courage. These qualities may be more inwardly than outwardly oriented when one perceives himself or herself vulnerable. These individuals may even appear excessively self-centered upon superficial observation. The nurse may be thinking, "He is such a stubborn, egotistic old duffer." Upon deeper thought it is apparent these are the trappings of hardiness. Reinforcing control, mastery, and commitment can be expected to bolster hardiness.

Problems of the Oldest-Old

The visualization of old age has most often been of a long slide down from a peak that occurs around the age of 35 years. One may crash on the way down or slide inexorably to oblivion and invisibility. This analogy is embedded in materialism and our excessive focus on the physical body. Therefore when examining the situation of the frail aged we most often hear what they can and cannot do physically. We are most interested in their survival strategies, and these should be discussed thoroughly as we learn from them to expand our repertoire of skills and our understanding of the very old.

Bone and Joint Problems. Problems with osteoarthritis are almost universal by the eightieth birthday. Mobility is greatly decreased in the oldest-old, largely because of degenerative joint disease (osteoarthritis) and osteoporosis (see Chapter 11 for discussion). These are often accompanied by severe discomfort. Because osteoarthritis affects weight-bearing joints and the spine, it is a key factor in instability and falls. Osteoporosis is another problem that is rampant among old women and increasingly among older men (Kessenich, 1996). Ninety percent of women over 75 years of age have some degree of osteoporosis. Fractures, falls, pain, and restricted mobility result (see Chapter 11).

Falls. Falls are a serious risk for the oldest-old because of chronic disorders, cognitive clouding, multiple medications, and difficulties with balance and proprioception. These are discussed in Chapter 11. A fall may presage immobility, decline, and death.

Visual and Hearing Problems. Half of the oldest-old report having trouble with their vision, even with glasses. Twenty-one percent have a lot of trouble seeing, and 12% report blindness in one or both eyes. Most very old elders have hearing loss that has not been adequately assessed. Sensory appraisal and augmentation when possible is critical to maximizing function (see Chapter 12) and prevention of accidents.

Cognitive Impairment. Cognitive impairment increases significantly in very old age. Among the oldest-old, 35% report that "senility" causes limitations for them. Statistics vary, but several sources agree that about 35% of persons 85 years and over who are living in the community are cognitively impaired, and 40% of these are severely impaired (see Chapter 22).

Energy Allotment. One of the issues with the oldest-old is their decreasing energy levels. Often this is seen only as a fatigue factor. Wells (1986, p. 21) discusses energy expenditure from an enlightened perspective:

> An elderly individual may be able to walk but prefers to use a wheelchair in order to travel a greater distance in less time and have more energy remaining. Although the ability to walk should be maintained, the desire to be more mobile should be respected and a wheelchair provided to permit a wider range of social opportunities . . . a person may prefer the privacy of self-toileting and may wish to use considerable energy in that activity but may request assistance in dressing.

The opportunity for choice in energy expenditure may be ignored if we have an all-or-none approach to the dependencies of the aged. Interdependence for the aged is a dynamic concept that implies they are not helpless recipients nor are they thrown into the expectation of variations of self-care that may be individually inappropriate. The goal of maximizing function and delaying decline while using and building on personal strengths and desires is the goal of wellness-oriented rehabilitation from our perspective. Unless we have a holistic understanding of the individual we may ruthlessly and inappropriately press for self-care.

Failure to Thrive. Periodically we have wondered whether there were similarities between marasmus babies, studied by Spitz (1945), that could not survive without human stimulation, interaction, and caressing and the very old, isolated, frail aged who lack companionship and caring. Braun et al (1988) found that failure to thrive (FTT) in adults had many corollaries with those of infants and symptomatically presented a mirror image. FTT is a rather indiscriminate diagnosis. It generally describes a person with unexplained weight loss, nutritional deficits, decline in physical and cognitive function, and depressive symptoms such as remaining in bed, isolating self, giving up, and feeling helpless (Kimball and Williams-Burgess, 1995).

There are many possible causes for these symptoms, so they must be evaluated carefully. Gaffney (1995) suggests FTT is the result of the "downward spiral" characteristic of the downward spiral of dependency conceptualized by Hess (1990). Newbern (1992) studied this and suggests the necessity of a thorough nutritional assessment first because many of the symptoms of FTT may be related to serious malnutrition. Mental assessment must be made to determine cognitive and depressive status. An attachment assessment is also important. It can be measured by the 24-item Lipson-Parra Adult Attachment Scale (1989). This tool allows the individual to identify special persons with attachment characteristics. Interestingly, the oldest-old reported long-standing attachments and higher scores than other older subjects.

For those suspected of FTT, interventions include physical stimulation through stroking, touching, rocking, and assistance to reestablish personal and social ties. There is little really known about FTT in the aged, and one must question whether the issue is a lack of meaning in one's existence and whether a spiritual deficit is the core problem (see further discussion in Chapter 27).

PRINCIPLES OF WORK WITH FRAIL VULNERABLE ELDERS

Working with older adults who are having serious difficulty coping with their lives demands a great deal of the nurse; sensitivity is needed to search out the exact difficulty. Because of reasons of pride or because of mental impairment, older people may not state their problem or problems directly. Tolerance and patience may be required to tease out the issues; often a great deal of trust must be present before a frail elder will confide in a nurse. Perhaps several visits will be needed. Working with this group of older people simply takes more time, and often the nurse will need to form a genuine relationship with her client to be effective. That relationship must include sincere caring and concern. The client will also care about the nurse, worry and possibly want to give gifts of some sort. It may be the older person's way of feeling less dependent and needy, an attempt to still have some control over the situation. It is important to remember always that these older adults are survivors, people who have lived through major world wars, social upheavals, and personal hardships.

These special old folks wherever they may be on the frailty/hardiness continuum have survival capacity, and there is little we understand at present of the elements of this endurance. Is it love of life, courage, determination, stubbornness? Perhaps a bit of each. We do know when one has nothing for which to look forward life ebbs away quickly, yet we see many very old frail folk asking to die but remaining alive. We must surmise that in some level of consciousness the life force remains strong. Current questions and concerns about assisted suicide will increase discussion of this important issue. While we can't anticipate all the questions or the answers, we do know that our mission is to add as much meaning as possible to these remaining months or years and assist the client in planning for a meaningful death (Ebersole, 1983).

Legal Protection for the Vulnerable Aged

Nurses have rarely had sufficient exposure to the legalities of the court system to make decisions regarding the protection of the vulnerable aged, especially in cases where there may be some mistreatment. For the most part these situations occur when the elder is either not strong enough or not competent enough to exert measures to protect his or her own interests.

In many states, guardianship over an incompetent person and the person's property is unified by a single legal determination. Under the Uniform Probate Code and in those states where it has been adopted, guardianship refers to control over the person and conservatorship refers to control over, and management of, the property. There are often overlapping powers such as the guardian's decision for nursing home placement and the conservator's contract to pay for the services. Mere memory impairment or physical deterioration does not provide a sufficient basis for the judgment of "incapacity" under the Uniform Probate Code; there must be a clear lack of understanding and inability to communicate (Quinn, 1989). A review of your state statutes on conservatorship and guardianship will clarify specifics. It may be necessary to contact a geriatric legal counselor in your area.

Many aged are judged incapable of managing their finances or their basic needs and are given adult protective services under the laws of conservatorship, which may vary from state to state. Conservatorship generally means that a court-appointed conservator (who may be a family member) makes decisions about where an individual lives and how his or her needs are met. Conservatorship hearings are presented in court at periodic intervals to determine necessity for continuation. Limits are set according to the degree of protection needed. Total dependency means the person cannot meet basic needs for survival and is unable to manage the environment in any self-sustaining way. Some dependency means the person may be able to manage certain challenges of life,—health or judgment may interfere with management of other needs.

The reliance on legal guardianships is increasing due to the numbers of vulnerable elders that are surviving and the effect on families and communities. However, even with the best of intentions, these can lead to further decline in the elders' capacities as they relinquish decision-making power and any remnant of autonomy (Thomas, 1994). Traditionally, it has been assumed that guardianships have been instituted for the protection of an elder who needs help. Now, system reforms are being instituted because it is increasingly realized that sometimes persons seeking guardianship of an elder are acting in their own interests that may result in taking advantage of the elder (Heisler and Quinn, 1993). Alternatives to guardianship are analyzed to identify limitations of several types of decision-making interventions as seen in Table 15-3 (Wilber and Reynolds, 1995).

The courts currently seem to be reluctant to judge people incompetent. Although this is a great improvement from 25 years ago, when old people were "railroaded" into institutions, it is sometimes detrimental to the client and family. When we err, it must always be in the direction of preserving client autonomy. Further discussion of cognitive impairment and clients' rights can be found in Chapters 14 and 22.

Adult Protective Services. The subspecialty in the field of aging that deals with frail elders is called "adult protective services." Adult protective services have evolved over the past 30 years in response to the immense growth in the numbers of older people who need assistance with ADLs. Although some public agencies carry the name Adult Protective Services, the term in general refers to a wide range of services that are delivered to frail endangered elderly: medical, social, and legal. Little is actually known about the specific utilization of adult protective services, but a research group in New Haven found that 73% of referrals over a period of 11 years involved reports from concerned persons of elder self-neglect (Lachs et al, 1996).

Because of the variability and comparative newness of the concept of adult protective services, programs in any given community are likely to be fragmented or have gaps in services. Lachs et al found that a variety of private and public agencies may be involved with a dependent older person. Complicating the picture even further is the fact that the frail, vulnerable old usually need several services at one time. The need for coordination among the various service providers—that is, community health nurses, social workers, physicians, clinic nurses, discharge planners, lawyers, clergy members, family, and friends—is obvious. Much more attention is being given to this in the present cost-saving milieu. Increasingly, overlapping services are seen as wasteful. Today, team coordination and case management form the cornerstones of care of the aged in health maintenance organizations (HMOs) and among similar medical care programs.

Adult protective services workers deal with people who tend to have complicated problems and many urgent needs, all of which present themselves at the same time. To deal with what seems like chaos, workers need guidelines. When intervening with frail, vulnerable elderly the following fundamentals must guide decisions:

1. When interests compete, the adult client is the only person you are charged with serving. This principle reaffirms the traditional primary loyalty nurses have always had to their patients.
2. When interests compete, the adult client is in charge of decision making until he or she delegates responsibility voluntarily to another or until the court grants responsibility to another.
3. Freedom is more important than safety; that is, the person can choose to live in harm or even self-destructively provided he or she is capable of choosing, does not harm others, and commits no crimes.
4. In the ideal case, protection of adults seeks to achieve simultaneously and in order of importance: freedom, safety, least disruption of lifestyle, and least restrictive care alternatives (Quinn, 1989).

Power of Attorney.   Power of attorney is a legal device that affords some assistance in handling legal affairs. It can be valid only if the person granting the power of attorney is capable of doing so. There are three types, one of which, the durable power of attorney, is valid even after mental impairment has set in. There is no bonding involved as there is with conservatorships, so there is less protection for the frail person. Nevertheless, it is helpful and appropriate for some people. It is possible to prepare a nomination of the person or persons desired to serve as conservator far in advance and to have that document kept with other legal papers. This can be a safeguard and give much peace of mind. Finding an attorney one can trust and put confidence in can be of great help in settling and keeping one's legal affairs in order. There are some attorneys who prefer older clients, usually attorneys who practice probate law.

Conservatorships.   Conservatorships (termed guardianships in some states) are the most legally restricting way that an individual's person and property can be handled short of imprisonment or commitment to a locked mental health facility. For that reason, and because it still is the legal device of first choice by many physicians and attorneys, it is discussed in some depth.

The law in one state, California, details criteria that must be considered to establish a probate conservatorship based on functional deficits:

A conservator of person may be appointed for a person who is unable properly to provide for his or her personal needs for physical health, food, clothing, or shelter.

Table 15-3   Legalities and Risks of Financial and Health-Related Services Available to Older People

Service	Required for execution	Survives incapacity	Personal risk: high, medium, low	Financial risk: high, medium, low	Responsible authority
Power of Attorney	Yes	No	Low	Medium	Oversight by family; legal action
Bill paying service	Yes	Not usually	Low	Medium	Agency audit; legal action
Joint accounts/joint tenancy	Yes	Yes	Low	Medium	Virtually none; legal action
Durable power of attorney	Yes	Yes	Low	High	Oversight by family; legal action
Durable power of attorney for health care	Yes	Yes	Medium	Low	Oversight by family; legal action
Representative payee	No	Yes	Medium	Medium	Virtually none by Fed. Govt. Agency
Personal trust	Yes	Yes, if drawn properly	Medium	High	Internal audit, banking commissioner, legal action
Guardianship	No	Yes	High	High	Court: legal action

Modified from Wilber KH, Reynolds SL: Rethinking alternatives to guardianship, *Gerontologist* 35(2):248, 1995.

A conservator of the estate may be appointed for a person who is substantially unable to manage his or her own financial resources or resist fraud or undue influence. Substantial inability may not be proved solely by isolated incidents of negligence or improvidence.

A conservator of the person or estate, or both, may be appointed for a person who voluntarily requests the appointment and who, to the satisfaction of the court, establishes good cause for the appointment (California Probate Code Division 4, Part 3, Chapter 1, Section 1801, 1802, Probate Codes, State of California, 1974).

The California legislature has moved over the years to view individuals needing substantial assistance in managing their affairs as persons in need of civil rights protections. And, there has been more focus on the actual daily functioning of the person as a criterion for conservatorship rather than a medical or psychiatric diagnosis. Conservatorship mechanisms are often ineffective for some of the reasons shown in Box 15-1.

Court Investigators. Probate conservatorship is aimed at protecting the rights of the individual in question and providing for full access to legal resources and safeguards. The position of the court investigator is central to the implementation of the law, ensuring that conservatees will receive the protections of due process. The court investigator must personally interview all subjects of proposed conservatorships when a medical certificate is filed alleging that the subject cannot attend the hearing. In some places it is the practice of the judge to order that every conservatorship be investigated before the appointment of a conservator even if the attorney and proposed conservator plan to bring the proposed conservatee to the hearing. A hearing is the public time for facts to be presented to the judge. At that time a decision is made by the judge as to the need for a conservatorship and who can best serve as the conservator.

At the time of the interview, the court investigator determines if the individual can attend the hearing without incurring physical damage as well as if the individual wants to come to the hearing; it is one of the person's legal rights to attend the hearing if he or she wishes to do so. The investigator may determine that the individual is able to attend the hearing even though the individual's physician may not agree.

As a result of the investigator's "watchdog" function and evaluation, more proposed conservatees are able to attend their hearings, at which time they can be more fully aware of their rights and the intent of the court in offering support and protection for their person and estate.

The investigator informs the proposed conservatee of the nature of the citation that should have been received before the arrival of the investigator, of the fact that there is a pending conservatorship, and who is proposing to be the conservator. The investigator also informs the individual of the nature, purpose, and effect of the hearing and the right to protest the proceedings, the right to be represented by legal counsel, and the right to oppose the proceedings up to and including a jury trial. The investigator determines if the proposed conservatee wishes someone other than the proposed conservator to serve.

Court investigators are required to follow conservatorships that have been established. This is done 1 year after appointment and then every 2 years, coinciding with the financial accounting that is required when there is a conservator of estate. At that time, in addition to discussing the conservatorship itself and evaluating the performance of the conservator, the investigator must determine whether the individual desires to have the conservatorship ended and whether termination would be in the best interests of the conservatee. Legal counsel, private or public, must be appointed when termination is sought. Court investigators respond to complaints from conservatees, from attorneys, and from the clinical community.

In addition to informing proposed conservatees of impending conservatorships and their rights and to following up periodically on these cases, investigators are required to update all conservatorship cases in which the attorney has failed to submit the required accountings. A great deal of judgment and persistence may be required to search out the facts of a situation and present them to the judge, who makes the final decision as to the need for a conservator. At times, certain interests may attempt to conceal relevant facts.

The goal of the court investigator is always to achieve that which is in the best interests of the conservatee. For instance, the proposed conservatee may protest the proceedings mightily but cannot remember his or her birth date, place of residence, what he or she ate for breakfast, where bank accounts are, or who paid the bills the previous month. That person is in need of a conservator. However, should that person request an attorney, he or she is entitled to one so that due process might be had. In another instance, an individual may suffer a stroke, be totally incapacitated, and be in need of a conservator. However, at the end of the year when the first annual investigation is performed, the person may be clear mentally and have regained full speech and gait functioning. Therefore a conservator is no longer needed.

In some situations, it can be quite a detective job to determine the mental status of an individual. There may be confabulation, a condition that can occur with some forms of dementia, in which stories are fabricated in response to questions about situations or events that are not recalled. In another instance, the individual may possess an elaborate paranoid system that involves detailed conspiracy, "facts" about people, or banks being after his or her money or belongings.

Because any claims, no matter how paranoid or irrational they sound, may have some basis in fact, the investigator must conduct a careful inquiry into all allegations. An investigator must also determine what properly constitutes sufficient food, clothing, shelter, and medical care, as well as determining (with the help of other trained court personnel) that the person's estate is being used in his or her best interest. The role of the court investigator has much in common with that of nurses, especially nurses who function in community settings.

Assessment

When older people are in need of adult protective services, they are upset and often deny the need. Further, family and friends are usually equally distressed. Perhaps they are exhausted from trying to help the impaired person over a long period of time. Maybe the elder is demanding, even hostile. People in need of help may be confused, frightened, dependent, and unwilling or unable to make decisions for themselves. Often, there is pressure on the worker to "do something—now." But help and services, except in emergencies, cannot be adequate without thoughtful, interdisciplinary conferences with family and client. Generally, assessment goes forward at the pace the client can tolerate, although some services may need to be put in place as the assessment proceeds. Priorities must be developed. Table 15-4 enumerates some factors contributing to an elder's vulnerability.

It is important to first address the problems most troubling to the client/family. In this way some trust can be established even in difficult situations. Working with frail elders is a balancing act in so many ways—pacing of the work, how much to intrude, what to push, when to leave the person alone. If the client is mentally clear and understands the situation but still refuses interventions, the case manager cannot legally intrude. In those cases, the only thing to do is to leave the person alone after first establishing a bond and making sure the person knows where to call if he or she desires assistance. If the client is not mentally clear and is refusing interventions, it may be necessary to take legal action, possibly proceeding to a conservatorship.

Establishing Competence. The issue of competency of an elder is a critical determination in his or her future rights to autonomy and the degree of restrictions imposed on his or her living situation. Heisler and Quinn (1993)

make the important distinction between legal competency and clinical competency. Legal competence is assumed until a court judgment declares an elder incapable in specific ways, whereas clinical competence relies on observations of health and social service providers' diagnoses, often arrived at in imprecise fashion, of an individual's abilities to maintain the BADLs as well as the IADLs. Further discussion of cognitive competence is found in Chapter 22.

Table 15-4	Assessment of Elderly Vulnerability
General assessment	**Specifics**
Physiologic	Diminished endurance/weakness
	Decreased mobility/ambulation/range of motion, unstable ambulation
	Bruises easily, often evidence of ecchymosis
	Decreased cardiac output
	Ineffective airway
	Shortness of breath interferes with activities of daily living (ADLs)
	Unstable blood glucose
	Inability to speak
	Altered vision
	Poor nutritional or fluid intake
	Incontinence
	Fragile skin integrity (breaks in skin or potential for)
	Potential infection
	Unable to see wound
	Numbness
	Dizziness
	Dysphagia
Environmental	Factors which create safety concerns in and outside the home
	Potential for falls
	Injuries from various sources in and outside of home
Cognitive	Knowledge deficit
	Signs of brain dysfunction/poor memory
	Confusion
Psychosocial	Lacks confidence in self-care abilities
	Absence of social supports
	Loneliness
	Overwhelmed by treatment
	Anxiety about caregiver's health
	Depression
Caregiver	Dependence on caregiver with limited physical abilities
	Dependence on caregiver with limited mental abilities
	Need for caregiver respite
	Nonacceptance of caregiver
Other	Need for physical assistance
	Self-care deficits
	Inability to adhere to medication or treatment regimens

Modified from Frost MH, Willette K: Risk for abuse/neglect: documentation of assessment data and diagnosis, *J Gerontol Nurse* 20(8):37, 1994.

Box 15-1	**Reasons for Ineffective Conservatorships**

1. Many people who need protection do not come to the attention of authorities, particularly if they are old and alone and their behavior is not bizarre.
2. Some people may appear alert and competent during court hearings but are a danger to themselves and others in their daily lives.
3. The appointed conservator, if a family member, may not be dependable or responsible; sometimes the family member is covertly or overtly destructive to the individual.
4. Public conservators may have an overload of cases and give them only cursory attention.
5. The discrimination between "eccentric" and "incompetent" is somewhat related to affluence. The wealthy are more likely to be judged eccentric.

Interventions

Nurses who deal with older adults in their caseloads can do much to help their clients protect themselves; however, few nurses have experience with the American legal system (Heisler & Quinn, 1993). It is imperative that clients be encouraged to seek counsel if uncertain about their rights.

It is the nurse who has the most direct and continuing contact with the frail elder. The challenge is to keep abreast of developments and to be aware of information from other disciplines that directly affects the frail elder. Consequently, nurses would do well to familiarize themselves with the laws that specifically affect older adults. This can be done by speaking with an attorney or selecting continuing education programs to update knowledge in the field of client legal protections.

Once informed of the laws affecting frail elders, nurses are in a position to assist elders and family members in seeking legal representation when necessary. For instance, knowing conservatorship and guardianship law would enable the nurse to guide family members and elders to appropriate individuals for assistance in the process of filing for conservatorship or guardianship when necessary.

Nurses can also help conservators and guardians fulfill their roles by their careful documentation of clients' status and family interactions. Further, families may need encouragement to assume increased responsibility for the affairs of aged members.

Some courts provide informational videotapes and handouts for newly appointed conservators and guardians that can be helpful for anyone dealing with conservatorships or guardianships (San Francisco Superior Court, 1989, see resources at the end of the chapter).

Least Restrictive Alternative. It is generally accepted by professionals working in the field of adult protective services that people in need of help should not be intruded upon any more than is necessary to keep body and soul together. This includes the personal care of persons as well as the handling of their material resources: bank accounts, real estate, stocks, bonds, jewelry. In considering which service to use when assisting an older adult, the least restrictive one should be the first choice.

Advocacy. An advocate is one who maintains or promotes a cause; defends, pleads, or acts on behalf of a cause for another; fights for someone who cannot fight; and often gets involved in getting someone to do something he or she would not otherwise do. Because so many older frail people cannot speak for themselves, nurses often find themselves in the position of having to do the "talking," being an advocate.

Many frail elders' situations seem globally desperate to middle-class workers not used to extreme hardships in life. In these situations the danger exists that workers will "over-advocate" and bring in services the client really does not want and cannot use. An advocate needs to be clear at all times just whose position and needs are being met. The client is the focus.

Topics for advocacy can include specific rights protections such as promoting the least restrictive alternative for a client, finding the best nursing home, or telling court personnel one's opinion of a proposed conservator. Other areas include the rights of medical patients, the right to have in-home supportive services and maintenance of government benefits such as veterans benefits, Medicare, Social Security (SS), and Supplemental Security Income (SSI), and food stamps.

Advocates function in various arenas: with their own and other disciplines within their own agencies, with other agencies, with physicians, with families, with neighbors and community representatives, with legislators, and with courts when conservatorships are at issue. In the latter case, the advocate might feel that the conservatorship is inappropriate, premature, or being used to deprive a capable older person of rights because of someone's interest in his or her money. Or, the advocate may feel that the conservatorship is needed and necessary even though the older person does not want it and thinks he or she is functioning beautifully. Interdisciplinary collaboration and teamwork will ensure that skewed opinions will be balanced by fact (see Chapter 14 for further discussion).

ABUSE AND NEGLECT OF THE AGED

The terms abuse and neglect of the elderly are used to describe situations in which individuals over the age of 65 experience battering, verbal abuse, exploitation, denial of rights, forced confinement, neglected medical needs, or other types of personal harm, usually at the hands of someone responsible for assisting them in their activities of daily living (Fulmer and O'Malley, 1987, p. 3).

In a society becoming increasingly more violent, it is reasonable to assume that abuse of elders and other vulnerable persons will continue to increase. Estimates are that from 1.5 to 2 million adults experience abuse or neglect each year in the United States (Aravanis et al, 1993). The National Center on Elder Abuse (1996) estimated the number from 820,000 to 1,860,000. It is impossible to get an accurate estimate because there is no place where elders are routinely exposed to scrutiny as in the case of children in school.

Abuse of elders has generated considerable interest in the last two decades as the prevalence of the problem has become more visible. Yet it is not given the attention needed. States on average spend $22 per child for youth protective services but only $2.90 per elder for protective services, though 40% of reported abuse involves elders (Lett, 1995). In an 11-year longtitudinal study of community elders, nearly 10% were at some point referred for adult protective services (Lachs et al, 1996).

In Canada a large survey of dentists revealed that 83% were aware of incidents of abuse and neglect related to dental care (Mayer and Galan, 1993). Of these, the greatest number were neglect of personal hygiene though 22% were for fractures, avulsed teeth, abrasions and lacerations. Treatment was provided to 53% of the cases, and 20% required emergency medical referrals.

In the Nordic countries of Sweden, Denmark, and Finland 8% to 17% of a random population sample reported knowing elders who were being abused in their homes by close kin (Hydle, 1993). In one of these surveys, conducted in Sweden, 12% of close family members admitted abusing an elder relative (Hydle, 1993). Not only families abuse elders; there are reports that elder abuse among nurses is on the increase (Casteldine, 1994). Perpetrators of elder abuse are shown in Figure 15-1.

While we often think of physical abuse as the most likely form, one study found that 46% of substantiated charges were of financial exploitation (Shiferaw et al, 1994). In Sweden the most frequently reported abuse was psychologic (Saveman et al, 1993), and most situations arose around family conflicts. In reality, neglect by self and other is by far the most frequent type of mistreatment (Figure 15-2).

In Britain a study was made of situations in which individuals were referred for respite care (Homer and Gilleard, 1990). Nearly half (45%) of the caregivers admitted to some form of physical or verbal abuse and neglect. Verbal abuse and neglect were significantly related to long-standing problems in the relationship and had occurred long before caregiving was necessary. Often the abuse was precipitated or augmented by alcohol abuse. The caregivers willingly talked about their difficulties, but the elders would rarely do so. This is extremely important for nurses to remember because the best source of information in these cases is apparently not the patient.

Increasing awareness of neglect and abuse of elders has led the American Medical Association (AMA) (1992) to is-

sue guidelines for the identification and treatment of abuse. The AMA has identified five classifications of elder abuse: (1) physical or sexual abuse, (2) psychologic abuse, (3) exploitation (misuse of assets), (4) medical abuse (withholding necessary treatment or aids for ADLs), and (5) neglect.

There are many reasons for abuse beyond the typically identified frustration and exhaustion of a caregiver. Some of the others include psychopathology of the abuser (often also includes alcoholism), extreme dependency of the elder, turbulent lifestyles, and lack of resources (financial, emotional, family, community). The AMA guidelines suggest practitioners ask direct questions to determine the presence and nature of abuse. However, elders often refuse to divulge information because of loyalty or fear of reprisal. The National Center on Elder Abuse has provided clear definitions and signs of the various types of abuse that provide guidelines for health professionals (see Appendix 15-D).

Dynamics of Abuse

Though there is little general agreement on the dynamics of abuse, Pillemer and Finkelhor (1988) found that men were just as likely to be abused as women (although the abused or neglected women were more severely damaged both physically and emotionally when abused). This is in contrast to numerous studies that have identified women as the most frequent victims (Figure 15-3).

The abuser is most usually thought to be an adult child, but this study found that 58% of the abusers were spouses. This raises the hypothesis that wives who are caregivers are abusing their frail husbands, possibly in retaliation for past abuse. Elder abuse may be spouse abuse grown old and reversed. On the other hand, it must be acknowledged that the

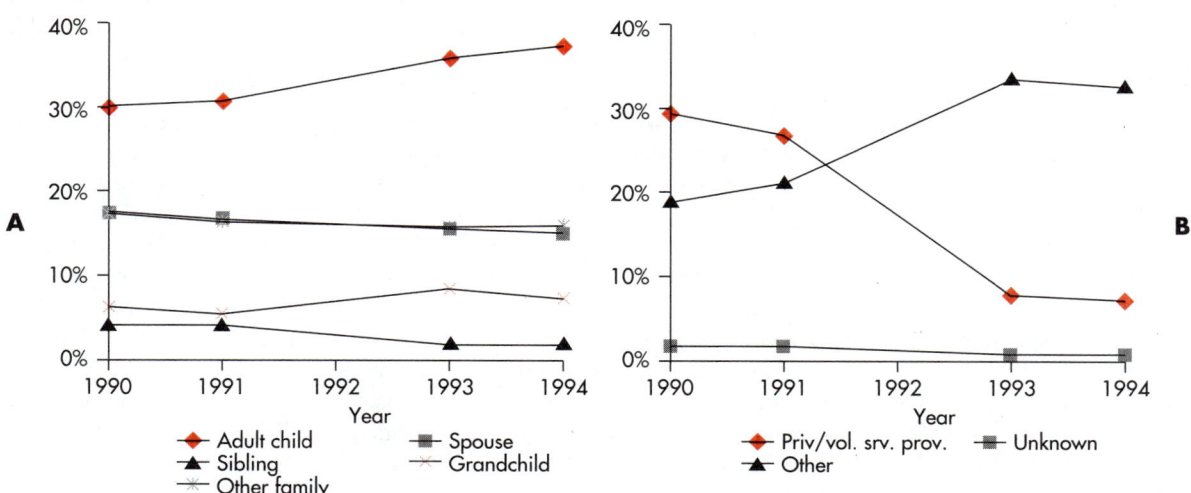

Figure 15-1. Perpetrators of domestic elder abuse. **A,** Family members. **B,** Other perpetrators. (From Tatara T, Blumerman LM: Elder abuse in domestic settings, *Elder abuse informational series,* No 3, Washington, DC, 1996, National Center on Elder Abuse.)

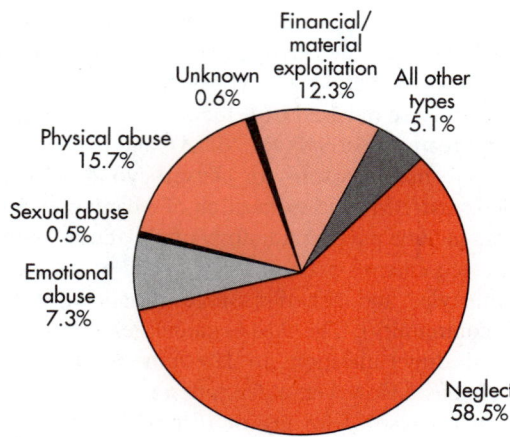

Figure 15-2. Types of domestic elder abuse. (From Tatara T, Blumerman LM: Elder abuse in domestic settings, *Elder abuse informational series,* No 3, Washington, DC, 1996, National Center on Elder Abuse.)

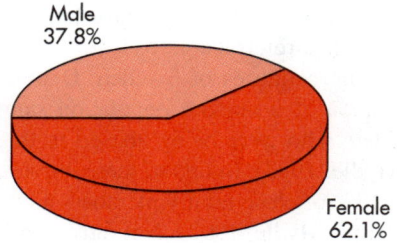

Figure 15-3. Sex of victims of domestic elder abuse. (From Tatara T, Blumerman LM: Elder abuse in domestic settings, *Elder abuse informational series,* No 3, Washington, DC, 1996, National Center on Elder Abuse.)

abuse or neglect could have commenced with old age and that elderly men are much more likely to be living with a spouse than are elderly women. Carlse (1987) notes that often the abusive person remains so and even when disabled may use manipulation and other forms of abuse. In other words, the abusive person may be the elder, the abuser grown old.

There are undoubtedly numerous cultural differences in identification and even of definitions of abuse. Given our diverse society, this must be taken under consideration. Moon and Williams (1993) obtained responses from African-American, White, and Korean-American elderly women regarding their perceptions of abusive situations. The Korean-Americans were much less likely than the others to perceive a given situation as abusive. Additional studies in this respect would be enlightening and particularly important in identification and intervention. There is no universal acceptance of actions that constitute abuse.

Frail elders are most often cared for in the home (see Chapter 17), and the demands of such care on family are thought to increase the incidence of abuse. Alzheimer's disease and other dementias are particularly intolerable. A recent study by Paveza et al (1992) found that the overall prevalence of severely violent behavior toward family members with Alzheimer's disease was 17.4%. Coyne et al (1993) sent anonymous questionnaires to 1000 caregivers who had called a telephone help line specializing in dementia. Of the 342 questionnaires that were returned, 33 indicated they had pinched, kicked, bit, struck, or shoved the elder in their care. The study concluded that the high physical and psychologic demands on caretakers of demented relatives became intolerable.

Anetzberger (1987) studied the perpetrators of elderly abuse in a small sample of Ohioans who abused their elderly

parents and identified certain predictive factors: socialization to abusive actions, pathologic or authoritarian personality characteristics that increased tolerance for abuse infliction or decreased tolerance for stress, inability to provide satisfactory care, intolerance for the intimacy of caregiving, and vulnerability of the victim. Although these individuals expressed love and filial obligation, they felt socially isolated and a lack of cooperation from the parent for whom they cared. Anetzberger's study did not reveal whether the adult children had in the past been physically or psychologically abused by their parents. There is speculation that some abusive persons are abused in retaliation as they become old and frail.

One dynamic of abuse that has not been seriously explored is that of the son who must care for an incontinent mother. The deep societal abhorrence of incest and particularly the taboo against a sexualized mother/son relationship may produce an irrationally strong response to the necessity of exposing a mother's perineum when giving care. Nurses may provide some anticipatory guidance and understanding when dealing with such cases. Even the reassurance that one understands how difficult this can be may reduce the revulsion and anxiety the caregiving son feels. Vulnerability factors have been summarized by Frost and Willette (1994) (see Table 15-4).

Studies provide profiles of abusive situations, family dysfunction, and abusive persons, but none could be found that address macro issues such as climatic conditions, seasons, culture, geographic differences, disaster situations, excessive political pressures, and stressors. For instance, are farm families more inclined toward abuse and neglect than urban or suburban families, in the South or North, in summer or winter, following floods or preceding tax deadlines? Will tax relief for the expense of caring for an elder change the prevalence of abuse? When a family depends upon the elder's Social Security or SSI, does that have an effect on how abusive they may be? These and many other questions that might shed light on the general topic of abuse seem not to have been asked or given serious consideration. We know only that the incidence is rising rapidly throughout society and toward all vulnerable persons.

Assessment

Risk factors include a history of mental illness, alcohol/drug abuse, a family history of violence, isolation of the victim, limited social network, minority status, stressful lifestyle of the victim and/or abuser, presence of dementia, behavioral problems, incontinence, and the need to be fed. To make an adequate assessment it is necessary to observe the living arrangements, evaluate the financial status, social supports, interactions of family members, and emotional stressors in the present situation (Paris et al, 1995; Lachs et al, 1994).

Elder abuse tends to be episodic and recurrent rather than an isolated event (Lett, 1995). Thus, it is also important to review past records of accidents and emergency room visits that may create a "high index of suspicion" when taken in total (Kingston and Penhale, 1995). Vinton (1993) studied clients referred to an intensive case management program and found numbers of elders had been subjected to physical and sexual abuse that had gone undetected because they had not been asked about such experiences. Assessment of mistreatment involves several components as noted in Box 15-2.

Dimensions of maltreatment include deprivation; verbal, physical, psychologic, material, and sexual abuse; violation of rights; passive and active neglect; and financial exploitation (Patwell, 1988). Ashley and Fulmer (1988) recommend that until a standardized method of identification and reporting is adopted, each case must be subject to the clinical judgment of experts in the field.

Interventions

The goals of intervention are to stop exploitation of elders, protect the victim and society from inappropriate and illegal acts, hold perpetrators of mistreatment accountable, rehabilitate the offender, and order restitution of property and payment for expenses incurred as a result of the perpetrator's conduct. The rules of the court dictate the procedures to accomplish these goals. Both civil and criminal law require that the accused is given notice of what they have allegedly done (Heisler and Quinn, 1993). This may create additional problems for the victim unless immediate removal from the abusive setting can be accomplished.

Few states have legal alternatives that can quickly be brought to play to immediately remove the elder to a protected situation. Those states with legal avenues operant often involve delay or placement in a nursing home. Neither of those may be effective actions. The American Society on Aging (1992) reports on a transitional home that has been established in Indianapolis for abused elders. The Elder Shelter provides emergency beds for elders during crises until a suitable arrangement can be made.

There are three basic dynamics of abuse: the psychopathologic, the learned, and situational stress causation. The design of appropriate interventions depends on understanding the dynamic, since each requires different strategies of intervention.

Box 15-2	**Evaluative Components of Mistreatment**

- Safety of the elder: Is the elder in immediate danger?
- What can be done immediately to increase safety?
- Are there barriers to reaching the elder (cognitive, family interference, emotional)?
- Are adequate physical, social, and financial resources available to properly care for the elder?
- What medical problems may make the elderly particularly vulnerable to abuse and neglect?
- What type of mistreatment has occurred, how frequently, and of what severity?

The psychopathologic presents the greatest challenge and generally requires removal of the offender or the elder from the situation, perhaps by legal intervention.

Learned abuse, theoretically, can be unlearned and may respond to a close working relationship with a mentoring professional who can demonstrate positive problem solving and new ways of managing difficult situations.

Most frequent are the stress-related situations. These are responsive to almost anything that eases the burden: removal of the stressor, often this is the elder; support groups for ventilation of frustrations and peer support; respite; crisis hot lines; professional consultation; victim support groups; victim volunteer companions and, above all, thoughtful and compassionate care for the victim and the perpetrator (Quinn and Tomita, 1997; Reis and Nahmiash, 1995; Wolf and Pillemer, 1994: Lachs and Fulmer, 1993).

Preventive interventions (Patwell, 1988) include the following:

- Make professionals aware of potentially abusive situations.
- Educate the public about normal aging processes.
- Help families develop and nurture informal support systems.
- Link families with support groups.
- Teach families stress-management techniques.
- Arrange comprehensive care resources.
- Provide counseling for troubled families.
- Encourage the use of respite care and day care.
- Obtain necessary home health care services.
- Inform families of resources for meals and transportation.
- Encourage caregivers to pursue their individual interests.

Reis and Nahmiash (1995) have developed a process protocol for the identification and subsequent actions to be taken in cases of elder abuse (Box 15-3). Their proposed intervention model seems to hold promise for the management of abuse and neglect. The essential elements are the availability of advice teams that can design health, financial, and legal supports for victims and an available "buddy" to

Box 15-3	**Identification and Subsequent Action for Elder Abuse**

Team

- BASE: *Brief Abuse Screen for the Elderly*—screens abuse: specifies types, sources of abuse, urgency for treatment.
- Abuse Checklist
- The Intervention Teams *Home-care team:* Trained Basic Intervention unit: screens using the Tool Package, intervenes.
  Multidiciplinary Team: about three to five Homecare team members: confirm/disconfirm abuse (using the BASE); brainstorm, plan, monitor and evaluate intervention strategies (using the AID).
- *Empowerment Support Group:* Victims discuss problems, strengths, solutions, resources, appropriate responses.
- *The Community Senior Abuse Committee* An independent group of volunteers: arrange programs and publications to educate/sensitize the community to abuse; advocacy functions; liaison with home-care team members.

Interventions

1. Abuse cases are tagged. The initial intervention strategies are planned and implemented. Screens abuse; specifies caregiver/care-receiver indicators for intervention focus.
2. Home care team members make initial home visits to further assess and make written (AID) plans. They brainstorm the case with the multidisciplinary team and consult with the expert consultant team for specialized advice and help. They enlist specialized advice and additional assistance as needed, e.g. buddies, empowerment group. They improve and continue the planned (AID) intervention strategies.
3. Empowerment group works to improve self-esteem, active responding, increase personal control and empowerment of victims.
4. Committee refers clients, volunteers to the intervention; provides community involvement in combating abuse.

Modified from Reis M, Nahmiash D: When seniors are abused: an intervention model, *Gerontologist* 35(5):667, 1995.

provide personal attention, assistance, companionship, and advocacy. In addition the "buddy" would quite obviously provide respite for the usual caregiver.

Quinn and Tomita (1997) have written the classic text on elder abuse and neglect that includes knowledge to date and diagnostic and treatment strategies in practical terms. These writers have not sensationalized the subject but presented case histories in all their complexity that clearly reveal the many facets of elder abuse. The unique quality of the text is that both writers are practitioners in the arena of elder abuse and bring a wealth of experience to their subject. The book is helpful to anyone who works with elders and is concerned about the possibility of abuse or neglect perpetrated by ignorance, by intent, or simply, as many cases demonstrate, by lack of resources and an exhausted caregiver.

Mandatory Reporting

Most states now have mandatory laws requiring the reporting of elder mistreatment.

A large (1521 subjects) interdisciplinary study was undertaken to determine factors that influenced clinicians' decision making regarding identification, reporting, and intervention with victims of family violence. Over one third indicated they had no education regarding abuse in their professional training programs and felt incapable of making such judgments (Tilden et al, 1994). Those who had some education were more inclined to suspect spouse abuse than child abuse and rarely suspected elder abuse. Many did not perceive themselves as responsible for reporting or intervening. In fact, elder abuse is most fre-

quently reported by doctors and nurses (Figure 15-4). It seems clear that there is much yet to be done to assure that professionals recognize and deal with the problems of abusive situations.

Nurses must be aware of the definitions and reporting policies within their area of practice. Even though the intent of mandatory reporting laws is protection of the abused person, at times it can create more abuse unless immediate action for removal is taken. The following case illustrates a few of the complexities:

Madge, a 64-year-old woman with crippling arthritis and advanced diabetes that resulted in neurologic deficits and almost total blindness, was admitted to the hospital for stabilization of her brittle diabetes. During her stay she was attended by a student nurse. In the course of their extensive interactions she confided that her husband often beat her. When the student reported this, the staff assured her that the husband was most attentive, and they discounted the student's report as if her inexperience had magnified Madge's confidences into a trauma. When the student was encouraged to determine the nature of the assaults and frequency, Madge said she did not want any intervention because on her last hospitalization someone had reported abuse and when she was discharged her husband beat her unmercifully for discussing it. The student was then in a dilemma . . . how to comply with the reporting law and yet avoid further abuse to the client, who had no intention of leaving the husband who beat her for the uncertain attentions of a nursing home. At least she knew the system and what to expect in her own home. On final report, the hospital administration made note of the abuse but did not report it to the police at the specific request of Madge.

Long-term relationships in which abuse has occurred are a thorny problem. It is estimated that abuse has occurred in 50% to 60% of marriages. The factors that sustain the rela-

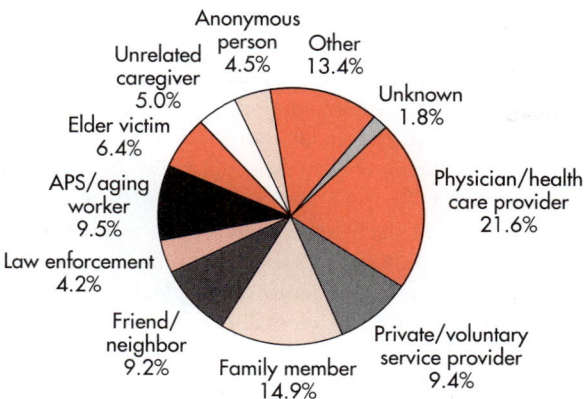

Figure 15-4. Reporters of domestic elder abuse. (From Tatara T, Blumerman LM: Elder abuse in domestic settings, *Elder abuse informational series,* No 3, Washington, DC, 1996, National Center on Elder Abuse.)

tionship may include dependency, poor self-esteem, social isolation, fear, and an overriding loyalty to the spouse.

The procedure for reporting suspected elder abuse is explained by DeLong (1995) and may entail any of the following actions:

- If you work in an agency or hospital, call the social worker or social service department to report the problem and manage the case.
- Call the elder abuse hot line listed in the front of the telephone book; advice and assistance is available and often counseling for the abused and abusers.
- If there is immediate danger to the victim, it is best to call the police.
- Contact Adult Protective Services to alert them to investigate.
- A written report, including the name, sex, race, and address of the abused and the type of abuse that occurred, must be filed promptly. Careful documentation is important. Some say to identify the suspected abuser, but we believe great caution must be exerted in this respect lest someone be accused inaccurately.

Abuse in Nursing Homes

Abuse of the aged in nursing homes has been documented and discussed for years, yet it still exists in many situations. Poor wages, overwork, and lack of cooperation from administration and physicians contribute to this mistreatment. Estimates of the extent of abuse of patients in nursing homes have been largely speculative and often based on isolated incidences.

Pillemer and Moore (1990) conducted a telephone survey of 577 nurses' aides and nurses working in 31 nursing homes in New Hampshire. Those persons interviewed were asked if they had observed incidences of physical or verbal

abuse of patients within the previous year and, secondly, if they had committed any such acts. The study showed that even with the possibility of underreporting, the incidences were significant. Thirty-six percent of the sample had observed physical abuse, and 10% reported they had committed one or more physically abusive acts. Even more appalling, 81% had observed psychologically abusive incidents, and 40% reported they had been psychologically abusive. The most frequent abusive actions were excessive restraints, pushing, grabbing, shoving, pinching, yelling, and swearing at the resident.

Based on the evidence of this study, it appears that maltreatment is a common part of institutional life. This study needs further replication, but the implications are that in spite of extensive state and federal regulation of nursing homes the quality of life from an interpersonal perspective may at times be deplorable.

In the most recent available study of elder abuse in nursing homes (U.S. Department of Health and Human Services, 1996), it was noted that the primary abusers of elders are aides and orderlies who have had no stress-management training. They sometimes view elders much as children needing punishment. Lynch (1997) provides an overview of elder abuse but mentions nothing about abuse by staff in various settings. However, some recent reports and articles have addressed the issue (Marr, 1995; Mullen, 1995; Nelson et al, 1995).

Abuse prevention programs must first attend to the quality of life of staff and the stresses of the work situation if more humane treatment is to trickle down to the dependent patient. Nursing home abuse is one of the "family secrets" that is kept within the walls as much as possible. Residents abuse staff and staff abuse residents.

Because of increased reports of such incidents, a national organization, The Coalition of Advocates for the Rights of the Infirm Elderly (CARIE), has developed educational materials to provide guidance and strategies for defusing the tensions (Hegland, 1992). CARIE has published a manual on abuse prevention training. It is primarily aimed at modifying the attitudes of the staff toward the elderly. In addition, aides are given stress-management classes and attention to their problems and frustrations (see resources at the end of the chapter for further information).

A common form of institutional abuse, fortunately on the wane because of legal and moral pressures, has been that of restraining individuals (see discussion in Chapter 11). Restriction of movement may be one of the most devastating of abuses and has been so embedded in nursing care that only recently has the enormity of such disregard for human dignity become an issue.

Abuse and Neglect in Home Care

Most abuse of elders occurs within the home by family, but with appalling frequency it is by hired caregivers in the home. Reports of problems include the following: inadequate supervision of patient care, poor coordination of services, inadequate staff training, theft and fraud, drug and alcohol abuse by staff, tardiness and absenteeism, unprofessional and criminal conduct, and inadequate record keeping. It appears that home care may vary from excellent to frightening, yet few enforcement actions have been taken.

The number and diversity of providers, both licensed and unlicensed, make monitoring of care extremely difficult (Institute for Health and Aging, 1989). Vilbig (1989) reports that home care workers hired to care for the disabled elderly are sometimes abusers and thieves. In a few recent cases they have murdered their clients. Although the home care industry at large is appalled at these events, there is no mechanism in place to avert them.

Theft of belongings seems to be the most common problem, and the aged who have complained are often dismissed as "confused" or "paranoid." A director of one home care agency in a personal conversation with the author said, "Yes, we know it happens, even though all our people are bonded. We really can't do much as we don't witness the abuse and we do not inventory homes, so what can we prove?"

Home care workers are paid on average $5.75 per hour, and the turnover rate of employees is 50% annually. Many simply do not show up or do the work when they do show up. It is clear that even though it may be costly, more care must be exerted in investigating the background of workers who are sent into the home to care for the dependent aged, and their work must be monitored more closely.

THE FRAIL AND VULNERABLE AGED AND THEIR FUTURE

The home is now and will continue to be the principal site of care for the frail elderly. Most of this is given by family members who may or may not be willing to assume the care. This is discussed in considerable detail in Chapter 17.

Home visitation by physicians and nurses is expanding for the following reasons: (1) to assess needs of patients and families within the context of daily living, (2) to enhance the use of multidisciplinary teams in the home, (3) to avoid premature institutionalization, (4) to provide more personalized and humane care, and (5) because much of the care has been priced out of the hospitals.

The needs of patients who have been discharged "quicker and sicker" are of the most sophisticated and complex nature. This is particularly true of the frail older adult. Not only the treatment related to the disease from which he or she is recuperating but also the personal and human needs must be attended if the individual is to recover necessary functions.

The hospital has in large part moved into the home. Some of the advantages include (1) assessment of patients and families within the context of daily living, (2) increased use of multidisciplinary teams in the home, (3) avoidance of premature institutionalization, and (4) the provision of more

personalized and humane care. The disadvantages are that more sophisticated knowledge is expected of caregivers and there is a higher probability of inadequate care and serious errors in caregiving, fragmentation and overlap of services, medical neglect, and financial abuse.

In addition, the number of very old ladies living alone is increasing yearly. In 1994, the greatest number of individuals living alone in the United States were women over 75 years of age (4,080,000) (U.S. Bureau of the Census, 1995). These are particularly subject to self-neglect and abuse and exploitation by hired caregivers. This problem is expected to increase.

Nurses may be the first to gain admittance to the home and to recognize a problem. Advocacy for individual rights and protections require considerable expertise. Consequently nurses will need to avail themselves of legal and financial consultation. The importance of multidisciplinary collaboration in these situations is critical while maintaining the highest level of concern for the autonomy and rights of the individual.

There will be a continued increase in the number of frail elderly being kept alive by advanced medical technology and experiencing more functional deficits. To meet their needs and maintain a stable economy, several trends have been identified. Multiple alternatives to institutional placement will be developed in communities. It is thought that alternatives to institutionalization are cost effective when offered in the context of comprehensive, coordinated health care that includes respite, home health care, domiciliary, and day-care components in combination with social supports in a case management model. Some of the alternatives to institutional care include the following:

- Self-help education
- Geriatric crisis outreach
- Neighborhood support networks
- Community nursing centers
- Telephone peer networks
- Adopt-a-Grandparent programs
- Foster family care
- Adult residential day care

Coordinated systems of long-term care delivering multiple services to the vulnerable elderly have been effectively demonstrated by the Alternative Health System in Georgia, the Mt. Zion Hospital and Medical Center in San Francisco, the On-Lok Senior Health Center in San Francisco, and the Hebrew Rehabilitation Center for the Aged in Boston. These model demonstration projects have shown that a full range of services reduces inappropriate institutional placement and mortality and increases functional status. Frail elders need the physical presence of another in a flexible manner in accordance with need. Such a capability should extend to the provision of funds to purchase this presence when necessary.

Nurses are the ideal advocates for the frail elderly and may assist them in actual provision or help them find suitable services to meet their needs. The need for help with daily activities increases sharply as people grow older, especially among the very old. Less than 10% who are 65 to 74 years old need help, compared with 40% who are 85 years or older.

In the future institutional costs and financial incentives to families may increase the number of elderly cared for at home. About 80% of care currently provided to the elderly is given by informal caregivers, usually family members, but federal policies have consistently been unsupportive of these families, denying the most minimum assistance and providing no support or recognition of their major contribution to the care of the frail elderly in our society.

Nurses particularly should be cognizant of the trends, the realities, and our place in influencing national aging policy. We can expect an increased recognition of our pivotal role in providing long-term care services, clinical research, and assessment data. Nurses are rapidly becoming the primary case managers for the frail aged.

Priorities for the long-term care of the frail and vulnerable elderly include the following:

1. Support functional independence.
2. Emphasize prevention at all ages.
3. Assist families caring for elders.
4. Seek increased public financing for long-term care and home-based care.
5. Involve physicians, nurses, social workers, aides, and others and provide incentives for these workers to master geriatric skills.
6. Encourage continuity of professional surveillance.
7. Provide adequate quality/cost controls for in-home care.
8. Ensure equal access to publicly funded benefits, regardless of economic status.

It has been said that the progress of civilization can be judged by the total fraction of human beings who achieve longevity while maintaining a life of meaning and purpose. In the care of the very old who are frail and vulnerable, subject to the whims of social policy and potential abuses and neglect, our human progress or lack of it is most visible. Thoughtful examination of social needs and deficiencies is a form of progress if we follow up with appropriate action. If not, we will reap the effects of our neglect. We urge nurses to look at the individual and beyond as we attempt to create a world where it is safe to depend on the good will and compassion of others.

KEY CONCEPTS

- Frail elders are generally considered to be those who are in tenuous physiologic, mental, or emotional balance and maintain their integrity within a small margin.
- Vulnerable elders are those who are placed under the legal protections of another who may or may not advocate or make decisions to their best advantage.
- Vulnerable elders are also those who live in situations that are potentially neglectful or outright abusive.

- Abuse may be physical, financial, psychologic, or extreme neglect, either intentional or unintentional.
- Adult Protective Services are usually public agencies who oversee the care of the vulnerable aged. There are some privately founded and funded adult protective services, and at times these have been found to take financial advantage of those under their protection.
- Nursing responsibilities are to be alert to signs of abuse and neglect of an elder and to report known cases to the appropriate state agency, as required by law.
- Abusive situations can emerge from overburdened caregivers who have little assistance, great frustration, and little respite.
- Abusive situations also often arise as a result of substance abuse by willing or unwilling caregivers.
- Elders rarely report family members who abuse them because they are uncertain whether an alternative situation would be an improvement.
- Nursing responsibilities include assisting caregivers to find resources to alleviate or partially relieve a stressful situation.

▲ **CASE STUDY**

Walter has lived with his 52-year-old son, Melvin, since his wife, Marie, died and his farm was sold 10 years ago. He never seemed to recover from those overwhelming losses. He has lost interest in everything, seldom goes anywhere, and gradually has become a shadow of his former self. Walter is now 84 years old and has been sleeping poorly, getting up several times each night to urinate, and has been steadily losing weight. Melvin never married and doesn't really mind having Walter live with him because he isn't home a lot. He works at the local telephone company, and evenings are usually spent with his cronies at the Last Chance pool hall. He does get annoyed when Walter complains about things. It seems as though Walter is always complaining and moaning, saying, "I just want to be with Marie, I just want to be with her." Walter's sister has offered to have him live with her, but Melvin discourages this because he suspects the sister is only after Walter's money. Walter has money stashed somewhere, but Melvin doesn't know where, and Walter seems to have forgotten where he put it. Several of the medicines that were prescribed over 3 years ago for Walter's cardiac and prostate problems are costly, and Melvin has not had the prescriptions filled for several months. He really doesn't see any purpose in them because Walter doesn't seem to care whether he lives or dies, and Walter's Social Security check helps pay expenses. One evening Melvin finds Walter unconsious when he arrives home at midnight. He takes him to the emergency room at the local hospital, and the admitting nurse asks, "Is he on any medications?" Melvin says, "No, but he seems really confused lately and may have fallen and bumped his head." Upon examination there is a bump on the occipital lobe of Walter's head, and he is extremely dehydrated.

Nursing Diagnoses

The following potential diagnoses must be considered as well as diagnoses unique to the particular individual:

Coping, defensive
Denial, ineffective
Family processes, altered
Health maintenance, altered
Risk for caregiver role strain
Home maintenance management, impaired
Knowledge deficit
Role performance, altered
Social isolation
Thought processes, altered
Trauma, risk for
Violence, risk for, directed at others

NURSING PROCESS AND NURSING DIAGNOSIS
Risk for Trauma, Unilateral Neglect

Etiologies and Related Factors
Physical, psychologic, economic action/inaction
History of violent/abusive family
Living arrangements
Family relationships

Defining Characteristics
Client
Bruises, welts, burns, fractures, dislocations, lacerations, abrasions, incompatible with normal injury, nausea with abdominal swelling
Unusual number of prior hospitalizations, surgeries, emergency room visits
Malnutrition
Poor hygiene
Property misuse
Violation of personal rights
Withdrawn
Fearful
Always in company of caregiver
Living arrangements
Caregiver:
Low stress tolerance
Authoritarian
Interest in elder's resources

Knowledge
Risk indicators
Types and forms of abuse and neglect
Signs and symptoms of abuse/neglect
Physical and psychologic, social assessment skills
Other reasons for sustaining injuries
State law requirements for reporting
Community resources and abuse prevention programs
Communication skills
Family dynamics
Counseling skills
Normal aging process
Nursing interventions for abused and abuser

Clinical Judgment and Related Skills
Risk assessment
Be direct and nonjudgmental
Provide client opportunity for privacy to validate abuse/neglect and talk about feelings
Provide caregiver privacy to discuss feelings
Encourage realistic appraisal
Assist in developing support system
Initiate health teaching to caregiver/community in the proper care of the elderly: nutrition, wheelchair transfers, etc.
Communication skills
Health history
Abuse assessment: physical, psychologic, support systems, alcohol and drug use, family relationships
Physical assessment of systems as necessary
Report abuse/neglect as required by law
Initiate community referrals

Evaluation
Altered living arrangement
Increased interaction
Improved health status
Family seeking or participating in supportive resources
Observed positive interaction with congruent responses
Decreased evidence of abuse or neglect

NEEDS ADDRESSED AND TASK STRENGTHS	
Need to respect own limitations; need to maintain dignity and to make choices (to meet needs for safety, security, belonging, and self-esteem)	Knows own limits Willing to seek and accept assistance Conserves energy for activities of personal significance Maintains balance in lifestyle demands

Based upon the case study, develop a nursing care plan using the following procedure*:

List comments of client that provide *subjective data.*

List information that provides *objective data.*

From these data identify and state, using accepted format, two *nursing diagnoses* you determine are most significant to this client at this time.

List two *client strengths* that you have identified from data.

Determine and state *outcome criteria* for each diagnosis. These must reflect some alleviation of the problem identified in the nursing diagnosis and must be stated in concrete and measurable terms.

Plan and state one or more *interventions* for each diagnosed problem. Provide specific documentation of source used to determine appropriate intervention. Plan at least one intervention that incorporates the client's existing strengths.

Evaluate success of intervention. Interventions must correlate directly with the stated outcome criteria in order to measure the outcome success.

STUDY QUESTIONS/ACTIVITIES

Discuss the meanings and the thoughts triggered by the student's and elders' viewpoints expressed at the beginning of the chapter. How do these vary from your own experience?

Discuss your concept of frail aged and develop a definition that provides clear distinctions.

What are the physiologic principles that best explain the concept of frailty in aging?

Discuss various legal mechanisms for protecting the frail aged.

What is the distinction between frail and vulnerable as used in connection with the aged?

Refer to the chapter on relationships (Chapter 17), and describe factors in a spousal relationship that may be functional or detrimental to the frail aged.

What are your responsibilities in reporting elder abuse in your state?

RESEARCH QUESTIONS

What is the distribution of symptoms in the FTT syndrome in the aged?

*Students are advised to refer to their nursing diagnosis text and identify possible or potential problems.

What is the demographic and sociocultural profile of elders who develop FTT?

How do health care agencies define frail elderly?

Which agencies offer services specifically designed for the aged, and what are these services?

What proportion of individuals over 80 are considered frail and based on what criteria?

Is the increasing population (over 85 years) shifting toward more durability or increasing frailty in recent decades?

How many elders have been victimized economically and legally by family members?

When is it appropriate to intervene?

RESOURCES

Films and Video

A Safer Place, L. Bloise, Terra Nova Films, Chicago, Ill, 20 minutes. A documentary about elder abuse that includes an interview with a woman who abused her mother and features two elderly victims of abuse who have made better lives for themselves.

Becoming a Conservator. A 20-minute videotape (VHS) that discusses the duties of the conservator of the person and the conservator of the estate. It can be ordered from Scott Thomas, Esq, 2700 Spear Street Tower, One Market Plaza, San Francisco, CA 94150, (415) 442-1211; (cost: $25; include payment with request).

Organizations

CARIE, (Beth Hudson), 1315 Walnut Street, Suite 1000, Philadelphia, PA 19107, (215) 545-5728

State Office of Protective Services

National Center for Elder Abuse, c/o American Public Welfare Association, 810 First Street, NE, Suite 500, Washington, DC 20002-4267; (202) 682-2470, fax (202) 289-6555. Source for statistics, publications, and newsletter.

Publications

U.S. Department of Health and Human Services, Special issue devoted to abuse and neglect of the elderly, *Aging Issue* N. 367, 1996.

◣ **Resources for You and Your Patient**

Whom to Contact	**Services They Provide**
Criminal Justice Services American Association of Retired Persons 601 E St NW Washington, DC 20049 202-434-2222	Self-instruction training program, pamphlets, and brochures on elder abuse prevention
National Association of State Units on Aging* National Eldercare Institute on Elder Abuse and State Long-Term Care Ombudsman Services 1225 I St NW, Suite 725 Washington, DC 20005 202-898-2578	Individual services, help for state and local programs, provider training
National Center on Elder Abuse* American Public Welfare Association 810 First Street NE, Suite 500 Washington, DC 20002-4267 202-682-2470	Information, provider training
National Organization for Victim Assistance 1-800-TRY-NOVA 202-232-6682	Referrals, resources in every state
National Coalition Against Violence* 202-638-6388 303-839-1852	Training and education on domestic violence, publications, and programs
Local resources • Adult Protective Services • Police • State elder abuse hot lines (consult local directory)	Protection

From Lynch SH: Elder abuse: what to look for; how to intervene, *AJN* 97(1):31, 1997.
*These organizations also have research or advocacy functions.

American Medical Association: *Guidelines for diagnosis and treatment of elder abuse and neglect,* American Geriatrics Society, 770 Lexington Avenue, Suite 300, New York, NY 10021, (212) 308-1414.

Douglass RL: *Domestic mistreatment of the elderly: towards prevention,* Washington, DC, 1992, AARP, 601 E Street NW, Washington DC 20049.

National Center on Elder Abuse: *Elder abuse: questions and answers,* Washington, DC, May 1995, National Center for Elder Abuse.

Handbook for Conservators. A 94-page handbook that describes the duties of the conservator of person and the conservator of estate in more detail than the preceding videotape and is considered to be a companion to the videotape. There are 23 appendixes, which include such issues as "Working Effectively with In-Home Service Organizations," "Sample Accounting Format," and "Suggested Readings for

Conservators." Order the handbook as follows: send a self-addressed, stamped manila envelope (10 × 13 inches) with $10 and the request to S.F. County Clerk, Probate Division, 400 Van Ness Avenue, Room 317, San Francisco, CA 94102. (Postage is $2.25.)

REFERENCES

American Medical Association: *AMA issues guidelines for physicians to treat abused, neglected elderly,* News release, Chicago, November 23, 1992, The Association.

American Society on Aging: Elder shelter: a transitional home for victims of abuse, *Aging Today* 13(5):15, 1992.

Anderson SJ, Johnson MA: Caring for patients on the edge of decline, *Am J Nurs* 96 (12):16B, 1996.

Anetzberger G: *The etiology of elder abuse by adult offspring,* Springfield, Ill, 1987, Charles C Thomas.

Aravanis SC, Adelman RD, Breckman R et al: Diagnostic and treatment guidelines on elder abuse and neglect, *Arch Fam Med* 2(4):371, 1993.

Ashley I, Fulmer T: No simple way to determine elder abuse, *Geriatr Nurs* 9(5):286, 1988.

Bowsher JE, Keep D: Toward an understanding of three control constructs: personal control, self-efficacy, and hardiness, *Issues Mental Health Nurs* 16(1):33, 1995.

Braun JV, Wykle MH, Cowling RW: Failure to thrive in older persons: a concept derived, *Gerontologist* 28(6):809, 1988.

Brown I, Renwick R, Raphael D: Frailty: constructing a common meaning, definition and conceptual framework, *Int J Rehabil Res* 18(2):93, 1995.

Buchner D, Wagner E: Preventing frail health, *Clin Geriatr Med* 8(1):1, 1988.

Carlse J: The abusive relationship, *NZ Nurs J* 12:16, 1987.

Casteldine G: Elder abuse by nurses is on the increase, *Br J Nurs* 3(13):675, 1994.

Castro FG, Hammond WR, John R et al: Risk taking and abusive behaviors among ethnic minorities, *Health Psychol* 14(7):622, 1995.

Clark PG: Quality of life, values, and teamwork in geriatric care: do we communicate what we mean? *Gerontologist* 25(3):402, 1995.

Coyne AC, Reichman WE, Berbig LJ: The relationship between dementia and elder abuse, *Am J Psychiatr* 150(4):643, 1993.

DeLong MF: Part I: Elder abuse, *NURSEweek* 8(4):11, 1995.

Ebersole P: *Gerontological nurse practitioners and the care of the aged.* Paper presented at the Annual Convocation of the American College of Health Care Administrators, Denver, 1983, Proceedings of the American College of Health Care Administrators.

Fries JF: Compression of morbidity 1993: life span, disability, and health care costs. In Vellas B, Albarede JL, Garry PJ, editors: *Facts and research in gerontology,* vol 7, New York, 1993, Springer.

Fries JF: Compression of morbidity/disease postponement. In Maddox GL, editor: *The encyclopedia of aging: a comprehensive resource in gerontology and geriatrics,* New York, 1995, Springer.

Frost MH, Willette K: Risk for abuse/neglect: documentation of assessment data and diagnoses, *J Gerontol Nurs* 20(8):37, 1994.

Fulmer T, O'Malley T: *Inadequate care of the elderly: a health care perspective on abuse and neglect,* New York, 1987, Springer.

Gaffney D: Commentary on failure to thrive: the silent epidemic of the elderly, *APNSCAN* 6:10, August, 1995.

Gloth FM, Walston J, Meyer J, Pearson J: Reliability and validity of the frail elderly functional assessment questionnaire, *Am J Phys Med Rehabil* 74(1):45, 1995.

Hegland A: Defusing conflicts: abuse prevention strategies, *Contemp Long Term Care* 15(11):60, 1992.

Heisler CJ, Quinn MJ: A legal perspective. In Johnson TF, editor: *Elder mistreatment: ethical issues, dilemmas, and decisions,* New York, 1993, Haworth Press.

Homer AC, Gilleard C: Abuse of elderly people by their carers, *Br Med J* 301:1359, 1990.

Hydle I: Abuse and neglect of the elderly: a Nordic perspective report from a Nordic research project, *Scand J Soc Med* 21(2):126, 1993.

Institute for Health and Aging: Home health services in California and Missouri, *Res Briefs* 6(1), Spring 1989.

Jarrett PG, Rockwood K, Carver D, Stolee P, Cosway S: Illness presentation in elderly patients, *Arch Intern Med* 155(10):1060, 1995.

Jones SR: Infections in frail and vulnerable elderly patients, *Am J Med* 88(3C):30S, 1990.

Kessenich CR, Rosen CJ: Osteoporosis: implications for elderly men, *Geriatr Nurs* 17(4):171, 1996.

Kimball MJ, Williams-Burgess C: Failure to thrive: the silent epidemic of the elderly, *Arch Psychiatr Nurs* 9(2):99, 1995.

Kingston P, Penhale B: Elder abuse and neglect: issues in the accident and emergency department, *Accid Emerg Nurs* 3(3):122, 1995.

Kobasa SC: Stressful life events, personality, and health: an inquiry into hardiness, *J Pers Soc Psychol* 37(1):1, 1979.

Kobasa SC, Maddi S, Kahn S: Hardiness health: a prospective study, *J Pers Soc Psychol* 42(1):168, 1982.

Lachs MS, Berkman L, Fulmer T, Horwitz RI: A prospective community-based pilot study of risk factors for the investigation of elder mistreatment, *J Am Geriatr Soc* 42(2):169, 1994.

Lachs MS, Fulmer T: Recognizing elder abuse and neglect, *Clin Geriatr Med* 9(3):665, 1993.

Lachs MS, Williams C, O'Brien S, Hurst L, Horwitz R: Older adults: an 11-year longtitudinal study of adult protective service use, *Arch Intern Med* 156(4):449, 1996.

Lett JE: Abuse of the elderly, *J Fla Med Assoc* 82(10):675, 1995.

Lipson-Parra HB: *Development and validation of the adult attachment scale: assessing attachment in older adults.* Presented at the Third Annual Conference of the Southern Nursing Research Society, February 1989, Austin, Texas, p 557.

Lynch SH: Elder abuse: what to look for, how to intervene, *Am J Nurs* 97(1):27, 1997.

Maddox GL, editor: *The encyclopedia of aging: a comprehensive resource in gerontology and geriatrics,* New York, 1995, Springer.

Marr JF: Poor wages and overwork can precipitate abuse, *Elder Care* 7(5):41, 1995.

Mayer L, Galan D: Elder abuse and the dentists' awareness and knowledge of the problem: a national survey, *J Can Dent Assoc* 59(11):921, 1993.

Moon A, Williams O: Perceptions of elder abuse and help-seeking patterns among African-American, Caucasian-American, and Korean-American elderly women, *Gerontologist* 33(3):386, 1993.

Mullen C: It doesn't happen here, *Elder Care* 7(4):36, 1995.

National Center on Elder Abuse: Elder abuse in domestic settings, *Elder abuse informational series,* No 3, Washington, DC, 1996, National Center on Elder Abuse.

Nelson HW, Huber R, Walter KL: The relationship between volunteer long-term care ombudsmen and regulatory nursing home actions, *Gerontologist* 35(4):509, 1995.

Newbern VB: Failure to thrive: a growing concern in the elderly, *J Gerontol Nurs* 18(8):21, 1992.

Pappas SH: Creating an environment to support hardiness and quality patient care, *Semin Nurse Manag* 3(3):115, 1995.

Paris BE, Meier DE, Goldstein T, Weiss M, Fein ED: Elder abuse and neglect: how to recognize the warning signs and intervene, *Geriatrics* 50(4):47, 1995.

Patwell T: Familial abuse of the elderly: a look at caregiver potential and prevention, *Home Healthcare Nurse* 4(2):10, 1988.

Paveza GJ, Cohen D, Eisdorfer C et al: Severe family violence and Alzheimer's disease: prevalence and risk factors, *Gerontologist* 32(4):493, 1992.

Pillemer K, Finkelhor D: The prevalence of elder abuse: a random sample survey, *Gerontologist* 28:51, 1988.

Pillemer K, Moore D: Abuse of patients in nursing homes: findings from a staff survey, *Gerontologist* 29(3):314, 1990.

Probate Code of the State of California, annotated and indexed by Bancroft-Whitney Co, San Francisco, 1974.

Quinn M: Probate conservatorships and guardianships: assessment and curative aspects, *J Elder Abuse Neglect* 1(1):91, 1989.

Quinn M, Tomita S: *Elder abuse and neglect: causes, diagnosis, and intervention strategies,* ed 2, New York, 1997, Springer.

Reis M, Nahmiash D: When seniors are abused: an intervention model, *Gerontologist* 35(5):666, 1995.

Savemen BI, Hallberg IR, Norberg A, Eriksson S: Patterns of abuse of the elderly in their own homes as reported by district nurses, *Scand J Prim Health Care* 11(2):111, 1993.

Shats VJ, Kozakov S, Kohn D: Critical age as the main parameter of deterioration of health in the elderly, *Harefuah* 128(10):615, 1995.

Shiferaw B, Mittlemark MB, Wofford JL, Anderson RT, Walls P, Rohrer B: The investigation and outcome of reported cases of elder abuse: the Forsyth county aging study, *Gerontologist* 34(1):123, 1994.

Siu AL, Hays RD, Ouslander JG et al: Measuring functioning and health in the very old, *J Gerontol* 48(1):M10, 1993.

Siu AL, Kravitz RL, Keeler E et al: Pastdischarge geriatric assessment of hospitalized frail elderly patients, *Arch Intern Med* 156(1): 76, 1996.

Spitz, R: Hospitalism: an inquiry into the genesis of psychiatric conditions in early childhood. In *The psychoanalytic study of the child,* vol 1, New York, 1945, International Universities Press.

Tennstedt S, McKinlay J: Frailty and its consequences, *Soc Sci Med* 7:863, 1994.

Thomas BL: Research considerations: guardianship and the vulnerable elderly, *J Gerontol Nurs* 20(5):10, 1994.

Tilden VP, Schmidt TA, Limandri BJ, Chiodo GT, Garland MJ, Loveless PA: Factors that influence clinicans' assessment and management of family violence, *Am J Public Health* 84(4):628, 1994.

Tsuji I, Whalen S, Finucane TE: Predictors of nursing home placement in community based long-term care, *J Am Geriatric Soc* 43(7):761, 1995.

US Bureau of the Census: *Statistical abstract of the United States: 1995,* ed 115, Washington, DC, 1995.

US Department of Health and Human Services: Special issue devoted to abuse and neglect of the elderly, *Aging* 367: 1, 1996.

Vilbig P: Elderly hiring caretakers often contract for abuse, *Senior Spectrum* 8(3):1, 1989.

Vinton L: Educating case managers about elder abuse and neglect, *J Case Manag* 2(3):101, 1993.

Wells T: Major clinical problems in gerontologic nursing. In Calkins E, Davis P, Ford A, editors: *The practice of geriatrics,* Philadelphia, 1986, WB Saunders.

Wilbur KH, Reynolds SL: Rethinking alternatives to guardianship, *Gerontologist* 35(2):248, 1995.

Wolanin MO: Mental frailty, personal communication, Feb 20, 1996.

Wolf RS, Pillemer K: What's new in elder abuse programming? Four bright ideas, *Gerontologist* 34(1):126, 1994.

Zusman RM: Oldest old. In Maddox GL, editor: *The encyclopedia of aging: a comprehensive resource in gerontology and geriatrics,* New York, 1995, Springer.

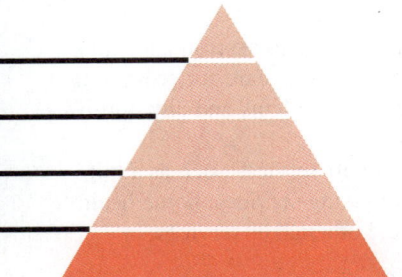

Screening Protocol for Identification of Abuse and Neglect of the Elderly

Definition: Abuse of the elderly is a continuum from simple inattention to needs to deliberate harm. It may be physical, psychological, medical, or material abuse.

DATA COLLECTION

Subjective

Interview with the patient alone in a calm, unhurried manner on the following points:

1. Description of a typical day
2. Recent crises in family life
3. Alcohol and drug use/abuse of family members
4. Amount of contact with persons outside the family
5. Patient's perception of his role in the family and family conflict over his role
6. Dependence on family alone for financial, physical and/or emotional support
7. Alternative shelter available
8. Can patient relate instances of:
   - Being shaken
   - Being shoved
   - Being hit
   - Being left alone, left tied to a chair, left locked in a room
   - Not being fed
   - Being threatened
   - Feeling fear of family member/caretaker
   - Not being given medicine, or other medical care
   - Being given too much medicine, sleeping pills or alcohol
   - Having money or property taken

Interview with the caretaker or family member in an empathic, nonaccusing manner on the following points:

1. Description of a typical day
2. Recent crises in family life
3. Alcohol and drug use/abuse of family members
4. Amount of contact with persons outside the family
5. Caretaker's perception of patient's role in the family; and family conflict over his role

From Johnson D: Abuse of the elderly, *Nurse Pract* 6:29, 1981.

6. Patient's dependence on family alone for financial, physical and/or emotional support
7. Alternative shelter available for the patient
8. Caretaker's knowledge of any medical conditions patient may have; care and medicine required
9. Support systems available to the caretaker in caring for the patient
10. Caretaker abused as a child, or exposed to other forms of family violence
11. Difficulties experienced in caring for the elderly patient
12. Commission of abusive acts, such as:
    - Shoving, shaking or hitting the patient
    - Leaving the patient alone, tying to a chair or bed or locking in a room
    - Withholding food or medicine
    - Giving too much medicine, sleeping pills or alcohol in order to make patient sleep
    - Inappropriate use of the patient's money or property
    - Threatening the patient with any of above or withholding support

Objective

Observation of the patient

1. Any injury incompatible with the history
2. Injury that has not been properly cared for
3. Hospital or health care provider "shopping"
4. Poor skin hygiene
5. Dehydration and/or malnourished without an illness-related cause
6. Evidence of inappropriate care (i.e., gross decubiti without seeking medical care)
7. Evidence of inappropriate medication administration (i.e., drowsiness or incoherence from sedative)
8. Bruising
   - Bilaterally on upper arms
   - Clustered on the trunk
   - Morphologically similar to an object
   - Presence of old and new bruises at the same time

Observation of the caretaker
1. Age
2. Physical and mental ability to withstand stress of caring for the patient

Observation of patient-caretaker interactions:
1. Fear shown by the patient
2. Excessive dependence on caretaker by patient
3. "Blaming" of patient by caretaker (i.e., accusation that incontinence is a deliberate act)

ASSESSMENT

Determine patient's status regarding abuse as:
1. No forms of abuse evident
2. Neglect and/or inappropriate care; determine causes as:
   • Age or frailty of caretaker
   • Caretaker's lack of knowledge of patient's condition
   • Caretaker's lack of knowledge of care needed
   • Illness, physical or mental, of the caretaker
   • Lack of support systems for the caretaker
3. Material abuse
   • Theft or misuse of money or property
   • Violation of patient's rights (i.e., forced removal from home or forced confinement to a nursing home)
4. Psychologic abuse
   • Verbal assault
   • Threat, inducing fear
   • Isolation
5. Physical abuse
   • Deliberate inappropriate care
   • Lack of food
   • Lack of medical care
   • Withholding medications
   • Direct beatings
   • Degree of physical abuse
   • Damaging—feasibility of alternative living situation should be investigated
   • Life threatening—alternative living situation needed immediately

PLAN

Take one or more actions appropriate to assessment status.
1. Appropriate medical and nursing care for presenting complaint, other identified problems and any injuries
2. Teach appropriate care
3. Refer to community support services such as adult day care, home health nursing services, home health aides for personal care, homemaker services, or meals-on-wheels
4. Refer for family counseling to clarify roles and reduce conflicts
5. Refer to appropriate social service agency available in the community, such as Adult Protective Services, for further investigation and possible placement of patient in alternative shelter
6. Refer for legal counsel such as Legal Aid Services or American Civil Liberties Union
7. Contact emergency services available in the community for immediate protection of the patient and removal from the home, such as a crisis intervention center or the local police department

PREVENTION

1. Public education to raise awareness of professional and lay members
2. Anticipatory guidance of the middle age family on care of elderly members
3. Increased resources, job and leisure opportunities for the elderly
4. Increased relief services for caretakers
5. Early recognition of abuse potential and referral to relief services by health professionals
6. Enactment of mandatory reporting legislation similar to child abuse legislation in every state
7. Mobilization of public resources for protection of the elderly similar to that afforded child abuse victims (i.e., a system of foster care, court-appointed guardians)
8. Further research to determine family characteristics which predispose to the potential for abuse

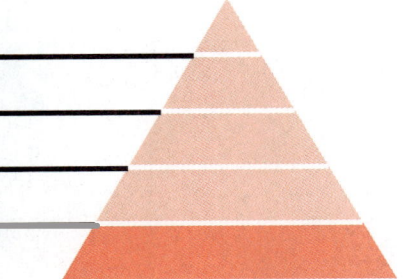

Harborview Hospital's Data Collection Form for Elder Abuse Cases

ELDER ABUSE/NEGLECT

Client last name _____ First _____ M.I. _____
Sex _____ Race _____ Birth date _____ HMC# _____ Referral date _____
Address: Street _____ City _____ State _____ Zip _____
Telephone number _____
LNOK _____ Relationship _____
LNOK Address: Street _____ City _____ State _____ Zip _____
Marital st. _____ Type of residence _____
Living with/name _____ Relationship _____
Referring agency/HMC dept. _____ Contact per. _____ Tel. # _____

PATIENT INFORMATION
New referral Yes ☐ No ☐   Repeat Yes ☐ No ☐

Presenting Complaint: _____
E.A. Protocol used: _____

	Yes	No	Date
Victim	☐	☐	_____
Alleged abuser	☐	☐	_____
Pictures taken	☐	☐	_____

HMC STAFF INVOLVED

Physician _____
Date of initial contact _____
Social worker _____
Date of initial contact _____
Other HMC staff involved _____
Referred to: _____ Prosecuting Attorney's Office
  (for legal action) Private Attorney
COMMENTS/ACTION TAKEN:
  Date

PURPOSE FOR REFERRAL

	Suspicious		Evidence	
	Yes	No	Yes	No
Physical abuse	☐	☐	☐	☐
Psychological/verbal abuse	☐	☐	☐	☐
Material abuse	☐	☐	☐	☐
Neglect/omission	☐	☐	☐	☐
Sexual abuse/sexual assault	☐	☐	☐	☐
Medical abuse/misuse	☐	☐	☐	☐

Alleged abuser _____
Relationship _____

Foundation for the Handicapped
Other:

_____
_____
_____

From Tomita S: Harborview Hospital and Medical Center, Seattle, 1982.

Where to Find State Ombudsman Offices

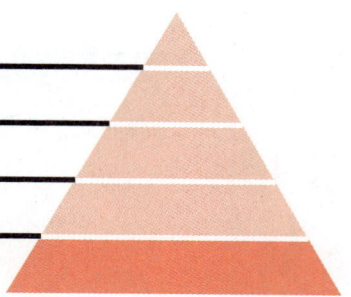

State Long-Term Care Ombudsman
COMMISSION ON AGING
RSA Plaza, Suite 470
770 Washington Avenue
Montgomery, AL 36130
(334) 242-5743

State Long-Term Care Ombudsman
OLDER ALASKANS
COMMISSIONER
3601 C Street, Suite 260
Anchorage, AK 99503-5209
(907) 279-2232

State Long-Term Care Ombudsman
AGING AND ADULT
ADMINISTRATION
Department of Economic Security
1789 West Jefferson, 950A
Phoenix, AZ 85007
(602) 542-4446

State Long-Term Care Ombudsman
DIV. OF AGING & ADULT
SERVICES
Arkansas Dept. of Human Services
PO Box 1437, Slot 1412
7th and Main Streets
Little Rock, AR 72203-1437
(501) 682-8952

State Long-Term Care Ombudsman
DEPARTMENT OF AGING
1600 K Street
Sacramento, CA 95814
(916) 323-6681

State Long-Term Care Ombudsman
THE LEGAL CENTER
455 Sherman St., Ste. 130
Denver, CO 80203
(303) 722-0300

State Long-Term Care Ombudsman
DEPARTMENT ON AGING
175 Main Street
Hartford, CT 06106
(203) 424-5200

State Long-Term Care Ombudsman
DIVISION ON AGING
Dept. of Health and Social Services
New Castle County
256 Chapman Rd.
Oxford Bldg. Suite 200
Newark, DE 19702
(302) 453-3820

State Long-Term Care Ombudsman
AARP - Legal Counsel for the Elderly
601 E Street NW, 4th Fl., Bldg. A
Washington, DC 20049
(202) 662-4943

State Long-Term Care Ombudsman
STATE LONG-TERM
OMBUDSMAN COUNCIL
Carlton Bldg-Office of the Governor
501 South Calhoun Street
Tallahassee, FL 32399-0001
(904) 488-2039

State Long-Term Care Ombudsman
OFFICE OF AGING
2 Peachtree St NW, 18th Floor
Atlanta, GA 30303
(404) 657-5319

State Long-Term Care Ombudsman
EXECUTIVE OFFICE ON AGING
Office of the Governor
335 Merchant St, Room 241
Honolulu, HI 96813
(808) 586-0100

State Long-Term Care Ombudsman
OFFICE ON AGING
PO Box 83720
Room 108 - Statehouse
Boise, ID 83720-0007
(202) 334-2220

State Long-Term Care Ombudsman
DEPARTMENT ON AGING
421 East Capitol Avenue
Springfield, IL 62701
(217) 785-3140

State Long-Term Care Ombudsman
BUREAU OF AGING/IN HOME
SERVICES
PO Box 7083-W454
Indianapolis, IN 46207-7083
(317) 232-7134

State Long-Term Care Ombudsman
DEPARTMENT OF ELDER
AFFAIRS
Jewett Bldg - Suite 236
914 Grand Avenue
Des Moines, IA 50319
(515) 281-5187

State Long-Term Care Ombudsman
DEPARTMENT ON AGING
Docking State Office Bldg, 122-S
915 SW Harrison
Topeka, KS 66612-1500
(913) 296-4986

State Long-Term Care Ombudsman
DIVISION OF AGING SERVICES
Cabinet for Human Resources
275 East Main Street, 5th Floor, West
Frankfort, KY 40621
(502) 564-6930

State Long-Term Care Ombudsman
OFFICE OF ELDERLY AFFAIRS
PO Box 80374
4550 N Blvd, 2nd Floor
Baton Rouge, LA 70806
(504) 925-1700

State Long-Term Care Ombudsman
160 Capitol St
PO Box 2723
Augusta, ME 04338-2723
(207) 621-1079

State Long-Term Care Ombudsman
OFFICE ON AGING
State Office Building, Room 1004
301 West Preston Street
Baltimore, MD 21201
(410) 225-1100

State Long-Term Care Ombudsman
EXECUTIVE OFFICE OF ELDER
AFFAIRS
1 Ashburton Place, 5th floor
Boston, MA 02108-1518
(617) 727-7750

State Long-Term Care Ombudsman
CITIZENS FOR BETTER CARE
416 North Homer St, Station 101
Lansing, MI 48912-4700
(517) 336-6753

State Long-Term Care Ombudsman
OFFICE OF OMBUDSMAN FOR
OLDER MINNESOTANS
444 Lafayette Road, 4th Floor
St. Paul, MN 55155-3843
(612) 296-0382

State Long-Term Care Ombudsman
DIV. OF AGING & ADULT SVCS.
750 North State Street
Jackson, MS 39202
(601) 359-4929

State Long-Term Care Ombudsman
DIVISION ON AGING
Department of Social Services
PO Box 1337
615 Howerton Court
Jefferson City, MO 65102-1337
(314) 751-3082

State Long-Term Care Ombudsman
OFFICE ON AGING
Department of Family Services
PO Box 8005
Helena, MT 59604-8005
(406) 444-5900

State Long-Term Care Ombudsman
DEPARTMENT ON AGING
PO Box 95044
301 Centennial Mall-South
Lincoln, NE 68509-5044
(402) 471-2306

State Long-Term Care Ombudsman
DIVISION FOR AGING SERVICES
Department of Human Resources
340 North 11th St, Suite 114
Las Vegas, NV 89101
(702) 486-3545

State Long-Term Care Ombudsman
DIV. OF ELDERLY & ADULT
SVCS
115 Pleasent St, Annex Bldg.
Concord, NH 03301-6508
(603) 271-4375

State Long-Term Care Ombudsman
OMBUDSMAN OFFICE FOR THE
INSTITUTIONALIZED ELDERLY
101 South Broad St
CN808, 6th Floor
Trenton, NJ 08625-0808
(609) 292-8016

State Long-Term Care Ombudsman
STATE AGENCY ON AGING
La Villa Rivera Bldg
228 East Palace Avenue, Suite A
Santa Fe, NM 87501
(505) 827-7640

State Long-Term Care Ombudsman
OFFICE FOR THE AGING
New York State Plaza
Agency Building #2
Albany, NY 12223-0001
(518) 474-0108

State Long-Term Care Ombudsman
DIVISION OF AGING
CB 29531
693 Palmer Drive
Raleigh, NC 27603
(919) 733-3983

State Long-Term Care Ombudsman
AGING SERVICES DIVISION
Department of Human Services
PO Box 7070
1929 North Washington Street
Bismark, ND 58507-7070
(701) 224-2577

State Long-Term Care Ombudsman
DEPARTMENT OF AGING
50 West Broad Street, 9th Fl
Columbus, OH 43215-5928
(614) 466-1221

State Long-Term Care Ombudsman
AGING SERVICES DIVISION
Department of Human Services
312 NE 28th
Oklahoma City, OK 73105
(405) 521-6734

State Long-Term Care Ombudsman
OFFICE OF THE LONG-TERM
CARE OMBUDSMAN
2475 Lancaster Drive NE, #B-9
Salem, OR 97310
(503) 378-6533

State Long-Term Care Ombudsman
DEPARTMENT OF AGING
400 Market Street, 6th Floor
Harrisburg, PA 17101-2301
(717) 783-7247

State Long-Term Care Ombudsman
GOVERNOR'S OFFICE FOR
ELDERLY AFFAIRS
Call Box 50063
Old San Juan Station
San Juan, Puerto Rico 00902
(809) 721-8225

State Long-Term Care Ombudsman
DEPARTMENT OF ELDERLY
AFFAIRS
160 Pine Street
Providence, RI 02903-3708
(401) 277-2858

State Long-Term Care Ombudsman
DIVISION ON AGING
202 Arbor Lake Drive, Suite 301
Columbia, SC 29223
(803) 737-7500

State Long-Term Care Ombudsman
OFFICE OF ADULT SVCS &
AGING
700 Governors Drive
Pierre, SD 57501
(605) 773-3656

State Long-Term Care Ombudsman
COMMISSION ON AGING
Andrew Jackson Bldg, 9th Floor
500 Deaderick Street
Nashville, TN 37243-0860
(615) 741-2056

State Long-Term Care Ombudsman
DEPARTMENT ON AGING
PO Box 12786, Capitol Station
1949 IH 35, South
Austin, TX 78711
(512) 444-2727

State Long-Term Care Ombudsman
DIVISION OF AGING & ADULT
SERVICES
Department of Social Services
Box 45500
120 North, 200 West, Rm 401
Salt Lake City, UT 84145-0500
(801) 538-3924

State Long-Term Care Ombudsman
VERMONT SENIOR CITIZENS
LAW PROJECT
18 Main Street
St. Johnsbury, VT 05819
(802) 748-8721

State Long-Term Care Ombudsman
VIRGINIA ASSOCIATION OF
AREA AGENCIES ON AGING
530 East Main Street, Suite 428
Richmond, VA 23219-2327
(804) 644-2804

State Long-Term Care Ombudsman
WASHINGTON STATE
OMBUDSMAN PROGRAM
1200 South 336th Street
Federal Way, WA 98003-7452
(206) 838-6810

State Long-Term Care Ombudsman
COMMISSION ON AGING
1900 Kanawha Blvd E
Charleston, WV 25305-0160
(304) 558-3317

State Long-Term Care Ombudsman
BOARD ON AGING AND LONG
TERM CARE
214 North Hamilton Street
Madison, WI 53703-2118
(608) 266-8944

State Long-Term Care Ombudsman
WYOMING SENIOR CITIZENS,
INC.
953 Water Street, PO Box 94
Wheatland, WY 82201
(307) 322-5553

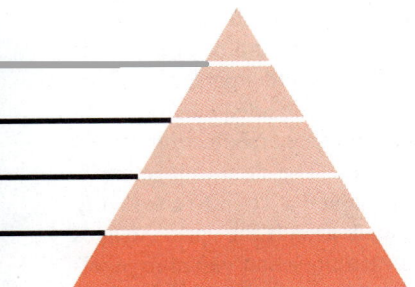

The National Elder Abuse Incidence Study

DEFINITIONS OF DOMESTIC ELDER ABUSE, EXPLOITATION, AND NEGLECT

The following definitions of domestic elder abuse, exploitation, and neglect pertain to elders living in domestic settings. The perpetrator of this abuse may or may not be the caregiver of an elderly person or a member of the elderly person's family. Furthermore, some signs and symptoms are characteristic of several kinds of maltreatment and should be regarded as indicators of possible maltreatment. The most important of these are:

- an elder's frequent unexplained crying; and
- an elder's unexplained fear of or suspicion of a particular person(s) in the home.

Physical Abuse is defined as the use of physical force that *may* result in bodily injury, physical pain or impairment. Physical abuse may include but is not limited to such acts of violence as striking (with or without an object), hitting, beating, pushing, shoving, shaking, slapping, kicking, pinching, and burning. In addition, the inappropriate use of drugs and physical restraints, force-feeding, and physical punishment of any kind also are examples of physical abuse.

Signs and symptoms of physical abuse include but are not limited to:

- bruises, black eyes, welts, lacerations, and rope marks;
- bone fractures, broken bones, and skull fractures;
- open wounds, cuts, punctures, untreated injuries, and injuries in various stages of healing;
- sprains, dislocations, and internal injuries/bleeding;
- broken eyeglasses/frames, physical signs of being subjected to punishment, and signs of being restrained;
- laboratory findings of medication overdose or under utilization of prescribed drugs;
- an elder's report of being hit, slapped, kicked, or mistreated;
- an elder's sudden change in behavior; and
- the caregiver's refusal to allow visitors to see an elder alone.

Sexual abuse is defined as nonconsensual sexual contact of any kind with an elderly person. Sexual contact with any person incapable of giving consent also is considered sexual abuse. It includes but is not limited to unwanted touching, all types of sexual assault or battery such as rape, sodomy, coerced nudity, and sexually explicit photographing.

Signs and symptoms of sexual abuse include but are not limited to:

- bruises around the breasts or genital area;
- unexplained venereal disease or genital infections;
- unexplained vaginal or anal bleeding;
- torn, stained, or bloody underclothing; and
- an elder's report of being sexually assaulted or raped.

Emotional or psychological abuse is defined as the infliction of anguish, pain, or distress through verbal or non-verbal acts. Emotional/psychological abuse includes but is not limited to verbal assaults, insults, threats, intimidation, humiliation, and harassment. In addition, treating an older person like an infant; isolating an elderly person from his/her family, friends, or regular activities; giving an older person a "silent treatment;" and enforced social isolation also are examples of emotional/psychological abuse.

Signs and symptoms of emotional/psychological abuse may manifest themselves in such behaviors of an elderly person as:

- being emotionally upset or agitated;
- being extremely withdrawn and noncommunicative or nonresponsive;
- unusual behavior usually attributed to dementia (e.g., sucking, biting, rocking); and
- an elder's report of being verbally or emotionally mistreated.

Neglect is defined as the refusal or failure to fulfill any part of a person's obligations or duties to an elder. Neglect may also include a person who has fiduciary responsibilities to provide care for an elder (e.g., pay for necessary home care services, or the failure on the part of an in-home service provider to provide necessary care). Neglect typically means the refusal or failure to provide an elderly person with such life necessities as food, water, clothing, shelter, personal hygiene, medicine, comfort, personal safety, and other essentials included in the responsibility or agreement to an elder.

Signs and symptoms of neglect include but are not limited to:

- dehydration, malnutrition, untreated bedsores, and poor personal hygiene;

From National Center on Elder Abuse.

- unattended or untreated health problems;
- hazardous or unsafe living conditions/arrangements (e.g., improper wiring, no heat or no running water);
- unsanitary and unclean living conditions (e.g., dirt, fleas, lice on person, soiled bedding, fecal/urine smell, inadequate clothing); and
- an elder's report of being mistreated.

Abandonment is defined as the desertion of an elderly person by an individual who has assumed responsibility for providing care for an elder, or by a person with physical custody of an elder.

Signs and symptoms of abandonment include but are not limited to:

- the desertion of an elder at a hospital, a nursing facility, or other similar institution;
- the desertion of an elder at a shopping center or other public location; and
- an elder's own report of being abandoned.

Financial or material exploitation is defined as the illegal or improper use of an elder's funds, property ar assets. Examples would include but are not limited to: cashing an elderly person's checks without authorization/permission; forging an older person's signature; misusing or stealing an older person's money or possessions; coercing or deceiving an older person into signing any document (e.g., contracts, a will); and the improper use of conservatorship, guardianship, or power of attorney.

Signs and symptoms of financial or material exploitation include but are not limited to:

- sudden changes in bank account or banking practice, including an unexplained withdrawal of large sums of money by a person accompanying the elder;
- the inclusion of additional names on an elder's bank signature card;
- unauthorized withdrawal of the elder's funds using the elders ATM card;
- abrupt changes in a will or other financial documents;
- unexplained disappearance of funds or valuable possessions;
- substandard care being provided or bills unpaid despite the availability of adequate financial resources;
- discovery of an elder's signature being forged for financial transactions and for the titles of his/her possessions;
- sudden appearance of previously uninvolved relatives claiming their rights to an elder's affairs and possessions;
- unexplained sudden transfer of assets to a family member or someone outside the family;
- the provision of services that are not necessary; and
- an elder's report of financial exploitation.

Self-neglect is characterized as the behaviors of an elderly person that threaten his/her own health or safety. Self-neglect generally manifests itself in an older person's refusal or failure to provide himself/herself with adequate food, water, clothing, shelter, personal hygiene, medication (when indicated), and safety precautions. The definition of self-neglect *excludes* a situation in which a cognitive/mentally competent older person (who understands the consequences of his/her decisions) makes a conscious and voluntary decision to engage acts that threaten his/her health or safety as a matter of personal preference.

Signs and symptoms of self-neglect include but are not limited to:

- dehydration, malnutrition, untreated or improperly attended medical conditions, and poor personal hygiene;
- hazardous or unsafe living conditions/arrangements (e.g., improper wiring, no indoor plumbing, no heat or no running water);
- unsanitary or unclean living quarters (e.g., animal/insect infestation, no functioning toilet, fecal/urine smell);
- inappropriate and/or inadequate clothing, lack of the necessary medical aides (e.g., eyeglasses, hearing aid, dentures); and
- grossly inadequate housing or homelessness.

NATIONAL CENTER ON ELDER ABUSE (NCEA)
Consortium Organizations

American Public Welfare Association (APWA)
810 First Street, NE
Suite 500
Washington, D.C. 20002-4267

National Association of State Units on Aging (NASUA)
1225 I Street NW
Suite 725
Washington, D.C. 20005

University of Delaware
College of Human Resources
Department of Textiles, Design, and Consumer Economics
Newark, Delaware 19716

National Committee for the Prevention of Elder Abuse (NCPEA)
c/o Institute on Aging
The Medical Center of Central Massachusetts
119 Belmont Street
Worcester, Massachusetts 01605

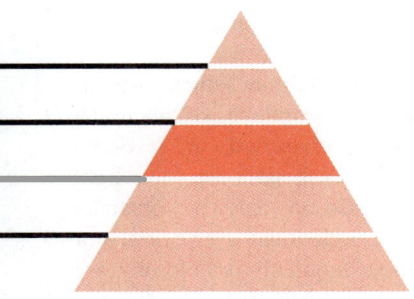

CHAPTER 16

Intimacy, Sexuality, and Aging

These early morning hours are terribly lonely . . . that's when I have such a longing for someone who loves me to be there just to touch and hold me . . . and to talk to.

Sister Marilyn Schwab From Schwab M: *A gift freely given: the personal journal of Sister Marilyn Schwab,* Mt Angel, Ore, 1986, Benedictine Sisters.

LEARNING OBJECTIVES

Upon completion of this chapter, the reader will be able to:

1. Define sexuality.
2. Describe the various approaches to sexuality assessment that may reduce nurse-client anxiety in discussing a sensitive area.
3. Discuss the physiologic alterations that affect the older adult's sexual function.
4. Collect data related to sexuality of the aged individual.
5. Identify the risks to sexual integrity.
6. Formulate and validate appropriate nursing diagnoses.
7. Discuss elders' need for closeness, touch, warmth, and sharing.
8. Discuss interventions that foster sexual integrity.

TOUCH

Touch affects almost anything we do. It is the oldest, most important, and most neglected of our senses. Touch is 10 times stronger than verbal or emotional contact. All other senses have an organ to focus on, but touch is everywhere. Touch is unique because it frequently combines with other senses. An individual can survive without one or more of the other senses, but one cannot survive and live in any degree of comfort without touch. In the absence of touching or being touched people of all ages can become sick and become touch starved (Ackerman, 1995). "Touch is a way to define self and experience the world . . . touch triggers a variety of responses that affect physiology, emotions, and behavior" (Miller, 1992, p. 3).

Mythology, magic, folklore, primitive medicine, and religion all affirm, through the centuries, the importance of touch in healing, destruction, communication, and personal power (Barnett, 1972a). The human yearning for physical contact is embedded in our language in such figurative terms as "keep in touch," "handle with care," and "rubbed the wrong way" (Huss, 1977). We will focus on touch as an overt expression of closeness, intimacy, and sexuality. We believe one must recognize the power of touch and its intimacy to fully comprehend sexuality. Touch and intimacy are integral parts of sexuality, just as sexuality is expressed through intimacy and touch. Together they can offer the aged a sense of well-being.

Touch is the first sensory system to become functional. Throughout life touch provides emotional and sensual knowledge about others: an unending source of information, pleasure, and pain. In all human cultures, gently touching another person conveys affection and friendliness (Barnett, 1972b).

Thayer (1982, p. 266) describes touch as follows: "like all nonverbal behavior, it rarely has unitary, unequivocal meaning. The message depends upon a host of factors."

We love and are loved by virtue of our skin sensation and appearance. How our skin is arranged affects others' willingness to touch us. Even though beauty is said to be only skin deep, skin is significant. The wrinkled skin of the old shows the beautiful lines of hard work and experience. Old hands and old faces tell us much of the bearer's capacity for intimacy. Sensations of old skin, clean, dry, and powdered or cologned, linger in the remote memories of many of us who were held by a grandmother or grandfather. These provide our foundation for intimacy with the old.

In the cases of the isolated or institutionalized aged, we may need to consider that higher death rates are more related to the quality of human relationships than to the degree of cleanliness, nutrition, and physical disabilities on which our attentions are focused. Montagu (1986) noted that "tactile hunger" becomes more powerful in old age when other sensuous experiences are diminished and direct sexual expression is often no longer possible or available. Further, he believes the cause of illness may be greatly influenced by the quality of tactile support received.

Ackerman (1995) equates touch to be as essential as sunlight. Colton (1983) cites tactile touch or touch hunger as analogous to malnutrition. Malnutrition results from the lack of adequate nutrients for body survival. Touch stimulates chemical production in the brain, which feeds blood, muscles, tissues, nerve cells, organs, and other body structures. Without this stimulation, like nutrients in food, the individual would be deprived of sustenance and would starve.

Intimacy Levels of Touch

Patterns. Jourard's cursory observation (1964) of touch in a hospital study revealed no physical contact during 2-hour observation periods. Barnett (1972b) found in a similar study that senior nursing students did not touch patients at all, but that after graduation, when they assumed the role of a registered nurse, touch was used as one means of communication. The absence of touch, or distancing, by the student nurses was thought to be their interpretation of professionalism. Barnett's study showed that women were touched more than men; the hands, forehead, and shoulders were touched, whereas the fingers, toes, ankles, and genitalia were not. The age group least touched was persons 66 to 100 years of age, while those in their late teens to 25 years old were touched the most.

Thayer (1982) describes five types of touch, the first of which, functional-professional touch, reflects Barnett's observations. In this mode, persons in their special roles (nurse, technician, aide) perform a task in which verbal, vocal, or kinesthetic signals of sexuality or disrespect are absent. Social-polite touch is formal or cordial. Friendship-warm touch allows physical demonstrations such as hugs, kisses, and hand-holding. The touch of love-intimacy reflects strong affection and intimacy and touching in areas that allow vulnerability. Sexual arousal is touch of the most physical and intimate form in a sexual context.

Cosgray and Davidhizar (1988) defined six types of touch that may be employed by nurses in the care of psychogeriatric patients: procedural, friendly, aggressive, limit setting, meeting own needs, and inappropriate touch. They found the vast majority of touch was procedural or related to limit setting. Friendly touch ranked third. No aggressive or inappropriate touch was observed. Many nursing implications can be drawn from their observations.

Response to Touch. Touch may calm or stimulate anxiety, fear, love, comfort, or rage. The subtleties of touch that convey these varied messages are learned early in life. Some people respond warmly to a firm touch and others to a light or casual touch. Useful information may be obtained through a handshake. Does the individual grasp firmly or hesitate? Does he or she relinquish quickly or hold on? Are the fingers intertwined or held together? Is the hand limp, passive, or responsive; tremulous, sweaty, or cold?

Touch except during illness, injury, or sexual encounters may be unacceptable to an individual. The use of touch by nurses should be based on the following considerations: Nurses should recognize the influence of their own personality, cultural expectations, and early exposure to touching. Everyone has definite feelings and opinions about touch based on his or her own life experience. Touch only if it is comfortable. Individuals quickly discern the discomfort of another if touch is not an integral part of behavior. It is important to remember that the comfort of touching depends on place, situation, social status, and age.

"Caring touch" has been used systematically in a nursing home setting as a cost-effective means to improve communication and quality of life of residents. Staff members were trained to use "caring touch" frequently as a means of becoming sensitive to the interaction between professional and client. The training model was based on the focusing technique of Gendlin (Sakauye and McDonald, 1987). The results not only showed significant increases in patient satisfaction but also had a positive impact on staff morale.

Touch Zones. Hall (1969) identifies different categories of touching—expanding or contracting zones around which every individual extends the sensory experience of touching, smelling, hearing, and seeing. It is the nurse's function to enter the zone of intimacy (Figure 16-1), which is identified to be an area within an arm's length of the individual's body and is the space used for comforting, protecting, and love-making. Illness, confinement, and dependency seen in institutionalization are stresses on the intimate zone of touch. Just as caregivers enter a room without knocking, so they often intrude into the intimate circle of touch without asking. We have attempted to examine the parameters of the intimate zone of touch to emphasize the importance of understanding behavior that might occur when the nurse enters this arena.

The social zone includes those areas of the body that are the least sensitive or embarrassing to have touched and that do not necessarily require permission to be handled. The consent zone requires the nurse to seek out or ask permission to touch or initiate procedures to these areas. The vulnerable zone is highly sexually charged and will be protected. The most intimate area, the genitalia, is the most personally protected and causes the most stress and anxiety when approached, touched, and viewed by the caregiver.

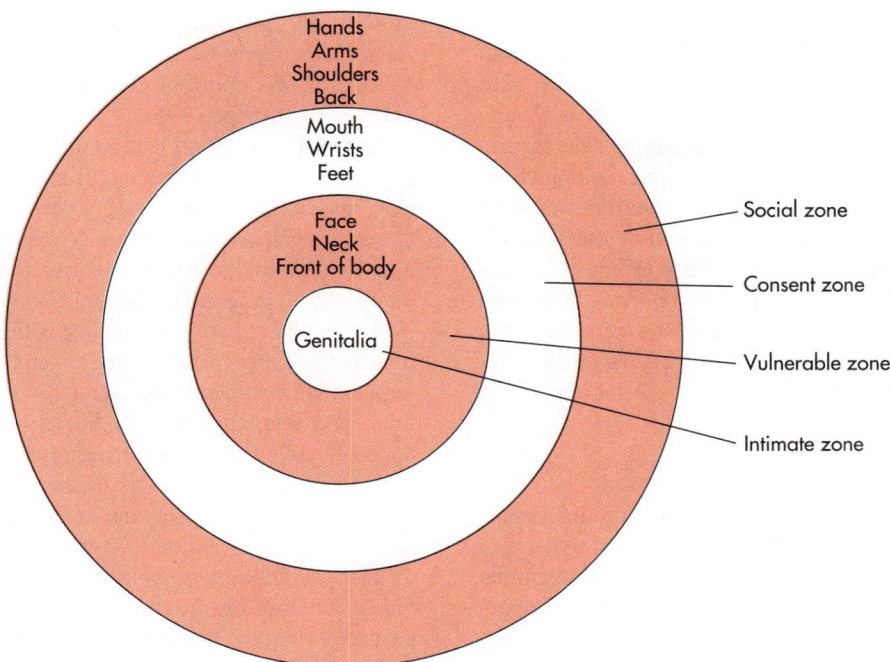

Figure 16-1. Zones of intimacy or sexuality.

A test of the person's readiness to be touched is to initiate a hand clasp or handshake. One can feel the tension or the welcoming relaxation that occurs. Later, a massage of tired neck or back muscles, hands, or feet will take the nurse into a closer area of intimacy. You will recognize in touching the front of the body, face, and the neck that these are sexually charged zones. Stroking the temples is a soothing intervention; stroking cheeks usually produces anxiety.

Fear of Touching. Many times a nurse will touch in a condescending way, a pat on the head or a tweak of the toe, or in a circumscribed nursing treatment. Of all health care professionals, nurses have the most frequent opportunities to provide gentle, reassuring, renewing touch, but the use of touch involves risk and may be misinterpreted by the nurse or patient. The intimacy of nurse/patient contacts may influence a nurse to be overly circumspect. Stirring sexual feelings, if that is a response to gentle touching, is a human response that need not frighten. Old women and old men have stated they miss the touching and holding of their earlier lives. They may seek such comfort by sexually provocative behaviors. Nurses need not encourage such overt behavior but must be cognizant of the underlying needs of intimacy.

Sometimes nurses respond negatively to a breach in the "status" of touch. There is a status system of touch that is significant to health care. One of the higher status may touch an inferior, but the reverse is frowned on; similarly, name familiarity may be used by one in a superior position but is greatly resented if the lower-ranking person presumes the same liberty. Since this notion is embedded in many hierarchic structures, it is wise to treat everyone with respect regarding their name and propensity for touch. Instant familiarity is seldom useful (Hall, 1969). When a patient reciprocates with the same level of intimacy as initiated by the nurse, it should not be surprising.

Touch Deprivation

Do old people suffer touch deprivation? Many do if they are separated from caring others. Old men, in particular, may find it hard to reach out to others for stroking and fondling. Their previous lifestyles often mitigated against this except in the intimacy of sexual contact, which may no longer be available to them (Montagu, 1986). It is not uncommon for old men to be wrongly accused of sexual offenses because they dared to give a child an affectionate pat on the head or on the buttocks. Old women are allowed considerably more freedom to touch, although they may lack the opportunity.

Adaptation to Touch Deprivation. Persons can survive extreme sensory deprivation as long as the sensory experiences of the skin are maintained. An outstanding feature of touch according to Ackerman (1995) is that it does not have to be performed by a person or other living thing. Some sustenance or peace for the old may be gained from the self-contained stimulation of a rocking chair or slowly stroking an animal's fur or wearing something that provides sensory stimulation. Thayer (1982) describes these as self-adapters.

Self-adapters are movements not intentionally used to communicate with others but that facilitate or block sensory input. For the aged, rocking in the chair or stroking oneself, the fur of a pet, or a child's silky hair may be self-adapters for touch. Emotionally disturbed people are often found rocking as if the motion is somehow soothing. People rock when grief stricken or when needing comfort. Montagu (1978) believes rocking stimulates and eroticizes skin through a complex series of motions and that it is a self-comforting measure. Perhaps the aged compensate for the lack of touch and closeness by the use of their rocking chair.

Music, perceived through the skin as well as the ears, may be another source of touch stimulation that is self-induced. Skin touched by the vibrations of music is enveloped and caressed. Music and dancing seem to be two important mechanisms of enjoyment of the aged. In later years they often return to dancing after decades of ignoring the pleasurable activity. Perhaps this is a response to the need for more touch.

Therapeutic Touch

Touch is a powerful healer and a therapeutic tool that nurses can use to satisfy "touch hunger" of the aged. Nursing has recognized the importance of touch and has the social sanctions to touch the body in the intimate and personal care of a person, an opportunity too often not fully used for the betterment of the aged person's adaptation to environment and location in time and space. Barnett (1972b) points out that *touch can serve as a means of providing sensory stimulation, reduction of anxiety, reality orientation, relief of physical and psychologic pain, and comfort in dying as well as sexual expression.*

Thayer (1982) cites the additional purposes of touch as relief of stress, cleansing, expression of joy, beautification, and sexual pleasure. The greater the sense of isolation, sensory deprivation, dependency, lack of self-esteem, and fear of death, the greater the need for touch. Conversely, the greater the need for privacy and distance, the less the person should be touched.

Kreiger's experiments with therapeutic touch (1975) demonstrate physiologic and psychologic improvement in patients who are exposed to consistent "doses" of touch. "Laying on of the hands" and the power of touch to heal had largely disappeared with the scientific revolution. Before that, divine powers of healing through touch were attributed to priests, religious leaders, and kings. Touch for healing remained a practice in many religions and was used in conjunction with prayer. The phenomenon has reemerged as "touch for health," "laying on of hands," and "therapeutic touch" movements.

Massage has gained acceptance as a touch therapy. Massage stimulates circulation, dilates blood vessels, relaxes tense muscles, and cleans toxins out of the body through the flow of lymph. Many nurses are convinced of the efficacy of touch to restore health and comfort and have begun to incorporate it into their care.

SEXUALITY

Sexuality provides the opportunity to express passion, affection, admiration, and loyalty. It is an affirmation that one's body functions well, maintains a strong sense of self-identity, and provides a means for self-assertion. Sexuality also allows a general affirmation of life (especially joy) and a continuing opportunity to search for new growth and experience (Lewis, 1995).

Sexuality, like food and water, is a basic human need. It goes beyond the biologic realm to include psychologic, social, and moral dimensions. The constant interaction between these spheres of sexuality work to produce harmony. The linkage of the four dimensions composes the holistic quality of an individual's sexuality.

The social sphere of sexuality is the sum of cultural factors that influence one's thoughts and actions related to interpersonal relationships, as well as sexuality related to ideas and learned behavior. Social sexuality is also influenced by television, radio, literature, and the more traditional sources of family, school, and religious teachings. The belief of what constitutes masculine and feminine is deeply rooted in one's exposure to cultural factors.

The psychologic domain of sexuality reflects one's attitudes, feelings toward self and others, and learning from past experiences. Beginning with birth, one is bombarded with cues and signals of how one should act and think about the use of "dirty words" or body parts. Conversation is self-censored in the presence of or in discussion with certain people.

The moral aspect of sexuality, the "I should" or "I shouldn't," makes a difference that is based in religious beliefs or in a pragmatic or humanistic outlook.

The final dimension, biologic sexuality, is reflected in physiologic responses to sexual stimulation, reproduction, puberty, and growth and development. Because of the inter-

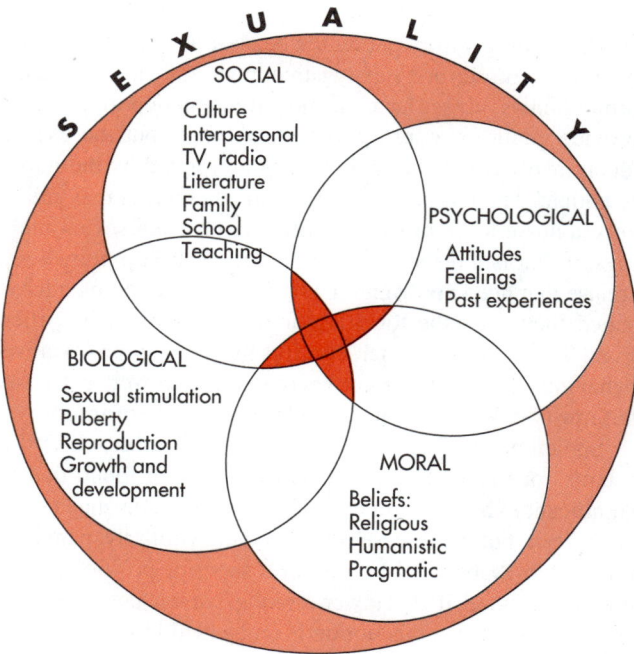

Figure 16-2. Interrelationship of dimensions of sexuality.

relatedness, these dimensions affect each other directly or indirectly whenever an aspect of sexuality is out of harmony. Figure 16-2 attempts to illustrate the interrelationship of the sexuality dimensions.

Sexuality has become an important theoretic issue of concern in the care of the aged. Kass (1979) has shown that caregivers agree that sexuality is important. Although they support this idea in theory, their actions do not. Rarely are aged persons in congregate living facilities (nursing homes, acute hospitals, homes for the aged, extended care, mental institutions, and other total care facilities) or residing in their own homes treated as sexual beings by health care professionals.

Sexuality is a vital aspect to consider in the care of the aged person regardless of the setting. Sexuality exists throughout life in one form or another in all persons. All of the aged have a need to express sexual feelings whether they are healthy and active or frail individuals. Sexuality is linked with one's personality and identity and has a significant role in the promotion of better life adaptation (Billhorn, 1994; Wiley and Bortz, 1996). At a time when the usefulness of the aged is questioned by others and by the aged themselves, this portion of one's identity can give meaning to life and bolster security, belonging, and esteem. One can envision sexuality as part of Maslow's hierarchy of needs, with physical reproduction the lowest level and a progression to the higer levels with increased communication, trust, sharing, and pleasure with or without a physical action. Figure 16-3 focuses on the hierarchy of sexuality.

Acceptance and Companionship

Sexuality validates the lifelong need to share intimacy and have that offering appreciated. Sexuality is love, warmth, sharing, and touching between people, not just the physical act of coitus. Margot Benary-Isbert in her book *The Vintage Years* (1968) expresses the essence of sexuality most eloquently:

Let us not forget old married couples who once shared healthy and happy days as they now share the unavoidable limitations of old age and grow even closer together in love and patience. When they exchange a smile, a glance, one can guess that they still think each other beautiful and loveable.

She continues with ". . . as long as we live with our companion all these seem worthwhile because each one desires to make life as easy as possible for the other" (Benary-Isbert, 1968, pp. 201-202). *The Hite Report* (Hite, 1977) identified touching at night, listening to the breathing and the heart beat, and open talking that occur in bed as important features of sexuality expressed by older women; a study by Nay (1992) confirms this. Berlin concludes: "Sexuality can mean anything which gives sexual or emotional pleasure, excitement, or comfort" (1978, p. 2).

Femininity and Masculinity

Males and females possess characteristic behavioral traits, which Jung refers to as the anima (female) and animus (male) (Fordham, 1970; Jacobi, 1973). Past social pressures did not often allow the appearance of sensitivity, gentleness,

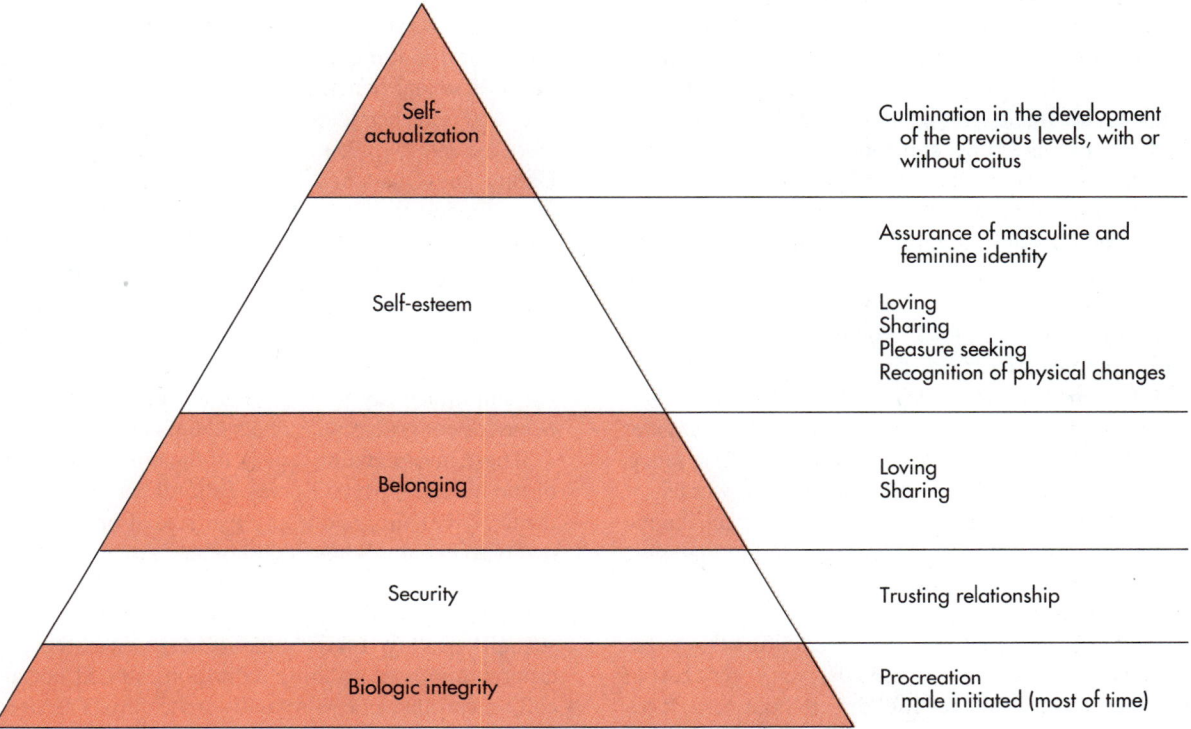

Figure 16-3. Progression of sexual emphasis through life.

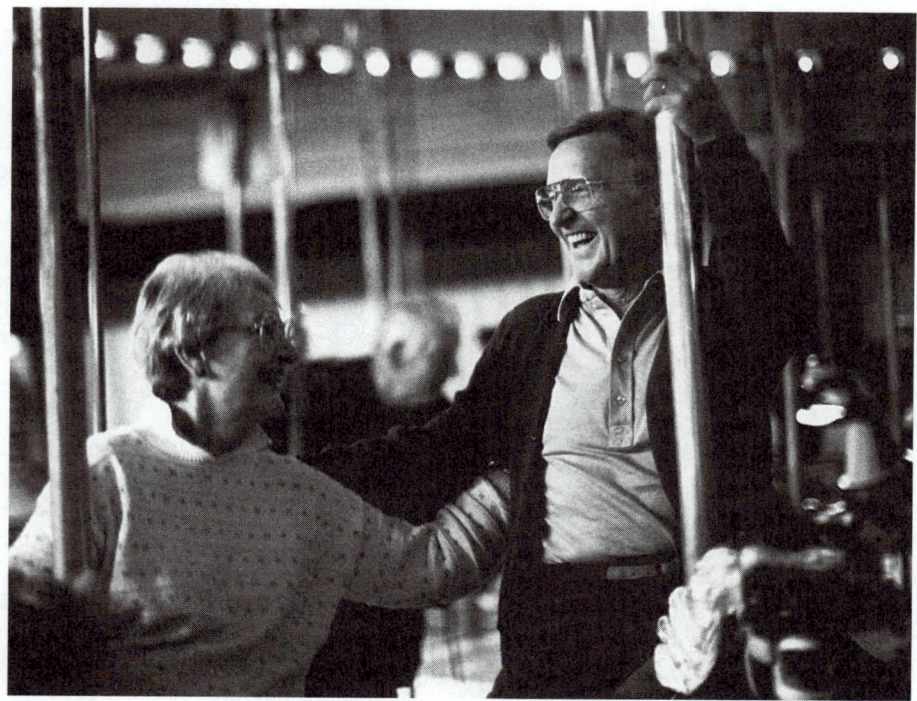

A special togetherness. (Courtesy Rod Schmall.)

and sentimentality in most men. Men were expected to be strong, to be in control of situations, and to handle their emotions. Likewise, women were not viewed as aggressive or the major decision makers.

What is often seen and perpetuated among the old are socially accepted standards characteristic of masculine and feminine behavior, which reflect male and female role models dominant in their formative years. Jung's work has shown this to be so, indicating that strong attitude types (male and female) and roles and functions associated with these attitudes are developed as adaptations of the person to the demands of the environment.

Man counted it a virtue to repress his feminine traits, and woman, until recently, repressed her animus. Both, however, are not consciously aware that they possess the opposite sexual identity. Goldblatt (1972) contends that neither gonads nor chromosomal sex are determinants of sexual behavior. Money and Tucker (1975) in their work *Sexual Signatures* believe that it is social stimulation that provides gender identity and limits one's concept of self. In essence, society expects men to be men and women to be women.

In the later part of life there is a deepening of self-knowledge. One tends to discover traits in one's nature that were previously suppressed or heretofore remained in the unconscious. At this time the emergence of the anima (in men) and animus (in women) may be seen. Jung identified this experience as the expression of the psyche that in the first half of life was turned inward. In later life, directed outward, it becomes indicative of the capacity for fuller living. Men be-

come more comfortable with tenderness and women with assertiveness. The person's ability to accord his or her other nature its due recognition will enhance sexuality (Box 16-1).

Sexual Health

The World Health Organization defines sexual health as "the integration of somatic, emotional, intellectual, and social aspects of sexual being, in ways that are positively enriching and that enhance personality, communication, and love" (Woods, 1979, p. 75). According to Maddocks (1975) and Denny and Quadango (1992), sexual health is a realistic phenomenon that includes four components: personal and social behaviors in agreement with individual gender identity, comfort with a range of sexual role behaviors and engagement in effective interpersonal relations with both sexes in a love or long-term commitment, response to erotic stimulation that produces positive and pleasurable sexual activity, and the ability to make mature judgments about sexual behavior congruent with one's beliefs and values.

These interpretations speak of the multidiciplinary nature of the biologic, psychosocial, cultural, and spiritual components of sexuality and imply that sexual behavior is the capacity to enhance oneself and others. However, these meanings, if literally applied, indicate that those who are neurologically impaired, celibate, transsexual, or ill are not sexually healthy. Taken in its broadest sense, the absence of criteria expressed in these definitions should not automatically mean that one is sexually unhealthy. The aged in the context of these criteria may not seek the erotic constancy or

- Masturbation is an immature activity of youngsters and adolescents, not older women.
- Since sexual desire and prowess wane during the climacteric, menopause is the death of a woman's sexuality.
- Hysterectomy creates a physical disability that results in the inability to function sexually.
- Sex has no role in the lives of the elderly, except as perversion or remembrance of times past.
- Sexual expression in old age is taboo.
- The elderly are too old and frail to engage in sex.
- The young are considered lusty or virile, the elderly are considered lecherous.
- Sex is unimportant or over.
- Elderly women do not wish to discuss their sexuality with professionals.

Adapted from Morrison-Beedy D, Robbins L: Sexual assessment and the aging female, *Nurse Pract* 14 (12):35, 1989.

prowess of the young and might be considered as experiencing poor sexual health. In truth one must look at these definitions as guidelines, not rules that govern all healthy sexual behavior. Sexual health is individually defined and wholesome if it leads to intimacy (not necessarily coitus) and enriches the involved parties. Old people may have a limited sexual life by some definitions, but the criterion of assessment and evaluation is their satisfaction.

Age Variables

Expectations. Sexual behavior of the aged is influenced by a number of cultural, biologic, psychosocial, and environmental factors. The aged may be confronted with barriers to the expression of their sexuality by reflected attitudes, health, culture, economics, opportunity, and historic trends.

The aged often internalize the broad cultural proscriptions of sexual behavior in late life that hinder the continuance of sexual expression. One learns early in life that permission for certain sexual behaviors is given and that what is acceptable and not acceptable changes with age. Permission for social and sexual initiative comes with maturity, status, and wealth. Much sexual behavior stems from incorporating others' reactions. Anderson and Newton (1966), Jarvik and Small (1988), and Butler and Lewis (1990) indicate that old people do not feel old until they are faced with the fact that others around them consider them old. Likewise, they do not feel asexual until they are continually treated as such. Kass (1979, p. 372) commented, "At any age sexual function is dependent on adaptation between physical capacities, societal mores, and individual desires."

Erikson et al (1986) found a large number of female octogenarians in their study to have been strongly influenced by the prudish, Victorian atmosphere of their youth. Many of them experienced difficult marital adjustments and serious sexual problems early in their marriages. Many of the couples found their old-age intimacy had transcended the painful differences they felt when they were young. Few elders acknowledged disharmony within their present marital relationship. Those that did were unhappy at the increased dependency of an ill spouse and in a sense were grieving the loss of the patterns and expectations that had become comfortable in the relationship and were now disrupted by illness and incapacity.

Incongruent needs and expectations may cause distress in older couples. Often these arise from discordant aging processes: the man may desire to be sexually active and the woman has lost interest, or vice versa. One couple who had long sustained a satisfactory sexual relationship could not conceive of engaging in the alternative modes of sexual expression (cunnilingus, mutual masturbation, and repositioning) suggested when the wife developed severe osteoarthritis. The old gentleman brought the worn and dog-eared illustrative pamphlet back to the nurse in the health clinic. "She just won't go for it, Nurse!" In such cases, the most well-meant advice may not be useful. To resolve such incompatible needs, the nurse may best counsel the most sexually active and liberal partner in ways to achieve orgasm while still remaining sexually comforting to the other partner.

Redefinitions. Sexuality in the aged shifts its focus from procreation to an emphasis on companionship, physical nearness, intimate communication, and a pleasure-seeking physical relationship. Some researchers have coined the phrase "from procreation to recreation," which refers to this change in sexual emphasis. This redefinition of sexuality within Maslow's hierarchical framework simply means the most basic level of function might be male-initiated sex for the purpose of reproduction, and the more complex levels involve a relationship of greater communication, trust, love, sharing, and the giving of pleasure with or without coitus. This change in sexual emphasis is also a reaffirmation of DeNigola and Peruzza's (1974) view that sexuality serves a comprehensive function in adaptation and is fulfillable in many healthy ways.

Sex can be a way of preventing social disengagement in old age. It can be a means of promoting intergenerational understanding. Both young and old share some of the same fears, insecurities, and pleasures afforded by sex. Sex can be a safe and valuable form of physical exercise. It can be a way of maintaining a healthy self-image in old age, and it can be a support in managing personal anxieties by serving as an outlet to defuse anxieties and by providing psychologic refueling and energizing. Sex may even be an escape from depression (Walz and Blum, 1987). Figure 16-3 reflects the changing emphasis and the totality of sexual behavior of later life in the framework of Maslow's hierarchy.

Activity Levels. No national comprehensive surveys of sexuality have been done for any age group. Historical and limited data of early studies of sexual behavior by Kinsey in the 1940s and 1950s and Masters and Johnson in the 1960s contained small samples of aged persons from which to draw conclusions. These studies did suggest that older persons continued to enjoy sexual relations into late life. The Duke Longitudinal Study and the Baltimore Longitudinal Study on Aging were questionnaires of self-reported sexual activity conducted by mail. These studies showed that a little more than 50% of the aged couples in the studies were sexually active. After the age of 75 years, there tended to be a significant drop in sexual activity. This cessation was primarily caused by illness of one or both partners or the death of one of the spouses. The studies also revealed that women tended to be less sexually active than men. Even though many old women retain a strong drive, the population imbalance of the sexes limits opportunity to engage in coitus. Aged women have been viewed by themselves and society (Burke and Knowlton, 1992; Nay, 1992) as sexually unattractive and are left out. There are more old women in proportion to old men and thus fewer opportunities. Statistics show that by the age of 85, there are 83 men for every 100 women in the United States (over 50% widows, 7% never married, 2% divorced, and 60% without spouses) (Lewis, 1995). The ratio of old men to old women becomes 1:4.

Men, on the other hand, remain relatively unscathed by social sanction and have none of the limitations imposed on them that women do. In fact, older men become newsworthy when they father a child in their later years. Older men tend to remarry sooner than do their female counterparts following the death of a spouse. Men marry an average of 3 years following the death, whereas women who remarry take an average of 7 years following widowhood (Burke and Knowlton, 1992). Besides gender variables, whites are less active than blacks, and higher socioeconomic groups are less sexually involved than persons of lower socioeconomic status (Woods, 1979).

Although her sample of aged women was a small segment of the total study, Hite (1977) helps emphasize that sexuality and the capacity to experience sexual pleasure are lifetime attributes for women. Such comments as the following were recorded, "I am 67, and find that age does not change sex much, circumstances determine it" (Hite, 1977, p. 510). A septuagenarian commented, "At my age and without responsibility I do not want matrimony but I have a continuing sex drive which keeps me looking 15 to 20 years younger than my chronological age" (Hite, 1977, p. 509).

Starr (1985) recognized that elderly persons' sexual activity and interest are consistent with those in early adulthood. For many, sexual response improves. The change in perception of the sexual activity of the aged is based on more recent studies of elderly sexual activity that have included an individual's experience and perception rather than just the physiologic and statistical changes characteristic of earlier studies.

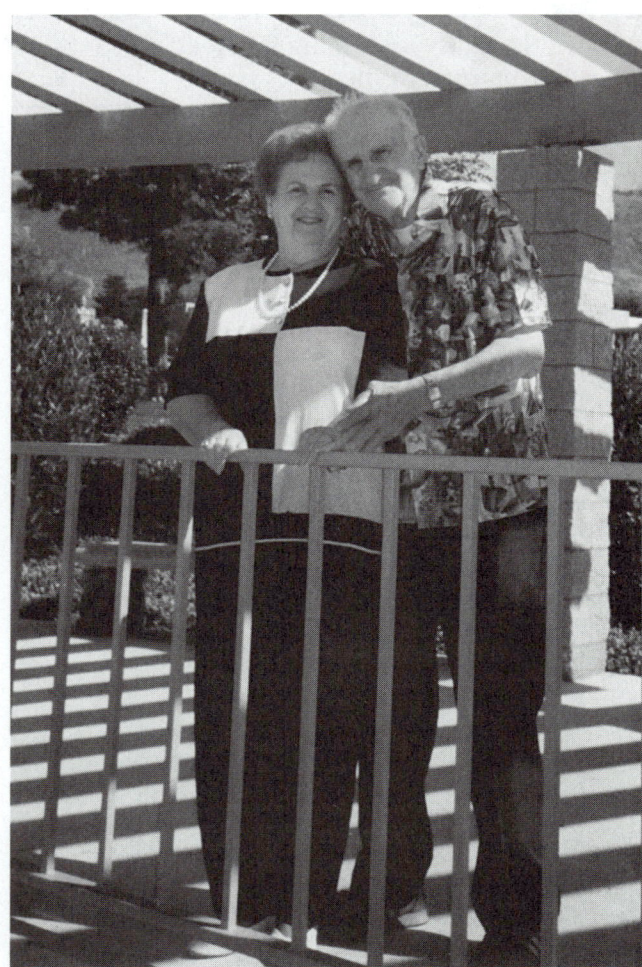

Redefining pleasures. (Courtesy Victoria DeZordo.)

Cohort Attitudes. History has shown that basic attitudes toward sexual expression have been venerated, openly accepted, or have been a subject of hostility. American society continues to struggle with open acceptance of sexual expression for the young but continues to remain hostile to the attempts of the aged to do the same. Sex interest and activity in the elderly are regarded as deviant behavior and described in such terms as "dirty old man," "lecher," and "old biddy." The same activity attempted by a younger person would be viewed as appropriate. The boomer generation interpretation may alter this perception as they find themselves experiencing sexuality beyond the age they assigned to their elders.

Biologic Changes with Age. Acknowledgement and understanding of the age changes that influence coitus may partially explain alteration in sexual behavior to accommodate these changes and facilitate continued pleasurable sex. Chapter 6 discusses the various physical changes that occur in men and women with age. Table 16-1 summarizes physical alterations that affect coitus in aging persons. This is one

Table 16-1	Physical Changes in Sexual Responses in Old Age	
	Female	**Male**
Excitation phase	Diminished or delayed lubrication (1 to 3 min may be required for adequate amounts to appear) Diminished flattening and separation of labia majora Disappearance of elevation of labia majora Decreased vasocongestion of labia minora Decreased elastic expansion of vagina (depth and breadth) Breasts not as engorged Sex flush absent	Less intense and slower erection (but can be maintained longer without ejaculation) Increased difficulty regaining an erection if lost Less vasocongestion of scrotal sac Less pronounced elevation and congestion of testicles
Plateau phase	Slower and less prominent uterine elevation or tenting Decreased muscle tension Decreased capacity for vasocongestion Decreased areolar engorgement Labial color change less evident Less intense swelling or orgasmic platform Less sexual flush Decreased secretions of Bartholin glands	Decreased muscle tension Nipple erection and sexual flush less often No color change at coronal edge of penis Slower penile erection pattern Delayed or diminished erectal and testicular elevation
Orgasmic phase	Fewer number and less intense orgasmic contractions Rectal spincter contractions with severe tension only	Decreased or absent secretory activity (lubrication) by Cowper gland before ejaculation Fewer penile contractions Fewer rectal sphincter contractions Decreased force of ejaculation (approximately 50%) with decreased amount of semen (if ejaculation is long, seepage of semen occurs)
Resolution phase	Observably slower loss of nipple erection Vasocongestion of clitoris and orgasmic platform quickly subsides	Vasocongestion of nipples and scrotum slowly subsides Very rapid loss of erection and descent of testicles shortly after ejaculation Refractory time extended (time required before another erection ranges from several to 24 hours, occasionally longer)

Data compiled from Miller CA: *Nursing care of older adults,* Glenview, Ill, 1990, Scott Foresman/Little Brown, Higher Education; Shippee-Rice R: Sexuality and aging. In Fogel C, Lauver D, editors: *Sexual health promotion,* Philadelphia, 1990, WB Saunders; Saxon SV, Etten MJ: *Physical changes and aging,* ed 3, New York, 1994, The Tiresias Press, Inc.

variable in the total picture of sexuality, and therefore we have included the main factors that influence the act of intercourse. Many texts explain biologic changes in depth.

Biologic factors include (1) adequate circulation to the genital area to support the vasocongestion that takes place; (2) functional neurologic pathways to conduct motor, sensory, and reflex impulses; (3) adequate and appropriate hormone availability to influence the integrity of the genital structure and function; and (4) intactness of the genitalia.

Aging individuals who do not understand the physical changes that affect sexual activity become concerned that their sex life is approaching its natural conclusion with the onset of menopause or, for men, when they discover a change in the firmness of their erection or the decreased need for ejaculation with each orgasm or when the refractory period is extended between episodes of intercourse. Morning intercourse is often more satisfactory because many aging men experience erection early in the morning.

Psychologic Factors. Given the gradual biologic changes in genital structures, there is potential for continued performance of the sex act among the old. However, psychologic factors such as guilt, depression, monotony, unresolved grief, anger, performance anxiety, and self-doubt may inhibit function (Box 16-2). The client or patient most often believes it is a biologic failure. Many health care professionals also conclude that it is age appropriate without consideration of a psychologic base.

Environmental Factors. Environmental barriers result predominantly from the lack of privacy available to the older person. Lack of privacy can occur when the aged person lives with adult children. It is rare that if a parent has a suitor in to visit they have a place to go by themselves without other family members around. Institutions tend to separate the sexes (less today than in past years, but this practice still exists), married elderly and single men from single women. There are specific places for mixed company to congregate, and there are rules about male residents going into women's rooms and vice versa. Medicaid, however, stipulates that married couples have the right to be housed together (Brier and Rubenstein, 1977).

Caregivers are surprised and become moralistic and, at times, angry with the elderly resident who is found in bed

<table>
<tr><td>Box
16-2</td><td>Psychologic Factors
in Elderly Sexuality</td></tr>
</table>

Misinterpretation of physical changes
Monotony, boredom with repetitious sexual relationship
Mental and physical fatigue
Increased expectations on retirement
Loss of role
Poor self-image
Fear of rejection
Freedom from fear of pregnancy
Freedom from scheduled activities

Compiled from Steffl BM: *Handbook of gerontologic nursing,*
New York, 1984, Van Nostrand; Ham RJ, Sloane PD: *Primary
care geriatrics,* St Louis, 1992, Mosby; Lewis MI: Sexuality. In
Abrams WB, Beers MH, Berkow R: *The Merck manual of
geriatrics,* ed 2, Whitehouse Station, NJ, 1995, Merck Research
Laboratories.

with another resident or who is sexually acting out or masturbating. Stevenson and Courtenay (1982) found that nurses' aides who were extremely religious had the most difficulty in accepting the sexual expression of older adults in nursing homes. It is not uncommon to hear a staff member talk to the aged person who has committed an indiscretion (in the staff member's eyes) as if he or she were a child, reprimanding the elder for the behavior.

Sometimes the staff members themselves unknowingly provoke a sexual response from the resident or patient. Comments about looking handsome or "Are you going to be my date?" seem harmless and "cute." However, for the elderly man who still has sexual desires but little opportunity to express them, this may initiate behavior that the staff finds offensive such as sexual statements or grabbing to fondle a staff member and that results in a reprimand to or punishment of the aged person. The same is true with the aged woman in an institutional setting. Comments made by male staff members about her appearance or about relationships with male residents can stimulate expressions of sexuality that are dealt with jokingly.

Alternative Sexual Lifestyles

Considering the restrictive attitudes within which many elderly were raised, it is understandable that any alternative sexual behaviors may be unacceptable to the old. Young people may be more accepting of peer variation but still intolerant of the same behavior in the old. It is estimated that gays and lesbians comprise 10% of the population in the United States; approximately the same proportion of the entire elder population is homosexual. No accurate figures are available, but the numbers are definitely no lower and may in fact be higher (Lewis, 1995; Freedman, 1995).

Older gay men and lesbians are as diverse as the remainder of the elder population. Many age successfully, are healthy, and are active with satisfied lives. Some are cou-

pled, have children, are open about their sexual orientation, and some are not. Some have only recently "come out;" others have been "out" most of their lives. Information about the aged homosexual continues to be limited except for the major works by Berger, *Gay and Gray: The Older Homosexual Man* (1982, 1995), and Kehoe's study of lesbians (1988), which provides major insight into the lifestyles of gay males and lesbians.

The studies of Kelly (1977, 1980) found homosexual activity of aged men varied from a low to moderate degree, depending on individual desire. By 65 years of age sexual satisfaction was still maintained, but the number of friendships had diminished. Both gays and lesbians used a self-selection process to establish friendships or friendship networks (Raphael and Robertson, 1980, Slusher et al, 1996).

Quam and Whitford (1992) noted that over half of the lesbians in their study reported most of their closest friends were lesbian, but only 27.5% of the gay men reported that their closest friends were gay men. Sixty-five percent of the study population indicated that their closest friends were a mix of gay and nongay men and women; about one third of the lesbian women described their friendships to be comparable. In the absence of kinship bonds, gays and lesbians develop homosexual friendship networks.

Lesbians over 60 years old live with the triple threat of being women, elderly, and having a different sexual orientation (Deevey, 1990). They tend to keep a very low profile, although conservative estimates are that over 2 million now reside in the United States. An intensive study of 100 lesbians between 60 and 86 years of age found that most lived alone, were retired from helping professions, and had college or advanced degrees. Nearly half were overweight and considered themselves restricted by health problems, although 72% considered themselves healthy, and 82% considered themselves emotionally healthy. Eighty-four percent felt positive about being lesbian, and almost half had at one time been married. Many described themselves as lonely, presently celibate, and desiring a relationship with a woman within 10 years of their own age. The majority desired special senior centers or retirement communities for lesbians (Kehoe, 1988).

Older lesbians often have practiced serial monogamy throughout life and in late life continue to anticipate the finding of a new mate if the need arises. According to Robertson (1979) lesbians who consider themselves feminists reject the monogamous love relationship. It is interesting to note that approximately one third of the lesbians "come out" after the age of 50. Before this time they often feel unable to deal with familial and societal pressures.

Gay men until the ages of 46 to 55 years have been found to have had multiple liaisons. However, with the impact of acquired immunodeficiency syndrome (AIDS) on this population, a decrease in multiple liaisons has become evident. Berger (1995) notes that sexual patterns tend to remain consistent over a lifetime. After 46 to 55 years of age partnerships are nearly nonexistent. The situation has been attributed to several factors: the death of a loved one and rejection of the idea of a single lifelong partner (Kelly, 1977).

It has been reported that gays and lesbians have less difficulty adjusting to aging because they have already faced difficult adjustments such as coping with the stigma of homosexuality. Adelman (1990) found adjustment to aging related to the lifestyle of being gay and satisfaction with being gay; the early developmental sequence of gay events correlated with high life satisfaction, low self-criticism, and few psychosomatic problems. Lesbians were found not to fear the prospect of being alone or isolated in old age. Conversely, older gays expressed fear of loneliness and isolation in later life. Some research indicates that more concern for the loss of youth and change in physical appearance occurred with gay men than with either lesbians or heterosexuals (Raphael and Robertson, 1980; Freedman, 1991). Problems that confront the aged homosexual are similar to those that face any aged person: loss of important people; presence of a stigma associated with being aged; and fear of institutionalization.

One problem unique to the aged homosexual is the lack of the economic, emotional, and physical security that occurs in most heterosexual relationships. Laws and rules governing *life insurance and estate benefits discriminate against the lover liaison.* Even with a legally recorded will that states that benefits should go to the lover, family members may successfully contest in probate hearings. In addition, use of health support services do not meet the needs of gay and lesbian elders (Slusher et al, 1995; Flaxman, 1996).

Lesbian and gay elders living in metropolitan areas may find organizations particularly designed for them, such as Senior Action in a Gay Environment (SAGE—SAGENet is now in nine states and Ontario, Canada), Gay and Lesbian Outreach to Elders (GLOE, San Francisco), Rainbow Project (Los Angeles), and Gay and Lesbians Older and Wiser (GLOW, Ann Arbor, Michigan).

Health care providers lack sufficient information and sensitivity when it comes to caring for older homosexuals. This sensitivity is of utmost importance when attempting to obtain a health history. The use of open-ended questions such as "Who is most important to you?" or " Do you have a significant other?" is much better than asking "Are you married?" This allows the nurse to look beyond the rigid category of family. Oftentimes euphemisms are used for a life partner (roommate, close friend). It is also better to ask individuals if they consider themselves as primarily heterosexual, homosexual, or bisexual. This conveys recognition that there is sexual variety. An older lesbian woman in a health care situation may refer to herself indirectly by saying "people like us." Nurses need to become more aware of these things and try to understand the fear of discovery that is apparent in the older gay man and lesbian woman. They are of a generation where they were and may still be closeted because of the homophobic experiences they had through their younger years.

Better support and care services for gays and lesbians by care providers should include working through one's homophobia and discomfort discussing sexuality, learning about special issues facing older gay men and lesbians, and becoming aware of the gay and lesbian resources in the community. Finally, a facility or agencies already in the community need to be assessed from the perspective of the client, patient, or resident, who may be gay or lesbian.

Homosexuality among older adults continues to be a subject ripe for research, since so little is known about these elders.

Procreation has been considered the sanctioned reason for sex and then only between those who were socially approved (married). Throughout the world, many of the elderly still believe this. For older women—single, divorced, or widowed—the only liaison permitted is with socially sanctioned partners. They are less free to seek sexual alternatives than men are.

The widow too may have an alternative life style. The sexual life of widows is a matter of great concern because so many older women will be widowed. Beresford and Barrett (1982) found that sexually active widows tended to be younger, widowed for a longer duration, and more liberal in their attitudes than sexually nonactive widows. Most widows indicated a desire for male companionship but possessed an ambivalent attitude toward remarriage. Widows report that they miss sexual relations with their husbands, but they have a great need for nongenital touching. These needs are not being met by friends and family.

AIDS and the Elderly. The compromised immune system of an aged individual makes him or her even more susceptable to human immunodeficiency virus (HIV) or AIDS than a younger person. As the geriatric population increases, so will the geriatric AIDS cases increase.

AIDS is not exclusively a young person's disease, but it is frequently underreported in the elderly because the symptoms of fatigue, weakness, weight loss, and anorexia are common to other elder disease conditions. In addition, the idea that elders are not sexually active limits physicians' and other care providers' objectivity to recognize HIV/AIDs as a possible diagnosis.

The Centers for Disease Control and Prevention (CDC) reported in September 1993 that more than 34,000 people over age 50 had full-blown AIDS, a number that has more than doubled since January 1991 (Baker and Crowley, 1994). Today, it is estimated that 10% of the individiuals over age 50, 3% over age 60, and 0.7% over age 70 have AIDS (Fletcher, 1995; Fletes, 1995). AIDS is rising faster among the older population than in those age 24 and younger.

Contrary to popular belief, HIV/AIDS in the elderly population is not due to blood transfusions alone. Research shows that elders are sexually active and thus at risk for HIV/AIDS. A study at the University of California, San

Francisco, of 3200 predominantly heterosexual Americans over age 50 found that about 10% had at least one risk factor for HIV infection. Those over 50 years of age were one sixth as likely to use condoms during sex and one fifth as likely to have been tested for HIV (Some older Americans, 1993). Though Diokno et al (1990) found frequency of sexual activity declined with age, a majority of persons over 60 remained sexually active (66.6% of the older men and 31.7% of older women). Homosexuality, bisexuality, and intravenous drug use are not exclusive to the younger population (Schuerman, 1994). The risk factors for the older age group include pre-1985 blood product recipients, spouses of those recipients, and persons who participate in unprotected anal and vaginal intercourse outside a monogamous relationship. Since procreation is not an issue with elders, they are least likely to use condoms. Elderly gay men who have spent a lifetime hiding their true sexual orientation may be reluctant to speak frankly with a health care provider. Others who know that they are HIV positive may hide the fact for fear of negative judgment from family, friends, and caregivers (Baker and Crowley, 1994).

Elders who are sexually active are not usually asked by physicians about their sexual activity and health. Elders usually do not confide in a health care provider or friends, because they are uncomfortable admitting to sexual activity "at their age." They have bought into the myth that old people do not have sex. Older women who are sexually active are at high risk for HIV/AIDS from an infected partner due in part to normal age changes of the vaginal tissue—a thinner and drier vaginal lining . Older men may frequent prostitutes (a potentially high-risk group for HIV/AIDS). Gay men may increase their risk of HIV exposure following the death of a long-term mate by turning to a more available younger partner, who may be more likely to have HIV. In general, elders lack adequate knowledge about about HIV/AIDS and believe that HIV/AIDS "just does not happen in their generation." This places elders at high risk for HIV /AIDS.

AIDS in the elderly has been called the "Great Imitator." In addition to the vague signs mentioned earlier, it presents as dementia with increased neurologic abnormalities and unexplained diffuse encephalopathy that is manifested in progressive and chronic dementia. Elders may be misdiagnosed as having Alzheimer's disease (AD) (Schuerman, 1994; Whipple and Scura, 1996) instead of the actual problem, AIDS. AIDS dementia is rapid in onset as opposed to the slow progressive decline associated with AD. Confusion and other cognitive difficulties may wax and wane. Aphasia, which is seen in AD, is usually absent in AIDS dementia. Extrapyramidal symptoms suggestive of parkinsonism may occur but without the tremors and ataxia. Leg tremors, peripheral neuropathy with progressive weakness, and a positive Babinski reflex may also be seen when diagnosing AIDS.

Other AIDS problems that the elder might manifest include opportunistic infections, malignancies, *Pneumocystis carinii* (PCP), tuberculosis, esophageal or recurrent genital candidiasis, toxoplasmosis, non-Hodgkin's lymphoma, Kaposi's sarcoma, or herpes zoster. Women may develop candidasis or human papilloma virus infections as a first sign of AIDS (Schuerman, 1994; Whipple and Scura, 1996). It is important to keep in mind that conditions that persist or reoccur should be suspect for HIV/AIDS and that the elder should be tested.

Elders need to get the message that they are at high risk for HIV/AIDS. Educational materials and programs need to be developed that include what HIV/AIDS is, how it is and is not transmitted, the need to use condoms to protect oneself and one's partner when engaging in sexual activity, symptoms to be aware of, and what treatments are available. Physicians, nurse practitioners, and other health professionals need to become comfortable taking a complete sexual history and talking about sex with the elderly. In addition the myth that elders do not engage in sexual activity must be put to rest.

The aged are different from other groups at risk for HIV/AIDS in that they have multiple acute and chronic illnesses and still can be highly functional. When hospitalized for multiple diagnoses, few health professionals consider them at risk for HIV. It is known that the time between acquiring HIV infections and the diagnosis of AIDS is shorter for elders, as is the time between diagnosis and death from AIDS.

Though no substantive research is available, it is an underlying assumption that many elders in nursing homes may be HIV positive. A limited number of long-term care facilities knowingly accept AIDS patients, and among those that do, the geriatric AIDS patient competes for extended care services with nongeriatric AIDS patients and non-AIDS geriatric patients. Finding appropriate services and facilities may be difficult, although in places in which this care is available, reports are positive. A major concern is that the needs of young persons dying of AIDS may be quite different from those of the old. If they are indiscriminately mixed in long-term care settings, neither group is likely to have its needs well met.

Because most communities do not have resources to establish separate systems for the aged and the AIDS patients who have some similar needs, long-term care providers must address these issues.

Sexual Dysfunction

Sexual dysfunction, which occurs in both men and women, has a physiologic or psychologic base or a combination of both. Psychologic dysfunction is more common than physical impairment (Ham, 1992; Butler and Lewis, 1990). A major problem confronting the aging man is the fear of impotence or the actual occurrence of impotence. What men generally call impotence is diminished potency and frequency of sexual activity. Impotence, according to Ham, is a psychogenic or organic pathologic condition that has its origins in excessive use of alcohol, preoccupation with work problems, monotony in the relationship, anger, fatigue, or neurologic or vascular conditions. Drug-related sexual dysfunction may be hard to distinguish from depression or disease.

Various medications that affect the sympathetic and parasympathetic nervous system interfere with the capacity of the penis to erect or ejaculate. Adrenergic agents block impulses that affect contractibility of the prostate gland and seminal vesicles and depress or interfere with ejaculation. The anticholinergic preparations affect penis erection by vasocongestion in the venous channels. The ganglionic blocking agents possess properties of both the adrenergic and anticholinergic preparations and affect both penis erection and ejaculation (Jarvik and Small, 1988; Sherman, 1992).

A few medications have been found to increase sexual desire. The phenothiazines and testosterone increase the libido in the aged woman, and L-dopa heightens sexual desire in the aged man (Sherman,1992; Testosterone and HRT, 1996). This situation can be extremely distressful to the individual and the caregiving staff if the person is institutionalized. Table 16-2 lists many drugs that alter sexual function.

Environmental agents, including industrial chemicals and exposure to electromagnetic fields used by some industries, can induce impotence. The effects of inadequate housing, lack of privacy, and feelings of psychologic inferiority are also contributory factors to impotence.

Most men who undergo surgical procedures such as transurethral resection and other types of prostatectomies, Y-V plasty of the bladder neck, resection of the colon for

Table 16-2   Potential Medication Effects on Sexual Function

Drug or drug category	Parameters of effect		Drug or drug category	Parameters of effect	
	Physiologic	Psychologic		Physiologic	Psychologic
Antidepressants			Antipsychotics		
Tricyclics	Central nervous system depression	Increased libido if depression reduced	Phenothiazines	Dry ejaculation	
Amitriptyline			Chlorpromazine	Erectile difficulty	
Desipramine	Impotence		Haloperidol	Gynecomastia	
Doxepin	Inhibited ejaculation		Thioridazine	Decreased vaginal lubrication	
Imipramine	Orgasmic difficulty		Thiothixene		
Nortriptyline			Trifluoperazine	Spontaneous milk flow from breasts	
Phenelzine					
Trazodone			Diuretics	Impotence	
Antihistamine and H$_2$ blockers				Gynecomastia	
				Breast tenderness	
	Central nervous system depression	Decreased libido	Antispasmodics	Vasoconstriction	Decreased libido
		Decreased erection ability		Ganglionic blockage of innervation of sex organs	
	Decreased vaginal lubrication			Impotence	
	H$_2$ blockers— impotence			Decreased vaginal lubrication	
Antihypertensives			Antiparkinsonism		
Clonidine	Peripheral blockage of innervation of sex organs	Decreased libido	Amantadine	Increased erectile function	Improvement of well being— may be responsible for increased libido
Enalapril			Benztropine		
Guanethidine			Bromocriptine		
Hydralazine	Decrease/absence of ejaculation		L-dopa		
Methyldopa			Selegiline		
Prazosin	Retrograde ejaculation		Other drugs		
Reserpine			Cytoxin		Decreased libido
Spironolactone			Androgens	Antiandrogenic effect	Decreased libido
Verapamil					
Beta-Blockers				Virilization of female	
Atenolol	Orgasmic difficulties	Decreased libido	Digoxin	Erectile failure	Decreased libido
Labetalol				Gynecomastia	
Metroprolol	Breast tenderness		Lithium		Increased libido
Propranolol	Gynecomastia		Opiates	Central nervous system depressant	Reduced inhibitions
Timolol					
			Morphine		
			Codeine	Impotence	Decreased sexual enjoyment

cancer, or a sympathectomy may find to their dismay that they have retrograde ejaculations, the result of interference with autonomic innervation in the pelvis (Boyarsky, 1983). Particularly after a prostatectomy, a space remains where the enlarged prostate had been. The principle that fluid travels the path of least resistance applies here. At the point of ejaculation, the semen moves backward into the bladder rather than forward through increased resistance, which produces a retrograde, or dry, ejaculation. Ignorance regarding this physiologic change further convinces men that their sexual activity is over, when in fact it is not. Erection can be attained and orgasmic pleasure achieved.

Most research on sexual dysfunction has been conducted by men on older men. Less knowledge of female sexual dysfunction is known, particularly drug effects.

Women worry more about youthfulness than problems of sexual performance. For heterosexual women frequency of intercourse is more dependent on the age, health, and sexual function of the partner or the availability of a partner rather than their own sexual capacity. However, women may experience pain on intercourse (dyspareunia) because of the thinning of the vaginal wall and the lack of lubrication. In many instances use of a water-soluble lubricant can resolve the difficulty. Hormone replacement therapy (HRT) has been an option for maintaining vaginal tissue integrity, but controversy continues regarding the benefits versus the potential danger of inducing endometrial or breast cancer (Schiff,1995). Prolapse of the uterus, rectoceles, and cystoceles can be surgically repaired to facilitate continued sexual activity.

Sex may be disrupted by acute illness while energy is directed toward regaining and maintaining homeostasis rather than toward physical sex. It is true that disuse decreases the ability of the aged to engage in sex, but when one has maintained regular sexual function before illness, sexual desire begins to return during convalescence.

Box 16-3	Causes of Impotence

Vascular insufficiency
Altered endocrine system
Altered nervous system
Structural abnormalities of the penis
Depression
Zinc defficiency
Alcoholism
Diabetes mellitus
Medication side effects
Psychogenic causes

Compiled from Gerchufsky M: Impotence: the problem men don't talk about, *Ad Nurse Pract* 3(3):13, 1995; Buczy B: Impotence in older men: a newly recognized problem, *J Gerontol Nurs* 18(5):25, 1992.

Impotence. Impotence is defined as the inability to develop and sustain an erection sufficient for satisfactory sexual intercourse. Impotence has become recognized as a common problem among men over the age of 50 (Buczny, 1992). Until now impotence has been a neglected area of health fraught with myths and superstition. Impotence transiently occurs to men of all ages at least once in their life; however, the prevalence of impotence increases with age. Morley (1988) estimates that 8% of men age 55 to 64 will experience impotence. Beers (1995) suggests impotence occurs in 25% of men age 65 and 50% in men age 80. Approximately 75% of men over the age of 85 experience impotence.

An erection is governed by the interaction among the hormonal, vascular, and nervous systems. A problem in any of these systems can cause impotence. There are of course multiple causes for this problem in older men (Box 16-3). These include psychologic causes such as multiple losses of cohorts (spouse or friends), which can lead to depression. Common medical causes include hypogonadism, thyroid dysfunction, and diabetes. Nearly one third of impotence is a complication of diabetes. Alcoholism, medication side effects, and zinc deficiencies are also causes of impotence in older men.

Assessment of impotence includes a history and screening for major psychologic problems of the man and spouse if possible. Physical examination generally is less revealing than a history but can detect structural problems. Testing for levels of testosterone, luteinizing hormone, zinc, thyroid function, alcoholism, and medication side effects is important. A workup for diabetes is also necessary. Once the assessment has identified the possible cause or causes, intervention is prescribed. This may take the form of sex therapy, psychosexual counseling (reeducation). Because society views sexual desires as unnatural in the elderly population, it can cause older people to feel guilty when they experience these desires. This is called geriatric sexuality breakdown syndrome. Therapy redirects and develops graded sexual experiences and is helpful as an adjunct to treatment when medical causes or a combination of causes are identified (Buczny, 1992).

One of the newer therapies accepted in 1994 is Pharmacological Erection Program (PEP) injections or the intracavernosal injection. The drugs of choice are papaverine and phentolamine, a vasoactive agent that reduces resistance of arteriolar and cavernosal smooth muscle tissue of the penis. This leads to increased arterial flow and subsequent venous trapping, facilitating an erection (Butler et al, 1994; Beers, 1995). The dose of the drug is determined by trial and error. PEP injections seem to help those with moderate vascular disease, which is most common in 80% of older men who are impotent. For others, with psychologically based impotence, PEP seems to bolster self-confidence, and after a few injections there is no longer a need for them.

Penile implants of the semirigid, adjustable-malleable or hinged and inflatable types are available when impotence does not respond to other treatments or is irreversible. The hinged and inflatable types, which are inserted in the testicular area, are the most popular types. Still in the experimental stage is penile revascularization surgery. This requires a highly skilled surgeon and is appropriate only for men with localized, identifiable lesions (Beers, 1995). Impotence Anonymous, which is a nationwide organization that emanated from the Impotence Institute of America, has been a helpful organization for those who experience impotence. It serves as a support group where individuals alone or with their spouses learn about and discuss all aspects of impotence and what can be done about it. It also facilitates expression of feelings about this problem.

The geriatric nurse working with clients who are impotent provides information and resources, serves as a client advocate, advises about assessment, and instructs in the use of prosthetic devices. The nurse's most important role is to provide support and guidance for this touchy subject.

Chronic Conditions and Sexuality. Sexual activity depends, under most circumstances, on the state of sex drive and performance before the illness or chronic conditions, on the function of the heart, and response to treatment.

Although pain, fatigue, and joint stiffness and limitation that occur with arthritis may interfere with sexual activity, it need not curtail enjoyment of sexual intercourse. Sexual activity may, in fact, enhance some arthritis therapies and be beneficial because it stimulates the release of cortisone, adrenalin, and other chemicals that are natural pain relievers. It is also posited that the act of intercourse is not only good exercise but a beneficial means of psychologic and physical tension reduction.

Individuals with heart disease or who have suffered a stroke often reduce their sexual activity because of fear and lack of knowledge about their condition. Caregivers often fail to discuss sexual matters with the aged person during recovery. The energy expenditure needed for intercourse is comparable to briskly climbing two flights of stairs or walking several blocks rapidly. If the individual can do this without adverse effects, he or she can resume normal sexual activity. Participation in a medically supervised exercise program can reduce oxygen requirements during sexual activity and improve the quality of sexual life.

Strokes should not be a cause for secession of sexual activity. Unless the stroke has resulted in severe brain damage, sexual activity is usually unimpaired, but sexual performance may be affected (some men experience impotence, some do not). The unaffected side should be the focus of lovemaking.

Diabetes often leads to impotence (two to five times greater in this group than in the general population), though interest and desire is still present. Once diabetes is properly controlled, impotence may disappear in some individuals. Loss of sexual function does not seem to be a problem with females who have diabetes.

Many misbeliefs abound about the aftermath of a prostatectomy. If these ideas are not clarified and corrected, the psychologic effect may contribute to impotence. Dry orgasms are normal following prostatic surgery.

Following hysterectomies, the abdomen may feel sore for 3 to 4 months and may interfere with resumption of normal sexual activity. Usually the individual abstains from intercourse for 6 to 8 weeks following surgery. A decrease in lubrication and sensation can occur in the lower genital tract. If the ovaries are removed with or without the removal of the uterus, sexual desire is lost.

Estrogen replacement therapy (ERT) remains controversial, but its benefits far outweigh the risks (Neyhart, 1995). ERT carries with it the possible side effects of headache, fluid retention, weight gain, vaginal discharge, breast swelling, and the possibility of endometrial and breast cancer. The risk of the latter effect can be reduced by opposing estrogen with progesterone. The benefits of ERT help protect against osteoporosis, which can lead to spinal and hip fractures, and heart disease. It also is a way of alleviating hot flashes, vaginal atrophy, and other manifestations of menopause that interfere with comfort, sexual function, and quality of life. Table 16-3 presents common conditions that can affect sexual function. Suggestions for interventions are also given.

Regaining Sexual Function. After heart attacks, strokes, and abdominal surgery the aged need not be categorically condemned to abstinence from coitus for the remainder of their lives. Recuperative time is usually 4 to 6 weeks or several months before sexual intercourse can be resumed. After a myocardial infarction intercourse can be initiated when scar tissue has formed (8 to 14 weeks) and if there is no evidence of ventricular arrhythmias or aneurysms. One method used to test if the individual is able to expend the energy necessary for intercourse is to evaluate the effect on the cardiopulmonary status of rapidly walking up two flights of stairs. Individuals with arrhythmias may need reassurance with a treadmill test to allay their anxiety regarding sexual activity.

Manual stimulation, masturbation, may be an alternative that can be used early in the recovery period to maintain sexual function, if not objectionable to the patient. It has been shown that masturbation is less taxing on the heart and makes less of an oxygen demand (Woods, 1983).

Masturbation is a common and healthy practice in late life. Persons without partners or with spouses who are ill or incapacitated find that masturbation is helpful. Self-stimulation is steeped in myth and fear. As children, today's aged population were stopped from practicing this pleasurable activity with stories of the evils of fondling one's genitals. Masturbation provides an avenue for resolution of sexual tensions, keeping sexual desire alive, physical exercise, and preserving sexual function in those individuals who have no other outlet for sexual activity and gratification of their sexual need (Butler and Lewis, 1990).

Table 16-3	Chronic Illness and Sexual Function: Effects and Interventions

Condition	Effects/problems	Interventions
Arthritis	Pain, fatigue, limited motion Steroid therapy may decrease sexual interest/desire	Advise patient to perform sexual activity at the time of day when least fatigued and most relaxed Suggest use of analgesics and other pain relief methods prior to sexual activity Encourage use of relaxation techniques prior to sexual activity such as warm bath/shower, application of hot packs to affected joints Advise patient to maintain optimum health through a balance of good nutrition, proper rest, and activity Suggest that he or she experiment with different positions, use pillows for comfort and support Recommend use of a vibrator if massage ability is limited Suggest use of water soluble jelly for vaginal lubrication
Cardiovascular disease	Most men have no change in physical effects on sexual function; one fourth may not return to pre–heart attack function, one fourth may not resume sexual activity Women do not experience sexual dysfunction following heart attack Fear of another heart attack or death during sex Shortness of breath	Encourage counseling on realistic restrictions that may be necessary Instruct patient/spouse alternative positions to avoid strain Suggest that patient avoid large meals several hours before sex Advise patient to relax, plan medications for effectiveness during sex

Cerebrovascular accident (stroke)	Depression
	May or may not have sexual activity changes
	Often erectile disorders occur; decrease in frequency of intercourse and sexual relations
	Possible problems:
	  Change in role and function of partners
	  Decreased physical endurance, fatigue
	  Mobility and sensory deficits
	  Perceptual and visual deficits
	  Communication deficit
	  Cognitive and behavioral deficits
	  Fear of relapse or sudden death
		Encourage counseling
		Instruct patient to use alternative positions
		Suggest use of a vibrator if massage ability is limited
		Suggest use of pillows for positioning and support
		Suggest use of water soluble jelly for lubrication
		Instruct patient to use alternative forms of sexual expression

The aged may or may not have difficulty discussing intimate areas with individuals who are comfortable and capable of dealing with it. The nurse has the responsibility to help maintain the sexuality of the aged by offering the opportunity to discuss. Rarely are sex histories elicited from the elderly patient. Physical examinations do not include the reproductive system unless it is directly involved in the present illness. However, when one does ask questions about sexual issues or when the elderly are examined, the nurse needs to be particularly cognizant of the era in which the individual has lived to understand the factors affecting conduct.

To assist and support the aged in their sexual needs nurses should be aware of their own feelings about sexuality. They must question their attitude toward old people (single, married, or homosexual) who hold hands or caress or fondle each other. Only after confronting one's own attitudes, values, and beliefs can the nurse provide support without being judgmental.

Sex in the Nursing Home

Expressions of sexuality are considered, in many nursing home settings, to be a disturbing or behavioral management problem. To consider them so is a measure of the taboo against sex and the elderly. White (1982) interviewed residents in 15 nursing homes and found that 91% were sexually inactive, although 17% said they would like to be active sexually. His study seems to reinforce the concept that sexual interest in the institutionalized is related to prior levels of activity and interest. If it has been an important method of coping, it is likely to remain so. Sexual education and discussion groups should be provided for staff and residents to decrease the overreactions that are commonly seen and to determine policies that allow consenting individuals to engage in sexual activity in private.

Federal nursing home regulations for intermediate care facilities (ICFs) mandate that a married resident must be given privacy during spousal visits. If both husband and wife are residents, they must be permitted to share a room.

Table 16-3	Chronic Illness and Sexual Function: Effects and Interventions—cont'd

Condition	Effects/problems	Interventions
Chronic obstructive pulmonary disease (COPD)	No direct impairment of sexual activity, though affected by coughing, exertional dyspnea, and activity intolerance Medications may lead to erectile difficulties	Encourage patient to plan sexual activity when energy is highest Instruct patient to use alternative positions Advise patient to plan sexual activity at time medications are most effective Suggest use of oxygen before, during, or after sex, depending when it provides the most benefit
Diabetes	Sexual desire and interest unaffected Neuropathy and or vascular damage may interfere with erectile ability. Fifty to 75% of men have erectile disorders, a small portion have retrograde ejaculation Some men regain function if diagnosis of diabetes is well accepted and/or if diabetes is well controlled Women have less sexual desire and/or vaginal lubrication (Katzm, 1991) Decrease in orgasms/absence of orgasm can occur; less frequent sexual activity; local genital infections	Recommend possible candidates for penile prosthesis Instruct patient to use alternative forms of sexual expression Recommend immediate treatment of genital infections
Cancers Breast	No direct physical affect. There is a strong psychologic affect: Loss of sexual desire Body-image change Depression Reaction to partner	Encourage individual or group counseling
Most other cancers	Men and women may lose sexual desire temporarily Men may have erectile dysfunction; dry ejaculation; retrograde ejaculation Women may have vaginal dryness, dyspareunia Both men and women may experience anxiety, depression, pain, nausea from chemotherapy, radiation, pelvic surgery, hormone therapy, nerve damage from pelvic surgery	

Skilled nursing facilities (SNFs) are under similar mandates unless medically contraindicated. But what of individuals in intimate relationships when they are not married? That has not been addressed. Few cases of sexual privacy invasion have reached the courts, but they are likely to increase as people become more aware of their rights. The institutionalized aged have the same rights as noninstitutionalized elders to engage in or abstain from sexual activity.

NURSING ROLES AND FUNCTIONS

Nurses have multiple roles in the area of sexuality and the aged. The nurse is a facilitator of a conducive milieu in which questions can be asked and in which the aged person's sexuality can be expressed. Most important is providing privacy and allowing the aged control over their sex lives. The nurse should be an educator and provide information as well as guidance to the aged who need it. The aged should be asked about their sexual satisfaction, since they may not mention it voluntarily. Anticipation of problems in aged persons' sexual experiences can ward off anxiety, misconceptions, and an arbitrary cessation of sexual pleasure. Validation of the normalcy of sexual activity may be needed, or a discussion of the physiologic changes that occur with age, or the effect of illness and treatment that may interfere with sexual activity by altering the routine or interfering with physical performance. Counseling may be needed for the aged to adapt to natural physiologic changes and image-altering surgical procedures.

The nurse may find that she is a consultant and counselor to others who give care to the aged.

Assessment

Discussion of sexuality and sexuality problems is uncomfortable for both nurse and elder. Yet it is important to learn the significance of sexual function to the elder and the perception of sexual function the elder has without bringing the nurse's own biases into the interaction. Box 16-4 provides guidelines for data collection.

Interventions

Interventions will vary depending on the needs identified from the assessment data. A variety of suggested interventions for maintenance of sexual function for the aged with chronic conditions has been presented in Table 16-3, and impotence has been discussed with available options of treatment. Perhaps one of the most important interventions is education regarding normal age changes related to sexual function and the dimensions of sexuality that provide pleasure.

Counseling and Advocacy. Old people do seek counseling on sexuality and sexual concerns, but we do not always hear them, and many of us are not well enough prepared to help them. Successful and continuing sexual activity is but one sign of healthy aging (Box 16-4).

Some nurses have extensive education in sexuality and are in a position to provide intensive therapy for persons with sexual problems. Although the nurse in the acute or long-term care facility may not be well prepared to engage in sex therapy, it is possible to provide information about sexual issues in anticipation of questions or in response to questions asked and to treat expressions of sexuality as normal and deserving of respect.

Box 16-4	**Guidelines for Obtaining Data about Sexual Needs and Concerns**

General

What do you think about romance at this stage of your life?

When you were growing up, did people you knew discuss sex and romance?

What were you told about sex when you were a child? How do you feel about discussing it now?

Do you think it is a very important part of life satisfaction for people of all ages?

What does sexuality mean to you?

How important has sexual activity been in your life?

What were you told about masturbation?

What values and morals influence your feelings about sex now?

How are your needs of intimacy being met now?

Sexual Satisfaction

Have you experienced any changes in your sexual relationships lately?

To what do you attribute this change?

What type of sexual activities have you usually enjoyed the most including such things as hugging, kissing, sleeping together, intercourse, and so on?

Do you or your partner take any prescription medications? What are they? How often do you take them? Have you experienced any changes in your level of energy since starting them? What about feelings of overall well-being? Any changes in sexual desire or activity?

Alterations in Self-Perception

How has growing old changed your life-style or things you enjoy doing?

How has the change in your health or the health of your partner altered your life-style or your goals?

How do you rate your general health?

On a scale of 1 to 10, how would you describe your satisfaction with your life?

On a scale of 1 to 10, how would you describe your satisfaction with your sexual relationships?

Relationships with Others

Have you ever discussed sexual topics with your spouse, friends, family, or health care professional?

Who do you talk to when you have problems of any kind or just want someone to talk to?

Environment

With whom do you live?

Does your present living situation foster opportunities to express your sexuality?

For men

Have you noticed any change in intensity of your ejaculation, orgasm, or ability to attain/maintain an erection?

Have you ever had an orgasm without ejaculation?

Has your level of enjoyment with sexual relations altered as a result of these changes?

Have you had any problems with urethral discharge or urination?

For women

Have you experienced any vaginal soreness or irritation after sexual intercourse? How long does it last? Any problems with urgency or with burning in urination after intercourse? Have you experienced abdominal contractions or back pain after intercourse?

Have you any problems with vaginal discharge or itching?

Have any of these problems interfered with your sexual pleasure?

Have you or your partner experienced any changes in your health status recently? How have these changes affected your sexual relationship?

From Burke MM, Walsh MB: *Gerontologic nursing: wholistic care of the older adult,* ed 2, St Louis, 1997, Mosby.

The nurse is also an advocate for the aged. It is important to look for ways to provide more home care to maintain the option of privacy and control over one's sexual life and to investigate possible directions to provide comfort without nursing homes and acute care hospitals exerting their authority over sexual expression.

Last, the nurse may become involved in considering issues that could enable the aged to remain in their own homes rather than be subjected to institutionalization.

Evaluation

Elders whose sexuality needs are fulfilled will consider their sexual life with satisfaction. This will be apparent through verbal and nonverbal expression, the individual's self-image, and involvement and concern about others.

In summary, the nurse has a variety of roles in assuring the sexuality of the aged: facilitator, educator, consultant, counselor, and advocate. Sexuality is an amalgamation of biologic, psychologic, and social moral elements that affect pleasure, adaptation, and a general feeling of well-being in the aged.

KEY CONCEPTS

- Touch provides sensory stimulation, reduces anxiety, facilitates reality orientation, pain relief, comfort, and sexual expression.
- The absence of touch, a powerful sense, threatens survival.
- Sexuality is love, sharing, trust, and warmth, as well as physical acts. It provides an individual with self-identity and affirmation of life.
- Sexual activity continues in old age, though adaptations are needed for the age-related changes of the male and female genital systems. Generally medications, ill health, and lack of a willing partner impact sexual activity.
- Older adults with alternative lifestyles such as gay men and lesbians are disenfranchised by govermental laws and rules that do not bestow the same economic, emotional, and physical security enjoyed by heterosexual couples.
- AIDS awareness and the practice of safe sex among older adults are still lacking. Health professionals, too, do not consider older adults at risk for AIDS. Though the incidence of AIDS in the older population is small compared to the numbers of younger adults, the aged population is rapidly increasing with a greater AIDS potential. Finding appropriate services for the older adult with AIDS may prove difficult.
- The major role of the nurse in older adult sexuality, in the community or long-term care settings, is education and counseling about sexual function, adaptations for age-related changes, chronic conditions, and the maintenance of sexuality for the older adult's health and pleasure.

▲ CASE STUDY

George was a 70-year-old man who had been widowed for 6 years. He lived alone in a lovely home in the hills of San Francisco. His many friends tried to introduce him to a lady that would be attractive to him, but they were unaware of his real concerns. George was attracted to young, energetic women, often barely older than his daughters, but he was justly cautious regarding their sincere attraction to him because he had a considerable estate. In addition, his sexual desire was waning, and his capacity for sexual performance was unpredictable. One thing he expressed fairly frequently was, "I don't like demands made upon me." To further complicate the picture, he had begun to take finasteride to reduce his benign prostatic hypertrophy (BPH) that had become increasingly troublesome. The medication further reduced his sexual desire. Also, his sleep pattern was disturbed by the need to arise three or four times each night to void. George came to the clinic for follow-up evaluation of his prostatic hypertrophy, and while talking with the nurse, he began crying uncontrollably . . . much to his embarrassment and the nurse's surprise because George had always seemed a rather stolid and stoic fellow, reluctant to discuss feelings.

Based upon the case study, develop a nursing care plan using the following procedure*:

List comments of client that provide *subjective data*.

List information that provides *objective data*.

From these data identify and state, using accepted format, two *nursing diagnoses* you determine are most significant to this client at this time. List two *client strengths* that you have identified from data.

Determine and state *outcome criteria* for each diagnosis. These must reflect some alleviation of the problem identified in the nursing diagnosis and must be stated in concrete and measurable terms.

Plan and state one or more *interventions* for each diagnosed problem. Provide specific documentation of source used to determine appropriate intervention. Plan at least one intervention that incorporates the client's existing strengths.

Evaluate success of intervention. Interventions must correlate directly with the stated outcome criteria in order to measure the outcome success.

STUDY QUESTIONS/ACTIVITIES

How would you begin discussing sexuality with George?

What are the factors that may be underlying George's sexual distress?

Discuss BPH and its prevalence and usual effects.

*Students are advised to refer to their nursing diagnosis text and identify possible or potential problems.

Nursing Diagnoses

Potential diagnoses unique to the particular individual must also be considered.

Sexual dysfunction related to:
  Role change
  Medication
  Motor, sensory, or cognitive deficits
  Self-concept disturbance
  Knowledge deficit
    Lack of education
Altered sexuality patterns related to:
  Lack of privacy
  Decreased activity tolerance
  Change or loss of body part
  Knowledge deficit
    Sexual experience since chronic condition

Anxiety related to:
  Unmet needs
  Sexual function
  Continued sexual desire
  Physical changes of aging
  Maintenance of present sexuality
  Inadequate touch (touch hunger)
  Self-image disturbance

NURSING PROCESS AND NURSING DIAGNOSIS
Personal Identity Disturbance, Social Isolation

Etiology and Related Factors
Physical loss
Extended separation
Threat of danger, illness, pain, death
Lack of privacy
Lack of touch
Institutional living
Placement in a long-term care facility
Loss of a loving, affectionate relationship
Loneliness
Isolation
Absence of significant other

Defining Characteristics
Mutual time spent together
Verbal expression of affection
Physical expression of affection
Seeking out others
Seeking and finding places and situations to be alone
  with another
Verbalization of loss and/or distress when separated for a
  period of time and/or when the important other is
  perceived to be threatened and/or in danger
Physical expression of loss and/or distress when
  separated for a period of time and/or when the
  important other is perceived to be in danger of illness,
  pain, death

Knowledge
Normal age changes
Chronic illness and aging
Progression of adult maturation
Importance of touch and intimacy to life and basic needs
Adaptive measures

Clinical Judgment and Related Skills
Communication skills: active listening
Obtaining an extended history of intimacy and sexuality
Discussion of concerns related to intimacy

Evaluation
Person identifies ways to facilitate intimacy
Has a place for privacy
Reports satisfaction with intimacy

NEEDS ADDRESSED AND TASK STRENGTHS

Need for intimacy and expressions of affection; need for
  release of sexual tensions (to enhance sense of
  belonging, self-esteem, and transcendence)
Open to various forms of sexual expression
Willingness to share thoughts and feelings

Able to reach out to others
Seeks to have own intimacy needs met
Sensually aware
Verbally and physically expresses affection

With a partner, role play and demonstrate your interpersonal interaction with George in this situation.

What resources or recommendations would you suggest for George?

RESEARCH QUESTIONS

What do women find are the most troubling changes in their sexuality as they grow older?

What do men find are the most troubling changes in their sexuality as they grow older?

What are the differences in sexual feelings and expression in the 60 year old, the 70 year old, the 80 year old, and the 90 year old?

What are the chronic disorders that most affect sexual performance of men and women, and how are they affected?

How many individuals over 60 have ever been given the opportunity to provide a thorough sexual history?

What community and health resources are available to meet the needs of older gay men and lesbians?

RESOURCES

Films and Videos

Love in Later Life. This is an explicit film about an elderly married couple, Mary and Keith, around 70 years old and together for more than 44 years. In the movie we get to know them through listening when they talk about their life and relationship and also by watching them in their day-to-day life, their work, and their intimacy, sexuality, and lovemaking. A moving image of two older persons still active and enjoying life in today's society. 30 minutes. Film available from Canadian Learning Company, 2229 Kingston Road, Suite 203, Scarborough, Ontario, M1N 1T8, (416) 265-3333.

The Blessing of Love, 9-minute color film, animated, nonverbal. Distributor: Audio Brandon, 1619 North Cherokee Street, Los Angeles, CA 90028.

Rose by Any Other Name, 15-minute color film by Judith Keller. Sole distributor: Adelphi University Center on Aging, Garden City, NY 11530, (516) 485-6730.

Silent Pioneers. Profiles the lives of eight older lesbians and gay men who have struggled in silence. Their heroism depicts the experiences of a generation who survived an intensely homophobic period in our culture. Filmmakers Library, 124 East 40th Street, New York, NY 10016 (212) 808-4980.

Sexuality and Aging, ¾-inch video, color, 35 minutes. Contact: Program on Gerontology, Milam Hall, Oregon State University, Corvallis, OR 97331 (503) 754-1765.

Sunday Is Okay Too, 32 minutes, producer: Ruth Davidow, University of California, San Francisco. Deals with privacy of couples and roommates in nursing homes. Trainex Corporation, 11016 Garden Grove Boulevard, Garden Grove, CA 92646.

Organizations

American Association of Sex Educators, Counselors, and Therapists
435 North Michigan Boulevard, Suite 1717
Chicago, IL 60611-4067
(312) 644-0828

National Institute on Aging
NIA Information Center
PO Box 8057
Gaithersburg, MD 20898-8057
(301) 495-3455
   Age Page: Should You Take Estrogen?
   Age Page: Sexuality in Later Life

Senior Action in a Gay Environment (SAGE)
208 West 13th Street
New York, NY 10011
(212) 741-2247

Sex Information and Education Council of the United States (SIECUS)
84 Fifth Avenue
New York, NY 10010
(212) 673-3850

National Association for Gay and Lesbian Gerontology (NALGG)
1853 Market Street
San Francisco, CA 94103

GLOE (Gay and Lesbian Outreach to Elders)
1853 Market Street
San Francisco, CA 94103
(415) 626-7000

Publications

AARP fact sheet, *AIDS: A Multigenerational Crisis,* stock no. D14942. Write AARP/SOS Dept. B, 601 East Street NW, Washington, DC 20049

AIDS and Aging: What People Over 50 Need to Know, program for small group discussion. Contact HealthCare Education Associates: (714) 240-2179.

The AIDS Hotline of the U.S. Centers for Disease Control and Prevention: (800)342-AIDS; Spanish-language hotline: (800) 344-7432; TTY hotline for hearing-impaired: (800) 344-7432. Calls are confidential and taken 24 hours a day. Answers all questions related to AIDS, offers free written materials, and provides referrals to services in your area.

The AIDS National Interfaith Network for information on pastoral counseling and support services: (800)288-9619.

American Red Cross (local chapter): *A Guide to Home Care for Persons with AIDS,* advice for both people with AIDS and for their caregivers, form no. 329542.

Berger RM: *Gay and Gray: The Older Homosexual Man,* ed 2, Binghamton, NY 1995, Hawthorn Press.

Family HIV/AIDS Support Helpline operated by Parents, Families, and Friends of Lesbians and Gays. Information on local groups: (202) 638-4200.

Journal of Gay and Lesbian Social Services, Hawthorn Press, 10 Alice Street, Binghamton, NY 13904-1580.

Kehoe M: *Lesbians over 60 Speak for Themselves,* Binghamton, NY, 1989, Hawthorn Press.

National AIDS Clearing House: (800) 458-5231

National Institute on Aging: *Fact sheet on AIDS and older adults,* call (800) 222-225.

OUTWord quarterly newsletter of the Lesbian and Gay Aging Issues Network (LGAIN). Contact Editor at American Society on Aging, 833 Market Street, San Francisco, CA 94103-1824.

Resource Guide: Lesbian and Gay Aging, updated periodically, published by and available from National Association for Gay and Lesbian Gerontology (NALGG).

Westheimer RK: *Sex for Dummies, A Reference for the Rest of Us!* IDG Books Worldwide, Inc. 1995.

Games

Sex and Aging: A Game of Awareness and Interaction. A board game that challenges players to examine their attitudes about sexuality in later life. Available from Extension Business Office, Extension Services, Oregon State University, Ballard 125, Corvallis, OR 97331-3604.

REFERENCES

Ackerman D: *A natural history of the senses,* New York, Vantage Books, 1995.

Adelman M: Stigma, gay lifestyles and adjustment to aging: a study of late-life gay men and lesbians, *J Homosex* 20 (3-4), 1990.

Anderson CJ, Newton K: *Geriatric nursing,* St Louis, 1966, Mosby.

Baker B, Crowley S: AIDS crisis reaches those 50 plus, *AARP Bull* 35(2):5, 1994.

Barnett K: A survey of the current utilization of touch by health team personnel with hospitalized patient, *Int J Nurs Stud* 9:195, 1972a.

Barnett K: A theoretical construct of the concepts of touch as they relate to nursing, *Nurs Res* 21:102, March/April 1972b.

Beers MH: Male hypogonadism and impotence. In Abrams WB, Beers MH, Berkow R, editors: *Merck manual of geriatrics,* ed 2, Whitehouse Station, NJ, 1995, Merck Research Laboratories.

Benary-Isbert M: *The vintage years,* New York, 1968, Abingdon Press.

Beresford JM, Barrett CJ: *The widow's sexual self: a review and new findings.* Paper presented at the meeting of the Gerontological Society of America, Boston, Nov 22, 1982.

Berger R: *Gay and gray: the older homosexual man,* Binghamton, NY, 1995, Hawthorn Press.

Berlin H: Your doctor discusses: sexuality in mature/late life, *Planning for Health* 21:2, fall 1978.

Billhorn DR: Sexuality and the chronically ill older adult, *Geriatr Nurs* 15 (2):106, 1994.

Boyarsky RE: Sexuality and the aged. In Steinberg FU, editor: *Cowdry's care of the geriatric patient,* ed 6, St Louis, 1983, Mosby.

Brier J, Rubenstein D: Sex for the elderly? Why not? *Perspect Aging* 2:7, 1977.

Buczny B: Impotence in older men: a newly recognized problem, *J Gerontol Nurs* 18(5):25, 1992.

Burke MA, Knowlton CN: Sexuality. In Burke MM, Walsh MB, editors: *Gerontological nursing,* St Louis, 1992, Mosby.

Butler R, Lewis MI, Hoffman E, Whitehead ED: Love and sex after 60: how to evaluate and treat the impotent man, *Geriatrics* 49 (10): 27, 1994.

Butler R, Lewis M: Sexuality. In Abrams WB, Berkow R, editors: *Merck manual of geriatrics,* Rahway, NJ, 1990, Merck Sharpe and Dohme Research Laboratories.

Colton H: *The gift of touch,* New York, 1983, Seaview/Putnam.

Cosgray R, Davidhizar R: *Touch among the elderly.* Report of unpublished research, Cincinnati, 1988, Jewish Hospital Third Annual Nursing Research Conference.

Denny NW, Quadango D: *Human sexuality,* St Louis, 1992, Mosby.

Deevey S: Older lesbian women: an invisible minority, *J Gerontol Nurs* 16(5):35, 1990.

Diokno AC, Brown MB, Herzog AR: Sexual function in the elderly, *Arch Intern Med* 150: 197, 1990.

DeNigola P, Peruzza M: Sex in the aged, *J Am Geriatr Soc* 22:380, 1974.

Erikson E, Erikson JM, Kivnick HQ: *Vital involvement in old age: the experience of old age in our time,* New York, 1986, Norton.

Flaxman, N: Personal conversation, June 13, 1996.

Fletcher JW: Sexually transmitted viral diseases in the elderly. In Cooper JW, editor: *Antivirals in the elderly,* New York, 1995, Pharmaceutical Products Press.

Fletes M: Human immunodeficiency virus infection. In Abrams WB, Beers MH, Berkow R, editors: *Merck manual of geriatrics,* ed 2, Whitehouse Station, NJ, 1995, Merck Research Laboratories.

Fordham F: *An introduction to Jung's psychology,* Baltimore, 1970, Penguin Books.

Freedman M: Diversity with a difference: Gay and lesbian aging, *Aging Today* 16(5):7, 1995

Freedman M: A good gay old age, *Aging Today* 12(2):9, 1991.

Gerchafsky M: Impotence: the problem men don't talk about, *Ad Nurse Pract* 3(3):13, 1995.

Goldblatt R: Factors influencing sexual behavior, *J Am Geriatr Soc* 20:49, Feb 1972.

Hall ET: *The hidden dimensions,* Garden City, NY, 1969, Doubleday.

Ham RJ: Sexuality. In Ham RJ, Sloane PD, editors: *Primary care geriatrics,* ed 2, St Louis, 1992, Mosby.

Hite S: *The Hite report,* New York, 1977, Dell.

Huss AJ: Touch with care or a caring touch, *Am J Occup Ther* 31:12, 1977.

Jacobi J: *The psychology of CJ Jung,* New Haven, Conn, 1973, Yale University Press.

Jarvik L, Small G: *Parent care,* New York, 1988, Crown.

Jourard S: *The transparent self,* New York, 1964, Van Nostrand.

Kass MJ: Sexual expression of the elderly in nursing homes, *Gerontologist* 18:372, 1979.

Katzm L: Chronic illness and sexuality, *Am J Nurs* 9(1):56, 1991.

Kehoe M: Have you ever seen a lesbian over 60? *The Aging Connection* 4(4):4, 1988.

Kelly J: The aging male homosexual: myth and reality, *Gerontologist* 17:328, 1977.

Kelly J: Homosexuality and aging. In Marmor J, editor: *Homosexual behavior: a modern reappraisal,* New York, 1980, Basic Books.

Kreiger D: Therapeutic touch: the imprimatur of nursing, *Am J Nurs* 75:784, 1975.

Lewis MI: Sexuality. In Abrams WB, Beers MH, Berkow R, editors: *Merck manual of geriatrics,* ed 2, Whitehouse Station, NJ, 1995, Merck Research Laboratories.

Maddocks J: Sexual health and health care, *Postgrad Med* 58:52, 1975.

Miller CA: *Nursing care of older adults,* Glenview, Ill, 1990, Scott Foresman/Little Brown Higher Education.

Miller J: The first language, *UCSF Magazine* 13(3):31, 1992.

Money J, Tucker P: *Sexual signatures: being a man or woman,* Boston, 1975, Little, Brown & Co.

Montagu A: *Touching: the human significance of the skin,* ed 2, New York, 1978, Harper & Row.

Montagu A: *Touching: the human significance of the skin,* ed 3, New York, 1986, Harper & Row.

Morrison-Beedy D, Robbins L: Sexual assessment and the aging female, *Nurse Pract* 14(12):35, 1989.

Nay R: Sexuality and the aged women in nursing homes, *Geriatr Nurs* 13(6):312, 1992.

Neyhart B: Estrogen therapy. In Ham RJ, Sloane PD: *Primary care geriatrics,* ed 2, St. Louis, 1992, Mosby.

Orlando PL: AIDS affects the older population, *Aging Connection,* 9 (2):1, 1988.

Quam JK, Whitford GS: Adaptation and age related expectations of older gay and lesbian adults, *Gerontologist* 32(3):367, 1992.

Raphael S, Robertson M: Lesbians and gay men in later life, *Generations* 6:16, 1980.

Robertson M: *The older lesbian,* master's thesis, Carson, Calif, 1979, California State University, Dominguez Hills.

Sakauye KM, McDonald WM: The impact of caring touch on quality of life in a nursing home (abstract), Chicago, *Proceedings of the Third Congress of the International Psychogeriatric Association* 3:131, 1987.

Saxon SV, Etten MJ: *Physical changes and aging,* ed 3, New York, 1994, Tiresias Press, Inc.

Schiff I: Menopause and ovarian hormone therapy. In Abrans WB, Beers MH, Berleow R, editors: *Merck manual of geriatrics,* Whitehouse Station, NJ, 1995, Merck Research Laboratories.

Schuerman DA: Clinical concerns: AIDS in the elderly, *J Gerontol Nurs* 20 (7):11, 1994.

Sherman D: Effects of medications on sexual function, *Contemp Long Term Care* 15(7):64, 1992.

Shippee-Rice R: Sexuality and aging. In Fogel C, Lavver D, editors: *Sexual health promotion,* Philadelphia, 1990, WB Saunders.

Slusher MP, Mayer CJ, Dunkle RE: Gay and Lesbians Older and Wiser (GLOW): a support group for older gay people, *Gerontologist* 36(1):118, 1996.

Some older Americans not practicing safe sex: *UCSF Health Letter* 19 (2):4. 1993.

Starr BD: Sexuality and aging. In Eisdorfer C, editor: *Annual review of gerontology and geriatrics,* vol 5, New York, 1985, Springer.

Stevenson RT, Courtenay BC: Old people, orgasms, and God: a replication determining the relationship between religiosity and attitudes of nurses' aides toward sexual expression among older adults in nursing homes (abstract), *Gerontologist* 22:261, 1982.

Testosterone and HRT, *Harvard Women's Health Watch* 3(10):1, 1996.

Thayer S: Social touching. In Schiff W, Foulke E: *Tactile perception: a source book,* Cambridge, 1982, Cambridge University Press.

Walz T, Blum N: *Sexual health in later life,* Lexington, Mass, 1987, DC Heath Co.

Wiley D, Bortz II WM: Sexuality and aging: usual and successful, *J Gerontol: Medical Science,* 51a(3)M142, 1996.

Whipple B, Scura KW: The overlooked epidemic: HIV in older adults, *Am J Nurs* 96(2):23, 1996.

White C: Sexual interest, attitudes, knowledge, and sexual history in relation to sexual behavior in the institutionalized aged, *Arch Sex Behav* 11:11, 1982.

Woods NF: *Human sexuality in health and illness,* ed 3, St Louis, 1983, Mosby.

Woods NF: Sexuality and aging. In Reinhardt AN, Quinn MD, editors: *Current practice in geronotological nursing,* vol 1, St Louis, 1979, Mosby.

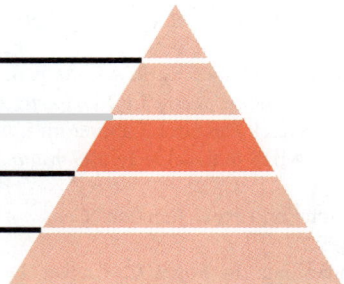

CHAPTER 17

Relationships and Their Significance

Grandparenting

A student learns

I have lived with my grandparents since the death of my mother almost 19 years ago. Living with them has had a great influence on my life. I do not look at older people the same way some of my peers do. Once you get past the myths that older people are unintelligent, physically unattractive shells of the people they once were, you begin to realize that they are one of the greatest unharnessed assets of our society. The knowledge and experience they possess are two of the greatest gifts a younger person will ever have the opportunity to receive.

Ross, age 25

Elders speak

I believe grandparents play a very important part in a child's life. We are raising two grandchildren ages 10 and 12 years; they have lived with us for 9 years. It has many rewards, but it is time consuming. Ten years ago we were free to do what we wanted, but now our lives are dictated by their school, sports, medical, dental, and social lives. However, under the circumstances, we wouldn't want it to be different.

Janice and Bill, age in late 60s

Caregiving

A student learns

My mother says I am not a good daughter. I am trying to finish my schooling, help my mother, take care of my two children and help my husband succeed in America. She has just moved here from Russia and left all her friends. I know she is lonely and wants me to spend more time with her, and I can't. I want to be a good daughter, but I don't know anymore who is most important—my mother, my children, my husband, or me? Sometimes I am so tired I just sit and cry.

Svetlana, age 33

Elders speak

I have no family except my dearest friends; several friends have live-in caretakers. My thoughts are to stay in close touch with my doctor and follow his recommendations. I have been caretaker to several: my mother, father, husband, and sister. All died within 5 years—all difficult—no rewards.

Clara, age 76

In Rwanda, prior to the genocide, I had occasion to ask, "How are elders cared for?" The pastor of a small village church said, "When they need a little help, the younger children in the family spend time with them each day; when they need more help, an older child will stay with them, and when they need a lot of help, they will come to live with their adult children." I realized that in spite of the vast differences in technologic development between Rwanda and the United States, we often do much the same when families are accessible and they have children. My grandchildren visit, run errands, water plants, find my glasses, and various other chores. As my needs become greater, they will grow older as well as I. They will do more for me as I will do less for them; the balance between the generations will shift, but the caring will remain.

Priscilla, age 68

Upon completion of this chapter, the reader will be able to:

1. Identify several types of primary relationships and describe the functions of each.
2. Relate several styles of grandparenting and contributions elders make to family life.
3. Specify factors that make caregiving of the aged particularly difficult.
4. Explain reasons why secondary support systems may be needed and useful for elders.
5. Discuss various types of groups that are supportive to elders.
6. Describe the nursing role in supportive networks serving elders.

BELONGING

Matilda White Riley, one of the earliest sociologic life course theorists, has throughout her career focused her studies on the interplay between institutions and individual lives and how each modifies the other. Some major changes that have greatly influenced our most fundamental institution, the family, are the increasing survival of numbers of the very old, late marriages of the young, late and limited childbearing, enduring relationships sans marriage, and the increasing rarity of one-income families in which the woman does not work outside the home. Although these are indicative of individual choices, these choices are in reponse to economic factors and technologic advances, as well as possibilities not available to earlier cohorts; thus the dialectic interplay in which society and individual are involved is continually modified. Riley (1996) notes that many of these individuals, collectively, have altered the meaning of mental health, work, and kinship structures.

In this chapter we are chiefly concerned with the impact of these numerous changes on the quality of life and range of possibilities for elders in their most important affiliations. Uhlenberg (1996a, b) addresses the impact of lives upon social structures and vice versa: as individuals live longer, the family adapts to the needs for caregiving, and this alters the lives of the middle aged, particularly of women. However, because most of the women are working, the industries and communities must respond with supports to meet the needs. Thus social change and individual need continue to change the nature of the life course and the affiliative inclinations.

This chapter will examine many facets of belonging: relationships with family, friends, groups, and community. Nursing interventions are included as they relate to each context.

The classic study of Lowenthal and Haven (1968) demonstrated the importance of caring relationships as a buffer against "age-linked social losses." The maintenance of a stable intimate relationship was more closely associated with good mental health and high morale than a high level of activity or elevated role status. In other words, one seems to be able to manage stresses if relationships are close and sustaining, and, if they are not, prestige and keeping busy may not prevent depression. An intimate, confiding relationship is a buffer against stress and illness. It is increasingly evident that a caring person may be a significant survival resource. Social bonding increases health status through as yet undetermined physiologic pathways.

This chapter will familiarize the reader with primary and secondary relationships as experienced in old age within generations and between generations. A network of kin, friends, and acquaintances can sustain the old and give life meaning. We might use the analogy of a tree that withstands storms and drought through an extensive root system, which provides stability and nourishment; such is old age. Often one must tend the ground around the tree to keep it thriving. We may find ourselves best caring for the aged by caring for those who are important to the aged.

The distinction between primary and secondary affiliations (Cooley, 1909) is based on the intensity and importance of relationships. Primary relationships are intimate, face-to-face associations that provide a strong sense of sharing and belonging; these are the deep roots of our tree analogy. The secondary relationships are more formal, impersonal, superficial, and often time limited. They are the surface network of roots that extend outward in many directions and sustain by their profusion. In old age the secondary network often diminishes, and the primary network may need more strength to bear the increasing demands. We will include specific nursing interventions toward this end.

Primary and Secondary Networks and Their Characteristics

Social networks are the vehicles through which social support and connections are maintained. The structure of these networks can be assessed by focusing on the individuals who provide various types of support. These individuals can be within an informal or formalized supportive role (Box 17-1). Characteristics of these various categories and the expectations that they form a support network must be examined closely to understand qualitative issues.

Living arrangements are the hub of the social network. In 1994 68% of older persons lived in a family (81% of older men and 58% of older women). Thirteen percent of those were not living with a spouse but with children, siblings, or other relatives (American Association of Retired Persons, 1996). The primary networks of individuals typically involve psychologic closeness, geographical proximity, and reciprocal supports.

The social networks of men and women are significantly different for singles but only slightly different for marrieds. Females, married or single, tend to maintain larger, more multifaceted networks and have more positive feelings about them than do men; married men tend to feel more satisfied with spousal support and less need for extensive social networks (O'Connor, 1993). There is a tendency for married men to maintain ties, particularly those with kin, through the wife's connections (Akiyama et al, 1996; Troll, 1994; Antonucci, 1990).

It is commonly presumed that the personal relationships of men are less intensive than those of women, though this is not borne out in recent studies (Akiyama et al (1996). In addition, there seems to be a distinct shift among older men from close relationships with men toward the development of more close relationships with women (O'Connor, 1993).

Married persons tend to have larger and more diverse networks than persons separated, divorced, widowed, or never married. Childless married persons tend to rely strongly on each other, whereas childless unmarrieds are more resourceful and have greater diversity in social networks. Widows generally have extensive support networks, and the role of children, particularly of daughters, is important (Brody et al, 1994).

Higher socioeconomic status, income, and education tend to be reflected in large and diverse social networks. Persons with lower income, status, and education tend to have smaller networks that consist mainly of family and close friends. Although the large, diverse networks may be more interesting, family and close friends may indeed be more reliable and more involved in providing instrumental and daily help. Lower income and less education are associated with increased contact with formal network providers such as physicians, clergy, and social workers.

A longitudinal study of the Berkeley older generation by Field and Minkler (1988) showed that social supports beyond the family decrease over time for the very old and for men but not for women and the oldest-old. The satisfaction with support from children tended to increase as elders relinquished involvement beyond the family. These data are significant because they confirm the constancy of family in the support network of the old.

Filial obligation toward parents is different than filial affection and seems to be somewhat related to proximity. The sense of obligation toward mothers tends to override role conflicts and even attenuated affections. Daughters involved in other roles seemed to feel less obligation toward fathers and in-laws, and the sense of obligation is somewhat related to affectional ties.

The dynamics of filial obligation in this study were related to sex, proximity, education, income, culture, and multiplicity of role demands (Welsh and Stewart, 1995). These factors need considerably more study before we will understand the complexity of issues that impact feelings about the significance and variables in close and superficial relationships.

There are many basic relationship possibilities among the aged: (1) spouse, (2) lover, (3) confidant, (4) friend, (5) parent, (6) grandparent, (7) great-grandparent, (8) sibling, (9) kin, (10) acquaintance, and (11) service provider. The first nine tend to be primary relationships and the last two, secondary and at times developing into primary. None or all of these may be a part of the sustaining network of the old. There are often several significant primary and secondary relationships at any given time and with overlapping characteristics.

The maintenance of primary and secondary relationships within one's own generation becomes more difficult with age. Cohorts die or age at such variable rates that they may be unable to provide the intimate exchange of earlier years. Territories shrink, and secondary networks are less available to an individual. The remaining relationships may become

---

Box 17-1   Networks

Formal	Informal
Church	Neighbors
Grandparenting	Maids, waitresses in small hotels
Foster Grandparents	Beauty salons, restaurants, bars, service personnel, shops
Vista	
Peace Corps	
Retired Senior Volunteer Program	Psychologic withdrawal—dreams, fantasies, hallucinations, daydreams
National Retired Teachers Association	
Unions	Fictive kin—soap operas
Friends of the Library Volunteers	Interest in celebrities
Public school	Laundromats
Senior centers	Sports
Title VII nutrition sites	Old people on bus
Involvement in social issues for seniors	Special tours
	Education, arts and crafts courses
	Trailer courts
	Retirement communities
	Pets
	Plants
	Dancing
	Physicians' offices
	Clinics
	Lobby gazers
	Vicarious participation
	Surrogate families—nurses, aides
	Nursing home—social corridor
	General social touching
	Radio shows
	Nostalgia
	Phone lines

burdened. It is not uncommon to find aged spouses or siblings living in relative isolation and struggling to maintain themselves with few supports. Therefore, maintenance of intergenerational affiliations is of great importance.

PRIMARY RELATIONSHIPS

Family members form the nucleus of primary relationships for the majority of the old. Cain (1996) surveyed recent literature to determine the strength of family ties to aged members. He found quite contradictory expectations that included increasing interdependence of the generations and the desire for more meaningful opportunities for the aged within the family and society, while yet identifying an existing "mismatch" between the expanding capacities of the aged and the shrinking opportunities.

The family relationships of the oldest-old tend to be characterized by cross-generational assistance, affection, and association (Troll and Bengtson, 1992). Calls, letters, gifts, visits, and evidences of concern and caring are highly valued. Relationships with children remain significant, but those with grandchildren sometimes weaken. Troll and

Bengtson (1992) surmise it may be related to limited energy to invest in maintaining the less necessary relationships.

Couple Relationships

The most significant and binding relationship is usually that of the couple. However, the chance of a couple going through old age together is exceedingly slim. In 1994 77% of older men were married, compared with 43% of older women; 47% of older women were widowed, compared with 13% of older men. Numerically, there are 5 times as many widows (8.5 million) as widowers (1.7 million) (American Association of Retired Persons, 1996). These statistics reflect the longer life span of women and other factors yet poorly understood.

The older they become, the more marked are the differences between the lives of men and women. After 75 years of age only 25.7% of women are living with a spouse (Table 17-1). These figures reflect the data most currently published by the U.S. Bureau of the Census. Compared with the previous data, slightly fewer very old are widowed, slightly more are divorced, and more are married. These shifting trends may be reflective of better general health in both men and women in late life.

Table 17-1   Marital Status of the Population, by Sex and Age: 1994

[As of March, Persons 18 years old and over. Excludes members of Armed Forces except those living off post or with their families on post. Based on Current Population Survey.]

Sex and Age	Number of Persons (1,000)					Percent Distribution				
	Total	Single	Married	Widowed	Divorced	Total	Single	Married	Widowed	Divorced
Male	**91,222**	**24,727**	**57,028**	**2,221**	**7,245**	**100.0**	**27.1**	**62.5**	**2.4**	**7.9**
18 to 19 years old	3,462	3,375	80	2	5	100.0	97.5	2.3	0.1	0.1
20 to 24 years old	9,221	7,469	1,658	5	89	100.0	81.0	18.0	0.1	1.0
25 to 29 years old	9,765	4,910	4,422	9	424	100.0	50.3	45.3	0.1	4.3
30 to 34 years old	11,108	3,298	6,940	6	864	100.0	29.7	62.5	0.1	7.8
35 to 39 years old	10,892	2,094	7,603	31	1,164	100.0	19.2	69.8	0.3	10.7
40 to 44 years old	9,651	1,255	7,104	31	1,262	100.0	13.0	73.6	0.3	13.1
45 to 54 years old	14,454	1,185	11,362	137	1,770	100.0	8.2	78.6	0.9	12.2
55 to 64 years old	9,933	539	8,034	327	1,033	100.0	5.4	80.9	3.3	10.4
65 to 74 years old	7,924	390	6,353	695	486	100.0	4.9	80.2	8.8	6.1
75 years old and over . .	4,812	211	3,471	980	150	100.0	4.4	72.1	20.4	3.1
Female	**98,765**	**19,458**	**58,113**	**11,073**	**10,120**	**100.0**	**19.7**	**58.8**	**11.2**	**10.2**
18 to 19 years old	3,454	3,152	278	3	21	100.0	91.3	8.0	0.1	0.6
20 to 24 years old	9,338	6,162	2,931	11	234	100.0	66.0	31.4	0.1	2.5
25 to 29 years old	9,861	3,476	5,689	29	667	100.0	35.2	57.7	0.3	6.8
30 to 34 years old	11,212	2,228	7,703	80	1,202	100.0	19.9	68.7	0.7	10.7
35 to 39 years old	11,078	1,420	7,959	135	1,563	100.0	12.8	71.8	1.2	14.1
40 to 44 years old	9,906	909	7,358	146	1,492	100.0	9.2	74.3	1.5	15.1
45 to 54 years old	15,068	892	10,977	705	2,494	100.0	5.9	72.8	4.7	16.6
55 to 64 years old	10,805	440	7,500	1,501	1,364	100.0	4.1	69.4	13.9	12.6
65 to 74 years old	10,163	386	5,520	3,476	781	100.0	3.8	54.3	34.2	7.7
75 years old and over . .	7,880	393	2,199	4,986	302	100.0	5.0	27.9	63.3	3.8

From U.S. Bureau of the Census: *Statistical Abstract of the United States,* ed 115, Washington, DC, 1995.

Half of the oldest-old men are married, but only 8% of their female cohorts are. Men who survive their spouse into old age ordinarily have multiple opportunities to remarry if they wish. It is less likely that a woman will have an opportunity for remarriage in late life.

About 52,000 older Americans marry each year; 94% of those are remarriages, yet it is notable that 6% marry for the first time in old age. Older men often marry younger women, and there is an increasing trend for younger men to marry older women. Couple relationships involve varying degrees of instrumental support, emotional support, and intimacy (Anderson and McCullough, 1993). This confirms our view that old people do not necessarily retreat from life and challenging situations. Developing an intimate, sharing relationship late in life between individuals who have had 75 or 80 years of varied experiences and often conflicting ideologies is an enormous challenge.

Couples in late life may have needs, tasks, and expectations that differ from those of their earlier postparental years. Those married 50 years or more may describe a happy marriage as related to congruence of perception. This does not necessarily mean the couples agree, but rather that they know what to expect from each other. However, people who stay together for a half century or more are not necessarily happy doing so.

Many of the following issues may put severe strain on couples in the last phase of life:

- Efficacy in task accomplishment
- Economics
- Health
- Previous marriages
- Relationships with children
- Sexuality
- Long-standing patterns of communication
- Matching of personal needs for activity or disengagement
- Ability to support each other through crises
- Attitudes about aging

Nurses may learn a great deal, as well as assisting couples in defining the value of the relationship, by discussing with the couple the strengths in their relationship as well as the difficulties. They may seldom have tried to articulate these clearly. See Chapter 20 for a discussion of divorce in late life.

Sibling Relationships

Moyer (1992) believes the sibling support system is underutilized. More studies are beginning to explore the significance of siblings as one grows old. There are many possible sibling relationships in old age: intimate, congenial, loyal, apathetic, distant, friendly and hostile. Others include the advisory, competitive, and envious. Siblings share a unique history; a similar biologic and cultural heritage, albeit with numerous variable personal interpretations.

The significance of these long-term parallel surviving relationships cannot be denied. They become particularly important when they are part of the support system, especially among single or widowed elders living alone. Sometimes they share living space (Connidis, 1994). Connidis (1994) found that the majority of siblings she studied (528)

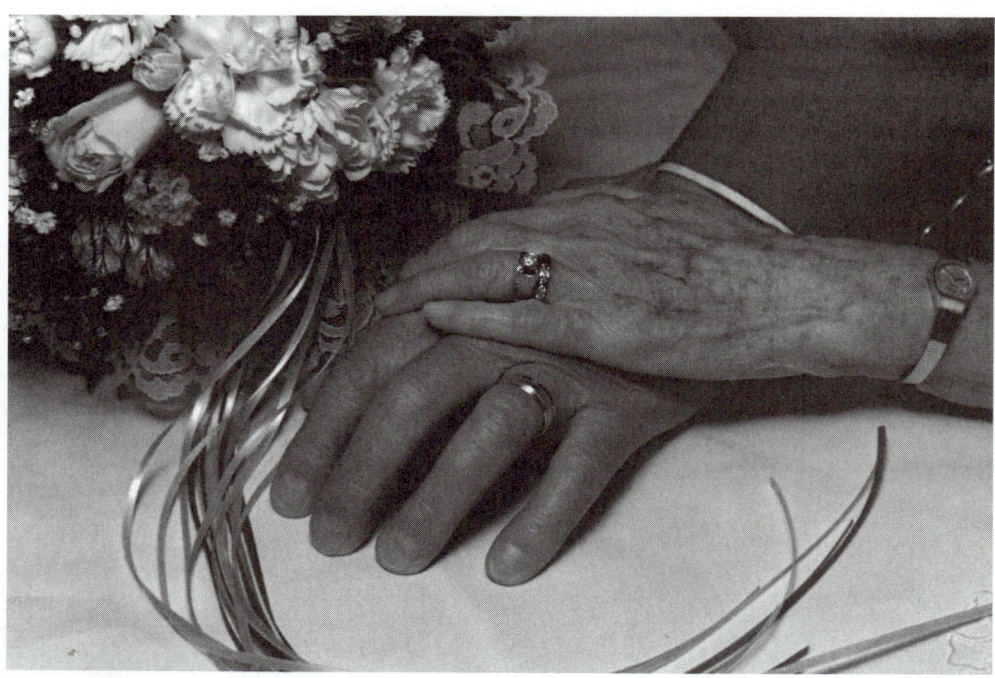

Late life marriage. (Courtesy Rod Schmall.)

would share their homes with a sibling if necessary and would go to them for help in a crisis.

Elders seldom rely on siblings for financial help or care during illness but, especially those from larger families, believe the siblings are a backup support that can be and is called upon for moral support and help in emergencies. As one would expect, unmarried and/or widowed siblings were more likely to go to each other for assistance and support. They harbor strong feelings of reciprocity in the relationships.

Avioli (1989) found that 74% of older adults considered at least one of their siblings to be a close friend. Siblings who live near each other often are confidants, especially those who are single or childless (Connidis and Davies, 1992). Freedman (1996) found that having even one sibling significantly reduced the likelihood of institutionalization.

When there are two or more siblings, they are likely to be a significant part of the support system and caregivers of each other and of very old parents. These relationships may be fraught with lingering resentments and competition for parental approval, or they may be particularly close and comforting. Scott (1992) suggests that resolution of old hurts or conflictual relationships may be necessary between siblings before they can work together in providing for parents' needs or in developing supports among themselves. They may help each other modify and refine early experiences that were troublesome (Moyer, 1992) by reminiscing and gaining new perspectives with which to interpret earlier events.

A sibling situation that seems to encompass special psychologic bonds is that of identical twins and triplets. On her seventy-eighth birthday, Ellen said, "You know, I was the only survivor of triplets. In those days it was rare for any to survive. I have always known something was missing. I have this longing I can't explain . . . a sense of loneliness so deep it can't be filled."

Another report that hints at a lifelong need for a missing twin is poignantly conveyed by Brandt (1996): "I am an identical twin, but my brother, Robert, was killed by electric shock when we were 20. It's now 47 years later, and it has been a constant struggle to continue alone." This gentleman has established a support group for those missing a twin (see resources).

In the future even more siblings of multiple births will grow old together, and it seems a fruitful area for longitudinal studies.

Parental Relationship

The role of elders with adult children is seldom considered except in relationship to caregiving issues. Adult children are often said to reverse roles with parents when the parents become old and dependent. This has a demeaning connotation, as if the elder becomes a child again. There is some evidence that adult children are shifted to the role of friend, companion, and confidant to the elder (Connidis and Davies, 1992). In illness and deterioration of the elder, the adult child may at times feel parental, but the inner child always remains in search of the protective and guiding parent. No matter how mature one becomes, the parent symbolizes security and acceptance regardless of the reality or facts. These dynamics often make the caregiving role very complex and difficult.

Grandparenthood

Grandparenting is a role instigated and often dictated by others. In many instances, and in the best of circumstances, the achievement and status of grandparenting is an enjoyable extension of parenting and totally subordinate to the parental role. Expected behavior from grandparents in those cases includes providing gifts, money, and access to certain places; traveling with grandchildren; having knowledge of family heritage, rituals, news, and folklore; aiding in raising children; and giving emotional comfort.

Jendrek (1994) found three major categories of grandparents assisting in the raising of children: the custodial, in which the child lives with the grandparents because of severe problems in the nuclear family; the live-in, in which the grandparent lives in the home of the grandchild and provides variable amounts of assistance to the family and the grandchild; and, the day-care provider, in which the grandparent cares for the child while parents work.

Grandparental functions may include any of the following:

Surrogate parent
Provider of support in times of crisis
Babysitter
Homemaker
Housesitter
Income provider/financial resource
Teacher
Confidant/wise counselor
Keeper of the family heritage

In recent years more grandparents have become, by default, the primary caregivers of grandchildren because parents are incapable of providing the care needed. Major antecedents to this situation are child abuse, imprisonment, joblessness, drug and alcohol addictions, illness, and social problems of the parents (Kelley, 1993). It is estimated that about 4 million children are in the care of grandparents, and this is 40% more than 10 years ago (Crowley, 1993).

These grandparents have been called the "silent saviors" (Jendrek, 1994). Most say they never intended to parent children again, but when the parents proved unable or unfit to do so, the grandparents stepped into the role. Grandparents are fast becoming a crucial resource on which society and the younger generation increasingly rely. Interestingly, the children raised solely by grandparents seem to maintain health and make good school adjustments (Solomon and Marx, 1995).

This surrogate parent phenomenon is historic among blacks and has been studied and reported on as early as

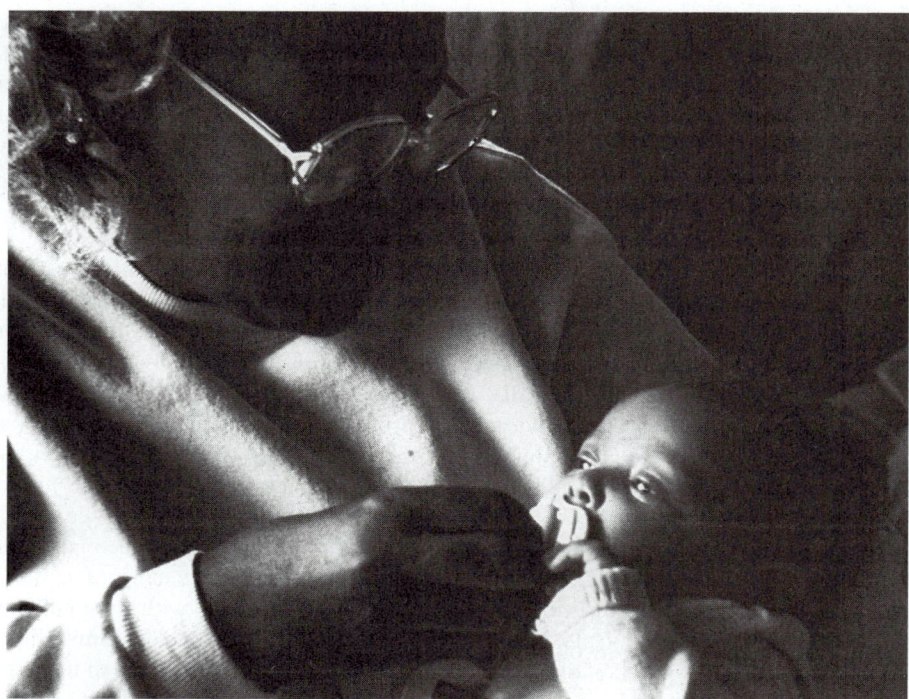

Grandparent as parent. (Courtesy Rod Schmall.)

the Civil War era (Jones, 1973; Jones, 1985; Kivett, 1991). These reports tended to romanticize a situation necessitated by a lack of other alternatives. Recent reports of grandparents who have acted as primary caregivers paint a less glorious picture. Often these older individuals have been the only ones available and have received no economic or social support in the role. Grandparents frequently report financial and health problems related to the additional burden of caring for grandchildren. Nearly half report increased stress, illness, anxiety, and depression (Burton, 1992). In spite of all that, grandmothers tend to report that the grandchildren provide purpose that keeps them going. As this situation becomes more prevalent, organizations are developing to provide resources and assistance for the grandparents (see resources at the end of the chapter).

Grandparenting is not a static state but a developmental status. The grandparent role can be a mutually significant one with the burden for making it so within the realm of the grandparent. The *Mayo Clinic Health Letter* (Good grandparenting, 1993) suggests several strategies that are helpful (Box 17-2). Grandparents, by their generational distance, may bring a sense of perspective in trying situations, often aligning their support with the grandchild and remembering (to the parents' dismay) similar problems occurring as their own children were growing up. They provide young adult grandchildren with advice, affirmation, and a sense of roots and continuity. The young often gain an understanding of aging and mortality through sharing with grandparents. Healthy youngsters and well-developed grandparents often

share a sense of immediacy and curiosity, tolerance of life as it is, and the capacity for appreciation.

It is a loss to everyone when grandparents are incorporated into family life only as they become feeble and ill. The child will then have a skewed view of what aging means, and it will be a source of dread and avoidance.

Grandparents' memories are stories and can be a special treasure for children. One woman in middle age wished that her grandparents had identified relatives in old snapshots, passed along their favorite recipes, told more about their school days, explained where they obtained the land they owned, and kept a family tree. These suggestions may be helpful in talking to elders about something useful they may do for their grandchildren. Grandparents' Day is observed the first Sunday after Labor Day. It is observed nationally, particularly in nursing home settings.

Nurses may find it interesting and useful to discuss the meaning and satisfaction older people find in the grandparenting role. Those who are not grandparents may wish to discuss their feelings about it. If they feel cheated, there are surrogate grandparent roles they may wish to assume, such as those in the Foster Grandparent programs. Grandparents are no longer just the "fun-seekers." The diversity of family lifestyles and cultural differences has resulted in numerous types of grandparenting.

Great-Grandparenting

Great-grandparenthood has been rarely studied, although 40% of the older people in the United States will live long enough to become great-grandparents. It is not unusual for a

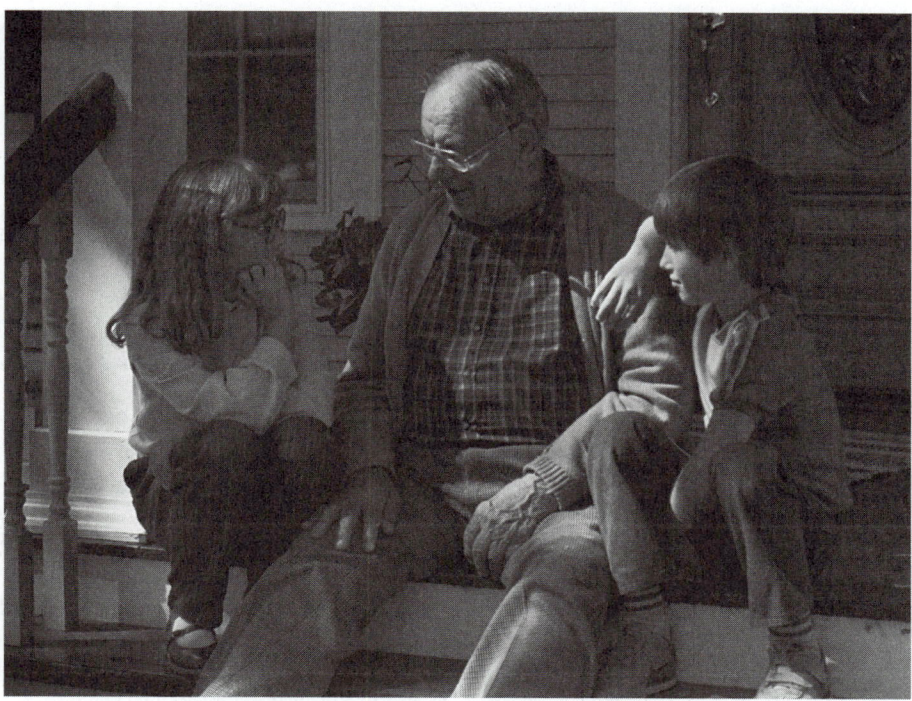

A grandparent listens. (Courtesy Rod Schmall.)

woman of 60 years old, still young and vital, to be a great-grandparent, and there are numerous great-great grandparents alive today. Stereotypically, great-grandparents have been consigned to a rocking chair and shawl.

Wentowski (1985) found considerable differences in great-grandmothers even among the older group she studied (average age of 86 years). In most cases the great-grandparental role was modeled after the role as grandparent, and the quality of the relationship was largely determined by the middle generation's attitudes and involvement with parents and grandparents. For most the intensity of the relationship was diminished compared with that of grandparenting. Many identified the great-grandchildren as children of their grandchild. They sent obligatory gifts and wanted to be loved and respected, but few had close relationships. Great-grandchildren seemed to validate the vitality and success of the family, and the great-grandparents enjoyed tracing the patterns of inheritance and personality traits.

Wentowski (1985) suggests that a study of age-matched grandparents and great-grandparents might better sort out the difference in grandparenting and great-grandparenting. She explored the perceptions great-grandparents have of their kinship role and found three significant trends: (1) it is not perceived as a primary kinship role but linked only in the generational context; (2) it is important emotionally, but there is little involvement in the daily lives of great-grandchildren; and (3) there is a diluted sense of obligation toward the great-grandchildren.

In advanced aged, the family role may be supplanted by a symbolic social role as representatives of living history. In

---

Box 17-2   Grandparenting

Don't give advice about childrearing.
Rules of behavior should relate only to your own home.
Give the child undivided attention during projects, games, and reading.
Be a link with the past; tell grandchildren about their parent and about you when you were a child.
Support the parents in their decisions; never undermine.
Create memories and traditions.
Offer the gift of your time: nature walks, baking cookies, etc.

Long-Distance Grandparenting

Brief and frequent letters and cards are useful; send clippings, cartoons, and riddles; use colorful stickers and stamps.
Audiotapes and videotapes that you produce are appreciated; storytelling, reading, or singing.
Celebrate special days and firsts (lost tooth, day of school, mastery of a new situation).
Telephone frequently.
Visit as often as you can.

From Good grandparenting, *Mayo Clinic Health Letter* 11(1):6, 1993.

some cases a great-grandparent outlives the grandparent and may assume some aspects of a grandparental role. Nurses may explore the meaning of being a great-grandparent with these clients, who rarely have role models and may be defining their function in a unique manner.

Other Kin

Interaction with collateral kin (cousins, aunts, uncles, nieces, and nephews) generally depends on proximity, preference, and the general availability of primary kin. Often maternal kin are emotionally closer than those in one's paternal line. These may provide a reservoir of kin from which to find replacements for missing or lost primary relationships or as single or childless people grow old. Elders often seem to be attached to a favorite niece or nephew whom they rely on to maintain some family connection and in some ways serve as a surrogate for the child they never had. Distant collateral kin become important to some elders as they seek to establish their place in the kin network and generational flow.

Marge has recently been scrimping to remain in the deluxe life-care community where she has resided for 20 years. Inflation and taxes have caught up with her investment returns. She often forgoes her evening meal to reduce her expenses but passes it off by saying, "I can do without those calories." Marge has no children, but her favorite nephew keeps in touch. Recently he called to request money for his graduate school tuition. Her nephew is 40 years old. Marge felt guilty that she couldn't provide it.

This is not an aberrant situation. We have heard many similar stories. The transfer of assets and funds to the younger generations is a frequent economic trend in families of today and seems to have important psychologic value for elders.

Friendships

Friends function in many ways: (1) to provide surrogate kin, (2) to ease the loneliness of widowhood, (3) to replace lost siblings, and (4) to validate one's generational viewpoint. Contacts with friends exceed all others in frequency. Considering the obvious importance of friendship, it seems to be a neglected area of exploration and a seldom-considered resource of professionals assisting the aged.

Sherman and Antonucci (1996) report on reciprocity in best-friend relationships with the interesting finding that feeling overbenefited or lessbenefited seemed to have little impact on the importance of the relationship. The critical issue for women seemed to be the opportunity for intimate disclosure within the relationship. This was less significant for men.

The study of the significance of friendships in old age has been extremely limited. Friendships across the life span can sustain in the face of overwhelming disasters. They often provide the critical elements of satisfactory living that family may not: commitment and affection without judgment, personality characteristics that are compatible because they are chosen, availability without demands, and caring without obligation. Friends may share a long-life perspective or may bring a totally new intergenerational viewpoint into one's life. Late life friendships often develop out of changing situations such as shared tenancies, widowhood, moves, and involvements in volunteer pursuits (O'Connor, 1993).

Adams (1987) studied the longitudinal patterns of friendship among elderly women and found that many changes occurred in the process of aging. The friendship network tended to enlarge in the later years, but the frequency and intensity of the relationships diminished. Widows tended to reach out to a new set of friends and diminished contact with friends who had spouses. Many developed new friendships in senior centers and retirement communities. The relative homogeneity in these settings may have contributed to the development of these relationships. On the other hand, many older individuals developed a sense of liberation from social constraint, and in turn friendships evolved that elders would never have considered in their youth.

Adams (1985) found that few women over 70 years old have male friends without romantic notions. The lack of male friends may be attributed to early socialization patterns and expectations (O'Connor, 1993) or to the absence of males from their network. If they have no legitimate contact with men through spouse or work, they may be reluctant to establish friendly relationships. On the other hand, the dearth of older men and their socialization to the sexualization of women may be an equally strong factor, although not addressed in this study.

Male friendships are even less frequently studied than those of females. Reisman (1988) assessed the value of friendship to a group of aging men and found that casual friends tend to increase in number during the leisure of retirement but close friendships remain few. Ongoing friendships were mentioned as significant by only 15% of married men, 12% of divorced men, and 6% of single men. These data obscure the fact that many men believed their wives or children to be their closest friends.

Akiyama et al (1996) found a distinct shift among older men from same sex alliances toward the development of more and closer relationships with women, possibly because there are more women in their network as they move out of work relationships and as male life expectancy diminishes. If married, they become more involved in their wives' activities; possibly because of frailty and dependency they are more comfortable with women. These data need further exploration. We do not yet know if for life satisfaction women need a broader network of friends than do men, but it is certainly a field ripe for investigation.

Nurses may help older people to maintain and revive old friendships by assisting them in letter writing, taking care to deliver phone messages, and discussing the nature of friendships. New friendships are facilitated by the opportunity for both closeness and distance. The impact of loss of a close friend seems dependent to some extent on the number of other close friends who remain in the network (deVries, 1995), particularly if the friend was mutual, and the remaining friends share the loss.

Adams (1983) makes helpful suggestions for service providers trying to keep an older person living independently. Consider the size, composition, and structure of the person's friendship network, the nature of the needed task, and the person's feelings about receiving certain types of help from friends. Friends are an excellent reservoir of strength, support, and help when needed.

Finally, the importance of intergenerational friendships should be mentioned. These often sustain the old and illuminate the young.

Families and the Aged

Families are the source of a great deal of material and emotional support across generations (American Society on Aging, 1992). The shifting need for supplies and demands among them helps establish a solid reciprocity that is comfortable in the giving and the receiving. Too often we think of the aged as only recipients. Even into advanced old age they often provide emotional and financial support, child care, and cultural and religious continuity. As the population shifts toward increasing numbers of frail aged with multiple problems, there is a danger that this balance will be neglected. Older family members, themselves impaired, may find themselves taking care of very old parents (Himes, 1992). This is already occurring for many but is expected to increase markedly in the future. As the age when "children" leave home continues to increase, it is likely we will again see many three-generational and four-generational households. Trends in mortality, fertility, marriage, divorce, and alternative family styles all affect the balance of generational needs and services.

The most enduring study of a cohort is that of the Berkeley Growth Study Group of children, begun in 1928. These children are now entering old age, and their parents, who are in advanced old age, form the sample for the Berkeley Older Generational Study. From a recent study of this group it was found that those in better health had greater contact with and felt closer to their families than those who were not well (Field et al, 1993). Some feel that as parents' needs for assistance intensify, the children's attitudes shift from affection to obligation (Abel, 1991). Women are in greater contact and feel closer in family relationships than men, although it appears from the Field et al study that widowhood may be a more important factor than gender in this observation.

It is equally as important to know how changes in feelings toward family can influence health. It is usually assumed that family relationships are desirable for the elderly to promote a sense of belonging. Such a generalization needs further examination. The quality, meaning, and importance of relationships with family members are significant factors in maintaining morale and experiencing life satisfaction (Connidis and McMullin, 1993).

Family History. A potent force, often overlooked in families with aged members, is the influence of the family history. Sibling position in a family profoundly influences relationships with parents and other siblings. From these early roots, sibling rivalry flourishes. Motivation, socialization, affiliation, and aggression are all related in some way to family configuration. Each child is destined to play out a facet of the parents' hopes and aspirations, albeit these dynamics are usually far beneath the surface of individual awareness of the parent or the child. From sibling relationships, parental expectations, and parental favoritism, later reactions to aged parents may arise. Little study has been done in this area, but it is known that the history of these early beginnings is never totally discarded (Whitbeck et al, 1994). It is known that one's placement and gender in the family configuration has signficant, though unpredictable, effects.

John was the eldest of a large family and was the good son. His brother, George, only 2 years younger, was a scrapper, and though he was frequently reprimanded for fighting, his father bragged to others about his ability to come out on top. The third son, Elmer, was studious, and his mother consistently praised him, though he felt as if his father hardly noticed. Finally a sister, Judy, arrived, and as she grew up she seemed more and more to resemble the sister her father has lost early in his childhood.

Matthews (1995) found that a lone sister among brothers was usually given charge of parents when they needed assistance, and, though the brothers contributed in many ways, neither they nor the sister considered their contributions important.

The sister moved the parents into her home in their later years. John was a professor at a nearby university and frequently brought books and recordings from the library that he knew his parents would enjoy. George functioned as advocate for his parents' medical care and seemed to be forever questioning, seeking other opinions, and resisting routinization of their care. Elmer managed their finances and helped them invest carefully.

Nurses might be helpful in pointing out to each family member how their contributions sustained and enriched the lives of their parents and were in their own unique ways demonstrations of their feelings of filial responsibility.

Parents in their old age may depend on the eldest child to care for them just as they depended on that child to care for younger siblings decades before, or each parent may have a different "favorite" child. Sometimes a "rejected" child may attempt to gain love and recognition by attending the aged parent or may unconsciously punish the parent for injustices experienced in the distant past. Nurses may help all family members understand the present situation as reflecting many conflicts from the past.

Caron et al (1996) have studied this to some extent and found that lingering perceptions of family conflict later influence the perception of caregiving burden. Simple awareness of the multiplicity of influences on interactions and recognition of the acceptability of feelings may provide sufficient reassurance. In more severe situations in which feelings are expressed in destructive ways, family counseling may be recommended (see Chapter 15).

Rivalry among family members for the approval of aged parents is most common when there is awareness of a potential inheritance. Many people are reluctant to admit to themselves that such thoughts enter their minds. It is helpful to recognize the reality of such considerations and that it may be just as natural to entertain such feelings as it was to attempt to gain more than one's share of the parental love in the early stages of childhood. Most close relationships are fraught with ambivalence. Learning to accept this fact will ease feelings of guilt or shame.

If the family has never been close and supportive, it will not magically become so when the parents are old. Resentments long buried may crop up and produce friction or psychologic pain. One of the tasks of middle-aged adults centers on their ability to work through youthful feelings and attitudes toward parents. The mature adult begins to see parents as individuals rather than extensions of one's own needs. However, submerged conflicts and feelings often return to surprise adult children (Townsend and Franks, 1995).

Mature acceptance of aged parents with all their foibles and personal idiosyncrasies is an ongoing task. Nurses may help family members accept their own idiosyncrasies as meaningful and valid, even though the relationships are always complex, clouded with ambivalence, and influenced by the past. Some families can be encouraged to express their feelings more openly, although if they have never done so, it may be difficult to break long-standing habits within the family relationships. Most important, each family member needs to be accepted and understood as significant to the family system.

Deference. Old people may play games with their children, perhaps ones they have always played or ones invented to avert fear and loneliness. Some manipulate, dwell on infirmities, belittle themselves, or use their money to wield power. Children may rightfully feel used and angry. Among health care providers it is common to believe that the old are maligned and neglected. Nurses can help people see their situation more clearly and recognize the validity of their view and also that one must not put up with games or avoid confrontation in deference to old age.

Scapegoating. We are aware of the detrimental effects of consistently being the scapegoat for others, although most people are given this role occasionally or cast it on others at times. Aged parents are often scapegoats. The focus of energy usually flows toward the younger generation as the bearers of unfulfilled dreams, whereas the elders are the carriers of disappointment and worn traditions. They may personify all the facets of life we are conditioned to avoid: death, illness, depression, and uselessness. It is easy to displace responsibility and project feelings onto an aged parent who may in fact have already internalized the social rejection of the generalized aged.

As nurses, perhaps the most useful approach to families who seem to scapegoat the aged members would be to explore the individual's fears and concerns related to his or her own aging; for example, "Having your parent in your home must stimulate a lot of thoughts about your own aging process." The dynamics of scapegoating the elderly have not been examined in the literature. It is recognized that when a family crisis occurs, the elderly member is likely to be removed from the family group and in some way seen as the source of the problem. If the older person has sapped the family energy system, the move may temporarily restore family balance even though solution of the real problem will only be deferred.

Crises. When an elder lives with adult children and there is a disruption in the family system, moving the elder may be seen as one way of restoring balance. Losing a member from a family system is a major crisis, particularly if by death or an abrupt undesired separation. This is the time when insidious scapegoating occurs.

A middle-aged woman dying of cancer is trying to make peace with herself and her family. Her aged mother has lived with the family for several years. She hovers over her daughter, as any mother would a dying child. The adult children of the dying woman are offended; the husband feels crowded out. Soon there is a spoken, or unspoken, desire: "Why isn't it Grandma? She has lived her life." Grandma is an object of resentment because she is surviving. It seems so unfair!

Nurses in contact with such families may help the family verbalize the unspoken and understand those feelings. The family, including Grandma, needs to talk about the needs each feels in relation to the dying woman and to each other. Helping each other through such trying times is difficult. External support, such as a nurse can give, will help each accept his or her pain without blaming.

It is thought that more than 8 million elders need, and get, some form of assistance from family and friends that allows them to live at home. These data must remain suspect because much help is given that never comes to the attention of data collectors or agency personnel. Yet, according to the American Association of Homes and Services for the Aging (AAHSA) (1996), nearly one in four Americans over age 50 feels responsibility for an elder needing long-term care (American Association of Homes and Services for the Aging, 1996). About 43% of noninstitutionalized elders over the age of 85 need assistance with basic activities of daily living. Relatives provide 84% of all care to males and 79% to females. More than 1 in 3 elderly men needing assistance is cared for by a wife, but only 1 in 10 disabled elderly women is cared for by a husband (American Association of Homes and Services for the Aging, 1996).

If an aged parent is beginning to need help, the following suggestions to family members may be useful:

1. Involve the parent in all decisions that affect care.
2. Assist the elderly parent to remain as independent as possible and provide assistance only for those things that are especially stressful or depleting.
3. Seek resources that provide options between independent living and a nursing home.
4. If the parent insists on promises never to be put in a nursing home, the family may promise that they will do everything possible to prevent it.

Before inviting an elder to move into the family's home consideration should be given to items in Box 17-3.

Caregiving. In the past three decades a plethora of studies and plans have arisen from the historic and enduring role of the family as caretakers of the old. It is as if this mode of care were recently discovered. At present families provide 80% to 90% of the long-term care of elders in the community (Family Caregiver Alliance, 1996). Numerically, 2.7 million adult children provide "hands-on care" for disabled elders (OWL, 1992); however, far more spouses provide care, and it is assumed they will do so when a spouse exists.

Historically, family support and care for older folk have always been voluntary, or tolerated because there were no other alternatives. Usually one adult child was expected to remain in the home of the parents while they were aging. Lone children and unmarried females are particularly vulnerable to the assumed expectation that they take care of the aged parents (Brody, 1994). In some cultures and subcultures family caregiving of elders appears to be more generally provided, but on closer examination it may be related to the unavailability of alternatives (Carpenter, 1996; Giarrusso et al, 1996; Burholdt et al, 1996; Constantino and Wykle, 1996; Lamphere et al, 1996).

In the past, families and individuals have had to rely on kin as their essential social base for assistance of various kinds (Hareven, 1992). Now, we are much more likely to expect the government to help and to develop programs to assist families with various social needs, including the burden of caregiving. Many families are clearly in need of assistance in the care of their elders. Changes in societal demands and expectations of families make it more difficult, if not impossible, for any one adult-child to be available around-the-clock.

Even when a caregiver is available, the burden may be onerous. Elderly spouses often find themselves available but not physically capable of the demands of constant caregiving. Psychiatric and physical morbidity of these caregivers have generated much study and concern (Schulz et al, 1995). Mittleman et al (1995) found that the continuous availability of ad hoc counseling and support group participation

---

Box 17-3   Planning to Add an Aged Member to the Household

Questions you need to ask:
- What are the needs of the new member and of the family?
- Where will space be allotted for the new member?
- How will this new member be included in existing family patterns?
- How will responsibilities be shared?
- What resources in the community will assist in the adjustment phase?
- Is the environment safe for this new member?
- How will family life change with the added member, and how does the family feel about it?
- What are the differences in socialization and sleeping patterns?
- What are the aged person's strong needs and expectations?
- What are the aged person's skills and talents?

Modifications you need to make:
- Arrange semiprivate living quarters if possible
- Consider a "granny flat" (see Chapter 13)
- Regularly schedule visits to other relatives to give each family times of respite and privacy.
- Arrange day-care and senior activities for the older person to help keep contact with members of his or her own generation.

Discuss potential areas of conflict:
- *Space:* especially if someone has given up his or her space to the aged relative.
- *Possessions:* old person may want to move possessions into house; others may not find them attractive or may insist on replacing them with new things.

- *Entertaining:* times when old and young feel the need or desire to exclude the other from social events.
- *Responsibilities and chores:* old may feel useless if they do nothing and in the way if they do something; young may feel that their position is usurped or may be angry if they wait on parent.
- *Expenses:* increased cost of home maintenance, food, clothing, and recreation may not be shared appropriately.
- *Vacations:* whether to go together or alone, the young may feel uneasy not taking older person but resentful if they must.
- *Child rearing:* disagreement over child rearing policies.
- *Child care:* grandparental babysitting may be welcomed by family and resented by older person, or if not allowed, older person feels lack of trust in capability (McGreehan and Warburton, 1978).

Decrease areas of conflict by:
- Respecting privacy.
- Discussing space allocations.
- Discussing elderly person's furnishings before move.
- Making it clear ahead of time when social events include everyone or exclude someone.
- Clearing decisions about household tasks—all should have responsibility geared to ability.
- Paying a share of expenses and maintaining a separate phone reduces strain and increases feelings of independence.

significantly reduced depression in aged spouse-caregivers. These and numerous other strategies, while reported as successful, are seldom available except as demonstration projects. Winbush (1992) suggests that families should be asked about their needs, and when resources are given, they should be tailored to the individual family type/style and situation. We would add that they should be reliable over time.

Stephens (1996) found that day care respite can be effective for some caregivers if it allows sufficient relief, creates no additional stress, is at least partially subsidized, and provides information about other resources that may be helpful. Audiotapes and videotapes that provide mild stimulation or entertainment for elders and respite for their caregivers have been developed and show some promise of being used effectively (Camberg et al, 1996).

The On Lok Senior Health Service Center in San Francisco has attempted to do this and to meet the needs of the elder and family in a supportive and supplementary manner "until death do us part" (Der-McLeod and Hansen, 1992). The interdisciplinary planning sessions with the family help accomplish these goals. Grants, Medicaid and Medicare waivers, and contributions have made these services possible in a manner affordable to the participants from the community surrounding On Lok. It is important to recognize that this model program could be provided across the United States and perhaps in an economic manner using some of the same strategies. However, in spite of the studies and efforts to pass legislation to give tax advantages and more

readily available respite care, families often indicate they do not want the services that are offered (Pillemer, 1996).

There are few studies to evaluate the effectiveness of services, and Pillemer suggests these should take precedence over the endless study of the caregiving situations. In fact, Nielsen et al (1996) found that when an elder was institutionalized, family members said there were no services that would have been sufficient to keep the elder in the home longer. It appears that most families manage as well as possible for as long as possible, but when insitutionalization is necessary, they have reached the end of their ability to continue as the primary caregivers. Long-range planning for health maintenance of the family caregivers has been sorely neglected.

Uhlenberg (1996) proposes an interesting paradigm of the shifting balance of caregiving and care receiving (Figure 17-1). This may be useful in allowing nurses, other professionals, elders, and their family members to more clearly see the complexities of supportive caring relationships. The elements to be considered are physical and mental status, skills and knowledge, opportunities and options for self-care, motivations, and access. We find this model has potential for appraisal throughout adult life of the reciprocal nature of the caregiving/care receiving balance and provides a framework for evaluating strengths and weakened areas that may need bolstering. From a systems perspective, strengthening one area of self-care may shift the balance to a more satisfactory level for all individuals involved in the equation.

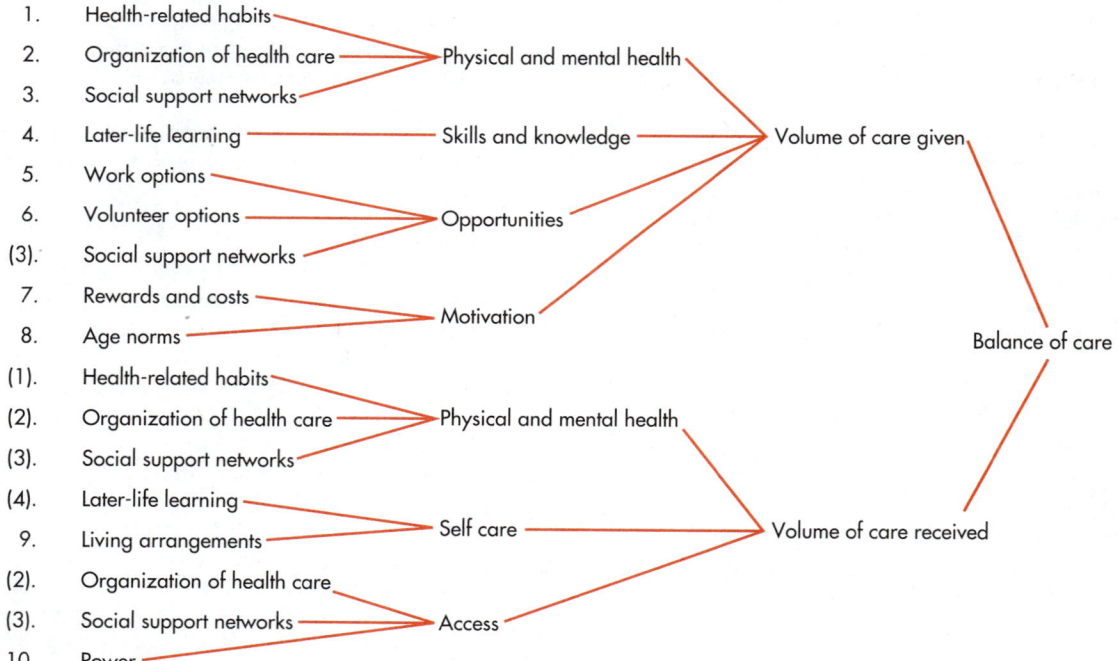

Figure 17-1.   The critical social variables affecting balance of care. (From Uhlenberg P: The burden of aging: a theoretical framework for understanding the shifting balance of caregiving and care receiving as cohorts age, *Gerontologist* 36(6):761, 1996.

Recently there have been questions about the real extent of the "sandwich" generation wedged between the obligations to children and those to elder parents. Dependency ratios published by the U.S. Bureau of the Census (1996) do not really represent family linkages (Soldo, 1996). On average there are 5 years between the ages of 50 and 55 when one is likely to have the care of both a parent and a minor child, though 20% have a child but no parents in the home, and 5% have parents but no children under their care (Figure 17-2). Soldo contends that the image of middle-aged adults balancing parental care duties and those of children gives an inappropriate picture for the majority of situations. Being caught in the middle is far from a typical experience (Rosenthal et al, 1996), though when it does occur, the pressures and conflicts are so tremendous it can be absolutely overwhelming.

Through the welter of descriptive studies of caregiving we need meta-analyses of similar issues such as gender, relationship type and quality, disabilities of elder and caregiver, ethnicity, living arrangement, and, perhaps most important, duration of care. Until some consistent parameters are defined and explored and studies are consistently

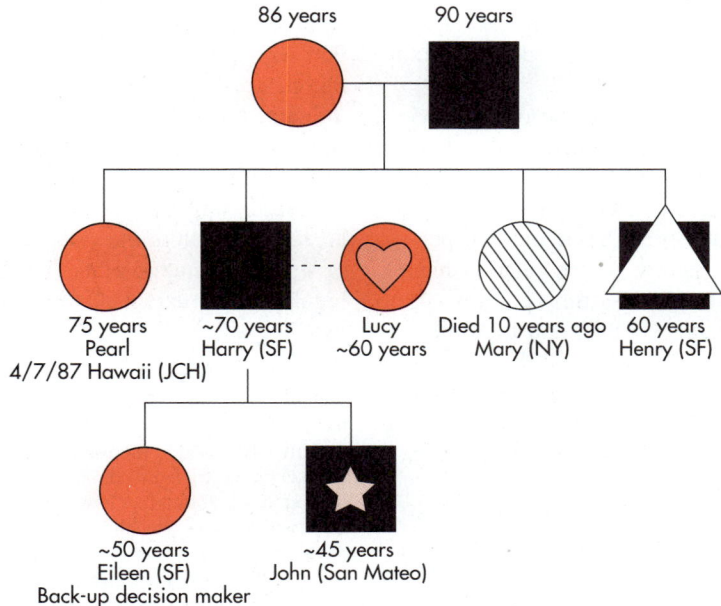

Notes
1. Prt. lives with husband in small room with shared bathroom and kitchen for 20 years.
2. Primary decision maker is grandson, John, who helped admit prt. to program. Handles finances.
3. 12/10/86 Durable Power of Attorney of health wishes signed and John designated.
4. Henry has been a very close friend and wants to be informed if something significant like death occurs.

Guidelines for Notes
a. Documentation is to be objective vs. impressions or subjective.
b. Include on diagram who would be the back-up decision maker (see comment on Eileen above).
c. If durable power of health care wishes and/or finances have been assigned, indicate in this area as well as in progress notes.
d. Any add-ons need to be initialed and dated (see comment on daughter Pearl above).

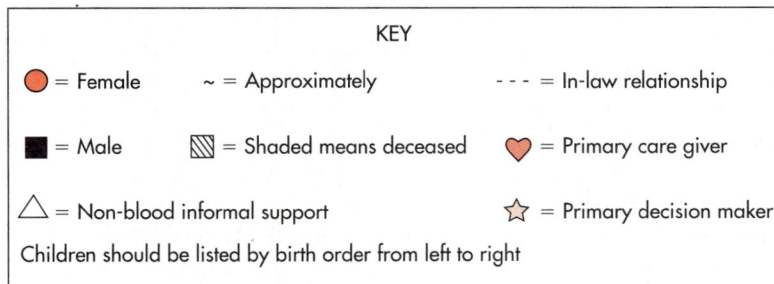

Figure 17-2. Family diagram (sample). (From Stanford Geriatric Education Center. Ethnogeriatric Conference, Jan 10, 1991, Stanford University, Palo Alto, Calif.)

replicated, we may be doomed to endless depictions of situations with little relief to the burdened caregivers.

Caregiving as a women's issue. Caregiving is a women's issue of crucial importance. It is estimated that 72% of care is given by females (Family Caregiver Alliance, 1996). One in four women become caregivers at some time between ages 35 and 44 and one in three between ages 55 and 64. Only 45% of the oldest cohort studied (born 1905 to 1917) were ever caregivers of elderly relatives compared with 64% of the present cohort (born 1927 to 1934) (Moen et al, 1994). To a large extent this is a result of the great increases in elderly women living to advanced old age, and we expect this trend to continue. Because of increasing numbers of frail elderly and strong trends toward their management in the home, policies must be adopted to provide supports for the female caregiver in the home.

There are two distinct categories of female caregiver: the spouse and the daughter. The single, never married daughter is particularly likely to be a caregiver for one or more parents (Brody et al, 1994). There are marked differences in wives and daughters in their adaptation, based on their perception of the role and prior quality of the relationship. Wives felt closer to the care recipient as time progressed, and daughters became more distant (Seltzer and Li, 1996). However, Cosbey and McMahon (1996) found that daughters caring for fathers often found that previously distant relationships became stronger and more intimate in the caregiving process, though some daughters found it difficult to give personal care to their fathers.

Spouse-caregivers may have no other major role to fulfill, whereas daughters often find their loyalties and energies split between husband, children, work, and aged parent. Daughters found difficulty when the demands of husband and father conflicted (Townsend and Franks, 1995). Most difficult for daughters is the pull between husband and parent, with all the conflicting roles and loyalties that are likely to occur, when there has never been a good relationship between them.

Psychologic well-being in the caretaker role has been correlated with high levels of social support and the ability to use a broad range of coping skills. Boucher et al (1996) found that many cognitively impaired spouses were attempting to care for a demented mate with few resources and marginal adequacy. Their coping skills were not sufficient for the demands placed upon them. These are important considerations for health care personnel who may be in the role of consultants or support persons to caregivers.

The older women's league (OWL). OWL was one of the first groups established specifically for the purpose of assisting older women in their caregiving roles. They have established a functional grass roots organization to respond directly to the concerns of caregivers in their own communities. Some volunteer groups, such as Sheehan (1989) reported, have developed to assist caregivers. "Natural" volunteer helpers from churches within a metropolitan

area were recruited for a training program in aging and caregiver support. From these efforts several programs were developed in various churches to reach out to community caretakers with assistance in problem solving and respite.

The needs of caregivers largely fall into a few categories: (1) support groups or allies, (2) knowledge of aging, (3) knowledge of resources, (4) respite, (5) financial assistance, and (6) recognition. George and Gwyther (1983, 1986) have designed a tool to assist the elderly and family in determining need for formal and informal supports (Figure 17-3). This is a simple questionnaire and the most practical that we have found.

Caregivers of elders with dementia. Caregivers of demented elders are thought to have the most difficult job, yet 96% agree it is a "labor of love" (Hoffman, 1996). Eighty one percent of these caregivers were women, 51% lived in the same household, and 30% were the sole caregiver. A "labor of love" may or may not mean the care is lovingly given, as the phrase seems to imply. "Labor of love" is often used to describe any labor that is unpaid. On the other hand it may be an indication of the caregiver's sense of duty, obligation, or simply having no other available alternative. Figure 17-4 highlights the extent of time involved in such a "labor of love."

A daughter, caring for her elderly mother afflicted with Alzheimer's disease, said she had previously thought it important to focus on reality. On one occasion, after trying unsuccessfully to convince her mother the month was May and not April, she went to get a calendar to show her. By the time she returned her mother had forgotten all about it. "It was then I realized that reality doesn't matter. That was the biggest breakthrough. If she thought it was April, what did it matter? I found that when I stopped correcting her and went along with her, it saved us both a lot of heartache. The content of the conversation did not matter as much as the feeling" (Hoffman, 1996).

A sense of humor helps.

Jane, an aide in a small facility, was trying to convince Bessie, an elder with dementia, to open her mouth for dental care. Bessie's mouth was tightly clamped shut. Jane remembered that Bessie frequently called for her dead father. Jane said, "Bessie, I hear your father, and he says you should open your mouth so you can have your teeth brushed." The registered nurse was aghast when she heard this, but Bessie compliantly opened her mouth. Jane cared about Bessie and her reality and used it to best advantage.

Elderly spouses caring for disabled partners have special needs. Often the spouse has significant health problems that are neglected in deference to the greater needs of the incapacitated partner. Most often the woman is in the role of caregiver and may be in dire need of caring and concern for herself. Life satisfaction tends to be limited when illness, low income, multiple demands, and the loss of intimacy and companionship converge on a conscientious mate. It is most difficult when the partner is aphasic or incontinent. Availability of children, relatives, and friends is significant in easing the load and increasing satisfaction. Respite from continuous care is essential (Feinberg and Kelly, 1995).

Women who care for a demented spouse seem to fare better if the relationship before illness had been close and remained so. Frustration was high for those wives who provided care based on a sense of obligation but perceived a significant change in the affectual tone of the relationship (Motenko, 1989). From a practical standpoint, nurses may encourage caregiving spouses to be alert to subtle signs of responsiveness. Periods when the patient is calm and content should be documented, and a log kept to help identify the times when the caregiver may feel gratified. These methods restore a sense of control and increase awareness of the positive aspects of caregiving. Jan said, "You know, I didn't think he knew me, but the other day I thought he said, 'I love you.' Of course, it was just a mumble, but I think that is what he said." Figure 17-5 illustrates the importance of small gains in maintaining the morale of a caregiving spouse.

The effects of caring for a cognitively impaired spouse are apparently quite different in men and women. Allen (1994) found that husbands are much more likely to have help with the hands-on care, whereas wives tend to be the sole caregivers. Moritz et al (1989) studied the responses of both sexes and found that men tend to become depressed to

---

Support for Caregivers

"Now I'd like to ask you about some of the ways your family and friends may help you out—either how they help you personally or the way they help you to care for your confused relative. For each question below, please check one column to indicate how often your family or friends give you that kind of help. Then please tell us the relationship of the person who gives you the most help of that type (for example, sister, friend, daughter-in-law)."

Type of Help Do your family or friends:	Never	Rarely	How often do you receive this help?			Relationship of helper
			Only if I ask	Now and then	Regularly	
1. Help you out when you are sick?						
2. Shop or run errands for you?						
3. Help you out with money or bills?						
4. Fix things around your house?						
5. Keep house for you or do household chores?						
6. Give you advice on business or finances?						
7. Provide companionship for you?						
8. Give you advice on dealing with problems?						
9. Provide transportation for you or your confused relative?						
10. Prepare or provide meals?						
11. Stay with your confused relative while you are away?						
12. Provide personal grooming services for your confused relative?						

13. Do you wish that your family and friends would give you more help with these kinds of things?
   1. No
   2. Yes

Figure 17-3. Informal support. (From George LK, Gwyther LP: *Duke University Caregiver Well-Being Survey,* Durham NC, 1983, Duke University Center for the Study of Aging and Human Development; Caregiver well-being: a multidimensional examination of family caregivers of demented adults, *Gerontologist* 26:253, 1986.)

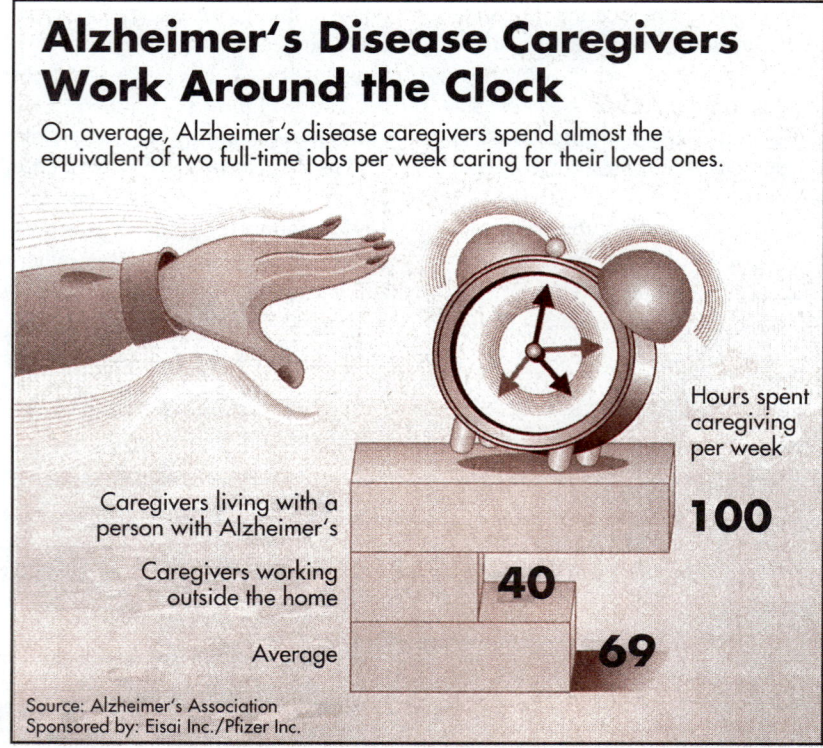

Figure 17-4. Time spent caring for patients with Alzheimer's disease.

a much greater degree than women caring for a demented spouse. Men responded with more concern to the lack of adequate financial support than to the loss of instrumental and emotional support or the decrease in intellectual and social participation.

Four sets of risk factors seem significant to the durability and acceptability of a caregiving relationship with a demented elder: the caregiving relationship, family life stressors outside of caregiving, individual and family coping styles, and the caregiver's perception of the situation (Rankin et al, 1992). In addition, tremendous tension is generated when caregiving interferes with highly valued activities (Stephens and Franks, 1995). The quality of life outside caregiving is important (Schott-Baer et al, 1995). These findings reinforce the importance of understanding and supporting the caregiver in efforts to care for the demented individual.

The ideal caretaker is one who:
- Is not threatened by the psychologic changes occurring in the patient
- Can facilitate effective communication by understanding the patient's increasingly tenuous connection with the phenomenal world
- Can use the relationship to strengthen the patient's sense of self
- Possesses the following characteristics:
  Compassion (most important)
  Flexibility (willingness to try the untried)

Sense of humor (keeping perspective)
Sense of timing (alteration of typical time expectations)
Acceptance (avoid arguing)
Ability to watch and touch (demonstrate genuine interest)
Capacity to talk without expecting an answer (recognize the individual even if he or she does not respond)

Five coping strategies were significant in reducing the perceived burden of care: (1) confidence in problem-solving ability, (2) ability to perceive the problems in alternative ways, (3) passivity in reference to things that could not be changed, (4) spiritual supports, and (5) an extended family (Pratt et al, 1985).

Caregiving: a cultural perspective. Blacks care for elders who are not related much more often than do whites (Lawton et al, 1992). Although there is no known explanation for that, it may be the residual of times past when survival itself depended on a close sense of community, whether related or not. This is a finding that bears further exploration with other ethnic groups.

Segall and Wykle (1988) studied the black family's experience caring for a demented parent. This is one of the few studies that has examined the ethnic perspective and is thus of considerable importance. Although blacks tend to live, on the average, 5 years less than whites and thus would

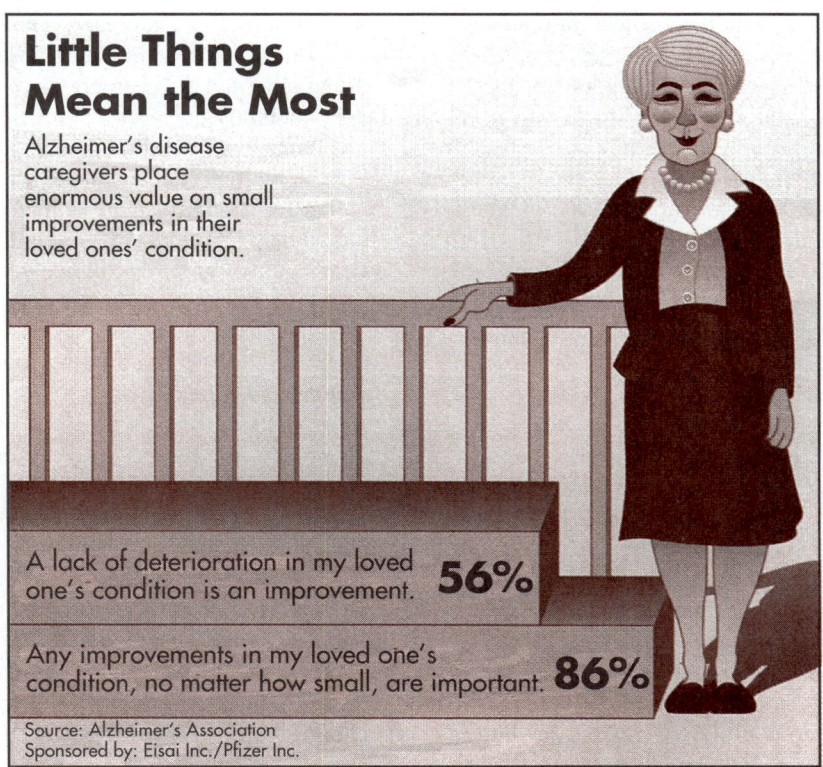

Little Things Mean the Most

Alzheimer's disease caregivers place enormous value on small improvements in their loved ones' condition.

A lack of deterioration in my loved one's condition is an improvement. **56%**

Any improvements in my loved one's condition, no matter how small, are important. **86%**

Source: Alzheimer's Association
Sponsored by: Eisai Inc./Pfizer Inc.

Figure 17-5. Little things mean the most for caregivers of patients with Alzheimer's disease.

have a lower number of elders surviving long enough to develop Alzheimer's disease, in the future we can expect significant numerical and percentile increases in the number of blacks living into late life. Mortimer et al (1981) found no racial or socioeconomic variation in the prevalence of Alzheimer's disease; therefore we may expect that as blacks live longer, the number developing Alzheimer's disease will increase.

Segall and Wykle focused their study on three issues: (1) what are the problems and stresses affecting caregivers of relatives with dementia? (2) what are the coping strategies used by the caregivers in response to the stress of care giving? and (3) what kind of help do the caregivers need in caring for the demented relative? Fifty-nine caregivers who were taking major responsibility for the care of a demented elder were interviewed in a semistructured manner and asked to respond to several instruments to measure stress and coping with the demands of caregiving.

Five categories of coping strategies were identified by Segall and Wykle (1988): accommodation, religious support (Taylor and Chatters, 1986), problem solving, wishful thinking, and emotional support. In spite of the fact that on average persons had been in the caregiver role for over 3 years, 80% assessed their overall health as good or excellent and reported moderately low levels of stress. Sixty-five percent said that prayer and faith in God were their major means of coping. Accommodating to the problems seemed to be

linked to the belief that there was a purpose and that they must do the best they could in the situation.

Haley et al (1995) found that black caregivers were less subject to depression than white caregivers. It is surmised that support and belief systems of blacks were more sustaining than those of whites.

Ozaki (1995), a retired Japanese nurse living in Chicago, has cared for her 97-year-old mother and lovingly expresses the cultural expectation of caring for the parent, pride in her ability to keep her mother comfortable and well, loving concern, and yet awareness of her own needs. The following are bits of her thoughts:

My mother has lived with our family for the past 36 years and has watched our three children grow up and reach maturity . . . All of my life I have liked caring for people, especially my mother . . . My mother compares her daughters and concludes that no one can take care of her "like Harue does." . . . She doesn't seem to realize that I need a break, time to rest and relax. . . . She doesn't often express thanks for the work I do. . . . I deal with the guilt when I do take time away by telling myself that it's for the good of all. The caregiver needs a day off and some freedom. The essense of freedom is essential to living. It is there for the taking. After all, if the caregiver cannot be a happy person, the care receiver will not be cared for at an optimum." (Ozaki, 1995.)

Emerging problems. Though we tend to think of caregivers as those middle-aged adults caring for elders, an unknown number of elders are caring for their middle-aged children who are physically and mentally disabled. Earlier in the century these developmentally disabled children usually died prior to reaching adulthood; now, with improved care they are surviving. Often this has been a burden carried by parents for their entire adult life and will end only with the death of the parent or the adult child. In a study of 115 older mothers (ages 58 to 96 years) caring for mentally retarded offspring, religion and prayer emerged as critical aspects of their coping, though they often questioned why God was letting them suffer so (Tobin et al, 1994). This problem as a mental health issue is discussed more fully in Chapter 21 and is an issue that the Society of Friends is giving serious attention to (Schwartz and Kelly, 1996).

There are 11 million blended families in the United States (Vinick et al, 1996), and this trend is expected to continue and perhaps increase. These stepfamilies and the long-range implications for elders needing care are stirring interest among gerontologists. The generational reciprocity so fundamental to our present system of survival of young and old may develop in entirely different ways or simply break down. A conceivable scenario would extend the "yours, mine, and ours" theme of blended families beyond childraising to elder caring: "My children could take care of me in their homes, your children could take care of you in their homes, but they will expect our children to take care of us in our own home." Prenuptial agreements regarding asset inheritance are common in later marriages, but agreements regarding inheritance of caregiving responsibilities are notorious by their absence.

Interestingly, the Asians, specifically Chinese, Malaysians, and Indians living in Singapore, are now able to sue their children for support and are doing so. In South Korea, adult children may be held legally responsible for the costs of their parent's care (Charging children for care of aging parents, 1996).

In countries that are seriously limiting population growth, such as China, filial responsibility will necessarily be attenuated. In addition, as more and more youth are dying of AIDS in their prime years, more elders will be left with one or no children to carry on. Costs of caregiving, emotionally and economically, are a worldwide problem that will continue to tax the ingenuity of world populations as longevity increases.

Assessment. Assessing the family's needs, strengths, and stresses as well as its support system and family diagram will assist the nurse in gaining a holistic picture of the interventions that may strengthen the family unit (Figure 17-6 and Box 17-4). A mutually constructed, written assessment of a family's needs and coping capacities can be com-

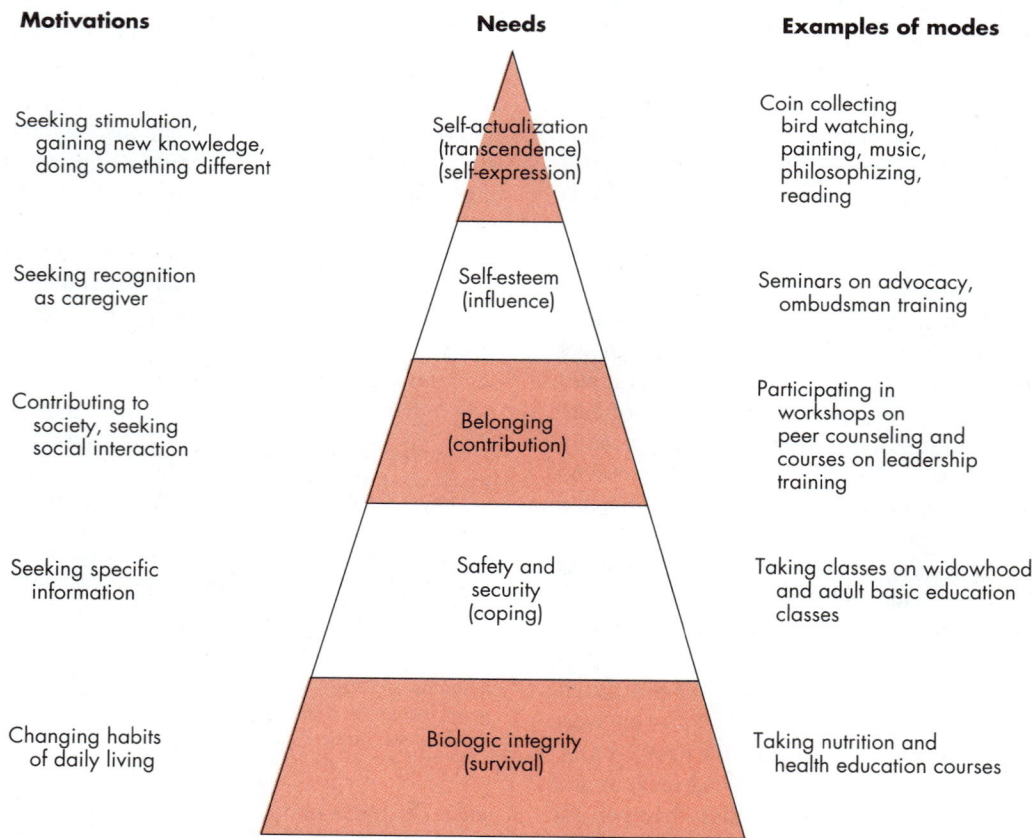

Figure 17-6. Family support problems and interventions.

prehensive and specific and becomes a document of their strengths in times of stress. Foci to be included are sources of stress, particular coping methods, resources that are used or can be used, and the rewards and problems of caregiving.

Although staff are cognizant of the need for written care plans and evaluation of patient progress, this may not be shared with or given to the family. Inclusion in the development of a nursing care plan and periodic evaluation may help family members assess their effectiveness even in the face of patient decline. Factors that are indices of coping in the caretaking role include perceived well-being, perceived social support, promotion of functional ability of the care receiver, and positive relationship to the care receiver (Georgemiller et al, 1987).

Counseling Families. Nurses may be instrumental in counseling families by encouraging all involved family members to discuss their needs and concerns. Including

young and aged family members is most likely to produce satisfactory results. Too often plans are made for the aged rather than with them. It is important to anticipate needs and crises and form contingency plans before they are needed (Wolanin, 1979).

Families may not know where to turn for support and guidance when needed. Nurses in contact with the middle-aged might ask about aged family members and their plans and expectations for the future and explore their awareness of possible resources or agencies to contact during times of crisis. Area Agency on Aging offices are located throughout the United States, and these are able to direct people to community services and agencies.

Health care workers consulting with middle-aged people might routinely ask, "What is happening with your aging relatives?" Adroit questions can explore functional state, quality of relationships, or tentative plans that have been discussed or stimulate some thought when the problems and issues have been ignored.

Sometimes people just need an opportunity to share the difficulties they are experiencing. Having an attentive listener without any emotional commitment may allow ventilation, release of stored-up feelings, and a restoration of energy to continue in a difficult situation. Some problems are not totally resolvable but may be borne if a supportive network is available, such as help from immediate and extended family. Recognizing this, nurses may see their function as ancillary and sustaining to family function.

Our greatest contribution to the care of the aged may be to modify our institutional and agency service delivery patterns toward sustaining the natural tendency of families to care for dependent members. Rice (1996) points out that families may refuse to provide this care if they feel incapable or not so inclined. However, many families do not know this and are reluctant to refuse. It is the nurse's responsibility to let them know they have this option.

Long-distance caring. A network of services is beginning to emerge to assist the geographically distant family member in ensuring that an elderly relative will be taken care of. In many cases a "case manager" approach is being used, in which the individual calls a care-coordinating entrepreneurial resource broker. Some nurses and social workers have seen the need and are developing this type of service. It is only available to those who are able to pay, since it is presently not covered by private insurance or public agencies of any kind.

City and county referral services or case managers through private agencies may assist family members in solving difficult problems in caring for an elderly parent. Often they may know of resources that can allow the elder to remain independent and yet assure the family that safety and other needs are being met. Case management services can be particularly useful to families who are geographically remote from the aging parent who needs assistance.

Issues for which the caregiver may need guidance are listed in Box 17- 5 (Heath, 1993). These must be covered by

Box 17-4	**Family Support System Assessment**	
Size	Number in extended family that are accessible	
	Number of daughters that are accessible	
	Number of sons that are accessible	
	Number of grandchildren, nephews, nieces, confidants, siblings	
Ability	Economic status of each	
	Poverty	
	Lower middle	
	Middle	
	Upper middle	
	Wealthy	
Willingness	Frequency of involvement	
	Monthly	
	Weekly	
	Daily	
	Constant	
Functions	Contributions to aged member	
	Money	
	Chores	
	Transportation	
	Listening/psychologic support	
	Functional assistance	
Deterrents	Other demands	
	Work	
	Travel	
	Adolescent children	
Recent stresses	Poor health	
	Job change	
	Moves	
	Deaths	

The strengths of the family or possible dysfunctional aspects can be assessed in a superficial but helpful manner by using the Family APGAR (Smilkstein et al, 1982). See Appendix 17-A for APGAR tool.

- How to handle emergencies
- How to prepare for scheduled and unscheduled visits
- How to quickly find people in your older relative's community to help with day-to-day needs
- How to get a handle on legal and financial issues
- How to organize and conduct a family meeting
- What to do when your job takes you to another state, or even another country
- And much more.

From Heath A: *Long distance caregiving,* Lakewood, Colo, 1993, American Source Books.

the case manager in advance of any evidence of problems. Well thought out plans and alternatives will prevent hasty decisions with unwanted ramifications. In many cases appropriate actions may forestall the need to move the parent into the child's home (see resources at the end of the chapter).

Employer assistance in the care of elders. Nearly one third of working adults have some caregiving responsibilities toward older parents or other relatives. Only 1% of a sample of working women between ages 21 and 50 actually left the labor force for a full year to provide care for an elderly relative (Sandell and Iams, 1996). The preponderance of middle-aged working women carry on the demands of caregiving in addition to work and other responsibilities (Boaz, 1996). Unfortunately, employee assistance programs (EAPs) that have provided some supports and assistance are being downgraded and attenuated in the restructuring and downsizing of corporations (Lechner and Neal, 1996).

Surveys conducted by several large companies indicate a link between employee productivity and care-giving responsibilities at home. In the 1990s, elder care has become as significant an issue as was child care in the 1980s. The age group most involved with elder care is between 40 and 49 years of age; many also have children for whom they are still responsible.

An elder care survey conducted by The National Alliance for Caregiving found that 22.4 million households provide caregiving to elderly friends or relatives; 64% of caregivers are working full or parttime. Three fourths report that they receive some help from others; a typical elder requires an average of 18 hours of care per week, most commonly with bathing, dressing, and eating. Other help commonly given involves household chores, transportation, and shopping. Half of all caregivers spend, out-of-pocket, an average of $171 a month. These data provide some basis for future investigation and planning for the needs of burdened employees (National Alliance for Caregiving, 1996).

Several companies are designing employee respite time, flextime, and unpaid personal leaves to assist the employee. Remington Corporation funds some respite care programs for employees, and Pepsi Company has a hot line and a community resource book for the support of working caregivers.

IBM has developed a network of 175 community organizations called Elder Care Referral Service (ECRS) to provide consultation, consumer information, and individualized referrals for IBM employees, retirees, and their spouses. It is employer supported, nationwide in scope, and focuses on the needs of the caregiver (Caregiving for elders gets corporate help, 1995). With information provided by experts with local knowledge, ECRS gives access to assistance in the community where the service is needed. Features include the following:

- Personalized consultation
- Information about the range of service options in the area
- Individualized referrals currently available
- Consumer education
- Guidance through the process of decision making
- Follow-up to determine whether needs were met

The service is especially helpful when the caregiver lives at a distance from the elder needing service. This model will undoubtedly generate similar efforts in other large corporations.

The corporate nurse working with the family and the aged person is in a unique position to maximize all of these supports. Human needs can be identified, and through empowering the support network, encouraging reciprocity within it, and linking the client system with the service system, goals can be accomplished.

Institutionalization. Families may feel defeated when a parent must be institutionalized. The efforts they have expended are rewarded with decline. It is imperative that nurses reinforce the family's adequacy and importance to the aged member.

Family support groups to deal with institutionalization. Richards (1986) found that family support groups for those who had placed an elder were important in adaptation and coping of the elder and the family. Goals of these groups can be seen in Box 17-6.

Caregiving issues are likely to remain in the forefront of discussions of public policy and concerns about family life. There is a continuing need for investigations which identify potentially modifiable features of caregivers' situations, and which contribute to the development and evaluation of interventions to assist families (Zarit, 1991).

Contributions of the Old to Family Life

The flow of help from adult child to parent is not unidirectional, although in the previous portion of this chapter our focus has been primarily related to the needs of the old in relation to their families. We will give attention now to the needs of adult children in relation to parents. The aged provide family historical perspective, models for growing old, assistance with grandchildren, a sense of continuity, and a philosophy of aging. In many cases the old continue to contribute money, gifts, status, and services to their adult children. Soldo and Hill (1993) contend that it is far more likely that elderly parents will give financial help to children and grandchildren than that they will receive it.

In addition, if one moves beyond the moment, it is apparent that the old have contributed their time and energy across the adult life span to provide opportunities for their children. Perhaps even more important, they appreciate the success of their children and convey their approval and pride. Although adults are motivated in the process of maturation by personal more than external motivation, there is still pleasure in knowing that one's parents are pleased with various accomplishments. Even at 50 years old, I felt a sense of sadness that my mother was unaware of certain significant events in my life. Just as Scott-Maxwell (1968) noted the tendency to always remain a parent concerned about the development of her child, so the adult child always needs the interest of the parent. Parental maturity supports adult-child maturation.

Not only mature adults but also their children benefit from the influence of a vital old person. They provide anticipatory socialization into old age. Not only that, but elders often tend to serve as "kin-keepers." *Kin-keeper* is a term used to denote a family member who arranges get-togethers, develops the family history and rituals, and in other ways promotes solidarity and unity among the kin (Rosenthal, 1985).

Grandma Daisy always merited a special visit from any of the kin in her vast Northwestern network. A pioneer settler in her small community, she knew the names, ages, and whereabouts of the children and spouses and the grandchildren and spouses of all her eight children. They seldom saw each other but always felt a connecting link through Grandma Daisy. When she died at age 94, a great portion of the family history and sense of solidarity died with her. She was a true kin-keeper.

Box 17-6	**Goals of Family Support Groups**

Learn to accept the elder as he or she is now; let go of the past.
Learn the balance between protectiveness and smothering.
Recognize one's own needs as fundamental to caring for others.
Learn to share and cope with disappointment.
Discuss resurgence of feelings of loss during holidays and anniversaries.
Share knowledge of how to deal with family and community.
Develop a caring and sharing network within the group.
Deal with feelings of guilt, helplessness, and hopelessness.
Identify realistic ways to assist in the care of the elder.

Modified from Richards M: Family support groups, *Generations* 10(4):68, Summer, 1986.

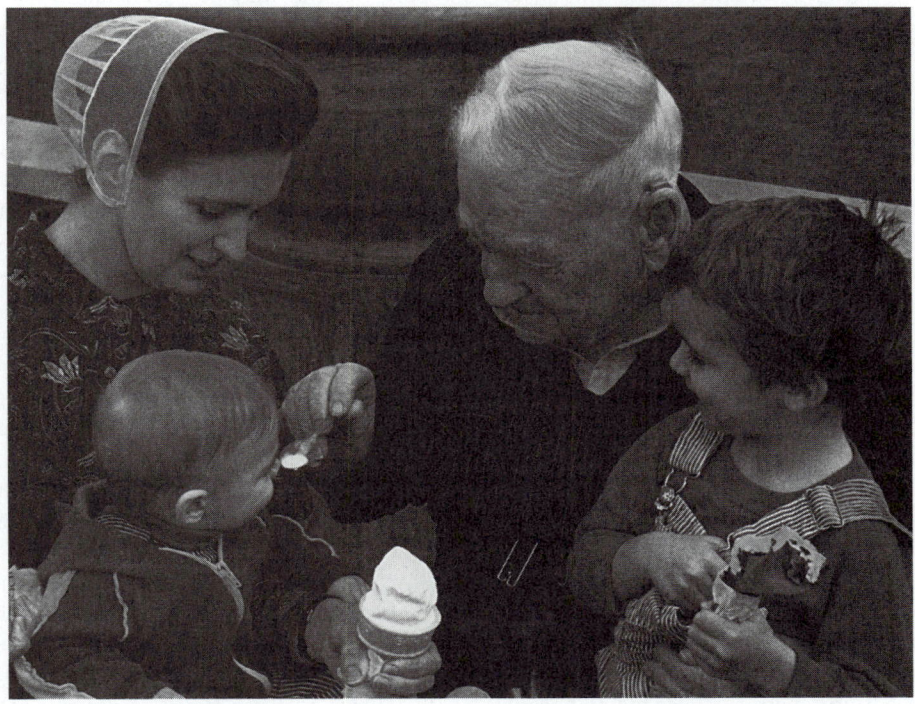

Strengthening family ties. (Courtesy Rod Schmall.)

Surrogate Family Forms

There are many nontraditional ways of viewing family, although these are less common among the old than the young. Some surrogate families of sufficiently absorbing nature to furnish primary ties might include the following:

1. The "share-a-home" concept, in which senior adults share a household
2. Integration of the elderly into a foster family
3. Boarding houses, which were common in the late nineteenth and early twentieth century industrial centers and provided a family surrogate for many single urban dwellers

There are many other such loosely defined substitute families functioning for old people. Additional discussion related to housing can be found in Chapter 13.

For many older people without families an effort could be made by the individual or service providers to develop a cadre of fictive kin. *Fictive kin* are nonblood kin who serve as "genuine fake families," as expressed by Virginia Satir. These become surrogate family and take on some of the instrumental and affectional attributes of family. Some elders alone adopt TV families and speak of them as if they were related (Genevay, 1992). Often primary care providers or case managers become fictive kin.

Genevay warns that nurses and other health care providers must understand their own needs and discourage the fictive kin role if they really cannot emotionally and professionally cope with it to the advantage of the elder and themselves. Potential problems are that the providers may become prone to self-sacrifice, and (2) the ethics and responsibilities are far more complex and unclear than in the professional role.

Gays and Lesbians

We are increasingly aware of the aged and the family styles they have developed as gays and lesbians. Kimmel (1992) believes gays and lesbians are often involved in three different family structures simultaneously: the family of origin, the family of spouse and children, and the family of friends and lovers. Though it is an issue before the courts, it is not legal in most states for same-gender couples to marry. However, many of them enter into marriage contracts and are legally registered as domestic partners. It is unknown how many of these involve old persons. We need much more knowledge of cohort and generational differences between age groups to understand the recent, dramatic changes in the lives of lesbians and gays in family lifestyles (Kimmel, 1992).

In terms of elderly parents and relationships with adult gay children, Allen and Wilcox (1996) found that coming to terms with the disclosure of the adult child involved several transitions. These were denial, acceptance, complacency, and in the majority of cases, the move toward political activism and advocacy for the civil rights of gays, as well as other groups suffering discrimination. These elders became stimulated to work for social change.

SECONDARY RELATIONSHIPS

Although family and friends seem to be most effective in acute, emergency situations and for affective sustenance, others are needed for long-term support, enjoyment, variety, services of various kinds, and augmentation of primary relationships.

Group Affiliations

Group affiliations are secondary and complementary to intense primary relationships that, by their very intensity and singularity, leave the aged vulnerable in the absence of secondary relationships. Secondary supports may also be more durable than primary because they are not bound by conflicting feelings. They do not have long-standing intimate histories and rarely involve constant exposure.

Secondary relationships are characterized by their parameters. Usually they are recreational or service oriented, somewhat superficial, and constrained by specific needs or goals. Professionals are often the instigators, facilitators, or connecting link to secondary networks. Fees for service are often a restricting element. Groups providing secondary support networks may be formal or informal. Either may function well or poorly, depending on the needs of the aged participants and the skill of the group leader.

Informal Groups. Informal groups are those that spontaneously arise and have few restrictions, expectations, or goals. They are secondary networks by virtue of their low intensity and lack of demands. In fact, we might call them tertiary groups (or those at a third level of importance) because they cannot be relied on to provide interpersonal support, but they may be significant in one's particular adaptation. Examples of such groups include informal groups of the aged that arise at nutrition sites, gatherings of old people observed in city parks, senior citizen activities (these have formal and informal components), groups that cluster together in long-term care or residential settings, or any group that occurs sporadically for the purpose of socialization, discussion, or participation in a particular activity.

Formal Groups. Formal groups are defined by their expectations, dependability, and goals. The intensity of interpersonal exchange varies in accordance with the members' and groups' goals. The development and maintenance of aged peer groups are particularly important when friends are no longer available. The great advantage of group affiliations for the aged is in the diffusion of relationship intensity and the constancy over time. A reliable group maintains its function despite the loss or addition of members. This is an important consideration when working with the aged.

Needs Assessment. Groups can be organized to meet any level of Maslow's hierarchy; obviously they often meet multiple needs. Using the assessment of social climate and human needs as basic guides, one can begin a determination of the type of group most suitable in a given situation.

There are three types of groups: (1) groups to accomplish something tangible, (2) groups meant for therapy, and

(3) groups that promote personal development and growth. The distinction between the second and third types is in the readiness of members. Therapy groups imply some psychologic deficit or conflict and should be led by qualified personnel. Nurses with training in psychotherapy often do an excellent job in such groups. The third type of group does not explore deep psychologic needs, but rather in helping persons extend and grow they often resolve some of the less-ingrained personality problems. By moving people through a series of group situations in a hierarchic fashion, we often discover latent growth potential (Figure 17-7).

Some basic assessment parameters may help define particular levels of need of the aged (Box 17-7).

This limited survey of needs, problems, and possible groups shows the versatility and potential of group work with the aged, which is a fertile area for creative nurses.

Group Goals. Functional goals for groups of aged include the following:

Socialization—interpersonal exchange
Therapeutic—healing through group
Entertainment
Cohort affiliation
Increased functional levels
Stimulation/environmental enrichment
Activation/movement
Behavioral management
Staff morale
Family morale
Autonomy

These might all be included in six overall goals, which Ebersole (1978) calls six R's for the aged:

1. Reality orientation
2. Remotivation
3. Reminiscence
4. Recognition
5. Recreation
6. Released potential

Group Structure. Implementing a group follows a thorough assessment of environment, needs, and potential for various group strategies. Major goal decisions are reached, and with those decisions several structural decisions are intrinsic. For instance, several aged diabetics in an acute-care setting may need health care teaching regarding diabetes. The nurse sees the major goal as restoring order (or control) in each individual's lifestyle.

Guide for Evaluation of Group Meetings. Some factors used to evaluate group meetings:

1. *Setting.* Seating arrangement, room comfort, activities carried on in area, facilities; note movement of chairs, reseating, and objects that facilitate or distract.
2. *Goal.* How established? Who included in decision about goal? Flexibility of goal.
3. *Participants.* List attendees, age, physical problems of importance to group, sex, mobility.

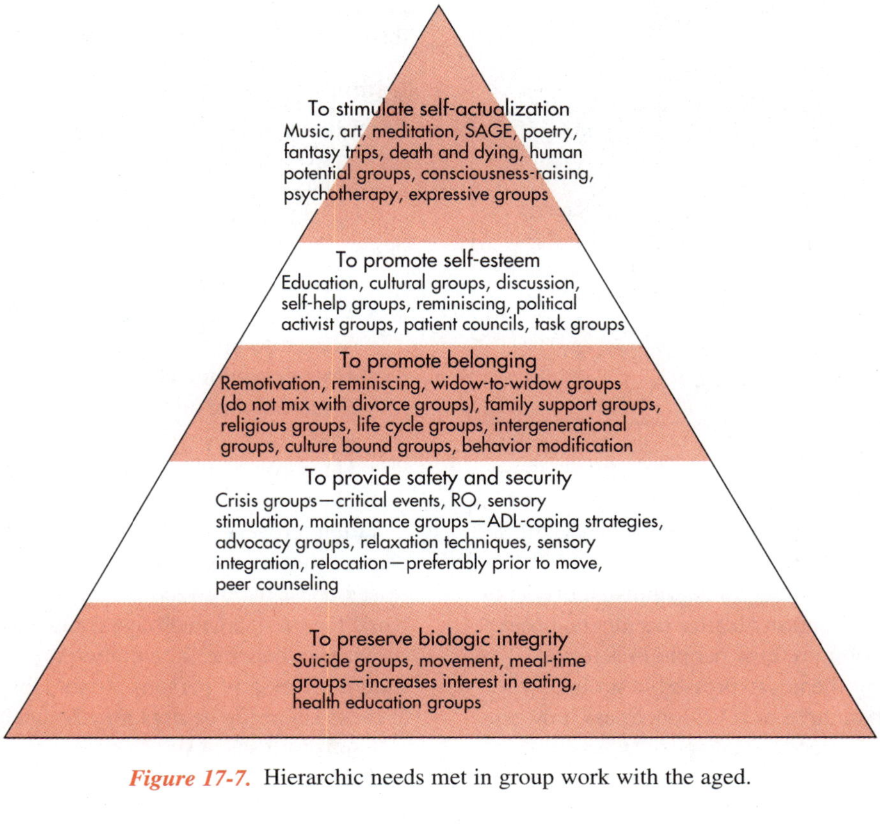

Figure 17-7. Hierarchic needs met in group work with the aged.

Box 17-7	**Choosing a Group According to Need**

Needs and Problems	Suggested Group
Biologic integrity	
Confusion—disorientation	Reality orientation
Loss of sexual satisfaction or opportunity	Male/female groups
Poor nutrition	Mealtime groups
Drugs—inadequate rest	Relaxation groups
Body preoccupation	Health monitoring groups (e.g., blood pressure or feet and mouth examinations)
Safety and security	
Impaired sensory perception	Sensory awareness training
Immobility	Movement groups
Translocation	Patient councils, environmental planning groups
Belonging	
Isolation	Socialization
Rejection of cohorts	Activities
Alienation from family	Family groups, cohort groups
Loss of significant others	Grief group
Self-Esteem	
Uselessness	Reminiscing groups
Lack of work	Productive groups
Lack of love objects	Remotivation groups
Lack of recognition	Discussion groups
Depression	Therapy groups, expressive groups
Self-Actualization	
Stimulation deprivation	Most groups, particularly those using touch
Apathy	Interest groups
Acceptance of cultural myths ("Old dogs can't learn new tricks.")	Discussions, debates, educational groups, creative/expressive groups

4. *Interactions.* Dyads? Triads? Miniconversations, monologues, effects of placement, role of leader, roles of members.
5. *Process.* Mood of group at beginning, unusual events in setting, in community, nation, deaths, accidents, upset in ward or agency routines, new people in setting.
6. *Themes.* Outstanding themes expressed in group, usually not more than three or four: loneliness, power or lack of autonomy, rejection, universality, independence.

7. *Problems.* How were they handled? Was the approach effective? If problems occur again, what could be done?
8. *Significant content.* One intervention that was goal directed and worked. One intervention that was unsatisfactory and what would have been more helpful.
9. *Evaluation of goal accomplishment.* Portions of goal accomplished; serendipity, evaluation of group progress, plans for next meeting related to evaluation of previous group meeting.

Groups of the aged have some unique aspects that require an extraordinary commitment on the part of the leader:

1. They often need assistance or transportation in getting to the group.
2. They may need more stimulation and are less self-motivating. (This is, of course, not true of self-help and senior activist groups such as the Gray Panthers.)
3. Many aged people likely to be in need of groups are depressed. The depression can be contagious, and leaders become depressed.
4. Leaders must be prepared for some members to become ill, deteriorate, and die.
5. Leaders are continually confronted with their own aging and attitudes toward it.

Group leaders need to plan in advance to incorporate a consistent support person in the group if possible. If not, someone must be available for planning and recapitulation of group sessions. Students should generally work in pairs and will need supervision. Skills in developing and implementing groups for the aged improve with experience. Even though the effort is sometimes draining, there are many rewards.

Community Affiliations

Community networks may not be visible to a casual observer. Even the aged individual may initially state he or she has no one to turn to when in need. The nurse must be specific to discover an existing network. Such questions as these may elucidate a secondary network in the community:

- How did you get to the doctor the last time you went?
- Where do you get your hair cut?
- Where do you buy your groceries?
- How do you manage your laundry?
- What did you do the last time you experienced a crisis?
- Have you called anyone for assistance recently?
- Have you been a member of any organizations?

Often grocery clerks, barbers, hotel managers, physicians, druggists, bankers, bus drivers, ministers, and waitresses are a barely recognized part of the community network for the "isolated" aged. Downtown shopping centers sometimes become the counterpart of the historical village square for elderly persons alone. Observing their behaviors in these shopping centers may be useful to nurses.

Communities of the Past. Celebrating shared memories of the communities in one's past through preservation of historic places, developing commemorative markers, seeking the places of youth and preserving the image in art and photo—all of these connect individuals' present to past and to the sense of community (Norris-Baker and Scheidt, 1996). A well-known example of this is the Vietnam Women's Memorial in the National Mall. The sense of communion with those involved is stirring when we gather in its presence. Another, more pertinent to the very old, is the raising of the flag on Iwo Jima, photographed by Joe Rosenberg in 1944. Aged men who fought in the Pacific have a particularly strong affinity for this.

Residential Communities. Old people in residential communities such as low-cost housing units and retirement complexes develop a sustaining network of contacts. Just as in other settings and stages of life, the women are more often the social agents. The implication for nurses is the recognition that old men living alone may need more assistance in making contacts than old women. Throughout life their relationships have been structured in a work setting, whereas women have learned to develop and maintain networks in myriad situations.

Retirement Communities. People who enter retirement communities are generally affluent and do so by choice. They necessarily sever some ties in the larger community, but many are maintained. Those who argue against the seclusiveness of these senior communities may not be fully aware of the advantages. Social events, friendships, and reliances abound in these exclusive settings. Security is maintained. Speakers, entertainers, and services are available in the community, and persons rarely need to leave the compound unless they wish. This is certainly one option for relatively wealthy old people who wish to relate to age peers and enjoy a country club atmosphere (see further discussion in Chapter 13).

Neighborhood Networks. Informal neighborhood support services for the frail elderly have been developed in many communities. The residents in these neighborhoods identify benefits such as opportunities for socialization, use of lifetime skills, and personal support in time of need.

In Riverdale, NY, a group has developed barter services. It involves people and agencies within a neighborhood arranging to exchange or share services, space, and equipment in behalf of the aged to promote community well-being. Bartering arrangements are established and publicized through a small service-swapping Yellow Pages directory. This model incurs no expense, does not rely on large organizations and policy restrictions, and seems a natural way of providing many needed services (Noberini and Berman, 1983). Some of the successful swaps:

1. College students studying foreign languages were matched with residents of a home for the aged who speak the same language, giving the older person an opportunity to converse and the student an opportunity to improve conversational language skills.

2. Fifth-grade public school children visited a group of elderly residents of an apartment complex on a weekly basis. In exchange, the administrators of the complex offered the children a six-session minicourse on the problems and concerns of institutional living.

3. Residents of a nursing home are serving as English tutors to elementary school youngsters from a Hispanic community. In exchange, the teenage siblings of these youngsters shop, provide escort services, and perform other personal chores for the nonambulatory institutionalized elderly.

Agencies. Chapters 13 and 14 provide many examples of how the lives of the elderly are interlocked and infiltrated with federal, state, county, and local agencies. Rather than providing a nourishing surface root system (relating to our tree analogy early in this chapter), their overlapping, intertwining nature may choke the life from an old tree. They are like the undergrowth that may hamper one from reaching the tree. The secondary relationships with specific agency personnel may in some cases be gratifying, but too often we hear of the frustration of the bureaucratic jungle. Policies that would integrate agencies and decrease the number of contacts within these networks would be more efficient and more meaningful to the old.

Nurses can assist in the task of helping old people identify key personnel in critical areas and consistently ask for the same person. This tends to create tentative supportive relationships between the personnel and aged clients. For example, advise old people to always obtain the name of an individual in phone or personal contacts and to consistently seek that person for further service. Obviously, continuity of personnel is not always predictable, but this is a move toward the establishment of accountability. The move toward case management and managed care can, if done well, serve to enlarge the network of elders in a gratifying manner.

NURSES AS MEMBERS OF NETWORKS

Throughout this chapter our intent has been to convey the sustenance derived from thriving primary and secondary relationships. Nurses often develop close ties with old people because we are with them during their most vulnerable moments. We have a privileged position in relation to the aged and must be aware of the quality of our relationships. Often we become like family, particularly to residents in long-term care situations. Our task is to help support existing relationships and attempt to find ways in which the old can find substitutes for those lost or no longer available. We might view nurses as providing transitional caring relationships that sometimes evolve into personal attachments of great significance to the nurse and the client or patient.

Nursing Diagnoses

The following potential diagnoses must be considered as well as diagnoses unique to the particular individual:

Communication, impaired
Conflict, parental role
Family processes, altered
Growth and development, altered
Risk for caregiver role strain
Parenting, altered
Role performance, altered
Self-esteem, disturbance
Sexuality patterns, altered
Social interaction, impaired

NURSING PROCESS AND NURSING DIAGNOSIS
Ineffective Family Coping: Declining Parent

Etiologies and Related Factors

Illness
Living arrangements
Change in functional ability
Loss of parent's spouse
Financial strain
Ethnicity/culture/filial responsibility
Ambivalent family relationships
Coping discrepancies

Defining Characteristics

Lack of mutual respect
Rigid family roles
Lack of space/privacy
Intolerance
Family unable to meet physical/emotional/spiritual needs
Inability to express and accept feelings
Inability to relate to each other
Ineffective decision making
Poor communication of family rules, rituals, symbols
Fears and doubts about elder's physical/emotional capabilities
History of sibling contention

Knowledge

Psychosocial/cultural aging
Family systems/family dynamics
Role theory
Maturational and situational crisis management
Areas of parental conflicts: space; possessions; entertaining; responsibilities and chores; expenses
Family assessment and tools (i.e., APGAR; FACE; Family Dynamic Measures)

Counseling skills
Group process
Coping strategies
Health education teaching
Caregiving patterns
Community resources

Clinical Judgment and Related Skills

Perform a family assessment
Assist family to focus on potential conflict areas
Avoid giving advice
Assist family to problem solve and develop contingency plans for unexpected events
Encourage family to verbalize feelings and share feelings and personal impact of dependent parent on them
Listen actively
Assist family in identifying causes and contributing factors to ineffective coping
Facilitate family strengths
Teach coping strategies, stress reduction techniques, communication skills, available resources (i.e., respite care)
Family counseling

Evaluation

Comfortable expressing feelings
Effective decision making
Anticipatory preparations in place for contingencies
Discusses adaptations made
Knowledge of available services
Utilization of available services as needed

NEEDS ADDRESSED AND TASK STRENGTHS

Need for connectedness with others, sharing and mutuality (to achieve and maintain a sense of belonging and self-esteem)
Develops reciprocal relationships

Establishes personally satisfying generational role
Balances own needs with those of others in relationships
Maintains contact with significant kin and friends
Is both self- and other-directed

KEY CONCEPTS

- Primary relationships are those that involve some degree of intimacy and reciprocity. Those ties due to kinship carry some rights, expectations, and obligations.
- Long-lasting couple relationships are becoming more and more frequent; numerous couples celebrate 50th and 75th wedding anniversaries. To some extent this may be a cohort phenomenon of the oldest generation.
- Marriage is beneficial to old men and somewhat less beneficial to old women. Single elderly women have great survival capacity while single elderly men are the most vulnerable.
- The aged and each of their family members carry a long history. Current family dynamics must be understood within the context of family history.
- Sibling relationships may increase in importance during old age as individuals cope with various losses.
- Grandparenting is a significant role among elders. Frequently grandparents are the primary provider for young children and function as parents.
- Caregiving of elderly parents is one of the major social issues of our times. Adult children most often will spend some time caring for aged parents.
- "Parenting" one's parents is a commonly used misnomer. Parents, no matter how vulnerable, do not become children. The life they have lived must be considered regardless of the present situation.
- Women most often provide the "hands-on" care while men are more frequently involved in the economic and practical aspects of caregiving.
- Groups and community activities may be relied on for supportive relationships when family and friends are not available. These can be considered secondary relationships although they may be the only ones the individual has. Quite often these evolve into meaningful primary relationships.
- A complex and extensive secondary relationship network may be sustaining and actually preferred by some elders over more intense and demanding primary relationships.

▲ CASE STUDY

Ivy and John were high school sweethearts. A few weeks before they celebrated their 50th wedding anniversary Ivy began to notice that John was becoming very forgetful. He went to the grocery store and came home empty-handed because he had no idea why he had gone. Other changes in his lifestyle and personality became apparent. He was becoming careless in his grooming, and he had always been meticulous. His usual sleeping pattern was disturbed, and he would often wander about during the night. Ivy wondered if these were normally expected changes because of aging. Their three children lived in opposite ends of the country, but when they came to the anniversary celebration, they noticed dramatic changes in their father's personality. He was irrita-

ble and was easily angered, which was not at all the way they remembered him. Upon the insistence of the children, Ivy agreed he should see a doctor. John refused because he felt there was nothing wrong with him. Ivy had always complied with John's wishes, so she persuaded the children that she could manage just fine and whatever was wrong was probably a temporary reaction to something. After the children returned to their homes and Ivy returned to her usual household routines, she realized she was feeling tired all the time and it seemed whatever she did would make John angry. There was just no pleasing him. She began to lose weight and was unable to sleep. John's rambling about worried her and just everything worried her. She struggled through the days. She told one of her church friends, "I feel like I'm carrying a sack of lead on my back." Somehow a year passed, and John was getting more difficult and forgetful each day. She rarely left the house because she was afraid he would do something dangerous or hurt himself. Finally, Ivy went to the doctor because her extreme fatigue made her fear she had leukemia or some other debilitating disease. She was given numerous diagnostic tests, but no particular problem was uncovered. As she was preparing to leave the doctor's office, the nurse noticed how teary and unnerved she appeared.

Based upon the case study, develop a nursing care plan using the following procedure*:

List comments of client that provide *subjective data*.

List information that provides *objective data*.

From these data identify and state, using accepted format, two *nursing diagnoses* you determine are most significant to this client at this time. List two *client strengths* that you have identified from data.

Determine and state *outcome criteria* for each diagnosis. These must reflect some alleviation of the problem identified in the nursing diagnosis and must be stated in concrete and measurable terms.

Plan and state one or more *interventions* for each diagnosed problem. Provide specific documentation of source used to determine appropriate intervention. Plan at least one intervention that incorporates the client's existing strengths.

Evaluate success of intervention. Interventions must correlate directly with the stated outcome criteria in order to measure the outcome success.

STUDY QUESTIONS/ACTIVITIES

If you were the nurse, how would you begin to deal with this lady?

What information would you seek from her?

Where might you refer her?

*Students are advised to refer to their nursing diagnosis text and identify possible or potential problems.

After discussing this case with a partner or a small group, determine the uppermost problem in this situation and develop an appropriate nursing care plan.

Discuss the various elements of support groups and the rationale for selecting one group over another.

Discuss the importance of siblings in your life and how you believe you will think of them or be involved with them when you are old.

Discuss the differences between primary and secondary relationships.

Identify the qualities that characterize primary relationships.

What are some of the things you would need to consider if your elderly parent or grandparent needed to come and live with you?

What are some of the most difficult aspects of caregiving of an elder?

What resources might be helpful to families who have a frail elder to care for?

Discuss the meanings and the thoughts triggered by the students' and elders' viewpoints expressed at the beginning of the chapter. How do these vary from your own experience?

RESEARCH QUESTIONS

How many gay or lesbian individuals over 65 years old live in a domestic, long-standing partnership they consider a marriage?

What are the various sibling configurations that can be identified among the elderly, and what are the problems and satisfactions?

What are the factors that influence grandparenting styles?

What are the reasons individuals give for seeking divorce after being married 40 or more years?

In what situations and for what reasons do friendships remain of primary importance to the old?

Older men form same-sex alliances less frequently in late life, whereas their relationships with females increase. Several reasons for this are possible: (1) there are more women in their surroundings as they move out of the work relationships with other men, (2) if married, they become more involved in the wife's activities; (3) because of frailty and dependency they are more comfortable with women. These data need further exploration. The question is, why does this occur, or is it the result of only one study of 700 individuals that needs replication for confirmation?

How many corporations offer material help or counseling to employees who are primary caregivers of aged parents?

What specific services do these corporations offer?

RESOURCES

Films and Videos

Humor Prescription: Care for the Caregiver, Produced by American Media; Distributor, Excellence in Training Cor-

poration, 11358 Aurora Avenue, Des Moines, IA 50322-7979, (800) 747-6569, (purchase, $395; rental, 5 d $110). Focuses on the need for humor to deal with difficult situations and respond creatively. Exercises and experiential opportunities to practice and implement ideas.

My Mother, My Father. This documentary takes a candid look at four families and their deep and often conflicting feelings as they deal with the stresses and changes involved in caring for an aging parent. Does not attempt to provide easy answers. Rather, it offers honest and compelling insight into the need for families to make individual decisions about caregiving. And it elicits a better understanding of and support for individuals and families involved in caregiving. Winner of five national awards. (Produced by Terra Nova Films, Inc., directed by James Vanden Bosch, 33 minutes, purchase, 16mm, $495.00; video, $395.00; rental, $50.00). Contact Terra Nova Films, Inc, 9848 South Winchester Avenue, Chicago, IL 60643, (312) 881-8491.

The Great Circle of Life: A Resource Guide to Films and Videos on Aging by Robert Yahnke (Owings Mills, Md, 1988, National Health Publishing) is a guide to the use of films and videos on aging for health care professionals, media librarians, and educators. The text is divided into six chapters: Portraits of Aging, Documentaries, Symbolic Statements, Intergenerational Relationships, Relationships in Old Age, and Responses to Loss. Updates will be issued periodically.

The following are available through Video Press, University of Maryland at Baltimore, School of Medicine, Suite 133, 100 Penn Street, Baltimore, MD 21201, (800) 328-7450 or (410) 328-5497, fax (410) 328-8471.

Grace. Nationally broadcast in 1991, *Grace* is available to nonbroadcast audiences for the first time this year. The program is a 58-minute composite of the previously released programs, *Living with Grace, Caregiving with Grace,* and *Glenn's Perspective on Grace. Grace* documents the different stages of progressive dementing illness and the challenges each presents to caregivers. Glenn, her husband and dedicated caregiver, provides a model for both home caregivers and professional service providers. (purchase, $400; rental, $100). (Note: Institutions that have already purchased two or more of the tapes in this series can receive a complimentary copy of this program by contacting Video Press.)

Marge and Walter. Presents life from the perspective of the family caregiver—the daily routine, the rewards, and the challenges. Printed materials and discussion questions for both professional and family groups prepared by Debra Wertheimer, MD; 30 minutes; (purchase, $400; rental, $100).

Marge: Supporting the Family Caregiver. Marge Lewandowski cared for her chronically ill husband for 10 years. Approximately 1 year after her husband's death, Marge Lewandowski recalls some of the difficulties associated with being a family caregiver. This program emphasizes the importance of health professionals working with family caregivers to educate them, to link them to available services, and to provide the emotional support needed for this role. Interview by Debra Wertheimer, MD, 14 minutes (purchase, $300; rental, $100).

Caregiver Stress. Expert panelists Beverly Baldwin, Georgia Stevens, Karen Kleeman, and Joyce Rasin, from the University of Maryland School of Nursing, explore the psychobiologic and mental health consequences of caring for family members with dementing illness. Primarily developed for home caregivers, this tape also provides important insights for institutional caregivers, 33 minutes (purchase, $300; rental, $100).

Organizations

Children of Aging Parents (CAPS); 1609 Woodbourne Road, Suite 302A, Levittown, PA 19056, (215) 945-6900. Provides resource information and referral services throughout the country for caregivers; helps to increase community awareness of the problems of aging and caregiving through educational programs, workshops, and seminars; produces and distributes literature for caregivers; acts as a clearinghouse for individuals and organizations serving families with aging parents or relatives; provides individual peer counseling for caregivers; publishes a national newsletter, *The Capsule,* with advice/current information for caregivers.

Sibling Network
Deborah Gold, PhD
Box 3003
Duke University Medical Center
Durham, NC 27710

Dementia Care and Respite Services Program
Bowman Gray School, Wake Forest University
Medical Center Blvd
Winston-Salem, NC 27157-1087

National Association of Private Geriatric Care Managers (a professional association) will send a list of members in your area. Send a self-addressed stamped envelope (SASE) to 655 North Alvernon, Suite 108, Tucson, AZ 85711; or call (602) 881-8008.

Children of Aging Parents (a nonprofit group) offers a brochure and list of materials. Send $5 and an SASE to Woodbourne Campus, Suite 302A, Dept MM, 1609 Woodbourne Road, Levittown, PA 19057.

AARP Health Advocacy has two booklets—*Miles Away and Still Caring: A Guide for Long-Distance Caregivers* (D12748), and *Care Management* (D13803)—available free by addressing a postcard to the title and number, AARP Fulfillment (EE0321), PO Box 22796, Long Beach, CA 90801-5796. Allow 6 to 8 weeks for delivery.

AARP Grandparent Information Center
(202) 434-2296

National Coalition of Grandparents
Ethel Dunn, 137 Larkin Street, Madison, WI 53705
or
Sylvie de Toledo, 2801 Atlantic Avenue, Long Beach, CA 90801

Rocking
Mary Fron
PO Box 96
Niles, MI 49120

Grandparents Raising Grandchildren
Barbara Kirkland
PO Box 104
Colleyville, TX 76034

National organizations that offer advice and assistance on grandparents' visitation rights

Equal Rights for Grandparents
7408 Vetnor Avenue
Margate, NJ 08402
(609) 822-3510

Foundation for Grandparenting
PO Box 31
Lake Placid, NY 12946

Grandparents Anonymous
536 West Huron
Pontiac, MI 48053
(313) 682-8384

Grandparents'-Children's Rights, Inc.
5728 Bayonne Avenue
Haslett, MI 48840
(517) 339-8663

Grandparents as Parents (GAP) is a support group for grandparents raising grandchildren. Contact Sylvie de Toledo, Psychiatric Clinic for Youth, 2801 Atlantic Avenue, Long Beach, CA 90801; (213) 595-3151.

The American Self-Help Clearinghouse is a nationwide computerized database that offers (1) tips on how to start your grandparent self-help group and (2) a listing of local self-help clearinghouses with resources in your area. Send a legal-size SASE to American Self-Help Clearinghouse, St Clares-Riverside Medical Center, Denville, NJ 07834; (201) 625-7101.

Publications

Answers: The Magazine for Adult Children of Aging Parents, Circulation Manager, PO Box 9889, Birmingham, AL 35220-0889, (800) 750-2199

Heath, Angela: *Long distance caregiving: a survival guide for far away caregivers,* PO Box 280353, Lakewood, CO 80228, (303) 980-0580, 1993, American Source Books.

REFERENCES

Abel E: *Who cares for the elderly? Public policy and the experience of adult daughters,* Philadelphia, 1991, Temple University Press.

Adams RG: Patterns of network change: a longitudinal study of friendships of elderly women, *Gerontologist* 27(2):223, 1987.

Adams RG: People would talk: normative barriers to cross-sex friendships for elderly women, *Gerontologist* 25(6):605, 1985.

Adams RG: Service support of elderly women by friends, *Gerontologist* 23:221 (special issue), 1983.

Akiyama H, Elliott K, Antonucci TC: Same-sex and cross-sex relationships, *J Gerontol* 51B(6):P374, 1996.

Allen SM: Gender differences in spousal caregiving and unmet needs of care, *J Gerontol* 49(4):S187, 1994.

Allen KR, Wilcox KL: *Becoming an activist: older parents of adult gay children.* Paper presented at the meeting of the Gerontological Society of America, Washington, DC, Nov 19, 1996.

Alzheimer's Association, 1996.

American Association of Homes and Services for the Aging: Burden weighs heavy on caregivers: study, *Currents* 11(4):2, 1996.

American Association of Retired Persons: *A profile of older Americans: 1995,* AARP PF3049 (1295), Washington, DC, 1996, The Association.

American Society on Aging: A new look at families and aging, *Generations* 17(3):1992. (Entire issue.)

Anderson TB, McCullough BJ: Conjugal support: factor structure for older husbands and wives, *J Gerontol* 48(3):S133, 1993.

Antonucci TC: Social supports and social relationships. In Binstock RH, George LK editors: *Handbook of aging and the social sciences,* ed 3, San Diego, 1990, Academic Press.

Avioli R: The social support functions of siblings in later life, *Am Behav Scientist* 33(1):45, 1989.

Boaz RF: *Full-time employment and informal caregiving in the 1980s.* Paper presented at the meeting of the Gerontological Society of America, Washington, DC, Nov 19, 1996.

Boucher L, Renvall MJ, Jackson JE: Cognitively impaired spouses as primary caregivers for demented elderly people, *J Am Geriatr Soc* 44(7):828, 1996.

Brandt RW: Twins no more, *Health* 10(7):10, 1996.

Brody EM, Litvin SJ, Albert SM, Hoffman CJ: Marital status of daughters and patterns of care, *J Gerontol* 49(2):S95, 1994.

Burkholt V, Wenger GC, Silverstein M: *The structures of parent child relations among very old parents in Wales and the United States: a cross-national comparison.* Paper presented at the meeting of the Gerontological Society of America, Washington, DC, Nov 19, 1996.

Burton LM: Black grandparents rearing children of drug-addicted parents: stressors, outcomes and social service needs, *Gerontologist* 32(6):744, 1992.

Cain LD: Loosening the binds that tie, *Gerontologist* 36(2):267, 1996.

Camberg L, Ooi W, Hurley A et al: *Methods to evaluate an audiotape intervention for Alzheimer's patients.* Paper presented at the meeting of the Gerontological Society of America, Washington, DC, Nov 19, 1996.

Caregiving for elders gets corporate help, *Longevity News* 3(9):6, 1995.

Caron W, Hepburn K, Ostwald SK: *Family accord and caregiver adjustment: family level measurement in caregiver research.* Paper presented at the meeting of the Gerontological Society of America, Washington, DC, Nov 19, 1996.

Carpenter BD: *Filial obligation, ethnicity and caregiving.* Paper presented at the meeting of the Gerontological Society of America, Washington, DC, Nov 19, 1996.

Connidis IA: Sibling support in older age, *J Gerontol* 49(6):S309, 1994.

Connidis IA, McMullin JA: To have or have not: parent status and the subjective well-being of older men and women, *Gerontologist* 33(5):630, 1993.

Connidis IA, Davies L: Confidants and companions: choices in later life, *J Gerontol* 47(3):S115, 1992.

Constantino L, Wykle M: *Comparing black and white daughter/non-daughter caregivers.* Paper presented at the meeting of the Gerontological Society of America, Washington, DC, Nov 19, 1996.

Cooley C: *Social organization: a study of the larger mind,* New York, 1909, Charles Scribner's Sons.

Cosbey J, McMahon S: *Adult daughters caring for their fathers.* Paper presented at the meeting of the Gerontological Society of America, Washington, DC, Nov 19, 1996.

Crowley SL: Grandparents to the rescue, *AARP Bulletin* 34(9):1, 1993.

Der-McLeod D, Hansen JC: On Lok: the family continuum, *Generations* 17(3):71, 1992.

Ebersole P: A theoretical approach to the use of reminiscence. In Burnside I, editor: *Working with the elderly: group processes and techniques,* North Scituate, Mass, 1978b, Duxbury Press.

Family Caregiver Alliance: Selected caregiver statistics, *Family Caregiver Alliance Newsletter,* San Francisco, Calif, 1996.

Feinberg LF, Kelly KA: A well-deserved break: respite programs offered by California's statewide system of caregiver resource centers, *Gerontologist* 35(5):701, 1995.

Field D, Minkler M: Continuity and change in social support between young-old and old-old or very-old age, *J Gerontol* 43(4):100, 1988.

Field D, Minkler M, Falk RF et al: The influence of health on family contacts and family feelings in advanced old age: a longitudinal study, *J Gerontol* 48(1):P18, 1993.

Freedman VA: Family structure and the risk of nursing home admission, *J Gerontol* 51B(2):S61, 1996.

Genevay B: "Creating" families: older people alone—what is the role of service providers? *Generations* 17(3):61, 1992.

George LK, Gwyther LP: Caregiver well-being: a multidimensional examination of family caregivers of demented adults, *Gerontologist* 26:253, 1986.

Georgemiller R, Iacono G, Browne E: Factors related to coping in caretakers of cognitively impaired elderly. (Abstract). *Proceedings of the Third Congress of the International Psychogeriatric Association,* 3:36, Chicago, 1987.

Giarrusso R, Feng D, Silverstein M, Chen X: *A cross-cultural comparison of the intergenerational stake phenomenon over the life course.* Paper presented at the meeting of the Gerontological Society of America, Washington, DC, Nov 19, 1996.

Global Aging Report: Charging children for care of aging parents: two Asian nations turn to family for cash, *Global Aging Report* 1(4):4, 1996.

Good grandparenting, *Mayo Clinic Health Letter* 11(1):6, January 1993.

Haley WE, West CAC, Wadley VG et al: Psychological, social and health impact of caregiving: a comparison of black and white dementia family caregivers and noncaregivers, *Psychol Aging* 10(4):S40, 1995.

Hareven TK: Family and generational relations in the later years: a historical perspective, *Generations* 17(3):7, 1992.

Heath A: *Long distance caring,* Lakewood, Colo, 1993, American Source Books.

Himes CL: Social demography of contemporary families and aging, *Generations* 17(3):13, 1992.

Hoffman D: Complaints of a dutiful daughter, *Alzheimer's Caregiver* 9(1):1, 1996.

Jendrek MP: Grandparents who parent their grandchildren: circumstances and decisions, *Gerontologist* 34(2):206, 1994.

Jones FC: The lofty roles of the black grandmother, *Crises* 80:19, 1973.

Jones J: *Labor of love, labor of sorrow: black women, work, and the family from slavery to the present,* New York, 1985, Basic Books.

Kelly SJ: Caregiver stress in grandparents raising grandchildren, *Image* 25(4):331, 1993.

Kimmel DC: The families of older gay men and lesbians, *Generations* 17(3):37, 1992.

Kivett VR: The grandparent-grandchild connection, *Marriage and Family Review* 16(3/4):267, 1991.

Lamphere JK, Dwyer JW, Franks MM: *Gender, age and race differences in intergenerational assistance and filial expectations.* Paper presented at the meeting of the Gerontological Society of America, Washington, DC, Nov 19, 1996.

Lawton MP, Rajagopal D, Brody E, Kleban MH: The dynamics of caregiving for a demented elder among black and white families, *J Gerontol* 47(4):S156, 1992.

Lechner V, Neal MB: *Future government and workplace support for employed caregivers.* Paper presented at the meeting of the Gerontological Society of America, Washington, DC, Nov 19, 1996.

Lowenthal MF, Haven C: Interaction and adaptation: intimacy as a critical variable, *Am Sociol Rev* 33:20, 1968.

Matthews SH: Gender and the division of filial responsibility between lone sisters and their brothers, *J Gerontol* B50(5):S312, 1995.

McGreehan D, Warburton S: How to help families cope with caring for elderly members, *Geriatrics* 33:99, 1978.

Michela NJ: Jumping the hurdles of high-tech home care, *Geriatr Nurs* 16(6):291, 1995.

Mittleman MS, Ferris SH, Shulman E et al: A comprehensive support program: effect on depression in spouse-caregivers of AD patients, *Gerontologist* 35(6):792, 1995.

Moen P, Robison J, Fields V: Women's work and caregiving roles: a life course approach, *J Gerontol* 49(4):S176, 1994.

Moritz D, Kasl S, Berkman L: The health impact of living with a cognitively impaired elderly spouse: depressive symptoms and social functioning, *J Gerontol* 44(1):S17, 1989.

Mortimer JA, Schuman LM, French LR: Epidemiology of dementing illness. In Mortimer JA, Schuman LM, editors: *The epidemiology of dementia,* New York, 1981, Oxford University Press.

Motenko A: The frustration, gratifications and well-being of dementia caregivers, *Gerontologist* 29(2):166, 1989.

Moyer MS: Sibling relationships among older adults, *Generations* 17(3):55, 1992.

National Alliance for Caregiving: *Family caregiver fact sheet,* 4720 Montgomery Lane, Suite 642, Bethesda, MD, 1996.

Nielsen J, Henderson C, Cox M et al: Characteristics of caregivers and factors contributing to institutionalization, *Geriatr Nurs* 17(3):120, 1996.

Noberini MR, Berman RU: Barter to beat inflation: developing a neighborhood network for swapping services on behalf of the aged, *Gerontologist* 23:171, 1983.

Norris-Baker C, Scheidt RJ: *Celebrating shared community memories of place.* Paper presented at the meeting of the Gerontological Society of America, Washington, DC, Nov 19, 1996.

O'Connor P: Same-gender and cross-gender friendships among the frail elderly, *Gerontologist* 33(1):24, 1993.

OWL: *Administration on aging awards support for national caregiving information project,* OWL Press Release, Washington DC, 1992, Older Women's League.

Ozaki H: The caregiver needs a day off, *Geriatr Nurs* 16(2):67, 1995.

Pillemer K: Family caregiving: what would a Martian say? *Gerontologist* 36(2):269, 1996.

Pratt C, Schall V, Wright S et al: Burden and coping strategies of caregivers to Alzheimer's Patients, *Family Relations* 34(1):27, 1985.

Rankin ED, Haut MW, Keefover RW: Clinical assessment of family caregivers of dementia, *Gerontologist* 32(6):813, 1992.

Reisman J: An indirect measure of the value of friendship for aging men, *J Gerontol* 43(4):109, 1988.

Rice R: *Home health nursing practice: concepts and application,* St Louis, 1996, Mosby.

Richards M: Family support groups, *Generations* 10(4):68, Summer, 1986.

Riley MW: Discussion: what does it all mean, *Gerontologist* 36(2):256, 1996.

Rosenthal CJ: Kinkeeping in the familial division of labor, *J Marriage Family* 47:965, 1985.

Rosenthal CJ, Martin-Matthews A, Matthews SH: Caught in the middle? Occupancy in multiple roles and help to parents in a national probability sample of Canadian adults, *J Gerontol* 51B(6):S274, 1996.

Sandell SH, Iams H: Caregiving and future social security benefits: a reply to O'Grady-LeShane and Kingson, *Gerontologist* 36(6):814, 1996.

Schott-Baer D, Fisher L, Gregory C: Dependent care, caregiver burden, hardiness, and self-care agency of caregivers, *Cancer Nurs* 18(4):299, 1995.

Schulz R, O'Brien AT, Bookwala J, Fleissner K: Psychiatric and physical morbidity of dementia caregiving: prevalence, correlates and causes, *Gerontologist* 35(6):771, 1995.

Schwartz D, Kelly C: Personal communication. Sept 16, 1996, Gwynedd, Pa.

Scott JP: Sibling interaction in later life. In Brubaker TH, editor: *Family relationships in later life,* Newbury Park, Calif, 1992, Sage Publications.

Scott-Maxwell E: *The measure of my days,* New York, 1968, Alfred A Knopf.

Segall M, Wykle M: The black family's experience with dementia, *J Appl Soc Sc,* Fall, 1988.

Seltzer MM, Li LW: The transitions of caregiving: subjective and objective definitions, *Gerontologist* 36(5):614, 1996.

Sheehan NW: The caregiver information project: a mechanism to assist religious leaders to help family caregivers, *Gerontologist* 29(5):703, 1989.

Sherman A, Antonucci T: *Reciprocity in best friend relationships.* Paper presented at the meeting of the Gerontological Society of America, Washaington, DC, Nov 18, 1996.

Soldo BJ: Cross pressures on middle-aged adults: a broader view, *J Gerontol* 51B(6):S271, 1996.

Soldo BJ, Hill MS: Intergeneration transfers: economic, demographic and social perspectives. In GL Maddox, MP Lawton, editors: *Annual review of gerontology and geriatrics,* vol 13, New York, 1993, Springer.

Solomon JC, Marx J: To grandmother's house we go: health and school adjustment of children raised solely by grandparents, *Gerontologist* 35(3):386, 1995.

Stephens MAP: *Day care and family strain: testing the effects of interventions.* Paper presented at the meeting of the Gerontological Society of America, Washington, DC, Nov 19, 1996.

Stephens MAP, Franks MM: Spillover between daughters' roles as caregiver and wife: interference or enhancement, *J Gerontol* 50B(1):P9, 1995.

Taylor R, Chatters L: Church-based informal support among elderly blacks, *Gerontologist* 26(6):637, 1986.

Tobin S, Fulimer E, Smith GC: Coping with a developmentally disabled offspring. In Thomas E, Eisenhandler S: *Aging and the religious dimension,* Westport, Conn, Auburn House, 1994.

Townsend AL, Franks MM: Binding ties: closeness and conflict in adult children's caregiving relationships, *Psychol Aging* 10(3):343, 1995.

Troll LE: Family connectedness of old women. In Turner BF, Troll LE, editors: *Women growing older,* Thousand Oaks, Calif, 1994, Sage Publications.

Troll LE, Bengtson VL: The oldest-old in families: an intergenerational perspective, *Generations* 17(3):39, 1992.

Uhlenberg P: The burden of aging: a theoretical framework for understanding the shifting balance of caregiving and care receiving as cohorts age, *Gerontologist* 36(6):761, 1996a.

Uhlenberg P: Mutual attraction: demography and life course analysis, *Gerontologist* 36(2):226, 1996b.

Uhlenberg P, Hammill B, Kirby JR: *The changing demography of grandparents over the twentieth century.* Paper presented at the meeting of the Gerontological Society of America, Washington, DC, Nov 20, 1996.

US Bureau of the Census: *65+ in the United States,* Current population reports, Special Studies, pp 23-190, Washington, DC, 1996, US Government Printing Office.

Vinick BH, Lanspery S, Hoy E: *Stepfamilies in later life: a neglected area of research.* Paper presented at the meeting of the Gerontological Society of America, Washington, DC, Nov 20, 1996.

Welsh WM, Stewart AJ: Relationships between women and their parents: implications for midlife well-being, *Psychol Aging* 10(2):181, 1995.

Wentowski G: Older women's perceptions of great-grandmotherhood: a research note, *Gerontologist* 25(6):593, 1985.

Whitbeck L, Hoyt DR, Huck SM: Early family relationships, intergenerational solidarity and support provided to parents by their adult children, *J Gerontol* 49(2):S85, 1994.

Winbush GB: Family caregiving programs: a look at the premises on which they are based, *Generations* 17(3):65, 1992.

Wolanin M: Personal communication, San Francisco, 1979.

Zarit SH: Methodological considerations in caregiver intervention and outcome research. In Lebowitz BD, Light E, Niederche G, editors: *Alzheimer's disease and family stress,* Rockville, Md, 1991, National Institute of Mental Health.

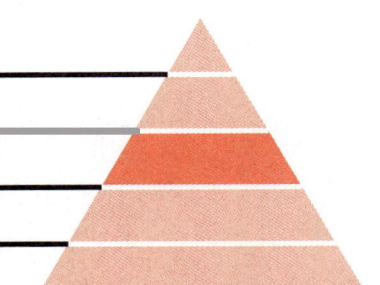

The Family APGAR

The following questions have been designed to help us better understand you and your friends. Friends are non-relatives from your school or community with whom you have a sharing relationship.

Comment space should be used if you wish to give additional information or if you wish to discuss the way the question applies to your friends. Please try to answer all questions.

The following questions have been designed to help us better understand you and your family. You should feel free to ask questions about any item in the questionnaire.

	Almost always	Some of the time	Hardly ever
I am satisfied that I can turn to my friends for help when something is troubling me. Comments:	☐	☐	☐
I am satisfied with the way my friends talk over things with me and share problems with me. Comments:	☐	☐	☐
I am satisfied that my friends accept and support my wishes to take on new activities or directions. Comments:	☐	☐	☐
I am satisfied with the way my friends express affection, and respond to my emotions, such as anger, sorrow, or love. Comments:	☐	☐	☐
I am satisfied with the way my friends and I share time together. Comments:	☐	☐	☐

Comment space should be used if you wish to give additional information or if you wish to discuss the way the question applies to your family. Please try to answer all questions.

"Family" is the individual(s) with whom you usually live. If you live alone, consider family as those with whom you now have the strongest emotional ties.

For each question, check only one box

	Almost always	Some of the time	Hardly ever
I am satisfied that I can turn to my family for help when something is troubling me. Comments:	☐	☐	☐
I am satisfied with the way my family talks over things with me and share problems with me. Comments:	☐	☐	☐
I am satisfied that my family accepts and supports my wishes to take on new activities or directions. Comments:	☐	☐	☐
I am satisfied with the way my family expresses affection, and responds to my emotions, such as anger, sorrow, or love. Comments:	☐	☐	☐
I am satisfied with the way my family and I share time together. Comments:	☐	☐	☐

Who lives in your home?* List by relationship (e.g., spouse, significant other,† child, or friend).

Please check below the column that best describes how you now get along with each member of the family listed.

Relationship	Age	Sex	Well	Fairly	Poorly
_____	___	___	☐	☐	☐
_____	___	___	☐	☐	☐
_____	___	___	☐	☐	☐

If you don't live with your own family, please list below the individuals to whom you turn for help most frequently. List by relationship, (e.g., family member, friend, associate at work, or neighbor).

Please check below the column that best describes how you now get along with each person listed.

Relationship	Age	Sex	Well	Fairly	Poorly
_____	___	___	☐	☐	☐
_____	___	___	☐	☐	☐
_____	___	___	☐	☐	☐

From Gallo J, Reichel W, Andersen L, editors: *Handbook of geriatric assessment,* Gaithersburg, Md, 1988, Aspen Publications.
*If you have established your own family, consider home to be the place where you live with your spouse, children, or significant other; otherwise, consider home as your place of origin, e.g., the place where your parents or those who raised you live.
†"Significant other" is the partner you live with in a physically and emotionally nurturing relationship, but to whom you are not married.

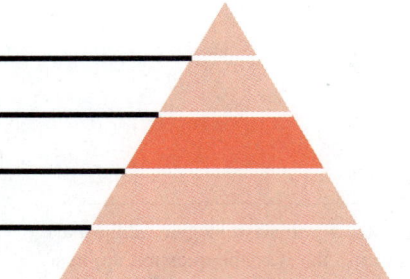

CHAPTER 18

Isolation, Loneliness, Alienation, and Stigmatization

Students learn

The fear of doing tasks such as cleaning the lower parts of a male, changing the briefs, or the dressing on deeply open ulcers is inexpressible. There are so many impressions and emotional feelings, and the aged to some extent suffer isolation because of this.

Thu Mong, age 21

I will be very frightened every time I look into the mirror because I will find myself getting old and uglier. My skin becomes thicker and darker, my eyes will start to have fat deposit under them. I will see wrinkles and crow's-feet on my face. I hate to think about aging because I don't know what will happen to me as well as what disabilities will occur next. I always want to look good and young, so I will dye my hair to make myself look younger. Hopefully, by using cosmetics, people won't be able to tell my real age.

Thao Thu, age 21

Elders speak

When I was young I was fat; as I grew older I developed addictions to things even worse for me than food. Now I'm a lonely old man with AIDS. I will die sooner than I might have without it, but does it matter? I've marched to a different drummer all of my life, but he has led me into ultimate isolation and loneliness.

James, age 60

Loneliness is a devastating illness—more so than any physical illness—and can be fatal. Some people can overcome a little, but the older the individual is, the more hazardous loneliness becomes. A hug or a touch is so important. Hospitals and nursing homes are destroying many people. There aren't enough nurses to go around.

Anne, age 87

When my husband developed something similar to Alzheimer's disease, the caregiving was exhausting, but when our associates didn't want to have anything to do with us socially, that was devastating.

Rose, age over 70

LEARNING OBJECTIVES

Upon completion of this chapter, the reader will be able to:

1. Identify several major social factors contributing to loneliness and alienation of the elderly.
2. Relate at least three factors that contribute to ageism and stigmatizing the elderly.
3. Discuss the alienating effects of neurologic disorders and sensory changes that interfere with communication.
4. Discuss interventions appropriate to achieving social integration of an alienated or stigmatized elder.

640

This chapter deals with conceptual issues of aging that occur for some elders and become acutely uncomfortable during crisis periods, transitional times, or when losses occur. Whenever the self-concept, feelings of efficacy, or social network is appreciably altered, these issues tend to emerge. The majority of elders confront them at various times in the aging process. For some they become constant companions of aging.

Because these concepts are subject to numerous interpretations and are largely immeasurable, the ideas set forth are often subject to question. I believe few ideas are truly original; many in this chapter combine the thoughts of numerous theorists. When the source of the idea is recognized, credit is given.

We challenge readers to observe elders, investigate, read, absorb, and develop your own thoughts on these critical issues. These are interpretations of life and its value in the later years. In the face of disease and impending death, isolation, loneliness, alienation, and stigmatization hamper the quality of existence for many.

Self-esteem is an inner assurance of personal worth based on feelings of being valued, loved, useful, and competent. The durability of the self-system depends to some extent upon the successful negotiation of the tasks of late life (Figure 18-1), and these are age and culture bound. They do not fit everyone because many elders fall outside the "normal" expectations. These persons are likely to be stigmatized and alienated. In addition, ageism and losses further alienate the individual. Isolation and loneliness may seem preferable to the struggle to remain socially involved.

The elder may require external shoring up to a greater extent than when younger and more energetic. The analogy of sandbags to strengthen foundations when floodwaters threaten to wash away a dwelling is apt. Nurses and other caring individuals provide the sandbags. One may have a solid foundation based on past achievements and personal integrity, but the durability of the self-system in later life will depend somewhat on personality, the successful negotiation of adult tasks, lifetime levels of social integration, and the number and duration of assaults. These are discussed in Chapters 2 and 21 more fully.

Depression may result from the absence of positive reinforcement by others, from rewards that are unrelated to behavior, and from reinforcement that is appropriate but infrequent. The loss of personal effectiveness in any important arena of living often results in alienation from the more effective or more valued members of the community. This, of course, ends in the individual feeling ineffective and unwanted.

Isolation may stem from alienation and stigmatization, which in turn lead to loneliness. Individual strengths and resources then go unrecognized, much less reinforced. Through discussion and observation we should identify and document areas of personal effectiveness of each elderly person we care for. Opportunities for expressing these

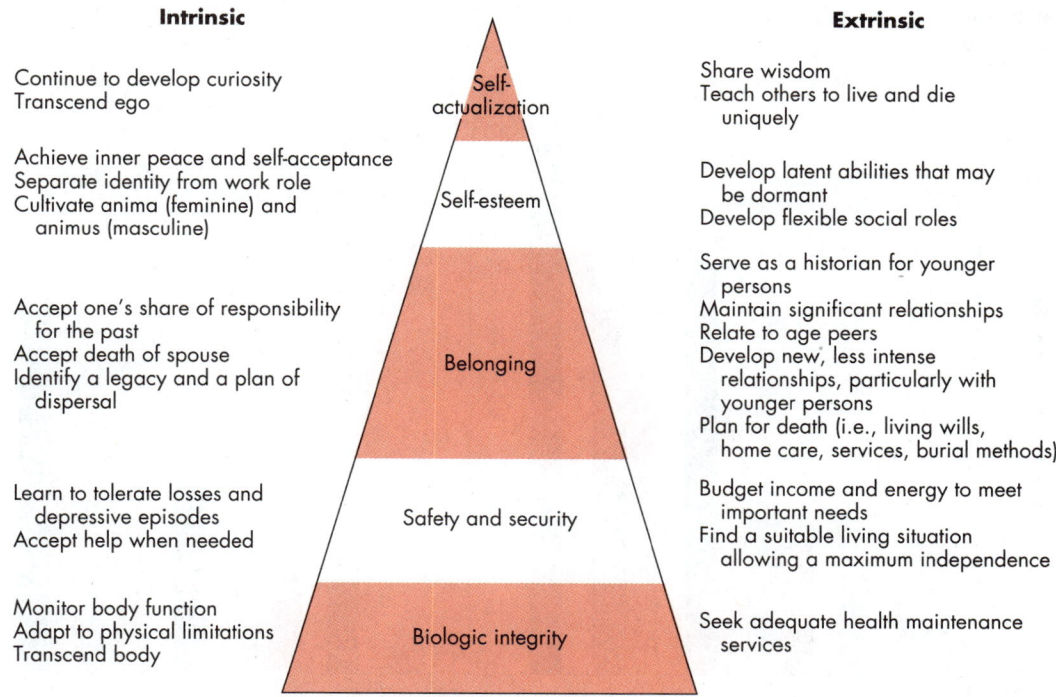

Figure 18-1. Developmental tasks of late life in hierarchic order. (Data from Peck R: Psychological developments in the second half of life. In Neugarten B, editor: *Middle age and aging,* Chicago, 1968, University of Chicago Press; Havighurst RJ: *Developmental tasks and education,* ed 3, New York, 1972, David McKay Co.)

strengths and for recognition need to be built into daily schedules. Feelings of personal efficacy provide some psychologic immunity against feelings of isolation, loneliness, alienation, and stigmatization.

ISOLATION

Isolation is a response to conditions that inhibit ability or opportunity to interact with others or is a result of the desire not to interact. It may be self- or other initiated. At times self-imposed isolation by individuals enhances creativity, individuality, and integrity, but when externally imposed by the aggregate mass, it can rarely be seen as a healthy or growth-promoting situation. When other initiated, it is to protect individuals or the group from contact with conditions that frighten them or threaten their security. Some individuals are isolated, quarantined, or set apart because of certain distinctive characteristics. The group no longer embraces the factor or person isolated. These are then alienated.

The classic study by Berkman and Syme (1979) showed that socially isolated individuals were more prone to certain diseases, such as ischemic heart disease, cancer, and cerebrovascular and circulatory disorders. They concluded that circumstances that create social isolation may have pervasive health consequences and that the lack of certain social factors may influence host resistance and disease vulnerability. Apparently, isolation increases vulnerability to disease, suicide, and death (Figure 18-2). We no longer quarantine individuals on Ellis Island because of suspected diseases or post yellow flags in front of homes to warn oth-

ers of the presence of individuals with contagious diseases. We are now more humane. Yet there are those who are isolated from the mainstream by age, color, culture, frailty, poverty, geography, appearance, sexual orientation, or stereotypical thinking.

Ageism Today

Ageism is a term coined by Robert Butler (1969) to describe the discrimination that often accompanies old age and is based solely on age. Cole (1992) examines the historic roots of ageism in American and concludes that some of the origins came about with the erosion of the patriarchal and hierarchical system in which male elders were held in high esteem because of their power of ownership and age. Early in U.S. history the general availability of land reduced the elder's power base and the intergenerational conflict so characteristic of the crowded and land-poor older countries, but old men were still venerated as symbols in a culture that was commited to the notion that the young were to serve and the old were to rule.

A more balanced society is one in which there are bright and energetic youth, secure middle-aged individuals, and wise old persons. With the shift to urban industrialism, emphasis on productivity, and shifting philosophies in government, old men with inflexible ideas became anachronistic and burdensome. In a consumer-oriented society it is inevitable that those who purchase less will receive less attention (Box 18-1).

In our society there is a specific type of ageist marketing. The old are aggressively marketed for health aids, funeral plans, and fraudulent schemes.

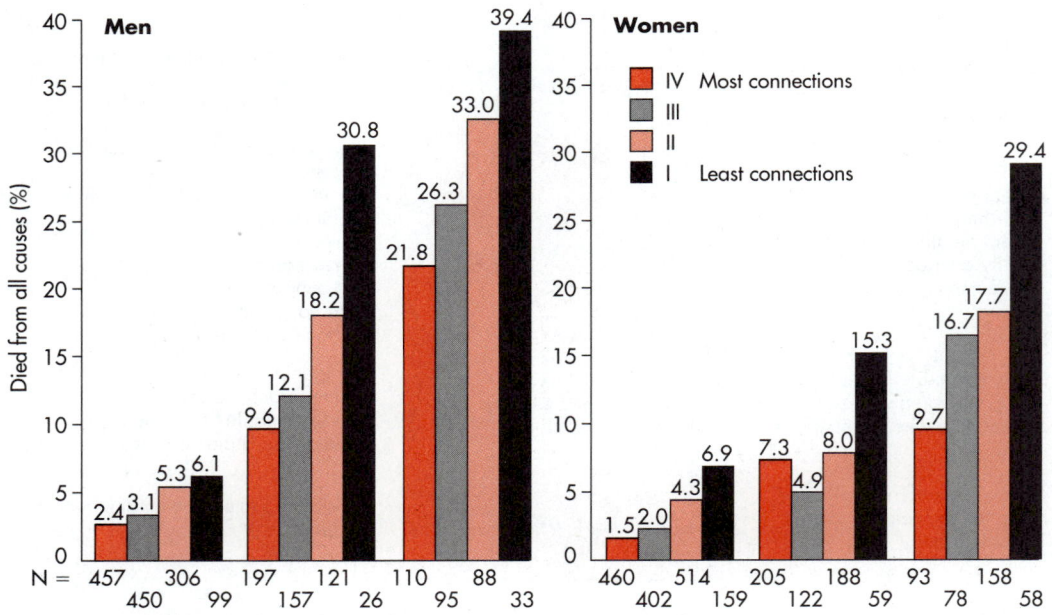

Figure 18-2.   Social network mortality index. (From Berkman LF, Syme L: Social networks, host resistance, and mortality: a nine-year follow-up study of Alameda County residents, *Am J Epidemiol* 109:186, 1979.)

Carl Djerassi(1996), a scientist who began writing fiction in his 70s, examines the particular ageism of scientists. In spite of the decline of ageism in many fields and among most groups, scientists as a whole hold fast to the notion that scientific endeavor peaks in the midthirties, and it is all downhill after that. He suggests that scientists are trained toward clear-cut, black-and-white questions and answers. With experience and wisdom older scientists recognize that important questions are complex and answers are gray, seldom black-and-white. Often there are no answers. Even though older scientists are considered to be past the prime of innovative thought, funding agencies and research teams generally tolerate and sometimes patronize their elder colleagues because they also want their image of maturity and stability and often the strength of their "track record."

Not only resources in the support of science but those in support of health smack of ageism. There are numerous questions about the impact managed care and restricted resources will have on the delivery of care to the aged. Rules are being put into place by the Health Care Financing Administration (HCFA) to insist that health maintenance organizations (HMOs) and managed care organizations cannot discriminate against those Medicare-covered individuals who are likely to consume more resources. This will also undoubtedly extend to the private insurers.

In the management of chronic disorders in which rehabilitation may be limited based on chronologic age, even though patients over 85 are especially likely to benefit from rehabilitation programs, nurses must function as advocates for the aged and be sure they have sufficient information to make wise decisions regarding their care.

Ageism still exists among many health care professionals. Duerson et al (1992) found that an increased amount of knowledge about aging, as reflected in higher scores on Palmore's Facts on Aging quizzes, resulted in significantly decreased biased responses of medical students. The influence of health professionals' negative perceptions of aging on potential therapeutic outcomes has been largely ignored.

Betty Friedan, to whom many attribute the spark that set aflame the feminist revolution, believes we are now on the brink of a radical change in attitudes on aging—just as 30 years ago a social revolution was launched by the feminist movement. She predicts a revolution in thinking about aging by the year 2000, with a transformation in consciousness about older persons and their role in society. She insists aging is not a problem but an adventure. But, as long as we refer to "them" rather than "us," aging is a problem. Friedan has become one of "us," and in her book, *The Fountain of Age*, she hopes to launch a new consciousness of the aged (Carlson and Crowley, 1992).

Her discovery that age is an adventure is not a new idea. In fact, her experience may be the essence of aging as it has always been for those who remain functional, wealthy, and reasonably healthy. The realization that it can be the greatest challenge one will ever face is a reality for the very old.

For some, the challenge is exciting, for others, a test of the human spirit. As long as old age represents proximity to death it will be embraced with some reluctance by those who love life.

Stereotypes. Stereotypes are isolating ideas that set individuals apart based upon supposed characteristic qualities. Positive stereotypes may be just as deleterious as those that are negative if they impose unrealistic expectations (McLerran, 1993). Stereotypes of the elderly held by young, middle-aged, and elderly adults vary significantly and become more complex as the individuals age (Hummert et al, 1994). In other words, the older one becomes the more likely one is to see old age as complex and with many more facets than younger persons view it.

When characteristics were clustered, the greatest differences in positive qualities were between the young, who had a benign, overly sentimental view of old age and the old, who saw themselves as activists and good neighbors. The differences are seen in the way young and old viewed the

> **Box 18-1   Seven Contributors to Ageism**
>
> Seven factors account for the majority of ageism in advertising, according to "Ageism in Advertising: A Study of Advertising Agency Attitudes Towards Maturing and Mature Consumers." According to the report's author, Richard A. Lee of High-Yield Marketing, based in Roseville, Minn, "Take them away, and ageism in advertising largely goes away with them."
>
> 1. The majority of advertising-agency professionals are in early adulthood, when empathetic understanding for people different generations is relatively uncommon.
> 2. Most agency professionals are most comfortable advertising to younger consumers like themselves.
> 3. Advertising-agency culture and output reflects the tastes and values of a relatively narrow slice of society—young adults in their 20s and 30s.
> 4. Advertising professionals don't believe that Baby Boomers are maturing (and will mature) as people always have.
> 5. Not wanting to be educated about older consumers, rather than lack of informational and educational resources, perpetuates common misperceptions among agency professionals about older consumers.
> 6. While ageism in advertising is most visible in relation to "seniors"—what we see is actually the culmination of a long process that starts with consumers in their 40s.
> 7. There is scant internal pressure within agencies to "break the lock" of ageism—and external pressure, while rising, is still at minimal levels.

From seven contributors to ageism, *Aging Today* 16(5):11, 1995.

shrew/curmudgeon factors. The young thought the old had more of these qualities, whereas the old felt some of the same qualities were indications of elitest, self-affirming behaviors. Other distinct differences in stereotypical thinking were that young adults thought elders were vulnerable, tired, and not eager to learn and experience, whereas elders had the opposite view of these factors (Table 18-1).

Women in another study viewed elders much more negatively than did men, but after interventions designed to help them identify with the old, the women had considerably more positive attitudes and the men became more negative (DeAngelis, 1994). The researchers believed that women are socialized to fear old age, based on appearance, whereas men see the potential for status and power, but upon closer examination of actual senarios of aging, the women become less fearful and the men more so.

Nursing students and others seeking health careers continue to hold stereotypes about old people in general, though they are more somewhat more positive than in the past (Lookinland and Anson, 1995).

Ageist images must be changed at many levels. It is naive to believe that "education" will transform deep emotional issues. Popular culture, media, work force relations, households, and intergenerational contacts must all avoid compartmentalizing "the old" by stereotyping. We find interpersonal contact with elders a continual illumination of their variability.

Social Isolation

Isolation may be chosen or imposed for a variety of reasons. It becomes a problem when involuntarily imposed.

Social isolation can be seen as having four layers: community, organization, confidants, and self (Biordi, 1995). In times past and in certain cultures isolation from the community served as the chief mechanism of control and punishment. Those who did not comply with community standards were socially ostracized; excluded from the group by common but often unspoken agreement.

On the organizational level, imposed isolation is perhaps most apparent in the treatment of religious heretics. Those who dissented from the organizational viewpoint, doctrine, or dogma were excommunicated.

On the more intimate level, a family might turn its back on an errant member, striking his or her name from the family Bible, literally or figuratively. Now, it is more common that the offender will simply be ignored.

Finally, self-isolation may occur because of shame and guilt or the inability to keep up appearances in public.

Social isolation has many causes and numerous defining characteristics: absence of supportive significant others; lacking purpose or challenges; aloneness imposed by others; or withdrawal because of hearing deficits, feelings of rejection, limited mobility, or vision impairment. Recognizable symptoms of the problem in individuals include personal withdrawal from interactions; institutionalization; sad, dull affect; preoccupation with own thoughts; insecurity in pub-

Table 18-1 Frequently Named* Traits in Additional Category

| | Age Group | | | |
Trait	Young (n = 40)	Middle-aged (n = 40)	Elderly (n = 40)	Trait Valence
Conservative	7.5	20.0	2.5	Positive
Depressed	12.5	20.0	7.5	Negative
Determined	2.5	20.0	17.5	Positive
Eager to learn and experience	0.0	17.5	25.0	Positive
Has sense of humor	12.5	15.0	12.5	Positive
Health-conscious	15.0	45.0	30.0	Positive
Independent	5.0	25.0	22.5	Positive
Likes social activities	25.0	20.0	17.5	Positive
Move after retirement	22.5	10.0	2.5	Positive
Politically aware and active	22.5	17.5	17.5	Positive
Pursues a hobby	30.0	30.0	27.5	Positive
Religious	12.5	32.5	20.0	Positive
Scared of becoming sick and incompetent	0.0	35.0	52.5	Negative
Successful	12.5	25.0	5.0	Positive
Timid	5.0	27.5	7.5	Negative
Tired	25.0	17.5	2.5	Negative
Travels often	10.0	20.0	32.5	Positive
Trustworthy	2.5	20.0	5.0	Positive
Well-groomed	5.0	17.5	20.0	Positive
Worried about finances	7.5	5.0	35.0	Negative

From Hummert ML, Garstka TA, Shaner JL, Strahm S: Stereotypes of the elderly held by young, middle-aged, and elderly adults, *J Gerontol* 49(5):P240, 1994.

*Named by 20% or more informants in at least one age group or by 10% or more of informants in all three age groups.

lic; poor eye contact; being uncommunicative; and seeking to be alone (Lien-Gieschen, 1992).

Social isolation and emotional isolation are not necessarily equivalent. Older adults are particularly susceptible to social isolation because of environmental strictures, loss of familiar friends, and inability to perform certain activities. In addition, they may voluntarily disengage from some activities and become more intensely involved in those that are more valued. This is characteristic of healthy adaptation, but enforced isolation is likely to have detrimental effects.

Emotional isolation involves needs for affiliation, degree of independence, and self-concept issues (Mullins et al, 1989) and often results from the loss of significant others.

Assessing elders for vulnerability to undesired social isolation and devising proactive measures to prevent or delay debilitating emotional isolation are nursing functions. Assessing vulnerability involves determination of sensory status and decrements that interfere with communication and participation, absence of interactional opportunities, degree and intensity of losses experienced, and alterations to the sense of self.

Interventions in general will involve compensation for sensory deficits, increasing opportunities for interaction with others, working through grief processes, and restoring self-esteem. These problems have been dealt with in depth elsewhere in the text (see index for specifics).

Biordi (1995) notes that there are also four patterns of social isolation with varying consequences: first, the individual who throughout life has been socially involved will find

isolation the most painful. A second pattern is of the individual who spent much of adulthood in isolated pursuits and may desire more involvement with others in retirement. He or she may not know how to effectively integrate into a social group. A third pattern is of the individual who has been actively involved and abruptly, voluntarily withdraws in late life because of events that cause shame. Finally, the lifelong isolate may find the social limitations of old age tolerable, expecting little else.

Care of the social isolate must be planned based on the source of the isolation, the level, the pattern, and the degree of vulnerability. Isolation conceptualized in levels of a hierarchy and life patterns provides a more accurate assessment of issues and possible interventions (Figure 18-3 and Box 18-2).

Institutionalization

Institutional life has been created for many reasons: to educate, to enhance opportunities, to create a collective identity, to protect from the demands of everyday life, to protect the community from exposure, to separate undesirables from less deviant members of society, and as a retreat from worldly concerns. Despite the varying reasons for institutional living, residents of institutions are alienated from the community at large, and their presence is not fully appreciated or understood by the larger community.

The old are usually institutionalized for care and protection. In addition to being isolated from the community by institutionalization, they are often isolated from significant personal interaction and validation within the setting. This

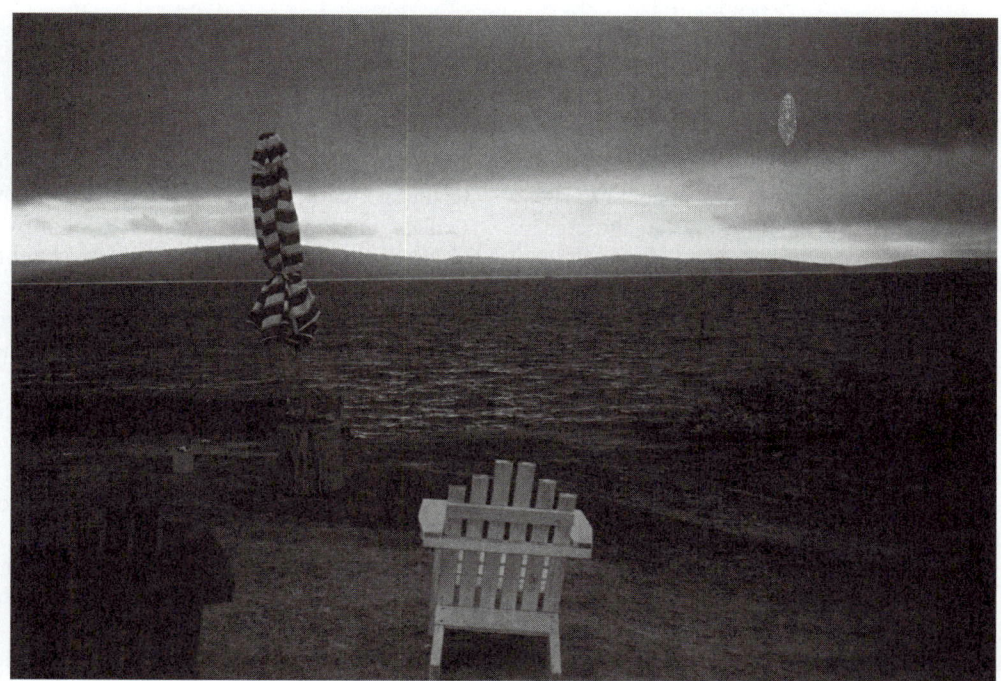

Abandoned. (Courtesy Priscilla Ebersole.)

Cause   **Interventions**

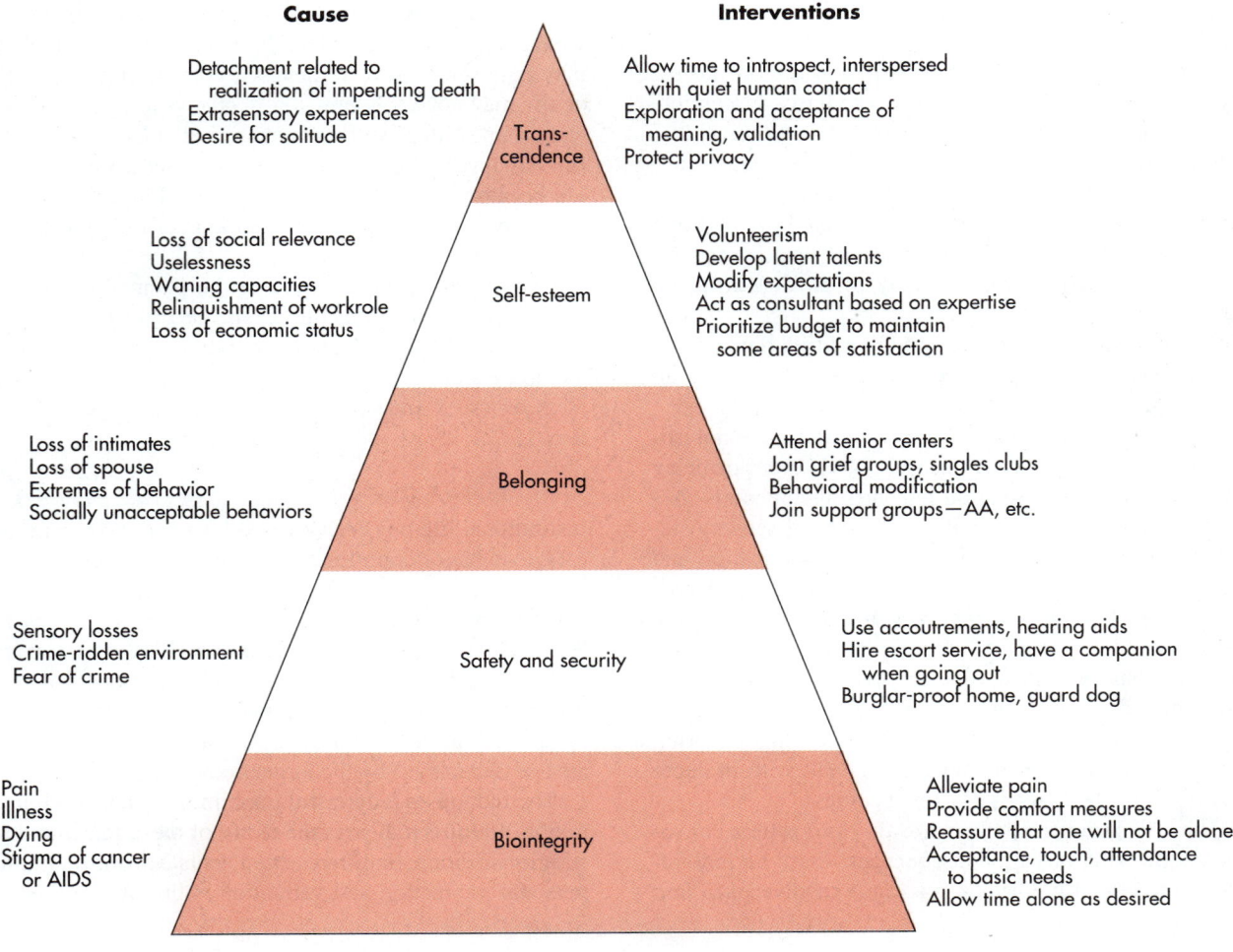

Figure 18-3. The hierarchy of isolation and loneliness. (Idea from Ravish T: *J Gerontol Nurs* 11(10):10, 1985.)

isolation produces depersonalization or loss of significance and influence as a person. One becomes a nonentity. The collective identity and pride cultivated in some institutional groups is rarely found among the institutionalized aged.

There can be little doubt that the community isolates the criminal offender and the deteriorating elder. Both threaten the health and vigor of the community. The impaired elder is more permanently isolated and has fewer guaranteed rights than the criminal.

Nursing homes, regardless of quality, carry stigma in the minds of the general population. People who work in institutions for the aged are tainted by the same exclusion and suffer some of the same stigma as residents. Much of the stigma lingers from the poorhouse concepts of the early part of the century.

Considerable efforts have been made toward enhancement of the experience of institutional living for aged residents and to provide opportunities for meaningful lives within the setting and individual limitations (DePaola and

Ebersole, 1995). Many nursing homes today are truly restorative care centers (Klusch, 1995). However, the individuals within them are usually ignored by the community at large and set aside from meaningful contributions. Even in the upscale "health care centers" of the life-care communities there are numerous residents who avoid going near the care center as if the disabilities of the residents were contagious.

Windriver(1993) suggests combating individual isolation and loneliness of institutionalized elders by offering a variety of activities for dyads and small groups and finding out from the residents which types of interaction they most enjoy. Observing spontaneous interactions and with whom they occur can give clues as to dyads or clusters of individuals where natural responses can be strengthened into friendships. This may address individual and organizational isolation, but much remains to be done to establish stronger ties between the long-term care institutions and communities.

Box 18-2	**Patterns of Isolation**

Type 1: Lifelong extrovert isolated by condition or situation
- Ameliorate the situation to the greatest extent possible.
- Seek to bring in contact with individuals and groups through Internet, distance learning.
- Assist to identify like individuals who may enjoy frequent telephone contact.
- Establish pen-pal network.

Type 2: Retiree whose contacts were mostly through work and who is now bereft of socialization opportunities
- Seek ready-made groups with some shared interests, often similar to work skills and expertise.
- Interest person in volunteer activities that will use particular skills.
- Opportunities to express particular skills in arenas where others will appreciate abilities.

Type 3: Active extrovert who withdrawals in late life due to events causing shame, e.g., divorce, alcoholism, poverty
- Assist with grief resolution, suggest counseling, seek support, self-help group.
- Help find resources addressing specific alienating condition.

Type 4: Lifelong isolate
- Assist in finding resources to augment areas of interest, hobbies.
- Initiate dyadic interactions if individual is willing.

Infusing nursing home life with companion animals, plants, gardens, and children allow residents richer opportunities to make connections and reactivate capacities for caring. Some remarkable examples of institutions providing such opportunities are the Benedictine Nursing Center in Mt Angel, Oregon, Southland Lutheran Home in Los Angeles, and the more than 100 nursing homes involved in the Eden Alternative concept developed by Dr. William Thomas of Sherburne, New York.

Combating Isolation and Depersonalization. Combating the effects of depersonalization in an institutional setting or community begins with the individual. Some suggestions for decreasing depersonalization include the following:
- Individuals may need assistance in developing a reciprocal relationship with at least one trusted person. Resources for "Friendly Visitors" and peer counselors can be found through suicide prevention centers, the mayor's office of the city, or senior centers. We seldom bring these resources into institutions, but they should be considered.
- In all situations options should be made clear in small and large matters.

- Legal aid should be sought for those whose rights have been or are being ignored. Legal aid for the elderly is available, also appeals to the human rights commission.
- Every person must have some personal items of importance and his or her own money.
- Contact with pets, plants, natural settings, and children can be renewing.
- Writing, taping, or telling life history can be a strong affirmation of identity.
- Aged persons should be given accurate information. Half-truths and concealment increase psychologic stress and confusion and refute individual worth.

The Rural Elder

Individuals in remote, sparsley populated, or inaccessible areas may be geographically and socially isolated. There is a great deal of concern about the lack of services and supports for very rural, very old individuals. In some states with vast ranches and large farms there are elders who seldom "get to town." These have been the objects of study and outreach by many geriatric nursing practitioners who may be the only health care providers for hundreds of miles.

We have had personal contact with nurse practitioners in Nevada, Arizona, Wyoming, and Montana, who have found that these elders demonstrate increasing reliance on self-care, alcoholism, stoicism, and individualism (Johnson, 1996a, 1996b). It is possible many of these fall into a category of lifelong semi-isolates, always having had a small network of affiliates that gradually shrinks even more as they age. They have a strong sense of pride and need for privacy. These isolated elders are unlikely to accept social agency assistance even if it is available (Stoller, 1993). They feel a strong need to reciprocate for any help they receive and may insist on paying or giving a gift even when depriving themselves.

Commonly reported stressors of the rural elderly include loss, isolation, financial concerns, and decreased ability to manage (Johnson et al, 1993). In addition, one of every three rural-residing elders are members of a racial or ethnic minority, compounding the problem of reaching them effectively.

One successful program reported by Boyd et al (1993) concerned the YES (Youth Exchanging with Seniors) program initiated in Texas with the cooperation of the Future Homemakers of America (FHA), Future Farmers of America (FFA), and 4-H youth organizations. These group members were uniquely suited to interact with isolated elders and, as grandchildren of neighbors and acquaintances, were not seen as intruders. More information regarding the YES project may be obtained from the Robert Wood Johnson Foundation.

Another area of concern is the consistent trend since 1960 for retirees to move to nonmetropolitan regions where the pace is slower and the costs of living lower (Fuguitt and Beale, 1993). These "recent isolates" may have trouble adjusting to the pace and the unavailability of services. In addition, long-term residents may not welcome their intrusion.

Poverty as an Isolating Factor

Throughout the text and particularly in Chapter 14 it is made clear that the very old, widowed females of color are among the most poverty-stricken individuals in our society. In this text we emphasize the needs of the elders while remaining well aware that children under 18 who are the progeny of single mothers of color are the poorest of the poor. However, the very old are more likely to be isolated because of infirmities that hamper their ability to obtain the services they need.

When thinking of ways to intervene with these isolated individuals, the nurse must seek supports that will not stigmatize the individual further because of the appearance of poverty. They rarely feel comfortable in the senior centers, even when the centers are available to them. The most likely acceptable resource will be within the churches of their ethnic group and affiliation. Transportation is a high priority and one seldom easily found. Calls to the regional Office on Aging or local Senior Centers should apprise the nurse of resources the elder may find acceptable.

ALONENESS

The United States has a large number of elders living alone (30%), mostly aged, white women (Figure 18-4). This reflects the affluence of our times, the likelihood of widowhood for women, the involvement of families willing to assist elders in maintaining an independent lifestyle, and the cultural value of individual independence that is highly treasured in our society. These are also influential factors in the numbers of elders internationally living alone and with family.

Most women must anticipate a period of living alone in late life (Table 18-2, A and B). Living alone does not equate with loneliness. The size and quality of the social network and the life patterns of the elder, as mentioned earlier, are far more significant than the number in a household. Foxall et al (1994) studied the effects on low-vision elders of living alone and found that loneliness was not a significant problem for them. Dykstra (1995) found that elders between 65 and 75 years old living alone indicated that lack of friends created loneliness but being unpartnered did not. They treasured their independence but found supportive friendships essential to their well-being.

There is little information on the effects of living alone as it pertains to survival and satisfaction. Males living alone or with someone other than spouse are thought to be at a disadvantage in terms of survival, whereas it seems to make less difference to women. Both sexes are affected by income, race, physical activity, and employment, but these are variables not necessarily related to being alone. To be alone is to be solitary, apart from others, and undisturbed. Many people have a strong need to be alone.

Assessing the Need to be Alone

Does the patient frequently close the door or turn toward the wall?
Does the patient wear earplugs or eyeshades?
Is the patient reluctant to engage in conversation?
Is there any time allowed for total privacy?
Does the patient seem absorbed in thought without agitation? Daydream?
Does the patient lie or sit with eyes closed frequently?

Interventions

Share your observations of behavior with patient.
Ask about the meaning.
Assure the patient of certain times of privacy.
Attempt to assign room with a quiet patient.
Minimize disturbances as much as possible.
Discuss the needs and perceptions of the patient in regard to being alone.

LONELINESS

There is a type of ageism that imposes the idea that old people are lonely and overcome by losses, that they are deprived and desolate. These may be attitudes of youth and middle age that change in the realities of the later maturing process.

Tornstam (1990) studied loneliness among Swedish people and identified four distinct variables of loneliness: intensity/quantity (how often and how painful), inner (personality introversion), and positive (isolation sought). Early developmental experiences and present situations remain

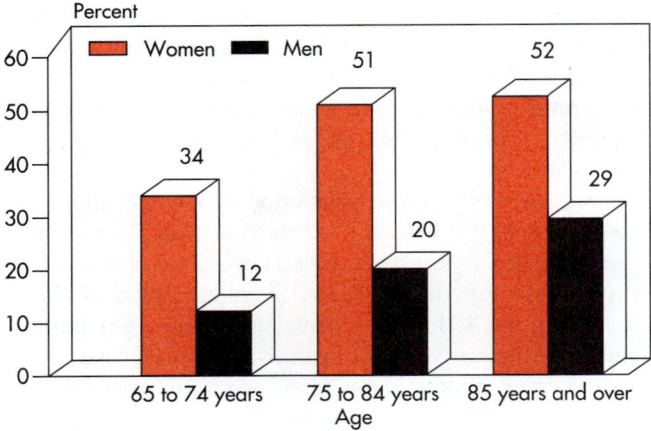

Figure 18-4. Percent of elderly living alone in the United States, 1987. (From Kinsella KG: *Living arrangements of the elderly and social policy: a cross-national perspective,* February 1990, Center for International Research, US Bureau of the Census, Washington, DC.)

important factors in the loneliness experienced by the aged. The important contribution of Tornstam's study is his attempt to show loneliness as a complex and multidimensional affect. It is not a categorical condition of the aged.

For nurses, this indicates the need to assess and discuss loneliness in depth rather than simply identify it as a possible factor in the existence of clients. Loneliness is a passive, possessive, and painful emotion, whereas aloneness, solitude, and isolation may be actively sought, enhancing, and creative. Nurses need to assess whether clients are lonely or like to be alone. Nursing care plans will be distinctly different for the alone and the lonely. To make an adequate assessment one must understand loneliness and being alone:

- Loneliness is an affective state of longing, emptiness, and feeling bereft.
- Lonely people may be physically alone or surrounded by others.
- People who are alone may be lonely or satisfied.
- Loneliness is a condition of human life that sustains, extends, and deepens humanity (Moustakas, 1961).
- Self-growth comes from one's ability to recognize and cope with loneliness.
- Factors of loneliness and aloneness change as one moves up Maslow's hierarchy of needs (Figure 18-3).

- Loneliness accompanies self-alienation and self-rejection.
- Loneliness is evidence of the capacity for love. The degree of attachment is directly correlated with the felt loss when detachment occurs.

Correlates of Loneliness

Psychologic, economic, sociologic, and physiologic factors contribute to loneliness in the elderly. A classic study by Sheldon (1948) has not been refuted. He found that the infirm widowed or single man over 80 years old and living alone was most prone to experiencing loneliness. Those well enough to exist without assistance in daily living were most lonely since others who were bedfast had some caregiver in attendance (Sheldon, 1948). Townsend (1973) found similar data but also that lifelong isolates were usually not lonely and that loneliness was attributable more to the desolation of lost companionship than to isolation.

Loneliness seems to rise in direct proportion to perceptions of physical incapacity for both men and women. Lonely persons visit the physician oftener, take more medications, and have lower energy levels and multiple psychosomatic illnesses. In support of Townsend's data, Cox et al (1988) found significant relationships between social

---

Table 18-2, A   Persons Living Alone, by Sex and Age: 1970 to 1994

[As of **March.** Based on Current Population Survey.]

Sex and age	Number of persons (1,000)					Percent distribution				
	1970	1980	1985	1990	1994	1970	1980	1985	1990	1994
Both sexes	**10,851**	**18,296**	**20,602**	**22,999**	**23,611**	**100**	**100**	**100**	**100**	**100**
15 to 24 years old*	556	1,726	1,324	1,210	1,126	5	9	6	5	5
25 to 34 years old	†1,604	†4,729	3,905	3,972	3,717	†15	†26	19	17	16
35 to 44 years old	(†)	(†)	2,322	3,138	3,518	(†)	(†)	11	14	15
45 to 64 years old	3,622	4,514	4,939	5,502	5,967	33	25	24	24	25
65 to 74 years old	2,815	3,851	4,130	4,350	4,199	26	21	20	19	18
75 years old and over ...	2,256	3,477	3,982	4,825	5,086	21	19	19	21	22
Male	**3,532**	**6,966**	**7,922**	**9,049**	**9,440**	**33**	**38**	**39**	**39**	**40**
15 to 24 years old*	274	947	750	674	570	3	5	4	3	2
25 to 34 years old	†933	†2,920	2,307	2,395	2,244	†9	†16	11	10	10
35 to 44 years old	(†)	(†)	1,406	1,836	2,115	(†)	(†)	7	8	9
45 to 64 years old	1,152	1,613	1,845	2,203	2,473	11	9	9	10	10
65 to 74 years old	611	775	868	1,042	1,031	6	4	4	5	4
75 years old and over ...	563	711	746	901	1,006	5	4	4	4	4
Female	**7,319**	**11,330**	**12,680**	**13,950**	**14,171**	**68**	**62**	**62**	**61**	**60**
15 to 24 years old*	282	779	573	536	557	3	4	3	2	2
25 to 34 years old	†671	†1,809	1,598	1,578	1,471	†6	†10	8	7	6
35 to 44 years old	(†)	(†)	916	1,303	1,401	(†)	(†)	4	6	6
45 to 64 years old	2,470	2,901	3,095	3,300	3,493	23	16	15	14	15
65 to 74 years old	2,204	3,076	3,262	3,309	3,168	20	17	16	14	13
75 years old and over ...	1,693	2,766	3,236	3,924	4,080	16	15	16	17	17

From U.S. Bureau of the Census: *Statistical abstract of the United States: 1995,* ed 115, Washington, DC, 1995.
*1970, persons 14 to 24 years old. †Data for persons 35 to 44 years old included with persons 25 to 34 years old.
Source: U.S. Bureau of the Census, *Current Population Reports,* P20-450, and earlier reports; and unpublished data.

| Table 18-2, B | Nonfamily Households, by Sex and Age of Householder: 1980 to 1994 |

[In thousands. As of **March.**]

Item		Male householder					Female householder			
	Total	15 to 24 yr old	25 to 44 yr old	45 to 64 yr old	65 yr old and over	Total	15 to 24 yr old	25 to 44 yr old	45 to 64 yr old	65 yr old and over
1980, total	**8,807**	**1,567**	**3,854**	**1,822**	**1,565**	**12,419**	**1,189**	**2,198**	**3,048**	**5,983**
One person (living alone) ..	6,966	947	2,920	1,613	1,486	11,330	779	1,809	2,901	5,842
Nonrelatives present	1,841	620	934	209	79	1,089	410	389	147	141
1990, total	**11,607**	**1,236**	**5,780**	**2,536**	**2,053**	**15,651**	**1,032**	**3,697**	**3,545**	**7,377**
One person (living alone) ..	9,049	674	4,231	2,203	1,943	13,950	536	2,881	3,300	7,233
Nonrelatives present	2,557	560	1,551	334	112	1,701	497	817	245	143
Never married	5,844	1,175	3,689	696	285	4,382	976	2,406	510	491
Married*	1,117	28	513	391	187	794	15	261	320	198
Widowed	1,417	—	29	221	1,166	7,428	4	52	1,333	6,038
Divorced	3,228	33	1,550	1,229	416	3,046	37	977	1,382	649
1994, total	**12,462**	**1,210**	**6,118**	**2,949**	**2,183**	**16,155**	**1,057**	**3,844**	**3,846**	**7,409**
One person (living alone) ..	9,440	570	4,359	2,473	2,037	14,171	557	2,872	3,493	7,248
Nonrelatives present	3,022	641	1,759	477	146	1,984	500	972	352	161
Never married	6,283	1,157	3,958	800	367	4,626	998	2,540	638	450
Married*	1,204	21	601	402	179	793	22	284	280	206
Widowed	1,411	—	15	211	1,185	7,097	1	75	1,064	5,958
Divorced	3,564	31	1,545	1,537	452	3,639	34	945	1,865	795

From U.S. Bureau of the Census: *Statistical abstract of the United States: 1995,* ed 115, Washington, DC, 1995.
—Represents or rounds to zero. *No spouse present.
Source: U.S. Bureau of the Census, *Current Population Reports,* P20-450, and earlier reports; and unpublished data.

network size, health status, and perceived loneliness. Persons who are lonely are at risk of poor health and deterioration.

The Geriatric Orphan

The "geriatric orphan" is an elderly person with no close friends or family members surviving or available to provide supports. He or she has had significant others and lost them to death, distance, and fractured relationships. He or she has not desired to be alone. In the event the individuals are the last surviving member of their clan, nurses may certainly encourage them to talk about those they have lost. Some have serious "survivor's guilt" that they need to express, particularly if the individual is the eldest and last survivor of a large sibling group. They can be assured this is an aspect of grief that is often experienced. Jennie said, "I was always the sickly one. I never expected to live so long. Why me and and not them?" The sensitive nurse will resist platitudes and will respond, "Tell me about them."

Boyack (1983) suggests it is imperative to establish a surrogate network, assist the individual through the grief, help resolve any unfinished business, and seek appropriate resources for maintenance in the community as long as the elder desires and is able. For some geriatric orphans it may be a relief to be among others in a congregate or institutional setting, though others may find it depressing and react much better to friendly visits from younger people. Nurses are urged to make a loneliness assessment

with their clients and discuss with them ways in which they could establish contact with others.

Assessing Loneliness

Luggen and Rini (1995) found it useful to assess the social network of community elders in order to predict those at risk of isolation. Almost half of the sample were found (based on the Lubben Social Network Scale) to be at great risk of isolation and detrimental loneliness. The greatest risk factor was childlessness.

Does the patient initiate contact?
Is the patient anxious, withdrawn, apathetic, or hostile?
Does the patient cling to others or attempt to detain them?
Is the patient unable to articulate his or her own needs?
Is the patient eager for visitors and distressed when they leave?
Does the patient exhibit contempt for his or her condition or self?
Has there been a major disruption in number of contacts with the patient?
How often does the patient feel lonely and under what circumstances?
Does the patient provoke to gain attention?

Interventions

Ask about loneliness.
Spend time with the patient in silence or in conversation.

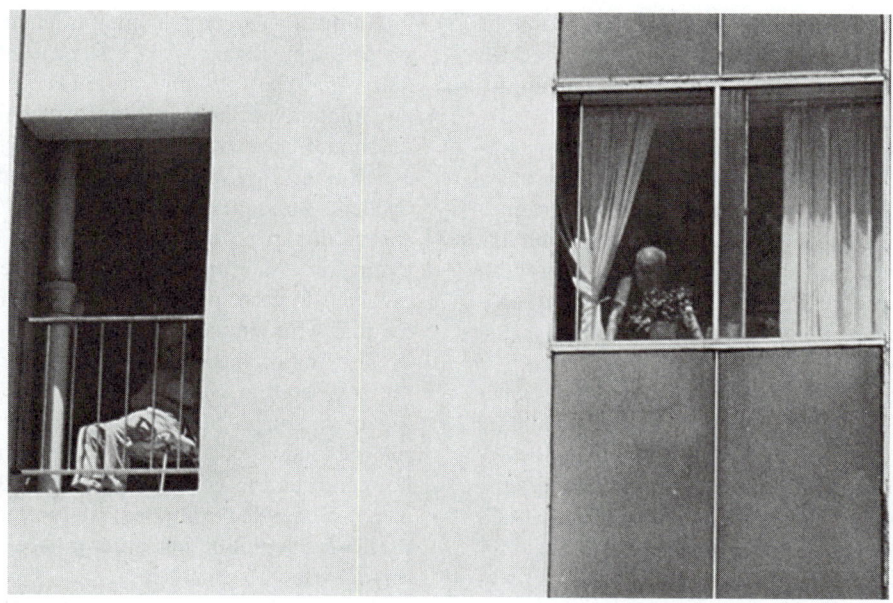

Loneliness. (Courtesy Stewart H. Bloom.)

Assist in keeping contact with people important to the patient.

Let the patient know when you will be available.

Explore the nature of the loneliness with the patient, also the phenomenon of loneliness.

Guide the person in reviewing life experiences related to loneliness to gain insight (for the patient) and data (for you).

See or call the client frequently for brief periods.

Combating Loneliness with Pets. In 1859 Florence Nightingale (reprint, 1992) wrote that pets were excellent companions for persons confined with long-term illnesses. Studies of the value of animals for the aged began to appear in 1980. Several articles and books on the topic have been well reviewed by Erickson (1985).

The most common reason people want pets is to combat loneliness. For stigmatized or isolated persons, pets may assume great importance because they are always available and nonjudgmental. Unquestioning, uncritical, and unconditional affection, seldom found in human relationships, may somewhat compensate for the lack of human contact. Some research suggests that a pet may even be the catalyst to establish relationships (Messent, 1983).

Touching and fondling a pet may provide a substitute for human touch. In addition, a dog may provide a sense of protection and safety. Tucker et al (1995) found in a retrospective longitudinal study that simply having a pet seemed to have little effect on an elder but those who had special needs for interaction, were recovering from a major loss, were institutionalized, or frequently played with a pet experienced beneficial effects and a greater sense of well-being.

In organizing and operating a volunteer community-based pet placement program for the community-dwelling elderly, consideration should be given to ethics, legalities, and pragmatic issues, including the desired organizational structure of the service process, criteria for client and animal selection, organization liability in placing pets, facilitation of bonding, development of support services for the elderly and their animals, and evaluation of the success or failure of the placements.

A consideration in the selection of a pet may be potential longevity because the loss of a pet can produce deep grief. Aged persons losing a pet often grieve intensely for a short period and find no socially sanctioned outlets for resolving their grief. Shirley and Mercier (1983) found that three fourths of them consider the pet a member of the family, and one half feel that the pet was a major part of their lives. Three fourths of the sample studied reported they had some type of funeral for the dead animal.

Recognizing the significance, nurses may inquire about pets and the attachment and validate the grief. At these times it would be important to make every effort to assist the elder in finding a support system. It may be useful to consider establishing grief groups for individuals whose pets have died. We sometimes become so preoccupied with "serious" issues that we do not fully understand the meaning of the loss of a pet in the life of a lonely elder.

Loneliness from Inability to Communicate

Speech is the major means of establishing and maintaining a satisfying network of relationships. Persons with speech disabilities will have many problems negotiating a personally acceptable milieu. Communication handicaps are among the most disastrous consequences of cerebrovascular accidents and disease in older adults. Having spent a lifetime relying on communication, sudden loss of this ability can be dehumanizing.

A 59-year-old radio broadcaster was struck by a left cerebrovascular accident. As his confusion lifted in the first few days of hospitalization, his nonverbal agony was heartrending. He sputtered meaningless sounds, pounded with his clenched left fist, and cried. His devastation was apparent to everyone who worked with him. Fortunately, an active rehabilitation team began working with him immediately, and his progress was rapid.

Another situation involved an aged man in a senior center who could speak quite intelligently 3 years after a cerebrovascular accident. He shared the feelings of agony he experienced for 2 years, before active rehabilitation efforts, when he understood everything going on around him but did not have the capacity to make himself understood. He said for those 2 years he was treated as an imbecile. Finally he was properly evaluated, and his potential for recovering speech was facilitated. It was an arduous task, but he was determined.

Nurses must insist that the care of aged persons with speech disorders is not adequate if a qualified speech pathologist has not been involved early in the care planning. This is not a frill but a necessity and should begin immediately. Communication is the single most important capacity of human beings, and there is little that is more dehumanizing than interference with verbal communication. The isolation and loneliness of the inarticulate can only be imagined by those who have not experienced it.

Language Disorders Associated with Aging. There are three major categories of impaired verbal communication: (1) reception, (2) perception, and (3) articulation. Reception is impaired by anxiety, hearing deficits, and altered levels of consciousness. Perception is distorted by stroke, dementia, and delirium. Articulation is hampered by dysarthria, respiratory disease, destruction of the larynx, and cerebral infarction. Specific difficulties (Ginsberg, 1988) include the following:

1. *Anomie:* word retrieval difficulties during spontaneous speech and naming tasks
2. *Aphasia:* an acquired impairment of language processes underlying receptive and expressive modalities caused by damage to areas of the brain that are primarily responsible for language processes
3. *Dysarthria:* impairment in the ability to articulate words as the result of damage to the central or peripheral nervous system

Difficulty in articulating words or selecting and comprehending appropriate words is caused by neuromotor disturbances that may be transient, long-standing, reversible, or irreversible. Prophylactic, or primary, prevention of these disorders is poorly understood, but much can be done in speech retraining programs to regain intelligible conversational ability.

Aphasia. The most common language disorder is aphasia following stroke; it is a significant problem for the elderly. Because communication is such a vital aspect of life, one might expect that great effort would be made to restore maximum speech abilities for individuals with aphasia. MacKay et al (1988) found in a sample of 95 community residents 6 months after stroke that 87% were not receiving speech therapy. Since stroke is one of the leading causes of long-term disability, it behooves nurses to become actively involved in assuring that the aged will receive appropriate treatment for language disabilities.

The importance of Broca's and Wernicke's areas of the left cerebral cortex in the expression and understanding of language has been recognized for over a century (Geschwind, 1965). These lie within the distribution of the left cerebral artery surrounding the sylvian fissure. Broca's area is associated with the posteroinferior frontal lobe (Figure 18-5). Wernicke's area lies adjacent to the primary auditory cortex.

The right hemisphere, unlike the left, cannot be compartmentalized into discrete functional roles. The more diffuse organization appears to adapt the right hemisphere to a more holistic, global processing of information. The skills of the right hemisphere include selective attention, visual perceptions, orientation to time and place, and understanding of the subtleties of communication. Research is increasingly em-

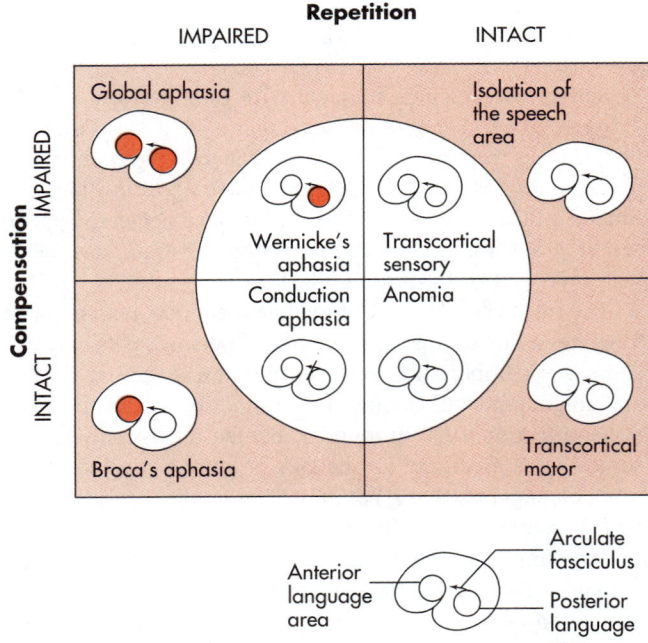

Figure 18-5. Aphasia diagram: The three components of language function to be tested are comprehension, fluency, and repetition. Aphasias depicted within the circle are the fluent aphasias. (From Gallo JJ, Reichel W, Anderson L: *Handbook of geriatric assessment,* ed 2, Gaithersburg, Md, 1995, Aspen Publications.)

phasizing the importance of the right hemisphere and the subcortical structures in language processing.

There are several types of aphasia that the nurse may encounter with elderly persons:

- *Wernicke's aphasia* is the result of a lesion in the superior temporal gyrus. Persons with Wernicke's aphasia speak easily but in a repetitive jargon that is poorly understood. Unrelated words may be strung together or syllables repeated. They also have difficulty understanding spoken language.
- *Broca's aphasia* typically involves damage to the posteroinferior portions of the dominant frontal lobe. Persons with Broca's aphasia understand others but speak very slowly and use minimum words. They often struggle to articulate a word and seem to have lost the ability to voluntarily control the movements of speech. This is often called "apraxia of speech."
- Persons with *conductive aphasia* understand speech and may speak fluently but may substitute sounds and words for the ones they wish to use.
- *Anomic aphasia* is associated with lesions of the dominant temporoparietal regions of the brain, although no single locus has been identified. Persons with anomic aphasia understand and speak readily but may have severe word-finding difficulty. They may be unable to remember crucial content words.
- *Global aphasia* is the result of large left hemisphere lesions and affects most of the language areas of the

brain. Persons with global aphasia are unable to understand words or speak intelligibly. They may use meaningless syllables repetitiously (InSpeech, Inc, 1988).

Behaviors of patients with right hemisphere stroke are often very similar to those diagnosed with dementia and include five major deficits: attention, orientation, perception, retention, and integration. These right hemisphere brain-damage reactions have been neglected.

When a cerebrovascular accident damages the dominant half of the brain (left side in right-handed people), some disruption will occur in the "word factory." There are two major types of aphasia: receptive and expressive (Figure 18-6). Receptive aphasic patients cannot understand language; it is as if they are in a foreign land. They may recognize objects and their uses. Expressive aphasic patients can understand verbal and written communication but cannot organize concepts into words or meaningful expressions. See suggestions in Box 18-3 for communicating with aphasic patients.

Nurses are responsible for accurate observation and recording of the speech and word recognition patterns of the client and for consistently implementing the recommendations of the speech pathologist. In each type of aphasia a qualified speech pathologist should be consulted to develop appropriate rehabilitative plans. The speech pathologist is able to identify the areas of language that remain relatively unimpaired and to capitalize on the

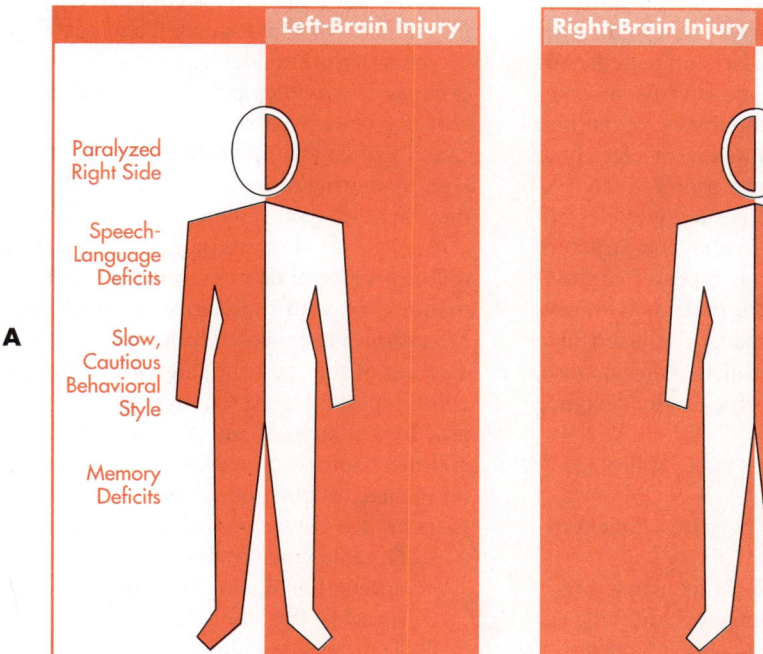

Figure 18-6. Receptive and expressive aphasia arising from left (**A**) and right (**B**) brain injury. (From American Heart Association: *How stroke affects behavior,* Dallas, 1994, American Heart Association.)

Box 18-3	**Communicating with Aphasic Patients**

- Explain situations, treatments, and anything else that is pertinent to the patient because he or she may understand; the sounds of normal speech tend to be rehabilitative even if the words are not understood. Talk as if the person understands.
- Avoid patronizing and childish phrases.
- The aphasic patient may be especially sensitive to feelings of annoyance; remain calm and patient.
- Speak slowly, ask one question at a time, and wait for a response.
- Ask questions in a way that can be answered with a nod or the blink of an eye; if the patient cannot verbally respond, instruct him or her in nonverbal responses.
- Speak of things familiar and of interest to the patient.
- Use visual cues, objects, pictures, and gestures as well as words.
- Organize the environment to be as predictable as possible.
- Encourage articulation even if words convey no meaning.
- Show interest in the patient as an individual.

Table 18-3   Prognostic Variables in Aphasia

Variable	Summary
Age at onset	Younger patients have a better prognosis
Premorbid education, intelligence, and language abilities	Undetermined influence on prognosis
Associated defects and health during recovery	Patients with no associated deficits or illness have a better prognosis
Social milieu	Undetermined influence on prognosis
Cause	Nonpenetrating trauma has a better prognosis than penetrating trauma, vascular accident, tumor, and infection
Size and site of lesion	Small lesions not in temporoparietal area have a better prognosis
Time after onset	Patients with brief duration of aphasia have a better prognosis
Severity and type of aphasia	Mild aphasia and the absence of significant auditory comprehension deficits and severe apraxia of speech are favorable prognostic signs
Nonlanguage behavior	Awareness, high motivation, and high aspiration are favorable prognostic signs
Length and intensity of treatment	Participation in a longer, more intense treatment program is more likely to achieve prognosis

From Ginsberg S: *Prognostic variables in aphasia,* Unpublished paper, Cleveland, 1988, Case Western Reserve University.

remaining strengths. The prognosis for recovery of speech is summarized in Table 18-3.

Staff tend to be less frustrated and show more incentive to work with clients when a means of communication is established and needs can be clearly identified. This enhances feelings of effectiveness for staff and patient. Additional techniques are developed that assist us in communicating with those who have temporarily or permanently lost verbal skills. There are an array of electronic tools available, but sometimes they are prohibitively expensive. Some that have proved effective include electro-mechanical boards, electronic boards, sentence structure boards, and computer programs. Various types of communication boards have been developed for patients with several levels of disability. For some, a particularly sensitive pressure switch can be activated by the touch of an ear, nose, or chin. The following are some types of specially designed switches:

1. Thumb-depressed switch: requires some ability to move thumb.
2. Minimum pressure switch: any finger is sufficient to activate switch.
3. Photoelectric switch: a beam of light interrupted by any object will activate switch (tongue, card, finger).
4. Superminimum pressure switch: may be touched from any angle at any place along bar, activated by slight contact with ear, nose, chin.
5. Probe switch: designed for a patient who cannot open his or her hand.

There are a number of commercially available switches for patients who have strength and dexterity in one hand. To be generally useful, devices must be simply constructed, inexpensive, portable, and connected to a signaling device to attract attention when the individual wishes to communicate. In situations in which electronic devices are not available, game boards with pointers and appropriate pictures may be developed (Figure 18-7).

Dysarthria. Dysarthria is a condition arising from central or peripheral neuromuscular disorders in which there is interference with the clarity of speech and pronunciation. Dysarthria is second only to aphasia as a communication disorder of the aged and may be due to neuromuscular flaccidity, spasticity, ataxia, hypokinesia, or hyperkinesia. It may be a mixture of any of these and will often involve several mechanisms of speech, such as respiration, phonation, resonance, articulation, and prosody (the meter, rhythm of speech). It is characterized by one or more of the following:

1. Organic voice tremor produces a quavering articulation arising from tremors of the larynx muscles, lips, tongue, and diaphragm.
2. Transient tremulous articulation may be the result of tranquilizers, particularly phenothiazines.
3. A slow, unsteady speech pattern may be the result of cerebellar degeneration. In this case the gait will also be halting and wide based.

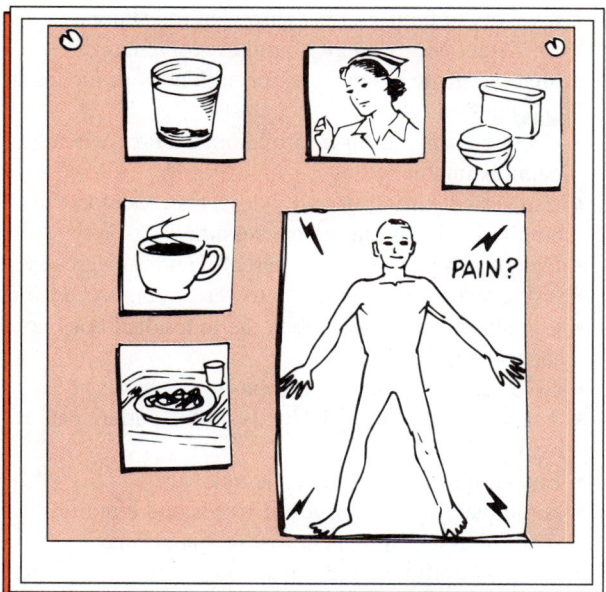

Figure 18-7. Communication board. (Illustration by Joseph Pierre.)

4. Uncontrolled movement of lips, face, and tongue may be an indication of Parkinson's disease. Speech may be slurred and jumpy, the expression flat, and the voice tone monotonous, sometimes hardly audible.
5. Spastic dysarthria is found in 12% of stroke patients. Words are correct, but flow of speech is tight, constrained, and laborious.

Treatment after an acute episode, such as stroke or surgery, requires a speech pathologist to develop a treatment program to retrain muscular coordination. In a progressive neurologic disease the treatment begins early and is ongoing while the person is encouraged to maintain speech as long as possible. The speech pathologist will assist in modifying speech patterns when necessary to maintain articulation (Lee and Itoh, 1990).

Laryngectomy. Following laryngectomy surgery, the patient has no voice. There are three options for the laryngectomy patient: reconstructive surgery, esophageal speech, or an electrolarynx. Some individuals may learn to master esophageal speech, and others may prefer the electrolarynx even though the sound emitted is robotic. All clients should be given the opportunity to talk to a member of the Lost Chord Club, a self-help group that offers advice and emotional support.

During the initial recovery period the patient will need guidance in dealing with intense feelings of loss of ability to make sounds. The patient cannot even cry audibly. The nurse will need to anticipate and articulate possible feelings, seeking corroboration by a nonverbal gesture. These early weeks and the efforts made by others to continue talking to the laryngectomee will assist greatly in keeping the individual motivated toward eventual speech training.

Bill's wife, Mary, was told by her physician that she just had a "sexy voice." Because her sore throat continued for several weeks, Bill insisted she get a second opinion. It was discovered that she had cancer of the larynx, and a laryngectomy was performed. She successfully learned laryngeal speech and was able to communicate, but the cancer had metastasized. As her physical condition deteriorated she was no longer able to exert the energy required for laryngeal speech. In the few weeks before her death she was unable to communicate with her husband verbally. His grief over losing her was compounded by his conviction that there were many important things she had wanted to say to him before her death.

A most compassionate intervention before laryngectomy would be to assist an individual to make an audiotape or videotape for family or significant persons expressing thoughts, feelings, or ideas that can be preserved. The subtleties, inflections, and tone of one's voice are major aspects of identity. Individuals can be identified by voice even when appearance has undergone major change. This part of one's identity must not be lost to those who love the person. Preservation of some intimate thoughts should not be neglected.

Verbigeration: incoherent or repetitious sounding. Verbigeration is described as meaningless repetition of words or sounds. We believe it has meaning. Sounding is a conscious or subconscious need to express one's inner life and an exertion of will that releases pent-up energy. It often occurs when meaningful communication has been interrupted. One groans or moans to release heart heaviness, just as one grunts and groans when lifting a heavy object. The release obtained by setting off sounding vibrations in the environment is gratifying.

Sounding has been used to measure the depth of water and to measure surface distances. Analogously, perhaps the aged are attempting to measure interpersonal distances and the depth of their isolation as they sound their environment with repetitious, often unintelligible utterances. Noises that emerge, bidden or unbidden, may be groans, chants, screams, sighs, mumbles, laughs, etc.

Sounding has several purposes for the old:
1. Reaffirmation of their presence among the living in the "sea of personalities," which means each must reestablish a field pattern of communication each day (Coulson, 1973)
2. Testing the caregiver's reaction to the sounds of need
3. Discharge of tension that is pent up in one's body
4. Self-stimulation
5. Establishment of one's personal space or territorial boundaries

For example, an old man in a nursing home chanted "who-who" most of his waking time. The staff would respond (if at all) with irritation or amusement, "There goes 'who-who' again." No one talked directly to him or tried to find out exactly what was his need. One resident summed it up nicely, "You know, 'who-who' gets a lot of attention around here, everyone knows about him."

Sounding has been coined as a word to cover all the "meaningless" babbling that often occurs in settings in which the impaired aged reside. We believe these sounds have meaning and are sometimes meant to make a loud statement, "I remain in the land of the living. Communicate with me."

Zachow (1984) worked with a very old lady (Helen) with dementia who constantly repeated "wa, wa, wa, wa" in a loud voice. A common and significant problem of communication in demented persons is their seeming inability to control these meaningless verbal perseverations. Zachow assumed that Helen wanted to communicate, which may be the first and most important assumption. She also determined that there must be a way to reach through the gray shroud of emotional chaos. Her method was planned multisensorial stimulation daily for 6 weeks. She used touch, talk, baroque music, body movement, and a combination of validation and fantasy to give meaning to all of Helen's actions. With continued work, Helen was eventually able to feed herself and to speak a few words that could be understood.

The success of the interventions may be based on some restoration of biorhythmicity. The dementias are believed to result in disturbances of biorhythmicity that are exhibited in perseverative babbling, sleep pattern disturbances, and basal metabolic rate disturbances. It is quite possible that selected music has the potential for restoration of body rhythm. The ancient Greeks and Egyptians gave full credence to the therapeutic power of music. We have yet to seriously study the use of music with demented persons. Most importantly, replications of Zachow's study have not been found and are still badly needed.

Recently it has been reported that playing recordings of loved ones' voices discussing pleasant memories has been beneficial in reducing agitation and verbigeration in demented elders (Woods, 1993).

Nursing Actions. In conclusion, some suggestions for working with the communicatively impaired elderly include the following:

- Establish hearing capacity by discussing with family or checking startle reaction to sounds in back of the person.
- Immediately engage a speech therapist.
- Establish rapport and demonstrate interest in the client's attempts to communicate.
- Establish a climate of acceptance and worth.
- Avoid artificial praise.
- Reduce client's anxiety by a relaxed approach and consistent expectations.
- Reassess the client often, and increase expectations as improvement is noted.
- When with the client, talk about what you are doing, name the act, and talk about the events in the daily routine.

- Involve the family in the care plan to ensure a consistent approach and family involvement.
- Share realistic gains and expectations with the client and the family.
- Use the family as an informational source when the client is unable.
- Use varied stimuli (touch, odors, tastes, colors) to emphasize ideas and words sessions.
- Demonstrate information verbally and nonverbally.
- Ask questions occasionally to verify comprehension.
- Use alternative words when the individual does not seem to understand.
- Give adequate time for response.
- Ask yes/no questions if that is all the patient can respond to.
- Encourage choices and decisions.
- Anticipate loss of control of words and emotions at times, reassure the client that this is normal.
- Keep a familiar and predictable environment to the extent possible.
- Encourage any attempts to communicate and give feedback about that which is understood.

ALIENATION

Alienation is intertwined with isolation and loneliness but has specific characteristics that can be recognized. Alienation encompasses powerlessness, normlessness, isolation, self-estrangement, and meaninglessness (Seeman, 1959). Alienation is also seen in social estrangement, hostility and exclusion. Alien is foreign, outside the accepted cultural norm, different, and often misunderstood.

Alienation often entails guilt because one is estranged from self, and the "not me" continually confronts the inner dialogue, battering self-concept. Actions, conditions, and situations that one knows are socially unacceptable challenge the inner child that has incorporated numerous shoulds and oughts in the course of growing to maturity. In old age, when the individual may have more time for reflection, these tend to emerge again in the life-review process.

Gays and Lesbians

At the White House Conference on Aging (WHCoA) in May 1995, there were delegates representing elder gay and lesbian individuals. With considerable effort and persistence they had gathered a sufficient number of signatures to merit inclusion of lesbian and gay elders in the language and substance of the recommendations of the WHCoA (Hamburger, 1996).

While young gay men have become a powerful political group, older homosexuals tend to remain hidden. As one young man put it, "Yes, I suppose there are some but I can't imagine my grandmother being a lesbian." Only recently, and largely through the efforts of the American Society on Aging, have they been given attention and recognition for their particular needs.

In a recent National Lesbian and Gay Health Conference (June 1996, Minneapolis) organized by Vincent Delgado, the founder of Senior Action in a Gay Environment (SAGE), one topic was "The Closet within the Closet." This highlighted the difficulty of breaking through age, sex, and cultural barriers. Reports were given of individuals diagnosed with depression and mental illness based on their sexual orientation (American Society on Aging, 1996). The fact that the diagnosis of homosexuality was removed from the American Psychiatric Association *Diagnostic and Statistical Manual of Mental Disorders* in 1975 seems in some cases to have resulted in only a diversion to an alternate diagnosis. This is reminiscent of the 50s, when numerous women were treated as narcissistic hysterics. Any powerless individual or group is likely to display symptomatic behaviors.

In the later years there are important issues to consider regarding partner's rights, advance directives, and availability of services (Henry, 1996). The price of invisibility may mean one must forgo important health services. Berger (1996) suggests that younger gay and lesbian individuals may want and need older role models. There is much research yet to be done to explore the capacities and contributions of elder homosexuals. Nurses are in a prime position to affirm elders' right to lifestyles of their choice and to strengthen their resolve to live in the light if that is their wish. Additional discussion of homosexuality can be found in Chapter 16.

The Homeless

The National Governors' Association characterizes a homeless person as one unable to secure permanent and stable housing without assistance. The homeless include many categories: the deinstitutionalized chronically mentally ill, skid row alcoholics, street people ("bag ladies" and "grate men"), and the situationally distressed (new poor). Many shelters focus on assisting the latter group (Damrosch and Strasser, 1988).

The drastic reduction in the budget for low-cost housing units and the gentrification of large urban areas have undoubtedly left many poor elders on the streets. Many were probably single-room occupants (SROs) of run-down inner-city hotels that have given way to urban beautification. Keigher (1989) found that among the Chicago aged homeless many had been evicted. Investigation revealed a substantial number of violent and tragic deaths. Thirty-eight percent of those in need of shelter had died within 1 to 3 years of their eviction. The current number of homeless aged is unknown but thought to be a growing problem.

Who are the street seniors, and what are their problems? This question was explored by Blakeney (1991), and the answers were based in her experience at the Long Island Shelter in Boston Harbor, Maine. One in 10 individuals in the shelter was over age 60. Other characteristics can be seen in Box 18-4. Of 30 homeless elders, it was found that three fourths were alcoholic, and many had pulmonary, neuro-

logic, and cardiovascular problems. In spite of the high incidence of alcoholism and physical problems, these elders had many survival skills and a far lower rate of mental illness than the younger homeless group.

Nurses at the Boston Harbor shelter encouraged attendance at Alcoholics Anonymous and better nutrition. In addition, they often accompanied elders to obtain emergency care when illnesses became serious enough to demand attention.

Elias and Inui (1993) found that among a group of homeless men in Seattle, alcoholism was a prevalent problem. They used the public shelters for safety, support, and a sense of community. Some also saw it as an opportunity to regain sobriety. This lends strength to the idea that many of the elderly homeless may be ready for social rehabilitation.

The large numbers of elderly homeless in our cities are a challenge to nurses, other professionals, and our society (Dolan, 1989). Many that need assistance may not find the form in which it is offered acceptable. Several groups of nurses across the United States have raised money for the homeless through fund-raising activities and direct contributions; others have contributed direct services in the form of meal preparation and health care in clinics.

One example of a homeless program in which nurses play a pivotal role is the Health Care for the Homeless Program in Baltimore. This program includes walk-in clinics, shelters, outreach sites, and a food van. They have arranged for dentistry, podiatry, and drug detoxification, as well as links with two hospitals (Damrosch and Strasser, 1988).

In Portland, Oregon, a comprehensive service program was developed for homeless mentally ill offenders (McFarland and Blair, 1995). Residential, health, mental health, and sobriety services were provided. Of the 47 individuals accepted into the program, 14 completed the program, attained sobriety, and were placed in community housing. Problems

---

Box 18-4	**Homeless Elders**

Mean age of 70.6 years
90% male, 10% female
Average of 4.5 years homeless, range 1 to 30 years
40% had families but were alienated from them
23% were widowed but had children
20% were single
16% unclear about status of families and children
53% were service veterans
70% received Social Security
30% had Medicaid benefits
25% had veterans benefits
33% had high school education
29% had attended college or graduate school

Summarized from Blakeney B: Old, homeless and sick, *Geriatr Nurs* 12(5):220, 1991.

encountered in delivering a comprehensive package such as this were costs, agency conflicts, and inconsistent staffing. However, this model seems to have potential.

Because of the increased vulnerability of the aged homeless to illness, death, and assault, Doolin (1986) recommends special shelters be established to meet their needs for protection, access to health care, and nutritious foods. Transportation and assistance in finding housing may be most important. Major economic and social changes, as well as new housing policies, are needed in order to assist these neglected elders. Many resist help because they fear losing their independence and freedom.

Divorce among Elders

Persons over the age of 60 are divorcing in greater numbers than ever before. As recently as 60 years ago, the divorce of an elderly lady from her spouse carried a great sense of shame with it. Even today for some of the older cohorts divorce carries the brand of failure.

One percent of women and 1.8% of men over age 65 seek and are granted divorce. This is a small but significant amount compared to the peak divorce ages of 30 to 34 years, when the divorce rate is slightly over 20% (National Center for Health Statistics, 1996). It is unclear from these data what percentage of elder divorces involve long-standing marriages and what percentage are shorter-term remar-

riages. However, the U.S. Bureau of the Census (1995) indicates that for women over age 50, 30% of the divorces are after first marriages and 34.5% are redivorced after remarriages. Apparently the remainder who remarry after divorce maintain the marriage.

Lanza (1996) states that each year at least 50,000 persons older than 60 dissolve marriages of 30 to 40 years' duration. Cain (1988) suggests that cohort effects and preexisting attitudes about the centrality of marriage to female roles often result in relentless despair and slow recovery from divorce. In any case, the impact of divorce upon women in later life has been poorly studied.

Psychologic and social consequences of divorce for women in later life can be seen in Box 18-5. If the male spouse seeks and marries a younger woman, self-esteem is seriously assaulted. There is in this an element of ageism as well as social devaluation of the older woman. Lanza suggests group affiliations with other late-life divorcees, restructuring interests and life patterns around singleness, and establishing social and economic stability all contribute to a successful resolution of these divorces, although the process and demands of aging itself may make adjustment more difficult. Gender differences in adjustment were not noted although we feel they may be significant.

Establishing an identity as a single individual may require redoing some elements of adolescence. The nurse may need to guide the ventilation process toward consideration of some options for beginning again while fully recognizing that divorce entails acute grief, anger, and shame for the victim and probable guilt as well as grief for the instigator. Ultimately, a new sense of freedom and self-direction is desirable. For those who remarry there may be considerable ambivalence and semiconscious comparisons with the strengths and weaknesses of the previous marriage.

Blatter and Jacobsen (1993) suggest interventions should focus on (1) methods to bolster self-esteem, (2) specific concrete and measurable goals the elder wishes to accomplish, (3) identification of particularly stressful situations and clear plans to ameliorate these stressors, (4) engagement of as much of the social support network as possible in providing social outlets and contacts, and (5) encouragement when any small gains are made.

The Alienation of Alzheimer's Disease

We cannot enter the world of the elder with Alzheimer's disease. No one on the outside can know the frustration of the inability to express pain, thirst, hunger, or loneliness—the most elemental of human needs. We suppose the limited awareness and reduced cognitive processing ability makes life less difficult for the victim of Alzheimer's disease, yet we know he or she responds to the affect and feelings of others. Those individuals, once greatly appreciated and loved, become a burden that must be borne with as much fortitude as possible. Small wonder that the inexpressible longings

Box 18-5	**Psychologic and Social Consequences of Divorce for Elderly Women***

Psychologic consequences
- Sense of loss, despair
- Increased anxiety
- Decreased self-esteem
- Impaired functioning
- Feeling of vulnerability during period of physical decline
- Guilt, self-recrimination

Social consequences
- Struggle to learn "instrumental" skills (e.g., how to manage finances, maintain a car, negotiate with a lawyer)
- Develop new ways to cope with own physical limitations due to absent husband
- Isolation, viewed as "out of step" with peers
- Difficulty finding same-age companions who shared similar levels of energy
- Dependent on adult offspring for residential help and daily companionship
- Care for rather than receive help from own parents

*Adapted from Cain (1988).
From Lanza ML: Divorce experienced as an older woman, *Geriatr Nurs* 17(4):166, 1996.

are made visible in obnoxious behaviors. Discussion of Alzheimer's disease is in Chapter 22, and further discussion of the caregiving aspects of these individuals can be found in Chapter 17.

STIGMATIZATION

Stigma may be the reason for loneliness, isolation, and alienation but is less the product of guilt and inner dissatisfaction than that of disgust and revulsion perceived from others. There is not, in my mind, a clear delineation in any of these conditions though stigma may carry a sense of victimization, perhaps feelings of anger and a sense of the unfairness of life that the others do not.

Goffman (1963) wrote the classic work on stigma. Stigma is a term used to refer to an attribute that discredits the individual. The historic roots of *stigma* referred to the body markings, such as brands, tatoos or cuts, that marked an individual and were designed to convey to the public the condition or moral status of the person (Saylor, 1995).

Some of the aged are discredited based on an alterations in appearance. An aged lady presented herself for a conservatorship hearing. She slowly shuffled forward, with voice quavering and grossly visible tremors. She appeared totally unable to manage her life, and the stage was set for a negative evaluation based on her appearance rather than competence. We are a visual society, and what we see forms strong opinions and emotional reactions.

The degree to which one is isolated by a disability is strongly correlated with the evidence of the disorder and the acceptability of its expression. Facial spider angiomas, often a sign of advanced liver disease and alcoholism, stir a negative response in many medical personnel. Diabetes stimulates concern or a neutral response. Obesity is not acceptable and incurs disgust; emaciation arouses sympathy. These examples illustrate the irrationality of stigma.

Cole (1992) makes the point that historically, those elders who were ill, afflicted, or had impaired function were stigmatized and thought to have earned their condition by indulging in poor life practices. Longevity was a reward for proper behavior. "The devastating implications of ageism lay not in negative images alone but in the splitting apart of positive and negative aspects of aging, along with the belief that virtuous individuals' souls achieve one and escape the other." (Cole, 1992, p. 91). Gradually, in this Victorian process, old age joined sex, death, and aggression as ideas held in check by repression and denial.

Today we are again approaching the notion that those who live right may live forever, and we are continually trying to determine all the aspects of "right living." In our obsession with healthful practices we build new stereotypes of good and bad and stigmatize individuals with certain appearances, conditions, and behaviors. Self-esteem is continually eroded if one feels out of control of the disorder or

guilty over lifestyle patterns that have contributed to the disorder. Depending upon the visibility or discomfort of a chronic disorder, one may feel stigmatized in direct relation to the self-revulsion experienced.

Alcoholism

Alcoholism is discussed as substance abuse in Chapter 21, but it needs to be brought to attention in this chapter as a condition that stigmatizes individuals. Much as Alcoholics Anonymous has consistently insisted alcoholism is a disease, possibly of genetic origin and altered metabolic processes, it is still generally viewed as indicative of emotional immaturity and self-indulgence or lack of control. The alcoholic is afflicted with self-revulsion and feelings of shame and guilt. The elderly late-life alcoholic may be particularly prone to these feelings.

It has been reported that as many as one third to one half of elderly individuals who develop problems with alcohol late in life do so as a result of life circumstances and changes that commonly accompany aging (Liberto et al, 1990). These data need considerably more investigation (Wood, 1995).

When alcoholism does develop in late life, there is great potential for recovery. Schuckit et al (1995) have found major alcohol-related life problems occur in both men and women. These will likely be the trigger to obtaining help. The hazards particular to the aged include dangerous interactions with medications, falls, fractures, activation of preexisting disease conditions, and further diminishing physical, emotional, and social functioning (Fink et al, 1996).

A nurse can be most helpful in assisting the individual to understand the alcohol abuse as symptomatic, often of loss, loneliness, isolation or alienation. Many HMOs and managed care programs now provide outpatient groups for alcohol abusers, and they are very effective. These give the elder needed contacts, structure, and group support.

One elderly bachelor spent considerable time fishing, playing solitaire, and sipping brandy. He had always been somewhat of a "loner." His nurse-neighbor frequently thought of the isolated existence he was living, but because she was not asked to intervene she did not do so. However, following a hospitalization for pancreatitis, he sought her advice. In a supportive manner she suggested he might try the alcohol program provided through the HMO, further explaining that the socialization in the groups was often helpful. After attending a few meetings he found the contacts interesting, made friends, and ultimately developed a special relationship with one of the ladies attending the group.

Another elderly gentleman became a serious alcoholic following the death of his wife and his son. He would routinely drink until he was stuporous. After a serious fall where he lay unconscious for several hours, he was hospitalized. Upon his discharge the family confronted him with his behavior and their concern for him. This shamed him even further.

Fortunately, his nurse-neighbor spoke to the family and helped them understand his acute grief. Alcoholics Anonymous was not appropriate for him. He was accompanied by a daughter to a grief support group, where his intense grief was recognized and he was encouraged to express his feelings and thoughts. He was an articulate man, and his self-esteem was gradually restored, as well as his grief process facilitated. The group support was an extremely important part of his recovery, but only because it was the appropriate group.

Nurses may be especially helpful in properly assessing an individual's need and directing the person toward appropriate resources. At times the nurse will need to accompany the individual and become the temporary bridge to recovery.

Mental Illness

Mental illness, homelessness, and alcoholism are a commonly existing triad of problems in individuals who roam the streets and alleys of cities across the nation, totally disenfranchised, seen as a blemish on the environment. In cities where there is room in jails they may be picked up for disorderly conduct; in most cities they are simply ignored.

Mental illness and alcoholism are addressed in Chapter 21, but persons with these problems must be mentioned here as examples of those who are stigmatized, alienated, and often lonely, though some are members of a loosely held, yet supportive subculture. The significance for nurses will be in the recognition that none of the problems of these individuals can be addressed effectively from only one corner of the triad. The Salvation Army has demonstrated the effectiveness of a three-pronged supportive model of rehabilitation. They provide shelter, alcoholic rehabilitation programs, and mental health counselors under one roof.

Human Immunodeficiency Virus (HIV) in Older Adults

HIV is not rare in the elderly population, but it is often overlooked because many health providers continue to believe the stereotype that most elders are sexually inactive. Elders who have spent a lifetime concealing their sexual orientation may not be inclined to discuss it. To complicate the problem, the most prevalent sign of HIV in elders may be HIV encephalopathy, which is likely to be misdiagnosed as Alzheimer's disease (Whipple and Scura, 1996).

As shown in Table 18-4, 2077 of elders are diagnosed with acquired immunodeficiency syndrome (AIDS), and in 1994 over 3% of deaths from AIDS were among those 60 years old and over (Table 18-5). Some think the real figures are much higher. An important consideration is the increased vulnerability of elderly women whose tissue friability and perineal dryness may lead to bleeding during intercourse.

In order to discuss the issue, Whipple and Scura recommend taking sexual histories of elders when health care is sought with questions such as, "How frequently do you engage in sexual activities with persons of the opposite sex?" and "How often do you engage in sexual activities with persons of the same sex?" To begin a history you may simply say, "Tell me about your sexual life."

Often the disease has been acquired through blood transfusions and tissue transplants. In any case, the elder may feel terribly stigmatized because cohort and age have often given them a very different orientation to sexuality and the discus-

Table 18-4   AIDS Cases Reported, by Patient Characteristic: 1981 to 1994

[**Provisional.** For cases reported in the year shown.]

Characteristic	Total	1981-1985	1986	1987	1988	1989	1990	1991	1992	1993	1994
Total*	427,392	15,331	13,083	21,503	30,703	33,631	41,762	43,776	45,964	103,360	78,279
Age:											
Under 5 years old ..	4,711	201	155	271	443	494	583	530	615	680	739
5 to 12 years old ...	1,184	23	27	56	127	103	144	149	142	202	211
13 to 29 years old ..	78,838	3,224	2,794	4,382	6,261	6,703	8,087	7,827	7,918	18,671	12,971
30 to 39 years old ..	195,304	7,214	6,078	9,826	14,176	15,555	18,994	20,026	20,760	47,148	35,527
40 to 49 years old ..	103,894	3,215	2,685	4,661	6,539	7,351	9,764	10,655	11,632	26,609	20,783
50 to 59 years old ..	31,319	1,143	966	1,594	2,142	2,418	2,940	3,248	3,442	7,455	5,971
Over 60 years old ..	12,142	311	378	713	1,015	1,007	1,250	1,341	1,455	2,595	2,077
Sex:											
Male	368,920	14,247	12,028	19,666	27,417	29,973	36,871	38,087	39,608	86,802	64,221
Female	58,472	1,084	1,055	1,837	3,286	3,658	4,891	5,689	6,356	16,558	14,058
Race/ethnic group:											
White†	214,061	9,125	7,769	13,253	17,050	18,597	22,378	22,163	22,507	48,039	33,180
Black†	146,159	3,981	3,392	5,435	9,141	10,292	13,250	14,684	16,103	38,424	31,457
Hispanic	62,419	2,133	1,810	2,608	4,236	4,371	5,685	6,446	6,789	15,642	12,699
Other/unknown	4,753	92	112	207	276	371	449	483	565	1,255	943

From U.S. Bureau of the Census: *Statistical abstract of the United States: 1995,* ed 115, Washington, DC, 1995.
*Includes other states not shown separately, and persons whose residence is unknown. †Non-Hispanic.
Source: U.S. Centers for Disease Control and Prevention, Atlanta Ga, unpublished data.

sion of sexual activities. One middle-aged lady was aghast when she discovered her father had AIDS, and her father was shattered to find he had given it to his wife. Nurses may be instrumental in assisting these individuals to join one of the numerous AIDS/HIV support groups.

Incontinence

Incontinence is a closet disorder and as such may be tolerable though isolating. We know that about half of the elderly women in nursing homes are incontinent of urine (Colling, 1996) but can only guess how many elders living in the community are also afflicted—and they are not likely to tell.

Incontinence is dealt with quite thoroughly in Chapter 8 but must be brought to attention here as a stigmatizing condition, as well as a source of self-revulsion and shame in many elders. A shopping cart with a large box of Attends, the need to cross one's legs tightly when coughing, the request for frequent stops to find a restroom, the bulky bulge noticeable under closely fitting pants and skirts, and the smell that one becomes inured to—all of these are the stigmata of the inability to control the flow of urine.

The nurse's function is as advocate. This problem can be corrected, or at least controlled, through training, medications, exercise, and/or surgery but, as with many other conditions, unless it is brought to attention and discussed, the individual may assume it is just something one must endure in the aging process. The nurse may introduce the topic in a nonthreatening manner, such as, "The loss of estrogen after menopause creates changes in the sexual organs and often results in the inability to control urine. Have you experienced any problems in this regard?" Or, for older men, "How frequently do you wake at night to urinate?" This then can lead to the discussion of prostate enlargement and the difficulty of starting and stopping the flow of urine.

Disfiguration

Acute disturbances producing rapid alteration in appearance will create an identity disturbance and self-devaluation. Erikson's concept of ego identity (1959) is pertinent to this discussion. The continuity of one's "felt" identity is sustained by socially validating interactions. However, even in the absence of external stigmatizing messages, internal perceptions of a disorder as punishment or an evidence of inferiority may produce disruption in one's felt identity and thus one's ability to relate to others. When a disability strikes suddenly, it is extremely difficult to reckon with an abrupt shift in identity. One feels trapped in the body of a stranger. It is as hard to relate to oneself as to another.

Elders with life-long disabilities, such as epileptic seizures, cerebral palsy, retardation, and other problems are becoming more visible as they age in numbers never before possible. Nurses and others must remain cognizant of the

---

Table 18-5 Deaths, by Selected Characteristics: 1982 to 1994

[Data are shown by year of death and are subject to substantial retrospective changes. For data on AIDS cases reported, see table 213. Based on reporting by State health departments]

Characteristic	Number									Percent distribution	
	Total 1982-1994*	1985	1988	1989	1990	1991	1992	1993	1994	1994	1992-1994
Total†	258,658	6,689	19,979	26,266	29,781	34,491	37,619	40,015	31,212	100.0	100.0
Age:											
13 to 19 years old	850	28	54	78	90	115	110	135	112	0.4	0.3
20 to 29 years old	44,770	1,311	3,812	4,795	5,246	5,846	6,073	6,409	4,868	15.6	17.3
30 to 39 years old	117,759	3,071	9,044	12,045	13,659	15,561	16,966	18,149	14,334	45.9	45.5
40 to 49 years old	64,639	1,426	4,499	6,188	7,312	8,916	10,059	10,718	8,396	26.9	25.0
50 to 59 years old	21,415	603	1,704	2,214	2,429	2,811	3,080	3,318	2,550	8.2	8.3
60 years old and over ..	9,225	250	866	946	1,045	1,242	1,331	1,286	952	3.1	3.6
Sex:											
Male	229,450	6,230	17,947	23,682	26,653	30,624	33,082	34,714	26,660	85.4	88.7
Female	29,619	468	2,050	2,616	3,177	3,920	4,599	5,392	4,620	14.8	11.5
Race/ethnicity:											
White	137,602	4,015	10,956	14,439	16,450	18,619	19,392	19,877	14,929	47.8	53.2
Black	82,556	1,754	6,061	7,941	8,989	10,706	12,493	14,084	11,453	36.7	31.9
Hispanic	36,244	889	2,798	3,647	4,105	4,828	5,404	5,691	4,488	14.4	14.0
Indian	537	6	25	40	49	87	73	117	97	0.3	0.2
Asian	1,750	29	129	180	195	240	246	281	280	0.9	0.7

From U.S. Bureau of the Census: *Statistical abstract of the United States: 1995,* ed 115, Washington, DC, 1995.
*Includes deaths prior to 1982. †Includes other race/ethnicity groups not shown separately.
Source: U.S. Centers for Disease Control and Prevention, *Surveillance Report,* manual.

stigma that is ingrained in them. To some extent this is a co-hort effect from the times when children with disabilities were shunned and their needs disregarded. Those early experiences of rejection may have made deep and lasting impressions that magnify the negative experiences of aging.

Body Image. Seeing the body as faulty often creates a disparity between the "me" and the "body." The body is the enemy that has betrayed "me." In extreme situations, one may become depersonalized and emotionally estranged from the body. "The older individual must make adaptations to an altered body image, especially in light of the American culture's emphasis on youth, beauty, and wholeness" (Janelli, 1986, p. 23).

In later life one becomes aware of changes in the body, and none are enhancing to self-concept and self-esteem. However, body image is both conscious and unconscious, composed of fantasy and reality. It is a dynamic process that involves culture, augmentations (such as wigs, makeup, prostheses, and clothing), comparison with others, and the functions required of the body.

Understanding the degree of body cathexis (personal investment in body image) is important in planning interventions. How far from the image of perfection is the individual? Has the individual always desired to be taller, thinner, or more muscular? Janelli (1986) found that posture, hair, eyes, and face were most significant indices of body acceptance in both young and old subjects. Old women rated poor posture as the least attractive feature, whereas young women were more concerned about wrinkled skin. Appearance for many indicated levels of competence.

In late life it is particularly important to shift focus from the external appearance to the inner beauty, but some persons have not been able to do this (Harvard Medical School, 1996). Nurses may assist elders, particularly women, to express their feelings and recognize the grief about the loss of their youthful image, particularly an ideal never achieved (the loss then is compounded by the perfect image never realized).

Body image is dynamic and constantly changing. Each person evaluates image through the eyes of culture, era, trends, and reflections from important others and mirrors. Internal messages of physiologic and psychologic origin form the depth dimensions of body image and self-concept.

Body image is the result of several processes:
1. Total perceptions of one's body and its performance form a self-view of acceptability or nonacceptability. Comparisons and contrasts with one's cohorts and close associates are significant.
2. Body image serves a definite function for each person. How one views one's body and its needs affects routine behaviors and lifestyle. Body monitoring may require more attention as one ages. For instance, special diets, medication regimens, elimination, and sleep patterns may intrude into daily schedules. When the body begins to limit valued activities, one's image of it changes.

Assisting clients to cope with the gradual and abrupt changes in body image that occur with aging is a very individual process. Some persons hardly notice the gradual changes until confronted with a specific limitation or a cohort they have not seen for years. Body image normally shifts in a constant series of minor revisions. Abrupt changes are always traumatic.

Interventions are in terms of whether or not the body image has produced a negative self-evaluation. Broad openings given to the client and a listening ear are most helpful. The following questions may be useful in assessing the individual's acceptance and integration of body and appearance:
How would you describe yourself?
How well has your body worked for you in the last few years?
Do you have any limitations that seem to annoy others?
How much can you trust your body?
How has your appearance changed with age?
Is physical appearance important in your circle of friends?

Major, traumatic shifts in body image often produce a revulsion to seeing oneself. Mirror viewing and acceptance of self may require time and a nurse who can support a patient during the process of viewing the reflected image. Nurses can help the individual work through the grief of the lost body image. Facial and sex organ disfigurations are among the most difficult to accept, and it may require considerable time. Total mastectomies are very difficult for many women. Using the "generalized other" approach is often useful, for example, "Many individuals experiencing a similar change in appearance find it useful to attend a group to support each other through the adjustment. Reach for Recovery is one such group."

Videotaping has been used to give depth and richness to body image. When one views oneself in the flat plane of a mirror, the image lacks animation, but during video self-viewing, appearance includes vitality and movement. The body image is less constricted. Some students working with institutionalized aged found that their interaction with each other increased when they were being videotaped. They were not devastated but rather enjoyed seeing themselves and made comments such as: "This is just like being in the movies!"

Obesity. Obesity is a growing problem in all segments of the population and is more prevalent in aging than in young adulthood (Centers for Disease Control and Prevention, 1995). If one has been obese during most of adult life, whatever adaptations have occurred are likely to be firmly embedded. Obesity is mentioned here only because it is such a stigmatizing condition that often creates revulsion in the observer that goes unrecognized. "Well, it took four of us to roll her onto the gurney!" or, "He looks like the Pillsbury dough-boy." Snide comments and openly expressed disgust are seen as socially acceptable. Fatness is laughable to those who are thin.

Only recently Disneyland executives decided the Pirates of the Caribbean will be gluttons, chasing maidens bearing trays of turkey and wine; lust is no longer amusing (Disneyland buccaneers to find new temptation: robot pirates to forgo women for food, 1997). "Disneyland spokesman, Tom Brocato, added, 'We're sensitive to issues that might be politically incorrect.'"

Why, of all the visible conditions that exist, does obesity incur no sympathy or empathy? Is it because it is seen as the just desserts of indulging oneself? The victim is suffering the visible results of "bad" behavior, yet we do not nearly understand the numerous reasons why one individual is overfilled with one Big Mac and another wants two Whoppers and is still not satisfied. Why is thin beautiful and fatness grotesque?

Alma stopped me in the hall of the retirement center and said, "What can I do about my fat? I have been fat all my life." She was fat, and I didn't have a real answer for this 75-year-old woman. Clearly, she had always felt stigmatized because of it.

Nursing interventions should be geared to refocusing on aspects of the individual's life that have been satisfactory and enjoyable but not before listening and discussing with the individual the misery of being laughed at about a condition that is not fully understood.

Baldness. Baldness may seem one of the lesser problems of appearance that affects self-esteem, and for some it is, but other individuals, both men and women, are very distressed by the loss of their hair. St Paul judged hair to be a woman's crowning glory (1 Corinthians 11:15). Men were admonished not to cover their heads when in prayer. The male's head was uncovered as a sign of respect or reverence, but men were not to have long hair (1 Corinthians 11:14).

We see the remnants of such thinking today: the "beat" generation made a statement of rebellion by the length of their hair; an old veteran of the Second World War is highly offended by youngsters wearing baseball caps turned backward and never removed except for sleep; some ladies still appreciate the man who doffs his hat in their presence; and I was greatly moved when I saw a very wizened old man remove his hat and place it over his heart during the playing of "The Star Spangled Banner" at a baseball game. Although these examples have little to do with male or female baldness, they signify the importance of the head and head coverings.

Hair continuously goes through cycles of loss and gain, normally producing about 7 miles total of hair each year (Morley, 1997). With aging the rate of replacement no longer equals the rate of loss. Women begin to lose hair faster than they replace it shortly after menopause, whereas men are more variable in the timing, rate, and pattern of hair loss. For both men and women hereditary factors are significant, but hormones seem to have the greatest effect (Randall, 1994).

When women begin to lose the hair on their head, they often also notice the increased growth of facial hair. For some it is sufficient to require shaving.

Men often attach sexual meanings to the hair and beard. Some of these are mythical but may have emotional significance none the less.

The importance of testosterone in hair growth was first recognized by Aristotle when he noted that castration of a boy before puberty resulted in baldness (Morley, 1997). Age-related baldness in men is thought to be a result of alterations in androgen receptors. However, baldness is likely to produce a variety of sexual/psychologic reactions in men, whereas in women it is more often an issue of appearance.

The significance to nursing is vague, but hair loss is mentioned here to alert us to the realization that it is one aspect of the aging process that may produce mild or severe reactions. The large industry involved in hair transplant, replacement methods of various types, toupees, wigs, and "snake oil" treatments attests to its importance.

Mobility Aids. Mobility aids are essential to locomotion for many elders and have been discussed quite thoroughly in Chapter 11. It is mentioned here because of the stigmatizing effects of using a walker or wheelchair. A cane, or walking stick, often lends a touch of dignity, class, and protection to an elder, but the walker or wheelchair signifies deterioration and dependency. Some are less offensive in appearance than others, but they form barriers that exclude the individual from certain places and events. In many retirement centers the walkers must be left outside the dining area, and in some life-care centers individuals needing a walker or wheelchair will not be accepted as a resident.

Some elders refuse to appear in public using a walker. It is insufficient for nurses to remind elders that it is a safety issue. It is likely to be more productive to discuss their feelings about the appliance, ask in what specific ways it has changed their lifestyle. Some externalize the aid by giving it a name, "Where's my Masserati?" and others incorporate it into their persona. One creative nurse said, "Let me try that and see how it feels." This not only increased the nurse's understanding but launched quite a discussion of meanings, feelings, and the expertise of the elder who was so able to get where she wanted to go, regardless of the encumbrance.

The meaning of mobility aids was explored by Rush and Ouellet (1997). A summary of client responses to their investigation is seen Table 18-6.

Grooming. Nurses are in a position to directly affect the image of the old. Matted, stiff hair; unkempt, food-stained beards; stained dentures; and urine-stained clothing are all readily corrected and yet often neglected. Old people may ignore appearances because they lack awareness, energy, incentive, and mirrors. If we care about the whole person rather than just the illness, we will see that he or she looks presentable.

Bernice took her mother to lunch when her mother's shoes didn't match, her hair was uncombed and her slip was showing. Bernice hadn't wanted to call attention to her mother's appearance, feeling it would distress her, but when others stared at them as they waited in the cafeteria line Bernice realized it would have been kinder to help her mother look more presentable before leaving home.

Table 18-6	Meaning of Mobility Aids
Categories	**Themes**
The stigma of mobility aids	
Client adjustment behaviors	a) Concealing
	b) Resisting
	c) Covering
	d) Withdrawing
	e) Accepting
Forces influencing responses to mobility aids	a) Duration of use
	b) Gender
	c) Health professional frame of reference
Potential benefits	a) Spatio-temporal dynamics
	b) Independence
	c) Energy conservation

From Rush KL, Ouellet LL: Mobility aids and the elderly client, *J Gerontol Nurs* 23(1):7, 1997.

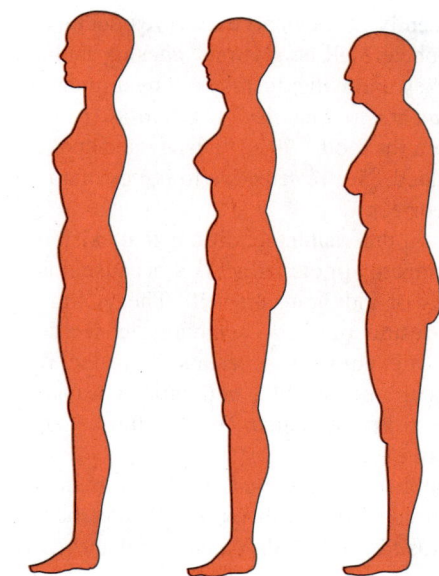

Figure 18-8. Changes in figure with age. (Illustrated by Joseph Pierre.)

Odors. Olfaction is a primitive, emotionally laden sense of great significance in acceptance or alienation. Unfortunately, we lose awareness of objectionable odors because olfactory cells adapt to a constant exposure. Nurses may become inured to the odor of feces, urine, and certain illnesses, but visitors will immediately be aware of them. Similarly, people are usually unaware of their own odors, but others are offended by them.

A nutrition center staff encountered a problem with an old man who had a strongly offensive body odor. People avoided him and did not sit near him during lunch. The staff solved this problem by telling the entire group that hot weather made body odors more intense and requesting that everyone bathe before coming to the nutrition site. A more direct approach might have been to privately give the same information to the offending individual.

Clothing and Self-Esteem. Clothing can be a demonstration of individuality and personality (Breen, 1983). Personal articles of clothing that express the individual's desires enhance self-esteem. When clothing must be worn for the convenience of the institution or the situation, the individual's needs are overlooked. Although the impact of clothing selection has been poorly investigated for the institutionalized elderly, it is part of one's identity throughout life and there is no reason to assume that it becomes less so in the later years.

Elderly people often have difficulty finding clothing that fits properly. Various biologic changes alter body shape (Figure 18-8). Ready-to-wear garments are not designed to enhance the appearance or comfort of the old. Old women complain that clothing is too long waisted, is loose across the back, is tight around waist and hips, and has back zippers that are hard to reach. Most prefer front zippers, few buttons, three-quarter length sleeves, and a comfortable fit. When nurses are involved in helping aged people choose clothing, we may guide them toward selecting garments for style, fit, comfort, and ease of dressing and removal.

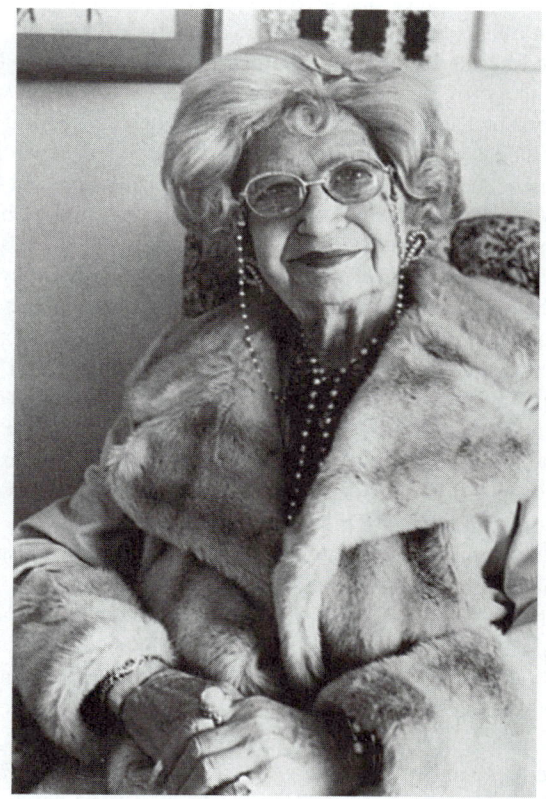

Personal presentation. (Courtesy Christine Becker, American Society on Aging.)

Judy Falk in Deerfield, Illinois, started designing specially adapted clothing when she was unable to buy such garments for her grandmother. Now her designs are available through the catalogs of nationwide department stores. They feature Velcro fastenings, raglan sleeves, and low wide-topped pockets. They are cut with extra material at the thighs. These garments help the physically impaired to look and feel better (Adams, 1987). Adaptive fashions are now available from many sources. Some care centers have organized workshops where volunteers bring patterns and ideas and create needed garments for residents.

Criminal Behavior in the Elderly

Criminal behavior in the elderly is a neglected field of study, perhaps because we are more conditioned to think of the aged as victims rather than offenders. The extent of crimes committed by the elderly has been largely ignored because of a reverse kind of ageism and myths we hold about the aged. A 92-year-old woman stabbed and killed her sister. Can you imagine her convicted of first-degree murder? A 70-year-old woman was arraigned for selling marijuana to schoolchildren. She was admonished to discontinue. An 80 year old threatened police with an axe when they attempted to evict her. Charges were not filed against her. These examples demonstrate that old deviants often receive preferential treatment.

The elderly, children, and the sick are not expected to fully adhere to performance standards of the remainder of society (Goffman, 1963). A lack of respect for them as full persons accounts for this. They are not held fully accountable because their actions are considered less significant and they are not accorded respect as full-fledged members of society (Goffman, 1963).

The legal system is presently unable to adequately distinguish older responsible violators from those unable to fully comprehend their crime, though conservatorship investigations as discussed in Chapter 15 may be very helpful. The criminal justice system will need to become even more adept at differentiating the competent from the impaired elderly offenders (Roesch et al, 1995).

Overall there has been a gradual decrease since 1975 in the number of persons over 55 years of age who have been arrested for crimes, and this group has the lowest crime rate of all adult age groups. Murder and nonnegligent manslaughter are infrequent but serious crimes of this group. Theft is categorized as a serious crime, and the aged comprise slightly over 1% of these offenders. Gambling, sex offenses, and drunkenness are the most frequent of the non-serious crimes (U.S. Bureau of the Census, 1995). For specific details regarding arrests of aged persons in relation to others in the population, see Table 18-7. It is interesting to note that gambling is the cause of most arrests in old age. Perhaps in gambling there is a germ of hope, and hope is a strong sustaining force. Surprisingly, arrests of females are not included in Table 18-7. These issues merit further gerontologic study.

Nurses working with old people who have a criminal record or deviant behavior may need support from peers and other professionals, depending on the nature of the crime and their own feelings. Personal values and beliefs often make it difficult to relate to the total person's needs.

Aging Prisoners. *Graying of the nation's prisons* is a term that has recently been bandied about. Of the more than 1 million state and federal prisoners, 3% are over the age of 65 (U.S. Bureau of the Census, 1995), and the number is increasing rapidly. These data will likely change under the impact of prison crowding, earlier paroles, and the "3 strikes program."

Most of the aged prisoners have been in the prison system for the majority of their lives and have grown old there. Between 1979 and 1988 the number of older inmates tripled, from 6000 to 18,000. This is attributed to the impact of longer sentences and limited parole eligibility. Many of these elders have already served 30 or 40 years, and the prison lifestyle is all they know. If they were paroled, they would have no place to go, and as they age in prison their increasing frailty ill equips them to deal with prison life.

Officers of departments of correction have concerns about the need for more medical care, provisions, and services designed for their needs and protection from victimization by younger, stronger prisoners (Anderson and Morton, 1989). Walsh (1996) reports that at Lakeland Correctional Facility in Coldwater, Michigan, a 61-year-old counselor, Robert Moore, has found his calling in serving the prison inmates in the 80-bed geriatric ward (Walsh, 1996).

Some prisoner advocates are seeking release for these older prisoners who are no longer considered dangerous; however, many would find living on their own in a world they have largely been isolated from even more difficult than the prison system that is essentially caring for them now.

Courts have ruled that prison inmates are constitutionally guaranteed a level of health care consistent with community standards. As an aside, it is incongruous that the old in nursing homes are not guaranteed the same rights. Less than 1% of prisoners in state prisons are over age 65 (Table 18-8) but they are beginning to create serious concerns within the system. Elders who are prisoners are not eligible for Medicaid or Medicare and thus become an expense to the overburdened state systems (Our gray-bearded ailing convicts, 1996).

The care of aged prisoners is an arena that geriatric nursing may begin to consider as a subspecialty practice. Rita Chow, the late Mary Jane Hennessey, and some other nurses of our acquaintance have worked in the prisons to provide hospice and other services to old and alienated prisoners.

Interventions

Goffman (1963) suggests the role of health care professionals working with stigmatized individuals is to assist them in the discovery of a new and valid self. Guidelines for this process can be seen in Box 18-6.

Table 18-7   Persons Arrested, by Charge, Sex, and Age: 1993

[Represents arrests (not charges) reported by 10,512 agencies (reporting 12 months) with a total 1993 population of 214 million as estimated by FBI]

Charge	Total (1,000)	Male	Under 15 years	Under 18 years	18-24 years	25-44 years	45-54 years	55-64 years	65 yr and over
					Percent distribution				
Total arrests	**11,766**	**80.5**	**6.0**	**17.1**	**27.5**	**47.6**	**5.4**	**1.7**	**0.7**
Serious crimes*	2,423	77.3	11.9	29.3	25.9	38.9	3.9	1.2	0.7
Murder and nonnegligent manslaughter . . .	20	90.6	1.9	16.2	41.2	35.6	4.5	1.6	0.9
Forcible rape	33	98.7	6.4	16.3	26.7	48.8	5.4	2.0	0.8
Robbery	154	91.3	8.1	28.2	33.7	36.2	1.6	0.2	0.1
Aggravated assault	442	84.3	4.9	15.3	26.8	49.9	5.5	1.7	0.8
Burglary†	338	90.1	13.9	34.3	28.5	34.7	2.0	0.4	0.1
Larceny-theft	1,251	67.3	14.1	31.3	23.4	38.2	4.4	1.5	1.1
Motor vehicle theft	169	88.2	13.2	44.6	28.7	25.0	1.4	0.3	0.1
Arson	16	85.3	32.3	49.3	17.0	28.0	3.7	1.3	0.6
All other nonserious crimes	9,343	81.4	4.4	14.0	27.9	49.8	5.8	1.8	0.7
Other assaults	965	82.1	6.7	16.2	24.8	51.8	5.2	1.5	0.6
Forgery and counterfeiting	89	65.3	1.2	7.3	32.8	54.6	4.2	0.9	0.3
Fraud	336	59.4	1.2	4.8	27.4	58.8	6.7	1.7	0.6
Embezzlement	11	59.5	0.7	5.6	34.1	51.7	6.3	1.8	0.4
Stolen property‡	135	87.1	7.7	27.0	34.0	35.3	2.8	0.7	0.2
Vandalism	261	87.8	21.9	45.6	24.2	27.1	2.2	0.6	0.3
Weapons (carrying, etc.)	224	92.2	7.1	23.3	35.9	34.7	4.1	1.4	0.6
Prostitution and commercialized vice	89	35.7	0.2	1.1	24.0	68.6	4.4	1.3	0.6
Sex offenses§	88	91.4	9.7	18.7	19.2	47.8	8.4	3.7	2.2
Drug abuse violations	969	83.8	1.5	9.6	31.9	53.8	3.8	0.7	0.2
Gambling	15	86.0	1.4	7.6	20.7	43.2	15.2	8.9	4.3
Offenses against family and children	89	80.7	1.4	4.4	21.7	65.2	6.7	1.5	0.5
Driving under the influence	1,230	85.9	(Z)	0.9	22.2	62.3	9.8	3.5	1.3
Liquor laws	419	80.7	2.3	21.9	52.0	21.1	3.3	1.3	0.5
Drunkenness	605	88.9	0.3	2.3	20.8	60.5	10.8	4.0	1.5
Disorderly conduct	607	79.3	6.7	20.0	30.3	42.9	4.7	1.4	0.7
Vagrancy	25	87.7	3.7	13.0	21.3	52.3	9.9	2.6	0.9
Suspicion	12	84.6	3.7	11.4	27.8	54.3	5.0	1.2	0.4
Curfew, loitering (juveniles)	85	71.9	30.3	100.0	(X)	(X)	(X)	(X)	(X)
Runaways (juveniles)	152	42.8	44.5	100.0	(X)	(X)	(X)	(X)	(X)
All other offenses, except traffic	2,935	82.1	3.0	10.9	29.7	51.7	5.4	1.6	0.7

From U.S. Bureau of the Census: *Statistical abstract of the United States: 1995,* ed 115, Washington, DC, 1995.
X, Not applicable. *Z,* Less then .05 percent. *Includes arson arrests, a newly established index offense in 1979. †Breaking or entering. ‡Buying, receiving, possessing. §Excludes forcible rape and prostitution, shown separately.
Source: U.S. Federal Bureau of Investigation, *Crime in the United States,* annual.

BUILDING SOCIAL NETWORKS

Throughout this chapter we have considered the various sources of social isolation. To assist in building relationship networks to increase physical and psychologic durability is the role of the nurse. Individual integration depends on strengthening the association with others through network bonds. People are tied into their society essentially through their beliefs, the groups they belong to, and the positions they occupy.

There is an accumulating body of evidence showing mortality related to lack of social contacts. Earlier in the chapter we referred to the Berkman and Syme (1979) longitudinal study of more than 5000 older who had lower mortality and morbidity (irrespective of factors such as health, socioeconomic status, smoking, alcoholism, obesity, physical activity, and use of health services) because of a stable positive support network. This study remains the most comprehensive and reliable one available. It appears that social networks are critical to survival (Figure 18-2).

Outreach

Outreach is a term used to describe myriad agency, institutional, and individual efforts to make contact with the isolated, alienated elderly. Chapters 13 and 17 discussed several methods of outreach presently used. Making contact

Table 18-8   State Prison Inmates—Selected Characteristics: 1986 and 1991

[Based on a sample survey of about 13,986 inmates in 1991 and 13,711 inmates in 1986; subject to sampling variability)

Characteristic	Number 1986	Number 1991	Percent of prison inmates 1986	Percent of prison inmates 1991	Characteristic	Number 1986	Number 1991	Percent of prison inmates 1986	Percent of prison inmates 1991
Total*	**450,416**	**711,643**	**100.0**	**100.0**	Never married	241,707	389,302	53.7	55.3
Under 18 years old	2,057	4,552	0.5	0.6	Married	91,492	127,389	20.3	18.1
18 to 24 years old	120,384	151,328	26.7	21.3	Widowed	8,343	13,036	1.9	1.9
25 to 34 years old	205,817	325,429	45.7	45.7	Divorced	81,264	129,913	18.1	18.5
35 to 44 years old	87,502	161,651	19.4	22.7	Separated	26,985	44,095	6.0	6.3
45 to 54 years old	23,524	46,475	5.2	6.5	Years of school:				
55 to 64 years old	8,267	16,997	1.8	2.4	Less than 12 years	276,309	†290,722	61.6	†41.2
65 years old and over ..	2,808	5,210	0.6	0.7	12 years or more	172,386	415,451	38.4	58.8
Male	430,604	672,847	95.6	94.5	Pre-arrest employment status:				
Female	19,812	38,796	4.4	5.5	Employed	309,364	476,068	69.0	67.3
White	223,648	349,628	49.7	49.1	Not employed	139,097	230,876	31.0	32.7
Black	211,021	336,920	46.9	47.3	Looking for work	80,750	115,590	18.0	16.4
Other races	15,412	25,094	3.4	3.5	Not looking for work	58,347	115,286	13.0	16.3

From U.S. Bureau of the Census: *Statistical abstract of the United States: 1995*, ed 115, Washington, DC, 1995.
*For 1986, includes data not reported for all characteristics except sex. For 1991, includes data not reported for marital status, re-arrest, employment status, and years of school. †In 1991, the survey question was revised; therefore, the response may not be entirely comparable with 1986 and before.
Source: U.S. Bureau of Justice Statistics, *Profile of State Prison Inmates, 1986;* and *Survey of State Prison Inmates, 1991.*

Box 18-6   Interventions to Combat Stigma

- Allow time for the client to talk extensively about perceptions of self. This review process is necessary before problem solving regarding the present situation can begin; for example, an elder newly diagnosed with AIDS must have considerable opportunity for ventilation and grief expression.

- Talk with the afflicted individual about prior experiences and knowledge of the condition: "Have you known anyone who had AIDS?" "How did it affect his or her life?" "What do you know about sexually transmitted diseases?"

- Generally follow the principles of grief work. When early grief has abated, it is often useful to introduce the person to someone dealing with a similar problem. Many organizations are established to support people with various kinds of stigmatizing disorders.

- Avoid overexposure of the individual to others with similar problems because they may begin to identify only with the problems, and the focus of the individual

may narrow. Self-help groups and similar supports should not constitute the sole social milieu.

- Identify the individual's self-perception, for example, "How do you see yourself now?" "How do you think others see you?" "Have you talked to your significant others about this?"

- Give specific feedback on present strengths: "I see that you are collecting information about this problem." or "You are expressing your feelings openly and this is important."

- Assist family members to accept the condition and relate to the person in other ways in addition to addressing the problem.

- Be aware that problems that affect facial structure or sexual capacities are the most difficult for the patient and intimate others.

- Develop reasonable expectations of the individual. Confidence is further eroded when one is catered to or given special privileges based on pity.

---

is the first step in rebuilding a social world, but it is not to be undertaken until the elder has determined the level of contact and the assistance desired.

KEY CONCEPTS

- Loneliness to some degree is a constant companion in late life as one's peers and family members die.

- A "geriatric orphan" is one who is the last remaining of the family tree.

- Choosing to be alone at times for personal renewal and reflection is a healthy sign and needs to be respected. When these needs are not met, personality aberrations may appear.

- Social isolation because of appearance or other personal characteristics may be detrimental and is accompanied by a loss of self-esteem.

Nursing Diagnoses

The following potential diagnoses must be considered as well as diagnoses unique to the particular individual:
- Anxiety
- Coping, ineffective
- Denial, ineffective
- Fatigue
- Grieving, anticipatory and dysfunctional
- Health maintenance, altered
- Nutrition, altered
- Personal identity disturbance
- Powerlessness
- Self-care deficit
- Self-esteem disturbance
- Sleep pattern disturbance
- Social isolation
- Spiritual distress

NURSING PROCESS AND NURSING DIAGNOSIS
Isolation/Loneliness

Etiologies and Related Factors
Change in living arrangement
Retirement
Physical/emotional illness
Chronic illness
Lack of shared language
Loss of social roles/relationships
Sensory deficits
Incontinence
Death of a spouse
Alcohol/alcoholism
Lack of transportation
Decreased mobility
Decreased cognitive function
Decreased social supports
Decreased financial resources

Defining Characteristics
Varies with client; each client basically defines own factors of loneliness/isolation
Expression of loneliness
Desires more people contact
Barriers to social contact
Lack of social supports
Sad affect
Withdrawn
Little or no eye contact
Few visitors or friends

Knowledge
Developmental theory of aging
Contributors to social isolation/loneliness
Basic interpersonal relation skills
Active listening
Social skills assessment
Therapeutic communication skills
Physical and psychologic assessment skills
Group process and training skills
Motivational therapy
Reminiscence therapy
Community resources

Clinical Judgment and Related Skills
Obtain a history related to social isolation/loneliness using available standard assessment tools
Consider prior lifestyle, communication style, impact of chronic illness, loss of spouse, etc.
Do a social skills checklist on client
Assess social isolation with standard isolation index
Employ appropriate interpersonal relations and listening skills
Conduct and lead therapeutic groups
Conduct socialization groups
Initiate family and community teaching
Design, implement, and evaluate a plan of care to prevent and manage social isolation/loneliness in community; in institutional setting

Evaluation
Client identifies reasons for feeling isolated/lonely
Discusses ways of increasing meaningful relationships
Identifies diversional activities
Participates in activities
States does not feel so isolated/lonely
Interacts with others
Resumes social activities and relationships
Makes new relationships

NEEDS ADDRESSED AND TASK STRENGTHS	
Depression	Recognizes normality of some depressions
Need to recognize mood fluctuations and affectual shifts	Recognizes symptoms of depression
Need to become aware of and express feelings	Seeks assistance when depression becomes disabling
Need for spiritual expression (to maintain self-esteem)	Seeks meaning in suffering
Tolerance of own moods and affectual changes	

- Isolation results in a lack of sufficient opportunities for feedback and often is the root of suspicious and paranoid behavior.
- Ageism is one of the most prevalent stigmatizing factors; even more than culture, race, or disfiguration.
- To combat isolation establish brief, scheduled times to meet with the individual to discuss items of the client's interest. Personal intrusions must be avoided; the client must set the pace of the developing relationship.
- Social networks may be deemed satisfactory only if the client feels a fit with the group.
- Provide choices and options in terms of activities and groups that may be of interest to the client.
- Respect an individual's choice of lifestyle, regardless of whether it seems healthy or gratifying to the observer.

▲ **CASE STUDY**

Clarence entered a life-care community at age 75, several years after his wife had died. His children lived on the West Coast and had repeatedly encouraged him to move from his Michigan home to be nearer them, but he had simply never made the decision to do so, though he frequently said it sounded like a good idea. However, when one of his lady friends moved into a life-care community on the outskirts of Chicago that was owned by a protestant religious organization, this inspired him to do so also. When his children came to help him move in, they were very pleased to see how comfortable his apartment appeared and the generally pleasant ambiance of the community. They knew of the reputation of this fine community, and they felt pleased for him and relieved of their concern for him. The solution seemed satisfactory in all ways because his lady friend was also there, and he knew he would have at least one friend. Clarence had never been a particularly social person, and one or two friends at a time seemed to be all he needed. He was financially well off and physically active, and the ladies in the community were delighted when he became a resident. His apartment was roomy, and there were numerous opportunities for activities and committee work, none of which really interested him. It seemed he had made a comfortable transition except that he was unable to bring his dog with him. He was somewhat satisfied when his son

agreed to take it. Initially he began going to meals with his lady friend and participated in some of the activities with her, but the remainder of the time he spent in his apartment, much of the time listening to classical music, which he loved. Some of the ladies were very friendly because there were few men in the community as healthy, active, and attractive as Clarence. However, he quickly dismissed their attentions because he felt his lady friend might get jealous. He soon realized that she had many friends in the community and was not available to him most of the time, but she continued to join him at mealtimes in the dining room. Several times she suggested they join a group at a table instead of the table for two, but he wasn't interested. She urged him to get acquainted with some other residents, but he didn't seem interested in doing that either. One day she called and said she had been invited to join a group of ladies for lunch, and she would join him for dinner. That day he didn't eat lunch or dinner. Of course, his friend felt sorry about it but did not feel she wanted to restrict her mealtimes to always being with him. The situation gradually deteriorated until Clarence missed many meals and often sat alone, glowering most of the time. One day when his friend walked into the dining room with some other friends, he shouted at her, "Well, you bitch, I can't believe after all I've done for you that you are so ungrateful and have abandoned me like and old shoe. I'm not just your pet poodle, you know!" He yelled a few obscenities and stomped out of the dining room. Of course, his friend was embarrassed, and the gossip in the community began. It was surmised that Clarence was probably drunk and perhaps drank a lot when in his apartment. Others mentioned various odd things he had done, such as ignoring them when they greeted him or simply looking vaguely at them without commenting. The administrator of the community sent the psychiatric nurse counselor to talk with Clarence, but she wasn't able to get any notion of what might be upsetting him. When asked, Clarence said he found everything satisfactory. For the next few days people avoided Clarence, and the counselor came to visit him each day. One day Clarence said, "I don't need a psychiatrist; you don't need to come to see me." If you were the psychiatric nurse counselor, how would you proceed with this case?

Based on the case study, develop a nursing care plan using the following procedure*:

List comments of client that provide *subjective data.*

List information that provides *objective data.*

From these data identify and state, using accepted format, two *nursing diagnoses* you determine are most significant to this client at this time. List two *client strengths* that you have identified from data.

Determine and state *outcome criteria* for each diagnosis. These must reflect some alleviation of the problem identified in the nursing diagnosis and must be stated in concrete and measurable terms.

Plan and state one or more *interventions* for each diagnosed problem. Provide specific documentation of source used to determine appropriate intervention. Plan at least one intervention that incorporates the client's existing strengths.

Evaluate success of intervention. Interventions must correlate directly with the stated outcome criteria in order to measure the outcome success.

STUDY QUESTIONS/ACTIVITIES

Discuss the variations in symptoms of alienation in the old and the young (refer to chapter 21 for additional information).

Describe some of the reasons we believe that elders are more vulnerable to loneliness than younger persons.

Describe a time when you were feeling out of step with others and as if you were different. What were your feelings? What did you do about it?

Itemize the conditions in society that contribute to ageist attitudes.

In what ways do you think society condones or contributes to the isolation and loneliness of elders?

RESEARCH QUESTIONS

Has ageism decreased in the past 3 decades of increasing knowledge and attention to the aging society?

What are the conditions that the aged feel are most stigmatizing or that make them feel the least valued?

Do the aged who are alone and isolated cope less well than those in families and in what ways?

Discuss the meanings and the thoughts triggered by the students' and elders' viewpoints expressed at the beginning of the chapter. How do these vary from your own experience?

RESOURCES

Crestwood Company, 6625 N Sidney Place, Milwaukee, WI 53209. Special gift catalog helps brighten lives of

---

*Students are advised to refer to their nursing diagnosis text and identify possible and potential problems.

---

disabled children and adults. Catalog contains numerous devices to assist those to communicate who have lost their voice.

J.C. Penney has a "special needs" catalog available through their regular catalog department. Another company that provides reasonable items is Buck and Buck, 3111 27th Avenue S, Seattle, WA 98144, (800) 458-0600. In the Buffalo, New York, area Rainbow Fashions of Orchard Park sells similar items.

Outward, a quarterly newsletter of the Lesbian and Gay Aging Issues Network of the American Society on Aging, 833 Market Street, Suite 511, San Francisco, CA 94103-1824.

Films and Videos

Because Somebody Cares. This film shows several real-life vignettes of volunteers, young and old, as they visit older persons who are homebound or in nursing homes. The amazing thing about them—these isolated elderly, as well as the volunteers—is their spirit, their coping abilities, the gifts they give, and the ones they receive. Capturing sensitive moments of exchange, this film shows the friendships that grow when people of all ages reach out to each other. (Produced by Terra Nova Films Inc, 9848 S Winchester Avenue, Chicago, IL 60643; directed by James Vanden Bosch; 27 minutes (purchase: 16 mm, $465.00; video, $375.00; rental, $50.00).

Reducing Resident Depression: Assessment and Intervention. This program may be used to teach geriatric nursing assistants how to identify and report symptoms of depression. It also identifies strategies geriatric nursing assistants can use when interacting with elderly persons with depressive symptoms (20 minutes; purchase, $300; rental, $100).

Both videos are available from Video Press, University of Maryland at Baltimore, School of Medicine, Suite 133, 100 Penn Street, Baltimore MD 21201, (800) 328-7450 or (410) 328-5497, fax (410) 328-8471.

The Wilson Crisis (Stroke). A 6-month documentation of the physical and psychologic rehabilitation after a stroke. Narratives from the stroke victim and his son, the caregiver, reveal the frustrations both experience. The final moments of the program document the reward of the long difficult months of rehabilitation—return to society. From Video Press, University of Maryland at Baltimore, School of Medicine, Suite 133, 100 Penn Street, Baltimore, MD 21202, (800) 328-7450 or (410) 328-5497, fax (410) 328-8471.

Organizations

Alcoholics Anonymous World Services
475 Riverside Drive
New York, NY 10613

Alcohol and Drug Problems Association of North America
444 N Capital Street, NW, Suite 706
Washington, DC 20001

American Parkinson's Disease Association, (800)223-2732

Lesbian and Gay Aging Issues Network of the American Society on Aging
833 Market Street, Suite 511
San Francisco, CA 94103-1824

AT&T Office on Devices for People with Disabilities, (800) 233-1222
AT&T Special Needs Center, (800) 833-3232.

The American Speech and Hearing Association (9030 Old Georgetown Road, Washington, DC 20014) compiles and publishes lists of speech pathology and audiology service programs and specialists in private practice in every state, (800) 638-8255.

The local university may have a speech and hearing clinic served by students in training. In some instances graduate students do practicums in senior centers for speech and language disorders.

The Easter Seal Society or United Way may sponsor clinics where speech pathologists work with adults.

The state committee on aging may have compiled a directory of speech and hearing services available for older people in your state.

The local Visiting Nurses Association (VNA) often has speech and language pathologists on staff who can provide excellent professional help to the homebound.

Information can also be obtained from the International Association of Laryngectomees, 219 East 42nd Street, New York, NY 10017.

You may want to use other community resources. The American Cancer Society provides varied information and resources for the laryngectomee; frequently it also sponsors local Lost Chord clubs for laryngectomees.

You may want to arrange for center stroke victims to attend local Stroke Club meetings. For information, write Stroke Club Coordinator, c/o American Heart Association, Texas Affiliate, Inc, PO Box 15186, Austin, TX 78761.

Publications

Resource Materials for Communicative Problems of Older Persons (1975) is available from the American Speech and Hearing Association, 9020 Old Georgetown Road, Washington, DC 20014, (cost: $4.95, 31 pp.).

Rehabilitation of the Laryngectomee. Conference at Mayo Clinic, Rochester, Minnesota, March 1975. Information can be obtained from the Mayo Clinic.

Guidelines: Animals in Nursing Homes. Available from California Veterinary Medical Association, 1024 Country Club Drive, Moraga, CA 94556 (cost: $3.00).

REFERENCES

Adams S: The relationship of clothing to self-esteem in elderly patients, *Nurs Times* 83(36):42, 1987.

American Society on Aging: Lesbian and gay health conference holds institute on aging, *Outward* 2(3):2, 1996.

Anderson JC, Morton JB: Graying of the nation's prisons presents new challenges, *The Aging Connection* 15(5):6, 1989.

Berger RM: *Gay and gray: the older homosexual man,* New York, 1996, Haworth Press.

Berkman LF, Syme L: Social networks, host resistance, and mortality: a nine-year follow up study of Alameda County residents, *Am J Epidemiol* 109:186, 1979.

Biordi D: Social isolation. In Lubkin I, editor, *Chronic illness: impact and interventions,* Boston, 1995, Jones and Bartlett.

Blakeney B: Old, homeless and sick, *Geriatr Nurs* 12(5):220, 1991.

Blatter CW, Jacobsen JJ: Older women coping with divorce: peer support groups, *Women Therapy* 14(1-2):141, 1993.

Boyack V: *The geriatric orphan: research and practice perspectives.* Paper presented at the annual convention of the Western Gerontological Society, Albuquerque, New Mexico, March 18, 1983.

Boyd SH, Stout BL, Volanty K: Youth exchanging with seniors: a rural Texas program, *Pride Institute Journal of Long Term Home Health Care* 12(3):21, 1993.

Breen J: Clothing for the elderly disabled person in the hospital, *Concord J Br Assoc Service Elderly* 24:9, 1983.

Cain BS: Divorce among older women: a growing social phenomenon, *Social Casework: The Journal of Contemporary Social Work* 69:563, 1988.

Carlson E, Crowley S: The Friedan mystique: feminist leader sees radical change in attitudes on aging, *AARP News Bull* 33(8):20, 1992.

Centers for Disease Control and Prevention: *National Health and Nutrition Examination Survey III,* 1995, National Center for Health Statistics.

Cole TR: Ageism and the journey of life in America, *Aging Today* 13(2):17, 1992.

Colling J: Noninvasive techniques to manage urinary incontinence among care-dependent persons, *J Wound Ostomy Continence Nurs* 23:302, 1996.

Coulson E: Introduction. In Keyes L, editor: *Toning: the creative power of the voice,* Marina Del Rey, Calif, 1973, Devorss and Co.

Cox C, Spiro M, Sullivan J: Social risk factors: impact on elders' perceived health status, *J Commun Health Nurs* 5(1):59, 1988.

Damrosch S, Strasser J: The homeless elderly in America, *J Gerontol Nurs* 14(10):26, 1988.

DeAngelis T: Researchers explore roots of ageism, *Aging Today* 15(1):12, 1994.

DePaola SJ, Ebersole P: Meaning in life categories of elderly nursing home residents, *Int J Aging Hum Dev* 40(3):227, 1995.

Disneyland buccaneers to find new temptation: robot pirates to forgo women for food, *San Francisco Chronicle,* p A3, January 4, 1997.

Djerassi C: A scientist/novelist examines ageism in science, *Aging Today* 17(5):17, 1996.

Dolan J: Fighting poverty: Social Security leads way, study finds, *AARP News Bull* 30(2):7, 1989.

Doolin J: Planning for the special needs of the homeless elderly, *Gerontologist* 26(3):229, 1986.

Duerson M, Thomas J, Chang J et al: Medical students' knowledge and misconceptions about aging: responses to Palmore's Facts on Aging quizzes, *Gerontologist* 32(2):171, 1992.

Dykstra PA: Loneliness among the never and formerly married: the importance of supportive friendships and a desire for independence, *J Gerontol* 50B(5):321, 1995.

Elias CJ, Inui TS: When a house is not a home: exploring the meaning of shelter among chronically homeless older men, *Gerontologist* 33(3):396, 1993.

Erikson E: Identity and the life cycle: selected papers, monogr no 1, *Psychol Issues,* 1959.

Erickson R: Companion animals and the elderly, *Geriatr Nurs* 6(2):92, 1985.

Fink A, Hays RD, Moore AA, Beck JC: Alcohol related problems in older persons: determinants, consequences, and screening, *Arch Intern Med* 156( ):1150, 1996.

Foxall MJ, Barron CR, Von Dollen K, Shull KA, Jones PA: Low vision elders living arrangements, loneliness, and social support, *J Gerontol Nurs* 20(8):6, 1994.

Fuguitt GV, Beale CL: The changing concentration of the older nonmetropolitan population, *J Gerontol* 48(6):S278, 1993.

Geschwind N: Disconnection syndromes in animals and man, *Brain* 88:237, 1965.

Ginsberg S: *Communication disorders,* Unpublished paper, Cleveland, 1988, Case Western Reserve University.

Goffman E: *Stigma: notes on the management of spoiled identity,* Englewood Cliffs, NJ, 1963, Prentice-Hall.

Hamberger LJ: Personal reflections on the 1995 WHCoA, *Outward* 2(3):1, 1996.

Harvard Medical School: Face lifts, *Women's Health Watch,* p 4, March 1996.

Henry ME: Serving invisible gay and lesbian elders, *Outword* 2(3):3, 1996.

Hummert ML, Garstka TA, Shaner JL, Strahm S: Stereotypes of the elderly held by young, middle-aged, and elderly adults, *J Gerontol* 49(5):P240, 1994.

InSpeech, Inc: *Understanding adult aphasia,* Valley Forge, Pa, 1988, InSpeech, Inc.

Janelli L: The realities of body image, *J Gerontol Nurs* 12(10):23, 1986.

Johnson J: Sleep problems and self-care in very old rural women: nursing implications, *Geriatr Nurs* 17(2): 72, 1996a.

Johnson J: Social support and physical health in the rural elderly. *Appl Nurs Res* 9(2):61, 1996b.

Johnson JE, Waldo M, Johnson RG: Stress and perceived health status in the rural elderly, *J Gerontol Nurs* 19(9):24, 1993.

Keigher S: Homeless study reveals preventable tragedy, *Aging Connection,* 10(1):11, 1989.

Klusch L: *Solutions in restorative care giving,* Des Moines, Iowa, 1995, Briggs.

Lanza ML: Divorce experienced as an older woman, *Geriatr Nurs* 17(4):166, 1996.

Liberto JG, Oslin DW, Ruskin PE: Alcoholism in older persons: a review of the literature, *Hosp Community Psychiatry* 43:975, 1990.

Lien-Gieschen T: *Nurse validation of social isolation related to maturational age,* master's thesis, Washington, DC, 1992, Georgetown University.

Lookinland S, Anson K: Perpetuation of ageist attitudes among present and future health care personnel: implications for elder care, *J Adv Nurs* 21(1):47,1995.

Lubkin IM: *Chronic illness: impact and interventions,* Boston, 1995, Jones and Bartlett.

Luggen AS, Rini AG: Assessment of social networks and isolation in community based elderly men and women, *Geriatr Nurs* 16(4):179, 1995.

MacKay S, Holmes D, Gersumky A: Methods to assess aphasic stroke patients, *Geriatr Nurs* 9(3):177, 1988.

McFarland BH, Blair G: Delivering comprehensive services to homeless mentally ill offenders, *Psychiatric Services* 46(2):179, 1995.

McLerran J: Saved by the hand that is not stretched out: the aged poor in Hubert von Herkomer's Eventide: a scene in Westminster Union, *Gerontologist* 33(6):762, 1993.

Messent P: A review of recent developments in human-companion animal studies, *CA Vet* 37:26, May 1983.

Morley JE: Update on men's health, *Generations* 20(4):13, 1997.

Moustakas C: *Loneliness,* Englewood Cliffs, NJ, 1961, Prentice-Hall.

Mullins L, Tucker R, Longino C et al: An examination of loneliness among elderly Canadian seasonal residents of Florida, *J Gerontol* 44(2):S80, 1989.

National Center for Health Statistics: Supplements to the monthly vital statistics report: advance reports, 1989, 1990, National Center for Health Statistics, *Vital Health Stat* 24(6), 1996.

The new analytical Bible and dictionary of the Bible, authorized King James version, Chicago, 1964, John A Dickson Pub Co.

Nightingale F: *Notes on nursing,* Philadelphia, 1992, Lippincott (originally published in 1859).

Our gray-bearded ailing convicts, *San Mateo County Times,* p A-10, July 25, 1996 (editorial).

Randall VA: Androgens and human hair growth, *Clin Endocrinol* 40(4):439, 1994.

Roesch R, Ogloff JR, Eaves D: Mental health research in the criminal justice system: the need for common approaches and international perspectives, *Int J Law Psychiatry* 18(1):1, 1995.

Rush KL, Ouellet LL: Mobility aids and the elderly client, *J Gerontol Nurs* 23(1):7, 1997.

San Francisco Examiner: "Lesbo" grandma murdered, but it's not a hate crime, *Outward* 2(3):2, 1996.

Saylor C: Stigma. In Lubkin I, editor: *Chronic illness: impact and interventions,* ed 3, Boston, 1995, Jones and Bartlett.

Schuckit MA, Anthenelli RM, Buckolz KK, Hesselbrock VM, Tipp J: The time course of development of alcohol related problems in men and women, *J Stud Alcohol* 56(2):218, 1995.

Seeman M: On the meaning of alienation, *Am Sociolog Rev* 24:783, 1959.

Sheldon J: *The social medicine of old age,* Oxford, England, 1948, Oxford University Press.

Shirley V, Mercier J: Bereavement of older persons: death of a pet, *Gerontologist* 23:276 (special issue), 1983.

Steadman HJ, Morris SM, Dennis DL: The diversion of mentally ill persons from jails to community based services: a profile of programs, *Am J Public Health* 85(12):1630, 1995.

Steinberg D: Some jokes about aging are funny, some ain't, *San Francisco Examiner,* p C-7, July 8, 1995.

Stoller EP: The price of pride: helping rural elders accept needed care, *Aging Today* 14(5):7, 1993.

Tornstam L: Dimensions of loneliness, *Aging* 2(3):259, 1990.

Townsend P: Isolation and loneliness of the aged. In Weiss R, editor: *Loneliness: the experience of emotional and social isolation,* Cambridge, Mass, 1973, MIT Press.

Tucker JS, Friedman HS, Tsai CM, Martin LR: Playing with pets and longevity among older people, *Psychol Aging* 10(1):3, 1995.

US Bureau of the Census: *Statistical abstract of the United States,* ed 115, 1995, Washington, DC.

US Federal Bureau of Investigation: *Crime in the United States,* (1986).

Walsh E: Geriatric care becoming a big concern for prisons, *San Francisco Chronicle,* p A7, July 15, 1996.

Whipple B, Scura KW: The overlooked epidemic: HIV in older adults, *Am J Nurs* 96(2):22, 1996.

Windriver W: Social isolation: unit based activities for impaired elders, *J Gerontol Nurs* 19(3):15, 1993.

Wood WG: Alcoholism. In GL Maddox, editor: *The Encyclopedia of aging,* ed 2, New York, 1995, Springer.

Woods P: *Simulated presence therapy: using selected memories to manage problem behaviors in Alzheimer's disease patients,* Unpublished manuscript, 1993.

Zachow K: Helen, can you hear me? *J Gerontol Nurs* 10(2):18, 1984.

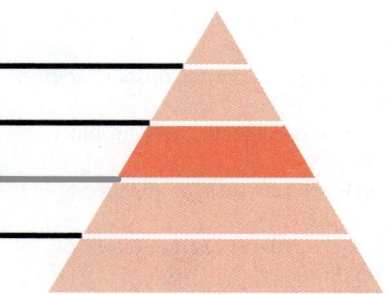

Lubben Social Network Scale

FAMILY NETWORKS

Q1. How many relatives do you see or hear from at least once a month?
(NOTE: Include in-laws with relatives.)   Q1 ____

    0 = zero   3 = three or four
    1 = one   4 = five to eight
    2 = two   5 = nine or more

Q2. Tell me about the relative with whom you have the most contact.
How often do you see or hear from that person?   Q2 ____

    0 = <monthly   3 = weekly
    1 = monthly   4 = a few times a week
    2 = a few times a month   5 = daily

Q3. How many relatives do you feel close to? That is, how many of them
do you feel at ease with, can talk to about private matters, or can call
on for help?   Q3 ____

    0 = zero   3 = three or four
    1 = one   4 = five to eight
    2 = two   5 = nine or more

FRIENDS NETWORKS

Q4. Do you have any close friends? That is, do you have any friends with
whom you feel at ease, can talk to about private matters, or can call
on for help? If so, how many?   Q4 ____

    0 = zero   3 = three or four
    1 = one   4 = five to eight
    2 = two   5 = nine or more

Q5. How many of these friends do you see or hear from at least once
a month?   Q5 ____

    0 = zero   3 = three or four
    1 = one   4 = five to eight
    2 = two   5 = nine or more

Q6. Tell me about the friend with whom you have the most contact. How
often do you see or hear from that person?   Q6 ____

    0 = <monthly   3 = weekly
    1 = monthly   4 = a few times a week
    2 = a few times a month   5 = daily

From Lubben I: Assessing social networks among elderly populations, *Fam Comm Health* 11(3):1988.

CONFIDANT RELATIONSHIPS

Q7. When you have an important decision to make, do you have someone you can talk to about it?   Q7 ____

Always	Very often	Often	Sometimes	Seldom	Never
5	4	3	2	1	0

Q8. When other people you know have an important decision to make, do they talk to you about it?   Q8 ____

Always	Very often	Often	Sometimes	Seldom	Never
5	4	3	2	1	0

HELPING OTHERS

Q9a. Does anybody rely on you to do something for them each day? For example: shopping, cooking dinner, doing repairs, cleaning house, providing child care, etc.

    NO—if no, go on to Q9b.

    YES—if yes, Q9 is scored "5" and skip to Q10

Q9b. Do you help anybody with things like shopping, filling out forms, doing repairs, providing child care, and so on?   Q9 ____

Always	Very often	Often	Sometimes	Seldom	Never
5	4	3	2	1	0

LIVING ARRANGEMENTS

Q10. Do you live alone or with other people?
(NOTE: Include in-laws with relatives.)   Q10 ____

    5 Live with spouse

    4 Live with other relatives or friends

    1 Live with other unrelated individuals (e.g., paid help)

    0 Live alone

                                              TOTAL LSNS SCORE: ____

SCORING:

The total LSNS score is obtained by adding up scores from each of the 10 individual items. Thus total LSNS scores can range from 0 to 50. Scores on each item were anchored between 0 and 5 to permit equal weighting of the 10 items. It is suggested that a score below 20 indicates an extreme risk for limited social networks.

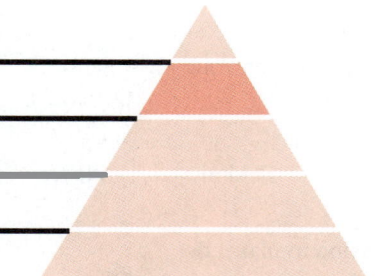

CHAPTER 19

Crisis and Stress Management

Students learn

I do look forward to growing old, to the process of learning more about myself and of growing in spirit and in mind. I do have fears, however, about growing old. My biggest fears are physical and mental changes I don't have control over; the possibility of an accident or an experience that scars me too deeply. Change can be a wonderful thing, an opportunity to grow, but it can also be quite painful and filled with pitfalls. My fear is that I will experience something too painful for my body or mind to handle.

Matthew, age 34

Essential to healthy aging is knowing what I can and cannot control. People spend their lives in stressful situations because they never learn this principle. Control gives one power, but with power comes worry and responsibility. It is a wise person who narrows his responsibilities to a manageable degree.

Daphne, age 36

Elders speak

I told my daughter, "Please don't hide the truth. At my age, I can cope with just about anything. It is being protected from truth that I can't stand."

Edna, age 80

Some of us just seem to live from one crisis to the next and not all of us succeed in managing them. The best examples of "managers" are those who have survived a series of crises offered by life. Experience is a great teacher. The critical events of my own life have given me a sense of inevitability bordering on fatalism, but I have had to compromise with each until I could accept the fact that not all realities were going to meet my expectations. Plenty of examples exist to convince me that I can live without attacking every small crisis as if it involved my whole existence. Sometimes it is best to walk away and forget it, which is not necessarily an admission of defeat. In such cases, it's possible the problem is not yours.

Lyn, age 85

Having to cope with the limitations of a stroke was the greatest crisis I have ever had. I have raised two sons, traveled and lived in Europe, studied Cantonese, and retired from teaching. The stroke was my greatest learning experience.

Aveline, over 70

LEARNING OBJECTIVES

Upon completion of this chapter, the reader will be able to:

1. Identify differences between crises and stress and describe the characteristics that would differentiate the two.
2. Relate crises and stressors that are likely to occur in the lives of the elderly in the community; list those that are likely for the institutionalized elder.

3. Discuss the concept of anxiety and explain several defense mechanisms that may be used to reduce the discomfort.
4. Discuss several coping styles of the elderly and compare their merits.
5. Specify the progression of helplessness exhibited in the spiral of dependency.
6. Explain methods of restoring a sense of control and averting excessive dependency.

EMOTIONS AND ILLNESS

There is much we do not yet understand about the connection between emotions and health and illness, though we know some emotions for some people result in illness. Though stress theorists often disagree, they are interested in understanding the process by which demands exceed the adaptive capacity of the organism and result in psychologic and biologic changes that place the person at risk of disease (Cohen et al, 1995). Cannon (1932), Meyer (1951), and Selye (1956), the fathers of stress theories, recognized that responses to life events often resulted in illness, and Holmes and Rahe (1967) attempted to quantify these into measurable psychic burdens.

Since that time numerous checklist life-event measurement scales with similar intent, but designed for special populations, have been generated. Those cited by Turner and Wheaton (1995) include 6 for children, 18 for adolescents, 20 for adults, and 3 for elders. Most of these require a retrospective analysis of the extent of the emotional burden in the prior 3, 6, or 12 months.

Now some researchers have found that early life events, such as parental loss, continue to exact an emotional price throughout life (Ensel et al, 1996; Wheaton, 1983; Rutter, 1989). In addition, the weighting of events at any given time is dependent upon concurrence of positive and negative events; recency of exposure; timing, interval, and duration of the event; number of roles occupied by the individual; affective state of the subject, and relevance and comprehensiveness of the scale to the particular population characteristics (Turner and Wheaton, 1995).

The scales designed for the elderly are cited in resources at the close of this chapter. We favor the Stokes/Gordon Stress Scale (1990) developed by nurses and elders specifically reflecting the stressors of the aged population (see Appendix 19-A).

Crises and stressful situations may produce emotions that erode the health of the frail aged. Demands upon the already vulnerable homeostasis, when they exceed a critical but individually undetermined level, are thought to elicit an array of harmful neuroendocrine responses (Kopin, 1995). Maladaptive neuroendocrine responses due to dysregulation of the stress response system may lead to autoimmune diseases such as arthritis, heart disease, and cancer (Stratakis and Chrousos, 1995; Vingerhoets et al, 1996; Ulmer, 1996), upper respiratory infections (Cohen, 1995), impaired response to influenza vaccine (Kiecolt-Glaser et al, 1996), and even memory loss (Modica, 1996; Krause, 1996). The impact of stress on the neurotransmitter, endocrine, and immune systems has generated a considerable amount of recent research (File, 1996).

Tricerri et al (1995) found significant impairment of immune function among elders who were depressed. In a survey by the Cancer Treatment Centers of America (1992) it was found that one in four nurses believed emotions and thoughts were the most important elements in a patient's health or recovery from illness.

Many studies in psychoneuroimmunology (PNI) are being conducted to more clearly determine the connection between mind and body. It was an artificial mechanistic thought mode that created the division between mind and body in the first place. Now, perhaps we will restore a more holistic perspective to health and illness. Zeller et al (1996) reviewed the few nursing studies that have focused on PNI and recommend that nurses conduct more studies grounded in the PNI framework because these are particularly relevant to the advancement of nursing science.

An example of the need for a more holistic approach is provided by the studies by Zotti et al (1991). They determined the need for psychologic assessment in the postinfarction patient. In a study of 168 unmedicated, postinfarction men between the ages of 36 and 69, those who exhibited a repressive style, denying anxiety, neuroticism, psychophysical symptoms, or depression had the highest levels of cardiac disturbances in response to mental stress tests (mental arithmetic and several concentration tasks). Half of the patients had high levels of cardiovascular response during the testing, but only 20% of the less responsive patients showed definite or possible electrocardiographic signs of significant arrhythmia or ischemia.

It is unclear if patients with low levels of emotional expression who had such cardiac responses during mental stress tests had similar characteristics before their infarction, because postinfarction patients are often in denial. However, the results emphasize the importance of psychophysical stress testing and comprehensive psychologic assessment in managing the postinfarction patient and identifying those at risk.

The relationship between mental stress testing and cardiovascular response was significant for heart rate, systolic and diastolic blood pressure, and skin conductance levels. Thus patients who have difficulty in acknowledging emotions or are too successful in controlling them may be coronary-prone individuals in need of assessment and risk management (Zotti et al, 1991).

During the course of the later years many situations and conditions occur that erode confidence in one's self and stir negative feelings. Restoration of a sense of control is basic to moving beyond the helplessness experienced during crises, stress, and illness.

This chapter is designed to engage students in the process of assisting elders to keep or rebuild feelings of control and competence. When elderly clients may be feeling helpless, hopeless, and dependent as a result of crises, overwhelming stress, and depleting illnesses, they will need emotional "splinting" (Wolanin and Phillips, 1981)—a temporary assist to keep the structure of their lives steady. Providing a framework nurses can use to assist clients to cope with stress and avert crises is our main purpose in this chapter.

Those clients who cling longer than necessary to a dependent role have lost faith in themselves and their capacities. They will need consistent encouragement and expectations as they gain confidence slowly. Yet we know that anyone who has survived this past 80 or so years has been inoculated numerous times by stressful events and must have tremendous resistance. No generation has faced so many changes or had its mettle so tested. This provides a beginning focus of discussion with elders feeling uncertain and incapable of making the changes necessary in their situation. Our task is to restore faith in one's adaptive capacity and self-directed action. These goals must be geared to the client's present situation and the realization that self-control, once relinquished, may be slow to return.

In this chapter we will not deal with all the situations that may assault one's self-worth because these have been quite thoroughly addressed in Chapter 18 and elsewhere. Our focus in this chapter will be on understanding stress and crises and the events, likely to occur in the process of growing old, that may create disruptions in daily life that drain one's inner resources or require the development of new and unfamiliar coping strategies.

CRISES AND STRESS

Crises and stressful situations occur throughout life but are thought to occur less frequently, although with more devastating effects, in the later years, when one may have less reserve adaptive capacity and often fewer available supports (McLean and Link, 1994). Psychologic homeostasis, comparable to and intertwined with physiologic homeostasis, fluctuates in the elderly within a reduced range of normal. The daily habits and rituals provide points of security and bolster stress immunity. When crises and cumulative stresses stretch the limits of coping capacity beyond one's individually established range, adaptive behavior temporarily deteriorates. Helplessness, lack of control, and dependency may emerge. It is important to remember this is a temporary condition and some degree of personal power can be restored.

Stress and crisis are not the same. Crisis events always create stress, but stressful situations do not necessarily precipitate crises. Some individuals have developed, through a lifetime of coping with stress, a tremendous stress tolerance, whereas others will be thrown into crisis by small changes in their life with which they feel unable to cope. The critical factor is personal perception of an event. The impact on one's self-esteem and sense of capability will be reflective of the degree of personal disorganization more than the magnitude of the event.

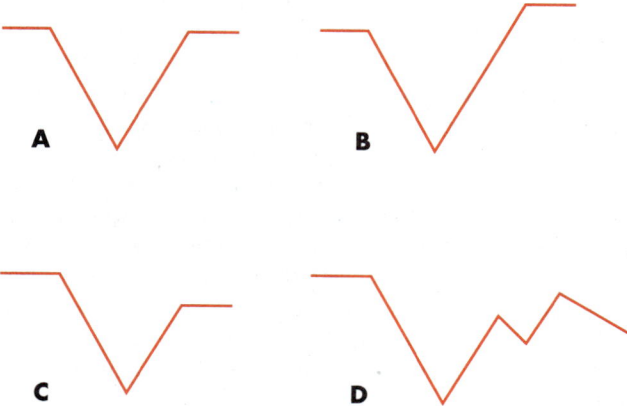

Figure 19-1. Crisis profiles. **A,** Same level of organization. **B,** Higher level of organization. **C,** Lower level of organization. **D,** Unstable after crisis. (From Koos E: *Families in Trouble,* New York, 1946, King's Crown Press.)

Box 19-1	**Crises Common to the Aged**

- Abrupt internal and external body changes and illnesses
- Other-oriented concerns: children, grandchildren, spouse
- Loss of significant people
- Acute discomfort and pain
- Breach in significant relationships
- Fires, thefts
- Injuries, falls
- Translocation
- Aphasia, abrupt loss following stroke
- Abrupt loss of mobility or source of transportation
- Major unexpected drain on economic resources; for example, house repair, illness
- Abrupt changes in housing, especially without warning, to a new location, home, apartment, room, or institution
- Death of roommates in institutions

Another distinction between crisis and stress is related to time. Crises are time limited and are always resolved as an individual initiates some action and reestablishes equilibrium on a higher or lower level of personal organization (Figure 19-1). The disequilibrium of crises cannot remain for more than a few weeks. Crises constitute a major, temporary disruption in coping capacity, whereas stress involves ineffectual or effectual coping and may be sustained over long periods. Ultimately it is expressed in higher levels of coping or deterioration in efficacy and feelings of failure, and is often then expressed through illness and eventual death.

Crises and Aging

The term crisis was first introduced by Erich Lindemann (1944). It is defined as the lack of defense or coping mechanisms to deal with sudden and unexpected intrusions into a life situation that was previously experienced as stable (Battegay, 1995). Crises common to the aged include those listed in Box 19-1.

Uncommon Crises and Post-Traumatic Stress Disorder (PTSD). Crises situations such as experienced by Second World War combat veterans, Jewish holocaust survivors, victims of torture, or those who have been imprisoned may seem intolerable, but the victims often settle into the rarified routine, not normal but ongoing, until the situation is experienced as a series of daily and constant high-level stressors. The influence of disciplined training, group trauma, and support in those situations has, to our knowledge, not been examined, but it seems likely that these factors defer the actual personal chaos and breakdown of coping activities, which then are deferred until a later time and emerge as post-traumatic stress disorder (PTSD).

These breakdowns may erupt later as personality disorders, nightmares, intrusive images, and physiologic disturbances such as arthritis and digestive disorders. These reactions are often activated by the weakened psychic defense system that may accompany the stressors of aging and the loss of loved ones (Buffum and Wolfe, 1995). One 75-year-old man noted that startle reactions and uncontrolled aggression had been an ongoing problem following his survival of the Battle of the Bulge over 50 years ago, though he noted these reactions had diminished somewhat in recent years. These data need considerably more study because the particular cohorts suffering these events are now well into their seventies and eighties, and some are in their nineties.

Benezra (1996) identified individuals who had experienced extremely traumatic events that created intense fear and helplessness. Those who coped successfully without enduring problems seemed to exhibit the following characteristics: secure and supportive relationships, ability to freely express or fully suppress the experience, avoiding dwelling on trauma, favorable circumstances immediately following the trauma, productive and active lifestyles, learning from the experience, strong faith/religion/hope, sense of humor, biologic strength, and endurance.

The numerous unexpected natural disasters that occur each year leave many elderly displaced or homeless (Tables 19-1 and 19-2). Tornadoes, hurricanes, cyclones, floods, tropical storms, firestorms, and earthquakes are examples of such events. In addition there are terrorist acts, bombings, killings, and accidents that occur suddenly and without

Table 19-1   Tornadoes, Floods, and Tropical Storms: 1984 to 1994

[See also *Historical Statistics, Colonial Times to 1970,* series J 268-278]

Item	1984	1985	1986	1987	1988	1989	1990	1991	1992	1993	1994, prel.
Tornadoes, number*	907	684	764	656	702	856	1,133	1,132	1,303	1,173	(NA)
Lives lost, total	122	94	15	59	32	50	53	39	39	33	(NA)
Most in a single tornado	16	18	3	30	5	21	29	13	10	7	(NA)
Property loss of $500,000 and over	125	69	75	38	48	60	91	64	108	72	(NA)
Floods: lives lost	126	304	80	82	29	81	147	63	87	101	(NA)
Property loss (mil. dol.)	4,000	3,000	4,000	1,490	114	415	2,058	1,416	800	16,400	(NA)
North Atlantic tropical storms and hurricanes:†											
Number reaching U.S. coast	12	11	6	7	12	11	14	8	7	8	7
Hurricanes only	1	6	2	1	1	3	—	1	1	1	—
Lives lost in U.S.	4	30	9	—	6	56	10	17	26	9	38
Property loss (mil. (1990) dol.)‡	77	4,457	18	8	9	7,840	57	1,500	25,000	57	973

From U.S. Bureau of the Census: *Statistical abstract of the United States: 1995,* ed 115, Washington, DC, 1995.
—Represents zero. NA Not available. *A violent, rotating column of air descending from a cumulonimbus cloud in the form of a tubular- or funnel-shaped cloud, usually characterized by movements along a narrow path and wind speeds from 100 to over 300 miles per hour. Also known as a "twister" or "waterspout." †Source: National Hurricane Center, Coral Gables, FL, unpublished data. Tropical storms have maximum winds of 39 to 73 miles per hour; hurricanes have maximum winds of 74 miles per hour or higher. ‡Source: Hebert, Jarrell, & Mayfield, "The Deadliest, Costliest, and Most Intense U.S. Hurricanes of this Century," NOAA Technical Memo, NHC-31, February 1993.
Source: Except as noted, U.S. National Oceanic and Atmospheric Administration, *Storm Data,* monthly.

Table 19-2   Deaths and Death Rates from Accidents, by Type: 1970 to 1992

[See also *Historical Statistics, Colonial Times to 1970,* series B 163-165]

Type of accident	Deaths (number)					Rate per 100,000 population				
	1970	1980	1990	1991	1992	1970	1980	1990	1991	1992
Total	**114,638**	**105,718**	**91,983**	**89,347**	**86,777**	**56.4**	**46.7**	**37.0**	**35.4**	**34.0**
Motor vehicle accidents	54,633	53,172	46,814	43,536	40,982	26.9	23.5	18.8	17.3	16.1
Traffic	53,493	51,920	45,827	42,621	39,985	26.3	22.9	18.4	16.9	15.7
Nontraffic	1,140	1,242	987	915	997	0.6	0.5	0.4	0.4	0.4
Water-transport accidents	1,651	1,429	923	851	837	0.8	0.6	0.4	0.3	0.3
Air and space transport accidents	1,612	1,494	941	1,000	1,094	0.8	0.7	0.4	0.4	0.4
Railway accidents	852	632	663	651	642	0.4	0.3	0.3	0.3	0.3
Accidental falls	16,926	13,294	12,313	12,662	12,646	8.3	5.9	5.0	5.0	5.0
Fall from one level to another	4,798	3,743	3,194	3,291	3,091	2.4	1.7	1.3	1.3	1.2
Fall on the same level	828	415	499	474	483	0.4	0.2	0.2	0.2	0.2
Fracture, cause unspecified, and other unspecified falls	11,300	9,136	8,620	8,897	9,072	5.6	4.0	3.5	3.5	3.6
Accidental drowning	6,391	6,043	3,979	3,967	3,524	3.1	2.7	1.6	1.6	1.4
Accidents caused by—										
Fires and flames	6,718	5,822	4,175	4,120	3,958	3.3	2.6	1.7	1.6	1.6
Firearms	2,406	1,955	1,416	1,441	1,409	1.2	0.9	0.6	0.6	0.6
Electric current	1,140	1,095	670	626	525	0.6	0.5	0.3	0.2	0.2
Accidental poisoning by—										
Drugs and medicines	2,505	2,492	4,506	5,215	5,951	1.2	1.1	1.8	2.1	2.3
Other solid and liquid substances	1,174	597	549	483	498	0.6	0.3	0.2	0.2	0.2
Gases and vapors	1,620	1,242	748	736	633	0.8	0.5	0.3	0.3	0.2
Complications due to medical procedures ..	3,581	2,437	2,669	2,473	2,669	1.8	1.1	1.1	1.0	1.0
Inhalation and ingestion of objects	2,753	3,249	3,303	3,240	3,128	1.4	1.5	1.3	1.3	1.2

From U.S. Bureau of the Census: *Statistical abstract of the United States: 1995,* ed 115, Washington, DC, 1995.

preparation. All of these are likely to generate crises and dysfunctional coping. They may or may not resolve quickly, depending upon the quality and immediacy of interventions.

Helplessness. Helplessness may be a result of repeated ineffective attempts to deal with stressors or crises. Seligman (1975) introduced the concept of "learned helplessness" into the vernacular of gerontologists. It is based on studies of mice that show they will continue to seek food through a maze even when they receive a predictable electric shock. However, when the shocks become unpredictable, they cease trying. Extrapolated to humans we believe that actions with unpredictable results over time will eventually result in the individual's retreat into helplessness.

Helplessness, powerlessness, and perceived lack of control erode the personality of individuals in uncertain and inconsistently demanding situations. Gordon (1991) has developed defining characteristics of this pervasive problem that will assist health care personnel in understanding the issues. Powerlessness is defined as "perceived lack of control over a situation and that actions will not significantly affect an outcome." Feelings of powerlessness and helplessness can arise from any of the sources identified in Box 19-2.

Learned helplessness may be the adaptive reaction of some elders living in a protected environment. Data reveal that, except in the areas of meals and privacy, these individuals are generally satisfied with the amount of control they have in their setting (Slimmer et al, 1987). This information alerts us to the fact that once helplessness becomes entrenched the unlearning process may not be desired by the elder and may create anxiety and unrest. We still ascribe to the belief that every effort should be made to increase independence to the maximum level, but staff must be aware of the process and have patience as the elder relearns to take charge of certain aspects of life of which they are capable.

Anxiety. Anxiety is a response to feelings of helplessness, isolation, alienation, and insecurity. Facilitative anxiety motivates one toward problem resolution whereas it appears that debilitative anxiety predisposes one to continue working on an inappropriate task rather than switching to a more effective one. Debilitative anxiety produces a diffuse feeling of panic, dread, and lack of control that can be insufferable in the acute stages.

Ongoing stressors may create moderate anxiety and be accompanied by unconscious alterations in behavior, such as repetitive actions, that transfer the anxious feelings to more specific and observable symptoms. Many changes and losses compounded may result in anxiety that has no specific trigger that the elder can identify. Hogstel (1990)

Sources of Feelings of Helplessness

- An unsuccessful illness-related regimen
- The implacable structure of the health care environment
- Interpersonal interactions
- A lifestyle of helplessness
- Repeated attempts to exert control that have failed
- Inability to predict a consistent outcome of certain actions

  The pervasiveness of the powerless feeling can be categorized from the most to the least severe in the following manner:

- Verbalization of lack of influence over outcome
- Depression when condition deteriorates in spite of compliance with health regimen
- Apathy
- Nonparticipation in care or decisions when opportunities are provided
- Expressed frustration over limitations
- Expressed doubt regarding role performance
- Passivity
- Disinterest in information regarding care
- Dependency on others with the accompanying feelings of resentment, anger, and guilt
- Reluctance to express true feelings
- Agreeing readily to whatever may be suggested
- Expressed uncertainty about fluctuations in energy and functional ability

makes an important point in noting that little is known about anxiety and its manifestations when it has not reached clinical proportions.

Madge was a 92-year-old lady of great dignity, self-sufficiency, and personality strength. Her adaptability to several moves, bereavement, and the loss of her belongings in a fire were remarkable demonstrations of her fortitude. Shortly after her ninety-second birthday she began telling her daughters she felt anxious and fearful but did not know why. Elements of the aging process, strength depletion, residual and chronic stressors, and a belated but mild post-traumatic stress reaction may all have been underlying her uncharacteristic anxiety.

Clinical levels of anxiety are seldom held for long periods because they are intolerable. They are commonly subverted into phobias or various other neuroses. Age-specific tools to determine the nature of anxiety in the old are not readily available. Evidence of anxiety in the elderly is often not as apparent as in younger clients.

Throughout life, anxiety is the motor that keeps people moving toward mastery of new and threatening situations. It usually runs with a soft, pleasurable purr that is not perceptible. Extreme or prolonged personal stress, however, is likely to bring on episodes of anxiety experienced as a noticeable, jittering hum within the epigastric

area. Anxious people often say they feel as if there is a motor running in them that they cannot stop.

Old people experience much stress but do not usually react in the same way as younger persons. It is thought that anxiety in the aged is likely to produce a state of hypervigilance. We have as often seen the retreat into apathy.

The following are some evidences of an anxiety state likely to occur in late life:

- Regression
- Disorganization
- Persistent use of a single behavior (sometimes called perseveration, for example, the patient may continually call for the nurse and then forget what was needed)
- Exaggerated emotional reactions to minor disturbances in routine
- Agitation
- Cardiac palpitation
- Disturbed memory
- Inability to concentrate
- Decreased problem-solving ability
- Suspiciousness
- Illusions, hallucinations, delusions, phobias
- Inability to carry out usual appropriate social behaviors

These reactions have often been labeled "dementia" in a person over 65 years old. Would the label be different in a person of 35 years of age?

Coping with anxiety. Severe, acute anxiety is rarely encountered among the aged. It seems those who survive must develop strategies for defending against this devastating discomfort. Jarvik and Russell (1979) suggest aged people do not fight or flee when endangered; instead they develop a passive "freeze" reaction. Fighting and fleeing require a heavy energy expenditure not appropriate or possible for most aged. Freezing does not imply giving up but rather energy conservation in response to overwhelming chronic insecurity. Inactivity, acceptance, contemplation, apathy, and neutrality may conserve energy for "vigilant watchfulness" (Jarvik and Russell, 1979).

Acute stresses often require action, but chronic stresses of aging call for long-term adaptive strategies. Some old-age strategies that might appear as maladaptive personality traits if predominant in other situations are effective in reducing anxiety in elders and should be respected (Box 19-3).

- Hanging onto pleasanter times through objects, reminiscing, and repetition of positive events
- Questioning others' motives and guarding self from emotional and physical intrusions
- Avoidance of change, resisting new activities or involvement in unfamiliar situations
- Endurance of drab surroundings that support independence rather than pleasanter surroundings and a forfeiture of independence

- Ritualistic behavior or repetitive actions that provide a feeling of sameness and comfort

All these can be used effectively to reduce insecurity to some degree.

Relaxation strategies such as deep, slow breathing, visualization, and progressive relaxation have been used to reduce anxiety effectively with elders. Significant positive changes in anxiety levels, psychologic symptoms, and relaxation ability persisted in subjects when a 1-year follow-up study of the training was conducted (Rickard, Scogin and Keith, 1994).

Crisis Assessment

Crisis assessment must take into account the recency of the event, effectual or ineffectual efforts to cope, and the available supports. The following are guidelines for determining the seriousness of a crisis:

0 = No crisis but rather a request for information.

1 = Mild crisis with ability to mobilize own resources after ventilating concern.

2 = Emerging crisis; client insightful but desiring specific help.

3 = Emergent crisis, second grade. Client recognizes need for assistance but uncertain what, where, or how to obtain. Counseling and referral necessary. Future crisis likely but client open and willing to use help when necessary.

4 = Moderate crisis. Decompensation impending, behaviors mostly ineffective, but client making attempts to resolve problem. Assistance can be deferred for a short time.

5 = Moderately severe crisis. Client agitated, disoriented, severely depressed.

6 = Severe crisis. Client presents likelihood of a life-threatening situation; client pleading for help, praying, trying ineffectively to escape the situation.

7 = Very severe crisis. Client in an immediate life-threatening situation; unable to focus on present situation; often engaged in irrelevant activities; for example, looking for makeup or comb when the house is on fire.

The elderly themselves and their families need more education in recognizing the early warnings of an impending crisis. Any of the reactions identified in stages 3 through 7 need immediate attention. Referrals are most often from family members or a nonrelative or professional. Rarely does the aged person seek crisis assistance. Therefore, the first action is to assess the degree of crisis and respond to the appropriate level of disorganization.

Long ago, Robert Butler (1967) identified four factors that significantly affect individual perception of crisis events in old age:

1. *Extrinsic factors.* The social or personal impact of losses and the degree of lifestyle reorganization required to adapt are significant in crisis resolution.

| Box 19-3 | Defense Mechanisms Used to Reduce Anxiety |

- *Denial* may be intrinsic to aging and necessary to maintain one's equilibrium in the face of major losses and impending demise of self.
- *Projection* is often used to give vent to inexpressible wishes and feelings; it signals high levels of internal stress.
- *Regression* may be temporarily necessary to mobilize energy and resources to cope with external stressors.
- *Displacement* may assist the elder to submerge feelings of anxiety and fasten on something more concrete and controllable.
- *Somatization* is a common means of dealing with psychosocial problems and is very hard to circumvent as it brings secondary gains if not overused.
- *Selective* memory tends to focus one on the memories that exemplify and corroborate present feelings, whatever they may be.
- *Compulsivity* allows one to keep control in a comforting way of certain aspects of life when the larger issues are overwhelming.

---

2. *Intrinsic factors.* Personality bents such as a pessimistic or optimistic outlook on life affect interpretation of events.

3. *Reserve capacity.* Depletion as a result of physical disabilities, chronic illness or stress, and brain damage may predispose one to experience small irritations as crises.

4. *Past history.* Capacity for surviving, adapting, and maintaining a positive self-view throughout life will influence ability to tolerate crises and stress in old age.

We have not found a better way of delineating the various influences on crisis impact for the aged. The important thing to remember is the great individual variability in definition of a crisis event. For some the loss of a pet canary is a crisis; others accept the loss of a limb as a challenge to their coping strategies.

Reactions to a perceived crisis include (1) anxiety, fear, a sense of unreality, and detachment; (2) restlessness, inability to sit still, searching for something to do, disorganized behavior, repetitiously performing behaviors that are no longer effective; (3) detachment and watchful waiting; (4) ruminating thoughts of guilt, incompetence, helplessness, questioning, confusion, paranoia; (5) physical reactions of exhaustion, anorexia, and other symptoms of grief as explained in Chapter 26; and (6) immobilization and apparent inability to take action. Recognizing characteristics of and reactions to crises will alert nurses to organize crisis intervention strategies. We have most frequently observed detachment, apathy, inability to make decisions, and disor-

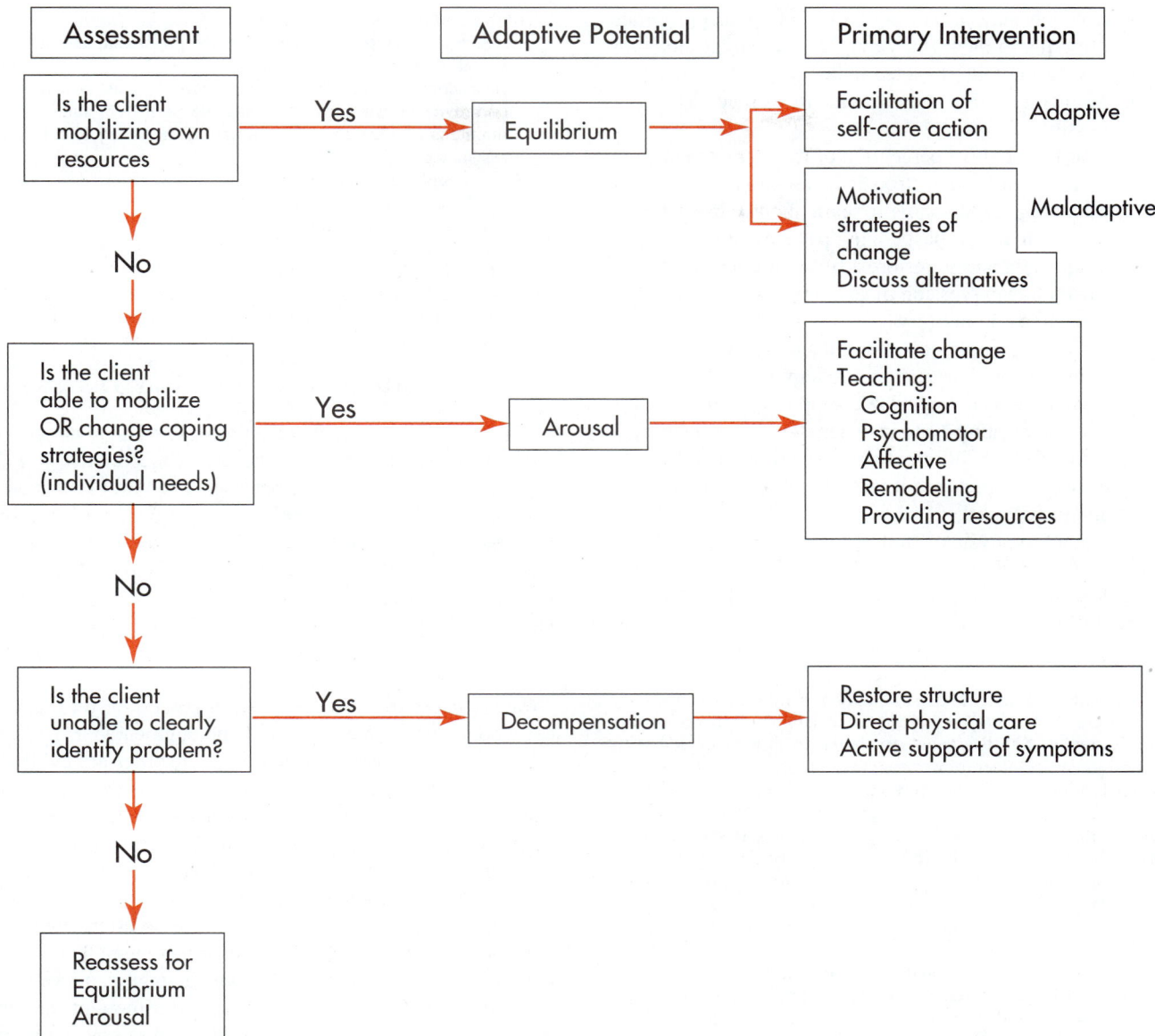

Figure 19-2. Adaptive potential for crisis management. (Modified from Bowman SB: The Fourth International Modeling and Role-Modeling Conference. Arcata, Calif, 1992, Humboldt State University.)

ganized behavior in elders experiencing a crisis. Any of the stressors that occur among the aged may actually be experienced as a crisis if the event occurs abruptly, is unanticipated, requires skills or resources the elder does not possess, and results in personality disorganization or psychic immobility.

Crisis Intervention Strategies

Crisis intervention is designed to resolve the immediate problem and to restore the person to the level of function that existed before the crisis occurred (Mosby, 1986). The immediate interventions must be geared to alleviating to some degree the anxiety (discussed previously) and the problem that most disturbs the elder. A crisis management model is shown in Figure 19-2. Immediate actions must decrease discomfort sufficiently to gain the elder's attention and cooperation.

Dealing with older persons in crisis is different from dealing with younger persons. The increased presence of chronic medical problems, decreased ability to manage independently, and the likelihood of living alone combine to produce a situation requiring more than brief therapy. Life crisis management may involve many referrals and ongoing case management as well as bolstering the informal care network, which may in fact be ineffective or inappropriate and contributing to the crisis. Some specific suggestions for crisis intervention with the aged include the following:

1. Maintain routine and usual habits as much as possible.
2. Clarify cognitive perception of the disruptive event.
3. Learn client's characteristic behavior.
4. Encourage reminiscing to learn about self-esteem, affect, character, past coping patterns, and uniqueness and to restore a sense of control.
5. Encourage expression of feelings toward tension discharge and mastery.
6. Listen to complaints; do not dismiss any as unimportant; help resolve predominant complaint.
7. Develop a readily available support system; identify and use existing systems when they are supportive.
8. Give adequate information to client but avoid overload; sometimes it will need to be written and/or repeated.
9. Attend to physical comfort measures.
10. Use touch as appropriate.
11. Identify resource person to be contacted if needed.

The following example enumerates crisis intervention functions:

Mrs. M is an 85-year-old Hispanic lady, recently moved from her home in Guadalajara to the home of her daughter and son-in-law in Los Angeles. She has been sent home from the hospital with draining lower leg ulcerations needing daily dressings, intermitten oxygen required to combat cerebral anoxia, and a gastrostomy tube for feeding. The decision to have her cared for at home was made by the physician, with the assistance of a Hispanic social worker and the patient, with the hesitant approval of her 60-year-old daughter and 67-year-old son-in-law. While in the hospital and discussing the plans with the doctor, visiting nurse, social worker and patient, the daughter and son-in-law thought the plan sounded feasible.

When Mrs. M arrived home by ambulance and was settled in her bed, she began to retch, and the gastrostomy tube exuded greenish, clotted fluid. They were not prepared sufficiently and had no coping skills for such a situation. Mrs M and her daughter and son-in-law panicked and called 911. Mrs M was returned to the hospital, and the crisis was quickly resolved, but the stress was enormous and though brief will influence the ability of the couple to continue supporting home care for Mrs. M. Their feelings of efficacy have been eroded.

Stressors often reach crisis proportions when the family with insufficient knowledge is confronted with life, death, and illness situations. The nurse will iterate all of the actions taken by the couple that were helpful and will explain those that are essential and will need to be taken in the future.

This example shows some of the vulnerability to crisis of the home care situation and the stress that is likely to occur when very old persons are sent home to be cared for and the family is inadequate or unable to understand the complex needs of the patient. The intervention to avert another crisis consists of the following:

- A visiting nurse with understanding of the Hispanic culture and Spanish language must be assigned to this case and must be available by phone until the care situation is stabilized.

- The family must be provided with emergency numbers by which to reach the visiting nurse, the physician, and the social worker when questions arise.
- Instructions for supportive care of Mrs. M must be written and reviewed carefully to be sure the caregivers understand maintenance care and when it may be necessary to call for assistance.
- The couple must be told that they are not required to care for the elder if they feel unable to do so.
- It will be helpful if the visiting nurse calls spontaneously for the first few days to reassure the family and the patient.
- The principles involve reinforcing available supports, assuring the individuals that there are resources to deal with emergencies and confirming their ability to employ strategies that will be effective in most circumstances. Comfort for Mrs M will be aimed at her physical condition and provided by an individual with whom she can converse.

Averting crises is an ongoing process in situations such as this. Nurses must understand the family's and client's anxiety and expect some anxiety reactions at times. Contact with consistent personnel will provide a sense of security, and concrete, carefully outlined care procedures will provide a sense of control and efficacy. Most importantly, contingency planning for major events that are likely to occur and formulating alternative preliminary plans will avert many crises.

Crisis as Growth

Growth occurs through crisis if the process is recognized, and coping efforts are supported and augmented as needed. Many of the symptoms of emotional disorder are evidence of an ineffective search for resolution of an earlier problem. Recognizing these symptoms may assist nurses in reassuring clients of their potential strength. Rather than attempting to ameliorate or ignore symptoms of crisis states, we might encourage recognition and acceptance.

Nurses may wish to pose alternative solutions long before the client has reached a state of readiness. This is not helpful. Timing is critical. Recognize stages and validate verbally, for example, "It seems as if your thoughts are going in circles. That is a necessary step before you can move on to resolution of the problem."

Much has been said of energy fields in scientific and pseudoscientific systems. In working through crisis stages toward integration, external positive energy facilitates the process. Nurses bring caring energy and effective actions at a time when the client's energy is at a low ebb. This infusion is critical and may significantly affect the ultimate outcome.

In addition, clients must be made aware of their personality qualities that serve as buffers. Benezra (1996) identified these, as discussed previously in the chapter. Clients may be unaware of their strengths and these must be enumerated and stated clearly.

Stress and Stressors of the Aged

The experience of stress is an internal state accompanying threats to self. Healthy stress levels motivate one toward growth, while a stress overload diminishes one's ability to cope effectively. Stressors may be external events and situations or inner dictates. Stress can be conceptualized as the result of poor tension management. Further, stressors may be distal or proximal (Ensel et al, 1996). Resistance resources are the factors that control anxiety, tension, and strain, precluding stress. In addition, accidents and the fear of accidents produce acute and chronic stress because the aged tend to experience more devastating consequences and are significantly more vulnerable to them (Table 19-3).

Among the aged stress is likely to appear as cognitive impairment (Krause, 1996). There are also particular gender differences in the effects of stress. Men are especially likely to seek the services of their physician when confronted by undesirable stressful events, whereas women, and particularly married women, who needed instrumental assistance during stress were unable to obtain it. Those in poor health had the most confidants under conditions of stress, but these did not act as buffers. In fact, married women in high-stress situations had poorer health than married men or unmarried individuals of either gender (Preston, 1995).

Proximal Stressors. Proximal stressors are those that are in the present, whether acute or chronic, and that require action and inner resources to avert crises. Some that are common to the aged include:

Caregiving of a demented spouse
Illness
Relocation
Loss of children
Loss of cohorts
Loss of siblings
Loss of friends
Dispersal of significant belongings

Incompetency proceedings
Inheritance conflicts
Abandonment: fear of dying alone/not being found/painful death
Hospitalization
Institutionalization
Separation from personal physician
Sensory changes (vision and hearing)
Housing and home maintenance
Lack of protection when frail and vulnerable
Limited mobility and lack of transportation
Unnamed concerns about the future
Fears of senility
Social losses, loss of driver's license
Acute and chronic pain
Medications
Abuse and neglect
Loss of pet
Rent increases

Several years ago student nurses interviewing community residing elders asked about stressors in their lives. The list of items in Box 19-4 were identified as stressors by those elders.

Acute Stressors. Acute stressors are those situations that are proximal and require adaptive energy on an ongoing, daily basis. The effects of these are mitigated by personality, available resources, environmental situation, contextual issues, and chronic stressors. They are likely to fluctuate from one month to the next as demands occur or recur and some situations are resolved. One issue that must be addressed is frequency of the stressor. Life event scales often make no allowance for frequency. For instance, if an elder has

Table 19-3   Death Rates from Accidents and Violence: 1990 to 1992

[Rates are per 100,000 population. Excludes deaths of nonresidents of the United States. Beginning 1980, deaths classified according to the ninth revision of the *International Classification of Diseases.* For earlier years, classified according to the revisions in use at the time.

| | White | | | | | | Black | | | | | |
| | Male | | | Female | | | Male | | | Female | | |
Cause of death and age	1990	1991	1992	1990	1991	1992	1990	1991	1992	1990	1991	1992
Total*	**81.2**	**78.7**	**76.2**	**32.1**	**31.5**	**30.4**	**142.0**	**143.9**	**134.5**	**38.6**	**38.4**	**36.7**
Motor vehicle accidents	26.1	24.4	22.4	11.4	10.8	10.2	28.1	25.6	24.0	9.4	8.7	8.8
All other accidents	23.6	23.3	23.4	12.4	12.6	12.4	32.7	34.2	30.9	13.4	13.5	12.7
Suicide	22.0	21.7	21.2	5.3	5.2	5.1	12.0	12.1	12.0	2.3	1.9	2.0
Homicide	9.0	9.3	9.1	2.8	3.0	2.8	69.2	72.0	67.5	13.5	14.2	13.1
15 to 24 years old	107.3	104.2	97.4	30.5	31.2	28.4	208.0	231.9	222.2	34.9	37.0	34.9
25 to 34 years old	97.4	94.2	90.4	26.0	24.7	23.6	218.1	213.8	193.6	48.1	47.7	46.1
35 to 44 years old	82.3	78.5	80.3	24.4	23.5	23.5	176.6	171.8	159.8	38.5	40.0	38.9
45 to 54 years old	73.5	72.9	69.8	25.3	25.2	24.2	138.5	132.4	132.9	30.7	33.1	29.5
55 to 64 years old	79.5	75.6	73.0	29.4	26.6	25.7	129.9	124.7	118.7	36.1	32.5	31.8
65 years old and over	150.7	147.4	145.4	80.1	79.6	78.6	175.5	182.2	165.7	81.6	78.6	72.6
65 to 74 years old	99.7	94.8	94.0	40.5	39.0	38.7	141.8	142.6	130.8	50.4	48.1	43.9
75 to 84 years old	195.7	190.5	186.2	89.4	87.1	83.9	206.1	213.5	201.4	95.8	89.7	89.5
85 years old and over	428.3	433.3	421.4	232.4	234.8	234.2	359.1	373.9	340.0	213.0	209.8	178.4

From U.S. Bureau of the Census: *Statistical abstract of the United States: 1995,* ed 115, Washington, DC, 1995.
*Includes persons under 15 years old, not shown separately.

Box 19-4	Stressors Identified by Community Elders

Sensory changes (vision and hearing)
Necessity to relocate
Housing and home maintenance
Protection when frail and vulnerable
Limited mobility and lack of transportation
Fears of senility
Social losses, loss of driver's license
Depression/bereavement
Management of acute and chronic pain
Medications
Protection from abuse and neglect
Retirement of physician
Loss of pet
Rent increases
Prevention of illness

From Ebersole P: Data obtained from nursing students' interviews of community elders, Holistic Nursing Course, San Francisco State University, San Francisco, 1988. Items not ranked or in order of significance.

received one moving violation in the previous year, it may be a mild stressor and engender overcautious behaviors when driving, but if he or she has received four tickets for violations, the consequences are quite different and highly stressful.

Chronic Stressors. Chronic stressors tend to be those categorized as distal, or remote events, and contextual, such as a nongratifying marriage or unrewarding work situation (Wethington et al, 1995). For elders contextual issues often involve a living situation that produces constant discomfort and dismay, enduring chronic illnesses and pain, abusive caregivers, and internalized ageism. Preston (1995) found that stress related to marital status, gender roles, and health was highest among married women in poor health. These findings need further investigation because it is unclear from the study how many may have been in demanding caregiving roles, which are among the most stressful situations elders experience.

Uncertainty of illness and outcome is seen as a particularly debilitating life event in which coping may be seriously undermined (Mishel, 1988). Inability to manage activities of daily living (ADLs) is also a major stressor for elderly persons. Individuals with unsupportive social relationships and low self-esteem are more likely to experience an increase in psychologic and somatic problems both on and following stressful days than are participants high in self-esteem and social support.

These data suggest that persons with low psychosocial resources are vulnerable to illness and mood disturbance when their stress levels increase, even if they generally have few current stressors in their lives. Chronic stress is most likely to activate depression, and this creates physiologic changes that result in illness and further exacerbate stress. This cyclic process may be the source of numerous illnesses; perhaps even the aging process itself is a result of a lifetime of numerous stresses and adaptive demands.

Hassles. Hassles are the small daily events, everyday stressors that are seldom given much thought. Gerontologists seriously consider the impact of "hassles" on stress levels, coping energy, and style of elders and of their caregivers (see Chapter 17). Hassles, according to *Funk and Wagnall's Standard Dictionary* (1983), are arguments, squabbles, or harassments. As used in gerontologic studies, hassles are minor and everyday irritants involving maintenance of home, finances, daily life, interpersonal relationships, and health. Hassles of this type may adversely affect well-being and health status even more than major life disruptions (Burks and Martin, 1985).

Older persons are thought to experience fewer hassles, but some produce more distress for them than for younger persons. Home maintenance and environmental and social hassles are particularly onerous for the elderly. Young people tend to confront most hassles head-on but avoid health irritations, whereas older individuals tend to avoid dealing with hassles unless they are health related.

Issues such as challenging versus senseless events and the range of pleasurable events one has to offset the noxious ones have not been adequately examined in relation to ultimate effects on coping.

DeLongis et al (1988) studied the effects of daily hassles and found that they affected mood for short periods but did not produce lasting negative effects if the individual had high self-esteem and social supports. Their data suggest that persons with low psychosocial resources are vulnerable to illness and lasting mood disturbances when stress levels increase, even if they generally have little stress. Individuals seem generally to adapt to daily hassles, but in combination with major stressful life events, hassles create psychologic problems.

The Daily Life Experience (DLE) 78-item checklist attempts to identify these hassles and the stress load (Stone, Neale and Shiffman, 1993). Earlier, Zautra et al (1986) modified the Inventory of Small Life Events (ISMLE) to be used to measure hassles of the elderly (see resources). It is also useful to keep a diary of daily events because many individuals are unaware of the small hassles; the diary may help to identify problems and patterns that are subject to solution and thus reduction of stress (Eckenrode and Bolger, 1995). Stetson (1997) uses these diaries to assist individuals to identify self-healing activities in which they select one element they wish to modify and develop a concrete plan to accomplish that with weekly, measureable goals.

Worry. A common perception about elderly people is that they worry excessively about the stresses associated with the aging process, such as declining health, limited finances, and decreased opportunities for social involvement. The feeling that the events in one's life are the result of fate, chance, or luck creates worry. The uncontrollability of thoughts and images is a central component of the worry process (Andrews, Borkovec, 1988). Worry has a negative impact on psychologic health. The emerging research on worry in the elderly, however, indicates that their worrying is limited. Powers et al (1992) developed a worry scale that may assist the elderly to make a more specific appraisal of their worries (Figure 19-3).

Instructions: Below is a list of problems that often concern many Americans. Please read each one carefully. After you have done so, please fill in one of the spaces to the right with a check that describes how much that problem worries you. Make only one check mark for each item.

THINGS THAT WORRY ME. . .

	Never	Rarely (1–2 times per month)	Sometimes (1–2 times per week)	Often (1–2 times a day)	Much of the time (more than 2 times a day)
Finances					
1. that I'll lose my home					
2. that I won't be able to pay for the necessities of life (such as food, clothing, or medicine)					
3. that I won't be able to support myself independently					
4. that I won't be able to enjoy the "good things" in life (such as travel, recreation, entertainment)					
5. that I won't be able to help my children financially					
Health					
6. that my eyesight or hearing will get worse					
7. that I'll lose control of my bladder or kidneys					
8. that I won't be able to remember important things					
9. that I won't be able to get around by myself					
10. that I won't be able to enjoy my food					
11. that I'll have to be taken care of by my family					
12. that I'll have to be taken care of by strangers					
13. that I won't be able to take care of my spouse					
14. that I'll have to go to a nursing home or hospital					
15. that I won't be able to sleep at night					
16. that I may have a serious illness or accident					
17. that my spouse or a close family member may have a serious illness or accident					
18. that I won't be able to enjoy sex					
19. that my reflexes will slow down					
20. that I won't be able to make decisions					
21. that I won't be able to drive a car					
22. that I'll have to use a mechanical aid (such as a hearing aid, bifocals, a cane)					
Social conditions					
23. that I'll look "old"					
24. that people will think of me as unattractive					
25. that no one will want to be around me					
26. that no one will love me anymore					
27. that I'll be a burden to my loved ones					
28. that I won't be able to visit my family and friends					
29. that I may be attacked by muggers or robbers on the streets					
30. that my home may be broken into and vandalized					
31. that no one will come to my aid if I need it					
32. that my friends and family won't visit me					
33. that my friends and family will die					
34. that I'll get depressed					
35. that I'll have serious psychological problems					
Other worries					
36.					
37.					
38.					
39.					
40.					

Figure 19-3. The Worry Scale. (From Powers CB, Wisocki PA, Whitbourne SK: Age differences and correlates of worrying in young and elderly adults, *Gerontologist* 32(1):82, 1992.)

One's sense of control or mastery over life events may be relevant in the assessment of worry-proneness. Research on the relationship between locus of control and coping indicates that individuals who are internally oriented are more effective copers than those who are externally oriented (Wheaton, 1983).

Those elders who focus on the past may use that as an adaptive strategy for coping with the stresses of life. They have survived much and are reminding themselves of that. This may provide an explanation for the low frequency of worry reported by the elderly individuals. In addition, when elders have confronted the major traumas of living and have survived, they often have a clearer perception of those things that are important and those that are not.

Dependency and loss of control as stressors. Impaired ability to maintain self-care is likely to deteriorate to the point of precipitating a dependency situation. Functional independence is the decisive factor in an old person's capacity to hold out at home and avoid family or institutional care. It is the basis of establishing the limits beyond which assistance and support become indispensable.

The aged person may, as part of a continuing lifestyle or pattern, be a dependent individual. The dependency need originated in early life but may remain dormant until physical, mental, social, or economic resources are threatened or lost. The impact directly affects the individual's capacity for mastery or gratification and activates feelings of helplessness. The aged person then exhibits loss of confidence; anticipates failure; and experiences shame, diminished self-esteem, and a sense of incompetence.

Anger, fear, and fear of retaliation can immobilize the aged person or mobilize him or her to seek help through a display of helplessness, hypochondriasis, or openly angry manipulation of others. This dependency is sometimes cultivated by caregiving staff who consciously or unconsciously are motivated by the assumed roles of healer, protector, and nurturant mother. Figure 19-4 depicts the spiral effect of dependency, which begins when the aged person seeks services from caregivers to solve a problem.

The question certainly arises, "What about those aged who continue in their dependency and are never restored to a state of autonomy?" We believe this occurs when supports are inadequate or missing during critical stress periods. Those aged who deteriorate mentally, emotionally, and physically exert a perverse kind of control through their dependency.

The nursing function is to redirect any evidence of control toward preserving the integrity, personality, and self-esteem of that individual. If power is properly redirected, some measure of life control can be restored. Even when people are unable to make decisions regarding their own personal care, they may still be able to participate if given direction and assistance. For example, giving the patient a washcloth and standing by to help if requested, rather than doing for the patient, reinstates an element of control.

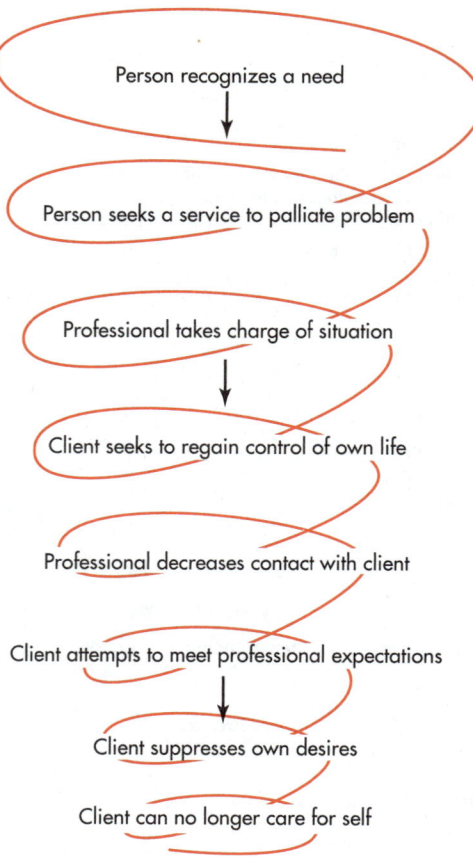

Figure 19-4. Spiral of dependency.

Nurses must examine their capacity to tolerate untidiness, inefficiency, and delay in the interest of promoting some measure of independence.

Regardless of the cause of the dependency of the aged person, the most constructive role the caregiver or nurse can assume is that of confidant, advocate, and counselor. These roles foster independence within the confines of the elderly person's capacity.

Assessment of Stress Levels

Early in the chapter, life event measurement tools were briefly discussed. However, assessing stress level is a very complex issue with many variables, both personal and environmental (Monroe and McQuaid, 1994). The confluence of daily hassles, distal and proximal stressors, worries, and functional capacities all create a stress load. Though many life event stress evaluation scales have been developed, none that presently exist can measure all these factors. We favor using them as tools to focus discussion of the various events and to suggest other factors that may be creating stress. Adolph Meyer's idea (1951) of evaluating numerous strands in a lifeline perspective is likely to be useful. A discussion of the clustering of events and situations at various times can be very revealing. Figure 19-5 can be used as a model.

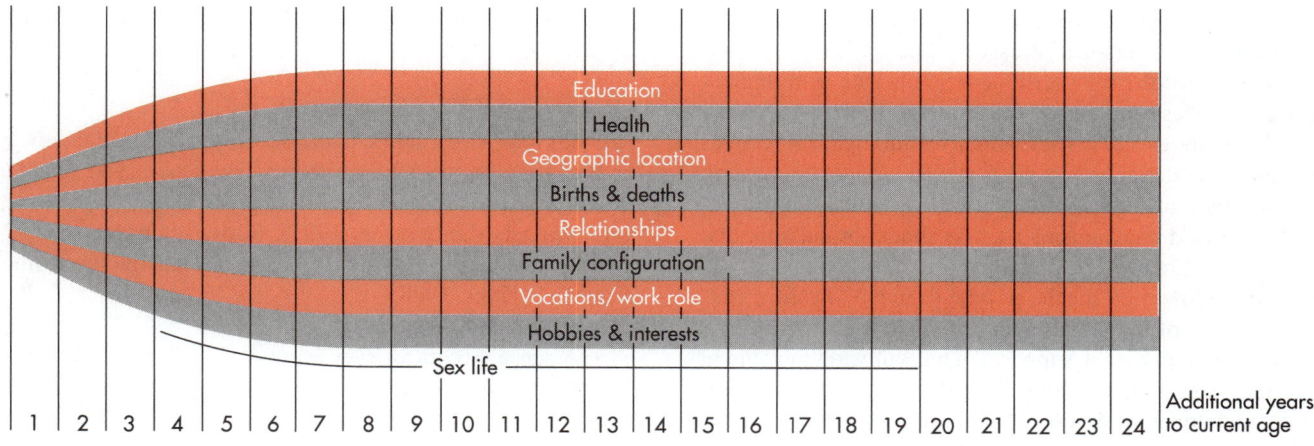

Figure 19-5. Life chart.

One factor that has seldom been given sufficient consideration is the stress created by positive events. Pasupathi et al (1996) used a modified Holmes and Rahe stress scale to determine the influence of age and socioeconomic status on the degree of stress in adapting to events ordinarily seen as positive. Age seemed to make little difference, but individuals of lower socioeconomic status who had experienced a positive event seemed to find it more stressful, perhaps more surprising and requiring alterations in lifestyle. The researchers suggest positive events have not been given sufficient attention as adaptive challenges and stress producers.

Stress Management

There has been a large body of research in the last 20 years on the effects of stress on aging and adaptation (Ensel, 1991; Hughes et al, 1988; Turner and Avison, 1992; Avison and Gotlib, 1994; Cohen, 1995). Researchers concerned with the effects of stress on the lives of elders have examined many moderating variables and have concluded that cognitive style, coping strategies, social skills, personal efficacy, support systems, and personality are all significant to the impact of stress (Folkman et al, 1987). Others have felt that control, power, sense of humor, and sensation seeking were significant variables. A critical age-related difference in stress management is the diminished ability to respond to stress and rapidly return to prestress levels of organismic homeostasis.

The following are factors to consider in stress management:

- Change is stressful; therefore interventions should impose as few changes as possible.
- Continuity of personnel and as few people as possible to administer services leave the client more energy to deal with the problem at hand.
- Timing is important. Individuals have personal time clocks that order their peak efficiency daily, monthly,

and developmentally; use best times to introduce change.
- Another aspect of timing to consider is the recency of stresses. More energy will be needed to integrate events that have occurred within the previous 6 weeks, 6 months, or year than those occurring in the remote past.
- The aged often experience multiple, simultaneous stresses, and reduction of anxiety is necessary before considering options for intervention.
- Some aged are in a chronic state of grief because losses are never fully resolved before another one occurs; stress then becomes a constant state of being.
- Discuss concepts of stress with the aged person, and assist him or her to understand that resolution may be slower than expected if he or she has recently been bombarded with change.
- Advise individuals in high-stress situations to increase rest and improve nutrition because the body chemistry changes and one is more vulnerable to illness.
- Acute stress is precipitated by change, whereas chronic stress is often a signal that change is needed.
- Teach relaxation strategies.

Martin (1996) has developed acronyms that are reminders of important tips in stress management:

S = Collect data with a stress scale.
T = Talk about upsetting situations.
R = Relax with imagery or visualization.
E = Exercise: gardening, walking, or window shopping (these also are distracters).
S = Support groups; join those that provide affirmation and problem solving.
S = Smile.

She further adds the HALT acronym, which specifies that decisions must never be made when one is *H*ungry, *A*ngry, *L*onely, or *T*ired.

Prevention and Treatment. Everyone is exposed to environmental and personal stressors. The question is, How does one reduce the long-term neuroendocrine disturbances induced by stress and emotional arousal? There are thought to be three modes: (1) conservation/ withdrawal, (2) relatedness, and (3) relaxation.

In the face of major stress an individual uses conservation/withdrawal mechanisms such as shock, projection, displacement, repression, rationalization, and depression. All these help allow time for the psyche to move toward a realistic appraisal of the situation and to move outward to connect with interpersonal supports. This outward movement of coping can then be followed by the relaxation so essential to maintenance of neuroendocrine regulatory mechanisms and protection from disease-producing disturbance. Forsythe and Compas (1987) believe efficacy in management of stressors immunizes the individual against emotional disruption.

Individuals with more personal and environmental resources use more active coping strategies when encountering difficulties (Holahan and Moos, 1987). A core set of attitudes, including optimism, self-efficacy, a sense of control, connectedness and coherence, and life sources of happiness and pleasure, resulted in positive outcomes (Sobel, 1995). The Harvard Community Health Plan found educational materials, relaxation-response training, and awareness training were all helpful in coping with stress (Sobel, 1995). Life experience in successful stress management may be the most important resource elders have.

In the future, nursing research should address personality impact, control, social supports, life experience, types of stressors, and gender differences in stress management. All of these and other unidentified factors may be significant, and as yet we do not know what combination is most effective in mediating stress in the lives of elders. We do know that 80% of health and stress management is self-initiated, so it is important to provide elders with an array of self-care tools.

Teaching the elderly stress reduction often begins with progressive muscle relaxation (PMR). This has several benefits in addition to stress reduction because it facilitates awareness of muscle groups and those that are weak, tight, stressed, or inactive. Weinberger (1991) found, in reviewing the literature, that elders given PMR training had beneficial results in stress reduction and enhanced immune function and memory.

The procedure for teaching progressive muscle relaxation and the sequential order of proceeding from one muscle group to another are shown in Boxes 19-5 and 19-6. These are modified from the work of Jacobson (1938). There are numerous books on the market for professionals and for lay persons that provide various techniques for managing stress (see resources at the end of the chapter).

Some provide detailed scripts to induce relaxation (Lusk, 1992).

Stress and Growth

Humans have two qualities that allow them to make the most or the least of stressful situations: awareness and choice. Stress mediators that are useful include religion, optimism, and hypnosis (Ishler et al, 1995). Stress filters are components in one's life that may be used to channel stress into growth (Schafer, 1978):

- Health and fitness
- A sense of control over events
- Awareness of self and others
- Patience and tolerance
- Support groups
- Personal stability zones or a strong sense of self
- Beliefs and values

Selye (1974) notes that stress inventories need to be more cognizant of individual differences. Self-knowledge allows us to judge whether we are running above or below the stress level that suits us best. The elderly are more prone to the adverse effects of stress and anxiety on the heart. Increased heart rate, blood pressure, insomnia, and irritability are some of the signs we have exceeded our optimum stress

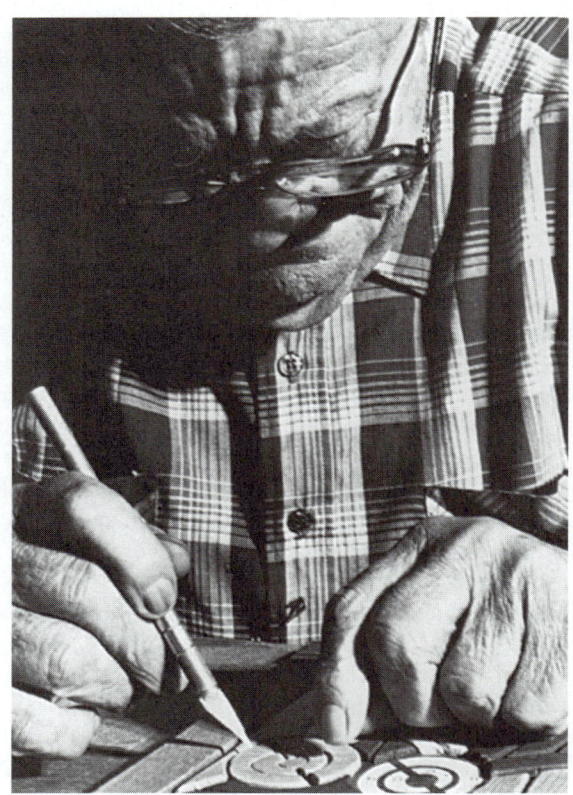

Eustress. (Courtesy Sally Wagner, American Society on Aging.)

level. In the frail old, confusion may be the signal of stress overload.

The term eustress is good stress engendered by challenging, demanding situations in which an individual still feels capable and in control (Selye, 1978). Attitudes may make an event a negative or a positive stress. Selye's recipe for good stress is (1) seek your own stress level, which fits you best; (2) choose your own goals, not ones imposed by others; and (3) altruistic egoism—look out for the self by being necessary to others and earning goodwill. Competence and usefulness make this feasible. Selye's recommendations are important to nurses as well as their aged clients.

Coping. "Buffering" and "hardiness" are terms that have captured the imagination of researchers interested in determining the differences in coping capacity of ostensibly similar elders. Buffers against decompensation with stress come from social supports and are usually seen as the most important coping resource (see Chapters 17 and 18).

Hardiness, the combination of personality characteristics of commitment, control, and challenge, apparently buffers the illness-related effects of stress (Ganellen and Blaney, 1984). Life goals and a sense of purpose or meaning undergird hardiness. Funk and Houston (1987) analyzed the research that has been done around the concept of hardiness and found many inconsistencies, but in general there is considerable support for the belief that hardy persons manage stress in a positive, growth-promoting manner more often than they experience its negative effects.

The relevance of hardiness to nursing practice is in assisting individuals to regain a sense of control over their lives, to feel committed or deeply involved with some activity that gives meaning, and to anticipate change as exciting. These may seem lofty goals, but they have been observed under the most extenuating circumstances.

Hardiness is a concept that explains the ability of some individuals to withstand enormous stress. The cornerstones of hardiness are control, competence, and compassion (Kobasa, 1979). Central to hardiness is the viewpoint that stress is a decision-making challenge and that meaning comes from making decisions. Stressful situations are seen as opportunities for growth. Clients should be apprised of any evidence of hardiness in their actions. These can reinforce their strength and coping abilities. Individuals should be asked the meaning of certain events in their lives and what they are learning from these challenging situations.

Coping strategies are the stabilizing factors that help individuals maintain psychosocial balance during stressful periods. More broadly, coping strategies are any efforts toward stress management, things that people do to avoid being harmed by life strains, or overt and covert behaviors to reduce or eliminate psychologic distress. Two major categories of coping behaviors are those that actively and directly deal with the problem and those that are designed for avoidance of the problem.

Lazarus and Folkman (1984) distinguish between problem-focused strategies and those that are emotion focused. For example, if one's elderly parent demands to be waited on, a direct method to solve the problem would be to discuss with the elder the assistance that can realistically be given and what is needed. In an effort to avoid the problem and reduce emotional frustration, one might take a Valium and go to bed, hoping that the problem would eventually resolve

---

Box 19-5	A Procedure for Teaching Progressive Muscle Relaxation

1. Provide a quiet environment.
2. Arrange for a comfortable chair; a recliner is ideal.
3. Instruct the client to wear comfortable clothes and remove any contact lenses
4. Instruct the client to focus attention on a muscle group
5. Instruct the client to tense that muscle group and focus on feelings of tension.
6. After 5 to 7 seconds of tension, instruct the client to relax that muscle group.
7. Allow the client to relax the muscle group for 30 to 40 seconds and instruct the client to focus on feelings of relaxation.
8. Repeat the tense and relax cycle.
9. Encourage the client to practice the complete procedure twice a day for 15 to 20 minutes.

From Weinberger R: Teaching the elderly stress reduction, *J Gerontol Nurs* 17(10):23, 1991.

Box 19-6	Sequential Order for Relaxation of Muscle Groups

Dominant hand and forearm
Dominant biceps
Nondominant hand and forearm
Nondominant biceps
Forehead
Upper cheeks and nose
Lower cheeks and jaws
Neck and throat
Chest, shoulders, and upper back
Abdominal region
Dominant thigh
Dominant calf
Dominant foot
Nondominant thigh
Nondominant calf
Nondominant foot

From Weinberger R: Teaching the elderly stress reduction, *J Gerontol Nurs* 17(10):23, 1991.

itself. Some emotion-focused strategies may be healthy, such as centering oneself or meditating, but are still an avoidance of the actual issue (Box 19-7).

Problem-oriented coping strategies have been shown to moderate the negative effects of adverse life events and to be associated with reduced depression (Mitchell et al, 1983). Those who were depressed used avoidance

coping increasingly as their depression became more profound. Holahan and Moos (1986) found that individuals who adapted to stress with little physical or psychologic strain were less inclined to use avoidance coping than were those who showed psychologic dysfunction under stress.

Coping Styles. There are many ways of coping and scales to measure styles of coping. The Ways of Coping Checklist (WCCL) devised by Aldwin et al (1985) focuses on seven styles of coping: (1) problem focused, (2) wishful thinking, (3) growth and learning, (4) minimizing the threat, (5) seeking support of others, (6) blaming self, and (7) using a mixture of strategies. Manfredi and Pickett (1987) studied the specific ways of coping used by 51 elders between 60 and 89 years of age and found the most and least frequent responses to the 66-item WCCL were those listed in Box 19-8.

Some evidence also shows that there is a maturation process in coping just as in other aspects of life. Irion and Blanchard-Fields (1987) did a cross-sectional comparison of coping behaviors in adolescents, young adults, midlife adults, and older persons and found that the elements of hostility, avoidance, and self-blame as aspects of coping consistently decreased over the life span of adults.

These data are significant for nurses as we identify and reinforce successful coping mechanisms. Because we often focus exclusively on the problem-solving mode, we may forget there are many ways to solve a problem besides resolving it. As elders confront many problems that cannot be reversed or logically resolved, they obviously resort to other mechanisms that help them successfully cope with the issue. Early memories are useful in comprehending the coping style of an elder. Ask about several early incidents that the elder remembers and listen carefully to the manner in which the elder tells the incident, as well as how he or she managed.

Box 19-7 **Coping Strategy Items**

Active-Cognitive Strategies

Prayed for guidance and/or strength
Prepared for the worst
Tried to see the positive side of the situation
Considered several alternatives for handling the problem
Drew on my past experiences
Took things a day at a time
Tried to step back from the situation and be more objective
Went over the situation in my mind to try to understand it
Told myself things that helped me feel better
Made a promise to myself that things would be different next time
Accepted it; nothing could be done

Active-Behavioral Strategies

Tried to find out more about the situation
Talked with spouse or other relative about the problem
Talked with friend about the problem
Talked with professional person (e.g., doctor, lawyer, clergy)
Got busy with other things to keep my mind off the problem
Made a plan of action and followed it
Tried not to act too hastily or follow my first hunch
Got away from things for a while
Knew what had to be done and tried harder to make things work
Let my feelings out somehow
Sought help from persons or groups with similar experiences
Bargained or compromised to get something positive from the situation
Tried to reduce tension by exercising more

Avoidance Strategies

Took it out on other people when I felt angry or depressed
Kept my feelings to myself
Avoided being with people in general
Refused to believe that it happened
Tried to reduce tension by drinking more
Tried to reduce tension by eating more
Tried to reduce tension smoking more
Tried to reduce tension by taking more tranquilizing drugs

From Holahan C, Moos R: Personal and contextual determinants of coping strategies, *J Pers Soc Psychol* 52(5):946, 1987.

Box 19-8 **Ways of Coping Checklist Responses**

Most Frequent Responses

- Pray.
- Remind self that things could be worse.
- Maintain pride.
- Look for the silver lining.
- Turn to work or activity.
- Keep feelings from interfering.
- Try to analyze the problem.

Least Frequently Used Coping Activities

- Talk with someone who can help.
- Get professional help.
- Apologize.
- Take it out on others.

Marge tells of being frightened by a big dog and throwing rocks for the dog to chase in order to distract him. Her voice sounds proud and triumphant as she tells the story. Mary tells of hiding under the bed when she was shown her new baby brother. She sounds ashamed and aware that she had retreated. Betty tells of a bull in a pasture that she would walk by on the way to her grandmother's house. Each time, she had to decide whether to run home crying or to go on to grandma's. She is somewhat amazed that she rarely ran home.

These incidents give clues to the personality of the individual and can be most helpful in determining coping style. Memories that remain over time serve an individual in various ways throughout life and have tremendous influence as reservoirs of problem solving. Conscious experience continually molds the way in which we perceive ourselves. The kaleidoscope of experience shifts into new patterns, but the source of the patterns remains the same.

Personal and Contextual Determinants of Coping. Factors that affect the choice of coping strategies have been categorized as sociodemographic, personal disposition, and contextual issues (Menaghan, 1983). Family support also had a significantly positive effect on adaptive coping. One might conjecture that families in better circumstances have more energy to invest in direct problem solving. Another contextual issue is that of marriage. Persons of higher education and socioeconomic status are reported to demonstrate more flexibility, logical choice, and problem-focused coping strategies than individuals of lower status and educational background (Holahan and Moos, 1987). Self-confidence and an inner locus of control are positively associated with active coping.

In situations amenable to change, persons who are internally motivated use fewer attempts at problem suppression than those who are externally motivated (Parkes, 1984). Individuals of an easygoing disposition seem more inclined to use active coping strategies and to maintain psychologic health (Holahan and Moos, 1986, 1987).

McCrae (1984) found that the type of stressful life event affected the coping response used. Individuals facing challenging life events chose active problem-solving strategies, and those facing loss or threat were more prone to use avoidance strategies.

If these results can be applied to the stresses experienced by the aged, we must consider that most are confronted with loss, threat, and deprivation at a time when their socioeconomic status is likely to be reduced and their health compromised. On the positive side they have developed over time survival strategies that have been effective to one degree or another, and they are more likely to have developed an internal locus of control.

In a study of over 400 randomly selected community subjects, Holahan and Moos (1987) found that active-cognitive coping was positively related to self-confidence, an easygoing disposition, and family support. Active-behavioral coping was positively associated with educational level, self-confidence, and family support. In contrast, avoidance coping was associated with few personal and environmental resources.

Although subjects reported coping responses to a single problem, their responses were affected by the broader life context and the ongoing demands of the situation. Up to a point, individually variable stressors engender an increase in coping efforts. Problems most frequently identified as stressful fell into the categories of interpersonal, financial or work related, and illness. In general, coping was found to relate more closely to ongoing current circumstances than to more remote and stable background factors.

Research on the importance of mastery and an internal locus of control in the use of active coping strategies is of significance in the care of the aged because it confirms the need to cultivate opportunities for autonomy and self-direction (Fleishman, 1984; Parkes, 1984).

All of these findings presume the use of certain coping strategies to be a result of situational or personality variables (Vitaliano et al, 1985). In fact, it may be that the coping style itself may result in the emergence of certain personality characteristics and situational effects.

Warheit (1979) conducted a study to measure stress factors and effective coping strategies. He found that people generally used a progressive pattern of resources in the following order:

1. Own inner resources
2. Assistance from spouse, children, parents, or family members
3. Interpersonal networks, friends
4. Assistance from professionals and agencies
5. Cultural beliefs, values, symbols, and myths

Depending on the effectiveness of these resources, three levels of response to stress were evoked. Transient symptoms of stress were present in most subjects; some developed psychologic or physiologic illness syndromes; and those most severely affected became socially dysfunctional. From this study it seemed that life event stressors were mitigated by the availability of a multileveled system of resources (Warheit, 1979).

CONTROL

The previous discussion of crises, stress, and coping has shown the importance of a sense of control in preventing illness, disability, and deterioration. Krause (1993) has for several years studied older adults and the effects of stress on their lives. Early parental loss seems to leave an individual with a life-long feeling of helplessness and diminished personal control (Krause, 1993). Isolation from supportive persons and financial stress are among the greatest stressors of the aged (Krause, 1991; Krause et al, 1991).

When dealing with long-term stress, some people simply lose incentive for effectively exerting control in their lives and are overcome with apathy and inertia. Crises, stress, chronic illness, and depression can erode self-esteem and the sense of mastery and induce feelings of "oldness." In these cases it is not uncommon for aged persons to seek an ally to whom they can relinquish control.

Aged people of both sexes, several races, various socioeconomic and education backgrounds, and varied degrees of self-esteem and life satisfaction all felt young and capable when they managed to maintain internal control (Linn and Hunter, 1979). These findings are important because they emphasize the importance of choices, options, and decisions.

It may be especially important to support the denial of old age because it seems to contribute to good psychologic function and vigor. The loss of health is often the precursor to loss of control and signals fatalistic acceptance of impairment, disability, discomfort, and old age. Nurses, remembering this, must make special efforts to reinstitute personal control, particularly with the ill aged.

Symbols of Control

Some people have symbols of control that suffice in the absence of real influence.

Catherine's cane conveyed her authority. She kept it near her at all times, slept with it, and threatened to use it to defend herself if necessary. It was lost in transferring to another facility. She said, "Well, I think they've about got me now. I'm lost without my cane."

When dealing with vulnerable patients, be alert to their symbols of control. Some common ones are money, presence of family, pictures of family, hoarding of supplies or food, refusal of meals, demanding small or large amounts of attention, compulsive placement of personal articles, and other ritualistic behaviors. Respond to the latent message of a need for control, and work with the patient to reinstate legitimate control.

In one facility a dying lady was extremely demanding about the details of her morning care. One student nurse was able to comply without resentment because she understood the need to establish some order in the events of the day to compensate for lack of control over impending death. This was a legitimate use of patient power, although sometimes inconvenient for staff members.

Nurses also have power symbols: uniforms, special equipment, records, standing above rather than sitting by a patient, closing and opening doors without permission, medications, addressing patients in familiar terms, and others. We might consider ways to diminish the overwhelming influence of our power symbols on vulnerable patients.

Establishing Control

Very specific suggestions for combating helplessness are provided by Aasen (1987):

1. Identify issues in which residents have control, such as arrangement of personal items and selection of clothing. Loss of some autonomy in a situation is often perceived as a global loss of control. Particular areas of control must be emphasized.

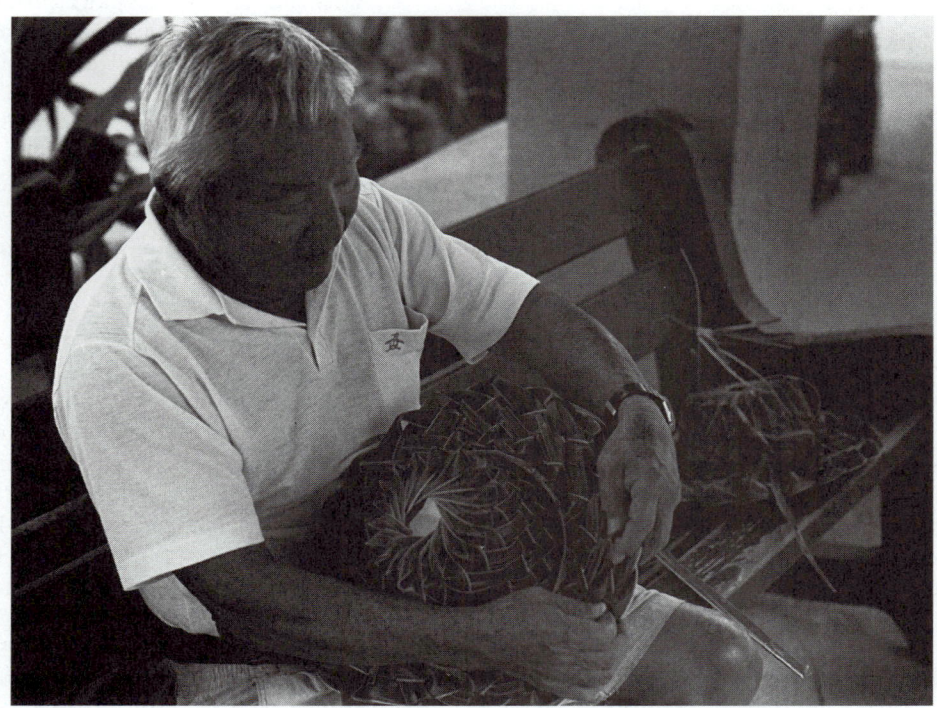

Exercising control through hand crafts. (Courtesy Rod Schmall.)

2. Provide realistic opportunities for choice of alternatives in areas of interest. Choices of books, music, newspapers, snacks, and music are always possible.

3. Too many choices may have the negative effect of making decisions difficult and confusing, which will further emphasize the feeling of loss of control.

4. Opportunities to share personal talents, hobbies, and interests can be made available. First efforts may be disappointing, but persistence is advised. Gentle encouragement and lack of pressure for performance are recommended. Singing, reciting poetry, and playing the piano are only a few of the talents some elders may be "hiding under a bushel."

5. Discuss and reinterpret irrational beliefs (cognitive restructuring) that one has no control.

6. Give information and rationale for situations in which resident does not have control.

It may be difficult to combat feelings of powerlessness that have been established over long periods of time. Generally, it is thought that beginning with small and valid choices is the most logical approach. As with all persons who are insecure about their position and uncertain of outcomes, the choices should be limited, be clear, and have visible results. For instance, bathing seems to be one of the inflexible expectations in many institutions. Logically we know elders' skin should be protected against drying, and yet we feel so much better if the individual is clean, dry, powdered, and tucked into a neatly made bed. Can we ask patients to identify their bathing habits and adjust our schedule to their expectations? Unfortunately, the Saturday night bath ritual from the childhood of many of our elders is no longer considered adequate.

An important event in institutional life is meal service. Could a buffet cart be available for persons to choose from when they are hungry or inclined to eat? One facility serves five small meals each day, which is physiologically healthier for most elders but hard on the kitchen help. There are many healthy and attractive foods that can be served cold or heated in a microwave oven. Undoubtedly, there would be concern about persons on special diets who might select foods that were banned.

Another area of choice that is significant is that of roommates. Unit supervisors may collaborate on ways that they can better match residents; in long-term living situations this is imperative. Perhaps there could be patient profiles of interests and abilities that could be shared with a new patient, thus involving him or her in selecting a compatible roommate.

All resident/patient choices may require extra effort and planning from staff, and the commitment to the goal of patient initiative and increased independence must be reinforced. Participation is invited in activities in which the client is unlikely to fail, such as making a collage with the assistance of the activity director. If the client adamantly re-

fuses, the activity director will need to discuss reasons. Together they can evaluate the validity of the reasons and try to pinpoint specifics and counteract problems realistically. This must be done in a nonjudgmental manner.

When some small gains are made in ADLs, the individual can be assisted to begin a daily log of events that produce momentary satisfaction. Each thing that was partially completed or attempted can be logged and discussed.

Exercising Control in the Health Care System

Recognizing the impact the aged could have as the largest body of health care consumers and also that, in fact, they exert little pressure to change health care delivery systems, a nursing function is to assist them in doing so. Elders should be given suggestions of resources they can use for self-care (Kiley, 1977) as the majority of care is actually self-generated. Beyond self-care, elders must learn how to use the health care system to best advantage. Alert the aged client to the following as important in obtaining satisfactory care from a physician:

1. Before engaging the services of a private physician provider, find out whether he or she follows Medicare fee schedules and will bill Medicare directly.

2. Get acquainted with the administrative personnel in the health care system; she or he can be a support person and assist in easing oneself through the system with best results.

3. Make notes of questions and symptoms before visiting the physician, since they are often forgotten during a visit.

4. Physicians in group practice are likely to be available. Ask about their familiarity with complex procedures. Remember, the client is the consumer.

5. Find out from the nurse whether the provider is following the laws regarding gag orders.

6. Ask about fees before receiving service.

7. Ask the physician to prescribe generic drugs when possible because they are less expensive.

8. If the physician does not answer questions in language that can be understood, let him or her know. If you leave feeling you do not have adequate knowledge about your condition, find another physician. If in a health maintenance organization (HMO), talk to the advice nurse. If still uncertain, insist on a consultation.

9. Do not accept "old age" as an explanation for any symptom.

10. Select a managed care program or HMO that best fits the individual's health needs. It is a competitive market, and the consumer has choices.

11. Does physician give orders, or does he or she ask what can be reasonably done by the individual? Clients should explain what they are or are not willing to do.

Health care providers confront numerous stressors, particularly in today's health care market. Some providers find the majority of their practice involves working with elders even though they have not chosen a geriatric specialty. They may find this stressful as they attempt to work through ageist attitudes and myths about elders that still persist in some situations.

In order to guide others through stressful and crisis situations, the nurse must maintain a reliable support system for his or her own needs and develop a range of stress reduction strategies effective for the self (Frisch and Kelley, 1996). Stetson (1997) has worked with faculty and student nurses in stress reduction classes to strengthen their coping skills and ability to relax as well as to gain personal insight. These sessions consist mainly of participants learning new stress management techniques each week, using the *Creating Wholeness* text (Peper and Holt, 1993). The exercises progress in complexity from muscle relaxation to imagery and cognitive reframing. Daily practice and logs were required to further embed skills and to facilitate skill mastery. Faculty involvement in these is more sporadic but nevertheless judged useful.

Finally, we emphasize, no matter where nurses are working with elders in this day and age, our first charge is, "Nurse, learn to take care of thyself!"

KEY CONCEPTS

- Disturbing emotions experienced over extended periods may result in depletions of the immune system and resulting illnesses.
- Crises and stressors are experienced by the aged less frequently than among younger adults but often have more devastating consequences.
- Crises have the potential for producing individual growth and higher levels of function as a result of successful mastery of the situation.
- If timely support and appropriate interventions are not activated during a crisis situation, the individual is likely to stabilize at a lower level of function than that prior to the crisis.
- Methods of assessing the impact of stressful events are inadequate if they do not consider chronic stressors that may exist over long periods of time, the particular population profile of the individuals being assessed, the individual's personality, the recency and frequency of events as well as very early traumatic events that erode the individual's sense of security.
- Stress management strategies must be designed to meet individual needs because some methods may in fact be experienced as an additional stressor; for example, a shy, reticent elder would unlikely find body massage soothing and relaxing.

- Though helplessness and dependency are often seen as negative qualities, they may be adaptive and stress reducers in certain situations within the family or institutions.
- Reestablishing feelings of adequacy and control are the sine qua non of crisis resolution and stress management.
- Health care providers must develop ways to manage personal stressors if they are to be effective in helping others through crisis and stressful situations.
- Psychoneuroimmunology is attracting considerable attention as the study of the actual relationship of emotions and disease and the particular physiologic responses involved are becoming clearer.

▲ CASE STUDY

Aaron and Anna had a very comfortable existence as the managers of a small hotel in upstate New York. They had downgraded from a large and lovely home when they retired but had been able to move most of their treasured possessions to the manager's cottage they occupied adjacent to the hotel. At 75 years old they felt fortunate to remain active, healthy, and generating an income. Their lives had provided much satisfaction, and this was a time to enjoy the rewards for long years of hard work and relative success. Their duties at the hotel were not strenuous because employees took care of all the work. They were in the control center—guiding, problem solving, and delegating—their dream retirement! One night while they were at a concert their cottage caught fire, and unfortunately, almost all their possessions were lost before the blaze was brought under control. Aaron repeatedly said, "I'm so glad we were not there and that we are safe." Anna wrung her hands constantly and chanted over and over, "My mother's photos are gone; my grandmother's quilts are gone; my Spode china is black." Clearly, for Aaron this was another hazard of living; for Anna it was the loss of the substance of her existence, definitions of her identity. Ordinarily one thinks of rape, traumatic injury, or cataclysmic events before worrying about the need to avert the later PTDS. In Anna's case this was truly a cataclysmic event. Fortunately, the firemen recognized the magnitude of the crisis reaction of Anna and called for assistance. This alert public servant called a crisis counselor to spend some time with Anna.

Based upon the case study, develop a nursing care plan using the following procedure*:

List comments of client that provide *subjective data*.
List information that provides *objective data*.

*Students are advised to refer to their nursing diagnosis text and identify possible or potential problems.

Nursing Diagnoses

The following potential diagnoses must be considered as well as diagnoses unique to the particular individual:

Adjustment, impaired
Anxiety
Coping, ineffective
Denial, ineffective
Fear
Hopelessness
Knowledge deficit
Personal identity disturbance

Post-trauma response
Powerlessness
Role performance, altered
Self-esteem, disturbance
Sleep pattern disturbance
Thought processes altered
Violence, risk for directed at others

NURSING PROCESS AND NURSING DIAGNOSIS
Relocation Stress Syndrome

Etiologies and Related Factors
Relocation from one living arrangement to another
Old age
Poor physical health
Emotional problems, illness
Social isolation
Confusion
Low socioeconomic resources

Defining Characteristics
Change in residence
Decreased social activity
Withdrawal
Decreased life satisfaction
Hyperirritability
Sleep disturbance (insomnia)
Disrupted interpersonal relations—distrusts people
Change in eating patterns
Passivity
Dependence
Emotional insulation/detachment
Declining health status
Aggressiveness
Alienation

Knowledge
Aging, stress and coping ability
Stress-adaptation theory
Risk factors

Collaboration skills with other disciplines
Therapeutic communication skills
Crisis intervention
Counseling skills
Discharge planning
Physical and psychologic assessments
Life satisfaction assessment
Interventions prior to and after relocation to new environment
Community resources

Clinical Judgment and Related Skills
Prepare client for relocation—premove visit
Elicit client's feelings
Assessment of physical and mental function prior to move
Include client/family in decision making
Provide sense of control
Conduct counseling sessions
Teach family about translocation
Design, implement, and evaluate a plan of care for the client

Evaluation
Few or no negative manifestations associated with move with least discomfort and emotional stress
Care continuity maintained
Regains maximum potential for a high level wellness with least discomfort and emotional stress

NEEDS ADDRESSED AND TASK STRENGTHS

Crises and Stress
Need to maintain a personally satisfactory threshold of stress; need to recognize own strengths and idiosyncracies (to maintain self-esteem)

Incorporates daily methods of relaxation/meditation
Anticipates and plans for crises that are predictable
Recognizes situations requiring new coping skills
Seeks assistance when crises occur

From these data identify and state, using accepted format, two *nursing diagnoses* you determine are most significant to this client at this time. List two *client strengths* that you have identified from data.

Determine and state *outcome criteria* for each diagnosis. These must reflect some alleviation of the problem identified in the nursing diagnosis and must be stated in concrete and measurable terms.

Plan and state one or more *interventions* for each diagnosed problem.

Provide specific documentation of source used to determine appropriate intervention. Plan at least one intervention that incorporates the client's existing strengths.

Evaluate success of intervention. Interventions must correlate directly with the stated outcome criteria in order to measure the outcome success.

STUDY QUESTIONS/ACTIVITIES

Discuss differences between crises and stress, and describe methods to discriminate between the two situations.

List crises and stressors that are likely to occur in the lives of elderly persons in the community and those that are likely for the institutionalized elder; list the crises and stressors you are likely to experience and compare differences and similarities in the three lists.

Discuss the concept of anxiety and explain several defense mechanisms that you may have used to reduce the discomfort.

Discuss several coping styles of the elderly and compare their merits.

Specify the progression of helplessness exhibited in the spiral of dependency, and describe the interventions you would use to interrupt the downward spiral.

Explain methods of restoring a sense of control and averting excessive dependency.

Discuss the meanings and the thoughts triggered by the students' and elders' viewpoints expressed at the beginning of the chapter. How do these vary from your own experience?

As a group project, develop a life events rating scale for an elderly population that includes the following considerations:
- Events and other possible sources of social stress
- Significance of event in relation to age, gender, cohort, and culture
- Desirable and undesirable events
- Comprehensivenss of events listed
- Roles occupied by the individual at the time of the survey
- Affect of the individual at the time of the survey
- Time frame, recency, and duration of event

RESEARCH QUESTIONS

What items would be important in the development of age-specific tools to determine the nature of anxiety in the old?

What are the events that are particularly malignant crises for elders?

In what areas of life do elders feel they have the least control?

What are the most common or frequent worries of elders?

What is the impact on stress management of various personality gender differences?

RESOURCES

Checklist Measures of Stressful Life Events of the Elderly

Amster L, Kraus H: The relationship between life crises and mental deterioration in old age, *Int J Aging Hum Dev* 5:51, 1974. Geriatric Social Readjustment Rating Scale.

Murrell SA, Norris FH, Hutchins GM: Distribution and desirability of life events in older adults: population and policy implications, *Am J Community Psychol* 12:301, 1984. Louisville Older Person Event Scale.

Zautra AJ, Guarnaccia CA, Dohrenwend BP: Measuring small life events, *Am J Community Psychol* 14:629, 1986. Inventory of Small Life Events (Modified for the Elderly).

Stokes S, Gordon S: *SGGS Stokes/Gordon Stress Scale,* Pace University, Lienhard School of Nursing, Bedford Road, Pleasantville, NY 10570.

Restoration Exercises

Lusk JT: *30 Scripts for relaxation, imagery and inner healing,* Whole Person Associates, 210 W Michigan Street, Duluth, MN 55802-1908, (218) 727-0500.

Film

Seniors' Esteem Issues, J. Rowe, Filmakers Library, New York, NY (30 minutes). A part of the Journey Into Self-Esteem series, this film shows personal stories of older persons who are able to deal with life's changes through the maintenance of healthy self-esteem.

REFERENCES

Aasen N: Interventions to facilitate personal control, *J Gerontol Nurs* 13(6):21, 1987.

Aldwin C, Folkman S, Shaefer C et al: *Ways of coping checklist: a process measure.* Paper presented at the annual American Psychological Association Meeting, Montreal, Sept 1985.

Andrews VH, Borkovec TD: The differential effects of inductions of worry, somatic anxiety, and depression on emotional experience, *J Behav Ther Exp Psychiatry* 19:21, 1988.

Avison WR, Gotlib IH: Future prospects for stress research. In WR Avison, IH Gotlib, editors: *Stress and mental health: contemporary issues and prospects for the future,* New York, 1994, Plenum.

Battegay R: Psychoanalytic aspects of crisis and crisis intervention, *J Psychosomatic Medicine and Psychoanalysis* 41(1):1, 1995.

Benezra EE: Personality factors of individuals who survive traumatic experiences without professional help. *Int J Stress Management* 3(3):147, 1996.

Buffum MD, Wolfe NS: Posttraumatic stress disorder and the World War II veteran, *Geriatr Nurs* 16(6):264, 1995.

Burks N, Martin B: Everyday problems and life change events: ongoing versus acute sources of stress, *J Human Stress* 11:27, 1985.

Butler RN: The crises of old age, *RN* 30:47, 1967.

Cancer Treatment Centers of America: *Nearly one of every four nation's nurses says emotions are the key to patients' recovery,* news release, Zion, Ill, Oct 12, 1992, Cancer Treatment Centers of America.

Cannon WB: *The wisdom of the body,* New York, 1932, WW Norton.

Cohen S: Psychological stress and susceptibility to upper respiratory infections, *Am J Respiratory Critical Care Medicine* 152(4):S53, 1995.

Cohen S, Kessler RC, Gordon LU, editors: *Measuring stress: a guide for health and social scientists,* New York, 1995a, Oxford University Press.

Cohen S, Kessler RC, Gordon LU: Strategies for measuring stress in studies of psychiatric and physical disorders. In Cohen S, Kessler RC, Gordon LU, editors: *Measuring stress: a guide for health and social scientists,* New York, 1995, Oxford University Press.

DeLongis A, Folkman S, Lazarus R: The impact of daily stress on health and mood: psychological and social resources as mediators, *J Pers Soc Psychol* 54(3):486, 1988.

Eckenrode J, Bolger N: Daily and within-day event measurement. In Cohen S, Kessler RC, Gordon LY, editors: *Measuring stress: a guide for health and social scientists,* New York, 1995, Oxford University Press.

Ensel WM: Important life events and depression among older adults, *J Aging Health* 3:546, 1991.

Ensel WM, Peek MK, Lin N, Lai G: Stress in the life course: a life history approach, *J Aging Health* 8(3):389, 1996.

Fleishman J: Personality characteristics and coping patterns, *J Health Soc Behav* 25:229, 1984.

File SE: Recent developments in anxiety, stress and depression, *Pharmacol Biochem Behav* 54(1):3, 1996.

Folkman S, Lazarus R, Pimley S et al: Age differences in stress and coping processes, *Psychol Aging* 2(2):171, 1987.

Forsythe C, Compas B: Interaction of cognitive appraisals of stressful events and coping: testing the goodness of fit hypothesis, *Cognitive Ther Res* 11:122, 1987.

Frisch NC, Kelley J: *Healing life's crises: a guide for nurses,* Albany, NY, 1996, Delmar.

Funk S, Houston K: A critical analysis of the hardiness scale's validity and utility, *J Pers Soc Psychol* 53(3):572, 1987.

Funk and Wagnall's Standard Dictionary, New York, 1983, Harper & Row.

Ganellen R, Blaney P: Hardiness and social support as moderators of the effects of life stress, *J Pers Soc Psychology* 47:156, 1984.

Gordon M: *Manual of nursing diagnosis, 1991-92,* St Louis, 1991, Mosby.

Hogstel MO: *Geropsychiatric nursing,* St Louis, 1990, Mosby.

Holahan C, Moos R: Personality, coping and family resources in stress resistance: a longitudinal analysis, *J Pers Soc Psychol* 51:389, 1986.

Holahan C, Moos R: Personal and contextual determinants of coping strategies, *J Pers Soc Psychol* 52(5):946, 1987.

Holmes TH, Rahe RH: The social readjustment rating scale, *J Psychosom Res* 11:213, 1967.

Hughes DC, Blazer D, George L: Age differences in life events: a multivariate controlled analysis, *Int J Aging Hum Dev* 27:207, 1988.

Irion J, Blanchard-Fields F: A cross-sectional comparison of adaptive coping in adulthood, *J Gerontol* 42(5):502, 1987.

Ishler KJ, Pargament KI, Kinney JM, Cavanaugh JC: *Religious coping, general coping and controllability: testing the hypothesis of fit.* Paper presented at the 48th Annual Meeting of the Gerontological Society of America, Los Angeles, Nov 18, 1995.

Jacobson E: *Progressive relaxation,* Chicago, 1938, University of Chicago Press.

Jarvik L, Russell D: Anxiety, aging and the third emergency reaction, *J Gerontol* 34(4):197, 1979.

Kiecolt-Glaser JK, Glaser R, Gravenstein S, Malarkey WB, Sheridan J: Chronic stress alters the immune response to influenza virus vaccine in older adults, *Proc Nat Acad Sci USA* 93(7):3043, 1996.

Kiley JC: *Self-rescue,* New York, 1977, McGraw-Hill.

Kobasa SC: Stressful life events, personality and health: an inquiry into hardiness, *J Pers Soc Psychol* 37(1):1, 1979.

Kopin IJ: Definitions of stress and sympathetic neuronal responses, *Ann NY Acad Sci* 771:19, 1995.

Krause N: Stress, gender, cognitive impairment, and outpatient use in later life, *J Gerontol* 51(1):P15, 1996.

Krause N: Early parental loss and personal control in late life, *J Gerontol* 48(3):p117, 1993.

Krause N: Stress and isolation from close ties in later life, *J Gerontol* 46:S183, 1991.

Krause N, Jay G, Liange J: Financial strain and psychological well-being among the American and the Japanese elderly, *Psychol Aging* 6:170, 1991.

Lazarus R, Folkman S: *Stress appraisal and coping,* New York, 1984, Springer.

Lindemann E: Symptomatology and management of acute grief, *Am J Psychiatry* 101:141, 1944.

Linn M, Hunter K: Perception of age in the elderly, *J Gerontol* 34:46, 1979.

Lusk JT: *30 scripts for relaxation, imagery and inner healing,* Duluth, Minn, 1992, Whole Person Associates.

Manfredi C, Pickett M: Perceived stressful situations and coping strategies utilized by the elderly, *J Community Health Nurs* 4(2):99, 1987.

Martin KS: S.T.R.E.S.S., *Home Health Focus* 2(11):81, 1996 (editorial).

McCrae R: Situational determinants of coping responses: loss, threat and challenge, *J Pers Soc Psychol* 46:919, 1984.

McLean DE, Link BG: Unraveling complexity: strategies to refine concepts, measures, and research designs in the study of life events and mental health. In Avison WR, Gotlib IH, editors: *Stress and mental health: contemporary issues and prospects for the future,* New York, 1994, Plenum.

Menaghan EG: Coping efforts as mediators of life stress: patterns of usage and effectiveness, *Gerontologist* 23:201 (special issue), 1983.

Meyer A: The life chart and the obligation for specifying positive data in psychopathological diagnosis. In EE Winters, editors: *The collected papers of Adolph Meyer,* vol 3, Baltimore, 1951, Johns Hopkins University Press.

Mishel M: Uncertainty in illness, *Image J Nurs Sch* 20(4):225, 1988.

Mitchell R, Cronkite R, Moos R: Stress, coping and depression among married couples, *J Abnorm Psychol* 92:433, 1983.

Modica P: Prolonged stress may lead to memory loss, *Medical Tribune News Service,* Aug 8, 1996.

Monroe SM, McQuaid JR: Measuring life stress and assessing its impact on mental health. In Avison WR, Gotlib IH, editors: *Stress and mental health: contemporary issues and prospects for the future,* New York, 1994, Plenum.

Mosby: *Mosby's medical and nursing dictionary,* St Louis, 1986, CV Mosby.

Parkes K: Locus of control, cognitive appraisal, and coping in stressful situations, *J Pers Soc Psychol* 45:655, 1984.

Pasupathi M, Sjostrom S, Richardson J: *Lifespan perspectives on stressful events.* Paper presented at the meeting of the Gerontological Society of America, Washington, DC, Nov 20, 1996.

Peper E, Holt CF: *Creating wholeness: a self-healing workbook using dynamic relaxation, images and thoughts,* New York, 1993, Plenum.

Powers CB, Wisocki PA, Whitbourne SK: Age differences and correlates of worrying in young and elderly adults, *Gerontologist* 32(1):82, 1992.

Preston DB: Marital status, gender roles, stress and health in the elderly, *Health Care for Women International* 16(2):149, 1995.

Rickard HC, Scogin F, Keith S: A one-year follow-up of relaxation training for elders with subjective anxiety, *Gerontologist* 34(1):121, 1994.

Rutter M: Pathways from childhood to adult life, *J Child Psychol Psychiatry* 30:23, 1989.

Schafer W: *Stress distress and growth,* Davis, Calif, 1978, Responsible Action.

Seligman M: *Helplessness: on depression, development and death,* San Francisco, 1975, Freeman.

Selye H: *The stress of life,* New York, 1956, McGraw-Hill.

Selye H: *Stress without distress,* Philadelphia, 1974, JB Lippincott.

Selye H: On the benefits of eustress. In interview by Cherry L, *Psychol Today* 11:60, March 1978.

Slimmer L, LeSage J, Ellor J, Lopez N: Learned helplessness experienced by elderly in long-term care (abstract). *Proceedings of the Third Congress of the International Psychogeriatric Assoc* 3:86, 1987, Chicago.

Sobel DS: Rethinking medicine: improving health outcomes with cost-effective psychosocial interventions, *Psychosom Med* 57:234, 1995.

Stetson B: Holistic health stress management program: nursing student and client health outcomes, *J Holistic Nurs* 15(2):143, 1997.

Stokes S, Gordon S: *SGGS Stokes/Gordon Stress Scale,* Pace University, 1990, Lienhard School of Nursing, Bedford Road, Pleasantville, NY 10570.

Stone AA, Neale JM, Shiffman S: Daily assessments of stress and coping and their association with mood, 1993, *Ann Behavior Med* 15(1):8-16, 1993.

Stratakis CA, Chrousos GP: Neuroendocrinology and pathophysiology of the stress system, *Ann NY Acad Sci* 771:1, 1995.

Tricerri A, Errani AR, Vangeli M, et al: Neuroimmunomodulation and psychoneuroendocrinology: recent findings in adults and aged, *Panminerva Med* 37(2):77, 1995.

Turner RJ, Wheaton B: Checklist measurement of stressful life events. In Cohen S, Kessler RC, Gordon LY, editors: *Measuring stress: a guide for health and social scientists,* New York, 1995, Oxford University Press.

Turner RJ, Avison WR: Sources of attenuation in the stress-distress relationship: an evaluation of modest innovations in the application of events checklists. In Greenley JR, Leaf P, editors: *Research in Community and Mental Health,* vol 7, Greenwich, Conn, 1992, JAI Press.

Ulmer D: Stress management for the cardiovascular patient: a look at current treatment and trends, *Prog Cardiovasc Nurs* 11(1):21, 1996.

US Bureau of the Census: *Statistical abstract of the United States: 1995,* ed 115, Washington, DC, 1995.

Vingerhoets AJ, Ratliff-Crain J, Jabaaij L, Menges LJ, Baum A: Self-reported stressors, symptom complaints and psychobiological functioning: cardiovascular stress reactivity, *J Psychosom Res* 40(2):177, 1996.

Vitaliano P, Russo J, Carr J et al: The ways of coping checklist: revision and psychometric properties, *Multivariate Behav Res* 20:3, 1985.

Warheit G: Life events, coping, stress and depressive symptomatology, *Am J Psychiatry* 136:592, 1979.

Weinberger R: Teaching the elderly stress reduction, *J Gerontol Nurs* 17(10):23, 1991.

Wethington E, Brown GW, Kessler RC: Interview measurement of stressful life events. In Cohen S, Kessler RC, Gordon LY, editors: *Measuring stress: a guide for health and social scientists,* New York, 1995, Oxford University Press.

Wheaton B: Stress, personal coping resources, and psychiatric symptoms: an investigation of interactive models, *J Aging Human Development,* 22, 147, 1983.

Wolanin MO, Phillips L: *Confusion: prevention and care,* St Louis, 1981, Mosby.

Zautra AJ, Guarnaccia CA, Dohrenwend BP: Measuring small life events, *Am J Community Psychol* 14:629, 1986.

Zeller JM, McCain NL, Swanson B: Psychoneuroimmunology: an emerging framework for nursing research, *J Adv Nurs* 23(4):657, 1996.

Zotti AM, Beltnardi O, Soffiantin F et al: Psychophysiological stress testing in post infarction patients, *Circulation* 83:25, 1991.

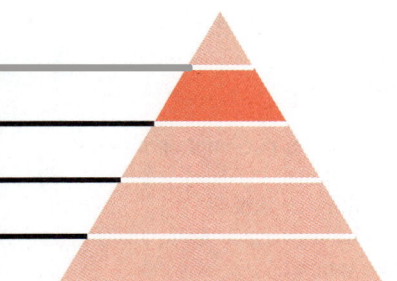

Stokes/Gordon Stress Scale

ADMINISTRATION

The Stokes/Gordon Stress Scale can be administered in person or by mail. Directions to the respondent are included on the front sheet of the scale. The scale (see below) requires approximately fifteen to thirty minutes to complete.

SCORING

A total "stress score" is obtained by adding the weights for individual items checked by each respondent. The weights are listed in descending order on an accompanying sheet entitled "Item Weights for Stokes/Gordon Stress Scale." A scoring sheet can be lined up with the test booklet for quick scoring. The sheet can be obtained from authors. See reference below.

Directions: Below are listed events and situations which occur in everyday life. Place an *X* next to any event or situation you are currently experiencing.

_____ 1. Change in your sleeping habits (such as ability to fall or stay asleep, change in place of sleep, etc.)

_____ 2. Decreasing number of friends or losing old friends

_____ 3. Giving up or losing driver's license

_____ 4. Personality characteristics of your husband or wife are more annoying than before

_____ 5. Time with children or grandchildren too short

_____ 6. Foreclosure of mortgage or loan

_____ 7. Change in behavior of family member

_____ 8. Taking relative or friend into your home to live

_____ 9. Fear of your own or your husband's or wife's driving

_____ 10. Change in your responsibilities at work

_____ 11. Major change in number of family get togethers

_____ 12. Fired from work or being laid off

_____ 13. Change in your diet or eating habits

_____ 14. Difficulty making new friends

_____ 15. Change in residence by moving to a new home

_____ 16. Concern for completing required forms (such as income tax, Medicare forms, etc.)

_____ 17. Thinking about your own death

_____ 18. Slowing down

_____ 19. Disturbing dreams

_____ 20. Difficulty dealing with children or grandchildren (such as noise, mess, etc.)

_____ 21. Minor violation of the law (such as traffic violation, jay-walking, disturbing the peace, etc.)

_____ 22. Feeling of remaining time being short

_____ 23. Feeling of being taken advantage of by "the system" (such as clinics, Medicare, social security, etc.)

_____ 24. Change in social activities (such as clubs, dancing, visiting, entertaining, etc.)

_____ 25. Constant or recurring pain or discomfort

_____ 26. Change in residence by moving in with children or other family members

_____ 27. Change in recreational activities (such as golf, tennis, walking, theatre attendance, etc.)

_____ 28. Change in your working hours or conditions

_____ 29. Making out a will

_____ 30. Holiday (such as Christmas, Rosh Hashonah, 4th of July, etc.)

_____ 31. Change to different line of work

_____ 32. Being away from home overnight or longer (such as vacation, visits, etc.)

_____ 33. Vacation

_____ 34. Anniversary

_____ 35. Retirement

_____ 36. Reaching a milestone year (becoming 65, 70, 75, 80, 85, 90)

_____ 37. Change in your sexual activity

_____ 38. Dependency on other people

_____ 39. Using your savings for living expenses

_____ 40. Needing to rely on cane, wheelchair, walker or hearing aid

_____ 41. Loneliness or aloneness

_____ 42. Inability to get out of the house

From Stokes S, Gordon S: *SGGS Stokes Gordon Stress Scale,* Pace University, 1990, Lienhard School of Nursing, Bedford Road, Pleasantville, NY 10570.

_____ 43. Minor or major car accident

_____ 44. Illness or injury of husband or wife

_____ 45. Illness or injury of son, daughter or grandchild

_____ 46. Illness or injury of close relative (such as sister, brother, parent, etc.)

_____ 47. Your own hospitalization (unplanned)

_____ 48. Your own hospitalization (planned)

_____ 49. Hospitalization of husband or wife

_____ 50. Hospitalization of son, daughter or grandchild

_____ 51. Not having enough money for food or medicine

_____ 52. Illness in public places (such as uncontrollable behavior, wetting, passing out, etc.)

_____ 53. Change in style of living because of lack of money

_____ 54. Fear of being a victim of a street crime

_____ 55. Decreasing mental abilities (such as forgetting, difficulty with decision-making, planning, etc.)

_____ 56. Being judged legally incompetent

_____ 57. Pressure for increased socializing

_____ 58. Son or daughter leaving home

_____ 59. Wife or husband begins or stops work

_____ 60. Uncertainty about the future

_____ 61. Trouble with your boss

_____ 62. Wanting events to go well with people seen infrequently (such as visits, parties, etc.)

_____ 63. Too much closeness or time with husband or wife (result of retirement, etc.)

_____ 64. Outstanding personal achievement

_____ 65. Your remarriage

_____ 66. Addition of a new family member (through birth, marriage, adoption, etc.)

_____ 67. Regret for not having done something you wanted to do in life (such as having children, getting a college education, etc.)

_____ 68. Change in religious activities

_____ 69. Death of a grandchild

_____ 70. Death of a son or daughter (unanticipated or unexpected)

_____ 71. Death of a son or daughter (anticipated or expected)

_____ 72. Death of a husband or wife (unanticipated or unexpected)

_____ 73. Death of a husband or wife (anticipated or expected)

_____ 74. Death of other close family member (such as sister, brother, parent, etc.)

_____ 75. Death of close friend

_____ 76. Death of loved pet

_____ 77. Change in ability to do own personal care (such as bathing, dressing, etc.)

_____ 78. Your own personal injury or illness

_____ 79. Change in residence by moving to an institution

_____ 80. Concern for children (such as out of work, divorce, arguments, etc.)

_____ 81. Inability to care for yourself

_____ 82. Decreasing eyesight

_____ 83. Loss of ability to get around due to illness or aging

_____ 84. Divorce or legally separating from your husband or wife

_____ 85. Being separated from husband or wife (such as admission to hospital or nursing home, vacation, etc.)

_____ 86. Having an unexpected debt (such as hospital bills, etc.)

_____ 87. Concern for grandchildren

_____ 88. Decreasing hearing

_____ 89. Fear of your home being invaded or robbed

_____ 90. Going to jail

_____ 91. Son or daughter moving back into house

_____ 92. Change in your financial state

_____ 93. Taking on a significant debt (such as mortgage, loan, etc.)

_____ 94. Not enough visits to or from family members

_____ 95. Wishing parts of your life had been different

_____ 96. Not feeling needed or having a purpose in life

_____ 97. Giving up long cherished possessions (such as home, dishes, pictures, etc.)

_____ 98. Longing for or missing children or grandchildren

_____ 99. Fear of abuse from others (such as family, associates, strangers, etc.)

_____100. Concern about elimination (such as constipation, diarrhea, difficulty urinating, etc.)

_____101. Concern for world conditions

_____102. Increase in arguments, bickering or disagreements with your husband or wife

_____103. Reconciliation with your husband or wife

_____104. Difficulty using public transportation system

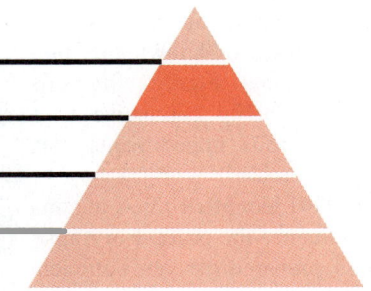

CHAPTER 20

Transitions and Role Changes

A student learns   **Retirement from work isn't retirement from life. I will have time to enjoy living as much as possible. I will have contributed decades of hard work to that. In order to fill the empty hours, to reduce loneliness and inactivity I would join centers for older adults where I could make social contacts.**

Ilona, age 36

Elders speak   **This is another stage of my life, and a most exciting one. I have the time and freedom to develop new interests that I have always wanted to pursue but never could fit in when my life was so full of other things.**

Lucile, age 70

A friend is developing a new life for herself after losing her husband of over 50 years. Her widowhood is only 2 years old now, but she is remarkably awakened to the possibilities of life after 88. Reviewing her life as it was with her husband, to whom she had devoted her entire existence, she now sees that she had been wife, mother, and child to him, her own identity completely subsumed under his. She looks upon her current popularity with amazement. As a human being, she is one of the best—her adjustment and late blooming is a surprise to her and a gift to us all.

Lyn, age 85

It is hard not to be the dominant member of the family and allow other family members to take over. My role was always to have the final say. I still have a say in whatever affects me, but most decisions are made by others.

Mary, over 70

The most difficult role change is from that of a primary caregiver to that of a recipient.

Dr. Leon Whitsell, over 70

LEARNING OBJECTIVES   Upon completion of this chapter, the reader will be able to:

1. Identify several important roles that elder members of society usually fulfill.
2. Discuss several "buffers" that make transitions to new roles somewhat easier.
3. Relate some of the factors that must be considered in the decision to retire.
4. Compare the differences you would expect in adaptation to retirement between an individual who retired because of ill health and one who chose to retire.
5. Compare some of the differences you would expect between the retirement adjustment of women and men.
6. Specify ways in which you would present a retirement planning seminar.
7. Explain the major issues in adaptation to a major role change such as retirement or widowhood.

TRANSITIONS

Developmental transitions are the mechanisms of movement by which individuals gradually and informally move through socially proscribed norms into new categories, roles, and statuses—the passage from one state of being to another. Social expectations and organizational dynamics form the frames within which transitions occur, and these often present strictures or challenges. For example, work life is dictated by retirement policies of companies and government and influenced by peer attitudes and family needs.

Transitions are typically seen as periods of instability, and because of this disruption in usual life patterns, they may result in personal growth or dissatisfaction. In this respect they are similar to crises (see Chapter 19) with the exception of timing and intensity.

Transitions often include marker events that alert one to the impending shift, define the passage, and signal the occurrence of the transition. Among elders, the most predictable of these, retirement and widowhood, often incorporate losses rather than gains in status, influence, and opportunity. The ideal outcome is when gains in satisfaction and new roles offset losses.

A major concern of nursing and the framework for interventions must be determined by particular conditions and individual needs that influence a healthy resolution of transitions (Schumacher and Meleis, 1994).

Transitions are processes that occur over time and that require changes in identities, roles, relationships, abilities, and patterns of behavior (Schumacher and Meleis, 1994). They embody a sense of personal movement and reorgani-

zation. Conditions that influence the outcome of transitions include meanings, expectations, level of knowledge, preplanning, and emotional and physical reserves. Supports and positive expectations are probably conducive to a smooth transition, whereas numerous impediments may mark a rocky path.

Schumacher and Meleis (1994) identified three nursing measures that can positively influence the process of transition. First is a state of readiness, preparedness, and sufficient anticipatory guidance.

Second and interwoven with the first is education. Nurses can provide background knowledge and information about methods others have successfully used to negotiate the situation. This also includes knowledge and practice of new skills that will be needed in the new situations.

Third, it is thought that environmental exposure and support influences the outcome. One example is moving into a retirement role 2 or 3 days a week, gradually testing the retirement setting. Another example is rehearsal of an anticipated event in the setting where it is likely to occur. This may occur by plan or subliminally when an elderly lady accompanies her friend to the funeral parlor to make funeral arrangements. Although probably not consciously identifying the possibility in her own life, she is nevertheless preparing in advance and vicariously experiencing the event. Figure 20-1 shows the nursing model of transitions.

ROLES

Numerous minor role changes occur in the aging process, but the expected transitions for most elders are related to the work role and the role of spouse. With few exceptions, all elders must adapt to these two major changes that occur with aging. These will be the focus of this chapter. Additional information about these roles will be found in Chapters 17 and 26.

In previous editions of this text we have considered the emergence of the grandparental role as a common transition of later life. However, we have moved this discussion to Chapter 17, where it seems more fittingly considered as a primary relationship because grandparents serving as parents is a major social phenomenon of the times.

Grandparenting requires a revival of remnants of a previous role and may or may not involve any personal developmental changes or significant life pattern shifts. Some grandparents do confront major situational transitions and role adaptations as they take on the function of parents. In cases where grandparents, and most especially a single grandparent, take on the full parenting role out of a sense of obligation, duty, or guilt, it is especially difficult. Some grandparents believe, correctly or incorrectly, that their deficiencies in parenting are the cause of their adult childrens' inability to parent. In those cases, grandparenting is not only a transition requiring reorganization of lifestyle, relationships, and patterns of behavior but also one in which thera-

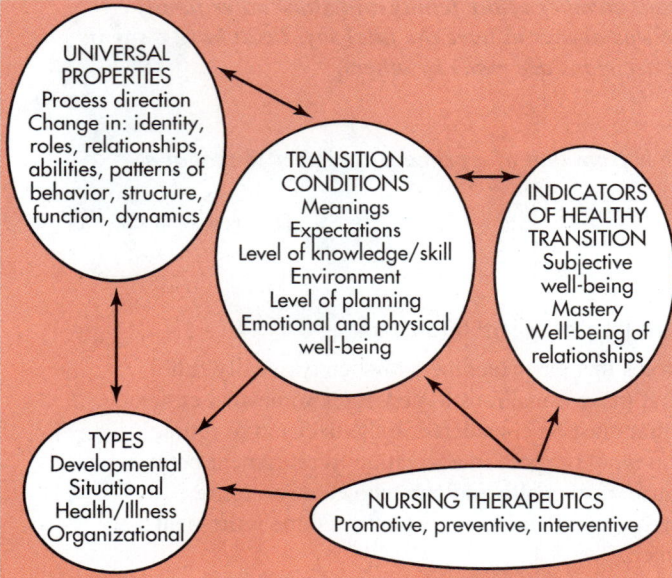

Figure 20-1. A nursing model of transitions. (Modified from Schumacher KL, Meleis AI: Transitions: a central concept in nursing, *Image J Nurs Sch* 26(2): 119, 1194.)

peutic support groups can be of enormous value. The wide range of involvement with grandchildren must be examined very individually to determine if the role of grandparent is actually transitional.

Mary's primary identity, role, and lifestyle remain unchanged, though she has experienced new opportunities, joys, and a recurrence of some previous interests as she spends some leisure time and special occasions with one or several of her grandchildren. Her neighbor, Bob, is definitely in transition because his 10-year-old grandson has moved in with him. Now he cannot afford to retire, has found it necessary to become involved in primary school activities again, has little time for old friends and golfing at his club, must be both mother and father to his grandson, and find child care for his grandson whenever he is not available and the boy is not in school. These cases exemplify the extremes of the continuum of grandparenting.

The socialization to roles supposedly comes from those who have experience and can retrospectively show others the way. At present, roles of the aged are much more variable and complex than in the past, and most older adults find themselves defining the successive roles they occupy in a manner different from their predecessors. Preparation for work roles is extensive, but there is inadequate preparation for marriage, parenting, "empty nest," divorce, widowhood, and retirement—all the major developmental shifts in adult life. The greatest problem is not that a new role may be ambiguous and the transition stressful, more often it is the loss of roles and the lack of gratifying replacement that is damaging to self-esteem in old age.

In cases of role accumulation, such as that of grandparent, some previous development will be applicable, with modification, to the new role. Likewise, the shifts in filial relationships are often gradual and do not require complete role deletion or role reversal. Those transitions that make use of past skills and adaptations may be least stressful. Some shifts, such as from functional independence to functional dependence, cut across many aspects of life and require several transitional shifts. Chapters 15, 17, and 19 address some of these issues.

From a life course perspective the transitions and adaptations required produce both stability and change in individual preferences, capacities, expectations, and behavior. Age-related transitions are socially created, shared, and recognized. A transition is socially recognized and entails a reorientation of perceptions and expectations of and by the individual. It is also important to remember that cohort and gender differences are inherent in all of life's major transitions.

The various role changes that occur during the aging process are often abrupt and undesired compared with role changes in young adulthood, which may be sought and strongly desired. In all role changes, adequate preparation and support during the transition can spell the difference between success and failure in satisfactory adjustment.

This chapter examines the various role functions, losses, reactions, and role replacements that occur most commonly during aging. Opportunities for the aged to occupy roles of significance and the support available during the transition from one role to another is also examined. Nursing interventions are suggested that will assist the aging person to maintain self-esteem and develop new and satisfying roles. The most common roles of the aged are retiree, parent, grandparent, great-grandparent, spouse, homemaker, widow, kin, friend, citizen, volunteer, church member, club member, acquaintance, patient, and service recipient.

Concepts Related To Transitions

An important concept is that of "life event timing synchrony" (Sorenson, 1995). This refers to the degree with which an event is perceived as harmonious and congruent with the individual's expectations. Appropriateness of timing as related to the individual's expectations is an important consideration. Those persons who must retire "too early" or are widowed "too soon" are examples of off-time events that elders may experience. It is as if, "I always knew it would occur, but I wasn't ready yet." In a judgmental manner onlookers and participants also often expect appropriate timing of movement through a transition. "Well, I thought I would be over it by now!" or "Isn't she over that yet?"

Some transitions may not be marked by disruptions and may be subtle and slowly shifting from one self-concept to another, only recognized retrospectively. Aging itself may be the most classic of these. The recognition that one is old in comparison to others in the social milieu is absorbed slowly and sometimes forgotten altogether. We wonder if we are not all in transition at all times. Perhaps it is only the *speed and intensity* of change that define the differences between crisis, transition, and gradual metamorphosis. We are continually changing, letting go and taking on, being and becoming. Considering transitions as a phenomenon to be addressed by nurses must then be restricted to those situations that are extended periods of personal disruption, the bridge between two quite different states of being.

Transitions may be crises or gradual periods of letting go of certain functions while simultaneously accumulating others. Role changes that produce crises (see Chapter 19) are usually abrupt losses of familiar functions at a time when meaningful substitute functions are not available.

Cohort effects and appropriate *role models* are critically important in how one makes the transition. Cohort effects are historic parameters that define a role in congruence with the times. (See Chapter 24 for further discussion of cohorts.) Young people watch role models during their impressionable years and may consciously or subconsciously expect those models to be fitting for them when they become old. This is certainly not the case in rapidly changing societies.

Environmental influence on role development in transition was explored by Laws (1995). He found that in retirement communities, such as Sun City, there is a form and structure that serves the retiree in identity formation. Such issues as security surveillance, easy access to support services, planned entertainment and activities, and an affluent consumer orientation contribute to the emergence of new skills and the abandonment of some that are no longer relevant. Additionally, there are numerous role models visible and readily available.

The ease of role transitions will depend on the following factors:

- Relevance of models
- Supportive milieu
- Presence of sustained roles not affected by particular role transition
- Age appropriateness of change
- Geographic and cultural milieu
- Personality and motivation in regard to constancy or change

We believe the potential for developing new, fulfilling life patterns is ever present and is enhanced during periods of transition. Influential dimensions promoting growth rather than stagnation during transitions are anticipatory planning, awareness of problems, positive or negative attitudes, and a sense of control (by far the most important).

Despite the diversity of transitions, Chick and Meleis (1986) have identified some commonalities, which they have defined as universal properties of transitions. These are summarized in Box 20-1.

Gender Considerations in Role Transitions

The roles of old women are generally judged less attractive than those of old men. They are considered "old" sooner than men and are more often economically and vocationally disadvantaged whether single, divorced, or widowed. However, throughout their lives women are confronted with more frequent and visible physical and social transitions and thus may be more adept at transitioning.

Mercer et al (1989) studied 80 women between the ages of 60 and 95 years. Some mentioned the menopause as a significant transition, but the years between ages 61 and 65 were ones of regeneration and redirection. They felt a new

---

| **Box 20-1** | **Definitions of Transition in the Nursing Literature** |

Bridges: A process that involves three phases: an ending phase (disengagement, disidentification, disenchantment), a neutral phase (disorientation, disintegration, discovery), and a new beginning phase (finding meaning and future, experiencing control and challenge).

Chick and Meleis: A passage from one life phase, condition, or status to another...transition refers to both the process and the outcome of complex person-environment interactions. It may involve more than one person and is embedded in the context and the situation. Defining characteristics of transition include process, disconnectedness, perception, and patterns of response.

Chiriboga: Marker events with discrete entries and exits.

Golan: A period of moving from one state of certainty to another, with an interval of uncertainty and change in between.

Meleis: The period in which a change is perceived by a person or others, as occurring in a person or in the environment. Commonalities that characterize a transition period: 1) disconnectedness from usual social network and social support systems, 2) temporary loss of familiar reference points of significant objects or subjects, 3) new needs that may arise or old ones not met in a familiar way, and 4) old sets of expectations no longer congruent with changing situations. A transition denotes a change in health status, in role relations, in expectations, or in abilities.

Meleis: A transition denotes a change in health status, in role relations, in expectations, or in abilities. It denotes changes in needs of all human systems. Transition requires the person to incorporate new knowledge, to alter behavior, and therefore to change the definition of self in social context, of a healthy or ill self, or of internal and external needs, which affects the health status.

Morris: A process of change from one activity or form of activity to another.

Murphy: Common themes in definitions of transition: disruption in routine, emotional upheaval, and adjustment required of individuals undergoing life changes.

Parkes: Processes of change that are lasting in their effects, force one to give up how one views the world and his or her place in it, and necessitate the development of new assumptions and skills to enable the individual to cope with a new altered life space.

Schlossberg: An event or nonevent that results in changes in relationships, routines, assumptions, and/or roles within the settings of self, work, family, health, and economics.

Tyhurst: A passage or change from one place or state or act or set of circumstances to another. Features common to all transitions: 1) a phase of turmoil, 2) disturbances in bodily function, mood, and cognition, 3) symptoms of psychologic distress, and 4) altered time perspective.

Webster: The passage from one state, condition, or place to another.

From Schumacher KL, Meleis AI: Transitions: a central concept in nursing, *Image J Nurs Sch* 26(2):119, 1994.

sense of personal freedom and time to do many things that had been deferred during their busier years, though the care of others still consumed the efforts of many.

The final transitional peak was at the age of 80. Having successfully negotiated the enormous developmental challenges, their strength and creativity were outstanding. At 84 years old, Thelma said, "Each day brings the possibility of new adventure." For her, adventure was in her mind. Her voracious reading led her into new thoughts and understanding. She was an avid student of world affairs and in discussion would place them in the context of history. It was a joy just to spend time talking with her, and thus she attracted daily visitors to her small apartment in the retirement community.

Many of the present generation of elderly women likely retained much of their homemaking role throughout their adult years, and therefore work roles may not have varied significantly.

Women in transition reported that it often took up to 2 years to complete the process and the supports were most helpful from other women experiencing similar life transitions (Harrison et al, 1995). Women are thought to have greater continuity in their late lives (Barer, 1994) and to occupy more roles than men (Adelmann, 1994).

Men may have major role disruptions and severe loss of status with the departure from the work role, which tends to be the one major transition in their lives that requires a total change in life patterns. The advantages that come from being a white male do not necessarily lead to a better adjustment (Danigelis and McIntosh, 1993). Men generally hold a less positive attitude toward retirement from paid work than do women (Hatch, 1992).

Antonovsky and Sagy (1990) have identified four central tasks of males in the transition to retirement: active planning, reevaluation of sources of satisfaction, reexamining one's world view, and attending to health maintenance.

In a study of 39 men and 111 women living in the community and over age 85, Barer (1994) found that the men had fewer functional limitations, a higher level of activity, and were more involved in hobbies, organizations, and household maintenance. However, one must interpret these differences thoughtfully because the very small proportion of men over age 85 are obviously a very select and undoubtedly outstanding group.

These men were disadvantaged in the fact that their well-being could be undermined by unanticipated events.

The Transition from Health to Illness

Recognition of and adaptation to a chronic illness (see Chapter 8) is likely to be a transition required of an aged person. For example, the move from being a "healthy" elder to that of an elderly "diabetic" requires changes in lifestyle, self-concept, and relationships. John was a highly sexual person. He adapted fairly well to the dietary changes and was able to tolerate his propensity to develop infections, but

as he became increasingly aware of his impotence, his whole self-image was threatened. He no longer felt "manly" and became quite suicidal. Early affiliation with a group confronting similar issues will usually assist in the adaptation to the altered role requirements necessitated by chronic illness.

The Work Role Transition

The major transition that is anticipated purely as a result of aging is that of retirement from the work force. Some elders continue to work long beyond the classic marker of 65 years because of necessity, devotion, enjoyment of challenge, need for structure, or simply a desire to hang on to the status that is part of the work role.

There has been an increase in younger retirees exiting and reentering the work force within the first year after retirement (Hayward et al, 1994). Hurd (1993) found that if they did not return to work within the first year of retirement, it was unlikely they would do so.

Some researchers are now focusing on the differences between "crisp" and "blurred" transitions from the labor force (Mutchler et al, 1997) (Figure 20-2). These patterns of retirement from the work force show variances by age in partial retirement (blurred), abrupt stoppage of work life (crisp), and those who continue working until age 73 or longer. The crisp transition is unidirectional and complete, whereas blurred transitions are characterized by repeated exits, entrances, and unemployment spells. These are likely related to economic status. This factor of retirement involves the entire career perspective. Is retirement more difficult for an individual who has been with one company for most of his or her adult life?

A problem with the studies of work and retirement is the lack of differentiation concerning the meaning of work to the individual. Blue collar/white collar/pink collar differentiations are simply inadequate to explain the meaning of any work role. Academics, nutritionists, rocket scientists, and auto mechanics may be equally bored or stimulated by their work. One man very succinctly stated the heart of the issue of work: "An orthopedic surgeon and a carpenter are basically doing many of the same things but using different materials." Either can be done by an artist or a plodder. The results and the level of satisfaction will differ. Work must be examined from a life and personality perspective rather than by job identification, though some jobs inherently carry more status and thus may be harder to give up.

It is commonly thought that physicians find it very hard to retire (Mandell, 1995), but a recent study of 878 Minnesota physicians (Seim and Mitchell, 1995) found that 73% retired in their 60s; most were healthy, comfortable, and enjoyed retirement. Activities most enjoyed were visiting family (86%), reading (79%), and travel (63%). Rural physicians tend to retire later (Lee et al, 1995). Among radiologists, only half intend to fully retire (Deitch et al, 1995).

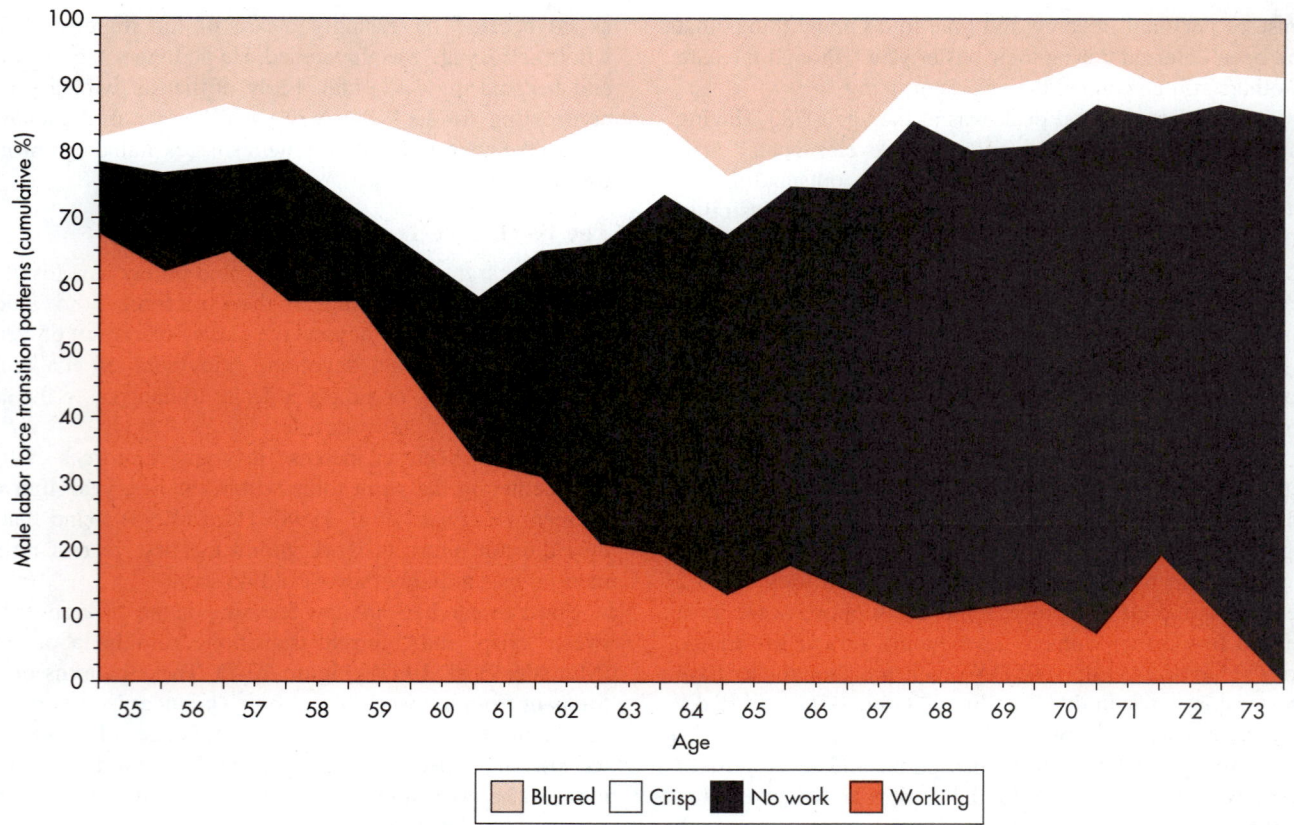

Figure 20-2. Labor force transition patterns by age. (Modified from Mutchler JE, Burr JA, Pienta AM, Massagli MP: Pathways to labor force exit: work transitions and work instability, *J Gerontol* 52 B(1):S4, 1997.)

It would be interesting to have similar studies of retirement plans among other specialty health practitioners. Studies of nurses' retirement plans are limited and focus primarily on the economic possibility of retiring (Moore and Biordi, 1995; Fellers, 1990; Halloran et al, 1996). Among Minnesota physicians in the study cited, only 14% had concern about income, feeling it was "barely adequate."

Work is a major social role for men, and increasingly for women, in our society. In 1994 16.2% of males over 65 were employed and 8.8% of females. There has been about a 1% gain in participation among women and slightly over a 2% drop among males in the work force (U.S. Bureau of the Census, 1995) since 1994 (Table 20-1). The trend of increased numbers of women working in their later years is expected to continue (Figure 20-3). The work scene continually changes and becomes more complex as technology and government policies continually destroy jobs and creates new ones. In the health care market this has been particularly noticeable in the last few years.

Labor Force Participation. There are at present approximately 4 million people over 65 years old who are working or looking for work (Population Reference Bureau, 1995). Although many people are retiring young, there re-

mains a sizable group of individuals who must work or wish to remain in the work force. These persons provoke particular concerns for employers (Box 20-2).

Zwerling et al (1996) studied the risk factors for occupational injury among older workers and found that impaired hearing and vision increased risk. Jobs requiring heavy lifting, mechanical and repair work were the most hazardous. An appropriate match between older workers' capabilities and the job demands is essential to continued safety in the workplace. Daly and Bound(1996) report that work-limiting health impairments are most often compensated for by altering the job demands or by the individual moving to a job that is more fitted to his or her capabilities.

Civilian labor force participation for individuals 65 years and older had been declining since 1970. In 1988 it began to rise slightly but overall has continued to drop and unemployment among those who wish to work has increased very slightly. However, because of the very complexitiy of work/nonwork, it is difficult to define increases or decreases in "leaving" the job force. It is not yet evident, but it is expected that there will soon be an increase of people working into the years beyond 65; it will be necessary because the age for retirement with full benefits and Social Security is

Table 20-1 Labor Force Participation Rates, by Marital Status, Sex, and Age: 1960 to 1994

[Annual averages of monthly figures. Based on Current Population Survey.]

Marital status and year	Male participation rate							Female participation rate						
	Total	16-19 years	20-24 years	25-34 years	35-44 years	45-64 years	65 and over	Total	16-19 years	20-24 years	25-34 years	35-44 years	45-64 years	65 and over
Single:														
1960 ..	69.8	42.6	80.3	91.5	88.6	80.1	31.2	58.6	30.2	77.2	83.4	82.9	79.8	24.3
1970 ..	65.5	54.6	73.8	87.9	86.2	75.7	25.2	56.8	44.7	73.0	81.4	78.6	73.0	19.7
1975 ..	68.7	57.9	77.9	86.7	83.2	69.9	21.0	59.8	49.6	72.5	80.8	78.6	68.3	15.8
1980 ..	72.6	59.9	81.3	89.2	82.2	66.9	16.8	64.4	53.6	75.2	83.3	76.9	65.6	13.9
1985 ..	73.8	56.3	81.5	89.4	84.6	65.5	15.6	66.6	52.3	76.3	82.4	80.8	67.9	9.8
1990 ..	74.9	55.1	81.5	89.9	84.6	67.1	15.7	66.9	51.8	74.7	81.2	81.0	66.1	12.2
1991 ..	74.2	52.6	80.6	89.6	84.8	66.8	14.0	66.5	50.3	73.5	80.3	81.2	68.4	12.7
1992 ..	74.6	52.9	80.7	89.8	84.9	67.6	16.3	66.4	49.2	73.7	80.5	80.6	68.2	11.3
1993 ..	74.2	52.5	80.5	89.2	84.5	68.2	15.0	66.4	49.8	74.2	79.1	79.1	68.8	12.5
1994 ..	73.9	53.6	80.5	88.4	83.1	67.8	17.8	66.7	51.4	73.6	78.9	78.7	68.8	12.7
Married*														
1960 ..	89.2	91.5	97.1	98.8	98.6	93.7	36.6	31.9	27.2	31.7	28.8	37.2	36.0	6.7
1970 ..	86.1	92.3	94.7	98.0	98.1	91.2	29.9	40.5	37.8	47.9	38.8	46.8	44.0	7.3
1975 ..	83.0	92.9	95.3	97.4	97.1	86.8	23.3	44.3	46.2	57.0	48.4	52.0	43.8	7.0
1980 ..	80.9	91.3	96.9	97.5	97.2	84.3	20.5	49.8	49.3	61.4	58.8	61.8	46.9	7.3
1985 ..	78.7	91.0	95.6	97.4	96.8	81.7	16.8	53.8	49.6	65.7	65.8	68.1	49.4	6.6
1990 ..	78.2	92.3	95.6	96.9	96.8	82.5	17.6	58.4	50.0	66.5	69.8	74.0	56.5	8.5
1991 ..	77.8	93.2	95.4	96.6	96.6	82.3	16.8	58.5	48.7	65.0	70.1	74.3	57.1	8.3
1992 ..	77.6	90.2	94.8	96.6	96.2	82.7	17.2	59.2	49.0	66.3	70.9	74.8	58.6	7.9
1993 ..	77.3	91.2	95.0	96.6	96.1	82.5	16.6	59.4	50.1	65.6	70.8	74.7	60.0	7.6
1994 ..	77.4	88.7	94.2	95.9	95.6	81.9	18.1	60.7	48.9	65.8	71.6	75.8	61.9	9.4
Other†														
1960 ..	63.1	(B)	96.9	95.2	94.4	83.2	22.7	41.6	43.5	58.0	63.1	70.0	60.0	11.4
1970 ..	60.7	(B)	90.4	93.7	91.1	78.5	19.3	40.3	48.6	60.3	64.6	68.8	61.9	10.0
1975 ..	63.4	(B)	88.8	92.4	89.4	73.4	15.4	40.1	47.6	65.3	68.6	69.2	59.0	8.3
1980 ..	67.5	(B)	92.6	94.1	91.9	73.3	13.7	43.6	50.0	68.4	76.5	77.1	60.2	8.2
1985 ..	68.7	(B)	95.1	93.7	91.8	72.8	11.4	45.1	51.9	66.2	76.9	81.6	61.0	7.5
1990 ..	68.3	(B)	93.1	93.0	90.8	74.6	12.0	47.2	54.4	65.6	77.3	82.3	65.0	8.5
1991 ..	67.7	(B)	93.9	92.1	90.5	73.5	12.3	46.8	45.8	63.3	74.8	82.1	65.2	8.4
1992 ..	68.0	(B)	91.8	93.5	90.3	74.7	12.2	47.0	47.8	66.9	75.7	81.6	66.4	8.4
1993 ..	67.4	(B)	91.7	91.9	89.6	74.2	12.0	47.1	53.3	65.2	75.2	81.6	66.9	8.2
1994 ..	66.8	65.1	91.0	90.3	88.6	72.6	11.9	47.5	46.2	66.6	74.3	80.4	67.6	8.7

From U.S. Bureau of the Census: *Statistical abstract of the United States: 1995,* ed 115, Washington, DC, 1995.
B for 1960, percentage not shown where base is less than 50,000; beginning 1970, 35,000
*Spouse present. †Widowed, divorced, and married (spouse absent).
Source: U.S. Bureau of Labor Statistics, Bulletins 2217 and 2340; and unpublished data.

gradually creeping upward. By the year 2010 it is likely one must work until age 70 to obtain full benefits.

Presently older men make up 3.1% of the civilian labor force and older women make up 2.7% (Table 20-2). Serious questions arise as to the availability of jobs in the future for those elders who wish to work. Some economists predict a great increase in the need for human service specialists, and others point to the developing technologies that displace workers rapidly. It is yet to be seen how these trends will affect the elderly work force.

Recent corporate cutbacks and mergers have resulted in numbers of older workers being "RIFFED" (reduction in personnel force). They are often from midmanagement positions that are quite specialized. Jobs requiring their particular skills and paying somewhat equivalent salaries are difficult to obtain.

AARP Works is a nationwide program of workshops to help older persons find suitable jobs (see Resources at the end of the chapter). Many retired individuals who would like to work are skilled professionals. They face

OLDER WORKERS

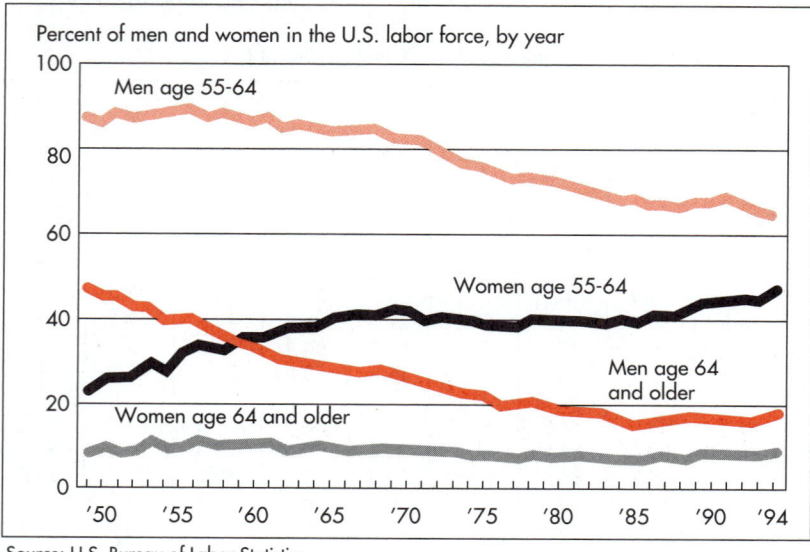

Source: U.S. Bureau of Labor Statistics

Figure 20-3. Percent of men and women in the U.S. labor force, by year. (Modified from Rogers FL: Older working men a vanishing species, *San Francisco Examiner,* p. A-13, July 9, 1995.)

Box 20-2	**Top 15 Business Issues**

How does business rank its concerns about dealing with the aging work force? Here is how a wide variety of firms throughout Colorado responded to the three-part Delphi method survey conducted last year by Colorado State University.

The most salient issues, scored by researchers and listed in order, were as follows:

1. Finding ways to effectively recognize, value and utilize the current skills of older workers.
2. Helping older workers deal effectively with technological change.
3. Designing and implementing health insurance programs and medical benefits to meet the needs of older workers.
4. Training and/or retraining older workers.
5. Facilitating career development and job change for older workers.
6. Dealing with company cost increases associated with benefits and programs designed to assist older workers and retirees.
7. Assisting older workers in financial planning in order to achieve security in retirement.
8. Designing and implementing retirement benefit packages for older workers.
9. Improving intergenerational relationships involving older and younger workers.
10. Developing wellness/preventive health programs for older workers.
11. Helping older workers deal with dependent care in their families.
12. Developing unbiased means for appraising the job performance of older workers.
13. Recruiting older workers.
14. Designing the work environment to accommodate the physical and psychological changes of older workers and to ensure their safety.
15. Dealing with age discrimination in the workplace.

From Barber CE: Top 15 issues, *Aging Today* 13(4):13, 1992.

---

subtle age discrimination and a lack of assistance because they are generally thought able to manage without help. A summary of persons not in the labor force is found in Table 20-3.

Nan McEvoy, age 75, filed an age discrimination suit when the Chronicle Publishing Company attempted to oust her from her corporate position (Trager, 1995). Though workers are protected by The Employment Retirement Income Security Act (ERISA) from mandatory retirement, corporations often have limits at age 72. Schulz (1994) states succinctly, "Everyone is in favor of keeping older people in the labor force except the union, government, business, and older people."

Table 20-2   Civilian Labor Force—Percent Distribution, by Sex and Age: 1960 to 1994

[For civilian noninstitutional population 16 years old and over. Annual averages of monthly figures. Based on Current Population Survey.]

Year and sex	Civilian labor force (1,000)	Percent distribution						
		16 to 19 years	20 to 24 years	25 to 34 years	35 to 44 years	45 to 54 years	55 to 64 years	65 yrs. and over
Total: 1960	69,628	7.0	9.6	20.7	23.4	21.3	13.5	4.6
1970	82.771	8.8	12.8	20.6	19.9	20.5	13.6	3.9
1980	106,940	8.8	14.9	27.3	19.1	15.8	11.2	2.9
1985	115,461	6.8	13.6	29.1	22.6	15.0	10.4	2.5
1990	124,787	5.9	11.1	28.7	25.5	16.4	9.5	2.8
1991	125,303	5.5	10.9	28.2	26.3	16.9	9.4	2.8
1992	126,982	5.3	10.8	27.6	26.5	17.6	9.3	2.8
1993	128,040	5.3	10.6	26.9	26.8	18.4	9.3	2.7
1994	131,056	5.7	10.8	26.2	26.9	18.6	8.9	2.9
Male: 1960	46,388	6.0	8.9	22.1	23.6	20.6	13.8	4.9
1970	51,228	7.8	11.2	22.1	20.4	20.3	13.9	4.2
1980	61,453	8.1	14.0	27.6	19.3	16.1	11.8	3.1
1985	64,411	6.4	12.9	29.2	22.5	15.3	11.0	2.7
1990	68,234	5.7	10.7	29.0	25.3	16.4	9.9	3.0
1991	68,411	5.2	10.6	28.6	26.1	16.8	9.8	2.9
1992	69,184	5.1	10.5	28.0	26.3	17.5	9.7	3.0
1993	69,633	5.1	10.3	27.4	26.6	18.1	9.5	2.9
1994	70,817	5.5	10.6	26.6	26.8	18.3	9.1	3.1
Female: 1960	23,240	8.8	11.1	17.8	22.8	22.7	12.8	3.9
1970	31,543	10.3	15.5	18.1	18.9	20.7	13.2	3.3
1980	45,487	9.6	16.1	26.9	19.0	15.4	10.4	2.6
1985	51,050	7.4	14.6	28.9	22.7	14.6	9.7	2.3
1990	56,554	6.3	11.6	28.3	25.8	16.5	9.0	2.7
1991	56,893	5.9	11.3	27.7	26.6	17.0	8.9	2.7
1992	57,798	5.5	11.2	27.2	26.7	17.8	8.9	2.6
1993	58,407	5.6	10.9	26.4	26.9	18.7	9.0	2.5
1994	60,239	6.0	10.9	25.7	27.0	18.9	8.8	2.8

From U.S. Bureau of the Census: *Statistical abstract of the United States: 1995,* ed 115, Washington, DC, 1995.
Source: U.S. Bureau of Labor Statistics, Bulletin 2307, and *Employment Earnings,* monthly, January issues.

Unlike McEvoy, Dorothy Eastman, at 75 years old, works as a maid because she has no pension and cannot afford to retire. She must supplement her $524 monthly Social Security check (Ferriss, 1994).

The Regional Coordinating Council for Older Workers (RCC) has been established in all nine federal regions to develop older worker programs. One of these, Operation ABLE (in several regions), offers seminars to assist the older professional in a job search. Other similar programs include Second Careers, Forty Plus, Experience Unlimited Job Club, The Los Angeles Council on Careers for Older Americans, and AARP Works. For further information see Resources at the end of the chapter.

Career transition programs have appeared in several universities across the United States. Senior Corp of Retired Executives (SCORE) has proved to be a dynamic organization using the talents of retired individuals. Many groups and communities have established job banks to match employers and older workers (see Resources).

Despite legislation many subtle pressures, such as the high unemployment rate among youth, may force individuals to retire when they wish to continue working. Many corporations would rather employ a young worker at a much lower rate of pay than retain the experienced older worker who commands a high salary. There has been an increase in age discrimination suits filed with the Equal Employment Opportunity Commission in the last few years, and some of these suits against major powerful companies have resulted in six-figure awards. It is expected that age discrimination suits will continue.

Before taking a complaint to a lawyer, one should ask the following questions: Are you in the right age group? Were you doing your job to the satisfaction of management? Were you dismissed without cause? Were you replaced by someone younger? An older worker who believes his or her employer is discriminating on the basis of age should contact the nearest Equal Employment Opportunity Commission office.

Table 20-3   Persons Not in the Labor Force: 1994

[In thousands. Annual average of monthly figures. For the civilian noninstitutional population 16 years old and over. Based on the Current Population Survey.]

Status and reason	Total	Age			Sex	
		16 to 24 years old	25 to 54 years old	55 years old and over	Male	Female
Total, not in the labor force	**65,758**	**10,937**	**18,720**	**36,101**	**23,538**	**42,221**
Do not want a job now	59,540	8,635	15,790	35,116	21,089	38,452
Want a job now	6,218	2,302	2,930	985	2,449	3,769
In the previous year—						
Did not search for a job	3,588	1,263	1,611	714	1,311	2,277
Did search for a job	2,630	1,040	1,319	272	1,138	1,492
Not available for work now	823	400	379	44	308	515
Available for work now, not looking for work	1,807	639	939	228	830	977
Reason for not currently looking:						
Discouraged over job prospects*	500	143	278	79	296	204
Family responsibilities	213	44	153	17	31	183
In school or training	267	213	52	1	137	129
Ill health or disability	150	21	92	36	69	81
Other†	677	219	364	94	298	379

From U.S. Bureau of the Census: *Statistical abstract of the United States: 1995,* ed 115, Washington, DC, 1995.
*Includes believes no work available, could not find work, lack necessary schooling or training, employer thinks too young or old, and other types of discrimination. †Includes such things as child care and transportation problems.
Source: U.S. Bureau of Labor Statistics, *Employment and Earnings,* monthly, January 1995.

Retirement Intentions. Decisions to retire are often based on attitude toward work, chronologic age, health, and self-perceptions of ability to adjust to retirement (Taylor and Shore, 1995). Retirement intentions are variable and include four types of "retirement": to retire from work, to change jobs, to partially retire, or to work for self (Ekerdt et al, 1996). When one speaks of retirement or analyzes research, it is important to know just what an individual means by retirement. Issues to consider are summarized in Box 20-3.

Partial Retirement. Part-time work during retirement is viewed by the working public of all ages as a desirable option. Temporary work agencies are now actively recruiting older workers who may wish to keep up their skills and decide when and where they want to work. Employers seek them because they are often more reliable and dependable. Seniors can earn up to a certain amount* annually without endangering Social Security benefits, and after 70 years of age they can earn an unlimited amount. Those seniors wishing part-time employment may benefit by the following suggestions:

- Register with more than one temporary agency.
- Tell the firm exactly what you wish to do and how often you would like to work.
- Document your skills.

A pattern is emerging in which many retired persons seek personally satisfying jobs they were previously unable to con-

*Earnings allowed without affecting Social Security are determined annually.

sider because the pay was not sufficient for their needs. Silver Foxes is an organization formed in 1986 by Alan Marzec of Oak Brook, Illinois. This organization offers part-time work to advertising executives who have retired. Clients are eager to tap the experience of these top-notch professionals, and the professionals are pleased with the opportunity to select assignments and work at their own pace. Although this program is limited to the Chicago area, it is a model that could be used by many professionals in other regions.

Some companies have developed retirees' job banks in which the experienced retiree may continue to work on special projects, as vacation relief, or in temporary jobs without endangering retirement benefits. This is advantageous for the retiree as well as the company that is able to use the accumulated expertise of years of experience (Older Americans program, 1987).

Most older workers indicate a wish to continue some form of employment beyond their expected retirement age.

Early Retirement. The median retirement age of Americans of all races has fallen from about 66 years in the period 1955 to 1960 to 62.7 in 1985 to 1990 (Gerontological Society of America, 1996). In 1950 43% of individuals over 55 were in the work force. In 1995 that figure had dropped to 30% (Rix, 1996). Gendell and Siegel (1996) found that, on average, men, women, blacks and whites have stopped working before collecting their retirement benefits. For many, the job reshuffling and subtle or not-so-subtle pressures have forced them out. Since 1949 older men between

---

Box 20-3
Issues in Retirement Potential

1. Financial need versus resources
2. Employability
3. Rewards derived from employment
   - Wages sufficient for needs and morale
   - Satisfaction level, possibility for resolution of job frustrations
   - Meaning of job, contact with friends, source of prestige
4. Psychosocial characteristics—attitudes toward retirement
   - Attitudes of significant others (advising? directing?)
   - Strength of work ethic
   - Effect of retirement on prestige
5. Personality factors
   - Time orientation (past, present, future)
   - Active versus passive in planning
   - Rationalism versus fatalism as life stance
   - Type-A versus type-B personality (hard-driving, easy-going)
   - Inner directed versus other directed (enjoyment of self or need for high level of external motivation)
6. Level of information about retirement
   - Planning programs on job, adult education, or community programs
   - Awareness of friends and family who have retired and how influenced by them
7. Pressures to retire
   - Compulsory, age discriminatory
   - Unemployment (how long?)
   - Job retrogression (being moved down the ladder)
   - Skill obsolescence (opportunities for developing other skills?)
   - Peer pressure, organized or informal
   - Employer pressure (reduced incentives to continue work, increased incentives to retire)
   - Family pressure (spouse's working status)
   - Health, discomfort, or disability interfering with job performance and dependability

---

ages 55 and 64 have left the work force at 1/2 % per year (Flinn and Rogers, 1995). Early retirement and multiple careers are becoming the norm and will probably increase in the future as companies try to increase profits and decrease overhead (Dennis, 1989). Early retirement incentive programs are often so attractive that individuals retire earlier than they had planned or expected (Hardy and Quadagno, 1995).

Most prospective retirees will be working couples and must plan together for retirement when both have been accustomed to working. Decisions will depend upon their career goals, shared future interests, and the quality of their interpersonal relationship. "Life planning" is replacing "retirement planning" as individuals recognize that future planning is a lifelong endeavor. Employers, retirement specialists, universities, professional associations, and advocacy groups can assist adults in "life planning" for their later years, but the ultimate responsibility remains with the individual (Dennis, 1989).

Early retirement may be a consequence of job dissatisfaction or boredom, unemployment, weeding out top wage and salary personnel, making room for advancement of younger personnel, outmoded skills, cost-effectiveness factors, poor health, or personal choice. Normal retirement age is more frequently occurring at 55 years old.

Although some people of late middle age choose to retire from the labor market, many are being forced out by unemployment. Regional, occupational, and personal variables account for unemployment in late middle age. Projections for the future have reported a higher labor force participation rate for these unemployed than has actually occurred or can be expected in the future. Many older workers declare themselves retired rather than remain in the ranks of the unemployed.

Many persons in early retirement made the decision because of ill health. Persons with work disability between 55 and 64 years of age make up 22% of the civilian work force population. Slightly more men than women and 50% more blacks than whites are disabled (U.S .Bureau of the Census, 1995).

Retirement

Between the years of 1955 and 1993 the labor force participation rates declined between 3 and 4 years, meaning individuals were retiring earlier. There was a major decline during the '70s. The decline has slowed somewhat through the late '80s and '90s (Gendell and Siegel, 1996). Increases in the disability rolls and involuntary job loss have also contributed to the declining participation (Henretta and Lee, 1996).

The variable consequences and the strategies individuals use to negotiate this event are the concern of health professionals. Retirement is no longer just a few years of rest from the rigors of work before death. It is a developmental stage that may occupy 30 years of one's life and may involve many stages. Individuals are increasingly retiring early as the option becomes more available and attractive to the majority of citizens.

Just as Social Security was initially seen as a mechanism for resolving unemployment, early retirement is now a means of regulating the labor supply. Employers encourage early retirement of older, more expensive workers by

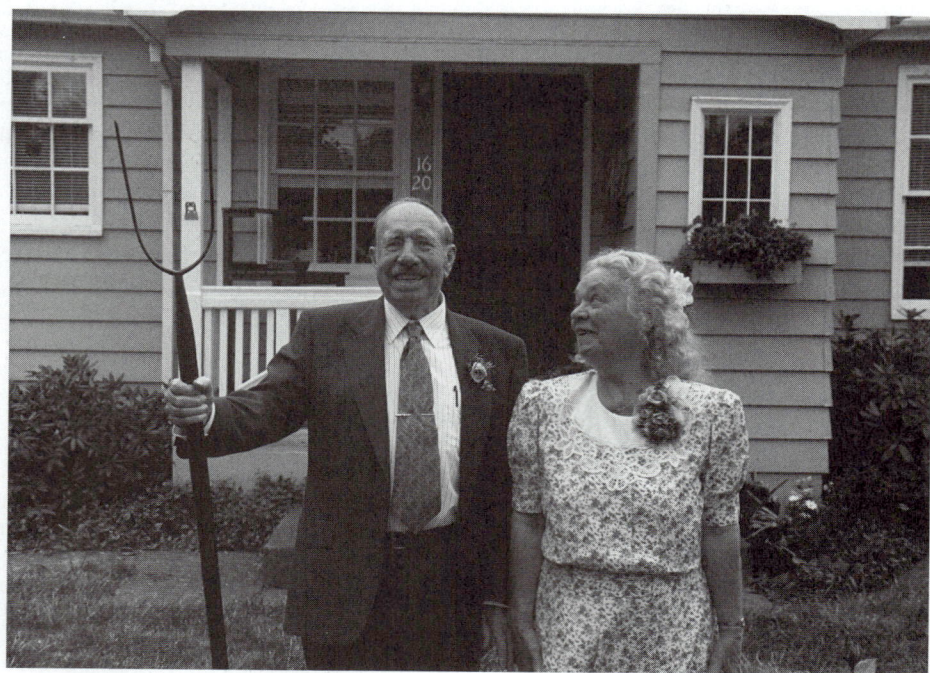

Retiring to the country. (Courtesy Rod Schmall.)

offering attractive incentives. Simultaneously, the government has developed policies to keep older workers in the labor market for longer periods by gradually delaying full Social Security benefits to 70 years of age (beginning in the year 2000) and abolishing forced retirement because of age. In 1986 the Age Discrimination in Employment Act (ADEA) eradicated any age ceilings on work participation except in a few very special circumstances.

It is clear that the goals of government and industry are in conflict related to the older work force. Government cannot afford a large body of nonworking individuals, and industry cannot afford to keep those individuals in top salaried positions. With pension security and portablity, workers no longer feel forced to remain in a position.

The complexity of the work-to-retirement transition is blurred by numerous variations in the process (Henretta, 1997). Retirement must be examined from several angles: a "post-career" job, exit from long-term job and return, partial retirement, ad hoc arrangements with long-term employers to meet changing work needs and capacities, retire to self-employment, and numerous variations. Some think that complex retirement patterns are becoming more common and others that retirement has become more standardized (Henretta, 1992).

A common assumption in the past was that retirement has a negative effect on health and mental health. This is emphasized by the subliminal reaction to retirement. When asked, "How are you enjoying retirement?" the inevitable response is, "I'm busier than ever." It is apparent that many

elderly individuals are still of the work ethic and cannot comfortably say, "I just love loafing."

In the large Kaiser Permanente Retirement Study (Midanik et al, 1995) it was found that retired members were less stressed and engaged in more regular exercise than those who were remaining in the work force. More nonretired women reported alcohol problems than those who were retired. In most respects it appeared that there were positive health and mental health benefits associated with retirement. Undoubtedly, the numerous patterns and styles of retiring have produced more satisfying experiences in retirement.

Concern must focus on the group of retirees who did not expect retirement at the time when they left the work force. These individuals are likely to suffer detrimental effects and be in need of counseling and assistance through the transition. They are likely to experience job separation as a crisis and have a traumatic role transition triggered by an unplanned job termination due to illness or company "downsizing," a euphemistic term for cutting out jobs. A recent study by Henretta et al (1992) reveals reasons for retirement among more than 1700 male retiree respondents to the Social Security New Beneficiary Study (Table 20-4).

Many elders desire to work as long as they are physically able, and the government has taken steps to make this possible. It is no longer the era of kind words and a gold fountain pen on the sixty-fifth birthday. In fact, by the year 2000 individuals must work until age 67 to receive full Social Security benefits. The retirement transition occurs at different ages and stages for each individual. For some, retirement is

Table 20-4 Cross-Classification of "Most Important" and "Important" Reasons for Leaving Last Job

Most important reason	N	%	Proportion mentioning other reasons								
			Wanted to retire	Health	Lost job	Compulsory	Social Security	Care for others	Pension	Didn't like job	Spouse retired
Wanted to retire	763	47.4	—	8.0	1.6	6.3	29.5	1.8	34.1	1.7	1.6
Health	401	24.9	25.4	—	2.7	5.5	12.5	4.0	13.2	0.2	0.7
Lost job	160	9.9	9.4	6.9	—	3.1	6.2	0	2.5	0.6	0
Compulsory	139	8.6	21.6	7.9	5.0	—	17.3	3.6	14.4	0	2.7
Social Security	49	3.0	47.0	12.2	2.0	10.2	—	2.0	40.8	0	2.0
Care for others	40	2.5	17.5	5.0	0	0	2.5	—	7.5	0	2.5
Pension	29	1.8	51.7	0	3.4	0	24.1	6.9	—	0	3.4
Didn't like job	24	1.5	54.1	0	4.2	0	8.4	4.2	20.8	—	0
Spouse retired	6	0.4	83.3	0	0	0	33.3	16.6	50.0	—	0
Other	123	7.6	22.0	8.9	4.9	4.1	11.4	2.4	12.2	3.2	0
Percent citing as a reason			56.6	28.5	11.2	12.4	21.8	4.7	23.4	2.5	1.5
Percent most important responses that are only response			48.2	59.8	76.2	56.1	30.6	75.0	37.9	37.5	16.7

From Henretta JC, Chan CG, O'Rand AM: Retirement reason versus retirement process: examining the reasons for retirement typology, *J Gerontol*, 47(1):S1, 1992. Permission granted by The Gerontological Society of America.

somewhat dependent upon the type of work, the status achieved, and the average job tenure.

Given the opportunity to work past retirement age, one must weigh the benefits. Older persons who wish to go into business for themselves have a few advantages over younger persons, such as more financial independence, established credit, knowledge, and a wide circle of contacts. Clients should be advised to contact the Social Security office 6 months before their sixty-fifth birthday to qualify for Medicare and to find out exactly how earned income and Social Security will be computed and the net benefit they will garner by continued employment.

Increasing numbers of individuals begin drawing Social Security benefits at age 62 and believe it is to their economic advantage in the long run. Others continue working for reasons of self-esteem as well as economic advantages. When this is done, earnings beyond the allowable amount (in 1996, $11,000 for those persons under 70 years of age) will reduce benefits. In an effort to encourage individuals to work longer, this law is changing. Individuals may now earn more without reductions in benefits.

The inequities inherent in various work roles compound over time, and thus cumulative progress or cumulative disadvantage result in major differences in retirement compensation and comfort. To our dismay it is found that the service industries that employ caregiving professionals are among the least likely to provide health care and adequate retirement for their employees (Hirshorn et al, 1996). Retirement decisions are based on a number of personal questions, including:

1. What do I want to do?
2. Who needs me, and what are my best opportunities?
3. What am I best able to do?
4. What is the meaning of my life?
5. What should my life accomplish or contribute?
6. Am I financially independent for the rest of my life if I live 30 more years?
7. Am I in excellent physical condition, and do I enjoy spending a great deal of time with my spouse?
8. Can I afford to completely retire from paid work?

Preretirement Planning. Retirement planning is advisable during middle age and essential in late middle age. However, people differ in their focus on the future, past, and present. Time orientation is an important consideration in assessing readiness for retirement planning. Although preretirement planning programs may be available, some will not participate in them because they are not "planners." Retirement preparation programs are usually aimed at employees with high levels of education and occupational status, those with private pension coverage, and government employees. A question preretirees must consider it, "Can I afford to retire?" A trial run is useful. Can the individual live comfortably on the anticipated retirement income? This self-test before retirement may influence critical decisions such as the following:

- Can the budget be altered and yet provide satisfaction?
- Would part-time work be a solution to budget and time problems?

Retirement education plans are supplied through group lectures, individual counseling, booklets, videocassettes, and computerized modules. Nurses need to be familiar with these sources of information and discuss the need for retirement planning with their clients (see Resources at the end of this chapter). Retirement planning must begin early in the work career. Typically, programs emphasize financial planning but neglect the issues of role change, use of time, relationship with spouse, and the psychologic and social impact of not working (Dennis, 1989).

Individuals who are retiring in poor health or are minority persons and those in lower socioeconomic levels need specialized counseling. These groups are neglected in retirement planning programs. Retraining for more satisfying positions and part-time work may be essential.

Many older persons preparing for retirement are also caring for elderly parents. Increasingly, large corporations are developing employee assistance programs that provide support and resources in coping with the needs of these elders (see Chapter 17 for discussion and resources).

Retirement research has often been implicitly biased toward sustained employment over time, with the assumption that the characteristics of the final employment from which one retires are a reliable indicator of lifelong work pursuits. Few if any studies investigate early work history or ongoing work history, with the result that much retirement research is skewed and incomplete (O'Rand, 1996). This common problem must be kept in mind as one plans the transition from work to retirement. It is especially important in this era when much of the future benefits of a retiree are intricately tied to the recent work history.

The adequacy of retirement income is dependent not only on work history but upon marital history as well. The poverty rates of divorced older women, as seen in Figure 20-4, are excessively high. Couples that have had previous marriages and divorces have significantly lower incomes than those in first marriages (Holden and Hui, 1996). This is

an ever-increasing impediment to retirement because among couples presently approaching retirement age less than one half are in a first marriage (Holden and Hui, 1996). Policies have been based on the traditional lifelong marriage, and this is no longer appropriate.

Nurses have rarely addressed the issue of nursing function related to retirement of self and clients. Studies do not agree on whether retirement contributes to deterioration of health, but nurses are aware that any major change is likely to be reflected in a client's physical status, tendency toward substance abuse, or deterioration of relationships. Anticipatory guidance regarding the feelings that accompany retirement may allow the client to cope with unexpected reactions. Preretirement education often neglects the emotional implications of the retirement experience. It has been shown that preretirement educational curricula that include preparation for psychologic reactions to retirement produce positive outcomes.

Postretirement counseling is also important. It is difficult for one to anticipate psychologic reactions to such a major event. Support groups for retirees might be particularly beneficial in the first year following retirement.

Retirement planning for women. Inadequate information is available regarding the status of older women in retirement because their work histories have been so spasmodic and diverse. Whereas most men have always worked outside the home, it has been only within the last 30 years that this has been the expectation of women. Therefore large cohort differences exist. The increased labor force participation of women has incited interest in their retirement, but little is yet known about the impact on their lives (Calasanti, 1996).

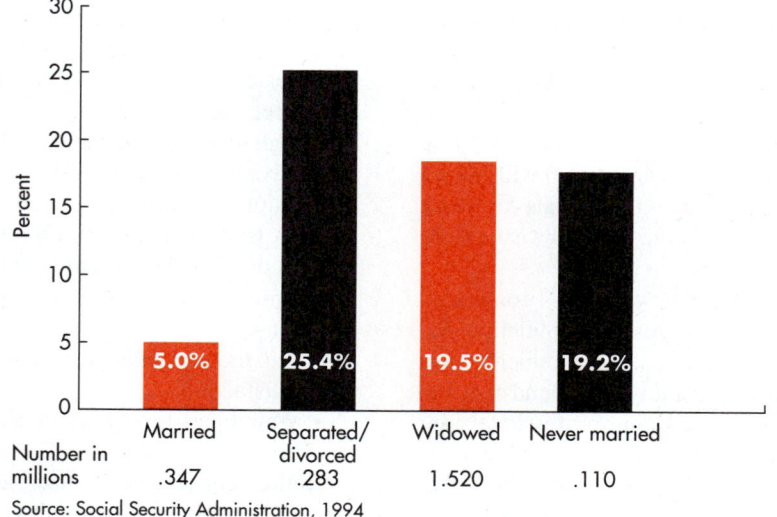

Figure 20-4. Poverty rates 1993—women Social Security beneficiaries by marital status. (Modified from *The path to poverty: an analysis of women's retirement income,* 1995 Mothers Day Report, Washington, DC, 1995, Older Women's League.)

Many older women have no understanding of the veterans pension or Social Security system and how these will or will not protect them. A news report in the *San Francisco Chronicle* (Confederate widow's pension restored, 1996) exemplifies the vagaries of the system:

Alberta Martin, possibly the only living Confederate widow, learned Tuesday that Alabama had agreed to renew her Confederate widow's pension and a supplement, 64 years after she became ineligible for the aid because she remarried. Martin was a 21-year-old widow with a young son in 1927 when she married 82-year-old William Jasper Martin, a former Confederate Army Private. Shortly after William Martin's death at age 87 in 1932, Alberta married Martin's grandson, Charlie Martin, making her ineligible to draw her late husband's pension. When Charlie Martin died in 1983, Alberta became re-eligible to collect a pension, but she did not know it.

Traditionally, the variability of women's work histories, interrupted careers, the residuals of sexist pension polices, Social Security inequities, and low-paying jobs created hazards for adequacy of income in retirement (The path to poverty: an analysis of women's retirement income, 1995). The scene is gradually changing in many respects, but the gender bias remains.

Older women are very likely to have several years of $00 earnings calculated in the averages that determine the amount of their Social Security benefits. Some find they will receive more if their Social Security benefits are calculated on their husband's earnings; this may be true even though widowed or divorced. The Social Security Administration must be contacted regarding these issues because there are many variables.

In addition, women are often ineligible for pensions because of the types of jobs they hold, and fewer are able to retire early. The number of women over 65 who are covered by pensions is less than half a million (U.S. Bureau of the Census, 1995) (Table 20-5). For those who do receive monthly benefits, the benefits are 55% of those received by men ($5,874 versus $10,645 annually) (The path to poverty: an analysis of women's retirement income, 1995).

Women are often called on to retire because of a spouse's illness or parents who need help rather than at the most expeditious time. Some are not yet old enough to collect Social Security (Gerontological Society of America, 1996).

The complexity of the issues includes differences between retirement patterns of single and married women. Single women are as likely as men to retire early, whereas married women, the larger portion of the female work force, are unlikely to do so. Single and married women differ in the degree of dependency on their own benefits and in work history. Pension coverage and health are useful predictors of retirement for men but not for women. The decision to retire for women is often based on the age and health of the spouse or the need to provide care for elder or younger dependents (Talage and Beehr, 1995). For single women, recent income is a more important factor in the decision to retire, and health was unrelated to retirement decisions (Table 20-6).

For women and men the most significant factors in adaptation to retirement are health, income, and social involvement.

Financial planning for retirement is quite a difficult matter for women who are discriminated against in pension plans and Social Security programs. It is now illegal to base retirement calculations on gender and projected survival statistics, though until the early '80s women were allotted less pension income based purely on their expected longevity in

Table 20-5   Pension Plan Coverage of Workers, by Selected Characteristics: 1993

[Covers workers as of **March 1994** who had earnings in year 1993. Based on Current Population Survey.]

Sex and age	Number with coverage (1,000)				Percent of total workers			
	Total*	White	Black	Hispanic†	Total*	White	Black	Hispanic†
Total	53,742	46,571	5,364	2,964	39.2	39.9	36.6	24.8
Male	29,923	26,440	2,506	1,739	40.8	41.8	35.6	24.4
Under 65 years old	29,331	25,913	2,451	1,713	41.6	42.7	35.6	24.5
15 to 24 years old	1,437	1,242	156	128	11.5	11.6	11.6	8.2
25 to 44 years old	17,190	15,100	1,466	1,133	45.0	46.5	36.9	27.5
45 to 64 years old	10,704	9,571	829	452	54.0	54.6	53.0	34.2
65 years old and over	592	528	55	25	21.5	21.0	34.5	20.4
Female	23,819	20,131	2,858	1,225	37.3	37.5	37.5	25.4
Under 65 years old	23,331	19,707	2,799	1,215	37.8	38.1	37.6	25.6
15 to 24 years old	1,193	1,030	137	104	10.5	10.8	10.4	9.6
25 to 44 years old	13,833	11,573	1,717	783	42.1	42.7	40.0	29.5
45 to 64 years old	8,305	7,103	945	328	47.6	47.4	51.4	32.7
65 years old and over	488	424	59	11	22.6	21.8	32.4	14.4

From U.S. Bureau of the Census: *Statistical abstract of the United States: 1995,* ed 115, Washington, DC, 1995.
*Includes other races, not shown separately. †Hispanic persons may be of any race.
Source: U.S. Bureau of the Census, unpublished data.

Table 20-6 Median Income of Year-Round Full-Time Workers with Income: 1980 to 1993

[Age as of **March of following year.** Prior to 1990 earnings are for civilian workers only.]

Item	Female					Male				
	1980	1990	1991	1992	1993	1980	1990	1991	1992	1993
Total with income	**$11,591**	**$20,591**	**$21,245**	**$22,093**	**$22,469**	**$19,173**	**$28,979**	**$30,332**	**$30,832**	**$31,077**
15 to 19 years	6,779	*13,944	*14,242	*14,662	*15,227	7,753	*15,462	*15,307	*15,658	*15,948
20 to 24 years old	9,407	(NA)	(NA)	(NA)	(NA)	12,109	(NA)	(NA)	(NA)	(NA)
25 to 34 years old	12,190	20,184	21,022	21,941	21,949	17,724	25,355	26,100	26,410	26,087
35 to 44 years old	12,239	22,505	23,385	24,125	25,282	21,777	32,607	33,588	34,714	35,233
45 to 54 years old	12,116	21,938	22,630	24,489	24,412	22,323	35,732	37,198	37,926	39,685
55 to 64 years old	11,931	20,755	21,325	22,581	22,587	21,053	33,169	35,720	35,537	35,736
65 years old and over ..	12,342	22,957	21,780	21,556	24,875	17,307	35,520	34,473	35,341	37,085
White	11,703	20,839	21,555	22,349	22,979	19,720	30,081	30,953	31,565	31,832
Black	10,915	18,544	19,134	20,258	20,315	13,875	21,481	22,628	22,991	23,566
Hispanic†	9,887	16,181	16,548	17,674	17,112	13,790	19,358	20,027	19,855	20,423

From U.S. Bureau of the Census: *Statistical abstract of the United States: 1995,* ed 115, Washington, DC, 1995.
NA Not available. *15 to 24 years old. †Persons of Hispanic origin may be of any race.
Source: U.S. Bureau of the Census, *Current Population Reports,* P60-188, and earlier reports; and unpublished data.

comparison to men. Though this is no longer true, those who retired 15 or 20 years ago remain penalized because of gender.

The economic situation, Social Security benefits, and pensions of retired women are more fully discussed in Chapter 14.

Retirement planning for domestic partners. Bartley (1996) quotes statistics indicating that from 2% to 10% of the United States population is not heterosexual. In New York, San Francisco, Los Angeles, and Dallas the percentage is thought to even greater. In total, there were an estimated 200,000 domestic partners over age 65 in the United States in 1994 (U.S. Bureau of the Census, 1995). Therefore Bartley believes that retirement planning programs must become more attuned to the needs of gay and lesbian couples.

Those couples who have lived together for years and have jointly acquired assets may suffer undue discrimination in retirement and death benefit planning. Because the automatic survivor benefits may not be in place in most states, it is important to have specific insurance policies or arrangements made that ensure the economic viability of the survivor. Bartley offers these tips: (1) the financial planner selected should not be prejudiced regarding sexual orientation or preferences, (2) advice must be given that is protective of clients' interests regardless of sexual orientation because some may not disclose their homosexuality, (3) keep in mind that a partner may be of first concern to the client even before children, and (4) retirement planners are ethically obligated to be sure clients have necessary legal documents on file to provide a smooth transition in the event of premature death or incapacity.

There is much yet that we do not know in regard to these issues, but nurses are in a position to introduce the idea of

future planning. Strangely, many older heterosexuals, homosexuals, and asexuals have not made adequate retirement or estate planning. Nurses may introduce the topic simply by asking, "Have you a will or living trust and advance directive on file and are they up to date?"

Nurse's Role in Retirement Preparation. Questions a nurse may introduce to clients considering retirement include the following:

Will retirement income be adequate to provide a lifestyle that includes items and activities that are currently most satisfying?

Are peer or health pressures significant factors in the decision?

Is the job depleting to health and energy?

Nurses counseling older adults might gather information and give anticipatory guidance related to retirement issues. Nurses interested in retirement preparation may:

1. Prepare proposals, documented with facts, for retirement programs.
2. Offer assistance to personnel departments with preretirement programs and encourage the development of programs where they do not exist. Large organizations are likely to be more receptive than smaller ones.
3. Develop and market a preretirement program suitable to individual or group participation. See list of suggested topics for retirement education in Box 20-4.
4. Support the development of community programs in a college or library for employees who do not have access to such services within their company.

On a more individual level, we would add the following:

1. What are the chief work-related satisfactions, and what might compensate for the loss of those?

| Box 20-4 | **Topics for Retirement Education** |

- Family and couple concerns
- Normal aging processes
- Maintenance of physical and mental health in the later years
- Financial planning: pensions, Social Security, investments, discounts, property tax rebates
- Budgeting
- Full- and part-time employment opportunities
- Housing and relocation
- Legal arrangements and estate planning
- Management of real estate
- Health care services; Medicare and Medicaid
- Death and dying
- Leisure and recreational pursuits
- Community organizations for elderly
- Government role in retirement

---

2. Are friendship networks tied to job?
3. How do spouse and family enter into the decision-making process?
4. Is there an opportunity to test partial work status or nonworking status before actual retirement?
5. Has sufficient information been available regarding retirement planning?
6. Is the work situation more stressful than satisfying?
7. How much of self is defined by job status?
8. Is competitive activity an important source of satisfaction?

Successful retirement adjustment depends on socialization needs, energy levels, health, variety of interests, amount of self-esteem derived from work, presence of intimate relationships, and general adaptability.

1. Talk to clients over 50 years of age about any retirement plans they may have.
2. Make clients aware that the transition to retirement is experienced as a crisis with manifestations of grief in many people.
3. Work with couples whenever retirement may be a possible stressor in their relationship.
4. Institute nursing research regarding the effects of retirement.

Nurses often consider the needs of clients and forget their own. Halloran et al (1996) note that though most hospitals provide retirement benefits for nurses, numerous factors prevent many nurses from enjoying these benefits. Downsizing, uneven career patterns, and poor representation often contribute to the problem. Moore and Biordi (1995) contend that current pension, benefit, and savings status of nurses suggest they will have inadequate income in retirement unless they actively manage personal finances or attend to the details of employee benefit packages.

The increasing numbers of nurses working in long-term care at various levels and numerous sites must band together and give retirement planning a high priority. The American Nurses' Association and other nursing organizations must expand their efforts beyond the "hospital" nurse. We as members must institute action. Nurses need to think of and plan for their own retirement needs. Just as we often say, "Physician, heal thyself," we would admonish, "Nurse, take care of thyself."

Retirement Transition. Atchley's (1975) classic definitions of the stages of retirement provide guidelines for nurses working with retirees. Just as we are aware of the significance of various stages of grieving and dying, we must become attuned to identifying stages clients are experiencing in the retirement process if we hope to serve them well (Box 20-5). There is some question about whether these phases progress in an orderly fashion.

Variables that emerge as critical to retirement adjustment are (1) the kind of work one has been involved in, (2) preretirement attitudes toward retirement, (3) health and social status before retirement, and (4) choices. The second variable is the most subject to alteration, and therefore the thrust of preretirement programs should be toward developing positive attitudes toward retirement and supportive social networks.

During the retirement transition, men who retire unwillingly are at risk. Alcoholism, depression, and suicide are three problems that may be particularly evident. Nurses may encounter such clients most frequently because their distress drives them to search for medical relief. Often they do not recognize the underlying depression. A nurse can be instrumental as a supportive, empathetic listener; by identifying the presence of depression (see Chapter 21); by instilling hope through assisting the client toward awareness of his or her transitory distress; by allowing the client time to fully review the work experience and its meaning to put it in order and gain closure; and by inquiring about other stressors that may add to the chaotic feelings.

Recent studies show increases in self-esteem and decreases in depression after retirement (Reitzes et al, 1996). One can speculate that society has changed in attitude toward work/nonwork, and present economic sustenance during retirement has improved.

"Bridge jobs" that provide part-time work in the move toward self-employment or nonemployment have proved to ease the retirement transition (Quinn and Kozy, 1996). These seem to be the wave of the future with increasing numbers of agencies, institutions, and corporations offering retirement incentive programs to workers with extensive seniority. These programs frequently involve gradual reductions in work.

Retirement and the Family. The effects of retirement on couples receive insufficient attention. How often are questions about the spouse's needs and interests included in preretirement planning? A couple whose relationship has

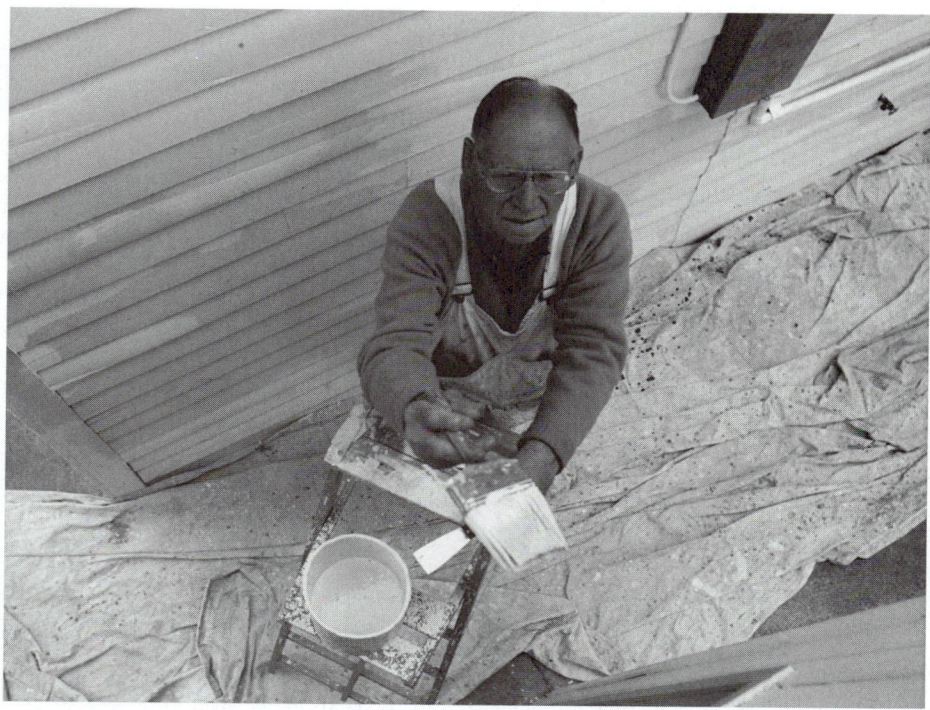

Part-time work. (Courtesy Rod Schmall.)

Box 20-5   Phases of Retirement

Remote: future anticipation with little real planning
Near: preparation and fantasizing regarding retirement
Honeymoon: euphoria and testing of the fantasies
Disenchantment: letdown, boredom, sometimes depression
Reorientation: developing a realistic and satisfactory lifestyle
Stability: personal investment in meaningful activities
Termination: loss of role due to illness or return to work

---

been warm and gratifying may find themselves able to tolerate increased interpersonal exposure. Conversely, those who have never enjoyed each other may find togetherness intolerable or an opportunity for growth as they face reconciliation with few ready distractions.

Vinick and Ekerdt (1991) found that when the husband retires there are severe feelings of impingement by the wife, but the acuity of these subside gradually as the couple develops new routines. Household tasks, companionship activities, and personal activities all must undergo alterations as the couple adapts. The retiree's adjustment may be equally difficult.

A pattern common to the present retired generation is that of the wife adapting to the husband's needs after re-

tirement: limiting her daytime social engagements, quitting her job to be with her husband, and fitting herself to his plans. It is important to let couples know each member needs time apart to maintain private lives as well as togetherness. Older women are becoming more assertive about their own retirement plans because many more are engaged in professions and positions of status than in previous decades.

Atchley (1979) has identified variables affecting couple adjustment to retirement: (1) effectiveness of communication; (2) decision-making patterns relating to money, space, and use of time; (3) role orientation (traditional or shared); and (4) level of affection and intimacy.

Follow-up contact by nurses involved in preretirement counseling to determine effects of retirement on a couple's relationship could be especially helpful. Nurses working with recent retirees might inquire about changes in communication patterns, decision making, and shared activities. Major personal adjustments are required of a spouse when the partner retires. Not enough attention has been given to this critical factor in retirement adjustment. Retirement often stimulates issues between spouses that had been submerged in the duties of child raising and occupational pursuits. Working couples often look forward eagerly to the companionship of the spouse in retirement.

Problems in adjustment usually are short lived and center around impingement on time or unrealistic expectations of the spouse. However, when either spouse is impaired, there are negative consequences for both partners. Those who have saved and planned for retirement activities and then find their companion unable to participate are particularly unhappy.

Other issues that emerge are the presence of an adult child in the home. "Boomerang" children are a common phenomenon in today's society because they find it financially impossible to establish their own homes. The couple who looked forward to time together may find the intrusion of children returning to the home a distinctly negative development. It is conceivable a couple in their late 60s will have both elderly parents and adult children depending upon them for material and psychologic support. In realistically planning for retirement an older couple should prepare to accommodate the needs of the generations above and below.

Retiring to a community.   More and more elders are retiring to senior communities. These are discussed in some detail in Chapter 13. Our concern in this chapter is with the transition and adaptation as they transpire. There have been numerous studies of these retirees because they form a collective group, in some ways homogenous and fairly available. In many of these secluded communities they are protected from intrusions by solicitors or researchers.

Silverstein and Zablotsky (1996) analyzed data from the Longtitudinal Study of Aging to identify the factors that led to moving from the general community to a retirement community. They found this most likely among elders who lived alone and had no children or none living nearby; some had moderate disabilities. They suggest that the move is often motivated not only by the social and amenity features but also by awareness of increasing frailty.

Adams (1995) surveyed residents of three retirement communities in Wisconsin and found that 38% of the 300+ who completed the questionnaires indicated they use both alcohol and high-risk medications. However, in a later study (1996), Adams found that the majority of individuals had decreased their alcohol intake after moving to the community.

Many elders retire to small towns and communities, sometimes in a hopeful retreat to the simpler rural life they remember from childhood. Unforeseen climatic conditions and the absence of readily available health care and social services often force them back to their original community within 2 or 3 years. Varied living situations in retirement are discussed in Chapter 13.

Satisfaction in Retirement.   The most powerful factors in retirement satisfaction are health status, sufficient income, and the option to continue working. Adequate income is often tied to the ability to continue some type of remunerative activity. Some companies and institutions in the United States are now encouraging part-time volunteer work among their preretirement personnel while paying them a full salary. The responsibility for initiating such action lies with the pre-retiree. Nurses may discuss this possibility with clients.

Other possibilities for the future include sabbaticals for workers of all ages, short work weeks, and serial careers.

Trends toward more flexible hours, reduction in work hours, and work sharing offer attractive options to some older persons. These accomodations are a means toward increasing job satisfaction and developing more options for the retirement years. Health conditions are the least subject to control by the retiree and apparently the most critical to perceived quality of life (Dorfman, 1995).

Preretirement programs are often helpful in terms of ultimate satisfaction postretirement, but few programs actually have any plan for follow-up assessment. Some companies, such as Corning, are doing so. We recommend nurses use a postretirement assessment tool such as the one in Figure 20-5 to determine how elders are adapting to retirement.

Gender and life satisfaction in retirement.   There appear to be distinct gender differences in the factors that contribute to satisfaction in retirement (Calasanti, 1996; Wolfson et al, 1993). Men seem to benefit more than women by being married when retired. The division of household chores creates dissatisfaction among women when they perceive little spousal support (Pina and Bengtson, 1995). These feelings are intensified among women who remained employed.

During preretirement planning these issues, which may seem small, should be discussed. Small annoyances over time become monumental as they accumulate. When these have not been addressed earlier, the nurse should inquire of the couple, "How are you dividing household chores?"

There is also a suggestion that retirement income is judged to be the reward for paid labor, and domestic labor is not considered within that equation (Meyer, 1990). This could create resentment if the male insists on holding tightly to the purse strings. Indeed, the structure of our Social Security benefit computation supports this inequity. Years that women are not being paid for work are entered as $00 in the benefit equation.

In a study of nearly 500 elders in rural Iowa, Dorfman (1995) found the presence of pulmonary disease was predictive of retirement dissatisfaction in both sexes, but men were more distressed by stroke and heart disease, whereas women were more upset by arthritis. We might speculate that the disorders that affect the ability to carry on most-valued activities contribute to the degree of the dissatisfaction of each.

Levels of preretirement commitment to the job, satisfaction with the spouse, and intrinsic self-esteem continue to influence postretirement self-esteem (Reitzes et al, 1996).

Overall, it appears that positive preretirement expectations are the greatest predictor of satisfaction in retirement, regardless of race, gender, or ethnicity (Honig, 1996).

Opportunities for New Development

Retirement is often thought of as a time to develop secondary interests—something to keep one interested in living. Our present elders are perhaps the only ones who have, in large numbers, the education, the health, the vitality, the opportunity, and the affluence to make retirement the most

Retirement Questionnaire

Date of birth _____
(month, day, year)

Sex: Male ☐   Female ☐

Total years in job from which you retired _____

Total years you have been retired _____

Marital Status:
☐ Never married
☐ Currently married
☐ Divorced & not currently married
☐ Spouse deceased & not currently married
☐ Not married; living with significant other

Current working status of self:
☐ Not working for pay/salary
☐ Working part-time (20 hrs/wk or less) for pay/salary
☐ Working part-time (more than 20 hrs/wk & less than 40 hrs/wk) for pay/salary
☐ Working full-time for pay/salary
☐ Looking for part-time job for pay/salary
☐ Looking for full-time job for pay/salary

If married, current working status of spouse (if not married skip this question)
☐ Not working for pay/salary
☐ Working part-time (20 hrs/wk or less) for pay/salary
☐ Working part-time (more than 20 hrs/wk & less than 40 hrs/wk) for pay/salary
☐ Working full-time for pay/salary
☐ Looking for work

My health is:
☐ Excellent
☐ Above average
☐ Good
☐ Fair
☐ Poor

How often do you do the following? If you answer yes, indicate the number of hours/week.

Watch television	☐ No	☐ Yes	_____ hrs/wk
Read	☐ No	☐ Yes	_____ hrs/wk
Travel within 100 miles	☐ No	☐ Yes	_____ hrs/wk
Do hobbies	☐ No	☐ Yes	_____ hrs/wk
Have sexual relations	☐ No	☐ Yes	_____ hrs/wk
Participate in religious activities	☐ No	☐ Yes	_____ hrs/wk
See relatives other than spouse	☐ No	☐ Yes	_____ hrs/wk
See former co-workers	☐ No	☐ Yes	_____ hrs/wk
See friends other than co-workers	☐ No	☐ Yes	_____ hrs/wk
Participate in social activities	☐ No	☐ Yes	_____ hrs/wk
Drink alcohol	☐ No	☐ Yes	_____ hrs/wk
Do regular physical exercise	☐ No	☐ Yes	_____ hrs/wk

What type(s) of retirement preparation did you have prior to retiring (Check all that apply)
☐ None
☐ Financial planning/investments
☐ Adjustment to retirement planning
☐ Retirement benefits
☐ Planning with family members for retirement
☐ Planning use of time in retirement
☐ Stress management
☐ Preparation of life after retirement

Figure 20-5. Postretirement assessment tool.

Check (√) any health problems that you *currently* have and if you are taking medication.

HEALTH PROBLEM	√ if currently have health problem	√ if taking medication for it	MEDICATION (indicate medication if known)
Heart Trouble			
Circulation Trouble			
Diabetes			
Arthritis			
High Blood Pressure			
Memory Loss			
Urinary Problems			
Cataracts			
Emphysema			
Cancer			
Nervousness			
Depression			
Hearing Loss			

Health Habits:
  Drink Alcohol
    ☐ Beer
    ☐ Wine
    ☐ Hard liquor
    ☐ Varies with situation
    ☐ Don't drink alcohol

  Exercise
    Type _____
    How many times a week _____

  Smoking
    ☐ Never smoked
    ☐ Yes
      Number of cigarettes/day _____
      Quit   ☐ Yes   ☐ No
      If yes, when _____

Diet
  How have your eating patterns changed?
    ☐ Unchanged
    ☐ Eat out more
    ☐ Eat at home more

Do you have the following (Check (√) all that apply)
  ☐ Advanced Directive
  ☐ A Living Will
  ☐ A personal Will
  ☐ None of the above

Continued

Figure 20-5, cont'd. For legend see opposite page.

What are your sources of transportation (Check (√) all that apply)
- ☐ Drive own vehicle
- ☐ Depend on others to drive
- ☐ Use public transportation
- ☐ Have no sources
- ☐ Do not go out
- ☐ Walk
- ☐ Bicycle

Check (√) your response to each of the following statements that most closely describe your feelings at this point in time. Use the key that follows: SA = Strongly agree, A = Agree, U = Undecided, D = Disagree, SD = Strongly disagree

STATEMENT	SA	A	U	D	SD
Retirement is what I thought it would be.					
I have plenty of things to do that I enjoy.					
I enjoy being active.					
I feel good about myself.					
I have people to rely on when problems occur.					
I enjoy retirement.					
I have enough to do with my time.					
I get up at the same time I did before I retired.					
Other people say that I am happily retired.					
I rarely feel lonely.					
A pet is currently an important part of my life.					
I have friends that I associate with on a regular basis.					
I have sufficient financial resources to meet my basic needs.					
People regularly visit my home.					
I am rarely bored.					
I enjoy life more now that I am retired.					
Other people tell me what to do.					
My living standards have declined since I retired.					
I worry about the future.					
I was adequately prepared for retirement.					
I feel that depression is a problem for me.					
Adjusting to retirement was easy for me.					
I worry about my health.					
Retirement is easier for me now than when I first retired.					
IF MARRIED, CONTINUE, IF NOT, STOP.					
My spouse and I have switched some roles since I retired.					
My marriage is more satisfying since I retired.					
My spouse and I get along better than we did before I retired.					
I sometimes feel in the way around the house.					
My spouse and I have better sexual relations than we did before I retired.					
My spouse says I am around the house too much.					
My spouse and I look forward to retirement together.					

Figure 20-5, cont'd. For legend see p. 722.

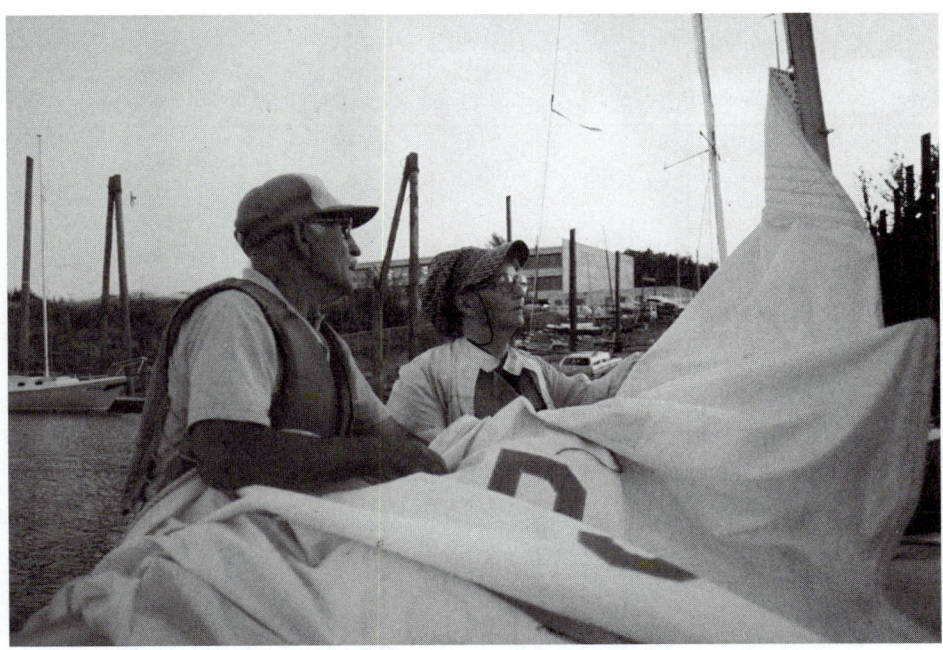

Going sailing. (Courtesy Rod Schmall.)

creatively productive and gratifying stage of life. Retirement can be the time when one is free to pursue a lifelong avid interest. Sara worked in a chemistry lab until retirement . . . then she began teaching creative writing and published her first book at age 80 (Ruffner, 1991). After spending much of his life as a prison officer, Joe built a trimaran and, with arduous study, became a certified celestial navigator through the U.S. Power Squadron. At age 63 he and his eager wife were ready to sail the seven seas (Pierre, 1992). Now, at age 67 he and his wife have settled into a comfortable routine with their Web pages, which occupy much of their waking time. The Bennetts left the utopia of Sun City, Arizona, to work on medical mission ships serving the South Pacific Islands (Mercy on the main, 1993). It appears that for the fortunate individuals retirement years can indeed be the best years of their lives and the most gratifying.

For individuals wishing to start new careers in paid work, there are many organizations throughout the nation that assist the elder to move into new areas of the work force (see Resources). Sum and Fogg (1991) discuss the concept of "bridge jobs" as designed for the older worker who retires or is laid off from the key work role and wishes to continue some kind of work before fully retiring. The Job Training Partnership Act (administered under Social Security Title III programs) is one option open to the elderly for retraining, though it is seldom used by them.

Cahn, a professor of law at the Columbia School of Law has developed a Time Dollar Network. The program combines networking, volunteering, and the barter system. Members offer volunteer services in numerous activities, and the time spent is "banked" for them. When they need

similar services, they can draw on the time they have accrued. For example, they may care for an elder so the caregiving spouse can have respite time. They can then draw on this time from some other member to provide a service such as home repair, shopping, or whatever assistance is needed (Greer, 1995)(see resources at the end of the chapter). The Robert Wood Johnson Foundation (Service credit banking in managed care, 1995) reports the completion of a similar program in which volunteers are given service credit in managed care organizations for providing nonmedical assistance such as transportation, medication monitoring, shopping, and light housekeeping services. They then receive credits from the organization toward similar services if and when they need them.

Volunteerism

Thirty-five percent of the population 65 and older are engaged in some type of volunteer work. It is estimated that seniors contribute 3.6 billion hours of volunteer service to organizations annually (Fischer, 1996). Volunteer service provides an attractive new role for many aged who have previously not had the luxury of investing time without monetary return. Interestingly, although women have traditionally volunteered, men have experienced the greatest increase in volunteerism among the elderly. The number of older women who are volunteers has remained relatively constant (Table 20-7). The heaviest current volunteer activity and potential activity are found among the college-educated and more affluent older citizens.

Most people involved in volunteer work feel they are contributing to the community and filling gaps in services

Table 20-7   Percent of Adult Population Doing Volunteer Work: 1993

[Covers persons 18 years and over. Volunteers are persons who worked in some way to help others for no monetary pay during the previous year.]

Age, sex, race, and Hispanic origin	Percent of population volunteering	Average hours volunteered per week	Educational attainment and household income	Percent of population volunteering	Average hours volunteered per week	Type of activity	Percent of volunteers involved in activity
Total	**47.7**	**4.2**	Elementary school	31.8	(B)	Arts, culture, humanities	4.4
			Some high school	29.9	(B)	Education	15.7
18-24 years old	45.3	4.0	High school graduate ..	40.4	3.6	Environment	6.2
25-34 years old	46.1	3.1	Technical, trade, or			Health	10.8
35-44 years old	54.5	4.8	business school	49.2	5.0	Human services	9.8
45-54 years old	53.8	5.2	Some college	56.9	4.3		
55-64 years old	46.6	4.1	College graduate	67.2	5.0	Informal	17.2
65-74 years old	42.9	4.8				International, foreign	1.3
75 years old and over ..	36.4	(B)	Under $10,000	34.0	(B)	Political organizations	3.7
			$10,000-$19,999	37.0	3.7	Private, community	
Male	43.9	4.3	$20,000-$29,999	52.5	4.2	foundations	2.2
Female	51.2	4.2	$30,000-$39,999	56.3	4.9		
			$40,000-$49,999	55.1	3.6	Public and societal benefit ...	5.4
White	51.1	4.2	$50,000-$59,999	56.9	4.1	Recreation - adults	5.4
Black	29.1	3.7	$60,000-$74,999	66.6	6.1	Religion	24.1
			$75,000-$99,999	58.1	(B)	Work-related organizations ..	6.9
Hispanic*	32.4	(B)	$100,000 or more	67.5	(B)	Youth development	11.7

From U.S. Bureau of the Census: *Statistical abstract of the United States: 1995,* ed 115, Washington, DC, 1995.
B Base figure too small to meet statistical standards for reliability. *Hispanic persons may be of any race.
Source: Hodgkinson, Virginia, Murray Weitzman, and the Gallup Organization, Inc.: *Giving and volunteering in the United States: 1994 edition.* (Copyright and published by INDEPENDENT SECTOR, Washington, DC, Fall 1994.)

that otherwise might be unmet. Thus self-esteem and a sense of usefulness prevail, though Fischer and Schaffer (1993) caution that some service programs exploit volunteers and deny them any status or authority. In her study, she notes that the most successful programs expect a lot from their volunteers and invest considerable time in training and sustaining their interest. Clear guidelines, periodic review, and feedback are critical to the success of any volunteer program.

Some of the programs that include or require senior volunteers are National Network on Aging (Nursing Home Ombudsman Program, National Nutrition Program), ACTION (Foster Grandparents [FGP], Retired Senior Volunteer Program [RSVP], Volunteers in Service to America [VISTA], Senior Companion, Peace Corps), Legal Service Corporation, Service Corps of Retired Executives (SCORE) (Small Business Administration), Department of Veterans Affairs, and National Volunteer School Program (teacher aides). Many of these volunteers are paid or are given other inducements to supplement low incomes. Though considered volunteer activity, all ACTION programs provide some minimal income.

Retired professionals have skills that are not being used. In these fiscally troubled times it may be possible to involve more of them in volunteer programs. The formulation of means to attract these persons into volunteerism requires

consideration of the special needs of retired professionals. Older volunteers serving the elderly indicate that the specific job responsibilities are the criteria for selection rather than a preference to work with a certain age group.

One of the predominant reasons for joining volunteer groups is the social contact with other volunteers. Weinstein et al (1995) found that retirees who volunteered more than 10 hours per week scored significantly higher in satisfaction and lower in boredom, as shown on the Purpose in Life test, than those who volunteered fewer than 10 hours weekly. This would seem to indicate that investment of self and contact with others needs to have a certain level of commitment to be most enriching.

Interfaith Volunteers. Communities nationwide have organized interfaith volunteer services to provide in-home services for isolated frail elders. These efforts have been organized and supported by the Robert Wood Johnson Foundation. The Interfaith Volunteer Caregivers Program (IVCP) demonstrates the commitment of religious congregations to serving the needs of elders in the community. Initially programs were funded through churches in 25 communities. Within 3 years, 900 participating congregations had recruited 11,000 volunteers and provided in-home service to 26,000 elders (Weisfeld, 1988). Individuals interested in developing or participating in such a program should see Resources at the end of this chapter.

Crime Busters. McLeod reports a volunteer program in which elders join the National Sheriffs' Association. They work for no pay and provide services primarily for small communities with insufficient police and sheriff's personnel. They aid in the fight against crime in myriad ways: locate criminal tracks on a computer trail, ride horseback with the sheriff's posse, participate in search and rescue efforts, and help with traffic control (McLeod, 1994). They have developed computerized crime analysis units and patrol neighborhoods with pagers. Most do not have police powers; they simply report anything that appears suspicious. They also assist in managing victims' assistance programs by contacting victims and informing them of their rights and providing whatever assistance they can. An officer in Alexandria, Virginia, says, "We use them in communications, we use them in patrol, we use them in records. We use them in every facet of the agency."

Health Care Volunteers. Elderly volunteers serving in hospitals find that not only do they help others, but, also their own health is improved in the process (Hospital volunteers: a hands-on job, 1993). They act as foster grandparents, tutor ill children, and write letters for or visit with ailing elders. Johns Hopkins Hospital has had such a volunteer program for 60 years and finds the services of elders invaluable.

There is a meaningful role for senior citizens as workers in nursing homes. Legislation that would train and pay older people who may wish to work in nursing homes would be desirable. Older volunteers have been used extensively in nursing homes without pay. One concern is the tendency for older adults to become depressed when constantly exposed to the limitations of their age peers. The support of a consistent coordinating individual is *essential* to the success of such programs and may produce a gratifying experience. Peer counseling training is important.

A newsletter from a long-term care facility posted in settings where senior citizens gather or reside, explaining various volunteer activities (such as entertaining, office work, transportation aide, cafeteria attendants, activity assistants, workshop assistants, boutique salespeople, gardeners, and friendly visitors) would be a useful method of recruiting volunteers.

Peer Counseling. Several institutions have peer counseling training programs in which volunteers learn interviewing skills and develop their ability to deal with patients who are lonely, depressed, or dying. These volunteer roles have potential for maintaining or elevating self-esteem of volunteers and patients and hold great potential for meeting the needs of many elderly. The older generation, often skeptical of professional counseling, will accept the help of peers.

A growing number of peer counseling programs are appearing across the United States. They train elders to help other elders deal with the major transitions of life: relocation, death of a spouse, retirement, or other crises that occur in the process of aging. Some counselors provide telephone counsel, and others go to the home or visit the institutionalized. The proviso is that the elder request help and the response be prompt. Some are based in churches, some are based in suicide prevention programs, and yet others make regular visits to retirement centers, senior centers, and institutions. For further information regarding development of peer counseling services see Resources at the end of the chapter.

Hoffman (1983) suggests that screening criteria be followed carefully in selecting peer counselors (Box 20-6). She found the ideal training period was a 2-hour class twice weekly for 5 weeks followed by a 10-week practicum. The students were placed in a number of agencies to provide services under the supervision of agency personnel. They identified themselves as volunteers rather than counselors and often helped their clients across several levels of care.

Typically the peer counselor has a case load of two to six clients and performs functions such as listening, providing information and referral, telephone reassurance, counseling families and groups, and making home visits. Based on their understanding of the painful experiences of old age, they add a dimension of friendship and empathy to the counseling function. Nurses assist in identifying clients most likely to benefit from peer counseling.

Volunteer Training and Roles

Training programs, supervision, and ongoing support are critical to the success of volunteer programs (Musson et al, 1997). The following considerations guide the development of successful volunteer programs:

- Administrative support of volunteers
- Clearly determined goals for the program
- A specific orientation program with printed support materials to give volunteers
- Buddy systems to orient and reinforce volunteer role and expectations
- Periodic evaluations and modifications as needs indicated by volunteer participants
- Determination of specific awards and rewards to sustain interest and involvment

Individuals should be encouraged to begin minimal participation in volunteer programs prior to work role discontinuation. This can serve as a bridge of continuity. There are certain identifiable steps in the full development of a role as a volunteer. These can be seen in Box 20-7. Group involvement and group meetings will solidify and strengthen the identification with the volunteer role.

Some people suggest that volunteering is an abuse and that individuals should be paid for what they do. Some of this thinking may be the outgrowth of a materialistic orientation that believes individual value is reflected in currency. Volunteers that we have contact with believe the payment comes in the enrichment of their lives. Some, such as the Foster Grandparents program, are particularly fulfilling.

Box 20-6

Screening Criteria for Peer Counselors

1. The applicant must be 60 years or older.
2. The applicant must show regular attendance at a senior center.
3. The applicant must be in good physical health.
4. The applicant must not have been seriously depressed in the preceding year.
5. The applicant must desire training and be able to attend all training sessions and a 10-week practicum placement.
6. The applicant must be motivated to work as a peer counselor for at least 6 months following training, with a time commitment of at least 3 hours per week (to compensate for training time).
7. The applicant must have an eclectic rather than a specific religious orientation toward helping.
8. The applicant must show evidence of flexibility.

Box 20-7

Steps in Development of Volunteer Role

1. Volunteer role uses skills from previous work or community experience. A gain in status, prestige, and community sanction is experienced.
2. Volunteer role improves interest in self and others. Dependence is reduced, and interdependence is created.
3. Feedback is gained from recipients of services. Self-view is improved, and resourcefulness is recognized.
4. Social and psychologic stimulation is found in volunteer settings. Personal growth and development occur as skills are refined.
5. Community rewards and recognition are awarded. New roles of social significance are internalized.

Box 20-8

Volunteer Community Services

Perform in a choral group in nursing homes
Sew for institutionalized children
Help deprived persons obtain entitlements
Provide widow-to-widow help
Perform American Cancer Society clerical work
Assist at nutrition programs
Make dolls for hospitalized children
Assist children in school remedial reading programs
Organize food co-op, sell to elders at discount prices
Raise money with bazaars, white elephant sales for nutrition programs
Serve as musicians for senior dances
Teach language classes in senior centers
Become "Fix it" men
Prepare kits for Red Cross Blood Mobile
Telephone for homebound
Present puppet shows to schoolchildren, bringing history alive
Serve coffee and act as language interpreters at geriatric centers
Help residents settle into new living arrangements, nursing or retirement homes
Assist with shopping, walking around
Teach remedial math to school children
Present slide shows as museum volunteers in churches and senior centers
Assist in child care shelters
Work with retarded—teach swimming, cooking, and activities of daily living
Alert isolated elderly to services and Supplemental Security Income (SSI)

It is important to remember that altruism never dies. Elders invariably wish to in some way be contributing members of society as long as they live. Nurses may explore the possibilities with elders and discuss latent interests they may wish to develop and ways they can contribute to others from their vast store of life experience and creative endeavors. Some of the myriad ways they may be involved are seen in Box 20-8.

LOSS OF SPOUSAL ROLE

Mavis and her husband, George, lived on a small rural farm and produced a large family. They were hard working and self-sufficient. Mavis was happiest when on Saturday night she had the childrens' shoes polished, clothing laundered and pressed, pies made, and everything prepared for Sunday church services. George made sure the car was clean, the garden watered and weeded, the vegetables harvested, eggs gathered, and chicken ready to prepare for Sunday dinner. As the children grew up they migrated to city jobs, but Mavis and George were able to maintain their rather isolated and somewhat anachronistic lifestyle. Mavis knew she was slowing down somewhat as she got older, but that really didn't alter her lifestyle, it just took a little longer to accomplish all she wanted to. George seemed as sturdy as ever, but one morning, at 75 years of age, he simply didn't get out of bed. A massive heart attack had occurred while he was sleeping. Soon the children insisted Mavis sell the farm, which she knew she must. Six months after George's death Mavis was living with her oldest daughter in the suburbs of a large city. There was little for her to do and nothing that made her feel needed. She was dependent on her daughter for transportation, so she rarely left her home. She had, within the course of a year, confronted developmental, situational, and health-illness transitions.

When nurses think of transitions, it is likely that several may be occurring simultaneouly that involve role change, status change, social change, and changes in self-image. Mavis was almost totally dependent on others, in an unfamiliar setting, and learning to be a widow.

Erikson et al (1986) identified the characteristics that tend to portend a satisfactory resolution after the loss of a spouse. Individuals who have been self-confident and competent seem to fare best. One woman said, "The crux of widowhood adjustment is how much you did for yourself before he died."

Losing a partner, when there has been a long, close, and satisfying relationship is essentially losing one's self and one's core. The mourning is as much for self as for the dead individual. Part of oneself has died with him or her, and even with satisfactory grief resolution, that self will never return. Even those widows who reorganize their lives and invest in family, friends, and activities often find that many years later they still miss their "other half" profoundly.

Widowhood

A student learns from her grandmother: "Both of my grandmothers lived alone since before I was born. Each were healthy, independent people who had learned to live alone. My maternal grandmother often said it was wonderful to do exactly what she wanted, when she wanted to do it" (Holiday Bruck, age 31).

By age 75, 63% of all women will be widows, and 20% of men will be widowers (U.S. Bureau of the Census, 1995). Each year about 645,000 women are widowed; most of these are elderly (Population Reference Bureau, 1995). For those who have been married for many years this is the most difficult adjustment one can face, aside from the loss of a child. This in itself exemplifies some of the principles of transitions. Older spouses are somewhat prepared for and expect that one must die before the other, but the loss of a child is not expected.

Robinson (1995) found that during the second year of spousal bereavement most widows were adapting to the new roles and had developed a supportive social network. Many studies have found widowers adapt more slowly to the loss and often marry quickly. Kanacki et al (1996) did not find this to be true. In a study of 31 widows and 35 widowers there were no significant gender differences in adaptation. Tudiver et al (1995) found that widowers involved in a support group used fewer health care resources than those who did not have such mutual support.

The Swedish twin study, which has followed over 2000 twins since 1984 (Lichtenstein et al, 1996), describes the recently widowed (less than 3 years) and the long-term widowed (more than 5 years). This gives some guidelines for expectations of the process of transition from bereaved widow to adjustment. In addition, these studies found that the young-old were more stressed than the oldest-old during the adaptational process, but both groups ultimately achieved a satisfactory adaptation.

Anxiety and fear are prevalent throughout the first 3 years of bereavement in women who were previously prone to anxiety and dependency (Sable, 1989). Imposed or externalized perceptions of religion tended to also increase distress and poor health after spousal death (Rosik, 1989). From these studies one might speculate that those individuals who felt less in control of their lives and more a victim of exter-

nal forces may have a more difficult adjustment to widowhood. These would be fruitful avenues of investigation.

Those who sought early help with their grief process were feeling depressed, unable to cope, and had poorer perceived health (Caserta and Lund, 1992). Other factors that seem to trigger the need for professional grief counseling are recent disability, having few friends, and having children who are not geographically and emotionally close (Goldberg et al, 1988).

Aber (1992) found that women who have been engaged in paid work during their married lives adapt to widowhood with fewer episodes of illness than those women who have focused solely on their homemaking role. Speculation is that working outside the home provides women with confidence, independence, and autonomy that may act as a buffer during the stress of grieving. On the other hand, because widowhood and poverty often go hand in hand, it is probable that working women have more resources to provide a healthier lifestyle.

Silverman (1987) found distinct differences in men and women in their successful adaptation to the death of a spouse. Women found satisfaction in freedom and newfound abilities while maintaining their connectedness to others. Men found themselves taking more responsibility for maintaining caring networks and other activities previously managed by the wife. Both men and women seemed to develop another, previously uncultivated, part of themselves. From Silverman's data we see that the study of widowhood must go beyond the first years of acute grief to truly understand the transformations that occur.

Transitions in Widowhood. Acute reactions usually subside by the second year, and it becomes possible to make the past a part of one's personal history. Maintaining an intact role in work or the community may attenuate the confrontation with a new reality at home.

Patterns of adjustment can be seen in Box 20-9. Stages of the transition to a new role as a widow or widower are proposed as guides to intervention rather than as predictive or prognostic indicators.

Widowhood is a stage in the life course that leads to a new identity. The transitional phase of grief if handled appropriately leads to the confirmation of a new identity. It is the end of one stage of life and the beginning of another. Seldom in life is there such an abrupt and distinct breach that creates the opportunity for the emergence of a new identity.

Personal interests and attributes long suppressed in the role of wife spring forth as a plant sprouting in the springtime. When the long-frozen winter is over, the woman emerges, shedding the widow's weeds, ready to cultivate her strength and independence to the fullest. Autonomy and individuation are avidly sought. The self, previously embedded in the identity of another, tries to emerge from the cocoon, not always successfully, but those who do emerge gain a new identity. An English widow said, "I am a different person than I was 14 years ago." Another widow said, "My friends, values, interests, understanding have all changed.

Box 20-9   Patterns of Adjustment to Widowhood

Stage One: Reactionary (first few weeks)

Early responses of disbelief, anger, indecision, detachment, and inability to communicate in a logical, sustained manner are common. Searching for the mate, visions, hallucinations, and depersonalization may be experienced.

INTERVENTION: Support, validate, be available, listen to talk about mate, reduce expectations.

Stage Two: Withdrawal (first few months)

Depression, apathy, physiologic vulnerability occur; movement and cognition are slowed; insomnia, unpredictable waves of grief, sighing, and anorexia occur.

INTERVENTION: Protect against suicide and involve in support groups.

Stage Three: Recuperation (second 6 months)

Periods of depression are interspersed with characteristic capability. Feelings of personal control begin to return.

INTERVENTION: Support accustomed lifestyle patterns that sustain and assist person to explore new possibilities.

Stage Four: Exploration (second year)

Individual begins new ventures, testing suitability of new roles; anniversaries or holidays, birthdays, and date of death may be especially difficult.

INTERVENTION: Prepare individual for unexpected reactions during anniversaries. Encourage and support new trial roles.

Stage Five: Integration (fifth year)

Individual will feel fully integrated into new and satisfying roles if grief has been resolved in a healthy manner.

INTERVENTION: Assist individual to recognize and share own pattern of growth through the trauma of loss.

I've developed a complete new way of life" (Silverman, 1987). "I sing in a stronger voice; it is no longer a duet. Yet, even with the new sense of self, on certain occasions the haunting melody of the past intrudes and for a few moments the desire to harmonize again is wrenchingly present" (Ebersole, 1989).

There is tremendous diversity in lifestyles of widows, but a new breed of older widow is emerging: the career-minded cosmopolitan, active in family, religious, recreational, and political groups and not geographically restricted. Better educated and financially sound, these widows are better able to reorganize their lives after the heavy grief is over. They are self-sufficient and manage their homes and lives with a sense of well-being. In age-segregated communities such as retirement villages the widows find activities and friendships with ease and largely enjoy their living situation. Many of these communities are ethnically and economically quite homoge-

neous. These women have loose but pleasurable ties with children and receive little from them in services or emotional support. Old friendships are maintained by correspondence, visits, and telephone calls (Neale, 1987).

Yet, the long-term effects of spousal loss pervasively influence the lives of many in terms of health, self-efficacy, life satisfaction, and future orientation (Arbuckle and deVries, 1995). Widowhood significantly increases the likelihood of being placed in a nursing home (Wolinsky and Johnson, 1992).

Variations in Widowhood. A very high proportion of widows do not wish to remarry and have no intention of giving up their independence. Gentry et al (1987) studied the differences in widows who do not wish to remarry, those who wish to but do not, and those who remarry.

Widows considering remarriage were on the average 10 years younger, were more educated, and had a higher income than those who did not consider it. Remarried widows were statistically similar to those who considered remarriage. The major reasons women gave for not wanting to remarry were valuing independence and inability to find a husband as nice as the deceased spouse. Other reasons included the following: still mourning husband, too old, economics, not enough men, and children's disapproval (Gentry et al, 1987). One third of the widows in the study liked being unmarried.

Widows who considered remarriage were primarily interested in love and companionship. Of the women who remarried, 69% reported thinking that marriage would solve problems for them. Half of the women reported conflicts with children and family over their decision to remarry. Remarried widows reported fewer concerns than those who did not wish to marry. The group with most concerns were those who wished to remarry but had not. All three groups experienced similar amounts of stress.

Erikson et al (1986) found that the widowed who remarried after the death of a long-term spouse often spoke of the youthful marriage as the most significant and the one that lasts forever. For those who believed in a reunion with the loved one after death, they expected it would be with the first spouse. Even those who considered a second marriage satisfactory in every way seemed to feel that the first love was most significant.

In the minds of our remarried subjects, marriage in youth and marriage in later life seem to represent two different kinds of intimacy. Marriage in youth appears to imply the fusion of individual identities in mutual intimacy, and those people view this fusion as permanent. In contrast, marriage in later life seems to represent a commitment to companionship. Although that commitment involves intimacy, sacrifice, compromise, and reciprocity, although it may be expected to last for the rest of life, it nonetheless remains separate from the early, intimate fusion that seems to transcend death and time.*

*From Erikson E, Erikson J, Kivnick H: *Vital involvement in old age: the experience of old age in our time,* New York, 1986, WW Norton.

There are also great cultural variations in the experience of widowhood.

Filipinos. Students, as they visit Filipino elders in the community, frequently find the aged widow has resumed the "housewife chores" and child care activities while all the adult members of the family work outside the home. Often the aged woman complains but feels it is her debt to the family for the resources they are providing.

Canadians. Canadian widows are much like those in the United States with some exceptions. They more often have lived in one locale, and siblings, friends, and church are notably present in their support systems. Factors identified that were significant predictors of positive morale were income, remarriage, education, health, small families, and solitary activities as well as social activities and religiosity.

African-Americans. Older African-American widows seem to have an enormous reservoir of emotional and religious strength and capacity for hope that has undergirded them from their slave ancestry. They are poorer than others and have fewer societal supports but stronger informal, reciprocal support systems (McDonald, 1987). The resurgence of the African-American multigenerational extended family, particularly in urban areas, often casts the widow as matriarch of the family. She may be the homeowner and chief provider for younger members, and thus much of her role remains unchanged even though the husband is gone.

Hispanics. Bereavement for the traditional Hispanic woman may be more difficult because of perceived cultural powerlessness. Those who have been dutiful wives have given over all decisions to their husbands and when widowed, must learn to make decisions. Rituals of grief, such as *luto,* exacerbate feelings of depression and loneliness as the widow goes into a strict period of social isolation and wearing black clothing. In addition, grief is complicated because Hispanic widows show outsiders the image of a perfect marriage when in reality the husband may have been unfaithful and abusive. Because of a sense of loyalty, this is rarely admitted. Segura (Fletcher-Stoelje, 1988) has established a Hispanic Widowed Person's Task Force and has written a book, *How to Survive an Unfaithful Husband, Before and After Death.* (See Resources at the end of the chapter for additional information.)

Widowers

Widowers are an elusive group, their grief often hidden in distorted "manliness." Widows' groups abound but not so for the widower. He is sometimes found in grief support groups but usually carries his pain alone. Historically, when maternal death rates were high, a man often had three or four wives and as many as 30 children. The old man, when widowed, remained the patriarch of the family with his needs attended by daughters, unmarried sisters, and other women within the family. Now, with the extended family dispersed, he is left to his own devices as long as he is functional.

Older widows receive considerable attention in the literature and among service providers because there are so many in late life. Widowers are seldom studied and even less frequently the recipients of services related to their bereavement.

Hogstel (1985) found that although their experience is in many ways similar to that of widows, there are some distinct differences. Widowers who must, for whatever reasons, reside with a son or daughter find the adjustment very difficult and threatening. They also report fewer physical manifestations of comfort are given; the hugs and holdings are much less frequent than those given to widows. Although many remarry precipitously, they often fear impotence and frequently experience it in the second marriage. This can most often be remedied but may, too often, simply be accepted fatalistically. Suggestions from Hogstel (1985) for working with widowers will be useful to nurses:

- Sponsor self-help groups in the community for widows and widowers.
- Discuss sexuality and recommend therapy when needed.
- Watch for signs of severe depression and make immediate contact with family and/or referral for mental health.
- Arrange classes for cooking and other homemaking skills.
- Provide information about homemaking services.
- Provide information about resources such as AARP and RSVP (Retired Senior Volunteer Programs).
- Encourage involvement in volunteer programs such as SCORE (Service Corps of Retired Executives).
- Encourage churches to sponsor programs, groups, and outings for older widowers.

Wives are the "kin-keepers" (Troll et al, 1979). They keep ties with relatives and friends and are usually the organizers of social and recreational activities. Even when the husband's career has been the central socializing force, the wife has been the social agent. When the wife dies, the husband is set adrift without his rudder. If he remains in the work role, he will immediately be seen as a potential candidate by single women and widows who are marriage minded. If he is retired, he is prone to isolation. In grief support groups, if he can find one not devoted only to widows, he is grossly outnumbered and less able to openly express grief, as well as being vulnerable to "women bearing pies."

Even though middle- and upper-class white men are seen as occupying the power base in society, they are among those most deprived of supports when grieving. To the extent they have occupied the role of provider they are further deprived by having no one left for whom to provide.

In search of patterns of adaptation among widowers we have gathered experiential and anecdotal data from friends, acquaintances, and colleagues. We are aware this has limited application, but it may enhance awareness and stimulate much-needed research on this subject.

Andrew was widowed at 60 years old after he had cared for his wife through a long and painful illness. His monogamous marriage of 40 years to a professional woman who had commandeered his life as she did her career left him with few internal or external resources. His career in the Army and the pattern of depending on his wife resulted in his having made few decisions about his own life. He was content to have others tell him what to do. His social life had been designed by her and his work life by his commanding officers. He had given some thought to what he would do when his wife died and immediately began searching for a female companion. His female companion was a professional woman, similar to his wife in many ways. A disinterested observer would have immediately seen his attempt as an object replacement. His friends and family misunderstood his lack of open grief and apparent disregard of a "decent period of mourning." They withdrew from him at the time he most needed their support. Unfortunately, his new companion did not like his dependency, which, exacerbated by grief, overwhelmed her. She also began to withdraw. Within 6 months after the death of his wife, Andrew was searching the "singles" advertisements and had joined several singles clubs. The saga of the search continued for years, always ending with the woman leaving, often because he was unable to really give himself to the relationship. He was unable to find his wife. He is now a lonely man of 70 years, still searching but with even less interest. He talks a lot about feeling old and wonders if he will live much longer. Materially he is well off, but socially he is poverty stricken.

Chester's wife died of a virulent and invasive cancer 6 weeks after it was diagnosed. This marriage, his second, had been one of mutual respect, love, and companionship. Both were writers and had lived in the rarified atmosphere of writers and publishers in New York City. They had dozens of friends and acquaintances but few intimates because they had lived for each other and their careers. Chester's psyche, frail at best, was grievously wounded. He was unable to function and eventually lost his job. He returned to his previous hometown on the West Coast and attempted to reestablish a bond with his first wife and his two children, who had become physically and emotionally distant over the years. Failing in that attempt was another blow to his ego. He found a nongratifying job and managed to keep it, although he spent his evenings isolated in a small apartment, drinking, crying, and sleeping. His neglect of his physical needs and lack of emotional support eroded his health. He was hospitalized several times. His grief consumed him for 3 years. He finally met a woman he thought he loved, a writer, somewhat like his wife, but his physical deterioration had left him impotent, and the relationship was short lived. He returned to New York City and found a job as an editor that demanded all his time and thought. His work has become his obsession, and he has become even more demanding of himself and others.

George was a traditional man, a successful lawyer, and a courtly gentleman. His family life had been as circumscribed and well planned as all the other elements of his existence. He nursed his wife through a long illness with the assistance of his daughters. He was dutiful and loving. When his wife died, he had many helpful friends and assistance from his family. After 2 years his grief subsided and he began to think of another relationship. Friends were helpful and introduced him to various women, but he found that women had changed in their expectations and relations with men. They were too liberated for him to understand. After the failure of two attempts to court women he began to develop self-doubts that were uncharacteristic of him. He attempted to meet other women, but his diffident approach was mistaken as lack of interest and was not successful. He is still trying to find a woman who will appreciate him, and he will with the help of his friends.

Abe was more fortunate than most widowers. His wife openly planned with him for his survival after her death. She found a grief therapist for him and a financial manager. She not only gave him

permission to find new female relationships but recommended it. In addition, they had a large network of friends and family among the Jewish community. He grieved openly after her death and sought solace with her sister's family. He was included in all of their activities and encouraged to make their home his emotional shelter. He saw his grief therapist weekly and more often when needed, and he left the management of his financial affairs to his advisor. He was thus able to work through his grief without other impediments. He found it very difficult to be at home alone and scheduled activities every evening of the week to avoid it. He finally realized that the home held too many memories for him, and he moved. After several brief relationships with women, he found one who was right for him. With the passage of 5 years and consistent support he has achieved a new life for himself in which he appreciates his new companion for herself.

Although these vignettes are limited in their application, it seems the following themes can be identified:

- The search for the lost mate
- The neglect of self
- The inability to share grief
- The loss of social contacts
- The struggle to view women as other than wife
- The erosion of self-confidence and sexuality
- The protracted grief period

Nurses may be instrumental in resolving some of these issues by encouraging the individual to share thoughts and feelings with friends and family, to emphasize the need for maintaining male friendships, to provide resources such as groups or grief therapists, to encourage delay in making female attachments, and to discuss the effects of depression on sexuality. Nurses who are empathetic and responsive may find the grieving man misunderstands their intentions. It must be made clear, sometimes repeatedly, that during grief the individual is vulnerable to inappropriate alliances with women and must recover before the energy to make a real investment is possible.

Nurse's Role with Widows and Widowers

Nurses working with the bereaved will need to review Lindemann's classic grief studies to understand the initial somatic responses of the bereaved (Lindemann, 1944). Supporting the grief requires an extension of self to reconnect the severed person with a world of warmth and caring. Each gesture crosses the void to bring the lost back to the land of the living. No one nurse nor one family member can do this alone. Hundreds of small caring gestures build strength and confidence in one's ability and willingness to survive.

Feelings of the bereaved are not orderly or progressive. They are conflicted, ambivalent, suicidal, full of rage, and often suspicious. Widows and widowers may exhibit personality disorganization that would be considered mentally aberrant or frankly psychotic under other circumstances.

In a study by Gallagher et al (1983) elderly widows and widowers were evaluated for the effects of bereavement on mental health 2 months after the death of a spouse. In general there was no evidence of a serious psychopathologic condition, but women reported greater distress than men.

Older women in both the bereaved and the nonbereaved group evidenced higher levels of depression than men. Decision making and focused attention on the details of living require psychologic energy that is not available.

Admittedly, some handle grief with less apparent decompensation. The reason for emphasizing extreme reactions is to avert mislabeling and focusing on pathologic conditions. It is critical that grief reactions be accepted as personally valid and useful evidences of healing.

How then does a nurse recognize an aberrant, mentally unhealthy grief reaction? We cannot immediately assess this because grief reactions are so individual. Persons with few familial or social supports are very likely to need professional help to get through the early months of grief in a way that will facilitate recovery. Therefore the nurse will need to assess the support network rather than focus on unusual symptomatology. If adequate support is available, reintegration can be expected in 2 to 5 years.

Divorce

Divorce is considered in Chapter 18 as a stigmatizing event, though so common today that one is inclined to forget the ostracizing effects of divorce 60 years ago. There are yet elders who are firmly tied to the adage, "until death do us part." Anything short of that is viewed as failure in the eyes of God and social expectations.

Although only 6% of older persons are divorced, this may be a cohort effect that is rapidly changing because in the past 6 years the numbers of divorced elders has increased more than 4 times as rapidly as the increase in the elderly population (AARP, 1996). There are large generational and individual differences in expectations from marriage, but older couples are becoming less likely to stay in an unsatisfactory marriage.

Health care professionals need to be alert to the possibility of marriage dissatisfaction in old age and avoid assumptions. Nurses need to ask, "How would you describe your marriage?"

John's arthritis, vision, and hearing deficits prevent him or his wife from enjoying the camping, skiing, and outdoor activities they shared most of their adult lives. They both love good food and have pleasant times together, though Jennie often feels hampered by John's disabilities. She has never believed a wife should pursue her own interests regardless of those of the husband. Her children say, "Come mother, go with us to the mountains." Her reply, "I can't leave Dad here alone." Jennie doesn't necessarily expect life to be the way she would like it. She remembers the struggles, the losses, and the pain she and John have shared throughout their lives. These bind her more strongly to him than the happy moments. It is unlikely that Jennie will divorce her husband of 55 years though they share few interests and abilities.

Margaret, her sister, says, "Why don't you get out and do something?" Margaret talks about divorcing her husband of 50 years. She has not told him yet because she feels like a traitor. But, she says, "We really never shared anything. He was always pursuing his interests but thought I should be there waiting whenever he wanted me. I felt like a widow most of my married life, so I have

decided to make a real break. I am concerned about finances, though. I might not have enough if I go out on my own." She may, in fact, not leave but remain in the situation because of guilt and fear.

Long-term relationships are varied and complex with many factors forming the glue that holds them together.

Lanza (1996) studied the divorces of older women and found them attributed to the husbands' infidelity, retirement, or simply growing apart; wives often tended to blame themselves and felt they were in some way deficient or the divorce would not have occurred. Few divorces were initiated because of the wives' dissatisfaction. Lanza concluded that marital breakdown is more devastating in old age because it is often unanticipated and may occur concurrent with other significant losses.

At age 65 and beyond, 11.5% of women and 9.2% of men are divorced (U.S. Bureau of the Census, 1995). Those who divorce in late life have been largely neglected in research and support services.

As health care workers, our concern is with supporting a client's decision to seek a divorce and assisting him or her in the transition. A nurse should alert the client that a divorce will bring on a grieving process similar to that of the death of a spouse and a severe disruption in coping capacity until an adjustment to a new life is made. The grief may be more difficult to cope with because there are no socially sanctioned patterns as in widowhood. In addition, tax and fiscal policies favor married couples, and many a divorced elderly lady is at a serious economic disadvantage in retirement (Holden and Hsiang-Hui, 1996).

A nursing care plan related to dealing with individuals who have lost the spousal role, whether through death or divorce, can be seen in Table 20-8.

ROLE REVERSAL

Developmental transitions in relationships have received insufficient attention. An interesting area of investigation would be that of the elder's experience of moving from caregiver to care recipient. Most attention has been given to the experience of the caregiver and little to that of the old person and their adjustment to the need to be a care recipient. When a strong and independent elder retires because of failing health, the reaction to dependency and role reversal with the spouse may sap the patience and energies of both.

Long-standing relationships may reverse in the illness of old age. Sometimes a passive/dependent spouse may be unable to make the transition without considerable help. (See Chapter 17 for additional discussion of caretakers.)

An elderly couple, both over 80 years old with no family or close friends, lived in San Francisco. The husband was head of the house, made decisions, and managed the money. A sudden stroke left him unable to walk without assistance. His memory was also affected, and he became increasingly dependent on his wife, who was overwhelmed with being the "stronger" of the two. She was

Table 20-8	Nursing Care Plan to Deal with Loss of Spousal Role	
Nursing diagnosis	**Expected outcomes**	**Interventions**

Loss of identity, spousal role, and balance in dependence and independence related to loss of spouse as evidenced by decreased self-concept and self-esteem
Manifestations: feelings of uselessness, hopelessness; decreased pride in appearance; uninterested in developing new skills, hobbies, and social interactions; lacks initiative to take part in previous roles and activities; unable to manage own affairs
	The survivor will:
	  Verbalize feelings of self-worth and self-esteem
	  Set realistic goals that are readily achievable
	  Replace spousal role with self-role
	  Actively participate in meaningful social relationships
	  Begin to accept independent role
		Emphasize positive aspects of behavior and appearance, ignore negative aspects.
		Encourage reminiscing if helpful.
		Assist in setting realistic, meaningful, attainable goals.
		Treat with respect and recognize as an individual of worth.
		Encourage volunteer work, hobbies, and crafts if desired.
		Assist in replacing lost roles with new ones.
		Encourage new relationships or the rekindling of old ones.
		Confirm that need for a sexual relationship is normal and healthy.

From Alexander J, Kiely J: Working with the bereaved, *Geriatr Nurs* 7(2):85, 1986.

physically healthy but could not see well. She became depressed and suicidal. Repeatedly, when he was admitted to the hospital, she was told he needed more care than she could provide. She agreed to nursing home placement two or three times but was very critical of nursing home care and took him home prematurely, without adequate supportive services.

Assuming an unfamiliar role is difficult for both parties. The nurse should be alert to situations in which health care personnel may be able to provide supports and resources that make it possible for an individual to assume new responsibilities without being totally overwhelmed. When a spouse is ill and the mate needs to take over functions for both, it is essential that someone be available to give reinforcment, encouragement, and relief. A day-care program, routine visits from a community health nurse, or periodic assistance from a home health aide or a housekeeper may make it possible for the couple to continue to live together. One important consideration is counseling the couple to maintain as much independent function as possible for both persons.

ROLES OF CLIENT AND NURSES

During the transition from familiar roles to new ones, an individual needs the freedom to try various possibilities in an accepting atmosphere that encourages success, tolerates failure, and recognizes that progress is not accomplished by slow, even steps. In real life, progress follows a more wayward, uneven course. One is easily distracted and often falls back to the familiar. A nurse is most helpful in providing an accepting milieu that encourages independence and exploration and the realization of the uncertainty inherent in transitions.

KEY CONCEPTS

- Roles define individual and societal expectations of function.
- In a rapidly changing society roles quickly become anachronistic.
- Transitions are akin to shedding one's skin as a new one is generated.
- Ability to successfully negotiate transitions and develop new and gratifying roles depends upon personal and environmental supports, timing, clarity of expectations, personality and degree of change required.
- Elders may perceive more losses than gains in the transitions of aging.
- A major transitional issue for an elder is moving from health to illness and redefining oneself in terms of a chronic disorder. Nurses must work to ensure that this does not become the identity of the individual.
- The work role transition is the major change for men and increasingly for women, though they often continue their homemaker/caregiver role without interruption.
- Numerous patterns of retirement exist at present, and therefore retirement per se cannot be viewed categorically.
- Preretirement planning and postretirement follow-up significantly affect positive adaptation to the transition.

Nursing Diagnoses

The following potential diagnoses must be considered as well as diagnoses unique to the particular individual:
Adjustment, impaired
Anxiety
Conflict, decisional
Coping, ineffective
Family processes, altered
Fear

Grieving
Knowledge deficit
Personal identity disturbance
Relocation stress syndrome
Role performance, altered
Self-esteem disturbance

NURSING PROCESS AND NURSING DIAGNOSIS
Ineffective Coping—Retirement, Role Loss, Ill Health, Transition

Etiologies and Related Factors
Transition from work to retirement
Poor physical health/functional decline
Emotional problems/illness
Social isolation
Cognitive changes
Low socioeconomic resources

Defining Characteristics
Change in status
Decreased social activity
Withdrawal/apathy
Decreased life satisfaction
Hyperirritability
Sleep disturbance/insomnia
Disrupted familial and interpersonal relations
Change in activity level
Passivity
Dependence
Emotional isolation
Declining health status

Knowledge
Past coping patterns
Stress-adaptation theory
Reactions to loss (grief process)
Risk factors
Collaboration skills with other disciplines
Therapeutic communication

Crisis intervention
Retirement counseling skills
Physical and psychologic assessments
Life satisfaction assessment
Interventions for prior to and after retirement
Community and national resources
Client's avocational interests

Clinical Judgment and Related Skills
Prepare client for retirement, preretirement counseling
Elicit client's feelings
Assessment of physical and mental function prior to retirement
Include client/family in preparation
Provide sense of control
Conduct counseling sessions
Teach family about expected reactions
Design, implement, and evaluate a plan for gradual retirement

Evaluation
Recognizes grief stages of role loss
Few or no negative manifestations associated with retirement
Care continuity maintained
Regains maximum potential for a high level of function with the least amount of discomfort or emotional stress
Develops new interests that are gratifying

NEEDS ADDRESSED AND TASK STRENGTHS

Need for flexibility and capacity for change; need for integration of life events and roles (to maintain self-esteem and self-concept)
Plans ahead for major role changes

Amenable to life changes
Recognizes elements of lost roles and grieves
Reminisces about previous activities and relationships
Accepts chaotic feelings and functions during transitions

- There are definite gender differences in the roles and transitions common to the aging process.
- Volunteerism is becoming increasingly attractive to elders who feel the need to express their altruistic motives; some opportunities also supplement retirement income.
- Loss of spouse is the role change that has the greatest potential for maladaptation, and nursing support can make a significant positive difference in the transition.
- Widowers are a neglected group in the literature and in the service arena. They are particularly vulnerable to maladaptive behaviors and deterioration.
- The role reversal from provider to dependent can be very difficult and needs to be recognized and explored with the individual.

▲ CASE STUDY

Sandy was a professor at a small, private college in a metropolitan area. She had taught nursing for 25 years and thoroughly loved her work, but it had been a demanding year and she was very tired. There had been a rumor recently that the college was in trouble financially. Some of the most affluent alumni could no longer be counted on for gifts and endowments because the football coach had not produced a winning team now for several years. The tuition was becoming exorbitant, and because of that the college had recently lost some students to one of the three state college campuses within driving distance of the city. The trustees of the college, in a move to cut expenses, offered an incentive to professors who were willing to retire early; an extra year of service credit for every 6 years worked. Sandy was only 55 years old but thought that the 4 years of extra credit would bring her near minimum retirement age for Social Security (an error, of course, as her age did not change with her service credit). Rather impulsively she decided to accept the offer, after telling colleagues, "Well, you know how I love to travel. Why wait until I'm too old to enjoy retirement? Why don't you think about the offer, too? This is a once-in-a-lifetime opportunity." Near the end of the academic year the celebrations began: recognition, plaques, expressions of gratitude from students, and envy from her associates. It was a wonderful send-off. In the summer Sandy withdrew her savings and booked a cruise to the Greek islands. It was lovely, and she enjoyed every moment. She began to feel depressed when she got off the ship but knew it was only because the elegant cruise was over. However, as fall came around she began to feel more depressed. Most of her friends were teachers, and they were all back at work. Sandy briefly thought of going to Pittsburgh to visit her sister but gave that idea up because she and her sister had really never been very compatible. Then she was hit with some of the realities of early retirement: she could not withdraw any of her considerable tax-deferred savings before she was $59\frac{1}{2}$ years old without significant penalty, her health insurance coverage was considerably less comprehensive upon retirement, her colleagues were all busy, and she was very bored. Then the real blow fell. The college, in desperation, had dipped into the retirement funds to remain solvent, and the retirees' pensions were now at risk. Sandy's sister, who was a nurse, called to announce she wanted to come and stay a few days while she attended a conference in the city. When she arrived Sandy overwhelmed her with the litany of her woes. If you were Sandy's sister what would you do?

Based upon the case study, develop a nursing care plan using the following procedure*:

List comments of client that provide *subjective data.*

List information that provides *objective data.*

From these data identify and state, using accepted format, two *nursing diagnoses* you determine are most significant to this client at this time. List two *client strengths* that you have identified from data.

Determine and state *outcome criteria* for each diagnosis. These must reflect some alleviation of the problem identified in the nursing diagnosis and must be stated in concrete and measurable terms.

Plan and state one or more *interventions* for each diagnosed problem.

Provide specific documentation of source used to determine appropriate intervention. Plan at least one intervention that incorporates the client's existing strengths.

Evaluate success of intervention. Interventions must correlate directly with the stated outcome criteria in order to measure the outcome success.

STUDY QUESTIONS/ACTIVITIES

Identify several important family and social roles that elder members of your family fulfill. Discuss how their roles differ from those of their parents.

What are the factors to consider in role transitions, and how can transitions be made smoother?

What factors must be considered in the decision to retire?

Discuss the differences you would expect in adaptation to retirement between an individual who retired because of ill health and one who retired because he or she desired to do so.

How do you think retirement differs for men and women?

Describe what you think would be an ideal retirement.

Plan specific ways in which you would present a retirement seminar to workers in a microchip computer factory.

Explain the major issues in adaptation to a major role change such as retirement and widowhood.

Discuss how you think one can prepare in advance for widowhood.

---

*Students are advised to refer to their nursing diagnosis text and identify possible or potential problems.

Discuss the meanings and the thoughts triggered by the student's and elders' viewpoints expressed at the beginning of the chapter. How do these vary from your own experience?

RESEARCH QUESTIONS

What are the differences in the retirement experience of men and women born in the 1910 to 1919 cohort, the 1920 to 29 cohort, the 1930 to 39 cohort, etc.?

What personality factors are critical to coping with transitions?

What role transitions present the most difficulty, and what are the factors identified as most difficult?

What nursing supports are the most significant to adaptation during role transitions?

How many individuals pursue a second career after retirement, and what careers are they most likely to pursue?

What advance preparation for widowhood is most helpful?

What personality or religious factors may influence one's adaptation to widowhood?

RESOURCES

Volunteer Opportunities

Many older Americans use their leisure by contributing volunteer service to day-care centers, hospitals, schools, and other agencies. They can do this by offering to help a particular agency or by contacting the volunteer office of their local health and welfare council. Also, the Area Agency on Aging may be able to provide information.

A federal agency, ACTION, sponsors Older American Volunteer Programs, including Foster Grandparents (FGP), Retired Senior Volunteer Program (RSVP), and Service Corps of Retired Executives and Active Corps of Executives (SCORE/ACE). Information about local sites of these programs may be obtained from ACTION, 806 Connecticut Avenue, NW, Washington, DC 20525, (202) 254-7310.

WPS Volunteers
WPS-JD, AARP
1909 K Street, NW
Washington, DC 20049

Silver Foxes
Marzec Communications
PO Box 1218
Oak Brook, IL 60521

Points of Light Foundation
PO Box 66534
Washington, DC 20035

The Robert Wood Johnson Foundation
Route 1 and College Road East
PO Box 2316
Princeton, NJ 08543-2316
(609) 452-8701

Those interested in starting a new Interfaith Volunteer Caregivers (IVC) project in their community can take heart from knowing what an enormous resource faith congregations have proved to be. According to Kenneth Johnson, these projects need "the proper stimulus and some $20,000 in seed money—the first dollars to recruit a full-time director and set up shop to train volunteers. With all the other claims on congregation funds, outside first dollars are required to put in place a project with substance . . .We know that given a sufficient lead time the project can demonstrate its effectiveness, then local continuing support will be forthcoming." People interested in exploring the possibility of starting Interfaith Volunteer Caregiver projects in their communities may call the National Federation of IVC at (914) 331-1358 or write:

Virginia Schiaffino
Executive Director
National Federation of IVC, Inc.
105 Mary's Avenue
PO Box 1939
Kingston, NY 12401

Resources from the national federation include the following:

Recommendations on funding sources

A rich network of experienced IVC directors

An extensive handbook including all aspects of developing and running an IVC project

Sources of further training expertise and materials

Time Dollar Network is an exchange program in which elders bank volunteer time for their own use at a later time for a needed service. This is available in 40 states. For information contact Time Dollar Network, Dept P, PO Box 42160, Washington DC 20015.

Films and Videos

Alleviating Stress Associated with Nursing Home Admission examines the stress and anxiety experienced by patients and their families when they are admitted to a long-term care facility. The adjustment to nursing home living begins prior to admission and continues through the first several weeks or months after admission. The program shows how nursing staff can facilitate a successful transition through a series of interviews with nursing home residents, families, and staff; (20 minutes) [purchase, $300; rental, $100). From Video Press, University of Maryland at Baltimore, School of Medicine, Suite 133, 100 Penn Street, Baltimore, MD 21201, (800) 328-7450 or (410) 328-5497, fax (410) 328-8471.

A Week Full of Saturdays. Utilizing a topical documentary format, this film emphasizes the importance of preretirement planning for active adults in particular. Three different vignettes are presented to the viewer. This film is 16 mm, 3/4-and 1/2-inch videocassette, 17 minutes, in color, produced in 1979. Producer is Alternate Choice, Inc. Distributor is Filmakers Library, Inc, 133 East 58 Street, New York, NY 10022, (212) 335-6565 (sale, $375 [videocassette, $325]; rent, $40 [discussion guide available]).

But Not for Lunch is the story of an older man and woman's struggle to adjust to each other and to retirement. The man retires from his job with apparently no preparation for the time when he will have 24 hours to fill each day. His wife also seems unprepared for the problems she will face when her husband is home all day. This film is 16 mm, 30 minutes, in color, produced in 1977. Producer is Ardon D. Albrecht. Distributor is Lutheran Television-LLL Films, 2232 Welsch Industrial Court, St Louis, MO 63141, (800) 325-4054, (rent, $25).

Pre-retirement Planning . . . It Makes a Difference uses the retirement experiences of three couples and a widow, as told by the retirees, to address several important topics in planning for retirement: financial security, choice of housing arrangements and location, and meaningful postretirement activities. This film is 16 mm, 15 minutes, in color, produced in 1981. Producer is Blacksides, Inc. Distributor is National AudioVisual Center, 8700 Edgeworth Drive, Capitol Heights, MD 20743-3701, (800) 638-1300, (purchase, $160; rental, $40).

So What If It Rains departs dramatically from *A Week Full of Saturdays* on several counts. In the sequel we are introduced to people from various walks of life experiencing greater and lesser degrees of financial strain. Emphasized throughout are some of the harsher realities of living on fixed income. This film is 16 mm, 3/4-and 1/2-inch videocassette, 17 minutes, in color, produced in 1980. Producer is Alternate Choice, Inc. Distributor is Filmakers Library, Inc, 133 East 58 Street, New York, NY 10022, (212) 355-6545. (Sale, $375 [videocassette, $325]; rent, $40 [discussion guide available].)

The Work I've Done presents a sensitive and powerful view of the feelings and concerns of blue-collar workers facing retirement. The film explains the psychologic and social aspects of retirement and their effect on three retiring autoworkers. This film is 16 mm, 3/4-and 1/2-inch videocassette, 56 minutes, in color, produced in 1984. Producer is Ken Fink. Distributor is First Run Features, 153 Waverly Place, New York, NY 10014, (212) 243-0600. (Sale, $850 [16 mm], $500 [video], $300 [35-minute video]; rent, $100 [16 mm and video], $50 [35-minute video].)

Toward Retirement is billed as a TV-style documentary that informs prospective retirees about basic concerns they must confront in planning for a successful retirement. *Toward Retirement* attempts to examine the role crisis that can often accompany this life transition by interviewing retirees who are described as coming from all walks of life and who have made successful adjustments. Four affluent, white, and well-educated married couples discuss their views on the relationship between income and lifestyle, the use of leisure time, the importance of good health practices, and the role changes they have experienced since retiring. This film is 16 mm, 3/4-and 1/2-inch videocassette, 14 minutes, in color, produced in 1982. Producer is Paul Henry. Distributor is Washington Courseware, 122 Willmont Avenue Cumberland, MD 21502-2630. (Sale, $475 [16 mm], $425 [video]; rent, $105 [15 days], $35 [3 days].)

Transitions. One of the most therapeutically precarious periods for elderly patients is the transition from institutional to home-based care. In this video program, Debra Wertheimer, MD, discusses how health professionals can facilitate transitions from institution to community. Topics addressed in the tape include the following: (1) assessing the psychologic, physical, functional, and environmental needs of the patient during hospitalization to allow appropriate comprehensive care plans to be developed for discharge; (2) assessing the home environment to determine if modifications are necessary for the patient, (3) evaluating family or community support available to the patient, (4) determining services needed to maintain the patient in the community, and (5) educating the patient and family caregiver prior to discharge. From Video Press, University of Maryland at Baltimore, School of Medicine, Suite 133, 100 Penn Street, Baltimore, MD 21201, (800) 328-7450 or (410) 328-5497, fax (410) 328-8471.

Waking Up Vanessa, is an educational videotape that documents the experience of older adults in training to work in child care. The producer is S. Newman, University of Pittsburgh, Pittsburgh, Pa, (20 minutes). Available from Video Press, University of Maryland at Baltimore, School of Medicine, Suite 133, 100 Penn Street, Baltimore, MD 21201, (800) 327-7450 or (410) 328-5497, fax (410) 328-8471.

Organizations

40 PLUS Clubs
1718 P Street, NW
Washington, DC 20036

Displaced Homemakers Network
1010 Vermont Avenue NW
Washington, DC 20005

AARP Works
Work Force Education
AARP Work Equity Department
1909 K Street, NW
Washington, DC 20049

Career Counseling
American Association for Counseling and Development
Washington, DC

For age discrimination on the job, file a complaint with the Equal Employment Opportunity Commission (EEOC, federal agency).

Listed below are two job banks that match employers and older workers.

Placement Services for Older Workers (PSOW)
541 East Colorado Boulevard
Pasadena, CA 91101

Job Alert
American Society on Aging
833 Market Street
San Francisco, CA 94103.

Points of Light Foundation
PO Box 66534
Washington, DC 20035
(800) 272-8306, fax (703) 803-9291

Provides information on opportunities in voluntary service, publications, videos and *Grapevine Newsletter.*

Widowed Services Program sponsored by the Center for Gerontology at the University of Oregon provides the following services: 24-hour "teleassurance," peer support groups, volunteer outreach, and Self Exploration and Life Planning (SELP) workshops. For more information, a publication entitled *Developing a Widowed Services Program* by Frances G. Scott, Director of the Center for Gerontology, and Hazel M. Foss, director of the Displaced Homemakers/Widowed Services Program, can be obtained for $3.00. Send requests to 1609 Agate Street, Eugene OR 97403.

For information on the AARP Hispanic Widowed Persons' Task Force, call (512) 659-4173.

Find PRO is a computer-assisted financial software program. Available from Life Planning Management, Irvine, Calif.

Two organizations focused on retirement planning needs of women in midlife are the National Council on the Aging and the Older Women's League (OWL).

Detailed earnings information and benefit estimates for all Social Security Administration programs for workers of all ages (particularly useful for financial planning for retirement) can be obtained from:

Personal Earnings and Benefit Estimate Statement (PEBES)
Social Security Administration
Social Security
Pueblo, CO 81009
(800) 937-2000

REFERENCES

Aber CS: Spousal death, a threat to women's health: paid work as a "resistance resource," *Image J Nurs Sch* 24(2):95, 1992.

Adams WL: Potential for adverse drug-alcohol interactions among retirement community residents, *J Am Geriatr Soc* 43(9):1021, 1995.

Adams WL: Alcohol use in retirement communities, *J Am Geriatr Soc* 44(9):1082, 1996.

Adelman PK: Multiple roles and psychological well being in a national sample of older adults, *J Gerontol* S277, 1994.

American Association of Retired Persons: *A profile of older Americans: 1995,* AARP PF3049 (1295), Washington, DC, 1996, The Association.

Antonovsky A, Sagy S: Confronting developmental tasks in the retirement transition, *Gerontologist* 30:362, 1990.

Arbuckle NW, deVries B: The long-term effects of later life spousal and parental bereavement on personal functioning, *Gerontologist* 35(5):637, 1995.

Atchley RC: *The sociology of retirement,* Cambridge, Mass, 1975, Schenkman.

Atchley RC: Issues in retirement research, *Gerontologist,* 19:44, 1979.

Barber CE: Top 15 issues, *Aging Today* 13(4):13, 1992.

Barer BM: Men and women aging differently, *Int J Aging Hum Dev* 38(1):29, 1993.

Bartley SK: Retirement planning for nonheterosexuals, *Aging Today* 17(5):8, 1996.

Calasanti TM: Gender and life satisfaction in retirement: an assessment of the male model, *J Gerontol* 51(1):S18, 1996.

Caserta MS, Lund DA: Bereaved older adults who seek early professional help, *Death Studies* 16(1):17, 1992.

Chick N, Meleis AI: Transitions: a nursing concern. In Chinn PL, editor: *Nursing research methodology: issues and implementation,* Rockville, Md, 1986, Aspen.

Confederate widow's pension restored, *San Francisco Chronicle,* p A3, August 23, 1996.

Daly MC, Bound J: Worker adaptation and employer accommodation following the onset of a health impairment, *J Gerontol* 51B(2):S53, 1996.

Danigelis NL, McIntosh BR: Resources and the productive activity of elders: race and gender contexts, *J Gerontol* 48:S192, 1993.

Deitch CH, Sunshine JH, Chan WC, Owen JB, Shaffer KA: How US radiologists use their professional time: factors that affect work activity and retirement plans, *Radiology* 194(1):33, 1995.

Dennis H: The current state of retirement planning, *Generations* 13(2):38, 1989.

Dorfman LT: Health conditions and perceived quality of life in retirement, *Health Soc Work* 20(3):192, 1995.

Ebersole P: Personal reflections, 1989.

Ekerdt DJ, DeViney S, Kosloski K: Profiling plans for retirement, *J Gerontol* 51(3):S140, 1996.

Erikson E, Erikson J, Kivnick H: *Vital involvement in old age: the experience of old age in our time,* New York, 1986, WW Norton & Co.

Fellers D: Care for yourself . . . save for retirement, *American Nurse* 22(1):44, 1990.

Ferriss S: Past retirement and still on the job, *San Francisco Examiner,* p B1, June 12, 1994.

Fischer LR: Respect—the key to valuing today's older volunteers, *Aging Today* 17(6):11, 1996.

Fischer LR, Shaffer KB: *Older volunteers: a guide to research and practice,* Newbury Park, Calif, 1993, Sage Publications.

Fletcher-Stoelje M: Hispanic bereavement: life after death, *Am Health* 7(6):120, 1988.

Flinn J, Rogers D: Older working men: a vanishing species, *San Francisco Examiner,* p A1, July 9, 1995.

Gallagher D, Breckenridge J, Thompson L et al: Effects of bereavement on indicators of mental health in elderly widows and widowers, *Gerontologist* 38:565, 1983.

Gendell M, Siegel JS: *Trends in retirement age in the United States, 1955-1993, by sex.*

Gentry M, Rosenman L, Schulman A: Comparison of the needs and support systems of remarried and nonremarried widows. In Lopata H: *Widows,* vol 2, North America, Durham, NC, 1987, Duke University Press.

Gerontological Society of America: Americans retiring earlier, even before their first SS check, news release *GSA,* p 1, May 15, 1996.

Goldberg EL, Constock GW, Harlow SD: Emotional problems and widowhood, *J Gerontol* 43(6):S206, 1988.

Greer C: What's an hour of your time worth? *Parade Magazine,* p 20, August 27, 1995.

Halloran EJ, Mullinix C, Van Der Puy N: Nurses' pensions: a need for change, *Nurse Manager* 27(6):43, 1996.

Hardy MA, Quadagno J: Satisfaction with early retirement: making choices in the auto industry, *J Gerontol* 50B(4):S217, 1995.

Harrison MJ, Neufeld A, Kushner K: Women in transition: access and barriers to social support, *J Adv Nurs* 21(5):858, 1995.

Hatch LR: Gender differences in orientation toward retirement from paid labor, *Gender and Society* 6:66, 1992.

Hayward MD, Crimmins EM, Wray LA: The relationship between retirement life cycle changes and older men's labor force participation, *J Gerontol* 49:S219, 1994.

Henretta JC: Uniformity and diversity: life course institutionalization and late-life work exit, *Sociological Quarterly* 33:265, 1992.

Henretta JC: Changing perspectives on retirement, *J Gerontol* 52B(1):S1, 1997.

Henretta JC, Chan CG, O'Rand AM: Retirement reason versus retirement process: examining the reasons for retirement typology, *J Gerontol* 47(1):S1, 1992.

Henretta JC, Lee H: Cohort differences in mens' late-life labor force participation, *Work and Occupations* 23:214, 1996.

Hirshorn BA, Tetrick LE, Sinclair RR: Understanding the provision of postretirement health care and pension benefits: which firm characteristics are most explanatory? *Gerontologist* 36(5):637, 1996.

Hoffman SB: Peer counselor training with the elderly, *Gerontologist* 23:358, 1983.

Hogstel M: Older widowers: a small group with special needs, *Geriatr Nurs* 6(1):24, 1985.

Holden KC, Hsiang-Hui DK: Complex marital histories and economic well-being: the continuing legacy of divorce and widowhood as the HRS cohort approaches retirement, *Gerontologist* 36(3):383, 1996.

Honig M: Retirement expectations: differences by race, ethnicity, and gender, *Gerontologist* 36(3):373-382, 1996.

Hospital volunteers: a hands-on job, *AARP Bulletin* 34(5):10, 1993.

Hurd MD: *The effect of labor market rigidities on the labor force behavior of older workers,* Working Paper Series No. 4462, Boston, 1993, National Bureau of Economic Research.

Kanacki LS, Jones PS, Galbraith ME: Social support and depression in widows and widowers, *J Gerontol Nurs* 22(2):39, 1996.

Lanza ML: Divorce experienced as an older woman, *Geriatr Nurs* 17(4):166, 1996.

Laws G: Embodiment and emplacement: identities, representation and landscape in Sun City retirement communities, *Int Jo Aging Hum Dev* 40(4):253, 1995.

Lee J, Lenzmeier T, Boulger J, Buck S, Bergeron D, Hill TJ: Retirement of senior physicians in rural Minnesota: factors influencing physicians' plans to retire, *Minn Med* 78(12):21, 1995.

Lichtenstein P, Gatz M, Pedersen NL, Berg S, McClearn GE: A co-twin control study of response to widowhood, *J Gerontol B: Psychology and Social Science* 51(5):279, 1996.

Lindemann E: Symptomatology and management of acute grief, *Am J Psychiatry* 101:141, 1944.

Mandell H: Physicians' retirement, *Conn Med* 5996):351, 1995.

McDonald J: Support systems for American black wives and widows. In Lopata H: *Widows,* vol 2, North America, Durham, NC, 1987, Duke University Press.

McLeod D: Older volunteers wield 'huge impact' on law enforcement, *AARP Bulletin* 35(7):1, 1994.

Mercer RT, Nichols EG, Doyle GS: *Transitions in a woman's life: major life events in developmental context,* New York, 1989, Springer.

Mercy on the main, *Modern Maturity* 36(1):6, 1993.

Meyer MH: Family status and poverty among older women: the gendered distribution of retirement income in the United States, *Social Problems* 37:551, 1990.

Midanik LT, Soghikian K, Ransom LJ, Tekawa IS: The effect of retirement on mental health and health behaviors: the Kaiser Permanente retirement study, *J Gerontol* 50B(1):S59, 1995.

Moore K, Biordi D: Nurses' retirement preparation, *J Nurs Adm* 25(6):62, 1995.

Musson ND, Frye GD, Nash M: Silver spoons: supervised volunteers provide feeding of patients, *Geriatr Nurs* 18(1):18, 1997.

Mutchler JE, Burr JA, Pienta AM: Massagli MP: Pathways to labor force exit: work transitions and work stability, *J Gerontol* 52B(1):S4, 1997.

Neale A: Widows in a Florida retirement community. In Lopata H: *Widows,* vol 2, North America, Durham, NC, 1987, Duke University Press.

Older Americans program, Hartford, Conn, 1987, The Travelers Companies.

O'Rand AM: The precious and the precocious: understanding cumulative disadvantage and cumulative advantage over the life course, *Gerontologist* 36(2):230, 1996.

The path to poverty: an analysis of women's retirement income, 1995 Mother's Day Report, Washington, DC, 1995, Older Women's League.

Pierre JH: Personal communication, Salem, Ore, 1992.

Pina DL, Bengtson VL: Division of household labor and the well-being of retirement-aged wives, *Gerontologist* 35(3):308, 1995.

Population Reference Bureau: What do people want to know about population aging? *Public Policy and Aging Report* 7(1):11, 1995.

Quinn JF, Kozy M: The role of bridge jobs in the retirement transition: gender, race, and ethnicity, *Gerontologist* 36(3):363, 1996.

Reitzes DC, Mutran EJ, Fernandez ME: Does retirement hurt well-being? Factors influencing self-esteem and depression among retirees and workers, *Gerontologist* 36(5):649, 1996.

Rix S: What do people want to know about older workers and an aging labor force? *Public Policy and Aging Report* 7(4):10, 1996.

Robert Wood Johnson Foundation: Service credit banking in managed care. *Advances* 8(4):3, 1995.

Robinson JH: Grief responses, coping processes, and social support of widows: research with Roy's model, *Nursing Science Quarterly* 8(4):158, 1995.

Rosik CH: The impact of religious orientation in conjugal bereavement among older adults, *Int J Aging Hum Dev* 28(4):251, 1989.

Ruffner SS: *A liberal education,* Santa Barbara, Calif, 1991, Fithian Press.

Sable P: Attachment, anxiety and loss of a husband, *Am J Orthopsychiatry* 59(4):550, 1989.

Schulz JH: Review of age, work and society, *Contemporary Gerontology* 1(3):83, 1994.

Schumacher KL, Meleis AI: Transitions: a central concept in nursing. *Image: J Nurs Sch* 26(2):119, 1994.

Seim HC, Mitchell JE: Life after medical practice: A retirement profile of Minnesota physicians, *Minn Med* 78(12):27, 1995.

Service credit banking in managed care, brochure, Princeton, NJ, 1995, Robert Wood Johnson Foundation.

Silverman P: Widowhood as the next stage in the life course. In Lopata H: *Widows,* vol 2, North America, Durham, NC, 1987, Duke University Press.

Silverstein M, Zablotsky DL: Health and social precursors of later life retirement-community migration, *J Gerontol* 51(3):S150, 1996.

Sorenson DLS: Life event timing synchrony, *Image J Nurs Sch* 27(4):297, 1995.

Sum AM, Fogg N: "Bridge jobs" for older workers, *Aging Today* 12(2):9, 1991.

Talage JA, Beehr TA: Are there gender differences in predicting retirement decisions? *J Appl Psychol* 80(1):16, 1995.

Taylor MA, Shore LM: Predictors of planned retirement age: an application of Beehr's model, *Psychol Aging* 10(1):76, 1995.

Trager L: How old is too old? *San Francisco Examiner,* p B-1, May 9, 1995.

Troll L, Miller S, Atchley R: *Families in later life,* Belmont, Calif, 1979, Wadsworth.

Tudiver F, Permaul-Woods JA, Hilditch J, Harmina J, Saini S: Do widowers use the health care system differently? Does intervention make a difference? *Can Fam Physician* 41:392, 1995.

US Bureau of the Census: *Statistical abstract of the United States: 1995,* ed 115, Washington, DC, 1995.

Vinick B, Ekerdt DJ: Retirement: what happens to husband-wife relationships? *J Geriatr Psychiatry* 24:23, 1991.

Weinstein L, Xie X, Cleanthous CC: Purpose in life, boredom, and volunteerism in a group of retirees, *Psychol Rep* 76(2):482, 1995.

Weisfeld V: *Interfaith volunteer caregivers: a special report,* Princeton, NJ, 1988, Robert Wood Johnson Foundation.

Wolfson M, Rowe G, Gentleman JF, Tomiak M: Career earnings and death: a longtitudinal analysis of older Canadian men, *J Gerontol* 48:S167, 1993.

Wolinsky FD, Johnson RJ: Widowhood, health status, and the use of health services by older adults: a cross-sectional and prospective approach, *J Gerontol* 47(1):S8, 1992.

Zwerling C, Sprince NL, Wallace RB, Davis CS, Whitten PS, Heeringa SG: Risk factors for occupational injuries among older workers: an analysis of the health and retirement study, *Am J Public Health* 86(9):1306, 1996.

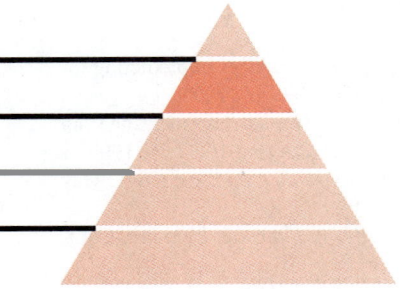

CHAPTER 21

Mental Health and Mental Disorders

Students speculate

The process of aging scares me. Aging brings up emotions such as low self-esteem, powerlessness and hopelessness. An old person has to accept the existing gap between the young and the old. I still remember telling my grandmother she was old-fashioned and out of touch. Now, I realize how rude I was to her. By the time I am about 75 years old I will be just as depressed as some of the elderly I work with.

Rossana, age 28

When I think of aging, I think of loss of friends and family through death, decreased visual acuity and hearing, loss of physical function, and changing body image, loneliness, social isolation, etc. It scares me to see myself growing older. I heard stories from my mom how her friend committed suicide. Her friend just jumped off the third floor from the YWCA senior home on Clay street. Her health had deteriorated for 2 years, and she was not able to do her daily activities. She was receiving SSI and also some money from In Home Supportive Services (IHSS) to use to hire someone to help her shop and cook. Her daughter took all the money and would not cook for her. Whenever her daughter did cook for her, she would scold her. One night she jumped from the third floor.

Huey, age 26

Elders speak

When I was a youngster, I had some notion that mental illness was a condition that descended on a person and they became so bizarre they frightened themselves and others. Now I know that almost everyone is "mentally ill" at various points in life and these episodes can lead to real growth, understanding, and compassion.

Jennie, 92

Of course I get depressed, but I am learning to live with those episodes. Who was it that said, "I never promised you a rose garden"? On the other hand, even roses have thorns. That is the biggest lesson I have learned in my 80 years.

Sarah, 82

LEARNING OBJECTIVES

Upon completion of this chapter, the reader will be able to:

1. Differentiate mental health from mental illness in older adults.
2. Name the three most common disturbances of the mental health of elders.
3. Assess the presence of depression in an elder.
4. Recognize elders at risk of suicide and conduct a suicide assessment of an elder.
5. Explain at least five therapies useful in the care of mentally disturbed elders.
6. Describe methods of communicating with the mentally disturbed elder.
7. Evaluate interventions aimed at promoting mental health in older adults.
8. Relate the nursing concerns in managing a resident with a communication disorder caused by a perceptual disturbance.
9. Develop an individualized nursing care plan for a client with a mental illness.

This chapter presents concepts of mental health and mental illness in old age and provides specific nursing strategies to maintain and promote mental health, self-esteem, and psychologic health of older individuals to the optimum of their capacity. The chapter is divided into three major sections: considerations in mental health of the aged, cognitive disturbances created by psychiatric problems, and therapeutic interventions. Developmental transitions, life events, and situations requiring psychic energy may interfere with the ability to concentrate in many older adults. These, though not unique to the old, very often influence adaptation. In previous chapters we examined these challenges in a Maslovian hierarchic fashion. We hope that nurses caring for the aged will first consider the status of their clients' basic human needs when attempting to assess mental health and illness.

MENTAL HEALTH IN OLD AGE

Mental health of the elderly is difficult to define because the increasing differentiation of personality throughout the life span results in idiosyncratic and sometimes eccentric adaptations in late life. Each individual becomes more uniquely himself or herself the older he or she becomes. The accumulation of life experience as well as particular situations emphasizes certain aspects of personality and appearance and diminishes others. Some apparently negative personality characteristics, such as being crusty, disagreeable,

grouchy, or grumpy, may be adaptive. Thus a cantankerous old man engaged in coping with a severe illness and stoically protecting others from awareness of his pain might be mentally healthy.

Mental health can be defined as a satisfactory adjustment to one's life stage and situation. We tend to believe certain cultural artifacts such as independence and assertiveness are indices of mental health when they may be maladaptive to certain lifestyles and stages. Using those criteria, it becomes apparent that a contented, but passive, institutionalized older person might be mentally healthy and adapted to the peculiar subculture that demands certain behaviors of those who best manage.

The *Diagnostic and Statistical Manual of Mental Disorders,* fourth edition, (DSM IV) provides categorical criteria for diagnosing mental disorders from a medical perspective but is of little help in assessing elders with mental illness because no special characteristics are noted except in age-related cognitive decline (see chapter 22 for further discussion). Actual geropsychiatric problems not related to cognitive pathologic conditions are neglected. We contend that some disorders in DSM IV should be defined more carefully in terms of symptomatology when considering the mental disorders of elders.

Qualls and Smyer (1995) note that mental health in the aged embodies effectiveness within sociocultural roles, cohort differences in expectations, positive relationships, and mature mental well-being. In later life, mental health

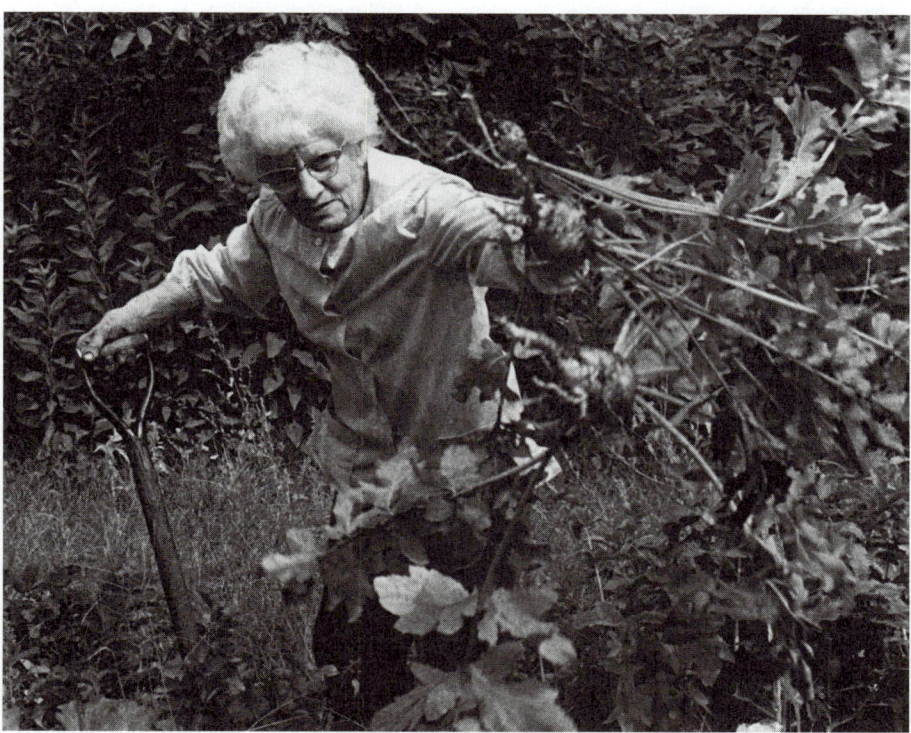

Work and play. (Courtesy Rod Schmall.)

is measured by the capacity to cope effectively with relationships and environment and by the satisfaction experienced in doing so. The individual's response to the environment can be used as a criterion of mental health only if the environment provides the potential for mental health. Theoretically, this view is useful. When someone is underrated, expectations of mental health are reduced, feedback is modified, and a danger of instigating a self-fulfilling prophecy exists. For example, many older people fear they will lose their intellectual powers as they age and are particularly vulnerable to any implication that confirms their fear. Thus in a community or society in which ageism is rampant and distribution of mental health resources to the aged has a low priority, as at present, we would expect many mental aberrations in the elderly. The development of holistic, humanistic, interactional, and individualistic models of psychiatric nursing care is critically important in the care of the aged at this time. Using Maslow's hierarchic need model, we might assume the higher one rises in terms of needs met, the more likely one is to be mentally healthy.

Mental health, like general health (Chapter 3), can be thought of on a fluctuating continuum from wellness to illness. The absence of mental illness does not mean one is mentally healthy, nor does the presence of psychologic symptomatology mean one is mentally ill. Individuals move back and forth on the continuum as stressors, supports, health, and resources are ample or scarce (Figure 21-1).

Freud believed the major determinants of mental health were the capacities to work and love, thus expressing the energies of aggression and eros. Freud's ideas regarding the centrality of work and love can be expanded in late life to include purposeful living as the work of aging and to include all evidences of altruism as love. In contemporary society we have added a third capacity, particularly significant to elders, and that is the ability to enjoy leisure.

Erikson thought autonomy, intimacy, integrity, and generativity were all aspects of mentally healthy adult adaptation. These concepts are culture bound and to some extent dependent upon semantics. Most importantly, no one is entirely mentally unhealthy, and no one is fully

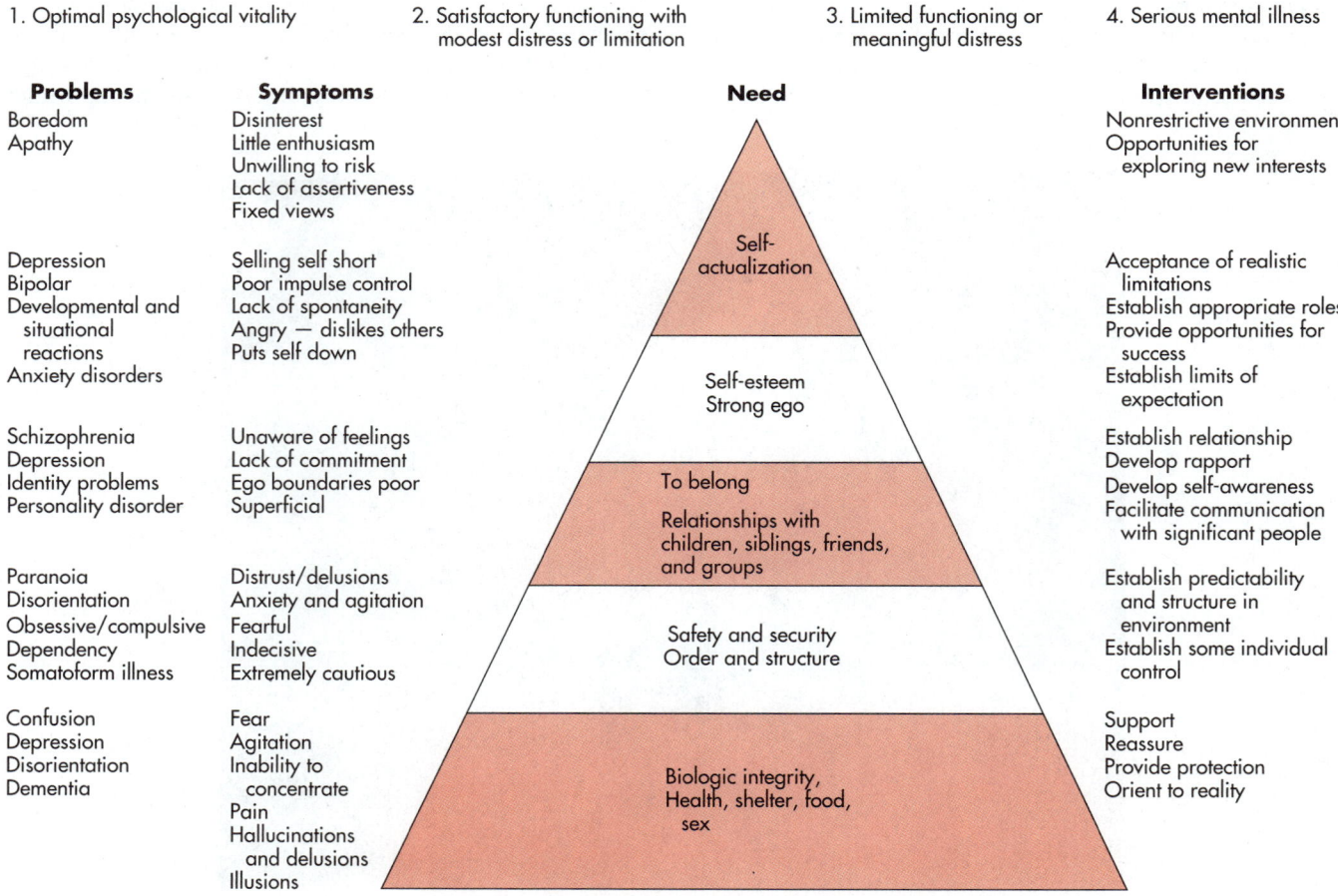

Figure 21-1. Continuum of mental health and illness.

healthy at all times. We can help the elder seek to maximize the healthiest self-attributes.

Mental Health Services for the Elderly

Severe gaps exist in the delivery of mental health services to the elderly seeking services. At this time federal policy and the Community Mental Health Centers Act both exclude the continuing care of persons with chronic disorders from reimbursment. In addition, there still remains a 190-day lifetime limit on treatment in mental hospitals. As of July 1990 psychiatric services by a psychologist, nurse practitioner or social worker became reimbursable, and many of the best health maintenance organizations (HMOs) provide mental health and counseling services, as well as programs for special problems, such as addictions. This portends somewhat better and more available care.

Primary health care services and case management usually employ a holistic approach to care and emphasize promoting health and reducing expense. In order to develop awareness of mental health needs within these broad but often basic service models, we must clearly identify risk profiles, toxic life situations, and recognition of the prevalence of certain problems (Gallo, 1995). In-depth assessment requires specialized expertise that is often not available.

Nursing homes, while not licensed as psychiatric facilities and seldom staffed to provide mental health assessment or care, are providing the majority of "care" given to elders with psychiatric conditions. Staff cannot treat them appropriately because of insufficient trained personnel. Some of the obtacles to mental health care in nursing homes are (1) shortage of trained personnel, (2) lack of in-service training in nursing homes related to mental health and illness, and (3) inadequate Medicaid and Medicare reimbursement for mental health services. Recommendations of the USHRSA report include additional funding for training, reimbursement, psychiatric and behavioral therapies, and consumer education. This is unlikely to happen given the shift to state fiscal responsibility. However, some progress is being made in nursing homes and long-term care facilities. The various revisions of the Omnibus Budget Reconciliation Act (OBRA) and the implementation of the Minimum Data Set (MDS.2) have resulted in more resident-oriented and holistic care and the reduction of chemical and physical restraints.

As part of OBRA 1989, Congress recognized nurse practitioners (NP) as direct providers of services to residents of nursing homes. The reimbursement varies by the type of NP, the health care setting, and the payment level (Mittelstadt, 1993). Medicare directly reimburses the services of NPs in nursing homes and in rural-area settings. Whether these NPs have geropsychiatric specialized training is always questionable.

Geropsychiatric nursing is the specialty care provided by nurses to elders with mental health disorders. There are few educational programs that focus on this specialty, and the mental health needs of elders are notoriously neglected by all of the professions. When this is available, geropsychiatric nursing consultation to facilities is recommended as one method of alleviating some of the lack of specific

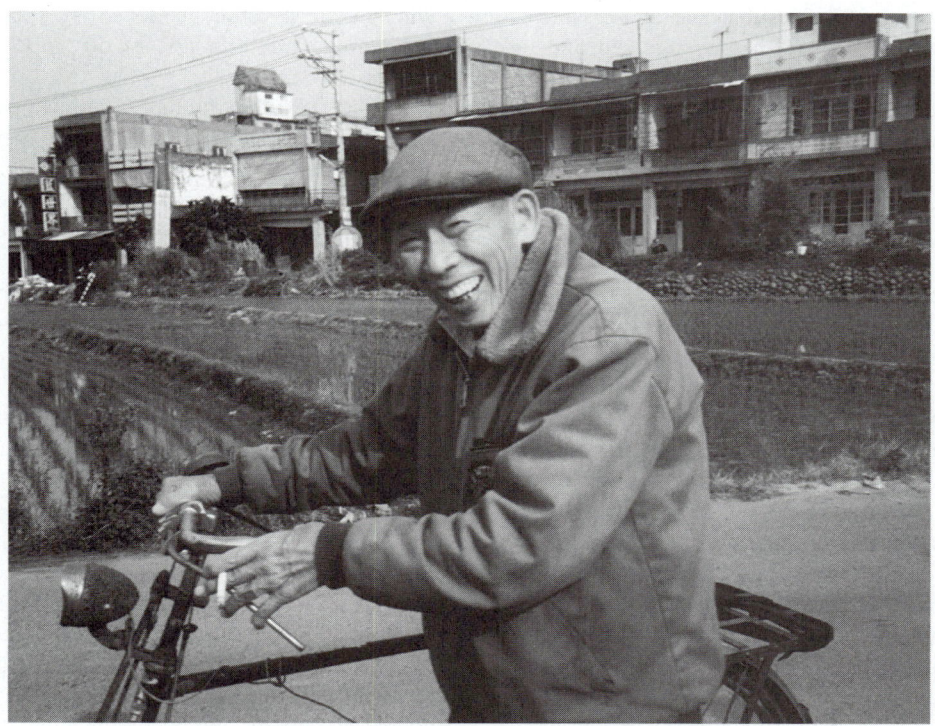

Joy in living. (Courtesy Priscilla Ebersole.)

expertise (Smith et al, 1995). However, because this is not the norm, nurses employed in long-term care must encourage the use of such consultation on an ongoing basis rather than only in occasional provocative situations.

Alternatives to hospital-based mental health care must be more fully developed as in-patient psychiatric units become more geographically and economically inaccessible. Community-based, multidisciplinary teams employing a variety of services and professionals instituted early on may prevent the eruption of serious mental health impairments. Case-finding mechanisms for targeting the seriously mentally ill in the community are needed (Kwakwa, 1995). At present, in home care few mental health services are reimbursable, and it requires great ingenuity on the part of the nurse to meet these needs.

To add to the difficulty of limited reimbursement and few adequately prepared personnel is the age bias of providers who do not wish to care for the age with mental problems (James and Haley, 1995). The elderly also often reject mental health services for reasons of finances, lack of transportation, dependence on family physicians, cohort biases, and lack of information. It is an even more significant problem for minority elders, who may experience culture and language barriers to care, as well as age discrimination (Scott and Polaca, 1996).

Psychologic Assessment of Elders

It is well known that depression in the elderly is highly prevalent and treatable but infrequently recognized or treated; however, Lish et al (1995) found substantial numbers of elders suffered anxiety, substance abuse, and somatoform disorders that were also unrecognized and untreated. These findings only serve to confirm the increasing prevalence and neglect of mental disorders in elders. Medical patients present with psychiatric disorders in 27% of cases (Silverstone, 1996) though they are unrecognized by medical staff 60% of the time. Yet the majority of nurses, psychiatrists, and primary care physicians can correctly diagnose personality and developmental disorders (Podgorski et al, 1996). Nurses were more able to recognize the coexistence of psychiatric disorders and had correctly identified these in 61% of the cases.

General issues in the psychologic assessment of older adults involve distinguishing between normal, idiosyncratic, and diverse characteristics of aging and pathologic conditions. Baseline data are often lacking from the individual's middle years. The use of standardized tools and functional assessment is valuable, but the data will be meaningless if not placed in the context of the client's past life and hopes and expectations for the future. Distinguishing normal from pathologic aging in a particular individual depends on these factors. Few standardized assessment tools included any old subjects in the development of the tool.

Assessment of mental health includes examination for cognitive function/impairment and the specific conditions of demoralization, depression, paranoia, substance abuse, psychopathology, and suicidal risk. Assessment of mental health must also focus on social intactness and affectual responses appropriate to the situation. Attention span, concentration, intelligence, judgment, learning ability, memory, orientation, perception, problem solving, psychomotor ability, and reaction time are assessed in relation to cognitive intactness and must be considered when making a psychologic assessment (see Chapter 22 for further discussion). Assessment includes specific processes that are intact as well as those that are diminished or compromised.

Obtaining data from elders is best done during short sessions after some rapport has been established. Performing repeated assessments at various times of day and in different situations will give a more complete psychologic profile. It is important to be sensitive to a client's anxiety, special needs, and disabilities. The interview should be focused so that attention is given to strengths and skills as well as deficits. A global assessment of functioning is very useful (Box 21-1) in the assessment of the old. It is also useful to take a psychologic inventory of the geriatric client (Box 21-2). See Appendix 21-A for Depression Rating Scales.

Defenses

"Defense mechanisms (or coping styles) are automatic psychological processes that protect the individual against anxiety and from the awareness of internal or external dangers or stressors" (DSM IV, 1994, p 751). Given the prevalence of anxiety and agitation among the aged, we must question whether the psychologic defensive processes become less efficient in later life just as do some of the physiologic processes.

In the DSM IV, the defenses have been grouped in the Defensive Functioning Scale. These hierarchial categories allow the practitioner to categorize coping styles and then indicate the predominant defensive level exhibited by the individual. A glossary of defense mechanisms, somewhat different and healthier than the classic definitions, assists in evaluation. This Defensive Functioning Scale holds promise for evaluating an elder's adaptation. As with all evaluative efforts, micro and macro timing are important as are fatigue, pain, and stress levels.

Some of the defensive mechanisms of the aged are very healthy and some inhibitory. We present some of the most predominant.

Denial. Denial of illness, aging, loss, death, or incapacity all helps ease one through some of the difficulties of aging. Denial may be difficult to assess because many older persons avoid discussion of major concerns and losses, not because they are unaware but rather because they have a strong enculturation to stoic endurance or have great courage. If denial is present, it is necessary and should be addressed directly only when the elder shows signs that it is weakening.

John (78 years old) went ahead and planned, scheduled, and prepaid for a cruise for himself and his wife the following month. His wife was in the process of divorcing him, his cardiac decompensation had nearly immobilized him, he had an unexplained seizure, and his doctor told him he would need to be closely monitored until his physical status was stabilized. The clinic nurse felt it would be impossible for him to surmount all those problems and take the cruise within the next month.

When he came to have his blood drawn for serum dilantin levels, he asked, "I must be well enough to go on my cruise by next month." She saw the opening and began asking astute questions: What is happening now between you and your wife? How far can you comfortably walk now without shortness of breath? What will be required of you on the cruise? What will you do if you have a problem while cruising? Are you worried about another seizure?

Box 21-1

Global Assessment of Functioning (GAF) Scale

Consider psychological, social, and occupational functioning on a hypothetical continuum of mental health-illness. Do not include impairment in functioning caused by physical (or environmental) limitations.

Code   (**Note:** Use intermediate codes when appropriate, e.g., 45, 68, 72.)

100
91 | **Superior functioning in a wide range of activities, life's problems never seem to get out of hand, is sought out by others because of his or her many positive qualities. No symptoms.**

90
81 | **Absent or minimal symptoms** (e.g, mild anxiety before an exam), **good functioning in all areas, interested and involved in a wide range of activities, socially effective, generally satisfied with life, no more than everyday problems or concerns** (e.g., an occasional argument with family members).

80
71 | **If symptoms are present, they are transient and expectable reactions to psychosocial stressors** (e.g., difficulty concentrating after family argument); **no more than slight impairment in social, occupational, or school functioning** (e.g., temporarily falling behind in schoolwork).

70
61 | **Some mild symptoms** (e.g., depressed mood and mild insomnia) **OR some difficulty in social, occupational, or school functioning** (e.g., occasional truancy, or theft within the household), **but generally functioning pretty well, has some meaningful interpersonal relationships.**

60
51 | **Moderate symptoms** (e.g., flat affect and circumstantial speech, occasional panic attacks) **OR moderate difficulty in social, occupational, or school functioning** (e.g., few friends, conflicts with peers or coworkers).

50
41 | **Serious symptoms** (e.g., suicidal ideation, severe obsessional rituals, frequent shoplifting) **OR any serious impairment in social, occupational, or school functioning** (e.g., no friends, unable to keep a job).

40
31 | **Some impairment in reality testing or communication** (e.g., speech is at times illogical, obscure, or irrelevant) **OR major impairment in several areas, such as work or school, family relations, judgment, thinking, or mood** (e.g., depressed man avoids friends, neglects family, and is unable to work; child frequently beats up younger children, is defiant at home, and is failing at school).

30
21 | **Behavior is considerably influenced by delusions or hallucinations OR serious impairment in communication or judgment** (e.g., sometimes incoherent, acts grossly inappropriately, suicidal preoccupation) **OR inability to function in almost all areas** (e.g., stays in bed all day; no job, home, or friends).

20
11 | **Some danger of hurting self or others** (e.g., suicide attempts without clear expectation of death; frequently violent; manic excitement) **OR occasionally fails to maintain minimal personal hygiene** (e.g., smears feces) **OR gross impairment in communication** (e.g., largely incoherent or mute).

10
1 | **Persistent danger of severely hurting self or others** (e.g., recurrent violence) **OR persistent inability to maintain minimal personal hygiene OR serious suicidal act with clear expectation of death.**

0   Inadequate information.

From American Psychiatric Association: *Diagnostic and statistical manual of mental disorders*, ed 4, Washington, DC, 1994, The Association.

Box 21-2   Inventory of Psychogeriatric Client: Function and Care Plan

1. List client's strengths:
   - Ability to take initiative in caring for self, finances, work project
   - Ability to express feelings
   - Ability to stand up for his or her rights
   - Ability to make decisions
   - Ability to care for self, for example, dressing, going to meals
   - Ability to share with others or show concern for others
   - Enjoyment of music and arts
   - Active participation in organizations
   - Interest in sports
   - Enjoyment of reading
   - Imagination and creativity
   - Special aptitudes, for example, mechanical ability, gardening

2. Identify predominant defensive coping styles:
   - Denial
   - Projection
   - Displacement
   - Passive aggression
   - Positive identification

3. Identify highly adaptive coping styles:
   - Affiliation
   - Altruism
   - Humor
   - Self-assertion
   - Sublimation

4. Identify defensive breakdown patterns:
   - Delusional projection
   - Psychotic suspiciousness
   - Psychotic denial
   - Immobilizing fears
   - Psychotic distortions
   - Apathetic withdrawal

5. Determine client needs and problems based on:
   - Reason for seeking assistance by patient, family, and others

- Medical history and findings (physical, mental, neurologic, and psychologic examinations and tests)
- Drug use profile (use of prescribed and nonprescribed drugs)
- Laboratory and diagnostic tests
- Psychiatric history
- Social history
- Mental status
- Other background information provided by patient, family, and each staff person who has interviewed the patient

6. Develop a nursing care plan considering:
   - Patient's problems, needs, and strengths
   - Mutually identified short-term goals
   - Mutually identified long-term goals

7. State expected outcome of care in terms that can be measured. The following are examples of goals stated in measurable terms:
   - Socializes more
   - Dresses appropriately—puts on coat or jacket when going outside in cold weather
   - Improves personal hygiene—brushes teeth daily without being reminded
   - Shows improvement in problem areas
   - Improves attitude—discusses problems or concerns instead of hitting or resisting
   - Increases functional independence
   - Reduces hostility—responds when spoken to in a friendly manner
   - Improves self-esteem—goes 1 day without self-criticism
   - Reduces depression—expresses interest in one outside activity
   - States increased enjoyment of activities
   - Reduces suspiciousness—eats a meal without expressing fear of poisoning

8. Review progress periodically and revise goals as necessary and appropriate.

Gently helping John consider the specifics of his situation may help him begin to accept the reality.

Projection. Projection is present when the individual attributes his/her own unacceptable feelings, impulses, or thoughts to another. Fear, anxiety, and anger accompanying uncertainty about one's situation are often not perceived as part of one's repertoire of feelings but rather are projected onto others with whom one comes in contact. The most common projection of elders is rejection of others who are aged or disabled; for example, "You won't catch me at the

Senior Center with all those old fogeys. All they do is complain about their illnesses—an organ recital I call it."

Altruism. Altruism is a highly valuable defense against meaninglessness. Elders often become involved in helping others or dedicating efforts to a good cause. The individual is gratified by the appreciation of others and by personal satisfaction. Laura volunteers to take school children on nature walks. Their clear observations and unique views restore her youth as she teaches them and all commune with nature. We find this one of the transcendent mechanisms and prefer to categorize it as quite beyond a defense mechanism.

Displacement. Displacement of feelings onto the intentions of others is quite common. The aged often become suspicious of others' intentions toward them because they may be quite vulnerable. Rather than feeling the vulnerability or precariousness of their existence, they may be wary and untrusting of others. This may progress to a pathologic paranoia and feelings that specific people are biased against them. The initial perceptions are often reality based. For example, one old man would not allow his wife to go anywhere without him because he feared other men would seduce her. He had no realization that this related to his own impotence.

Passive Aggression. Passive aggression is used when outright aggression would be dangerous, or unacceptable to self-concept or others' opinions. This is commonly used by elders who are feeling unable or unwilling to carry out expectations of others. Compliance is often a mask for resentment and hostility. Mary, widowed last year, is expected to move into the cottage her son is having built for her on his property. She doesn't want to leave the community where her long-time friends are, and she doesn't like her son's wife. She continues to agree with his proposal but quietly resists sorting out the things in her home, always feels ill, and can't be available when the real estate agent wants to show her home. In addition, she never calls back when her daughter-in-law leaves telephone messages regarding the plans they need to make.

Positive Identification. Positive identification is not listed among the defensive mechanisms in the DSM IV, but it appears to be a healthy coping activity. Heidrich and Ryff (1993) found that some aged individuals in poor health identified strongly with others who were physically and psychologically more intact, and because of this identification, appraised themselves as more able. It seems to be a process embodying both hope and affiliation. If Bob Hope or George Burns could be clever, rich, and functional at their ages, then the elder can claim their success through cohort affiliation. They are contemporaries and make the elder feel more effective because of affiliation with the respect they generate.

All of us use defensive strategies, some quite conscious and others that are far below our awareness. The more vulnerable we become, the more these are needed. If the individual is maintaining sufficient supports and life satisfac-

tions in the situation he or she is in, let us not disturb the balance, no matter how precarious. Shore up the foundations of strength.

NONORGANIC PSYCHIATRIC DISORDERS OF AGING

The incidence of psychiatric disorders in old age has been studied since the 1950s and has shown a rather consistent prevalence rate of 15% to 25% in those over 65 years of age. These data reflect a conglomerate of disorders. Cognitive changes and psychiatric disturbances often go hand-in-hand in aging, but because they are so frequently considered synonymous, we have separated them for more precise understanding. Normal cognitive function and the problems of cognitive dysfunction that arise from brain pathologic conditions are addressed in Chapter 22.

Adjustment Disorders

Adjustment disorders are diagnosed when one develops significant emotional or behavioral responses to an identifiable psychosocial stress or stressors (DSM IV, 1994, p. 623). Clinical significance is noted when the distress exhibited by the elder is in excess of that expected by the nature of the stressor (Box 21-3). The stressors may be single or multiple, recurrent or continuous, and some are more prominent in certain developmental periods, such as frequent moves into increasingly dependent situations experienced by many elders.

Assessment of excessive emotional reactions to certain adjustments required of the aged may be difficult because personality, gender, and cultural factors must be considered, as well as the availability of supportive relationships. Adjustment disorders may be exhibited by profound depression, with or without anxiety, and behavioral disturbances.

Nursing interventions should include anticipatory rehearsal of the event and instigation of a reliable and ongoing support system available to the individual prior to and following the occurrence. In addition, options and alternatives related to the particular adjustment should be thoroughly discussed and considered. This will reduce the sense of helplessness and irreversibility.

Lester had all his teeth removed and both upper and lower dentures put in place in one day. The analgesics made him nauseated, pain kept him awake, and, of course, he lost interest in food. These not unusual occurrences continued to be a focus of attention and complaint for him for several months. Whenever anyone said, "How are you?" he would go into a litany about his teeth. Insomnia and weight loss became serious problems, and he became increasingly nonfunctional.

When this persisted for several months and after many visits to the dentist because the teeth "didn't fit properly," the prosthodontist recognized an extreme adjustment reaction and referred Lester for a psychiatric consult. The geriatric nurse practitioner who saw him convinced him to accompany her to the senior center, which he had previously avoided because of "all the old folks there." She

Box 21-3 **Diagnostic Criteria for Adjustment Disorders**

A. The development of emotional or behavioral symptoms in response to an identifiable stressor(s) occurring within 3 months of the onset of the stressor(s).

B. These symptoms or behaviors are clinically significant as evidenced by either of the following:
  (1) marked distress that is in excess of what would be expected from exposure to the stressor
  (2) significant impairment in social or occupational (academic) functioning

C. The stress-related disturbance does not meet the criteria for another specific Axis I disorder and is not merely an exacerbation of a preexisting Axis I or Axis II disorder.

D. The symptoms do not represent Bereavement.

E. Once the stressor (or its consequences) has terminated, the symptoms do not persist for more than an additional 6 months.

Specify if:
  Acute: if the disturbance lasts less than 6 months
  Chronic: if the disturbance lasts for 6 months or longer

American Psychiatric Association: *Diagnostic and statistical manual of mental disorders,* ed 4, Washington, DC, 1994, The Association.

introduced him to some of the elders in her case load that attended the center meals and activities. Fortunately, she was able to establish a tentative relationship between Lester and a lady who had experienced similar difficulties adjusting to dentures. Much later he told her she had literally saved his life. He found others who had been as distressed as he about adjusting to dentures, and he established a friendship with the lady he had first been introduced to. To avoid such an intense adjustment there should have been much preparatory work and discussion of options by Lester and his dentist and sufficient time elapsed to incorporate the idea of this major change in appearance, self-perception, and sensual pleasure.

Anxiety Reactions

The DSM IV delineates three categories of anxiety disorder: phobic disorders, post-traumatic stress disorders (PTSDs), and anxiety states. Phobic states are seldom seen in late life, and there are few data available regarding them in geriatric literature (Blazer, 1995a). A current literature search produced only one study, done in Spain (Saz et al, 1995), that addressed phobias in the aged and then only to point out that symptomatic patterns of phobias were different in the British and the Spanish. This would lead to the conclusion that the expression of phobias in the United States would also be somewhat culture bound. PTSD, probably more common than has been recognized, is dealt with in the next section.

Anxiety states are common in late life, and up to 5% of community-dwelling elders experience generalized anxiety disorder (Blazer, 1995a). Frequent symptoms include shakiness, trembling, inability to relax, palpitations, worry or anticipated disaster, a sense of impending doom, distractability, poor concentration, insomnia, and excessive vigilance. In the aged anxiety is most frequently expressed in somatic concerns (Boerner, 1995). The threat of illness is very real as is the confrontation with mortality. Illness may precipitate loss of self-trust, changes in self-concept, alteration in interpersonal relationships, and fears of death and permanent dependency. Thus anxiety is frequently experienced as forebodings of illness.

In reality, medical problems such as cardiac arrhythmias, hypoglycemia, hypotension, pulmonary emboli, pulmonary edema, and shortness of breath may be mistaken for anxiety states and thus must be investigated prior to the common tendency to prescribe medications to quell the anxiety. Assessment of anxiety must first rule out physical disorders presenting as anxiety states and secondary anxiety.

Anxiety is frequently accompanied by agitation. Agitation in itself is visible as the inability to remain still, but in itself rarely includes the sense of foreboding so characteristic of anxiety. Both anxiety and agitation often coexist with major depression.

Stress levels and excessive demands or cognitive impairment may trigger anxiety reactions. Often there are coexisting disorders such as delirium or early Alzheimer's disease that produce anxiety. Sympathomimetic drugs, anticholinergics, caffeine, and withdrawal from alcohol and anxiolytics will produce secondary anxiety.

In other cases, precipitants of anxiety reactions may be obscure and difficult to identify. Disturbances in daily routine or ritual that form the basis of security and control may be trigger events. One aged man said, "If I can just have my newspaper in the morning and find out what's going on in the world, then I can get moving."

When dealing with anxiety reactions, look for daily disturbances such as staff or caregiver changes, room changes, and other events over which the individual feels a lack of control or influence. By themselves, these seldom provoke an anxiety reaction, but they may be the "straw that breaks the camel's back." Anxiety embodies an overwhelming sense of being out of control of one's life and destiny. It is critical to restore the individual's sense of influence as quickly as possible. Discuss feelings and actions that can be taken. In a room change, for instance, how can the individual be alerted in sufficient time to incorporate the idea? How can the new room be personalized? Is there a choice of rooms? We can assist by focusing attention away from the body and onto feelings and problem solving. One old man said, "Just stay with me and let me talk. Please don't interrupt or try to help." Principles of crisis intervention are useful (see Chapter 19).

Medications to control anxiety should be short-acting and prescribed for brief periods. Antipsychotics are not appropriate for generalized anxiety (Blazer, 1995a).

Posttraumatic Stress Disorder in Older War Veterans

PTSD has been recognized for some time as an outcome of overwhelmingly stressful experiences of individuals in the Vietnam War. It has been realized only recently that many World War II veterans have lived the majority of their lives under the shadow of PTSD without it being recognized as such (Buffum and Wolfe, 1995).

According to the DSM IV, PTSD is a syndrome characterized by the development of symptoms following an extremely traumatic event, which involves experiencing, witnessing, or unexpectedly hearing about an actual or threatened death or serious injury to oneself or another closely affiliated person. Individuals often reexperience the traumatic event in episodes of fear, helplessness, flashbacks, terror, and uncontrolled impulses. These episodes may occur periodically for years, though they frequently remain submerged until activated by the losses of aging. These individuals may have ongoing sleep problems, somatic disturbances, anxiety, depression, and restlessness. Over the long term they are typically impaired in work, have maladaptive lifestyles, and do not develop close relationships.

Ernie may have had PTSD though it was only speculative following his suicide. On his eighteenth birthday he joined the U.S. Army Air Corps (precedent to our present U.S. Air Force) in 1941. He was quickly trained and sent to Burma to "fly the hump," the Himalaya mountains between Burma, China, and India. During his 3-year stint he survived two airplane crashes, saw several of his companions mutilated in crashes, watched the torture of captured Japanese, and witnessed the capture of some of his friends. When he returned to the United States his hair had turned from deep auburn to pure white. He retired from the service after 20 years but never really was able to work after his retirement. His life was filled with episodes of alcoholic binges, outbursts of anger, and episodes of abusing others, all seemingly quite out of his control. One friend remained from his "service" days and visited him periodically until his death in 1996. Other relationships seemed to have been superficial and to have had little meaning for Lester. On his seventy-eighth birthday, which he spent alone, he shot himself. One must wonder how many of the aged veterans of World War II, the most highly suicidal group in the United States, are suffering from PTSD.

The care of the individual with PTSD involves awareness that certain events may trigger inappropriate reactions, and the pattern of these reactions should be identified when possible. Current losses may unexpectedly unearth feelings long suppressed. Aging and the numerous losses that often accompany the process may create a full-blown reaction to the past. The nurse will need to provide emotional comfort and a place and time for the expression of the feelings that have gone unexpressed for years. Depending upon the background and the individual personality, the elder may feel victimized, slighted, and lacking control. The nurse will encourage the elder to tell his story, reminisce, and express feelings. Psychiatric referral may be necessary. If there is a family involved, they will need knowledge and assistance in understanding the disorder, and coping resources should be suggested. Ragsdale et al (1996) worked with PTSD patients in both inpatient and outpatient groups and found sustained positive psychologic changes occurred only in the group that had the support of the inpatient unit.

Obsessive/Compulsive Disorders

Obsessive/compulsive disorders are those recurrent thoughts or actions that significantly impair function and consume more than 1 hour each day (DSM IV, 1994, p. 417). These disorders are exaggerated manifestations of a need for control and order and a way of warding off anxiety. They are common in the aged though very often not sufficient to seriously disrupt function and thus not truly considered a disorder; rather they are a coping strategy. If they progress to the point where they disrupt the lifestyle, they will need clinical attention (Jenike, 1989).

In the aged these disorders are often displayed as obsessions about body functions and morbid fears. The compulsive rituals that accompany these thoughts are an effort to ward off anxiety and discharge tension. In the process of carrying out these tension-relief behaviors the individual may ignore important aspects of life.

Interestingly, the two most consuming compulsive disorders I have observed were related to the control of clocks. One lady had numerous clocks with alarms set for different times of day and night. In dealing with her, staff considered the symbolic significance of clocks and time and death from an existential perspective. The elder was gradually weaned, one clock at a time, and other gratifying activities were introduced into her schedule, one at a time and on a precise timetable that staff assured her would not vary. She was also shown her chart to show that she was checked each half hour at night to be sure she was all right.

A most common issue, with both obsessive and compulsive components, is that of bowel management. Jim moved in with his daughter's family and distressed the household by his endless talk about his bowel function and continual preoccupation with the rituals of medications, laxatives, and prune juice. If his prune juice was not available, he became extremely upset. His concern about bowel function literally dominated his life and obscured the pleasure and pain that might be encountered living within his daughter's family. It is seldom helpful to discuss the annoyance produced by an obsessive compulsive individual or to attempt to interrupt the behavior. In this case, nurses may be most helpful in assisting the family and Jim to talk about the stresses for Jim and the family related to the move and to develop a plan that allows the family and Jim certain privileges and areas of control within the household. As all parties involved feel more secure in the new relationship, the obsessive/compulsive coping style should diminish in intensity.

Substance Abuse and Addictions

Substance abuse often arises in old age as a coping mechanism to deal with loss, anxiety, depression, or boredom. While alcohol alleviates the distress temporarily in some situations, it has been found to create significantly more problems in carrying out important social roles (Krause, 1995). Alcohol-related problems in the elderly often go unrecognized, though the residual effects of alcohol abuse complicate the presentation and treatment of many chronic disorders of the aged. In the general population, abuse of alcohol is readily recognized because of social and work problems; however, elders may not come under observation as frequently and may essentially hide out when they are drinking. It is estimated that between 1% and 3% of women and 12% of men over 60 have severe problems related to alcohol abuse (Atkinson, 1992) and that 20% of persons in nursing homes are alcoholics (Kaplan and Sadock, 1994).

It is thought that heavy drinking gradually subsides until age 70, at which time an increase occurs (Swanson, 1993), suggesting that the stresses of aging trigger alcohol abuse, and in turn this may increase the stresses of aging. Women tend to attribute increased drinking to stress, whereas men are more likely to say the cause is boredom (Kety, 1993).

Less than half of primary care physicians correctly diagnose alcohol abuse (Wenrich et al, 1995). One study found that more than half of physicians ask an alcohol screening question of three quarters of their patients but rarely go beyond that even if patients report drinking more than one drink daily. Only 50% of the doctors in this study included alcohol abuse in the diagnosis of individuals who drank four or more drinks per day (Wenrich et al, 1995).

It is recommended that a brief questionnaire be used routinely during a physical assessment of new clients. The CAGE questionnaire, consisting of four questions, is commonly used and is thought to be reliable, but it seems a bit judgmental. We have incorporated the basic ideas in Box 21-4 in what we feel is a more acceptable form.

Elderly individuals who are drug abusers are most likely addicted to prescribed anxiolytics or misusing over-the-counter (OTC) analgesics. Nicotine and caffeine may be misused by the elderly, but the most common offenders are OTC analgesics (35%) and laxatives (30%) (Kaplan and Sadock, 1994). Unexplained gastrointestinal, psychologic, or metabolic problems may be signs of the abuse of OTC products.

Assessment and Treatment. It is estimated that 40% of all adverse drug reactions occur in those over 65 years old, and many are the result of over-the-counter (OTC) drugs and alcohol (McMahon, 1993). A summary of facts regarding alcohol abuse (American Association of Retired Persons,

1994a) states that an estimated 70% of hospital admissions in 1991 were for alcohol-related problems, widowers over age 75 have the highest rate of alcoholism of any population and this contributes to the frequency of suicide among this group, and more older people were hospitalized in 1993 for alcohol-related problems than for heart attacks.

These data are provided to alert nurses to the extent of the abuse because nurses are often the first to recognize problems and are most likely to see clients in a variety of situations—most importantly, at home. Morning drinking is seen as particularly indicative of problems in the elderly female (Schuckit et al, 1996). The more frequent and diverse contact of nurses with clients gives them the advantage of recognizing subtle changes in a client's behavior and appearance.

Symptoms of alcohol abuse include difficulties with gait, balance, and cognition (Clement, 1995). In addition, frequent falls and bruises may alert the nurse to the possibility of alcohol and drug abuse, though these may also indicate abuse by others. Often these are overlapping. An elder may abuse alcohol and also be abused by alcoholic family members. Detection guidelines are seen in Box 21-5.

Changes in drinking patterns should alert nurses to potential coping problems or deterioration of health and/or social outlets. Emphasizing the disease model of alcoholism, especially when it is not proven, may result in continual focus on the symptom rather than the underlying cause. Just as interventions for physical pain are most effective before the pain fulminates, so it is with psychic pain. Depression and mental oblivion induced with drugs and alcohol can lead progressively to suicide or apathetic withdrawal. In the arena of drug and alcohol abuse the tendency of health care providers to judge the behavior as the problem results in a judgmental attitude. Particularly in the case of substance abuse, nurses must search for the pain beneath the behavior. Elderly individuals entering treatment programs report they do so because they had more problems because of drinking, were feeling more symptoms of depression, experienced more negative life events and stressors, and were self-derogating as they found alcohol becoming a problem more than a solution (Finney and Moos, 1995).

Treatment programs for elders show high rates of success, especially when social outlets are emphasized and long-term self-help groups and cohort supports are available (Blazer, 1995b). Acute alcoholic withdrawal in an elder is a serious and sometimes life-threatening issue. Recommended treatment includes frequent determination of vital signs, maintaining fluid balance without overhydrating, and providing regular dosage with oxazepam (Serax) every 1 to 2 hours (Ketcham and Hayner, 1992).

Many of the traditional ways of dealing with alcoholism have a punitive sound, for example, "Have you ever thought you were drinking too much?" It would be far more productive to discuss the issue factually. For example, "Many elders find that the stresses, loneliness, and losses of aging are very hard to bear. Some retreat into alcohol use as a way of coping. There are treatments and groups that assist individuals in these difficult adjustments. If this is a problem for you or if it becomes a problem, please let us know so we may provide resources or referrals for you." Elders are likely to feel excessively guilty and regretful about alcohol misuse, and it is important to reach out to them with understanding. The notion that alcoholism is a genetic or metabolic disorder that can be cured only by a return to God may be useful to some, but we find elders responsive to activity enrichment and group support.

Risks of alcohol and medication mixtures have not been sufficiently emphasized with most elders. A primary goal of geriatric nurse practitioners should be prevention through the education of the provider community, families, and elders about these risks (McMahon, 1993).

Excessive Suspicion and Paranoia

Many older people without previous history of mental disturbance develop a suspicious or paranoid viewpoint. Various estimates of the prevalence of paranoia range from 5% to 10% of the aged population. These reactions are sometimes induced by alcoholism or medications, particularly male hormones in combination with antidepressants. The majority, however, originate in attempts to exert control in an unsatisfactory situation or to feel capable. Inability to correctly evaluate the social milieu because of isolation or degrees of cognitive disturbance is a significant factor (Blazer, 1995a). Forgetfulness may result in an elder being convinced items are being stolen. Fear and a lack of trust originating from a reality base may become magnified, especially when one is isolated from others and reality feedback.

Men are more subject than women to those reactions. The male dilemma of expecting to be in control and gain recognition may be a factor. Women (of the present older generation) were subject to control by others and by their body reactions through their adult lives and have had more experience coping with events beyond their control. (See Chapter 19 for discussion of the importance of control.)

In addition to these dynamics, there are an unknown number of elders who have a paranoid personality disorder

that has simply grown old and more pronounced. They have had a pervasive distrust and suspiciousness of others' motives all of their adult life, assuming that others will harm, exploit, or deceive them even though they have no basis to support these beliefs (DSM IV, 1994, p. 634).

Assessment and Treatment. Paranoia is characterized by suspiciousness and insecurity (Riley, 1990). Deafness or hearing impairment may accentuate these feelings. Delusions often incorporate significant persons rather than the global grandiose or persecutory delusions of younger persons. It is sometimes difficult to determine the reality of an apparent paranoid reaction. Many cases have been encountered in which plots against an older person were real. In the case of simple paranoid psychoses the delusions appear to serve an adaptive function. When an individual becomes incapable of obtaining life's satisfactions or of maintaining function or adequate supplies, the delusions may allow the individual to avoid depression and self-blame and maintain self-esteem by projecting blame onto others or society.

Direct confrontation is likely to increase agitation, a sense of vulnerability, and the need for the delusion. A more useful approach is to establish a trusting relationship that is nondemanding and not too intense and to identify the client's strengths and build on them (Box 21-6). Paranoid behavior may be present in the absence of any cognitive loss but may also be the first symptom noted in the development of dementia. Individuals who develop paranoia for the first

---

Box 21-4

Questions Regarding Abuse of Alcohol

Are you upset when people criticize your drinking? How do you handle that?

Do you feel you sometimes drink too much? Are there particular occasions when that occurs?

Do you feel disturbed about your alcohol consumption?

Do you drink when you are feeling lonely?

Have you identified a pattern regarding your drinking?

Would you like to stop drinking?

Box 21-5

Alcohol Abuse Detection Guidelines

The following list of detection guidelines can help nurses and other healthcare providers recognize alcohol abuse in the elderly.

- Falls or accidents: Elders under the influence of alcohol may suffer more frequent mishaps, such as tripping on stairs or falling from bed while trying to get up.
- Poor nutrition: Some elderly patients may gain weight if alcohol increases their appetite. For others, consumption may inhibit or suppress appetite; alcohol becomes a substitute for food, causing excessive weight loss.
- Poor hygiene and self-care: Older alcoholics may lose track of time and the need for personal hygiene, such as bathing and changing clothes. This may be the most obvious of indicators for a nurse to observe.
- Lack of physical exercise: Many elderly who drink regularly are not interested in physical activity such as walking, gardening, or other light exercise.
- Social isolation: Friends or family may report that an elderly person declines invitations to socialize and generally displays a lack of interest in people.

From Clement M: Recognizing dependence on alcohol in the elderly, *Nurseweek* 8(20):8, 1995. Reprinted with permission.

Box 21-6 Guidelines for Nursing Care of Suspicious Patients

Remember that anger is pervasive and is not meant for the nurse per se.

Anger is a legitimate expression of feeling.

Suspicious persons will look for flaws or indications of injustice.

Attempt to accept criticism without resentment or defensiveness.

Arguing only increases the struggle for control.

The quality of nursing care may not be measurable by patient progress, particularly if the goals are unrealistic or not relevant to the patient. In other words, paranoia may lift slowly or not at all.

Nursing care should provide for the following needs:

1. Suspicious persons need to learn to trust themselves. Allow the patient to function independently in areas in which success can be achieved and identified.

2. Suspicious persons need to be able to trust others. Nurses should state what they are willing and able to do. Vague promises such as, "I'll be around whenever you need me," only increase opportunities for distrust and disappointment.

3. Suspicious persons need to test reality. When the larger reality is distorted, focus on smaller aspects of reality, for example:

   Mrs. J: The whole world is against me.

   Nurse: What in this room gives you that feeling? Are there certain times when you feel that most strongly?

   Contact with the nurse and her accepting responses reassure the person and decrease the need for a protective delusion.

4. Suspicious persons need outlets for their anger.

---

time in old age are usually very receptive to helping agencies as long as the shared goal is medical care (Jenike, 1989).

The presence of paranoid ideation is a problem only if it disturbs the patient or others in his or her environment. Paranoia may act as an effective shield against intrusion into one's vulnerable state and as such may be a useful defensive posture. When encountering suspicious elderly, the nurse's primary concern is first directed at establishing the reality of the feeling, but if the suspicions are not substantiated, the elder should not be challenged.

Nurses need to reduce the alienation and feelings of insignificance that underlie paranoid ideation. It is important that the nurse be trustworthy, that clear information be given, and that clear choices always be presented to the patient. When offering food, medication, treatments, or resources, relevant information should be given. When patients refuse "necessary" treatments, their decision must be respected. Focusing on decision-making power is most likely to be beneficial, for example, "Mrs. S, it seems you are reluctant to take these medications. I respect the fact that you are cautious about such things. I will get you more information about these drugs. Are there particular reactions you are concerned about? Let me know if you decide to take them"; or "Mrs. J, many people feel angry or afraid when they are ill. Is there anything I can do to make you more comfortable?"

Delusions

A delusional disorder is one in which conceivable ideas, without foundation in fact, persist for more than one month. These beliefs are not bizarre and do not originate in psychotic processes (DSM IV, 1994, p. 296). Common delusions are of being poisoned, being followed, or being deceived by a spouse or lover. Delusional disorders in the absence of psychoses usually begin between the ages of 40 and 55 when psychologic and physical stressors and major personal and social problems occur (Kaplan and Sadock, 1994). Delusions are intellectual mechanisms for maintaining a sense of control when security is threatened. They are beliefs that guide one's interpretation of events and help make sense out of disorder. The delusions may be comforting or threatening but always form a structure for understanding situations that otherwise might seem unmanageable. One old lady persistently held onto the delusion that her son was coming to get her, although her son had been dead for 10 years. The events of her day, her hopes, and her status were all organized around this belief. It is clear that without her delusion she would have felt forlorn, lost, and abandoned. I have encountered many delusions related to family members and their actions or intentions among the institutionalized aged.

The assessment dilemma is often one of determining the truth of the delusional belief and avoiding assumptions. It is never safe to conclude someone is delusional unless you have thoroughly investigated his or her claims. In one case an old man insisted he must go and visit his mother. His thoughts seemed clear in other respects (often the case with people who are delusional), and I suspected he had some unresolved conflicts about his dead mother or felt the need of comforting and caring. I did not argue with him about his dead mother, since arguing is never a useful approach to persons with delusions. Rather, I used the best techniques I could think of to assure him I was interested in him as a person and recognized that he must feel very lonely sometimes. He continued to say he must leave and go to his mother. When I could delay his leaving no longer, I walked with him to the nurses' station and found that his 103-year-old mother did indeed live in another wing of the institution and he visited her every day.

Frightening delusions such as those that the world is coming to an end or that one is being poisoned are usually in response to anxiety-provoking situations and are best handled by reducing situational stress, being available to the client, and attending to the fears more than the content of the delusion.

Hallucinations

Hallucinations are best described as sensory perceptions of nonexistent object stimulus and may be spurred by the internal stimulation of any of the five senses (Sprinzeles, 1992). Although they are not attributable to environmental stimuli, they may well occur because of the total environmental impact. Hallucinations arising out of psychologic conflicts tend to be less predominant in old age, while those generated as security measures tend to increase. These hallucinations are thought to germinate in situations in which one is feeling alone, abandoned, isolated, or alienated. To compensate for insecurity, an hallucinatory experience, often a companion, is imagined. Imagined companions may fill the intense void and provide some security, but they may become accusing and disturbing.

The character and stages of hallucinatory experiences have not been adequately defined in terms of the aged. Many are in response to physical disorders such as dementias, Parkinson's disease, physiologic and sensory disorders, and medications. Most often hallucinations of the aged seem mixed with disorientation, illusions, intense grief, and immersion in retrospection, the origins being difficult to separate. Almeida et al (1995) found that psychotic states arising in late life were predominately associated with cognitive decline.

It is important for nurses to determine whether the hallucinations are the result of dementia, psychoses, deprivation, or overload because the treatment will vary. An isolated old person who is admitted to the hospital in an hallucinatory state must be carefully and thoroughly assessed physically and then gradually brought into socializing experiences. He or she should be allowed peripheral participation and retreat when necessary. Persons in the community who develop hallucinations must be assessed in terms of threats to security, severe physical or psychologic disruptions, withdrawal symptoms, medications, and overload of stimuli. They will need a subdued environment with staff continuity and availability, and comprehensive assessment and care. Psychotropic medications are a significant aspect of management for most hallucinations (see Chapter 23).

Schizophrenia

The onset of schizophrenia after age 50 is extremely rare (Kaplan and Sadock, 1994).

Chronic schizophrenia tends to show beneficial changes in late life. Many of the symptoms remit entirely or diminish in intensity with a concomitant improvement in social adaptation (Jonas, 1987). When encountered in the aged, schizophrenia more likely appears as a schizoaffective disorder. Emergence of florid symptoms may be indicative of a relapse caused by undue stress and pressure (O'Connor,

1994). Putnam et al (1996) found increased negative symptomatology in aged schizophrenic patients who were institutionalized and little difference in symptoms between young and aged schizophrenic patients. These data need further study in terms of effects of environment as well as extent of chronicity.

It is suspected that many elderly homeless persons may have chronic schizophrenia; discharged from state hospitals years ago after spending their young adulthood institutionalized, they were simply unable to develop satisfactory living situations. Other elderly persons who have schizophrenia and take medication can maintain an adequate lifestyle in the community. When an individual's condition deteriorates and medication reevaluation is needed, hospitalization may be required. O'Connor (1994) emphasizes the importance of establishing a strong social support group, emphasizing activities that avoid use of alcohol or drugs, and developing specific strategies for dealing with troublesome symptoms.

Bipolar Disorders

The essential features of a bipolar disorder are characterized by the experience of one or more manic episodes and one or more major depressive disorders (DSM IV, 1994). Mania does occur in old age and may be an exacerbation of a previous disorder, a result of drug therapy (L-dopa, steroids), illness (encephalitic influenza), or head trauma (Masters, 1996). Bipolar disorders tend to decrease in the intensity of the extremes of depression and elation in the later years and sink more frequently into the depressive mode. The standard treatment has been with lithium, though this may not be tolerated well, particularly in the elderly. Irritable and agressive manics are least responsive to lithium treatment.

Commitment by the patient to the treatment regimen may be minimal because of insufficient understanding of the medications and inability to tolerate symptoms of the disease and side effects of the drugs. The patient needs relief from the most troublesome side effects of medication and can be encouraged to discuss these rather than simply accepting them. Medication management of an elder with manic episodes is often difficult, and it is necessary to individualize medication dosages and to monitor lithium levels regularly. When lithium is ineffective or poorly tolerated, anticonvulsant agents and calcium channel blockers may be better choices (Masters, 1996). Medications for the elderly with mania must be very carefully prescribed, monitored, and adjusted.

Patient and family education is essential. The family needs help to understand that the individual is not able to control mania and irritating behaviors because of a chemical imbalance in the brain. They also need a great deal of support and information. The individual who has dealt with bipolar swings throughout most of adult life is usually quite self-aware and often knows the best methods for managing. Pollack (1996) studied self-management strategies of individuals who had been hospitalized with bipolar disorders. There were no persons over 65 years old included in the study, yet many of the strategies may be applicable to elders. Most interestingly, the participants identified information they felt needed to be imparted to others with the disorder, indicating a sound understanding of the critical components of a self-management program. Given the decreased availability of mental health resources, their ideas may be very useful for professionals to incorporate in self-management teaching plans for families and individuals (Tables 21-1 and 21-2).

Depression

Depression is the mental health problem of greatest frequency and magnitude in the aged population. Estimates of prevalence vary radically depending on the qualitative variables being considered and the definition being used. Although it is estimated that between 1% and 2% of the population over age 65 meet the DSM IV criteria for a major depressive disorder (Alexopoulos, 1995b), numerous others have dysthymic conditions of varying degrees. Katona (1994) reports that though relatively few meet the DSM IV criteria for depression, many of those considered dysthymic are equally severely distressed. It is useful to think of depression as on a continuum from mild, brief sadness through intense reaction to loss, to severe psychotic depression, and then to the profound regression of pseudodementia (Alexopoulos, 1995).

Depression in the aged differs in several ways from that of younger adults. One of the major differences is the insidious manner in which it develops and the concurrency with other events, which results in depression frequently going unrecognized and untreated. Some even attribute symptoms of depression to "aging."

Aged persons tend to see their physicians often, and though at least 20% of them have various degrees of depression, they are seldom assessed, diagnosed, advised, or given specific antidepressant treatment (Williams et al, 1995). Most often they are given tranquilizers, which may actually exacerbate the problem. In addition, unfortunately, when one is profoundly or clinically depressed, the frustration and helplessness of caregivers, whether family, friends, or professionals, is often expressed as irritation, which compounds the problems. Poor performance by the elder often appears as stubborn resistance. Fortunately, depression is one of the most manageable and remedial of psychogeriatric problems once it is recognized. However, there is a high incidence of relapse after treatment, especially in the very old who have concurrent physical disorders and unrewarding life situations.

Depression is the most frequent psychiatric reason that elderly persons are admitted to the hospital, yet both diagnosis-related groups (DRGs)–based prospective payment systems in acute hospitals and the flat fee provided the exempt psychiatric units, are incentives for reduced intensity of services (Davis et al, 1995). However, though treatment days under DRGs are shortened, patients are more frequently transferred to psychiatric units, and the intensity of services are increased (Davis et al, 1995).

Etiology of Depression. Depressive symptoms in an older adult are complex and may arise from several intersecting situations and conditions: biologic changes of age, sleep cycle changes, neurotransmitter reduction, and alterations in neuroendocrine substances are thought to con-

---

Table 21-1 Factors in the Self-Management Process

| Motivators | Self-management efforts | | Self-assessment parameters |
	Successful	Unsuccessful	
Wanting to live	Follow professional advice	Deny there's a problem	How you feel
Wanting mental wellness	Talk with people	Overextend self	Intervention frequency
Wanting to get along with others	Take medication	Expect too much from misinformed	Common sense
Wanting love	Set goals		How people treat you
To become productive	Follow schedule	Stay to oneself	How you treat people
To feel better about self	Be prepared	Be open with family*	Positive results
To avoid problems in family	Stay active	Do street drugs	Decreased hospital stay
Self-love	Seek information	Rely on others for information	Behavior
Because of barriers	Read	Self-start/stop medication	Able to manage daily activities
Receiving help	Groups	Let problems overwhelm	
Finally knew what was wrong	Therapy	Get angry	
Costs (e.g., relationships, jobs)	Selective disclosure	Watch TV all the time	
Duration of illness	Don't let things get to you	Not coping with stress	
Symptoms	Hospitalization	Not seeking help	
Being hospitalized		(A particular hospitalization)	
Self-management not an option		(A prison group)	

From Pollack LE: Inpatient self-management of bipolar disorder, *Appl Nurs Res* 9(2):71, 1996.
*An unsuccessful intervention for one person may be helpful for another in differing circumstances.

tribute to predispositions toward depression. The old are thought to be more vulnerable to depression because of the reduced production of and dysregulation of mood-controlling neurotransmitters (Kaplan and Sadock, 1994). Multiple losses, illness susceptibility, and despair related to the expenditure of one's mortal time are all factors common to the depressions of the old. The helplessness of observing one's slowly deteriorating physical capacities is also undoubtedly depressing. Some factors that have been found to have a high correlation with depression are stroke, physical impairment, B vitamin deficiencies, hearing loss, and pain. Kalayam et al (1991) found a correlation between late-onset depression and hearing loss. Degenerative neurosensory changes may predispose one to depression. Frequently, medications add to or initiate depression (Box 21-7).

Contributing Factors. Many factors contribute to and influence development and patterns of depression. Factors

of health, gender, developmental needs, socioeconomics, environment, personality, and losses are all significant to the development of depression in later life. The range of these can be seen in Box 21-8.

Age and gender. Age and gender differences in incidence and expression of depression in very old age are important to consider. We do not yet know why women survive the ravages of aging better than men. In the young and middle adult years women seek help for depression twice as frequently as men. By age 65 the gender gap of depression closes somewhat, though women still seek relief more quickly than men and may abuse medications more frequently in order to seek relief (Weissman and Olfson, 1995). Suicide statistics (seen later in the chapter) indicate that there are also significant age differences in the frequency of depression among the very old.

Illness. Illness is often coexistent with depression, which may intensify illness and delay recovery through effects on the immune system and other unknown factors (U.S. Department of Health and Human Services, 1991). Patients with chronic medical illnesses are frequently subject to secondary depressions related to the disease processes. Older persons with serious medical problems are at high risk of developing depression. Estimates are that from 10% to 45% become significantly depressed (Waxman and Carner, 1984; Borson, 1987; Rapp et al, 1988). Even though depression related to the failure of physical functions is always suspected, there are particular illnesses and drugs that may produce depressive symptoms in the elderly (Box 21-9). Blazer (1995b) suggests the elements of a diagnostic workup of the elderly person with depressive symptoms (Box 21-10). Studies have shown that the presence of depression impedes healing in hip fractures and myocardial infarctions (Barker, 1990; Fielding, 1991).

Table 21-2 Self-Management Information Needed for Bipolar Group Patients

Area of concern	Information needed
Understanding bipolar disorder	Education for self and others
	Importance of medication
	Importance of groups
	Importance of therapy
	How to deal with the disorder
	How to manage yourself
	Follow medical advice
	The need to get help
Managing daily life	Set goals
	Schedule self
	Seek support
	Manage stress
	Daily functioning
	Enjoy life
	Importance of exercise
Living in society	Stress management
	Money management
	Society reentry
Relating to others	Anger management
	Need for support
	Be self-aware and independent
Relating to self	Need for good self-esteem
	Avoid substances
	Think positively
	Take responsibility for your life
	Assess self
	Problem solve
	Help self
	Attend groups
	Seek spiritual strength
	Deal with situations
	Seek support
	Meditate
	Exercise mind and body

From Pollack LE: Inpatient self-management of bipolar disorder, *Appl Nurs Res* 9(2):71, 1996.

Box 21-7 **Drugs That Are Common Contributors to Depression**

Benzodiazepines
Alcohol
Antipsychotics
Beta-blockers
Chemotherapeutic agents
Cimetidine
Digitalis
Excess or deficiency of potassium, sodium, calcium, glucose
Hypoxemia
Uremia
Vitamin B and folic acid deficiencies
Metabolic alkalosis

From Koenig HG, Blazer DG: Depression and other affective disorders. In Casell CK, Riesenberg DE, Sorenson LG et al: *Geriatric medicine,* New York, 1990, Springer-Verlag.

| Box 21-8 | **Related Factors in Onset of Depression in Older Adults** |

Illnesses

- Hypothyroidism
- Hyperthyroidism
- Cushing's disease
- Infections
- Lymphoma
- Cancer: pancreatic, breast, prostate
- Other malignancies

Medications

- Reserpine (Serpasil)
- α-methyldopa (Aldomet)
- Clonidine (Catapres)
- Hydralazine (Apresoline)
- Propranolol (Inderal)
- Digitalis
- Cimetidine (Tagamet)
- Steroids
- Estrogens
- Progestational agents
- Indomethacin (Indocin)
- Propoxyphene (Darvon)
- Codeine
- Antibacterials
- Levodopa (Larodopa)
- Tamoxifen (Nolvadex)
- Vincristine (Oncovin)
- Vinblastine (Velban)
- Benzodiazepines
- Barbiturates

Nutritional Deficits

- Lack of B vitamins
- Tooth loss

- Malfitting dentures
- Loss of interest in eating alone

Neurologic Changes

- Reduction in norepinephrine
- Reduction in dopamine
- Reduction in serotonin brain concentrations
- Increase in monoamine catabolic enzyme monoamine oxidase

Psychosocial Stressors

- Restricted social contacts
- Reduced vocational, social, and recreational activities
- Financial impoverishment with poor living conditions
- Widowhood
- Separation from children and others
- Lack of adequate social supports
- Loss of "beauty" in western world
- Loss of status in western world
- Loss of employment and "self-worth" in western world
- Lack of stimulating environment

Physiologic Changes

- Sleep disturbances
- Slowed gait
- Decreased eyesight
- Decrease in hearing
- Chronic illnesses as loss (eg, benign prostatic hypertrophy and surgery leading to loss of potency)

From Groh C, Whall AL: Geriatric depression. In Burggraf V, Barry R: *Gerontological nursing: current practice and research,* Thorofare, NJ, 1996, SLACK, Inc.

Mossey et al (1996) note that subdysthymic depression occurs in 20% to 50% of hospitalized elderly associated with physical and social disabilities. This delays recovery and increases costs. They found interpersonal counseling provided for elders by psychiatric clinical nurse specialists following discharge from the hospital reduced depression and had a positive effect on recovery. Moreover, these gains were sustained in a periodic follow-up. Studies replicating these findings would be useful to demonstrate cost savings sufficient to interest HMO providers in the routine employment of these methods.

Poststroke depression is so common it is virtually ignored in treatment because symptoms parallel those of the stroke itself: apathy, amnesia, and pathologic crying (Black, 1995). Borson (1987) found that patients with chronic obstructive pulmonary disease (COPD) are particularly vulner-

able to depression. The depression is often accompanied by anxiety and panic. Often physicians do not recognize these as symptoms of depression, and when they do, they may be reluctant to treat it because of the adverse reactions to antidepressant drugs. This is a significant problem and often related to routine assessment practices that ignore depression as a possible deterrent to recovery. Older individuals are likely to be judged hypochondriacal when the complications of depression slow their recovery from illness. For these reasons we feel the U.S. version of the Cambridge General Health Questionnaire (1979) may be the most useful of the brief symptom checklists. We encourage nurses to use the simple and reliable tools provided in Appendix 21-A and to alert physicians when there is evidence of depression. The Zung Self-Rating Depression Scale (1965) is similar and preferred by some, though it contains more

Illnesses That Cause Depression

Parkinson's disease
Amyotrophic lateral sclerosis
Gliomas (intracranial tumors)
Multiple sclerosis
Hypothyroidism
Hypoparathyroidism
Addison's disease (hypoadrenal function)
Cushing's disease (hyperadrenal function)
Anemia (particularly pernicious anemia)
Pancreatitis
Hyperinsulinism
Pancreatic cancer
Uremia
Congestive heart failure
Lymphoid leukemia
Systemic lupus erythematosus

"physical" symptoms than some and tends to produce a false positive in elders who have normal physical changes of aging.

Hypochondriasis. Hypochondriasis is a diffusion of health concerns that seems to increase when there is a real health problem but is often a cardinal symptom of depression. Elderly people tend to express depression through somatic symptoms. Thus the hypochondriacal preoccupation of the elderly may be a signal of the presence of depression as are frequent visits to general practitioners. Mild, transient bouts of hypochondriasis are frequent and serve as a means of coping with the stress of real illness and loss. The patients are far less likely to view problems as psychologic, interpersonal, or situational; chief complaints are usually of various physical discomforts (e.g., "constipation," "gas pain," or "heartburn"). These sorts of complaints are too readily dismissed as hypochondriacal when a more holistic approach to the patient would reveal the extent and complexity of problems.

Fortunately, physicians are beginning to address the psychologic and interpersonal reasons why elders feel symptomatic and seek medical attention (Barsky, 1996). Depressed individuals using more medical services than the nondepressed had experienced marital separation and divorce, were of lower socioeconomic status, and had chronically disabling physical illnesses. Nonrecognition of depression in the elderly may in fact be costly, since these patients tend to overuse medical services (Borson, 1989).

Grief. Grief as a predominant aspect of depression and vice versa must be explored with all elders. Chronic grief and multiple losses may result in profound depression, apathy, and withdrawal from life. Farberow et al (1992) studied the grief process in people over 55 through comparisons of spouses of suicides and spouses who lost their mate through illness. This longitudinal study (2.5 years) challenges some previous ideas about the grief process in elders as well as confirms some concepts already in the literature. Rather than specific, identifiable stages of resolution, they found a gradual adaptation to the loss, which was facilitated by a supportive network and prior good coping skills. Those in an environmental setting that was stressful and those with other concurrent losses had a more difficult adaptation. The biggest problems were loneliness and managing the tasks of daily living. At the completion of the 2.5-year study it was found that both groups were significantly more composed, enthusiastic about life, and relaxed.

Guilt, so predominant among younger spouses of suicides, was not as great a factor in the adaptation of elderly survivors as one might have expected. The major variation between the two groups was in the instability of emotions of the spouses of the suicides and their more intense grief for the first year. The other group seemed to follow a steadier course toward healing.

Adjustment to bereavement is an ongoing life process with no precise point when grieving is over and mourning ends. The pain of loss may remain for a lifetime, felt in a different manner as time passes. Schmall, Lawson, and Stiehl (1990) have thoughtfully examined the aspects of grief in the elderly. They itemized the various intersecting factors that often result in depression: heredity, biochemical changes of aging, drugs, illnesses, personality types, sensory impairments, stressors, and even the seasons of the year.

Anticipatory grief for self. Anticipatory grief for self arises with the recognition of old age. There may be a depression related to anticipation of death. One becomes cognizant of time lived balanced against time left. There is an urgency: so much yet to learn, to experience, to share, and so little time. Those who love life the most may feel the acuity of it. Joe said, "Do I have to die with so many stories still untold?" He will leave this world and take with him all the hidden hopes and fears, the small pleasures, the inexpressible thoughts, the small child, and the inner man that was never let out.

It is even more painful to contemplate a life only partially lived with the full awareness that time precludes recapture.

Arthur had lived an ordinary life with few demands and few adventures. As he was dying he invented, in his delirium, adventures that he could have had. It was as if his psyche were expressing that element of his nature that had lain dormant for so long.

Charles, who had seemed so superficial and lacking in the capacity for inner exploration, became visibly different following his seventieth birthday. He began to speak of his past experiences with some insight and to express his uncertainties. He, who had appeared so blasé, expressed his tender feelings. Tears would fill his eyes as he speculated about the future of his grandchildren: Would they remember him? Would they care? Would they wonder about him?

This distinct type of depression is born of the existential loneliness each feels when confronted with the ultimate relinquishment of self. The great drama is ending, and there

Diagnostic Workup of the Elderly Patient with Depressive Symptoms

History
Symptoms
Present history, including onset, duration, and change in symptoms over time
Past history of depressive or manic episodes and other psychiatric and medical disorders
Presence or absence of symptoms of a thought disorder such as schizophrenia, organic brain disease, or significant physical illness
Medication history
Family history of depression, other psychoses, or alcoholism

Physical Examination
Special attention paid to the evaluation of possible endocrine disorders, occult infection, neurologic deficits, cardiac function, and evidence of occult malignancy

Mental Status Examination
Disturbances of consciousness
Disturbances of mood and affect
Disturbances of motor behavior
Disturbances of perception
Presence or absence of hallucinations
Disturbances of thinking
Self-esteem and guilt
Suicidal ideation

Disturbances of memory and intelligence (usually should be tested on at least two or three occasions)
  Memory, e.g., "Do you know the date today?"
  Ability to abstract, e.g., "In what way are a pear and a banana alike?"
  Ability to perform simple calculations, e.g., "Subtract 3 from 20 and keep subtracting 3 from each number you get until you reach 0."
  Knowledge of important current events, e.g., "Who is the president of the United States now?"

Laboratory Tests
Complete blood cell count
Urinalysis
Thyroxine level determination
VDRL
Electroencephalogram
Computerized tomography scan (when indicated)
Vitamin B_{12} and folate assays

Psychologic Tests
Experimental Tests
Plasma and spinal fluid assays for neurotransmitters and neurotransmitter metabolites
Evoked potentials
Specialized neuropsychologic testing

From Blazer D: *Depression in late life,* St Louis, 1982, Mosby.

will be no sequel. Even those who believe firmly in an afterlife or reincarnation must let go of this particularly unique life and personality.

Social and cultural factors. Social and cultural factors influence the appearance and course of depression. In spite of deep and profound misery, some older individuals may not seek treatment for depression because they, like so many people, believe that it is a character weakness that must not be given in to and that they should be able to pull themselves out of the "doldrums" by their own efforts. Some families and professionals share this view. The problems most frequently causing reactive depressions have been identified by Müller-Spahn and Hock (1994) and are enumerated in Box 21-11.

Institutions. Institutions cause depression as well as harbor those who are depressed. Commerford and Reznikoff (1996) found that neither religiosity nor social support were significant to reduction of depression in nursing home residents. In other words, it appears that depression is a result of the impact of the environment regardless of the quality of external and internal supportive resources. Issues of control may be at the crux of these depressions. Barder et al (1994) found that after 6 or 7 weeks in a nursing home elderly

males, even though without a history of mental illness or cognitive impairment, developed depression and learned helplessness. This suggests that immediately upon admission to long-term care strategic patient care planning must include ways in which the individual will be given control of the situation.

Biorhythmicity. Biorhythmicity and the emotional effects of disruptions in light must be considered. Temporal patterns of exposure refers to the length of exposure to solar radiation that maintains health and avoids overexposure. Seasonal affective disorders (SADs) have been given attention by psychologists and others as the source of annual depressive episodes in some individuals. There is growing evidence that light-dark cycles are critical to these.

Evidence suggests some individuals have strong psychophysiologic responses to artificial light. Bright, artificial light has been shown to increase calcium absorption in healthy elderly men and to enhance synthesis of vitamin D while simultaneously lowering plasma bilirubin (Kolanowski, 1992). In addition, Lovell et al (1995) found that bright light administered 2 hours each morning for two 10-day periods reduced agitated behaviors in six demented subjects living in a skilled nursing home. The National In-

---

Box 21-11   **Depression in the Elderly: Most Frequent Problems**

1. Social isolation, loss of important social support systems
2. Loss of autonomy (psychiatric and physical illness, physical disability)
3. Inactivity (retirement)
4. Loss of reputation, financial problems
5. Relocation of residence
6. Severe insomnia

From Müller-Spahn F, Hock C: Clinical presentation of depression in the elderly, *Gerontology* 40(suppl 1):10, 1994.

---

stitute of Mental Health follow-up studies of individuals suffering winter SAD (Schwartz et al, 1996) found that light treatment was safe and effective for most, but severely affected persons were nonresponsive to light therapy. Wirz-Justice et al (1996) found that morning walks in natural light were more effective than treatment with low-dose artificial lighting.

Assisting residents of institutions to get outdoors or to use solariums should be a part of the daily care plan because it becomes more and more apparent there are physiologic and psychologic needs that respond to appropriate amounts of sunlight. Nurses are largely responsible for the contact a resident has with environmental and natural lighting.

Kolanowski (1992) suggests the need for more clinical nursing research into the optimum amounts of light to achieve inner harmony and a sense of well-being. More study needs to be done on the specific uses of light therapy with the elderly.

Symptoms of Depression. DSM-IV defines a major depressive disorder as the persistence of five of nine symptoms for most of the time during a 2-week period. (One of the five symptoms must be depressed mood or loss of interest in usual activities.) The main characteristics of depression fall into categories of thought disturbance, mood disturbance, behavioral disturbance, and body complaints (Table 21-3). Individuals with chronic health problems are at high risk of depression. Depression in the elderly is often seen as low self-esteem, feelings of helplessness, hypochondriasis, complaints of forgetfulness, difficulty concentrating, low energy, weight loss, and anorexia (Kaplan and Sadock, 1994).

Questions have been raised concerning specific differences that may be expected in the presenting symptoms of older adults. It is not at all clear that depressive symptomatology is the same in the later years. The characteristics of older adults may alter the facets of depression. For instance, the classic early morning waking so characteristic of depression in youth is often a normal part of growing older (see Chapter 6). The diagnosis of depression in the elderly is particularly difficult because many of the symptoms that are

---

Table 21-3   Symptoms and Signs of Depression in Late Life

Symptoms	Behavioral signs
Mood	**Social**
Dejected mood or sadness	Uncooperativeness
Decreased life satisfaction	Social withdrawal
Loss of interest	Hostility
Impulse to cry	Suspiciousness
Irritability	Confusion and clouding of consciousness
Emptiness	Diurnal variations of mood
Fearfulness and anxiety	Drooling (in severe cases)
Negative feelings toward self	Crying or whining
Worry	
Helplessness	
Hopelessness	**Physiologic**
Sense of failure	Occasional ulcerations of skin secondary to picking
Loneliness	Occasional ulcerations of cornea secondary to decreased blinking
Uselessness	
Loss of motivation or "paralysis of will"	
Thoughts	**Psychomotor retardation**
Low self-esteem	Slowed speech
Pessimism	Slowed movements
Self-blame and criticism	Gestures minimized
Rumination about problems	Shuffling slow gait
Suicidal thoughts	Mutism (in severe cases)
Delusions	Stupor or semicoma (in severe cases)
Of uselessness	Cessation of mastication and swallowing (in severe cases)
Of unforgivable behavior	Decreased or inhibited blinking (in severe cases)
Nihilistic	
Somatic	
Hallucinations	**Psychomotor agitation**
Auditory	Continued motor activity
Visual	Wringing of hands
Kinesthetic	Picking at skin, which may lead to ulcerations
Doubt of values and beliefs	Pacing
Difficulty concentrating	Restless sleep
Poor memory	Grasping at others
Physical	**Bizarre or inappropriate behavior**
Loss of appetite	Suicidal gestures or attempts
Fatigability	Negativism such as refusal to eat or drink and stiffness of the body
Sleep disturbance	Outbursts of aggression
Initial insomnia	Falling backward
Terminal insomnia	
Constipation	
Loss of libido	
Pain	
Restlessness	
Weight loss	
Bowel impaction	
Appearance	
Stooped posture	
Sad face	
Unkempt appearance (in severe cases)	

From Blazer D: *Depression in late life,* St Louis, 1982, Mosby.

used as diagnostic criteria fall under the vegetative signs of depression that include disturbance of sleep, appetite, libido, attention and concentration, easy fatigability, and psychomotor retardation or agitation. Likewise, constipation and slower movements may be caused by physiologic changes rather than psychologic stress.

Melancholia. A particular type of depression seen as melancholia is particular to the elderly. It is a complex of feelings that includes depression, low-self esteem, feelings of worthlessness, hypochondria, self-accusatory thoughts about sex and sinfulness, and often includes suicidal and paranoidal ideation (Kaplan and Sadock, 1994). Melancholic depression is exhibited by total disinterest in environment, diurnal variation, and psychomotor agitation or retardation (Blazer, 1995b)

Pseudodementia. One of the major difficulties in determining the presence of a clinically significant depression in the aged is the frequent misdiagnosis as dementia. Many of the presenting symptoms are similar. To complicate this problem, dementia is frequently concurrent with severe depression. A depression so severe it appears as dementia is classified as pseudodementia.

Pseudodementia is a syndrome in which dementia is mimicked or caricatured by functional psychiatric illness. The most common psychiatric illness presenting in this manner is a major depressive episode. The diagnosis is generally made by exclusion when no organic pathologic condition can be found. Trials of antidepressants may be useful, although there are high nonresponse rates even in clear-cut depressive illnesses. Social withdrawal, global errors of omission, acuteness of onset, past psychiatric history, and the tendency of the patient to point out errors rather than hiding them are all suggestive of a depressive pseudodementia. The separation of dementia and major depression is one of the first assessment tasks. Symptoms of profound depression (pseudodementia) as they are differentiated from dementia are seen in Table 21-4.

Assessment of Depression. Primary care physicians are the professionals who encounter the majority of aged individuals with depression, and the physician is sought because

---

Table 21-4   Features Distinguishing Pseudodementia from Dementia

Pseudodementia*	Dementia
Characteristics	
Variability in symptoms	Consistent symptoms in stable situations
Recent and remote memory loss	Recent memory loss more severe than remote
Orientation vague	Disorientation present
Attention intact	Distractability
Sleep patterns fragmented, early waking	Sleep pattern reversal common
Diurnal patterns, worse in morning	Diurnal pattern, sundowner syndrome
Great distress regarding cognitive impairment	Often unaware of cognitive dysfunction
Refusal to attempt activities	Attempts to perform as requested, often unable
Judgment intact	Judgment impaired
Verbalizations limited	Verbalizations repetitious, often incomprehensible
Focus on failure	Responds to praise and encouragement
Melancholic	Irritable, easily disturbed
Somatic complaints, hypochondriasis	Often unaware of bodily needs/reactions
Demonstrates "learned helplessness"	Attempts to do more than capable of
Complaints of inability to remember	Seldom seems aware of memory deficits
Symptoms immobilize client	Symptoms slowly progressive
Psychomotor retardation severe	Excessive movement, agitation common
Failings highlighted by individual	Failings highlighted by family
Caregiver input is necessary and helpful	Caregivers may be in denial/angry
May respond to antidepressants	No improvement noted with course of antidepressants
Nursing Care Plans	
Identify precipitants of disorder	Identify pattern of personality decline
Encourage expression of feelings	Focus on feelings may produce agitation
Gradually increase expectations of client	Maintain consistent expectations of client
Explore and revive old interests	Provide immediate comforts and gratifications
Provide opportunity for return of social skills	Support remaining social skills
Encourage assertiveness regarding needs/wants	Encourage cooperation with caregivers
Encourage caregivers to expect improvement	Locate resources to support caregivers

From Wells CE: *Am J Psychiatry* 136:898, 1979; National Institute of Mental Health: *Individualized treatment planning for psychiatric patients,* Washington, DC, 1977, NIMH; Teri L, Truax P: Assessment of depression in dementia patients: association of caregiver mood with depression ratings, *Gerontologist* 34(2):231, 1994; Foreman MD, Fletcher K, Mion L, Simon L: Assessing cognitive function, *Geriatr Nurs* 17(5):228, 1996; Ebersole, clinical experience.
*Refer to glossary for definitions of pseudodementia and dementia.

of hypochondriacal concerns. In one study of 2000 persons in managed care systems and fee-for-service practices it was found that 26% of nonpsychiatric patients had "double depression," that is, major depression as well as dysthymia (mild depression and anxiety) lasting more than 2 years (Wells et al, 1995). It was concluded that improving detection of depressive disorders by general physicians, both in managed care and private practice, is a high priority.

It may be even more critical in the home. One study showed that 27.5% of home-bound clients scored in the depressed range on the Geriatric Depression Scale, but none had been documented by home health nurses as depressed (Dalton and Busch, 1995). Covinsky (1996) recommends the screening of all hospitalized elders for depression because it has been found that the risk of increasing dependency in activities of daily living (ADLs) was directly related to depressive symptomatology. We would suggest this is just as important in home care.

The Zung Self-Rating Depression Scale (Zung, 1965; see Appendix 21-A) has had more trials with older adults than any other depression instrument, although it is not specifically constructed with norms derived from an aged population. One criticism is that physiologic factors are predominant in this tool, and therefore it may inaccurately reflect normal physiologic slowing of aging or subclinical and clinical disease as depression.

The Beck Depression Inventory has become rather popular, since it has demonstrated a moderate degree of reliability and validity (Beck et al, 1961; see Appendix 21-A and Box 21-13). The gradients of each question are rated from 1 to 4, and the sum total indicates the level of depression.

The Geriatric Depression Scale was developed by Yesavage et al (1983; see Appendix 21-A). It is a 30-item assessment tool designed for geriatric patients and based almost exclusively on psychologic discriminators. It has been

markedly effective in determining the presence of significant depression because the confounding features (physical complaints, libido, and appetite) are deemphasized. It is presently seen as a more accurate measure of depression in the elderly than the various other tools (Vezina and Laprise, 1995). Davis (1996) summarizes the components of an assessment for depression (Box 21-12).

Goals of Treatment. The goals of treatment for depression include (1) decreasing symptoms, (2) reducing risk of relapse and recurrence, (3) increasing quality of life, (4) improving medical health status, and (5) decreasing health care costs and mortality (U.S. Department of Health and Human Services, 1991). The changes in the health care delivery system, the emphasis on cost savings and the increasing numbers of frail elderly make these goals even more pertinent today than when they were formulated almost a decade ago. Mann (1996) reports an interview with Dr. David Kupfer, professor and chair of the department of psychiatry at the University of Pittsburgh School of Medicine, in which he reiterates the treatability of depression and emphasizes the need to intervene as promptly as possible and to continue treatment 4 to 6 months beyond the relief of symptoms.

Treatment considerations. In treating depression in the aged, consider the following:

1. There are several types of depression. It is important that a comprehensive evaluation is made before a conclusion is reached.
2. Biochemical and hormonal changes of aging may intensify depression in the aged (e.g., neurotransmitters change with aging); most hormones are reduced, particularly thyroid hormones.
3. Drugs that are used for medical problems may intensify depression (e.g., hypotensives, psychotropics, cardiotonics, hypnotics).
4. Antidepressant drugs may have idiosyncratic effects, toxic accumulation, and/or paradoxical effects. They should be used with expert knowledge, discrimination, and adequate observation.
5. Knowledge of the presence of depression may be helpful in assisting the older person to understand and cope with some of the unexplained symptoms he or she is experiencing. Clients should be involved in assessment and discussion of depression. Having the individual assess the level of depression immediately engages the person actively in examining his or her own feelings. The "Stepladder of Depression" (Box 21-13) is one of the tools that can be used in that manner.
6. Recognize the importance of restoring a sense of control, choice, and mastery.
7. Often increased socialization and relief from physical discomfort and ailments will significantly lift depression.
8. Vigorous treatment of the elderly depressed patient and adequate aftercare clearly improve treatment outcome (Burvill et al, 1991).

Box 21-12   Assessment for Depression

To assess for depression
1. Observe affect, speech, behavior, and sleeping and eating patterns
2. Review medications
3. Appraise circumstances and health history
4. Use brief, standardized tools that measure depression
5. Observe for sad countenance, forgetfulness, poor concentration, withdrawal, hypochondriasis, decreased appetite, minimal participation in the therapeutic regimen, negligence in grooming, and insomnia or hypersomnia
6. Listen for evidence of low self esteem, self blame, helplessness, hopelessness, guilt, or spiritual emptiness

From Davis B: Rx for teaching: depression and the elderly, *Home Health Focus* 3(2):14, 1996.

9. Be alert to early signs of recurrent depression because this is common in major depressions.

10. To decrease depression and raise self-esteem, defensive structures should be supported unless they are clearly detrimental to the client or family.

Interventions. Interventions are primarily medical (drugs and electroconvulsive therapy [ECT]), social (family and social support), grief management, and behavioral conditioning. Seldom is anything said about rediscovering meanings and renewing spirituality, but we believe those are significant to recovery. We would suggest the use of the JAREL scale for initiating discussions regarding spirituality (Stollenwork et al, 1996) (see appendixes to Chapter 27). The scale is used only to focus attention and stimulate discussion, not to judge how spiritual another may be.

Richman (1995) has found humor useful because it increases a sense of sharing and is highly interactive and stress reducing. Obviously, humor must be used with extreme care. Clients must never believe that their misery is taken in a light-hearted manner.

A strategy we developed fully in one of our earlier editions was the use of dreams for self-expression, understanding, and reestablishing control. We have found this useful because many very depressed people seem to live more in their dream time than while awake. We have not corroborated this with studies. Reminiscing serves somewhat the same functions, though a very depressed elder may not reminisce spontaneously. Always, in all interventions with depressed elders, the goal is to stimulate them to take control and make the decisions, explain what they want, and what they enjoy or appreciate.

Medications. Despite much research, it is not known exactly how antidepressant drugs exert their effects, though it is known they influence numerous neurotransmitter systems (Figure 21-2). Nevertheless, the chief intervention being used for depression is the prescription of antidepressants despite numerous negative side effects experienced by the el-

derly. Glassman and Roose (1994) report that tricyclic antidepressants (TCAs) are notoriously poor selections for the elderly. TCAs fall into the category of class I antiarrhythmic drugs, which have been responsible for increased cardiac disorders and deaths in persons with ischemic heart disease. It is not yet known whether the same effects may exist with the use of serotonin specific reuptake inhibitors (SSRIs).

In about 60% of cases, antidepressant medication is helpful in reducing depression. (To produce effects in elderly patients 6 to 12 weeks of medication regimen may be necessary.) Active participation in the treatment plan and compliance with medication dosage must be encouraged because clients' motivation may be very low (see further discussion in Chapter 23).

Electroconvulsive therapy. ECT has been useful, but relapse is frequent. Risk factors that suggest caution are concurrent medical illnesses, certain medications, and cognitive deficits. Recent retrospective research found the safety, effectiveness, and survival of elders who were treated with ECT superior in efficacy to those treated with conventional pharmacotherapy (Philibert et al, 1995).

Cognitive-behavioral therapy. Cognitive-behavioral group therapy, focused visual imagery group therapy, and education/discussion groups on cognition, depression, and hopelessness have been used with moderate improvement in cognitive function but no significant change in depression in nursing home residents (Abraham, et al, 1992). One must then wonder if depressive symptomatology is amenable to thought control because depressive thoughts are clouded and pessimistic. Cognitive-behavioral therapy focuses on

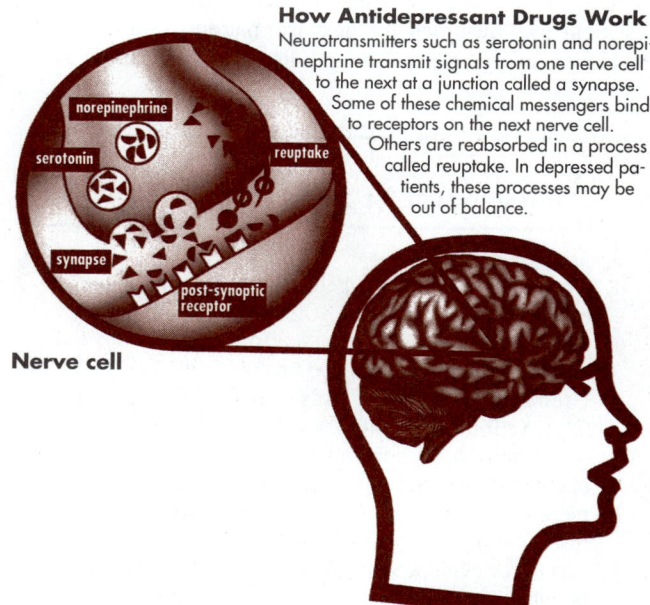

How Antidepressant Drugs Work
Neurotransmitters such as serotonin and norepinephrine transmit signals from one nerve cell to the next at a junction called a synapse. Some of these chemical messengers bind to receptors on the next nerve cell. Others are reabsorbed in a process called reuptake. In depressed patients, these processes may be out of balance.

Figure 21-2. Workings of antidepressants. (Courtesy SmithKline Beecham Pharmaceuticals, Paxil Access to Care program, Philadelphia.)

Box 21-13	**A Stepladder of Depression**

1. I am not particularly discouraged about the future.
   I feel discouraged about the future.
   I feel I have nothing to look forward to.
   I feel the future is hopeless and things cannot improve.
2. I do not feel like a failure.
   I feel I have failed more than the average person.
   As I look back on my life, all I can see are failures.
   I feel I am a complete failure as a person.

Example from Beck Depression Inventory. © 1978, 1993 by Aaron T. Beck. Reproduced by permission of the publisher, The Psychological Corporation. All rights reserved. "Beck Depression Inventory" and "BDI" are registered trademarks of the Psychological Corporation.

negating cognitive errors that are common to depressed elderly: (1) overgeneralizing; (2) awfulizing; (3) exaggerating own importance; (4) demanding of others; (5) expecting mind reading; (6) self-blame; and (7) unrealistic expectations. Mann (1996) reports that Kupfer specifies cognitive-behavioral therapy as efficacious in the treatment of depression.

Healing in nature. Groh and Whall (1996) propose the use of natural environments to restore psychologic well-being. Bombardment with noise, expectations and demands, and the constant distractions of our environment creates mental fatigue; elders may be especially prone to this. Birds, plants, animals, flowers, flowing water, and fresh air are all proposed as restorative. This is an intervention that feels instinctively right, but we know little about why that is so. Winnie said, "I hate being 85. I climbed mountains and explored valleys when I was 70, and now I need help to get around my small apartment." We must wonder if the physical limitations of aging may contribute to depression by hindering access to the mountains and the sea, by limiting contact with nature.

Social supports. Family interventions may consist primarily of shoring up their tolerance, knowledge, and understanding. Chapter 17 discusses caregivers.

The following is a summary of interventions that have been found effective with depressed elders:

- Structured, noncompetitive activities
- Opportunities for decisions and to exercise control
- Focus on spiritual renewal and rediscovery of meanings
- Guided autobiography (Birren and Deutchman, 1991)
- Self-analysis through journals and dreams
- Reactivation of latent interests
- Validation of depressed feelings as aiding recovery, not trying to bolster patient's mood or deny his or her despair
- An accepting atmosphere and an empathic nursing response

Encourage the individual to recognize depression as a treatable illness and to seek help. It is most helpful to discuss the nature of the depression with the client. Help the client become aware of the presence of depression, the nature of the symptoms, and the time limitation of depression. For example, do not talk him or her out of being depressed; do not console with "life is worth living" or other clichés that only confirm the nurse's inability to comprehend the pain.

Present depression as a dynamic process of choosing to experience the depression rather than avoiding it by overactivity, suicide, psychosomatic illness, or substance dependence. All of these can be seen as less healthy options than dealing directly with depression.

Encourage and validate feelings of family, friends, and professionals as they deal with anger, hostility, and rejection. These feelings intensify the sense of loss and rejection the client is experiencing, further increasing self-deprecation. To the extent possible, the feelings should be defused before approaching the depressed elder.

Reminiscence is believed to have particular diagnostic and therapeutic potential for elderly patients. It can be used as a means to resolve old conflicts, guilts, and disappointments; for socialization experiences; and as a way to capitalize on the preserved memories of those who may have lost some cognitive capacity. Maintenance of self-esteem and self-continuity are some of the benefits of reminiscence therapy. Reminiscence as a therapeutic strategy is summarized in Box 21-14. Additional discussion of reminiscence is presented later in the chapter.

Nurses may help themselves and the client by being present, accepting the client's limited amount of interaction, and continually giving the client choices and clear feedback. When there are certain expectations of the client, state them in the form of options, for example, "It is important for you to get up and get dressed. Movement will increase your circulation and your energy levels. Do you want to get up before breakfast or after breakfast?" The client may respond that he does not want to get up. In that case the nurse might reply, "You do have the right not to participate. I will return in 30 minutes, after you have given it more thought." On returning the nurse may ask, "What is your decision?" Sometimes humor restores perspective, if used gently rather than aggressively, "Do I understand you intend to remain in bed? Remaining in bed ensures that you won't get up on the wrong side!"

Getting into a power struggle over involvement in activities only ensures that the nurse will lose. If this occurs inadvertently, stop as soon as you recognize it and bring it to the attention of the client, "You will win this game; you can choose to remain in bed and there is little I can do about that."

There are many ways of treating depression, and none is consistently effective. The following have all been used with varying degrees of success (Figure 21-3):

1. Activity therapy, which restores smooth and striated muscular function
2. Rest and recreation, which promotes recuperative ability

Box 21-14	**Reminiscence as a Developmental and Therapeutic Strategy**

Maintain continuity
Extract meaning
Define and develop personal philosophy
Identify cycles and themes
Recapitulate learning and growth
Evolve identity
Provide insight and growth
Integrate and accept regrets and disappointments
Perceive universality

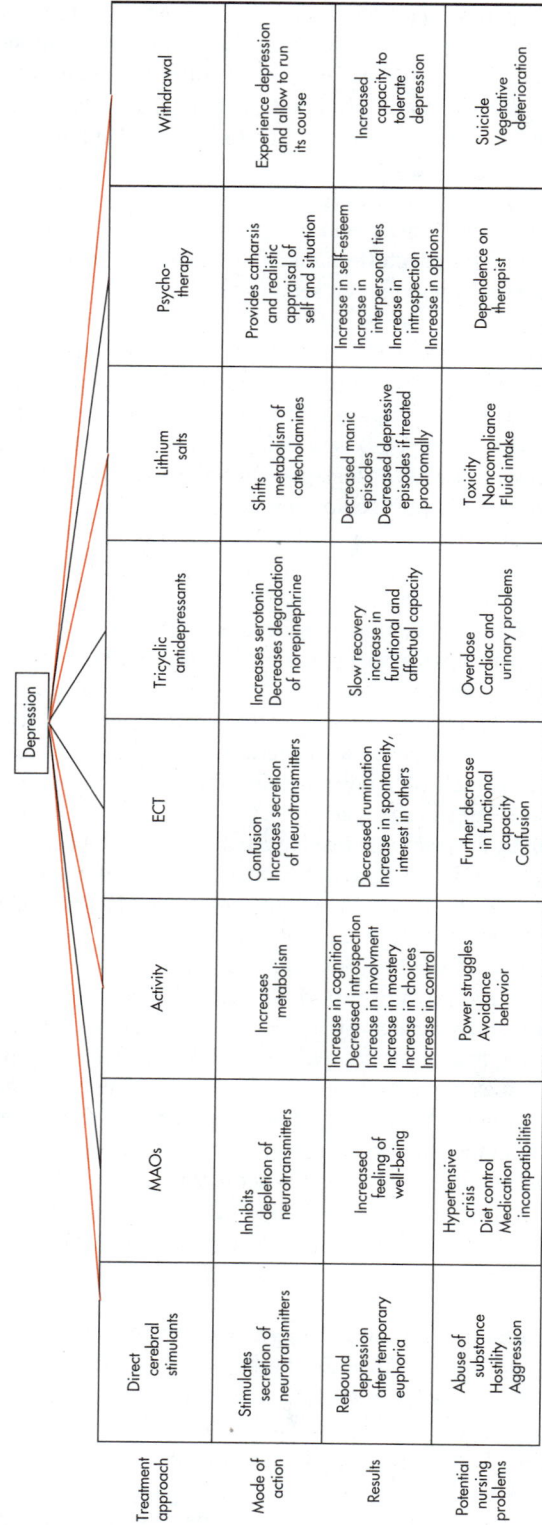

Treatment approach	Direct cerebral stimulants	MAOs	Activity	ECT	Tricyclic antidepressants	Lithium salts	Psycho-therapy	Withdrawal
Mode of action	Stimulates secretion of neurotransmitters	Inhibits depletion of neurotransmitters	Increases metabolism	Confusion Increases secretion of neurotransmitters	Increases serotonin Decreases degradation of norepinephrine	Shifts metabolism of catecholamines	Provides catharsis and realistic appraisal of self and situation	Experience depression and allow to run its course
Results	Rebound depression after temporary euphoria	Increased feeling of well-being	Increase in cognition Decreased introspection Increase in involvment Increase in mastery Increase in choices Increase in control	Decreased rumination Increase in spontaneity, interest in others	Slow recovery increase in functional and affectual capacity	Decreased manic episodes Decreased depressive episodes if treated prodromally	Increase in self-esteem Increase in interpersonal ties Increase in introspection Increase in options	Increased capacity to tolerate depression
Potential nursing problems	Abuse of substance Hostility Aggression	Hypertensive crisis Diet control Medication incompatibilities	Power struggles Avoidance behavior	Further decrease in functional capacity Confusion	Overdose Cardiac and urinary problems	Toxicity Noncompliance Fluid intake	Dependence on therapist	Suicide Vegetative deterioration

Figure 21-3. Depression: treatment and nursing problems.

3. Individual psychotherapy, which allows self-expression and resolution of despair
4. Group psychotherapy, which allows one to reestablish social connections
5. Hypnotism, which allows the surfacing of unconscious blocks to self-realization
6. Antidepressant medications and lithium, which alter cerebral physiologic condition
7. ECT, which seems to temporarily restore neurotransmitter secretion

To be successful, the treatment of depression must include considerations of the individual's premorbid personality, determination of reactive or endogenous origins, symptom relief, social support manipulation, and the importance of a positive relationship with health care providers. The ability to tolerate depression enhances one's coping capacity in later years. All aged people will be depressed at some time and may better survive those episodes if they can develop a perspective that allows depression to be viewed as a

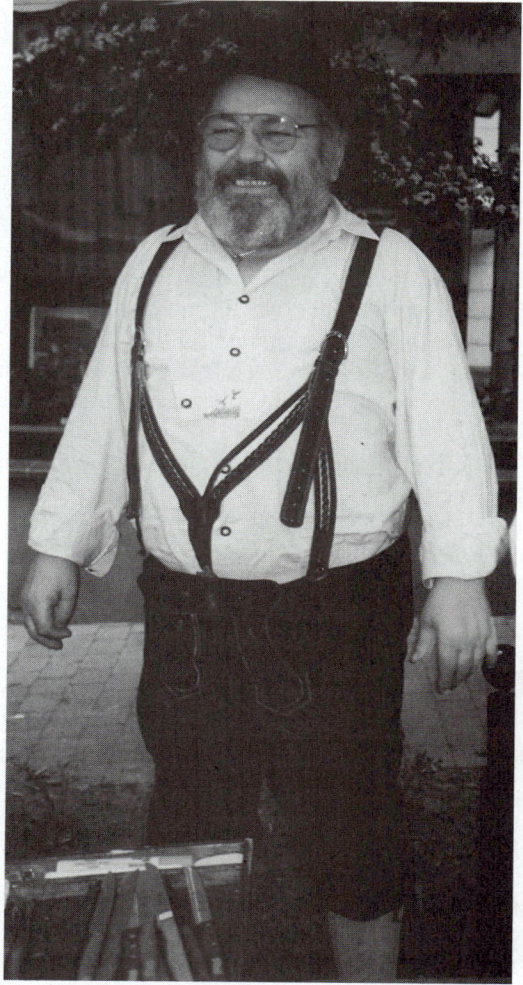

Mental health and individuality. (Courtesy Priscilla Ebersole.)

valid and healing life process. It is time needed for psychologic wound repair, cleansing tears, protection of the wounded psyche by withdrawal, and the facilitation of repair and restoration of vitality, enthusiasm, and spontaneity. Nurses can facilitate this process by validation. Ronsman (1987) developed an extensive nursing care plan based on Maslow's hierarchy of needs to be used in the care of a depressed patient (Table 21-5).

Suicide

Lying dormant within all of us is an extremely personal equation that determines the point where the quality of our lives would be so pathetically poor we would no longer wish to live. This "line of unbearability," as it might be called, usually exists only subconsciously, and we are therefore not normally cognizant of it. However, when we actually find ourselves in an intolerable situation, even for the first time in our lives, we become conscious of our "line of unbearability." Once the line of unbearability is crossed, a crisis is triggered. Those who still maintain hope cry out for help. Those who don't are likely to kill themselves (Miller, 1979, p. 8).

White men over 85 years of age commit suicide at an annual rate of 67 per 100,000. In contrast, white women of the same age category commit suicide at an annual rate of 6 per 100,000. Women are most suicidal between ages 45 and 54 with an incidence of 8 per 100,000. Suicide rates for white men and white women over age 75 have slightly but steadily increased since 1980. Old blacks have much lower suicide rates (men, 18 per 100,000, and women, less than 1 per 100,000); however, suicide rates of elderly black males have almost doubled since 1980 (U.S. Bureau of the Census, 1995). One of the significant differences in suicidal behaviors in the old and young is the lethality. Eight of ten suicides of males over age 65 were with firearms, and most were successful (Kaplan et al, 1994).

Suicide is an act of deliberate self-destruction that has been variously condemned as immoral or exalted as a highly ethical act that allows an individual to maintain control, even of death itself. Cultural and religious beliefs are deterrents to suicide for some. The aged who are ill may seek suicide as a means of control and death with dignity. Diogenes of Sinope, the renowned cynic of the fourth century BC wrote, "A wise man will quit life when oppressed with severe pain, or deprived of any of his senses, or when laboring under desperate diseases" (Dublin, 1963, p. 194).

In primitive societies it was often expected that the old would commit suicide when their existence was considered a burden to the community. Stories of assisted suicide and mutual suicides are being reported more frequently, and society generally condones the suicide of an aged person who is ill and in pain. In fact, in the current climate of increasing interest in "assisted suicide" there may be a time when we regress to the primitive mode. Then it was the distribution of food that was at stake; now it is money.

Suicide, overt or covert, may be the ultimate expression of dignity and autonomy or of rage, disgust, and mobilized depression. Or, it may be the method of avoiding a frightening eventuality (Loebel et al, 1991). It has been found that most aged individuals who commit suicide are depressed but not necessarily ill or in pain (Clark, 1992). In the case of 18 elders who committed suicide and left notes or revealed reasons for suicide to a relative, the fear of nursing home placement was highest on the list (Loebel et al, 1991). A summary of reasons appears in Box 21-15.

Aged white men in America suffer the most status loss because American white male society is almost wholly devoted to occupational success, often to the neglect of other social roles. Women in all countries have much lower suicide rates. As more women identify themselves with the work role and abstain from having children, statistics may shift. The variations between country, sex, and age are intriguing and given sufficient study would undoubtedly yield fascinating information about roles, expectations, and sociologic factors (U.S. Bureau of the Census, 1995).

Manton et al (1987) found that cohort affiliation, historic period, and age are all significantly related to suicide rates, as shown in Figure 21-4. Given the increased interest in the eruption of PTSD in elderly war veterans discussed earlier in the chapter, we may be able to identify some cohort stressors that are significant.

Common precipitants of suicide include physical or mental illness, death of spouse, substance abuse, and pathologic relationships. The *San Francisco Chronicle* (New study on suicide by older people, 1991) reported that, contrary to general opinion, the majority of elderly suicides were not physically ill. Most were depressed (65%) or had other mental health problems. Depression was a potential underlying cause in 53% of cases studied by Haring et al (1987). Twelve percent of the suicides investigated were patients of long-term care.

Suicide of widows and widowers has been attributed by Durkheim (1951) to "domestic anomie." That is a deregulation of behavior by the loss of spouse that results in a vague and unstructured state of being that lacks guidelines, status, and clear expectations. Widowers are most vulnerable because they are unfamiliar with domestic chores and have often depended on the wife to maintain the comforts of home and the social network of relatives and friends.

Assessing the Suicidal Risk of an Elder. The lethality potential of an elder must always be assessed when elements of depression, disease, and spousal loss are evident. Delusional and hypochondriacal thinking are risk factors (Lester and Tallmer, 1994). Many studies have shown that, with few exceptions, a suicidal individual has seen a physician within a month before the suicide attempt (American Association of Retired Persons, 1994b). Unfortunately, few physicians make a suicide assessment.

Nurses are often in a position to assume responsibility for assessing lethality potential. The clues that are common signals of suicidal intent may be absent, disguised, or misinterpreted in the elderly. However, any direct, indirect, or enigmatic references to the ending of life must be taken

Table 21-5   Dealing with Depression: The Nursing Process and Maslow's Hierarchy of Need

Needs	Assessment	Identifying problems	Establishing goals	Intervention	Evaluation
Physiologic needs Food/fluid Shelter/warmth Air Rest/sleep Avoidance of pain Sex	Usual and present nutritional, elimination, sleep, and sexuality patterns Physical activity—exercise pattern Emotional pain and discomfort Suicide potential Physical health Medications	Nutritional deficit Dehydration Constipation Sleep pattern disturbance Sexual dysfunction Self-destructive behavior Medications or physical illnesses that may cause depression	Establishing and maintaining adequate biologic functioning in areas of sleep, nutrition, and elimination Relief from emotional pain and discomfort Elimination of drug or disease-induced depression	Assist with ADLs Support of self-care abilities Encouragement to start a physical activity regimen Teach side effects of antidepressants Treat medical problems under poor control Change medications that may cause depression	Feelings of physical satiation Homeostasis Optimal physical health
Safety and security needs Feel free from danger Need for a predictable, lawful, orderly world Need to feel in control	Home environment assessment Mental status examination Assessment of visual acuity and hearing Knowledge of disease process Physical mobility	Perceived inability to control feelings or behavior Perceived powerlessness Translocation syndrome Cognitive impairment Alteration in sensory perceptions Impaired physical mobility	Establish predictability and structure in environment Maintenance of a safe environment Realistic understanding of disease course and expected outcome Reversal of treatable confusion	ECT, hospitalization, antidepressive medications for the severely depressed Avoid relocations when possible Correct environmental hazards Encourage a structured daily routine Instruct about disease course and prognosis	Feeling in control of one's disease and optimistic about the future Confidence in the future Feelings of safety, peace, security, protection, lack of danger and threat

From Ronsman K: Therapy for depression, *J Gerontol Nurs* 13(12):21, 1987.

seriously and discussed with the elder. Many, having grown up in the era when suicide bore stigma and even criminal implications, may not discuss their feelings in this respect. It is often helpful to depersonalize the subject and discuss it on a more philosophic basis, using questions such as the following:

"Under what conditions do you think a person has a right to take his life?"

"What are your opinions about the present interest in active euthanasia and assisted suicide?"

"Do you think suicide is a sign of weakness or strength?"

"Suicide is a taboo subject that many people are uncomfortable discussing, but as a health professional I feel it is very important. Have you ever felt like you would be better off dead?"

Typical behavioral clues such as putting personal affairs in order, giving away possessions, and making wills and funeral plans are indications of maturity and good judgment in late life and cannot be construed as indicative of suicidal intent. Other things such as self-neglect, erratic behavior, suspiciousness, hoarding pills, and personality change are more likely the side effects of illness or progressive dementia than

of suicidal intent. Even such statements as "I won't be around long" may be only a realistic appraisal of the situation in old age. Requests to die and statements that life has no meaning may indicate despair and hopelessness but often lack the conviction of planned suicide.

In evaluating lethality potential, the informed nurse will recognize the high-risk patient: male, old, widowed or divorced, white, in poor health, retired, alcoholic, with a family history of unsatisfactory relationships and mental illness. A cluster of these factors should be a red flag of distress to all health professionals. Recent traumatic changes, mild dementia, depression, or cerebrovascular disease also increase the danger. Present relationships that are unsatisfactory, critical, or rejecting greatly enhance the potential for suicide.

The straightforward aspects of a suicide assessment include the following:

- Frequency of suicidal ideations
- A formulated plan for suicide
- Availability of means to complete plan
- Specificity regarding details (time, place)
- Lethality of the method chosen

Needs	Assessment	Identifying problems	Establishing goals	Intervention	Evaluation
Need for love, belonging, and affection Need for contact and intimacy Need for friends Need for a feeling of having a place, "belonging" Need for interactions with others	Family relationships and members Friends that are supportive Recent losses Present and past social interactions	Disruption in significant relationships Social isolation Lack of contact with or absence of significant others Alterations in socialization with reduced social interactions	Maintenance of significant relationships with family and friends Establish community support system Resumption of previous level of social activity	Encourage social interactions that have been enjoyed in the past Encourage interactions with family members, friends, and health care givers Provide reassuring, supportive atmosphere	Feelings of loving and being loved, of being one of a group, of acceptance
Need for esteem and self-respect Need for achievement, mastery, and competence Need for reputation or prestige, appreciation, and dignity Need for love of self	Amount of pleasurable pursuits Emotional or mood assessment Role patterns Coping—stress tolerance pattern Attitude about self, the world, the future	Negative feelings or conception of self Loss of significant roles Unrealistic self-expectations Anxiety Life-style change Dependency on others	Acceptance of realistic limitations Establish appropriate roles Achieve self-acceptance Accept ownership of consequences of one's own behavior	Teach problem-solving skills Cognitive therapy Promote self-care Counseling Behavior therapy Relaxation techniques	Feelings of self-confidence, worth, strength, capability, and adequacy, of being useful and necessary in the world
Need for self-actualization Need for beauty Need for self-expression Need for new situations and stimulation	Occupation, job history Value-belief patterns	Distress of human spirit Loss of zest for life	Expression of self through meaningful recreational activities Exploring new interests	Encourage a nonrestrictive environment Provide beauty in environment Read to the sick or hard of hearing Music	Autonomy Freshness of appreciation Creativeness Spontaneity Feelings of self-fulfillment

Three other factors must be considered in assessing lethality potential:

- Internal resources (personality factors and coping strategies)
- External resources (money, family, friends, services)
- Communication skills (ability to ask for help and express feelings)

Suicide is a taboo topic for most of us, and there is a lingering suspicion that the introduction of the topic will be suggestive to the patient and may incite suicidal action. Precisely the opposite is true. By introducing the topic we demonstrate interest in the individual and open the door to honest human interaction and connection on the deep levels of psychic need. Superficial interest and mechanical questioning will not, of course, be meaningful. It is the nature of our concern and ability to connect with the alienation and desperation of the individual that will make a difference. No matter how much empathy and concern are conveyed, there will be a number of old people who will quietly and methodically kill themselves with never a clue to their intent.

Box 21-15   Reasons for Suicide

	n	%
Fear of nursing home placement	8	44.4
Pain	4	22.2
Interpersonal difficulties	2	11.1
Incapacity	2	11.1
Finances	1	5.6
Remorse	1	5.6
Total	18	100.0

Note: Eighteen decedents represent 31.6% of the total series. From Loebel JP, Loebel JS, Dager SR et al: Precipitants to elder suicide, *J Am Geriatr Soc* 39:407, 1991.

Interventions with a Suicidal Elder. Community health nurses, visiting nurses, and other professionals have a case-finding role in the community that extends beyond traditional boundaries: first, awareness and use of resources within the high-risk populations, and second, providing depression screening clinics at nutrition sites, senior centers, industrial health sites, churches, and community clubs.

Establishing lifesaving connections with individuals and groups that can be available on demand and provide ongoing, long-term counseling, emotional support, and reassurance is the approach to the suicidal elder (Arbore, 1995). Arbore established a 24-hour "Friendship Line" designed especially for elders under the umbrella of Suicide Prevention. Phone call-in counseling is always available by specially trained volunteers, as well as telephone outreach reassurance and a visiting service. The goal is to intervene before suicide becomes a seriously considered option. Suicide risk and recovery factors are seen in Box 21-16.

Aged suicidal clients are encountered in many settings. It is our professional obligation to prevent whenever possible an impulsive destruction of life that may be a response to a crisis or a disintegrative reaction. In other words, we must be concerned about immediate protection for the highly lethal individual while respecting the individual's right to make the most significant remaining decision open to him or her; namely, whether to live or to die. For some, our well-planned interventions may restore a sense of self and purpose so that the suicidal individual will deem preservation worthwhile. For others, their final statement of dignity will be in the control of their death.

Actions to deal with the suicidal elderly include:

- Build trust and rapport.
- Overcome fear of responsibility for client suicide.
- Come to terms with own suicidal impulses and feelings.
- Recognize and handle resentment of client who wants to die.
- Listen intently and empathically.
- Focus on the individual's perception of problem.
- Begin to help establish or restore a supportive network.

If suicidal intent has been established, the following interventions, arranged in order of immediacy, are necessary:

1. Reduce immediate danger by removing hazardous articles.
2. Evaluate the need for constant attendance and arrange for family, friend, or professional to be present during the period of imminent danger.
3. Evaluate the need for medication.
4. Focus on the current hazard or crisis that gives the client the most present distress.
5. Extract a promise from the client not to attempt suicide before your next meeting.
6. Mobilize internal and external resources by getting the individual reinvolved with external supports and reconnected with internal capacities. The caregiver may have to find activities, support systems, transportation, and other resources for the individual.

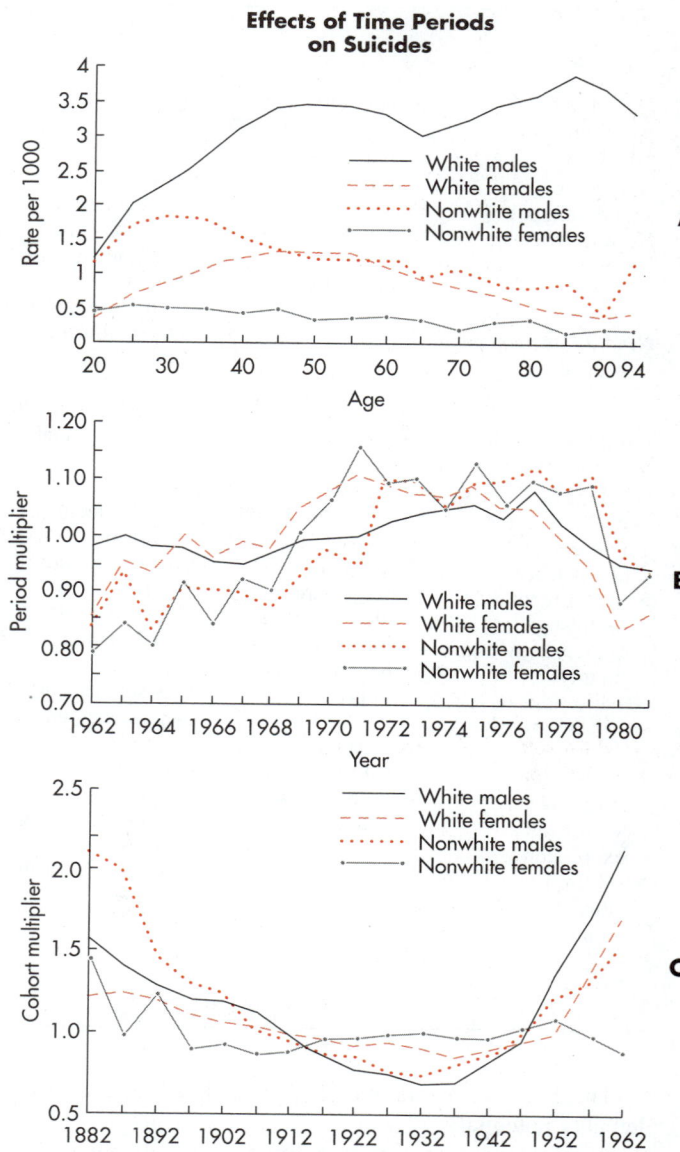

Figure 21-4. A, Effects of age on suicide in the U.S. elderly population with cohort and period effects controlled. **B,** Effects of periods on suicide in the U.S. elderly poulation with age and cohort controlled. **C,** Effects of cohorts on suicide in the U.S. elderly population with age and period controlled. (From Manton KG, Blazer DG, Woodbury MA: Suicide in middle age and later life: sex and race specific life table and cohort analyses, *J Gerontol* 42(2):219, 1987.)

7. Implement a specific plan of action with an ongoing structured program to obviate long periods alone; develop a "lifeline" of individuals who can be called at any hour of distress, and plan regular calls to the individual.

Box 21-16	**Recognition of Risk Recovery Factors of Suicide**

Risk Factors

Depression

Paranoia or a paranoid attitude.

Rejection of help; a suspicious and hostile attitude towards helpers and society.

A major loss, such as the death of a spouse.

A history of major losses.

A recent suicide attempt.

A previous history of suicide attempts.

A major mental, physical, or neurological illness.

Major crises or transitions, such as retirement or imminent entry into a nursing home.

Major crises or changes in others, especially among family members.

Typical age-related blows to self-esteem, such as loss of income or loss of meaningful activities.

Loss of independence, when dependency is unacceptable.

Expressions of feeling unnecessary, useless, and devalued.

Increased irritability and poor judgment, especially after a loss or some other crisis.

Alcoholism or increased drinking.

Social isolation: living alone; having few friends. The social isolation of the couple is also associated with suicide.

Expression of the belief that one is in the way, a burden, or harmful to others.

Expression of the belief that one is in an insoluble and hopeless situation.

Communication of suicidal intent: the direct or indirect expression of suicidal ideation or impulses. Included, too, are symptomatic acts, such as giving away valued possessions, storing up meds., or buying a gun.

Intractable, unremitting pain—mental, or physical—that is not responding to treatment.

Feelings of hopelessness and helplessness in the family and social network.

Feelings of hopelessness in the therapist or other helpers, or a desire to be rid of the patient.

Expression of a belief in ageism, especially that the aged should not be.

Acceptance of suicide as a solution.

Recovery Factors

A capacity for:

Understanding

Relating

Benefitting from experience

Benefitting from knowledge

Acceptance of help

Loving

Wisdom

A sense of humor

Social interest

A caring and available family

A caring and available social network

A caring, available, and knowledgeable professional and health network

From Richman J: A rational approach to rational suicide. In Leenars AA, Maris RW, McIntosh JL et al, editors: *Suicide and the older adult,* New York, 1992, The Guilford Press.

In many cases, interventions with depressed elders can be extrapolated to suicidal elders, since they are often depressed (see discussion earlier in the chapter). Suicide is often a distorted method of regaining control of one's life. Prevention of suicidal behavior is related to alleviation of depression and restoration of a sense of control in one's life. Working with isolated, depressed, and suicidal elders continually challenges the depths of nurses' ingenuity, patience, and self-knowledge.

THERAPEUTIC STRATEGIES TO PROMOTE MENTAL HEALTH

Mental health promotion and treatment strategies for the elderly are primarily based in the community and nursing homes, though there are some geropsychiatric units and some mental health units providing excellent care for elders with mental disorders. Individual integration into the relevant community and family activities with suffi-

cient supports to remain vital and esteemed are the overriding goals of all therapeutic efforts.

Most articles about the mental health of older adults focus on the presence of organic brain disorders as a primary issue. Extensive psychotherapy is rarely reported, and most treatment is somatic. Problems labeled psychotic or neurotic in the young are most often labeled senile in the old. Although many psychologic problems of aging may be accompanied by a cerebral deficit, active therapeutic psychodynamic interventions can be expected to produce some improvement in most cases because dementia seldom exists without some overlay of mental health problems that are potentially reversible or that can be ameliorated. Effective treatment modes include psychoanalysis, psychotherapeutic reminiscence, brief psychotherapy and crisis intervention, somatotherapy, behavioral therapy, family therapy, reality orientation, resocialization, and remotivation. The choice of therapy depends on the needs of the client and method of reimbursement (McDougall, 1995).

Community-Based Psychiatric Care

Elderly psychiatric patients have been treated with "Band-Aids" and then misplaced and all too frequently forgotten. Now, with the trend of all health care to move the majority of care provision to the community, the mental health providers are creating new comprehensive community psychogeriatric care systems (Cyr and Peppler, 1995). Canadians in Ontario have found this method most satisfactory. Case finding may be from a number of sources, and initial screening is often in response to a crisis call from a client, family member, or professional in the community or based in an institution. The assessment of the situation involves a multidisciplinary team of health professionals and includes components listed in Box 21-17.

When completed, the assessment provides the base for a holistic plan of care. The client and care planning team determine what is both desired and feasible. The range of options is thoroughly examined. Only then is it decided what level of supports is needed and whether a move may be necessary. Wherever the site in which the care plan is activated, the client is still provided access to the community-based services that have been identified in the care plan. Periodic assessment of progress toward goals involves all team members, the client, and the family. This community case-managed model can be effectively implemented in any community.

Stolee et al, (1996) report on the same program as it has become integrated into the community. As the program has more fully developed, increasing numbers of caregivers and local resources have been involved. Overall the program has proved economically and humanistically effective. Institutions and community groups have worked together to maintain continuity of efforts and consistency of service.

Goldberg and associates (1996) studied the cost-effectiveness of a similar program and found it considerably more cost-effective than institutionalization.

Psychotherapy

Goldfarb and Turner (1953,1955), pioneers in psychogeriatric care, first reported serious attempts at psychotherapy with the aged. They carried out brief (15-minute) semiweekly therapeutic sessions aimed at increasing self-esteem and reinforcing a therapeutic alliance between psychiatrist and client. In an average of six to eight sessions 78% improved in their social adaptation and psychologic functions. Interestingly, two thirds of the sample had some cerebral impairment, yet all but 22% of them improved or stabilized. Of the subjects who were psychotic in the absence of organic mental disorders, only one in five improved. Of those with psychoneuroses or personality disorders in the absence of organic mental disorders, all either stabilized or improved. Goldfarb and Turner emphasized the point, made by so many others since their pioneer studies, that treatment is

helpful even in cases in which severe dementia is present. They found repeatedly that emotional disorganization often exaggerates the picture of dementia. In addition, they advocate warm interactions and focusing on positive transference as helpful to most elderly. In contrast to traditional psychotherapy, the therapist often interjects thoughts, opinions, and personal experiences when relevant (Nowak and Wandel, 1997).

Brief Psychotherapy and Crisis Intervention

These modalities are often surprisingly successful because the elderly are acutely aware that their time is limited and their problems are often clearly apparent. Crisis intervention was discussed thoroughly in Chapter 19. Brief psychotherapy is often the treatment of choice for the elderly who need to resolve interpersonal problems and develop more effective coping strategies. Issues of transference and resistance, which are the essence of a long-term therapeutic alliance, are not developed in brief psychotherapy. Generally, brief psychotherapy is limited to less than 15 weeks. The emphasis is on important problems in the person's life; goals are limited. The therapist is active in providing direction, guidance, and environmental manipulation. Some therapists recommend a philosophical approach to psychotherapy with older adults (McDougall, 1992).

Brief psychotherapy with the elderly can be successful when conducted by experienced psychotherapists who use brief psychodynamically oriented psychotherapy, psychologic testing, and diagnostic interviews. Psychotherapists are advised to focus on issues of major concern or on ones that will restore a sense of mastery and self-esteem. Nurses, acting as client advocates, are often in the position of encouraging both physician and client to include psychotherapeutic support in the treatment regimen.

Benefits from verbal psychotherapy for aged individuals cannot be predicted from current tests. Individual long-term psychotherapy for the aged in the community is theoretically beneficial but seldom seen in actual practice. The distance between therapists and potential aged clients is mutually maintained for many reasons. Despite these impediments, several modes of psychotherapy with the aged have been effectively demonstrated (McDougall, 1993a).

Psychodrama

Psychodrama has been infrequently used with aged individuals because they have been thought poor candidates for development of insight and personality change, but in a study reported by Johnson (1985), it was used effectively. Residents of nursing homes (ages 64 to 96 years) were involved in expressive groups for the purpose of dramatizing physical limitations, death of self and loved ones, and dependencies. These topics, frequently avoided when working with the aged, were potent issues that were handled openly and in depth. The participants confronted conflictual issues and developed insight into anxieties. The dramatic role-playing not only resolved past issues but brought about reinvestment in the present relationships in the group. Johnson contends that groups of this type increase spontaneity and hopefulness and may even decrease morbidity.

Psychodrama and life-review have been used successfully to enhance adaptation and life satisfaction. Psychodrama emphasizes the reenactment of troublesome memories that are consuming psychic energy and producing incongruence in an individual's self-concept. The life-review and reminiscence activity can be effectively implemented using the techniques of psychodrama (Stepath and Martin, 1987). Though used with adolescents, dreams have also been incorporated into psychodrama for further understanding (Verhofstadt, 1995). Imagery-based cognitive training techniques have also been used successfully with elders. The particular techniques used include visual imagery elaboration, verbal judgment, and relaxation. Elders who are intuitive seem to benefit most from psychodrama, life-review, and the use of imagery.

Box 21-17   Comprehensive Psychogeriatric Assessment

The Department of National Health and Welfare, in its document *Guidelines for Comprehensive Services to Elderly Persons with Psychiatric Disorders* (1988), stated that assessment is the cornerstone of good psychogeriatric care. It was further suggested that assessment "is necessary for determining priority of needs, for establishing competency, for client monitoring, for outcome or program evaluation, and hence for resource allocation." A comprehensive assessment should follow a holistic approach that promotes "harmony in the person's whole self including the mind and body and their interaction within the environment." Assessment embraces the domains of physical and mental health, social and economic status, behaviour and self-care abilities, and the individual's physical environment in addition to the determination of the client's wishes and preferences.

Components of a Comprehensive Psychogeriatric Assessment

Assessments would take place in the client's place of residence, if possible, and would be conducted by a multidisciplinary team of health professionals. As indicated by the Department of Health and Welfare, it may not be necessary for all members of the multidisciplinary team to go on all or most home visits given that the whole team is represented by the type of assessment conducted. It is possible for one or more team members to conduct a preliminary comprehensive psychogeriatric assessment to determine the need for further specialized assessment—neurophysiological, psychiatric, legal, financial, medical, and so on. Therefore, the model can be applied across the province based on availability of appropriately trained professionals.

Comprehensive multidimensional psychogeriatric assessment includes: • **demographic characteristics:** age, marital status, children, education, previous occupation, ethnicity, languages spoken and understood, place of residence, sources of support; • **perceived needs and client preferences:** client's perceived strengths and problem areas, desired interventions, perception of health; • **physical health:** client's current and past physical illnesses, sensory functions, communication, dental care, elimination, mobility, medication use, substance abuse; • **family history:** age of parents at death and cause of death, size of family, surviving family, childhood experiences, history of psychiatric illness in family members; • **mental health:** mental state, cognitive abilities, psychiatric symptoms, affective state, behavioural problems, coping skills; • **physical environment:** barriers, hazards, cleanliness, safety features or problems, pets, pests, water supply, heat, condition and existence of appliances and tools, type of neighbourhood, access to shopping, transportation for client and family; • **functional status (ADL and IADL):** bathing, grooming, toileting, transferring, ambulation, eating, dressing, appearance and manner, ability to perform household tasks; • **social functioning and social resources:** extent, quality, availability and satisfaction with social interactions, experiences of discrimination, available supports from the ethnoracial community, availability of trusted friends, type of relationship with relatives/friends (loving, concerned, hostile, indifference, manipulative), the willingness and availability of a person to regularly assist if needed, access to community social/recreational resources; • **recreational resources:** past interests, ability to participate in activities of interest, frequency of participation in recreational activities, exercise habits, accessibility and availability of recreational resources; • **financial and legal resources:** sources and amounts of income, homeownership and other assets, the person's subjective financial analysis, persons who have legal authority to act on behalf of the person for both financial and care decisions; • **support network:** relationships of the caregivers to the client and his/her satisfaction with their availability, willingness to help, capabilities, regularity of assistance and specific roles, health and social service supports and resources available, specific services and frequency of visits, client satisfaction with services, financial resources needed, receptivity of the client to services and services pending.

Further assessment may be indicated if one or more of the assessed areas show moderate to severe impairment. Following the multidimensional assessment, an individualized care plan would be developed based on the assessment findings.

From Cyr JJ, Peppler C: A comprehensive community-based model of psychogeriatric care, *Perspectives* 19(1):14, 1995.

Institutionally Based Care

Typically, as mentioned earlier, nursing homes have, by default, been given the task of caring for the mentally disturbed elder. Many have done quite an excellent job in implementing reality orientation (RO), remotivation, and resocialization using group therapy strategies. RO is presented in Chapter 22 because it is primarily used for those who have some cognitive impairment. Remotivation and resocialization can be adapted to those with dementias or psychologic disturbances (see Table 21-6).

Remotivation Technique. This approach was designed for long-term, chronic psychiatric residents and for use in extended care facilities and nursing homes. Avoidance of emotionally laden issues and a focus on extending opportunities for varied successful experiences are characteristic of remotivation techniques. Butler et al (1991) emphasize five steps in the remotivation technique:

1. The climate of acceptance—establishing a warm friendly relationship in the group
2. A bridge to reality—reading of simple poetry, current events, and so on
3. Sharing the world—development of the topic, introduced above, through planned objective questions, use of props, and so on
4. An appreciation of the work of the world—designed to stimulate the residents to think about work in relation to themselves
5. The climate of appreciation—expression of enjoyment at getting together, and so on

Remotivation for the aged in long-term care situations may be successfully used by individuals with little training. Student projects in applying remotivation techniques are useful and often result in youth forming relationships with the aged. The students learn to appreciate the aged, and the elders, in turn become more interested in life, less irritable, better groomed, and motivated toward interpersonal contacts. The therapeutic value of contact between young students and the psychiatrically disabled aged is thought to be important. Table 21-6 provides some guidelines and comparisons of RO, remotivation, and resocialization.

Pet Therapy. Pet therapy in nursing homes is generally used to bridge the gap between the resident and the therapist. The dog or cat helps the resident break through apathy and depression. The resident is then better able to respond to caregivers and interact with others. Pet therapy consists of a brief session each month in which well-behaved cats and dogs are brought to nursing homes for residents to play with and hold. Animals are selected based on their good temperament and ability to withstand the confusion and the number of people who will hold and play with them. Volunteers from the animal shelter usually accompany pets to ensure the safety of both animals and residents. Sometimes nursing homes adopt an animal who becomes the mascot,

and various residents take responsibility for caring for the animal. The Humane Society of the United States offers the following points that should be considered before initiating pet therapy in a nursing home (Wright and Dribben-Butman, 1981):

1. How does the staff feel about the project?
2. Will the facilities lend themselves to such a program?
3. Is there space where the animal can retreat and also be kept out of the way of residents who have no interest in pets or are afraid of them?
4. Can a program schedule be set up to include an animal on a routine basis?
5. Is the local humane society or animal shelter willing to become involved in such a project?
6. If adopting a resident mascot, are there adequate food, shelter, and water at all times, and will there be persons consistently responsible for the care of the animal?

Reminiscing and Life-Review

Reminiscing has been viewed as a particularly adaptive function at the last stage of life. Reminiscence is an activity that can allow clients a sense of security through rehearsal of comforting memories, belonging through sharing, and self-esteem through confirmation of uniqueness. Box 21-18 lists several ways memories and reminiscences can be used effectively for the enrichment of the aging process. For the nurse it is a tool of assessment and understanding.

The concept of reminiscence fits well with mechanisms of crisis and grief resolution and seems a fitting tool to accomplish some of the work in these situations (see Chapters 19, 20, and 24). It is versatile because it is ubiquitous and natural and embodies the whole of one's conscious life experience. Goals of reminiscing are related to enhancing one's identity, socialization skills, sense of continuity, and coping. There are many ways the tendency to reminisce can be applied therapeutically: socialization, remotivation, integration, assessment, and as part of RO. Webster (1993) has tested a reminiscence functions scale that can be used to assess some of these. Although this was used with all ages, the scale demonstrated a significant increase in death preparation functions in those 80 years old and beyond (Table 21-7). Interestingly, the function of teaching and informing remained steady through the forties and beyond.

Parker(1995) has developed, based on literature review, seven theoretical propositions regarding reminiscence (Box 21-19). These need further testing and verification.

Life-review. Psychotherapeutic reminiscence is akin to psychoanalysis and forms the conceptual base for life-review. The life-review concept is only one aspect of reminiscence that may decrease depression with some resolution of disappointments, ventilation, or closure. It involves the review of remote memories (self-revelation), the expression of related feelings (catharsis), the recognition of conflicts (insight), and the relinquishment of viewpoints that are self-inhibiting (decathexis).

Parker (1995) found that life-review occurs most frequently as an internal review of memories, an intensely private soul-searching activity, while reminiscing is for pleasure. Sharing and self-expression occurs most in an interpersonal context. It often occurs sporadically in a long-term trusted relationship. During periods of crisis and transition, it occurs quite naturally for many persons. This approach is appropriate for any aged person, and Butler (1963) has called this process *life-review*. Butler and Lewis (1983) provide the following guidelines for the use of life-review therapy:

1. Mastery of the past is the basis for adaptation to the present.
2. Encourage spontaneous life-review.
3. Support the search for meaning, problem-solving, and emotional gratification.
4. Use an eclectic approach.
5. Confront conflicts and anxieties regarding death, guilt, and dependency.
6. The therapist's stance is that of a dependable confidant.

The psychologically disturbed elderly may be reluctant or unable to reminisce fluently in dyadic or group situations. Self-view is often distorted, distressed, or suppressed. Group sharing may be useful because it is less intense than dyadic communication and tends to provide balance to extreme feelings. Some nurses are reluctant to stir the memories of older persons who seem psychologically vulnerable. We would not advocate confrontation or interpretation but rather exploration of all the meanings and feelings relevant to the situation being shared. If anxiety or agitation seems to become an inhibition factor, we would verbally validate the discomfort and move the focus to another group member. Crying, guilt, or regret expressed by group members can be reinforced as an evidence of self-affirmation. We believe the full range of human emotions and experiences

Table 21-6   Differences in Reality Orientation, Resocialization, and Remotivation

Reality orientation	Resocialization	Remotivation
1. Correct position or relation with the existing situation in a community; maximum use of assets	1. Continuation of reality living situation in a community	1. Orientation to reality for community living; present oriented
2. Called reality orientation, RO and classroom reality orientation program	2. Called discussion group or resocialization to differentiate a social function from a therapeutic need	2. Called remotivation
3. Structured	3. Unstructured	3. Definite structure
4. Refreshments and/or food may be served for identification	4. Refreshments served	4. Refreshments not served
5. Appreciation of the work of the world; constantly reminded of who he is, where he is, why he is here, and what is expected of him	5. Appreciation of the work of the world; reliving happy experiences; encourages participation in home activities relating to subject	5. Appreciation of the work of the group stimulates the desire to return to function in society
6. Class range from 3-5, depending on degree/level of confusion or disorientation from any cause	6. Group range from 5-17, depending on mental and physical capabilities	6. Group size: 5-12 patients
7. Meeting ½ hour daily at same time in same place	7. Meetings three times weekly for ½ to 1 hour	7. Meeting once to twice weekly for an hour
8. Planned procedures: reality-centered objects	8. No planned topic; group centered feelings	8. Preselected and reality-centered objects
9. Consistency of approach/response of resident responsibility of teacher	9. Clarification and interpretation in responsibility of leader	9. No exploration of feelings
10. Periodic reality orientation test pertaining to residents' level of confusion or disorientation	10. Periodic progress notes pertaining to residents' enjoyment and improvements	10. Progress ratings
11. Emphasis on time, place, person orientation	11. Any topic freely discussed	11. Topic: no discussion of religion, politics, or death
12. Use of portion and mind function still intact	12. Vast stockpile of memories and experiences	12. Untouched area of the mind
13. Resident greeted by name, thanked for coming, and extended handshake and/or physical contact according to attitude approach in group	13. Resident greeted on arrival, thanked him, and extended handshake upon leaving	13. No physical contact permitted; acceptance and acknowledgment of everyone's contribution
14. Conducted by trained aides and activity assistants	14. Conducted by RN, LPN/LVN, aides, and program assistants	14. Conducted by trained psychiatric aides

From Barns E, Sack A, Shore H: Guidelines to treatment approaches, *Gerontologist* 13:513, 1973.

Life story recording for family
Legacy identification
  Products
  Contributions
  Qualities of character
  Talents
Scrapbooks
Photo albums
Establish rituals of security and comfort
Work history
Life's turning points—can be mapped out as a road map
Fantasy trips—follow the alternate road
Grief resolution
History of homes
Map life geographically
Historic events—cohort identification
Life history of significant persons—why significant
Sensory stimulation
Develop memory chains
Inventory significant items—why significant
  To whom would he or she like to give them?
Dietary history—significant foods of the past may stimulate appetite
Resolve disappointment
Entertainment

Table 21-7	Reminiscence Functions Scale

Factor 1:	Boredom Reduction
Q20	To reduce boredom (.83)*
Q47	For something to do (.80)
Factor 2:	Death Preparation
Q41	Because I feel less fearful of death after I finish reminiscing (.77)
Q43	Because it helps me see that I've lived a full life and can therefore accept death more calmly (.76)
Factor 3:	Identity/Problem-Solving
Q40	To try to understand myself better (.73)
Q49	To see how my strengths can help me solve a current problem (.73)
Factor 4:	Conversation
Q42	To create ease of conversation (.71)
Q28	To create a common bond between old and new friends (.68)
Factor 5:	Intimacy Maintenance
Q6	To keep alive the memory of a dead loved one (.84)
Q32	To remember someone who has passed away (.83)
Factor 6:	Bitterness Revival
Q53	To keep memories of old hurts fresh in my mind (.82)
Q50	To rekindle bitter memories (.80)
Factor 7:	Teach/Inform
Q29	In order to teach younger persons about cultural values (.78)
Q1	To teach younger family members what life was like when I was young and living in a different time (.72)

From Webster JD: Construction and validation of the reminiscence functions scale, *J Gerontol* 48(5):P256, 1993.
*Values in parentheses are factor loadings.

are acceptable, and group validation may allow each member to move toward expression and resolution of psychologic pain.

A memory is a gift to the nurse, a sharing of a part of oneself when one may have little else to give. The more personal memories are saved for persons who will patiently wait for their unveiling and who will treasure them. Of course, a recitation of life history may be a boring affair. When a nurse finds boredom setting in, it may be helpful to confirm the feeling; "It sounds like life became pretty monotonous for you at that time," or "The small details of life may keep one from thinking of larger problems."

Depressed individuals may ruminate about past inadequacies or illnesses. Often there is an unspoken message: "See how sad and helpless I feel. Please take care of me." Nurses fear depression because we begin to feel helpless too. Fromholt et al (1995) found that depressed individuals tended to recall negative memories but after successful treatment and the recovery from depression the memories recalled were more positive.

Restoring adequacy and a sense of being cared for requires patience and tolerance of depression. One nurse listened attentively to a long recitation of painful events and then interrupted the flow with "Who helped you get through these difficult times?" Another comment might also be helpful: "You must have a tremendous tolerance for discomfort. How did you survive such trauma?" At times a nurse must also restore perspective with a comment such as "When you are depressed, everything you remember seems to have been miserable. As you recover, you will begin to remember happier times in your life." Nurses demonstrate caring by willingness to listen to sad and disappointing memories as well as the joyful, entertaining ones.

A most effective life-review would resolve (at least partially) some past conflicts in a manner that would hold significance for the present and future. For instance, a group of elders might indicate some regret about insufficient planning for retirement. Ideally, the group would assess the supremacy of other needs that prevented them from making such plans and arrive at an acceptance of their needs and motives then and now. When working with the elderly in a life-review process, it is important to have a clear understanding of goals:

1. Is the person reviewing the life course preparatory to letting go? If so, the main goal is acceptance of what has been.

2. Is the individual facing a major crisis in self-esteem or need? The goal will be to identify past coping

Box 21-19	**Assumptions Regarding Reminiscence and the Elderly**
Proposition 1:	Individuals reminisce more frequently during periods of personal transition than during periods of personal stability.
Proposition 2:	The lower the level of functioning of an individual, the greater the tendency to reminisce.
Proposition 3:	Life-review reminiscence occurs more frequently in intrapersonal contexts, while simple reminiscence occurs more frequently in interpersonal contexts.
Proposition 4:	The more positive the content of the reminiscence, the greater the therapeutic benefit.
Proposition 5:	Negative life stories are more likely to be intrapersonally reminisced, while positive life stories are more likely to be interpersonally reminisced.
Proposition 6:	Decline in short- and long-term memory leads to an increased reliance upon remote memory systems.
Proposition 7:	Increased use of remote memory in older adults improves general cognitive functioning.

From Parker RG: Reminiscence: a continuity theory framework, *Gerontologist* 35(4):515, 1995.

strategies and from them gather strategies that will be currently effective. Evaluating times when one was effective will sustain confidence in future effectiveness.

3. Is the individual bound in a morass of regret? The goal will be to reenergize the person for present and future function by developing alternative views of past failures.
4. Is the individual suffering the effects of institutionalization? The goal will be to stimulate clear memories of what one has been and has accomplished to reaffirm uniqueness and individuality.
5. Has the person held long-standing grievances against significant others? The goal will be to explore the complexity of those relationships and provide opportunities for interpersonal resolution with the individuals involved.

Life-review occurs periodically throughout the life span. It is most often used to achieve resolution and identify potential for new directions. In the very old it is most likely to alter views of what has been rather than what will be. There are many uses of reminiscence in addition to cognitive stimulation, reduction of depression, and psychologic restitu-

tion. The nurse can learn much about a resident's history, communication style, relationships, coping mechanisms, strengths, fears, affect, and adaptive capacity by thoughtful listening.

A caring nurse will want to protect herself and others from boredom. The resident must learn how to relate in a manner that does not drive people away. On occasion the garrulous chatter is a warm-up for a life-review. In those cases the nurse can facilitate meaning by directing the resident toward critical life passages; for example, "Mrs. J, tell me what it was like for you when you began school." "Mrs. J, do you remember your first date?" "Mrs. J, who was with you when your first child was born?"

Other questions that may guide away from perseveration and circumstantiality are as follows:

What was your most fearful experience?
In your life, when did you feel most proud of yourself?
Are there any events in your life you would like to have handled differently?
If you could change anything about your past, what would it be?
What is the greatest lesson life has taught you?
Who was most influential in your life?
If you could choose a time and place to live your life, when and where would it be?
Did you have any major disappointments in your life?

These and many other exploratory statements will facilitate the life-review. It is usually helpful to begin with descriptions of events, since those are less threatening than sharing fears, failures, and feelings. During any interview it is important to comment on increasing evidence of anxiety and tension and ask if the interviewee wishes to continue, to sit quietly, or to be left alone. The cathartic release experienced in life-review therapy may be less intensely experienced in old age but is nonetheless therapeutic. Guidelines for life-review therapy are provided in Box 21-20.

An old person is a living history book, but unlike written history, the story remains flexible and changeable, similar to a kaleidoscope—each shift, however minor, in the person's self-esteem displays another pattern and colorful image. The most exciting aspect of working with the aged is being a part of the full emergence of the life story. Impatience with the early garrulous or tentative process may reduce the possibility of resolution in the resident and inspiration in the nurse.

Group Psychotherapy

This approach may be more practical and acceptable than individual psychotherapy for those with limited incomes and psychologic distress resulting from the aging process. Cohort groups sharing common problems reduce feelings of alienation and ineffectiveness. Intergenerational groups are also successful in promoting understanding of common human needs and conflicts. The importance of group affiliations for the aged were discussed in Chapter 17. Some guidelines for conducting group therapies are provided in Table 21-8.

Goals of group therapy with the aged are as follows:
1. Reduction in stress-related anxiety
2. Short-term treatment of specific disorders
3. Acceptance of the aging process
4. Resolution of conflicts

Grief Support Therapy. The most common problem of aging, grief resolution, is seldom addressed in the care of the institutionalized elderly. Staff avoidance, lack of skill, ignorance, and lack of concern are a few of the reasons this may occur. Worley (1996), an experienced grief therapist, has contracted with several long-term care facilities in California to provide grief counseling and has found the response encouraging. With continuation of these efforts and measurement of efficacy, we hope greater interest will develop in implementing grief counseling in nursing homes on a national level.

In addition, similar groups are conducted on a weekly basis for community residents recovering from losses. These are provided by hospitals as part of community outreach efforts. These "drop-in" groups are open to all community residents and are focused on warm acceptance, immediate support, sharing of feelings, provision of specific information, guidance, and resources in written form, and referral for individual therapy when needed. Although these groups are not limited to the aged, the great majority of participants are over 60 years old. Some attend weekly for several years, and some attend a few times or drop in sporadically as they feel the need. The individual is not "expected" to follow any particular pattern.

Somatotherapies. The promotion of health, nutrition, activity, and rest is crucial to the success of any psychotherapeutic venture. These activities have been discussed in many ways throughout this text. We would emphasize the importance of a balance of sleep and activity in maintaining mental health. Sleep is not only essential to daily restoration of function, it is the domain of the psyche. Interference with sleep delays the integration and resolution of daily events. Psychologic work is accomplished during dream sleep (REM), and this work may not proceed efficiently during drugged sleep. The dilemma for nurses is to support the need for rest and dream sleep. At times individuals may need a hypnotic, but the continued reliance on such substances is physically and psychologically ill advised. Activity during the day and anxiety reduction exercises before sleep may have beneficial results in promoting the natural healing tendencies of the psyche during sleep. (See Chapter 6 for discussion of sleep and activity.)

Activity is useful in discharging anxiety and reducing agitated movement. In addition, exercise improves physical reserves, increases bone density, and reduces serum cholesterol (Fries, 1990). Nurses might consider providing some opportunity for exercise before verbal therapies.

Somatic therapies are often heavily reliant on drugs. Drugs must be used judiciously in the care of the aged. Major and minor tranquilizers often create more problems than they resolve (see Chapter 23).

ECT may be recommended for middle-aged and elderly severely depressed persons. It can be effective and alters the entire affectual response of a severely depressed patient (Mulsant et al, 1991; Katona, 1994). Clinical experience clearly demonstrates that judicious use of ECT lifts depression and reduces the guilty ruminations that often accompany involutional depressive disorders. The problem is that no one understands exactly what all the cerebral consequences are. ECT has generally fallen out of favor as a treatment mode as more effective antidepressants have been developed. Many consider it prudent to discontinue its use entirely until mechanisms of the brain are more fully understood and the potential recipients can truly make an informed choice.

Nursing Home Consultation. Monthly psychiatric consultation in nursing homes is another method of attempting to serve the mental health needs of residents. The consultations are primarily useful in increasing staff understanding and acceptance of the emotional problems of residents. Better understanding will also encourage staff to increase the number of therapeutic programs offered.

Lowe (1987) contends that obtaining immediate psychologic evaluation of residents in long-term care settings facilitates rapid and successful adjustment. The information obtained may assist caregivers in structuring care and activities to enhance the resident's strengths and to reduce anxiety.

Information from the resident's family is integral to accurate assessment. The family can be asked about personal-

---

Box 21-20	**Guidelines for Life-Review Therapy**

1. Alert aged persons to the characteristics and normality of the life-review process.
2. Provide opportunities for aged persons to recapitulate events in their lives; e.g., "What has most influenced the course of your life?" "Who has most influenced the course of your life?"
3. Assist aged persons to view their life experiences in a broader or different context; e.g., "As you explain your regrets, can you think of other factors that contributed to those events?" "How would you have changed your life then?" "What factors influenced your course of action?" "What would you do differently now?"
4. Facilitate connections between past hopes, present events, and future expectations.
5. Be aware that the process may be carried out sporadically over several months. It is a painful examination of the past and is sometimes avoided.

ity characteristics, cognitive abilities, patterns of response to stress and anxiety, history of psychopathology, and pervasive emotional tone. The resident's perspective and mental status must also be assessed.

Providing continuity of care for geropsychiatric patients across a variety of institutional and community-based settings has not been given adequate attention. Relocation stress and trauma can be reduced significantly by prior preparation, preservation of autonomy, and follow-up by persons from the prior setting to assist in problem solving and adjustment to the new setting. Providing programs for information and preparation of individuals and their families when a move is necessary may facilitate the adaptation. Introduction to a "patient pal" from the new unit can ease the way and may increase the self-esteem of both residents (McDonough, 1987).

In dealing with individuals who are experiencing their first admission to a psychogeriatric ward it is particularly important to assess their life stresses and functional capacity before the emergence of the current problems. Most commonly, a major loss precedes the first admission. Although most of these residents have lived independently, they are often discharged to nursing homes. Symptomatology or diagnosis alone is not sufficient to determine the need for a protected setting. This determination should be made with

great caution and sensitivity to the self-concept implications, and every effort made to restore the residents to the setting of their choice.

NONTRADITIONAL THERAPY AND COUNSELING

Nontraditional therapies are nonthreatening and designed to enhance coping, self-esteem, and respect for individuality. Developing an individualized nursing care plan is essential (Box 21-17). Motivating the aged to use traditional counseling and psychotherapy has always been a factor in underuse of mental health facilities. Nontraditional programs and approaches that are therapeutic may be more acceptable to older persons than those that have the mental illness stigma.

Peer Counseling

In peer counseling, people without professional training but of similar age and experience help another. It is appealing to both the helper and the helpee and is nonthreatening. The peer concept can facilitate the development of a genuinely supportive relationship and a special rapport. The older person providing service enhances his or her own mental health through the opportunity to engage in productive,

Table 21-8   Guidelines for Group Therapies

	Cognitively impaired	Psychologically disturbed	Depressed
Patient selection	No more than five members Age cohorts Both sexes	10 members Varied ages Both sexes	8-10 members Those with similar problems, for example, grieving, retired Both sexes
Structure	Consistent place and time Frequent 30-minute meetings Coleaders	Consistent place and time Biweekly 1-hour meetings One leader consistently	Varied meeting places Weekly 1-hour meeting Variable leadership
Process	Connect specific events, things, and places common to group	Connect members through shared feelings and survival strategies	Focus members on successful coping during life span; encourage mutuality
Goals	Stimulate memory Enhance identity Raise self-esteem Increase socialization skills	Recognition of feelings and meaning of suppressed conflicts Enlarge coping strategies Integrate self-view Promote universality	Reduce feelings of hopelessness Restore personal control Increase affectual responsiveness Develop a sense of integrity and acceptance of life as lived Promote caring between members
Nurse's function	1. Provide a comfortable, mildly stimulating environment 2. Select props that will stimulate memories 3. Assist members by giving specific information, reminders, and clues 4. Give praise and recognition for any participation	1. Establish a private meeting and a closed group 2. Plan to focus on specific developmental stages or critical life events 3. Accept and validate all expressions of feeling 4. Clarify multiple meanings of events 5. Reduce anxiety	1. Provide a comfortable, stimulating environment 2. Appeal to sensory memories 3. Focus members' attention on evidence of caring and sharing 4. Demonstrate a caring attitude 5. Allow time to complain

other-directed activities. Some ways elders have been used to provide services for other elders include the following:

- Counseling persons in retirement transition about benefits, income tax, insurance and investment, and retirement adjustment
- Counseling elders about legal issues and social and personal problems
- Providing for developmentally disabled adults
- Providing senior companions, visitation, and support to residents in nursing homes and to the homebound
- Providing aged advocacy by indigenous elders for minorities

Volunteers in peer support programs need special training in the following:

- Empathic interviewing and listening skills
- Aspects of normal aging
- Special problems of the elderly
- Self-awareness
- Problem-solving methods
- Information and resources available to the aged

Particular topics that may be introduced in peer counselor training sessions include the following:

- Assertiveness training
- Management of depression
- Death and dying; grief
- Evaluation of institutional care
- Working with the disabled
- Use of reminiscence
- Human sexuality

Self-Help Programs. Self-help programs have flourished in the last two decades, as has the use of peer counselors and volunteers. Self-help programs usually follow a "train-the-trainer" model and recruit from churches, community colleges, and universities in which vital and engaged older persons can be found. Community and news announcements are also effective in recruiting trainees.

Screening of volunteers is a sensitive issue and must not in any way erode the self-esteem of the individual volunteer. Throughout the process of selection and training the emphasis must be on the strengths the volunteer brings. If the qualities necessary for counseling are not present, the person must be routed early to an activity fitting his or her skills.

Providing scheduled supervision and support is necessary, as are providing tokens and awards of appreciation and planning activities in which the peer counselors have opportunities to share and learn from each other. The failure to plan for these needs of the peer counselor or volunteers is likely to result in less than satisfactory results from them as counselors.

Mobile Clinics

In Ottawa a psychogeriatric clinic has become a vital addition to the elder services (King, 1987). The clinic offers multidisciplinary assessment and treatment services. Home assessments, follow-up visits, and psychosocial, nursing, medication, and occupational therapy consultation are included in the comprehensive care plans. Referrals are accepted from anyone in the community. The clinic also provides consultation to nursing homes and ongoing support groups for elders at risk, including such foci as relaxation, memory strengthening, and peer counseling.

Roy et al (1987) report similar services provided in Middletown, New York, through a mobile geriatric treatment team. The team has been able to avert inpatient psychiatric hospitalization for 77% of cases. Comparable efforts have been made in communities throughout the nation and should certainly be given consideration.

Within the home, providing such services is not only cost-effective but also more attendant to the holistic perspective of an individual's needs. Older persons account for only 5% of visits made to mental health clinics and less than 2% of visits to private psychotherapists (Nesbit, 1987). Given that most elders consult their internist when encountering an emotional problem, it is imperative that acceptable and comprehensive methods of meeting their needs are used. The mobile mental health clinics seem a step in the right direction. Additionally, identifying high-risk individuals such as those living alone, homebound, recently bereaved, or suffering from repeated falls or hospitalizations and mental deterioration and providing preventive supports could best be accomplished by mobile mental health units.

A similar model in Ventura, California, has been reported by Knight (1984, 1986). The services of a psychologist, nurses, geriatric nurse practitioner, and psychiatrist provide individuals with comprehensive physical and mental health assessments and problem management.

Multidisciplinary community mental health teams will continue to grow because of the multiple health and social needs of the older population and the limited availability of appropriate psychogeriatric institutional care. The geropsychiatric nurse's role is becoming a critical component of human services.

KEY CONCEPTS

- Mental health in old age is difficult to determine as the accrual of life experiences makes for great variations. Mental health must be determined by the gratification or satisfaction individuals feel within their particular situation.
- Mental health is a fluctuating situation for most individuals with peaks and valleys of happiness and pain.
- Elders are not well served within the mental health system as it exists today. Neither practitioners nor reimbursement mechanisms are adapted to their needs.
- Psychologic assessment of elders based upon the common psychometric instruments will usually show deficits because these instruments, with few exceptions, have been designed to test the mental health of young adults.

Nursing Diagnoses

The following potential diagnoses must be considered as well as diagnoses unique to the particular individual:

Denial, ineffective
Knowledge deficit
Noncompliance
Poisoning, risk for
Sensory/perceptual alteration

Sleep pattern disturbance
Social interaction/impaired
Spiritual distress
Thought processes altered

NURSING PROCESS AND NURSING DIAGNOSIS
Ineffective Coping: Alcoholism

Etiologies and Related Factors
Stresses
　Environmental changes
　Losses
　Chronic illness
　Finances
Lack of purpose
Physiologic changes (neurotransmitter depletion)
Physiovulnerability to depression

Defining Characteristics
Denies alcohol use is problematic
Justifies use of alcohol
Argumentative with mate/friends/authority
Unreasonable resentments
Paranoia
Impulsive judgment
Impatience
Daytime fatigue
Unsteady gait
Impaired memory
Apathy
Disorientation
Confusion
Slurred speech
Self-neglect
Social isolation
Blackouts
Falls
Physical pathology: myopathy, diarrhea, malnutrition, gout, decreased lower extremity sensation, tremors
Visual/tactile hallucinations

Knowledge
Alcohol abuse/alcoholism
Effects of alcohol on the older adult
Percentage of alcohol in various alcoholic beverages and over-the-counter medications
2 oz alcohol

= 2 shots = 4 oz 100 proof whiskey
= 4 glasses = 16 oz wine
= 4 mugs = 48 oz beer
Physical and psychologic assessment skills
Standard alcohol screening tests (i.e., CAGE)
Signs and symptoms of withdrawal
Therapeutic communication skills
Crisis intervention skills
Group therapy
Coping strategies
Treatment of alcoholism
Community resources

Clinical Judgment and Related Skills
Maintain a nonjudgmental approach
Administer a standard alcohol screening tool
Perform a physical and mental status examination
Monitor nutritional status
Assist client to gain an understanding of alcoholism as an illness, its progressiveness, effects on the body and interpersonal relationships
Set realistic short-term goals
Discuss alternative coping strategies
Involve family (if there is one)
Conduct group sessions with recovering and recovered persons
Educate family and community groups on the older adult and alcoholism
Provide information of resources
Make referrals as needed

Evaluation
Admits is alcoholic
Abstains from alcohol use
States recognizes need for continued treatment
Explains the physical and psychologic effects of alcohol
Uses alternative coping mechanisms for stress
Takes pride in appearance
Reintegrates into social activities

NEEDS ADDRESSED AND TASK STRENGTHS

Need for stimulation, comfort and management of feelings (to maintain safety, security, sense of belonging and self-esteem); for some, substances are used to achieve spiritual enlightenment (to meet need for transcendence)	Recognizes impact of substances on personality Avoids reliance on medications as a coping strategy Takes responsibility for informing physicians of total medication regimen Recognizes transient nature of medication induced affectual changes

- Classic defense mechanisms, such as denial, displacement and identification, when used by the elderly are often life enhancing and necessary to their function.
- Anxiety disorders are common in late life and are best managed by restoring some sense of control to the situation the individual perceives as out of control.
- Post-traumatic stress disorder is finally being recognized in the aged who have been subjected to extremely traumatic events. Programs are now available to provide support and insight for these individuals.
- Substance abuse and addictions may be distorted adaptational methods used by some aged to cope with losses and end-of-life concerns. These individuals have been successfully treated by providing supportive groups and relationships
- Depression is the most common emotional disorder of aging and likewise the most treatable. Unfortunately, it is often neglected or assumed to be a condition one must "learn to live with." Nurses may be instrumental in assuring that elders are assessed properly and treated for depression.
- Grief is a component of aging for most individuals as they confront various losses. Grief is not a mental illness, but it often requires grief counseling and support for resolution.
- Suicide is *not* prevalent among the aged. Women vastly outnumber men in late life, and they are rarely suicidal. *Very old white men are highly suicidal and must be assessed for suicidal intent whenever they confront a trauma or catastrophe.*

▲ CASE STUDY

Depressive Disorder with Suicidal Thoughts

Elmer had cared for his wife, Emma, during a long and painful illness until she died 4 years ago. He found alcohol provided a way to cope with the stress. Within a year after her death he met a lady that he was very attracted to, and a few months later Reva moved in with him. He managed to move his things about until there was some space for hers, but neither of them were very comfortable with this . . . he, because he really didn't like to move his things from their usual place, and she because her allotted space was so small she felt like an intruder. He collected guns, and she shuddered when she saw them. He was an avid fan of John Wayne movies, and she preferred going to the symphony. He liked meat and potatoes, and she was a vegetarian. She also disapproved of his increasing reliance on alcohol. The blending of two such different lifestyles proved difficult. In a few months Reva moved out, and Elmer blamed himself. He said over and over, "I should have done more for her. I'm not good for anything anymore." His friends began to pull away from him, just when he needed them most, because he seemed to talk of nothing but his various aches, pains, and pills and his general discouragement with life. His consumption of alcohol increased markedly. He had some health problems: a mild congestive heart, a lack of exercise, dairy products gave him diarrhea, he was somewhat obese, and his knees were painful most of the time. He routinely visited his allergist, his internist, his orthopedist, and his cardiologist. But it seemed the more he went to the doctors, the worse he felt. He was taking several medications, and each time he saw one of his doctors he came away with another prescription. None asked about his drinking and he never mentioned it. He awoke one morning feeling very dizzy, and so he went to his internist later in the day. He began to share the litany of his discomforts, and the physician reminded him that at 76 years of age he could not expect to always feel in top shape. When he returned from seeing the doctor, he called his daughter and surprised her by saying he had just decided he would take a week off and go to Hawaii to see if the sun and sand would revive him. Elmer was not usually impulsive. His daughter, fortunately, was a psychiatric nurse and was concerned about the change in his behavior.

Based upon the case study, develop a nursing care plan using the following procedure*:

List comments of client that provide *subjective data.*
List information that provides *objective data.*

---

*Students are advised to refer to their nursing diagnosis text and identify possible or potential problems.

From these data identify and state, using accepted format, two *nursing diagnoses* you determine are most significant to this client at this time. List two client strengths that you have identified from data.

Determine and state *outcome criteria* for each diagnosis. These must reflect some alleviation of the problem identified in the nursing diagnosis and must be stated in concrete and measurable terms.

Plan and state one or more *interventions* for each diagnosed problem.

Provide specific documentation of source used to determine appropriate intervention. Plan at least one intervention that incorporates the client's existing strengths.

Evaluate success of intervention. Interventions must correlate directly with the stated outcome criteria in order to measure the outcome success.

STUDY QUESTIONS/ACTIVITIES

Discuss the variations in symptoms of depression in the old and the young.

Describe some of the reasons we believe that elders are more vulnerable to depression than younger persons.

Describe a time when you were depressed and the feelings you had. What did you do about it?

Given the situation in this case, discuss what your thoughts would be if you were his daughter.

Given his daughter's background, what are her responsibilities in this case?

What is the responsibility of a student nurse in the case of suspected suicidal thoughts?

Would you address the possibility of suicidal thoughts if you were the nurse in the physician's office? When and how would you do this?

What action should be taken for Elmer's protection?

Would you expect that Elmer is still grieving the death of his wife? What are your thoughts about this?

What are the clues or indications that an elder is thinking of committing suicide?

What are some of the signs of suicidal intent in young adults? How are they different from those of elders?

Under what conditions do you think a person has a right to take his or her life?

What are your thoughts about Elmer's use of alcohol?

Do you think suicide is a sign of weakness or strength?

Work together in small groups and discuss whether the following statements are true or false (see bottom of column for answers):

1. Normally older people feel depressed much of the time.
2. Older people are more likely than young people to admit to depression.
3. Most older people talk about suicide but rarely try to kill themselves.

4. Depressions of the elderly are helped by medications.
5. Depression may be the cause of forgetfulness.
6. Depression in the elderly is often linked with disease and alcoholism.

▲ CASE STUDY

Bipolar Disorder

June is a 67-year-old white female admitted to the geropsychiatry inpatient unit for alcohol abuse and noncompliance with her lithium, which had been prescribed for a diagnosed bipolar disorder. June's primary mode of coping with her depression and mood swings has been to drink alcohol, meet abusive men, and play bingo. However, when she stops taking her lithium dosage, she begins to have flights of ideas, argues with her daughters, and tries to pick up men in her apartment complex. Upon seeing her at home you discover that she has a long history of being physically abused by her husband, now deceased for 12 years, and has been living with one daughter who has also emotionally and physically abused her, causing her to be hospitalized. June's ability to test reality is compromised because of years of denial and low self-esteem. She says, "I used to have lots of times when I felt really good in between the depressions. Now I feel depressed most of the time." She tells you that her daughters harass her and interfere in her life. Your goals as a community-based nurse are to facilitate her independence; that is, being able to live in her own apartment, to assist her with medication compliance, and to intervene with June to improve relationships with her daughters. Home visits are approved through Medicare for 2 months after hospital discharge.

Based upon the case study, develop a nursing care plan using the following procedure*:

List comments of client that provide *subjective data*.

List information that provides *objective data*.

From these data identify and state, using accepted format, two *nursing diagnoses* you determine are most significant to this client at this time. List two client strengths that you have identified from data.

Determine and state *outcome criteria* for each diagnosis. These must reflect some alleviation of the problem identified in the nursing diagnosis and must be stated in concrete and measurable terms.

Plan and state one or more *interventions* for each diagnosed problem. Provide specific documentation of source

(1. F, 2. F, 3. F, 4. T, 5. T, 6. T.)

*Students are advised to refer to their nursing diagnosis text and identify possible and potential problems.

used to determine appropriate intervention. Plan at least one intervention that incorporates the client's existing strengths.

Evaluate success of intervention. Interventions must correlate directly with the stated outcome criteria in order to measure the outcome success.

STUDY QUESTIONS/ACTIVITIES

How will you evaluate June's ability to live independently?

What particular strategies are necessary to meet the goals of the nursing care plan?

Given that June's primary coping strategy is drinking alcohol, how will you facilitate her sobriety and help her deal with stress?

How much involvement with June's daughters do you believe is necessary to assist with her transition back into her own apartment?

Given the short number of visits covered by Medicare, what information is needed by June to provide self-care? In other words, the nurse must be teaching June how to live independently upon discharge from home health care. What does June need to know?

Discuss the meanings and the thoughts triggered by the students' and elders' viewpoints expressed at the beginning of the chapter. How do these vary from your own experience?

RESEARCH QUESTIONS

What is the prevalence of mental disorders in community-dwelling older adults? What mental health care is nursing able to provide in the home?

How common is alcohol abuse a strategy of self-care used by the mentally ill elderly?

What types of assessment instruments best determine an individual's ability to provide self-care?

Is psychiatric home care a more cost-effective alternative than institutional care?

Discriminate more clearly the types of geriatric depression and develop specificity of treatment based on these findings.

Clarify cause-and-effect relationship between various illnesses and depression.

Identify risk factors, prodromal signs, and their relationship to depressive symptomatology.

Determine in what circumstances antidepressants are useful in grief reactions.

What are the cardinal symptoms of depression in the oldest-old?

To what extent can depression be identified as a major precipitant to suicide?

Although the general status of aged white males is thought to be the best it has been from a socioeconomic perspective, inexplicably, suicide has begun to increase since 1981. What factors may be contributing to this?

Do degenerative neurosensory changes predispose one to depression?

What are some factors that explain the great age difference in peak suicidal behaviors in men and women?

How many physicians consider or evaluate for the presence of depression in the elders who see them for physical complaints?

What is the most reliable tool for identifying depression in the elderly?

In what present cultures are the aged most comfortable and honored?

What is the earliest sign of depression that an elder experiences?

RESOURCES

Video

Depression in the Long Term Care Setting discusses the nurse's role in assessment and management of depression, including medical, pharmacologic, and psychologic approaches. Available from Geriatric Video Productions, PO Box 1757, Shavertown, PA 18708-0757, (800) 621-9181.

Organizations

Alcohol and Drug Problems Association of North America
444 N Capital St NW
Suite 706
Washington, DC, 20001

Alcoholics Anonymous World Services (AA)
475 Riverside Dr
New York, NY 10613

American Association for Geriatric Psychiatry
1440 Main St
Waltham, MA 02254-9132

Anxiety Disorders Association of America
6000 Executive Blvd
Rockville, MD 20852

Depression and Related Affective Disorders Association
Johns Hopkins Hospital, Meyer 3-181
600 N Wolfe St
Baltimore, MD 21205

Mental Health Law Project
1101 15th NW, Suite 1212
Washington, DC 20005

National Association of Developmental Disabilities Councils
1234 Massachusetts Ave NW
Suite 103
Washington, DC, 20005

National Council on Alcoholism and Drug Dependence (NCADD), (800) 622-2255.

National Mental Health Association
1021 Prince St
Alexandria, VA 22314-2971

Publications

The Zung Self-Rating Depression Scale (SDS) is probably the most widely used test of depression in the elderly. The SDS is a self-administered questionnaire consisting of 20 items that measure areas associated with depression such as mood, well-being, optimism, and somatic symptoms (Zung, 1965). The scale incorporates both positive and negative responses. The items are scored on a 4-point scale ranging from "none or a little of the time" to "most or all of the time." The score is derived by dividing the sum of the 20 items (which are rated from 1 to 4) by the maximum score of 80 to arrive at a number expressed as a decimal. Scores above 0.38 (or a raw score of 50 and over) were associated with depression requiring hospital treatment (Zung, 1965).

The Beck Depression Inventory (BDI) consists of 21 categories of symptoms and attitudes describing the cognitive, behavioral, and vegetative manifestations of depression (Beck et al, 1961). The items require the rating of symptom severity on a 4-point scale. The BDI can be self-administered or given in an interviewer-assisted manner. A total score is obtained by summing the severity levels and cutoff levels that have been established. The BDI has been found to be highly reliable with older adults (Gallagher et al, 1982), with good concurrent validity (Gallagher et al, 1983, 1986). It should prove to be a useful scale for identifying depression in older adults and for assessing treatment effectiveness.

The Geriatric Depression Scale (GDS) exists in both short and long forms (Yesavage et al, 1983). The original 30-item form of the GDS has been shown to be an effective screening test for depression in a variety of settings. The short, 15-item version of the GDS was developed primarily for brevity and, in particular, for use in populations such as the medically ill or those with dementia, where the longer form might be burdensome. How well this short form works in these populations, however, is largely undetermined. The short version of the GDS, like its longer predecessor, is an effective screening tool in the cognitively intact. However, in a population of subjects with mild dementia of the Alzheimer's type (DAT), it does not appear to retain its validity.

REFERENCES

Abraham IL, Neundorfer MM, Currie LJ: Effects of group interventions on cognition and depression in nursing home residents, *Nurs Res* 41(4):196, 1992.

Alexopoulos GS: Difficult to diagnose: the special challenges of identifying depression in the elderly, *Hebrew Home Res Newsletter* 1(3):1,7,1995a.

Alexopoulos GS: Mood disorders. In Kaplan H, Sadock B, *Comprehensive textbook of psychiatry,* ed 6, vol 2, Baltimore, 1995b, Williams & Wilkins.

Almeida OP, Howard RJ, Levy R, David AS, Morris RG, Sahakian BJ: Cognitive features of psychotic states arising in late life, *Psychol Med* 25(4):685, 1995.

American Association of Retired Persons: *Alcohol abuse among older people,* Washington, DC, 1994a, American Association of Retired Persons.

American Association of Retired Persons: *Suicide by the elderly,* Washington DC, 1994b, American Association of Retired Persons, PF5053(694).

American Psychiatric Association: *Diagnostic and statistical manual of mental disorders,* (DSM IV), ed 4, Washington DC, 1994, The Association.

Arbore P: *Suicide in the elderly.* Presentation at Gerontological Society of America, 48th Annual Scientific Meeting, Los Angeles, Nov 20, 1995.

Atkinson P: *Alcohol and drug abuse in old age,* New York, 1992, American Psychiatric Press.

Barder L, Slimmer L, LeSage J: Depression and issues of control among elderly people in health care settings, *J Adv Nurs* 20:597, 1994.

Barker S: Does depression impede hip-fracture recovery? *Contemp Senior Health* 2(2):10, 1990.

Barsky AJ: Hypochondriasis: medical management and psychiatric treatment, *Psychosomatics* 37(1):48, 1996.

Beck A, Ward C, Mendelson M et al: An inventory for measuring depression, *Arch Gen Psychiatry* 4:561, 1961.

Birren JE, Deutchman DE: *Guiding autobiography groups for older adults: exploring the fabric of life,* Baltimore, 1991, Johns Hopkins University Press.

Black KJ: Diagnosing depression after stroke, *South Med J* 88(7):699, 1995.

Blazer DG: Anxiety disorders. In Abrams WB, Beers MH, Berkow R, editors: *The Merck manual of geriatrics,* ed 2, Whitehouse Station, NJ, 1995a, Merck Research Laboratories.

Blazer DG: Depression. In Abrams WB, Beers MH, Berkow R, editors: *The Merck Manual of Geriatrics,* ed 2, Whitehouse Station, NJ, 1995b, Merck Research Laboratories.

Boerner RJ: Anxiety disorders in the elderly: diagnostic problems and therapeutic prospects, *Z Gerontol Geriatr* 28(6):435, 1995.

Borson S: Secondary depression in the medically ill, (abstract), *Proceedings of the Third Congress of the International Psychogeriatric Association* 3:133, 1987, Chicago.

Borson S: Symptomatic depression in the elderly medical outpatient: prevalence, demography and health service utilization, *J Am Geriatr Soc* 34:341, 1989.

Buffum MD, Wolfe NS: Posttraumatic stress disorder and the World War II veteran, *Geriatr Nurs* 16(6):264, 1995.

Burvill PW, Hall WD, Stampfer HG, Emmerson JP: The prognosis of depression in old age, *Br J Psychiatr* 158:64, 1991.

Butler RL: Life review: an interpretation of reminiscence in the aged, *Psychiatry* 26:65, 1963.

Butler R, Lewis M: *Aging and mental health: positive psychosocial approaches,* ed 3, St Louis, 1983, Mosby.

Butler RN, Lewis MI, Sunderland T: *Aging and mental health: positive psychosocial, and biomedical approaches,* ed 4, New York, 1991, Macmillan.

Centers for Disease Control and Prevention, National Center for Health Statistics, 1996, Hyattsville, Md.

Clark DC: "Rational" suicide and people with terminal conditions or disabilities, *Issues Law Med* 8:147, 1992.

Clement M: Recognizing dependence on alcohol in the elderly, *NURSEweek* 8(20):8,1995).

Commerford MC, Reznifkoff M: Relationship of religion and perceived social support to self-esteem and depression in nursing home residents, *J Psychol* 130(1):35, 1996.

Covinsky K: Depressive symptoms and disability progression, *Pepper Review* 3(3):4, 1996.

Cyr JJ, Peppler C: A comprehensive community-based model of psychogeriatric care, *Perspectives* 19(1):14, 1995.

Dalton JR, Busch KD: Depression: the missing diagnosis in the elderly, *Home Healthcare Nurse* 13(5):31, 1995.

Davis B: Depression and the elderly, *Home Health Focus* 3(2):14, 1996.

Davis L, Wells K, Rogers W: Effects of Medicare's prospective payment system on service use by depressed elderly inpatients, *Psychiatric Services* 46(11):1178, 1995.

DSM IV (See American Psychiatric Association.)

Dublin L: *Suicide,* New York, 1963, Ronald Press.

Farberow NL, Gallagher-Thompson D, Gilewski M et al: Changes in grief and mental health of bereaved spouses of older suicides, *J Gerontol* 47(6): 357, 1992.

Fielding R: Depression and acute myocardial infarction: a review and reinterpretation, *Soc Science Med* 32:1017, 1991.

Finney JW, Moos RH: Entering treatment for alcohol abuse: a stress and coping model, *Addiction* 90(9):1223, 1995.

Fries JF: Medical perspectives upon successful aging. In Baltes PB, Baltes MM, editors: *Successful aging: perspectives from the behavioral sciences,* Cambridge, 1990, Cambridge University Press.

Fromholt P, Larsen P, Larsen SF: Effects of late-onset depression and recovery on autobiographical memory, *J Gerontol* 50B(2):P74, 1995.

Gallagher D: Assessment of depression by interview methods and psychiatric rating scales. In Poon L, editor: *Clinical memory assessment of older adults,* Washington, DC, 1986, American Psychological Association.

Gallagher D, Breckenridge J, Steinmetz J et al: The Beck depression inventory and research diagnostic criteria: congruence in an older population, *J Consult Clin Psychol* 51:945, 1983.

Gallagher D, Nies G, Thompson L: Reliability of the Beck depression inventory with older adults, *J Consul Clin Psycho* 50:152, 1982.

Gallo JJ: Epidemiology of mental disorders in middle age and late life: conceptual issues, *Epidemiol Rev* 17(1):83, 1995.

Glassman AH, Roose SP: Risks of antidepressants in the elderly: tricyclic antidepressants and arrhythmia-revision risks, *Gerontology* 40(1):15, 1994.

Goldfarb A, Turner H: Psychotherapy of aged persons. II. Utilization and effectiveness of "brief" therapy, *Am J Psychiatry* 109:916, 1953.

Goldfarb A, Turner H: Psychotherapy of aged persons, *Psychoanal Rev* 42:916, 1955.

Groh C, Whall AL: Geriatric depression. In Burggraf V, Barry R: *Gerontological nursing: current practice and research,* Thorofare, NJ, 1996, SLACK, Inc.

Haring C, Miller C, Barnas C et al: Suicide in the elderly (abstract). *Proceedings of the Third Congress of the International Psychogeriatric Association* 3:17, 1987, Chicago.

Heidrich SM, Ryff CD: The role of social comparisons processes in the psychological adaptation of elderly adults, *J Gerontol* 48(3):P127, 1993.

James JW, Haley WE: Age and health bias in practicing clinical psychologists, *Psychol Aging* 10(4):610, 1995.

Jenike MA: *Geriatric psychiatry and psychopharmacology: a clinical approach,* St Louis, 1989, Mosby.

Johnson D: Expressive group psychotherapy with the elderly: a drama therapy approach, *Int J Group Psychother* 35:109, 1985.

Jonas E: Aging and developmental trends in the long term course of schizophrenia (abstract). *Proceedings of the Third Congress of the International Psychogeriatric Association* 3:31, Chicago, 1987.

Kalayam B, Alexopoulos GS, Merrell HB et al: Patterns of hearing loss and psychiatric morbidity in elderly patients attending a hearing clinic, *Int J Geriatr Psychiatr* 6:131, 1991.

Kaplan MS, Adamek ME, Johnson S: Trends in firearm suicide among older American males: 1979-1988, *Gerontologist* 34(1):59, 1994.

Kaplan HI, Sadock BJ: *Synopsis of psychiatry,* ed 7, Baltimore, 1994, Williams & Wilkins.

Katona CLE: Approaches to the management of depression in old age, *Gerontology* 40(1):5, 1994.

Ketcham ML, Hayner GN: Safe withdrawal from acute alcohol abuse in the aged, *Geriatr Nurs* 13(5):281, 1992.

Kety, S: *New perspectives in alcoholism: beyond reductionism,* Boston, 1993, Beacon Press.

King H: A community psychogeriatric clinical model (abstract). *Proceedings of the Third Congress of the International Psychogeriatric Association* 3:7, Chicago, 1987.

Knight B: *Psychotherapy with older adults,* Beverly Hills, 1986, Sage.

Knight R: Multidisciplinary crisis assessment and home management, *Gerontologist* 24:147, 1984.

Kolanowski AM: The clinical importance of environmental lighting to the elderly, *J Gerontol Nurs* 18(1):10, 1992.

Krause N: Stress, alcohol use, and depressive symptoms in later life, *Gerontologist* 35(3):296, 1995.

Kwakwa J: Alternatives to hospital-based mental health care, *Nursing Times* 91(23):38, 1995.

Lester D, Tallmer M: Now I lay me down to sleep, *Contemp Gerontol* 1(3):91, 1994.

Lish JD, Zimmerman M, Farber NJ, Lush D, Kuzma MA, Plescia G: Psychiatric screening in geriatric primary care: should it be for depression alone? *J Geriatr Psychiatr Neurol* 8(3):141, 1995.

Loebel JP, Loebel JS, Dager SR et al: Precipitants to elder suicide, *J Am Geriatr Soc* 39:407, 1991.

Lovell BB, Ancoli-Israel S, Gevirtz R: Effect of bright light treatment on agitated behavior in institutionalized elderly subjects, *Psychiatr Res* 57(1):7, 1995.

Lowe B: A call for psychological evaluation for residents in long-term care facilities, *Aging Network News* 3:9, 1987.

Mann D: Battling depression, *Medical Tribune News Service,* Aug 26, 1996.

Manton K, Blazer D, Woodbury M: Suicide in middle age and later life: sex and race specific life table and cohort analyses, *J Gerontol* 42(2):219, 1987.

Masters JC: When lithium does not help: the use of anticonvulsants and calcium channel blockers in the treatment of bipolar disorder in the older person, *Geriatr Nurs* 17(2):75, 1996.

McDonough S: Intrainstitutional relocation (abstract). *Proceedings of the Third Congress of the International Psychogeriatric Association* 3:124, Chicago, 1987.

McDougall GJ: What role philosophy in psychotherapy? *Perspectives Psychiatr Care* 28(2):3, 1992.

McDougall GJ: *Existential psychotherapy with older adults* (under review, 1993a).

McDougall GJ: *Memory strategies utilized by older adults* (manuscript in progress, 1993b).

McMahon AL: Substance abuse among the elderly, *Nurse Practitioner Forum* 4(4):231, 1993.

Miller M: *Suicide after sixty: the final alternative,* New York, 1979, Springer.

Mittelstadt PC: Federal reimbursement of advanced practice nurses' services empowers the profession, *Nurse Pract* 18:1, 1993.

Mossey JM, Knott KA, Higgins M, Telerico K: Effectiveness of a psychosocial intervention, interpersonal counseling, for sub-dysthymic depression in medically ill elderly, *J Gerontol* 51A:M172, 1996.

Müller-Spahn F, Hock C: Clinical presentation of depression in the elderly, *Gerontology* 40(1):10, 1994.

Mulsant BH, Rosen J, Thornton JE, Zubenko GS: A prospective naturalistic study of electroconvulsive therapy in late life depressions, *J Geriatr Psychiatr Neurol* 4:3, 1991.

Nesbit D: Attitudinal barriers to delivery of mental health services to the elderly (abstract). *Proceedings of the Third Congress of the International Psychogeriatric Association* 3:16, Chicago, 1987.

New study on suicide by older people, *San Francisco Chronicle,* April 8, 1991.

Nowak KB, Wandel JC: Sharing of self in geriatric clinical practice, *Geriatr Nurs* 1997 (in press).

O'Connor FW: A vulnerability-stress framework for evaluating clinical interventions in schizophrenia, *Image J Nurs Sch* 26(3):231, 1994.

Parker RG: Reminiscence: a continuity theory framework, *Gerontologist* 35(4):515, 1995.

Philibert RA, Richards L, Lynch CF, Winokur G: Effect of ECT on mortality and clinical outcome in geriatric unipolar depression, *J Clin Psychiatr* 56(9):390, 1995.

Podgorski CA, Tariot PN, Blzina L, Cox C, Leibovici A: Cross-discipline disparities in perceptions of mental disorders in a long-term care facility, *J Am Geriatr Soc* 44(7):792, 1996.

Pollock LE: Inpatient self-management of bipolar disorder*, Appl Nurs Res* 9(2):71, 1996.

Putnam KM, Harvey PD, Parrella M et al: Symptom stability in geriatric chronic schizophrenic inpatients: a one year follow-up study, *Biol Psychiatr* 15(39):92, 1996.

Qualls SH, Smyer MA: Mental health. In GL Maddox, editor: *The encyclopedia of aging,* ed 2, New York, 1995, Springer.

Ragsdale KG, Cox RD, Finn P, Eisler RM: Effectiveness of short-term specialized inpatient treatment for war-related posttraumatic stress disorder: a role for adventure based counseling and psychodrama, *J Trauma Stress* 9(2):269, 1996.

Rapp S, Davis K: Geriatric depression: physicians' knowledge, perceptions and diagnostic practices, *Gerontologist* 29(2):252, 1989.

Rapp S, Parisi S, Walsch D, Wallace C: Detecting depression in elderly medical inpatients, *J Consult Clin Psychol* 56:509, 1988.

Richman J: The lifesaving function of humor with the depressed and suicidal elderly, *Gerontologist* 35(2):271, 1995.

Riley B: Schizophrenia, paranoid disorders, anxiety disorders, and somatoform disorders. In MO Hogstel, editor: *Geropsychiatric nursing,* St Louis, 1990, Mosby.

Ronsman K: Therapy for depression, *J Gerontol Nurs* 13(12):19–23, 1987.

Rosenkoetter M: Changing life patterns of the ECF resident, *Geriatr Nurs* 17(6):267, 1996.

Roy B, Obaid M, Rudick S: Patterns of psychiatric illness in elderly and the role of a mobile geriatric treatment team-management outcome and cost effectiveness (abstract). *Proceedings of the Third Congress of the International Psychogeriatric Association* 3:9, Chicago, 1987.

Schmall VL, Lawson L, Stiehl R: *Depression in later life: recognition and treatment,* Eugene, Ore, 1990, Oregon State University.

Schuckit MA, Anthenelli RM, Bucholz KK, Hesselbrock VM, Tipp K: The time course of development of alcohol-related problems in men and women, *J Stud Alcohol* 56(2):218, 1995.

Schwartz PJ, Brown C, Wehr TA, Rosenthal NE: Winter seasonal affective disorder: a follow-up study of the first 59 patients of the National Institute of Mental Health seasonal studies program, *Am J Psychiatr* 153(8):1028, 1996.

Scott RW, Polacca M: Staying in balance on the fourth hill of life: mental health and elderly native Americans, *Dimensions, American Society on Aging* 2(4):1, 1995-1996.

Silverstone PH: Prevalence of psychiatric disorders in medical patients, *J Nerv Men Dis* 184(1):43, 1996.

Smith M, Mitchell S, Buckwalter KC, Garand L: Geropsychiatric nursing consultation as an adjunct to training in long-term care facilities: the indirect approach, *Issues Mental Health Nurs* 16(4):361, 1995.

Sprinzeles L: Hallucination: the phantom reality, *Parkinson's Disease Foundation Newsletter,* p 5, Summer, 1992.

Stepath S, Martin R: Psychodrama and life-review for the geriatric psychiatric patient (abstract). *Proceedings of the Third Congress of the International Psychogeriatric Association* 3:107, Chicago, 1987.

Stolee P, Kessler L, Le Clair JK: A community development and outreach program in geriatric mental health: four years' experience, *J Am Geriatr Soc* 44(3):314, 1996.

Stollenwerk RM, Hunglemann JA, Kenkel-Rossi E et al: Focus on spiritual well-being: harmonious interconnectedness of mind-body-spirit, *Geriatr Nurs* 17(6):262, 1996.

Swanson D: Geriatric alcohol abuse: a clinical perspective, *Mayo Clin Proc* 48:30, 1993.

US Bureau of the Census: *Statistical abstract of the United States: 1995,* ed 115, Washington, DC, 1995.

US Department of Health and Human Services: Diagnosis and treatment of depression in late life, *Consensus Statement,* 9(3):1991. (Reprinted from NIH Consensus Development Conference, Bethesda, Md, Nov 4-6.)

U.S. Health Resources and Services Administration: Nursing. In Klein S, editor: *White papers: a national agenda for geriatric education,* USDHHS, 1995, Public Health Service, pp 176–195.

Verhofstadt-Deneve LM: How to work with dreams in psychodrama: developmental therapy from an existential-dialectical viewpoint, *Int J Group Psychother* 45(3):405, 1995.

Vezina J, Laprise R: *A comparison of the diagnostic performance of the Beck depression inventory and the geriatric depression scale using ROC analysis.* Paper presented at the 48th Annual Scientific Meeting of the Gerontological Society of America, Nov 15-19, 1995, Los Angeles, Calif.

Waxman H, Carner E: Physicians' recognition, diagnosis, and treatment of mental disorders in elderly medical patients, *Gerontologist* 24:23, 1984.

Webster JD: Construction and validation of the reminiscence functions scale, *J Gerontol* 48(5):P256, 1993.

Weismann MM, Olfson M: Depression in women: implications for health care research, *Science* 269:799, 1995.

Wells KB, Burnham MA, Camp P: Severity of depression in pre-paid and fee-for-service general medical and mental health specialty practices, *Med Care* 33(4):350, 1995.

Wenrich M, Paauw M, Carline J: Do primary care physicians screen patients about alcohol intake using CAGE questions? *J Gen Intern Med* 10:631, 1995.

Williams JW, Kerber CA, Mulrow CD: Depressive disorders in primary care: prevalence, disability, and identification, *J Gen Intern Med* 10:7, 1995.

Wirz-Justice A, Graw P, Krauchi K et al: Natural light treatment of seasonal affective disorder, *J Affect Disord* 37(2-3):109, 1996.

Worley A: *Grief group counseling in nursing homes and community "drop-in" grief support groups,* Unpublished manuscript, 1996.

Wright P, Dribben-Gutman B: Animal facilitated therapy in nursing homes, *Nurs Homes* 30:2, 1981.

Yesavage J, Brink T, Rose T et al: Development and validation of a geriatric depression screening scale: a preliminary report, *J Psychiatr* 12:63, 1983.

Zung W: Zung self-rating depression scale, *Arch Gen Psychiatr* 12:63, 1965.

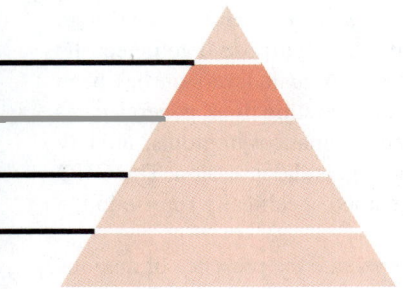

APPENDIX 21-A

Depression Rating Scales

The *Zung Self-Rating Depression Scale* (SDS) is probably the most widely used test of depression in the elderly. The SDS is a self-administered questionnaire consisting of 20 items that measure areas associated with depression such as mood, well-being, optimism, and somatic symptoms (Zung, 1965). The scale incorporates both positive and negative responses. The items are scored on a 4-point scale, ranging from "a little of the time," "some of the time," "a good part of the time," to "most of the time." The responses are given a score of 1 to 4, arranged so that the higher the score, the greater the depression: the statements designated with (+) are given "1" for response "most of the time," while those with (−) are given a "4" for "most of the time." The score is derived by dividing the sum of the 20 items (which are rated from 1 to 4) by the maximum score of 80 to arrive at a number expressed as a decimal. Scores above 0.38 (or a raw score of 50 and over) were associated with depression requiring hospital treatment (Zung, 1965).

Zung Self-Rating Depression Scale

1. (−) I feel down-hearted and blue.
2. (+) Morning is when I feel the best.
3. (−) I have crying spells or feel like it.
4. (−) I have trouble sleeping at night.
5. (+) I eat as much as I used to.
6. (+) I still enjoy sex.
7. (−) I notice that I am losing weight.
8. (−) I have trouble with constipation.
9. (−) My heart beats faster than usual.
10. (−) I get tired for no reason.
11. (+) My mind is as clear as it used to be.
12. (+) I find it easy to do the things I used to.
13. (−) I am restless and can't keep still.
14. (+) I feel hopeful about the future.
15. (−) I am more irritable than usual.
16. (+) I find it easy to make decisions.
17. (+) I feel that I am useful and needed.
18. (+) My life is pretty full.
19. (−) I feel that others would be better off if I were dead.
20. (+) I still enjoy the things I used to do.

From *Archives of General Psychiatry* (1965; 12:65), Copyright © 1965, American Medical Association, with permission.

All depression checklists from Gallo JJ, Reichel W, Andersen LM: *Handbook of geriatric assessment,* ed 2, Gaithersburg, Md, 1995, Aspen Publishers.

The *Center for Epidemiologic Studies Depression Scale* (CES-D) was developed by the Center for Epidemiologic Studies at the National Institute of Mental Health for use in studies of depression in community samples. The CES-D contains 20 items. Respondents are asked to report the amount of time they have experienced symptoms during the past week. Typically, a threshold of 17 and above is taken as defining "caseness," although higher cutoff points (e.g., 24 and above) have been suggested.

The *General Health Questionnaire* (GHQ) is a 60-item self-administered instrument whose purpose is to detect the presence of psychiatric distress. A scaled version has been devised; it consists of 28 items testing four general categories (seven questions each): somatic symptoms, anxiety and insomnia, social dysfunction, and depression. The GHQ is unusual in that it was developed specifically for use in the primary care setting.

Using the GHQ, respondents rate the presence of anxious and depressive symptoms "over the past few weeks" into one of four categories: "not at all" (coded 1), "no more than usual" (coded 2), "more than usual" (coded 3), or "much more" (coded 4). There are four responses for each question: score 1 for either of the two answers consistent with depression and 0 for the other two.

Center for Epidemiologic Studies Depression Scale

INSTRUCTIONS FOR QUESTIONS: Below is a list of the ways you might have felt or behaved. Please tell me how often you have felt this way during the past week.

Rarely or None of the Time (Less than 1 Day)
Some or a Little of the Time (1–2 Days)
Occasionally or a Moderate Amount of Time (3–4 Days)
Most or All of the Time (5–7 Days)

During the past week:
1. I was bothered by things that usually don't bother me.
2. I did not feel like eating; my appetite was poor.
3. I felt that I could not shake off the blues even with help from my family or friends.
4. I felt that I was just as good as other people.
5. I had trouble keeping my mind on what I was doing.
6. I felt depressed.
7. I felt that everything I did was an effort.
8. I felt hopeful about the future.
9. I thought my life had been a failure.
10. I felt fearful.
11. My sleep was restless.
12. I was happy.
13. I talked less than usual.
14. I felt lonely.
15. People were unfriendly.
16. I enjoyed life.
17. I had crying spells.
18. I felt sad.
19 I felt that people dislike me.
20. I could not get "going."

From Center for Epidemiologic Studies, National Institute of Mental Health.

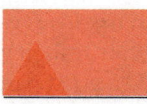

Items from the Scaled U.S. Version of the General Health Questionnaire

A. Somatic symptoms
A1. Been feeling in need of some medicine to pick you up?
A2. Been feeling in need of a good tonic?
A3. Been feeling run down and out of sorts?
A4. Felt that you are ill?
A5. Been getting any pains in your head?
A6. Been getting a feeling of tightness or pressure in your head?
A7. Been having hot or cold spells?

B. Anxiety and insomnia
B1. Lost much sleep over worry?
B2. Had difficulty staying asleep?
B3. Felt constantly under strain?
B4. Been getting edgy and bad-tempered?
B5. Been getting scared or panicky for no reason?
B6. Found everything getting on top of you?
B7. Been feeling nervous and uptight all the time?

C. Social dysfunction
C1. Been managing to keep yourself busy and occupied?
C2. Been taking longer over the things you do?
C3. Felt on the whole you were doing things well?
C4. Been satisfied with the way you have carried out your tasks?
C5. Felt that you are playing a useful part in things?
C6. Felt capable of making decisions about things?
C7. Been able to enjoy your normal day to day activities?

D. Depression
D1. Been thinking of yourself as a worthless person?
D2. Felt that life is entirely hopeless?
D3. Felt that life isn't worth living?
D4. Thought of the possibility that you might do away with yourself?
D5. Found at times you couldn't do anything because your nerves were too bad?
D6. Found yourself wishing you were dead and away from it all?
D7. Found that the idea of taking your own life kept coming into your mind?

From *Psychological Medicine*, Copyright © 1979, Cambridge University Press.

In scoring the *Social Dysfunction Rating Scale,* the rater assigns a score based on the following six gradations: not present (score 1), very mild (score 2), mild (score 3), moderate (score 4), severe (score 5), and very severe (score 6). This instrument, while not designed to measure degrees of depression, is very useful when assessing the impact of depression on quality of life.

The Geriatric Depression Scale (GDS) exists in both short and long forms (Yesavage et al, 1983). The original 30-item form of the GDS has been shown to be an effective screening test for depression in a variety of settings. The short, 15-item version of the GDS was developed primarily for brevity and, in particular, for use in populations such as the medically ill or those with dementia, where the longer form might be burdensome. How well this short form works in these populations, however, is largely undetermined.

The short version of the GDS, like its longer predecessor, is an effective screening tool in the cognitively intact. However, in a population of subjects with mild DAT, it does not appear to retain its validity.

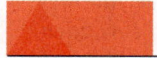 Social Dysfunction Rating Scale

Self-esteem

1. Low self-concept (feelings of inadequacy, not measuring up to self-ideal)
2. Goallessness (lack of inner motivation and sense of future orientation)
3. Lack of a satisfying philosophy or meaning of life (a conceptual framework for integrating past and present experiences)
4. Self-health concern (preoccupation with physical health, somatic concerns)

Interpersonal System

5. Emotional withdrawal (degree of deficiency in relating to others)
6. Hostility (degree of aggression toward others)
7. Manipulation (exploiting of environment, controlling at other's expense)
8. Overdependency (degree of parasitic attachment to others)
9. Anxiety (degree of feeling of uneasiness, impending doom)
10. Suspiciousness (degree of distrust or paranoid ideation)

Performance System

11. Lack of satisfying relationships with significant persons (spouse, children, kin, significant persons serving in a family role)
12. Lack of friends, social contacts
13. Expressed need for more friends, social contacts
14. Lack of work (remunerative or nonremunerative, productive work activities that normally give a sense of usefulness, status, confidence)
15. Lack of satisfaction from work
16. Lack of leisure time activities
17. Expressed need for more leisure, self-enhancing, and satisfying activities
18. Lack of participation in community activities
19. Lack of interest in community affairs and activities that influence others
20. Financial insecurity
21. Adaptive rigidity (lack of complex coping patterns to stress)

From Linn MW et al: A Social Dysfunction Rating Scale, *J Psychiatr Res* 6:300, 1969. Copyright © 1969, Pergamon Journals Ltd.

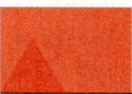 The Short Form of the Geriatric Depression Scale

1. Are you basically satisfied with your life?
2. Have you dropped many of your activities and interests?
3. Do you feel that your life is empty?
4. Do you often get bored?
5. Are you in good spirits most of the time?
6. Are you afraid that something bad is going to happen to you?
7. Do you feel happy most of the time?
8. Do you often feel helpless?
9. Do you prefer to stay at home, rather than going out and doing new things?
10. Do you feel you have more problems with memory than most?
11. Do you think it is wonderful to be alive?
12. Do you feel pretty worthless the way you are now?
13. Do you feel full of energy?
14. Do you feel that your situation is hopeless?
15. Do you think that most people are better off than you?

From Yesavage J, Brink T, Rose T et al: Development and validation of a geriatric depression screening scale: a preliminary report, *J Psychiatr Res* 17(1):37-49. 1982-1983.

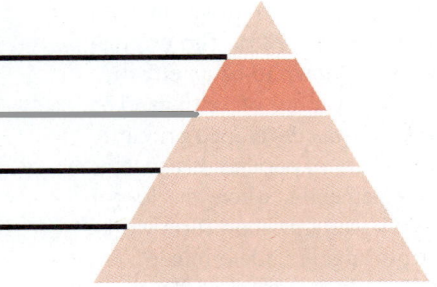

Cognition: Function and Dysfunction in Old Age

Graham McDougall
Priscilla Ebersole

A student speculates

I imagine I am in my late eighties and my husband and I live with our daughter. I am experiencing an unpleasant physical change; I am losing my memory. I can sharply remember all details about events that happened a long time ago, but often fail to recall what happened 2 hours ago. Although this situation scares me and I wonder what will happen if my family gets tired of my forgetfulness, I remind myself that I live with the people who love and care for me very much and will not desert me at the time when I need them the most.

Tatyana, age 30

Elders speak

Dear P: Here's something you will appreciate, author unknown, "A friend knows the song in my heart and sings it to me when my memory fails."

Luv, B (age 75)

It has been quite a relief to be in this retirement home . . . everyone here forgets names and words, and I don't feel alone when I'm forgetful.

Liz, 78

LEARNING OBJECTIVES

Upon completion of this chapter, the reader will be able to:

1. List five purposes of a cognitive assessment.
2. Explain reasons nurses may provide a most accurate assessment of cognitive status.
3. Describe similarities and differences between dementia and delerium.
4. Relate six ways in which cognitive impairment is measured.
5. Describe the parameters and methods used in a comprehensive assessment of cognitive function.
6. Develop a nursing care plan for an individual with irreversible dementia.
7. Develop a nursing care plan for an individual with reversible dementia.

COGNITIVE FUNCTION

This chapter will address normal cognition of the aged and the various situations, disorders, and diseases that influence cognitive processes and at times produce temporary or permanent cognitive decline. We remain oriented to the healthy aging model while we examine each of the states of mentation in old age as having the potential for comfort and pleasures (though sometimes only momentary) and deserving of active nursing intervention to maintain the highest practicable level of function and satisfaction.

We have artificially separated cognitive function from mental health, though they are in most ways interdependent. The mind is in some ways limited by the capacities of the brain, yet just as in medicine, there is a danger of evaluating the person by the measured and tested efficiency of cells and organs. The postmodernist thought, particularly appealing to us, is that objective, reliable, and scientific knowledge based upon a set of humanly constructed paradigms is not the measure of universal truth. No one, scientist or researcher, directly or objectively knows reality, but each actively constructs meanings that influence that which is called reality (Ray, 1996). Nowhere is this more important than in examining the cognition of the aged. Baltes (1993) confirms that cognitive mechanics, genetically and biologically controlled, show definite loss with aging, but pragmatic cognition, adapting to culture and life stage, shows positive change in elders who have no specific brain pathologic condition. Citing John Morris, professor of neurology at Washington University in St Louis, Crowley (1996) says if brain function becomes impaired in old age, it is a result of disease, not aging.

Models of Adult Cognition

Cognitive development of the aged is often measured against the norms of young or middle-aged people, which may not be appropriate to the distinctive characteristics of the aged. More and more theorists are now speculating about the possibility of unique cognitive powers of old age, as did Plato.

The great Erik Homburger Erikson in his seventy-third year, when writing of Freud, noted that in Freud's sixty-eighth year he became aware of a phase of regressive development and the "all-enveloping duality of life and death" (Erikson, 1975, p. 33). This awareness of reflective regression seems to be a stage of cognitive development characteristic of late life. Individuals become absorbed with memories and meanings.

Berry provides a good example in Old Jack who sat in a rocking chair on the veranda of the general store, immersed in the span of his years and the meanings of events. He failed to see what was going on around him or recognize people, not because of cognitive decline but immersion in memories (Berry, 1974). It is doubtful he would remember, if asked, what he ate for breakfast, or even if he ate breakfast. Various cognitive activities may appear impaired if we are not alert to differences that occur in the process of aging.

The determination of intellectual capacity and performance has been the focus of a major portion of gerontologic research. The period from ages 65 to 74 has been identified as one in which decrements in visual memory and verbal intelligence become apparent in those individuals with less favorable cognitive backgrounds, though there is considerable variance (Giambra et al, 1995). In general, cognitive performance in testing is poorer for the very old than for those 60 or 80 years old (Poon et al, 1992). Interrelationships between intelligence quotient (IQ) and mental and physical health are exceptionally strong. The data from this study showed that instrumental activities of daily living (IADLs) were compromised in those elders with low fluid intelligence scores. High fluid intelligence seems to ameliorate the effects of age on daily chores. These findings are significant to satisfaction in old age because the capacity for effective lifestyle management and cognitive resources contribute to adaptation and enjoyment in old age.

Woodruff-Pak (1989) summarized 100 years of research on aging and intelligence into four phases. Phase I reflected the research literature between 1920 and the mid-to-late 1950s as a unidimensional model emhasizing age-related decline. Even though this research contributed a beginning understanding of cognitive aging, it was devised in an attempt to screen out male candidates for the U.S. Army who might not have enough mental capacity to perform in the military. This was the beginning of the belief that older individuals performed more poorly than younger individuals.

Phase II was initiated as the result of a 30-year longitudinal research study published in 1953 that proposed the notion of stability versus decline. Many other longitudinal studies were conducted during this phase, and scholars continue to debate over various study designs, the number of age functional relationships that actually exist, and the usefulness of describing the relationships between age and intelligence. Results of this period indicated that adult age functions in intelligence are not singular or unidirectional.

Phase III began during the 1970s of the post-Great Society and emphasized interventions to ameliorate intelligence decline in the aged and is represented by manipulation of adult IQ. During this phase it was discovered that "practice" may improve intelligence in older adults through familiarization on tasks that might have been considered novel to them. While this phase of intervention research provided a positive outcome, data were not available to compare other age groups of adults participating in the same interventions during the same period. During Phases I through III information about intelligence in old age was based on tests initially designed for children or young adults at best.

Phase IV, which began in the late 1970s, may be considered to be a reexamination of the psychometric approach to testing older adults. It is during this phase that the terms *ecological validity* and *context* are introduced into traditional testing methods. Ecological validity and context imply relevance to cognition in everyday life; that is, psychometric tests of intelligence must have relevance to the daily lives of older adults if they are to be useful. Cognitive aging research implies that intelligence in old age is dynamic and that certain abilities change and even improve with age (Figure 22-1).

During Phase IV late adulthood is no longer seen as a period of growth cessation and arrested cognitive development but as a life stage programmed for plasticity and the development of unique capacities. It is quite clear from several studies that young adult intelligence levels, education, pulmonary health, general health and activity levels, and self-efficacy are significant to the maintenance of high levels of cognitive activity in later life (Albert et al, 1995; Gold et al, 1995; Diehl et al, 1995).

This summary review of developments in cognition provides excellent background understanding of the issues that are still being explored.

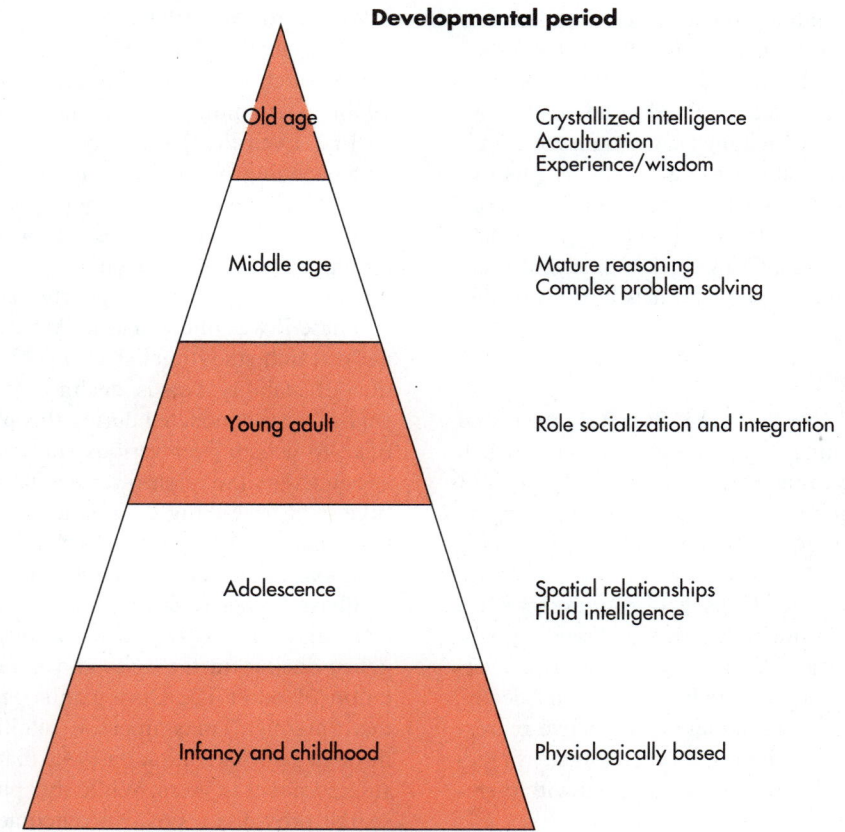

Developmental period

Old age	Crystallized intelligence Acculturation Experience/wisdom
Middle age	Mature reasoning Complex problem solving
Young adult	Role socialization and integration
Adolescence	Spatial relationships Fluid intelligence
Infancy and childhood	Physiologically based

Figure 22-1. Life span cognitive developmental strengths. (Developed by Priscilla Ebersole.)

The Aging Brain

It has been generally assumed that cognitive function declines in old age because of morphologic changes in cerebral tissue and decreases in circulatory capacity and neurotransmitters. In the past 15 years studies have appeared that refute this conclusion, but it remains a generally held assumption. Other reasons have been advanced for the variations of intellectual performance of the elderly being tested (Box 22-1).

On autopsy it becomes clear that visible morphologic cerebral cellular changes cannot be directly correlated with previous level of function. We now understand the necessity of stimulation and that continued development requires appropriate levels of challenge throughout life. There is untapped potential for patterning and learning through stimulating alternate cerebral cells to expanded function. This is shown most remarkably in the retraining of speech and other functions following a stroke.

Regeneration. There is potential for regeneration of cerebral cell loss. The adult central nervous system was once considered unable to generate new growth. In 1978 Diamond refuted the myth that one loses brain power over time due to the shrinkage of brain weight. Because neurons in adult brains were believed not to replicate themselves and many older people do lose mental acuity, generations of people believed that the brain stopped growing early in childhood. As early as 1964 Diamond presented evidence that rats in stimulating environments showed increases in brain size, which provided the first anatomic evidence that the structure and chemistry of the brain could be influenced by the environment. In the cerebral cortex, nerve cells grew larger, changed chemically, and increased in complexity in response to enriched living conditions.

Diamond continues to study the aging human brain and has shown increases in neuron size and in the number of dendrites, or the neuron branches, that transmit information to other cells. She contends that nerve cells are designed to receive stimuli and will very quickly shrink when in a boring, unstimulated environment (Basu and Diamond, 1983).

Researchers from the University of Rochester found that severed axons can regenerate and that these repaired cells may be able to restore communication with other cells, which may be significant (Phelps and Sladek, 1983). "The ability of the brain to repair itself after the onset of dementia, stroke and other ailments, as well as trauma, would be of enormous importance," said Phelps, one of the investigators. Phelps and Sladek (1983) discovered that certain types of damaged nerve fibers in rodents and monkeys could regrow across scar tissue.

Complexities of Accurately Assessing Intellect in Old Age

- The old are most frequently compared with college students, whose chief occupation is proving their intellectual capacity.
- Young adults are in the habit of being tested and have developed test wisdom, a skill never developed by the elderly or one that has grown rusty with disuse.
- Test material may not be relevant to the world of the aged.
- The ability to concentrate is inversely related to anxiety.
- Intellectual function declines differentially. The old are assumed deficient in encoding during learning, storing information for retention, and/or speed of retrieving stored information (Figure 22-1).
- Adrenal or stress hormones may be responsible for some of the gradual changes in the brain during aging.
- A distinct relationship may exist between cognitive function and nutritional status.
- Older persons always perform more slowly than younger people in tasks involving neuromuscular learning because of slower reaction time and an increase in cautious behavior.
- Aged clients often perform poorly on test items because they are less likely to guess and more likely not to answer any items that seem ambiguous to them.

- Cautiousness has often been described as the reason why older adults do not perform as well as younger people in memory tasks. Other personality traits such as greater activity levels, less impulsiveness, and greater emotional stability also seem to influence how well older people perform on memory tests.
- Old people may have difficulty focusing attention and ignoring irrelevant stimuli.
- Subject attrition in longitudinal studies of the aged shows evidence of the survival of the intellectually superior.
- There is no evidence of general slowing of central nervous system activity in old age as had been commonly presumed and reported by researchers.
- Intellectual performance relying on verbal functions shows little or no decline with age, but speeded tests using nonverbal psychomotor functions show a great decline.
- Social cognition and social context are related in terms of elder function. The elderly who maintain the best cognitive function are also those with a high social interactional level.

Sladek believes that an unknown growth factor may stimulate regeneration, and some people may lose their growth factor more readily than others. By learning about the growth factor, it will be possible to determine whether the regrowth of brain tissue can be stimulated. This self-reparative process is known as reactive synaptogenesis. When neuronal input to a neuron or a group of neurons is lost, the nerve fibers from undamaged neurons may sprout and form new connections to replace the lost connections. This phenomenon is known as axon sprouting. Reactive synaptogenesis is now known to be part of a general process known as synapse turnover. This process of synaptic turnover is a stimulus-induced loss and replacement and not part of the normal growth and development processes. The stimulus may vary, and examples of documented cues are (1) an injury, (2) a metabolic insult, (3) a subtle modification in behavior, such as learning a new task, and (4) a physical or chemical stimulus (Cotman, 1990).

The regeneration and rebuilding of lost circuits in the brain has been termed plasticity and has been thought limited to the immature brains of children and adolescents (Weikel, 1989). Cotman (1990) has shown that this plasticity continues, with training, into very old age. He has even reported this regenerative process in the brains of elderly Alzheimer's victims. When brain cells die and the connections are lost, the healthy cells rebuild those connections. Harris has found that elders learn, with maturity, to remember the things that they must or want to remember (Weikel, 1989).

Researchers are becoming more interested in the regenerative aspect of brain function. Although it has long been thought that cerebral cell death is irreversible, the compensatory actions of the remaining cells is less well known. Svanborg has been studying a group of individuals 70 years and older (Weikel, 1989). He has found that living in isolation with little input is detrimental to their brain function and that with intellectual stimulation these individuals' cognitive function is markedly improved.

These findings are significant and indicate that when working with the elderly to improve cognitive functions, there must be regular input and "exercise" of the brain around ideas that are significant and interesting to the older person. It also tends to mitigate the notion that loss of cognitive capacity is irreversible.

Memory Retrieval. Memory, according to the information processing (IP) model of adult cognition, is the process of storing and retrieving information. The computer is the metaphor for human cognition and relies on the methods of experimental psychology.

Memory includes a number of capacities that make up the system enabling us to remember. Scientists using the IP model speak of the sensory register, which can maintain a literal copy of a stimulus for up to 2 seconds, short-term memory (STM), which requires attention and retention of information from 30 seconds to 30 minutes, and long-term memory (LTM), which stores and retains information for long periods.

The practicality of these distinctions in everyday life are that even though older subjects show some decrements in processing information, reaction time, perception, and attentional tasks, the majority of functioning remains intact and sufficient. Familiarity, previous learning, and life experience compensate for the minor loss of efficiency in the basic neurologic processes. In unfamiliar, stressful, or demanding situations these changes may be more marked.

An interesting phenomenon was found by Byrd (1986-1987). Older adults, when required to retrieve recent textual information, may have difficulty differentiating recently learned information from that acquired over the course of their lives. Byrd's study suggests that older adults have a high probability of remembering new knowledge about which they have a great deal of prior knowledge, but recent textual knowledge that is not sufficiently unique blends with previously acquired knowledge and is not recalled as new information.

Research by Guttentag and Hunt (1988) shows that older adults are less able to discriminate imagined functions from those that are actually performed. The practicality of this study is in the recognition that some older individuals may be unable to remember clearly whether an action has been performed or has only been imagined. In their study individuals were asked to perform several simple actions and to imagine performing several other actions. Most of the actions that were performed were clearly recalled, but those that required imaginary performance were more difficult to recall. Generally, older adults seem to demonstrate slowing of nonverbal information processing (Hale et al, 1987).

The most significant finding in this group of studies was that the use of motor activity, thought to greatly enhance recall, may be less significant than the integration of actions into the context of previous knowledge. Elders seem to learn best when new information or expectations can be braided into familiar concepts. Mood is extremely important in terms of what individuals (old and young) will recall. In other words, when we attempt to measure recall of events that may have occurred under duress or anxious states, the events are less likely to emerge when the present state is not congruent with that of the past event.

Age-Associated Memory Impairment. Age-associated memory impairment (AAMI) is a term used to describe recall deficiencies that occur with aging. This condition was previously termed benign senescent forgetfulness and erroneously expected among the old. A longitudinal study of more than 3000 women, funded by the National Institute on Aging, shows that less than 1% of women are cognitively impaired prior to age 65, nearly 5% by age 84, and 14% after age 85 (Fried et al, 1995).

Mental Frailty. An interesting concept proposed by Wolanin (1997) has to do with "mental frailty." The concept is rooted in the triad of change, stress, and support. The elder has a sense of continuity of self that persists throughout life and must be maintained to properly filter and integrate events into the persona. When undesired, unexpected, or overwhelming changes occur—sociologically, psychologically, or physiologically—the elder needs stress relief and familiar supports to maintain the disturbed balance of self-perception. When these are not available at the appropriate time and degree to maintain the sense of the continuity of the predictable self, the elder's mentation goes awry and various psychologic and cognitive disturbances emerge. Nurses are in a position to restore the personal continuity of the elder by focusing on the familiar, obtaining the support of those within the individual's comfort zone, and immediately reversing to the extent possible the overwhelming changes and relieving stress. This concept needs considerably more attention.

Cognitive Impairment

Cognitive impairment (CI) is a term describing a range of disturbances in cognitive functioning. Cognitive functioning is a broad construct that includes a number of categories: attention span, concentration, intelligence, judgment, learning ability, memory, orientation, perception, problem solving, psychomotor ability, reaction time, and social intactness (Kane and Kane, 1981; McDougall, 1990; McDougall, 1995) (Table 22-1). Assessment of cognitive function and a complete mental status examination are essential components in the diagnosis of CI. A Venn diagram is included in Figure 22-2 that shows the relationship among the nine descriptors used in the literature review.

In view of the numerous terms used to describe CIs, definitions are necessary for clarification. The following descriptions and conditions of CI were taken from the *Diagnostic and Statistical Manual of Mental Disorders,* fourth edition (DSM IV) when possible. Discrimination is important. If a patient is misdiagnosed, the treatment prescribed may be grossly inadequate or the patient may be written off as a hopeless or untreatable case.

Confusion

Confusion is a broad and imprecise term that conveys little specific meaning. A more precise term or description of clinical behavioral manifestations must be used to guide management (Inouye, 1993). Confusion is a clinical term used to describe a patient's behavior. According to Wolanin, nurses use the nursing diagnosis "confusion" synonymously with the medical diagnosis of "organic brain syndrome." Sometimes, however, confusion may be used to refer to an acute state, and organic brain syndrome to a chronic state. Therefore the two terms are used in different contexts based on the acuity of the confusional state. This imprecision of meaning among nurses leads to inconsistent reporting of patients' behavioral manifestations. In addition, the *Diagnostic and Statistical Manual of Mental Disorders* revises acceptable terminology with each edition, which further adds to professionals' confusion with terminology.

In a review of the literature Foreman (1986) defined acute confusional states (ACS) as "an organic brain syndrome characterized by transient, global cognitive impairment of abrupt onset and relative brief duration, accompanied by diurnal fluctuation of simultaneous disturbances of the sleep-wake cycle, psychomotor behavior, attention, and affect." Foreman's definition of an acute confusional state and its associated clinical features describes "delirium."

Delirium is the proper term for the clinical assessment of an ACS and is intended to include the broad spectrum of clinical states having in common the essential features described previously. Any alteration in mentation may be loosely labeled confusion, and thus comparisons of delerium, dementia, and depression may be helpful in making a cursory judgment. These can be seen in Table 22-2.

Delirium. While the official nomenclature of the syndrome is delirium, it has been called many other names: acute confusional state, acute brain syndrome, confusion, metabolic encephalopathy, and toxic psychosis. Delirium is a transient mental disorder with a relatively rapid onset, a course that typically fluctuates, and a brief duration.

The essential features of delirium are "reduced ability to maintain attention to external stimuli and to appropriately shift attention to new external stimuli, and disorganized thinking, as manifested by rambling, irrelevant, or incoherent speech" (DSM III-R, 1987, p. 100). There is difficulty in shifting, focusing, and sustaining attention to both external and internal stimuli, sensory misperception, and a disordered stream of thought. Irrelevant stimuli can easily distract the delirious individual.

Also common are perceptual disturbances that result in misinterpretations, illusions, and hallucinations. In addition, disturbances of sleep-wakefulness and psychomotor activity are present.

The DSM IV identifies many of these factors but defines delirium as "a disturbance of consciousness that is accompanied by a change in cognition that cannot be better accounted for by a preexisting or evolving dementia" (1994, p. 124). The diagnosis of dementia cannot be made if delirium is present.

Delirium is a commonly occurring global cognitive disorder in the elderly. The causes of delirium usually lie

---

Table 22-1	Domains Assessed in Mental Status, Cognitive Function, and Dementia		

Mental status	Cognitive function	Dementia
	Attention span	Attention span
Affect and mood		
Level of consciousness		Level of consciousness
General speech		
	Learning ability	
Intellectual performance	Intelligence	Intellectual performance
Abstraction		Abstraction
Attention		
Concentration	Concentration	
Insight		
Judgment	Judgment	Impaired judgment
Memory	Memory	Memory impairment
Orientation	Orientation	Disorientation
Thought content		
	Perception	Perceptual disturbances
		Personality changes
	Problem solving	
Physical appearance and behavior		
	Social intactness	
Psychomotor behavior	Psychomotor ability	Psychomotor activity
	Reaction time	
		Sleep-wake cycle disturbances

From McDougall GJ: A review of screening instruments for assessing cognition and mental status in older adults, *Nurs Pract* 15:11, 1990.

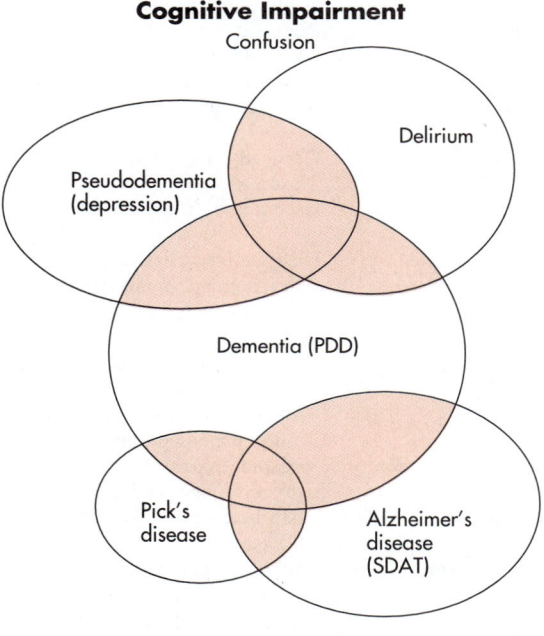

Cognitive Impairment

Assessment of Cognitive Functioning Includes

1. Attention span
2. Concentration
3. Intelligence
4. Judgment
5. Learning ability
6. Memory
7. Orientation
8. Perception
9. Problem solving
10. Psychomotor ability
11. Reaction time
12. Social intactness

Figure 22-2. Relationship of Alzheimer's disease to other manifestations of cognitive impairment.

outside the nervous system. Acute organic mental disorders are so labeled because they are not chronic conditions, are organic in origin, and are potentially reversible (Box 22-2). "Acute" in these cases has no connotation of abrupt onset. The onset of disturbance may be rapid or gradual but is usually resolved within 7 days to the degree it can be reversed (Foreman, 1993).

These states occur at all ages but more frequently in the elderly. They occur in 30% to 50% of elderly medical-surgical patients. These statistics may be even higher because they do not include patients who are quietly confused and overlooked because they are cooperative.

Acute brain disorders are often accompanied by overwhelming anxiety; florid delusions; frightening illusions; and tactile, visual, and olfactory hallucinations. In younger people they are assumed to be transient and reversible. Older people are often labeled "senile" and not actively treated to reverse the underlying physiologic or psychologic problems.

Any interruption in biologic processes is likely to produce perceptual disorganization in the elderly. Common causes can be seen in Box 22-3. Delirious states may be hypokinetic (characterized by somnolence and apathy), hyperkinetic (characterized by excitability, hallucinations, and

Table 22-2   A Comparison of the Clinical Features of Delirium, Dementia, and Depression

Clinical feature	Delirium	Dementia	Depression
Onset	Acute/subacute, depends on cause, often at twilight or in darkness	Chronic, generally insidious, depends on cause	Coincides with major life changes, often abrupt
Course	Short, diurnal fluctuations in symptoms, worse at night, in darkness, and on awakening	Long, no diurnal effects, symptoms progressive yet relatively stable over time	Diurnal effects, typically worse in the morning, situational fluctuations, but less than with delirium
Progression	Abrupt	Slow but uneven	Variable, rapid or slow but even
Duration	Hours to less than 1 month, seldom longer	Months to years	At least 6 weeks, can be several months to years
Awareness	Reduced	Clear	Clear
Alertness	Fluctuates, lethargic or hypervigilant	Generally normal	Normal
Attention	Impaired, fluctuates	Generally normal	Minimal impairment, but is easily distracted
Orientation	Generally impaired, severity varies	Generally normal	Selective disorientation
Memory	Recent and immediate impaired	Recent and remote impaired	Selective or "patchy" impairment, "islands" of intact memory
Thinking	Disorganized, distorted, fragmented, incoherent speech, either slow or accelerated	Difficulty with abstraction, thoughts impoverished, judgment impaired, words difficult to find	Intact but with themes of hopelessness, helplessness, or self-depreciation
Perception	Distorted, illusions, delusions, and hallucinations, difficulty distinguishing between reality and misperceptions	Misperceptions usually absent	Intact, delusions and hallucinations absent except in severe cases
Psychomotor behavior	Variable, hypokinetic, hyperkinetic, and mixed	Normal, may have apraxia	Variable, psychomotor retardation or agitation
Sleep/wake cycle	Disturbed, cycle reversed	Fragmented	Disturbed, usually early morning awakening
Associated features	Variable affective changes, symptoms of autonomic hyperarousal, exaggeration of personality type, associated with acute physical illness	Affect tends to be superficial, inappropriate and labile, attempts to conceal deficits in intellect, personality changes, aphasia, agnosia may be present, lacks insight	Affect depressed, dysphoric mood, exaggerated and detailed complaints, preoccupied with personal thoughts, insight present, verbal elaboration
Assessment	Distracted from task, numerous errors	Failings highlighted by family, frequent "near miss" answers, struggles with test, great effort to find an appropriate reply, frequent requests for feedback on performance	Failings highlighted by individual, frequently answers "don't know," little effort, frequently gives up, indifferent toward test, does not care or attempt to find answer

From Foreman MD, Fletcher K, Mion LC et al: Assessing cognitive function, *Geriatr Nurs* 17(5):228, 1996.

Box 22-2   Disorders Causing or Simulating Dementia

Disorders Causing Dementia

Degenerative diseases:
  Alzheimer's disease
  Pick's disease
  Huntington's disease
  Progressive supranuclear palsy
  Parkinson's disease (not all cases)
  Cerebellar degenerations
  Amyotrophic lateral sclerosis (ALS) (not all cases)
  Parkinson-ALS-dementia complex of Guam and other
    island areas
  Rare genetic and metabolic diseases (Hallervorden-
    Spatz, Kufs', Wilson's late onset metachromatic
    leukodystrophy, adrenoleukodystrophy)
Vascular dementia:
  Multi-infarct dementia
  Cortical micro-infarcts
  Lacunar dementia (larger infarcts)
  Binswanger disease
  Cerebral embolic disease (fat, air, thrombus fragments)
Anoxic dementia:
  Cardiac arrest
  Cardiac failure (severe)
  Carbon monoxide
Traumatic dementia:
  Dementia pugilistica (boxer's dementia)
  Head injuries (open or closed)
Infectious dementia:
  Acquired immune deficiency syndrome (AIDS)—
    dementia and opportunistic infections
  Jakob-Creutzfeldt disease (subacute spongiform
    encephalopathy)

Progressive multifocal leukoencephalopathy
Post-encephalitic dementia
Behçet's syndrome
Herpes encephalitis
Fungal meningitis or encephalitis
Bacterial meningitis or encephalitis
Parasitic encephalitis
Brain abscess
Neurosyphilis (general paresis)
Normal pressure hydrocephalus (communicating
  hydrocephalus of adults)
Space-occupying lesions:
  Chronic or acute subdural hematoma
  Primary brain tumor
  Metastatic tumors (carcinoma, leukemia, lymphoma,
    sarcoma)
Multiple sclerosis (some cases)
Auto-immune disorders:
  Disseminated lupus erythematosus
  Vasculitis
Toxic dementia:
  Alcoholic dementia
  Metallic dementia (e.g., lead, mercury, arsenic,
    manganese)
  Organic poisons (e.g., solvents, some insecticides)
Other disorders:
  Epilepsy (some cases)
  Post-traumatic stress disorder (concentration camp
    syndrome-some cases)
  Whipple disease (some cases)
  Heat stroke

Disorders That Can Simulate Dementia

Psychiatric disorders:
  Depression
  Anxiety
  Psychosis
  Sensory deprivation
Drugs:
  Sedatives
  Hypnotics
  Anti-anxiety agents
  Anti-depressants
  Anti-arrhythmics
  Anti-hypertensives
  Anti-convulsants
  Anti-psychotics
  Digitalis and derivatives
  Drugs with anti-cholinergic side effects
  Others (mechanism unknown)
Nutritional disorders:
  Pellagra (B_6 deficiency)

Thiamine deficiency (Wernicke-Korsakoff syndrome)
Cobalamin deficiency (B_{12}) or pernicious anemia
Folate deficiency
Marchiafava-Bignami disease
Metabolic disorders (usually cause delirium, but can be
  difficult to differentiate from dementia):
  Hyper- and hypo-thyroidism (thyroid hormones)
  Hypercalcemia (calcium)
  Hyper- and hypo-natremia (sodium)
  Hypoglycemia (glucose)
  Hyperlipidemia (lipids)
  Hypercapnia (carbon dioxide)
  Kidney failure
  Liver failure
  Cushing syndrome
  Addison's disease
  Hypopituitarism
  Remote effect of carcinoma

From Office of Technology Assessment: *Losing a million minds: confronting the tragedy of Alzheimer's disease and other dementias,* Washington, DC, 1987, U.S. Government Printing Office.

Box 22-3	Common Causes of Confusion in the Elderly*

- Drug intoxication
- Circulatory disturbances
- Metabolic imbalances
- Fluid imbalance
- Major medical and surgical treatments
- Neurologic disorders
- Infectious processes
- Nutritional deficiencies
- Abrupt loss of significant person
- Multiple losses in short span of time
- Moves to radically different environments

*Shown in rank order of occurrence.

delusions), or mixtures of these factors. Although acute confusion is generally considered transient and self-limiting, its presence concomitant with illness is associated with higher mortality rates and longer hospital stays (Foreman, 1993).

The severity of delirium is related to the level of physiologic disturbance and degree of cerebral edema. Illusions are often evident in conjunction with acute organic brain disorder and may be the most significant signals of toxic states.

Frightening misinterpretations of the environment when under physiologic stress and in unfamiliar situations are common for many aged persons. Immediate attention to prevention of confusion is therefore critical. Identifying and removing the underlying causes and providing supportive and symptomatic care are essential.

Previous psychiatric history and antecedent history of head trauma may indicate a susceptibility or vulnerability to CI. An accurate diagnosis of delirium, dementia, depression, and pseudodementia is a challenge because all present symptoms of CI. If the condition is an abrupt confusional onset, then it is probably not a dementia but delirium and may be reversible.

Nursing interventions are useful in reducing the discomfort of delirium. One study found simple interventions such as continuity of personnel, correcting sensory deficits, providing orienting stimuli, and encouraging family attendance were helpful (Francis, 1992).

In our experience, we have found the most effective intervention to be the continuous presence of one reliable family member or friend who will provide ongoing reassurance that the experience is caused by toxicity and will subside in a few hours or days. We have also used students in this manner and found it effective.

In addition to psychologic manifestations of acute cerebral impairment, physical symptoms such as vasomotor instability; elevated pulse and respiration; temperature fluctuations; tremors of fingers, hands, lips, and facial muscles; headache; and generalized weakness are often present. An individual with acute organic brain disorder is physically ill as well as cerebrally impaired.

Any condition that compromises the cellular function at the brain will cause an acute organic brain disorder. Delirium is a common psychiatric complication of physical illness and of treatments for physical illness in the elderly. It is a more common signal of physical illness of the elderly than body symptoms such as fever, pain, or tachycardia (Lipowski, 1986). Elderly individuals with some degree of dementia are particularly apt to develop transient delirium in response to physical illness, drug intoxication, and psychosocial stressors. Delirium is typically of abrupt onset and brief duration.

Pseudodelirium is a delirium-like state that occurs as a result of psychosocial stressors, depression, mania, or severe anxiety.

It is estimated that 50% of persons more than age 65 who are admitted to medical or surgical units will display delirium on admission or in the course of hospitalization. Delirium results from a combination of reduced cerebral oxidation and cholinergic activity, disturbances in the sleep-wake cycle, and physical or psychosocial stress. It usually ends in either full recovery or death, although it may result in some degree of permanent dementia if the causal factors go unattended (see Nursing Diagnoses box at the end of the chapter).

Prevention of acute confusional states. Approximately 16% of all older patients admitted to hospitals exhibit some symptoms of acute confusion (Foreman, 1993). Acute confusional states often occur during hospitalizations. The exacerbation of delirium during hospitalization depends upon the patient's illness and care management while hospitalized. Preventing or minimizing these occurrences is often possible through judicious use of short-term medications, especially the benzodiazapines (Marcantonio et al, 1994; Buffum and Buffum, 1997), preventing nosocomial infection, maintaining fluid balance, and promoting electrolyte balance.

Irreversible Dementia

In contrast to delirium, usually a reflection of physiologic disturbance or depression (see Chapter 21), dementia is an irreversible mental state characterized by decreased intellectual function, personality change, impairment of judgment, and often change in affect caused by permanently altered cerebral metabolism. Dementia has three basic components: (1) CIs, including memory deficit, (2) neuropathologic changes underlying these CIs, and (3) clinical manifestation and outcomes resulting from these CIs. Dementia is a syndrome consisting of loss of intellectual abilities of sufficient severity to interfere with social or occupational functioning.

There are two types of dementia, the cortical and the subcortical, which may appear somewhat different. In cortical dementia there is aphasia, agnosia, and apraxia as it progresses, whereas the subcortical dementias (aquired immunodeficiency syndrome [AIDS], Huntington's disease, normal pressure hydrocephalus, and progressive supranuclear palsy) feature movement disorders, tremor, rigidity, and depression (Scharnhorst, 1992). The non-Alzheimer's dementias include multi-infarct, Parkinson's disease, Pick's disease, Creutzfeldt-Jakob disease, human immunodeficiency virus (HIV) dementia. There are several other uncommon conditions that produce irreversible dementias (Berkow et al, 1995).

The essential feature of dementia is impairment in short-term and long-term memory. This syndrome is multifaceted and involves memory, judgment, abstract thought, higher cortical functions, and changes in behavior and personality. The diagnosis is not made if these features are due to clouding of consciousness, as in delirium (defined below); however, delirium and dementia may coexist (DSM IV, 1994, p. 123). The most common reasons for coexistence of delirium and dementia in elderly patients are multiple medications, fluid and electrolyte imbalance, systemic disease, and malnutrition. There are, of course, numerous other disorders causing or simulating dementia that were noted in Box 22-2.

In a study of over 7500 elders in Rotterdam between ages 55 and 106 years, 6.3% were found to have dementia and 72% of those had dementia of the Alzheimer's type (DAT) (Ott et al, 1995). The percentage increased exponentially with age from 0.4% (55 to 59 years old) to 43.2% (95 years and older). Vascular dementia (16%), Parkinson's disease (6%), and other dementias (5%) decreased with age. However, this may be interpreted as reflecting the morbidity associated with the other disorders and the relative physical health of many elders with Alzheimer's disease.

Dementia has biopsychosocial components that produce disruption in behavior, cognition, affect, and socialization. The tendency to equate dementia and chronic organic brain disorders with a fatalistic approach to care is unwarranted. Irreversible dementia, by the nature of the label, promotes the belief that "nothing" can be done. This is rooted in our mechanistic approach to illness. Recovery and growth are not the options, but often careful evaluation of all factors involved, both primary and secondary, will reveal that improvement in function and enjoyment, may be facilitated (Persson and Skoog, 1992).

Criteria for Dementia Syndrome. Dementia is the decline of memory and other cognitive functions in comparison with the patient's previous level of function. Components of a dementia syndrome include the following: a history of decline in cognitive and functional performance, abnormalities in thought processes noted from clinical examination, and neuropsychologic tests indicating deficits in recall, attention, spatial perception, and psychomotor performance. The diagnosis of dementia is based on behavior and cognitive responses and cannot be determined by computerized tomography (CT), electroencephalogram (EEG), or other laboratory instruments, although specific causes of dementia may sometimes be identified by these means. When consciousness is impaired by delirium, drowsiness,

stupor, or coma, or when other clinical abnormalities prevent adequate evaluation of mental status, a diagnosis of dementia cannot be made until these conditions are reversed to the maximum possible degree.

Alzheimer's Disease or Senile Dementia of the Alzheimer Type. Alzheimer's disease (AD) was described by Alzheimer in 1906 and is a cerebral degenerative disorder of unknown origin. It is not just a disease of the old, but the incidence increases concomitant with aging. AD destroys proteins of nerve cells of the cerebral cortex by diffuse infiltration with nonfunctional tissue called neurofibrillary tangles and plaques. The disease is progressive and is accompanied by increasing forgetfulness, confusion, inability to concentrate, personality deterioration, and impaired judgment. The cause of the disorder is still unknown, although there is some genetic factor that doubles the occurrence within susceptible families to 4% as opposed to 2% of the general population.

Senile dementia of the Alzheimer type (SDAT) was the term used to describe the Alzheimer's disorder as diagnosed by clinical research criteria but not histologically verified. SDAT was the usage suggested by the National Institute of Neurological and Communicative Disorders and the Alzheimer's Disease and Related Disorders Association Work Group. In the more recent publication of the DSM IV, senile dementia of the Alzheimer type is no longer considered an appropriate category. Rather, it is classified as dementia of the Alzheimer's type (DAT) with subsets of early onset or late onset. It is further refined into subtypes such as with delerium, with delusions, with depressed mood, with behavioral disturbance, or uncomplicated.

Because more people are living into the seventh, eighth, and ninth decades, the number of diagnosed cases of AD is estimated to increase. Approximately 6% of the population over the age of 65 may suffer from this disorder (Fenn et al, 1993). However, estimates of incidence vary greatly because AD is mentioned almost interchangeably with the generic term dementia, which includes both AD and other related and unrelated conditions. Terminologic confusion makes the accuracy of statistics difficult to assess.

Diagnosis of Alzheimer's disease. The only accurate method of diagnosing AD is to perform a brain biopsy or autopsy, though some promising gene research and single photon emission computed tomography (SPECT) magnetic resonance imaging (MRI) predict or diagnose with a high level of accuracy. The clinical criteria for the diagnosis of probable, possible, and definite AD are presented in Box 22-4.

Probable AD can be clinically diagnosed if there is a typical insidious onset of dementia with progression and if there are no other systemic or brain diseases that could account for the progressive memory and other cognitive deficits. Histopathologic confirmation is required for a diagnosis of definite AD. The diagnosis of possible AD is made in the presence of other significant diseases when AD is suspected to be the cause of the progressive dementia. If the course of the disease is aberrant, the clinical diagnosis of possible rather than probable AD is used.

AD is diagnosed on the basis of tests ruling out other disorders that may mimic Alzheimer's disease and the globally progressive nature of the disease (Box 22-5).

The characteristic changes (found on autopsy) in the brain are neurofibrillary tangles in cellular matrix, senile plaques (depositions in cerebral cells), atrophy of cortical tissue (brain shrinks in size), and a loss of cholinergic neurons in the limbic system. Plaques are focused most densely in the hippocampus and the cortex. Tomlinson et al(1970) established the actual pathologic picture of senile dementia as it is known today.

At present, no major differences have been found either clinically or pathologically between AD occurring in middle age or in the old. The course of this disease ranges from 1 to 15 years, with death usually occurring because of pulmonary infections, urinary tract infections, decubitus ulcers, or iatrogenic disorders. Current research focuses on many aspects of AD: anatomy, biochemistry, diagnosis, genetics, language, memory, nutrition, perception, pharmacology, physiology, psychosocial issues, virology, and vitamin therapy. A summary of theories of AD is provided in Table 22-3.

Genetics. There is no doubt that genetic transmission is one strong factor in the development of AD. In one large family in Belgium, 21 members developed the disease before the age of 45 years, and it was transmitted in autosomal-dominant fashion (Gomme et al, 1987). A rare, early onset form of Alzheimer's disease has been traced to heritable mutations of an amyloid precursor protein (APP) gene, but the more common late-onset form is associated with the inheritance of an apolipoprotein allele, Apo E4 (Roses, 1995; Beffer and Poirier, 1996). Even more exciting is the discovery that while Apo E4 is a susceptibility gene, Apo E2 lowers the risk of the disease. The Apo Es (Apo E2, 3, and 4) play an important role in triglyceride-rich lipoprotein metabolism and cholesterol homeostasis. There is much work to do to uncover the interplay among these factors and preventive or treatment modes. Questions regarding the influence of genetics on AD are continually being investigated.

Researchers in the School of Medicine at Case Western Reserve University have made some fundamental observations concerning the origin of the amyloid deposited in the senile plaques of brain cells of patients with AD. Younkin et al (1988) report that increased levels of amyloid protein precursor lacking the protease inhibitor may play an important role in amyloid deposition in AD. This finding has more recently been confirmed by Roses (1995).

Viral and other theories. Viral residue from remote disorders is providing researchers with questions about a

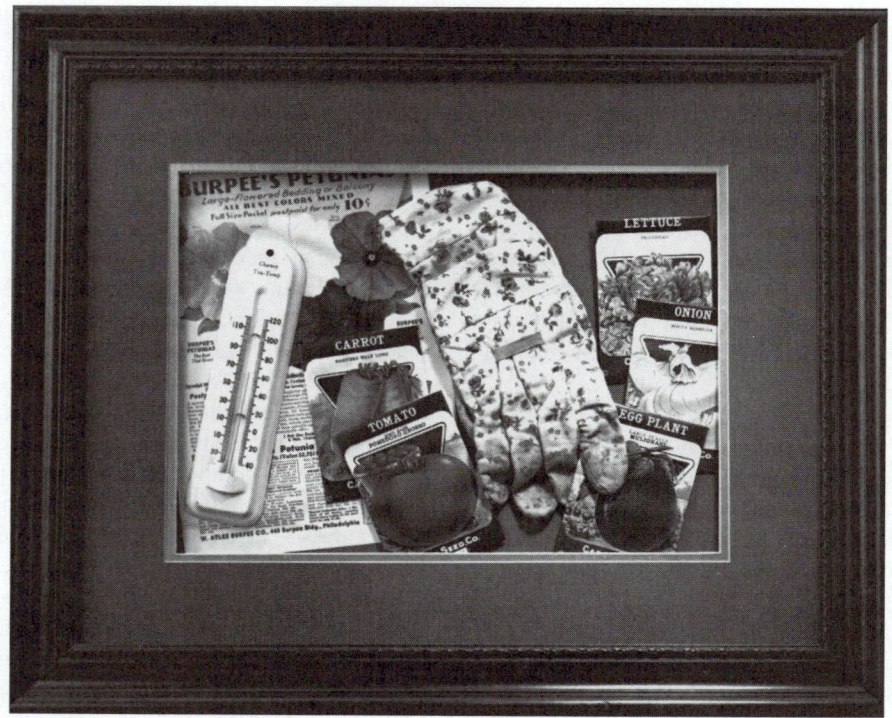

Shadow box frame holds various items that stir memories for Alzheimer's patients and others with dementia-related illnesses. "My Garden" holds seed packets, gardening gloves, planting instructions, and other items. (Courtesy ArtLine, Ltd.)

possible relationship to later development of AD and some other dementias. British researchers have detected the herpes simplex virus type 1 (HSV1) in the brains of people who have AD. They believe the virus interacts with apolipoprotein E4 (Apo E4) to increase the risk of AD or perhaps to trigger the formation of the characteristic filamentous protein aggregates that form the neurofibrillary tangles and senile plaques, lesions characteristic of AD (La Voie, 1997).

A 25-year epidemiologic case-control trend analysis of dementia conducted at the Mayo Clinic has determined that general medical conditions, previous head injury, thyroid disease, exposure to therapeutic radiation, anesthesia, and blood transfusions are not risk factors for AD. Sociodemographic factors and gender showed no significant differences, although the presence of depression may increase the risk for the development of AD (Kokmen et al, 1996).

Recently, atherosclerosis and AD were linked because researchers in the Netherlands found individuals with atherosclerosis three times more likely to have AD (Christensen, 1997). This suggests that changes in blood

---

Box 22-4

Criteria for Clinical Diagnosis of Alzheimer's Disease

I. **Probable** Alzheimer's disease include:

Dementia established by clinical examination and documented by the Mini-Mental Test, Blessed Dementia Scale, or some similar examination, and confirmed by neuropsychologic tests

Deficits in two or more areas of cognition

Progressive worsening of memory and other cognitive functions

No disturbance of consciousness

Onset between ages 40 and 90, most often after age 65

Absence of systemic disorders or other brain diseases that in and of themselves could account for the progressive deficits in memory and cognition

II. The diagnosis of **probable** Alzheimer's disease is supported by:

Progressive deterioration of specific cognitive functions such as language (aphasia), motor skills (apraxia), and perception (agnosia)

Impaired activities of daily living and altered patterns of behavior

Family history of similar disorders, particularly if confirmed neuropathologically

Laboratory results of:

Normal lumbar puncture as evaluated by standard techniques

Normal pattern or nonspecific changes in EEG, such as increased slow-wave activity

Evidence of cerebral atrophy on CT with progression documented by serial observation

III. Other clinical features consistent with the diagnosis of **probable** Alzheimer's disease, after exclusion of causes of dementia other than Alzheimer's disease, include:

Plateaus in the course of progression of the illness

Associated symptoms of depression, insomnia, incontinence, delusions, illusions, hallucinations, catastrophic verbal, emotional, or physical outbursts, sexual disorders, and weight loss

IV. Features that make the diagnosis of **probable** Alzheimer's disease uncertain or unlikely include:

Sudden, apoplectic onset

Focal neurologic findings such as hemiparesis, sensory loss, visual field deficits, and incoordination early in the course of the illness; and

Seizures or gait disturbances at the onset or very early in the course of the illness

V. Clinical diagnosis of **possible** Alzheimer's disease:

May be made on the basis of the dementia syndrome, in the absence of other neurologic, psychiatric, or other systemic disorders sufficient to cause dementia, and in the presence of variations in the onset, in the presentation, or in the clinical course

May be made in the presence of a second systemic or brain disorder sufficient to produce dementia, which is not considered to be the cause of the dementia

Should be used in research studies when a single, gradually progressive severe cognitive deficit is identified in the absence of other identifiable causes

VI. Criteria for diagnosis of **definite** Alzheimer's disease are:

The clinical criteria for probable Alzheimer's disease

Histopathologic evidence obtained from a biopsy or autopsy

VII. Classification of Alzheimer's disease for research purposes should specify features that may differentiate subtypes of the disorder, such as:

Familial occurrence

Onset before age of 65

Presence of trisomy-21

Coexistence of other relevant conditions such as Parkinson's disease

From McKhann G, Drachman D, Folstein R et al: Clinical diagnosis of Alzheimer's disease: Report of the NINCDS-ADRDA Work Group under the auspices of Department of Health and Human Services Task Force on Alzheimer's disease, *Neurology* 34:940, 1984. Copyright the American Academy of Neurology. Used with permission of Lippincott-Raven Publishers.

vessels in the brain may trigger the deterioration that causes AD. This is complicated by the fact that the likelihood of developing any kind of dementia increases as atherosclerosis progresses.

The most promising theory is based on a concept of a deleterious network of factors that together form the key components of AD, resulting in the characteristic abnormalities of brain tissue. These are increased free radical damage, impaired energy metabolism, abnormalities of calcium homeostasis, and alterations in amyloid precursor protein metabolism (Ying, 1996). Various risk factors may trigger the network by activating one or more of these key factors. At present no one theory adequately explains the complex biochemical and pathologic factors of the disease (Smith et al, 1995).

HIV-Related Dementia. HIV is the most notorious of the five known human retroviruses. Four of them (including HIV) are associated with degenerative diseases of the nervous system. Weiler (1988) reports several cases of mistaken diagnoses of AD that on autopsy were found to be AIDS-related dementia. He contends that clinicians must consider HIV infection as a possible cause of dementia in elderly persons even when they are not initially known to be in any high-risk group for AIDS. HIV-related dementia is the neurologic impairment that occurs in up to 75% of people with AIDS (Baumann, 1993).

HIV-related dementia is of two types, depending on whether it is the result of direct or indirect involvement of the central nervous system (CNS). Indirect effects on the CNS are the result of tumors, malignancies, and abscesses that occupy cerebral space. Symptoms include lethargy, confusion, headaches, focal neurologic deficits, and seizures. However, recent studies indicate that the HIV can infiltrate the CNS directly and produce a distinctive AIDS dementia complex. It is thought to do so early in the disease or even before onset of other symptoms and may be the earliest and only sign of HIV infection (Navia and Price, 1987).

AIDS dementia complex is characterized by cognitive, motor, and behavioral changes. Only rudimentary intellectual and social functioning remain intact, and psychomotor retardation is evident. Overall verbal and motor slowing are prominent characteristics as well as gait ataxia and hyperreflexia (Scharnhorst, 1992). Depression, agitation, delusions, hallucinations, grandiosity, and paranoia are common symptoms. The end result of AIDS dementia complex closely resembles AD (Havarth et al, 1995). Nurses must be aware that, in some cases of dementia that progress more rapidly than is typical of AD, the AIDS dementia complex must be considered.

The AIDS epidemic is not restricted to younger persons and intravenous (IV) drug users. Although statistics are available for these groups, issues of privacy preclude accurate demographic data about the prevalence of the disease in the general population and particularly in the geriatric population. Feltes (1995) estimates that 10% of AIDS cases oc-

cur in those over 50 years old and 4% in those over 70. An ageist attitude exists regarding the potential for acquiring HIV through sexual activity. The compromised immune system of an aged individual may make him or her even more susceptible to AIDS than a younger person. The aged AIDS patient is likely to die soon after diagnosis because the diagnosis is often delayed (Scharnhorst, 1992). As the geriatric population increases, so will the geriatric AIDS cases increase.

It is an underlying assumption that many elders in nursing homes may be HIV positive, although not identified as such. The aged are very likely to have undergone massive blood transfusions (before the advent of careful monitoring of blood products) during surgeries before transfer to long-term care. A few older persons have publicly discussed their acquisition of AIDS through transfusion. Others will be identified as the public becomes less biased and more inclined to accept HIV testing as a routine procedure. Those presently identified comprise 3.6% of all U.S. AIDS cases (U.S. Bureau of the Census, 1995).

A limited number of long-term care facilities knowingly accept AIDS patients, and among those that do, the geriatric AIDS patient competes for extended care services with nongeriatric AIDS patients and non-AIDS geriatric patients. Finding appropriate services and facilities may be difficult, although in places in which this care is available, reports are

---

Box 22-5 | **Clinical Diagnostic Work-up and HIV Testing**

The basic evaluation should include a CBC, electrolyte panel measurements, SMA-12/60 (Sequential Multiple Analyzer) tests, thyroid function tests, folate and vitamin B_{12} levels, VDRL test, urinalysis and HIV testing; ECG and chest x-ray may be useful in some patients. Assessment tools such as the Hachinski Ischemic Score can be used to differentiate multiinfarct dementia from Alzheimer's disease. A CT or MRI scan should be done when the history suggests a mass, when focal neurologic signs exist, or when the dementia is of brief duration to rule out tumors, infarcts, subdural hematoma, and normal-pressure hydrocephalus. Magnetic resonance imaging is more sensitive than CT for detecting small infarcts and mass lesions. A lumbar puncture is rarely needed but should be considered if a chronic infection is suspected as the cause of cognitive impairment. Apo E4 can be identified in the blood, making it likely that a blood test will become available to help diagnose Alzheimer's disease. Recent data suggest that persons with Alzheimer's disease have a strong pupillary response to very dilute anticholinergic eyedrops.

From Abrams WB, Beers MH, Barkow R, editors: *The Merck manual of geriatrics,* ed 2, Whitehouse Station, NJ, 1995, Merck Research Laboratories.

Table 22-3 Alzheimer's Theories

Factors	Action/theory	Results	Progress
Neurotransmitters			
Acetylcholine	Acetylcholine levels drop by about 90%	Decline in memory	Drug therapies aimed at post-synaptic receptor sites: vitamin E and Deprenyl being tested in clinical trials
Serotonin; somatostatin; noradrenaline	Levels lower than normal	Sensory disturbance; aggressive behavior; neuron death	
Phospholipids	Shape and action of the receptors may be role	Abnormalities transmit garbled messages from one neuron to another due to dysfunction or blockage of relay points	
Proteins			
Beta amyloid	Forms insoluable plaque	Possible neuron death	Studies link the disruption of K^+ and Ca++ levels; link between cholinergic neuron death and beta amyloids
Tau	Neurofibrillary tangles	Twisted paired helical filaments destabilize the microtubule structure	
Genes			
1, 14, 19 (Apo E4)	Protein and amyloid become insoluble, leading to deposition of plaque	Linked to late onset of Alzheimer's; increases deposits of beta amyloid	
	Tau protein allows structure of microtubules to become undone causing tangles	Directly regulates apolipoprotein (Apo E4) and quickly binds with beta amyloid	How tau and beta amyloids react to APP
21	Neurons with short dendrites; carries code for mutated amyloid precursor protein (APP) familial Alzheimer's disease (FAD)	Early Alzheimer's	Supports theory that beta amyloids play a role in Alzheimer's disease; also gene found in Down syndrome
Metabolism			
Glucose and O_2 molecules	Altered glucose metabolism	Dramatic decline in glucose and oxygen as neurons degenerate and die or neuron degeneration causes glucose decline	Neurons having problems with metabolism react abnormally to another neurotransmitter "glutamate"
Calcium	A rise in Ca++ level inside the cell	Series of cascades of biochemical events, allowing a rise in calcium channels admit in excess Ca++	
	Levels rise because of energy level crisis in neurons	A defect in structure leads to an increase in storage or pumping calcium out	
		Chronically high levels of neurotransmitter glutamate disrupts metabolism causing an influx of Ca++	
	Hormone glucocorticoid	Neuron death and dysfunction caused in hippocampus	
Environment			
Aluminum	Trace metal in brain	Turns up in more than normal amounts in many brain autopsies of AD patients	Nothing confirmed
Zinc	Too little or too much	Found on brain autopsy of AD patients	

Modified from *Alzheimer's disease: unraveling the mystery,* NIA, NIH No. 95-3782, 1995.   *Continued*

Table 22-3 Alzheimer's Theories—cont'd

Factors	Action/theory	Results	Progress
Food-borne poisons	Food toxins	Causes soluble beta amyloid of the cerebral spinal fluid to clump together similar to plaque of AD patients; may cause neurologic damage and enhance the action of neurotransmitter glutamate	Current studies are looking at this
Viruses	A virus or other infection		

positive. One of the major concerns we have is that the needs of young persons dying of AIDS may be quite different from those of the old. If they are indiscriminately mixed in long-term care settings, neither group is likely to have its needs well met.

Linsk et al (1993) surveyed 54 Illinois nursing facilities to find that AIDS and HIV-related illness is extremely rare within long-term care facilities. In fact, only 6 of the 54 facilities received an actual referral from hospital discharge planners; however, no admissions were completed.

Because most communities do not have resources to establish separate systems for the aged and the AIDS patients who have some similar needs, long-term care providers must address these issues.

Parkinson's Dementia. Parkinson's disease (PD) describes a constellation of symptoms arising from disorders of the basal ganglia, the islands of gray matter in the cerebral hemispheres. Though the etiology of primary parkinsonism is unknown, the death of substantia nigra cells within the basal ganglia results in a marked reduction in dopamine and is the cause of symptoms of tremor, muscular rigidity, akinesia, and loss of postural reflexes (Berkow et al, 1995; Kaszniak, 1995). It is the most common of neurologic syndromes and has an average onset at age 68. The incidence peaks at age 75 and then seems to decline in frequency.

Secondary PD is caused by several medications (see Chapter 23 for discussion), metabolic and degenerative disorders. Depression and anxiety are common in individuals with primary or secondary parkinsonism and may occur in 80% of these individuals. The most common initial symptom is tremor of one hand and the pill-rolling motion of the fingers.

It remains controversial whether the dementia that occurs in about 25% of patients with PD is related to the pathologic findings of the disease or whether it is a disorder quite distinct from PD without dementia (Hazzard et al, 1994). However, the DSM-IV states that the dementia is a direct result of pathophysiologic changes that occur in the presence of PD. Early signs of dementia are subtle and are somewhat related to age and age of onset, though specific cognitive

changes commonly occur early in the course of PD (Levin and Katzen, 1995). Incidence of dementia in PD is associated with depression, institutionalization, older age at onset of PD, and atypical neurologic features (Aarsland et al, 1996).

Nurses will best serve the clients dealing with the mood disorders because these may mimic dementia and must be relieved to the greatest extent possible. Medications and individualized treatment plans are critical to the care of the person with PD. No curative therapy is available, and the challenge to client, family, and nurse is to maintain the highest possible level of hope. At times the progress is rapid but most patients remain functional for many years (Berkow et al, 1995).

Vascular Brain Disorders. Dementia of vascular disease origin is marked by several distinguishing characteristics: remission and fluctuation, preservation of personality, insight, lability of emotion, and epileptiform attacks (Box 22-6). Intracerebral hemorrhage and the interruption of an adequate supply of blood and nutrients to the brain, resulting in tissue damage, accounts for about 80% of strokes in the elderly (Caplan, 1995). It is now thought that immediate treatment, within 6 hours of the cerebrovascular accident, may prevent some of the brain cell death (Krieger, 1995). The prevalence of cerebrovascular disease varies with race and gender but averages about 7% of the population over age 75 (Caplan, 1995).

In addition to major brain attacks, there are transient ischemic attacks (TIAs) caused by impaired circulation. The attacks occur suddenly and are completely resolved within 24 hours (Kelly, 1995) but leave lacunae of nonfunctional cerebral tissue. Numerous TIAs result in multi-infarct dementia that may appear symptomatically as AD and are often prodromal to major brain attacks. Strokes and the chronic symptoms and needs are discussed more fully in Chapter 8. In addition, the impairments in communication are an alienating factor that is considered in chapter 18.

Because of the numerous ways in which circulation to cerebral cells can be impaired and the multiplicity of sites in which this may occur, vascular disease may be initially seen with varied symptoms and run an unpredictable course (Figure 22-3). These two factors are especially threatening. An individual may feel as if he or she were living with an internal time bomb. The following may restore some sense of security to the patient:

1. Install a telephone with a long cord or a portable phone and post emergency numbers on the phone.
2. Advise client to wear antiembolic hose and avoid rising rapidly from a lying to a standing position.
3. Engage family, friends, or agencies in a daily telephone check to determine client's status.
4. Subscribe to "Lifeline" through a community hospital.

Traumatic Brain Injury (Dementia due to Head Trauma). Traumatic injury causes disarray in the complex synchronized systems of the brain and most usually results in anger, agitation, and aggression (Patrick and Hebda, 1996). These changes in behavior and personality interfere with all aspects of life and are intensified when the demands of daily living become more complex. Neurologists have identified certain sites within the brain that, when injured, express themselves in anger and aggression. Antiseizure medications and serotonin specific reuptake inhibitors (SSRIs) are often helpful. As the chemistry of the brain is modified, the individual is more capable of managing daily challenges and learning. However, interpersonal relations may still be difficult. It is important to recognize that the problems in this respect always involve both parties in the exchange. Solutions must take into account the context and all the individuals involved in the exchanges that result in loss of control of impulses (Patrick and Hebda, 1996).

Pick's Disease. Pick's disease is a rare progressive degenerative brain disorder involving atrophy of the frontal and temporal lobes of the cerebral cortex. Pick's disease is an uncommon type of progressive dementia with clinical features similar to AD and is often misdiagnosed. It was discovered by a Czechoslovakian physician, Arnold Pick (1851-1924) and has a distinctive histopathology of degenerating neurons that contain globular intracytoplasmic filamentous inclusion bodies. The clinical distinction between AD and Pick's disease is often difficult; however, Pick's disease shows a more rapid progression than AD, generally occurs more abruptly and at younger ages, and presents some unique signs, such as the "mirror sign." In the "mirror sign" the patient stands in front of the mirror and tries to engage his image in conversation (Jung and Solomon, 1993). The differences between Pick's disease and AD can be seen in Table 22-4.

Creutzfeldt-Jakob Dementia. Creutzfeldt-Jakob disease (CJD) is a rare dementing disorder that seems to be on the increase and has been linked to bovine spongiform encephalopathy ("mad cow disease") (McKnight and Rockwood, 1996). It is an infectious disorder thought to be transmitted by prior transfer through contact with blood products and other body fluids (Vaughn, 1996). It produces rapidly progressive dementia, ataxia, myoclonus, degeneration of the

---

Box 22-6   Vascular Brain Disease

Vascular brain disease may result from any of the following:

- Arteriosclerotic plaques blocking circulation to cerebral cells
- Blood dyscrasias interfering with platelet and clot formation
- Cardiac decompensation, resulting in insufficient perfusion to the brain
- Cerebrovascular hemorrhage (strokes) of small or large magnitude.
- Diabetic deterioration of blood vessels
- Primary hypertension causes deterioration of capillary walls because of sustained pressure; cerebral cells dependent on the deteriorated capillaries no longer function. Over time, hypertensive persons show greater decrements in cognitive performance than persons with normal blood pressure.
- Rupture of cerebrovascular or aortic aneurysms
- Sustained severe anemia
- Systemic emboli lodging in cerebrovascular pathway
- Transient ischemic attacks (TIAs) lasting up to 24 hours, resulting from spasms of blood vessels in certain segments of the brain, which produce temporary disturbances in sensation, cognition, and motor activity, and are often a warning of impending stroke

---

CNS, neuromuscular disturbances, electroencephalographic changes, and other neurologic signs. The clinical diagnosis is confirmed through immunohistochemistry assay and various other laboratory diagnostic techniques (Kretzschmar et al, 1996). The course of the disease is typically 3 to 6 months. The patient is hypersensitive to sound, bright lights, sudden movement, and touch.

Nursing care is centered on family support, avoiding transmission of the disease, supporting patient respiration, nutrition, hydration, and comfort and medication management of seizures and myoclonic movement (Rotkoff et al, 1997). There is concern that this dementing disorder may go unrecognized, and therefore the necessary infectious precautions may not be observed as stringently as required.

Huntington's Disease. Dementia originating in Huntington's disease is seldom considered a problem of the aged because it usually occurs at younger ages, is heritable, and is exhibited with characteristic choreiform movements. However, Shulman et al (1996) find late-onset Huntington's disease more common in the elderly than has been supposed and presenting with unique clinical features. It should not be dismissed from consideration as a cause of dementia in the aged but does remain rather rare.

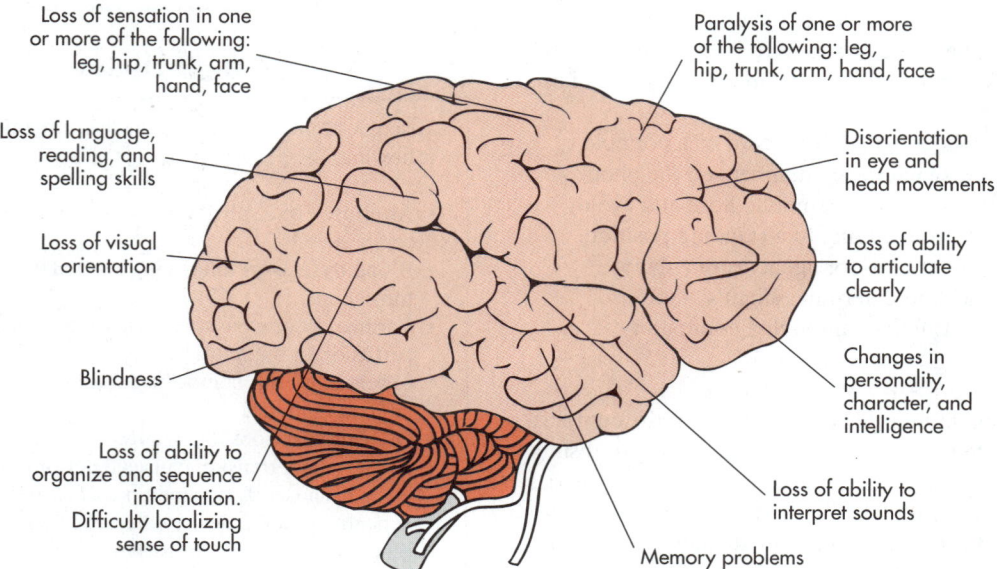

Loss of sensation in one
or more of the following:
leg, hip, trunk, arm,
hand, face

Loss of language,
reading, and
spelling skills

Loss of visual
orientation

Blindness

Loss of ability to
organize and sequence
information.
Difficulty localizing
sense of touch

Paralysis of one or more
of the following: leg,
hip, trunk, arm, hand, face

Disorientation
in eye and
head movements

Loss of ability
to articulate
clearly

Changes in
personality,
character, and
intelligence

Loss of ability to
interpret sounds

Memory problems

Figure 22-3. Brain areas affected by strokes.

Developmentally Disabled Elders. The number of developmentally disabled elders (DDE) is rapidly increasing primarily because of medical advances and healthier living conditions that maintain them longer than in previous generations. Interestingly, all individuals with Down syndrome (trisomy 21) who survive until old age develop the pathogenic hallmarks of AD (Royston et al, 1996). Functional limitations in the biologic, social, and psychologic spheres may be a major cause of frailty in the DDE. Those elders are particularly dependent on their environment for stimulation, and in its absence behaviors suggestive of dementia may emerge.

Many aspects of the aging process apparently are prematurely experienced by the developmentally disabled. Thus they may experience musculoskeletal changes, sensory decline, and certain disease states earlier. Retirement needs and responses to relocation present special considerations. Box 22-7 suggests issues in need of further study.

In Ohio a study of the needs and characteristics of the aged mentally retarded (developmentally disabled) found that of those who survived to old age, three fourths were only mildly or moderately retarded. They required little supervision, were able to communicate, and were free from maladaptive behaviors. Their physical health was similar to others of the same age. As would be expected because of their earlier lifestyle, social and academic skills were limited. Three quarters of them lived in group homes.

More recently, Maisto and Hughes (1995) found that both previously institutionalized and noninstitutionalized adults with mental retardation adapted to group homes at higher levels than were previously evident (Maisto and Hughes, 1995). Elderly mentally retarded persons may be kept in a more restrictive setting than necessary because no one has carefully assessed their abilities. A more humanistic and individualized model of care is emerging (Mooney et al, 1995).

Assessment of Cognitive Impairment

Cognitive function encompasses the processes by which an individual perceives, registers, stores, retrieves and uses information (Foreman et al, 1996, p. 228). Memory testing may be used primarily for establishing the presence of dementia and assessment of other cognitive functions for determining the severity of CI. Though extremely common in individuals over 75 years of age, CI is not diagnosed by primary care providers even for those with moderate to severe impairment (Callahan et al, 1995). Even among younger clients it was found during routine office visits that 15.7% of patients over 60 years of age were cognitively impaired (Callahan et al, 1995).

Foremost in assessment of CI is a thorough medical workup to rule out factors that may be clouding consciousness. Following that an evaluation for depression is necessary because the confounding effects of severe depression are a significant problem and frequently are severe enough to mimic dementia. Nurses' recognition and assessment of CI is most likely to be accurate if appropriate instruments are employed. Nurses see the patient throughout the course of the day and observe mentation and behavior in many circumstances.

Self-appraisal is also important and will be discussed with the client and family by the nurse. However, it is known that individuals with dementia may overestimate their capacities, whereas those with depression are inclined to underestimate them (McDougall, 1996).

Table 22-4	Pick's Disease versus Alzheimer's Disease	
	Pick's	**Alzheimer's**
Personality change	Early; before cognitive change	Late; after cognitive change
Deterioration of ADLs	Early; before cognitive change	Late; after cognitive change
Memory loss	Late	Early; often first symptom
Disordered language	Early	Late
Socially inappropriate behavior	Early	Late
Stereotypies	Early	Mid or late
Non-paranoid delusions	Rare	Common
Hallucinations	Never	Common
Apraxias, agnosias, alexia	Late	Early in patients with family history; otherwise variable
Alcohol abuse	Common	Rare
Hypersexuality	Common	Rare
Criminal behavior	Common	Rare
Visuo-spatial disorientation	Rare	Common
Emotional distress	Rare	Common, especially early
Moria/*Witzelsucht*	Common	Rare
Mirror sign	Rare	Never
Age of risk	Mean: 50s up to 80	Increases into 90s
Length of illness	2-11 years	5-25 years

From Jung R, Solomon K: Psychiatric manifestations of Pick's disease, *Int Psychogeriatr* 5(2):187, 1993.

Changes in function that persist may be indicators of CI. An overview of cognitive assessment is provided in Box 22-8 and assessment of cognitive function in Table 22-5.

Piaget's influence (1952) was important in the understanding of cognitive development in childhood. He characterized a gradual progression of cognitive development and the idea that each stage must be evaluated by tools appropriate to the stage and task. The observation that aged individuals with dementia may go through a similar process in reverse is being given serious consideration and study (Matteson et al, 1996) (Table 22-6).

Orientation. Many nurse clinicians use the patient's orientation to time, place, and person as a quick evaluator of cognitive function; however, orientation items are inaccurate indicators of degree and severity of CI. In a nursing study, Palmateer and McCartney (1985) found that when reviewing the charts, 87% of the time the nurses' only comment regarding cognitive functioning was the word "oriented." Orientation screening is unacceptably insensitive.

Perception. Perception is one criterion used to assess a person's level of CI. Investigations reveal a relationship between quality of the sensory apparatus and cognitive functioning. Auditory status and cognitive functional decline may be associated. Hearing impairment not only interferes with comprehension but significantly reduces stimulation needed to maximize cerebral function.

Psychomotor Ability. Psychomotor behaviors pertaining to motor effects of cerebral or psychic activity do not lead to purposeful behaviors and are observed in patients with CI. Sundown syndrome (SS) was first identified by Cameron in 1941 and was called "nocturnal neurosis and wandering." SS resembles delirium, and nurses often see the agitation, rest-

Box 22-7	**Information Gaps Related to the Needs of DDE**

Identification of the population and their special needs
    Biologic and clinical aspects of aging
    Relationship between Down syndrome and AD
    Issues related to these needs
    Epidemiology of the population
    Population's characteristics and needs
Health-related issues
    Service approaches
Community and social policy
Perspectives for the future

lessness, confusion, and wandering behavior of older adults when the sun goes down. Evans (1987) identified risk factors for SS in institutionalized elderly. Physiologic factors were dehydration, mental impairment, frequent night awakening for nursing care, dementia, and odor of urine. Psychosocial factors were being in room less than 1 month, recent admission to facility, and fluctuating levels of orientation.

Reaction Time. Reflex elicitation is a routine part of a neurologic examination to determine psychomotor ability, as well as degree of CI. Nurses use reflex elicitation as a quick indicator to help determine cognitive functioning in neurologic patients. This is essential in the clinical diagnosis of CI and other dementias. The presence of primitive reflexes represents severe cerebral degeneration, particularly of the frontal lobes, and is closely associated with dementia. The primitive reflexes routinely tested are corneomandibular, gegenhalten, glabellar, hand grasp, palmomental, snout,

Box 22-8	**Overview of Cognitive Assessment**

A. Concepts and categories
 1. Definition: cognitive function: the processes by which an individual perceives, registers, stores, retrieves, and uses information
 2. Categories of cognitive change/decline
   a. The dementias (e.g., Alzheimer's, vascular) are chronic, progressive, insidious, and permanent states of cognitive impairment
   b. Delirium/acute confusion: an acute and sudden impairment of cognition that is considered temporary, generally an identifiable, biophysical cause
   c. Impairment in thought processes

B. Assessment
 1. Methods of assessment
   a. Formal—cognitive testing using standardized instruments
     i. Advantages: standardized; enables comparison across individuals and nurses
     ii. Disadvantages: individual performance influenced by pain, education, fatigue, cultural background, and perceptual and physical abilities
   b. Informal—through structured observations of nurse-individual interactions
     i. Advantages: may have greater meaning about individual's actual cognitive ability/performance
     ii. Disadvantages: difficult to make judgments regarding change in individual condition; variability in interpretation
 2. Other considerations for assessment
   a. Characteristics of the environment for assessment
     i. Physical environment
       —Comfortable ambient temperature
       —Adequate lighting but not glaring
       —Free of distractions; e.g, should be conducted in the absence of others and other activities
       —Position self to maximize individual's sensory abilities
     ii. Interpersonal environment
       —Use individual's self-paced rate for assessment
       —Emotionally nonthreatening
   b. Timing considerations
     i. Timing should reflect the actual cognitive abilities of the individual and not extraneous factors
     ii. Times of the day to generally avoid
       —Immediately on awakening from sleep, wait at least 30 minutes
       —Immediately before or after meals
       —Immediately before or after medical diagnostic or therapeutic procedures
       —When patient has pain or discomfort

From Foreman MD, Fletcher K, Mion LC et al: Assessing cognitive function, *Geriatr Nurs* 17(5):228, 1996.

and suck. Research on primitive reflexes has produced conflicting results because they occur in normal elderly, in adults with signs of brain disease, in demented patients, and in patients with psychiatric disease.

Social Intactness. Inappropriate behaviors, particularly abusive and violent behaviors that may be present in CI, let nurses know that a patient may be unable to conform to the routines and rules of the environment. In a descriptive study of agitated nursing home residents, Cohen-Mansfield (1986) identified three behavioral categories: (1) physical aggressive behavior—biting, spitting, hitting, and throwing objects; (2) verbal aggressive behavior—cursing and verbal aggression; and (3) nonaggressive behavior—pacing, dressing or disrobing inappropriately, and constant requests for attention.

Functional Ability. Allen and Allen (1987) have developed a taxonomy of cognitive levels and task analyses that is useful for assessing functional abilities in patients with AD. Numerous uses are suggested for this taxonomy, including measurement of the severity of mental disorders, measurement of changes in temporal levels that reflect needed changes in treatment, assessment of need for hospitalization and/or community placement, determination of readiness for discharge from hospital, and evaluation of the effectiveness of treatment.

Researchers at Duke Universtiy constructed a Functional Dementia Scale (FDS) designed for completion by caretakers of persons with dementia to monitor objectively the disease course and to evaluate treatment. The items of the

Box 22-8	**Overview of Cognitive Assessment—cont'd**

3. Parameters of assessment
   a. Alertness/level of consciousness: the most rudimentary cognitive function and level of arousal, or responsiveness to stimuli determined by interaction with individual and determination of level made on the basis of the individual's best eye, verbal, and motor response to stimuli
      i. Alertness—able to interact in a meaningful way with the examiner
      ii. Lethargy or somnolence—not fully alert; individual tends to drift to sleep when not stimulated, diminished spontaneous physical movement, loses train of thought, ideas wander
      iii. Obtundation—transitional stage between lethargy and stupor; difficult to arouse, meaningful testing futile, requires constant stimulation to elicit response
      iv. Stupor or semicoma—individual mumbles/groans in response to persistent and vigorous physical stimulation
      v. Coma—completely unable to be aroused, no behavioral response to stimuli
   b. Attention: ability to attend/concentrate on stimuli: can follow through with directions, especially a three-stage command; is easily distracted
   c. Memory: ability to register, retain, and recall information both new and old; does individual remember your name? Is individual able to learn and remember new information?
   d. Orientation to time, place, and person
   e. Thinking: ability to organize and communicate ideas; thoughts should be organized, coherent, and appropriate
   f. Perception: presence/absence of illusions, delusions, or visual or auditory hallucinations
   g. Psychomotor behavior: ability to comprehend and perform simple motor skills. Relative to execution ability to ask the individual to perform certain ADLs/IADLs, or to perform a three-step command, and to copy a figure
   h. Insight: ability to understand oneself and the situation in which one finds oneself
   i. Judgment: ability to evaluate a situation (real or hypothetical) and determine an appropriate action

C. Outcomes of assessment
   1. Individual
      a. Detection of deviations will be prompt and early with appropriate care and treatment instituted in a timely manner
      b. Plans of care will appropriately address corrective and supportive cognitive function
   2. Health care provider
      a. Assessment and documentation of cognitive function
      b. Appropriate strategies to address any deviation in cognitive function
      c. Competence in cognitive assessment
      d. Evidence of ability to differentiate among the different types of cognitive change/decline
   3. Institution
      a. Documentation of cognitive function will increase
      b. Referral to appropriate advanced practitioners (e.g., geriatrician, geriatric/gerontological or psychiatric clinical nurse specialist or nurse practitioner, or consultation-liaison service) will increase

ADL, Activities of daily living; IADL, instrumental activities of daily living.

Functional Dementia Scale were selected to assess the major problems associated with dementia, such as emotional lability, wandering, agitation, incontinence, memory loss, and need for supervision. This scale may be useful to clinicians and families caring for demented patients and is easily administered by nursing home personnel or families (Moore et al, 1983) (Box 22-9). The Functional Dementia Scale is a brief scale capable of distinguishing varying degrees of functional limitation and is useful in establishing the level of impairment and assessing the impact of interventions over time.

A Mini-Mental State examination revised from Meyers' initial formulations can assess orientation, immediate and recent memory, attention, calculation, and language and motor skills (Box 22-10). The Mini-Mental State examination is unique because it allows assessment of fluid and crystallized intelligence. Symptoms in AD usually progress in five stages: (1) loss in memory, (2) loss in powers of reasoning, (3) loss in comprehension, (4) deterioration in personality, and (5) a terminal vegetative state (McDougall, 1990).

Affectual Disturbance. Affect is often unstable, heightened or flattened; in some, emotional incontinence is characteristic. In the later, severe stages of dementia affect seems totally lacking.

Depressed mood among persons who later developed dementia has been studied longtitudinally in over 1000 elders residing in Washington Heights community of North Manhattan (Devanand, 1996). The frequency with which depression existed prior to the development of dementia has

Table 22-5 Assessment of Cognitive Function

Domain	Definition	Assessment
Attention span	The ability to focus, in a sustained manner or for a period of time, on one activity or object.	Is the individual able to move freely in time between past, present, and future? This is judged to be psychologically adaptive skill.
Concentration	The ability to concentrate is manifested by the individual's ability to answer questions, ignoring unimportant or irrelevant external stimuli.	Are memories spiced with perceptions and feelings or consistently filled with descriptions of things and events? Persons with readiness for insight would more likely demonstrate the first style.
Intelligence	Broadly defined, intelligence is the ability to comprehend or understand. General intelligence usually includes verbal aptitude, calculation skills, and spatial relationship skills. There is evidence that as people age, noncognitive factors such as motivation, response speed, and sensory deficits play increasingly significant roles in intellectual performance. When referring to older adults, a distinction must be made between the terms "intelligence" and "competence." Intelligence is described as an inference of underlying traits, based on observations in many situations. Competence is a more situation-specific combination of intellectual traits that with adequate motivation will permit adaptive behavior. Intelligence is usually determined by similarities and vocabulary tests, and mathematical tests, e.g., calculations that require the individual to add or substract using serial sevens or serial threes and/or digit span forwards and backwards. The individual is required to add or subtract three or seven from 100 five consecutive times.	What is the entertainment or teaching value of the memories shared? Those who use memories to teach may have a capacity for caring and ego transcendence.
Judgment	Judgment is the mental ability to perceive and distinguish the relationship between two objects. An individual is evaluated for appropriate and realistic behavior that is based on an awareness of the environment and the consequences of his or her behavior. Parameters usually assessed include physical and psychologic needs, ability to form appropriate goals and plans, and ability to act on these goals and plans. Other important indicators of judgment are the individual's ability to handle financial matters or drive a car.	Is the person unable to reminisce? This is often a sign of depression or of action orientation versus verbal orientation.
Learning ability	Learning is a sustained, highly deliberate effort to acquire knowledge or a skill. An important learning difference for older adults is the increasing time required for acquisition of knowledge or skills and retrieval of information from memory. Older adults' ability to learn may be improved with a longer acquisition and response period, with a particular emphasis on a self-paced approach. The amount of material and the number of task demands presented during instruction may also influence learning ability.	Are the memories quite outlandish or grandiose? This may signify low self-esteem and a bid for attention.

*Modified from McDougall GJ: A review of screening instruments for assessing cognition and mental health in older adults, *Nurs Pract* 15:11, 1990.

generated interest among researchers in the possibility that depressed mood may be an early manifestation of AD or increases susceptibility to it.

Interventions: Caring for the Person with Dementia

Much of dementia care takes place in the home and is provided by an aging spouse (see Chapter 17) or in a nursing home where it is provided by aides. Therefore nurses will be most effective when they assist the caregivers in whatever setting to understand the nature of dementia and the interventions likely to be most effective. Overall, interventions must match expectations with capacities, incorporate earlier life skills and interests, and provide a calm, caring, and structured environment. These

	Table 22-5	Assessment of Cognitive Function—cont'd

Domain	Definition	Assessment
Memory	In a broad sense, memory implies the ability to recall previously experienced ideas, impressions, information, and sensations. It is clinically helpful to differentiate between immediate retention (memory for the recent past) and recall (memory for the remote past). Memory is usually assessed by an individual's ability to remember and recall specific words during an interview.	Are the remembrances vague and global or filled with names, dates, and specific data? Cognitive function can often be assessed by the specificity of information.
Orientation	Orientation usually consists of an individual's knowledge of person, place, and time. Orientation is evaluated from an individual's ability to answer self-referent questions, i.e., questions with the who, what, where, and when of a situation. Does the person recognize the function of and awareness of those around him or her?	What are the events one never mentions? These may be conflict-laden areas of one's life that need exploration.
Perception	Perception generally refers to the processes involved in the acquisition and interpretation of information from one's environment. There is a relationship between quality of the sensory apparatus and cognitive functioning. Assessment is usually accomplished through observation of an individual's capacity to accurately reproduce the design drawn by the examiner, and to do this with a reasonable degree of coordination and speed.	How does one describe other people during reminiscence? Clues to interpersonal awareness and egocentricity may be gained by asking one to describe a significant other.
Problem-solving	Problem-solving comprises the set of cognitive activities required to transform one state or condition into another. Reaching a solution involves three steps: analyzing the given set or condition, determining what new condition is desired, and generating and weighing alternative strategies for getting from the given condition to the desired condition. A naturalistic example of problem-solving would be to ask grocery shoppers to determine the best buys on a particular set of products.	What is the general affectual tone of memories shared? Present situations and feelings are often mirrored in events recalled.
Psychomotor ability	Psychomotor behaviors pertain to motor effects of cerebral or psychic activity that lead to purposeful or goal-directed behaviors.	Are there recurrent themes in memories that may symbolize present needs? Themes frequently encountered include the importance of food, travel and adventure, territory, nature, family, trauma and pain, skills and talents, and traditions and rituals. One might order themes as expressions of hierarchic need.
Reaction time	Reaction time in the purest sense is the time that elapses between the application of a stimulus and the resulting reaction. Reaction time is assessed by determining response time to abstract shapes, letters, visual stimuli, and words.	Does the reminiscence resemble a record played again and again? This may indicate rigidity, a comforting ritual, poverty of thought, or a conflicted event. The attending affect will assist the nurse in correctly judging repetitious reminiscence.
Social intactness	Socialization is a process of individual integration into society and learning to behave in socially acceptable ways. Social intactness as an adult includes a narrow range of skills and attitudes that are necessary to perform social roles such as occupational skills. Social intactness is usually determined by assessing the quality and quantity of an individual's social support network and the appropriateness of one's social interactions.	Does the remembrance of an event change over time? A growing personality will continually see past events in the light of new knowledge and self-perception.

are mighty challenges to nurses and direct caregivers wherever they may be.

Determining the strengths of the dementia-afflicted older person requires staff commitment and patience. Too often the obvious deficits create an unwarranted assumption that the individual has nothing left of personality that is valuable. In an atmosphere of acceptance individuals will show their maximum potential. Staff can reinforce independence and prevent shame by helping the patient only with things he or she has tried and is unable to accomplish. This requires patience and hope and providing assistance at the minimum level necessary.

Basic Nutrition. Individuals with dementia exhibit numerous behaviors that interfere with adequate nutritional intake. The nursing challenge is to increase functional

| Table 22-6 | Piaget's Developmental Levels and Stages of Alzheimer's Disease |

Piaget developmental level	Alzheimer's stage
1. **Sensorimotor Period** (*first 2 years of life*): **Substage 1-Use of Reflexes** Automatic innate or reflex responses to external stimuli **Substage 2-Primary Circular Reactions** Effort to reproduce behavior that was first achieved by chance; development of habits **Substage 3-Secondary Circular Reactions** Beginning association of events that occur close together; dawning recognition of symbols; beginning recognition of causality; object permanence **Substage 4-Coordination of Secondary Circular Reactions** Simple problem-solving using behaviors that have already been mastered; anticipatory behavior; object permanence **Substage 5-Tertiary Circular Reactions** Rudimentary trial and error; manipulation of objects; object permanence **Substage 6-Invention of New Means through Deduction** Well developed understanding of the nature of objects; concepts of causality; use of mental symbols and words to refer to absent objects; ability to remember, plan and imitate someone else's previous actions; object permanence	**Late Dementia:** Speech and motor dysfunction; few words spoken; inability to walk; incontinence; inability to eat **Middle Dementia** (moderately severe Alzheimer's disease): Recall own name; recent memory loss; little remote memory; disturbed diurnal rhythm; generally unaware of surroundings; personal hygiene dysfunction; fear of bathing—requires assistance; difficulty putting clothes on properly; inability to handle mechanics of toileting; urinary incontinence; fecal incontinence; agitation, wandering; obsessive symptoms; loss of willpower; difficulty counting to 10
2. **Preoperational Period** (*age 2 to 7 years*): **Stage 1-Preconceptual Stage** Formation of mental images (symbolic thought); imitation of previously viewed activities; parallel play; instructions taken literally **Stage 2-Perceptual or Intuitive Stage** Prelogical reasoning experiences and objects judged by outside appearances and results; selective attention (centration)—can only concentrate upon one characteristic of an object at a time; beginning use of words, but thoughts still acted out; more social; transductive reasoning	**Early Dementia** (moderate Alzheimer's disease): Unable to recall phone number; can recall own name and names of spouse and children; no assistance required with eating or toileting difficulty choosing proper clothing; coaxing required for bathing; difficulty subtracting 3s from 20
3. **Concrete Operational Period** (*age 7 to 12 years*): Think and reason with inductive logic at beginning, deductive later; conservation and reversibility; capable of decentration (ability to focus on multiple aspects of an object, event or situation at the same time); understand the value of rules; judgment based on reason; inability to comprehend the future and the abstract.	**Early and Late Confusional** (borderline to mild Alzheimer's disease): Decreased ability to perform in demanding employment and social interactions; deficit in memory and ability to concentrate; difficulty with serial 7s
4. **Formal Operational Period** (*age 12 onward*): Logical reasoning and ability to think about hypothetical and abstract	**Normal Forgetfulness:** No impairment but subjective concern about memory loss

From Matteson MA, Linton AD, Barnes SJ: Cognitive developmental approach to dementia, *Image J Nurs Sch* 28(3):233, 1996.

behaviors during the process of eating or being fed (Van Ort and Phillips, 1992). Norberg et al (1987) described the feeding of a demented patient as an act of communication and as an art. The caregiver must develop a sensitivity to the subtle cues the patient gives and must respond in kind. These investigators compared the feeding situation to a waltz in which the patient is in the lead.

Common problems encountered in the feeding process include the following:

- Refusal to open mouth without extra stimulation such as coaxing it open with a spoon
- Closing mouth inappropriately; extrusion and disturbed tongue movements; hoarding food in mouth
- Inability to swallow

- Coughing when swallowing
- Spitting out food.

Van Ort and Phillips (1992) suggest general interventions should include: leaning toward person, addressing person by name, touching person, explaining content of each bite, offering sips of fluid between bites, holding spoon ready while verbalizing to and touching resident, hugging resident when successfully taking and swallowing bite. There are for each resident particular behaviors of the nurse that will facilitate the process. The caregiver with sensitivity to the individual's eating patterns, preferences, life history, and present symptoms, can respond more effectively to the patient's eating preferences.

Dealing with Agitation. Agitation is pervasive among individuals suffering from SDAT. They become agitated eas-

Box 22-9	**Functional Dementia Scale**				

Circle one rating for each item:
1 None or little of the time
2 Some of the time
3 Good part of the time
4 Most or all of the time

Patient _____

Observer _____

Position or relation to patient _____

Facility _____ Date _____

1	2	3	4	(01)	Has difficulty in completing simple tasks on own, e.g., dressing, bathing, doing arithmetic.
1	2	3	4	(02)	Spends time either sitting or in apparently purposeless activity.
1	2	3	4	(03)	Wanders at night or needs to be restrained to prevent wandering.
1	2	3	4	(04)	Hears things that are not there.
1	2	3	4	(05)	Requires supervision or assistance in eating.
1	2	3	4	(06)	Loses things.
1	2	3	4	(07)	Appearance is disorderly if left to own devices.
1	2	3	4	(08)	Moans.
1	2	3	4	(09)	Cannot control bowel function.
1	2	3	4	(10)	Threatens to harm others.
1	2	3	4	(11)	Cannot control bladder function.
1	2	3	4	(12)	Needs to be watched so doesn't injure self, e.g., by careless smoking, leaving the stove on, falling.
1	2	3	4	(13)	Destructive of materials around him, e.g., breaks furniture, throws food trays, tears up magazines.
1	2	3	4	(14)	Shouts or yells.
1	2	3	4	(15)	Accuses others of doing him bodily harm or stealing his possessions—when you are sure the accusations are not true.
1	2	3	4	(16)	Is unaware of limitations imposed by illness.
1	2	3	4	(17)	Becomes confused and does not know where he/she is.
1	2	3	4	(18)	Has trouble remembering.
1	2	3	4	(19)	Has sudden changes of mood, e.g., gets upset, angered, or cries easily.
1	2	3	4	(20)	If left alone, wanders aimlessly during the day or needs to be restrained to prevent wandering.

From Moore JT et al: A functional dementia scale, *J Fam Pract* 16:498, 1983.

ily and frequently, and caregivers often have great difficulty knowing the cause or how to intervene. A systematic and individualized approach is necesary because agitation is often a multidimensional problem. It is often demonstrated in aggressive behaviors, motor restlessness, aberrant vocalizations, and resistance to care (Gerdner and Buckwalter, 1994). The BARS, Brief Agitation Rating Scale, may be useful in assessing agitation (Table 22-7). Most difficult behaviors often occur at bathtime (Bergener et al, 1992).

Frequent causes of agitation are hypoxia, delirium, urinary tract infection, fatigue, or pain (Box 22-11). Small environmental changes and psychologic stress must also be considered. All of these factors should be explored. Too often the agitation is considered just another demonstration of dementia.

Agitation, which is a common problem observed in institutionalized elders, may result from idiosyncratic reactions to medications, anxiety related to an overload of adaptational stresses for which the elder does not have the psychic reserve or available supports, and disturbances in biologic

rhythmicity. The first two have been written about rather extensively, but the third, disturbance in rhythmicity, needs more study. It is quite possible that the aged individual is less integrated biorhythmically when stressed, and that providing a routine, structured environment that is clearly understood and is designed according to the individual's lifestyle patterns is essential to reduction of agitation. Norris (1986) states that restlessness that seems random is really an indication of the individual's coping efforts, and even though ineffective, it signals the potential for coping when appropriate assistance is provided.

Care must be individualized to preserve dignity. In spite of cognitive deficits and behavioral aberrations, these clients are sensitive to attitudes and seem to know instinctively whom they can trust. Body language sets an emotional climate; facial expression, eye contact, gestures, and fluidity of movement convey messages (Bartol, 1979). Moments of pleasure and joy must not be overlooked as sources of brief satisfaction, distraction, and respite from the underlying anxiety. Affection,

Box 22-10	Mini-Mental State Inpatient Consultation Form

Maximum Score	Score	Orientation
5	( )	What is the (year) (season) (date) (day) (month)?
5	( )	Where are we (state) (country) (town) (hospital) (floor)?

Registration

| 3 | ( ) | Name three objects: 1 second to say each. Then ask the patient all three after you have said them. |
| | | Give one point for each correct answer. Then repeat them until he learns all three. Count trials and record. |

Attention and Calculation Trial

| 5 | ( ) | Serial 7s. Give one point for each correct. Stop after five answers. Alternatively spell "world" backwards. |

Recall

| 3 | ( ) | Ask for three objects repeated above. Give one point for each correct. |

Language Trial

9	( )	Name a pencil and a watch (two points).
		Repeat the following: "No ifs, ands, or buts" (one point).
		Follow a three-stage command: "Take a paper in your right hand, fold it in half, and put it on the floor" (three points).
		Read and obey the following:
		"Close your eyes" (one point).
		"Write a sentence" (one point).
		"Copy design" (one point).
		Assess level of consciousness along a continuum.

Alert	Drowsy	Stupor	Coma

TOTAL ( )

From Folstein MF, Folstein S, McHugh PR: Mini-mental state: a practical method for grading the cognitive state of patients for the clinician, *J Psychiatr Res* 12:189, 1975.

Table 22-7   The Brief Agitation Rating Scale (BARS)

	None	Once in 2 weeks	2 or 3 times in 2 weeks	Once a week	2 or 3 times a week	Once a day	Several times a day
Hitting	1	2	3	4	5	6	7
Grabbing	1	2	3	4	5	6	7
Pushing	1	2	3	4	5	6	7
Pacing/aimless wandering	1	2	3	4	5	6	7
Repetitious mannerisms	1	2	3	4	5	6	7
Restlessness	1	2	3	4	5	6	7
Screaming	1	2	3	4	5	6	7
Repetitive sentences or questions	1	2	3	4	5	6	7
Strange noises	1	2	3	4	5	6	7
Complaining	1	2	3	4	5	6	7

From Finkel S, Lyons J, Anderson RL: A brief agitation rating scale (BARS) for nursing home elderly, *J Am Geriatr Soc* 41:50, 1993.

---

appreciation, and touch may provide some moments of meaning. Bergener et al (1992) found the most significant calming effect was achieved by a relaxed, smiling caregiver.

Coping with Problem Behaviors. Management of common problems such as incontinence, immobility or constant wandering, shouting, spitting, and aggressive actions becomes a heavy burden for nursing personnel (Ryden, 1988). Nursing responsibilities include the following:

1. Carefully observe and record mood, behavior, and memory. Erratic changes in the last two areas would be less indicative of AD than would a slowly progressive loss of functional abilities.

<table>
<tr><td>

Box 22-11 Antecedents of Agitation

Cognitive Impairment
Acute and chronic brain syndrome (delirium, dementia)

Psychiatric Disorders
Depression
Manic-depressive illness (bipolar disorder)
Agitated depression
Involutional depression
Schizophrenia
Paraphrenia

Internal and External Stimuli Situational Anxiety
Unresolved past stressors
Intracerebral or extracerebral stress
Sensory isolation
Invasion of personal space

Sensory Impairment
Impaired hearing
Impaired sight
Communication losses

Physical Disorders
Acute hypoxia
Pain or discomfort
Infectious processes
Parkinsonism
Fatigue
Cardiovascular disorders
Renal disorders
Neurologic disorders
Electrolyte disturbances
Endocrine disturbances

Pharmacologic Effects
Antipsychotic medications
Drug toxicity
Drug withdrawal
Psychotropic drugs

</td></tr>
</table>

From Gerdner LA, Buckwalter KC: A nursing challenge: assessment and management of agitation in Alzheimer's patients, *J Gerontol Nurs* 20(4):11, 1994.

2. Manage behaviors with the use of as few psychotropic medications as possible. They tend to increase the patient's difficulty negotiating the environment.
3. Avoid changing routines: make surroundings as predictable as possible.
4. Groom patient carefully; encourage independence in this area, but if he or she is unable, do not leave him or her untidy.
5. Provide occupational therapy geared to patient's abilities.

<table>
<tr><td>

Box 22-12 Communicating with the Cognitively Disturbed

Be patient; the individual may lack comprehension but may respond to repeated and varied attempts to communicate.

Keep routines the same and provide written reminders. Repetition is often necessary.

Introduce one idea and allow time for response. A demented person may require inordinate amounts of time to respond.

Use the active tense when speaking; e.g., "Eat this apple."

Demonstrate and give pictures of eating the apple or whatever you wish the person to do.

Additional and specific information may tap some element of comprehension. Use redundant cueing; e.g., "Bite the apple with your teeth."

Ask closed, specific questions; e.g., "Do you want to eat the apple?" If the individual does not answer, offer another alternative after waiting for a response; e.g., "Are you hungry?"

Remember: the patient is likely to become even more frustrated than you when messages are not understood. Intersperse verbal activities with periods of quiet touch or stroking.

</td></tr>
</table>

6. Work with family toward premorbid grief resolution. Support family and instruct in particular ways to interact in a helpful manner.
7. Provide patient with consistent reality orientation.
8. Avoid using physical or chemical restraints.
9. Provide a mildly stimulating environment.
10. Interact in a caring and supportive manner.
11. Make every effort toward consistency of caregivers.

Improving Communication. Bartol's pioneering studies in the nursing care of individuals with dementia (1979) alerted nurses to the extreme difficulties of communicating with a patient in the advanced stages of SDAT. Memory loss, aphasia, apraxia, agnosia, and overwhelming disorientation make verbal communication quite meaningless. Communicating with the cognitively disturbed elderly patient requires special skills. When the environment is misperceived and one feels threatened, the following signs are noted (Bartol, 1979): (1) threatening gestures, (2) increased voice volume, (3) increased restlessness, (4) agitation, (5) hostility, and (6) striking out.

The nurse's calm concern will do much to alleviate anxiety and cultivate client and family responsiveness (Box 22-12). Actions, however, will have more influence than words in such situations. This does not imply that one should not speak to the patient. The sound of communication is a humanizing factor, even though words may not be understood. Proulx (1996) has provided some guidelines for communicating with individuals who have memory problems but remain able to respond verbally (Box 22-13).

Preventing Catastrophic Reactions. Goldstein (1952) coined the term *catastrophic reaction* to describe the overreaction toward minor stresses that occurs in demented patients. It is precipitated by fatigue, overstimulation, inability to meet expectations, and misinterpretations. Interventions to avert or minimize this reaction include those proposed by Wolanin and Phillips (1981) in their classic work on confusion (Box 22-14).

Recognize that the feelings of distress may linger in a patient after he or she has forgotten the precipitant. Time spent with an uninvolved person may help. The nurse present during the reactions may instinctively respond with anger or irritation. It is important for the nurse to express her annoyance or impatience to another staff member. We believe it is futile to talk of caring, patience, and gentleness with patients without learning to handle irritating behaviors.

Even grossly disoriented persons, often seen as helpless and hopeless, may briefly respond with warmth and pleasure when stimulated. For those persons the goal is not orientation but rather human contact. Care should be directed toward fostering good general health and maintaining locomotor skills and functional preservation in all areas of behavior. Reality orientation and environmental awareness may be futile. Listening with respectful attention to any attempts to communicate is most important. This can lead to reminiscing, even though patients may not remember the names of their spouse or children. The care is based on the premise that what is left that is uniquely human should be preserved as long as possible (Hellebrandt, 1978).

Bartol's thorough nursing care perspective is a beacon to those working with the extremely cerebrally impaired. Her work was conducted in a research unit well staffed with physicians, clinical specialists, and primary care nurses. A major nursing function for those in less ideal settings will be toward obtaining qualified personnel. The quality of life provided the patient depends directly on the skill and interest of care providers. There are currently no known cures, an overabundance of descriptive data, and few medical treatments; thus the meaning of those last years lies with nursing personnel.

The management of ambulatory institutionalized patients with dementia presents many problems to the staff and the institutional milieu. Disorientation, wandering, rummaging, irritability, and combativeness are difficult for other patients and for staff. In a demonstration project at the Blumenthal Jewish Home in Clemmons, North Carolina, residents with AD were removed from the setting for 2 hours each afternoon 4 times a week into another protected environment in which a structured program of activity, music, exercise, memory recall, sensory stimulation, and nourishment were provided. This allowed the staff respite from the difficulty of managing their behaviors, and, more important, the partici-

pating residents rapidly became more manageable; had fewer episodes of rummaging, combativeness, and incontinence; and demonstrated more acceptable social behavior. For some, wandering decreased slightly, and they were able to sleep uninterrupted through the night (Sawyer and Mendlovitz, 1982).

Cohen (1996) focuses his attention on the treatment of AD in the absence of cure and prevention strategies. The growing attention to considerate pharmacologic, behavioral, and psychosocial approaches to care of both family and the individual are promising. For example, the catastrophic reaction of certain patients responds quite readily to distraction. The infectious nature of agitated behaviors often results in overreactions of caregivers as well. Slow, calm, deliberate action is much more likely to be effective.

It is becoming more common in the care of the patient with AD to design a facilitative environment, a special care unit that supports the remaining functions of the afflicted. Cohen suggests a three-pronged approach to care: (1) identify the range of the patient's problems, (2) identify the range of the patient's strengths, and (3) identify the range of individualized interventions needed to capitalize on strengths and minimize problems.

Reality Orientation. *Reality orientation* is a term much used and abused. Approximately 30 years ago a specific program of reality orientation (called RO) was begun in Tuscaloosa, Alabama, to stimulate staff members' interest and hope for the profoundly disoriented patients in their care. This program was useful because it provided caregivers with a specific program and structure that resulted in increased interaction with patients and some hopeful interventions. In the intervening years it has been found that some of the expectations were unrealistic, but the interest in communicating with the individual resident has been sustained. At present the thrust of programs is toward identifying with elements of the individual's past and helping them and staff to appreciate the connections and the feelings. It remains important to retain the following concepts that evolved out of the RO programs:

1. A calm, caring atmosphere
2. Dependable routines and structured expectations
3. Clear communication in simple words; brief and consistent instructions
4. Consistent caregivers
5. An RO board containing information about date and place consistently maintained to give residents an opportunity to remain oriented to dates, times, and important events
6. Connecting present situations with past similar experiences to accentuate strengths and capitalize on the tendency for remote memories to be more intact than retention of recent events

Box 22-15 provides guidelines for working with the confused elderly.

Morton and Bleathman (1988) question the blanket application of RO procedures to confused patients and suggest the judicial use of RO in combination with validation therapy (Feil, 1982) as more realistic and more humane. Rather than insistently reminding an apparently confused individual of time and place, it may be far more revealing and therapeutic to join the individual in his or her time and place. Validating his or her inner orientation as expressive of a particular need or feeling can restore self-esteem and give staff members a deeper understanding of the individual. Thoughtfully considering repetitious or unusual behaviors and applying the principles of validation therapy links behavior to previous life activities and may provide reassurance and increase staff understanding.

Validation Therapy. Validation therapy was developed by Naomi Feil (1982) and involves following the patient's lead and responding to the issues of importance to the patient rather than interrupting to supply factual data. Even the most bizarre misinterpretations and actions carry a message if we will listen. This does not mean that we reinforce the client's action or misinformation but only means that we respond sensitively and reorient the client only when there is legitimate reason for doing so.

Joe was dying of invasive cancer that had metastasized to his brain. He was disoriented, inattentive, and unable to make reasonable judgments about most events that were transpiring; at least, that was the way it appeared to an observer. But was Joe able to meet his needs? The need to die, the need to say goodbye to those he would not see again, and the need to inform those "on the other side" that he was on his way were of overwhelming significance to him. He spoke to people who were not visible to anyone else, he accused a family member of interrupting a Cheyenne death ceremony, and he became irate when told that no one had been there. From his viewpoint, many people had been there. A sensitive nurse need only have said, "Tell me about the ceremony."

Box 22-13

Communication Guidelines: Do's and Don'ts

1. Orient yourself to the individual. Make sure you are at eye level with the person. Look for signs of agitation or withdrawal.
2. Assume the person understands more than he or she is able to express. Watch how the person communicates and use that knowledge to converse.
3. Recognize the misperceptions and misunderstandings. Avoid complicated issues.
4. Avoid noisy and busy environments. Find out if the person has a hearing or visual disorder and compensate for it.
5. Convey messages through touch, expressions, posture, head movement, eye contact, gesture, and position relative to the person with dementia. Speech should be in a low, audible tone.
6. Be concrete and direct.
7. Use short sentences or questions. Ask questions that are yes/no or either/or answers.
8. Try again and be redundant.

From Proulx G: When someone you know has a memory problem: some of the "do's and don'ts" to help you communicate, *Baycrest Bulletin* 8(1):3, 1996, Baycrest Centre for Geriatric Care, Toronto, Canada.

Box 22-14

What to Do for Catastrophic Behavior

The patient with Alzheimer's may exhibit a sudden temporary worsening in behavior related to buildup of stress, fatigue, and/or physical discomforts. Thinking deteriorates (cognitive inaccessibility) and the patient becomes unable to communicate (social inaccessibility). The patient experiencing a catastrophic episode is generally frightened or panicked, unsafe, and exhibits strong potential for injuring himself or others.

How to prepare for it: A person's catastrophic episodes are usually the same each time. Ask the caregiver how the patient usually acts when tired or overwhelmed: Does he become fearful? Agitated? Wander? Act more confused? Become combative? Ask what the caregiver does to calm the patient.

Immediate measures: Place the patient in a quiet room, eliminating all extraneous stimuli, including people. Regard the patient as frightened. Focus your interventions on returning his sense of mastery or control over his environment.

- Assess for and eliminate all potential stressors, such as full bladder, restraints, catheters, pain.
- Provide a "time out" of at least one-half to one hour. If possible, ask the caregiver to sit quietly with the patient. (No TV or talking except quiet, gentle reassurance.)
- If the patient's combative behavior poses an immediate hazard to himself or others, provide physical or chemical restraints in the least restrictive manner possible. *However,* if the patient is not combative unless approached, simply supervise while maintaining a safe distance, using the "time out" to defuse the situation.
- Remain calm: this is a time-limited event. Talk in low, calm, reassuring tones to help the patient feel safe and secure. Do not attempt to argue with the patient's belief. ("They are not constructing that building in your yard, you are in the hospital!") Usually the patient will not believe such a comment; instead, it will heighten his anxiety.
- Chart the symptoms of the event, time of onset, duration, and successful interventions.
- Prevent further episodes by simplifying the daily schedule, increasing rest periods, evaluating environmental stressors, limiting visitors, controlling pain, and using other interventions.

From Wolanin, MO, Phillips LR: *Confusion: prevention and care,* St Louis, 1981, Mosby.

Environment Alterations. For mildly confused people, clocks and calendars and an indoor sign naming the institution would allow people to orient themselves. How often have you seen anything visible in patients' rooms that indicates the name of the hospital they are in? In mental health units it is common to have rooms that appear "homelike" and staff members in street clothes. How could you find out

---

Box 22-15	**Orientation Guidelines for Working with Confused Elderly**

1. Add as many visual cues to the setting as you can. When patient's vision is impaired, heavy reliance on consistent auditory input is essential. Check patient's hearing aids and eyeglasses for effective function.
2. Make the environment as predictable as possible by using anticipatory planning, printed schedules, and a safe, routine schedule. When changes must be made, introduce them slowly and rehearse expected performance with the individual involved.
3. Insist on a thorough physical and neurologic examination of the patient to rule out organic bases of confusion. Remember that too many intrusive or diagnostic procedures in a short time will increase confusion.
4. Assess the stresses the patient has experienced recently and within the last 2 years.
5. Either a lack of stimulation or an overload of changes can result in confusion. If sensory deprivation or lack of stimulation is the problem, add color, texture, flavor, and noncompetitive activity to the daily schedule. If an overload of new expectations and adaptations has occurred, providing environmental stability, reduced expectations, rest, and continuity of supportive personnel is essential.
6. When confusion is extensive and organically based, reduce expectations to those that can be accomplished and give consistent, immediate praise for any degree of success. This must be done by all personnel, and long-term consistent efforts are essential.
7. No matter what degree of confusion is present, individuals remain sensitive to warm affect and caring gestures. Providing a relationship that conveys the value of each human regardless of functional capacity is of the utmost importance. Achieving the patient's recovery may not be realistic, but caring in the presence of deterioration and decline is high-level nursing.
8. Finally, when working with individuals whose ability to give accurate feedback and warm gratitude is impaired, the nurse may develop a solid personal, peer-support system. Those peers who understand the disappointments and struggles are in the best position to listen to each other. Sharing feelings, anger, exasperation, and humor allows the nurse to continue in a very difficult task.

---

where you were if you awoke in such a setting? Would you believe you were in a hotel (one of the most common misperceptions of place)? We must be more careful in assessing disorientation. Perhaps environmental cues are lacking. When RO is considered necessary, there are several ways it can be facilitated.

Memory Enhancement. Cutler and Grams (1988) found that 15% of persons 55 years of age and older had experienced memory problems within the previous year. The treatment for negative self-evaluation of memory in healthy elderly persons takes two forms. The most frequent intervention is to simply tell the individual, "Don't worry, there is nothing wrong with you." This advice is rarely heeded, and the person continues to seek help or silently remains concerned. The second approach is for the older adult to attend memory training programs.

Memory training programs designed for older adults operate on two basic assumptions: (a) older adults with less than optimal performance will benefit from intense exposure to memory aids; and (b) participation in training will increase the use of these memory aids. The aim of memory training is teaching older adults to use internal memory strategies such as elaboration and rehearsal and external strategies such as using calendars, and lists to enhance remembering (Dellefield and McDougall, 1996).

A review of 39 published studies of memory training with older adults documented that the elderly may improve their memory performance on episodic memory tasks (Verhaeghen et al, 1992). The training was most effective when it was carried out in groups, sessions were relatively short (less than 90 minutes), and pretraining in imagery and relaxation techniques was provided. The review indicated that treatment gains were largest when subjects were younger. These conclusions are only valid for memory performance on classical episodic memory tasks; however, nothing can be inferred about the impact of memory training on everyday memory performance or on metamemory (memory awareness).

Clearly, more research is needed in this area, and older adults should be encouraged to continue learning. The old adage, "Use it or lose it," certainly applies to elders and their memory performance.

Support Groups. Most of the intervention strategies suggested can be applied in small groups of no more than three or four individuals. These are particularly useful with those who have mild to moderate dementia. Snyder et al (1995) report success with larger groups of mildly demented individuals and their caregivers. The groups focused on memory problems, daily tasks, relationships, health, and legal and financial concerns. Group techniques and guidelines can be found in Chapter 21. However, expectations must be geared very thoughtfully to the capacities of the group to avoid agitation and catastrophic reactions.

Caring for the Developmentally Disabled with Mental Retardation. Developmental disabilities are pathologic conditions that start developing before the age of 18, and most persist throughout life, though some can be effectively treated. Those individuals with developmental disabilities that have produced cognitive deficits have special needs. Caring for those who have been mentally impaired throughout their lives is somewhat different than caring for the elderly person who has developed dementia late in life. While the individual with DAT may not remember what happened yesterday, they have a lifetime of experiences and skills that may remain to some degree until the later stages of the disease.

The aged who have developmental disabilities have often spent the majority of their lives in institutions and may have had very limited exposure to the community outside. Moving out of a state institution into a group home and involvement in sheltered workshops have been comparatively recent phenomena. Roberts and Davis (1988) provide one of the few studies that report the particulars of success in reintegrating these individuals into community life and activities. They are first assigned an escort, or buddy, to accompany them into each new activity but are soon able to launch into some activities unescorted. They attend senior meals and senior programs in which they are involved in music, art, and other activities that stimulate interest and self-expression. Most importantly, they have the opportunity to make friends with other seniors.

These community-oriented programs provide a model for other states, and training materials have been developed (see Resources at the end of this chapter for address). We believe this model deserves replication.

More attention must be given to delineating the characteristics of this population. Those experienced in working with them believe the following:

- The profoundly retarded rarely survive to old age because they often have multiple physical incapacities. In general, retarded persons experience greater deficits in vision, hearing, and strength than other aged persons. Accurately assessing and enhancing their sensory capacities as necessary is extremely important.
- The educable (mildly) retarded may not have had the advantage of any education in youth, and their potential has been undeveloped. Most grew up in a time and place in which programs for the developmentally disabled were unavailable. Many were given no formal schooling, remaining sheltered by the family or spending a lifetime inappropriately institutionalized.

The mentally retarded in nursing homes are usually physically and mentally impaired and physically and socially dependent and have an excess of empty time. They readily adapt to the nursing home environment, possibly because their expectations are lower than those of other aged persons and because they were institutionalized before aging. Nurses may effectively use Maslow's hierarchy as a guide to needs assessment. Those patients who are congenitally cerebrally impaired may have limited hopes and expectations, but their human needs remain: comfort, protection, security, acceptance, pride, and self-expression.

Creative nurses will seek to enhance sensual pleasures; promote personal ties; and provide an orderly, predictable environment. One might think of retardation as a condition in which an individual is sensorially ill-equipped for the place and time in which he lives. For example, imagine a medieval peasant set in the middle of New York City or one transported through time and space to a place where the mode of communication is through thought transference, and intellect depends on tuning in to electromagnetic waves through antennas we do not possess. One might expect fear, anxiety, and attempts to conform or mimic what others are doing. Anger and mood swings could be expected to accompany such feelings of vulnerability.

Working with the retarded is somewhat more difficult than working with those who have had social skills and lost them. Retarded older women may wish to play with dolls. We suggest substituting a living pet. Both older men and women may never have developed a sense of modesty. They should be trained to interact in an appropriate manner to promote interpersonal acceptance. Rather than behavioral modification programs depending upon tangible rewards, we favor those that provide immediate rewards of warmth and praise for each small success. Both methods are useful.

Some innovative programs have been found that are designed for the retarded elderly. One psychologist shared her experience working with retarded adults in a program designed to tap nondominant (nonintellectual) cerebral activity (Murphy, 1979). Arts, music, and movement conducted in an atmosphere of acceptance and noncompetitiveness aroused feelings of pleasure and self-esteem in the program participants.

The increased attention being given to the developmental problems of retardation is the focus of an entire issue of the *Journal of Applied Gerontology* (The elderly person with mental retardation, 1989). Such work requires patience in the caregiver and an ability to appreciate small pleasures.

Another aspect of aging and retardation is encountered quite frequently. We have known several cases in which an elderly parent has become disabled and unable to continue the care of a retarded adult child. In those cases, the retarded adult has been placed in a long-term care institution, and the aged parent is worried and grief stricken over the inability to continue sheltering and protecting the adult child. Retarded adults living with the frail elderly, in institutions and at home, often assume a helping role if they have such skills. Some are abusive of the aged parent. The Friends of Philadelphia are particularly concerned about assisting the aged parents to deal with developmentally disabled adult children and have developed a booklet of helpful guidelines (Schwartz and Kelly, 1996).

Families of Patients with Dementia

There are special problems with caring for severely demented individuals because they are psychologically absent and physically present. Ambiguity and ambivalence exist in all aspects of their care. Some caregivers with the capacity for retrospective reverie can sustain themselves with memories of the individual: others who do not stray into the past but focus entirely on the present often find the burden intolerable.

Madeline L'Engle (1980), writer of children's books, found herself in charge of the management and care of her mother, who was in a moderately advanced stage of AD. The poignant description of her mother holding the twin babies, the brief moments of lucidity when she would apologize, and the pain of seeing the beautiful and regal woman deteriorate are all conveyed with great honesty and passion in her book. We would recommend it to those who need to remember the beauty and the meaning of the beloved elder who has vacated the premises and left only the shell without the curtains, carpets, and lights.

We can feel the pain of caring for a loved one who has AD. The help is derived from encouraging the caregiver to recite incidents from the better times. Seventy years of living leave a legacy of love. What do we say to the tree when ravaged by parasitic mistletoe? You are the bearer of a gift of love. Can we know that the gift the demented elder gives is the endurance of the aberration that terrorizes? Must we be held hostage by this dread threat of old age? Can we remember that life is more than momentary cerebral synapses? It is the total piece that has been woven, and if at the end there are ragged edges, are they fault or fringe? We know full well the strain that loved ones endure when the beloved is out of touch with reality and incapable of behaving in socially acceptable ways. Yet, when in the depths of despair, can we be reminded of the better times? For further discussion of caregivers and their needs see Chapter 17.

Caregivers and Coping. Families report that the greatest source of stress is watching the deterioration and being unable to help. The process of caregiving has been studied by numerous individuals, and these studies are discussed in Chapter 17, but some studies are particularly relevant to this section.

Lichtenberg and Barth (1989) and Lovett and Gallagher (1988) found that depression in the caregiver is influenced by the changing condition of the elder. These investigators emphasize the importance of reducing the burden on the caregivers. Belgrave, Wykle and Choi (1994) determined that black caregivers have significantly lower levels of knowledge about the caregiving situation than a comparable group of white caregivers. The distress experienced by caregivers includes their perception of burden and is evidenced by depression, anxiety, hostility and other manifestations of negative affect (Knight et al, 1993). The coping strategies used by caregivers of Alzheimer's patients have a strong influence on the mental health of the caregiver and the patient. Groups to support the providers of care for those with AD

have formed throughout the United States. Knight et al (1993) determined that psychosocial support and respite were helpful.

There is currently an increasing emphasis on the cognitive function of the caregiver. Lichtenberg et al (1992) found that caregivers not only have depression but perform below expectation on memory tasks, a common problem with depressed persons of all ages. There is a clear need to treat depression and to provide counsel, education, and other psychosocial interventions to the family caregivers of cognitively disturbed persons. Interventions with the family are enabling of their capacity for caregiving, as well as taking care of themselves (Ripich et al, 1995; Wykle, 1994) (Figure 22-4).

When families must finally be separated by institutionalization, the maintenance of some mutually shared activities can ease the pain and guilt. Group and recreational activities in which family members and elders participate are useful. Open communication with and accurate information for the family and the elder cultivate an atmosphere of trust. Encourage sharing feelings of anxiety, powerlessness, role changes, and alterations in intimacy (Rosenkoetter, 1996). Spouses in particular need special consideration when separated by dementia.

With understanding staff, shame is diminished in the community-residing spouse, and acceptance will gradually emerge. In the ideal nursing home setting the feelings, attitudes, communication, and actions of the staff are the cornerstones of the milieu that tap the wellspring of dignity in each individual, no matter how impaired.

Day Care. The use of day-care units to care for the disabled demented elderly is increasing. Day-care units provide a safe and supportive environment that can give family members respite while providing a positive emotional atmosphere for the elder. The foremost guiding principles for all activities were prevention of harm to self and others and maintaining competence in areas in which the individual is most capable (Hasselkus, 1992). These units require heavy staffing (usually a ratio of 1:3) and do not prevent the inevitable cognitive decline of the patient, but they do enhance quality of life and reduce psychosocial dysfunction. Restlessness, anxiety, and agitation that often occur in the demented patient are kept to a minimum by the calm, nonthreatening environment provided in these centers. The main goals for such programs are the following:

1. To provide respite and support of caretakers
2. To provide socialization and stimulation appropriate for the demented patient
3. To help family members keep the individual in the community as long as is appropriate
4. To assist family with placement of patient when necessary

Day-care units include such features as the following:
- Therapeutic and recreational activities
- Mental and social stimulation
- Exercise and movement therapy

- Music therapy and entertainment
- Nursing and social work consultation
- Caregivers' support group
- Nutritious hot meal
- Transportation

Respite care, foster care, and assisted living settings are other methods that families may use to relieve the pressures of caregiving. These are discussed in Chapter 13.

Legal Issues in Geriatric Psychiatry

In 1986 the American Psychiatric Association Task Force on Forensic Issues in Geriatric Psychiatry was organized to develop a guide for the evaluation of the older patient and to review the legal issues that psychiatrists would encounter in their work with geriatric patients (Baker et al, 1986). Nurses must be cognizant of these issues to ensure legal protection of self and patient.

Establishing Competence. The evaluation of a patient's cognitive capacity and judgment is at the core of most legal dilemmas that health care personnel face, whether an issue of consent, commitment, or civil or criminal law. Five general factors must be considered in the evaluation of competence:

1. Psychodynamic factors
2. Accuracy of historical information conveyed by the patient

3. Accuracy of information disclosed to patient by others
4. Stability of patient's mental status over time
5. Environmental factors

It is always important to clarify where the question of competence has originated. The family may have ulterior motives, the physician may be distressed by noncompliant behaviors, the health care system may be responding to difficulties in patient management, and the patient may be concerned about proving legal competence. All of these sources have different reasons for wishing competence to be evaluated.

Many schemes and protocols have been proposed to judge competence, but at best there may be ambiguity about the patient's cognitive capacity and judgment. Most important, the patient must be informed that when cognitive capacity is being evaluated for legal purposes, there is no confidentiality. Data gathering to establish competency will ideally include the following:

1. Thorough neuropsychiatric evaluation
2. Physical functioning
3. Mental status examination
4. Depression assessment
5. Anxiety state assessment

Cautions are needed related to source and accuracy of data. As mentioned earlier, the source of the data, accuracy

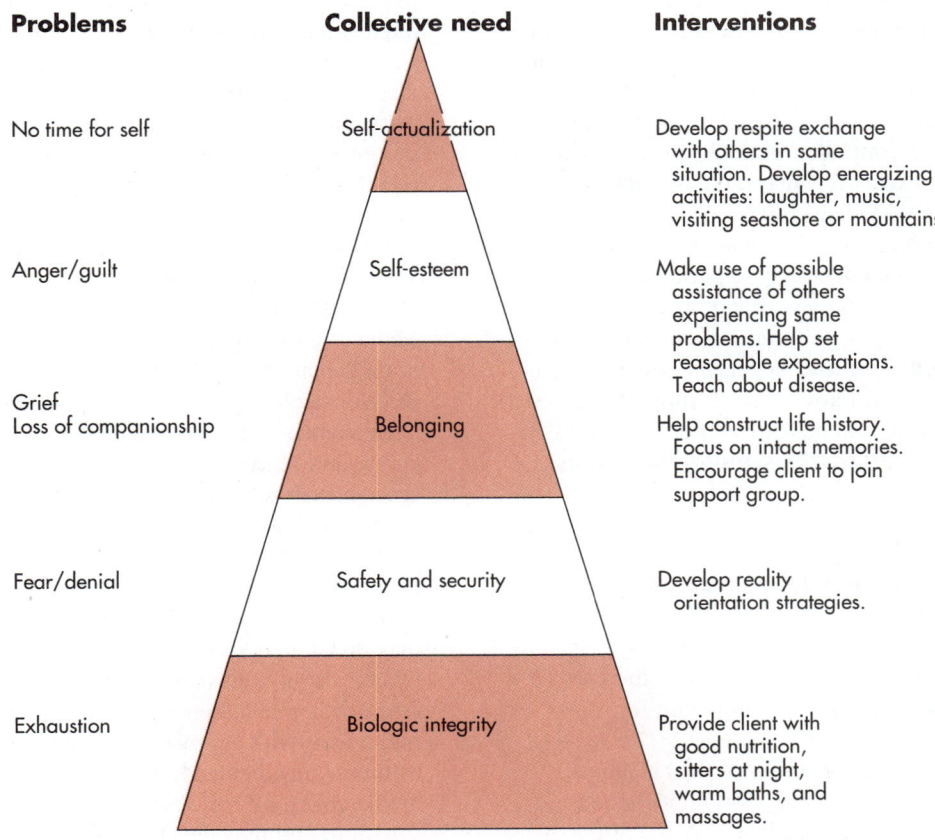

Problems	Collective need	Interventions
No time for self	Self-actualization	Develop respite exchange with others in same situation. Develop energizing activities: laughter, music, visiting seashore or mountains.
Anger/guilt	Self-esteem	Make use of possible assistance of others experiencing same problems. Help set reasonable expectations. Teach about disease.
Grief Loss of companionship	Belonging	Help construct life history. Focus on intact memories. Encourage client to join support group.
Fear/denial	Safety and security	Develop reality orientation strategies.
Exhaustion	Biologic integrity	Provide client with good nutrition, sitters at night, warm baths, and massages.

Figure 22-4. Hierarchy of needs of families caring for family members with SDAT.

of informant, observational skills of the appraiser, and the time, place, and pacing of the interview are of critical importance. The presence of depression or anxiety states has a significant influence on the quality of patient response. Criminal issues of the elderly most often involve drunken driving, shoplifting, exhibitionism, and occasionally homicide. In all these situations, competency may be called into question. Additional discussion of competence, guardianship, powers of attorney, and the legal ramifications can be found in Chapter 15.

End-of-Life Decisions and Physician-Assisted Suicide.

At present there is a move, with much controversy, to legally support assisted suicide, presently only truly legal in Australia. This has been condoned in some cases for devastating and painful illnesses when an individual felt unable to endure life any longer. Media reports have kept the public aware of the controversy over assisted suicide for individuals who are incapable of deriving sufficient meaning from continued existence.

Attention to advance directives (see Chapter 26) and quality of life is a concern for families of individuals with progressive and unremitting dementia. Usually, it has been assumed that decisions for persons suffering dementia would be made by a court-appointed conservator or family member, but this has not included any decisions regarding assisted dying. However, Sansone (1996) reported a study in which it was demonstrated that some individuals with dementia can decide appropriately regarding treatments they wish at the end of their lives. Thirty percent of demented residents at the Frances Schervier Home in the Bronx, New York, were consistent in their decisions about naming a proxy, and 27% were consistent in decisions regarding resuscitation. We may expect this may at some time extend to decisions regarding assisted suicide.

The numerous ethical and humane issues involved in planning and caring for the mentally impaired individual are not nearly fully addressed in view of individual and societal needs. We can expect ongoing discussion and concern about these devastating situations and hopefully some real solutions. The nursing role will always be to support and assist families of these victims and provide all possible means toward comfort and momentary pleasures for the victims.

KEY CONCEPTS

- Cognitive function has been the most studied topic in age-related research.
- It has long been assumed that cognitive decline is a necessary concomitant of aging, but recent studies demonstrate the potential of the aging brain for regeneration.
- The distinctive cognitive capacities of the aged have hardly been investigated and are poorly understood.
- Age-associated memory impairment (AAMI) refers to the common forgetfulness that many elders experience.

This is usually attributed to distraction, preoccupation, or performance anxiety. It is poorly understood but must be met with reassurance that this is not an evidence of impending dementia.

- Cognitive impairment that is significant is a disease process and must be regarded as such. Some of the dementias are treatable, and some are not. Nurses need to advocate for thorough assessment of any elder who appears to be experiencing genuine cognitive decline and inability to function in important aspects of life.
- Delirium, sometimes referred to as acute confusional states, is the result of physiologic imbalances and may be caused by a variety of biologic disturbances. Delirium is characterized by fluctuating levels of consciousness, sometimes in a diurnal pattern, and frequent misperceptions and illusions.
- Medications are frequently the cause of delirious states in the aged.
- Irreversible dementias follow a pattern of inevitable decline accompanied by decreased intellectual function, personality changes, and impaired judgment. The most common of these is Alzheimer's disease.
- Alzheimer's disease has been the subject of enormous amounts of research in attempts to understand the causes. Genes, latent viruses, enzyme and neurotransmitter deficiencies, environmental toxins, and psychosocial stressors have all been implicated to some degree. Research is continuing in attempts to discover ways to protect against or halt the progress of the disease. At this time there is no known cure, though some medications being developed seem to slow the progress of the dementia for a time.
- HIV-realated dementia is often overlooked in the aged; there is an ageist assumption implicit in this neglect.
- Vascular brain disorders (brain attacks) are caused by interruption of the blood supply to the brain because of clots, hemorrhages, and vascular spasm or occlusion. Many of these situations can be remedied and serious brain damage prevented if treatment is immediate.
- Developmentally disabled elders are a rather new phenomenon because these individuals usually died long before they reached old age. Those who have survived have special needs related to the levels of development they may or may not have achieved. These individuals should not be treated as if demented but given opportunities carefully matched to the level of their abilities.
- Assessment of cognitive impairment is complex. Nurses may do a cursory assessment with any number of brief mental status exams and need to request more thorough assessment when there is an indication of dementia.
- Individuals who are mentally impaired respond best to calmness, few demands, clear communication, and predictable routines. They are hypersensitive to chaotic situations and may develop catastrophic reactions when demands exceed their ability.

Nursing Diagnoses

The following potential diagnoses must be considered as well as diagnoses unique to the particular individual:

Adjustment, impaired
Anxiety
Communication, impaired
Coping, ineffective
Denial, ineffective
Diversional activity deficit
Fear
Grieving, dysfunctional
Growth and development, altered
Knowledge deficit

Noncompliance
Personal identity disturbance
Post-trauma response
Powerlessness
Self-esteem, chronic low
Sensory/perceptual alteration
Sleep pattern disturbance
Thought processes, altered
Trauma, risk for
Violence, risk for: directed at others

NURSING PROCESS AND NURSING DIAGNOSIS
Altered Thought Process: Delirium

Etiologies and Related Factors

Chemical
Depression (emotional illness)
Metabolic/endocrine
Environmental (sensory-vision/hearing)
Nutritional
Physiologic (serious underlying illness)
Psychopathology

Signs and symptoms of delirium
Assessment of client/family
Physical and mental status testing MSQ; OARS or
   similar test; ADLs; neurologic tests
Diagnostic tests
Therapeutic interventions
Legal rights of client
Community resources

Defining Characteristics

Perceptual disturbance:
   Misinterpretation
   Illusions
   Hallucinations
Occasional incoherent speech
Shortened attention span
Disturbance of sleep/wake patterns
Altered psychomotor activity
Agitation
Anger
Restlessness
Hyperexcitability
Disorientation
Dazed frightened expression
Fear of self or others

Clinical Judgment and Related Skills

Obtain a client history or history through
   family/caregiver; including analysis of a symptom
Assess mental status and physical abilities with
   standardized tools
Perform a physical assessment with focus on the
   neurologic system and other systems as appropriate
Implement nursing interventions for environmental
   safety
Reality orientation with audio and visual cues and/or
   immediate environment
Allow sufficient time for information processing
Provide sufficient time for client to complete tasks and
   ADLs
Teach family/caregiver about delirium
Make appropriate referrals

Knowledge

Causational factors
Differentiation of delirium, dementia, depression

Evaluation

Underlying cause of delirium resolved
Client returns to previous physical and mental state

NEEDS ADDRESSED AND TASK STRENGTHS

Need for pride and feelings of self-worth; need for
   intellectual stimulation (to maintain self-esteem and
   self-concept)
Recognizes own personality idiosyncracies

Accepts personality foibles in others
Consciously exercises memory
Incorporates memory cues in life patterns as needed

▲ CASE STUDY

John was 67 years old and had been a successful contractor until his retirement from business 4 years ago. His wife, Janet, of 30 years was a primary school teacher. Their marriage had been minimally gratifying, but both enjoyed their work and had felt they led a full and satisfying life. They had no children but had developed a large social network over the years, most were friends that were in some way work related. Six months ago John began to seem restless, he was easily angered and embarrassed himself and his wife several times by being verbally abusive during a social function with their friends. John was also less careful about his grooming; because he had always been most meticulous about his appearance, his wife was quite alarmed that he seemed not to notice or care. After returning from one particularly exhausting vacation trip, John became enraged when he thought someone had stolen his wallet. He ignored his wife's efforts to calm him and seemingly became angrier. Later his wife found his wallet in an inner suit jacket pocket. He ordinarily kept his wallet in the back pocket of his trousers. His wife began to feel anxious and frightened of him, though he had never physically abused her. She urged him to see the doctor for a "general checkup" but was not surprised that he refused. She went to the doctor for tranquilizers to quell her anxiety. He gave her a prescription for Prozac and sent her on her way. Her nurse-neighbor dropped by one day and found her in tears saying, "I just can't stand it anymore. John is not like himself. We used to have such fun and now he is angry all the time." As the nurse-neighbor how would you help Janet and John?

Based upon the case study, develop a nursing care plan using the following procedure*:

List comments of client that provide *subjective data*.

List information that provides *objective data*.

From these data identify and state, using accepted format, two *nursing diagnoses* you determine are most significant to this client at this time.

Determine and state *outcome criteria* for each diagnosis. These must reflect some alleviation of the problem identified in the nursing diagnosis and must be stated in concrete and measurable terms.

Plan and state one or more *interventions* for each diagnosed problem. Provide specific documentation of source used to determine appropriate intervention.

Evaluate success of intervention. Interventions must correlate directly with the stated outcome criteria in order to measure the outcome success.

---

*Students are advised to refer to their nursing diagnosis text and identify possible or potential problems.

STUDY QUESTIONS/ACTIVITIES

Discuss ways in which you might help an individual who is complaining of memory loss.

Is there any evidence that cerebral cells may regenerate?

What are some of the differences between delirium and dementia?

Discuss some reasons you might suspect an elder with dementia to have HIV dementia.

Identify several signs of early dementia.

How can Alzheimer's disease be diagnosed accurately?

Develop a nursing care plan for dealing with an individual with agitated dementia.

How could you communicate best with an individual who is perseverating?

What is the essense of validation therapy?

What memory aids might you suggest for a person who was forgetful?

What is the most difficult thing for a family dealing with a demented elder? Why do you think this is so?

Discuss elders you have known who are between 85 and 90 years old and evidences of their intact cognition or signs of dementia.

RESEARCH QUESTIONS

What is the prevalence of dementia in community-dwelling older adults?

What methods of memory enhancement are most effective in the long term?

RESOURCES

Films and Videos

Blazo A: *Symptoms of Senility: Recognition and Management,* Sandoz Pharmaceuticals, East Hanover, NJ 07936.

Camochan D: *Memaw,* David Camochan, 4571 River Road, Scottsville, NY 14546. This film is about an 88-year-old woman who has AD and presents the problems that children must cope with when dealing with aging parents with AD.

Communication Strategies for Alzheimer's Patients. Presents methods of maintaining patient dignity and self-respect while communicating effectively. Utilizes actual scenes with patients, family, and staff. Available from Geriatric Video Productions, PO Box 1757, Shavertown, PA 18708-0757, (800) 621-9181.

The Glass Curtain: A Poem in Prose, D. Chase, producer, Doris Chase, 222 West 23rd Street, No 722, New York, NY 10011. A personal film that tells the story of a daughter who must deal with her mother, a patient with AD.

Dementia in Middle and Later Years, Medical Films Library, Sandoz Pharmaceuticals, East Hanover, NJ 07936. Dementia in middle and later years is actually four short films under one title. Each film has a short commentary, followed by actual case histories of patients with Alzheimer's disease.

Managing with Alzheimer's Disease, West Associates, No 287, Kingsway Garden Mall, PO Box 11028, Edmonton, Alberta, T5/3K3. A lively and rewarding program that focuses on solutions to the problems encountered by anyone caring for a person with this neurologically degenerative disease. This program includes valuable information on when and how to choose a nursing facility; 30 minutes.

Problem Behaviors in Geriatrics: Agitation and Restlessness. Discusses triggers and preventive strategies to eliminate the behaviors without the use of physical and chemical restraints. Available from Geriatric Video Productions, PO Box 1757, Shavertown, PA 18708-0757, (800) 621-9181.

Problem Behaviors in Geriatrics: Wandering. Discusses types of wandering and nonrestrictive management techniques. Available from Geriatric Video Productions, PO Box 1757, Shavertown, PA 18708-0757, (800) 621-9181.

The Silent Epidemic: Alzheimer's Disease, Filmmakers Library, Inc, 138 East 58th Street, No 703A, New York, NY 10022. The film presents two case studies of patients with AD and comments by their spouses, nursing home administrator, and a social worker.

Someone I Once Knew, J Walter Thompson Producers, 160 Lexington Avenue, New York, NY 10020.

Working with the Confused Elderly, Dr. Joyce Colling, Oregon Health Sciences University, Nursing School, 3181 SW Sam Jackson Park Road, Portland, OR 97201. A 29-minute video that presents verbal and nonverbal techniques that increase skills in coping with problem behaviors associated with chronic confusion in the elderly. The work presents some revolutionary methods to deal with problems such as wandering, paranoia, and disorientation.

A three-part series that addresses the design, operation, and successes of the small unit for Alzheimer's patients that was housed within a larger long-term-care facility, Terra Nova Films, 9849 S Winchester Avenue, Chicago, IL 60643. Each of these works comes with an excellent user's manual.

1. *Wesley Hall: A Special Life* is a 28-minute overview of a pilot project aimed at creating an environment in which institutionalized victims of AD thrive, live with dignity, minimize functional loss, and maximize functional ability.
2. *Designing the Physical Environment for Persons with Dementia* addresses the design issues that demand consideration if one is contemplating opening an Alzheimer's unit or (re)designing an existing or newly committed Alzheimer's unit.
3. *Helping People with Dementia in Activities of Daily Living* is a 22-minute video describing methods that foster independent functioning in the confused elderly. It focuses on the technique of task-breakdown and contrasting approaches to persons exhibiting varying degrees of confusion.

A series of excellent videos are available from Video Press, University of Maryland at Baltimore, School of Med-

icine, Suite 133, 100 Penn Street, Baltimore, MD 21201, (800) 328-7450 or (410) 328-5497 or (410) 328-8471. The following are a few of their productions:

Managing the Resident with Dementia: Specific Nursing Strategies. This program presents case studies that illustrate the potentially difficult behaviors associated with dementing illnesses or other conditions. At the conclusion of each case vignette, a positive management strategy is provided. Taped in a nursing home setting, this program presents the viewer with a realistic picture of both the problems and solutions of behavioral management. This program provides an excellent staff development training tool for paraprofessionals and professional staff in all health care disciplines; 19 minutes, (purchase, $300; rental, $100).

Behaviors Associated with Dementia: Case Presentations. This program, shot on location in a nursing home, documents the daily experiences of residents who exhibit difficult behaviors associated with dementia and other conditions. Behaviors include disorientation, confusion, delusions, withdrawal, depression, agitation, hostility, and aggression. There is no explanatory narration with this program. It may be used for training or staff development in all health professions or social work.

The actual patient presentations provide the viewer with a reality-based experience of situations that may escalate if staff is not trained in appropriate interventions and patient interaction skills. The video provides an excellent stimulus for discussion in staff development training seminars addressing positive management of difficult behaviors; 28 minutes, (purchase, $300; rental, $100).

Nursing Care for Elderly Dementia Patients. National experts present a discussion of the cognitive and behavioral manifestations of dementia syndromes. Emphasis is on the utilization of the nursing process to develop, implement, and evaluate a comprehensive patient care plan. Special considerations include combativeness, agitation, wandering, pacing, crying, and sleeplessness. A very important program for nursing home and hospital staff; 33 minutes, (purchase, $300, rental; $100).

Medication and Dementia. Dr. Peter P. Lamy, author of *Prescribing for the Elderly,* clearly describes the role and the important responsibilities of all health professionals working with medicated elderly patients having symptoms of dementia. Nurses, nursing assistants, and family caregivers must be active observers and reporters of information.

Although drugs cannot prevent or cure Alzheimer's disease, there are drugs that can help patients live with dementia. These medications are frequently prescribed. The physician must be informed of the side effects in order to regulate medications appropriately. Physicians need accurate observations from nursing staff and family members. Appropriate use of medication can improve quality of life only if the health care provider observes and reports patient response to medication. Interview, 22 minutes, (purchase, $300; rental, $100).

Assessing the Mental Status of the Older Person. Why is it important to do a mental status assessment on all elderly patients? In introductory remarks, Dr. Rabins explains the many reasons why assessing the mental status of elderly patients is essential. Then through structured patient interviews he demonstrates the use of the Mini-Mental State Examination, a tool that can be used by nurses, physicians or social workers.

Dr. Rabins emphasizes that geriatric patient assessment should include an objective assessment of cognitive function. This assessment can identify problem areas and provide information that can show improvement or decline. This video program provides the unique opportunity to observe Dr. Rabins interacting with normal elders and with dementia patients. Patients interviewed range from normal to severely impaired. Behaviors documented include confusion, loss of memory, hallucination, loss of cognitive skills, and depression.

This program provides a useful guide on how to do a mental status exam. Print materials accompany the videotape, listing the mental status examination questions, describing scoring, and discussing scoring ramifications. This tape is appropriate for staff development in hospitals and long-term care and professional training programs in all health-related fields and social work. Interviews, 34 minutes, (purchase, $300; rental, $100).

Organizations

Alzheimer's Disease and Related Disorders Association. Nation's leading organization dedicated to finding a cure and pursuing public policy that addresses the physical and financial burdens faced by Alzheimer's families. Has chapters around the country. Regularly helps organize conferences. 919 N Michigan Avenue, Suite 1000, Chicago, Ill 60611.

National Associatin of Developmental Disabilities Council, 1234 Massachusetts Avenue, NW, Suite 103, Washington, DC 20005.

Institute for Health & Aging, University of California, San Francisco, Room N53 1, San Francisco, CA 94143-0646; (415) 476-5902. Currently involved in a number of research studies involving public policy, AIDS, and Alzheimer's.

National Institute on Aging, Federal Building, Room 6C12, Bethesda, MD 20892; (301) 496-1752.

Respite Programs for Caregivers of Alzheimer's Disease Patients. A national hot line available through the Brookdale Center for Aging of Hunter College. The service is designed to give technical assistance to individual people or groups across the country who are trying to organize a community respite program. Call (800) 648-COPE.

Publications

Alzheimer's Disease: A Guide to Federal Programs. Published by Alzheimer's Disease Education & Referral Center, PO Box 8250, Silver Spring, Md 20907-8250, (800) 438-4380, NIH Publication No. 93:3635.

Office of Technology Assessment: *Losing A Million Minds: Confronting the Tragedy of Alzheimer's Disease and Other Dementias* (OTA Publication No. OTA-BA-324), Washington, DC, 1987, U.S. Government Printing Office.

Brief Symptom Inventory (BSI) (Derogatis and Spencer, 1983). The BSI is a 53-item scale designed to measure nine dimensions of psychopathology and takes approximately 20 minutes to administer. Its primary use is as a research instrument; however, clinicians may also find it a useful screening device for identifying potential problem areas for further assessment. All of the items have been described as appropriate for elderly populations, and norms are available for adults over the age of 65 (Hale et al, 1984). The validity and reliability of the BSI are good, and its use is likely to increase in both clinical and research efforts.

Mental Status Questionnaires

Mental Status Questionnaire (MSQ) (Kahn et al, 1960). This 10-item MSQ is one of the shortest and most widely used instruments of its kind. Its validity as a rough screening measure is generally equivalent to most other MSQs (Lesher and Whelihan, 1986), yielding, like the others, unacceptably high false-negative rates. Internal consistency, test-retest, and split-half reliability for the Kahn MSQ are all adequate. Use of this MSQ should be limited to the identification of moderate to severe cognitive impairment (Ferris et al, 1984) and should be followed with a detailed assessment.

Mini-Mental State (Folstein et al, 1975). As an extended version of a Kahn-like MSQ, MMS measures only orientation and cognitive function. It has a maximum score of 30, with cut-off scores designed to identify four levels of impairment. It can be administered in 10 minutes or less and has been moderately successful in discriminating among demented, depressed, and healthy elderly persons. However, it cannot be used to discriminate among the different fog-faun of dementia, and persons with low intellectual, educational, or motivational levels may score in the impaired range (Fine et al, 1986). If a mental status questionnaire is to be used as part of a clinical screening procedure, the MMS will likely be the most reliable and valid measure. It too may yield false-positives or false-negatives with regard to the identification of a dementing illness. However, if its use is limited to the evaluation of current functional performance and if it is accompanied by a careful evaluation of more detailed cognitive abilities before a diagnosis, the MMS can be a useful component of a comprehensive screening evaluation.

Short Portable MSQ (Pfeiffer, 1975). The FINN is a part of the OARS battery but has been validated and normed as a separate instrument. It consists of nine orientation and re-mote memory items, along with an item that requires the se-rial subtraction from 20 by threes. It is somewhat more chal-lenging than the Kahn MSQ, and its norms have been adjusted for race and education (Kane and Kane, 1981).

Behavioral Rating Scales for Dementia

Brief Cognitive Rating Scale (BCRS) (Reisberg, 1983): The BCRS was designed to provide a brief, structured assess-ment of cognitive decline for use in clinical work with aged patients. It has five major axes: concentration, recent mem-ory, remote memory, orientation, and daily functioning. The older person is rated for severity of impairment on a scale of 1 to 7 on each axis. The ratings are derived from information obtained during a structured interview with the client and a family member or caregiver. Concurrent validity and coeffi-cients with the Guild Memory Test have been high, but other validity measures are lacking, and there are, as yet, no re-ports of test-retest or interrater reliability for the BCRS. It can, however, be a useful guide to obtaining, organizing, and quantifying data gathered in clinical interviews and should prove helpful in the functional assessment and differential diagnosis of SDAT.

Dementia Rating Scale (DRS) (Mattis, 1976). The DRS consists of five subscales with items arranged in order of dif-ficulty. It is relatively easy to administer and has the advan-tage of incorporating items that can elicit useful information from moderately to severely impaired persons. Adequate content and concurrent validity coefficients have been re-ported (Poon, 1986), but further data are needed on these and other measures of validity and reliability. The DRS will probably prove most useful in assessing the functional ca-pacity of individuals for whom the diagnosis of dementia has already been established, and the clinician may also find it helpful in assessing behavioral change over time.

Global Deterioration Scale (Reisberg, 1983). The GDS is similar to the BCRS in that it organizes and quantifies data gathered in clinical interviews. It provides seven clinical phases of cognitive decline, which also carry labels for the authors' characterizations of the stages of primary degener-ative dementia. Its usefulness lies primarily in describing the global functional deterioration seen in dementia, and the GDS is unlikely to be useful in assessment or differential di-agnostic efforts. From Riley K: *Interdisciplinary geriatric assessment: a psychological perspective,* 1987, Cleveland Western Reserve Geriatric Education Center.

REFERENCES

Aarsland D, Tandberg E, Larsen JP, Cummings JL: Frequency of dementia in Parkinson's disease, *Arch Neurol* 53(6):538, 1996.

Abrams WB, Beers MH, Berkow R, editors: *Merck manual of geri-atrics,* ed 2, Whitehouse Station, NJ, 1995, Merck Research Laboratories.

Albert MS, Jones K, Savage CR et al: Predictors of cognitive change in older persons: MacArthur studies of successful aging, *Psychol Aging* 10(4):578, 1995.

Allen CK, Allen RE: Cognitive disabilities: measuring the social consequences of mental disorders, *J Clin Psychol* 48(5):185, 1987.

American Psychiatric Association: *Diagnostic and statistical man-ual of mental disorders,* ed 3 (revised), Washington, DC, 1987, The Association.

American Psychiatric Association: *Diagnostic and statistical man-ual of mental disorders, fourth edition,* Washington, DC, 1994, The Association.

Arie THD: Acute confusional states. In Abrams WB, Beers MH, Berkow R, editors: *Merck manual of geriatrics,* ed 2, White-house Station, NJ, 1995, Merck Research Laboratories.

Baker F, Perr I, Yesavage J: *An overview of legal issues in geriatric psychiatry,* Washington, DC, 1986, American Psychiatric Asso-ciation.

Baltes P: The aging mind: potential and limits, *Gerontologist* 33(5):580, 1993.

Bartol M: Dialogue with dementia: nonverbal communication in patients with Alzheimer's disease, *J Gerontol Nurs* 5:21, 1979.

Basu JL, Diamond MC: Challenging the myths of aging, *San Fran-cisco Focus* 30:43, 1983.

Beffer U, Poirier J: Apolipoprotein E, plaques, tangles and cholin-ergic dysfunction in Alzheimer's disease, *Ann N Y Acad Sci* 777:166, 1996.

Belgrave L, Wykle M, Choi J: Health, double jeopardy and culture: the use of institutionalization by African-Americans, *Gerontol-ogist* 33(3):379, 1993.

Bergener SC, Jirovec M, Murrell L, Barton D: Caregiver and envi-ronmental variables related to difficult behaviors in institution-alized, demented elderly persons, *J Gerontol* 47(4):P242, 1992.

Berkow R, Butler RN, Sunderland J: Cognitive failure: delirium and dementia. In Abrams WB, Beers MH, Berkow R, editors: *Merck manual of geriatrics,* ed 2, Whitehouse Station, NJ, 1995, Merck Research Laboratories.

Berry W: *Memory of Old Jack,* New York, 1974, Harcourt Brace Jovanovich.

Buffum M, Buffum J: Medication usage in the elderly, *Geriatr Nurs* 17(3), 1997.

Byrd M: The effects of previously acquired knowledge on memory for textual information, *Int J Aging Hum Dev* 24(3):231, 1986-1987.

Callahan CM, Hendrie HC, Tierney WM: Documentation and eval-uation of cognitive impairment in elderly primary care patients, *Ann Intern Med* 122(6):422, 1995.

Caplan LR: Cerebrovascular disease. In Abrams WB, Beers MH, Berkow R, editors: *Merck manual of geriatrics,* ed 2, White-house Station, NJ, 1995, Merck Research Laboratories.

Christensen D: Hardening of the arteries linked to Alzheimer's dis-ease, *Medical Tribune News Service,* Jan 16, 1997.

Cohen G: Treatment of Alzheimer's disease in the absence of cure and prevention, *High Notes Newsletter,* Spring 1996.

Cohen-Mansfield J: Agitated behaviors in the elderly. I. A concep-tual review, *J Am Geriatr Soc* 34(10):711, 1986a.

Cohen-Mansfield J: Agitated behaviors in the elderly. II. Prelimi-nary results in the cognitively deteriorated, *J Am Geriatr Soc* 34(10):722, 1986b.

Cotman CW: Synaptic plasticity, neurotrophic factors, and transplantation in the aged brain. In Schneider EL, Rowe JW, editors: *Handbook of the biology of aging,* San Diego, 1990, Academic Press.

Crowley SL: Aging brain's staying power, *AARP Bulletin* 37(4):1, 1996.

Cutler SJ, Grams AE: Correlates of self-reported everyday memory problems, *J Gerontol* 43(3):S82, 1988.

Dellefield KS, McDougall GJ: Increasing metamemory in community elderly, *Nurs Res* 45(5):284, 1996.

Devanand DP, Sano M, Tang MX, et al: Depressed mood and the incidence of Alzheimer's disease in the elderly living in the community, *Arch Gen Psychiatry* 53(2):175, 1996.

Diehl M, Willis SL, Schaie KW: Everyday problem solving in older adults: observational assessment and cognitive correlates, *Psychol Aging* 20(3):478-491, 1995.

DSM III-R (See American Psychiatric Association: *Diagnostic and statistical manual of mental disorders,* ed 3 [revised].)

DSM IV (See American Psychiatric Association: *Diagnostic and statistical manual of mental disorders,* ed 4.)

The elderly person with mental retardation (topical issue), *J App Gerontol* 8(2), June 1989.

Erikson E: *Life history and the historical moment,* New York, 1975, WW Norton.

Evans LK: Sundown syndrome in institutionalized elderly, *J Am Geriatr Soc* 35(2):101, 1987.

Feltes M: Human immunodeficiency virus infection. In Abrams WB, Beers MH, Berkow R, editors: *Merck manual of geriatrics,* ed 2, Whitehouse Station, NJ, 1995, Merck Research Laboratories.

Fenn H, Luby V, Yesavage JA: Subtypes in Alzheimer's disease and the impact of excess disability: recent findings, *Int J Geriatr Psychol* 8(1):67, 1993.

Fielo S, Rizzolo M: Handle with caring: meeting elderly client's special method for grading the cognitive state of patients for the clinician, *J Psychiat Res* 12:189, 1979.

Finkel S, Lyons J, Anderson RL: A brief agitation rating scale (BARS) for nursing home elderly, *J Am Geriatr Soc* 41:50, 1993.

Folstein MF, Folstein S, McHugh PR: *Mini-mental state: a practical method for grading the cognitive status of patients for the clinician,* 1975, Pergamon.

Foreman MD: Acute confusion in the elderly, *Ann Rev Nurs Res* 11:3, 1993.

Foreman MD, Fletcher K, Mion LC et al: Assessing cognitive function, *Geriatr Nurs* 17(5):228, 1996.

Francis J: Delerium in older patients, *J Am Geriatr Soc* 40:829, 1992.

Fried L, Kasper J, Guralnik J, Simonsick E: The women's health and aging study: an introduction. In Guralnik J, Fried L, Simonsick E, Kasper J, Lafferty M, editors: *The women's health and aging study: health and social characteristics of older women with disabilities,* Bethesda, 1995, National Institute on Aging, Pub No 96-4009.

Gerdner LA, Buckwalter KC: A nursing challenge: assessment and management of agitation in Alzheimer's patients, *J Gerontol Nurs* 20(4):11, 1994.

Giambra LM, Arenberg D, Zonderman AB, Kawas C, Costa P: Adult life span changes in immediate visual memory and verbal intelligence, *Psychol Aging* 10(1):123, 1995.

Gold DP, Andres D, Etezadi J, Arbuckle T, Schwartzman A, Chaikelson J: Structural equation model of intellectual change and continuity and predictors of intelligence in older men, *Psychol Aging* 10(2):294, 1995.

Goldstein K: The effect of brain damage on the personality, *Psychiatry* 15:245, 1952.

Hale S, Myerson J, Wagstaff D: General slowing of nonverbal information processing: evidence for a power law, *J Gerontol* 42(2):131, 1987.

Hasselkus BR: The meaning of activity: day care for persons with Alzheimer's disease, *Am J Occup Ther* 46(3):199, 1992.

Havarth TA, Patsdaughter CA, Bumbalo JA, McCann MK: Dementia-related behaviors in Alzheimer's disease and AIDS, *J Psychosoc Nurs/Ment Health Serv* 33(1):35, 1995.

Hazzard W, Bierman E, Blass J, Ettinger W, Halter J, editors: *Principles of geriatric medicine and gerontology,* ed 3, New York, 1994, McGraw Hill.

Hellebrandt F: Comment: the senile dement in our midst—a look at the other side of the coin, *Gerontologist* 18:67, 1978.

Inouye SK: Delirium in hospitalized elderly patients: recognition, evaluation and management, *Conn Med* 57(5):309, 1995.

Jung R, Solomon K: Psychiatric manifestations of Pick's disease, *Int Psychogeriatri* 5(2):187, 1993.

Kane RA, Kane RR: *Assessing the elderly: a practical guide to measurement,* Lexington, Mass, 1981, Lexington.

Kaszniak AW: Parkinson's disease. In Maddox GL, editor: *The encyclopedia of aging,* ed 2, New York, 1995, Springer.

Kelly M: Transcient ischemic attack, *Am J Nurs* 95(9):42, 1995.

Knight BG, Lutzky SM, Macofsky F: A meta-analytic review of interventions for caregiver distress: recommendations for future research, *Gerontologist* 33(2):242–248, 1993.

Kokmen E, Beard CM, O'Brien PC, Kurland LT: Epidemiology of dementia in Rochester, Minnesota, *Mayo Clin Proc* 71(3):275, 1996.

Kreiger LM: Drugs cushion brain from stroke, *San Francisco Examiner,* p A-12, Aug 14, 1995.

Kretzschmar HA, Ironside JW, DeArmond SJ, Tateishi J: Diagnostic criteria for sporadic Creutzfeldt-Jakob disease, *Arch Neurol* 53(9):913, 1996.

La Voie A: Cold-sore virus linked to Alzheimer's disease, *Medical Tribune News Service,* Jan 23, 1997.

L'Engle M: *The summer of the great-grandmother,* San Francisco, 1980, Harper and Row.

Levin BE, Katzen HL: *Arch Neurol* 65:85, 1995.

Lichtenberg PA, Barth JT: The dynamic process of caregiving of elderly spouses: a look at longtitudinal case reports, *Clin Gerontol* 9(1):31, 1989.

Lichtenberg PA, Manning CA, Turkheimer E: Memory dysfunction in depressed spousal caregivers, *Clin Gerontol* 12(1):77, 1992.

Linsk NL, Cich PT, Cianfrani L: The AIDS epidemic: challenges for nursing homes, *J Gerontol Nurs* 19(1):11, 1993.

Lipowski Z: A comprehensive view of delirium in the elderly, *Geriatr Consult* 7:26, 1986.

Lovett S, Gallagher D: Psychoeducational interventions for family caregivers, *Behavior Ther* 19:321, 1988.

Maisto AA, Hughes E: Adaptation to group home living for adults with mental retardation as a function of previous residential placement, *J Intellect Disabil Res* 39(1):15, 1995.

Marcantonio ER, Goldman L, Mangione CM, et al: A clinical prediction rule for delirium after elective noncardiac surgery, *JAMA* 27:134, 1994.

Matteson MA, Linton AD, Barnes SJ: Cognitive developmental approach to dementia, *Image J Nurs Sch* 28(3):233, 1996.

McDougall GJ: A review of screening instruments for assessing cognition and mental status in older adults, *Nurse Pract* 15:11, 1990.

McDougall GJ: A critical review of research on cognitive function/impairment in older adults, *Arch Psychiatr Nurs* 9(1):22-33, 1995a.

McDougall GJ: What role philosophy in psychotherapy? *Perspectives Psychiatr Care* 28(2),3, 1992.

McDougall GJ: Existential psychotherapy with older adults, *J Am Psychiatr Nurs* 1(1):16, 1995b.

McDougall GJ: Predictors of memory improvement strategy use in older adults, *Rehab Nursing* 21(4):202–209, 1996.

McKnight C, Rockwood K: Bovine spongiform encephalopathy and Creutzfeldt-Jakob disease: implications for physicians, *Can Med Assoc J* 155(5):529, 1996.

Miller NE, Cohen GD: *Schizophrenia and aging,* New York, 1987, Guilford Press.

Mooney RP, Mooney DR, Cohernour KL: Applied humanism: a model for managing inappropriate behavior among mentally retarded elders, *J Gerontol Nurs* 21(8):45, 1995.

Moore JT et al: A functional dementia scale, *J Fam Pract* 16:499, 1983.

Morton I, Bleathman C: Does it matter whether it's Tuesday or Friday, *Nurs Times* 84:25, 1988.

Murphy M: Personal communication, 1979, Living Arts Center, Oakland, Calif.

National Institute on Aging: *Alzheimer's disease,* Pub No 85-1646, Bethesda, Md, 1985, The Institute.

Navia B, Price R: The AIDS dementia complex as the presenting or sole manifestation of HIV infection, *Arch Neurol* 44:65, 1987.

Neely AS, Backman L: Long term maintenance gains from memory training in older adults: two 3 1/2 year follow-up studies, *J Gerontol* 48(5):P233, 1993.

Norberg A, Alhlin E, Asplund K: Feeding problems in severely demented patients (abstract). *Proceedings of the Third Congress of the International Psychogeriatric Association* 3:64, Chicago, 1987.

Norris C: Restlessness: a disturbance in rhythmicity, *Geriatr Nurs* 7(6):302, 1986.

Office of Technology Assessment: *Losing a million minds: confronting the tragedy of Alzheimer's disease and other dementias,* Washington DC, 1987, US Government Printing Office.

Ott A, Breteler MM, van Harskamp F: Prevalence of Alzheimer's disease and vascular dementia: association with education, *BMJ* 310(6985):970, 1995.

Orlando P: AIDS affects the older population, *Aging Connection* 9:1, 1988.

Palmateer LM, McCartney JR: Do nurses know when patients have cognitive deficits? *J Gerontol Nurs* 11(2):6, 1985.

Patrick P, Hebda D: Neurobehavioral limitations: managing aggression, *Re-Learning* 3(3):5, 1996.

Persson G, Skoog I: Subclinical dementia: relevance of cognitive symptoms and signs, *J Geriatr Psychiatr Neurol* 5:172, 1992.

Phelps J, Sladek R: Neuron growth in cerebral cells, *Gerontologist* 27:310, 1983.

Piaget J: *The origins of intelligence in children,* New York, 1952, International Universities Press.

Pinching A: Clinical and immunological aspects of the acquired immunodeficiency syndrome and related disorders, *J Hosp Infect* 6 (suppl C):1, 1985.

Proulx G: When someone you know has a memory problem: some of the "do's and don'ts" to help you communicate, *Baycrest Bulletin* 8(1):3, 1996.

Roberts R, Davis G: Expanding options for seniors with mental retardation, *Aging* 357:17, 1988.

Rosenkoetter M: Changing life patterns of the ECF resident, *Geriatr Nurs* 17(6), 1996.

Roses AD: Apolipoprotein E and Alzheimer's disease, *Scientific Am Science Med* (September/October):16, 1995.

Rotkoff N, Labosky S, Dobson J, Groman AM: Nursing care of the resident with Creutzfeldt-Jakob disease, *Geriatr Nurs* 18, 1997.

Royston MC, Mann D, Pickering-Brown S: Apo E2 allele, Down's syndrome and dementia, *Ann N Y Acad Sci* 777:255, 1996.

Ryden M: *Behavioral problems in dementia: a review of the literature,* Unpublished manuscript, 1988.

Sansone P: Elderly with dementia can decide treatment at end of lives.

Sawyer JC, Mendlovitz AA: *A management program for ambulatory institutionalized patients with Alzheimer's disease and related disorders.* Paper presented at the meeting of the Gerontological Society of America, Boston, Nov 21, 1982.

Scharnhorst S: AIDS dementia complex in the elderly, *Nurse Prac* 17(8):37, 1992.

Schwartz D, Kelly C: *A guide for hospital staff working with adult patients with developmental disabilities,* Gwynedd, Pa, 1996, Elders with Adult Dependents.

Sherman D: Avoiding and treating drug-induced delirium, *Cont Long Term Care* 15(3):76, 1992.

Shulman KI, Lennox A, Karlinsky H. Late-onset Huntington's disease: a geriatric psychiatric perspective, *J Geriatr Psychiatr Neurol* 9(1):26, 1996.

Smith MA, Sayre LM, Monnier VM, Perry G: Radical aging in Alzheimer's disease, *Trends Neurosci* 18(4):172, 1995.

Snyder L, Quayhagen MP, Shepherd S, Bower D: Supportive seminar groups: an intervention for early stage dementia patients, *Gerontologist* 35(5):691, 1995.

Taulbee L, Folsom J: Reality orientation for geriatric patients, *Hosp Community Psychiatr* 17:133, 1966.

US Bureau of the Census: *Statistical abstract of the United States: 1995,* ed 115, Washington, DC, 1995, US Government Printing Office.

Vaughn P: Creutzfeldt-Jakob disease latest unknown in struggle to restore faith in blood supply, *Can Med Assoc J* 155(5):565, 1996.

Verhaegen P, Marcoen A, Goossens L: Improving memory performance in the aged through mnemonic training: a meta-analytic study, *Psychol Aging* 7(2):242, 1992.

Weiler P: Medical perspectives on Alzheimer's disease and AIDS, *Aging Connection* 9:8, 1988.

Wolanin M: Mental frailty, *Geriatr Nurs* 18(2), 1997.

Wolanin MO, Phillips LR: *Confusion: prevention and care,* St Louis, 1981, Mosby.

Woodruff-Pak DS: Aging and intelligence: changing perspectives in the twentieth century, *J Aging Studies* 3(2):91, 1989.

Wykle ML: The physical and mental health of women caregivers of older adults, *J Psychosoc Nurs* 32(3):41-42, 1994.

Ying W: Deleterious network hypothesis of Alzheimer's disease, *Med Hypotheses* 46(5):421, 1996.

CHAPTER 23

Psychotropic Drug Management

Martha D. Buffum, RN, DNSc, CS
John C. Buffum, PharmD

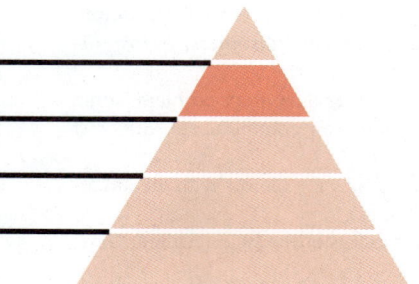

An elder speaks

I was beside myself with grief after my husband had his heart attack and died. I didn't know what to do with myself. I went to bed at night hoping I wouldn't wake up. After a couple of weeks on the antidepressant, I felt totally different. I don't know what happened to those feelings, but they're gone. I'm more like myself now. I don't like pills, but one that could take away those awful feelings is worth taking.

Anonymous widow, 72 years

LEARNING OBJECTIVES

Upon completion of this chapter, the reader will be able to:

1. Identify diagnoses or symptoms for which psychotropic drugs are prescribed.
2. Discuss issues about psychotropic medication management in the elderly population.
3. Identify several neurotransmitters and their influence on mental illness and mental health.
4. Discuss OBRA '87 guidelines for psychotropic medication use in institutionalized patients.
5. Develop a nursing care plan for patients prescribed psychoactive medications.

Psychotropic medications are drugs that alter brain chemistry, emotions, and behavior. They include antipsychotics or neuroleptics, antidepressants, mood stabilizers, antianxiety agents, and sedative/hypnotics. This chapter provides an overview of psychotropic medications used to treat symptoms that occur in disorders of behavior, cognition, arousal, and mood in the geriatric population. A section is devoted to treating the movement disorders that may occur as a side effect from the use of neuroleptics. Because each individual experiences symptoms in a unique way, several types of drugs are frequently prescribed for any particular illness. Hence, medications are used to target specific symptoms. Nursing care of patients taking psychotropic medications is also discussed.

The aged are active consumers of psychotropic drugs. A recent study of 1360 community-dwelling elderly in rural Pennsylvania determined that women were taking significantly more antidepressants and benzodiazepines than men ($p = <.002$ and $p = <.06$, respectively) and the same number of antipsychotics (Lassila, Stoehr, Ganguli et al, 1996). Urban dwellers, who have a 19% higher rate of tak-

ing daily prescribed medications than their rural counterparts, may also have more access to non-prescription medications, that have psychoactive effects (Darnell, Murray, Martz, and Weinberger, 1986). When patients were admitted to an urban geriatric psychiatric unit, Zisselman and others (1996) found, through a retrospective chart review of 131 admissions, that 58 persons (44.3%) were receiving benzodiazepines before admission. Of the 76 patients diagnosed with depression, 30 patients (39.5 percent) were receiving benzodiazepines as the only treatment for their symptoms before admission. Elderly persons institutionalized in skilled nursing facilities may be prescribed more than eight medications at any one time, which is twice the number of medications prescribed for the noninstitutionalized elderly (Beers, Avorn, Soumerai et al, 1988; Beers, Ouslander, Rollingher et al, 1991). As an important part of treatment in the vulnerable geriatric population, medications require scrutiny to be sure they are being appropriately used for specific symptoms.

Thinking in terms of Maslow's hierarchy, we might conclude that the primary need met by the use of psychotropics is basic comfort, security, or transcendence. Patients may have varying reasons for taking their medications. From the health care provider's point of view, the goal of medicating patients with psychotropic medications is the improvement of quality of life (Keltner and Folks, 1993).

Many older patients are ambivalent about medications, feeling they must take them while simultaneously resenting and welcoming them. Some persons will want to regulate medication themselves, often not understanding purposes, side effects, timing of dosages, or drug/food interactions. Still others wish to be compliant and will take medications regardless of the results they may be experiencing. Resistance may occur when a person is fearful that the psychoactive medication is prescribed for "craziness" or that the medication is addictive. The patient's understanding about his or her psychiatric disorder and the rapport established with the health care provider will influence reactions to medications including behaviors about taking them. In most situations, a psychotherapeutic approach includes both medication and psychotherapy.

A patient should be prescribed a psychotropic medication only after thorough medical, psychologic, and social assessments are done. Nursing assessment before medication intervention contributes knowledge and baseline information that can optimize the patient's medical and psychologic improvement. Issues to consider include the patient's medical status (and other medications that might interact with psychotropics), mental status, ability to carry out activities of daily living, ability to conduct social activities and relationships with others, and the potential for patient or caregiver compliance with any pharmacologic or nonpharmacologic recommendations (Keltner and Folks, 1993). Additionally, the cost of medications may determine whether the patient will comply with taking them.

Some of the nursing activities directed to the patient taking psychotropic medications include advocacy, education, assessment, observation, monitoring, documenting, and communicating. Listening to the patient's feelings, observing for behavioral improvements, and participating in team decisions about the patient's medications must be part of the nurse's repertoire. Interdisciplinary communication and collaboration are components in advocating for the patient's needs. Some general guidelines for nurses to consider include the questions in Box 23-1. The information generated from these questions should be shared with the patient to improve patient understanding and safety. Discussing psychotropic medications with patients is often difficult because side effects are frightening. Many states across the United States require informed consent from patients prescribed psychotropic medication, and this process mandates communication and education. Brown and associates (1987) found that psychiatric patients given instructions regarding the side effects of their medications actually experienced a decreased number of such effects. Judgment is important in knowing how and when to teach the patient

and caregiving family. Such discussions are often therapeutic, enhancing trust and rapport among the patient, family, and nurse.

NEUROTRANSMITTERS

Biochemical processes in the brain influence all activities including behavior, emotion, mood, cognition, and motor movement. Categorizing drugs by their receptor activities assists in identifying side effect profiles. Boxes 23-2 and 23-3 illustrate potential side effects with the different receptors. Since most psychotherapeutic agents do not affect a single neurotransmitter system, a wide range of side effects or adverse effects may result. Unidentified neurotransmitters may be the cause of some adverse effects. Simple side effects are considered unpleasant consequences of taking drugs, but adverse effects are usually more serious. Both types of effects can be cause for discontinuing the drug.

Age-related changes in neurotransmission may affect the number and response of receptors. For example, decreased production of dopamine and a decreased number of dopamine neurons are responsible for the increased responsiveness to haloperidol treatment and for causing parkinsonian

Box 23-1	**Questions to Consider about the Drug and the Specific Patient**

1. Is the drug working to improve the patient's symptoms?
   A. What are the therapeutic effects of the drug? (What symptoms are targeted?)
   B. What is the time frame for the therapeutic effects?
   C. Have the appropriate drug and dose been prescribed?
   D. Has the appropriate time been tried for therapeutic effects?
2. Is the drug harming the patient?
   A. What physiologic changes are occurring?
   B. What lab values are changing?
   C. What mental status changes are occurring?
   D. What functional changes are occurring?
   E. Is the patient experiencing side effects?
   F. Is the drug interacting with any other medication?
3. Does the patient understand the following?
   A. Why he or she is taking the drug?
   B. How the drug is supposed to be taken?
   C. How to identify side effects and drug interactions?
   D. How to reduce or manage side effects?
   E. Limitations imposed by taking the drug? (sedative effects)

Box 23-2	**Potential Adverse Effects Caused by Blockade of Muscarinic Acetylcholine Receptors**

Blurred vision
Constipation
Decreased salivation
Decreased sweating
Delirium
Hyperthermia
Memory problems
Narrow-angle glaucoma
Photophobia
Sinus tachycardia
Urinary retention

Modified from Kaplan HI, Sadock BJ: *Pocket handbook of psychiatric drug treatment,* ed 3, Baltimore, 1996, Williams & Wilkins, p 21.

Box 23-3	**Potential Adverse Side Effects of Psychotherapeutic Drugs and Associated Neurotransmitter Systems**

Dopamine Blockade
Endocrine dysfunction
   Hyperprolactinemia
   Sexual dysfunction

Movement Disorders
   Dystonia
   Parkinsonism
   Tardive dyskinesia

Norepinephrine Blockade (Alpha₁)
   Dizziness
   Postural hypotension
   Reflex tachycardia
   Delayed or retrograde ejaculation

Histamine Blockade
   Sedation
   Weight gain

Modified from Kaplan HI, Sadock BJ: *Pocket handbook of psychiatric drug treatment,* ed 2, Baltimore, 1996, Williams & Wilkins, p 22.

symptoms (Sunderland, 1992). Since older people are frequently on multiple drugs that affect the neurotransmitters, the receptors may have increased or decreased capacities for producing responses to particular agents.

ANTIPSYCHOTICS
History

Historically, chemotherapeutic approaches to psychiatry began in the last half of the 20th century with the discovery that chlorpromazine, originally synthesized for use in anesthesia, was effective in treating severe agitation and psychosis (Kaplan and Sadock, 1996). Chlorpromazine became available in 1954. In 1958, Janssen synthesized haloperidol, a butyrophenone antipsychotic. In the past 40 years, other similarly effective drugs have become available to treat psychotic behaviors. In 1990 the atypical neuroleptic, clozapine, was introduced in the United States as a drug that offers improvement in treatment of neuroleptic-resistant cases (Lohr, Jeste, Harris, Salzman, 1992). It produces few, if any, of the movement disorders that characterize use of the other antipsychotics. Newer antipsychotic medications approved for use in the U.S. market since 1990 include risperidone, sertindole, and olanzapine. Antipsychotics in varying developmental stages include ziprasidone and seroquel (Kaplan and Sadock, 1996). Box 23-4 highlights some historical events in psychopharmacology between 1845 and 1960.

Definitions and Target Symptoms

Antipsychotics, also formerly known as major tranquilizers and frequently known as neuroleptics, are drugs used to treat psychotic symptoms. (Originally given in high doses, these drugs produced loss of initiative, blunted affect, lethargy, somnolence, and movement disorders; hence, they were called major tranquilizers. In contrast, antianxi-

ety agents have been called minor tranquilizers—usually benzodiazepines—which produce only sedation without most of the effects of the major tranquilizers. The development of newer drugs with different effects has made obsolete the terms "major" and "minor" tranquilizers.) Psychosis covers a range of thinking and behavioral characteristics that are based on responses of the ill person to a private reality—a reality that is distressing and problematic for the patient and those around him or her.

Characteristically, psychosis occurs in schizophrenia but can also occur in mania, depression, delirium, dementia, and paranoid states. Psychosis manifests itself as delusional thinking and hallucinations, both of which can cause extreme anxiety and bizarre behavior. Other target symptoms include illogical thinking, loose associations, and ideas of reference. Antipsychotics are also used in the geriatric patient to relieve agitation, belligerence, assaultiveness, and nighttime sleep problems (Lohr, Jeste, Harris, Salzman, 1992).

Issues for Elderly

Issues for using these medications in the geriatric population involve indication, drug selection, and patient response. First, an antipsychotic drug may be indicated for the patient's psychotic symptoms if possible organic causes of the symptoms are investigated. However, other medical, psychologic, social, and environmental influences can cause thinking and behavioral changes. Behavior changes can also

<table>
<tr><td>Box 23-4</td><td colspan="2">Significant Points in the Evolution of Psychotrophic Drugs</td></tr>
</table>

1930s	Benzodiazepines are first synthesized by Sternbach.
1948	Rapport, Green, and Page isolate "serotonin" from beef serum.
1949	John Cade, an Australian psychiatrist, reports on the efficacy of lithium in mania.
1949	The U.S. Food and Drug Administration bans lithium because of deaths in patients with cardiac disease.
1951	Chlorpromazine is developed as a nonsedating antihistamine. Laborit and others report diminished surgical anxiety in conscious patients.
1952	Delay and Deniker, two psychiatrists working with Laborit, administer chlorpromazine to a manic patient with successful results.
1952	Iproniazid, a derivative of the anti-tuberculosis agent isoniazid, is identified as a monoamine oxidase inhibitor (MAOI).
1953	Bein isolates reserpine from *rauwolfia*. Reserpine, effective in treating psychosis, causes severe depression related to depletion of norepinephrine.
1954	Lehman publishes the first American article on chlorpromazine in the *Archives of Neurology and Psychiatry.*
1955	Researchers alter the molecular structure of chlorpromazine, developing new antipsychotic agents, e.g. haloperidol and fluphenazine.
1957	The first papers appear on MAOIs as antidepressants.
1957	Haloperidol (Haldol) is developed.
1958	Kuhn publishes the first article on tricyclic antidepressants in the *American Journal of Psychiatry.*
1960	Harris presents the first paper on the effectiveness of benzodiazepines in *The Journal of the American Medical Association.*
1970	The ban on lithium is lifted in the United States.
1980s	A new class of antidepressants is developed, the selective serotonin reuptake inhibitors (SSRIs).
1980s	The antiepileptic drugs carbamazepine and valproate are reported to have mood-stabilizing properties.
1990s	Clozapine (Clozaril) and risperidone (Risperdal), the first truly antipsychotic agents in 40 years, are released in the United States.
1990s	Tacrine (Cognex), a drug used to treat patients with Alzheimer's disease, is made available. Studies indicate that about 20% to 30% of cases improve.

From Ayd FJ: The early history of modern psychopharmacology, *Neuropsychopharmacology* 5(2):71, 1991; Kuhn R: The treatment of depressive states with G 22355 (imipramine hydrochloride), *Am J Psychiatr* 115(5):459, 1958; Rifkin A: Extrapyramidal side effects: a historical perspective, *J Clin Psychiatr* 48(9):3, 1987.

Table 23-1 Classes and Relative Potencies of Antipsychotics

Generic name	Trade name	Class	Approximate Equivalent dose (mg)
Low potency			
Chlorpromazine	Thorazine	Phenothiazine	100
Thioridazine	Mellaril	Phenothiazine	95
Intermediate potency			
Perphenazine	Trilafon	Phenothiazine	10
Loxapine succinate	Loxitane	Dibenzoxazepine	15
Molindone HCl	Moban	Dihydroindolone	10
High potency			
Haloperidol	Haldol	Butyrophenone	2
Thiothixene	Navane	Thioxanthene	5
Fluphenazine HCl	Prolixin	Phenothiazine	2
Trifluoperazine HCl	Stelazine	Phenothiazine	5
New antipsychotics			
Risperidone	Resperidal	Benzisoxazole	1.5
Clozapine	Clozaril	Dibenzodiazepine	50

From Ayrd FJ: The early history of modern psycopharmocology, Neuropsychopharmacology 5(2):71, 1991; Kuhn R: The treatment of depressive states with G 22355 (impramine hydrochloride), Am J Psychiatr 115(5):459, 1958; Rifkin A: Extrapyramidal side effects: a historical perpective, J Clin Psychiatr 48(9):3,187.

occur suddenly from reversible causes such as infection, fever, electrolyte imbalance, addition of a new drug to an established regimen, or stress. For example, admission to the hospital can cause disorientation and fear that others will take the person's possessions. Reassurance, consistency of staff, familiarity with objects in the environment, and visits from family and friends are interventions that will help such thinking more than antipsychotic medication. The need for staff to medicate a patient because of loudness or other agitated behaviors must be evaluated in light of the context of conditions influencing the patient. Likewise, the nurse must safeguard the patient whose caregiver is requesting sedation for the patient.

A second consideration for the geriatric patient is selection of the medication. There are different classes and potencies of antipsychotics, as illustrated in Table 23-1. The side effect profile influences selection. Strong antipsychotics (high potency), such as haloperidol, are less sedating but cause more extrapyramidal reactions. The elderly are susceptible to developing extrapyramidal reactions, particularly neuroleptic-induced parkinsonian symptoms. Weak antipsychotics (low potency), such as chlorpromazine, are sedating and cause orthostatic hypotension, thereby precipitating falls. Further, the anticholinergic properties in the weaker antipsychotics can cause dry mouth, constipation, urinary retention, hypotension, and confusion. Table 23-2 illustrates comparison of sedative, extrapyramidal, anticholinergic, and cardiovascular side effects of the different potencies of antipsychotics.

Authors differ on which drug is best in the elderly. Many clinicians feel that low dose high potency (haloperidol) is best in the elderly. Management of the agitation of dementia usually requires different doses than that required for treating delusions or psychosis (see Table 23-8). Strome and Howell (1991) observed 150 patients and concluded that the elderly best tolerate mid-potency drugs, such as molindone and loxapine, because these patients seldom need anticholinergic drugs for extrapyramidal side effects. These mid-potency agents also avoided the anticholinergic, sedative, and hypotensive side effects commonly seen with the low potency drugs. An individual's history with a particular antipsychotic may assist with drug selection. *Also, the other drugs that the patient takes for medical conditions should be considered for interactions with any selected antipsychotic.*

Careful nursing observation is essential for monitoring side effects and drug interactions whenever any of these medications is given.

Response to treatment is the most important consideration when geriatric patients are taking psychotropics. Clearer, logical thinking and less distressed behaviors are targeted. Subjective patient comments about feelings and symptoms and objective observations about the patient's behavior are important data for evaluating effectiveness of a drug. The nurse should ask patients about their feelings, symptoms, and side effects. Generally, calmness is the first noticeable beneficial sign. Hallucinations may or may not respond to medication, and delusions do not usually respond. However, the patient's calmness and improved restfulness will change perceptions about the hallucinations and delusions; usually these symptoms become less distressing. Although side effects are usually cause for changing to another class of drug, an adequate trial of a drug cannot be assessed until a therapeutic response is seen. Such a response can vary from 24 hours to 5 days or longer in individuals.

Using new drugs is tempting, but caution is warranted for treating the elderly. Clozapine (Clozaril) has a lower profile of extrapyramidal effects, but side effects include sedation and fatigue, sialorrhea, weight gain, hypotension, gastrointestinal symptoms, tachycardia, fever, seizures (with high doses), electrocardiographic changes, and leukopenia or agranulocytosis (Gelenberg and Katz, 1993). Although tachycardia and hypotension may dissipate over time, death

from cardiorespiratory complications has been documented in case reports when clozapine was given in high doses (up to 400 mg/day) (Leo, Kreeger, and Kim, 1996). Although cause and effect relationships are not possible with small numbers of case reports, pre-existing cardiac disease should preclude the use of clozapine. Certainly, the deleterious cardiovascular effects make this drug less desirable in the elderly. The general rule for safety, comfort, and minimization of side effects—particularly in the elderly—is to "start low and go slow."

How Antipsychotics Work

Most antipsychotics are dopamine type 2 (D_2) receptor antagonists that affect various pathways within the brain. Dopamine blocking produces most of the extrapyramidal side effects associated with the antipsychotics. Most D_2 receptor antagonists affect other neurotransmitters, but the significance of this is not known. Some of these transmitters are GABA, histamine, serotonin, neurotensis, substance P, and endorphins (Gelenberg and Katz, 1993). Again, what is known is that antipsychotics have side effects because of these receptor activities. For example, blockage of the muscarinic acetylcholine receptors produces autonomic effects that are anticholinergic, such as dry mouth, blurred vision, and urinary retention. Further, dopamine blockage in the hypothalamus results in weight gain, hyperprolactinemia, and impaired temperature regulation, which may result in hypo- or hyperthermia. Blockade

Table 23-2   Comparison of Side Effects of Antipsychotics

Generic name	Side Effects			
	Sedative	**Anticholinergic**	**Extrapyramidal**	**Hypotensive**
Low potency				
Chlorpromazine	High	High	Low	IM: High PO: Low
Thioridazine	High	High	Low	Moderate
Intermediate potency				
Perphenazine	Moderate	Moderate	Moderate	Low
Loxapine succinate	Moderate	Moderate	Moderate	Low
Molindone HCl	Moderate	Moderate	Moderate	—
High potency				
Haloperidol	Low	Low	High	Low
Thiothixene	Low	Low	High	Moderate
Fluphenazine HCl	Low	Low	High	Low
Trifluoperazine HCl	Moderate	Low	Moderate	Low
New Antipsychotics				
Risperidone	Low	Low	Dose related	Low
Clozapine	High	High	Low	High
Olanzapine	Moderate	Moderate	Low	Moderate

Modified from Bloom HG, Shlom EA: *Drug prescribing for the elderly,* New York, 1993, Raven Press, p. 62; Jenike MA: *Geriatric psychiatry and psychopharmacology: a clinical approach,* Boston, 1989, Year Book Medical Publishers; and Semla TP, Beizer JL, Higbee MD: *Geriatric dosage handbook,* ed 2, Cleveland, 1995, Lexi-Comp Inc.

of the alpha$_1$ adrenergic receptors produces orthostatic hypotension, dizziness, and delayed or retrograde ejaculation.

Side Effects of Antipsychotics

Anticholinergic Side Effects. The low potency antipsychotics are more strongly anticholinergic. These side effects, which are also called *atropine-like,* result from the blockage of the muscarinic type of cholinergic receptor. The side effects are illustrated in Box 23-5 and are divided into peripheral and central effects. Peripheral effects are the symptoms affecting the peripheral nervous system and central effects are those that affect the central nervous system (Gelenberg and Katz, 1993).

The elderly are more sensitive to anticholinergic effects than younger persons. Medical illnesses can be worsened by addition of anticholinergic side effects. For instance, patients with glaucoma, prostatic enlargement, cardiac problems, gastrointestinal problems, and dental problems may be compromised by taking antipsychotics and experiencing such side effects. Additionally, the health care provider who prescribes and the nurse who cares for the patient should learn the patient's list of medications because the synergistic effects of anticholinergic side effects can result in life-threatening toxic states. In assessing the risk of delirium, Tune et al (1992) assayed the anticholinergic drug levels of 25 of the most commonly prescribed drugs. Drug levels in excess of 0.83 ng/ml of atropine equivalents are associated with impairment in the capacity for self-care in elderly, particularly in demented persons. Table 23-3 lists the assayed drugs with anticholinergic levels.

Monitoring for anticholinergic delirium is an important nursing activity. The behaviors occurring in delirium can be mistaken for agitation and worsening psychosis because the patient becomes confused, disoriented, and may become agitated. However, the onset of anticholinergic delirium is rapid and physiologic signs are evident. These are typically large pupils, dry mucous membranes, hot and flushed skin, tachycardia, and markedly diminished bowel sounds. The best treatment is withdrawal of causative agents.

Cardiovascular Side Effects. Two major concerns about side effects of antipsychotics, particularly in the elderly, are orthostatic hypotension and arrhythmias. More common with the low potency antipsychotics like chlorpromazine, postural hypotension can also occur with clozapine. It occurs more frequently in those with pre-existing vascular instability or postural hypotension. Keeping the patient horizontal, arising slowly after sitting at the edge of the bed for a few minutes, and maintaining fluid volume (hydration) may help. Epinephrine must be avoided because it could create a paradoxic drop in blood pressure (alpha receptors are blocked and the unopposed beta stimulation, with dilation of muscle capillary beds, leads to further hypotension). Norepinephrine or phenylephrine can be safely administered (purely alpha adrenergic) (Gelenberg and Katz, 1993).

Patients with pre-existing cardiac disease require close monitoring for arrhythmias and should avoid low potency

Table 23-3	Anticholinergic Drug Levels in 25 Medications Most Frequently Used By the Elderly

Drug*	Anticholinergic drug level (ng/ml of atropine equivalent)
Furosemide	0.22
Digoxin	0.25
Dyazide	0.08
Lanoxin	0.25
Hydrochlorothiazide	0.00
Propranolol	0.00
Salicylic acid	0.00
Dipridamole	0.11
Theophylline anhydrous	0.44
Nitroglycerin	0.00
Insulin	0.00
Warfarin	0.12
Prednisolone	0.55
Alpha-methyldopa	0.00
Nifedipine	0.22
Isosorbide dinitrate	0.15
Ibuprofen	0.00
Codeine	0.11
Cimetidine	0.86
Diltiazem hydrochloride	0.00
Captopril	0.02
Atenolol	0.00
Metoprolol	0.00
Timolol	0.00
Ranitidine	0.22

*At a 10^{-8} M concentration.
From Tune L, Carr S, Hoag E, Cooper T: Anticholinergic effects of drugs commonly prescribed for the elderly: potential means for assessing risk of delirium, *Am J Psych* 149(10):1393-1394, 1992.

Box 23-5	**Anticholinergic Side Effects of Antipsychotics**

Peripheral Anticholinergic Effects

Warmth, flushing of skin
Decreased sweating
Mydriasis, difficulty accommodating
Increased intraocular pressure
Xerostomia
Tachycardia
Constipation from decreased intestinal motility
Urinary retention

Central Anticholinergic Effects

Memory deficits
Confusion
Delirium

Modified from Bressler R, Katz MD: *Geriatric pharmacology,* New York, 1993, McGraw-Hill.

agents, particularly large doses and, specifically, thioridazine and clozapine. Physical assessments, vital signs, ECGs are among the monitoring methods. Combinations of antipsychotic drugs and tricyclic antidepressants can produce additive cardiotoxic effects.

Hematologic Side Effects: Agranulocytosis and Clozapine.

Low potency antipsychotics are possibly weakly toxic to bone marrow elements, often producing a transient leukopenia. Occasionally a patient will develop agranulocytosis. This life-threatening hematologic problem occurs at a general rate of 1 in 500,000 (1 in 3000 to 4000 taking chlorpromazine); in those taking clozapine, a new atypical antipsychotic, it occurs in 1 in 50 persons, or 2% (Gelenberg and Katz, 1993; Kaplan and Sadock, 1996).

Weekly monitoring of leukocyte count is required for clozapine treatment. Monitoring for agranulocytosis means observing for signs of infection and teaching the patient to report sore throat, fever, malaise, or other symptoms of infection. If the white count is low, the antipsychotic should be discontinued. The count should return to normal within several weeks unless an infection occurs. Infection in the presence of agranulocytosis is life-threatening.

Movement Disorders.

Neurologic side effects manifest as extrapyramidal syndrome (EPS) (acute dystonia, akathisia, and parkinsonian symptoms), tardive dyskinesia, or neuroleptic malignant syndrome. Ganzini and colleagues (1991) studied 19 elderly patients and reported incidences of movement disorders, as follows:

- 52% had signs of parkinsonian symptoms 2 weeks after being withdrawn from antipsychotic agents
- None developed acute dystonias
- 19% developed akathisia
- 71% developed dose-related parkinsonian symptoms
- 10% developed incontinence associated with the parkinsonian symptoms

This work demonstrates that parkinsonian symptoms are the most frequently occurring movement disorder in the elderly who are prescribed antipsychotics.

Acute dystonias. An acute dystonic reaction is an abnormal involuntary movement consisting of a slow and continuous muscular contraction or spasm. One hypothesis for why this reaction occurs is the acute increase in dopamine neurotransmission in the basal ganglia. Perhaps this suddenly occurs as dopamine transiently supervenes the dopamine blockade brought about by the antipsychotics (Gelenberg and Katz, 1993).

An acute dystonic reaction may occur hours or days following antipsychotic medication administration or after dosage increases and may last minutes to hours. Episodic and recurrent incidents occur. Involuntary muscular contractions of the mouth, jaw, face, and neck are common. The jaw may lock (trismus), the tongue may roll back and block the throat, the neck may arch backward (opisthotonus), or the eyes may close. In an oculogyric crisis, the eyes are fixed in one position. Often this creates a feeling of needing to look up constantly without an ability to make the eyes come down.

Dystonias can be painful and frightening. Caregivers or others unfamiliar with EPS reactions also become alarmed. Although frightening, these incidents are not usually dangerous. They are acutely responsive to anticholinergic medication, such as benztropine (Cogentin), trihexyphenidyl (Artane), or diphenhydramine (Benadryl), providing relief within minutes if given intravenously, 10 to 15 minutes if given intramuscularly, and up to 30 minutes if given orally. These medications should be readily available to treat an EPS and are usually given for a brief time following a reaction. Within several weeks without an EPS, these medications should be tapered off. Especially in the elderly, the anticholinergic properties of some of these medications are not desirable. Anticholinergics and amantadine (Symmetrel), a dopamine agonist, are useful in preventing dystonic reactions, but because of slow onset of action should not be used for acute treatment.

These EPSs occur most often with the high potency antipsychotics and in young males. From the patient's perspective, the painful and frightening dystonic reaction is cause for rejecting a drug, and many patients will say they are allergic to the drug that caused the reaction. Rapid attention is reassuring while a patient is in the hospital. Sometimes the reaction happens quickly, and the patient has no time to prepare. For example, one patient described having a "problem with my eyes" while driving a car. She was unable to look down. Fortunately, she was able to pull to the side of the road and wait until the reaction passed. She thought her "bad thoughts" were causing this to happen. Medications relieve the EPS, and the risk of dystonic reactions wanes with continued antipsychotic therapy. Clearly, patients need education about these phenomena when taking antipsychotic medication.

Akathisia. Contrary to the finding of Ganzini and colleagues (1991) about drug-induced parkinsonian symptoms, Lohr et al (1992) reports that the most common drug-induced EPS in the elderly is akathisia. Akathisia is the compulsion to be in motion. Patients describe feeling restless, being unable to be still, having an unrelenting desire to move, feeling "like crawling out of my skin." This symptom is uncomfortable, and the patient looks agitated. Often this symptom is mistaken for worsening psychosis. Pacing, aimless walking, fidgeting, shifting weight from one leg to the other, and marked restlessness are characteristic behaviors for a person experiencing akathisia. This side effect does not appear to wane as therapy progresses, unlike the dystonic reaction. Akathisia may occur at any time during therapy.

Treatment response is variable. Usually, approaches include lowering the antipsychotic dose, changing to a less potent drug, or adding a drug to counteract the akathisia. Although results are less successful than treating acute dystonias, the same drugs are tried: anticholinergics, antiparkinsonians, antihistamines, and benzodiazepines (Lorazepam). Propranolol and clonidine have also been used and do improve the subjective complaints of akathisia. However, hypotension and sedation are often unacceptable side effects and can be dangerous in the elderly.

Parkinsonian symptoms. In neuroleptic-induced Parkinson's syndrome, a bilateral tremor (as opposed to a unilateral tremor) is often seen. More commonly, bradykinesia and rigidity are seen, which may progress to akinesia. Rigidity is the most common symptom associated with drug-induced parkinsonism. The patient may have an inflexible facial expression and, with the slow movements also occurring, appear bored and apathetic and be mistakenly diagnosed as depressed.

More common with the higher potency antipsychotics, parkinsonian symptoms may occur within weeks to months after beginning antipsychotic therapy. Women and elderly are more frequently affected by this syndrome, and some become tolerant to the effects while others need ongoing treatment (Gelenberg and Katz, 1993).

One approach to treatment is lowering the dose of the antipsychotic drug, which should decrease the amount of dopamine blockade at the synaptic receptor. Other approaches include counterbalancing the decreased dopamine transmission by either blocking acetylcholine transmission (anticholinergic antiparkinson drugs such as benztropine and trihexyphenidyl) or by increasing dopamine transmission (dopamine agonist such as amantadine). The lowest effective dose should be used, as all of these counterbalancing agents have undesirable side effects for the elderly. Anticholinergic antiparkinson drugs may impair memory, cognition, time perception, and cause dry mouth, blurred vision, urinary retention, and constipation (Gelenberg and Katz, 1993). Amantadine may be used when anticholinergic drugs have been ineffective; despite having a long half-life of about 24 hours, it can be given in doses of 100 mg two to three times daily. However, it is excreted unchanged in the urine, making elderly persons at risk for toxicity if they have impaired renal function. Worsening of psychiatric symptoms can occur. Finally, low-dose clozapine, particularly in patients with pre-existing Parkinson's disease, may be an alternative strategy for antipsychotic use because of its extremely low incidence of parkinsonian symptoms (Baldessarini and Frankenburg, 1991).

Tardive dyskinesia. Exposure to neuroleptics continuously for at least 3 to 6 months raises the risk of developing the delayed dyskinetic side effect known as tardive dyskinesia. Both low and high potency agents are implicated. Tardive symptoms usually appear first as wormlike movements of the tongue, and other facial movements include grimacing, blinking, and frowning. Slow, maintained, involuntary twisting movements of the limbs, trunk, neck, face, and eyes (involuntary eye closure) have been reported (Burke, Fahn, Jankovic, et al, 1982). These unusual movements were described shortly after the introduction of antipsychotics and have occurred progressively since the advent of these agents. Perhaps newer drugs, lower doses, and faster detec-

tion may promote less of this disturbing side effect. Lohr et al (1992) describe risk factors, outlined in Box 23-6.

Why tardive dyskinesia occurs is not fully known. The dopamine excess theory purports that the chronic blockade of dopamine receptors within the basal ganglia leads first to underactivity and then to overactivity. Hence, the excess dopaminergic activity is thought to cause the tardive dyskinesia types of abnormal movements. Studies of prolonged exposure to neuroleptics produce different results when animals and humans are compared. Specifically, supersensitivity seems to develop less in older animals (less tardive dyskinesia) than in older patients (more tardive dyskinesia). Some authors suggest that the dopamine excess theory may be too simplistic and that alternative neurotransmitters may contribute to tardive symptoms, such as GABA, acetylcholine, and norepinehprine (Gelenberg and Katz, 1993).

Treatment is based on prevention, early detection, and medication manipulation. Antipsychotic use in the nonpsychotic patient should be avoided unless necessary, and then should be used only for brief periods of time. Treatment of schizophrenia necessitates continuous antipsychotic use, but at the lowest possible dose that will prevent relapse. Early detection means screening and monitoring. The Abnormal Involuntary Movement Scale (AIMS), which was designed by the National Institute of Mental Health (NIMH, 1976), should be used before therapy and after initiation of therapy. Table 23-4 offers recommended scales for monitoring movement disorders (see also Barnes Rating Scale for Akathisia, Simpson Angus Rating Scale for EPS, and the AIMS, Appendices 23-A to 23-C.) Always, the benefit of the drug must be weighed in relation to the intensity and

---

Box 23-6	**Risk Factors for Tardive Dyskinesia**

Advanced age
Length and amount of neuroleptic exposure
Medical conditions
   Edentulousness
   Decreased estrogen
Female gender
Mood disorder
History of EPS
Treatment with antidepressants or anticholinergics
Use of depot neuroleptics (IM administration, slow
   release drug over 10 days to 2 weeks; not commonly
   used in elderly)
History of drug interruptions ("drug holidays")
Smoking
Dementia
Brain damage
Mental retardation

Modified from Lohr JB, Jeste DV, Harris MJ, Salzman C: Treatment of disordered behavior. In Salzman C, ed: *Clinical geriatric psychopharmacology,* ed 2, Baltimore, 1992, Williams and Wilkins, p. 90.

seriousness of the psychotic symptoms. For some, tardive dyskinesia is less bothersome than psychosis. Withdrawing the drug may temporarily worsen the symptoms, but will make greater the likelihood that the tardive symptoms will improve. Lower doses of neuroleptics should be used, and anticholinergics should be discontinued (Salzman, 1992). There is no standard accepted treatment for tardive dyskinesia, and drugs that have been tried include benzodiazepines, lecithin, baclofen, sodium valproate, and propranolol (Gelenberg and Katz, 1993; Lohr et al, 1992).

A recent development is the idea that increased free radical formation may play a role in tardive dyskinesia. The antioxidant, vitamin E, may be useful in reducing some of the symptoms. However, the longer the patient has had tardive dyskinesia the less likely vitamin E will help. Suggested dosage ranges of vitamin E have been from 400 to 1600 IU/day (Lohr and Caligiuri, 1996).

Neuroleptic Malignant Syndrome (NMS). Neuroleptic Malignant Syndrome (NMS) is mainly a syndrome that occurs in younger patients; occuring at a rate of .5 to 1% and evolving over a period of 1 to 3 days. This potentially lethal disorder makes early detection an important part of the nurse's knowledge base. It has occurred in patients in their sixties (Salzman, 1992). The clinical picture involves both extrapyramidal and autonomic dysfunctions. NMS begins with motor abnormalities such as rigidity or dyskinesia and is quickly followed by high fever and cardiovascular abnormalities. Other symptoms include dystonia, tremor, tachycardia, diaphoresis, tachypnea, fluctuating blood pressure, urinary incontinence, and confusion leading to stupor. Abnormal laboratory values include elevated creatine phosphokinase levels, leukocytosis, and myoglobinuria. The medical complications that may occur are cardiac problems, pneumonia, pulmonary emboli, renal failure, and death.

Although the etiology is unclear, the characteristic symptoms are caused by a blockage of dopamine at the basal ganglia, precipitated by a massive overloading at the receptor site (Pelletier, Dailey, and Bennett, 1992). Dopamine receptor blockade is thought to occur in the temperature-regulating centers of the brain leading to an inability to regulate temperature associated with heat-generating muscular contractions.

Treatment is aimed at supportive medical management. The neuroleptic drug must be discontinued. Some young patients respond favorably to dantrolene or bromocriptine, but these may be toxic in the elderly. Admission to intensive care is usually necessary for maintenance of hydration and respiratory function. Cooling blankets, ice packs, and even iced enemas may be necessary to reduce fever, and oxygen and a respirator may be needed to maintain gaseous exchange. Several days may pass before improvement is clearly evident because of the long half-life and slow metabolism of most antipsychotics (Dresser, 1992).

Neuroleptic-related heatstroke. Antipsychotics impair the body's hypothalamic dopaminergic thermoregulatory pathways. Hence, patients taking neuroleptics cannot tolerate excess environmental heat. Heatstroke has very high associated mortality and morbidity rates. Even mild elevations of core temperature can result in liver damage. The nurse or caregiver must protect the elder from hyperthermia by making sure the environment is cool enough. The problem is more likely to occur during hot weather. Appropriate interventions include adequate hydration, relocation to a cooler area away from direct sunlight, and use of a fan or sponge

---

Table 23-4   Recommended Scales for Monitoring Movement Disorders

Movement disorder	Rating scale	Time to administer	Frequency of monitorig
Neuroleptic-induced akathisia	Barnes Akathisia Scale (see Appendix 23-A)	10 minutes	Daily to weekly during first 3 months after initiating or increasing neuroleptic; may be done for other meds (SSRI) that cause akathisia; patients in acute care hospital may need daily assessment
Neuroleptic-induced parkinsonism	Simpson-Angus EPS (see Appendix 23-B)	5-10 minutes	Daily for first 2 weeks, then weekly for 3 months after initiating neuroleptic; patients in acute care hospital may need frequent assessment
Tardive dyskinesia	Abnormal Involuntary Movement Scale (AIMS) (see Appendix 23-C)	5-10 minutes	Monthly during first 2 years after intiating neuroleptic, then semiannually; at each admission to hospital

Modified from Sweet RA, Pollock BG: Neuroleptics in the elderly: guidelines for monitoring, *Harvard Rev Psych* 2:327-335, 1995.

bath. The patient may or may not share his or her discomfort about the heat, so assessment of body temperature is essential. Any circumstance resulting in dehydration greatly increases the risk of heatstroke. Diuretics, coffee, alcohol, lithium, and uncontrolled diabetes may decrease vascular volume, thereby decreasing the body's ability to sweat. Anticholinergics inhibit the sweating and lead to further heat retention (Lazarus, 1989).

Geriatric Dosing. Physiologic changes associated with aging necessitate dosage regulation. Some of the changes that affect antipsychotic drug therapy are presented in Table 23-5. Historically, physiologic changes in aging have not been translated into dosing guidelines, and the elderly have been an overmedicated population. Based on the overuse and potential risk if psychotropic drugs are not used judiciously in the elderly, particularly in nursing homes, federal regulations were enacted. The Health Care Finance Administration and the Congressional Omnibus Budget Reconciliation Act of 1987 mandated that the elderly in long term care settings receive psychotropic drugs for specific diseases or symptoms and that the uses be monitored, reduced, or eliminated when possible (OBRA, 1987). Behaviors requiring neuroleptic use are defined in Box 23-7. "Organic mental syndromes" refer to behaviors not diagnosed as psychotic-psychiatric disorders, such as agitation associated with dementia. Further, OBRA guidelines delineate the recommended dosages (Table 23-6) for such behaviors. (Table 23-8 differentiates doses for psychoses and dementia.)

Physicians may exceed the recommended doses if documentation reasonably explains the rationale for the benefit of the higher dose in restoring function and/or preventing dangerous behavior (Stoudemire and Smith, 1996). Likewise, there are guidelines for dosage reduction, behavioral interventions for reducing or eliminating the medications, and directions for documentation about adequacy of treatment for symptom reduction.

The impact of the OBRA legislation has been reported in the literature. Educational interventions offered to physi-cians and nurses by pharmacists have reduced rates of antipsychotic use by 36% in 17 nursing homes (Rovner, Edleman, Cox et al., 1992), 72% in two experimental sites, and 13% in two control sites (Ray, Taylor, Meador, et al., 1993). According to Rovner et al., OBRA requirements reinforced the educational intervention so that the rate was maintained. In one longitudinal study of 9432 elderly in nursing homes over 30 months, antipsychotic drug rates dropped by 27%; one quarter of the facilities had no change or had increased usage, and another quarter of the facilities had decreases of up to 46% (Shorr, Fought, and Ray, 1994). The role of nursing in monitoring antipsychotic use has been described (Table 23-7).

Considerations about Behavior Management in Patients with Dementia

Careful examination of the patient with dementia enables determination of the type of dementing process (Cummings, 1996). Alzheimer's disease patients present language, memory, and visuospatial skill deficits with normal neurologic and laboratory findings and atrophy on neuroimaging. Vascular dementia is characterized by history of cerebrovascular incidents, positive neurologic findings, and deficits on neuroimaging. Patients with movement disorders such as Parkinson's disease have positive neurologic findings, normal laboratory findings, and normal neuroimaging findings. With toxic and metabolic disturbances, mental status changes and changes in laboratory findings are evident. Neuroimaging is helpful in identifying brain tumors. Patients with depression show negative findings and exhibit behavioral changes. Certainly, pre-existing medical conditions must also be evaluated, assessed, or ruled out.

All patients with dementia exhibit behavioral manifestations at some point in the course of the disease (see Chapter 22 regarding dementias). Frequent behaviors that have been described include apathy, agitation, anxiety, irritability, dysphoria, motor activity, disinhibition, delusions, and hallucinations (Mega, Cummings, Fiorello, and Gornbein, 1996). The role of the nurse is first to attempt nonpharmacologic approaches to the patient's behaviors. If these methods are ineffective alone, pharmacologic intervention should be attempted in tandem with psychotherapeutic and behavioral interventions. Table 23-8 lists medications in appropriate geriatric dosages used for agitation in demented elders.

Severe side effects of neuroleptics have resulted in the clinical uses of non-neuroleptic treatment of agitation in dementia patients. Currently, literature is mostly from case reports. Well-controlled clinical trials are needed. To date, medications used for agitation in Alzheimer's disease and other types of dementia include propranolol, trazodone, buspirone, fluoxetine, carbamazepine, and lithium (Salzman, 1992; Schneider and Sobin, 1992). Monitoring must include, respective to the drug, vital signs, sedation, lithium levels (with thyroid and renal function tests) and

---

Table 23-5	Impact of Age-Related Changes on Antipsychotic Drug Therapy

Physiologic Change	Effect
More body fat	Effects and side effects persist longer, even after the drug is stopped
Less plasma albumin	Less drug is protein-bound; more drug is free to circulate
Less body water	Less drug is needed to achieve a given blood level
Fewer brain cells	Less drug is needed to produce the desired effect
Slower liver metabolism	Drug remains in the body longer
Slower renal clearance	Drug remains in the body longer

From Strome T, Howell T: How antipsychotics affect the elderly, *Am J Nurs* 91(5):46-49, 1991.

Box 23-7   Defined Indications and Behaviors for Appropriate and Inappropriate Use of Neuroleptics in the Nursing Facility, According to OBRA Guidelines

Unnecessary drugs; each resident's drug regimen must be free from unnecessary drugs.

Antipsychotic drugs are given *only as necessary* therapy to treat the following specific conditions as diagnosed and documented in the clinical record:

Schizophrenia
Schizoaffective disorder
Delusional disorder
Psychotic mood disorder (mania, depression with psychotic features)
Acute psychotic episode
Brief reactive psychosis
Tourette's disorder
Huntington's disorder
Organic mental syndromes (dementia and delirium included) with associated psychotic and/or agitated behaviors
Short-term (7 days) symptomatic treatment of hiccups, nausea, vomiting, or pruritus

Behaviors for which antipsychotic medication *is* appropriate:

Agitated psychosis (biting, kicking, hitting, scratching, assaultive and belligerent behavior, sexual aggressiveness) presenting a danger to self or care providers or interfering with ability to provide care
Hallucinations, delusions, paranoia
Continuous crying out and screaming

Behaviors less responsive to antipsychotics; antipsychotic therapy should *not* be used if one or more of the following is/are the *only* indication:

Repetitive, bothersome behavior (pacing, wandering, repetitious statements or words, calling out, fidgeting)
Poor self-care
Unsociability
Indifference to surroundings
Uncooperativeness
Restlessness
Impaired memory
Anxiety
Depression (without psychotic features)
Insomnia
Agitated behaviors that *do not* represent danger to the patient or others

Data compiled from Semla TP, Beizer JL, Higbee MD: *Geriatric dosage handbook,* ed 2, Cleveland, 1995, Lexi-Comp Inc; United States Statutes, Omnibus Budget Reconciliation Act (OBRA) of 1987, 101 Stat. 1330-160, U.S. Health Care Financing Administration: *Medicare and Medicaid: requirements for long-term care facilities,* Federal Register 54(21):5316-5373, 1989; Stoudemire A, Smith DA: OBRA regulations and the use of psychotropic drugs in long-term care facilities: impact and implications for geropsychiatric care, *Gen Hosp Psych* 18:77-94, 1996.

carbamazepine levels (with CBC), and effectiveness in controlling aggressive or assaultive or agitated behaviors.

Treatment for Cognitive Aspects of Dementia

Recent drug development has been in progress for persons with Alzheimer's Disease to enhance memory, stall cognitive deterioration, or stimulate remaining functional neurons to increased activity. One compound that has shown some promise is tacrine (tetrahydroaminoacridine, THA, Cognex). Physostigmine, bethanechol, and lecithin have also been touted, with mixed results. All of these substances are used to stimulate the synthesis of the neurotransmitter acetylcholine, which is abnormally low in these patients. In 1987 Ban reported a class of psychotropics dubbed "nootropics" purported to improve efficiency of higher ner-

vous system function without affecting other body systems. Little has been heard about these in the intervening years.

The newest drug approved specifically for Alzheimer's disease is tacrine (Cognex), which has been found effective for improving cognition in about one third to one half of all persons who can tolerate high doses of the drug (Davis and Powchik, 1995). The reported improvement is the equivalent of returning the patient to a functional level 7 to 12 months before taking the medication (Cummings, 1996). It appears to be most effective in the early stages of the disease when the person is experiencing mild to moderate symptoms. So far, it is difficult to determine which patients will demonstrate improvement.

Tacrine is a cholinesterase inhibitor that increases brain acetylcholine levels, the neurotransmitter deficient in pa-

Table 23-6   Maximum Dosages of Selected Antipsychotics, According to OBRA Guidelines

Generic	Brand Name	Usual max daily dose for age ≥65	Usual max daily dose	Daily antipsychotic oral dosage for residents with organic mental syndromes
Chlorpromazine	Thorazine	800 mg	1600 mg	75 mg
Haloperidol	Haldol	50 mg	100 mg	4 mg
Loxapine	Loxitane	125 mg	250 mg	10 mg
Thioridazine	Mellaril	400 mg	800 mg	75 mg
Molindone	Moban	112 mg	225 mg	10 mg
Thiothixene	Navane	30 mg	60 mg	7 mg
Fluphenazine	Prolixin, Permitil	20 mg	40 mg	7 mg
Mesoridazine	Serentil	250 mg	500 mg	25 mg
Trifluoperazine	Stelazine	40 mg	80 mg	8 mg
Chlorprothixene	Taractan	800 mg	1600 mg	75 mg
Acetophenazine	Tindal	150 mg	300 mg	20 mg
Perphenazine	Trilafon	32 mg	64 mg	8 mg
Trifluopromazine	Vesprin	100 mg	200 mg	—

From Semla TP, Beizer JL, Higbee MD: *Geriatric dosage handbook,* ed 2, Cleveland, 1995, Lexi-Comp Inc, p 757.

Table 23-7   Nursing Role in Monitoring Medication Use: Sample Antipsychotic Medication Flow Sheet

Name:
Psychiatric diagnosis: **Patient's birthdate:**
Target symptoms:

Date med started, reviewed, or changed	Name of medication	Dose, frequency	Signed informed consent (date)	Frequency of patient reported target symptoms/day	Frequency of staff observed target symptoms/day	Frequency of observed patient distress/day	Side effects: AIMS score; Simpson-Angus score; anticholinergic effects; other
1/21/96	Haldol	1 mg bid	1/21/96	3x/day	5x/day	7x/day, crying, yelling at voices	AIMS = 0
1/26/96	Haldol	1.5 mg AM 1 mg HS		2x/day	4x/day	4x/day, angry outbursts	AIMS = 0
1/30/96	Haldol	1.5 mg bid		1x/day	2x/day	1x/day, tearful, yelling at voices	AIMS = 0

Modified from Strome T, Howell T: How antipsychotics affect the elderly, *Am J Nurs* 91:46-49, 1991.

tients with Alzheimer's disease. Before beginning tacrine, a complete physical and laboratory examination should be done with special regard to liver function and hematologic indices. Since the half-life of the drug is only 3 to 4 hours, three times daily dosing is necessary. The patient should be started on 40 mg per day and raised slowly, by 40 mg per day every 6 weeks, until 160 mg per day is reached. Ideally, tacrine should be given an hour before meals because absorption is reduced by about 25% when taken with or 2 hours after meals (Kaplan and Sadock, 1996).

Recent reports state that up to 70% of all patients will be able to tolerate long-term treatment with tacrine.

Troublesome side effects include nausea, vomiting, diarrhea, headache, dizziness, myalgia, anorexia, and rash. The major problem with high doses of tacrine is hepatotoxicity, seen in about 40% to 50% of patients. Serum alanine transaminase (ALT) levels become elevated and should be monitored weekly for at least 6 weeks after the last dose increase. Since late hepatotoxicity can occur, monthly testing is recommended. If jaundice occurs, tacrine should be discontinued (Kaplan and Sadock, 1996).

Tacrine enhances cholinergic transmission. The tricyclic antidepressants should be avoided. The action of cholinomimetics (bethanecol) and cholinesterase inhibitors (neostigmine) might be enhanced. Davis and Powchik (1995) report increased tacrine blood levels from concurrent cimetidine use and decreased blood levels from smoking tobacco. Patients with a history of gastric bleeding should not take tacrine because it stimulates gastric secretion, which may cause irritation. Tacrine has been found to increase serum theophylline levels to more than twice normal values, so dosage reduction in theophylline and monitoring are recommended.

Tacrine is an expensive drug, and the patients who can most benefit are not clearly characterized at this time. Despite the adverse effect of hepatotoxicity, the drug may be of value for some patients and their families. The effectiveness of tacrine should be evaluated in discussion with the patient and caregiver to determine improvement in mental status and quality of life (Davis and Powchik, 1995).

ANTIDEPRESSANTS
History

In the late 1940s Hafliger and Schindler synthesized imipramine, a dibenzazepine compound (Baldessarini, 1996). Clinical investigation in the late 1950s revealed that it did not sedate agitated psychotic patients like the phenothiazines, but it had a remarkable effect on improving depression. Since the 1960s tricyclic antidepressants (TCA), such as imipramine and amitriptyline, have been widely used for treating depression. Clomipramine (Anafranil) is a TCA, the most serotonin-selective of the TCAs, and is specifically used to treat obsessive-compulsive disorder. High mortality associated with overdose is a major safety concern. Alcohol potentiates the TCAs, and, even alone, they are potentially lethal with overdose. Depressed persons with suicidal ideation or impulsivity are particularly at high risk if taking TCAs (see Danger in Overdose section p. 848).

The monoamine oxidase inhibitors were developed for treating tuberculosis (TB), beginning with isoniazid in 1951. TB patients treated with iproniazid, a derivative of isoniazid, had mood elevations. Monoamine oxidase (MAO) was discovered as having an influence on mood; in 1952 MAO inhibitors were used effectively to treat depression

Table 23-8 Pharmacotherapy for Agitated Behavioral Disturbances in Dementia Patients

Behavior	Agent	Approximate daily dosage range (maximum dose not usually recommended for treatment)
Agitation	Haloperidol	.25 - 4 mg (max)
	Trazodone	25 - 300 mg (max)
	Carbamazepine	50 - 800 mg (max)
	Valproate	125 - 1000 mg (max)
	Lorazepam	.5 - 2 mg (max)
	Buspirone	5 - 30 mg (max)
	Propranolol	10 - 100 mg (max)

Data from Cummings JL: Differential diagnosis and medical management of dementia patients. In *Federal Practitioner (supplement)* Birmingham, AL, 1996, Birmingham Regional Medical Education Center, pp 10-16, Liptzin B: Treatment of mania. In Salzman C, ed: Clinical geriatric psychopharmacology, Baltimore, 1992, Williams & Wilkins, pp 175-188; Semla TP, Beizer JL, Higbee MD: *Geriatric dosage handbook,* ed 2, Cleveland, OH, 1995, Lexi-Comp Inc; Watsky E, Salzman C: Prescribing information. In Salzman C, ed: *Clinical geriatric psychopharmacology,* Baltimore, 1992, Williams & Wilkins, pp 303-307.

(Baldessarini, 1996). It was not until the 1960s however, that MAO inhibitors were studied intensively, found to cause mania in some patients, and had dangerous drug interactions and reactions with foods containing tyramine. MAO inhibitors continue to be used but are not considered as safe as the newer agents (see Danger in Overdose section p. 848).

In 1987, a serotonin reuptake inhibitor (SSRI) was introduced. Fluoxetine (Prozac) was the first of this type, with sertraline (Zoloft), paroxetine (Paxil), and fluvoxamine (Luvox) following it. The SSRIs are popular currently because the side effect profile is different from that of the TCAs and the MAO inhibitors; they are also safer in overdose.

Other new agents include the "atypical" antidepressants, such as trazodone (Desyrel), nefazodone (Serzone), venlafaxine (Effexor), mirtazapine (Remeron), and bupropion (Wellbutrin). The neuropharmacology of these agents is less well-defined. Studies in the elderly are limited. Specifically, nefazodone, introduced in 1995, has no published data on efficacy in elderly in comparative trials with other antidepressants. In the treatment of mild to moderate major depression, all antidepressants are equally efficacious. In the treatment of severe major depression with melancholia, tricyclics and venlafaxine are superior to SSRIs. Atypicals and SSRIs are generally better tolerated and have fewer serious side effects than TCAs. More research appears to be needed regarding antidepressants and the elderly, particularly in persons over 70 years old. The classes of antidepressants that are available in the United States and their side effects are listed in Table 23-9.

	Table 23-9	Classes and Side Effects of Antidepressants Available in the United States

Class	Examples	Side Effects
Tricyclic antidepressants (TCA)	• Amitriptyline, doxepin, imipramine, clomipramine	Dry mouth, constipation, urinary retention, orthostasis, sedation
	• Nortriptyline, desipramine	Less of above side effects
Selective serotonin reuptake inhibitors (SSRI)	• Fluoxetine, sertraline, paroxetine, fluvoxamine	Nausea, vomiting, dry mouth, headache, sedation, nervousness, anxiety, dizziness, insomnia, sweating, ejaculatory/orgasmic dysfunction
Atypical blockers (phenethylamine type)	• Bupropion, venlafaxine	Nausea, dry mouth, headache, dizziness, nervousness
Serotonin-2 antagonists/serotonin reuptake inhibitors	• Trazodone, nefazodone	Sedation, orthostasis, nausea, dizziness, headache
Monoamine oxidase inhibitors (MAOI)	• Phenelzine, tranylcypromine	Orthostasis, weight gain, sexual dysfunction (anorgasmia), edema, insomnia

Data compiled from Kaplan HI, Sadock BJ: *Pocket handbook of psychiatric drug treatment,* ed 2, Baltimore, 1996, Williams & Wilkins; Schatzberg AF: Course of depression in adults: treatment options, *Psych Ann* 26(6):336-341, 1996; and Semla TP, Beizer JL, Higbee MD: *Geriatric dosage handbook,* ed 2, Cleveland, 1995, Lexi-Comp Inc.

Definitions and Target Symptoms

Antidepressants, as their name implies, are drugs that counter depression. Depression is defined according to the DSM-IV (1994), to which readers are referred for a detailed description.

Patients may have some depressive symptoms without having a major depressive episode. Sometimes the symptoms will respond to psychotherapy alone. Since the suicide rate rises with increasing age, untreated and inadequately treated depression in the elderly has serious consequences (Newhouse, 1996).

Target symptoms include depressed mood, lack of energy, fatigue, lack of interest in usual activities, inability to concentrate, loss of appetite, weight changes, sleep problems (difficulty falling asleep or staying asleep or early morning awakening), feelings of worthlessness, and suicidal thoughts.

Issues for Elderly

Depression and depressive symptoms occur commonly in the elderly. In the Epidemiologic Catchment Area study, 15% of community residents over 65 years were found to have depressive symptoms (NIH, 1992). This same study reported rates of depression among the elderly ranging between 5% for those in primary care to 15% to 25% for those in nursing homes. Other authors report depressive disorders in up to 31% of the medically ill elderly (Okimoto, Barnes, and Veith, 1982) and up to 45% in hospitalized elderly (Kitchell, Barnes, and Veith, 1982). This high prevalence lends credence to the fact that the majority of prescribers of antidepressants for elderly persons are nonpsychiatrists (Dewan, Huszonek, Koss et al., 1992).

Diagnosing depression in the elderly is complex and problematic. Depression is frequently underdiagnosed in this population (NIH, 1992). The classic symptom of depression—depressed mood—may be less prominent in the elderly than loss of appetite, sleeplessness, loss of energy, loss of interest or pleasure in usual activities, and somatic preoccupation (Rothschild, 1996). Complicating the diagnosis, psychosocial factors and medical problems play contributory roles. That is, depressive symptoms can be thought to be related to the financial, personal, and social losses associated with aging. Likewise, health problems that occur with age limit mobility and enjoyment of usual or special activities. Depression may be the actual illness (a biochemical process), part of a medical illness, an adjustment to changing life circumstances, or response to medications. A past history or a family history of depression may be helpful in determining a current episode. Despite the complexity of diagnosis, inadequately treated depression will markedly compromise the person's quality of life by causing feelings of despair and hopelessness. One of the clinician's challenges is to determine whether the depressive symptoms or a major depression will respond to medication.

Once a diagnosis is made, medication selection requires careful consideration. Prior treatment responses will indicate whether a drug should be tried for subsequent depressive episodes. Age is an important factor because the elderly are more sensitive to anticholinergic and cardiovascular properties of drugs. Dosing low and slowly titrating medication increases are prudent practices for medicating the elderly with antidepressants.

Medical conditions and the type and number of medications currently taken are considerations in selecting an antidepressant medication. For example, a person with glaucoma or with benign prostatic hypertrophy should not be taking medications with anticholinergic effects; hence, the tricyclic antidepressants should be avoided in these persons. The chances for drug interactions and toxic reactions are great in the elderly because they are generally prescribed more medications than are younger patients. Further, most newer antidepressant agents inhibit specific liver-metabolizing enzyme activity (cytochrome P450), resulting in increased plasma levels of concomitantly administered drugs (Ereshefsky, 1996). Fluoxetine, fluvoxamine, paroxetine, and nefazodone have the highest potential for drug interactions because of this enzyme inhibition whereas venlafaxine and bupropion do not inhibit the metabolism of other drugs.

Dementias, including Alzheimer's disease, can worsen with certain antidepressants. That is, anticholinergic properties of TCAs will worsen cognitive abilities and should be avoided in patients with all types of dementia-related (vascular and nonvascular) cognitive impairment. Newhouse (1996) reports effective management of depression with SSRIs in Parkinson's patients without exacerbating the disease but cautions about drug interactions with such drugs as selegiline. Because SSRIs can cause Parkinsonian symptoms, caution is warranted in using SSRIs in patients with Parkinson's disease.

SSRIs cost considerably more than the other, older, antidepressants. If effective against depression, the cost will be much lower than the consequences of inadequately treated depression. The drugs that least interfere with the elderly person's quality of life should be considered. Many sexually active men and women may be concerned about the negative impact SSRIs have on their sex lives but may be unable or unwilling to discuss their concerns. Letting them know that sexual dysfunction (primarily anorgasmia and ejaculatory delay) can occur and can be treated may give patients the permission they need to talk about their concerns.

How Antidepressants Work

All antidepressant medications alter the availability and/or metabolism of the neurotransmitters, norepinephrine and/or serotonin. The TCAs can affect several monamine neurotransmitters, including serotonin, norepinephrine, histamine, and acetylcholine. The MAOIs increase norepinephrine, serotonin, and dopamine by inhibiting monoamine oxidase. The SSRIs inhibit the reuptake of serotonin. These actions or inhibitions occur as soon as the drugs are absorbed, yet it takes 2 to 4 weeks before any antidepressant action occurs. The current explanation of this phenomenon is that antidepressants down-regulate, or make less sensitive, neurotransmitter receptors. This down-regulation occurs over 2 to 4 weeks (e.g., CNS, beta, adrenergic, and $5HT_2$ receptor down-regulation). The newer drugs affect the neurotransmitters in different ways. Briefly, the pharmacodynamics (receptor activity, dose-response, plasma levels and steady state, tolerance, dependence, withdrawal) and pharmacokinetics (drug absorption, distribution, metabolism, excretion) are described in the following sections.

Pharmacodynamics. The pharmacodynamics of how particular antidepressants function will be discussed in the following sections.

TCAs. TCAs reduce the reuptake of norepinephrine and serotonin and block muscarinic acetylcholine and histamine and $alpha_1$ adrenergic receptors. The different tricyclic drugs vary in their pharmacodynamic effects; nortriptyline and desipramine (and others) have the least anticholinergic activity and doxepin has the most antihistaminergic activity. Clomipramine is serotonin-selective, but its primary metabolite is norepinephrine-selective.

MAOIs. MAOIs inhibit monoamine oxidase. Inhibition of MAO prevents degradation of norepinephrine, serotonin, and dopamine (Schatzberg, 1996). Platelet MAO activity needs to be reduced about 80% for achievement of antidepressant effects, which takes 3 to 6 weeks. When the drug is discontinued, the body requires about 2 weeks to replenish its monoamine oxidase (Kaplan and Sadock, 1996).

SSRIs. The SSRIs inhibit the reuptake of serotonin without significant effects on the reuptake of norepinephrine and dopamine although sertraline inhibits dopamine reuptake and is one fourth as potent as amphetamine. The SSRIs, although they differ from each other, have the potential to inhibit cytochrome oxidases. This means that drug interactions can occur with coadministration of other drugs, resulting in reduced clearance with drug accumulation (Newhouse, 1996).

Atypical blockers (Phenethylamine type) (Venlafaxine, Bupropion). Venlafaxine and its metabolite (o-desmethylvenlafaxine) are potent reuptake inhibitors of serotonin and norephinephrine.

One of bupropion's metabolites, hydroxybupropion, is a norepinephrine reuptake inhibitor (Kaplan and Sadock, 1996).

Serotonin-2 antagonists (Trazodone, Nefazodone). Trazodone is a serotonin$_2$ reuptake inhibitor and weak serotonin reuptake inhibitor with one active metabolite. Trazodone has alpha adrenergic antagonist activities and antihistaminergic activity.

Nefazodone antagonizes the serotonin$_2$ receptor and is a weak inhibitor of serotonin reuptake. It has mild short-term norepinephrine reuptake blocking activity. Trazodone and nefazodone have the same $alpha_1$ blocking activity (Cusack, Nelson, and Richelson, 1994).

Presynaptic alpha$_2$ receptor antagonist with $5HT_2$ and $5HT_3$ antagonist properties (Mirtazapine). Mirtazapine is a presynaptic alpha$_2$ receptor antagonist with $5HT_2$ and $5HT_3$ antagonistic properties and acts as an antihistamine. It does not block reuptake of norepinephrine or serotonin nor is it anticholinergic.

Pharmacokinetics. The pharmacokinetics of particular antidepressants will be discussed in the following sections.

TCAs. Over 75% of the TCA drug is protein bound, and the lipid solubility is high. TCAs are metabolized in the liver. They have long half-lives, ranging from 10 to 70 hours or more. These long half-lives mean that once-daily dosing is possible, but 5 to 7 days are required to reach steady state plasma levels (Kaplan and Sadock, 1996).

MAOIs. The only current drugs in this category for antidepressant usage are phenelzine (Nardil), which is a derivative of hydrazine, and tranylcypromine (Parnate), which is a derivative of amphetamine. The hydrazine derivative is metabolized by an acetylation process. The significance of this is that about half of North American and European persons and a higher percentage of Asian persons are slow acetylators; theoretically, this may explain why some persons experience more adverse effects when given usual doses of phenelzine (Baldessarini, 1996; Kaplan and Sadock, 1996). Little is known about the pharmacokinetics of the MAOIs. Maximum inhibition of monamine oxidase occurs within 5 to 10 days. Also clinical efficacy appears best when the drug is given more frequently than once daily.

SSRIs. Plasma protein binding ranges from 80% (fluvoxamine) to 99% (sertraline). SSRIs are metabolized in the liver. Half-lives for the parent drug range from 15 hours (fluvoxamine) to 6 days (fluoxetine). The metabolites of the drugs range in half-lives from 2 to 4 days (sertraline) to 4 to 16 days (fluoxetine); paroxetine and fluvoxamine do not have active metabolites. The long half-life of the metabolite of fluoxetine is the reason that steady state plasma levels are not reached until 7 to 8 weeks of continuous dosing has occurred. While the long half-life minimizes any possible withdrawal symptoms when the drug is discontinued, the risk for drug interactions continues after the drug has been stopped (Kaplan and Sadock, 1996). Usually SSRIs are given once a day, in the morning to minimize risk of insomnia.

Atypical blockers (Phenethylamine type) (Venlafaxine, Bupropion). Venlafaxine has a half-life of about 5 hours. Its active metabolite has a half-life of about 9 to 11 hours (Schatzberg, 1996). Divided dosing is recommended. It is metabolized by the liver, takes 3 days to reach steady state, and is 27% protein bound (Ereshefsky, 1996). The low percentage of protein-binding makes this drug preferable in debilitated patients or those with renal or hepatic failure. Other drugs that are highly protein bound are less likely to interact with the antidepressants that have low protein-binding potential. Venlafaxine causes a dose-related increase in blood pressure and must be used cautiously in patients with hypertension.

Bupropion is metabolized by the liver and has two active metabolites. The half-life is about 12 hours (Kaplan and Sadock, 1996). Dosing should be two to three times daily with no single dose exceeding 150 mg. Because of drug accumulation, bupropion is not recommended for patients with hepatic and renal diseases or a history of seizures.

Serotonin-2 antagonists (Trazodone, Nefazodone). Trazodone has a half-life of 6 to 11 hours, is metabolized in the liver, and 75% of its metabolites are excreted in the urine (Kaplan and Sadock, 1996). It must be given in divided doses.

Nefazodone has a half-life of 2 to 4 hours, and its two active metabolites have half-lives of 4 to 9 hours and 18 to 33 hours, respectively (Schatzberg, 1996). It should be given in divided doses.

Presynaptic alpha$_2$ receptor antagonist with 5HT$_2$ and 5HT$_3$ antagonistic properties (Mirtazapine). Mirtazapine's half-life is 20 to 24 hours; it is metabolized in the liver with 85% of its metabolites excreted in urine. The metabolites are inactive. Steady state is achieved in 5 days following once-a-day dosing. Clearance is reduced 30% in liver disease and 30% to 50% in renal failure.

Side Effects of Antidepressants. The side effect profiles differ between the classes of drugs and are summarized in Table 23-9. Generally, the side effects of the TCAs include dry mouth, constipation, urinary retention, arrhythmias, tachycardia, cardiac conduction defects, blurred vision, sedation, dizziness, and weight gain. Many of these problems are concomitant with aging and become increasingly troublesome when exacerbated by medication.

The MAOI side effects include hypotension, edema, tachycardia, drowsiness, nervousness, paresthesias, skin rash, dry mouth, constipation, urinary retention, impotence, anorgasmia, and peripheral neuropathy. These drugs require medication restrictions and dietary restrictions related to tyramine, tryptophan, and other vasopressors. Elders may find dietary restrictions unpleasant or may not realize the importance of compliance; this is an important pre-treatment discussion and a reason to select another drug. Disregard of these restrictions can produce a life-threatening hypertensive crisis. Tyramine-containing foods include aged cheeses (Camembert, Liederkranz, Edam, Cheddar, Brie, Bleu); soy sauce; fermented, pickled, or tenderized meats or fish; fermented beverages (some beers on tap; some wines). Caffeine products (coffee, colas, tea, chocolate) should be used in moderation because they raise blood pressure, which can be worsened when MAOIs are taken. (Walker, Shulman, Tailor, and Gardner [1996] offer a complete and updated list of tyramine-containing foods, particularly those previously restricted.) Some of the drugs that interact with MAOIs to produce a hypertensive crisis include L-dopa, amphetamines, cocaine, phenylephrine, pseudoephedrine, and epinephrine. (Over-the-counter cold remedies often contain phenylephrine or pseudoephedrine.) Drugs interacting with MAOIs to produce serotonin syndrome include SSRIs, venlafaxine, nefazodone, and trazodone. (Serotonin syndrome is a state of serotonergic hyperstimulation. Clinical features include confusion, restlessness, myoclonus, hyperreflexia, diaphoresis, shivering, and tremor. These symptoms do not specifically indicate serotonin syndrome.) To prevent dangerous crises when a patient changes antidepressants, a drug-free period is recommended. If an MAOI is discontinued, a waiting period of up to 15 days precludes initiation of a TCA. Similarly, if a TCA is discontinued, a 1-week waiting period must elapse before an MAOI can be initiated. If fluoxetine is discontinued and an MAOI trial is planned, 7 to 8 drug-free weeks are needed (Alexopoulos, 1992).

Also 15 days should elapse before starting mirtazapine following MAOI therapy.

The side effects of the SSRIs include nausea, vomiting, diarrhea, insomnia, tremor, nervousness, headache, sexual dysfunction, and dry mouth.

Three of 2796 patients developed agranulocytosis when treated with mirtazapine, which remitted when the drug was stopped. There is a warning to discontinue the drug should fever, sore throat, and decreased white blood cell count occur.

Side effects can be minimized with attention to drug and dose selection. In a review of actual prescribing practices for the elderly in 1986 and 1989, Dewan et al. (1992) recommended elimination of medications with greater side effects. According to several authors (Buffum, 1996; Dewan et al., 1992) the drugs to eliminate included amitriptyline and doxepin. Geriatric Dosage Guidelines (Buffum, 1996) for one Veterans Affairs Medical Center, based on the facility's formulary, are listed in Table 23-10. These include antidepressants and all other types of psychiatric medications.

Danger in Overdose. Suicidal feelings and impulsivity pose safety concerns when the TCAs are prescribed. That is, an overdose can produce QRS (quinidine-like) arrhythmias, tachycardia, and hypotension that are all unresponsive to

Table 23-10	Geriatric Dosage Guidelines for one Veterans Affairs Medical Center	
Drug	**Dosage recommended**	**Comments**
Antipsychotics		
Chlorpromazine	Psychosis: 800 mg/day	Divided doses
	Dementia: 75 mg/day	
Fluphenazine	Psychosis: 20 mg/day	Doses exceeding 7.5 mg/day do not improve therapeutic outcome, but only increase
	Dementia: 7.5 mg/day	side effects
Haloperidol	Psychosis: 50 mg/day	Doses exceeding 7.5 mg/day do not improve therapeutic outcome, but only increase
	Dementia: 4 mg/day	side effects
Loxapine	Psychosis: 125 mg/day	Doses exceeding 37.5 mg/day do not improve therapeutic outcome, but only increase
	Dementia: 10 mg/day	side effects
Perphenazine	Psychosis: 32 mg/day	Doses exceeding 37.5 mg/day do not improve therapeutic outcome, but only increase
	Dementia: 20 mg/day	side effects
Thioridazine	Psychosis: 400 mg/day	Doses exceeding 375 mg/day do not improve therapeutic outcome, but only increase
	Dementia: 75 mg/day	side effects
Thiothixene	Psychosis: 30 mg/day	Doses exceeding 19 mg/day do not improve therapeutic outcome, but only increase
	Dementia: 7 mg/day	side effects
Trifluoperazine	Psychosis: 40 mg/day	Doses exceeding 19 mg/day do not improve therapeutic outcome, but only increase
	Dementia: 8 mg/day	side effects
Antidepressants		
Amitriptyline	—	All use should be avoided
Desipramine	10-25 mg/day initially; titrate up to 150 mg/day	Titrate dose up by 10-25 mg/day every 2-4 days (every week for outpatients) to a maximum of 150 mg/day
Doxepin	— Dermatologic use: 10-25 mg/day initially; titrate up to 150 mg/day	All psychiatric use should be avoided; care should be used when required for dermatologic use: 10-25 mg/day initially; titrate dose up by 10-25 mg/day every 3-4 days (every week for outpatients) to a maximum of 150 mg/day
Imipramine	10-25 mg/day initially; maximum of 150 mg/day	Titrate dose up by 10-25 mg/day every 2-4 days (every week for outpatients) to a maximum of 150 mg/day
Nortriptyline	25 mg/day initially	Titrate dose up by 25 mg/day every 3 days (every week for outpatients) to a maximum of 75 mg/day or serum levels of 50-150 ng/ml
Trazodone	25-50 mg/day initially; titrate up to 150 mg/day	Titrate dose up by 25-50 mg/day every 3 days (every week for outpatients) to a maximum of 300 mg/day
Antianxiety agents		
Alprazolam	.125-.25 mg twice daily; maximum of .75 mg/day	Higher doses permissible if necessary for maintenance of functional status; dosage reduction should be attempted twice within 1 year before it can be concluded that dosage reduction is clinically contraindicated

From Buffum J: *Geriatric Dosage Guidelines,* VA Medical Center, San Francisco, 1996.

treatment. The average lethal dose of imipramine is 30 mg/kg (Kaplan and Sadock, 1996). Prescriptions should be limited to a 1-week supply if the patients is at suicide risk.

Overdose with the MAOIs is fatal with single doses of 1.75 to 7g. (Kaplan and Sadock, 1996). Symptoms at lethal levels include hypotension, mental confusion, and tachycardia.

Lethal doses of the SSRIs have not been established. They are considered safer than the TCAs; the MAOIs are rarely used in elders. There have been no reported deaths from overdose on mirtazapine alone.

How Long to Treat? Recurrence of depression can occur at any age and the consequences can be lethal. Length of treatment for the elderly is not well documented in the research literature, but some authors recommend treatment for 6 months for a first episode in patients over 60 years of age (Newhouse, 1996). Longer treatment should continue up to 1 to 2 years if the person has had a prior depressive episode. Lifetime maintenance is considered when the person has had three or more episodes that have been severe enough to warrant hospitalization. Doses should be tapered to prevent withdrawal symptoms when the person stops the medication.

Decisions regarding treatment for depression must go beyond the decision of which medication is best. Actual situational adjustments that create depression must be dealt with as grieving processes that have healing properties if dealt with supportively. For a discussion of depression from the psychosocial perspective, see Chapter 21.

Treatment with Stimulants. Patients who suffer from depressive symptoms (but are not clinically depressed),

Table 23-10   Geriatric Dosage Guidelines for one Veterans Affairs Medical Center—cont'd

Drug	Dosage recommended	Comments
Antianxiety agents—cont'd		
Chlordiazepoxide	— If lorazepam is unsuccessful, maximum of 20 mg/day	All use should be avoided, unless lorazepam has been tried unsuccessfully; daily use should be less than 4 continuous months unless an attempt at gradual dosage reduction has been unsuccessful; higher dosage than 20 mg/day if necessary for maintenance of functional status; dosage reduction should be attempted twice within 1 year before it can be concluded that dosage reduction is clinically contraindicated.
Clonazepam	— If lorazepam is unsuccessful, for control of acute manic agitation, maximum of 1.5 mg/day in divided doses	All use should be avoided; daily use should be less than 4 continuous months unless an attempt at gradual dosage reduction has been unsuccessful; exceptions are for seizure disorder, nocturnal myoclonus, tardive dyskinesia, or maintenance of functional status; dosage reductions should be attempted twice within 1 year before it can be concluded that dosage reduction is clinically contraindicated.
Diazepam	— If lorazepam unsuccessful, maximum of 5 mg/day	All use should be avoided unless lorazepam has been tried unsuccessfully; daily use should be less than 4 continuous months unless an attempt at gradual dosage reduction has been unsuccessful; exceptions are for seizure disorder, tardive dyskinesia, or maintenance of functional status; dosage reduction should be attempted twice within 1 year before it can be concluded that dosage reduction is clinically contraindicated.
Lorazepam	.5-1.0 mg/day, divided doses initially, maximum of 2 mg/day, maximum hypnotic dose of 1 mg/day	Higher dose than 2 mg/day if necessary for maintenance of functional status; dosage reduction should be attempted twice within 1 year before it can be concluded that dosage reduction is clinically contraindicated.
Diphenhydramine	25 mg/three times a day	All hypnotic use should be avoided; increase dose as needed for other indications.
Sedative/hypnotic agents		
Chloral hydrate	Maximum of 500 mg	Daily hypnotic use should not exceed 10 consecutive days unless an attempt at gradual dosage reduction has been unsuccessful; gradual dose reductions should be attempted at least three times within 6 months before it can be concluded that dosage reduction is clinically contraindicated.
Temazepam	7.5 mg initially; maximum of 15 mg/day	Daily hypnotic use should not exceed 10 consecutive days unless an attempt at gradual dosage reduction has been unsuccessful; gradual dose reductions should be attempted at least three times within 6 months before it can be concluded that dosage reduction is clinically contraindicated.
Triazolam	Maximum of .125	Daily hypnotic use should not exceed 10 consecutive days unless an attempt at gradual dosage reduction has been unsuccessful; gradual dose reductions should be attempted at least three times within 6 months before it can be concluded that dosage reduction is clinically contraindicated.

might demonstrate apathy or disinterest in their surroundings, lack of energy, and withdrawal. These symptoms in the elderly respond to central nervous system stimulants such as amphetamine or methylphenidate. These agents are effective in chronically medically ill elderly who have become demoralized and refuse participation in rehabilitation. These stimulants are not antidepressants.

Methylphenidate (Ritalin) and d-amphetamine (Dexedrine) should be given only in the morning and early afternoon to prevent insomnia at night. Like all psychotropic medications, dosing should start low (2.5 to 5 mg/day) and titrate slowly, increasing every 2 or 3 days (by 2.5 to 5 mg) until a total of 20 mg/day is reached (Lohr et al., 1992). Side effects are tachycardia, mild blood pressure increases, agitation, restlessness, and confusion. Methamphetamine (Desoxyn) has similar effects. Patients on these medications should be encouraged to resume all daily activities. Responses should include motivation, interest, attention, and sense of well-being.

Elders are at risk for depression from a variety of causes. Declining physical health or a medical condition, loss of friends and family, adjustment to retirement, medication interactions or side effects, or a major depressive episode are possible causes. The antidepressants available include TCAs, MAOIs, SSRIs, and the newer atypical medications. The selection of the appropriate drug for the particular person should be based on prior successful treatment with the medication, family history, medical conditions, and other medications. Side effects may be dose-related and must be closely monitored; they can be unpleasant and dangerous. Nursing concerns include assessing and monitoring physical, emotional, and social changes, and patient and family education.

MOOD STABILIZERS

Mood stabilizers are the group of agents used for the treatment of mania associated with bipolar disorder. They are also used for schizoaffective disorder, major depression, schizophrenia, and impulse control disorders. Pharmacologic treatments include lithium, anticonvulsants such as carbamazepine and valproic acid, and calcium channel blockers such as verapamil. Ancillary medications for use in acute mania before onset of mood stabilizers include benzodiazepines (lorazepam and clonazepam are most studied but have no specific antimanic properties) and antipsychotics.

Particular features are prominent in the elderly who suffer from mania. That is, the person may demonstrate confusion, paranoia, labile affect, pressured speech and flight of ideas, morbid or depressive content, increased psychomotor activity resembling agitated depression, long period between depressive episode and appearance of mania, and altered orientation and attention span (Liptzin, 1992).

History and Target Symptoms

Past treatments of mania have included sedatives, neuroleptics, and electroconvulsive therapy. In 1970, lithium became the drug of choice for treating mania, preventing episodes of mania and depression in bipolar illness. Lithium continues to be the favored drug. However, if rapid cycling, mixed mania, or substance-induced mania is present, valproic acid or carbamazapine is the drug of choice. The addition of these latter drugs occurred in the 1980s. Mood stabilizers such as lithium target explosive behaviors and mood fluctuations. As the drug of choice, lithium is discussed in the following section. Geriatric dosing, side effects, and nursing actions are listed for lithium, carbamazepine, and valproic acid in Table 23-11.

Issues for Elderly

The safe use of lithium requires pretreatment medical workup. Baseline thyroid function tests should be performed. Although the evaluation should focus on cardiac, renal, and thyroid functions, mental status is another important assessment. Some authors suggest an electroencephalogram before and during treatment to determine the baseline and to observe for lithium-related changes in the brain. Evaluating for evidence of dementia, memory loss, or confusion is essential because lithium can cause these changes. Likewise, tremor or lack of coordination should be evaluated. A baseline creatinine level should be obtained because lithium may cause an elevated level in the elderly; this may not mean renal function is impaired but may indicate an age-related skeletal muscle tissue breakdown. Further evaluation would be indicated if levels are elevated.

Evaluation should include a list of medications and an assessment of the type of diet. Lithium interacts with other medications and certain foods. For example, a low salt diet will elevate and a high salt diet will decrease the lithium level. Likewise, thiazide diuretics and nonsteroidal antiinflammatory agents (NSAIDS) will elevate serum lithium level.

How Lithium Works

Pharmacodynamics. Lithium's exact therapeutic mechanism remains uncertain (Kaplan and Sadock, 1996). Theoretically, lithium blocks an enzyme (inositol-1-phosphatase) within neurons, which results in decreased cellular responses to neurotransmitters.

Pharmacokinetics. Lithium is rapidly absorbed by the gastrointestinal tract. Because it is not plasma protein bound, it is not affected by variations in protein levels secondary to aging, nutritional state, or physical illness. Distributed throughout total body water, lithium levels are higher in the elderly because of the age-related reduction in body water; this is particularly true for women. Lithium is excreted by the kidneys. Decreased renal function in the elderly results in a 30% to 60% decrease in creatinine clearance. This age-related change causes less lithium clearance, prolonging the half-life from 20 hours in young adults to 34 hours in elderly (Liptzin, 1992).

Side Effects. Side effects are the same for the young and old in spite of the use of lower dosage and serum levels in the geriatric population. Although toxicity is not usually a problem, those at risk for serious side effects include the physically ill, very old, frail, cognitively impaired, and those on multiple medications. Side effects include the following: confusion, disorientation, memory loss; flattening of T-waves on the electrocardiogram; polyuria and polydipsia; nausea, vomiting, diarrhea; fine resting tremor; benign goiter; ataxia. Lithium-induced hypothyroidism, more common in women than men, may resemble dementia or depression. Thyroid levels should be checked every 3 to 6 months. Fortunately, careful monitoring can prevent toxic reactions. At toxic concentrations, the lithium level is elevated (>2 mEq/l) and all of the symptoms mentioned previously worsen. For example, resting tremor becomes a gross tremor.

Dosing. Starting dose for the elderly manic patient should be 300 mg twice daily. The dose may be increased weekly in increments of 300 mg/day to achieve a maximum dose of 900 to 1200 mg/day (Semla, Beizer, and Higbee,

1995). Serum concentration and clinical response determine proper dose. Serum concentrations must be monitored frequently, with an interval of 12 hours after the last dose before blood can be drawn. Therapeutic effects in acute mania may be seen in the elderly when the level is .6 to 1.2 mEq/L (Semla, Beizer, and Higbee, 1995). Maintenance for relapse prevention can be achieved with lower levels of .6 to .8 mEq/L. Although this is a low level in younger persons, it is therapeutic for the elderly if symptoms of mania are improved. As with other psychotropic medications, the rule for the elderly applies: start low and go slow. As always, the nurse must monitor for side effects. Lithium has a narrow margin between therapeutic and toxic levels in the blood. Frequent serum lithium levels should be determined until the patient is stabilized and then checks should be done monthly. The patient needs to learn symptoms of minor toxicity (nausea, vomiting, weakness, diarrhea, drowsiness). Also the patient needs to maintain adequate hydration.

Table 23-11   Lithium, Carbamazepine, Valproic Acid: Dosages, Side Effects, and Nursing Actions

Drug	Geriatric dose	Side effects	Nursing actions
Lithium	300 mg twice daily initially; increase by 300 mg increments weekly according to clinical state and therapeutic serum range; maximum dose of 900-1200 mg/day in divided doses Serum concentration .6-1.2 mEq/L for therapeutic effects Serum concentration .6-.8 mEq/L for maintenance	Confusion Polyuria Polydipsea Nausea Vomiting Diarrhea Tremor Ataxia Thyroid changes Renal changes (Narrow margin between therapeutic and toxic blood levels)	Take drug with food Monitor mental status Monitor fluid intake and output Monitor salt intake Weight gain/loss Avoid excess caffeine Observe for electrolyte imbalance Observe for resting tremor and coarseness Observe motor coordination, ensure safety in case of fall Monitor blood level frequently (weekly, then monthly) Teach patient symptoms of toxicity
Carbamazepine	200 mg twice daily initially, with meals; increase by 200 mg/day at 2-3 week intervals; maximum dose for acute mania of 800-1200 mg/day in divided doses or 7-15 mg/kg/day to attain therapeutic blood level Blood level of 6-12 µg/mL is therapeutic	Confusion Memory loss Ataxia Hepatotoxicity Impaired water excretion Depression of bone marrow—leukopenia	Take drug with food Monitor mental status Observe for oversedation Monitor motor coordination, ensure safety in case of fall Monitor fluid intake and output Observe for infection Monitor blood levels weekly for 6 wks, then monthly
Valproic acid, divalproex	125 mg/day initially; increase as tolerated and as necessary Research in elderly limited; maintenance dose for anticonvulsant action of 30-60 mg/kg/day in divided doses Blood level of 50 to 100 µg/ml recommended	GI symptoms (anorexia, nausea, vomiting, dyspepsia, diarrhea) Neurologic symptoms (tremor, sedation, ataxia) Alopecia Increased appetite Weight gain Hepatotoxicity Decreased platelets	Take drug with food (except divalproex) Monitor for side effects Monitor liver function tests and platelets Avoid in patients with liver dysfunction Do not crush enteric-coated drug (divalproex) or capsules Watch for signs of bruising or bleeding

From Liptzin B: Treatment of mania. In Salzman C, editor: *Clinical geriatric psychopharmacology,* Baltimore, 1992, Williams & Wilkins, pp 175-188, and Semla TP, Beizer JL, Higbee MD: *Geriatric dosage handbook,* ed 2, Cleveland, 1995, Lexi-Comp Inc.

ANXIOLYTICS

Drugs used to treat anxiety are referred to as anxiolytics or antianxiety agents or sometimes as sedatives. These agents include benzodiazepines, buspirone, beta-blockers, and antihistaminics. In the early 1900s, barbiturates, such as phenobarbital, were used, and in the 1950s meprobamate was popular. These drugs are hazardous for elderly persons because of increasingly toxic sedative properties, psychological and physical dependence, withdrawal seizures, confusion and delirium, and lethal overdoses. These drugs are no longer used.

Anxiety is a universal human emotion, which ranges from a normal mild apprehension to an emotionally disabling disorder. Causative factors can be situational, psychosocial, personality-related, medically related, psychiatric illness, or other drugs. Examples of contributory drugs are caffeine, phenylpropanolamine (cold remedies), MAOIs, desipramine, and fluoxetine (Salzman, 1992). Persons who have been anxious most their adult lives might be anxious to an even greater degree as geriatrics. An elder who has a debilitating medical illness may become anxious about facing death. Further, anxiety can appear without apparent reason. In the elderly, anxiety can appear similar to depression because the person has depressed mood, difficulty concentrating, difficulty sleeping, and appetite changes. Symptoms might also include dizziness, memory changes, feelings of impending faintness or heart attack, and a feeling of "going crazy" (Salzman, 1992). The decision to treat anxiety pharmacologically must be based on the person's degree of impairment, extent of preoccupation, inability to perform activities of daily living, and subjective feelings of discomfort.

Benzodiazepines

Although benzodiazepines have been available for almost 30 years, only minimal research has been done in the el-

| Table 23-12 | Benzodiazepines and Half-Lives in the Elderly |

Benzodiazepine	Half-life
Oxazepam (Serax)	5-20 hours
Lorazepam (Ativan)	10-20 hours
Alprazolam (Xanax)	12-15 hours
Chlordiazepoxide (Librium)	30-96 hours (not recommended for elderly)
Clonazepam (Klonopin)	20-50 hours (not recommended for elderly)
Diazepam (Valium)	100 hours (not recommended for elderly)
Flurazepam (Dalmane)	>100 hours (not recommended for elderly)
Temazepam (Restoril)	11 hours
Triazolam (Halcion)	2 hours

Data compiled from Semla TP, Beizer JL, Higbee MD: *Geriatric dosage handbook,* ed 2, Cleveland, 1995, Lexi-Comp Inc.

derly. What is evident, however, is that there are toxic effects in the elderly. Specifically, the toxic effects include sedation, unsteady gait, confusion, disorientation, cognitive impairment, memory impairment, agitation, and wandering. Because these symptoms resemble dementia, elderly persons can easily be misdiagnosed once begun on benzodiazepines. Another danger about this class of drugs is the central nervous system depression that results when they are combined with alcohol, hypnotics, analgesics, narcotics, and some antidepressants and neuroleptics. Unsteady gait can lead to risk of falls and hip fractures.

If possible, the benzodiazepines should be avoided. If necessary, lorazepam can be prescribed in doses up to 1 mg; these doses have been shown to have negligible effects on memory (Sunderland, Weingartner, Cohen et al., 1989). Some patients have reported no problems with benzodiazepines while others object to the sedation and memory problems. Guidelines for using benzodiazepines include use of a short half-life agent, brief treatment period, and careful monitoring for safety. Elderly persons on benzodiazepines for lengthy periods of time (longer than 1 year) will experience withdrawal symptoms should they discontinue use. Mild withdrawal symptoms include irritability, headache, muscle twitching, tremor, insomnia, anxiety, difficulty concentrating; sensory hypersensitivity, depersonalization, nausea, and abnormal movement sensations are distinctive withdrawal symptoms; serious withdrawal symptoms include depression, paranoia, delirium, hallucinosis, and seizures (Roy-Byrne, 1988).

Pharmacodynamics. Benzodiazepines potentiate the effects of GABA and other inhibitory neurotransmitters. These agents bind to specific benzodiazepine-receptor sites in various areas of the central nervous system (Semla, Beizer, and Higbee, 1995).

Pharmacokinetics. Intravenous administration is for seizure activity, and intramuscular absorption is slow and irregular and not recommended; lorazepam is available in parenteral form and is the only one that has rapid and reliable absorption from an intramuscular route (Kaplan and Sadock, 1996). With the exceptions of lorazepam, temazepam, and oxazepam, the benzodiazepines are metabolized in the liver, bind extensively to plasma albumin (diazepam is 98% protein bound), and have metabolites that are both therapeutic and toxic (chlordiazepoxide, diazepam, halazepam). Since the time required to reach steady state is related to the elimination half-life, the elderly require a long time to reach steady state when the half-lives are long. See Table 23-12 for the different drugs and half-lives in geriatrics.

Side Effects. Although there are various short, intermediate, and long-acting benzodiazepines, the side effects are similar. The most common side effect is drowsiness. Other effects include dizziness, ataxia, mild cognitive deficits, and memory impairment. The high potency drugs (small dosage drugs: triazolam, lorazepam, alprazolam, midazolam, clonazepam) have been associated with anterograde amnesia.

Disinhibition is common, and triazolam received media attention for association with aggressive behavioral manifestations. Since toxicity develops easily in the elderly, only short-term treatment is recommended with agents with relatively short half-lives. However, triazolam, the agent with the shortest half-life, is associated with rebound insomnia and abrupt withdrawal symptoms.

Some authors recommend against the following specific benzodiazepines for use in the elderly: chlordiazepoxide, clorazepate, diazepam, prazepam, flurazepam, and quazepam (Semla, Beizer, and Higbee, 1995). Others suggest avoiding those agents with long half-lives, several active metabolites, strong sedative effects, or those causing morning drowsiness (Salzman, 1992). Lorazepam, which has a short half-life and no active metabolites, is a safe choice in the elderly.

Buspirone

Pharmacodynamics. Buspirone selectively antagonizes central nervous system serotonin $5HT_1A$ receptors without affecting the benzodiazepine-GABA receptors. Decrease in anxiety occurs after 1 week; full effects are evident after 3 to 4 weeks.

Pharmacokinetics. Research in the elderly is limited. Buspirone is 95% protein bound and is metabolized by the liver. Its half-life is 2 to 3 hours (range 2 to 11 hours), thus requiring multiple daily dosing.

Side Effects. Common side effects include dizziness, light headedness, nervousness, headache, nausea, diarrhea, and dry mouth.

Dosing. Geriatric dosing is more than half of adult dose. Initially, 5 mg twice daily should be given with increases by 5 mg/day every 2 to 3 days to 20 to 30 mg/day. The maximum daily dose is 60 mg/day.

Other Agents

Propranolol and diphenhydramine have been used as antianxiety agents but have disadvantages in the elderly. Propranolol (Inderal), a beta-blocker, is indicated for hypertension, arrhythmias, tremors, migraine headaches, and sometimes anxiety. Its usefulness in the elderly is not well documented as an antianxiety agent. However, it is used for parkinsonian tremor, aggressive behavior, akathisia, anxiety, and schizophrenia. Propranolol is contraindicated in conditions such as congestive heart failure, asthma, chronic obstructive pulmonary disease, diabetes, and Raynaud's syndrome. Caution is advised and careful monitoring is necessary when administering to patients with renal or hepatic impairment. Hypotension, congestive heart failure, cardiac conduction defects, bradycardia, and depression are adverse effects that can easily occur in the elderly.

Diphenhydramine (Benadryl) is an antihistamine that is useful for antianxiety properties. It is sedating but has anticholinergic properties. By itself, diphenhydramine can produce dry mouth, blurred vision, urinary retention, and con-stipation. (As discussed in the antipsychotic and antidepressant sections previously, anticholinergics in the elderly can be cumulative and produce confusion, disorientation, oversedation, agitation, and delirium.) As specified in the *Geriatric Dosage Guidelines* (Table 23-10) its use requires caution.

HYPNOTICS

Sleep problems are common in elderly persons, and many medicate frequently or daily to ensure a good night of sleep. The underlying cause of sleeplessness must be assessed. Three distinguishing classifications include: dyssomnias (internal or external problems, circadian rhythm problems), parasomnias (abnormal behaviors during sleep), and medical/psychiatric sleep disorders (anxiety, sleep terror, depression, psychoses) (Gillin and Ancoli-Israel, 1992). The usual medications prescribed for insomnia are benzodiazepines. (Their pharmacodynamic and pharmacokinetic actions are covered in the anxiolytic section presented previously.) Other medications include chloral hydrate, antihistamines, aspirin, neuroleptics, and antidepressants.

Some persons have been on specific medications, such as barbiturates, for years or even decades. Tolerance, dependence, and withdrawal symptoms are reasons for selecting sleep medication carefully and for brief periods of time. Barbiturates are currently not the first drug of choice.

Benzodiazepines are recommended with caution. Rebound insomnia and excitation on withdrawal can occur with short half-life agents such as oxazepam, triazolam, and lorazepam. Only temporary use of up to 1 week is recommended. Temazepam (Restoril) has a short half-life (10 to 20 hours), is intermediate-acting, and produces some morning hangover but less rebound insomnia than oxazepam. Triazolam is a short half-life agent (2 to 5 hours) that causes fast onset of deep but brief sleep and produces less next-day sedation; however, it is associated with daytime anxiety, agitation, anterograde amnesia, and delirium (Regestein, 1992). If used, the Geriatric Dosage Guideline (Buffum, 1996) should be followed with a low dose of .125 mg. There are no reasons for using long half-life benzodiazepines (flurazepam, diazepam, clonazepam) in the elderly.

Sedating drugs, such as the benzodiazepines, contribute to confusion and gait disturbances. Many elderly awaken during the night to use the bathroom or to move about their homes. They are at risk for falls during the night—the time when medicated. The patients and their families or caregivers need information about this effect.

Chloral hydrate is an older inexpensive hypnotic, which is effective in elderly persons. Its half-life is 8 hours and it acts quickly. However, it interacts with other drugs by inducing hepatic enzymes (it increases rates of metabolism of other agents, such as anticoagulants) or by displacing drugs from proteins (diuretics) (Regestein, 1992). The dose, usually 500 mg, is not fixed. That is, some elders require higher doses, up to 2 g.

Drug Regimen Review Checklist

Does the Patient and His or Her Family or Responsible Party

Understand their rights to know the particular disease state or condition?

Understand the need for each of the patient's medications?

Understand the risks and benefits of each drug?

Understand the laboratory and physical assessments being done to monitor responses to treatment?

Understand that the nurse, physician, and pharmacist are responsible for following the patient's care and are available for any questions.

Modified from Cooper JW: *Drug-related problems in geriatric nursing home patients,* New York, 1991, Pharmaceutical Products Press.

Antihistamines, as discussed previously, are not ideal for elderly persons. However, those who can tolerate anticholinergic properties may benefit from the recommended small dose (diphenhydramine, 25 mg).

Some persons find aspirin useful for insomnia. Regestein (1992) reports that it loses effectiveness with chronic use. It produces no withdrawal or sleep pattern alterations.

Low doses of sedating antipsychotics may be helpful, but side effects must be monitored in the elderly. Thioridazine is preferable with doses of 25 to 75 mg. Side effects to monitor include anticholinergic effects, orthostatic hypotension, confusion, next-day drowsiness, altered cognitive ability, tardive dyskinesia, and parkinsonian symptoms.

Low doses of antidepressants are also used in the elderly for sleep problems. Trazodone 25 to 75 mg may be effective and less habituating than the benzodiazepines.

Zolpidem (Ambien) is a BZ_1 agonist useful in treating insomnia. It has a short half-life (9.9 hours in elderly) and no active metabolites. Initial doses of 5 mg are recommended in

Table 23-13	Nursing Interventions for Side Effects of Psychotropic Medications

Type of drug	Common side effects	Nursing interventions
Antipsychotic	Sedation	Reassure patient/family that this side effect subsides in 5-10 days; prevent falls; avoid work requiring alertness, such as driving; dosing only at hour of sleep (HS) may decrease sedation during day.
	Orthostatic hypotension (more pronounced with low potency medications)	Teach patient to dangle feet at bedside for 1-2 minutes before rising; rise slowly; support stockings may be helpful; prevent falling or tripping on obstacles.
	Photosensitivity Photophobia	Protect skin from sun with clothing and sunscreen; sunglasses may be more comfortable because of dilated pupils.
	Hyperthermia	Maintain adequately cool environment; teach patient to avoid hot temperatures and to increase water intake; ensure adequate hydration.
	Weight gain	Discuss with patient/family that this is a side effect; consult with dietitian for dietary planning; encourage avoidance of fattening foods; sweets may be craved to counteract sedation.
	Acute dystonic reactions (more common with some high potency medications)	Simpson-Angus testing at regular times of day; Cogentin 0.5 mg IM for immediate relief (may repeat if .5 ineffective); observe for confusion associated with anticholinergic properties of Cogentin; reassure patient of immediate and full recovery with injection; for prevention thereafter, use Amantadine; monitor for repeat EPS reactions; assess need for changing medication; assess patient compliance related to EPS.
	Parkinsonism	Same as above; may give Cogentin po; reassurance needed.
	Tardive dyskinesia (may occur after 3-6 months of continuous treatment)	Assess for signs using AIMS test; observe for tongue movements and involuntary movement early in treatment; decrease dose of medication, change drug, consider Vitamin E; if antipsychotic discontinued, tardive will get worse; if give Cogentin, tardive will appear worse. Much support is needed, as this is not always reversible.
	Akathisia	Assess for signs using Barnes Scale; decrease dose, change drug, consider propranolol. Reassure patient that this is a side effect and will subside; difficult and uncomfortable to tolerate; monitor for safety and impulsive behavior related to anxiety and distress.

Data compiled from Keltner NL, Schwecke LH, Bostrom CE: *Psychiatric nursing: a psychotherapeutic approach,* St Louis, 1991, Mosby.

patients over 65 years (Semla, Beizer, and Higbee, 1995). For quickest onset, the nurse should give this drug to the patient on an empty stomach. The debilitated and frail elderly should be observed for impaired cognitive or motor performance.

NURSING CONSIDERATIONS

All of the medications presented in this chapter have indications, side effects, interactions, and individual patient reactions. The nurse's advocacy role includes education for the patient and family or caregiver. Box 23-8 lists questions for the nurse to consider when reviewing the drug regimen with the patient and family. Further, the nurse can determine whether side effects are minimal and tolerable or serious. Asking the patient produces subjective data and observing the patient's interactions, behavior, mood, emotional responses, and daily habits provides objective data. From this compilation of data, patient problems can be delineated, nursing diagnoses developed, outcome criteria planned, and

interventions initiated. Nursing actions for the side effects associated with each drug class are presented in Table 23-13. These actions will help guide care planning for individual elderly persons.

Nursing care planning can be applied to the following case study. Students are advised to refer to their nursing diagnosis text and identify possible or potential problems.

KEY CONCEPTS

- Biochemical processes in the brain influence all activities including behavior, emotion, mood, cognition, and movement.
- Neurotransmitters, of which there are many yet only partially identified or understood, are the chemicals that stimulate these processes.
- The side effects of psychotropic medications vary significantly and thus must be selected with care when prescribed for the aged.

Table 23-13   Nursing Interventions for Side Effects of Psychotropic Medications—cont'd

Type of drug	Common side effects	Nursing interventions
Anticholinergic effects of antipsychotics, antidepressants, antiparkinson agents	Blurred vision	Encourage use of magnifying glass and adequate lighting; reassure that the side effect subsides (up to 2 weeks); refer to physician if continues.
	Urinary hesitancy (particularly in elderly men with benign prostatic hypertrophy)	Consider less anticholinergic drug; encourage patient to report this symptom; provide privacy, run water in the sink, warm water over perineum.
	Urinary retention	Encourage frequent voiding, whenever urge exists; teach patient to monitor output; catheterization may be indicated; observe for discomfort, pain.
	Dry mouth	Give water, ice, sugar-free lozenges or candy or gum; often a disturbing side effect and may be associated with bad breath; provide materials for adequate oral hygiene; explain that this is a side effect.
	Constipation	Often a problem in elderly without medication; add fluids, fruit, vegetables to diet; prune juice at HS or in AM, (patient preference); stool softener can be helpful. Monitor for bowel movement frequency and bowel sounds to prevent obstruction or ileus.
	Dizziness	Teach patient to change positions slowly, especially from stooping or sitting to standing (tying shoes, lying in bed).
	Tiredness/sedation	Teach to avoid activities requiring alertness and concentration; decrease dose or increase dose more slowly if this occurs with TCAs; give medication at HS if possible; each patient that alcohol and other CNS depressants worsen sedative effect.
Anxiolytics	Sedation Confusion Memory loss Amnesia	Prevent accidents by teaching patient and family to avoid activities requiring alertness; keep patient oriented to environment; assess level of confusion by checking mental status qd; use drug with short half-life and no active metabolites (Lorazepam); teach patient that sedative effects are worsened with alcohol or other CNS depressants.
Lithium	GI effects	Take medication in divided doses with food; observe for worsening of diarrhea (fluid loss).
	Polydipsia	Explain side effect; tendency is to overhydrate; teach patient to maintain adequate hydration (particular vigilance needed if patient exercises vigorously); encourage fluids up to 3000 ml daily.
	Polyuria	Observe for diabetes insipidus; teach patient that frequent urination is a side effect.
	Tremors	Small tremor may be harmless; observe for worsening tremor; can determine whether increased salt intake (lowers lithium level) improves tremor.

Nursing Diagnoses

The following potential diagnoses must be considered as well as diagnoses unique to the particular individual:

NURSING PROCESS AND NURSING DIAGNOSIS
Risk for or Actual Poisoning: Drug Toxicity

Etiologies and Related Factors

Aging process of liver and renal function: metabolism or biotransformation of drugs excretion of drugs
Polypharmacy
Self medication (OTC and Rx)
Inadequate or misunderstood instructions for prescribed medications

Defining Characteristics

Internal (individual) factors
    Reduced vision
    Cognitive or emotional difficulties
    Insufficient finances
External (environmental) factors
    Effects of polypharmacy
    Variables of drug administration
    Effects of drugs in the aging body

Knowledge

Therapeutic ranges of medication
    pharmacokinetics
    side effects
    toxicity
Safe administration of drug
    polypharmacy
    medication/dietary interactions

Clinical Judgment and Related Skills

Administer drugs—all routes in institutional settings
    Plan and implement "drug holidays"
    Act as resource when use of "PRN" medication is being considered
    Plan and implement drug administration routines in home settings for aged individual or family to maintain
    Monitor for effectiveness, side effects, and record
    Patient/family teaching
    Family/community teaching (health maintenance)

Evaluation

Medications correctly taken
Dosage prescribed is congruent with liver and kidney function
Clear instructions provided and evidence of client understanding demonstrated.

NEEDS ADDRESSED AND TASK STRENGTHS

Need to cope with acute and chronic health disorders; need to make own choices (to meet need for basic survival, safety, and security)

Healthy skepticism
Inquisitive regarding effects of medications
Body awareness and monitoring ability
Follows directions but questions untoward effects

- The response of the elder to treatment with psychotropic medications should show reduced distress, clearer thinking, and more appropriate behavior.
- Newer drugs should be prescribed for the elderly with caution as the long-term effects, side effects, and efficacy may vary significantly with the aged.
- The aged are particularly vulnerable to developing movement disorders (extrapyramidal symptoms, parkinsonism, akathisia, dystonias).

- The Health Care Financing Administration and the Congressional Omnibus Budget Reconciliation Act (OBRA) have severely restricted the use of psychotropic drugs for the elderly unless truly needed for specific disorders. Then they must be carefully monitored.
- Antidepressant medications must be tailored to the elder with careful observation for side effects.
- Dosage levels must be carefully titrated for elders, and their responses accurately and consistently recorded.

▲ CASE STUDY

A Patient on Antidepressant Medication

Dr. T., a 69-year-old married father of five, was admitted to the inpatient psychiatric unit for evaluation of suicidal ideation. He had been a physician all of his adult life and retired 3 years ago. He and his wife have enjoyed good health, spend time with their adult children and seven grandchildren, and began attending classes at the community college 2 years ago. Over the last 6 weeks, the patient has become disinterested in activities, refuses to participate in daily walks with his wife, cannot fall asleep at night and naps during the day, and has lost interest in food. In the past month he has lost 15 pounds. He has no past history of depression. His wife is worried about him, as his personality has changed and he is sometimes irritable, acts depressed, and states that life is not worth living. The family brought him to the hospital when they discovered the he was collecting pills from samples he had accumulated over past years and making vague statements about ending his life.

Dr. T's admitting psychiatrist ordered trazodone 50 mg per day at bedtime to increase by 50 mg every 3 days until 300 mg is reached. The patient is skeptical but willing to take the medication: "Well, these newer medications are quite different. I wonder if it will work as well as some of the older ones. Of course, they were often not as effective as one would hope."

Based upon the case study, develop a nursing care plan using the following procedure*:

List comments of client that provides *subjective data.*

List information that provides *objective data.*

From these data, identify and state, using accepted format, two *nursing diagnoses* you determine are most significant to this client at this time.

Determine and state *outcome criteria* for each diagnosis. These must reflect some alleviation of the problem identified in the nursing diagnosis and must be stated in concrete and measurable terms.

Plan and state one or more *interventions* for each diagnosed problem. Provide specific documentation of source used to determine appropriate intervention.

Evaluate success of intervention. Interventions must correlate directly with the stated outcome criteria in order to measure the outcome success.

STUDY QUESTIONS/ACTIVITIES

Develop a specific plan for teaching the patient about his medication using the following information:

- The medication will not work right away. Onset of therapeutic effects may appear in 1 to 3 weeks. It may

take up to 4 weeks to achieve maximal therapeutic benefit. However, the trazodone should help him sleep, and that is why it is given at bedtime. He may get dizzy upon arising so he should sit on the bed for a few moments. He should report dizziness to the staff if it occurs. Priapism is rare, but it has occurred, and the patient should be informed so that he seeks treatment immediately. He should report symptoms he experiences.

- Be sure patient receives physical exam before medication. Monitor blood pressure and pulse for orthostatic changes. Monitor sedation and ability to perform activities of daily living, providing assistance as needed. Assess sleeping changes. Continue to monitor target symptoms and assess closely for suicidal ideation. Invite communication about any aspect of his care. Involve patient in his care. Involve family to extent that patient is willing. Educate about medication, referring patient to pharmacist for more information and psychiatrist for questions about his care.

What nursing activities must be carried out before administering the medication?

Describe how, when, and why you will monitor blood pressure and pulse.

What effect may this medication have on the patient's abilities to carry on daily activities?

What effect will it have on his sleep patterns?

Discuss recommendations you might make to family members.

▲ CASE STUDY

A Patient on Psychotropic Medication

Mrs. S., a 75-year-old widow of 1 year, was admitted to an unlocked psychiatric unit by her family for symptoms over the past 2 weeks of delusional thinking, agitation, and refusal to eat. Before the 2-week period she had been functioning well and was actively pursuing interests recently acquired with a friend in her apartment complex. She had been married for 50 years until her husband died suddenly of a heart attack during their vacation. She had a history of psychosis in her thirties after the birth of her second child. At that time she was hospitalized for a month and had a 4-week course of chlorpromazine. She recovered fully and has led a productive life as a homemaker and mother of three children. Mrs. S. is close to her two sons and one daughter, all of whom are now in their forties and living in the same town. Her behavior became confusing for her family when she accused them of wanting to be with her for inheritance money. She escalated into thinking that others were after her and she refused entry to her family and friends, some of whom offered food. Mrs. S. was angry at her family for tricking her into going with them to the doctor.

Her daughter reported that Mrs. S. was planning a vacation with her friend, a woman living next door who was also

*Students are advised to refer to their nursing diagnosis text and identify possible or potential problems.

widowed. Also, she had fallen recently but told her daughter she was fine. The daughter wondered whether taking a vacation was too stressful and too much of a reminder of her husband's traumatic death.

Mrs. S. was diagnosed with psychosis and the psychiatrist ordered chlorpromazine (Thorazine) 100 mg three times daily and diphenhydramine (Benadryl) 50 mg every 4 hours for agitation and for sleep. She states: "Well, I really don't like the effects of some of these medications. I don't really need them anyway."

On your assessment, you noted that she appeared frightened, tired, disheveled, had dilated pupils, and exhibited poor hygiene. According to her family, she was 15 pounds lighter than her usual weight. Her vital signs were within normal limits, but her heart rate was elevated. Her skin was warm and dry. She told you her family was trying to poison her, but she accepted a glass of water from you.

Based upon the case study, develop a nursing care plan using the following procedure*:

List comments of client that provide *subjective data.*

List information that provides *objective data.*

From these data, identify and state, using accepted format, two *nursing diagnoses* you determine are most significant to this client at this time.

Determine and state *outcome criteria* for each diagnosis. These must reflect some alleviation of the problem identified in the nursing diagnosis and must be stated in concrete and measurable terms.

Plan and state one or more *interventions* for each diagnosed problem. Provide specific documentation of source used to determine appropriate intervention.

Evaluate success of intervention. Interventions must correlate directly with the stated outcome criteria in order to measure the outcome success.

STUDY QUESTIONS/ACTIVITIES

Discuss nursing priorities regarding her medications.

Why do you think the psychiatrist ordered Thorazine rather than some of the newer antipsychotics?

Is Thorazine appropriate for an elderly person? Discuss reasons why it may or may not be appropriate.

What are your concerns about the combination of medications she is receiving?

What are the reactions they may trigger?

As a nurse, what would your responsibility be regarding these reactions and what actions would you take?

What do Thorazine and Benadryl have in common that could be problematic in the elderly?

Would a fall influence psychosis?

*Students are advised to refer to their nursing diagnosis text and identify possible or potential problems.

RESEARCH QUESTIONS

What percentage of elders develop serious side effects related to particular drugs?

What are the circumstances that most frequently precipitate the institution of psychotropic drug therapy?

What are the circumstances and percentage of elders who commit suicide?

Under what conditions do elders commit suicide through drug overdoses?

How frequently do nurses discuss psychotropic drugs, their actions, interactions, and side effects with elders for whom they are providing care?

How can a nurse know when the elder has understood medication education?

Is the reliance on psychotropic drugs increasing or decreasing among the elderly within the last decade? How does this relate to the increasing services and attention that have been devoted to elders' care?

What are the long term effects of the SSRIs in the elderly? What is the frequency of drug interactions in persons prescribed SSRIs?

How is quality of life assessed in the elderly? What is quality of life in the nursing home for patients over 65 years? What is the quality of life for those on psychotropic medications? Is there change over time?

Are the OBRA 1987 guidelines applicable in hospital and community settings? What are the frequencies of agencies following OBRA guidelines outside of institutional settings?

How do elders describe adjusting to age-related sleep changes?

RESOURCES

Mail order pharmacies are numerous. Inquire at your local pharmacy or HMO regarding this service. The following are known to be reliable:

AARP Pharmacy Service
500 Montgomery Street
Alexandria, VA 22341
(703) 684-0244

Walgreen Health Care Plus
8350 South River Parkway
Tempe, AZ 85284
(800) 345-1985

Medicines and You: A Guide for Older Americans
Council on Family Health
(212) 598-3617

National Council on Patient Information and Education
666 Eleventh Street, Suite 810
Washington, DC 20001
(202) 347-6711
Fax: (202) 638-0773

Council offers services including provision of an individualized wallet card identifying the patient and medications. Information updates related to drugs and public service campaigns to improve the use of medication.

Age Page: Safe Use of Medications for Older People
Informational page designed for laypersons' education
National Institute on Aging
Building 31, Room 5C35
Bethesda, MD 20892
(301) 496-1752
E-Mail: www.nia.gov-nia.

Paxil Access to Care
SmithKline Beecham Pharmaceuticals
P.O. Box 7929
One Franklin Plaza
Philadelphia, PA 19101
E-Mail: www.sb.com

APREX, A Division of Apreia Health Care, Inc.
1430 O'Brien
Menlo Park, CA 94025
(415) 614-4100; (800) 916-3535 dosing partner
E-Mail: Janice@aprex.com

A product and a handbook to help patients to take their medication on time. Their customers are usually referred by physicians. Provides commercial in-home electronic medication monitoring system and compliance support services.

REFERENCES

Alexopoulos GS: Treatment of depression. In Salzman C, ed: *Clinical geriatric psychopharmacology,* ed 2, Baltimore, Md, 1992, Williams & Wilkins, pp 137-174.

American Psychiatric Association: *Diagnostic and statistical manual of mental disorders,* ed 4, Washington, DC, 1994, The Association.

Baldessarini RJ: Drugs and the treatment of psychiatric disorders: depression and mania. In Hardman JG, Limbird LE, Molinoff PB, Ruddon RW, Gilman AG, eds: *Goodman and Gilman's The pharmacological basis of therapeutics,* ed 9, New York, 1996, McGraw-Hill, pp 431-461.

Baldessarini RJ, Frankenburg FR: Clozapine. A new antipsychotic agent, *N Engl J Med* 324:746-754, 1991.

Ban T: *Therapeutic indications for nootropics within the current classifications of psychiatric disorders,* Paper presented at the Third Congress of the International Psychogeriatric Association, Chicago, Aug 28-31, 1987.

Barnes TRE: A rating scale for drug-induced akathisia, *Br J Psych* 154:672-676, 1989.

Beers M, Avorn J, Soumerai S, Everitt DE, Sherman DS, Salem S: Psychoactive medication use in intermediate-care facility residents, *J Am Med Assoc* 260(20):3016-3020, 1988.

Beers MH, Ouslander JG, Rollingher I, Reuben DB, Brooks J, Beck J: Explicit criteria for determining inappropriate medication use in nursing home residents, *Arch Inter Med* 151:1825-1832, 1991

Bloom HG, Shlom EA: *Drug prescribing for the elderly,* New York, 1993, Raven Press.

Brown CS, Wright RG, Christenson DB: Association between type of medication instructions and patients' knowledge, side effects, and compliance, *Hosp Com Psych* 38(1):55-60, 1987.

Buffum J: *Geriatric dosage guidelines* (unpublished document to be placed in Decentralized Hospital Computer Program [DHCP]), San Francisco, 1996, VA Medical Center.

Burke RE, Fahn S, Jankovic J, Marsden CD, Lang AE, Gollomp S, Ilson J: Tardive dystonia: late onset and persistent dystonia cause by antipsychotic drugs, *Neurology* 32:1335-1346, 1982.

Cooper JW: *Drug-related problems in geriatric nursing home patients,* New York, 1991, Pharmaceutical Products Press.

Cummings JL: Differential diagnosis and medical management of dementia patients, *Federal Practitioner (supplement),* Birmingham, AL, 1996 Birmingham Regional Medical Education Center, pp 10-16.

Cusack B, Nelson A, Richelson E: Binding of antidepressants to human brain receptors: focus on newer generation compounds, *Psychopharmacology* 114:559-565, 1994.

Darnell JC, Murray MD, Martz BL, Weinberger M: Medication use by ambulatory elderly: an in-home survey, *J Am Geriatr Soc* 34:1-4, 1986.

Davis KL, Powchik P: Tacrine, *Lancet* 345:625-630, 1995.

Dewan MJ, Huszonek J, Koss M, Hardoby W, Ispahani A: The use of antidepressants in the elderly: 1986 and 1989, *J Geriatr Psych Neurol* 5:40-44, 1992.

Dresser J: *Neuroleptic malignant syndrome: early identification and intervention,* Presentation at the Annual Conference on Psychiatric Nursing, 1992, Las Vegas, sponsored by Resource Applications, Mosby.

Ereshefsky L: Drug interactions of antidepressants, *Psych Ann* 26(6):342-350, 1996.

Finkel SI: Efficacy and tolerability of antidepressant therapy in the old-old, *J Clin Psych* 57(suppl 5):23-28, 1996.

Ganzini L, Heintz R, Hoffman WF, Keepers G, Casey DE: Acute extrapyramidal syndromes in neuroleptic-treated elders: a pilot study, *J Geriatr Psych Neurol* 4: 222-225, 1991.

Gelenberg AJ, Katz MD: Antipsychotic agents. In Bressler R, Katz MD, eds: *Geriatric pharmacology,* New York, 1993, McGraw-Hill.

Gillin JC, Ancoli-Israel S: The impact of age on sleep and sleep disorders. In Salzman C, ed: *Clinical geriatric psychopharmacology,* Baltimore, 1992, Williams & Wilkins, pp 213-234.

Jenike MA: *Geriatric psychiatry and psychopharmacology: a clinical approach,* Boston, 1989, Year Book Medical Publishers.

Kaplan HI, Sadock BJ: *Pocket handbook of psychiatric drug treatment,* ed 2, Baltimore, 1996, Williams & Wilkins.

Keltner N, Folks DG: *Psychotropic drugs,* ed 2, St Louis, 1997, Mosby.

Keltner NL, Schwecke LH, Bostrom CE: *Psychiatric nursing: a psychotherapeutic approach,* St Louis, 1991, Mosby.

Kitchell MA, Barnes RF, Veith RC: Screening for depression in hospitalized geriatric medical patients, *J Am Geriatr Soc* 30:174-177, 1982.

Lassila HC, Stoehr, GP, Ganguli M, Seaberg EC, Gilby JE, Belle SH, Echement DA: Use of prescription medications in an elderly rural population: the MoVies project, *Ann Pharmacother* 30:589-595, 1996.

Lazarus A: Differentiating neuroleptic-related heatstroke from neuroleptic malignant syndrome, *Psychosomatics* 30(4):454-456, 1989.

Leo RJ, Kreeger JL, Kim KY: Cardiomyopathy associated with clozapine, *Ann Pharmacother* 30:603-605, 1996.

Liptzin B: Treatment of mania. In Salzman C, ed: *Clinical geriatric psychopharmacology,* Baltimore, 1992, Williams & Wilkins, pp 175-188.

Lohr JB, Caligiuri MP: A double-blind placebo-controlled study of vitamin E treatment of tardive dyskinesia, *J Clin Psych* 57(4):167-173, 1996.

Lohr JB, Jeste DV, Harris MJ, Salzman C: Treatment of disordered behavior. In Salzman C, ed: *Clinical geriatric psychopharmacology,* ed 2, Baltimore, 1992, Williams & Wilkins, pp 79-113.

Mega MS, Cummings JL, Fiorello T, Gornbein J: The spectrum of behavioral changes in Alzheimer's disease, *Neurology* 46:130-135, 1996.

Morton WA, Sonne SC, Verga MA: Venlafaxine: a structurally unique and novel antidepressant, *Ann Pharmacother* 29:387-395, 1995.

Newhouse PA: Use of serotonin selective reuptake inhibitors in geriatric depression, *J Clin Psych* 57(suppl 5):12-22, 1996.

NIH Consensus Development Panel on Depression in Late Life: Diagnosis and treatment of depression, *J Am Med Assoc* 268:1018-1024, 1992.

NIMH Psychopharmacology Research Branch: Abnormal involuntary movement scale. In Guy W, ed: *ECDEU assessment manual for psychopharmacology, revised,* Rockville, MD, 1976, National Institute of Mental Health, pp 534-537.

Okimoto JT, Barnes RF, Veith RC: Screening for depression in geriatric medical patients, *Am J Psych* 139:799-802, 1982.

Omnibus Budget Reconciliation Act of 1987, Washington, DC, 1987, US Government Printing Office. House of Representatives, 100th Congress, 1st Session, Report 100-391.

Pelletier L, Dailey D, Bennett D: Neuroleptic malignant syndrome: identification and treatment, *NURSEweek* 5(6): 10-11, 1992.

Ray WA, Taylor JA, Meador KG et al.: Reducing antipsychotic drug use in nursing homes: a controlled trial of provider education, *Arch Inter Med* 153:713-721, 1993.

Regestein QR: Treatment of insomnia in the elderly. In Salzman C, ed: *Clinical geriatric psychopharmacology,* ed 2, Baltimore, 1992, Williams & Wilkins, pp 235-253.

Rothschild, AJ: The diagnosis and treatment of late-life depression, *J Clin Psych* 57(suppl 5): 5-11, 1996.

Rovner BW, Edelman BA, Cox MP et al: The impact of antipsychotic drug regulations on psychotropic prescribing practices in nursing homes, *Am J Psych* 149:1390-1392, 1992.

Roy-Byrne PP, Hommer D: Benzodiazepine withdrawal: overview and implications for the treatment of anxiety, *Am J Med* 84:1041-1052, 1988.

Salzman C: Treatment of anxiety. In Salzman C, ed: *Clinical geriatric psychopharmacology,* ed 2, Baltimore, 1992, Williams & Wilkins, pp 189-212.

Schatzberg AF: Course of depression in adults: treatment options, *Psych Ann* 26(6):336-341, 1996.

Schneider LS, Sobin PB: Non-neuroleptic treatment of behavioral symptoms and agitation in Alzheimer's disease and other dementia, *Psychopharmacol Bull* 28(1):71-79, 1992.

Semla TP, Beizer JL, Higbee MD: *Geriatric dosage handbook,* ed 2, 1995, Cleveland, Lexi-Comp, Inc.

Shorr RI, Fought RL, Ray WA: Changes in antipsychotic drug use in nursing homes during implementation of the OBRA-87 regulations, *J Am Med Assoc* 271:358-362, 1994.

Simpson GM, Angus JWS: A rating scale for extrapyramidal side effects, *Acta Psychiatri Scand* 212:11-18, 1970.

Stoudemire A, Smith DA: OBRA regulations and the use of psychotropic drugs in long-term care facilities. Impact and implications for geropsychiatric care, *Gen Hosp Psych* 18:77-94, 1996.

Strome T, Howell T: How antipsychotics affect the elderly, *Am J Nurs* 91(5):46-49, May 1991.

Sunderland T: Neurotransmission in the aging central nervous system. In Salzman C, ed: *Clinical geriatric psychopharmacology,* ed 2, Baltimore, 1992, Williams & Wilkins, pp 41-59.

Sunderland T, Weingartner H, Cohen RM, Tariot PN, Newhouse PA, Thompson KE, Lawlor BA, Mueller EA: Low-dose oral lorazepam administration in Alzheimer subjects and age-matched controls, *Psychopharmacology* 99:129-133, 1989.

Sweet RA, Pollock BG: Neuroleptics in the elderly: guidelines for monitoring. *Harvard Rev Psych* 2:327-35, 1995.

Tune L, Carr S, Hoag E, Cooper T: Anticholinergic effects of drugs commonly prescribed for the elderly: potential means for assessing risk of delirium, *Am J Psych* 149(10): 1393-1394, 1992.

United States Statutes, Omnibus Budget Reconciliation Act (OBRA) of 1987, 101 Stat. 1330-160, US Health Care Financing Administration: *Medicare and Medicaid: requirements for long-term care facilities,* Federal Register 54(21):5316-5373, 1989.

Walker SE, Shulman KI, Tailor SAN, Gardner D: Tyramine content of previously restricted foods in monoamine oxidase inhibitor diets, *J Clin Psychopharmacol* 16(5): 383-388, 1996.

Watsky E, Salzman C: Prescribing information. In Salzman C, ed: *Clinical geriatric psychopharmacology,* Baltimore, 1992, Williams & Wilkins, pp. 303-307.

Zisselman MH, Rovner BW, Shmuely Y: Benzodiazepine use in the elderly prior to psychiatric hospitalization, *Psychosomatics* 37:38-42, 1996.

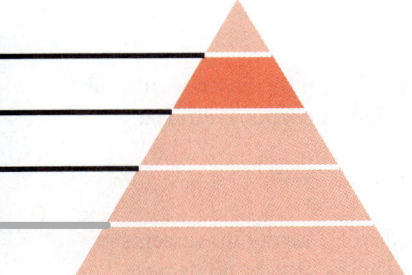

Barnes Rating Scale for Drug-Induced Akathisia

For each item circle the number identifying the response which best characterizes the patient:

Patients should be observed while engaged in neutral conversation while they are seated, and then standing (for a minimum of two minutes in each position). Symptoms observed in other situations, e.g., engaged in activity on the ward, may also be rated. Subsequently, the subjective phenomena should be elicited by direct questioning.

OBJECTIVE

0   Normal, occasional fidgety movements of the limbs.
1   Presence of characteristic restless movements: shuffling or tramping movements of the legs/feet, or swinging of one leg, while sitting, and/or rocking from foot to foot or "walking-on-the-spot" when standing, BUT movements present for less than half the time observed.
2   Observed phenomena, as described in (1) above, which are present for at least half the observation period.
3   The patient is constantly engaged in characteristic restless movements and/or has the inability to remain seated or standing without walking or pacing during the time observed.

SUBJECTIVE
Awareness of restlessness

0   Absence of inner restlessness.
1   Non-specific sense of inner restlessness.
2   The patient is aware of an inability to keep the legs still, or a desire to move the legs, and/or complains of inner restlessness aggravated specifically by being required to stand still.
3   Awareness of an intense compulsion to move most of the time and/or reports a strong desire to walk or pace most of the time.

DISTRESS RELATED TO RESTLESSNESS

0   No distress
1   Mild
2   Moderate
3   Severe

Continued

From Barnes TRE: A rating scale for drug-induced akathisia, *Br J Psych* 154:672–676, 1989.

GLOBAL CLINICAL ASSESSMENT OF AKATHISIA

0 **Absent**

No evidence of awareness of restlessness. Observation of characteristic movements of akathisia in the absence of a subjective report of inner restlessness or compulsive desire to move the legs should be classified as pseudoakathisia.

1 **Questionable**

Non-specific inner tension and fidgety movements.

2 **Mild akathisia**

Awareness of restlessness in the legs and/or inner restlessness worse when required to stand still. Fidgety movements present but characteristic restless movements of akathisia not necessarily observed. Condition causes little or no distress.

3 **Moderate akathisia**

Awareness of restlessness as described for mild akathisia above, combined with characteristic restless movements such as rocking from foot to foot when standing. Patient finds the condition distressing.

4 **Marked akathisia**

Subjective experience of restlessness includes a compulsive desire to walk or pace. However, the patient is able to remain seated for short periods of at least 5 minutes. The condition is obviously distressing.

5 **Severe akathisia**

The patient reports a strong compulsion to pace up and down most of the time. Unable to sit or lie down for more than a few minutes. Constant restlessness which is associated with intense distress and insomnia.

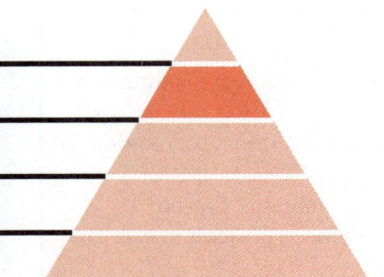

Simpson-Angus Rating Scale

For each item circle the number identifying the response which best characterizes the patient:	
1. Gait: The patient is examined as he or she walks into the examining room—his gait. The swing of the arms, the general posture all form the basis for an overall score for this item.	0 = Normal 1 = Mild diminution in swing while patient is walking 2 = Obvious diminution in swing suggesting shoulder rigidity 3 = Stiff gait with little or no arm swing noticeable 4 = Rigid gait with arms slightly pronated; this would also include stooped, shuffling gait with propulsion and repropulsion
2. Arm dropping: The patient and the examiner both raise their arms to shoulder height and let them fall to their sides. In a normal subject, a stout slap is heard as the arms hit the sides. In the patient with extreme Parkinson's syndrome, the arms fall very slowly.	0 = Normal, free fall with loud slap and rebound 1 = Fall slowed slightly with less audible contact and little rebound 2 = Fall slowed, no rebound 3 = Marked slowing, no stop at all 4 = Arms fall as though against resistance, as though through glue
Cogwheel rigidity may be palpated when the examination is carried out for items 3, 4, 5, and 6. It is not rated separately and is merely another way to detect rigidity. It would indicate that a minimum score of 1 would be mandatory.	
3. Shoulder shaking: The patient's arms are bent at a right angle at the elbow and are taken one at a time by the examiner who grasps one hand and also clasps the other around the patient's elbow.	0 = Normal 1 = Slight stiffness and resistance 2 = Moderate stiffness and resistance 3 = Marked rigidity with difficulty in passive movement 4 = Extreme stiffness and rigidity with almost a frozen joint
4. Elbow rigidity: The elbow joints are separately bent at right angles and passively extended and flexed with the patient's biceps observed and simultaneously palpated. The resistance to this procedure is rated.	0 = Normal 1 = Slight stiffness and resistance 2 = Moderate stiffness and resistance 3 = Marked rigidity with difficulty in passive movement 4 = Extreme stiffness and rigidity with almost a frozen joint
5. Wrist rigidity: The wrist is held in one hand and the fingers held by the examiner's other hand with the wrist moved to extension, flexion, and ulnar and radial deviation, or the extended wrist is allowed to fall under its own weight, or the arm can be grasped above the wrist and shaken to and fro. A zero score would be a hand that extends easily, falls loosely, or flaps easily upwards and downwards.	0 = Normal 1 = Slight stiffness and resistance 2 = Moderate stiffness and resistance 3 = Marked rigidity with difficulty in passive movement 4 = Extreme stiffness and rigidity with almost a frozen wrist

From Simpson GM, Angus JWS: A rating scale for extrapyramidal side effects, *Acta Psychiatr Scand* 212:11-18, 1970.

6. Head rotation: The patient sits or stands and is told that you are going to move his or her head from side to side; that it will not hurt and that he or she should try and relax. (Questions about pain in the cervical area or difficulty in moving the head should be obtained to avoid causing any pain.) Clasp the patient's head between the two hands with the fingers on the back of the neck. Gently rotate the head in a circular motion three times and evaluate the muscular resistance to this movement.	0 = Loose, no resistance 1 = Slight resistance to movement although the time to rotate may be normal 2 = Resistance is apparent and the time of rotation is shortened 3 = Resistance is obvious and rotation is slowed 4 = Head appears still and rotation is difficult to carry out
7. Glabellar tap: Patient is told to open eyes wide and not to blink. The glabellar region is tapped at a steady, rapid speed. The number of times the patient blinks in succession is noted. Care should be taken to stand behind the subject so that he or she does not observe the movement of the tapping finger. A full blink is frequently not observed; more often there will be contraction of the infraorbital muscle producing a twitch each time a stimulus is delivered. Variations in the speed of tapping ensures that the muscle contraction is related to the tap.	0 = 0-5 blinks 1 = 6-10 blinks 2 = 11-15 blinks 3 = 16-20 blinks 4 = 21 or more blinks
8. Tremor: Patient is observed walking into examining room and then is reexamined for this item with arms extended at right angles to the body and the fingers spread out as far as possible.	0 = Normal 1 = Mild finger tremor, obvious to sight and touch 2 = Tremor of hand or arm occurring spasmodically 3 = Persistent tremor of one or more limbs 4 = Whole body tremor
9. Salivation: Patient is observed while talking and then asked to open the mouth and elevate the tongue. (Once the patient has received antiparkinson agents, this sign is unlikely to be present.)	0 = Normal 1 = Excess salivation to the extent that pooling takes place 2 = Excess salivation is present and might occasionally result in difficulty in speaking 3 = Speaking with difficulty because of excess salivation 4 = Frank drooling
10. Akathisia: Patient is observed for the presence of observable restlessness. After a determination of observable restlessness is made, the patient should be assessed by asking, "Do you feel restless or jittery inside; is it difficult to sit still?"	0 = No restlessness reported or observed 1 = Mild restlessness observed during the exam; e.g., occasional jiggling of the foot occurs during the sitting part of the exam 2 = Moderate restlessness observed; e.g., on several occasions, jiggles foot, crosses and uncrosses legs, or twists a part of the body 3 = Restlessness is frequently observed during the exam; e.g., the foot or legs move most of the time 4 = Restlessness persistently observed during the exam; the patient cannot sit still and may get up and walk

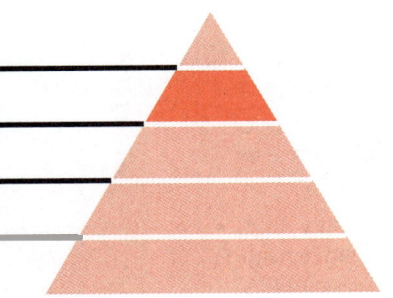

Abnormal Involuntary Movement Scale (AIMS)

Instructions: MOVEMENT RATINGS:	Complete Examination Procedure (see p. 866) before making ratings. Rate highest severity observed. Rate movements that occur upon activation one value less than these observed spontaneously.	Code for #1-7
		0 = None 1 = Minimal, may be extreme normal 2 = Mild 3 = Moderate 4 = Severe

FACIAL AND ORAL MOVEMENTS	1. Muscles of facial expression e.g., movements of forehead, eyebrows, periorbital area, cheeks; including frowning, blinking, smiling, grimacing.	☐
	2. Lips and perioral area e.g., puckering, pouting, smacking.	☐
	3. Jaw e.g., biting, clenching, chewing, mouth opening, lateral movement.	☐
	4. Tongue rate only increases in movement both in and out of mouth. NOT inability to sustain movement.	☐
EXTREMITY MOVEMENTS	5. Upper (arms, wrists, fingers) Include choreic movements (i.e., rapid, objectively purposeless, irregular, spontaneous) and athetoid movements (i.e., slow, irregular, complex, serpentine). Do NOT include tremor (i.e., repetitive, regular, rhythmic).	☐
	6. Lower (legs, knees, ankles, toes) e.g., lateral knee movement, foot tapping, heel dropping, foot squirming, inversion and aversion of foot.	☐
TRUNK MOVEMENTS	7. Neck, shoulders, hips e.g., rocking, twisting, squirming, pelvic gyrations.	☐

GLOBAL JUDGEMENTS	8. Severity of abnormal movements: Mark one				
		[0] None	[1] Minimal	[2] Mild	[3] Moderate	[4] Severe
	9. Incapacitation due to abnormal movements: Mark one				
		[0] None	[1] Minimal	[2] Mild	[3] Moderate	[4] Severe
	10. Patient's awareness of abnormal movements (Rate only patient's report)				
		[0] No Awareness	[1] Aware, No Distress	[2] Aware, Mild Distress	[3] Aware, Moderate, Distress	[4] Aware, Severe Distress

DENTAL STATUS	11. Current prolems with teeth and/or dentures	Yes = 1 No = 0	☐
	12. Does patient usually wear dentures?	Yes = 1 No = 0	☐

From Guy W, editor: *ECDEU assessment manual for psychopharmacology, revised,* Rockville, MD, 1976, National Institute of Mental Health, pp. 534–537.

AIMS EXAMINATION INSTRUCTION

Step 1:   Ask the patient whether there is anything in his or her mouth (such as gum or candy), and if there is, to remove it.

Step 2:   Ask about the current condition of the patient's teeth. Ask if he or she wears dentures. Ask whether teeth or dentures bother the patient now.

Step 3:   Ask whether the patient notices any movements in his or her mouth, face, hands, or feet. If the answer is yes, ask the patient to describe the movements and do what extent they currently bother the patient or interfere with activities.

Step 4:   Have the patient sit in a chair with hands on knees, legs slightly apart, and feet flat on the floor. (Look at the entire body for movements while the patient is in this position.)

Step 5:   Ask the patient to sit with hand hanging unsupported for a male patient, hands hanging between legs, and for a female patient wearing a dress, hands hanging over her knees. (Observe hands and other body areas.)

Step 7:   Ask the patient to protrude his or her tongue. (Observe abnormalities of tongue movement.) Do this twice.

Step 8:   Ask the patient to tap his or her thumb with each finger, as rapidly as possible for ten to fifteen seconds, first with the fingers of the right hand, then with the left hand. (Observe facial and leg movements.)

Step 9:   Flex and extend both arms out in front, with palms down. (Observe trunk, legs, and mouth.)

Step 10: Ask the patient to stand up. (Observe the patient in profile. Observe all bodily areas again, hips included.)

Step 11: Ask the patient to extend body arms out in front, with palms down. (Observe trunk, legs, and mouth.)

Step 12: Have the patient walk a few paces, turn, and walk back to the chair. (Observe hands and gait.) Do this twice.

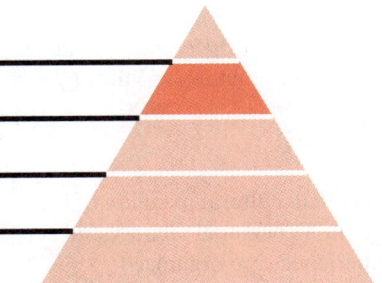

Gender, Cohort, and Culture

The old ones, in their seventies or eighties, with long memories of hardships faced and perhaps only partially (if at all) surmounted, deprived of education, made to feel hopelessly inarticulate, and obviously out of "the American mainstream," they are nevertheless men and women who seem to have held stubbornly to a peculiar notion: that they are eminently valuable and important human beings, utterly worth the respect, even admiration, not to mention the love, of their children and grandchildren.

Description of the Chicanos of New Mexico in Coles R: *The old ones,* Albuquerque, 1973, University of New Mexico Press.

LEARNING OBJECTIVES   Upon completion of this chapter, the reader will be able to:

1. Identify personal factors contributing to ethnic and cultural sensitivity.
2. Relate major historic events that have affected each cohort of elders.
3. Compare several different ethnically based approaches to health care.
4. Specify some gender characteristics that have been identified in recent studies.
5. Explain various ways in which ethnic groups may be incorporated into the larger culture.
6. Discuss approaches that facilitate an appreciation of diverse cultural and ethnic experiences.
7. Formulate a care plan incorporating ethnically sensitive interventions.

DIFFERENCES RELATED TO BIRTH CIRCUMSTANCE

Geographic origin, historic events, cohort position, and gender create significant individual differences within any culture. As our aged become more diverse and heterogeneous we are constantly challenged to understand their needs and assist them to appropriate resources. Competent role enactment requires a bio-psycho-socio-political-spiritual-cultural perspective. The increasing specificity and accumulation of knowledge on any of these topics make this charge appear not only impossible but one of sheer grandiosity. If we hope to approach this commitment to persons of various cultures, cohorts, and social strata we must learn to be expert listeners . . . to fact and innuendo, to nonverbal messages, to the subjects that are avoided, to messages acted out, to group statements as well as those of individuals. We must become skilled in deciphering the unstated agenda in political and

economic communication. And we must certainly try to understand the messages some of our minority citizens receive through the structure of our health care system.

In this chapter we consider old people from other cultures and subcultures; those whose childhoods were marked by distant social and world events; youth of another time and place and the marked gender differences that existed. We suggest ways that nurses may help the elderly preserve their individuality.

Cohorts

A cohort (in geographic circles) is a group of people born within the same time span, most often a decade. Thus a cohort would contain all the people born in the United States between 1900 and 1909. These rigid boundaries fit nicely with statistical and actuarial tables but not so well with people. However, it is useful to consider the "cohort" effects of major national and world events. How would a child of 7 be affected by the Great Depression? A youth of 17? A man of 27? Each would be influenced to a different degree by the same event. Usually political ideology and wars affect adolescents and young adults profoundly; health patterns and educational changes significantly affect children's lives. Mature adults are affected most by relocation and financial and natural disasters. They have accumulated more, have established extensive personal networks, and have much to lose. Wars, economic disasters, great discoveries, shifts in moral values, and progress in health care will alter how one experiences life.

Birth cohort effects have been recognized as significant, but few intensive/extensive, qualitative longitudinal studies exist to actually elucidate the impact on one's life of his or her cohort. Even more difficult is to account for the effects of geography and cohort. Seigler et al (1992) briefly discuss this phenomenon as it has affected centenarians of Georgia. Segregation, population composition, religious predominance, differences in opportunity for formal education, and numerous other factors interrelate with cohort, raising far more questions than answers.

Elders are the embodiment of living history. The tell it like it was from their vantage point and in the process, if we listen, they tell us about themselves; how and why they grew up as they did. Reminiscing has been one of the most entertaining means elders have for sharing their life story and enriching the young. Each cohort has a different view, and each individual within the cohort carries innumerable variations of the story. Older persons will vary greatly in how they view the world, and part of this variance results from the impact of historic eras and beliefs surrounding them.

The study of the aged is anthropologic. Our aged citizens and immigrants form a mosaic of multicultural backgrounds and decade differences. Each decade closes the door on a vanishing breed. A civilization disappears with the death of each cohort. The urgency of meeting their needs and preserving the heritage they carry becomes more pressing as technologic advances propel us forward with ever-increasing speed. To properly serve them and learn from them, we must stop to listen.

In the United States today there are the rural aged in communities; the rural aged on farms; the urban aged in ghettos; the urban aged in exclusive penthouses; the suburban aged living with families, spouse, or alone; the retired aged who have sought warm climates; the migrant aged; the settled aged; the immigrant aged; the native born; and the first-, second-, and third-generation aged from countries around the world. The aged can also be described by their state of health or illness, by their marital and family status, by cohort, and by gender.

Many studies focus on generational differences and the conflicts or alliances between generations. We suggest that each generation has a unique perspective of life based on its historic spot in time, and although the individual's view may shift and change, some remnant of cohort effect will always remain. Cohort as well as gender differences, in addition to the discussion here, have been addressed throughout the text.

Gender

Gender, which refers to the personal, cultural meaning of biologic differences, is fundamental to personal identity and is the primary way in which experiences are organized.

There are some definite gender variations in demographics (Table 24-1). Gender incorporates those and other less measurable characteristics that are the result of a coalescence of cohort, culture, and genetics. Environmental influences, social expectations, and early training, as well as innate capacities, all seem to fall within the purview of these three categories. Interestingly, in the previous editions of this textbook we did not have a category related to gender alone as there was so little to be found that identified gender characteristics in the old. We are now finding more studies related to gender. In 1990 an entire issue of *Generations* (the journal of the American Society on Aging) was devoted to gender and aging (American Society on Aging, 1990). And, some gender-focused research centers have developed. The goals of a gender-focused research center include such aims as the following:

- Basic and clinical research related to gender-specific needs and characteristics.
- Developing and testing gender-specific therapeutic strategies.
- Providing gender-appropriate health recommendations.
- Disseminating research findings that promote understanding of gender-specific issues.

To identify the relevance of gender is exceedingly difficult and requires a breadth of perspective and objectivity not easily achieved by either sex. In the last 2 decades we have moved from simply describing biologic differences to an emphasis on the shaping of gender roles by socialization patterns, and we are now in a phase of describing gender in terms of social structure and cultural patterns (Hendricks, 1990; Hooyman and Kiyak, 1996).

Gender-specific information, while accruing, remains limited. The important message is do not make presumptions about the aged and their needs. Be cognizant that culture, cohort, and gender have all influenced the client's values, perceptions, and needs. Discuss these issues.

Survival and the Gender Gap.
At every age, beginning in embryo, females outlast males. In later life it is thought that female hormones protect against hypercholesteremia and heart disease. They also tend to enhance the immune system. However, women have a higher incidence of autoimmune diseases and nonfatal conditions that contribute to frailty and functional decline. Although females have fewer suicides in old age, they are more likely to suffer from anxiety and depression. These data are confounded by the

fact that women seek help for physical and emotional disorders more frequently than do men. It has been thought the male is more stoic and less likely to express feelings and, in the work setting, was subject to stressors that had particularly devastating effects on his survival. Clearly, many of these assumptions were cohort based and were never backed by solid evidence. Speculations regarding the contributions of the Y and the X chromosome to sex/gender differences abound. So far, nothing conclusive can be shown, although obviously these account for some inherent differences.

Gender Issues. One of the major issues in late life is that of caretaking. Numerous studies have shown caretaking as primarily a woman's role. Many frail old ladies take care of a frail old spouse to the detriment of their own health. And after years of subverting their own needs, they become so intermingled with those of the spouse that on the death of the spouse, they are at a loss for filling the empty time and heart (Ebersole, 1996). Interestingly, a recent study done by Kaye and Applegate (1995) provided strong support for the unwavering devotion and direct caregiving capacity of old men, most often caring for a spouse with a disabling chronic illness. Because of our gender stereotypes, we may not have looked closely enough at the actual caregiving situation with old couples.

Another gender statistic that has been widely accepted must be examined; that is, that a significantly greater number of older women are afflicted with Alzheimer's disease. The incidence of Alzheimer's disease increases exponentially with age so that the extended survival of women skews the statistics. Age-adjusted statistics show that men have Alzheimer's disease more frequently than women (National Institute on Aging, 1995). Now some of the most recent research on Alzheimer's disease seems to support the action of estrogen in preserving cognition (National Institute on Aging, 1995).

Women. "In neither the women's movement nor the old age movement have concerns of older women been centrally featured" (Hudson and Gonyea, 1990). Women, in numbers sufficient to influence policy, have never been a part of our governing bodies. For older women, cohort socialization and socioeconomic status have played a large part in subduing activism. Older women are becoming more active politically but considering they were the first generation given the right to vote, there is much yet to be done.

The Older Women's League (OWL) grew out of the White House Mini-Conference in Des Moines in 1980. The organization continues to be a strong political advocate for the needs and concerns of older women (see Resources at the end of the chapter). The major goals of the organization are to improve the status and image of older women while achieving economic and social equity and building a mutually supportive network.

Woods and Shaver (1992) describe the launching of a Center for Women's Health Research at the University of Washington, under the aegis of the National Center for Nursing Research.

Women are not given as intense or immediate cardiac care as men. Older women with a heart disorder can expect to be treated less energetically than men. More women than men die of heart attacks each year. There are several possible reasons: hormonal protection before menopause may give a false sense of security to women, as well as their physicians; heart drugs have not as yet been tested on older women, so the normal reactions and side effects are unknown. The risk of death for women who have coronary artery angioplasty is 5 times that of men of the same age with similar medical histories, and they are 2 to 3 times less likely to survive coronary artery bypass (FDA Consumer, 1996). A study of "clot-busting" drugs found that the drugs worked just as well with both men and women except that 1 month later 13% of the women, compared to 5% of the men, died. It was thought that this occurred because the women in the study were at least 10 years older than the males of the sample and had more cardiac risks factors such as high blood pressure and diabetes, yet they were not able to completely explain the gender differences in death (Christiensen, 1997). Throughout adult life, before age 65, men are much more at risk for heart disorders.

Many topics related to concerns unique to women have been identified. Those most related to older women include breast self-exam and female aging experiences in various ethnic groups. Journals devoted to women's health issues tend to focus on few topics relevant to older women except breast cancer, menopause, and osteoporosis. Some medical

Table 24-1	Gender Significant Statistics (Not including ethnic variations)		

At age 65 and over	Male	Female
Population	13.5 million	19.7 million
Life expectancy at birth	73.2 years	79.8 years
Life expectancy at 65	14 years	18 years
Married	77%	43%
Widowed	13%	47%
Live in family	81%	58%
Live alone	16%	40%
Median income	$15,250	$8950
Below poverty level	7%	15%
Employed	17%	9%
Need Help with ADLs	18%	26%
Need Help with IADLs	19%	35%
Annual days of restricted activity	30	36
Suicide/100,000	152.6	19.2
Alzheimer's deaths per 100,000 (age adjusted)	30.8	28.1
Heart disease-related deaths per 100,000	2058.5	1712.0

Data from U.S. Bureau of the Census: *Statistical abstract of the United States: 1995,* ed 115, Washington, DC, 1995, US Government Printing Office; American Association of Retired Persons: *A profile of older Americans: 1995,* Washington, DC, 1995, The Association.
ADL, Activities of daily living; IADL, instrumental activities of daily living.

centers have now developed special health history forms for women that include, in addition to basic health history and physical exam, detailed information about reproductive organs, sexual history, lifestyle factors, psychologic well-being, and special health support services that are desired (Seton Medical Center, 1992). In reality, aside from the specificity of questions regarding reproductive organs, these special histories should be useful for males as well. Little is actually known about the characteristics of very old women.

We often hear about unequal distribution of economic resources between men and women. Yet there are numbers of old women who inherit vast estates on the death of their husbands. It is possible that the maldistribution of resources within the gender is a critical problem that gets little attention. However, it is clear that very old women who have not worked outside the home and did not have wealthy husbands are likely to be poverty stricken if they survive to outlive their limited savings.

Studies specific to women have been appearing in recent years. Wagnild and Young (1990), in an attempt to describe the characteristics of resilient older women, found five underlying themes through using a grounded theoretical research approach. Equanimity, self-reliance, existential aloneness, perseverance, and meaningfulness all seemed to constitute resilience and gave evidence of successful psychosocial adjustment. Grounded theory must be rigorously replicated if it is to be relevant.

A longitudinal study of over 500 remarkable women born between 1900 and 1910 was conducted by Day (1992). She has identified three characteristics common to all: a strong sense of independence, dedication to interests outside of self, and gratifying social relationships.

The women's issues that are prominent and will follow society into the next millennium include the following:

- An aging society primarily of women since they are the fastest growing segment of society
- Inadequate health and long-term care
- Economic jeopardy with the threat to Social Security, and insufficient pensions

Males. It is difficult to find studies devoted to describing any abiding characteristics of aged males. A largely male veteran sample has formed the basis for a mass of research on "the aged." These data form the basis for conclusions about aging that, when presented, often lack gender specificity but were applied as if they were appropriate. A case in point is the oft-repeated statistic that the aged are more highly suicidal than any other group. This is untrue. Aged males, particularly white males, have the highest suicide rates. Women do not. Gender-significant variations are presented in Table 24-1 and 24-2.

A number of questions arise when discussing gender issues. Some questions to ponder include the following:

- Why, if older women have so many disadvantages, do they survive longer and seemingly maintain morale, in spite of being old, poor, and alone?

- Why is it so difficult for men to seek medical help before serious, life-threatening conditions occur?
- What effect will the baby boomers have on gender parity or disparity?

Population Diversity

The United States continues to experience a "gerontologic explosion" of ethnically diverse adults 65 years of age and that which will persist for at least the next 60 years (Angel and Hogan, 1991). There were approximately 14% of the population age 65 and older in 1995. The year 2000 will see a decrease to 12% in the aged population as those born during and following the depression reach age 65. By the year 2010 the "baby boomers" will have increased the older population to 14%. By the year 2025 the older population will comprise about 20% of the population (U.S. Bureau of the Census, 1995; American Association of Retired Persons, 1995). In approximately 30 years, minority elders will represent 25% of the total aged population. The U.S. Bureau of the Census (1995) projects that Hispanics will represent 13%; blacks 17%; Asian and Pacific Islanders, 12%; and Native Americans, Eskimos, and Aleuts 11% of the elder population. White elders will constitute only 47% of the older population.

The present and expected growth and diversity of the elderly population means that nurses will be caring for a significant number of minority elders, new immigrants and citizens, immediately and in the future. Standard care approaches will not necessarily be appropriate for the emerging group of elders and the subgroups who are ethnically and culturally diverse in needs, abilities, and resources. Figure 24-1 illustrates the expected population growth and distribution by ethnicity of the aged, 65 years of age and over, by the year 2050.

Minority Elders. The number of minority elders in the United States has increased faster than white elders (Figure 24-2). There are now more than 2.75 million blacks over 65 years old, one and a half million Hispanics, three quarters of a million Asian/Pacific Islanders, and just under 150,000 Native Americans (U.S. Bureau of the Census, 1995). Each has special social and cultural needs.

The status of minority elders in the United States reflects the social, economic, and discrimination barriers. In 1994 one fifth (19%) of the older population was poor or near poor (American Association of Retired Persons, 1995). Thirty-two percent of blacks in urban areas live in poverty, and 50% are in poverty in rural areas. Sixty-eight percent of rural black women are poor. Overall, 32% of Native Americans live below the official poverty line. The percentage of elderly Hispanics living in poverty is close to 37%, and the poverty rates of the Asian/Pacific Rim elderly are similar to those of the white elderly population (14%) (Richardson, 1990; Cuellar, 1990a,b; Morioka-Douglas and Yeo, 1990; American Association of Retired Persons, 1990).

Sharing a home with an adult child is more common among the ethnic elderly than among whites. Black elderly persons commonly live with family members or family members live with them, and only 4% are institutionalized. Hispanic elderly persons often (72%) live with a family member (3% institutionalized), and among the Asians, 96% live in the community, 77% live with someone, and 2% live in institutions. Among the Native American elderly, at least one fourth live on reservations. Sixty-six percent live with family members, some live alone, and only 3% were institutionalized (Cuellar, 1990a, b). The question arises as to whether this is due to cultural or economic necessity.

The sex ratio increases with age, ranging from 146 women for every 100 men for the 65 to 69 age group to 259 women per 100 men for the 85 and older age group (American Association of Retired Persons, 1995). The ratio of men to women is highest among whites at 65 years of age, but by 75 years of age, it is the lowest. By 85 years and over it is 43:100 for whites, 50:100 for blacks, 61:100 for Hispanics, 60:100 for Asians/Pacific Islanders, and 59:100 for Native Americans (U.S. Bureau of the Census, 1995). For additional statistics about various minority groups, see Resources. Figure 24-3 shows the projected density of the general ethnic population by the year 2090.

Immigration in late life. There was a great wave of European immigration in the early part of the twentieth century. The influx of aged Asians, Filipinos, and other individuals from the Pacific Rim to the western states has been significant in the past 20 years (Figure 24-4). European immigration consisted of many youth and families, but the immigration from Asia and the Pacific islands is often of elders who have come to the United States to join their children. They mourn the "old country" and wish to return, but their children want to watch over and care for them. Relocation to a new culture and language in late life has not been thought-fully examined in the literature, but from anecdotal information the relocation seems to impinge on the sense of personal continuity and security. Resources that are available are underused, and the transplanted individual may lack the social and cultural nourishment necessary for satisfaction even though survival needs may be met at a higher level than in the mother country.

Sarina came to the United States in 1986 at the urging of her oldest son. He provided home, security, and love, but she missed the farm in the Philippines, and she worried about her son and grandchildren who remained in the Philippines and pleaded to return. She was alone during the day while her family all worked or went to school. She consciously avoided learning English because her Tagalog was her last link with the past and her roots. Her isolation and depression were clearly related to the discontinuity of lifestyle and relationships.

Language. We seldom think of language as the foundation of self-concept, but the self is continuously constructed and inextricably bound up with the linguistic categories available in a given culture (Berman, 1991). We can only conceive of ourselves within the language we know. To make each contact with the elderly fully meaningful, shared communication is essential. Communication with persons of a different culture, ethnic group, or geographic region is an issue not only of language but also of idiom, style, and jargon. Even if it were possible for a nurse to learn all these

Table 24-2	Gender Differences	
	Male	**Female**
Mental disorders	Addiction	Neuroses
	Personality disorders	Depression
Cognitive function (specific capacities)	Spatial ability	Processing information
	Accuracy	
	Mathematics	Verbal skills
Personality	Both sexes are thought to become more androgenous—"gender free"	
Role behaviors (most likely troublesome)	Work transition	Poverty
Living situation		
With spouse	74.3%	40.1%
Alone	15.9%	40.9%
With relative(s)	8.4%	17.8%
With nonrelative	1.4%	1.2%

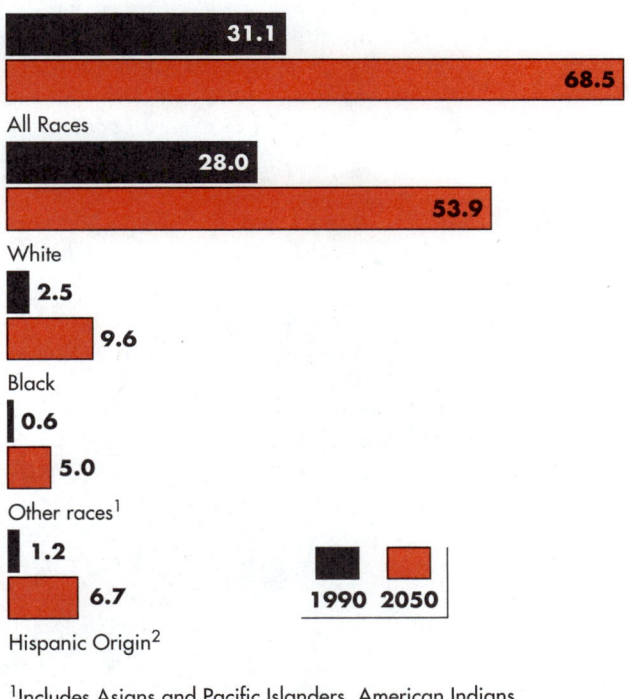

[1]Includes Asians and Pacific Islanders, American Indians, Eskimos, and Aleuts.
[2]Hispanic origin may be of any race.

Figure 24-1. Racial diversity of persons 65 and older, 1990 versus 2050 (in millions). (From U.S. Bureau of the Census: *Sixty-five plus in America,* Washington, DC, 1992.)

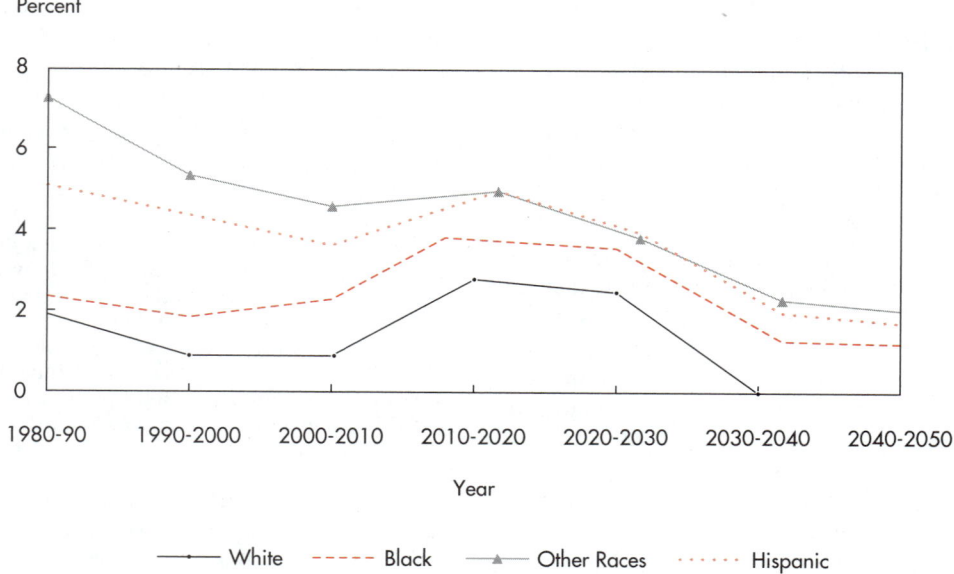

Figure 24-2. Annual rate of increase in elderly population by race and ethnicity: 1980–2050. (Modified from Angel JL, Hogan DP: The demography of minority aging populations. In *Minority Aging,* The Gerontological Society of America, Washington, DC, 1994, The Society.)

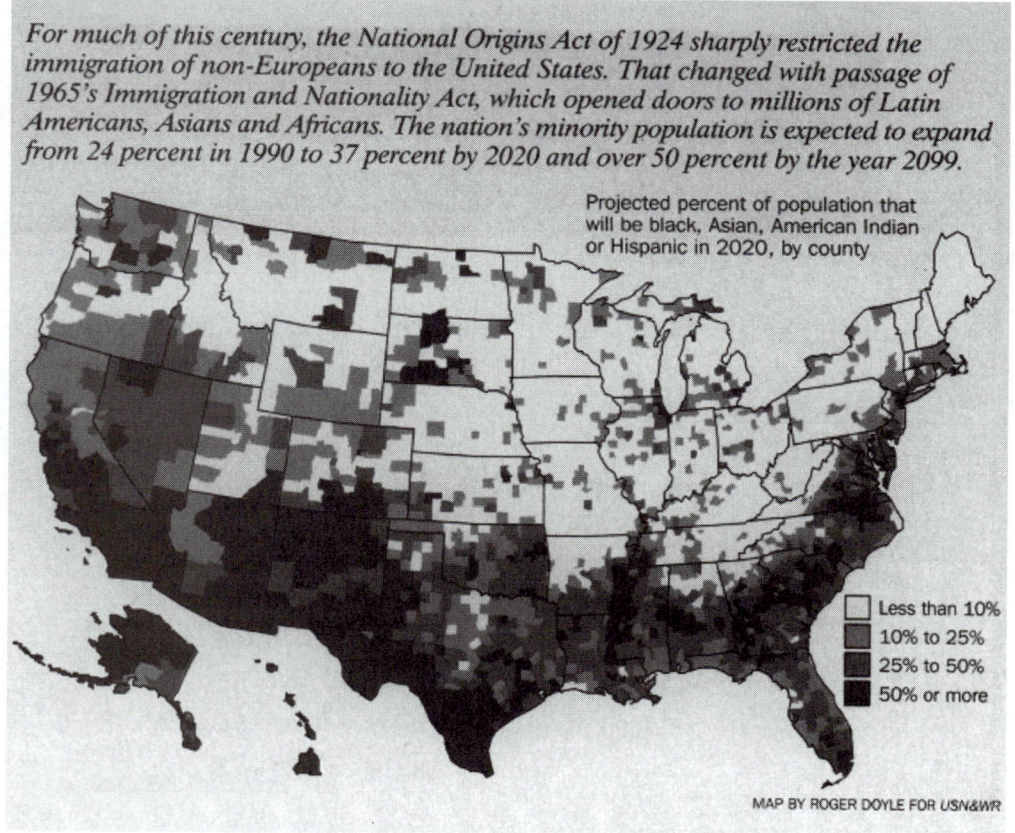

Figure 24-3. Future distribution of the American minority population. (From U.S. Census Bureau.)

vagaries, it would likely not be useful. It would be similar to entering a family and using all the pet names and phrases treasured by the family. In most cases the artificiality and intrusive nature of such an action would be irritating. Asking the individual about a phrase can be illuminating. In turn, we must remember that as health professionals our jargon and idiomatic expressions may be perceived as frightening or threatening. They will most certainly increase the social distance between the provider and the client.

Never assume you know what an aged person means. Ask him or her. If the person speaks a foreign language, every effort should be made to find an interpreter. In old age people find comfort in their mother tongue. However, when family members are used as interpreters, they may be unable to aid a care provider because of role conflicts or inability to use medical terms appropriately. Often messages to the client and the provider are based on the interpreter's perception of the situation, and vital information may be withheld or omitted to shield the client from family embarrassment.

In working with these elders, nurses must recognize the importance of their identification with past patterns and relationships. They are often living on the edge of anonymity. The most significant intervention is to find someone who speaks their language and can discuss their previous lifestyle. (Refer to Box 24-1 regarding the use of interpreters.) They may also enjoy senior centers designed specifically for their cultural needs. Churches may be another important source of other elders of the same ethnic background. Families need to understand that no matter how

pleasant the surroundings the displaced individuals long for the old ways and are experiencing a grief process. If they can be encouraged to talk about the losses, they may experience the relief that comes with ventilation in the presence of a concerned listener. These individuals often neglect health care because they may not know what is available to them; language is a barrier to information and expression of health needs. In addition they may be frightened by the health care system.

Ethnicity. Ethnicity and culture are frequently used interchangeably. In reality, a distinct difference exists in meanings. Ethnicity is a complex phenomenon. It is a social differentiation based on cultural criteria. (Gunter, 1991; Giger and Davidhizar, 1991, Spector, 1996). Most important, there is a shared identity.

An ethnic group may share common geographic origins, migratory status, race, language, and dialect. Religious factors (ties that transcend kinship, neighborhoods, and community boundaries) are also important in ethnicity. Traditions, values, symbols, literature, folklore, and diverse food preferences should be considered a part of ethnicity too. Settlement and employment patterns, special interests or politics in the homeland and in the United States, as well as an internal sense of distinctiveness or perception of external distinctiveness are additional facets of ethnicity that must be considered (Gunter, 1991; Giger and Davidhizer, 1991, Spector, 1996).

Thus ethnicity involves three components: culture, social status, and support systems. These components influence the

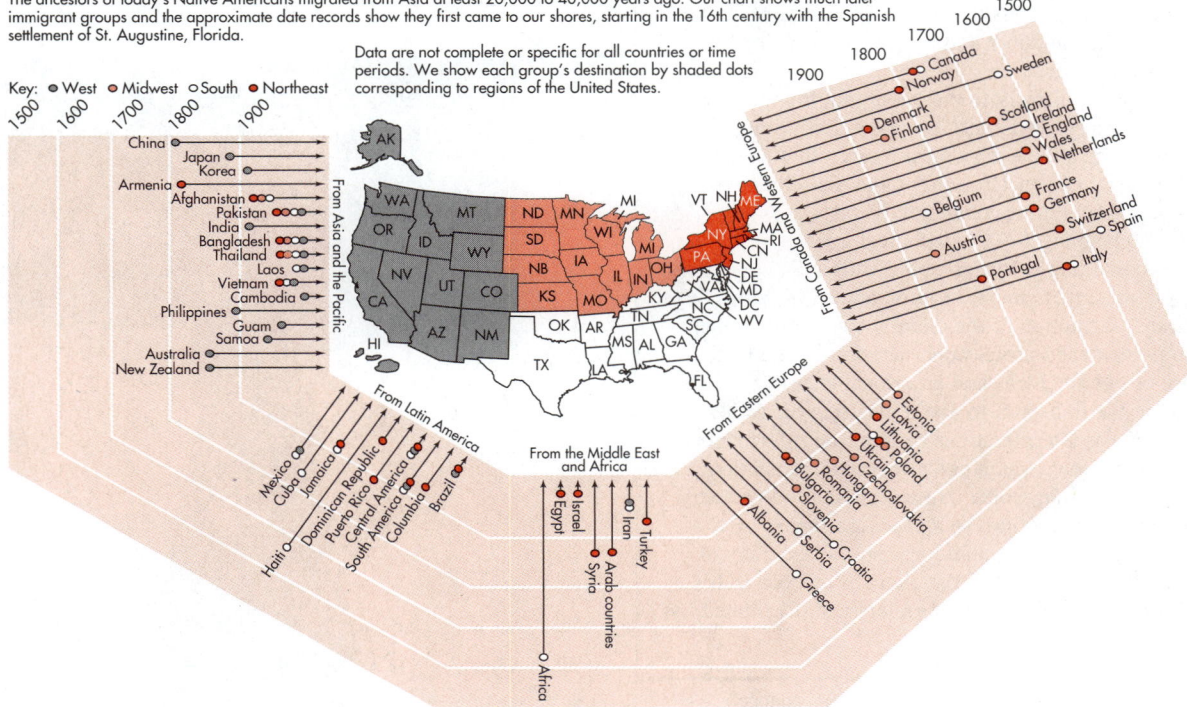

Figure 24-4. Migration patterns. (Modified from *Modern Maturity* 35(3):30, 1992.)

way people feel about themselves and how they interact with their environment (Hooyman and Kiyak, 1996). Moore (1971) cites five characteristics that constitute an ethnic minority:

- Each group has a specific history.
- The history has been accompanied by discrimination.
- A subculture develops.
- Coping structures develop.
- Rapid change occurs.

Our obligation is not to seek out minutiae of rituals and folkways, differences in habits of living, but to respect those important to the individual. When we insist on regimented care, we infringe on an individual's ability to maintain his or her own cultural orientation.

Writers often focus on nutritional patterns, folk medicine, death rituals, and specific cultural beliefs of ethnic groups. These generalities may not meet individual needs and may serve only to stereotype a person into artificial boundaries. It is therefore difficult to write about or do justice to the Mexican-American (also referred to as Chicano), Raza Latina (Latin American), black American (African

American), Native American (American Indian), or Asian and other groups because of the internal heterogeneity that exists within each ethnic community.

For example, it is estimated there are 1.6 million American Indians who speak 250 different languages besides English. Each of the more than 500 federally recognized tribes, nations, bands, and native villages or groups have different customs, mores, and needs (Cuellar, 1990a, Spector, 1996, Kramer, 1996). Spanish-speaking persons are often lumped together as if a homogeneous group, but there are Mexican-Americans, Puerto Ricans, Cubans, Central and South Americans, and Spaniards. All these people may be labeled Hispanic, which tells little about individual and group differences. Yet each major category shares certain distinctive cultural aspects. For this reason, general information is presented, which may help the caregiver develop an elemental and broad understanding basic to various cultural groups.

Ethnic elders prefer programs and services where the staff reflect the ethnic background and speak the language of the elderly clientele. Adequate and quality health care for the minority elders of today and tomorrow revolve around the issues of appropriate programs for them and cultural relativism. One of the most pervasive barriers to improving services has been the failure of caregivers to recognize race as a critical factor in the provision of such services. Others have noted that effective service delivery to ethnic elders requires a conscious effort to be responsive to the cultural uniqueness of these elderly populations. An example of just what cultural relativism in a senior center can do is described by Ochoco and Shimamoto (1987). They found that

---

Hints to Working with Interpreters

Prior to an interview or session with a client, try to meet with the interpreter to explain the purpose of the session.

Encourage the interpreter to meet with the client before the session to identify the educational level, attitudes toward health and health care, and for the interpreter to determine the depth and type of information and explanation needed.

Look and speak directly to the client, not the interpreter.

Be patient. Interpreted interviews take more time because long explanatory phrases are often needed.

Use short units of speech. Long, involved sentences or complex discussions create confusion.

Use simple language. Avoid technical terms, professional jargon, slang, abbreviations, abstractions, metaphors, or idiomatic expressions.

Encourage translation of the client's own words rather than paraphrased professional jargon to get a better sense of client's ideas and emotional state.

Encourage the translator to avoid inserting his or her own ideas or interpretations or omitting information.

Listen to the client, watch nonverbal communication (facial expression, voice intonation, body movement) to learn about emotions to a specific topic.

Clarify the client's understanding and the accuracy of the translation by asking the client to tell you in his or her own words what they understand, facilitated by the interpreter.

Modified from Lipson JG, Dibble SL, Minarik PA, editors: *Culture and nursing care: a pocket guide,* San Francisco, Calif, 1996, UCSF School of Nursing Press.

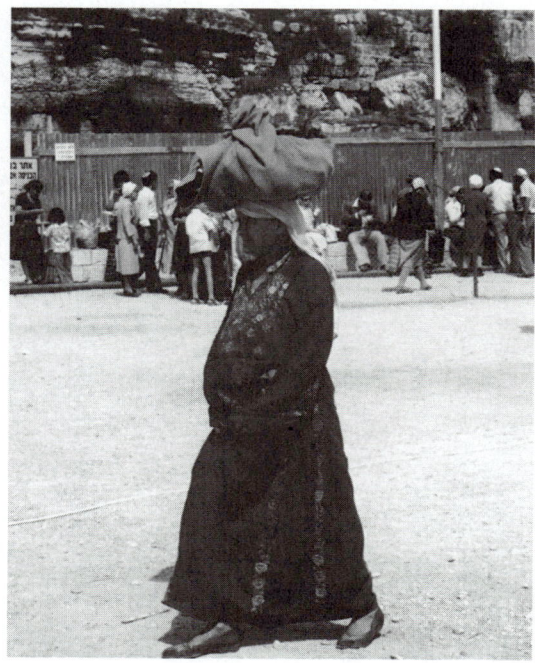

Uniqueness. (Courtesy Patricia Hess.)

by introducing ethnic-related activities at a senior center in Hawaii they were able to increase patient self-esteem, independence, and satisfaction. Many of the participants had been passive, dependent, and depressed. Two thirds were widowed women who had originally emigrated from Japan. Because a language barrier existed, some of the widows lived with children and deferred to their wishes to the neglect of their own self-esteem and self-concept. The community health nurse who activated the group wished to strengthen the sense of self in group members through a focus on cultural heritage. In addition to health teaching sessions and education about the aging process, the nurse used reminiscence and construction of a collective oral history to stimulate interaction and the sense of accomplishment. This model is adaptable to many community and institutional settings.

Culture

Rousseau, an eighteenth century romantic, believed human nature to be noble and essentially scarred and distorted by civilization and culture. But when Victor, the Wild Boy of Aveyron, was found at the end of the century, sociologists and anthropologists were confronted with the reality that the "noble savage" does not exist apart from a culture and an organizing experience represented by symbols. The capacity to develop these and the degree to which they are developed is the essence of human nature. Geertz (1973) says that we are incomplete or unfinished animals who finish ourselves through culture. Culture is, in its simplest concept, bonding with a group through collective interests or concerns, and thus the capacity for communicating these concerns becomes the root of culture. It then becomes easier to understand the origins and development of a culture that in vanished ages was at the mercy of certain geographic formations and natural resource availability (Geertz, 1973).

Culture, on the other hand, is an integrated pattern of behavior, a learned way of acting, communicating (language), and thinking of a particular group that is transmitted to others (Gunter, 1991; Giger and Davidhizar, 1991). Culture guides thinking, decision making, and actions (Leininger, 1978).

Fejos (1959) defines culture as "the sum total of socially inherited characteristics of a human group that comprises everything which one generation can tell, convey, or hand down to the next; in other words, the non-physically inherited traits we possess." Culture is something each of us carries around for a lifetime.

Habayeb (1995) suggests culture is a complex concept of interrelationships among beliefs, values, language, social relationships, and other factors. Habayed goes on to state that culture is usually narrowly defined in terms of "color, religion, and geographic location" and "when cultural diversity is discussed in nursing, it is only in terms of minority or ethnic clients."

The nature of culture provides personhood and social relationships. It is the means of creating and limiting human choices and is expressed and identified by interlaced symbols; culture is an extension of biologic capabilities and can be two places at once—in the person's mind and also in the environment as artifacts or spoken word.

Any one definition of culture is too circumscribed, omitting salient aspects of culture and becoming too global to have any substantive meaning (Spector, 1996). For the purpose of having some definition, culture is the social process that is learned, changed, and taught. It is the matrix that influences consciously and unconsciously successive generations. Particular aspects of culture such as knowledge, beliefs, art, law, morals, and customs are retained and passed on unaltered from one generation to the next, or fall by the wayside depending on the social, political, and economic forces in our lives (Bohannan, 1992).

The cultural matrix influences the self-concept and interactions of the individual in coping with and adjusting to life circumstances. It is the sum of intellectual, behavioral, and emotional expressions of living formed by a group of persons and transmitted to succeeding generations. Culture is the substratum that nourishes ethnic expressions. For example, the aged Jewish (culture) immigrants clustered together in Venice, California, form a subculture based on their ethnicity and expressed characteristically by certain ceremonies and language idiosyncrasies that convey their collective generational and cultural identity. Variations exist in all cultures in all groups; some hold strong traditional values, and others are more contemporary.

Many of the differences in the elderly attributed to cultural variation may in reality be indications of educational differences, socioeconomic status, language limitations, misunderstanding or unawareness of potential resources, and wariness of the white middle-class professional agency personnel.

To fully understand another culture, one must enter into an unknown conceptual world in which time, space, religion, tradition, and wellness are expressed through a unique language that conveys these formulations about the nature of the world and humanity. Heritage consistency is a component of many features: communications, space, time, socialization, environment, and biology. These in turn affect culture, religion, and ethnicity. Collectively, the personal uniqueness is established. Figure 24-5 illustrates the relationship of the components of heritage consistency. Terms that are associated with cultural consistency such as assimilation, acculturation, socialization, ethnicity, ethnocentrism, and xenophobe are important to understanding cultural diversity and acquiring cultural sensitivity. Box 24-2 provides term definitions.

Assimilation and Adaptation

Four forms of assimilation occur, according to Spector (1985). These are culture, marital, primary, and secondary structural assimilation. Culture assimilation is reflected in the ability to speak excellent English. Marital assimilation is recognized through the intermarriage of persons of different groups. Primary and secondary structural assimilation are determined by the extent of social mingling and friendship between groups. Primary assimilation reflects relationships that are warm and friendly in all settings (home, social groups, church), whereas in secondary structural assimilation, there is a nondiscriminatory sharing, but it is cold and impersonal in nature.

There has been much concern about aged immigrants and how culture facilitates or hinders their adjustment to old age. Pierce et al (1978-1979) and Spector (1985) believed various kinds of acculturation were more critical to functional adaptation than others. For instance, outward adaptation to the Anglo culture that incorporates language, dress, and behavior was seen as superficially important. On a deeper level, traditional personal value orientations, including concepts of time, man to nature, and relationships, were more likely to remain in the original cultural context. Individually, it was found that most people had very unique patterns of acculturation, each incorporating certain aspects of the Anglo culture and retaining some from the original homeland. This study demonstrated the difficulty in making conclusive statements related to one culture or another, and we should hesitate to make assumptions. Nurses need to spend time finding out those aspects of culture that remain significant to the individual (cultural relativism). If a language barrier exists, it is imperative to find an interpreter. In most universities and some high schools there are students of language who may be flattered to assist. (Refer to Box 24-1 regarding the use of interpreters.)

Cultural Competence and Sensitivity. Nurses must avoid an ethnocentric stance; that is, the belief that the values and practices of one's own culture are the best ones (Gunter, 1991; Spector, 1996).

Cultural competence and sensitivity is being aware of the issues related to culture, race, gender, sexual orientation, so-cial class, economic situations, and many other factors (Meleis et al, 1995) through knowledge and the ability to intervene appropriately and effectively. In sum, cultural competence encompasses a complex combination of knowledge, attitudes, mutual respect, skill, and negotiation (Chrisman, 1992?). Attitudes are affected by experience, flexibility, empathy, and language facility. Skill includes cross-cultural communications, cultural interpretation, assessment, cultural interpretation of the assessment, and intervention (Lipson, 1996).

Knowledge is what the nurse learns and knows about the client, family, and community and their behaviors. Essential is knowledge of the person's way of life, ways of thinking, believing, and acting—knowledge obtained through personal experiences. Over time, the nurse builds up a reservoir of information about the beliefs of his or her clients and how they behave. An additional reservoir of knowledge comes from the clients and their families. Often nurses turn to these sources for information about ways they cope with chronic conditions and past health problems. Members of the health community who come from specific cultural backgrounds can also afford valuable data. A final source of knowledge comes from the literature. Books, pamphlets, articles, and journals can be significant sources of information about cultures different from that of the nurse. This knowledge needs to be taken and related to professional principles of nursing care. A common example of this is when a client adheres to their food customs, which are contrary to their therapeutic regimen. The nurse must weigh the nutritional value of the customs in order to recommend a reasonable substitute that will conform to the client's health state.

Mutual respect is closely allied with knowledge. It is working "with" the client rather than "on" the client. Knowledge allows the nurse to recognize and react more positively to seemingly strange and even bizarre health beliefs and practices. A nonjudgmental reaction due to knowl-

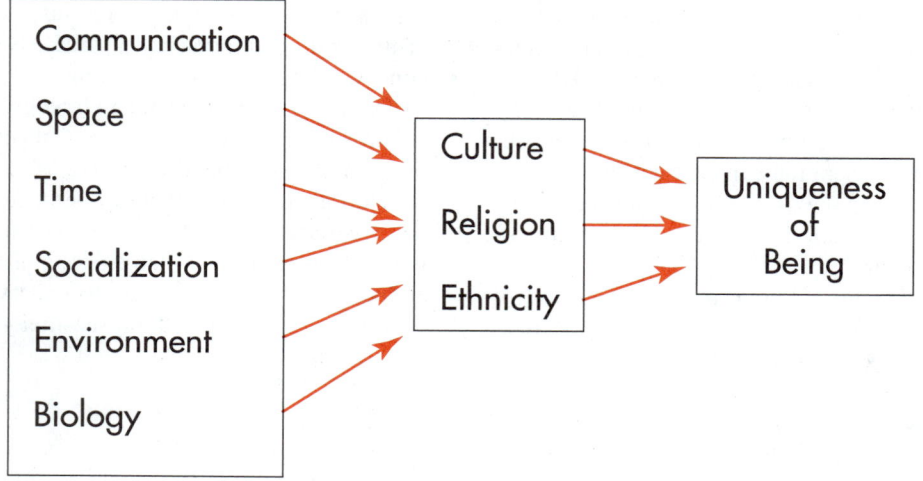

Figure 24-5. Heritage consistency. (Modified from Spector RE: *Cultural diversity in health and illness,* ed 4, East Norwalk, Conn, 1996, Appleton & Lange.)

edge about the ethnic group can signal to a client that the nurse trusts and respects the individual. Mutual respect is fundamental to culture-sensitive care because it opens opportunities for innovative planning of care that depends on trust between client and nurse (Chrisman, 1992).

Negotiation should attempt to preserve helpful beliefs and practices, accommodate beliefs that are neither helpful or harmful from the viewpoint of Western medicine, or repattern harmful beliefs or practices (Jackson, 1993). When repatterning is necessary, it is important to try and make the change without compromising underlying belief systems. When there is an impasse between client and nurse with each person perceiving the issue as nonnegotiable, the foundation of knowledge and trust or mutual respect that has been achieved will be helpful in seeking a goal that will optimize health outcomes beneficial to the client and still support the nurse's technical and ethical concerns.

In summary, Grossman (1994) and Spector (1996) suggest steps to cultural sensitivity and competence.

- **Know yourself:** examine your own values, attitudes, beliefs, and prejudice and your cultural heritage and identity.
- **Confront biases and stereotypes.**
- **Don't judge:** don't measure others' behavior against your beliefs and values.

- **Keep an open mind:** attempt to look at the world through other cultures' perspectives.
- **Respect differences among people:** each group has strengths and weaknesses. Appreciate inherent worth of diverse cultures, value them equally, and do not consider them inferior to one's own.
- **Listen!** Develop the ability to hear things that transcend language, and foster understanding of the client and his or her cultural heritage and the resilience that supports family and community that comes from within the culture.
- **Be willing to learn:** this requires interest in people's beliefs, values, and practices. Travel, read, and attend events in the local ethnic or cultural events in the community.
- **Develop an awareness and understanding for the complexities of the health-care delivery system—** its philosophy, problems, biases and stereotypes,— and become keenly aware of the socialization process that brings the care provider into this complex system.
- **Be resourceful and creative:** there are many ways to accomplish the same thing. Adapt your nursing interventions to suit different cultures and individuals.

Cultural Groups

Demographic and descriptive data about various cultural groups are useful in helping nurses to understand how and where they appear in the host culture. In many instances now there are printed and audiovisual materials available to assist the ethnic elder.

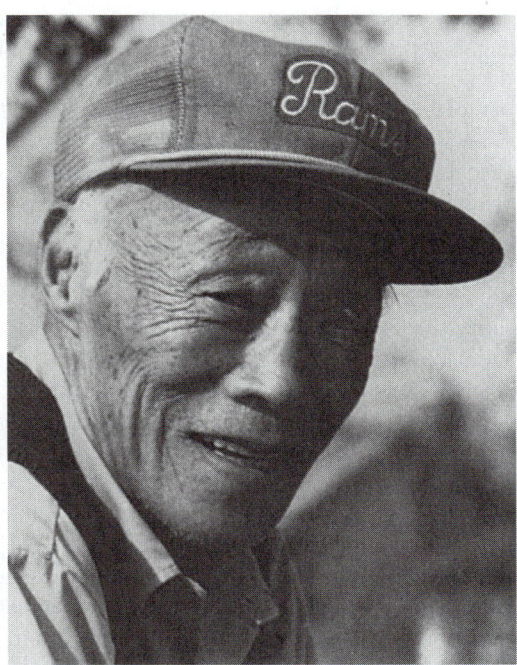

Adaptation to Anglo culture. (Courtesy Marie Walter, American Society on Aging.)

Box 24-2	Definition of Terms Associated with Culture

Heritage Consistency
　　The degree to which a person's lifestyle reflects his or her traditional culture; determination of one's culture, ethnic and religious background
Socialization
　　The process of being raised within a culture and acquiring the characteristics of that group
Acculturation
　　Becoming a competent participant in the dominant culture, even though one will always be identified as a member of a minority culture
Assimilation
　　The process of giving up or rejecting one's current cultural identity to develop a new cultural identity
Ethnicity
　　Belonging to a particular ethnic group within a cultural and social system based on such traits as religion, linguistics, ancestral or physical characteristics
Ethnocentrism
　　The belief in the superiority of one's own ethnic group
Xenophobe
　　One unduly fearful or contemptuous of strangers or foreigners, especially as reflected in his or her political and cultural views

Asian/Pacific Island Americans. There are at least 30 different languages and cultures subsumed under Asian/Pacific Islanders. Statistical data lump the Chinese, Japanese, Asian Indians, Cambodians, Filipinos, Guamanians, Hawaiians, Samoans, Vietnamese, and others under the category of Asian/Pacific Islanders. This extremely diverse group contains elders who immigrated to the United States during the turn of the century, children born to these immigrants, and elderly refugees, primarily from Southeast Asia, who entered the United States in the 1970s and 1980s. Approximately 640,000 (6.5%) Asian/Pacific Islanders are 65 years of age and older. Of these, 44,000 (6.9%) are 85 years or over. As of the 1995 census, 16% were concentrated in the Pacific Northwest and Pacific states. California has the largest single concentration of Asian/Pacific Islanders in that region (6%) and in the United States (40%). Smaller enclaves reside in other states, mainly in metropolitan areas, with only 10% living in rural areas (U.S. Bureau of the Census, 1995).

Although Asians vary immensely, they share certain characteristics that include a cyclic view of time, careful and orderly management of space, religious views that reinforce the importance of ancestry and tradition, languages written in imagery and expressed in subtleties, health practices that focus on vital balances within the organism, and traditionally, a greater concern for collective goals than for individual pursuits, though this is changing among the young. Table 24-3 lists health problems, risk factors, and areas for health education for Asian/Pacific Island elderly.

Chinese. The aged Chinese who emigrated to the United States have special needs, and it is suggested that to serve them best the health care providers should communicate through the youth in the family, who are often within the U.S. educational system and conversant with the ways of the elders as well as those of the dominant culture (Lin, 1988). One of the frequent errors whites have made in attempting to respond to cultural needs is to assume that Chinese is Chinese, black is black, and so on. We are becoming more discriminating now and are beginning to understand the vast differences within racial and cultural groups of the same generation but of different geographic roots. Lin (1988), a Chinese nursing student from Taiwan, refused to speculate about the needs of elderly Chinese who were not from Taiwan because she felt they were so distinctly different.

The Chinese are often known as quiet and noncomplaining patients. Caregivers interpret this as ideal behavior, but it may indicate conflict over modern treatment practices versus the traditional therapies and their tendency to hide feelings. Medical care may not be sought, or it may be rejected because of lack of funds, location of services, and lack of culturally sensitive health care services and personnel. The absence of bilingual staff creates a language barrier, often preventing adequate expression of these concerns. The strong belief in maintaining harmony may also be a factor in compliant behavior.

The traditional Chinese believe health is physical and spiritual harmony, which originates from ancient Taoist religion and philosophy. The individual must seek harmony within the environment. Wood, fire, earth, metal, and water are the guiding principles for human beings. Yin, the female negative energy (symbolized by cold, dark, and emptiness), and Yang, the male positive energy (symbolized by light, warmth, and fullness), must be in balance for health to prevail. Yin protects vital strength of life, and Yang protects the body from outside forces. The body is viewed as a gift of the parents and forebears, which should be well cared for and maintained. Any procedure that is intrusive detracts from body harmony. Any disruption of harmony is regarded as the sole cause of disease.

Traditionally diagnosis was made by inspecting, listening, smelling, asking questions, and palpating for pulses. Male physicians were not allowed to touch women; diagnosis was made by using a figurine on which the woman indicated the malady. From this background, diagnostic studies performed in modern medical practice are not understood. Painful procedures may create confusion. The Chinese, however, accept immunization and x-ray examinations willingly.

Treatments by moxibustion, acupuncture, and herbal medicine to restore the balance of Yin and Yang are used by those Chinese who refuse modern medical assistance or are used in conjunction with today's medical practices. Health-seeking behavior is based on "whatever works." Western medicine is used for acute conditions, whereas Eastern medicine and cultural healers are used for chronic problems.

There are few left of the Chinese elderly who as young men immigrated to the United States early in the twentieth century with intentions of bringing the family later but, because of restrictive immigration laws, could not. When immigration laws relaxed after World War II, the Chinese were again thwarted by China's restrictive laws; people could not return to or leave China. However, by 1965, large numbers of refugees who had relatives in the United States were able to come to this country (Spector, 1996).

Japanese. Although increasingly acculturated to the United States, the feelings and attitudes of the older Japanese are strongly rooted in the cultural values and norms of their homeland. The Japanese Nisei (first American-born children of Japanese immigrants) were routinely sent to Japan by their parents (Issei) to be educated and socialized and as a means of cultural perpetuation. The Japanese immigrants did not expect much in terms of assimilation, equality, or expanded job opportunities; instead of demanding change, patience prevailed until opportunities arose.

Most Issei live in areas designated "Little Tokyo" or Nihonmachi, which remain relatively safe havens for the Japanese elderly. Traditional filial piety, *koko,* keeping problems to themselves, face-saving behaviors, limited fluency in the English language, and unfamiliarity with the social service bureaucracies are reasons for not using the larger community's resources. Discriminatory and hostile behaviors of health care providers are further barriers.

The Nisei adopted values and expected behaviors of American culture, but they were slow to be accepted and included in personal or social relationships with whites. The worst discrimination suffered by this group occurred during World War II, when over 70,000 American-born Japanese were confined to "relocation camps." Simultaneously, many of the young male Nisei were serving in the US Army and stationed in Europe. There is probably a residue of bitterness, even among the Sansei (third generation) and Yonsei (fourth generation), although their devotion to politeness may cover these feelings. In the early 1990s the US government acknowledged the inequities and disruption to the lives of the Japanese Americans and made monetary restitution to those who had been interned in the relocation camps.

As part of cultural behavior, the elder may refuse an offer or offered object out of a sense of overpoliteness before accepting the offer. In the hospital, the Japanese patient may not turn on the call light until in dire need so as to not bother the staff. One perceives his or her own needs as less important than others (Morioka-Douglas and Yeo, 1990). The elders who speak only Japanese are more responsive to caregivers, friends, and family who speak their language.

Most importantly, the Japanese elder expects respect and tact when interacting with caregivers. Giving a command to a Japanese elder is an insult. The aged person needs only respect and understanding of expectations to comply. Attention to the specific manifestations of these cultural values will lead to better assessments, interpretations, and conclusions.

African (Black) Americans. Approximately 2.7 million (8.2%) of the black population are 65 years or over. Nine percent (268,000) of black elders are 85 years of age or older (U.S .Bureau of the Census, 1995). Work history of the black elders has seldom produced Social Security and pension benefits adequate to meet their needs in late life. Old black women in rural areas are triply disadvantaged, and about 65% of them live in poverty. Within the black population, ethnic diversity is complex. Immigrant blacks come from African countries, the West Indies, Dominican Republic, Haiti, and Jamaica and bring with them the varied beliefs and customs of these regions as well as their commonalties.

Health in black cultures is generally viewed as harmony with nature, and illness is viewed as disharmony. The mind, body, and spirit are not viewed separately. The black health belief system is an amalgam of ethnic origins, remnants of folk and formal medicine practiced 100 years ago and influenced by Christianity, nativistic religions, sympathetic magic (Snow, 1974), and selected beliefs from modern scientific medicine. Many black elderly continue to use folk medicine practices when orthodox medicine and procedures do not work. Urban blacks are known to occasionally visit black cultural or religious healers.

| **Table 24-3** | Leading Health Problems of Asian/Pacific Americans, Modifiable Risk Factors, and Education Areas |

Diseases	Modifiable factors	Education areas
Filipinos, Japanese, Native Hawaiians, Chinese		
High blood pressure	Lack of exercise, smoking, obesity, diet (high sodium)	Proper use of medications Nutrition: Sodium, cholesterol recipe modification
Japanese, Native Hawaiians		
Coronary heart disease	High blood pressure, high cholesterol levels, smoking, diabetes, alcohol	Exercise Preventive services/screening for hypertension and diabetes
Japanese, Chinese, Native Hawaiians		
Cancer	Smoking, diet, alcohol	
Japanese, Filipinos, Chinese, Koreans, Native Hawaiians		
Diabetes	Diet, obesity, lack of exercise, alcohol	

From American Association of Retired Persons: *Healthy aging: making health promotion work for minority elders,* Washington, DC, 1990, The Association.

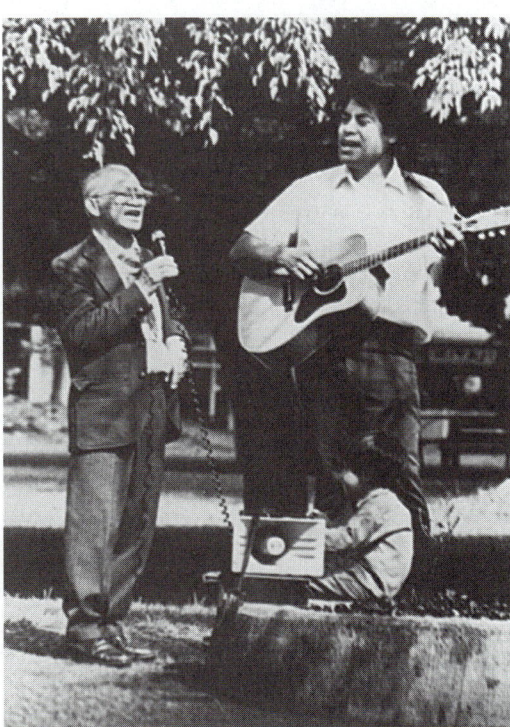

Issei, Nisei, and Sansei. (Courtesy American Society on Aging.)

Caregivers who do not understand beliefs and practices or have their own fears, insecurity, or misinformation may approach the black client with a demeaning action or tone of voice. The client may be told about problems in medical jargon, which produces fear of manipulation, feelings of alienation, and a sense of being talked down to and subjugation.

Elderly blacks usually react with patience, perseverance, and fatalistic acceptance of their fate. Time orientation differs between blacks and whites, with blacks functioning on a more flexible time orientation. Awareness of this difference in perspective dictates greater flexibility when providing care to the black elder. Another issue requiring some insight is the use of black English, which evolved from West Africa during the period of slavery. A combination of English words and West African language patterns creates a highly oral, stylized, rhythmic, and spontaneous language. Meaningful interaction is conveyed by the intonations and inflections of speech. Caregivers may gain some understanding of the specific health beliefs and practices important to a particular black client simply by careful observation and discussion with the individual.

We frequently hear of disadvantaged African-Americans and their shorter life expectancy when compared with whites. A study by Manton et al (1979; Gibson, 1994) demonstrates the hardiness of very old blacks. Those who live past 75 years of age are likely to outlive their white cohorts. This is called the mortality crossover (Markides and Mindel, 1987). After age 85, both African-American men and women have a lower incidence of heart disease, arteriosclerosis, and cancer. Blacks who survive to 85 years of age are considered "old-old." They are sturdier than whites, have a lower mortality, and often appear much younger. According to Stokes (1979), the black elderly seem to accept old age better and maintain higher morale than the white elderly.

It is estimated that one third of the African-American community has no form of health care reimbursement, and the large majority of that group do not receive attention to health problems until they become critical. During the Reagan administration, a task force to study the health status of black Americans was established (Pinkleton, 1988). The six major problems identified were (1) cancer, (2) heart disease and stroke, (3) infant mortality, (4) diabetes, (5) homicide, suicide, and unintentional accidents, and (6) chemical dependency. Table 24-4 lists the present health problems, risk factors and areas for health education for the elderly. The report of the task force indicated an excess of deaths in the African-American population, a disparity between the number of deaths in this minority population compared with a similar group in a nonminority population. A large number of African-Americans are dying because of their life histories, current economic situation, and impaired access to health care. The task force identified the following social characteristics that particularly influence health status of minorities: (1) demographic profiles, (2) nutritional status and dietary practices, (3) environmental and occupational exposures, and (4) stress and other coping patterns. It is thought that some coping patterns engendered by substandard housing, education, and employment have put elders at risk or have been singularly etiologic to the identified major health problems. It is known that the life expectancy of African-Americans is 5.6 years less than for whites. Pinkelton, a black professor at Hampton University, in 1988 made a plea for increased numbers of competent, autonomous, African-American nurses to provide comprehensive health services for the increasing numbers of black elders. African-American nurses are likely to "speak their language" and in so doing increase their comfort and responsiveness.

Black elders have unique histories and adaptive patterns that are often neglected because their cultural and social needs are not recognized. Recognizing typical patterns of behavior, while not to be used as stereotypes, will help nurses work more sensitively. Compared to the majority of individuals, the education of African American elders has been neglected, and these elders are poorer, have less adequate housing, and a shorter life span. They experience more chronic health problems, illnesses, and injuries than similar groups of whites. All of these factors must be given special consideration.

Table 24-4   Leading Health Problems of Black Americans, Modifiable Risk Factors, and Education Areas

Diseases	Modifiable factors	Education areas
Heart disease, cardiovascular Stroke	High blood pressure, high cholesterol levels, smoking, diabetes, diet, obesity, lack of exercise	Nutrition: salt, cholesterol levels, weight loss and control, exercise
Cancer	Smoking, diet, alcohol	Smoke cessation, nutrition, referral for alcohol abuse
Diabetes	Diet, obesity, alcohol, lack of exercise	Exercise
		Preventive services/screening for hypertension, diabetes
Cirrhosis of the liver	Alcohol	Referral for alcohol abuse

From American Association of Retired Persons: *Healthy aging: making health promotion work for minority elders,* Washington, DC, 1990, The Association.

Church members are an important source of support to the elderly African-American. They develop a hierarchy of assistance, from family to friends and then neighbors and church members, before they seek help from formal organizations. Findings from the extensive National Survey of Black Americans (NSBA) show that over 80% of blacks receive support from church members (Dilworth-Anderson, 1992; Walls, 1992). This study found that elderly African-Americans have an extensive support network of family, friends, and church. Belgrave et al (1993) suggest that the multigenerational households may be a function of age, mental and socioeconomic status, and health. In addition, the African-American is less likely to be in a nursing home with only 3% after age 65 and 12% aged 85 and older.

A young black nursing student chose, for her community elder assignment, to work with "Auntie Grace" . . . not a relative, but a member of the church community. Auntie Grace was old, poor, and obese, lived alone in a deteriorating home, and had great difficulty ambulating. The student's major assignment was to learn about aging and adaptation from Auntie Grace. Auntie Grace gave art lessons to several young children, and when the student realized how much she loved them, the talk turned to children. She was astonished to find that Auntie Grace never had children because she had inherited her father's dark color rather than her mother's lighter complexion, and she was afraid the same would happen to her children. The student and I discussed the impact of the previous generational perspective and the great sacrifice the old lady had made to protect unborn children from segregation and injustice. Auntie Grace did not regret her decision but took pleasure in enriching the lives of others' children. This old black lady, with a family history of slavery, enriched our lives as well.

Hispanic Americans. Hispanics are culturally diverse with unique cultural heritage, histories, and dialects. Hispanics come from Mexico, Central and South America, Cuba, Spain, and Puerto Rico. Mexican-Americans are the largest group of Hispanic people in the United States. This highly diverse population includes native born, legal and undocumented immigrants. Over 1.5 million (8%) are 65 years old or older. Of this group, 9%, or approximately 140,000 Hispanic elders, are 85 years of age or over (U.S. Bureau of the Census, 1995).

Though Hispanic Americans live in every state in the nation, the vast majority (73%) of these elders live in barrios and groups of 100,000 to 300,000 in four states. California (34%) and Texas (10%) attract Hispanic groups from Central America and Mexico; Florida (7.2%) seems to attract Cubans; and New York (8.8%) attracts Hispanics from the Caribbean Islands and Puerto Rico (U.S. Bureau of the Census, 1995).

Many Hispanics, particularly Mexican-Americans, believe that health and illness are "God's will," and they are expected to maintain their own equilibrium in balance with the universe by proper behavior, proper nutrition, and work. Illness may be prevented by praying, adorning one's self with religious medals and amulets, and maintaining religious symbols in the home. Illness, when it occurs, is the result of imbalance or is a punishment for an evil deed. Illness occurs because of (1) imbalance of cold, hot, wet, or dry humors; (2) dislocation of body parts, the "evil eye" (magic or supernatural); (3) fright or envy; or (4) wrongdoing. Illness is seen as punishment. When illness is very serious, magic or religious practices are used.

Caregivers often become annoyed with Mexican-Americans because they do not respond to time the way Anglos do. Time orientation for the Mexican-American is relative, and time is measured by day and night and need (Monrroy, 1980; de Paula et al, 1996).

A Mexican-American nurse, Carmen Altamirano Wilson (1988), wrote of elderly Hispanic people as a unique and culturally special group particularly sensitive to evidence of respect or lack of it. They are intensely proud. She shares the following evidence, "Pobres pero orgullosos. El orgullo si podemos tener porque eso no se compra en las boticas!" Her translation is, "Poor but proud. Pride is something we can possess because it is something we don't have to buy." Respect is evidence to the aged Hispanic of his or her worth and merit. When not treated respectfully, the elder assumes he or she is in some way undeserving of respect. Health providers must address elderly Hispanics formally and avoid familiarity until (if ever) the elder indicates differently. Elders have a strong sense of privacy and feel they are able to handle their own problems within the family with the help of church and faith. Many believe that God will not give them a cross too heavy to bear and that if they follow His will He will take care of them. Daily prayer sustains them, and their faith provides comfort and peace. They are cautious, nonaggressive, and humble when giving and receiving. They give as a thanksgiving to God and expect nothing but His blessing in return (Wilson, 1988).

A Hispanic's evaluation for health care may be influenced by these attitudes. For instance, outright criticism is seldom given because the individual may feel he or she is somehow getting what is deserved and is unworthy of anything better (Wilson, 1988). Keeping in mind that the profile given by Wilson cannot be applied to all aged Hispanics, it can do no harm to anyone to give respect, consider privacy, and proceed with formality until the client indicates otherwise.

Many old persons of all cultures value their faith and tend to feel fatalistic about "the burdens God has given me to bear." It will rarely be possible or useful to convince them otherwise. If you suspect this may be true of your client, ask him or her about the story of Job and thoughts about it.

It would be helpful if caregivers demonstrate interest in the Hispanic subgroup with which the elder is affiliated, and it would be a beginning of respect, understanding, and sensitivity. The Hispanic usually prefers to be addressed by his or her last name. Ask what is preferred. Respect and courtesy toward elders are important in the Hispanic culture, as are privacy and modesty.

Hispanics do not want to hurt anyone's feelings, so they will not readily express dissatisfaction. Even when the individual does not understand what is said, he or she will usually respond with a polite affirmative reply. It is important for the caregiver to be aware of this and be sure that the individual truly understands.

Respect for life, family structure, hard work, and involvement in the care and education of the children are expectations in Hispanic culture (Spector, 1996; Hooyman and Kiyak, 1996; de Paula et al, 1996). Aged Hispanics are increasingly without a role. Their children have increased social status and educational levels, whereas their own status and respect have decreased. Their children do not seem to need their knowledge and wisdom to survive today. The aged live either in small towns far away from their children or in cities surrounded by a system that does not need their skills. The role they had envisioned in their old age has not materialized.

Table 24-5 provides insight into the leading health problems of Hispanic Americans, the risk factors, and areas of health education. It appears that some of these factors relate directly to the degree of enculturation rather than to ethnicity or poverty (Espino and Maldonado, 1990). Hooyman and Kiyak (1996) point to social and cultural barriers that interfere with care. Mistrust of white medical providers, stigma associated with mental health services, reliance on folk medicine, religious healing, and less health insurance coverage are seen as significant issues.

Native Americans. The Native American elders include the American Indians and the Alaskan natives (Eskimos and the Aleuts). This combined group has the fastest growing elderly population. It is expanding at about twice the rate of white and black elders. By the end of the century, the number of those over 75 year of age will have doubled, and by the year 2050 this population will have reached 38% of the Native American population. One quarter of the Native American elders live on American Indian reservations or in Alaskan native villages. Over half of the Native American elders reside in California, Arizona, New Mexico, Texas, and Oklahoma with the remainder living throughout the other states (U.S. Bureau of the Census, 1995). Native Americans comprise the largest group of elders to reside in rural areas.

Health means living in harmony with nature and the ability to survive under exceedingly difficult circumstances for the approximately 500 recognized tribal groups with 200 native languages (Hooyman and Kiyak, 1996). The earth and the self are tied; what affects one affects the other. The body is treated with respect and is viewed as having two parts, a positive and a negative energy.

Every sickness or pain that occurs results from something that happened in the past or will in the future, representing a cause-and-effect relationship. Some tribes, however, relate illness to evil spirits.

| Table 24-5 | Leading Health Problems of Hispanic Americans, Modifiable Risk Factors, and Education Areas |

Diseases	Modifiable factors	Education areas
High blood pressure	Lack of exercise, obesity, eating habits	Nutrition: Balanced diet, salt, sugar, cholesterol Weight loss and control
Diabetes	Lack of exercise, obesity, eating habits, alcohol	Prevention services/screening for hypertension and diabetes
Cancer	Eating habits, smoking, alcohol	Referral for alcohol abuse, smoking cessation

From American Association of Retired Persons: *Healthy aging: making health promotion work for minority elders,* Washington, DC, 1990, The Association.

| Table 24-6 | Leading Health Problems of Native Americans and Alaskan Americans, Modifiable Risk Factors, and Education Areas |

Diseases	Modifiable factors	Education areas
Heart disease	High blood pressure, smoking, high cholesterol levels, diabetes, obesity, diet, lack of exercise	Preventive services/screening/inoculations Support groups or referral for alcohol Smoking cessation Nutrition: fats, fiber Weight loss and control Exercise
Cancer	Smoking, alcohol, high animal fat, low fiber diet	
Accidents	Alcohol and alcoholism	
Chronic liver disease and cirrhosis	Alcohol and alcoholism	
Diabetes	Diet, obesity, lack of exercise, alcohol	
Pneumonia/influenza	Malnutrition, alcoholism, smoking, diabetes	

From American Association of Retired Persons: *Healthy aging: making health promotion work for minority elders,* Washington, DC, 1990, The Association.
*All education areas noted are interrelated.

A Native American converses in low tones and expects to be listened to with attentiveness. To ask the person to repeat or to say "huh" is inappropriate. Notes should not be taken; they are taboo. The nurse must develop acute mental processes for retaining information such as assessment data. Questions are not well received. Instead, declarative statements such as, "You have a pain that keeps you awake" are seen as evidence of respect. The American Indian elderly expect the caregiver to deduce the problem by intuition rather than by questioning (Wilson, 1988). In addition, one must be aware of the strong importance of nonverbal communication (Cuellar, 1990a; Spector, 1996; Kramer, 1996).

Self-esteem is based on the ability to help others by giving advice to younger members of the tribe and being regarded as a source of wisdom. Cooperation is a source of pride, and competition is discouraged (Martin, 1977).

Table 24-6 lists the leading health problems with the risk factors and areas of health education for native American elders.

Various tribes may have specific rituals that are performed at death, such as burying certain personal possessions with the individual. Consulting with members of the specific tribe to gain insight into special rituals during sickness and at death would be advantageous for nurses working with Native American patients.

MULTICULTURAL NURSING PERSPECTIVES

Most universities now have an international division or section to represent and attend to the needs of students of foreign backgrounds or ethnic study programs. Nursing schools and nursing students may find valuable ideas and assistance toward providing appropriate care through cultivating ties with persons of a particular culture or country or through collaboration with representatives of university ethnic study programs. In addition, cross-cultural research that is conducted by investigators representing both cultures is desperately needed. As Lin noted (1988), professionals visiting a country for short periods rarely discover the real needs and problematic issues. It is interesting to note how few studies of ethnic or foreign elders have been conducted by persons indigenous to the group.

If nurses are unfamiliar with a particular ethnic group, churches or associations (for example, Polish American Alliance, Celtic League, Jewish Family and Children's Society, Slovak League of America) can be helpful in identifying interpreters or persons who can serve as a cultural resource. Consulates for various countries may provide a list of organizations specific to a cultural group. Schools of nursing have recently started to address cultural aspects in their curriculum. Nurses who graduated prior to this time and who are working may need to individually seek these experi-

ences. Suggestions for upgrading knowledge about the minority aged include the following:

1. Develop interest in and commitment to the needs of minority groups.
2. Become involved in experiences with diverse ethnic and cultural groups.
3. Learn about historical and cultural roots of ethnic variations.
4. Respond to the diverse needs within your community.

Cultural and Health Belief Systems

There are a number of health belief systems that fall into three categories and are actively practiced today as they have been in the past. These are the biomedical or Western system, the personalistic or magicoreligious system, and the naturalistic or holistic system. The diversity of the population has brought the strong potential for a clash of health belief systems, language, and attitudes about health and illness between the care provider and the client. Many of the beliefs and practices do not fit into the traditional format of health care as most care providers know it.

The biomedical, scientific, or Western medical belief system espouses that disease is the result of abnormalities in structure and function of body organs and systems. It is still a dominant belief that permeates the thinking of those educated in Western health care. The objective term *disease* is used by care providers, and *illness* is a subjective term to describe symptoms of discomfort or sickness. A personal state of illness has distinct social dimensions. Assessment, and diagnosis are directed at identifying the pathogen or process causing the abnormality and removing or destroying the cause or at least repairing or modifying the problem through treatment. Highly skilled clinicians use the scientific method, and sophisticated laboratory and other procedures to stem the disease or disease process. Prevention in this belief system is to avoid pathogens, chemicals, activities, and dietary agents known to cause malfunction.

Personalistic or magicoreligious beliefs may have originated in groups that were relatively small, isolated, illiterate and lacked contact with ancient high civilizations (Jackson, 1993). Those who follow the beliefs of the personalistic or magicoreligious system believe that illness is caused by active, purposeful intervention of agents of the supernatural, such as gods, deities, non-human beings. Ghosts, ancestors, evil spirits, or humans in the form of witches or sorcerers are responsible for sickness. The individual is considered a victim, an object of aggression or punishment. Someone may be put under a spell by a disgruntled neighbor so that they can't eat or sleep. A dead relative may be angry that his or her wishes were not followed and send an animal to bite the person, cause a growth, or cause a woman to be infertile.

Identification of the agent behind these events and rendering it harmless, lifting a spell, or reversing the method used by the agent is the aim of treatment. Once the agent is

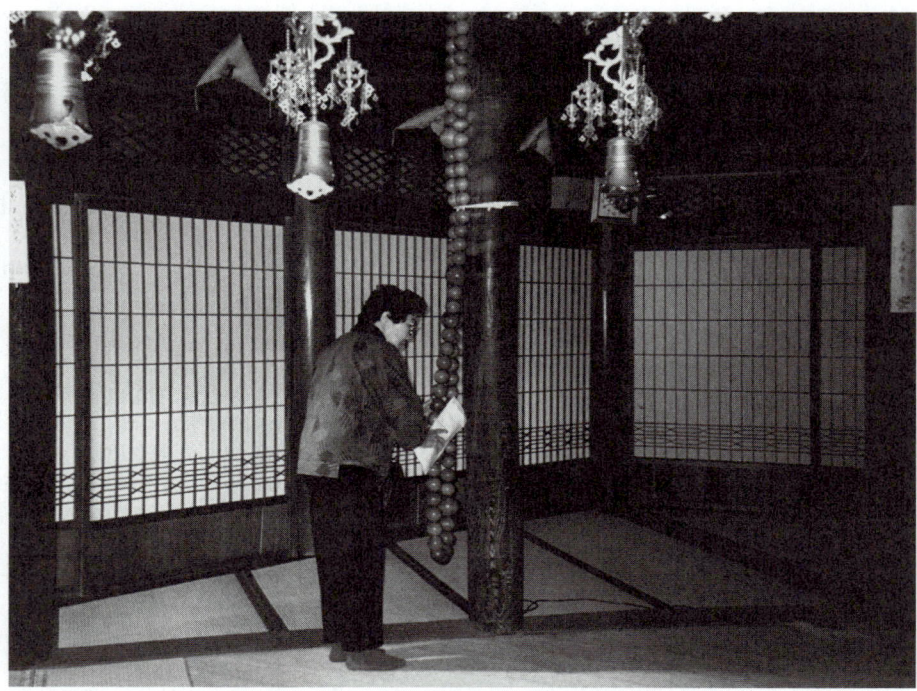

Healing beads. (Courtesy Priscilla Ebersole.)

known, the curer or person can take steps to resolve the situation. Physical symptoms are secondary to finding the initial cause of the dilemma. Making sure that social networks with their fellow humans are in good working order is the essence of prevention in this health belief system. Therefore avoiding angering family, friends, neighbors, ancestors, gods, etc.; adherence to and the correct performance of rituals are very important. Etiologies of the personalistic beliefs may be intertwined with religious beliefs. Entities that cause illness may be expanded to explain that the deities, ghosts, etc. are the cause of crop failures, accidents, financial reversals, and so on.

Naturalistic or holistic health beliefs consider sickness an impersonal systemic term. Health is due to equilibrium of the elements of the body such as hot and cold. These must be in balance or harmony. When this is not so, illness is present. The current naturalistic beliefs stem from the ancient civilizations of China, India, and Greece (Jackson, 1993).

Traditional Chinese medicine is the basis for the health belief system and practices today of such countries as Japan, Vietnam, Korea, Taiwan, Singapore, Hong Kong, and China. In India and some of its neighboring countries, Ayurvedic medicine, which arose in ancient India, is still practiced. Humoral pathology, practiced by the ancient Greeks was disseminated both east and west and was embraced by the Moslem culture, Spanish and Italian explorers. Variations of humoral pathology can be found in the medical systems of rural and some urban people in Latin America, Philippines, in some low-income blacks and whites in the southern

United States. These beliefs are also found in sophisticated and unsophisticated populations in Iran, Pakistan, Malaysia, and Java (Jackson, 1993). In the United States or countries that are steeped in the biomedical system, the aforementioned beliefs are considered "folk medicine."

Though the origins of naturalistic beliefs are different, they all consider illness the result of an excess of heat or cold that enters the body and causes an imbalance. Hot and cold is generally metaphoric, although at times temperature is an aspect. Various foods, medicines, environmental conditions, emotions, and bodily conditions such as menstruation, pregnancy, etc., may posses the characteristics of either hot or cold (Jackson, 1993; Spector, 1996).

Diagnosis is concerned with identifying the cause of the disease as either hot or cold in origin. Remedies are divided into hot and cold. Treatment then is focused on using the opposite element; if the disease is the result of excess hot, then treatment will be with something which has cold properties and vise versa. The treatments may take the form of herbs, food, dietary restrictions, medications from Western medicine that have hot and cold properties such as antibiotics, massage, poultices, and other therapies. Naturalistic curers are physicians or herbalists who specialize in symptomatic treatment and know which medicines will restore the body's equilibrium. Prevention is directed at protecting oneself from extremes of heat and cold in both the literal and metaphoric sense.

One may recognize a melding of the various health system beliefs in oneself and others. Therefore, it behooves care providers to become sensitive to and versed in these

Table 24-7	Explanations of Illness: Biomedical and Behavioral	
	Biomedical model	**Behaviorally ethnic model**
Etiologic beliefs		
Social causes of illness	Usually limited to the stress model or attributed to paranoia.	Many social indiscretions can cause illness. Blaming oneself or others for symptoms is common.
Environmental causes of illness	Exposure to known pathogens, toxins, and social stress may cause symptoms.	Dietary indiscretion can cause hot-cold imbalance in the body. Drafts may cause symptoms.
Blood conditions as causes of illness	Limited to specific hematologic disorders or hypertension.	Many conditions of the blood (too thick, thin, high, low, or stagnant) can cause illness.
Symptom presentation and interpretation		
Altered states of consciousness (trance, visions)	Likely to be considered abnormal.	Often considered to be normal or desirable.
Attitudes toward pain	Stoicism expected unless complaints are congruent with clear organic pathology.	Either total stoicism or emotional expression of pain is healthy and expected.
Focus on physical symptoms	May be considered a psychiatric syndrome.	Expected, proper way of showing distress.
Treatment expectations		
Who is the patient?	Individual is focus of decision making and care.	The family must be involved in decision making.
Beliefs about self-medication and alternative practitioners	Considered potentially dangerous or undesirable.	Self-medication and consulting with traditional healers are common.

Modified with permission from Johnson TH, Hardt EJ, Kleinman A: Cultural factors in the medical interview. In Lipkin M Jr, Putnam SM, Lazare A, editors: *The medical interview,* New York, 1994, Springer-Verlag.

systems to better understand, not necessarily agree, with persons for whom they are providing care, while recognizing their own ethnocentristic tendencies. Table 24-7 illustrates variations in illness beliefs between the biomedical and other ethnically based models.

Culture and Health Practices

Attempts to discover and assess health practices and preferences within various groups often yield fascinating results. Elders who grew up in remote areas of any country, including the United States, where traditional health services were scarce or unavailable, developed quite a number of unusual health practices. Some are physiologically sound, and others may have been beneficial because of the placebo effects. It is important to include this type of information in a health assessment. Even though the client may not admit to presently using any historic folk remedies or unusual practices, awareness of the possibility is important. Encourage and incorporate these practices unless the practice is clearly detrimental. We know belief and hope have therapeutic benefits. Alternative healers must also be discussed and encouraged if the client believes they are important. Some of the barriers ethnic elders experience can be seen in Figure 24-6.

Many questions have been raised about the advisability of using indigenous health care providers and agency personnel to serve the elderly of ethnic minorities. We believe this is ideal but not always possible. A sensitive nurse needs to become aware of her own cultural roots, embrace and enjoy them, but keep them in proper perspective in the nurse-client relationship. As with clients of all backgrounds, one

nursing function of great importance is to support the ties with family or reference group that maintain the aged person's sense of solidarity. Encourage family members to prepare specially enjoyed foods and perform significant rituals. Locate priests, monks, rabbis, or ministers who may comfort the aged person. When alternative healing methods are used, respect them as judiciously as the traditional. A sense of caring is conveyed in these gestures of personal recognition. Caring can surmount cultural differences.

Assessment

A cultural history is one way to understand where the aged adult's health beliefs lie. There are few tools or instruments that assist the nurse to elicit health care beliefs and at the same time identify to the nurse his or her own perceptions of the beliefs. Given the necessary data, the nurse is able to use this information to negotiate a clear understanding of problems and solutions with the client or the individual who is the appropriate support figure in the client's life. One must keep in mind that there may be great generational cohort and cultural differences between practitioner and client. To provide quality care to ethnic elders, a comprehensive cultural assessment is important. This type of assessment takes time. It is clear that not all situations allow for this, but even if it must be done bit by bit over time, it will be valuable to the caregiver in better understanding how to work with and within the culture of the client. The Exploratory Models developed by Kleinman (1980) and Pfeifferling (1981) have helped caregivers obtain needed information in a culturally sensitive manner (Appendix 24-A). Box 24-3 offers

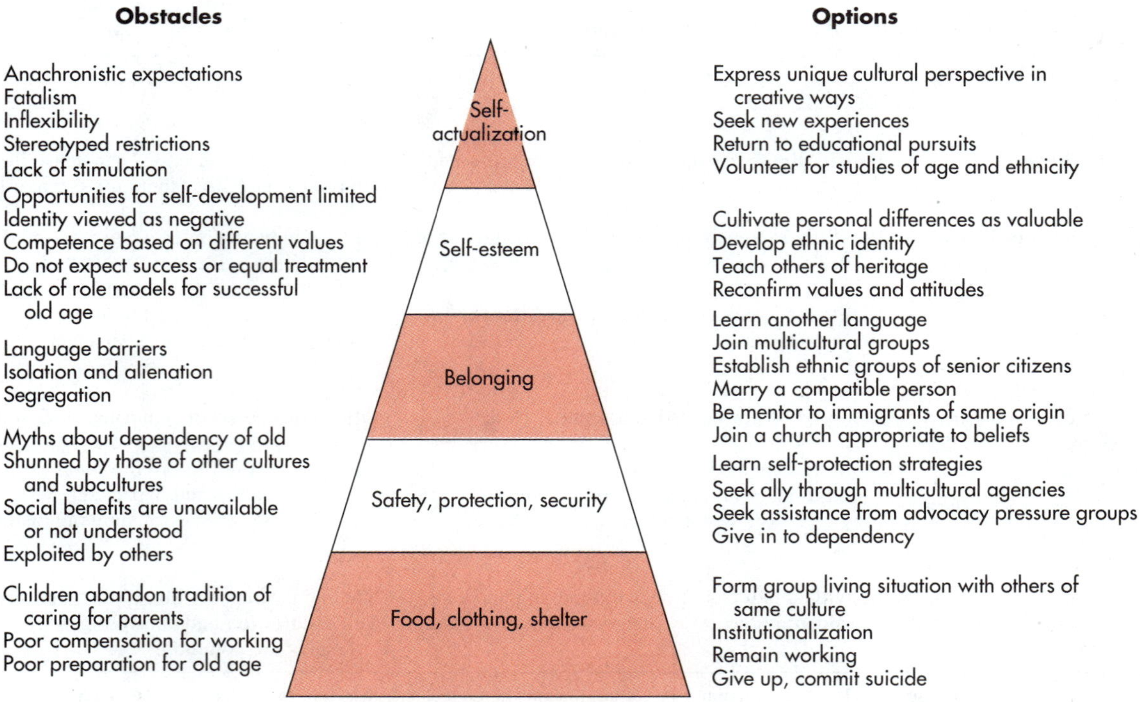

Obstacles

Anachronistic expectations
Fatalism
Inflexibility
Stereotyped restrictions
Lack of stimulation
Opportunities for self-development limited
Identity viewed as negative
Competence based on different values
Do not expect success or equal treatment
Lack of role models for successful
   old age

Language barriers
Isolation and alienation
Segregation

Myths about dependency of old
Shunned by those of other cultures
   and subcultures
Social benefits are unavailable
   or not understood
Exploited by others

Children abandon tradition of
   caring for parents
Poor compensation for working
Poor preparation for old age

Options

Express unique cultural perspective in
   creative ways
Seek new experiences
Return to educational pursuits
Volunteer for studies of age and ethnicity

Cultivate personal differences as valuable
Develop ethnic identity
Teach others of heritage
Reconfirm values and attitudes

Learn another language
Join multicultural groups
Establish ethnic groups of senior citizens
Marry a compatible person
Be mentor to immigrants of same origin
Join a church appropriate to beliefs

Learn self-protection strategies
Seek ally through multicultural agencies
Seek assistance from advocacy pressure groups
Give in to dependency

Form group living situation with others of
   same culture
Institutionalization
Remain working
Give up, commit suicide

Pyramid levels (top to bottom): Self-actualization; Self-esteem; Belonging; Safety, protection, security; Food, clothing, shelter

Figure 24-6. Cultural barriers to meeting needs. (Modified from Smith D et al: *A multicultural view of drug abuse,* Boston, 1978, GK Hall & Co.)

Box 24-3

Cultural Assessment Related to Client's Health Problem

The clinician may need to identify others who can facilitate the discussion of the client's problem(s).

1. How would you describe the problem that has brought you here? (What do you call your problem; does it have a name?)
   A. Who in the community and your family helps you with your problem?
2. How long have you had this problem?
   A. When do you think it started?
   B. What do you think started it?
   C. Do you know anyone else with it?
   D. Tell me what happened to them when dealing with this problem
3. What do you think is wrong with you?
   A. What does your sickness do to you?
   B. How severe is it?
   C. What might other people think is wrong with you?
   D. Tell me about people who don't get this problem.

4. Why do you think this happened to you, and why?
   A. Why has it happened to the involved part?
   B. Why do you get sick and not someone else?
   C. Will it have a long or short course?
   D. What do you fear most about your sickness?
5. What are the chief problems your sickness has caused you?
6. What do you think will help clear up this problem? (What treatment should you receive; what are the most important results you hope to receive?)
   A. If specific tests, medications are listed, ask what they are and do.
7. Apart from me, who else do you think can make you feel better?
   A. Are there therapies that make you feel better that I don't know? (May be in another discipline.)

Adapted from Kleinman A: *Patient and healers in the context of culture: an exploration of the borderland between anthropology, medicine, and psychiatry,* Berkeley, 1980, University of California Press; Pfeifferling JH: A cultural prescription for mediocentrism. In Eisenberg L, Kleinman A, editors: *The relevance of social science for medicine,* Boston, 1981, Reidel.

an adaptation of these models for use in a cultural health assessment. Evans and Cunningham (1996) offer specific assessment topics and items to be assessed in Table 24-8.

Usually information gleaned about minority elders concerns the type of practitioners, rituals, and medications, but little attention is given to the activities of daily living that are so vital to care of the aged (Gunter, 1991). In order to plan for immediate and long-term care Gunter (1991) offers an assessment of personal care practices of minority aged. These are depicted in Table 24-9. Some of these orientations literally cannot be expressed in another language and cannot be fully understood outside the culture. As stated earlier, nurses must avoid an ethnocentric stance; that is, the belief that the values and practices of one's own culture are the best ones (Gunter, 1991). Ethnocentrism will be discussed again later in this chapter.

Table 24-8   Nursing Care for the Ethnic Elder

	Assessment	Interventions
Ethnicity	Number of years living in United States. Age at immigration (immigrant vs refugee). Degree of affiliation with ethnic group or assimilation to U.S. culture.	Be sensitive to historical events that influence elders' perception of self and authority of health care providers. Demonstrate respect for elder by using surname and providing care in a manner sensitive to cultural norms.
Communication	English as primary or secondary language. Level of fluency. Barriers to communication such as sensory deficits, lack of privacy, distractions. Meaning of nonverbal gestures.	Use of translator for exchange of health information. Document system for communicating basic needs between patient and staff. Provide patient access to sensory aids (glasses, hearing aids, pocket talkers). Eliminate background noise and provide optimum lighting. Smile, offer gestures of assistance with basic needs (warm blanket, glass of water).
Health perception	Perception of health problem, causes, and prognosis. Response to pain, illness and death.	Educate patient/family about disease process and medical treatments. Identify and document reasons for behavior. Develop system for identifying and rating pain.
Folk practices	Use of cultural healers, herbal medicines, alternative health practices and beliefs.	Obtain order for use of folk remedies as indicated. Educate patient regarding contraindications for folk remedy and discourage use if dangerous.
Health care system	Previous hospitalization experiences. Current hospitalization planned or emergency?	Encourage patient to express fears regarding hospitalization and treatments. Keep patient/family informed of patient's progress.
Religion	Spiritual practices and beliefs. Level of incorporation of spiritual practices into healing/dying process.	Allow privacy and space for religious articles and practices. Arrange for visit from spiritual leader. Refer patients to hospital chaplain. Document beliefs about death and burial.
Food	Beliefs regarding food and healing. Use of hot/cold system. Specific food preferences.	Obtain consultation with dietician. Incorporate food preferences into menu selection. Ask family to supply familiar foods. Document use of hot/cold practices as they relate to nursing care.
Social support	Current living situation. Support of family and/or community.	Encourage family participation in care. Encourage visits or phone calls with peers.
Decision making	Primary decision maker for health care. How does the patient make decisions? Who is needed for decisions?	Involve family when providing patient with health care information. Arrange for family conference if disparity exists between goals of patient, family, and/or health care team.
Discharge planning	Expectations for care after hospitalization and during future years of aging. Financial status that affects discharge planning and long-term health status. Ability of patient/family to support discharge needs.	Involve family in discharge planning. Obtain consult for social services. Refer patient to community resources for legal advice, transportation, meals, shopping, and emotional support.

From Evans CA, Cunningham BA: Caring for the ethnic elder, *Geriatr Nurs* 17(3):105, 1996.

Brislin and Pederson (1982) approach this dilemma by taking a "culture-general" approach. Rather than focus on eating habits, religious customs, interpersonal etiquette, and decision-making styles, they train the caregiver in self-awareness and sensitivity. This is a wise approach for health care providers who daily encounter clients from extremely different cultural backgrounds with varied levels of assimilation into the host culture. Gaining insight into one's own values and assumptions encourages a perspective that respects the validity and tenacity of others' values and assumptions. For instance, a missionary in Japan experienced a severe identity crisis when she realized that her religious myths and traditions were no more rational than those of Shintoism or Buddhism.

This segment of the chapter combines both "culture-general" and "culture-specific" approaches to assist the caregiver in recognizing adaptations that influence responses to care, while simultaneously hoping the student will remain aware of self and avoid stereotypic expectations.

Nursing concerns must focus on overall health care for minority elders by assisting them to gain access to needed services through ascertaining affordability, efficacy, accessibility and availability of information, client satisfaction, respect for their health beliefs, illness perspective, and informal support systems.

Caring for the Minority Elderly

The consumers of health care are increasingly being cared for in the home, and providers must adapt strategies to the beliefs and culture of the individual if we hope to be useful. Folk remedies abound among the various ethnic elders and among the dominant culture. We, the dominant cultural group, also embrace many of the beliefs brought in from other shores and welcome the relief from the mechanistic approaches of our Western, technology-dominated culture. We listen with interest to the efficacy of mind control over body ailments and aches. We embrace acupressure, acupuncture, and other modes of relief that would have been anathema to our thinking as we entered the age of human mechanical efficiency. We may have matured to the awareness of the human mind and meanings as a counterbalance to our extreme efficiency. This small world, in the expanding universe, has not yet lost its anthropomorphic orientations. We have much to learn from those ancient and enduring civilizations that bring from their history another cognitive mode of existence.

The nurse and the health care system have strong ethnocentric tendencies. That is, individual's or the group's (the health care system) beliefs and ways of providing care is considered the most desirable when dealing with illness or health care. In essence, Western medicine and nursing care are considered superior to others. This latter statement is ethnocentrism (Leininger, 1978; Gunter, 1991, Grossman, 1994, Spector, 1996). In order to combat this and provide sensitively designed care many components of the individual's life system must be considered (Table 24-8; Box 24-4).

We must also become acutely aware of the influence of our own values, beliefs, and prejudices before we can hope to understand another's. If we do not become sensitive to the influence of values and beliefs on health we will be unable to provide effective care. Scientific problem solving, the foundation of nursing care planning, is necessary but not inclusive. Intuition, superstition, belief, faith, and hope are necessarily woven into effective care packages. Jackson (1993), Grossman (1994), and Spector (1996) believe provider self-awareness is fundamental to this process.

In caring for the aged a knowledge of history and culture is necessary. The nature of diseases is changing, and new health problems have emerged. Fads and fashion in health care have changed significantly, as has the delivery of care. Many elders remember when the family physician would advise an ocean voyage to combat illness, would accept eggs in payment for services, would taste or smell urine as a diagnostic test, and would remain with a laboring woman for several hours before delivering the infant at home.

A particularly sensitive physician recently asked if one of my Chinese students could act as interpreter for an elderly Chinese woman who had just been admitted to the hospital.

Table 24-9 Areas of Assessment of Personal Care Practices of Minority Elderly

Activities of daily living	Coping strategies	Environment	Family or significant support	Attitudes toward care givers/professionals
Eating Feeding Nutrition	Problem solving	Home Housekeeping	Availability	Preferences
Bathing Dressing Toileting Continence	Stress Pain/discomfort Loneliness Religion, prayer, meditation	Safety and support/reassurance Institution arrangements Artifacts	Acceptance	Rejections
Mobility/disability				

This form may be used as a comparative assessment of minority elders. From Gunter LM: Cultural diversity among older Americans. In Baines EM, editor: *Perspectives on gerontological nursing,* Newbury Park, Calif, 1991, Sage Publications.

The student, having been in the United States only 2 years, was delighted to speak in her mother tongue, and the old lady became noticeably calm as they talked. The physician was grateful and praised the student for her assistance. It was only later I learned that the student's mother had died a few months before and her last days were spent in physical and psychologic misery because she was unable to understand what was being done to her in the hospital. This became the student's motivation for entering nursing. In schools such as ours where varied ethnic groups abound, it is wise to make students' language skills known to the professionals in the clinical settings in which they practice. A nursing administrator might keep a computerized list of the various language skills of all personnel and have this service as readily available as the technologic services in the health care system.

A number of measures suggested by Spector (1996) have already been addressed earlier in this chapter that will assist nurses to deal sensitively with people from other cultures (Box 24-5).

Ethno-Geriatric Health Care. The term *ethno-geriatrics* has entered the vernacular of health care professionals; it is a specialty in which we hope to work sensitively with ethnic elders. The prediction of a significant increase in ethnic elders suggests that they will have considerable impact on service needs and delivery. It is expected that 41% of elders in California will be non-Anglo by the year 2020. Other states will also experience this upsurge in non-Anglo elders (Figure 24-3). In light of this, it will be impossible to think of ethnic elders as incidental to the elderly population as a whole.

When we speak of traditional versus nontraditional medicine we must clarify these terms. Mitchell (1989) believed popular versus professional is more accurate. In most parts of the world there is a formal system of health care and the informal system of "folk medicine" or "popular medicine." Anglos are no exception. We quickly adopt one fad after another that we think may preserve health. The difference between our "popular medicine" and that of many ethnic elders is that theirs is steeped in tradition and ritual. Theirs is truly traditional, and ours is not. In all of health care, from whatever culture, we must recognize the power of the mind in healing and incorporate the significant beliefs and rituals in the pattern of health care if we hope to be successful. And we often discover scientifically that the folk remedies were indeed beneficial.

The basis for much folk medicine is purely making the most of whatever was available. We speak in the past tense because most ethnic elders have now incorporated Western

---

Box 24-4   Guidelines to Nursing Interventions for Ethnic Elders

Respect the cultural preferences in food, music, and religion.

Design teaching to the vocabulary and attitude of the individual.

Listen attentively to complaints because these may be the clues to health problems.

In people of color, the signs of some disorders may be masked by color (pallor, cyanosis, ecchymosis); buccal cavity coloration is significant.

Base physical assessment on norms for the ethnic group:

Adequate light is especially important in skin assessment for turgor, blemishes, and cyanosis; eye lens, nail beds, palms of hands, and soles of feet can be revealing.

Listen for signs of depression, often in the form of hypochondriasis and apathy.

Inquire about losses and the individual's adaptation to them.

Gather information about lifestyle preferences and incorporate into care plans.

Inquire about health practices the individual finds effective.

Identify spiritual resources and incorporate in care plan; contact minister and church friends.

Box 24-5   Culturally Sensitive Health Care

Ethnic studies are essential in the curricula required of health care providers. Students may be required to interview aged individuals of other cultures. Guest speakers from representative cultures may be invited to classes.

Health care providers must be sensitized to their own perceptions and practices related to health and illness. Consciousness-raising exercises include interviewing family about health beliefs and health practices that have been or are part of the family heritage.

Health care providers should become aware of the complex issues of health care from the client's viewpoint: cost, religious beliefs, interpretation of services, inequality of treatment, and many others of which even the client may be unaware.

More minority persons must be recruited into health care professions. Support services for students entering professional education programs must be made readily available to compensate for deficits experienced in early education and language differences.

Health services must be accessible to ethnic minorities and delivered with respect to cultural beliefs and practices. Neighborhood health centers with indigenous providers are most effective for entry into the health care system and appropriate guidance and referral.

Summarized from Spector RE: *Cultural diversity in health and illness,* East Norwalk, Conn, 1985, Appleton-Century-Crofts.

medicine into their care and rarely rely totally on their traditional cures. However, they do often cling to some of these and supplement their professional care as they see fit. Separation of cultural beliefs from economic resources and educational background is exceedingly difficult, and additional "education" related to health care rarely changes individual habits and rituals (Chavira, 1989).

Some guidelines for dealing with ethnic elders who are using a mixture of Western and traditional methods to cure their ills are offered by Mitchell (1989):

- Realize that many ethnic elders do not have a concept of chronic illness that cannot be cured and will continually search for a method to alleviate the problem experienced.
- Determine what the problem is from the client's perspective: what does he or she think is wrong?
- What does the client think caused the problem?
- Does the client understand the treatment plan and how it relates to symptoms?
- Try to find out if the elder is supplementing prescriptions and what is the expected result.
- Alert the individual to signs of adverse reactions to treatment.
- Always try to discover the underlying logic of the client's belief.
- Incorporate folk medicine beliefs if they are not harmful.

Scott and Polacca (1995-1996) also note that a definition of pathologic condition and diagnosis in one culture may be different in another culture. For example, mental illness may be seen as dysfunctional in one culture but normal or a spiritual phenomenon in another culture.

We live in a medicalized society where it is not uncommon to "ask the doctor" what to eat, how and when to have sex, how to discipline children, when to go on a diet, if it is safe to travel, and many other issues of living. This is a rather recent phenomenon. In many other societies and eras a physician was sought only for serious problems, and although we have thought that seeing a physician routinely somehow prevents serious problems from developing, we have found that this is not true. It is becoming evident that the daily decisions one makes and the attitudes one has about life are more important than a yearly visit to a physician.

For many ethnic elders (particularly the Hispanic and Asian) life is viewed as a balance of energy and forces; intrusion into body systems and drawing off vital fluids are viewed with alarm. Also, the family and environment are intrinsic to the energy systems and must not be excluded from consideration. Thus we can understand how hospitals, diagnostic procedures, and other noxious elements that disturb the peace can be interpreted as producing more harm than good.

Interestingly, there are some racial differences identified in drug metabolism (Zhou et al, 1989). For instance, blacks with hypertension do not respond to beta-blockers, and Chinese men are twice as sensitive to them as are whites. Studies have focused on hypertension because it is easy to measure.

Isoniazid rapidly inactivates in Native Americans, Asians, and blacks but can be slowed to some degree with the taking of pyridoxine. It has been suggested that there are many other metabolic differences in ethnic groups that are not as easily identified (Goldstein, 1989, Giger and Davidhizer, 1991).

Mexicans are prone to diabetes and blacks to hypertension. We usually think of these as fundamentally dietary problems, but they may not be. In other words, there is much we do not yet know. As we work with ethnic elders we are learning with them and about them. We are not the experts with all the answers.

Nurses should not attempt to change the client's beliefs. It is difficult if not impossible and usually is counterproductive. What is helpful is negotiating options with the client. This can be done with knowledge and mutual respect. The nurse should attempt to preserve helpful beliefs and practices, accommodate beliefs that are neither helpful or harmful from the point of Western medicine, or repattern harmful beliefs or practices. If the nurse has little or no knowledge of a belief or practice, the nurse should study and evaluate it to determine its helpfulness or its potential harm. The nurse should also keep an open mind, learn about practices, encourage their use, be flexible, creative, and persistent. In this way preservation of beliefs and practices can be achieved. Respectfully explaining concern about harmful client practices with the offer of possible alternatives may show the client that the nurse is taking the client's beliefs and practices into consideration. It is less likely that the client will be dissatisfied and not return for future care (Chrisman, 1992, Grossman, 1994).

Self-Care. Coulton (1988) presented preliminary evidence regarding the use of medical care among blacks, Hispanics, and Eastern European immigrants. Osteoarthritis is present in 85% of individuals between 75 and 79 years of age and thus becomes a focus of self-care practices for many. Ethnic groups differ in their preferential methods of self-care and the extent to which they use medical care versus traditional healing methods and alternative health practices. Coulton found that Hispanics, although poorest and least educated, were most likely to use medical care and prescription drugs for joint symptoms. They also had more chronic health conditions and generally rated their health poorer than blacks or Eastern Europeans. Crisis/health advice lines to serve specific ethnic populations have proved effective when publicized well within the select group.

Implications of Ethnicity in Long-Term Care. Jones and van Amelsvoort Jones (1986) studied the interactions of nursing staff with groups of elderly persons in a long-term care facility to determine the nature of verbal interactions. Immigrants, Canadian-born elders, and American-born elders were included in the study. Although the study was done in only one small nursing home and the sample was of only 41 elders, it is significant to alert us that we may unwittingly be influenced by subliminal stereotypes and discriminatory feelings. Tape recorders were discreetly placed to determine the nature of verbal content: commands, words, statements, and questions. Most of the verbalization (42%) was in the form of commands. The Canadian group was communicated with most frequently, the ethnic Europeans the least, and the American-born in between. Men were spoken to less frequently than women and were more frequently given commands. Relating to ethnic elders in long-term care may be more difficult than has been thought. The most important finding of this study was that during the entire 72 hours in which it was conducted only 850 words were spoken in all to the entire group of subjects—20 words per person! It appears that elders in this long-term care facility, of whatever ethnic background, were severely deprived of communication. Box 24-6 gives Jones and van Amelsvoort Jones' suggestions (1986) for more meaningful care and communication.

Ethnicity may be one of the major elements of self-concept, and when age and institutionalization make one vulnerable, ethnic heritage becomes even more important. To the Chinese, achieving old age is a blessing, and the elderly are held in high esteem. The old are respected and sought for advice. The family unit is expected to take care of its elder members, and thus there may be a reluctance to utilize long-term care even when badly needed.

Originally, nursing home placement for elderly parents was not considered by the Japanese, but the modern Nisei and Sansei (third generation) face the same dilemmas as others when caring for their elderly parents, despite Issei expectations of *oya koko* or "care for parents." Thus nursing home placement is becoming more common. Nursing homes specifically for the aged Japanese are rare. One does exist near Los Angeles in which familiar traditions are maintained by Japanese staff.

Box 24-6	**Approaches to Caring for the Ethnic Aged in Long-Term Care Facilities**

Construct monocultural facilities where population
　　demographics warrant.
Develop transcultural programs in facilities by the
　　incorporation of existing community culture-specific
　　activities, groups, and clubs.
Establish hiring policies whereby the ethnic roots of
　　staff reflect the resident ethnic population as closely
　　as possible.
Increase cross-cultural long-term care content in
　　nursing school curricula.
Select roommates with careful consideration of
　　individual's needs and preferences.

There is an increasing cultural diversity in physicians and nurses who are choosing geriatrics and long-term care. These providers of geriatric care are an increasingly heterogeneous cultural group. The countries from which these providers come vary from one part of the United States to another. Some large groups have come from the Philippines, Haiti, and India (Yeo, 1996-1997). There are positive aspects to this trend: (1) they may bring respect for the elder, found in other cultures and less in the youth-driven society of the American, and (2) they may have the language skills and understanding to better care for the elders and families of their own cultural background. There are concerns as well: (1) the complexities of cross-cultural communications and decision making when second languages are used, and (2) the use of cultural norms not well understood by each other.

Human Need Hierarchy

Maslow's hierarchy may not be relevant to all cultures. As it stands, the hierarchy is applied to all without regard for cultural diversity. Brooks and Nisberg (1974) looked at the hierarchic framework from the black business world perspective and developed the Brooks/Nisberg Need Hierarchy. The import of this approach might serve as a basis for a broader look at human need hierarchies in cultures other than Euro-American.

The Brooks/Nisberg framework presents these levels: (1) staying alive, (2) enjoying life, (3) praising God, (4) getting ahead, and (5) upgrading the race or ethnic group (Figure 24-7). Staying alive; seeking better conditions; basic life necessities of food, clothing, and health care; and recreation are at the first level of human need in the Brooks/Nisberg hierarchy. Economic factors in many ethnic communities interfere with the ability to obtain these survival basics. Interethnic differences exist in eligibility for Social Security and public assistance benefits. Few ethnic groups had survival rates equal to white Americans, so benefit eligibility was not sufficiently considered. Although adjustments have been made and future generations of aged will fare better, the present elderly must cope with this economic inequity.

Enjoyment of life and security within one's own group is the second level of the Brooks/Nisberg hierarchy. The inner community provides an escape from tensions experienced with white society. Major cities tend to have their nihonmachi, Chinatown, and barrio in which the elderly remain. Traditional ties and cultural identity support the familiar, which has brought pleasure in the past. Here the language, common interests, and interpersonal relationships can remain relatively unchanged.

The third level of which Brooks and Nisberg speak is praising God. Some groups are steeped in deep religious beliefs. At times it is difficult to distinguish that which is culture from that which is religion. Hispanic, Native American, and black cultures look at life as harmony of self with environment sustained through religious practice or following

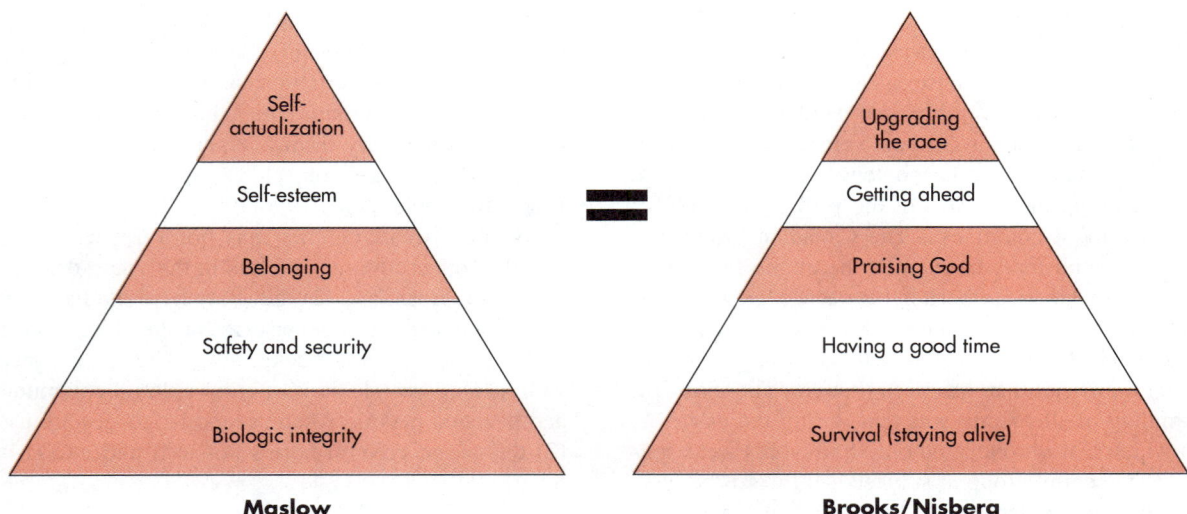

Figure 24-7. Need hierarchies compared.

specific tenets. White Americans do not clearly understand the significance of this intense religious foundation in culture. For the average Anglo-American, the religious affiliation seems to surface at times of births, weddings, and deaths.

Getting ahead and upgrading the race or ethnic group occupy levels four and five, respectively. This may not be as significant for the aged of today as for the younger representatives of the particular ethnic community, who will be the aged of tomorrow. The potential and desire for self-actualization may not be the highest attainment for persons of certain cultures. In fact, the greatest goal may be to subjugate the needs of the self to others; for example, the Navajo elderly do all they can to help the young "make it" in the new society. Self-esteem may be intricately tied to belonging and contingent on the success of the group rather than on productivity or independent identity.

The ethnic-cultural systemic framework of Orque et al (1983) uses the concepts of Maslow and also seems to incorporate the Brooks/Nisberg hierarchy. Orque's system is holistic and comprehensive in scope and can be used to understand elders in any culture (Figure 24-8). The core of the system contains the basic human needs, which are cyclic in nature because people are continually adapting to their environment. The extent to which each aspect of culture is reflected in meeting these needs depends on the individual's ethnic/cultural system. Although all the components are universal, the nuances of the components indicate the diversity that exists between groups or individuals.

INTEGRATING CONCEPTS

Family, religion, community, and history are important reference points for self-worth and identity for any ethnic group. Familial supports are variable between groups, social classes, and subcultures, yet the nuclear or extended family is the chief avenue of transmitting cultural values, beliefs, customs, and practices. The family provides orientation, stability, and sanctuary. In a simplistic sense we may say Asians value familial piety; Hispanics, the extended family (*compadres* translates to co-parents); blacks, extended or fictive kin supports; and Native Americans, a system of kinship and line of descent.

Church or religiosity plays a major role in defining many cultures. Religion may function as a consistent experience that affords psychic support in the individual's life. In the black community, religion is a pervasive force and the place to instill self-determination toward change (Moriwaki and Kobata, 1983; Walls, 1992). The Issei seek religious tradition in the face of aging and death (Kitano, 1969). Padilla and Ruiz (1976) note that Hispanics tend to seek Spanish-speaking clergy rather than mental health professionals when they have emotional problems.

The ethnic community (barrios, nihonmachi, and Chinatown) serves as a buffer and a means of strengthening cohesiveness for elders and others of various cultural groups. Within the community, members are protected from discrimination and strange language and customs of the dominant society.

Changes are threatening the historic role of the aged and the traditional family. Economic independence and mobility of the younger members of the family are chipping away at the insulation afforded by the community. Intergenerational discontinuities of assimilation create a communication gap between the young and the old. Often the elderly are not proficient in the language of the dominant culture, and the younger members tend not to retain the language of their parents. This may cause isolation and estrangement between the oldest and youngest generations. Members of ethnic mi-

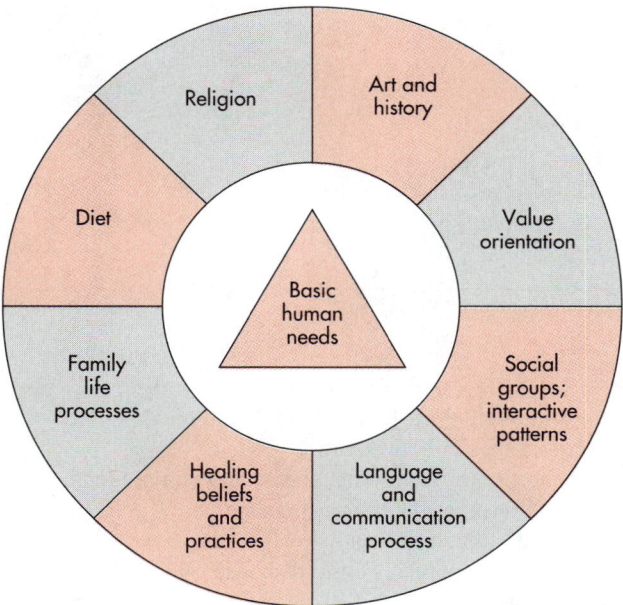

Figure 24-8. Components of Orque's ethnic-cultural systemic framework. (Modified from Orque M, Bloch B, Monrroy L: *Ethnic nursing care: a multicultural approach,* St Louis, 1983, Mosby.)

norities are extremely vulnerable in old age. They may be devalued because of age and ethnicity. Attitudes and economic inequality contribute to their problems.

• • •

Throughout this chapter the aged have been viewed, individually and collectively, as they have been defined and developed by the influence of their time and place in history, their gender, and distinctive group practices and beliefs that have served as the foundation for the self system. The study of the uniqueness and individuality of each surviving elder is one of the most complex and intriguing opportunities of our day. Realistically it will almost be impossible to become familiar with the whole range of clinically relevant cultural differences of older adults one may encounter, but to attempt to serve them holistically and sensitively is the most challenging opportunity.

KEY CONCEPTS

- Cohort groups are convenient for statistical analysis, but such factors as geography, composition, and religion reflect the heterogeneity within groups.
- Gender impacts values, perceptions, and the approach to health care assessment and treatment.
- Population diversity is rapidly increasing and will continue to do so for many years. This suggests that nurses will be caring for a greater number of minority elders than they have in the past.

- Culture, social status, and support systems are essential components of ethnicity.
- Programs staffed by persons who reflect ethnic elders' background and speak their language are preferred by the elders.
- Culture is a complex concept reflecting the interrelationship of many components.
- Cultural competency and sensitivity require awareness of issues related to culture, race, gender, sexual, orientation, social class, and economic situations.
- Stereotyping negates the fact that there is significant heterogeneity within cultural groups.
- Health beliefs of various groups emerge from three general belief systems: biomedical, magicoreligious, and naturalistic. Elders may adhere to one or more of these systems.
- Nurses caring for minority elders must let go of their ethnocentrism before effective caring can occur.
- Family, history, religion, and community are the core of the ethnic elder's self-worth and identity.

▲ CASE STUDY

Georgia was a misfit. She had always been a misfit. She felt she was born in the wrong time and most of the time was in the wrong place. She was born in China in 1920, the child of missionary parents. Her parents had built and managed a school for orphaned children in Shanghai. There were many problems and uprisings in China, and when she was 15 the political situation and threat of war was so intense her parents were asked to leave the school and return to the United States. They were then sent to an Appalachian mining village to manage a small school and clinic. Having grown to adolescence in China she felt more Chinese than Anglo. She had a difficult adjustment in the poverty-stricken rural mining village in Appalachia, so unlike where she had been. In a few years her parents sent her to a private religious college, mainly attended by the children of the affluent elders of the church. She married a young Army officer, and they were immediately sent to France. Her life from then on seemed comprised of nothing but moves as she followed her husband about. She was grateful she never had children as she said, "My life has always seemed so unsettled, I don't think I could have provided any stability for children." As she aged she developed crippling arthritis, and her husband provided much of her care. When she was widowed at 80, she almost immediately entered a nursing home. There she found most of the staff were Filipino and talked among themselves in Tagalog. Again, she felt out of step with the prevailing culture she found herself in. She became very difficult to get along with, and the staff were at their wits end trying to please her. You recently went to work as Director of Nursing in the facility Georgia is in. How will you help her and the staff maximize their life satisfactions?

Nursing Diagnoses

The following potential diagnoses must be considered as well as diagnoses unique to the particular individual:
Coping, ineffective
Personal identity disturbance
Powerlessness
Self-esteem, situational low
Social isolation
Spiritual distress

NURSING PROCESS AND NURSING DIAGNOSIS
Impaired Communication: Language Barrier

Etiologies and Related Factors
No or limited language fluency of dominant health care givers
Professional jargon
Illiteracy
Cohort disparity in idioms
Regional variations in terminology

Defining Characteristics
Response inappropriate to spoken words
Body language predominant means of communicating
Family member accompanies client and translates
Social isolation
Anger
Fear
Anxiety

Knowledge
Others' perceptions of health care
General ethnic/cultural diversities
Ethnic health assessment tools
Basic medical/surgical/psychiatric theory and interventions
Resources

Clinical Judgment and Related Skills
Sensitivity to cultural beliefs/customs/perception of health care

Assess individual for language in which most comfortable for conversing
Assess ability to read, write, speak, and comprehend English or other dominant language
Face client, talk clearly and slowly
Validate with rephrasing if no response of comprehension
Use alternative forms of communication: gestures, pictures, drawings, written messages
Obtain/provide a translater
Learn some important words that will help communication and make client feel acceptance
Adjust theory to integrate cultural belief system as much as possible
Keep directions simple
Have directions translated into native language and give to client in written form (when possible)

Evaluation
Able to communicate basic needs
Relates feelings
Reduced anxiety/fear
Attempts to ask questions
Complies with therapy
Relates to caregivers with positive emotion

NEEDS ADDRESSED AND TASK STRENGTHS

Cultural and Cohort Needs
Need for recognition, social interaction and dignity; affiliation (to meet need for security, belonging and self-esteem)
Claims and cultivates own heritage
Recognizes shifting perspectives of cohorts
Recognizes generational differences
Identifies with major concerns of own cohort
Takes pride in distinctive characteristics
International interests
Nonverbal communication skills

Based upon the case study, develop a nursing care plan using the following procedure*:

List comments of client that provide *subjective data.*

List information that provides *objective data.*

From these data identify and state, using accepted format, two *nursing diagnoses* you determine are most significant to this client at this time.

Determine and state *outcome criteria* for each diagnosis. These must reflect some alleviation of the problem identified in the nursing diagnosis and must be stated in concrete and measurable terms.

Plan and state one or more culturally relevant *interventions* for each diagnosed problem. Provide specific documentation of source used to determine appropriate intervention. Plan at least one intervention that incorporates the client's existing strengths.

Evaluate success of intervention. Interventions must correlate directly with the stated outcome criteria in order to measure the outcome success.

STUDY QUESTIONS/ACTIVITIES

Define the terms *culture, ethnicity, ethnocentricity, cultural sensitivity and competence.*

Identify several personal values/beliefs that are derived from your ethnic and cultural roots.

Relate major historic events that have affected your birth cohort and explain in what way.

Discuss several different ethnically based approaches to health care.

Describe characteristics that you believe are specific to your gender.

Construct a cultural genogram and discuss your roots.

Discuss ways in which you have learned to appreciate cultural and ethnic differences.

Privately list your stereotypes and "ethnocentrisms" for various ethnic groups and explore the basis of these beliefs (taught, fear, experience, lack of knowledge). Then consider what can be done to be more culturally sensitive and competent.

Select a food or particular behavior and examine differences in custom that arise from ethnic/cultural interpretations.

Describe the advocacy role of nurses who care for ethnic elderly.

Formulate a care plan incorporating ethnically sensitive interventions.

Plan strategies to provide care that is culturally sensitive and acceptable without losing a focus on the individual's own aging experience.

*Students are advised to refer to their nursing diagnosis text and identify possible or potential problems.

RESEARCH QUESTIONS

What are the chief difficulties in providing nursing care for individuals from an entirely different background from one's own?

Which personalities thrive best in a homogenous environment, and which in a heterogeneous environment?

What are the factors that identify a group as an ethnic minority?

What are the enduring cohort differences that are unlikely to change throughout life?

How is cultural sensitivity incorporated into curriculum?

What are the outcomes of an integrated cultural curricular approach verses a separate course approach in curriculum?

All aspects of differences in the aging male and the aging female need to more clearly understood. No comprehensive comparative studies exist that factor in cohort, culture, and gender.

RESOURCES

Films

A Portrait of Older Minorities, AARP Fulfillment, 1909 K Street, NW, Washington, DC 20049.

These films are available in local video stores:

Toto Le Heros 90 minutes, color, 1991, produced by Pierre Drouot and Dany Geys, Triton Pictures.

Toto Le Heros, from Belgium, is the reconstructed tale of an old man looking back upon his life. Told primarily in flashbacks, the movie follows the key characters from childhood through old age.

The Wash, 85 minutes, color, 1988, produced by Calvin Skaggs, Skouras Pictures.

The character in *The Wash* is in many ways the very model of the traditional spouse, but she learns new skills and what it is like to be "too happy" in a new relationship. While her husband remains mired in the past, recalling past events and dredging up old slights, she embraces change even when it means breaking with socially sanctioned roles and the conditioning that comes with culture, gender, and age.

Babette's Feast, 102 minutes, color, 1988, Produced by Just Betzer and Bo Christensen, Orion Films.

Babette's Feast, based on a story by Isak Dinesen, takes place in Denmark in the 1870s. It portrays the life of two old sisters, daughters of a pastor who headed a small Lutheran sect. The daughters are devoted to their late father's legacy and faith, holding services and doing "good works" for a dwindling community of elders. The disciples have aged in place and become increasingly testy and querulous over time: old grievances are revived and intolerance reigns.

Videos

A Place of Our Own, B. Josea Kramer, Department of Community and Senior Citizens Services, Los Angeles,

California (12.5 minutes). This videotape documents the lives of older American Indians living in Los Angeles and illustrates important issues, such as social isolation.

Responsive Health Care for Minority Elderly. A series of actual patient interviews demonstrates the need for health professionals working with elderly minority patients to expand the traditional concept of assessment to include psychosocial, cultural, educational, economic, and environmental factors. Emphasized is the importance of integrating the patient into the health care system, patient education, and preventive medicine.

This program is important viewing for physicians, physician's assistants, nurses, nurse practitioners, social workers, physical and occupational therapists, and students in professional training programs. Staff development and in-service seminars in hospitals, senior centers, and community health centers servicing minority elderly should definitely include this program. From Video Press, University of Maryland at Baltimore, School of Medicine, Suite 133, 100 Penn Street, Baltimore, MD 21201, (800) 328-7450 or (410) 328-5497, (410) 328-8471.

Triple Jeopardy (The Hispanic Elderly in the United States). Videocassette, 3/4 inch or 1/2 inch, $50; filmstrip version with cue-signaled cassette, $30. Asociacion Nacional Pro Personas Mayores, National Association for Hispanic Elderly, 3325 Wilshire Boulevard, Suite 800, Los Angeles, CA 90010.

Barriers (Service Delivery to the Hispanic Elderly of the United States). Videocassette, 3/4 inch or 1/2 inch, $50; filmstrip in either Spanish or English, $30. Asociacion Nacional Pro Personas Mayores, National Association for Hispanic Elderly, 3325 Wilshire Boulevard, Suite 800, Los Angeles, CA 90010.

Minority aging organizations

The Center on Aging, San Diego State University School of Social Work, 348 Cedar Street, San Diego, CA 92101, annually sponsors the National Institutes on Minority Aging to raise and discuss issues relevant to ethnic minority older people. Technical assistance, training and consultation are available.

National Center on Black Aged (NCBA), 1730 M Street, NW, Suite 811, Washington, DC 20020, provides a comprehensive program of education, information dissemination, coordination, and consultative services to the public and private sectors. Their goal is to improve policies, programs, and the delivery of services to black and low-income elderly.

Japanese: Seattle Keiro, Issei Concerns, 1700 24th Avenue, S, Seattle, WA 98144.

Chinese: On Lok, Day Health Center, 1333 Bush Street, San Francisco, CA 94108.

National Asian Pacific Center on Aging, Melbourn Tower, Suite 914, 1511 Third Avenue, Seattle, WA 98101, has developed "FAX-IT" (Facsimile Information in Trans-

lation). FAX-IT is online. The NAPCA health care and social service pamphlets, booklets, and brochures are cross-indexed by broad topical areas under headings such as health, wellness, nutrition, culture, etc. Currently there are more than 300 documents in Cambodian, Chinese, Hindi, Hmong, Ilocano, Japanese, Korean, Laotian, Punjabi, Samoan, Tagolog, Tai Dam, Thai, Tongan, and Vietnamese. The whole catalog is stored in the computer and can be requested by fax, or holdings in individual languages can be listed separately. A particular document can be ordered by entering the four-digit number corresponding to its listing in the catalog. FAX-IT is accessible at (206) 624-0185.

Asian Pacific Center on Aging, 1511 Third Avenue, Seattle, WA 98101.

Pacific/Asian Coalition (PAC), 1760 The Alameda, Suite 210, San Jose, CA 95126, is a national organization acting on behalf of Pacific/Asian Americans. The coalition functions as a resource clearinghouse and advocacy research coordination center. Although its focus is not specifically on aging, the coalition can provide aging contacts and resources to local areas. PAC publishes a monthly newsletter *(PAC Memo),* and regional conferences are held at various times.

National Association for Spanish Speaking Elderly (Asociación Nacional Por Personas Mayores), 3875 Wilshire Boulevard, Suite 401, Los Angeles, Ca 90005, (213) 487-1922, or 1801 K Street NW, Suite 1021, Washington, DC 20006, is a national organization acting on behalf of the social service needs of Spanish-speaking senior citizens. The association works to inform the Hispanic community of current legislation or existing programs, to encourage the recruitment and development of Hispanic professional employees by universities and social welfare and public administration programs, and to testify before state and federal committees.

National Hispanic Council on Aging, 2713 Ontario Road, NW, Washington, DC 20009.

National Indian Council on Aging (NICOA), PO Box 2088, Albuquerque, NM 87103, provides advocacy for Indian and Alaskan native elderly. The council works to bring about remedial action in the areas of income, personal environment, legal problems, and special health problems including spiritual well-being, recreation, and legislation. NICOA publishes a newsletter, *The NICOA News.*

U.S. Department of Health and Human Services, Public Health Services, Health Administration, Indian Health Service, 5600 Fisher Lane, Rockville, MD 20857.

Older Women's League, 666 11th Street, NW, Suite 700, Washington, DC 20001, (201) 783-6686, fax (202) 638-2356.

Publications

A home care training manual, *Taking Care of Others: A Personal Guidebook for Home Care Workers,* has been published by Chicago's Coalition of Limited English

Speaking Elderly (CLESE) in Arabic, Chinese, English, Korean, Polish, and Spanish. For information, contact CLESE, "Taking Care" Guidebooks, 327 S. LaSalle Street, Suite 920, Chicago, IL 60604, (312) 922-5890. Development of the guides was funded by the Retirement Research Foundation.

REFERENCES

American Association of Retired Persons: *Healthy aging: making health promotion work for minority elders,* Washington, DC, 1990, The Association.

American Association of Retired Persons: *A profile of older Americans 1995,* Washington DC, 1995, The Association.

American Society on Aging: Gender and aging, *Generations* 14(3): 1990.

Angel JL, Hogan DP: *The demography of minority aging populations: Minority elders—longevity, economics, and health,* Washington, DC, 1991, Gerontological Society of America.

Belgrave LL, Wykle ML, Chio JM: Multigenerational households more a function of aging, mental and socioeconomic status and health, *Gerontologist* 33(3):379, 1993.

Berman HJ: From the pages of my life, *Generations* 15(2):33, 1991.

Bohannon P: *We, the alien: an introduction to cultural anthropology.* Prospect Heights, Ill, 1992, Waverly Press.

Brislin RS, Pederson P: *Cross-cultural orientation programs,* New York, 1982, Cardier Press.

Brooks WC, Nisberg JN: Effects of cultural differences on motivation, *Personnel Administrator* 51:28, Oct 1974.

Chavira J: *Common remedies used by Mexican American elders: their source and use: Traditional and nontraditional medication use among ethnic elders.* Conference sponsored by the Stanford Geriatric Education Center, San Jose, Calif, April 28, 1989.

Chrisman NJ: Culture-sensitive nursing care: In Patrick et al: *Medical-surgical nursing,* Philadelphia, 1992, JB Lippincott.

Christensen D: Heart attack shows gender bias, study finds, *J Am Coll Cardiol* 29: 35, 1997.

Cole SR: *The old ones,* Albuquerque, 1973, University of Mexico Press.

Coulton C: *Ethnicity, self care and use of medical care among the elderly with joint symptoms.* Paper presented at the Veterans Hospital and Medical Center Gerontology Resource and Educational Center, Cleveland, Oct 1988.

Cuellar J: Aging and health: American Indian/Alaska native, Stanford Geriatric Education Center Working Paper Series, No 6, *Ethnogeriatric Reviews,* Stanford, Calif, 1990a.

Cuellar J: Aging and health: Hispanic American elders, Stanford Geriatric Education Center Working Paper Series, No 5, *Ethnogeriatric Reviews,* Stanford, Calif, 1990b.

Day AT: Remarkable survivors: insights into successful aging among women, *Aging Today* 13(6):10, 1992.

dePaula T, Lagana´ K, Gonzalez-Ramirez L: Mexican Americans. In Lipson JG, Dibble SL, Minarik PA, editors: *Culture and nursing: a pocket guide,* San Francisco, 1996, UCSF Nursing Press.

Dilworth-Anderson P: Extended kin networks in black families, *Generations* 17 (3):29, 1992.

Ebersole P: Editorial, *Geriatr Nurs* 17(4):149 July/Aug 1996.

Espino DV, Maldonado D: Hypertension and acculturation in elderly Mexican Americans: results from 1982-84 Hispanic males, *J Gerontol* 45(6):M209, 1990.

Evans CA: Cunningham BA: Caring for the ethnic elder, *Geriatr Nurs* 17(3):105, 1996.

FDA Consumer 29(9):4, 1996.

Fejos P: Man, magic, and medicine. In Goldstone I, editor: *Medicine and anthropology,* New York, 1959, International University Press.

Geertz C: *The interpretation of cultures,* New York, 1973, Basic Books.

Gibson R: The age-by-race gap in health and mortality in the older population: a social science research agenda, *Gerontologist* 34: 454, 1994.

Giger JN, Davidhizar, RE: *Transcultural nursing,* St Louis, 1991, Mosby.

Goldstein M: *Overview of geriatrics and medications. Traditional and nontraditional medication use among ethnic elders.* Conference sponsored by the Stanford Geriatric Education Center, San Jose, Calif, April 28, 1989.

Grossman D: Enhancing your cultural competence, *Am J Nurs* 94(7):58, 1994.

Gunter LM: Cultural diversity among older Americans. In Bains EM, editor: *Perspectives on gerontological nursing,* Newbury Park, Calif, 1991, Sage Publications.

Habayeb GL: Cultural diversity: a nursing concept not yet reliably defined, *Nursing Outlook,* 43:224, 1995.

Hendricks J: Gender and aging: making something of our chromosomes, *Generations* 14(3):5, 1990.

Hooyman N, Kiyak HA: *Social gerontology,* Boston, 1996, Allyn & Bacon.

Hudson RB, Gonyea JG: A perspective on women in politics: political mobilization and older women, *Generations* 14(3):67, 1990.

Jackson LE: Understanding, eliciting, and negotiating clients' multicultural health beliefs, *Nurse Pract* 18(4):30, 1993.

Jones D, van Amelsvoort, Jones G: Communication patterns between nursing staff and the ethnic elderly in long-term care facility, *J Adv Nurs* 11:265, 1986.

Kaye LW, Applegate J: Men's style of nurturing elders. In Sabo D, Gordon D, editors: *Men's health and illness,* Thousand Oaks, Calif, 1995, Sage Publications.

Kitano H: *Japanese Americans,* Englewood Cliffs, NJ, 1969, Prentice-Hall.

Kleinman A: *Patients and healers in the context of culture: an exploration of the borderland between anthropology, medicine, and psychiatry,* Berkeley, 1980, University of California Press.

Kramer J: American Indians. In Lipson JG, Dibble SL, Minarik PA: *Culture and nursing care: a pocket guide,* San Francisco, 1996, UCSF School of Nursing Press.

Leininger M: *Transcultural nursing concepts; theories, and practices,* New York, 1978, John Wiley & Sons.

Lin H: Personal communication, Case Western Reserve University, Cleveland, 1988.

Lipson JG: Culturally competent nursing care. In Lipson JG, Dibble SL, Minarik PA, editors: *Culture and nursing care: a pocket guide,* San Francisco, Calif, 1996, UCSF School of Nursing Press.

Manton K, Poss SS, Wiing S: The black/white mortality crossover: investigation from the perspective of the components of aging, *Gerontologist* 19:291, 1979.

Markides KS, Mindel CH: *Aging and ethnicity,* Sage Library of Social Research, vol 163, Newbury Park, Calif, 1987, Sage Publications.

Martin K: Native American customs bear on service delivery, *Generations* 1(2):24, summer 1977.

Meleis A, Isenberg M, Koerner J, Stern P: *Diversity, marginalization and culturally competent health care: issues in knowledge development,* Washington DC, 1995, Academy of Nursing.

Mitchell F: *Folk beliefs and health practices of ethnic elders. Traditional and non-traditional medication use among ethnic elders.* Conference sponsored by the Stanford Geriatric Education Center, San Jose, Calif, April 28, 1989.

Monrroy LA: Nursing care of Raza/Latina patients. In Orque MS, Block B, Monrroy LSA: *Ethnic nursing care: a multicultural approach,* St. Louis, 1983, Mosby.

Moore JW: Situational factors affecting minority aging, *Gerontologist* 11:88, 1971.

Morioka-Douglas N, Yeo G: Aging and health: Asian/Pacific Island American elders, Stanford Geriatric Education Center Working Paper Series, No 3, *Ethnogeriatric Reviews,* Stanford, Calif, 1990.

Moriwaki S, Kobata F: Ethnic minority aging. In Woodruff R, Birren J, editors: *Aging,* ed 2, Monterey, Calif, 1983, Brooks/Cole.

National Institute on Aging: *Progress report on Alzheimer's disease,* US Institutes of Health NIH publication #95-3994, 1995.

Ochoco L, Shimamoto Y: Group work with the frail ethnic elderly, *Geriatr Nurs* 8:185, 1987.

Orque MS, Block B, Monrroy LSA: *Ethnic nursing care: a multicultural approach,* St Louis, 1983, Mosby.

Padilla A, Ruiz R: Prejudice and discrimination. In Hernandez CA, Haug MJ, Wagner NN, editors: *Chicanos: social and psychological perspectives,* ed 2, St Louis, 1976, Mosby.

Pfeifferling JH: A cultural prescription for mediocentrism. In Eisenberg L, Kleinman A, editors: *The relevance of social science for medicine,* Boston, 1981, Reidel.

Pierce R, Clark M, Kaufman S: Generation and ethnic identity: a typological analysis, *Int J Aging Hum Dev* 9:19, 1978-1979.

Pinkleton N: The status of black health care, 1988: implications for the health management of the elderly, *GNP Newsletter* 21:2, summer 1988.

Richardson J: Aging and health: black American elders, Stanford Geriatric Education Center Working Paper Series, No 4, *Ethnogeriatric Reviews,* Stanford, Calif, 1990.

Scott RW, Polacca M: Staying in balance on the fourth hill of life: mental health and elderly Native Americans, *Dimensions* 2(4):1, 1995-1996.

Seton Medical Center: The Woman's Health Test, *Health Scene,* Fall 1992, Seton Medical Center, Daly City, Calif.

Siegler IC, Longino CF, Johnson K: The Georgia centenarian study: comments from friends. In Poon LW, editor: *The Georgia centenarian study,* Amityville, NY, 1992, Baywood.

Snow LF: Folk medicine beliefs and their implications for patient care: a review based on studies among black Americans, *Ann Intern Med* 81:82, 1974.

Spector RE: *Cultural diversity in health and illness,* East Norwalk, Conn, 1985, Appleton-Century-Crofts.

Spector RE: *Cultural diversity in health and illness*, ed 4, East Norwalk, Conn, 1996.

Stokes LG: Growing old in the black community. In Reinhardt AM, Quinn MD, editors: *Current practice in gerontological nursing,* St Louis, 1979, Mosby.

US Bureau of the Census: *Statistical Abstract of the United States: 1995,* ed 115, Washington, DC, 1995, US Government Printing Office.

Wagnild G, Young HM: Resilience among older women, *Image J Nurs Sch* 22(4):252, 1990.

Walls CT: The role of church and family support in the lives of older African Americans, *Generations* 17(3):33, 1992.

Wilson C: Health care and the Hispanic elderly: dehumanization or what, *GNP Newsletter* 21:3, Summer 1988.

Woods NF, Shaver JF: The evolutionary spiral of a specialized center for women's health research, *Image J Nurs Sch* 24(3):223, 1992.

Yeo G: Ethnogeriatrics: Cross-cultural care of the older adult. In Geriatrics: a clinical care update, *Generations* 20(4):72, 1996-1997.

Zhou HH, Koshakji RP, Silberstein DJ et al: Racial differences in drug response: altered sensitivity to and clearance of propranolol in men of Chinese descent as compared with American whites, *N Engl J Med* 320:565, 1989.

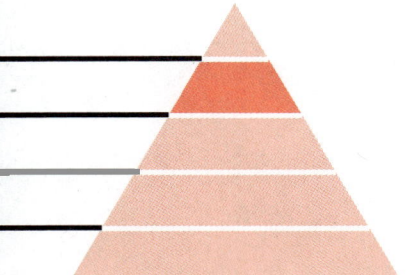

Cultural Status Examinations

PFEIFFERLING MODEL*

1. How would you describe the problem that has brought you here?
   NOTE: The clinician may need to identify others who can facilitate the discussion of the client's/patient's problem.
   a. Who in the community and your family helps you with your problem?
2. How long have you had this problem?
   a. Do you know anyone else with it?
   b. Tell me what happened to them when dealing with this problem.
3. What do you think is wrong with you?
   a. What might other people think is wrong with you?
   b. Tell me about people who don't get this problem.
4. Why has it happened to you and why now?
   a. Why has it happened to the involved part?
   b. Why do you get sick and not someone else?
5. What do you think will help clear up this problem?
   a. If specific tests or medications are listed, ask what they are and what they do.
6. Apart from me, who else do you think can make you feel better?
   a. Are there therapies that make you feel better (some discipline) that I don't know about?

KLEINMAN EXPLANATORY MODEL†

1. What do you call your problem? What name does it have?
2. What do you think caused it?
3. When do you think it started?
4. What does your sickness do to you?
5. How severe is it? Will it have a long or short course?
6. What do you fear most about your sickness?
7. What are the chief problems your sickness has caused for you?
8. What treatment should you receive? What are the most important results you hope to receive?

*Modified from Pfeifferling JH: *In service provider briefings.* Material prepared by Gutierrez-Mayka M, Henderson JN, Poiley EF, editors; University of South Florida Geriatric Education Center, Suncoast Gerontology Center, funded by Bureau of Health Professions, Health Resources and Services Administration (#DHHS AH64019-04), 1981.
†From Kleinman A: *In service provider briefings: ethnic minority elderly—better understanding for better care.* Material prepared by Gutierrez-Mayka M, Henderson JN, Poiley EF, editors, University of South Florida Geriatric Education Center, Suncoast Gerontology Center, funded by Bureau of Health Professions, Health Resources and Services Administration (#DHHS AH64019-04), 1981.

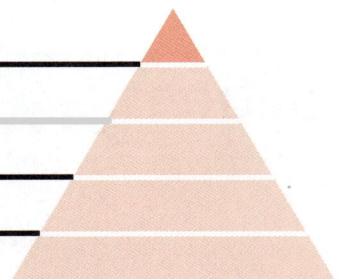

CHAPTER 25

Actualizing the Self

Students learn

The image of my own aging grows increasingly simpler. The list of things I like to do becomes shorter yet more refined. I finally have the courage and wisdom to let the unimportant issues go and fully concentrate on the important ones. I gradually attain wisdom by constantly learning from and valuing the past, while staying open so as not to let the past become the present.

Margit, age 22

To me, experience is a series of lessons we must learn to reach maturity. I think healthy aging means learning those lessons, gaining experience about how life works. Part of this learning process is accomplished by making mistakes. As long as we learn how to do things differently next time, making mistakes can make us better people.

Daphne, age 36

Elders speak

No, I am not caught in a revolving door but rather climbing a circular stairway, maybe, with each landing affording a new aspect of the view out there of truth and beauty.

Anna at 90

From where I stood at 40 the long road to the horizon continually seemed to become narrower until all I saw toward the end was a bleak and barren future, but as I progressed forward the bleak became lovely and I could see things I could not imagine from a distance.

Muriel at 70

Someone once said that old age is the accumulation of unsolved problems. For me, old age is the challenge of continuing to solve the problems. It's important for me to think increasingly about the "you" and not so much about the "me."

Aveline, over 70

LEARNING OBJECTIVES

Upon completion of this chapter, the reader will be able to:

1. Provide a comprehensive definition of self-actualization and identify several qualities to be expected in self-actualized elders.
2. Compare self-actualized and inhibited elders and discuss the fundamental differences in their capacities and abilities to enjoy life.
3. Describe several learning opportunities that are available to elders and the special characteristics and growth factors predominant in each.
4. Specify several types of creative self-expression, including those less often visible to the public. Relate creativity to self-development and describe how this can be stimulated or augmented by various activities the staff may institute.
5. Relate numerous possibilities for creativity and self-expression.
6. Discuss the nursing role in relation to the self-actualization of elders.

ACHIEVING SELF-ACTUALIZATION

Self-actualization is the highest level of human function defined by Maslow (1959) and implies inner motivation freed to express the most unique self. The crux of self-actualization is defining life in such a way as to allow room for continual growth and expansion. We must emphasize that growth and expansion of the aged, from our perspective, carries no mandate from society but embodies the full freedom to be oneself. Inner development cannot be measured by actions, and thus we may not know the extent of an elder's growth. It is not subject to measurement. Martha Holstein (1996) expresses it well: "Establishing a new—and desired—image of productive aging could foreclose needed conversation about what other normative possibilites for old age can be imagined. A public dialogue might reveal cultural images that move us far beyond the ruling continuity of middle-aged values" (p. 12). Maslow believes self-actualization is seldom achieved among the young because it requires experience and maturity acquired through facing the realities of life, especially those beyond one's control, and choosing to be fully oneself. The self-actualized person has inner convictions that may be somewhat removed from ordinary daily concerns and is more absorbed in ideas and ideals than in people and things. The traits of self-actualized persons are summarized in Box 25-1.

Our faithful readers who have continued to purchase updated versions of the text will find much of the material remains cogent and relevant today. We continue to seek new ways that elders express the styles and components of self-actualization.

Characteristics of the Self-Actualized

Young (1983) expressed the changes in her life and thought that occurred after 70 years, "There is an intensified consciousness of having crossed an invisible barrier, entered into another area of being. What was once of paramount importance has receded into relative insignificance. Although my deep involvement with life and people remains, there is now also an urgency, a call if you will, clear and insistent, to move inward; to undertake, in some sense a journey. Its nature is still partly unclear, except that it calls for greater depth, for detachment."

There is an evolution of maturity and emotions that many writers have identified in one way or another. We have chosen Maslow's model because it moves one forward in continual self-development. It can be viewed as a development model, a need model, and is both a macrosystem and microsystem.

A child's first need is to be given food, shelter, safety, security, and love. This need is fulfilled by an adult, who has

Box 25-1	**Traits of Self-Actualized Persons**

- Time competent: Uses past and future to live more fully in the present.
- Inner directed: Source of direction depends on internal forces more than on others.
- Flexible: Can react situationally without unreasonable restrictions.
- Sensitive to self: Responsive to own feeling.
- Spontaneous: Able to and willing to be self.
- Values self: Accepts and demonstrates strengths as a person.
- Accepts self: Approves of self in spite of weaknesses or deficiencies.
- Positively views others: Sees both the bad and the good in others as essentially good and constructive.
- Positively views life: Sees the opposites of life as meaningfully related.
- Acceptance of aggressiveness: Able to accept own feelings of anger and aggressiveness.
- Capable of intimate contact: Able to develop warm interpersonal relationships with others.

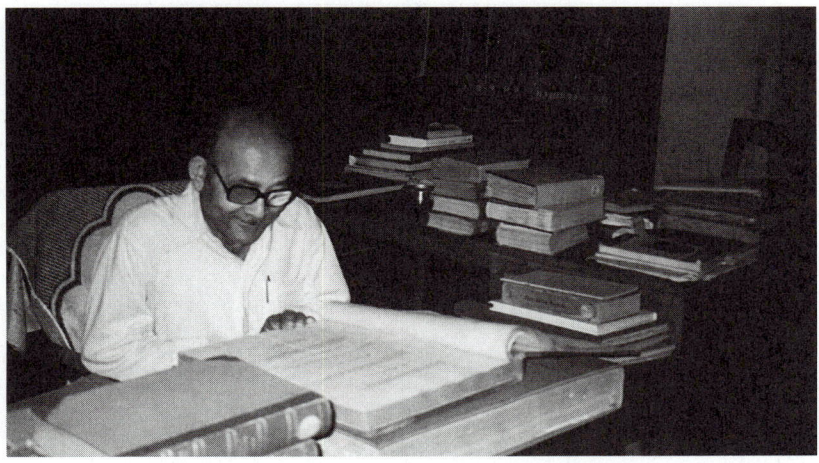

The scholar. (Courtesy Priscilla Ebersole.)

moved to sufficient levels of self-esteem and mastery to give to the child. In adolescence the focus on self reaches narcissistic proportions, and development is powered by the need to be accepted. As one experiences love outside the family, goals enlarge. World concerns and ethics transcend self, family, community, and nation.

Anywhere along the developmental continuum concerns may again become constricted. A self-actualized person may, under threat of illness, become self-centered and narrow. On the other hand, many old people whom I would call self-transcendent live out their last years in a "home" rather than disturb the adult children whom they love enough to release.

A pyramidal model appears to convey a narrowing, rising principle. True human development might be viewed as an inverted triangle. We might conceptualize energy focused in an intense, narrow manner on lower level needs, becoming less focused and intense as one moves upward in maturity. The inverted pyramid concept shows development as a process of enlarging concerns (Figure 25-1).

Only with self-transcendence, do humans emerge to a state high enough to see the needs of others as important as those of self. According to Maslow, few people are self-transcendent, and those are the elite. The mass of humanity restricts its concern to self and a small circle of others. The circle enlarges, and the concern becomes more diffuse as one becomes less self-absorbed.

In old age, threats to self-esteem are strong if value is measured only by attainment, containment, power, and influence. Ethics, values, humor, courage, altruism, and integrity flourish in those who continue to grow.

Courage.   Courage is the quality of mind or spirit that enables a person to conquer fear and despair in the face of difficulty, danger, pain, or uncertainty. We believe facing a long, painful, and restricted existence is the highest level of courage. An old man, diabetic, with amputations and failing vision, sits in his room at the retirement home, looking out the window for hours each day, for weeks, months, and years. That is courage. An old lady crippled with arthritis attends her ailing spouse, who no longer recognizes her. That is courage.

When asking old people how they keep going day by day, there are various answers. None has ever said to me, "It is because I am courageous." They need to be told. A gold star could be given to those who have lived and survived the long battle of a mediocre existence. In current vernacular mediocre means "ordinary." These individuals are not ordinary. The origins of the word *mediocre* translate to "halfway up a stony mountain" (Merriam-Webster, 1974). Many elders are enduring the climb up a stony mountain, and they are the epitome of courage. Memorials are made for those who die in battle, but few monuments are raised to those who courageously wake every morning with no great purpose or challenge to push them out of bed. Yet they endure

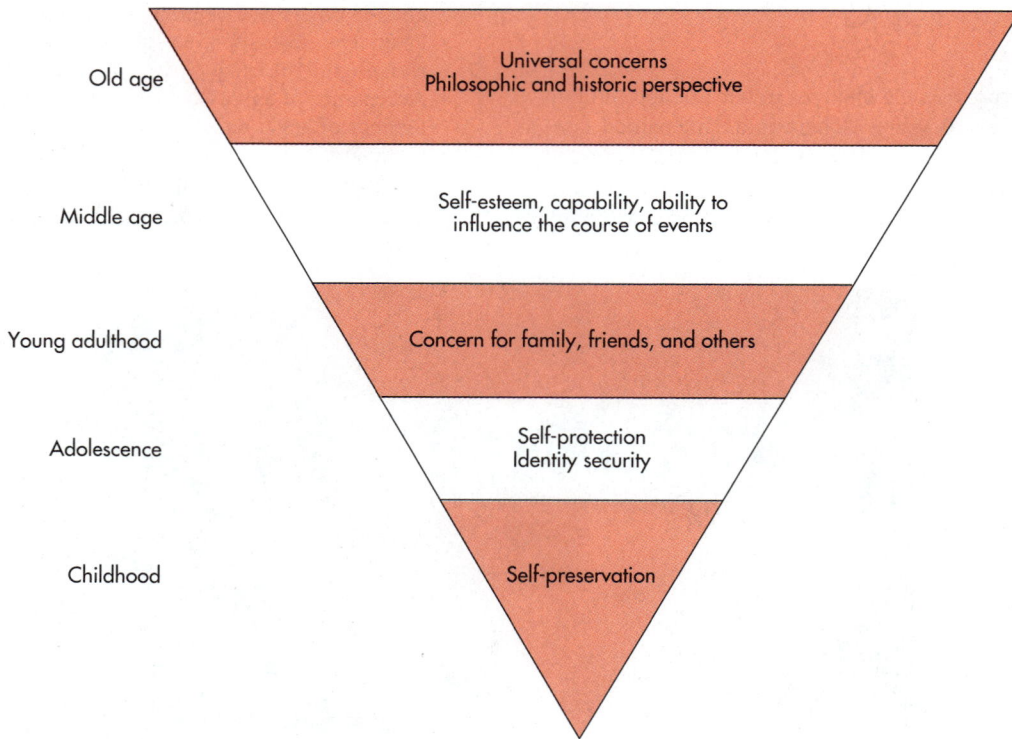

Figure 25-1. Development: expansion of concerns.

the seemingly purposeless, monotonous hours and somehow find meaning. It is a mistake to believe the aged are unable to be self-actualized unless they are energetic, healthy, and wealthy. The capacity of the spirit to find meaning in existence is often remarkable.

Catherine was self-actualized. Her physical constraints were enormous; she had no material assets, her range of activity was limited to her small cubicle in a skilled nursing facility, and her body was frail. But her spirit was strong.

Her creativity was expressed at each meal when she rearranged, mixed, and added to her food. She carefully chopped a pickle and sprinkled it on her cottage cheese and added a little honey to her applesauce. Each meal was a small adventure.

Several friends would visit regularly and bring her small items she enjoyed. They could always count on being entertained with creatively embroidered tales of the past. The gifts they brought were always used in extraordinary ways. A scarf might be tied around her head. Powder, perfume, books, and other things would be bartered for favors from staff members or given as gifts. Her radio brought news of the day interspersed with classical music.

She created a milieu in which she enjoyed life and maintained her self-esteem. There was never any doubt that she was self-actualized. Her artistry overflowed in myriad small gestures. A felt hanging was presented to her on her birthday by hospital volunteers. She stripped off its gigantic red heart and yellow daisy. The words "enjoy life" were all that remained on the forest-green felt (Figure 25-2).

Altruism. In a study of persons of all ages and their willingness to contribute to a worthy cause, Midlarsky et al (1983) found that the elderly were consistently more altruistic. In a summary of charity contributions (U.S. Bureau of the Census, 1995) it is clear that individuals between ages 65 and 74 are the heaviest contributors (Table 25-1). A high degree of helping behaviors is present in many aged. The very old will remember the Great Depression and the altruism that kept people physically and spiritually alive. Neighbor helped neighbor long before the government came to the rescue.

More recent researchers have found the helping experience fundamental to high morale (Trice, 1990). It appears that a sense of meaning in life is strongly tied to survival and

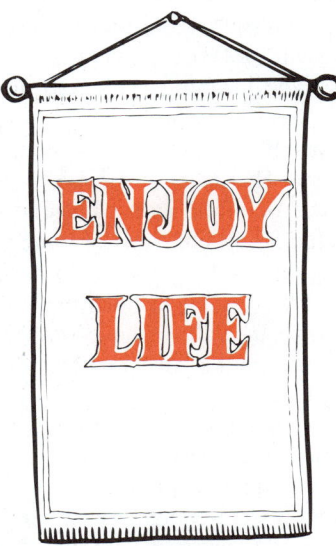

Figure 25-2. Enjoy life. (Illustrated by Joseph Pierre.)

Table 25-1   Charity Contributions—Average Dollar Amount and Percent of Household Income, 1987 to 1993, and by Age of Respondent and Household Income, 1993

[Estimates cover households' contribution activity for the year and are based on respondents' replies as to contribution and volunteer activity of household. Based on a sample survey conducted during the spring of the following year and subject to sampling variability]

Year and age	All contributing households		Contributors and volunteers		Household income	All contributing households		Contributors and volunteers	
	Average amount (dol.)	Percent of household income	Average amount (dol.)	Percent of household income		Average amount (dol.)	Percent of household income	Average amount (dol.)	Percent of household income
1987	790	1.9	1,021	2.4	**1993—**				
1991	899	2.2	1,155	2.6	Under $10,000	207	2.7	(B)	(B)
1993, total	**880**	**2.1**	**1,193**	**2.6**	$10,000-$19,999	332	2.3	460	3.1
18-24 years	514	1.2	(B)	(B)	$20,000-$29,999	668	2.7	862	3.4
25-34 years	520	1.4	666	1.6	$30,000-$39,999	715	2.0	824	2.3
35-44 years	978	1.8	1,376	2.5	$40,000-$49,999	572	1.3	713	1.6
45-54 years	1,241	2.5	1,766	3.3	$50,000-$59,999	632	1.1	758	1.4
55-64 years	1,037	2.4	1,222	2.6	$60,000-$74,999	1,572	2.3	2,006	3.0
65-74 years	1,135	3.9	1,832	4.8	$75,000-$99,999	1,720	2.0	(B)	(B)
75 years and over ...	666	3.2	(B)	(B)	$100,000 and over ...	3,213	3.2	(B)	(B)

From U.S. Bureau of the Census: *Statistical abstract of the United States: 1995,* ed 115, Washington, DC, 1995.
B, Base too small to meet statistical standards for reliability.

is derived from the conviction of in some way being needed by others. Luchs and Growald (1988) discuss the physiology of altruism and propose that doing good, or even thinking about it, may boost immunity.

Many elders find helping behaviors a mode of personal transcendence. There are ways for even the most isolated and impaired elderly to reach beyond themselves. In a classic study, residents of a nursing home who had responsibility to care for individually placed bird feeders demonstrated more feelings of autonomy and happiness and were more active than those residents who did not have responsibility for a bird feeder (Banzinger and Rousch, 1983).

Humor. Metcalf (1993) explains humor: originating in the Latin root *umor,* meaning "fluid and flexible," able to flow around and wear away obstacles. In the same way that water sustains our life and well-being, humor sustains our mental well-being. Humor is transcendent because it momentarily removes one from an isolated ego state to join in surprise at the ludicrous situations of human beings. It requires the ability to step back from oneself and see the total context of an event. Maslow has identified humor as a high level of awareness. Indeed, we have wondered if strength and inner resources can be measured by one's appreciation of the humor in life.

Cousins (1979) and many others have recognized the importance of humor in recovery from illness. The physiologic effects of humor stimulate production of catecholamines and hormones and increase pain tolerance by the release of endorphins. Cardiac, respiratory, and muscle metabolism is improved (Fry, 1979).

Psychological elements of humor can be cognitive/perceptual, social/behavioral, or psychoanalytic. The cognitive/perceptual aspect deals with incongruities, the social/behavioral aspect disparages others and may be used aggressively or to express superiority and derision, and the psychoanalytic aspect expresses taboos and thoughts that may be repressed or suppressed.

Sullivan and Deane (1988) found that patients became more willing to share concerns of deeper significance and the quality of the nurse-patient relationship improved when humor was used thoughtfully.

Humor as an intervention must be individualized to the elder's preferential style. Careful observation of the elder's tolerance or appreciation of varied situations will give clues that are useful in assessing appreciation of humor. Humorous songs, jokes, cartoons, or slapstick movies may generate laughter. Healthy humor must not be tasteless or offensive or give the impression of disregard of a patient's concerns. Teasing or mocking is totally unacceptable.

The nurse must also remember that often the elder initiates humor, and in our seriousness we may overlook the dry wit or, worse, perceive it as confusion. The aged are not a humorless group and frequently laugh at themselves. Objections to jokes about old age seem to emanate from the young far more than the old. Perhaps the old, from the vantage point of a lifetime, can more clearly see human predicaments. Ego transcendence (Peck, 1955) allows one to step back and view the self and situation without the intensity and despair of the egocentric individual.

Humor is often mentioned as an attribute of wisdom and self-actualization, but Steffl (1994) found that even elders with cognitive impairment respond to humor. This echoes the experience of Oliver Sachs (1987), reported in *Awakenings,* when he heard a group of mentally disturbed patients laughing uproariously at a polititian's speech. He concluded that when content was irrelevant, they sensed the false posturing and found it entertaining. We do know that many confused or disturbed elders are extremely sensitive to the mood and affect of others.

High Morale. Clark and Anderson (1967) in their pioneering studies found six factors that contributed to high morale among the aged:

1. Stimulation of mind and imagination
2. Avoidance of physically overtaxing activities
3. Autonomy
4. Personal comfort
5. Vanity in surroundings
6. Passionate involvement with life

Scott-Maxwell exemplifies the passion:

Age puzzles me. I thought it was a quiet time. My seventies were interesting, and fairly serene, but my eighties are passionate. I grow more intense as I age. To my own surprise I burst out with hot conviction (Scott-Maxwell, 1968, p. 13).

Scott-Maxwell was undoubtedly one of the elite, self-actualized elderly.

In this unit, we hope to expose the nurse to the myriad evidences of self-actualization in old age and suggest ways in which the nurse can assist older persons to seek their own unique way of living and growing.

Continuous Moral Development. The moral development of mankind on an individual and collective basis has been of interest to philosophers and religious leaders throughout history. The driving forces of morality are love (Plato) and intellect (Aristotle). Augustine viewed moral development as the process of conquering self and sin.

Kohlberg's early conceptualizations (see Chapter 2) defined discrete stages of moral development based upon growing intelligence and linked these to Piaget's stages of cognitive development and reasoning (Jecker, 1990). Kohlberg's refinements of his original theories have focused on the evidence, derived from autobiographies, that in maturity there are transformations of moral outlook. This can be demonstrated in Katharine Hepburn's autobiographical statement:

I hope you realize that I am remembering all this now. I am looking back and realizing what the truth was. The motives back of my action. I don't think that it was all as cold-blooded as it sounds. I hope not. But the truth has to be that I was a terrible pig. My aim was ME ME ME. All the way—up—down—all about (1991, p. 158).

Kohlberg has posited old age as a seventh stage of moral development that goes beyond reasoning and reaches awareness of one's relative place in universal morality. This stage of moral development involves identification with a more enduring moral perspective than that of one's own life span (Kohlberg and Power, 1981). This involves moral expansion and the exemplary impact of the fully developing elder upon the following generations, born and unborn. We have come to believe that at present this may be the most important task of elders as we see honor and recognition given to individuals who seem to have little integrity or reliability. Each individual carries a mass of motivations and desires. Some are stunted and some will flourish. Youngsters must have models of honorable, truthful, and honest individuals if we hope to cultivate these qualities in human experience.

SUCCESSFUL AGING

We have much yet to learn about those who age successfully. Successful aging is an individualistic pursuit, and success is evaluated almost entirely in the eye of the beholder. The *Mayo Clinic Health Letter* (Aging Successfully, 1992) gives suggestions for "how to succeed at the business of growing older." Box 25-2 lists guidelines for successful aging. The essential outcomes seem to be continual learning, growing, questioning, creating, and enjoying.

The concept of "hardiness" is significant in successful aging (Pappas, 1995). Qualities of control, competence and compassion are the cornerstones of hardiness, as well as the qualities that support satisfaction and personal growth in the later years. Ward and Mroczek (1995) confirm what many have speculated for some time: that basic personality characteristics may have a positive or restrictive effect on health and satisfaction. Holistic health practices, while dealt with in depth in chapter 3, are somewhat relevant to self-actualization because they are the first step in acknowledging one's active participation in becoming whole.

Learning and Growing in Later Life

The formal education of elders has significantly increased in the 20 years since serious attention began to be focused on the situations of the aged. Age is no longer a barrier to education. Individuals in their 80s and 90s seek graduate degrees (Guttmann-Gee, 1995-1996). In 1980 43% of the over 65 population had 8 years or less schooling. Presently, 22% are in that category, and nearly twice as many have had some college (U.S. Bureau of Census, 1995). Between 1970 and 1994 the percentage who had completed high school rose from 28% to 62% (American Association of Retired Persons, 1996).

These statistics are a reflection of cohort differences as well as increased involvement in late life education. Following World War II there was a major change in higher education in America. Veterans returning from the war were given the opportunity to gain a college education. Prior to that only the relatively affluent elite had higher degrees. The common individual could not afford the time or the money. These young men entered universities in droves. Now, 50 years later, these elders are still learning and pursuing knowledge.

Some elders remain who have special learning needs based upon education deprivation in their early years and consequent anxiety about learning in an organized setting. Box 25-3 summarizes some of the ways to overcome these problems.

Opportunities for elders to learn are available in many formal and informal modes: self-teaching, college attendance, participation in seminars and conferences, public television programs, videotapes, courses via telecommunications, and countless other modes. A program of more than 100 courses, sponsored by Saddleback College near Leisure World Laguna Hills (1996) is designed to meet the

Box 25-2	**Guidelines for Successful Aging**

Plan for retirement.
Balance solitary activities with social activities.
Try something new; adapt interests.
Accept limitations.
Budget finances to cover items of personal importance.
Draw on friends and kin for support and
  encouragement.
Maintain a faith that gives peace of mind.
Maintain an optimistic outlook.
Engage in activities in the world and community.
Practice good health habits.

Summarized from Aging successfully, *Mayo Clinic Health Letter* 10(11):6, 1992.

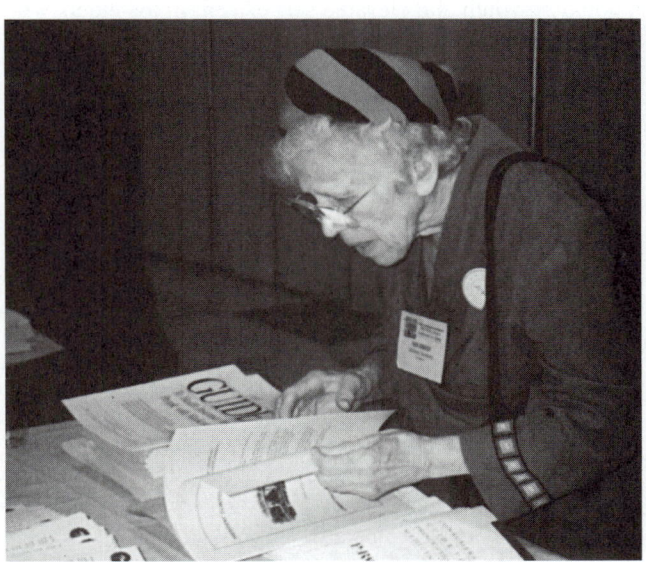

Keeping informed. (Courtesy Priscilla Ebersole.)

educational needs and desires of seniors. More than 8000 residents of Leisure World are enrolled in the courses; arts and physical education are the most popular. Television is a particularly important avenue of learning because statistics indicate almost universal viewing by adults over age 65, whereas radios and newspapers are less often a source of information (U.S. Bureau of the Census, 1995) (Table 25-2).

Ten percent of individuals over age 65 participate in some form of adult education and usually purely for personal satisfaction (Table 25-3).

This portion of the chapter introduces only a few of the ways in which elders are learning new skills and arts, health management, and personal enrichment. The nurse's function is to be informed and assist an elder in finding the learning mode and setting appropriate to his or her need or desire (Figure 25-3).

In most universities there are older persons taking classes of all types. Fees are usually lower for individuals over 60 years of age, and they may choose to work toward a degree and complete all assignments or audit classes just for enrichment and enjoyment.

Adults who have been away from the competitive atmosphere of 4-year colleges and universities may first need to enroll in a study skills course before pursuing a baccalaureate degree. Older adults returning to the classroom after many years may need orientation to academia and special encouragement. Many educators are beginning to recognize a need to revise traditional educational approaches if they hope to serve more older citizens. As college youth enrollments decrease nationwide, educators will begin to court the older learners.

The intergenerational classroom provides the aged with an opportunity to share their perspective from a long-range view and the youth to interject immediacy and energy. The results are increased positive attitude toward the aged among the youth and elevated self-esteem in the elders who compete and achieve academic success.

Numerous opportunities exist for older learners within the established educational institutions or in very special programs such as the Academy of Life Long Learning in Delaware or the Learning in Retirement programs. *Regenerational learning,* a term coined by McConatha (1983), is a process designed to encourage and facilitate the full development of individual potential in mature and older adults. The activities are based on the concepts of lifelong learning, the human potential movement, and positive wellness. To tap the often ignored abilities and resources of adults, regenerational learning concentrates on stimulating creativity and expressivity while encouraging the exploration of new fields of endeavor through "venture learning exercises." Some of the techniques used to facilitate this process include self-talk, visualization and imagery, role playing, biofeedback, and forced positive expression.

Many universities have "senior scholars" (Case Western Reserve University) programs designed especially for el-

---

Box 25-3	**Elderly Client's Special Learning Needs**

- Make sure the client is ready to learn before trying to teach. Watch for clues that would indicate that the client is preoccupied or too anxious to comprehend the material.
- Sit facing the client so that he or she can watch your lip movements and facial expressions.
- Speak slowly.
- Keep your tone of voice low; elderly persons can hear low sounds better than high-frequency sounds.
- Present one idea at a time.
- Emphasize concrete rather than abstract material.
- Give the client enough time in which to respond because elderly persons' reaction times are longer than those of younger persons.
- Focus on a single topic to help the client concentrate.
- Keep environmental distractions to a minimum.
- Defer teaching if the client becomes distracted or tired or cannot concentrate for other reasons.
- Invite another member of the household to join the discussion.
- Use audio, visual, and tactile cues to enhance learning and help the client remember information.
- Ask for feedback to ensure that the information has been understood.
- Use past experience; connect new learning to that already learned.
- Compensate for physical discomfort and sensory decrements.
- Support a positive self-image in the learner.
- Use creative teaching strategies.
- Respond to identified interests of learners.
- Emphasize and integrate emotional and personal values in the acquisition of skills and ideas.

Modified from Fielo S, Rizzolo M: Handle with caring: meeting elderly clients' special learning needs, *Nurs Health Care* 9(4):193, 1988.

---

ders. At the McGill Institute for Learning in Retirement, students design their own course of study (Clark, 1995-1996).

Travel. Travel is a route many elders take to achieve knowledge while simultaneously increasing pleasure. The number of traveling elders is a reflection of the increased affluence and energy of the aged of today. It is estimated that over 20% of all trips in the United States were taken by individuals over 55 years old (Hudson and Rich, 1993).

Intergenerational travel seems to be increasing with many elders traveling with grandchildren. The Grandtravel agency offers vacations specially designed for grandparents and grandchildren (see Resources at the end of the chapter).

For those people who have a strong desire to travel, and to seek new lands and scenes, there are many opportunities available if they are physically and economically able. The Senior Travel Exchange Program gives elders the opportu-

Table 25-2   Multimedia Audiences—Summary: 1994

[In percent, except as indicated. As of spring. For persons 18 years old and over. Represents the number of people viewing/listening during a specified time period. Based on sample and subject to sampling error; see source for details]

Item	Total population (1,000)	Television viewing	Television prime time (viewing)	Cable viewing	Radio listening	Newspaper reading
Total	**188,654**	**92.1**	**78.4**	**61.6**	**84.7**	**82.9**
18 to 24 years old	24,247	91.0	73.0	59.6	93.5	80.0
25 to 34 years old	43,548	91.0	76.8	60.2	92.3	81.5
35 to 44 years old	40,581	90.7	77.4	64.4	89.7	85.6
45 to 54 years old	27,501	91.3	78.8	66.1	87.7	85.6
55 to 64 years old	21,394	93.6	81.0	63.4	77.8	84.6
65 years old and over	31,383	95.9	83.8	56.3	63.0	80.0
Male	90,177	91.7	76.9	63.5	86.6	83.0
Female	98,478	92.4	79.8	59.9	83.0	82.8
White	160,581	91.7	78.0	64.0	84.8	83.6
Black	21,415	94.5	81.1	48.1	84.7	82.2
Other	6,658	92.8	79.7	47.0	82.9	68.5
Spanish speaking	16,247	93.6	81.1	49.1	88.0	75.2
Not high school graduate	37,489	93.7	81.1	48.3	72.7	65.0
High school graduate	65,896	92.7	80.0	62.8	84.9	82.8
Attended college	47,506	91.3	76.3	66.4	90.1	88.5
College graduate	37,763	90.3	75.5	66.6	89.4	93.8
Employed:						
Full-time	102,971	90.6	76.1	65.6	91.6	86.4
Part-time	16,348	91.2	74.4	60.2	90.5	88.1
Not employed	69,335	94.6	82.8	56.0	73.2	76.5
Household income:						
Less than $10,000	19,620	92.3	81.1	42.3	70.9	62.9
$10,000 to $19,999	29,530	93.6	80.5	49.4	77.3	75.3
$20,000 to $29,999	29,135	93.5	80.4	57.0	82.7	80.4
$30,000 to $34,999	13,658	94.0	80.3	63.1	85.6	83.5
$35,000 to $39,999	13,087	92.2	78.1	62.6	87.6	84.8
$40,000 to $49,999	22,163	92.1	78.7	67.3	89.2	88.4
$50,000 or more	61,461	90.1	75.0	73.2	91.3	91.6

From U.S. Bureau of the Census: *Statistical abstract of the United States: 1995,* ed 115, Washington, DC, 1995.
Source: *Multimedia audiences,* New York, NY, Fall, 1994, Mediamark Research, Inc (copyright).

nity to travel to other nations, develop friendships, and really get to know the people. These are organized into groups of 20 to 25 elders and are very economical. Travelers stay in the homes of locals, and at a later time the hosts and guests reverse roles when the original hosts travel to the United States (Leitner and Leitner, 1996) (see Resources at the end of the chapter).

For those elderly who are less affluent and content to stay closer to home territory, many organized low-cost tours explore unusual sites near one's area. The American Bed and Breakfast Association can provide information regarding providers nationwide who belong to the organization and offer inexpensive lodging and breakfast. They also give information to elders who wish to establish a bed and breakfast (see Resources at the end of the chapter).

The personal effects of travel are as variable as the individuals and the places they select to see. Nursing involvement will be most useful in addressing potential problems and assisting elders to plan ahead for contingencies. Pets must be placed appropriately, house sitting services are sometimes necessary, and physical limitations must be considered. The following questions should be asked and resolved prior to departing:

- Whom will you contact in an emergency? Is their number in your billfold? Is your blood type also noted?
- What health care and travel insurance coverage do you have? Is it adequate for unforseen illness? Do you have sufficient medications, hearing aid batteries, extra eyeglasses?

Table 25-3   Participation in Adult Education: 1990-91

[For the civilian noninstitutional population 17 years old and over not enrolled full-time in elementary or secondary school at the time of the survey. Adult education is considered any part-time enrollment in any educational activity at any time in the prior 12 months. Based on a telephone survey and subject to sampling error; see source for details]

| | | Participants in Adult Education | | | | | |
| | | | | | Reason for taking course (percent)* | | |
Characteristic	Adult popu-lation (1,000)	Number taking adult ed. courses (1,000)	Per-cent of total	Per-sonal/ social	Advance on the job	Train for a new job	Complete degree or diploma
Total	**181,800**	**57,391**	**32**	**30**	**60**	**9**	**13**
Age: 17 to 24 years old	21,688	7,125	33	30	38	18	29
25 to 34 years old	47,244	17,530	37	25	63	12	14
35 to 44 years	38,565	17,083	44	27	66	8	12
45 to 54 years old	25,375	8,107	32	29	70	6	7
55 to 64 years old	19,967	4,516	23	35	61	5	5
65 years old and over	28,960	3,031	10	73	22	4	3

From U.S. Bureau of the Census: *Statistical abstract of the United States: 1995,* ed 115, Washington, DC, 1995.
*Reason for taking at least one course. Includes duplication. Excludes "to improve basic skills," cited by no more than 4% of participants.
Source U.S. National Center for Education Statistics, *Adult Education Profile for 1990-91;* and unpublished data.

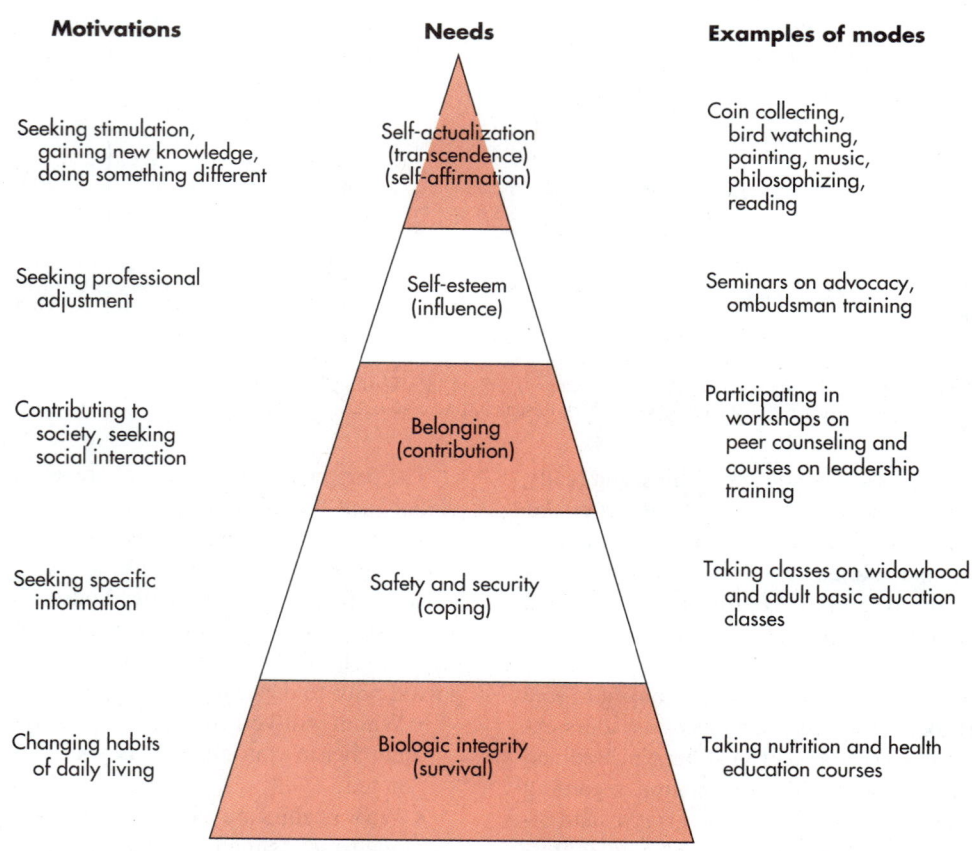

Figure 25-3.   Learning and growing in later life. (Developed by Priscilla Ebersole.)

- What immunizations will you need, and where can you obtain them?
- Do you have a safe place on your body for money?
- Where are you obtaining prior information about the places you intend to go?
- Are the areas you wish to see accessible in terms of your mobility and energy?
- Do you desire accomodations similar to those used by locals or Western type hotels?
- What is the usual weather during the time you will be visiting?

Changes in water, altitude, and climate can produce distressing reactions. Individuals must allow themselves time to adjust to the changed condtions, and many people obtain bottled water.

Often people find travel after retirement a vehicle for learning and growing. Careful planning will make travel safer and more enjoyable. Suggestions for travel are summarized in Box 25-4.

Elderhostel. The Elderhostel program, an adult education program originally based on the youth hostel concept, was originated by Marty Knowlton in 1974 at the University of New Hampshire and now offers programs at 2000 educational and cultural institutions in 70 countries throughout the world in addition to the United States and Canada (Elderhostel, 1997).

Elderhostel is a nonprofit international program that provides low-cost room and board and specially designed classes for elders on college campuses, conference centers, state and national parks, museums, theaters, environmental outdoor education centers, and other sites. The program mails its catalogs to over a half million people, and each year there are nearly 300,000 persons over age 55 or who have a spouse over age 55 that participate in this phenomenally successful educational program for older adults. About half of those who participate in the Elderhostel program live in dormitories and eat in college dining halls while taking brief noncredit college courses taught by regular faculty members or specialists in a particular field.

The national Elderhostel concept is a response to the awareness that the elderly want to continue learning in their later years. Some scholarships are offered for programs within the United States. Some of the reasons for attending Elderhostel are (1) change (opportunity to go somewhere or do something different), (2) time (short time frame for learning), (3) cost (low fixed cost), (4) courses (suitable course content), (5) absence of evaluation (no tests or homework), and (6) learning (opportunities to develop new interests and reexplore old ones). Programs of special interest include hiking and biking trips, historic houses, folk colleges, and study cruises. The opportunities for study address almost every interest one could imagine. Classes, taught by academics, specialists and local experts, cover a broad range of

subjects such as jazz, art, religion, astronomy, history, and mythology. Older citizens who may wish intellectual stimulation and personal enrichment should be encouraged to investigate these programs (see Resources at the end of the chapter).

Community Colleges and Adult Education. Community colleges assume much of the responsibility for providing low-cost, accessible educational programs for citizens within their boundaries. They have been a boon to older persons who want to develop a specific skill or knowledge base. Community colleges offer preretirement programs, job reentry skills, second-career guidance counseling, vocational training and general education. In many cases retired elderly teach the community college classes.

We encourage nurses to become aware of programs that their community colleges offer and assume some responsibility in developing classes and courses to close the gap in service to the older members of the community. The community college emphasis on practical knowledge serves one group of older learners. Knowledge gained purely for personal enrichment may be equally as important to some

---

Box 25-4	**Travel Tips for Elders**

- Many organizations offer special group rates and tours planned for elders.
- Travel agencies can give information about reduced rates for charter flights or in less popular travel months. Choose off-season to avoid crowds and get best rates.
- Some air carriers have reduced rates for the aged or handicapped.
- Many countries offer special rates to older travelers. Information should be obtained from the tourist bureau of the countries on itinerary.
- Social Security benefits continue indefinitely.
- Medicare coverage does not extend outside the United States and its territories; however, many European countries have national health services that are extended to travelers. Supplementary health insurance is a good idea.
- Passports should be applied for well in advance if birth certificates are not readily available. Visas are required for many countries.
- Immunizations are required to travel in certain countries. Check with the U.S. Public Health Service.
- Take a medical travel kit containing sufficient medication for any chronic condition; first aid equipment; medications for diarrhea, dyspepsia, and nausea; an extra pair of glasses; and records of medication problems, allergies, and blood type.
- Take extras of equipment needed such as hearing aid batteries, eye glasses, braces, and orthopedic shoes.

or the opportunity to meet general education requirements as a stepping stone to higher education and academic credentials.

Convenience, accessibility, scheduling of classes, and the opportunity to audit if desired are important to the aged. Many community colleges now offer courses on television or the internet that are inexpensive, fully accredited, and available to elders with impaired mobility or lower energy levels. They also frequently offer weekend courses to familiarize residents with local areas of interest or special projects.

Education for Those with Special Needs

The homebound elderly. Education has become accessible to many homebound persons through public television, telephone, and radio. Public libraries throughout the United States provide videotapes and audiotapes to the confined elderly. There are many methods for implementing educational outreach programs; for example, telephone seminars in which individuals are connected with each other and the instructor through a central telephone monitor. Such teleconferencing approaches may be particularly valuable in reaching the rural, isolated elderly. With increasingly adaptable telecommunications technology and cost reductions, these adaptations are becoming more common.

Stanley-Muchow and Poe (1988) report the use of audio teleconferencing to provide a college course for nursing home residents. The course focused on personality development, values, self-concept, coping, and communication. Packets of materials were prepared for the students that were used during the conference call discussions. An on-site staff person was available to assist and facilitate discussion in each of the participating nursing homes. At the completion of the course all students met at one of the nursing homes for a graduation ceremony. This experiment has implication for future courses that may use similar strategies. Other topics to consider are memory enhancement, interpersonal relationships, health management, death and loss, hearing loss, and family relationships.

A creative method of tapping the growth potential of seniors has been devised by two hospitals in Pittsburgh that conduct semi-annual Town Meetings for Seniors. The seniors learn about health care, legal rights, insurance, and numerous other items of general interest to elders. The outgrowth of these meetings has been a sense of empowerment and the creation of several new community programs (Rubin and Black, 1992).

Reading for Self-Development.

Bond and Miller (1987) call reading an ageless activity and find that institutionalized elders often much prefer the individual, passive involvement in reading to the group activities that are planned for them. Group reading and discussion can also be enjoyable as demonstrated in the Great Books discussion groups that meet routinely in many libraries. Suffice it to say that when an array of books is available, many aged find them sustaining. They extend boundaries imposed by physical limitations, allow exploration into untouched arenas of thought, and enrich the individual. For many elders, reading has been a major pleasure throughout life and, common as it seems, should not be underestimated as a form of self-discovery and actualization.

Many libraries across the country have developed creative programs to serve elders. Some of these programs include talking books for the blind, large-print books and magazines, mail delivery to the homebound, low-vision reading aids, 24-hour audio reader service through a closed-circuit radio station (through the University of Kansas), kits designed to provoke reminiscing, and one-to-one reading service in several languages. To provide these services they rely on intergenerational projects through schools, grants, gifts, bequests, volunteers, and close-out book sales. For more information see Resources at the end of the chapter.

Peer Teaching/Learning

Peer teaching projects have served as a means to allow individuals to share their expertise while meeting the academic interests of retired persons. These may be the first step in launching individuals into the pursuit of higher education that may have been closed to them earlier. In our diverse culture this is an ideal way of including individuals who may not have the academic credentials or cultural comfort to pursue conventionally structured subjects.

To keep costs low, elderly persons are enrolled as students but also teach some classes in which they are knowledgeable. Sometimes retired professional teach courses in their particular area of expertise as a volunteer activity. In some classes students set their own objectives, and a coordinator is chosen to find appropriate resources and instructors. Class members may prepare special topics and lead class discussions, which in addition to inquiry is a method of learning. The success of these programs is attributed to low cost, accessibility, hours and location adapted to elders' needs, and using older persons as instructors.

Such a unique learning/teaching exchange opportunity has been developed at Eckerd College on Florida's gulf coast. It is called the Academy of Senior Professionals and boasts a unique mix of high-achieving professionals who are retired or semiretired and enjoy sharing their knowledge (Trussell, 1992). (See Resources at the end of the chapter for further information.) These individuals concomitantly learn from and teach each other in seminar style.

Learning and the Humanities.

There has been a great revival of interest in the humanities in what is considered the postmodern phase of our social culture. New Age phenomena are not of interest only to youth. The study of the humanities in old age may enlarge horizons, transcend limitations, and strengthen the connection between old age and wisdom. The old have always been involved in the dialogue of humanities and history as they become vitally interested in the exploration of life's meanings. The epic of a generation can be elaborated with the wisdom of those who lived it, and we find more and more individuals involved in seeking the wisdom and life experience of the old in numerous ways.

The tie between the humanities and life history becomes even more clear when we recognize the significance of the aged in the progression of culture through the ages of time. For a time there seemed to be little interest in the "story-telling" function of elders, because the printed and electronic media were accessible to almost everyone, but this interest has been revived in the new appreciation of the personal interpretation of myths, legends, and experience. The National Council on Aging (NCOA), with a grant from the National Endowment for the Humanities, has developed a method to capture the elusive threads of human experience that the aged hold. Program themes are developed around local history, family, the land, particular eras in history, work life, immigrant experience, and other topics. Information for those interested in starting such a program can be obtained from NCOA (see Resources).

Volunteering

Volunteering is important to elders and may fill their need for altruistic endeavors (Table 25-4). Volunteering often involves new role development; this was discussed in Chapter 20. From the perspective of health care providers, volunteer service must be planned appropriately if it is to become gratifying to the participants. Aspects of planning volunteer activities were also noted in Chapter 20.

The focus in this chapter is on nursing actions that may encourage elders to seek new avenues of self-actualization. When volunteer services are considered as a means of personal enrichment and an expression of altruism, it is important for the elder to seek to augment some latent interest areas and launch into pursuits perhaps unavailable earlier because of time constraints or other commitments. Nurses may question elders about interests and talents that they may want to perfect.

COLLECTIVE ACTUALIZATION

The collective power of self-actualized older persons has already brought about many changes in society. Power is a term describing the capacity of an individual or group to accomplish something, to take command, to exert authority, and to influence. The self-actualized aged are powerful, and power is the gateway to resources and recognition.

The age equality movement, older citizens returning to school, and the revolution of older people in movements such as the Gray Panthers have made major changes in the status and recognition of the aged. Gray Panthers

---

Table 25-4   Percent of Adult Population Doing Volunteer Work: 1993

[Covers persons 18 years and over. Volunteers are persons who worked in some way to help others for no monetary pay during the previous year.]

Age, sex race and Hispanic origin	Percent of population volunteering	Average hours volunteered per week	Educational attainment and household income	Percent of population volunteering	Average hours volunteered per week	Type of activity	Percent of volunteers involved in activity
Total	**47.7**	**4.2**	Elementary school	31.8	(B)	Arts, culture, humanities	4.4
			Some high school	29.9	(B)	Education	15.7
18-24 years old	45.3	4.0	High school graduate . .	40.4	3.6	Environment	6.2
25-34 years old	46.1	3.1	Technical, trade, or			Health	10.8
35-44 years old	54.5	4.8	business school	49.2	5.0	Human services	9.8
45-54 years old	53.8	5.2	Some college	56.9	4.3		
55-64 years old	46.6	4.1	College graduate	67.2	5.0	Informal	17.2
65-74 years old	42.9	4.8				International, foreign	1.3
75 years old and over . .	36.4	(B)	Under $10,000	34.0	(B)	Political organizations	3.7
			$10,000-$19,999	37.0	3.7	Private, community	
Male	43.9	4.3	$20,000-$29,999	52.5	4.2	foundations	2.2
Female	51.2	4.2	$30,000-$39,999	56.3	4.9		
			$40,000-$49,999	55.1	3.6	Public and societal benefit . . .	5.4
White	51.1	4.2	$50,000-$59,999	56.9	4.1	Recreation-adults	5.4
Black	29.1	3.7	$60,000-$74,999	66.6	6.1	Religion	24.1
			$75,000-$99,999	58.1	(B)	Work-related organizations . .	6.9
Hispanic*	32.4	(B)	$100,000 or more	67.5	(B)	Youth development	11.7

From U.S. Bureau of the Census: *Statistical abstract of the United States: 1995,* ed 115, Washington, DC, 1995.
B, Base figure too small to meet statistical standards for reliability. *Hispanic persons may be of any race.
Source Hodgkinson V, Weitzman M, and The Gallup Organization, Inc: *Giving and volunteering in the United States: 1994 edition.* (Copyright and published by INDEPENDENT SECTOR, Washington, DC, Fall 1994.)

recognized that issues of aging were not narrow or exclusive but rather were representative of human rights for persons of all ages.

Kuhn (1979), founder of the Gray Panthers, died April 22, 1995 at the age of 89 but her beliefs survive. She perceived that the issues confronting older persons are not those of self-interest, but rather, as "elders of the tribe," the old should seek "survival of the tribe." She outlined steps by which old people can be advocates of the public interest (Kuhn, 1979, p. 3):

- Identify and document the social issue/problem/need. Providers delivering services to individuals should record cases, instances of critical need, scope, extent of deprivation, alienation; what needs to be changed?
- Bring together the victims of discrimination, abuse, and oppression to discuss their problems, understand their situation, and the interaction between personal need and public response.
- Raise the consciousness of victims, educate them about the societal aspects, roots, and causes of their dilemmas.
- Organize victims to develop support groups for mutual support and empowerment, to confront oppressors, and to find local support from established bodies and agencies (insiders!).
- Map strategies for action, including new models for dealing with particular issues, legislative initiatives, court action, and forming coalitions of groups with similar problems.
- Go public: organize a rally with posters, speeches, marches to public places where public officials, interested persons, agency heads, and boards can become aware and be held accountable. Go before television cameras with street theater. Go to press with well-prepared press releases.
- Present testimony in public hearings: set up telegram, telephone campaigns pressing for redress and change.
- Take stock of your advances or setbacks, evaluate results, and consider the next steps.
- Report back to groups for their information and encouragement. Keep communication open with members and coalitions.
- Draft legislation or prepare for legal action in the courts. Marshal arguments, collect "cases" including "horror stories," evoke interest.
- Celebrate victories, even the small ones. Coverage in the press and on television may be significant successes. Even failures should be recognized and evaluated.
- Regroup to fight on with increased knowledge, broader impact, and enlarged constituencies!

Though Kuhn is gone, others, such as Harry Moody of the Brookdale Center on Aging, continue to build upon her ideals. Their thoughts challenge the old to reach beyond themselves. Realistically, the plights of the young, the poor, and the ill are presently of greater concern than the lack of opportunity for the mass of well aged. However, it is clear that there is a lag between the capacities of long-lived people and opportunities for them to challenge those capacities.

Politics and Power

The aged are a powerful political group. Over 31 million individuals over 65 are eligible to vote, three fourths of them are registered, and 70% voted in the 1996 election (Table 25-5). Throughout adult life individuals tend to shift toward Democratic party affiliation, though the more educated are more likely to be strong Republicans (Table 25-6 and Figure 25-4). Roughly 30% are Republicans, 35% are Democrats, and the remainder are independents. Three quarters of people over 65 years old vote compared with less than half of those individuals under 35 years of age. The older voters generally recognize their power, as do politicians (MacManus, 1996).

Elders can be counted on to vote, but their voting behaviors demonstrate their diversity. However, sacrosanct programs such as Social Security and Medicare must be manipulated very gently by any politician who wishes to remain in office. Aside from issues of Medicare and Social Security elders do not form strong voting blocks as they are very individualistic. The contingent of those who label themselves independent has grown in recent years. Older voters are often more concerned about a candidate's character and experience than the party affiliation. Younger voters tend to look for leadership qualities and focus on particular issues.

There are numerous issues of concern to seniors. The following indicates the range of concerns of politically minded elders in California. The California Senior Legislature convened in Sacramento in 1995 and presented 10 proposals they wanted the regular legislators to address:

- Allocate a Senior Special Fund to support the administration of various senior programs in California
- Increase food stamp eligibility for seniors in need
- Establish rural mental health facilites for elders
- Increase opportunities for geriatric training for physicians
- Make public transportation available to rural and nonurbanized areas
- Require geriatric training for administrators of senior centers and residences
- Establish better controls of HMOs and require regular audits
- Require itemized bills for hospital care within 3 days of discharge and prior to billing the insurer
- Require rapid legal resolution of criminal actions involving witnesses or victims over the age of 65 years (California Association of Health Facilities, 1995).

Table 25-5 Voting-Age Population, Percent Reporting Registered, and Voted: 1980 to 1994

[As of November Covers civilian noninstitutional population 18 years old and over. Includes aliens. Figures are based on Current Population Survey.]

| Characteristic | Voting-age population (mil) | | | | | | | | Percent reporting they registered | | | | | | | | Percent reporting they voted | | | | | | | |
| | | | | | | | | | Presidential election years | | | | Congressional election years | | | | Presidential election years | | | | Congressional election years | | | |
	1980	1982	1984	1986	1988	1990	1992	1994	1980	1984	1988	1992	1982	1986	1990	1994	1980	1984	1988	1992	1982	1986	1990	1994
Total[a]	157.1	165.5	170.0	173.9	178.1	182.1	185.7	190.3	66.9	68.3	66.6	68.2	64.1	64.3	62.2	62.0	59.2	59.9	57.4	61.3	48.5	46.0	45.0	44.6
18 to 20 years old	12.3	12.1	11.2	10.7	10.7	10.8	9.7	10.3	44.7	47.0	44.9	48.3	35.0	35.4	35.4	37.2	35.7	36.7	33.2	38.5	19.8	18.6	18.4	16.5
21 to 24 years old	15.9	16.7	16.7	15.7	14.8	14.0	14.6	14.9	52.7	54.3	50.6	55.3	47.8	46.6	43.3	45.5	43.1	43.5	38.3	45.7	28.4	24.2	22.0	22.3
25 to 34 years old	35.7	38.8	40.3	41.9	42.7	42.7	41.6	41.1	62.0	63.3	57.8	60.6	57.1	55.8	52.0	51.5	54.6	54.5	48.0	53.2	40.4	35.1	33.8	32.2
35 to 44 years old	25.6	28.1	30.7	33.0	35.2	37.9	39.7	41.9	70.6	70.9	69.3	69.2	67.5	67.9	65.5	63.3	64.4	63.5	61.3	63.6	52.2	49.3	48.4	46.0
45 to 64 years old	43.6	44.2	44.3	44.8	45.9	46.9	49.1	50.9	75.8	76.6	75.5	75.3	75.6	74.8	71.4	71.0	69.3	69.8	67.9	70.0	62.2	58.7	55.8	56.0
65 years old and over	24.1	25.6	26.7	27.7	28.8	29.9	30.8	31.1	74.6	76.9	78.4	78.0	75.2	76.9	76.5	75.6	65.1	67.7	68.8	70.1	59.9	60.9	60.3	60.7
Male	74.1	78.0	80.3	82.4	84.5	86.6	88.6	91.0	66.6	67.3	65.2	66.9	63.7	63.4	61.2	60.8	59.1	59.0	56.4	60.2	48.7	45.8	44.6	44.4
Female	83.0	87.4	89.6	91.5	93.6	95.5	97.1	99.3	67.1	69.3	67.8	69.3	64.4	65.0	63.1	63.2	59.4	60.8	58.3	62.3	48.4	46.1	45.4	44.9
White	137.7	143.6	146.8	149.9	152.9	155.6	157.8	160.3	68.4	69.6	67.9	70.1	65.6	65.3	63.8	64.2	60.9	61.4	59.1	63.6	49.9	47.0	46.7	46.9
Black	16.4	17.6	18.4	19.0	19.7	20.4	21.0	21.8	60.0	66.3	64.5	63.9	59.1	64.0	58.8	58.3	50.5	55.8	51.5	54.0	43.0	43.2	39.2	37.0
Hispanic[b]	8.2	8.8	9.5	11.8	12.9	13.8	14.7	17.5	36.3	40.1	35.5	35.0	35.3	35.9	32.3	30.0	29.9	32.6	28.8	28.9	25.3	24.2	21.0	19.1
Region[c]																								
Northeast	35.5	36.4	36.9	37.3	37.9	38.1	38.3	38.4	64.8	66.6	64.8	67.0	62.5	62.0	61.0	60.9	58.5	59.7	57.4	61.2	49.8	44.4	45.2	45.2
Midwest	41.5	41.9	42.1	42.8	43.3	43.9	44.4	44.5	73.8	74.6	72.5	74.6	71.1	70.7	68.2	68.7	65.8	65.7	62.9	67.2	54.7	49.5	48.6	48.8
South	50.6	55.4	57.6	59.2	60.7	62.4	63.7	66.4	64.8	66.9	65.6	67.2	61.7	63.0	61.3	60.7	55.6	56.8	54.5	59.0	41.8	43.0	42.4	40.5
West	29.5	31.9	33.4	34.6	36.2	37.7	39.3	41.0	63.3	64.7	63.0	63.6	60.6	60.8	57.7	58.1	57.2	58.5	55.6	58.5	50.7	48.4	45.0	46.4
School years completed																								
8 years or less	22.7	22.4	20.6	19.6	19.1	17.7	15.4	14.7	53.0	53.4	47.5	43.9	52.3	50.5	44.0	40.1	42.6	42.9	36.7	35.1	35.7	32.7	27.7	23.2
High school																								
1 to 3 years	22.5	22.3	22.1	21.4	21.1	21.0	[d]21.0	[d]20.7	54.6	54.9	52.8	[d]50.4	53.3	52.4	47.9	[d]44.7	45.6	44.4	41.3	[d]41.2	37.7	33.8	30.9	[d]27.0
4 years	61.2	65.2	67.8	68.6	70.0	71.5	[e]65.3	[e]64.9	66.4	67.3	64.6	[e]64.9	62.9	62.9	60.0	[e]58.9	58.9	58.7	54.7	[e]57.5	47.1	44.1	42.2	[e]40.5
College																								
1 to 3 years	26.7	28.8	30.9	33.0	34.3	36.3	[f]46.7	[f]50.4	74.4	75.7	73.5	[f]75.4	70.0	70.0	68.7	[f]68.4	67.2	67.5	64.5	[f]68.7	53.3	49.9	50.0	[f]49.1
4 years or more	24.0	26.9	28.6	31.3	33.6	35.6	[g]37.4	[g]39.4	84.3	83.8	83.1	[g]84.8	79.4	77.8	77.3	[g]76.3	79.9	79.1	77.6	[g]81.0	66.5	62.5	62.5	[g]63.1
Employed	95.0	97.2	104.2	108.5	113.8	115.5	116.3	122.6	68.7	69.4	67.1	69.9	65.5	64.4	62.6	62.9	61.8	61.6	58.4	63.8	50.0	45.7	45.1	45.2
Unemployed	6.9	10.8	7.4	6.6	5.8	6.7	8.3	6.5	50.3	54.3	50.4	53.7	49.8	50.6	44.6	46.4	41.2	44.0	38.6	46.2	34.1	31.2	27.9	28.3
Not in labor force	55.2	57.5	58.4	58.8	58.5	59.9	61.1	61.2	65.8	68.1	67.2	66.8	64.3	65.4	63.4	61.9	57.0	58.9	57.3	58.7	48.7	48.2	46.7	45.3

From U.S. Bureau of the Census: *Statistical abstract of the United States: 1995*, ed 115, Washington, DC, 1995.
[a]Includes other races not shown separately. [b]Hispanic persons may be of any race. [c]Composition of regions. [d]Represents those who completed 9th to 12th grade, but have no high school diploma. [e]High school graduate. [f]Some college or associate degree. [g]Bachelor's or advanced degree.

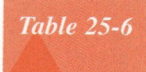

Table 25-6   Political Party Identification of the Adult Population, by Degree of Attachment, 1972 to 1994, and by Selected Characteristics, 1994

[In percent. Covers citizens of voting-age living in private housing units in the contiguous United States. Data are from the National Election Studies and are based on a sample and subject to sampling variability; for details, see source]

Year and selected characteristic	Total	Strong democratic	Weak democrat	Independent democrat	Independent	Independent Republican	Weak Republican	Strong Republican	Apolitical
1972	100	15	26	11	13	11	13	10	1
1980	100	18	23	11	13	10	14	9	2
1984	100	17	20	11	11	12	15	12	2
1986	100	18	22	10	12	11	15	11	2
1988	100	18	18	12	11	13	14	14	2
1990	100	20	19	12	11	12	15	10	2
1992	100	18	18	14	12	12	14	11	1
1994, total*	**100**	**15**	**19**	**13**	**10**	**12**	**15**	**16**	**1**
Age:									
17 to 24 years old	100	9	20	22	10	8	19	10	1
25 to 34 years old	100	11	19	14	12	11	16	16	1
35 to 44 years old	100	13	18	14	12	11	14	18	—
45 to 54 years old	100	15	16	15	7	16	12	17	1
55 to 64 years old	100	18	22	8	8	16	12	15	—
65 to 74 years old	100	28	17	6	8	13	14	15	—
75 to 99 years old	100	19	26	9	9	5	17	13	2
Sex:									
Male	100	13	17	12	11	14	14	18	1
Female	100	18	21	13	10	9	15	13	1
Race:									
White	100	12	19	12	10	13	16	17	1
Black	100	38	23	20	8	4	2	3	1
Education:									
Grade school	100	26	26	7	13	7	11	6	4
High school	100	15	22	14	13	10	13	11	1
College	100	14	16	13	7	13	16	21	—

From U.S. Bureau of the Census: *Statistical abstract of the United States: 1995,* ed 115, Washington, DC, 1995.
—Represents zero. *Includes other characteristics, not shown separately.
Source Center for Political Studies, University of Michigan, Ann Arbor, MI, unpublished data. Data prior to 1988 published in Miller WE, Traugott SA: *American National Election Studies Data Sourcebook, 1952-1986,* Cambridge, MA, Harvard University Press, 1989 (copyright).

CREATIVITY

Creativity transcends time and limitations through selfless absorption in universal meanings. The creative self is the God in man, the spiritual self (Csikszentmihalyi, 1990; Watson, 1988) (Table 25-7). Creativity is a bridge between the growing self and transcending the self. It may be the transit mechanism between self-actualization (the reaching of one's highest potential) and the step beyond, to transcend the limitations of ego (Table 25-8). Creativity is risking a leap across the chasm of the known to reach the unknown.

Kastenbaum (1991) believes the end of life often stimulates creativity, "It's then, when people are right about to jump into the void, that they can sometimes be more creative, the most able to transform their situation. At times like

this, people can be more intense, actually more alive" (p. 4). Folklore has it that the swan sings but once in its life, as death approaches. Creativity may triumph over the debilitation of an aging body as it has in many individuals (Box 25-5). Mercer, Nichols and Doyle (1989) found that among some of the women they studied a response to loss and loneliness was an increase in creativity. Simonton (1990) has studied the aged and their creative genius and concludes that creative productions are not tied to chronology but to successive acts of self-actualization.

Products of creativity are less important than creative attitudes. Curiosity, inquisitiveness, wonderment, puzzlement, and craving for understanding are creative attitudes. Much of the natural creative imagination of childhood is subdued

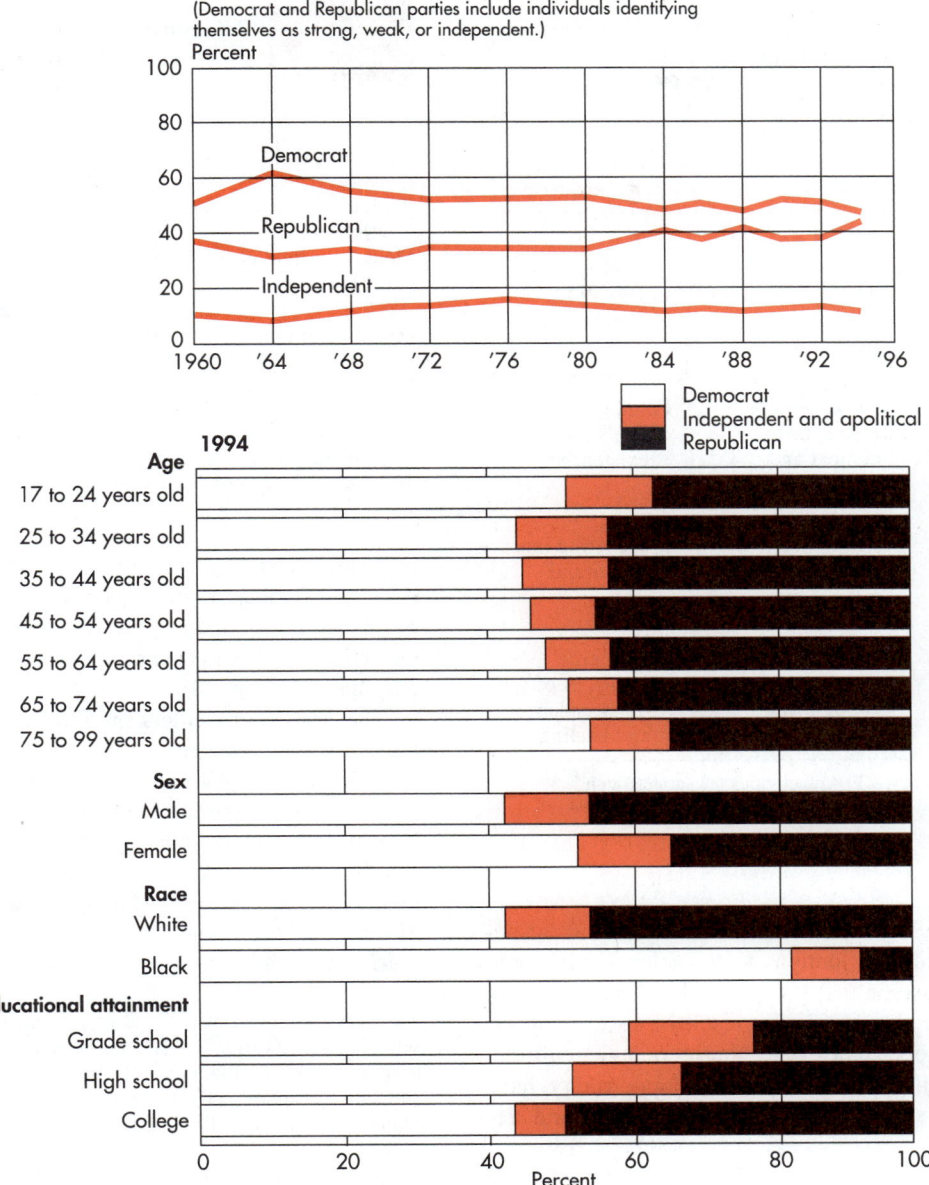

Figure 25-4. Political party identification of the adult population: 1960 to 1994. (Democrat and Republican parties include individuals identifying themselves as strong, weak, or independent.) (Redrawn from chart prepared by U.S. Bureau of the Census: *Statistical abstract of the United States: 1995,* ed 115, Washington, DC, 1995.)

by enculturation. In old age some persons seem able to break free of excessive enculturation and again express their free spirit when practical matters no longer demand their sole attention.

Creative Contributions and Age

The peak years of creativity have been a subject of inquiry among many developmental psychologists. Lehman (1953) found a peak at 35 years of age, measured by creative contributions in historical biographies of notable people.

Lehman's classic work (1953) considered a wide range of individuals and achievements and correlated them with frequency and age.

An important factor that may have been overlooked by those who refer to Lehman's work is that the world of middle-aged and older adults is much different now than it was 40 years ago. Factors of health, opportunity, and ageism have shifted markedly. A fine corollary would be to examine the contributions of men versus women in the same method as was done by Lehman. We would see that women

| Table 25-7 | Interrelationships of Central Concepts of Flow, Creativity, and Watson's Theory of Human Care |

Commonalities of flow experiences	Components of creativity/play	Goals of Watson's theory of human care
Growth, meaning		
Contributes to growth of the self	Leads to learning and evolution; expands one's field of action	Mental-spiritual growth for self-others
Reintegration; empowerment		
Promotes ordering of experience	Creative process relates us to context and environment	Finding meaning in one's own existence
Self-esteem		
Returns control to the individual	Freedom to explore without rules or restrictions	Discovering inner power and control
Transcendence		
Selfless state of absorption yields altered sense of time	Delight and enjoyment in the present moment/suspension of time	Potentiating instances of self-transcendence and healing

From Sterritt PF, Pokorney ME: Art activities for patients with Alzheimer's and related disorders, *Geriatr Nurs* 15(3):155, 1994.

| Table 25-8 | Relationship of Patient Intervention Responses to Goals of Watson's Theory |

Goals of Watson's theory of human care	Patient responses to art activity common themes
Finding meaning in one's own existence	Increased life review and reminiscence
Mental/spiritual gorwth for self/others	Increased interaction, expression of feelings and exercise of abilities
Discovering inner power and control	Overcoming limited abilities and exercising choices
Potentiating self-transcendence and healing	Increased absorption and concern about others

From Sterritt PF, Pokorney ME: Art activities for patients with Alzheimer's and related disorders, *Geriatr Nurs* 15(3):155, 1994.

historically, at any age, were almost totally devoid of accomplishments and contributions to the sciences. It would be a mistake to assume that this was related to age or sex when we are well aware it was a result of sexual oppression and lack of opportunity. Age, socioeconomic, cultural, and sexual discrimination and lack of opportunity have been, and still are, significant deterrents to scientific and creative work.

Older researchers have two important assets: a developed retinue of disciples and the ability to integrate and synthesize ideas into broad perspectives rather than remaining absorbed in minutiae. A few examples of such major creative contributions might include those of Einstein, Freud, Adolph Meyer, and Darwin. These men completed their more profound works in their 60s and 70s and clearly showed the maturation of their creative abilities.

The creative act emerges from the consolidation of energies of thought, feelings, and imagination. The stages of creativity are preparation, frustration, incubation, illumination, and elaboration. Elders excel in illumination and elaboration.

The Creation of Self through Journaling

The central activity of human beings is creating meaning. Through the personal journal one can, in thoughtful reflec-

tion, discover meaning and patterns in daily events. The self becomes a coherent story with successive revisions as old events are reread and perceived in new contexts. "The self is not fixed, but rather is continuously reconstructed over time" (Berman, 1991, p. 38).

The journals of elders provide rich descriptions of the interior lives of the authors. May Sarton (1984) and Florida Scott-Maxwell (1968) are two of the most well-known. The study of these journals and of the journals of less well-known and less articulate elders assists nurses in understanding the inner experience of the aged and, perhaps, their own. For example, Sister Marilyn Schwab of the Benedictine Sisters, a pioneer in gerontic nursing, and not yet old, kept a journal of her dying process. An excerpt states:

"What is healing anyway?" . . . [her doctor] . . . "knows how to go with the mystery of it" . . . he told his nurse of her decision to forgo bone marrow transplant . . . "Bob told her about where I am and she said not many people live their lives or make their decisions really in touch with all the dimensions of life" (Schwab, 1986).

To read her journal is a profound experience in learning the interior landscape of death with meaning. The common themes Berman (1991) identified in journals of the old and dying (individuation, cathectic flexibility, and attitudes toward death) are apparent in Sister Marilyn's writing.

Creating a Life History. Becoming whole requires one to integrate all of life's remembered experience into the self-concept in a way that sustains or enhances self-esteem. Numerous gerontic nurses have used reminiscence, individually and in groups, as a therapeutic strategy to achieve these goals. Because it is such a natural function of many elders it is one of the simplest and most enriching for elder and nurse. Rigorously controlled studies of its effects, however, are seriously lacking, and the few that exist are often contradictory.

Life-review, the recall of "not me" life events, is painful and is the real psychotherapeutic work of reminiscing.

<table>
<tr><td>

Box 25-5   **The Old and Their Contributions**

Cervantes completed Part II of *Don Quixote* at age 68.
Chevreul began the study of gerontology at age 90 and published his last scientific paper at age 120.
George Bernard Shaw was 94 when one of his last plays was first produced.
Benjamin Franklin was a framer of the Constitution of the United States when he was 81.
Humboldt finished his last volume of *Cosmos* at age 89.
Alice Roosevelt Longworth could kick higher than her head at age 90.
Golda Meir was 71 when she became Prime Minister of Israel.
Heinrich Schutz composed *Schwanengesang* at age 84.
Richard Strauss at 83 composed *Metamorphosen*.
Titian painted *Christ Crowned with Thorns* when almost 90 years old.
Verdi composed *Falstaff* at age 80.

</td></tr>
</table>

Haight (1992) studied the long-term effects (1 year after intervention) of a structured life-review process with homebound elders. She found no significant change but a trend toward lesser depression and higher levels of life satisfaction. Carefully controlled studies similar to Haight's to determine the actual benefits of reminiscing with elders and in what circumstances it is most effective are needed.

Possibilities grow out of life history. One's life history is a product of multiple histories: (1) the timing, duration, spacing, and order of events; (2) multiple, independent, and interdependent roles; and (3) the intermingling with paths of intimates, friends, and acquaintances (Elder, 1974). To work with the aged in the most mutually satisfying manner, knowledge of life history is essential. Moloney (1995) found that older women, when developing their life stories seemed to focus on themes of surviving, finding strength, gathering memories, and seeing the patterns. In addition to information about life history, Back and Bourque (1970) have found it useful to have clients graphically represent life in terms of highs, lows, and plateaus experienced at various ages. Development of a lifeline in which each decade is marked and important events placed at appropriate times and places is also useful; note the feelings and impact of these events.

If this method is used, the nurse may match life history against the graphic representation to gain a clearer understanding of events, patterns, and the impact of experiences. Development is facilitated by examining the peaks and valleys in one's life. When both inner and outer structures are changed, reorganization becomes possible. The period of disequilibrium is necessary for growth. (See Chapter 20 for additional discussion.) People are not born self-actualized. They learn through the changes in their lives to become more fully human. Periods of stability, crisis, and joy are

necessary. Some theorists believe the spacing of these elements is critical to the possibility for continued growth.

The use of life history and reminiscence for older learners in classroom settings is useful in many ways. The reminiscing of elders attending classes in adult education or community college programs may reveal connections between early life and present interest in education. For many it is a return to an interrupted education or a youthful intention that had waited 50 or more years for fulfillment. Often they recall a latent interest, a parent's hope, or a teacher's appraisal. Almost all older students can connect their current educational experience with the past. Taped interviews that focus on childhood and early experiences in school can be intriguing; encourage details and elaboration. A group in Mill Valley, California, enrolled in a course, "Tales Told From Memory," for persons over 60, sponsored by the College of Marin's Emeritus College Program (Steinberg, 1993). There are many similar programs throughout the country.

Reminiscence of places where one has lived, drawing these, reexperiencing the effect of events attached to place; all are significant to stability of self. The social and physical settings of remembered episodes are potent. Chaudhury (1996) expresses place as the "container of lived experience." Developing a residential life history may have unexpected benefits in revealing surroundings significant to individuality and attachment. During these activities the awareness of self as continually growing and learning can be affirmed.

Creative Arts for the Elderly

Many projects across the country have brought art to elders in senior centers, nursing homes, and retirement complexes. Often these are organized through community colleges and have the distinct advantage of intergenerational participation. Students may, as class projects, teach or assist the elder; they may learn together. At the Hebrew Home for the Aged in Riverdale, New York, the works of resident artists are often featured (Zimmer, 1995). The opportunities are as broad as the imagination of the elders but often begin with very small ventures.

Maximizing the use of self in the later years in unique ways might be termed creative self-actualization. Many persons will need the stimulus of an interested person to uncover latent interests and talents. Others will need encouragement to try new avenues of self expression—some will be fitting for them and others not. Several ideas are presented here for nurses working with the aged who may need an introduction to creative use of leisure time.

Elders' participation in various art activities is variable, though needlework, modern dancing, and playing classical music tend to remain rather stable activities throughout adult life for those who were inclined (Table 25-9). Attendance at art activities, including musical performances, art museums, and historic parks, remain important, though

Table 25-9   Participation in Various Arts Activities: 1992

[In percent, except as indicated. Covers activities engaged in at least once in the prior 12 months.]

Item	Adult population (mil.)	In the past 12 months percent engaged at least once in—							
		Playing classical music	Modern dancing*	Pottery work†	Needle work‡	Photography§	Painting‖	Creative writing	Buying art work
Total	**185.8**	**4**	**8**	**8**	**25**	**12**	**10**	**7**	**22**
Sex: Male	89.0	3	8	8	5	13	9	7	22
Female	96.8	5	8	9	43	10	10	8	22
Race: White	158.8	4	8	9	26	12	10	7	24
Black	21.1	3	8	8	15	11	5	6	12
Other	5.9	5	9	5	24	9	10	11	8
Age: 18 to 24 years old	24.1	6	11	9	18	11	19	14	13
25 to 34 years old	42.4	3	10	10	24	15	10	7	19
35 to 44 years old	39.8	4	7	10	25	13	10	8	27
45 to 54 years old	27.7	5	6	9	26	13	8	7	29
55 to 64 years old	21.2	5	6	6	27	10	6	5	26
65 to 74 years old	18.3	4	9	6	29	7	6	5	20
75 to 96 years old	12.3	3	5	3	26	2	4	2	17
Education: Grade school	14.3	1	4	2	22	3	1	(Z)	4
Some high school	18.6	1	4	7	25	5	5	3	11
High school graduate	69.4	2	8	8	25	9	9	4	15
Some college	39.2	6	10	12	26	15	13	11	27
College graduate	26.2	8	8	9	26	16	12	12	32
Graduate school	18.1	9	10	8	21	22	13	16	49
Income: Under $5,000	8.6	2	7	7	22	6	8	7	10
$5,000 to $9,999	15.2	2	7	4	27	7	8	7	10
$10,000 to $14,999	19.2	3	7	8	26	8	8	6	14
$15,000 to $24,999	32.9	4	9	8	26	9	10	7	17
$25,000 to $49,999	62.2	5	8	10	25	13	10	7	22
$50,000 and over	32.1	6	8	8	23	17	11	9	40
Not reported	15.6	4	8	8	24	12	11	9	24

From U.S. Bureau of the Census: *Statistical abstract of the United States: 1995,* ed 115, Washington, DC, 1995.
Z, less than .05 percent. *Dancing other than ballet (e.g. folk and tap). †Includes ceramics, jewelry, leatherwork, and metalwork. ‡Includes weaving, crocheting, quilting, and sewing. §Includes making movies or videos as an artistic activity. ‖Includes drawing, sculpture, and printmaking.
Source U.S. National Endowment for the Arts, *Arts Participation in America: 1982 to 1992.*

reading surpasses all other activities (Table 25-10). Factors that impinge on these statistics are income, education, health, and age above 75 years. One must realize that all statistics reflecting age differentials are flawed when health and comparable age intervals are not calculated in the equation. Thus the interests of the aged are extremely varied and cannot accurately be categorized. Program planning to involve older adults in the arts involves the steps listed in Box 25-6.

Many aspects of the developmental needs of the aged are met by artistic expressions. Among them are (1) conflict resolution, (2) clarification of thoughts and feelings, (3) creation of balance and an inner order, (4) a sense of being in control of the external world, (5) the creation of something positive from defeating experiences or in the face of paralyzing depression, (6) artistic communication as an integral part of human experience, and (7) the sustenance of human integrity. Sterritt and Pokorney (1994) found art activities with patients suffering Alzheimer's disease enhanced communication, decreased isolation, and provided an opportunity for personal control and expression of feelings.

The choice of art presentations in settings where residents have various degrees of dementia is being addressed by vendors who provide art works for nursing homes. One of these, Interactive Therapeutic Art, designed by ArtLine Limited (1997), combines aesthetics with therapeutics. (See photos, *My Garden* and *Clothesline.* These shadow boxes are designed to stir early memories that may be preserved).

Stimulating Creative Activity. The importance of creative expressions for the elderly was emphasized when in 1977 the National Endowment for the Arts established an

Table 25-10   Attendance Rates for Various Arts Activities: 1992

[In percent. For persons 18 years old and over. Excludes elementary and high school performances. Based on 1992 household survey Public Participation in the Arts conducted January through December 1992. Data are subject to sampling error; see source.]

Item	Jazz perfor-mance	Classical music perfor-mance	Opera	Musical play	Non-musical play	Ballet	Art museum	Historic park	Reading litera-ture*
Total	11	13	3	17	14	5	27	35	54
Sex: Male	12	12	3	15	12	4	27	35	47
Female	9	13	4	20	15	6	27	34	60
Race: White	10	13	3	18	14	5	28	37	56
Black	16	7	2	14	12	3	19	18	45
Other	6	12	5	11	10	6	29	23	42
Age: 18 to 24 years old	11	10	3	16	13	5	29	33	53
25 to 34 years old	14	10	3	16	12	5	29	36	54
35 to 44 years old	13	12	3	19	14	5	30	40	59
45 to 54 years old	11	17	4	22	17	5	29	41	57
55 to 64 years old	8	15	4	19	15	5	25	33	53
65 to 74 years old	7	14	4	17	13	4	20	29	50
75 to 96 years old	2	8	2	9	7	2	10	12	40
Education: Grade school	1	2	1	3	2	1	4	8	17
Some high school	2	3	1	5	4	1	7	15	32
High school graduate	6	7	1	12	8	2	16	26	49
Some college	14	14	3	21	16	6	35	43	65
College graduate	20	23	6	30	23	9	46	52	71
Graduate school	25	36	12	37	35	12	59	64	79
Income: Under $5,000	6	5	2	8	8	2	12	17	37
$5,000 to $9,999	5	6	1	7	6	3	14	16	40
$10,000 to $14,999	5	6	2	8	7	2	13	20	43
$15,000 to $24,999	9	11	2	14	11	3	23	31	50
$25,000 to $49,999	11	13	3	18	14	5	29	40	58
$50,000 and over	18	23	8	33	24	10	44	51	71
Not reported	11	13	4	18	15	5	28	33	50

From U.S. Bureau of the Census: *Statistical abstract of the United States: 1995,* ed 115, Washington, DC, 1995.
*Includes novels, short stories, poetry, or plays.
Source U.S. National Endowment for the Arts, *Arts Participation in America: 1982 to 1992.*

office to review the grant applications of projects involving the elderly, the institutionalized, or the handicapped. At present the Older Americans Act specifies that all the arts are classified under Recreational Services and administered through the Department of Health and Human Services. President Clinton in his State of the Union address, February 4, 1997, reiterated his commitment to support for the arts and humanities.

Each person has a private, symbolic, feeling world that can be brought out by certain expressive activities. Art workshops were introduced into some nursing homes in Vermont, and residents produced art that has been exhibited nationally and internationally (Mooney, 1992).

The creative process is any activity in which the unconscious can be expressed in an integrated unique manner. To do this, an atmosphere of trust is essential. Trust is attained through rules, structure, and acceptance of all efforts without approval or disapproval. When this atmosphere is provided, creative expressions begin to occur. At that time the facilitator needs to relax rules and structure and cultivate individualistic expressions. Useful concepts and guidelines for those wishing to involve the elderly in creative artistic expressions are noted below.

Art
Using oil pastels, create a drawing that represents self; or select three colors you like and three colors you dislike, using all six colors to create a self-portrait.
Draw a representation of your world.
Create a collage or mobile out of an assortment of materials and pictures that can represent subjects such as the self, part of self you like or dislike, the family, etc.

In small groups using clay, create an "art piece" or a statement.

Music

Play a variety of music, center discussion around imagery and any feelings that music evoked.

Discuss, or have clients bring in, music that elicits feelings of sadness, happiness, etc.

Show a picture (can be cut from a magazine) and ask members to see if they can imagine the sounds that might go with the picture.

Express self or group through dance and movement to selected music.

Imagery

Use guided fantasies and imagery to facilitate stress reduction and relaxation, awareness, the power of one's own healing capability, and self-expression through symbols and symbolisms.

Movement

Create a movement to fit how you are feeling while introducing self to group.

Have members stand and initiate a slow swaying motion (good exercise to end the group with).

Have members mirror each others' movements, such as hands, or the entire body, creating a duet.

Writing

Encourage journals, diaries, set a group time available to write and share ideas.

In small groups, create a "group poem."

Read selected poems or stories in group, then share reactions and feelings from what is read.

Create a "book" to be distributed to group consisting of a collection of members' writings.

Activities may need to be modified for some elders. Consider the following when an activity is not enjoyable or successful:

Shift the expected outcome to meet individual and/or group needs.

Modify equipment and supplies to make the activity easier.

Provide intermittent rest and relaxation periods frequently.

Deep breathing can be useful physiologically and psychologically.

Partner or small group activities are usually less stressful than individual expectations.

Leitner and Leitner (1996) provide an extensive list of resources that may be helpful in generating activities, and obtaining donated items and volunteer assistance to provide stimulation and opportunities for elders in institutional or community settings (Box 25-7).

Creative Arts and Theater. Recent monographs on the arts and older Americans report Arts Endowment grants to ensure the continued contributions of elders as artists, teachers, mentors, students, volunteers, patrons, and consumers of the arts (Sherman, 1996). Some of the programming grants have supported drama groups, storytelling, dance, painting, weaving, writing, and singing. These are designed for aged people of all levels of ability; some are teachers and mentors, some are entertainers, some are participants,

---

> **Box 25-6** **How to Begin Involving Older Adults in the Arts**
>
> Develop program ideas using a range of older adults as advisors.
>
> Plan specific ways that older adults can participate.
>
> Survey Office of Aging, senior centers, nursing homes, adult day care centers, and community-dwelling elders regarding their needs, sources of talent, and possible contributions.
>
> Contact local resource people who may be of assistance.
>
> Consider access issues such as cost, transportation, and time of day.
>
> Seek local and national funding.
>
> Publicize.
>
> Orient elders who are interested in participating.
>
> Provide incentives for participating: awards, receptions, refreshments, etc.

purely for the joy of living. Hillary Rodham Clinton says, "Some of our most powerful works of art have been produced by older Americans by hands that have engaged in years of hard work, eyes that have witnessed decades of change, and hearts that have felt a lifetime of emotions. Our whole society benefits when older Americans use their talents and experiences to become involved in the arts as creators, teachers, mentors, volunteers and audiences." (Sherman, p. 1)

Theater. McDonough (1996) reports the rapid emergence of numerous senior adult theater groups that have been flourishing because of national conferences, increased awareness of and interaction among the various groups. A particular boost occurred as these older adults met in a mini-conference of the arts held during the White House Conference on Aging in 1995. Oral histories have formed the substance of many performances as have some classics and numerous life issues of elders portrayed in humorous fashion. Steinberg (1996) reports that theater has in many cases formed a bridge between the generations as young and old work together portraying historic and other significant events and relationships. Temporarily shedding the constraints of one's life role and donning the garb of hopes, dreams, and imagination has a healing and growing effect for many elders. Earlier reports by Thurman and Piggins (1982) and Clark and Osgood (1985) identified many psychologic benefits of drama for elders. For further information, see resources at the end of the chapter.

Creative Expression through Music, Poetry, and Dance. Rhythms infiltrate life on every level from individual cellular functions to the constantly expanding/contracting universe. Unseen and unfelt oscillating waves surround us. Felt waves, pulsating, vibrating, undulating, stimulate us. They are intrinsic to existence and may somewhat explain

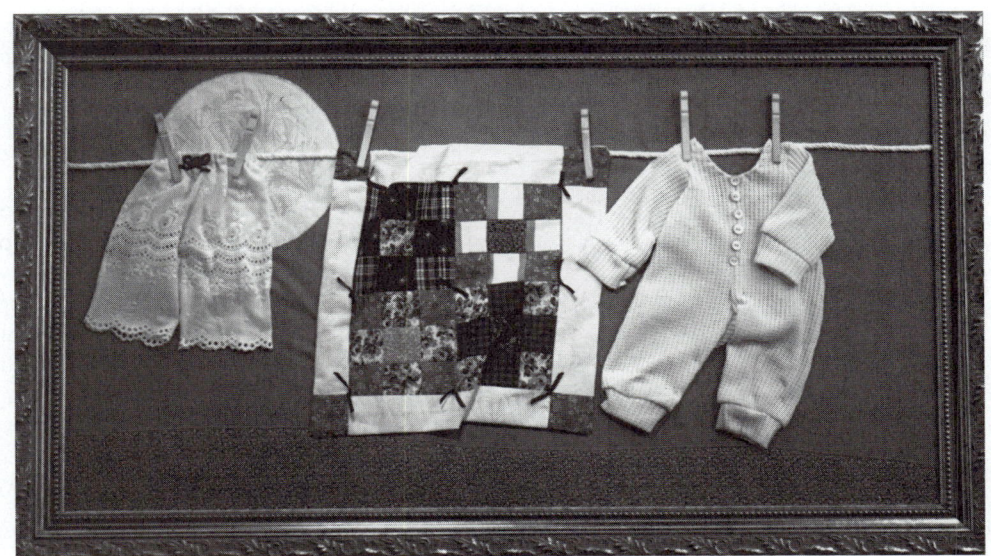

This tactile art has garments hanging from a clothesline. The clothespins can be manipulated and removed; each garment can be taken down from the piece and reapplied. Items such as the quilt add visual interest, texture, and tactile stimulation for patients. (Courtesy ArtLine, Ltd.)

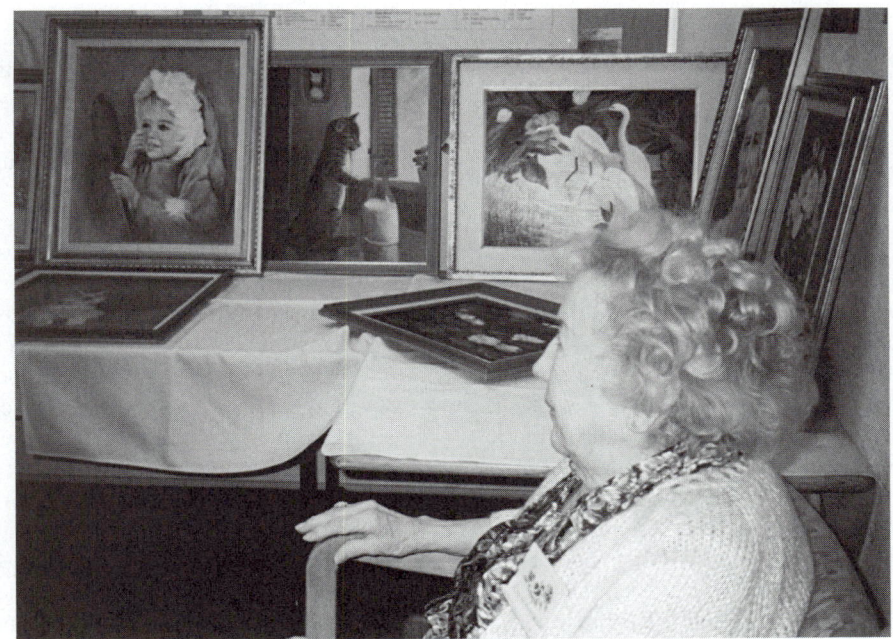

Displaying creative works. (Courtesy Priscilla Ebersole.)

the healing power of music, poetry, and repetitive movement. Life itself is an ongoing dance. One is reminded that the Polynesians express themselves beautifully with hand as well as body movements. In many countries today song, dance, and poetic history flow as naturally as breath and are inextricably interwoven in daily existence. It seems sad that for many of us these must be scheduled events.

Dance can be a commercial enterprise featuring the talents of elders. A report by Markowitz (1996) in *Modern*

Maturity features a troupe of "show girl" dancers, all over 60 years of age, in the Fabulous Palm Spring Follies. One of the dancers says, "I've been dancing since I was 14. I ride my bike to the theater each day and do my own exercises." Another says, "We're showing people that it's absolutely not over at 60. This show is proof of that." "People tell us we don't look our age, but I think we do. It's the rest of the world that looks awful at its age." (pp. 52, 53).

Music. Music is a familiar and universal experience. Even the tone-deaf person expresses himself or herself in rhythmic patterns. Tonal or rhythmic music can be an inward experience or an outward expression. As such, music is adaptable to each individual. Deanna Edwards was one of the first nurses to use music to assist the ill and the dying to cope with and transcend their physical limitations (1977). Many have used it in myriad ways since that time.

In Milwaukee a group of very old, retired nuns choreograph hoop movements to music because their bodies are too frail for major movement. Oliver Sacks, author of *Awakenings,* found music smooths motor functions in patients with movement disorders such as Parkinson's disease (Crowley, 1992). Vecchione (1994) states that elders with dementia respond well to music and movement. Sambandham and Schirm (1995) found that some elders with Alzheimer's disease responded to music with increased communication and memory improvement. There are many such ways to use music. Music can be a comforting, structured expression, a therapeutic tool, or it can provide the opportunity for creative and imaginative self-expression.

Music has kept many an elder going. Pablo Casals, the great cellist, played each morning in his 90s to limber the fingers bound by rheumatoid arthritis. Albert Schweitzer played Bach or a concerto before dinner each night, although he told his staff both he and the piano were frail and old. Music is a remarkable rejuvenator for those who have learned to appreciate its mystical power.

Music therapy is an individual music program prescribed by a professional music therapist to bring about desirable changes in behavior. The self-determined use of music as a means of enjoyment and personal expression can be achieved by listening, meditating, improvising, relaxing, moving to music, creative dancing, composing, learning new songs, studying music history, rhythmic patterning, mastering an instrument, building an instrument, or in any other manner an individual chooses to adapt music toward self-fulfillment.

Music has always been revered. Kings, clerics, and philanthropists have endowed musicians. Youth sometimes idolizes them. Musical tastes and talents vary historically and personally.

Nurses using music as a springboard for client self-development must first find out the interests and talents of the client. One old man improvised lyrics to old tunes, expressing himself poetically. An old lady pleaded for some Baroque chamber music to ease her pain. A very regressed old man came alive when handed a banjo. Another aged man restored valuable violins and played them lovingly before returning them to their owners. An aged blind man taught pipe organ to university students and played the organ for chapel services. All of these were means of using music toward self-fulfillment.

Moore (1977) developed guidelines for using music with groups of seniors. They remain the most specific and useful we have found:

1. Respect a music activity by providing an environment free of extraneous noise.
2. Use music in small therapy groups in addition to large, recreational ones. Goals can be individualized and interaction maximized in small groups. Small groups also enable the therapist to combine music with the techniques of reality orientation, sensory training, and reminiscence.
3. Use themes for music sessions. Establish the theme with a special song or rondo (used as a secondary opening and closing), with visual aids or props, with sensorily stimulating articles that can be passed among the group, and with interactional activities.
4. Include group members in planning themes, songs, and activities. Members may also be trained as coleaders.
5. Use team leaders. One person can be responsible for the music, while the other can handle the activities. Team leaders can also share observations and ideas.
6. Capitalize on the security and memories afforded by familiar music, but challenge the group occasionally with recent and/or classical material.

ment income or for professional reasons. Ideally, patterns of leisure should begin long before retirement in order to provide a smoother transition (Thompson and Cruse, 1993).

There are several conceptual models of leisure:

- Humanistic: a celebration of life, an end in itself
- Therapeutic: an instrument of control and healing
- Quantitative: uncommitted time after work is done
- Institutional: segments of time committed to various interests: religious, marital, educational, or political
- Epistemologic: activities that provide meanings and aesthetic appreciation
- Assumptive: activities based on affirmation, legend, and folklore
- Analytic: to understand, question, and experiment; is present oriented
- Aesthetic: transformative, future oriented, involves creative action, and reordering ideas, objects, social institutions and organizations

Statistics tell us that elders' attendance at leisure events gradually drops off from age 35 on, though home improvement activities and gardening increase rather markedly after age 35 (Table 25-11). To cultivate the tendency of many elders to enjoy gardening, Bassen and Baltazar (1997) insti-

tuted an extensive horticulture program at the Hebrew Home for the Aged in New York. They incorporated the ideas reported earlier by Olszowy (1978) and other horticulture publications (see Resources at the end of the chapter), as well as developing their own. Some of the activities are noted in Box 25-8. They found many resources and volunteers within the surrounding community eager to assist them in their efforts. They developed activities appropriate for all levels of cognitive and physical abilities. They found increased psychologic well-being, gross and fine motor agility, and social interaction among the participants. The Canadian Horticulture Therapy Association has developed numerous programs for institutions and the homebound elderly.

Bernstein (1995) dealt with loss by going into the heart of her garden for healing.

Here it is a knee high weed. I grab clumps of stems with my two fists and yank them out, taproots and all. I can feel my muscles tense in my arms and shoulders and back. I balance myself by spreading my feet wider apart as I bend down to the ground. Centered, I realize I can meet my anger and use it constructively, tearing through section after section of the garden, ousting the intruder. It feels good to release the tension I have stored in my body for so long (p. 27).

Table 25-11   Participation in Various Leisure Activities: 1992

[In percent, except as indicated. Covers activities engaged in at least once in the prior 12 months.]

Item	Adult population (mil.)	Attendance at—			Participation in—				
		Movies	Sports events	Amusement park	Exercise program	Playing sports	Outdoor activities*	Home improvement/ repair	Gardening
Total	**185.8**	**59**	**37**	**50**	**60**	**39**	**34**	**48**	**55**
Sex: Male	89.0	60	44	51	61	50	39	53	46
Female	96.8	59	30	50	59	29	29	42	62
Race: White	158.8	60	38	51	61	40	37	50	57
Black	21.1	54	32	45	51	32	10	32	39
Other	5.9	62	20	46	51	38	28	31	42
Age: 18 to 24 years old	24.1	82	51	68	67	59	43	33	31
25 to 34 years old	42.4	70	47	68	67	52	41	47	51
35 to 44 years old	39.8	68	43	58	62	44	42	58	57
45 to 54 years old	27.7	58	35	44	62	34	36	57	64
55 to 64 years old	21.2	40	23	30	56	21	21	53	63
65 to 74 years old	18.3	34	20	29	50	18	21	42	63
75 to 96 years old	12.3	19	7	14	34	7	5	20	55
Education: Grade school	14.3	16	9	24	24	10	11	24	44
Some high school	18.6	35	19	35	39	18	21	34	50
High school graduate	69.4	54	33	51	55	34	31	47	53
Some college	39.2	21	45	59	71	49	42	53	55
College graduate	26.2	77	51	58	75	55	42	52	61
Graduate school	18.1	81	51	54	79	57	51	65	65

From U.S. Bureau of the Census: *Statistical abstract of the United States: 1995,* ed 115, Washington, DC, 1995.
*Camping, hiking, and canoeing.
Source U.S. National Endowment for the Arts: *Arts Participation in America: 1982 to 1992.*

At 65 and older, exercise walking and swimming are the most common sports activities (Table 25-12). It is unclear the effects of income on sports participation, though some type of regular fairly strenuous activity is important (Goleman, 1994). McAuley and Rudolph (1995) report that less than 40% of elders engage in any leisure time physical activity. This must be a concern of nurses when we consider the benefits of leisure and exercise. Creative nursing care calls for identifying or designing activities that do not become chores but rather are renewing. For example, Tai Chi has become popular with elders because it interjects humor, relaxation and control into movement.

Individuals who have led extremely active professional lives and have strongly identified with work roles may feel somewhat like a ship without a rudder when they find themselves with large amounts of leisure time. (See further discussion of retirement in Chapter 20.) It is even more difficult for those who lose a mate just before retirement and find they must begin to develop satisfying leisure time activities without the secure and safe companionship of the spouse. Carpenter (1987) experienced these situations and has provided suggestions for persons in similar circumstances. Retirees who have limited amounts of money to spend on leisure may find Carpenter's suggestions useful (Box 25-9).

Various types of leisure are engaged in based on need fulfillment (Figure 25-6). Other factors influencing leisure patterns are social networks, age, time, work role, health, income, location, and family situation. Some senior day-care programs provide opportunities for physically and mentally impaired persons to regain satisfaction at all levels of need. A full range of services and activities are shown in Figure 25-7.

Modifications in leisure activities may need to be made for elders with visual deficits (Kelly, 1995). Simple changes such as brighter lighting, magnifying devices, needle threaders, and large print materials can increase the enjoyment and participation of those with visual deficits.

The importance of contact with the natural landscape is seldom mentioned as a need of the aged. The revitalization that occurs for many persons at the seashore or in the mountains may become more important in the later years. An aged man in San Francisco took a daily trip to the beach. As a sailor from the rugged coast of Norway, contact with the sea remained essential to him. Old people often feel a special intimacy toward plant and animal life. Laura walked in the woods each day, and each new sprout or flower she noticed was viewed as a personal reward from a bountiful nature. She felt very much a part of it all.

Wilderness areas are not accessible to all older persons, but some opportunities for contact with nature should be made for those so inclined. Spiritual stimulation and stress relief may be important aspects of contact with the natural landscape. Carson (1970) believed this will become increasingly important to each cohort of aged. One elderly lady took an intensive course in order to become a docent at the

Box 25-8	Activity Ideas for a Horticulture Program

Drying plants and flowers
Pressing flower and plant arrangements
Flower arranging
Making terrariums
Window box gardening
Tub gardening
Boxed herb gardens
Hanging baskets
Forcing bulbs
Vegetable garden plots
Flower garden plots
Hydroponics
Annual plant and flower sales
Developing hybrids
Presenting flower arrangements to elders confined to bed

marine reserve. She now guides small groups of elders through the tidepools where they learn the myriad varieties of tiny sea life, often overlooked.

Senior adult camping has been organized and sponsored by several groups (Winfrey, 1977; Armstrong, 1979; Chenery, 1987). Benefits reported included sensory stimulation for those with some impairments, refreshing of memories of earlier times, renewal of confidence in physical abilities, and spiritual elevation. The esthetics of dew on grass, the smell of water and willows, the clear views of the heavens at night all bring one closer to union with the earth and our origins. Many use these opportunities for photography. Elders particularly respond to bird walks, horticulture walks, and other opportunities to learn more about the environment around them. The American Camping Association offers several camping experiences especially designed for seniors (see Resources at the end of the Chapter).

Leisure and recreational opportunities for the elderly. The 300 senior centers federally funded through the Administration on Aging (AOA) Title XIX in 1965 now exceed 15,000 (NCOA, 1993). Area Agencies on Aging are designated in each state to provide senior centers and information about local recreational programs for the aging. These have been a great boon for the aged. The arts, trips, activities, and assistance of numerous varieties are available. Some of the more innovative programs include teleconferencing programs for homebound elders, internet computer contact through "Senior Net," and interactive television programs (Mattimore, 1993). The National Council on Aging (NCOA) outlines steps in program planning for senior centers (Box 25-10). These often reflect the local needs and culture. Area offices can be located through the U.S. Department of Health and Human Services. Nonfederal affiliated programs can be located through city and county park and recreational

Table 25-12 Participation in Selected Sports Activities: 1993

[In thousands, except rank. For persons 7 years of age or older. Except as indicated, a participant plays a sport more than once in the year. Based on a sampling of 10,000 households]

Activity	7-11 years	12-17 years	18-24 years	25-34 years	35-44 years	45-54 years	55-64 years	65 years and over
Total	18,773	21,579	25,846	42,225	41,264	29,001	21,132	33,166
Number participated in:								
Aerobic exercising*	464	1,083	4,566	6,945	4,994	2,236	1,280	1,633
Backpacking†	859	1,427	1,501	2,769	2,073	519	367	293
Badminton	1,073	1,099	733	1,104	778	447	165	24
Baseball	5,107	4,148	1,548	1,820	1,623	418	203	229
Basketball	5,554	7,951	5,165	4,768	3,462	797	287	208
Bicycle riding*	11,403	9,363	4,707	8,460	7,580	3,750	2,202	2,353
Bowling	4,501	4,833	6,476	9,215	6,185	2,846	1,346	1,954
Calisthenics*	1,178	1,259	1,414	1,654	1,239	682	371	738
Camping‡	6,100	5,566	4,280	9,580	8,832	4,258	2,420	1,896
Exercise walking*	2,218	2,850	5,870	13,032	14,336	11,198	8,596	12,695
Exercising with equipment*	770	3,063	6,984	10,975	9,145	5,795	3,379	3,672
Fishing—fresh water	4,883	4,632	3,548	9,408	7,599	4,791	2,581	3,035
Fishing—salt water	855	1,037	1,026	2,532	2,668	1,353	784	1,260
Football	3,021	4,958	3,255	2,484	1,105	271	228	253
Golf	670	1,885	2,868	5,988	4,901	3,283	2,207	2,748
Hiking	2,710	2,811	3,125	5,690	5,440	2,808	1,432	1,285
Hunting with firearms	297	2,130	1,693	4,292	3,674	2,206	1,245	831
Racquetball	255	438	1,637	1,634	821	351	191	12
Running/jogging*	1,661	3,399	4,614	4,782	3,112	1,844	759	470
Skiing—alpine/downhill	646	1,966	2,493	2,683	1,620	931	173	107
Skiing—cross country	216	467	395	599	861	518	396	176
Soccer	5,494	3,536	1,394	1,023	778	157	59	67
Softball	3,292	3,567	3,070	4,340	2,667	893	246	68
Swimming*	10,669	9,335	6,565	10,645	10,470	5,261	2,742	4,591
Table Tennis	1,056	1,283	1,517	1,600	1,124	702	276	258
Target shooting	878	1,401	1,484	3,427	2,394	1,420	603	624
Tennis	941	2,083	2,155	2,655	1,725	1,172	480	378
Volleyball	1,739	4,222	3,374	4,538	2,551	591	314	55

From U.S. Bureau of the Census: *Statistical abstract of the United States: 1995,* ed 115, Washington, DC, 1995.
X, Not applicable. *Participant engaged in activity at least six times in the year. †Includes wilderness camping. ‡Vacation/overnight.
Source National Sporting Goods Association, Mt Prospect, Ill, *Sports Participation in 1993: Series I* (copyright).

facilities. In addition, several national organizations promote recreational and sports opportunities specifically designed for seniors (see Resources at the end of the chapter).

Some literature seems to indicate that elders seek activities that are comfortable and nonchallenging. A good number of elders seek active sports and high-risk activities. Numerous organizations have arisen just for these elders, limiting the lower age levels for membership, usually to age 55. The Over the Hill Gang is primarily geared to skiers but also organizes groups for high mountain hiking, and biking; Senior Tennis Programs and "70+" are designed for elders who remain athletic and competitive; National Veterans Golden Age Games and Senior Olympics promote competitive sports events for national exhibition. The goals of the organization are noted in Box 25-11.

Bringing Young and Old Together

Recognizing the developmental significance of contact between the generations, many plans and projects have flourished in attempts to bring them together. The thrust of these efforts has been toward those old and young who may be isolated from the continuum of life by illness, institutionalization, or isolation. MacPhail (1993) reported a particularly delightful effort to bring young and old together in her

---

Box 25-9   Leisure Activities for Persons with Limited Money

"Splurge and starve, some of both, which accommodates my financial seesaw. The trick is to find a way to make time a pleasure for myself and others while staying within my budget" (Carpenter, 1987, p. 226). Other suggestions include the following:

Never say "no" to an invitation even though it may be for an unfamiliar activity. Something new can be challenging and stimulating and open new interests.

Treat yourself to a massage; it is relaxing and good for the circulation. Invite a friend for dinner and a massage afterward.

Take a youngster, grandchild if possible, to a movie and rehash it later (a good way to bridge the years and gain a totally different perspective).

Browse through a farmer's market, bring home some unusual produce, and invite a friend to help you conjure up a meal.

Develop an interest in city politics or civic affairs. Spend a few hours each week in the campaign office of your favorite candidate.

Volunteer to assist in annual town events, act as a docent at a local museum, make recordings for the blind, or deliver meals on wheels.

Get involved in churches. They may offer classes, choirs, singles groups, and social events.

Plan and give a house party around a particular theme. Create an ambiance; obtain help by involving friends in planning and preparation, and they may also share the cost. Invite people of different backgrounds, interests, and talents. Make use of their talents. Do not worry about keeping a balance between the number of men and women.

Take a trip and visit an old friend. Make plans well in advance and notify the friend of exact arrival and departure dates. Arrive with a gift that is a usable contribution such as a ham, a roast, or a case of wine. Take a camera and when the visit is completed make a small album as a host appreciation gift.

Have a cook-fest with friends; can or freeze and share the results. In some areas it is possible to pick fruits and vegetables from the field...this can also be a very sociable activity with a few friends.

Arrange a special outing with a grandchild. That provides respite for the parent, joy for the grandparent, and memories for the grandchild.

Summarized from Carpenter L: *Getting better all the time,* New York, 1987, Simon & Schuster.

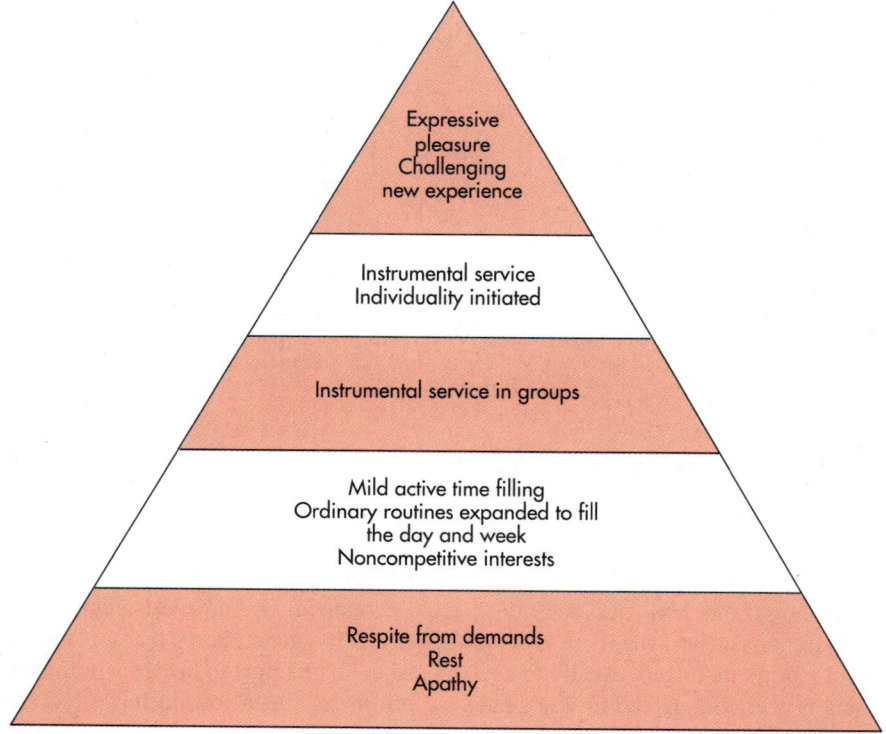

Figure 25-6. Leisure hierarchy.

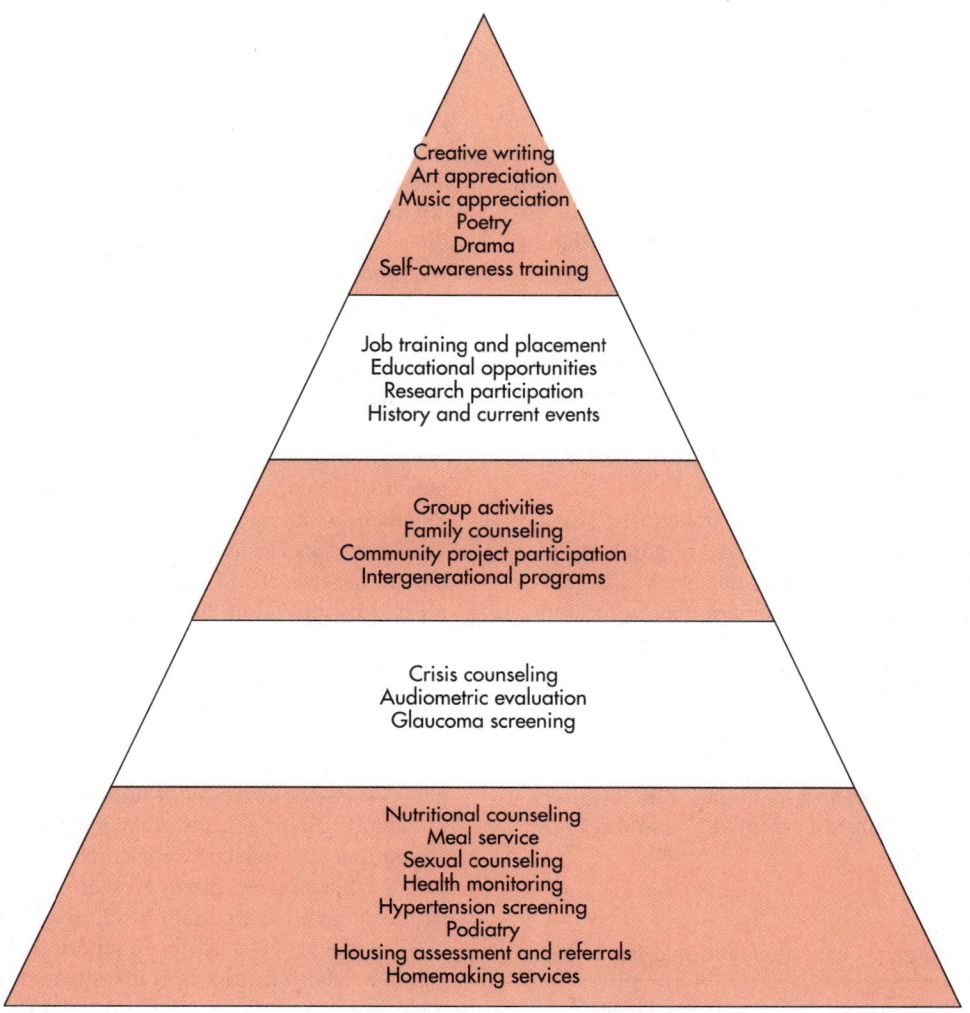

Figure 25-7. Opportunities available in multiservice centers for the aged.

According to the NCOA (1975), program planning should follow the following steps:
1. Assess individual needs;
2. Identify criteria and indicators of need fulfillment;
3. Identify barriers to need fulfillment;
4. State objectives and action steps to attain these needs;
5. Monitor and assess the objectives; and
6. Examine the impact, measure the data, and evaluate the program.

From Leitner MJ, Leitner SF: *Leisure in later life,* ed 2, New York, 1996, Haworth Press.

| Box 25-11 | **Goals of the Senior Olympics** |

To encourage regular exercise among senior adults
To promote better health and higher productivity
To give recognition to elder athletes
To advance international relations and friendships with athletes of other countries
To bring adults and youth together in positive interactions

Data from Provost CS: *The Senior Olympics: preventive medicine with findings pertaining to health and longevity,* Los Angeles, 1981, Warren W Blaney.

profession. She is a gerontology education coordinator and her husband a family physician with a largely geriatric urban practice in Toronto. On Tuesday afternoons she, her husband, their infant, and their toddler make home visits to select elders, who appreciate the brief contact with the children while they are getting the medical and health education they need. As she says, "we decided to concentrate our energies on providing a solid foundation for our contribution to the next generation. At the same time, we wanted to continue to devote our knowledge, skills and experience to caring for the elderly. This balancing of priorities evolved into a schedule of part-time work for me both in and outside the home" (p. 104). The summary of benefits and pitfalls in these home visits can be seen in Table 25-13.

Many institutions have included children in their milieu in various ways:

- As visitors or entertainers (usually not consistent)
- As residents (children with profound retardation or severe neurologic disabilities); elders rock, stroke and cuddle these children, providing stimulation for both
- As a service to employees (day-care centers for children of employees); elders sometimes assist in the care and special programs for the children, such as reading stories or teaching basic skills (tying shoes, telling time)
- In adopt-a-grandparent programs (one child affiliates with one institutionalized person with periodic visits, cards, and inclusion of grandparent in some special family events)

The noninstitutionalized aged are often involved in class projects for schools or community programs. The federal ACTION program uses the services of retired Americans with low incomes to help disadvantaged children in a variety of institutional settings. Foster Grandparents are paid for their work in addition to the benefits gained from contact with the young (see Chapter 20).

As community health nurses, exploration of potential intergenerational experiences within your community may be rewarding. Although we recommend intergenerational contact, when desired by the aged, there are certain pitfalls one must consider. The very young energetic child must be taken in small doses, or the elder is likely to be exhausted, and the benefits will decrease in direct relation to uninterrupted time together. In intergenerational programs young people need consistent supervision, support, and training in the developmental aspects of old age. In other words, more is accomplished by providing an opportunity for young and old to meet when an intermediary support person is available to hear about the experiences and maximize understanding and learning in the situation.

Martee developed skits to present to schoolchildren that conveyed aging concepts in a humorous and positive manner. Genevieve interested a high school social studies class in exploring their genealogy. Whole families were soon contacting her for assistance in searching out their family history. Arthur revived his interest in music and developed a "kitchen band" to entertain local groups and senior citizens.

A model program has been reported (Schulman, 1996) in which a school district in Kansas was short of teachers and the community had a high proportion of elders. The solution was to bring the two together. The elders provided living history experiences for the children, tutored those who needed extra help, worked as classroom aides and music education assistants, and functioned in many other ways to enrich the school experience for children. Both the youngsters and the elders were so enthusiastic about the program it has now been expanded to include connections with the park system, the library and local church groups.

Teaching and assisting youngsters in other ways seems to fill many needs for some elders who find it very personally gratifying. Some volunteer activities evolve into income-generating businesses or skills.

Creative Health Care

Belief is often stronger than any medicine known and more effective than any treatment. The normal body processes can be transcended. Although we would not advocate instilling unfounded expectations, we would hope nurses would openly share with clients the limits of our knowledge and the unknown potential that lies within them. We can then say to an ill or dying person, "There is much within the human body and spirit we don't understand. Almost anything is

Table 25-13 Summary of Intergenerational Home Visits

	Benefits	Pitfalls
Seniors	Touch Mobility, speech, and ADL practice Social stimulation Life review/reminiscing Positive behavior changes Mood elevation Reality orientation	Fatigue Inconvenient scheduling of visit Overstimulation
Juniors	Touch Speech practice Social stimulation Another world view Experience with a person with a deficit Empathy practice Inclusion in parent's work	Disruption of schedule Foreign environment and social responses
Middle-aged generation	Opportunity to "show-off" children Share personal and professional lives	Time management No remuneration Hinders objectivity of caregiver

From MacPhail J: Intergenerational caring in professional and family life, *Geriatr Nurs* 14(2):104, 1993.

possible. Holding onto one's own hopes and beliefs will undoubtedly affect the course of illness and recovery."

The Academy of Parapsychology and Medicine (1975) states several fundamental beliefs that encompass an enlarged view of the treatment of disease and potential for health.

- That man is a multidimensional being whose experience and ultimate purposes are inextricably and meaningfully related, and that that meaning is made manifest in patterns of health and disease
- That medicine must adopt a new view of man: one that recognizes the unity of body, mind, and spirit, and the importance of the interrelationship of these dimensions in health and disease
- That all physical and mental disease is directive experience in human development, and that they must be viewed as a manifestation of conditions existing on subtler levels—whether mental, emotional, or spiritual
- That the treatment of disease must be directed to the whole man, and that no lasting healing of the physical body can be achieved where the mental, emotional, and spiritual elements have been untouched
- That there is no condition or disease in the human body that cannot be successfully treated if a means is discovered for treating on the appropriate level

Bill Moyers, a widely known journalist, has recently joined the large cadre of people, scientists, and mystics, who believe in the healing power of the mind.

NURSING AND NURTURING CREATIVITY

This chapter should stimulate thoughts about what aging can be and present the hope and belief that the last years can be truly transcendent and the culmination of hopes and beliefs. Human potential movements are springing up throughout the United States like mushrooms and may be just as unpredictable. Nurses might caution people not to participate until the credibility of a group has been established. The trend, however, is heartening because it indicates a general belief that humanity has much yet to learn about the capacity for self-actualization. For the aged reaching for transcendence through a higher level of consciousness, courses and workshops are offered throughout the United States. The goals are integrative: the connection of the finite and the infinite, mortality and immortality, matter and spirit, physics and metaphysics, humans and God. Unfortunately, many of them are expensive. For further information, resources are included at the end of this chapter.

Our functions as health care workers valuing self-actualization are (1) to continually spur our clients to ask, "What is possible and suitable for me?" and (2) to assist them in finding appropriate resources and, when needed, assist in the implementation of activities toward self-actualization. The nature of self-actualization is self-determination and direction. Nurses are ancillary to the process.

Self-actualization implies that one actualizes the potential of self through various mechanisms. We have mentioned only a few of these in a somewhat cursory manner, knowing that these individually instituted actions have a force of their own that once activated goes far beyond the professionals' involvement. Such things as yoga, focused meditation, the discipline of karate, and other forms of centered concentration are segued into transcendence, and these are explored more fully in Chapter 27 as related to altered states of consciousness. We have touched on these briefly in Chapter 9 as related to pain control. In reality we know little of the capacities of the transcendent self that are on the margin of the next evolution of humankind.

Ginny is 87 years old, alert and somewhat officious about managing her own affairs and those of others, whenever possible, in the life care center in which she has resided for the past 10 years. She is comfortable in her setting, belongs to numerous committees, chairs several of them, and feels rather negative about the individuals who prefer to remain in their own apartment with little involvement in the workings of the center. She is particularly distressed because one of her friends has recently been admitted to the care center and has expected her to be available to carry complaints to the administrator or director of nursing at the care center about various irritations. Ginny believes, and frequently tells her friend, "Well, tell them what you are unhappy about. It is not my job." Unfortunately, Ginny fell while in the supermarket and broke both wrists and was admitted to the care canter after her casting and stabiliziation at the nearby community hospital. Her roommate was none other than her friend whom she felt was not assertive regarding her own care. Ginny believes she is a very practical person and must manage her own situation but cannot abide those who seemingly passively accept whatever fate has in store. She says to her roommate, "Well, just look at me, totally helpless with two broken wrists and I manage. I don't feel very sorry for those who cannot take care of themselves." The roommate is occasionally heard mumbling the rosary but seldom asks for anything or complains. Ginny says, "I always thought God takes care of them who take care of themselves."

If you were the nurse, how would you begin to actualize the potential of these roommates?

KEY CONCEPTS

- Self-actualization is a concept articulated by Abraham Maslow that he believes is the pinnacle of human development.
- Self-actualization is most clearly embedded in Eurocentric cultures.
- Continued learning, creativity, and rising beyond egocentric concerns are characteristic of self-actualized individuals.
- Wisdom is an expression of self-actualization and is the ultimate achievement of old age.
- The expression of higher human attributes, such as creative endeavors, are impeded by unmet needs on the lower levels of need.
- Individuals need opportunities for exposure to various experiences and diverse ideas in order to achieve self-actualization.

Nursing Diagnoses

The following potential diagnoses must be considered as well as diagnoses unique to the particular individual:
Diversional activity deficit

Growth and development, altered
Self-esteem disturbance
Spiritual distress

NURSING PROCESS AND NURSING DIAGNOSIS
Self-esteem disturbance

Etiologies and Related Factors
Self-perception: inadequate, unable
Losses: body part(s)
    function(s)
    significant other(s)
    support systems
Disfigurement (disease/surgery)
Institutionalization
Relocation
Dependent on others for ADLs and/or IADLs
Incontinence

Defining Characteristics
Depends on others' opinions
Passive
Nonassertive
Excessive reassurance sought
Minimal or no eye contact
Hesitant to try new or different things or situations
Negative verbalizations about self
Hypersensitive to comments and criticisms
Diminished socialization

Knowledge
Therapeutic communication skills
Interpersonal relation skills
Problem solving, social skills
Positive health behaviors
Maturational development and changes
Group therapy
Assessment of social skills, coping
Physical and psychologic assessment

Crisis management
Reminiscence
Relaxation techniques, tension-relieving strategies
Aging process
Community resources

Clinical Judgment and Related Skills
Listen
Respect personal space
Appreciate individual's uniqueness
Encourage positive and negative self-expression
Employ art and music for self-expression
Use open-ended questions when conversing
Teach social skills as needed
Encourage participation with others who share same
    interest
Reduce anxiety
Help verbalization of what client finds difficult to
    express
Encouragement as task/skill attempted
Avoid competitive activities

Evaluation
Realistic self-perception
Accepts maturational changes
Identifies positive aspects of self
Expresses a positive outlook of future
Identifies ways to exert control and influence outcomes
Makes decisions alone
Interacts positively with others
Participates in activities
Begins to make suggestions and voice opinions

NEEDS ADDRESSED AND TASK STRENGTHS

Self-actualization
Need for intellectual stimulation and spiritual expression
    (to maintain self-esteem and seek self-actualization)
Inner-directed personality

Spontaneity
High self-esteem
Optimistic
Ego balance and acceptance of shadow self

- Creativity is the product of the self-actualized. Creativity can appear in many forms.
- Creativty is evident in any activity that is conducted in an exploratory manner.
- Intergenerational contact between elders and youth tend in many instances to bring out the creative qualities in each of the generations.
- The life history of an individual is a story to be developed, integrated, and treasured. This is particularly important toward the end of life.
- Nursing functions related to learning and creativity are mainly focused on providing resource information, encouragement to individuals expressing certain interests, assistance toward self-expression when there are impediments in function, and assuring, to the extent possible, that basic needs are met.
- In order to avoid ageist attitudes and a focus on medical problems, it is important for nurses, and other health care professionals, to maintain contact with some highly creative and self-actualized elders.

▲ CASE STUDY

Lee was born in 1896, the grandson of a slave. At the age of 96 years he is still actively farming his own land by horse and plow as he has been doing for more than 50 years. He states that a "hoss is better for a poor man than a tractor," since a tractor can break down and cannot be used as readily for going into town or to church meetings on Sunday. His childhood experiences as a hired hand kept him from attending school, and it is not known whether he now can read and write. He continues to live in the house that he built when he bought his farm land in Jasper County, Texas, in 1940. He had been married 58 years before his wife's death and states, "We never spent a day apart in our entire married life. She was a good wife and a religious woman." He affirms his love of God and his respect for the land and his belief that a man who is willing to work can "make a good life off the land." He indicates that it is his active life and enjoyment of work that has kept him well and able to sleep at night without worry about what the next day may bring. He feels he has kept peace with God and when it is his time to leave this world he is ready to go. He cares for his horse, chickens, and several cows. He enjoys relating stories about the Civil War to his great-granddaughter and takes her to locations where battles were fought and soldiers could find hiding. He does this while walking over irregular country ground and climbing over fencing. He walks to and regularly attends his local church. He taught himself to play the piano at the age of 92 after the death of his wife; she had been the one to play religious hymns on the piano and he would sing with her and play his guitar. Lee had rarely been ill enough to interfere with his day's work and had never been hospitalized. One morning when his granddaughter came to bring some homemade bread she found Lee half-conscious, as if dozing, in his favorite chair. She immediately called her father and they took Lee to the hospital. It was determined he had a mild stroke that left him weakened on the left side. As his nurse case manager, begin to develop a plan for his discharge.

Based upon the case study, develop a nursing care plan using the following procedure*:

List comments of client that provide *subjective data.*

List information that provides *objective data.*

From these data identify and state, using accepted format, two *nursing diagnoses* you determine are most significant to this client at this time.

Determine and state *outcome criteria* for each diagnosis. These must reflect some alleviation of the problem identified in the nursing diagnosis and must be stated in concrete and measurable terms.

Plan and state one or more *interventions* for each diagnosed problem. Provide specific documentation of source used to determine appropriate intervention. Plan at least one intervention that incorporates the client's existing strengths.

Evaluate success of intervention. Interventions must correlate directly with the stated outcome criteria in order to measure the outcome success.

STUDY QUESTIONS/ACTIVITIES

Identify one old person that you consider self-actualized and discuss the qualities he or she possesses that you feel indicate his or her self-actualization.

Provide a comprehensive definition of self-actualization and identify several qualities to be expected in self-actualized elders.

Discuss the fundamental differences in the self-actualized and those who are not and identify some of the reasons you believe this to occur.

Describe several learning opportunities that are available to elders and the special characteristics and growth factors predominant in each.

Discuss the types of creative self-expression you have seen among the very old and how this relates to their age.

Discuss how you can provide opportunities for elders to express their creativity.

Discuss the nursing role in relation to the self-actualization of elders.

Discuss the talents, qualities, and interests you have that you believe will help you continually grow to higher levels of self-actualization.

Discuss the meanings and the thoughts triggered by the students' and elders' viewpoints expressed at the beginning of the chapter. How do these vary from your own experience?

*Students are advised to refer to their nursing diagnosis text and identify possible or potential problems.

List your leisure activities and those of the elders you know. Discuss the commonalities and differences you discover.

Discuss with an elder how his or her leisure and recreation needs may have changed or remained the same as he or she aged.

Interview three elders and list all of the creative activities they are engaged in that you can identify. Discuss these and their effects.

RESEARCH QUESTIONS

Is there a need for reliable instruments to measure the various creative qualities of the very old?

What is the functional significance of self-actualization?

What are the variations in themes of reminiscence in elders who are socially active in the community and those who are socially restricted or institutionalized?

What factors in a formal learning situation are most important to the elderly? In an informal situation?

What are the creative contributions most frequently found among the very old in the community?

What creative opportunities are most often provided for the institutionalized elder? Which are the least often available?

What are the most frequent creative contributions of old men? Old women? Comparisons?

How can wisdom be measured, and is it an achievement of the majority of well-adjusted aged?

Investigate types of humor elders find amusing.

RESOURCES

Films and Videos

Seasons of the Mind, J. Rowe, Filmmakers Library, New York. A concise and excellent report on two septuagenarians who, on entering the university, relish the intensity, face the difficult challenges, and perhaps most surprisingly, find that they are welcomed and accepted by their younger fellows. To watch the expression of an 82-year-old lady accepting her Bachelor of Arts degree after 7 years of study is to know the truth (21 minutes).

Emil and Fifi: The Story of My Grandfather, J. Rowe, Filmmakers Library, New York, NY (50 minutes). An image of aging videotaped by a grandson of Emil Synek, a Czech playwright, journalist, and statesman, and Emil's constant companion, Fifi, a poodle.

Giants of Time, J. Rowe, Filmmakers Library, New York, NY (57 minutes). This film celebrates elders whose lives have already spanned two centuries, and are approaching their third.

Fools' Dance, Baxley Media Group, 110 West Main St, Urbana, IL (30 minutes). This film deals sensitively and symbolically with the heart of old age from the experiencer's perspective and promotes insight into how to enrich life at any age. It is a very effective and wonderful experience. It has lots of potential uses in gerontology education and inservice training in a variety of areas: death, ethnicity, and the role of philosophy and spirituality in the caring process.

National Organizations

Five national organizations representing older persons have local units in many parts of the United States. The local units schedule meetings and plan activities that often include recreational or social components. Information can be obtained from the national headquarters of these groups, which are as follows:

American Association of Retired Persons
1909 K St NW
Washington, DC 20049
(202) 872-4700

National Council of Senior Citizens
1511 K St NW
Washington, DC 20005
(202) 783-6850

National Council on the Aging
600 Maryland Ave SW
W Wing 100
Washington, DC 20024
(202) 479-1200

National Association of Retired Federal Employees
1533 New Hampshire Ave NW
Washington, DC 20036
(202) 234-0832

Elderhostel
50 Federal St
Boston, MA 02110
(617)-426-8056 To receive catalogs write ELDERHOSTEL, PO Box 1959, Wakefield, MA 01880-5959.

Publications

Intergenerational Idea Book by the American Association of Retired Persons, 601 E St NW, Washington DC 20049, 1993. Describes and gives sources for more information related to special intergenerational programs for education, arts, history, service, and other activities.

Chase Annual Events Calendar. Significant events, local and national celebrations, notable birthdays, historic anniversaries, theme months, and trivia are all included in a day-to-day calendar. This calendar would be useful to construct activities, to trigger discussions, and as a general focus of interest. Contemporary Books, Inc. (312) 782-9181 or Fax (312) 782-2157.

Creative Services for Elders through Libraries, a monthly newsletter, L. Nelson, American Library Association, (312) 280-4295 or Fax (312) 280-3256.

Focus: Library Services to Older Adults, People with Disabilities, 216 N Frederick Ave, Daytona Beach, FL 32114; annual subscription, $12.

If an educational environment sounds idyllic, you'll be interested in writing for AARP's free *Directory of Centers for Older Learners.* The state-by-state listing includes the names, addresses, phone numbers, and sponsors of 254 educational programs around the country designed for older students. For a copy of *Directory of Centers for Older Learners,* send a postcard requesting stock number D13973 to AARP Fulfillment, EE0233, PO Box 2400, Long Beach, CA 90801-2400.

Lifelong Learning: The Adult Years. Journal contains articles on adult education and is published monthly (except July and August) by the Adult Education Association of the USA, 810 18th St NW, Washington, DC 20006.

Senior Learning Times. Journal is published by the College Board and AARP and is available to individuals and groups. Single copies are $1.50; multiple orders are available for $12 per set of 50. Make checks payable to the College Board, and mail to the College Board, PO Box C749, Pratt Street Station, Brooklyn, NY 11205.

Institutes for Lifetime Learning. A service of the American Association of Retired Persons (AARP)/National Retired Teachers Association (NRTA), it provides classes at institute centers throughout the country and a series of radio programs allowing members of AARP/NRTA to pursue independent study at their own pace in their own fields of interest. Contact AARP, (202) 872-4700.

American Association of Community and Junior Colleges, No. 1 Dupont Circle, Suite 410, Washington, DC 20036, (202) 293-7050.

Adult Education Association: Aging Section publishes a quarterly newsletter, *Education for Aging News.* The association conducts seminars and has published *Old Gold,* a guide to financing in adult education. Contact Adult Education Association: Aging Section, Brookdale Center on Aging, Hunter College, 129 E 79th St, New York, NY 10021.

Recreation and Travel

Grandtravel: destinations include Washington, DC, Alaska, France, Holland, New England, England, and Scotland. Contact Grandtravel, 6900 Wisconsin Avenue, Suite 706, Chevy Chase, MD 20815, (800) 247-7651.

Senior Travel Exchange Program: contact Walt Stanley, Senior Travel Exchange Program, PO Box H, Santa Maria, CA 93456.

American Bed and Breakfast Association: 16 Village Green, Suite 203, Crofton MD 21114, (301) 261-0180.

70+: Lloyd Lambert, 104 Eastside Dr, Ballston Lake, NY 12019.

Over the Hill Gang International: 3310 Cedar Heights Dr, Colorado Springs, CO 80904, (719) 685-4162.

Senior Tennis Programs/USTA Education and Research Center: 729 Alexander Rd, Princeton, NJ 08540.

National Senior Sports Association: 317 Cameron St, Alexandria, VA 22314.

Men's Senior Baseball League: 8 Sutton Terr, Jericho, NY 11753.

National Association of Senior Citizens Softball: PO Box 1085, Mt Clemens, MI 48046.

Senior Olympics: Warren Blaney, Senior Sports International, Wilshire Blvd, Suite 360, Los Angleles, CA 90026.

National Veterans Golden Age Games: Department of Veterans Affairs, (202) 273-5736.

International Senior Games Headquarters: 460 Summer St, Stamford, CT 06801, (800) 223-6106 or (203) 352-0532.

US National Senior Sports Classic: US National Senior Sports Organization, 14323 S Outer Forty Rd, Suite N300, Chesterfield, MO 63017.

American Horticultural Therapy Association: 9220 Wrightman Rd, Suite 300, Gaithersburg, MD 20879, (301) 948-3010.

Growing with Gardening: A Twelve Month Guide for Therapy, Recreation and Education, Moore B, Chapel Hill, NC, 1989, University of North Carolina Press.

Gardening in Raised Beds and Containers for the Elderly and Physically Handicapped, Relf PD, Blacksburg, Va, 1989, Cooperative Extension Service, Virginia Polytechnic University.

Horticulture Therapy for Senior Centers, Nursing Homes, and Retirement Living, Rothert E, Daubert J, Glencoe, Ill, 1981, Chicago Horticultural Society.

American Camping Association: Martinsville, Ind, (765) 342-8456; *Guide to Camps,* $16.95, lists numerous camps for seniors.

Library of Congress. Through its Blind and Visually Handicapped Division, the Library of Congress offers certain services for persons with a visual handicap. Special materials can be provided to any person who is certified by a competent authority to be unable to use conventional print material. Braille publications, cassettes, talking books on phonodiscs, and open-reel tapes may be selected. These are obtainable through regional and subregional libraries. In most cases, local public libraries can provide information, or contact may be made with the Division at 1291 Taylor St, NW, Washington, DC 20011, (202) 707-5100.

National Recreation and Park Association. The National Recreation and Park Association, 1108 Jessica St, Alexandria, VA 22209, (703) 838-4343, has established a national task force committee to improve and expand its services for the aging. This committee develops technical resources of all aspects of services for the aging at the local community level. The association has two publications for sale that are of interest: *Management Aid No. 88: Recreation in Nursing Homes* and *Senior Citizen Program Manual.*

National Park Service. The National Park Service, U.S. Department of the Interior, offers to persons 62 years old and older a Golden Age Pass, which allows the holder free access to any park that charges a fee. The pass may be obtained by any older person who presents proof of age at any national park that charges a fee. The National Park Service also has recognized the special needs of handicapped and infirm persons and has published the *National Park Guide for the Handicapped.* For further information, contact Public Inquiries, National Park Service, Interior Building, Washington, DC 20240, (202) 343-1100.

The Discovery through the Humanities Program is a life and community-enriching venture. Write or call for a free introductory packet containing further details and order forms: Discovery through the Humanities Program, The National Council on the Aging, Inc, 600 Maryland Ave, SW, West Wing 100, Washington, DC 20024, (202) 479-1200.

American Alliance for Health, Physical Education, Recreation and Dance. This program offers model education and service approaches in health, fitness, and leisure for older Americans and is intended to increase the number and quality of programs preparing students for careers in health, fitness, and leisure services for the aging. It also conducts workshops, and publishes materials developed by the project. AAH-PER-IVEA Center, 1201 16th St, Washington, DC 20036.

The following sources give detailed information for older travelers:

A Foreign Language Guide to Health Care, Blue Cross Association, 840 North Lake Shore Dr, Chicago, IL 60611.

Helpful Hints for the Older Traveler (and other information), Consumer Information, United States Travel Service, U.S. Department of Commerce, Washington, DC 20230.

Your Medicare Handbook, Social Security Administration, Baltimore, MD 21235.

Your Social Security Check . . . While You're Outside the United States, Social Security Administration, PO Box 1756, Baltimore, MD 21203.

Creative and Theater Arts

National Senior Adult Theater Festival, Ann McDonough, (702) 895-4248.

The Golden Stage: Dramatic Activities with Older Adults, Ann McDonough, Kendall-Hunt Publishing, Del Vecchio Communications, Inc, 2865 Sorrel St, Las Vegas, NV 89102, (702) 876-6747.

Seniors Acting Up: Humorous New One-Act Plays and Skits for Older Adults, Ted Fuller, Pleasant Hill Press, 241 Greenwich Dr, Pleasant Hill, CA 94523.

Come Step Into My Life: Life Drama with Youth and Elders, Rosilyn Wilder, New Plays, Inc, PO Box 5074, Charlottesville, VA 22905, (804) 979-2777.

Americans for the Arts, 927 15th St NW, 12th Floor, Washington, DC 20005-2304, (202) 371-2830.

REFERENCES

Academy of Parapsychology and Medicine: First National Congress on Integrative Health, Tucson, Ariz. Oct 1975.

Aging successfully, *Mayo Clinic Health Letter* 10(11):6, 1992.

American Association of Retired Persons, 1996, p7.

Armstrong CH: *Senior adult camping,* Martinsville, Ind, 1979, American Camping Association.

Artline Ltd: *Interactive therapeutic art,* p18, Waukesha, WI, 1997.

Asmuth MV: Reaction reading: a tool for providing fantasy imagery for long-term care facility resident, *Gerontologist* 35(3):415, 1995.

Back C, Bourque L: Life graphs: aging and cohort effects, *J Gerontol* 25:249, 1970.

Banzinger G, Rousch S: Nursing homes for the birds: a control-relevant intervention with bird feeders, *Gerontologist* 23:527, 1983.

Bassen S, Baltazar B: Flowers, flowers everywhere: creative horticulture programming at the Hebrew Home for the Aged, *Geriatr Nurs* 18(2):53, 1997.

Berman HJ: From the pages of my life, *Generations* 15(2):33, 1991.

Bernstein A: *Growing season,* Berkeley, Calif, 1995, Wild Canyon Press.

Bond C, Miller M: Reading: the ageless activity, *Geriatr Nurs* 8(4):910, 1987.

Carpenter L: *Getting better all the time,* New York, 1987, Simon & Schuster.

California Association of Health Facilities: Seniors list top 10 priorities, *CAHF Long Term Care News,* Oct 27, 1995.

Carson D: Natural landscape as meaningful space for the aged. In Pastalan L, Carson D, editors: *Spatial behavior of older people,* Ann Arbor, Mich, 1970, University of Michigan.

Chaudbury H: *Self and reminiscence of place: toward a theory of re-discovering selfhood in place-based reminiscence for people with dementia.* Paper presented at the meeting of the Gerontological Society of America, Washington, DC, Nov 19, 1996.

Chenery MF: Camping and senior adults, *Camping Magazine,* p. 50, March 1987.

Clark F: Learning thrives when seniors take responsibility for their own program, *The Older Learner* 4(1):1, 1995-1996.

Clark M, Anderson B: *Culture and aging: an anthropological study of older Americans,* Springfield, Ill, 1967, Charles C Thomas.

Clark P, Osgood NJ: *Seniors on stage: the impact of applied theater techniques on the elderly,* New York, 1985, Praeger.

Cousins N: *Anatomy of an illness,* New York, 1979, WW Norton.

Crowley SL: The amazing "power of music," *AARP Bulletin* 32(2):20, 1992.

Csikszentmihalyi M: *Flow: the psychology of optimal experience,* New York, 1990, Harper & Row.

Edwards D: Presentation at American Nurses' Association Gerontological Nurses Conference, St Paul, Apr 1977.

Elder G: *Children of the depression: social change in life experience,* Chicago, 1974, University of Chicago Press.

Elderhostel: *Elderhostel international catalog: 1997,* Boston, 1997, Elderhostel.

Fry W: Humor and the human cardiovascular system. In Mindness H, Turek J, editors: *The study of humor,* Los Angeles, 1979, Antioch University.

Goleman D: Mental decline in aging need not be inevitable, *New York Times,* p. B5, April 26, 1994.

Guttmann-Gee B: The power of education for the older learner, *The Older Learner* 4(1):1, 1995-1996.

Haight B: Long term effects of a structured life review process, *J Gerontol* 47(5):P312, 1992.

Hepburn K: *Me,* New York, 1991, Ballatine Books.

Holstein M: Unintended consequences of "productive aging," *Aging Today* 17(6):9, 1996.

Hudson SD, Rich SM: Group travel programs: a creative way to meet the leisure needs of older adults, *J Phys Educ Recreat Dance* 64(4):38, 1993.

Jecker NS: Adult moral development: ancient, medieval, and modern paths, *Generations* 14(4):19, 1990.

Kastenbaum R: Guest editorial, entire issue devoted to creativity in later life, *Generations* 15(2):4, 1991.

Kelly M: Consequences of visual impairment on leisure activities of the elderly, *Geriatr Nurs* 16(6):273, 1995.

Koch K: *I never told anybody,* New York, 1977, Random House.

Kohlberg L, Power C: Moral development, religious thinking and the question of a seventh stage. In Kohlberg L, editor: *The philosophy of moral development,* vol I, San Francisco, 1981, Harper and Row.

Kuhn M: Advocacy in this new age, *Aging* 3:297, July/Aug 1979.

Lehman H: *Age and achievement,* Princeton, NJ, 1953, Princeton University Press for the American Philosophical Society.

Leisure World Laguna Hills: *Emeritus program offers education in its purest sense for active seniors,* Leisure World Laguna Hills, 23522 Paseo de Valencia, Laguna Hills, CA 92653, (800) 711-9273.

Leitner MJ, Leitner SF: *Leisure in later life,* ed 2 New York, 1996, Haworth Press.

Luchs A, Growald ER: Doing good—or even thinking about it—may boost your immunity, *Am Health Care* 7(2):51-53, 1988.

MacPhail J: Intergenerational caring in professional and family life, *Geriatr Nurs* 14(2):104, 1993.

MacManus SA: Older voters: what we know, what to expect, *Aging Today* 17(5):1, 1996.

Markowitz R: Showtime, *Modern Maturity* 39(5):52, 1996.

Maslow A: Creativity in self-actualizing people. In Anderson H, editor: *Creativity and its cultivator,* New York, 1959, Harper & Row.

Matsumoto M: *Class presentation in Gerontological Certificate Program,* Division of Continuing Education, San Francisco State University, San Francisco, 1978.

Mattimore H: Seniors and computers, *CPRS Magazine* 49(2):24, 1993.

McAuley E, Rudolph D: Physical activity, aging and psychological well-being, *J Phys Activity Aging* 3(1):67, 1995.

McConatha D: Regenerational learning: a model for expanding the potential of older adults (abstract), *Gerontologist* 23:156 (special issue), 1983.

McDonough A: The changing scope of senior adult theater, *Aging Today* 17(6):18, 1996.

Mercer RT, Nichols EG, Doyle GC: *Transitions in a woman's life: major life events in developmental context,* New York, 1989, Springer.

Merriam-Webster: *Merriam-Webster dictionary,* New York, 1974, Simon & Schuster.

Metcalf CW: *Lighten up,* Niles, 1993, Nightingale Conant, (audiotapes).

Midlarsky E, Hannah ME, Kahana E: Who cares? naturalistic studies of altruism, *Gerontologist* 23:131 (special issue), 1983.

Moloney MF: A Heideggerian hermeneutical analysis of older women's stories of being strong, *Image* 27(2):104, 1995.

Mooney G: An arts program in Vermont that draws people out, *Smithsonian* 23(8):76, 1992.

Moore E: *Hints for using music with senior groups.* Class presentation, Group Work with the Aged, Division of Continuing Education, San Francisco State University, San Francisco, 1977.

NCOA-National Council on Aging: *Senior centers: 50 years of progress—1943-1993,* Washington, DC, 1993, NCOA.

Olszowy D: *Horticulture of the disabled and disadvantaged,* Springfield, IL, 1978, Charles C Thomas.

Pappas SH: Creating an environment to support hardiness and quality patient care, *Sem Nurs Manag* 3(3):115, 1995.

Peck CF: From deep within: poetry workshops in nursing homes, *Activities Adaptation Aging* 13(3):153, 1989.

Peck R: Psychological developments in the second half of life. In Anderson J, editor: *Psychological aspects of aging,* Washington, DC, 1955, American Psychological Association.

Riordan RJ, Williams CS: Gardening therapeutics for the elderly, *Activities Adaptation Aging* 11(1/2):103, 1988.

Rubin FH, Black JS: Health care and consumer control: Pittsburgh's town meeting for seniors, *Gerontologist* 32(6):853, 1992.

Rubinstein RL: *Feelings for the past: reminiscences about former residences.* Paper presented at the meeting of the Gerontological Society of America, Washington, DC, Nov 19, 1996.

Sacks O: *Seeing voices: a journey into the world of the deaf,* Berkeley, Calif, 1989, University of California Press.

Sacks O: *Awakenings,* revised ed, New York, 1987, Alfred A Knopf.

Sambandham M, Schirm V: Music as a nursing intervention for residents with Alzheimer's disease in long term care, *Geriatr Nurs* 16(2):79, 1995.

Sarton M: *At seventy: a journal,* New York, 1984, WW Norton.

Schulman K: Older Kansas volunteers go back to school, *Aging Today* 17(5):19, 1996.

Schwab M: *A gift freely given: the personal journal of Sister Marilyn Schwab, OSB,* Mt Angel, Ore, 1986, Benedictine Sisters.

Scott-Maxwell F: *The measure of my days,* New York, 1968, Alfred A Knopf.

Sherman J: The arts and older Americans, *Monographs: National Assembly of Local Arts Agencies,* Americans for the Arts 5(8):1, 1996.

Simonton DK: Creativity in the later years: optimistic prospects for achievement, *Gerontologist* 30(5):626, 1990.

Stanley-Murchow J, Poe B: Teleconferencing: an avenue for college coursework in nursing home settings, *Int J Aging Hum Dev* 26(3):201, 1988.

Steffl BM: Group work and professional programs. In Burnside I, Schmidt MG, editors: *Working with older adults: group process and techniques,* ed 3, Boston, 1994, Jones and Bartlett.

Steinberg D: More than theater—an intergenerational connection, *Aging Today* 17(6):19, 1996.

Steinberg D: Satisfying the urge to write, *San Francisco Examiner,* pB-7, Nov 13, 1993.

Sterritt PF, Pokorney ME: Art activities for patients with Alzheimer's and related disorders, *Geriatr Nurs* 15(3):155-159, 1994.

Sullivan J, Deane D: Humor and health, *J Gerontol Nurs* 14(1):20, 1988.

Thompson R, Cruse D: Leisure awareness and education: preparing for retirement, *J Phys Educ Recreat Dance* 64(4):35, 1993.

Thurman AH, Piggins CA: *Drama activities with older adults: a handbook for leaders,* New York, 1982, Haworth Press.

Trice LB: Meaningful life experience to the elderly, *Image* 22(4):248, 1990.

Trussell T: More fun in the sun: high achievers find haven on campus, *AARP Bulletin* 33(2):2, 1992.

US Bureau of the Census: *Statistical abstract of the United States: 1995,* ed 115, Washington, DC, 1995.

Vecchione KM: A recreational therapist's perspective. In Burnside I, Schmidt MG, editors: *Working with older adults: group process and techniques,* ed 3, Boston, 1994, Jones and Bartlett.

Voelkl JE, Fries BE, Galecki AT: Predictors of nursing home residents' participation in activity programs, *Gerontologist* 35(1):44, 1995.

Voelkl JE: Activity involvement among older adults in institutional settings. In Kelly JR, editor: *Activity and aging: staying involved in later life,* Newbury Park, Calif, 1993, Sage.

Ward KD, Mroczek DK: Personality and the incidence of hypertension among older men: longtitudinal findings from the normative aging study, *Health Psychol* 14(6):563, 1995.

Watson J: *Human science and human care: a theory of nursing,* New York, 1988, National League of Nursing.

Wax TM: Poetry efforts by aged deaf: expression of life cycle experience, *Gerontologist* 23:462, 1983.

Winfrey C: For the aged, camp life's slower, but much like that for the young, *New York Times,* p 26, July 16, 1977.

Young CI: One person's journey, *Generations* 8:26, fall 1983.

Zimmer W: An artist with a sharp eye for the seams between two ages, *NY Times,* Sunday, May 21, 1995, p. 18.

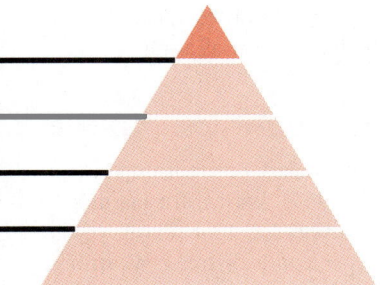

CHAPTER 26

Death, Dying, and Grief

An elder speaks   **Losses are the hardest of all experiences. Losing parents is expected, deaths of children hurt. If one lives as long as I have, increasingly others my age and younger are expiring, and then there is the experience of real loneliness. I sometimes feel like the proverbial last leaf clinging to the tree. When I was 50, numerous uncles, aunts, cousins; in the past 5 years my only brother, last week his daughter-in-law. Since living at the Meadows I have made and lost many friends; we are constantly reminded of the proximity of death.**

Lyn, 85

LEARNING OBJECTIVES   Upon completion of this chapter, the reader will be able to:

1. Differentiate between loss and grief.
2. Explain the different types of grief and the dynamics of the grieving process.
3. Explain the attributes required of the nurse to be able to effectively intervene in grief/mourning.
4. List interventions that are helpful to the newly bereaved and those whose grief is established.
5. Discuss the process of dying and the pros and cons of the various theories/frameworks for the dying process.
6. Identify and discuss the needs of the dying and appropriate interventions.
7. Differentiate between the types of advance directives and explain the role and responsibilities of the nurse related to each of them.
8. Discuss the pros and cons of suicide and physician-aid in dying.

Loss, dying, and death are universal incontestable events of the human experience that one is unable to stop or control. The numerous physical, psychologic, and behavioral responses that are manifested are known as grief, mourning, or bereavement.

Loss, like death, is an event, whereas dying and grief and mourning are dynamic processes. Loss for elders generally relates to loss of relationships through death (spouse, friends, at times adult children), and life transitions (retirement, role change, relocation from home to nursing care facility) (Box 26-1). Dying may be the elder's own or that of a significant other. Regardless, grief and grief work or mourning are important to facilitate elders in maintaining their lives.

Grief and *mourning* (bereavement) are usually used synonymously. However, in its purest form, grief refers to the individual's response to the event of loss. Mourning represents those behaviors that the bereaved uses to incorporate the loss experience into his or her ongoing life. Mourning is an active process rather than one that is reactive to an event. The behaviors associated with mourning are determined by social and cultural norms that prescribe the appropriate ways of coping with loss in a given society.

The approach in this chapter may lean toward a modernistic perspective, due to the amount of research that has been disseminated during the twentieth century. However, it is important to emphasize that there is no single way to grieve or respond to loss. Responses will vary widely among individuals and across cultures.

The experience of death (age, place, and manner of death) has been profoundly altered during the twentieth century. Seventy-three percent of deaths each year are of the aged (Vital Statistics Report, 1995), with the leading cause of death attributed to chronic disorders. Increasingly, it is the old who die, making it a predictable and an expected function of old age (Hooyman and Kiyak, 1988). The elderly are considered the only group of individuals in which death is culturally acceptable (Godow, 1987). The numbers of elders surviving into very old age have influenced the experience of death and bereavement. Death, unfortunately, is a form of ageist discrimination, a subtle denigration of aging.

CONCEPTUAL UNDERPINNINGS OF GRIEF

Theorists have suggested that grief work or mourning occurs in three to ten stages. Bowlby (1961), known for his theory of attachment and bonding theory, offers four phases of the grief process: numbness, anger, and distress; yearning, searching for the lost figure; disorganization and despair; and reorganization (Figure 26-1). Raphael (1983), using the work of Bowlby and Freud, suggested that there was a need to review relationships and a release of the bonds that tied one to the dead. It also required the living to form new attachments. Engel (1967) and Parks (1972) noted five stages of grief: shock, awareness of loss, withdrawal, healing, and renewal. Regardless of who the theorist is, it is clear that grief has a beginning with physical and psychologic manifestations, a middle (considered the work of grieving or mourning) during which time the individual is breaking the bonds that tied them to the deceased, and an end with the individual emerging refocused, having *severed* the ties to the dead person.

The theories or models are based on the Euro-American perspective of breaking the emotional ties between the bereaved and the dead (DeSpelder and Strickland, 1995). The majority of these grief theories evolved between the early 1900s and early 1980s and have been the foundation of what caregivers and society in general have been taught about the grieving process.

Recently the stages or phases of grief have again been looked at with a critical eye. The implication of stages/

Box 26-1	**Losses of the Aged**

Loss of Relationships
    Significant others
    Social contacts through
        Illness
        Death
        Distance
        Decreased mobility
Life Transitions
    Significant roles
    Financial security
    Independence
    Physical health
    Mental stability
    Life-death

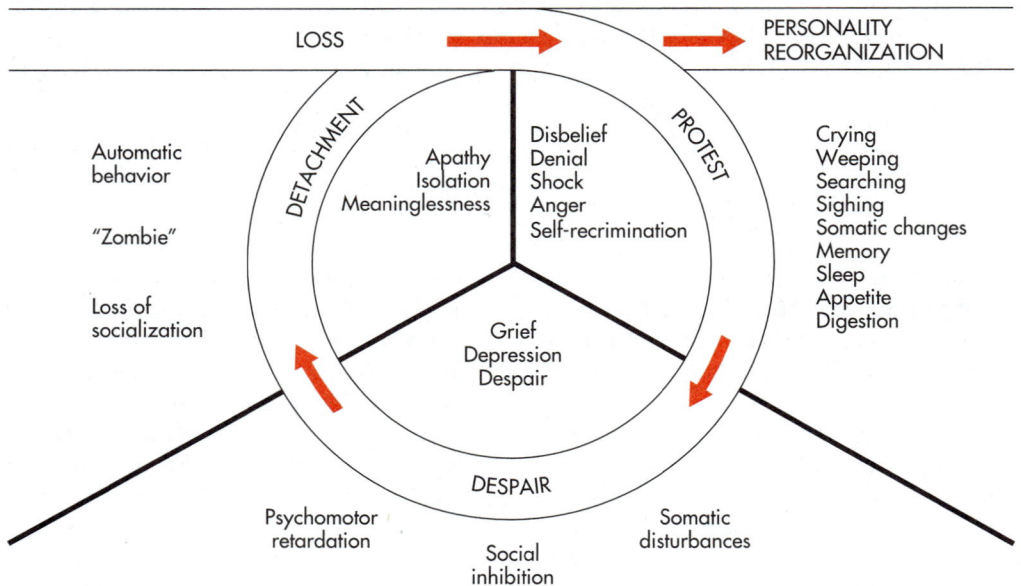

Figure 26-1. An illustration of John Bowlby's approach to loss. (From Beare PG, Myers JL: *Adult health nursing,* ed 3, 1998, Mosby.)

phases is that young and old grieve alike and that the progression through grief or mourning occurs in a linear pattern. This suggests that each stage must be achieved sequentially or else one has not grieved well. To this end, misunderstanding or misinterpretation of the models implies to caregivers that all who grieve should experience each stage/phase, all the reactions contained therein must occur in a neat chronological order, and individuals progress toward an ending, completion, or resolution of the grief. If this is not accomplished, the individual has grieved poorly or has not adjusted to the loss. Figure 26-2 summarizes successful and unsuccessful directions of grieving.

Current concepts about grief recognize that it is not rigidly structured and is without a predictable pattern of responses. Some responses to grief occur internally and are not visible, whereas other aspects of grief may not occur at all. From Gorer's work (1965) the following styles of grief were identified by their length of time: (1) little or no grief—inclusive of denial and absence of grief, anticipatory

grief, and hidden grief; (2) time-limited grief—intense grief followed by a return to the pregrief state; (3) unlimited grief—"I'll never get over this," suggestive of a continuing grief that does not interfere appreciably with daily life; and (4) mummification—the making of a shrine of the deceased's room, indicative of never-ending, deeply painful grief.

Taking Gorer's unlimited grief and expanding on that premise, current thought suggests a newer model that looks at reactions or tasks rather than stages. Worden (1991) modified previous perspectives by offering tasks of grieving. These tasks require (1) accepting the reality of the loss; (2) working through the pain (both physical and emotional, as well as behavioral pain), the intensity of which will vary with the individual; (3) adjusting to a change in environment; and (4) emotionally relocating the deceased and moving on with life. Doka (1993) added a fifth task, spiritual, to rebuild faith and philosophical systems that challenge loss.

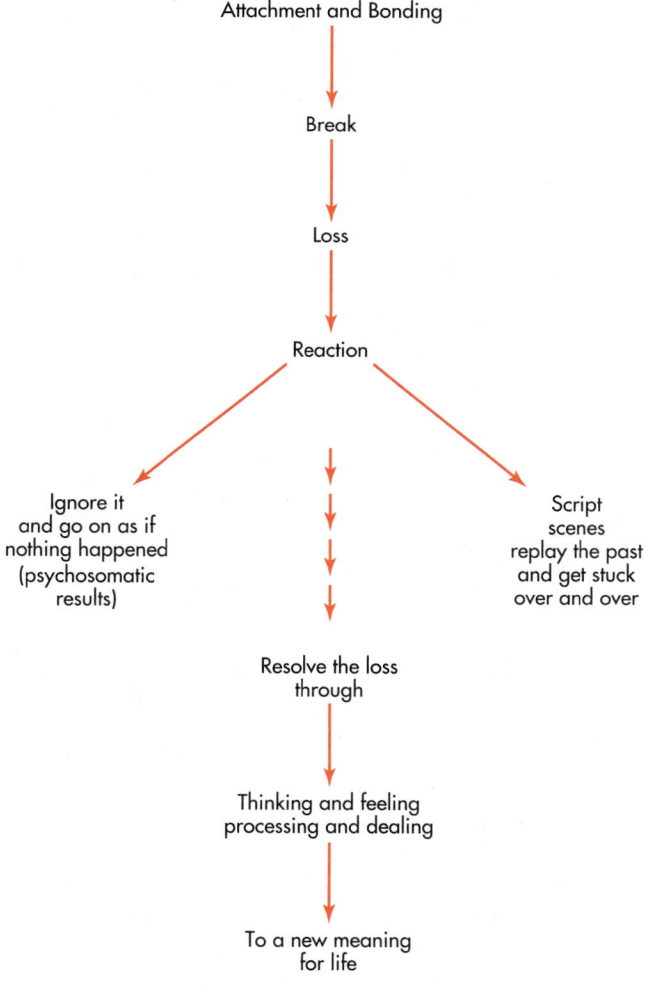

Figure 26-2. Progression through grief.

Accepting the reality of the loss can be measured by the use of present or past references to the dead. The individual "is" or "was."

Working through the pain, while individual, requires that there is a support network for the individual who is bereaved. The danger in this particular task of mourning is the potential for the misuse of pain killers such as alcohol or prescription and nonprescription drugs. *The pain needs to be experienced, not deadened.*

Adjusting to a changed environment may take a considerable period of time, especially if the relationship with the deceased had been a long and close one. Changes in the environment may be physical, emotional, and spiritual: rearrangement of furniture, a different seating pattern at the dinner table, or taking a trip at holiday time rather than observing a celebration as it always had been.

The emotional relocation of the deceased and moving on with life produces considerable anxiety. An individual may feel that this is a dishonor to the dead. They may develop a high degree of anxiety about investing emotional energy in other relationships (a letting go of former attachments). It is important to impart to the mourner that letting go does not mean that the individual loved the deceased any less but that there are also others still to be loved. This is also true with other losses: there are new avenues to explore.

Modernistic or Romanticistic Approaches

The modernistic and romanticistic approaches to grief have been offered by Stroebe et al (1992). They suggest that there is a romanticistic and a modernistic approach to grief. The modernistic approach proposes that there are specific stages or steps to the grieving process that everyone must go through to become whole again. In addition, the focus of life in Western society is to be direct, efficient, and rational. In short, *functionality is the key essential in Western society.* Therefore, when grief occurs, people need or are expected to recover from their intense feelings (grief) and return to normal function and effectiveness as quickly as possible. The theories of Lindeman (1944), Engel (1967), Bowlby (1969), and others suggest this and the relinquishing of the ties that bind one to the dead. Grief is seen as debilitating and an interference with daily routine.

This is clearly evident in the workplace when death occurs. An individual is given a short period of time away from the job but is expected to return and function normally; anything less is an impediment to the smooth workings of the organization in which the individual is employed. One has often heard others say, "snap out of it," "life goes on." The same applies to the aged whether they work or not; functionality is expected rather quickly. What often occurs is that individuals publicly appear to have resolved their grief, but in the privacy of their own environment, behind closed doors, they continue to grieve, often with little support.

The romanticistic perspective of the grief response facilitates the maintenance of bonds with the dead. It represents fidelity of memories and the essence of the relationship. Ties are deeper than death. To grieve shows everyone the significance of the relationship and the depth of one's spirit. To dissolve the bonds indicates the superficiality of the relationship and denies one's self-worth and suggests the relationship was a sham. Evidence of romanticistic grief is expressed in the naming of a child after one who has died as a way of bringing back or perpetuating the deceased. Reference to a reunion in heaven implies a continual wish to resume contact. Wishes of the deceased often guide one's actions and decisions, and seances or spiritual mediums are sought, in the hope of remaining in spiritual contact with the dead.

This approach to grief would cause the followers of the modernistic point of view to question the normalcy or emotional adequacy of the grieving process of the person who exhibited romanticistic beliefs. The grief would suggest aberrant, inadequate, or pathologic grieving, thus making an unproblematic response to grief problematic. Modernistic thought does not seem to facilitate cultural differences in the grief process.

Contemporary studies show grief resolution to be more complex than just letting go and moving on with life. Examples of ongoing attachments (which to some would be labeled as unhealthy or problematic) are pilgrimages to the Vietnam War Memorial, the Wailing Wall, and to family grave sites. Each year individuals visit the Vietnam War Memorial in Washington, DC, to remember and leave items that connect them to the their deceased. Similarly, individuals make pilgrimages to the Wailing Wall in Jerusalem, praying and placing little prayer papers in the crevices of the wall. Other cultures, at least once a year, visit the grave of their family to clean the grave, leave food, and commune with their dead relatives.

Perhaps integration of both modernistic and romanticistic approaches would be more desirable or appropriate. This would allow for an internal dialogue and respect for culturally imbedded practices. One could then deal with unfinished business, reflect on the relationship, and prepare for the future.

Postmodern Era

Today we live in what is being called a postmodern era (DeSpelder and Strickland, 1995). Awareness of the entire experience of the human race heretofore was not available to previous generations. This postmodern influence is reflected in social, political, lifestyle, and art expression. It opens the possibilities to select ideas from all historical periods and cultures.

In light of the opposite thoughts on the approaches to grieving, it is important to also consider the appropriate therapies. Rather than strict adherence to modernistic or romanticistic dictums, the expression of grief needs to move toward growth, flexibility, and appropriateness within the cultural context.

The newest interpretation of grief and grief work is a conceptual approach offered by Solari-Twadell et al (1995) called the pinwheel model of bereavement. Grieving is seen as a dynamic process, the central theme or core being the personal history of the griever. This history is surrounded by the care themes: (1) being stopped, (2) pain and hurting, (3) missing, (4) holding, (5) seeking, and (6) valuing. These care themes are deeply rooted in the inner experience of bereavement. Change, expectations, and inexpressibility rotate around the core of inner experiences. The unique, individually lived loss experience with its subsequent grief is symbolized by the pinwheel. Figure 26-3 illustrates the pinwheel model.

Loss is the "initial wind" that spins the pinwheel. The intensity and power of this wind sets in motion the life-changing process of bereavement. Throughout life the winds of loss will gently stir recurrent episodes of grief through sights, sounds, smells, anniversary dates, and other triggers. The arms of the pinwheel suggest movement by the be-reaved, reaching out of the circular experience of grief by surrendering. Surrendering in the context of this model implies resting or the lowering of one's defenses toward life and being open to reality or the acceptance of the life event through reaching out to others and rejoining life through change. With each gust of wind the grief experience may reoccur.

It is important to remember that *theories are attempts to specify dynamics of the grieving process. They are helpful to our understanding of grief, but they should not be imposed on the survivor. Thus there are similarities and differences: the behavior is the same, but the process is explained differently.*

TYPES OF GRIEF

There are several types of grief that need to be addressed briefly. These include acute grief, chronic grief, anticipatory grief, and disenfranchised grief.

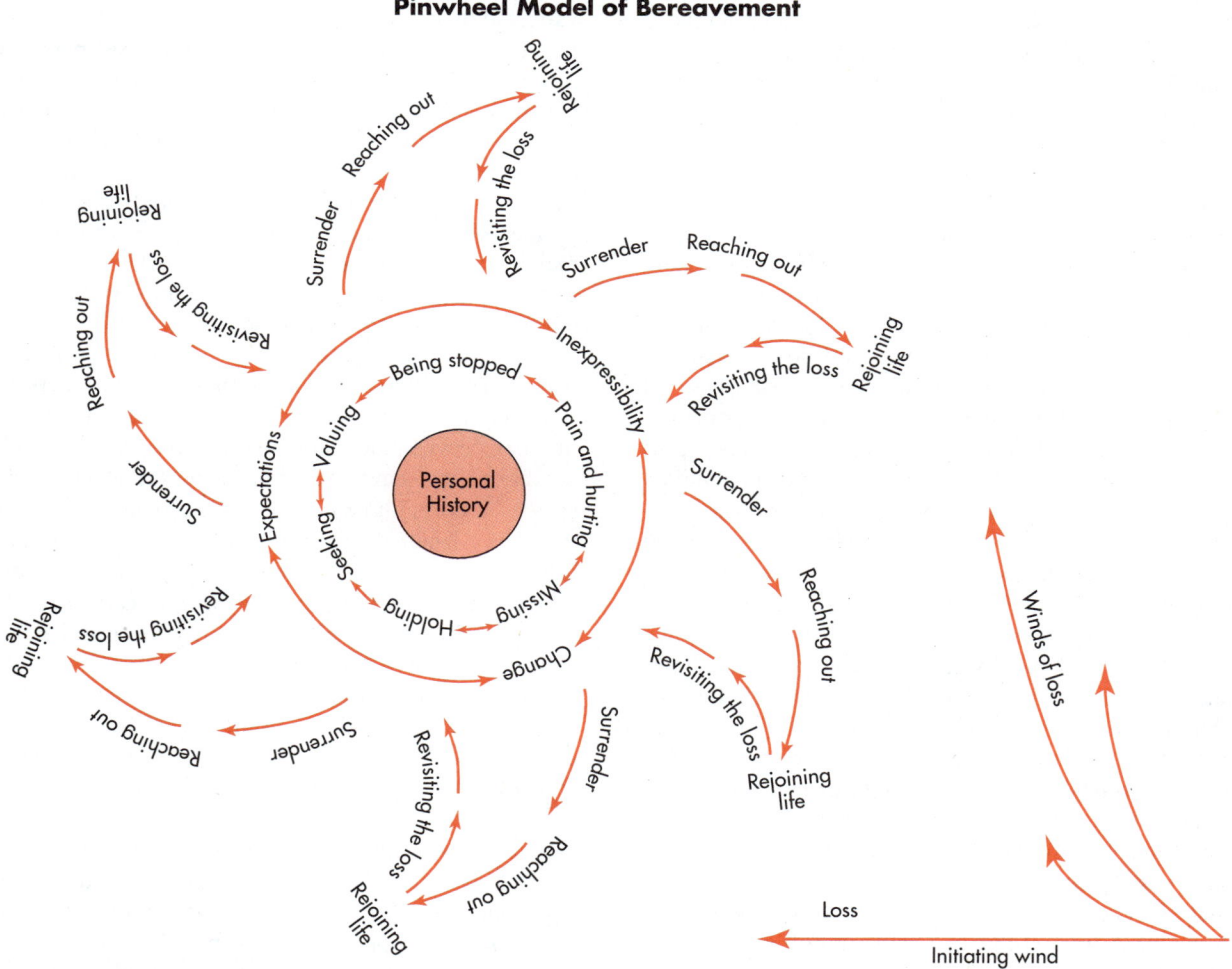

Pinwheel Model of Bereavement

Figure 26-3. Pinwheel model of bereavement. (From Solari-Twadell PA, Schmidt-Bunkers S, Wang CE, Snyder D: The pinwheel model of bereavement, *Image J Nurs Sch* 27[4]:323, 1995.)

Acute grief is like a crisis, lasting approximately 4 to 6 weeks. Acute grief has a definite syndrome. Various theorists have identified somatic symptoms of distress that occur in waves lasting varying periods of time, usually 20 minutes to 1 hour. These symptoms occur every time the loss is acknowledged. Preoccupation with the image (of the deceased, as well as a loss of body function or loss by relocation) is a phenomenon similar to daydreaming and is accompanied by a sense of unreality. Feelings of self-blame or guilt, are often present. These feelings of guilt may remain unstated, or a verbalized attempt is made to seek validation. Hostility or anger toward usual friendships may occur as a result of the griever's inner struggle. The lack of warmth toward others is another internal struggle that also occurs. Outward behavior may be stiff or formal in interactions with persons with whom the griever was previously relaxed socially.

People usually have typical ways of accomplishing activities of daily living, tasks, and responsibilities. The distraction and restlessness created by acute grief causes feelings of being at "loose ends." Motivation and zest disappear; tasks and activities take considerable effort to accomplish. Activities such as dressing that normally took 30 minutes now may take hours, and every moment may seem exhausting. The griever becomes overwhelmed with ordinary decisions and activities that have to be performed. These feelings and behaviors are considered loss of patterns of conduct.

Anticipatory grief is the response to a real or perceived loss before it occurs . One observes this grief in preparation for potential loss of belongings, friends moving away, and knowing that a body part or function is going to change. It is also evident when a person anticipates the loss of a spouse through death. In a sense it is insulation against what will be, a dress rehearsal for the actual event that is destined to occur. Behaviors similar to acute grief are experienced, including preoccupation with the particular loss and anticipation of the mode of adjustment that might be necessary.

Futterman et al (1972) conceptualized anticipatory grief as having five functionally related aspects: (1) acknowledgment—convinced the inevitable will occur; (2) grieving—experiencing and expressing the emotional impact of the anticipated loss and the physical, psychologic, and interpersonal turmoil associated with it; (3) reconciliation of the situation; (4) detachment—withdrawal of the emotional investment from the situation; and (5) memorialization—developing a relatively fixed conscious mental representation of that which will be lost. One frequently sees the struggle of anticipatory grief in families with elders who have been diagnosed with Alzheimer's.

There are negative aspects of anticipatory grief that should be mentioned. If the loss does not occur when or as expected, those awaiting the actual loss or death may become hostile and impatient. In the event of a relocation, individuals may become angry or hostile toward the agency,

institution, or others who are responsible for the delay. Anticipatory grief can result in premature detachment from an individual who is dying. If there is premature detachment, it prevents the family or others from reinvesting in the dying individual. This is known as the Lazarus syndrome. It may deprive family and friends from a final close relationship and prevent resolution of unfinished business.

Researchers have found that grief after anticipatory grief is no less painful than unanticipated loss, but it does allow for less of an assault on the mourner's adaptive capacity (Parks and Weiss, 1983). It has sometimes been assumed that anticipatory grief work among widows helped them adjust to bereavement when the spouse died. Studies by Dessonville et al (1983) revealed that expectancy of death was not related to adjustment to bereavement. Further rehearsal for the role of widowhood was not related to better adjustment and in some cases was actually associated with a poor adjustment (see additional discussion in Chapter 20). Anticipatory grief, then, can be helpful or harmful to the griever but is recognized as a legitimate phenomenon.

Disenfranchised grief is grief that is not recognized or validated by others. This type of grief occurs when the relationship between the mourner and the dead person is not recognized or the griever is not recognized by others. This has frequently been associated with domestic partnerships in which the family of the deceased does not acknowledge the partner of the dead person. It can also occur in the "black sheep" of the family in situations of family discord, in family members who have not provided support to other family members who cared for the individual who has died, or in a participant in secret trysts, where the involved party cannot tell others of the strong relationship.

The aged can experience this disenfranchisement when persons associated and close to them do not understand the full meaning of a retiree's retirement, the impact of the death of a pet, or when there are gradual losses caused by chronic conditions that have great impact on the elder but are not seen as important to others. Families coping with a member who has Alzheimer's may also experience disenfranchised grief, particularly when others perceive death of the elder as a blessing but fail to support the griever/caregiver who has struggled for years with anticipatory grief and now must cope with the actual death.

Chronic grief has often been called impaired, pathologic, abnormal, or maladaptive grief. It has been thought that chronic grief begins with normal grief responses, but obstacles occur that interfere with the normal evolution of grieving. Where there should be normal responses, there are exaggerated responses. This type of grief may be fostered by the lack of social involvement with others. Individuals who live alone, socialize little, and have few close friends or have an ineffective support network will be more at risk for chronic grief. Issues of guilt, anger, and ambivalence toward the individual who has died are factors that will impede the grieving process until they are resolved. Behaviors such as irrational anger, social outbursts, and insomnia that linger for an extended time or surface months or years later, or the appearance of mental or physical ailments should be suspected as potential inability to grieve in a healthy, constructive manner. Other behaviors describe maladaptive grief, depending on the interpretation applied to them. This type of grief requires professional intervention of a clinical nurse specialist or hospice nurse trained to deal with it or a psychologist or psychiatrist. Guidelines for psychotherapy for bereaved older adults appears in Box 26-2.

GRIEF WORK

The process or experience of mourning takes time, much longer than any one anticipates. The pangs of grief continue for years, even though the intensity and the resurgence of the grief may become less frequent. In loss by death it is not unusual for grief to remain with us. Lund et al (1986) and Arbuckle and deVries (1995) demonstrated that older widows' and widowers' grief is not completed or ended in the prescribed period of time usually considered for grief completion. Horacek (1991) referred to this lingering grief (a form of chronic grief) as *shadow grief*. It may inhibit some normal activity but may be a common response that is not thought to be abnormal. The pain of grief is often exacerbated on anniversary dates (birthdays, holidays, and wedding anniversaries). Grieving or mourning is often viewed as a "weakness," a self-indulgence, a reprehensible bad habit rather than a psychologic necessity (Parks, 1972).

Grief work takes enormous amounts of physical and emotional energy. It is the hardest work anyone can do. All cultures seem to observe a certain set of behaviors after death, but there do not appear to be a set of behaviors when the loss is of another type. For example, an individual who is seriously ill, who is moved from his or her home (or loses the home), who retires willingly (or is forced to retire), may not realize that feelings being experienced and behaviors displayed in the weeks that follow are natural and normal responses to loss. In most instances the individual is labeled "depressed" rather than grieving. The essential point is that after any significant loss or change some degree of grief and grief work will occur.

Grief for the older adult may be longer than others might expect. Confusion, depression, preoccupation with thoughts of the deceased may be mistaken for other conditions as dementia, deterioration, or depression. Initially there may be positive feelings about the ability to cope, but over time the grief response may be exhibited. An attempt to get the older person into routine activities too soon after a significant loss may complicate the grieving process rather than help it.

Multiple loss experiences through acute and chronic illness may be superimposed on relocation, a shrinking support network, economic changes, and role change. This can lead to a continual state of grieving, known as bereavement overload. No sooner has the individual begun to grieve for

Box 26-2	**Guidelines for Psychotherapy for the Bereaved Older Adult**

Permit and help the patient to put into words and nonverbal expression the pain, sorrow, and finality of bereavement.

Review the relationship of the patient with the decreased, i.e., a life history approach.

Encourage the patient to discuss feelings of love, guilt, and hostility toward the deceased.

Help the patient recognize the alterations in cognition, affect, and behavior secondary to bereavement.

Work with the patient to find an acceptable balance for the future incorporated memory of the deceased.

Avoid interpretations of long-dormant, highly charged intrapsychic conflicts.

Support existing coping mechanisms.

Reassure the patient that the intense suffering and pain are transient.

Allow a positive, even parental transference to evolve.

Facilitate the transfer of dependency from the deceased to other sources of gratification when necessary.

Decrease sessions with the patient on improvement but avoid abrupt termination.

one loss than another occurs and so forth. An individual must grieve one loss before he or she can go on to grieve the next.

Grief Assessment

Mortality of the bereaved during the first year of mourning is greater than for those who have not experienced a loss through death. Rees and Lukin (1967) found the mortality rate of the aged surviving spouse to be 7 times greater than the average population. A higher mortality rate for widowed males after the age of 75 was also noted by Bowling (1989). Another concern is that diseases such as cancer, ulcerative colitis, asthma, congestive heart failure, leukemia, and diabetes may develop or exacerbate during this time (Carr and Schoenberg, 1970). Mittleman (1996) found that heart attack risk was 5 times higher than normal 2 days after the death of a significant person and remained elevated for about a month following the death. Pietruszka (1992) notes that bereaved elders may present clinical symptoms that mimic the signs and symptoms of serious medical and psychologic conditions and present a diagnostic challenge to primary care providers. Therefore to anticipate the problems that grief may precipitate, it is important to do a grief assessment.

Assessment is based on knowledge of the grieving process and the subsequent mourning. Data are obtained through observation of behavior of the individual elder, keeping in mind cultural context. Questions should include losses and gains that have occurred within the past year (gains also bring with them some losses), strengths the aged person brings to the situation, what the person values in life, and how grief is unique to the individual. These will help the nurse to develop a plan with the older person that will facilitate physiologic and psychologic manifestations of grieving, regardless of whether they are transient or continuing. Inherent in developing intervention strategies is knowledge about the elder's coping mechanisms (effective and ineffective) and support systems upon which he or she can rely. Box 26-3 provides physical, psychologic, and social factors that influence grieving.

A risk factor profile for bereaved spouses was developed by Steele (1992) to identify persons whose behaviors are suggestive of risk for physical or emotional disturbances due to the loss of a loved one. For example, a 70-year-old, middle class, female widow might exhibit despair/optimism, loss of vigor, depersonalization, physical and somatic symptoms, anger, and social isolation (Table 26-1).

Interventions

One of the goals of intervention is to assist the individual (or family) attain a healthy adjustment to the loss experience. Actions that can meet this goal are basic and simple; however, the emotional overlay makes the simple often difficult. For the nurse who is confronted with a person's grief for the first time, there is intense discomfort, fear, and insecurity.

The tendency is to be sympathetic rather than empathetic. Questions arise in one's mind: What do I say? Should I be cheerful or serious? Should I talk about or even mention the dead person's name?

The nurse requires four strengths to help someone cope with grief. First, the nurse must have spiritual strength, or strength from within. This does not mean that the nurse must have a specific religious orientation or affiliation but that the nurse must have a positive belief in self. Second, the nurse must find meaning in life. One needs a philosophy to sustain oneself during difficult times. With age, life experiences grow, and a person's philosophy may change or be amended; but at any particular time, the individual should have a philosophy. Third, the nurse must develop emotional maturity. The individual who has always gotten his or her way will most likely have trouble when confronted with deprivation or loss. Lastly, comfort with one's own mortality is essential for working with loss and grief.

The nurse must be ready to listen. Active listening is an important skill for the nurse who serves as a support person for the griever. It is far easier to give advice on how to solve a problem than it is to allow a grieving person time and space to express feelings.

When listening, the nurse soon discovers that it not the actual loss that is of utmost concern, but the fear associated

---

Box 26-3   Factors Influencing the Grieving Process

Physical
Illness involves numerous losses
Each loss must be identified
Each loss prompts and requires its own grief response
Importance of the loss varies according to meaning by individual
Sedatives—deprive experience of reality of loss that must be faced
Nutritional state—if inadequate, leads to inability to cope or meet demands of daily living, and numerous symptoms caused by grief
Rest—inadequate leads to mental and physical exhaustion, disease, unresolved grief
Exercise—if inadequate, limits emotional outlet, aggressive feelings, tension, anxiety, and leads to depression

Psychologic
Unique nature and meaning of loss
Individual qualities of the relationship
Role body part/self-image/aspect of self was to the individual and/or family
Individual coping behavior, personality, mental health
Individual level of maturity and intelligence

Past experience with loss or death
Social, cultural, ethnic, religious/philosophic background
Sex-role conditioning
Immediate circumstances surrounding loss
Timeliness of the loss
Perception of preventability (sudden vs expected)
Number, type, quality of secondary losses
Presence of concurrent stresses/crises

Specific to Dying/Death (in addition to above)
Role deceased occupied in family or social system
Amount of unfinished business
Perception of deceased's fulfillment in life
Immediate circumstances surrounding death
Length of illness before death
Anticipatory grief and involvement with dying patient

Social
Individual support systems and the acceptance of assistance of its members
Individual sociocultural, ethnic, religious/philosophic background
Educational, economic, occupational status
Ritual

From Beare PG, Myers JL: *Adult health nursing,* ed 3, 1998, Mosby.

with the loss. If the nurse listens carefully to both the stated and the implied, what will be heard may be phrases such as, " How will I go on?" "What will I do now?" "What will become of me?" "I don't know what to do." "How could he (she) do this to me?" Because the nurse knows there is resolution, such statements may seem exaggerated or melodramatic, but to the one who is grieving there seems to be no resolution. The griever cannot yet look ahead and know that the despair and other feelings will resolve. Therefore, in the process of active listening, the nurse will seek to clarify what is said to help the person confront their fears about the future.

It is difficult for the nurse and others to listen to the same thing endlessly repeated, but reminiscing is important to the griever. It allows for the working through of the loss. Reminiscence is a means by which denial can fall by the wayside and allow reality of the loss to filter slowly into the conscious mind. Reminiscence helps the griever acknowledge that indeed the loss is real and that life can go on even though it will be difficult.

Kelly (1992) talks about re-forming one's life story. By incorporating the loss, and putting the deceased into the life story in a new way (re-forming the story), energy can be invested in all other relationships that exist or may come to be. Drawing out anecdotes and vignettes of the relationship help's the griever keep control over the story and over his or her own life. Encourage the griever to talk and tell the story of the relationship as it had been. Keeping the continuity of the presence of the deceased alive gives permission for the griever to feel the presence of the dead in life. Spirituality (mystical, beyond humans) is linked with specific beliefs or religions. This is a basis for faith and religious beliefs. Critical to recovery is the ability of the nurse/caregiver to allow the griever to remain in control. Control is crucial to recovery!

A three point approach that the nurse might employ to facilitate the grieving process is "talk out," "feel out," and "act out."

Talking it out requires active listening when the griever is encouraged to talk about his or her grief and express feelings. When feelings are ventilated or shared with others, the momentary panics, hysteria, and other sensations accompanying the grief are less frightening. The belief that those who are grieving want to be left alone is incorrect; in actuality, it is not the usual desire. The person in grief wants to talk about the loss with people who care.

Feeling it out is a cathartic experience. In many instances it is the nurse who guides the griever to express hurt, anger, crying, etc. The nurse may have to say "It's okay to . . ."—whatever feelings the griever has.

Acting out is a natural extension of feelings. Intense physical activity gives one some control over emotions. Ancients used to rend their clothes or tear their hair. Today, there are numerous ways of acting out feelings from throwing things to taking a walk, to busying oneself with tasks, to

expressing feelings in creative works. In situations where acting out predominates, it is important to provide a safe means of acting out and a safe environment in which to do so to prevent self-harm.

Krohn (in press) suggests that the nurse's role is as an advocate who displays the behavioral qualities of responsiveness, authenticity, commitment, and competence. Table 26-2 correlates caring behaviors with caring actions or interventions.

Outliving those one loves may create an emptiness that can never be fully assuaged. Table 26-3 provides a nursing care plan for survivors, whether the survivor is a spouse, sex partner, friend, companion, or confidant, with suggested interventions. The nurse must be prepared for this most difficult task.

Table 26-1	Risk Factor Profile of Bereaved Spouses
Demographic category	**High-risk bereavement behavior & feelings**
Age	
66-85	Despair
76-85	Denial
	Loss of vigor
Sex	
Female	Depersonalization (shock, numbness, hopelessness)
	Somatization
	Physical symptoms
	Loss of vigor
	Optimism/despair (loss of meaning/ hopelessness)
	Anger/hostility
Male	Guilt
	Social isolation
	Rumination
	Social desirability
Socioeconomic status	
Upper-middle class	Anger/hostility
Lower class	Guilt
	Rumination
	Depersonalization (shock, numbness, confusion)
	Physical symptoms, loss of vigor
Middle class	Optimism/despair
Quality of relationship	
Extremely close to deceased	Guilt
	Rumination
	Depersonalization
	Physical symptoms, loss of vigor, somatic complaints
Somewhat close to deceased	Anger/hostility
	Social isolation
	Optimism/despair

Modified from Steele L: Risk factor profile for bereaved spouses, *Death Studies* 16(5):387, 1992.

Evaluation

As the mourning proceeds toward an integration of the loss, and a new beginning or re-forming of the life story occurs, a change in language used by the bereaved often occurs that is suggestive of progress and growth (Table 26-4).

What is actually helpful to bereaved older persons? Rigdon et al (1987) interviewed 30 older widows to determine the attitudes and actions that they found helpful in coping with grief and that they advised other widows to consider:

- Keep busy; accept and extend social invitations.
- Help someone else.
- Learn to enjoy some solitary activities.
- Accept your own grief process as unique and individual.
- Talk to others and express feelings.
- Have faith in recovery and maintain beliefs.
- Take one day at a time, and do not expect to follow a timetable of recovery.

Often help received is crisis oriented and soon dissipates. Rigdon et al suggest help over time is much needed. Rather than asking, "What can I do?" a person should simply do something. Accompany the bereaved in a new activity or a new situation, and by action invite them toward the building of a new life.

The Newly Bereaved. Crisis intervention with the newly bereaved is commonly provided by nurses, since the majority of deaths occur in the institutional setting and most of these deaths are of the aged. Richter (1987) sought information from newly bereaved persons to determine what nursing actions they found most helpful during the death or immediately thereafter. These data may assist nurses in gaining a clearer perspective of comfort interventions:

- Kept me informed
- Asked how I was doing and offered support
- Put an arm around me when I cried
- Brought me food
- Knew my name
- Cried with me
- Brought a bed and encouraged me to stay in the room with my dying husband
- Told me to hold my husband's hand while he was dying
- Held my hand
- Got the chaplain for me
- Let me take care of my husband
- Stayed with me after their shift was over

Although we do not know the impact of action as related to overall grief recovery, it is clear these events stood out as significant for individuals in their immediate grief. Grief survivors report great variance in the recovery process and deeply resent a professional's efforts to hurry them through it. Even other widows can be a source of distress when imposing their timetable on a grieving widow. The lesson for nurses is to accept whatever the individual is experiencing

Table 26-2	Caring Behaviors
Behavior	**Caring Action**
Advocacy	Extend oneself to find proper help
	Work to grant reasonable requests
Authenticity	Sharing feelings appropriately
	Honesty
	Use of healing
	Touch
Responsiveness	Be available
	Interact verbally
	Provide comfort
	Provide privacy
	Be nonjudgemental
Committment and presence	Provide the little extras
	Grooming
	Quiet for talking
	Time
	Presence
Competence	Perform tasks consistently
	Radiate self-assurance in care giving
	Teach simply and completely
Give positive meaning to another's life	Listen
	Touch
	Point out reactions to family
	Praise when appropriate
	Help them gain a sense of control

From Krohn B: When death is near, *Geriatr Nurs* (in press).

and exert extreme caution in urging the person to "get going."

Dysfunctional grief can be assessed only holistically. Is the individual able to maintain self-care? Is the person reaching out to others? Does the individual have a hope for recovery? Is the person searching for meaning in the event? Gass (1987) found that widows using the greatest number of resources were more functional. Caserta and Lund (1993) found that one's intrapersonal resources had more of an impact in reducing negative effects of spousal bereavement among older adults. Self-help groups seemed to assist those who did not possess the intrapersonal skills helping them toward self-esteem and an optimistic meaningful outlook.

Effects of Grief on Sexuality. The absence of a sexual partner following the death of a spouse temporarily cancels an important expressive role of feelings of femininity or masculinity. The intimacy and closeness of a mate provide strong self-affirmation. The loss of this important role results in asexuality for many of the old. Seldom are they thought to be full sexual beings even when married. When widowed, most older women are effectively neutered. Men may seek and find new sexual partners but are vulnerable to "widower's impotence," a result of guilt, depression, long periods of abstinence from sexual activity, and the strangeness of a new sexual partner. All of these factors may hinder an aged man from consummating a new marriage.

Grief and Gender Differences. Three of four women

Table 26-3   Nursing Care Plan for Survivors

Nursing diagnosis	Expected outcomes	Interventions

Depression, loneliness, social isolation related to loss of spouse, sexual partner, friend, companion, or confidant

Manifestations: teariness, crying, sleep disturbance, weight gain, compulsive eating, weight loss, anorexia, fatigue, confusion, forgetfulness, withdrawal, disinterest, indecisiveness, inability to concentrate, guilt feelings; displays feelings of detachment, inferiority, rejection, alienation, emptiness, isolation; unable to initiate social contacts; seeks attention	*Short-term/intermediate goals:* The survivor will: Develop or use immediate support systems; Express feelings of security; Exhibit meaningful social relationships; Show decreasing signs of depression. *Long-term goal:* The survivor will demonstrate readiness to build a new life as a single person.	Attempt to develop a therapeutic relationship through touch, empathy, and listening. Listen to perceived feelings. Help person realize that grief is a painful but normal transitional process. Encourage use of other women, daughters, widows, men, and friends as support systems. Encourage balance between linking phenomena (mementos, photographs, clothes, furniture) associated with the deceased and the bridging phenomena (new driving skills, evening classes, new job). Establish contact with Widow to Widow Program for counseling if appropriate. Refer to appropriate agencies.

Anxiety related to increased legal, financial, and decision-making responsibilities

Manifestations: anger, nervousness, palpitations, increased perspiration, face flushing, dyspnea, urinary frequency, nausea, vomiting, restlessness, apprehension, panic, fear, headache	*Short-term/intermediate goals:* The survivor will demonstrate adequate decision-making skills in financial and legal matters as evidenced by: Seeking legal aid; Writing or calling appropriate agencies; Formulating a realistic budget. *Long-term goals:* The survivor will: Cope with legal, financial, and decision-making responsibilities with only a moderate degree of anxiety; Make rational decisions about single life.	Assist in obtaining attorney if necessary. Encourage to contact Social Security and/or spouse's employer to assure receipt of all benefits. Encourage to contact insurance agencies if applicable. Discourage immediate decision making regarding assets (e.g., home, stocks, etc.). Encourage to seek advice from individuals who are trusted. Contact proper social agencies if indigent or in need. Assist in seeking employment if health permits and client so desires. Offer alternatives for decision making. Refer to any other proper community agencies that offer needed assistance.

From Alexander J, Kiely J: Working with the bereaved, *Geriatr Nurs* 7(2):85, 1986.

will be widowed at one time or other due to women living longer and frequently marrying older men. It has been suggested that widowhood is less difficult for women than retirement is for men because there are other widows with whom to share leisure time and activities. In many instances, a woman's status increases with widowhood, whereas a man's decreases with retirement (DeSpeleder and Strickland, 1996).

The abundance of literature on bereavement, loss, and mourning sheds little light on the bereavement of men, particularly in spousal loss where males are the survivors. The assumption is that men are less emotionally involved in the conjugal relationship than women and therefore less likely to grieve or express their grief. This was found not to be true (Brabants, Forsyth and Melanon, 1992). Evidence showed that men hurt and knew they hurt but did not reach out to others for help. The magnitude of the loss was felt in hurt, pain, and anger. Men also carried deep lasting attachments to the deceased spouse (Schreck, 1993).

Coping with the Death of a Child. It is often thought the death of an adult child may be the most difficult grief an elder must bear. A small study of 12 Jewish and 17 non-Jewish elders whose child died seemed to indicate that the Jewish women accepted and went on with their lives (Goodman et al, 1991). Although we question this interpretation, the study points out that the manner in which one integrates the death of a child has to do with the centrality of that child to one's existence, the ability to express grief, aspects of generativity in the lifestyle, and general health and well-being.

Grief and Sibling Death. Death of siblings are particularly hard to integrate because the close affiliation and identification threaten one's mortality to a greater degree

Table 26-4   Language Changes as a Function of Growth after Loss

Before	After
Function/cope/survive	Grow/discover/live
Adjust	Center/balance
Control	Flow with
Pain	Hurt
Pain/illness as negative	Hurt/illness as a sign/signal
Enduring	Reliable
Anxiety (diffuse)	Scared (focused)
Guilt as responsible	Guilt as not fulfilling
Loneliness	Solitude/aloneness
Explain/judge	Understand
Expectations	Wants
Hopelessness	Discouraging
Problems	Challenges
Winning	Succeeding
Time as past, now, or future	Time as a continuum, a flow
Losing	Not realizing potential
Mistake, error	Limited awareness
Assume	Question, reformulate
Tragedy	Tragic opportunity
Pathology	Natural healing/restoration
Responsibility	Awareness of consequences
Symptoms	Reminders
Specialized	Balanced
Search for meaningful existence, happiness	Search for wholeness
Peak or "peek" experience	Fulfilling awareness
Awareness of limits & strengths	Awareness of potential
What is probable	What is possible
Helplessness = weakness, incompetence	Helplessness = a sometimes condition of being alive
Positive or negative feelings	Feelings are signs of being alive
Operate "as if" immortal or in mortal fear of death	Operate "as if" death can occur at any time but without fear or without self-fulfilling prophecies
Death as failure, tragedy, termination, the ultimate loss	Death as transition
Self = individual physical being who is sometimes social & sometimes solitary, but clearly separate from other individuals	Self = all things which have significance for the individual

Developed by Sisneros J for N112, San Francisco State University School of Nursing, 1994.

than most relationships. In addition, the death of each sibling removes one more member from childhood, those who can confirm youth and energy (Moyers, 1992). On the other hand, the first sibling who dies may teach the others more about death and coping.

Bereavement as a Growth Opportunity.   Survivor coping ability improves when there is awareness that death and bereavement can lead to growth. A change in thinking from

limits to potential, from coping to growth, from problems to challenges are perceptual mind sets that help move one toward growth. Resolution of loss and working through the grief provide incentives enabling possible important life changes. Transformation from intense focus on self-awareness evolves into a new sense of identity. The loss is placed within the context of growth and life cycles: the lost relationship is changed not ended. By turning to the inner resources, creativity arises from the experience of grief. Table 26-4 lists the transformation of language used prior to loss (if dying is occurring) or early in bereavement and the terms used later in the bereavement process with the resolution of the loss.

THE PROCESS OF DYING
The Nature of Dying

Dying is the most challenging of life experiences and a very individual and private one. Most of all, dying is coming to terms with being alone. How one reacts to extreme stress, bad news, disappointment, loss, or change governs attitudes and coping with dying. An individual's coping patterns and personality are established early in life, thus most people die as they have lived.

The dying of young and middle-aged persons is perceived as tragic, a loss of a not fully lived life. Dying and death of an aged person is frequently regarded as a blessing, a culmination of a full and rich life. That of course is presumptive! Many aged have not fulfilled their lives, nor are they ready to die. The dying process for one of advanced years can be a period of positive forward movement, a time of fulfillment and growth, *a completion of life orchestrated by the individual* with support, understanding, and assistance of those around him or her.

Elders seek to make sense of their lives in the face of impending death. The remaining time may become a time of life review or a time to try and repair former failures, such as resolution of parent-child or sibling-sibling conflict or completing a task that has been left undone.

The Dying Process

Dying may take weeks, months, or years and can be anticipated, in some instances predicted. For the aged dying often arises from degenerative diseases typical of mortality in our society. However, the dynamics of experiencing dying vary greatly based on age, experiences, and culture.

The literature on coping with terminal illness and dying has appeared over a 20-year period from the 1960s to the 1980s, during which time stages and phases associated with dying were identified. As with the grieving process, the descriptions or expectations were linear structured progressions. The literature is replete with different yet similar variations of the dying process. Persons use these frameworks often as a panacea for dealing with the dying. These stage-based approaches lead to obstacles stereotyping the individual when the person is vulnerable and is coping with dying.

Health professionals should not force the terminally ill into preestablished stages; rather they should take into account the experiences of the individual (Lindley, 1991). The previously established works provide a useful vehicle to facilitate sharing of information about dying.

The benchmark work of Kübler-Ross (1969) focused on untimely dying and death. Those in her study were mainly middle-aged, confronted with an abrupt cessation of their careers, relationships, and tasks that had been planned. The framework continues to suggest a cognitive grid or guideline of possible moods and coping mechanisms, but it does not provide direction for interventions that would be helpful to a caregiver trying to support the dying individual. In addition, most of the research studies on dying were not focused on the aged. Retsinas (1988) points out that model responses such as Kübler-Ross might not be appropriate for the aged because the aged have completed many of the developmental tasks ascribed to adulthood and advanced age.

Keleman (1974) incorporated Kübler-Ross's anger, denial, and bargaining into the first of his three phases of the dying process. These phases were the resistive phase; the review phase, which dealt with unfinished business and the reclaiming of a part of the self by becoming more in tune with the present rather than the past; and the unconscious phase, in which the individual talked about their dying with calm and which is comparable to acceptance.

Corr (1993) suggests three concepts that can be gleaned from the previous interpretations of the dying process, especially that of Kübler-Ross: those who are coping with dying are still living and often have unfinished needs that must be addressed; one cannot become an effective provider of care without listening actively to those who are coping with dying and identifing with them and their needs; and finally, one needs to learn from those who are dying and coping with dying in order to come to know oneself better. Corr also points out that there are more than five ways in which individuals cope with anything as fundamental as dying. People cope with living and dying in more varied and individualistic ways. One should not assume that the five stages or types of coping are somehow obligatory or prescriptive in how one must or should cope with dying. Insistence on the individual dying in a particular way, considered to be the correct way by others, imposes additional external burdens on the one who is dying.

It is suggested that any approach to coping with dying should consider a basic understanding of all dimensions and all of the individuals involved. The approach should foster empowerment by emphasizing the options available while they live on, emphasize participation or shared aspects of coping with dying (interpersonal network), and provide guidance for care providers and helpers. To date, there is no such model.

Corr (1995) proffers a task-based concept that addresses coping with dying from an individual's own perspective and with coping tasks grounded in situational tasks that are fundamental markers of human living. The dimensions of coping—physical, psychologic, social, and spiritual—

each have a specific function and afford development of interventions.

The physical realm addresses satisfaction of bodily needs and minimization of physical distress in ways that are consistent with other values. These needs include nutrition, hydration, elimination, and shelter. Maslow also considers these as fundamental. Pain, nausea, vomiting, and constipation are among the physical distresses that must be managed. The physical dimension is extremely important because there still remains inadequate understanding of the management of pain and other symptoms, misplaced fear of addiction, overemphasis on cure, fear of failure, concern about one's own mortality (caregiver's), and feelings of frustration and inadequacy in the presence of dying.

The psychologic dimension promotes three features: freedom from anxiety, fear and apprehension; autonomy (security); and self-governance or control of one's life (often supported by others) and the texture of one's life that makes it satisfying or bountiful, such as serenity, activity, creativity, and risk or danger (richness).

Relationships with others and society as a whole are the two aspects of the social dimension. Relationships with others—individuals or groups—sustains and enhances interpersonal attachments. Significant ties continue, others fall by the wayside as death nears. These relationships are ones that the dying person feels are important, not those that others think are important. No matter how much individuals think that they are alone, they are connected to society as a whole through family, culture, congregations, and governmental entities. The dying individual may need to call upon these resources at some point.

The spiritual dimension from which one draws spiritual vigor and vitality is dependent on the individual's fundamental values and moral commitments of acceptance, reconciliation, self-worth, meaning, and purpose in living. The latter is reflective of Erickson's integrity or wholeness (1963). The spirituality may be formal or informal religiosity, or it may be a life-review or both. Hope is a key element in coping. Hope involves faith and trust, which may or may not have a religious basis. Hope may be related to a cure, a holiday, the birth of a grandchild, or reconciliation. What the definition of hope is to the dying individual requires one to listen carefully and identify what the meaning of life is to him or her.

Based on task analysis, Corr (1993, 1995), Doka (1993), and Coolican et al (1994) focused on living with life-threatening illness and developed tasks that address the initial diagnosis, the living-dying interval, recovery or death, and the aftermath. These tasks confront general issues and acute, chronic, and terminal phases of the life-death cycle (Table 26-5).

Much of what Corr, Doka, and Coolican et al offer elaborates on the living-dying trajectory of Pattison (1967). The trajectory explains patterns of coping with a diagnosis of a terminal illness that abruptly confronts an individual. Pattison describes this as a crisis.

Living While Dying. The time between the diagnosis and the point of death is the living-dying interval, composed of acute, chronic, and terminal phases. Science may extend the length of terminal illness for a number of years, thus lengthening the living-dying interval.

The acute phase is associated with recent diagnosis of the terminal illness and is usually the peak time of crisis because there is great uncertainty. Crisis intervention is most effective here because the individual, family, and caregivers are struggling to come to terms with impending death. Impending death or the chronic living-dying phase, a segment of the trajectory, is a time when work-activity patterns, entertainment, and relationships should be maintained as normally as lifestyle permits. Martocchio (1982) describes patterns of living-dying as peaks and valleys, descending plateaus, and downward slopes. The patterns may be singular or in combination and may or may not be related to the pathology of the disease. The terminal phase is ushered in by withdrawal or turning away from the outside world in response to internal body signals that tell the dying person to conserve energy.

The dying process affects all involved. Glaser and Strauss (1963) observed a process of interactional dynam-

ics between those who are terminally ill, family, friends, and health professionals that still can be observed today. The interactions identified are closed awareness, suspicious or suspect awareness, mutual pretense, and open awareness.

Closed awareness is described as "keep the secret." Medical personnel and the family know that the patient will die prematurely, but the patient does not know it. Generally caregivers invent a fictitious future for the patient to believe in, in hopes that it will boost the patient's morale.

In *suspicious awareness,* the patient suspects that he or she is going to die. Hints are bandied back and forth, and a contest ensues for control of the information. In truth, the patient wants his suspicions to be wrong.

Mutual pretense is basically called "let's pretend." Everyone knows the patient has a terminal illness and will die, but neither the patient, family, friends, or medical personnel talk about it—real feelings are kept hidden. *Open awareness* acknowledges the reality of approaching death. The patient, family, friends, and medical staff openly acknowledge the eventual death of the patient. The patient may ask, "Will I die?" and "How and when will I die?" The

---

Table 26-5   Tasks in Life-Threatening Illness

General	Acute phase	Chronic phase	Terminal phase
1. Responding to the physical fact of disease	1. Understanding the disease	1. Managing symptoms and side-effects	1. Dealing with symptoms, discomfort, pain, and incapacitation
2. Taking steps to cope with the reality of disease	2. Maximizing health and lifestyle	2. Carrying out health regimens	2. Managing health procedures and institutional stress
3. Preserving self-concept and relationships with others in the face of disease	3. Maximizing one's coping strengths and limiting weaknesses	3. Preventing and managing health crisis	3. Managing stress and examining coping
4. Dealing with effective and existential/spiritual issues created or reactivated by the disease	4. Developing strategies to deal with the issues created by the disease	4. Managing stress and examining coping	4. Dealing effectively with care givers
	5. Exploring the effect of the diagnosis on a sense of self and others	5. Maximizing social support and minimizing isolation	5. Preparing for death and saying goodbye
	6. Ventilating feelings and fears	6. Normalizing life in the face of the disease	6. Preserving self-concept
	7. Incorporating the present reality of diagnosis into one's sense of past and future	7. Dealing with financial concerns	7. Preserving appropriate relationships with family and friends
		8. Preserving self-concept	8. Ventilating feelings and fears
		9. Redefining relationships with others throughout the course of the disease	9. Finding meaning in life and death
		10. Ventilating feelings and fears	
		11. Finding meaning in suffering chronicity, uncertainty and decline	

From Coolican MB, Stark J, Doka KJ, Corr CA: Education about death, dying, and bereavement in nursing programs, *Nurs Educa* 19(6):38, 1994.

patient becomes resigned to dying, and the family grieves with the patient rather than for the patient.

NURSING THE DYING

In reviewing the literature, a major question arises: When is an aged person dying? The consensus is that physical deterioration is the prime indicator of dying. The less visible, subtle, and frequently misinterpreted indications of an aged person's terminal process are based on psychologic clues. The aged individual without perceptible physical changes that indicate dying may have a sudden and abrupt change in thought or behavior. Coded communication such as saying good-bye instead of the usual good night, giving away cherished possessions as gifts, urgently contacting friends and relatives with whom the person has not communicated for a long time, and direct or symbolic premonitions that death is near are indications that the aged individual is approaching or is experiencing death. Anxiety, depression, restlessness,

and agitation are behaviors frequently categorized as manifestations of confusion or dementia but in reality may be responses to the inability to express feelings of foreboding and a sense of life escaping one's grasp.

Speculation regarding terminal drop has been recognized as a 1- to 4-year period prior to death during which time an alteration in psychologic or performance ability, vocabulary, or verbal ability occur (Botwinick et al, 1978; White and Cunningham, 1988; Lentzner et al, 1992). However, this remains unclear as to its accuracy, and no conclusive studies have emerged.

The elderly do not have a clearly marked dying trajectory as do the young and middle-aged. They may harbor multiple illnesses or pathologic conditions; the list may get longer as the person grows older. Elders become accustomed to chronic disorders and repeatedly make adaptations in their lifestyle to remain active and defy death.

Institutional settings tend to dissect an individual into component parts, dealing with segments rather than with the living whole. Nurses are caught in the biologic and physical aspects of patient care. It is easy and nonthreatening to relieve physical symptoms associated with dying, but to permit oneself to become involved in a meaningful interpersonal relationship to support the dying aged is extremely difficult for most nurses and other caregivers (Box 26-4).

Perhaps because the nurse brings his or her experience with death, perpetuated myths, and values regarding life, and death, caring for the aged is very difficult. It is also possible that the philosophy of acute care settings, whose goal is to effect cure, governs to some extent care outcomes expected by the nurse. Long-term care facilities, of which there are more than 1 million, are places where the aged are supposed to die and where the decision is made to evaluate or treat a medical problem as the aged face death. It is not an uncommon occurrence for an elder not to be allowed to die in the long-term care facility but to be transferred to the acute facility.

The individual who is dying is a symbol of every person's fears and that which the nurse knows she or he must eventually face: aging and mortality. The nurse follows a social code of living but has none sufficient for dying. The negative cultural norms provide little help in facing death. Many are still not educated in state-of-the-art caring for the dying. The way caregivers perceive the act of dying, as painful, upsetting, indifferent, or a blessing, influences the treatment the dying patient will receive in the last days whether in the acute hospital or in a long-term care facility. A study of nursing home personnel demonstrated that nursing personnel who had more negative attitudes toward the aged had a higher death anxiety. Therefore they were less able to deal with death of the elderly (Depaola et al, 1992).

Whatever the reason, the nurse may show avoidance behavior when ministering to the dying aged. The nurse must begin to acknowledge the feelings that have been suppressed. When the nurse is able to deal with his or her fears,

---

Box 26-4   Bill of Rights for the Dying

Nursing Care in Acute Care Hospital

I have the right to be treated as a living human being until I die.

I have the right to maintain a sense of hopefulness, however changing its focus may be.

I have the right to be cared for by those who can maintain a sense of hopefulness, however changing this may be.

I have the right to express my feelings and emotions about my approaching death in my own way.

I have the right to participate in decisions concerning my care.

I have the right to expect continuing medical and nursing attention even though "cure" goals must be changed to "comfort" goals.

I have the right not to die alone.

I have the right to be free from pain.

I have the right to have my questions answered honestly.

I have the right not to be deceived.

I have the right to die in peace and dignity.

I have the right to retain my individuality and not be judged for my decisions, which may be contrary to beliefs of others.

I have the right to expect that the sanctity of the human body will be respected after death.

I have the right to be cared for by caring, sensitive, knowledgeable people who will attempt to understand my needs and will be able to gain some satisfaction in helping me face my death.

From The terminally ill patient and the helping person workshops, Lansing, Mich, Jan 1975.

recognize them honestly, acknowledge the behavior they produce, and begin to act on such behavior, the nurse will be able to approach the dying aged in a more honest and caring way.

The development of the art of being with the dying necessitates inner strength, a strength that may or may not have its basis in religious teachings but that definitely stems from a positive belief in oneself. Formulation of a philosophy and belief about life will help the nurse through difficult times. Emotional maturity and the ability to deal with disappointment and postponement of immediate wants or desires will have a bearing on the nurse's ability to cope with the deprivation that loss brings. Knowledge of the grieving process and the human responses it elicits is also essential for the nurse to effectively and empathetically care for the aged, the family, and himself or herself during the patient's death.

Some nurses are unable to care for the dying because of their own unresolved conflicts and should not be expected to function in these situations. It is important, however, that someone more able to deal with the situation be asked to intervene in the care.

Needs of the Dying

The needs of the dying aged are like threads in a piece of cloth. Each thread is individual but necessary to the integrity and completeness of the fabric. If one thread is pulled, it touches the other threads, affecting the material's appearance, the thread placement, and the stability of the piece. It is difficult to separate the physical and psychologic needs of the dying aged to identify specific interventions and approaches because they are interwoven. Freedom from pain, freedom from loneliness, conservation of energy, and maintenance of self-esteem are four major needs that are most often neglected in the dying older person and when unfulfilled,

impede the ability to reconcile the remainder of life. The needs of the terminally ill individual in hierarchic order are shown in Figure 26-4.

Freedom from Pain. Pain may be acute or chronic. Acute pain is limited in duration, is diagnostic, and can be relieved by the administration of analgesics given properly (McCaffrey and Beebe, 1989), by positioning, and by other physical measures. Chronic pain is a situation, not an event. It is pain that lasts 6 months or longer. The pain becomes the patient's pathologic condition. It frequently expands to occupy the patient's whole attention, isolating him or her from the world. Patients with chronic pain do not respond to the usual methods of relief like those with acute pain. *Most nurses make no distinction between the two types of pain.*

With any dying person, not just the dying aged, the nurse is placed in conflict. Pain requires the nurse to use a double standard. In the acute pain situation, in which pain is expected to dissipate, the nurse is concerned that the patient is weaned from a narcotic analgesic and given a nonnarcotic drug as soon as possible. Chronic pain cannot be treated this way. It requires a regimen of narcotic and adjuvant drug therapy administered around-the-clock and on time, not just as requested by the patient. *Narcotic addiction of a dying patient is not the issue;* relief of pain is paramount (refer to Chapter 9). A study by Cleeland et al (1994) found 42% of cancer outpatients still had pain inadequately treated. Patients over the age of 70 were at increased risk of undertreatment of pain because of fears of addiction, hastening death, and incurring legal liability.

Saint Christopher's Hospice, London, demonstrated over the years the effectiveness of a regimen of pain control as hospices and oncology units here in the United States continue to do today. When physical pain is controlled proactively, the amount of narcotic medication required by the dying patient does not endlessly increase. The sooner the nurse realizes that imposing his or her values and fears about ad-

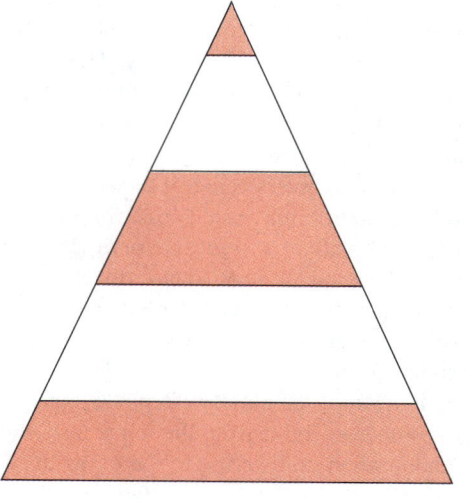

To share and come to terms with the unavoidable future
To perceive meaning in death

To maintain respect in the face of increasing weakness
To maintain independence
To feel like a normal person, a part of life right to the end
To preserve personal identity

To talk
To be listened to with understanding
To be loved and to share love
To be with a caring person when dying

To be given the opportunity to voice hidden fears
To trust those who care for him or her
To feel that he or she is being told the truth
To be secure

To obtain relief from physical symptoms
To conserve energy
To be free of pain

Figure 26-4. Hierarchy of the dying person's needs.

diction on the dying patient is negative care, the sooner physical relief for the dying will be effectively met. The key to effective care is knowledge of pain control and management. With the methods available today there are few patients whose pain cannot be relieved.

Only in recent years has a focus on comfort by treating pain and other symptoms associated with dying (palliative care medicine) come into its own. In addition, religious and spiritual concerns are also receiving more attention. There are still too few who heed the needs of the dying.

One tends not to think of psychologic pain, but pain induced by depression, anxiety, fear, and other unresolved emotional concerns of the dying is just as strong and just as real. When emotional needs are not met, the total pain experience, physical and psychosocial, may be exacerbated or intensified. Medication alone cannot relieve this pain. Instead, empathetic listening and allowing the dying person to verbalize what is on his or her mind are important interventions that must be based on the energy level of the one who is dying. If tears and sadness are present, silence and touch are worth more than words could ever convey. Gentleness of touch, closeness, and sitting near the person are appropriate. The acknowledgment and sharing of the nurse's own emotions may be meaningful to the dying person.

Sometimes diversional activity can be helpful when there is pain: a backrub to ease tension, a foot massage, or access to a radio or television set. If hearing is impaired, perhaps an amplifier close to the patient's ear would help. If vision is impaired, talking books can be obtained, or arrangement for a volunteer reader might be made. Often all that the dying elder needs to feel safe is someone close by to talk with, to listen, and to touch.

Freedom from Loneliness. Loneliness can come from within as well as without. The dying aged have sustained many losses: loss of friends through death, perhaps loss of spouse, loss of control by institutionalization, loss of meaningful possessions, and loss of physical abilities (sight, hearing, and body functions). Loneliness can also be generated by language barriers and cultural differences.

In the hospital setting the nursing staff can easily intensify loneliness by caring for the aged person with detachment, by surrendering to the mechanical technology of the profession, and by avoiding the death situation. In these ways the nurse truly isolates the old person. Offensive odors emanating from the patient's room or body keep people away. Unrelieved pain, physical or psychologic, intensifies loneliness. Behavior meant to attract attention may in fact distance people. The dying person is frequently placed in a single room or curtained off as it becomes more apparent that death is approaching; care is reduced with decreased tactile and audio stimulation. Lighting in the room is dim, curtains or shades may be drawn, and people speak in hushed tones or not at all. The dying person perceives this as abandonment, the ultimate loneliness. No one wants to die alone; yet knowingly or unknowingly nurses foster this loneliness and aloneness.

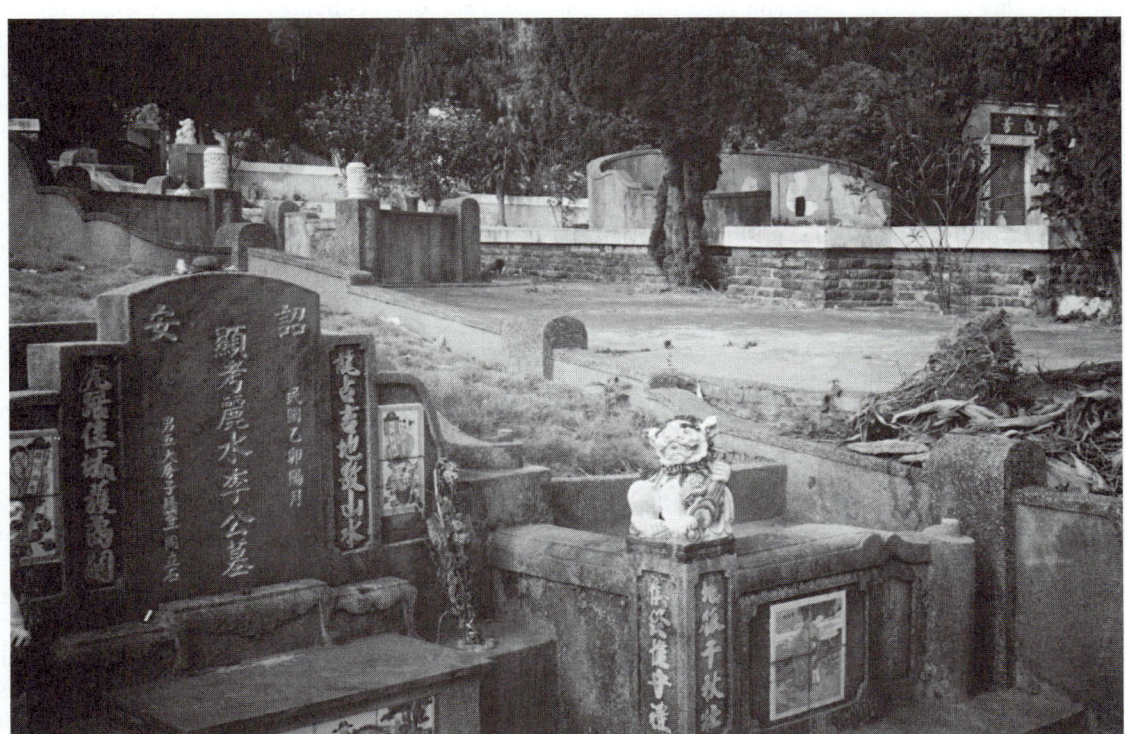

Cemetery. (Courtesy Priscilla Ebersole.)

Room location and environment are important considerations to reduce or eliminate loneliness. It is critical to assess the rationale for isolating the dying person in a single room. For whose benefit is it . . . the patient, the staff, or to protect the uncomfortable visitors to the hospital unit? For some elders, it is reassuring to see activity when one is confined to bed. Placing the dying older person in a room with several other persons can provide the opportunity to share conversation and companionship and security that he or she will not die alone. The patients who remain in the room after a death have the support and solace of each other. When there are only two persons in a room, the remaining occupant is left alone, a situation that can be frightening and a negative experience. These considerations are very individual and must be based upon patient preference.

If the energy level of the dying elder allows ambulation, he or she should be free to leave the confines of his or her room and associate with other patients, visitors, and staff. When physical tolerance is limited to sitting in a chair, a wheelchair can provide mobility and accessibility to the larger environment with the least energy expenditure. Sitting by the nurses' station or desk is sometimes preferable to sitting alone in one's room. If possible the patient should be encouraged to wear his or her own clothing.

A pleasant room atmosphere with bright colors and diffuse, high-intensity lighting not only protects the aged from visual discomfort but also affords a clearer visual contrast of objects. Gray (1976) noted that in the last hours of the dying process individuals turned toward light. Perhaps this supports the value of using bright colors and adjusting lights to keep the patient in touch with life until the end of living.

Live plants and flowers are a way of bringing the outside world in. Memorabilia, pictures, cherished objects, or any thing that brings solace should be recognized as important in the care of the dying aged. These tangibles are a means of coping with anxiety and furnish a modicum of security and familiarity in an alien environment. A portable radio is easy to reach or one with headphones conserves energy, staves off loneliness, and provides contact with the outside world. Television, if available, can also be a beneficial outlet.

Visitors should be allowed to be with the dying aged any time of the day or night. Night is the most lonely and painful time for the aged. It is a time of least attention, a time when one thinks and reviews the sorrows and joys of life past and what is to be. It is a time of fear of dying alone and no one will know. When a friend or relative cannot stay with the dying person, a mature sitter might be the answer. *The sitter's prime responsibility would be psychologic support, not nursing care.* If the dying person is part of a hospice program, a volunteer may be available to stay with him or her. Not all elderly dying patients want this attention, but if they do, it should be available.

Everyone who cares for the dying elderly should be aware of the isolation and loneliness evoked by the dying process. Treating the dying aged person as an intelligent adult, holding a hand, or putting an arm around a shoulder says, "I care" and "You're not alone."

A little time spent listening to the elderly person relieves some of the loneliness of impending death. When caregivers cut the patient off as he or she begins to recall days of long ago, an avenue that helps relieve loneliness has been deliberately blocked. Reminiscence is a means of putting one's life in order. It is a valuable way for the elder to evaluate the pluses and minuses of life. It is a means of achieving closure to life by resolving conflicts, giving up possessions, and making final good-byes. It can create a new meaning in life.

Some elderly persons have developed a lifestyle around aloneness. These individuals do indeed prefer solitude. Thrusting any of the nursing care approaches at them would only serve to aggravate the patient. It is important to be sensitive to the patient's clues and to assess and act on them accordingly.

Because of the interactive nature of loneliness and pain (pain may precipitate loneliness and loneliness can exacerbate pain), the nurse may need to deal with physical and psychologic discomfort separately or together, depending on assessment of the situation.

Conservation of Energy. The dying aged use great amounts of energy in attempting to cope with the physical assault of illness on the body and in the emotional unrest that dying initiates.

Nursing interventions should be directed toward the conservation of patient energy. How much can the individual do without becoming physically and emotionally taxed? What activities of daily living are most important for the aged person to do independently? Would it be best to bathe the person so he or she could eat alone or feed the patient so he or she could wash or receive visitors? How much energy does the patient need to talk with visitors or staff without becoming exhausted? The aged person should be involved in answering such questions and making these decisions. The emotional turmoil and anxiety saps the energy that might have been conserved by manipulating the patient's physical requirements when the patient receives care without explanation or is excluded from decision making.

Anxiety binds energy. Energy can be spared and anxiety reduced by listening, touching, and providing rest and an environment that permits the patient to be dependent when it becomes necessary.

Perhaps conservation of energy is the most tangible patient need the nurse faces when caring for the dying aged. By meeting the needs for freedom from pain, freedom from loneliness, and conservation of energy, the nurse has already begun to intervene in behalf of the maintenance of self-esteem.

Maintenance of Self-Esteem. Pride in oneself is a composite of the physical and psychologic attributes of one's years of living. For the aged person, it is difficult to watch self-image dissolve through loss of independence, loss of the potential for doing (a result of physical disabilities), or loss of body functions such as hearing, seeing, eating, urinating, defecating, or cleaning self. The aged person begins to feel ashamed, humiliated, and like a "burden."

Institutions and caregivers (by their approach and attitude toward the aged) can erode an elder's self-esteem. The aged patient's privacy and dignity are invaded by the number of physicians and others who come to look, prod, and poke in search of diagnoses and learning. Additional insults are imposed by calling the aged person "Mom," "Pop," or "Dearie." Bows are put in women's hair, and the old person is treated as if he or she has the mentality of a child. Behavior such as this by caregivers compounds the situation for the dying aged. Withdrawing from the dying aged reinforces the aged person's feeling of worthlessness.

When self-esteem is at an ebb, other factors such as psychologic and physical pain, aloneness, and depletion of energy are intensified. Depression aggravates pain and further isolates the individual. One cannot deny that the way the elderly respond to dying is influenced by their background, past experiences, religious and philosophic orientation, and the prior degree of life involvement. If experiences have been negative, the lack of care and attention by caregivers creates a pathetic state of affairs.

Self-esteem and dignity complement each other. Dignity involves the individual's ability to maintain a consistent self-concept. Caregivers frequently take control and dignity away from the dying and impose their expectations on the patient. Essential to the facilitation of self-esteem is the premise that the values of the patient must figure significantly in the decisions that will affect the course of dying.

The important concept for the caregiver to master is that *the dying aged individual is a living person with the same needs for good and natural relationships with people as the rest of us.* If this concept can be fully accepted, incorporation of the value of the patient to himself or herself will significantly affect the course of the person's dying process. Including the person in decisions about care encourages the patient to control the most important event in life.

What can be done to help maintain and bolster self-esteem of the dying aged? Focus on the present and the opportunities that exist in the immediate future. Attention must be paid to the person's hygiene: cleanliness, lack of odors, and personal appearance (without hair ribbons unless asked for). Physical comfort is vitally important because with comfort comes security. Caregivers must become good listeners to allow the dying aged to express their fears of pain, aloneness, and the struggle with the separation and grief over losses. Caregivers may assume the management of necessary body and ego functions for the aged. This requires emphasis on respect and helpfulness rather than encouraging dependency, guilt, or conflict. Human contact is vital. One quickly falls into the confusional syndrome of human deprivation: loneliness. As early as 1967, it was shown in sensory deprivation experiments (i.e., touch) that a disintegration and loss of ego integrity (dignity) occurred (Pattison,

1967). It is therefore of utmost importance for the caregiver to use auditory, visual, and tactile stimulation appropriately to nurture and foster self-esteem in the dying aged. Verbal and nonverbal communication is necessary to convey positive messages; handholding, placing an arm around the shoulder, or sitting on the edge of the bed conveys to the dying person that the nurse or caregiver is prepared to meet the person on his or her own terms and that the aged person is an individual unique unto self and appreciated.

Reconciliation. Many individuals seek reconciliation with God and other persons as death approaches. Pain and other disabilities may interfere with this reconciliation. Symptomatic control in a milieu that responds to psychologic, social, and religious needs can facilitate this process of adjustment. This requires a multidisciplinary team that includes pastoral care of the dying as a high priority. Schuman (1987) reports on such an undertaking that developed in response to the expressed needs of patients and families. This approach deserves serious consideration because an individual must feel involved and in control of treatment and care as long as life persists. Pastoral care seems to facilitate this humanistic approach. Depressed and dying elders often express concerns that have religious overtones. When this is the case, the need for pastoral counseling should be seriously considered and every effort made to assist the elder toward spiritual peace.

• • •

Communication and control are the borders necessary to complete the fabric of needs of the dying aged. Their influence is omnipresent in the other needs. Without them the cloth can fray, and attempts to meet the needs will be limited.

Talking helps relieve anxiety; it fills time and fosters the sharing of feelings. The dying aged should never be lied to nor should they be ignored. Lying is betrayal, not listening is interpreted as emotional abandonment, and avoiding the person's room is perceived by the dying as physical abandonment.

Control over one's time of death is a phenomenon that occurs everywhere. If care and institutionalization in life are seen as overwhelming negatives by the dying aged person, death can be hastened through the person's own control. The exact physiologic mechanism is unknown, but it is suggested that hypersensitivity of the sympathetic adrenal system or responses of the parasympathetic nervous system is involved in persons willing their own death (Watson and Maxwell, 1977). Neglect of the needs of the dying aged encourages the aged person to indeed use this last source of control over life, namely, the willing of death.

Conditions have begun to change as death education for health care personnel has become more available; patients insist on being informed about their illnesses; and the public in general exercises the "right to know" and "right to die."

The nurse has great influence on what happens to a dying patient. She or he can influence the social milieu by regulating drug use, controlling interactions between the patient and the family, and influencing feelings of patient importance by talking with or ignoring the patient. The nurse can also assume the roles of supporter, facilitator, and advocate of the dying aged.

Spirituality and Hope. Spirituality is the basic human quality for hope. Without one's own spiritual nourishment, one cannot meet the same needs in others. There is a transcendental relationship between a person and a higher being but not necessarily a religious being. In most instances spirituality is two dimensional: that being between God and between others. Spirituality may be met through religious acts and/or through human caring relationships. A person's internal beliefs, personal experiences, and religion are expressions of spirituality.

Hope is expectancy of fulfillment, an anticipation, or relief from something. It is based on the belief of the possible, support of meaningful others, a sense of well-being, overall coping ability, and a purpose in life. Generally speaking, hope is an overall feeling of future good. "Enabling hope" empowers and is an integral thread in one's life. Erickson equates hope with integrity, and it is comparable to Maslow's self-actualization.

The multidimensional nature of hope is expressed through thoughts, feelings, and actions. Hope is activated when a crisis occurs and personal resources are exhausted (Herth, 1990). Hope empowers, generates courage, motivates action and achievement, and can strengthen physiologic and psychologic function. Forbes (1994) describes six characteristics of hope that reflect the affective (emotional and sensation); cognitive (imaging, having a future); affiliative (sense of relatedness to others); temporal (time, future, change); and contextual (placing experiences within one's life situation) domains. The characteristics according to Forbes are the following:

- Confidence that change and adaptation is possible
- Relating to others
- A belief in the future
- Spiritual belief
- Active involvement
- Trust

Box 26-5	**Hope in Aging**

Love from others
Interaction with others
Freedom to make choices
Growth through discovery
Future orientation
Active movement toward goals
Life after death

The degree of hope that the dying possess is dependent on caring relationships with others and with caregivers such as health professionals. Love from others is a message of hope (Box 26-5).

DYING AND THE FAMILY

Aged persons today may be a member of a multigenerational family. Though they do not necessarily live under the same roof or may be geographically separated, there is some degree of filial tie.

When an elder becomes seriously or terminally ill and cannot uphold his or her role or obligation, the family balance or dynamics can be significantly altered. Even the aged person who is single and relies on friends and neighbors finds a change in the relationships. Depending on the role the individual has in the family constellation, problems often begin at the time of diagnosis or shortly thereafter. Roles and traits of the person who is now considered to be dying may create adjustment difficulties in the to-be survivors whether they are the spouse, the adult children, or the grandchildren. Adult children often begin to see their own mortality through the death of their parent, with the appearance of a new family order.

It can be a constant struggle for a family to remain involved with the dying person as they try to withdraw and try to readjust their lives without the dying member. This requires enormous energy by family members who are already burdened with their own anticipatory grief, daily living, and in many cases raising their own children. The conflict is not only grieving for the dying but for a part of themselves that will be lost with the death of the parent or significant family member. A number of adaptive tasks are required to facilitate healthy resolution of the dying of a family member.

Family members need to remain involved with the patient. This means sharing and responding to the patient's experiences. At times family members have to separate their own identities from that of the patient's and learn to tolerate the reality that this family member will die while they live on. The ability of the family members to truly support, love, and provide intimacy may lead to exhaustion, impatience, anger, and a sense of futility as the patient's illness drags on and on. Often family members may be at different points in grief than the patient. This can hinder communication between the patient and family members. As the illness worsens, physical disability increases, and the patient complains more often, intensifying feelings of helplessness and frustration in family members.

Role changes require adaptation and accommodation to new demands within the family of new responsibilities and permanent change. For example, an adult child has to deal with the death of one parent and assumes responsibility for the welfare of the remaining parent.

Bearing the effects of grief requires acknowledgment of the current feelings that surface in anticipatory grief. Coming to terms with the reality of the impending loss means that family members must go through many emotional responses in achieving acceptance of the loved one's approaching death. Because people are supposed to die in old age, the grief responses may not be exceptionally intense, but then, too, many filial relationships that seem superficial can result in very deep and acute grief responses.

Family members may feel extremely pressured during the final days of an aged relative's life. They may be caught between experiencing and remembering the patient as he or she is and was, between pushing for more or letting nature take its course, and at times not wanting to be involved because of a discordant relationship with the patient. These discussions will profoundly affect them for the rest of their lives. Many times families feel guilt-ridden because they are thinking more about their needs instead of those of the dying patient.

Despite the family's grief and pain, the family must give the patient permission to die, let the patient know that it is allright to let go and leave. It is the last act of love and dignity the family can offer the dying patient. There are times when there is no family to say, "It's okay to let go." The task then falls to the nurse who has developed a meaningful relationship with the patient throughout care. Rando (1984) summarizes grief work of families with the six "Rs" of grieving: recognition, reaction to separation, recollection and reexperience of the deceased and relations, relinquishment of old attachments, readjustment to moving into a new world without forgetting the old, and reinvestment.

DYING AND THE HEALTH PROFESSIONAL

Whenever an individual invests in something or someone and it leaves, is gone, or is lost, there is a need to grieve. Similarly, nurses in their daily work environment are confronted with dying patients. By the very nature of the population whom nurses serve, they are forced to confront loss, not only of patients and families, but personal loss as well. Caring for dying patients over time, or watching patients go home and repeatedly return, involves a degree of emotional investment and a feeling of grief that requires resolution.

A social factor that has long affected the nurse's ability to grieve is the assumption that the role of the caregiver is to be emotionally strong. The nurse has been told that feelings of ambivalence or guilt toward the patient are inappropriate. The nurse attempts to control those feelings by remaining detached, thwarting the acknowledgment or resolution of feelings. The nurse, too, can experience conflict between wanting the dying patient to live and yet wanting the patient to be relieved of suffering, if it is a lingering death. A study of nurses in a rehabilitation center found a greater chance of being affected negatively by patient deaths the longer the nurses were employed at the facility or if they were recently grieving a loss (O'Hara et al, 1996). The study also suggested that some nurses are at higher risk for negative im-

pact if they had a high personal tendency toward immersing themselves in nursing care. This is an example of an earlier discussion of investing oneself without adequate support systems.

Harper (1977) identified a process of adaptation through which health professionals must pass to cope with the stress of caring for the dying. Intellectualization, which focuses on professional knowledge and facts and at times emphasizes philosophical issues, is the first stage of adapting. At this time conversation with the dying is distant, and a flurry of activity ensues as the caregiver busies himself or herself with physical tasks and reading about the patient's illness in an attempt to allay their own anxieties.

The professional, in the second stage of adapting, is jolted out of this intellectual haven into a confrontation with the realities of the patient's impending death and their personal mortality. Grieving is triggered for oneself and at the same time by genuine compassion for the dying patient. Caregivers can feel guilty, frustrated, and hostile. Hostile feelings are not uncommon for caregivers to experience when they attempt to fight their feelings, a situation Harper calls emotional survival. Depression, pain, mourning, and grief are crucial in this period for the health professional.

The health professional is said to have arrived at self-mastery when he or she is free from identification with the patient's symptoms and is no longer occupied with personal mortality. Self-mastery allows greater sensitivity to the patient without the incapacitating effects on the caregiver. This phase is called emotional arrival: moderation, mitigation, and accommodation.

The culmination of previous growth and development enables the caregiver to relate compassionately to the patient and fully accept the impending death. The enhanced dignity and self-respect that the caregiver feels allow him or her to give respect and dignity to the dying patient. Through this growth process, the health professional has learned that living can be more painful than dying. Now concern for the dying can be translated into constructive and appropriate care activities for both the patient and the family. Needless to say, the caregiver must have outside interests and a support network beyond the work setting to maintain a balanced perspective on life. Without this equilibrium, it will be difficult to grow and accept the death of others and oneself.

Assessment

The Dying Aged. Few, if any, tools are available to assess dying patients. Caregivers, for the most part, have to depend on their understanding of the grieving and dying processes and draw carefully from the literature behavioral responses outlined in the literature. A danger exists among health professionals of superimposing what they think the patient should feel and do in the dying process. The purpose of knowing about grief and dying theories is to recognize what emotions and behaviors can offer and to plan interventions accordingly as they appear. Rando (1984) presents an extensive list of items to assess for the dying patient and the illness (Box 26-6).

As an individual nears the final days and hours of life, physical, psychologic, and emotional events occur that provide clues to the impending death. Too often nurses, families, and patients are unaware and unprepared for these signs and responses. Tables 26-6 and 26-7 provide guidance for these responses.

The Family of the Aged.   The family, whether biologic or chosen by the aged individual, is often neglected when the aged person is dying. Attention paid to family members revolves around their presence as an obstacle or a nuisance to the caregiving staff. As institutions downsize and there are fewer available professional staff to care for patients, patients' families may find themselves begin to assume more care responsibility. More often than not, animosity toward the family develops, and prejudgments are made about their behavior during this stressful time.

The ability to do a detailed assessment depends on the willingness, availability, and degree of stress of the family, as well as the time constraints of the nurse who may be caring for a group of patients. Using available time, the nurse can make an attempt to acquire information early in the dying patient's illness to help the family cope with the dying process as it progresses. Rando (1984) outlines assessment data that are important to obtain if effective intervention is to be developed (Box 26-6).

Values, norms, beliefs, and priorities of the family must be recognized and accepted. Rarely do major changes in behavior and communication patterns occur just because a family member is dying. However, if a health professional plans realistic interventions and outcomes consistent with the existing family system, he or she may be able to foster positive growth.

Intervention

Interventions have many facets and range from the simple act of hand holding to dealing with a multitude of emotions. The core of interventions focus on communication, pain and symptom relief, knowledge of available resources, and fostering involvement in and control of decision making by the patient as long as possible. Many interventions have been mentioned throughout the discussion of the

---

Box 26-6	**Assessment of the Dying Patient and Family**

Patient
Age
Gender
Coping styles and abilities
Social, cultural, ethnic background
Previous experience with illness, pain, deterioration, loss, and grief
Mental health
Intelligence
Life-style
Fulfillment of life goals
Amount of unfinished business
The nature of the illness (death trajectory, problems particular to the illness, treatment, amount of pain)
Time passed since diagnosis
Response to illness
Knowledge about the illness/disease
Acceptance/rejection of the sick role
Amount of striving for dependence/independence
Feelings/and fears about illness
Comfort in expressing thoughts and feelings and how much is expressed
Location of the patient (home, hospital, nursing home)
Relationship with each member of the family and significant other since diagnosis
Family rules, norms, values, and past experiences that might inhibit grief or interfere with a therapeutic relationship

Family
Family makeup (members of family)
Developmental stage of the family
Existing subsystems
Specific roles of each member

Characteristics of the Family System
How flexible or rigid
Type of communication
Rules, norms, and expectations
Values, beliefs
Quality of emotional relationships
Dependence, interdependence, freedom of each member
How close to or disengaged from the dying member
Established extrafamilial interactions
Strengths and vulnerabilities of the family
Style of leadership and decision making
Unusual methods of problem solving, crisis resolution
Family resources (personal, financial, community)
Current problems identified by the family
Quality of communication with the care givers
Immediate and long-range anticipated needs

From Hess PA: Loss, grief, and dying. In Beare P, Myers J: *Adult health nursing,* ed. 3, St Louis, 1998, Mosby.

Table 26-6 Physical Signs and Symptoms Associated with the Final Stages of Dying, Rationale, and Interventions

Physical signs and symptoms	Rationale	Intervention (if any)
Coolness, color, and temperature change in hands, arms, feet, and legs, perspiration may be present	Peripheral circulation diminished to facilitate increased circulation to vital organs	Place socks on feet; cover with light cotton blankets; keep warm blankets on person, but *do not use electric blanket*
Increased sleeping	Conservation of energy	Spend time with the patient; hold the hand; speak normally to the patient even though there may be a lack of response
Disorientation, confusion of time, place, person	Metabolic changes	Identify self by name before speaking to patient; speak softly, clearly, and truthfully
Incontinence of urine and/or bowel	Increased muscle relaxation and decreased consciousness	Maintain vigilance, change bedding as appropriate, utilize bed pads, try not to use an indwelling catheter
Congestion	Poor circulation of body fluids, immobilization, and the inability to expectorate secretions causes gurgling, rattles, bubbling	Elevate the head with pillows and/or raise the head of the bed; gently turn the head to the side to drain secretions
Restlessness	Metabolic changes and decrease in oxygen to the brain	Calm the patient by speech and action; reduce light; gently rub back, stroke arms, or read aloud; play soothing music; *do not use restraints*
Decreased intake of food and fluids	Body conservation of energy for function	Do not force patient to eat or drink; give ice chips, soft drinks, juice, popsicles as possible; apply petroleum jelly to dry lips; if patient is a mouth breather, apply protective jelly more frequently as necessary
Decreased urine output	Decreased fluid intake and decreased circulation to kidney	None
Altered breathing pattern	Metabolic and oxygen changes of respiratory system	Elevate the head of bed; hold hand, speak gently to patient
		Additional general interventions
		Learn to be "with person" without talking; a moist washcloth on the forehead may be soothing; eye drops may help soothe the eyes

From Hess PA: Loss, grief, and dying. In Beare P, Myers J: *Adult health nursing,* ed 3, St Louis, 1998, Mosby.

Table 26-7 Emotional/Spiritual Symptoms of Approaching Death, Rational, and Interventions

Emotional/spiritual symptoms	Rationale	Intervention
Withdrawal	Prepares the patient for release and detachment and letting go of relationships and surroundings	Continue communicating in a normal manner using a normal voice tone; identify self by name; hold hand, say what person wants to hear from you.
Vision-like experiences (dead friends or family, religious vision)	Preparation for transition	Do not contradict or argue regarding whether this is or is not a real experience; if the patient is frightened, reassure them that is normal.
Restlessness	Tension, fear, unfinished business	Listen to patient express his or her fears, sadness and anger associated with dying; give permission to go.
Decreased socialization	As energy diminishes, the patient begins making his or her transition	Express support; give permission to die.
Unusual communication: out of character statements, gestures, requests	Signals readiness to let go	Say what needs to be said to the dying patient; kiss, hug, cry with him or her.

From Hess PA: Loss, grief, and dying. In Beare P, Myers J: *Adult health nursing,* ed 3, St Louis, 1998, Mosby.

needs of the dying patient. Tables 26-5 and 26-6 address interventions that can be taken as death nears.

Communication includes the verbal and nonverbal exchange between the nurse, the elder, and possibly the family. Talking with the dying is full of emotional land mines, but it is a vehicle for establishing a trust relationship that can help relieve anxiety. Talking is a way to instruct, explain, divert attention, and amuse. Humor can be very therapeutic. Nonverbal responses are expressed in facial expressions, touch, and behavior. "Touch hunger," or the lack of human contact through tactile stimulation such as holding hands or receiving and giving hugs, is often experienced by the dying. Procedural touch used in bathing and treatments does not fulfill the touch need.

Knowledge of community resources will help the nurse give direction to the patient and family and help them cope with the physical, emotional, socioeconomic, and religious and spiritual problems that might occur. A list of resources appears at the end of this chapter.

Loss of health or deterioration due to chronic problems, loss of independence, social contacts, finances, and energy threaten control over oneself and the environment. The nurse's role is that of supporter, facilitator, advocate, and caregiver. Nurses can facilitate meeting patient needs through patient empowerment and control and by providing choices in care, so that the patient remains an active participant. Environmental stimulation through social contacts and diversional activities often relieves the sense of isolation and abandonment.

It is not feasible for all patients to choose to be cared for at home, but they should be supported if they choose it. Ancillary services must be provided that will cooperate with the patient and family. The patient and family should be aware that if they get into difficulty, they should not consider it defeat to return to the hospital for care. The nurse must realize that some emotions and experiences are inexpressible, but that the nurse's role is his or her presence, being with the person and the family and being able to detect feelings of these individuals.

Hospice: An Alternative

The hospice movement, which began in the United States and Canada in 1971, has made "hospice" a familiar word to health care professionals and the lay public. However, the meaning attached to it is still subject to a variety of interpretations. The model for hospice and its concepts was resurrected more than 35 years ago and implemented at Saint Christopher's Hospice in London under the direction of Dr. Cicely Saunders.

Since then the number of hospices has expanded enormously, and these are now over 2000 in the United States; at least 800 of these are affiliated with community hospitals (U.S. Bureau of the Census, 1995). Others are operated by public health agencies, home health agencies, or volunteer groups. The variations in origins and style reflect the partic-

ular needs of the community, the style of leadership, funding sources, political forces, available resources for health and social services, and the spiritual care in each community where hospices are established. Long-term care facilities often have difficulty reconciling the hospice approach to care because of their own rigid interpretation of regulations meant to protect residents from neglect.

Most provide services that incorporate hospice ideals and are developed using the guidelines of the National Hospice Organization (NHO) (Box 26-7). This organization, formed in 1978, has been in the forefront of promoting standards of hospice care that ensure the purposes and intents are met. Some facilities offering hospice care may not have appropriately trained staff. Nurses would do well to investigate the quality and staffing of a hospice against the standards of the organization. The NHO is committed to the development of education in the hospice concept and to promoting appropriate legislation, regulation, and reimbursement.

Hospice care is usually free to the patient and has been supported by volunteers, public and private funds, and memorial donations. Efforts to incorporate hospice care into health insurance payments and other third-party reimbursement mechanisms resulted in the implementation of hospice benefits under Medicare in November 1983, under the Tax Equity and Fiscal Responsibility Act (TEFRA). In 1986 Congress passed legislation making hospice a permanent Medicare benefit and granted a modest increase in reimbursement rates. Since then, the number of private insurance companies and health maintenance organizations (HMOs) offering a hospice option has increased. The hope is that in this age of accelerating costs hospice care will save money while making more humane care available to terminally ill patients and their families. It is hoped that hospice care eventually will be generally available to all who wish it.

The hospice process or ideology is unique. Hospice is described as the link between the needs of the terminally ill and their families and a staff that employs the medieval concept of hospitality in which a community assists the traveler at dangerous points along his journey. It returns nursing to its roots: humane compassionate care, an ideal that has been the basis of nursing for centuries. The dying are indeed travelers—travelers along the continuum of life—and the community is friends, family, and specially prepared people to care—the hospice team.

The philosophy of hospice care is, "The last stages of life should not be seen as defeat, but rather as life's fulfillment. It is not merely a time of negation, but rather an opportunity for positive achievement . . . " (Ulrich, 1978, p. 20).

Hospice care is a reorientation in health care for the patient and family. The home usually becomes the primary center of care, and care is provided by family members or friends who are taught basic nursing care, including diet, exercise, and medication needed to care for the dying individual. The patient generally wishes to die at home; the family fears this because they do not know what to do, and they want the patient to die in the hospital. Given the necessary tools and orientation, much anxiety is eliminated, and families with the emotional support of the hospice team, are able to care for the dying at home.

Hospice is available 24 hours every day of the year for its clients, providing, as needed, the services of physicians, nurses, mental health specialists, therapists, social workers, and chaplains.

Hospice facilitates a redefinition of relationships. The spouse may not always be the caregiver; it could be a friend or child. For those without family, hospice staff and, at times, friends become the patient's family. Someone from hospice is readily available to stay with the patient or family whenever the need occurs. Neither the dying person nor the family is alone during the dying process or during the months of bereavement that follow. There is a great amount of contact, interaction, and sharing between the family and hospice team. Hospice volunteers provide direct or indirect assistance. They perform chores and provide friendship and companionship to the patient and family.

The unprecedented contribution of hospice continues to be reestablishment of control for the dying person. Through polypharmaceutic means, control of distressful symptoms and pain has been accomplished without denying the patient full alertness and the ability to communicate to others. This gift, so to speak, allows normality for the patient. The crux of accomplishing this end is the anticipation of symptoms and intervention by the caregiver before problems occur (Tables 26-6 and 26-7).

Pain control, the issue that is discussed most frequently when hospice is mentioned, is not exclusively physical pain but also relief of psychologic, social, and spiritual pain. Heightened physical pain may be the only tangible clue to the existence of the others. Psychologic pain emerges when loss of control over one's life occurs. The equilibrium is disturbed, and usual coping mechanisms may not be effective. Social pain can be summed up as "man's inhumanity to man," problems stemming from loss of interpersonal relationships, unfinished business, unsaid good-byes, and nonclosure of life.

Spiritual pain may be tied to cultural, racial, and religious aspects from which the dying person feels alienated, for example, rituals or participation in group prayers.

Acceptance of death is thought to be easier for individuals with a strong religious faith regardless of whether they believe in an afterlife (Cartwright, 1991). Siegel and Kuykendall (1990) found corroborating evidence that membership in a church or temple moderated the impact of death. Mickley et al (1992) found with women diagnosed with breast cancer that internally defined religious beliefs contributed significantly to spiritual well-being. This was characterized by affirmation and satisfaction with life, a relationship with God, and perception that one's life has meaning. Those extrinsically religious expressed less spiritual well-being.

Reeducation of the patient and family is another dimension of hospice care. Before teaching is initiated, the hospice team finds out what the patient and family already know, what functional abilities are operant, what unfinished goals remain for the family, and what kind of rehabilitation will facilitate the achievement of the patient's and family's goals.

Pain control and the opportunity to die at home are the key ideas and activities that people associate with hospice. In actuality hospice represents much more. It supports and

---

Box 26-7   **Principles of Hospice Care (NHO)**

1. Hospice offers palliative care to all terminally ill people and their families regardless of age, gender, nationality, race, creed, sexual orientation, disability, diagnosis, availability of a primary caregiver, or ability to pay.
2. The unit of care in hospice is the patient/family.
3. A highly qualified, specially trained team of hospice professionals and volunteers work together to meet the physiologic, psychologic, social, spiritual, and economic needs of patient/families facing terminal illness and bereavement.
4. The hospice interdisciplinary team collaborates continuously with the patient's attending physician to develop and maintain a patient-directed, individualized plan of care.
5. Hospice offers a safe, coordinated program of palliative and supportive care, in a variety of appropriate settings, from the time of admission through bereavement, with the focus on keeping terminally ill patients in their homes as long as possible.
6. Hospice care is available 24 hours a day, seven days a week, and services continue without interruption if the patient care setting changes.
7. Hospice is accountable for the appropriate allocation and utilization of its resources in order to provide optimal care consistent with patient/family needs.
8. Hospice maintains a comprehensive and accurate record of services provided in all care settings for each patient/family.
9. Hospice has an organized governing body that has complete and ultimate responsibility for the organization.
10. The hospice governing body entrusts the hospice administrator with overall management responsibility for operating the hospice, including planning, organizing, staffing, and evaluating the organization and its services.
11. Hospice is committed to continuous assessment and improvement of the quality and efficiency of its services.

From The National Hospice Organization: *Standards of a hospice program of care,* 1993, Arlington, Va.

guides the family in patient care and ensures that the patient will not die alone and that the family will not be abandoned. Bereavement services for the family extend for a period of time on an emergency and regular basis after the death of the patient. Hospice staff help family members learn care techniques, dietary approaches, medication management, and how to handle an assortment of problems that occur in a family in which a member is dying. Life is made as meaningful as possible.

Nurse's Role in Hospice Care. Nursing practice and hospice incorporate the mind-body continuum. Cicely Saunders refers to nursing as the cornerstone of hospice care. The nurse provides much of the direct care and functions in a variety of roles: as staff nurse giving direct care, as coordinator implementing the plan of the interdisciplinary team or as executive officer responsible for research and educational activities, and as an advocate for the patient and hospice in the clinical and political arena.

Thomas (1983) and the American Nurses' Association's Standards and Scope of Hospice Nursing Practice (1987) enumerate the special skills, knowledge, and abilities needed by a hospice nurse:

1. Thorough knowledge of anatomy and physiology and considerable familiarity with pathophysiologic causes of numerous diseases
2. Well-grounded skill in physical assessment and in various nursing procedures such as catheterization, colostomy, and traction care
3. Above-average knowledge of pharmacology, especially of analgesics, narcotics, antiemetics, tranquilizers, antibiotics, hormone therapy, steroids, cardiotonic agents, and cancer chemotherapy
4. Skill in using psychologic principles in individual and group situations
5. Great sensitivity in human relationships

Box 26-8   Principles for Measuring the Quality of Care at the End of Life

1. Physical and emotional symptoms
   Pain, shortness of breath, fatigue, depression, fear, anxiety, nausea, skin breakdown, and other physical and emotional problems often destroy the quality of life at its end. The focus should be on these needs and ensuring that people can count on a comfortable and meaningful end to their lives.
2. Support of function and autonomy
   It is extremely important to maintain a patient's personal dignity and self-respect.
3. Advance care planning
   Planning ahead allows for decisions to be made that reflect the patient's preferences and circumstances rather than only a response to crises.
4. Aggressive care near death—site of death, CPR, and hospitalization
   Although aggressive care is often justified, most patients would prefer to have avoided it when the short-term outcome is death.
5. Patient and family satisfaction
   Both patient and family satisfaction should be measured by these elements: the decision-making process, the care given, and the outcomes achieved.
6. Global quality of life
   Overall well-being can be good despite declining physical health. Care systems that achieve this should be valued.
7. Family burden
   When possible, serious financial and emotional effects from the costs of care and the challenges of direct caregiving should be reduced.
8. Survival time
   There is reason to worry that death may be too readily accepted. Purchasers and patients need to know that survival times vary across plans and provider systems.
9. Provider continuity and skill
   Providers must have relevant skills, including rehabilitation, symptom control, and psychological support. Care systems must demonstrate competent performance on continuity and provider skill.
10. Bereavement
    Survivors may benefit from relatively modest interventions when immediately available.

Modified from American Geriatrics Society: Measuring quality of care at the end of life, a statement of principles, *AGS Newsletter* 25(3), May/June/July, 1996.

6. Personal characteristics such as stamina, emotional stability, flexibility, cooperativeness, and a life philosophy or faith

7. Knowledge of measures to comfort the dying in the last hours

A summary of principles for measuring the quality of care at the end of life are presented in Box 26-8.

The Hospice Nurses Association provides guidance in end-of-life care (see resources). They bring geriatric theory, nursing concepts, and knowledge of medical management of acute and chronic conditions of elders together to provide the most sensitive and comprehensive care.

Hope. Hope changes as one is dying. Hope for a cure is never abandoned, but the focus of care is on creating an environment that encourages honesty, compassion, and mutual support. The intimacy of everyone working together establishes an environment where it is safe for the patient, family, and hospice personnel to share sad and wonderful moments with one another.

CURRENT ISSUES IN DEATH AND DYING

Decision making on life-prolonging procedures when death is inevitable have become legal, ethical, medical, and professional issues today. The blurring of the lines between living and dying result from technological advances, the ambivalence of whether death is to be fought or accepted, and the dilemma brought about by medical technologies. Decision making at the end of life has become increasingly complex because most people die in advanced age from chronic illnesses, dying over a period of years, slowly declining from degenerative conditions, including Alzheimer's and Parkinson's. Seventy-three percent of the deaths each year are elders, making end-of-life decisions a frequent part of this group's needs (U.S. Census, 1995; Mezey, 1996).

Self-determination is at the core of protecting patients from the medical system. Many physicians are unaware of or ignore patients' advance directives. They are inadequately trained to care for the dying and economically deterred from providing humane compassionate care.

Advance Directives

The Patient Self-Determination Act (PSDA), under which the durable power of attorney (DPA) for health care (DPAHC), the living will (LW), and the directive to physician (DTP) are subsumed, was created by the United States Congress in October 1990 and implemented in all states in December 1991. The intent of the PSDA is based on belief in the preservation of individual rights in decisions related to personal survival. A durable power of attorney for health care can relate to any medical situation in which the individual becomes unable to communicate his or her own choices.

All agencies that receive Medicare and Medicaid funds are mandated to disseminate PDSA information to their clients (Mezey et al, 1994; Mezey, 1996; Berrio and Levesque, 1996). Hospitals and long-term care facilities are responsible for providing written information at the time of admission about the individual's rights under law to refuse medical and surgical care and the right to initiate this in a written advance directive. HMOs and home health care agencies are required to do the same at the time of membership enrollment or before the patient comes under the care of the agency. Hospices are obliged to inform patients of their self-determination rights on the initial visit (Parkman, 1996; Berrio and Levesque, 1996; Mezey, 1996).

Durable Power of Attorney. A DPA enables an individual to appoint a trusted person as "attorney in fact." It gives the person named the power to represent the elder in all legal matters. This should be carefully considered in later life and should be entered into with complete understanding of the risks and benefits. In 1979 the Commissioners on Uniform State Law (a federally appointed commission) adopted the Uniform Durable Power of Attorney that will survive a person's incapacity (Cohen, 1987). The DPA can be drawn up to include specific legal capacities within a specified period of time, or it may be broad and have no time limits. The principal may also express the intent to have the power of attorney survive the incompetency or incapacity of the principal. One can also draft a DPA that does not take effect until the principal becomes incapacitated. Such durable powers are called "spring powers" (Gilfix, 1987). The DPA can be regarded as a substitute for a funded revocable trust or as an alternative to court-oriented procedures such as conservatorship and guardianship (Cohen, 1987). A few states give the "attorney in fact" the power to make health care decisions through a document known as the durable power of attorney for health care (DPAHC).

Durable Power of Attorney for Health Care. The DPAHC or health care proxy is a legal, notarized or witnessed document by which an individual can express his or her wishes regarding care in acute illness and in dying. The proxy authorizes someone of the individual's choosing (a proxy) to make medical decisions for him or her in case he or she is unable to do so. The proxy may be next of kin, a friend, significant other, or in some cases a conservator (Delong, 1995; Weenolsen, 1996; Berrio and Levesque, 1996; Mezey, 1996).

Emanuel and Emanuel (1989) of Harvard developed a medical directive describing hypothetical scenarios to which persons creating this directive could respond (see Appendix 26-A). Many states have their own forms for the execution of a DPAHC. The forms are available from many agencies, including the state medical association and personal physicians. A resource list of agencies is provided under Resources at the end of this chapter. An example of one state's DPAHC or health care proxy appears in Appendix 26-B.

Autopsy as an Advance Directive. Advance directives may include the individual's wishes regarding autopsy. For some this is an insignificant consideration, but for others it may be very important. Rarely is this topic discussed in nursing literature, and nurses have nearly as many misconceptions as do patients. The informed and sensitive nurse can do a great service to patients by discussing the idea and the procedures, clarifying misconceptions, and advocating for the client's wishes. Importantly, autopsy is a method of quality control that assures that misdiagnosis is recognized. Interestingly, even with all the sophisticated diagnostic technologies we now have, autopsy confirms about a 10% error rate, which has remained constant for over 40 years. The lowest rate of autopsy is among the very old (2.4% at age 90). Common reasons for refusing an autopsy are concern about disfigurement, religious beliefs, cost, and lack of good reason to conduct an autopsy. Individuals are rarely approached regarding autopsy, and more than 50% of the time it is not mentioned to the family after the death of a loved one. There is little to be gained by the physician in promoting autopsies, and the number done consistently decreases.

Living Will (LW). Introduced in 1970, the LW is a personal statement of how and where one wishes to die. This document sets forth the treatment choices and instructions for personal end-of-life care. It is not as specific as the DPAHC, nor is it as readily recognized by many states as a legal document (Weenolsen, 1996). It does not acknowledge decisions by a proxy and is activated only when the person is terminally ill and incapacitated. The LW is comparable to the Directive to My Physician, also known as instructional directives or treatment directives. Two states—Alabama and Alaska—recognize only the LW (see Appendix 26-C).

Wills Not Related to Health Care. Wills and living trusts are needed to express one's wishes regarding the disposition of assets on death. A will simply states how the estate will be distributed. A revocable trust is more costly and sophisticated but will avoid probate and many management problems. It ensures ongoing management of the estate without a court-supervised conservatorship because it can incorporate asset preservation and tax planning.

Christian Affirmation of Life. The Catholic Hospital Association approved the Christian Affirmation of Life in 1994. Consistent with Catholic doctrine, the person need not accept extraordinary medical care, but must accept ordinary care such as food, water, pain relief, and hygiene care (Weenolsen, 1996). It is similar to the LW but expresses wishes consistent with the religious faith.

Studies by Emanuel et al (1991) showed that about 70% of individuals decide against life-sustaining treatments if they become incompetent and have a poor prognosis for survival. Danis et al (1991) found that care followed the advanced directive in 75% of the cases they studied retrospectively. These figures were compiled prior to the implementation of the Patient Self-Determination Act. Three years after the PSDA, Berrio and Levesque (1996) reviewed patient records at their facility and discovered only 17% (N = 51) of the patients had completed an advance directive. Johns Hopkins Hospital found only 31% (N = 26) of patients had completed an advance directive (Berrio and Levesque, 1996). Other studies have shown rates of 4% completion. It is hoped that in the future the completion rate for advance directives will be higher.

Gilfix (1987) makes a point that legal planning is essential for the protection of Alzheimer's victims and their families. Unless taken well in advance there may be serious financial and legal repercussions. Because no one can predict future capacities, *everyone* should consider establishing certain legal protections. For the elderly this is exceedingly important.

MacKay (1992) discusses the several methods by which elders may dictate desires regarding control of their medical care and introduces the pros and cons of each (Table 26-8).

Table 26-8 Strengths and Limitations of Advance Directives for Nursing Home Use

Requirements	Advance directives		
	LW	DTP	DPAHC
Patient must be competent to initiate this type of advance directive.	Yes	Yes	Yes
Patient must be competent to revoke this type of advance directive.	No	No	Yes
Two witnesses are required.		Yes	Yes
One witness must be a patient advocate/ombudsman designated by the state.		Yes	Yes
Notary public can be substituted for the required witnesses.		No	Yes
Special form is required.	No	Yes	No
Advance directive lasts up to 5 years	Yes	Yes	Yes
Advance directive lasts at least 7 years.	No	No	Yes
Advance directive requires the patient to have an agent or surrogate decision maker.	No	Yes	Yes
Attending physician is required to be the agent or surrogate decision maker for the patient.		Yes	No
Patient can select a friend or family member as agent.		No	Yes
Legal liability.		Yes	Yes
Advance directive used only for terminal illness/when death is imminent.	Yes	Yes	No
Agent can become guardian.		No	Yes
Advance directive can go into effect immediately.	No	No	Yes
Advance directive requires 14-day waiting period after terminal illness is determined.	Yes	Yes	No

From MacKay S: Durable power of attorney for health care: is DPAHC the best advance directive for patients residing in long-term care facilities? *Geriatr Nurs* 13(2):105, 1992.

Nurse's Role and Advance Directives. The nurse serves as a resource person ready to answer questions openly and honestly about available options, which requires knowledge and understanding of the Patient Self-Determination Act. The nurse is one of the health care professionals who is responsible for ensuring that the individual has the opportunity to learn about and to make an advance directive. The nurse must also ascertain proper disposition of the advance directive if it is completed. For the patient who enters a facility with a directive, the nurse needs to ascertain that it is current and contains directives reflective of the person's choices. The document must be easily available to caregivers (placed on the chart where all can see it).

Nursing home residents with cognitive ability have an opportunity to discuss their thoughts regarding life and death decisions with someone. Residents perceived to have a lack of cognitive capacity do not get the opportunity to do so nor do those residents with communication disorders. *All residents should be given the opportunity to execute an advance directive.*

In a small study of elder patients who were diagnosed as demented by standard tests, 30% were found to possess the mental ability to understand the nature of a health care proxy and designate a relative as their decision maker. Twenty seven percent of the group were able to express their preference for or against a Do Not Resuscitate (DNR) option; 21% could do both a DNR and health care proxy (Schmitt, 1996). Although this is a limited study, it suggests that decision-making capacity is not always accurately predicted by screening tests such as the Folstein Mental Status Exam (MMSE) or the Global Deterioration Scale (GDS-2). Further, it raises the question of who is making the decision

of mental capacity? The implication for elders in long-term care facilities is that these elders should not be excluded from consideration in executing an advance directive.

As a provider of information, the nurse needs to be aware of the types of directives that are legally recognized in the state in which the nurse practices and the terminology associated with directives; for example, surrogate is not recognized as interchangeable with proxy or agent (Weensolen, 1996). The nurse should also be familiar with the advance directive form(s) used by the organization in which he or she is employed. Forms vary from state to state, institution to institution, and still may be recognized as legal documents (Figure 26-5). It is also important to know that if one is taken ill in a state other than where the directive was executed, reciprocal legislation usually recognizes the original document. The nurse must also be cognizant of the barriers to completion of an advance directive (Box 26-9). This will aid in clarifying patient misunderstanding.

The nurse is expected to be able to answer an elder's questions, such as "Can I just talk about my wishes, or do I have to put it in writing?" or "Does this type of form have to be witnessed?" In addition, the nurse must know how a directive is accomplished. Elders in long-term care facilities usually need two witnesses for their directive, one witness being the ombudsman from the department of aging, who serves as a patient advocate.

The nurse may be a patient advocate by bringing family members and the elder together to discuss the difficult issues addressed in making a directive or to just discuss the elder's wishes. It may be the nurse who brings the patient and the physician together to ensure that the patient and the doctor agree on terms of the directive and whether the physician

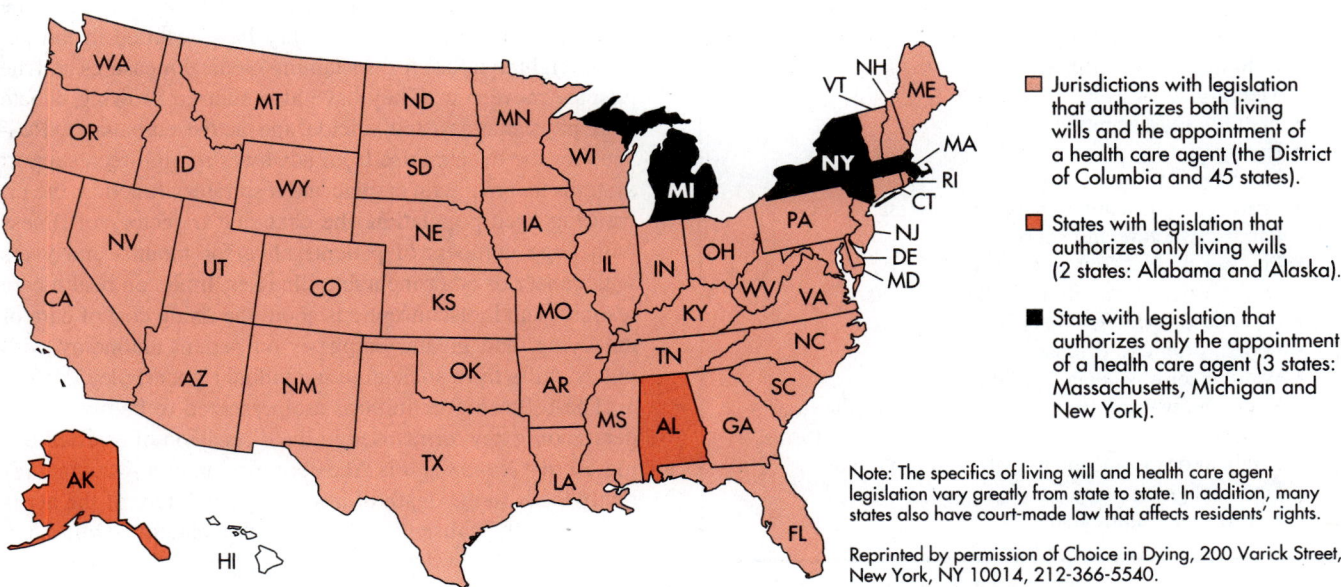

□ Jurisdictions with legislation that authorizes both living wills and the appointment of a health care agent (the District of Columbia and 45 states).

■ States with legislation that authorizes only living wills (2 states: Alabama and Alaska).

■ State with legislation that authorizes only the appointment of a health care agent (3 states: Massachusetts, Michigan and New York).

Note: The specifics of living will and health care agent legislation vary greatly from state to state. In addition, many states also have court-made law that affects residents' rights.

Reprinted by permission of Choice in Dying, 200 Varick Street, New York, NY 10014, 212-366-5540.

Figure 26-5. State statutes governing living wills and appointment of health care agents. (Courtesy Choice in Dying.)

can honor the patient's wishes. It may also be the nurse who obtains the appropriate advance directive form for the elder who is well or ill. Several studies have concluded that counseling by hospital representatives, nurses and others, of hospitalized patients is an effective and generalizable way of improving recognition and execution of advance directives (Meier et al, 1996).

As a facilitator, the nurse encourages the elder to think about end-of-life decisions before becoming a patient. However, it is not unusual that necessity requires this to be done while one is a patient. Elders in long-term care may be vulnerable to loss of control in their life. Advance directives enable them to have some control over care issues at the end of life.

A values assessment, learning what the elder holds important in his or her life and how this relates to his or her desires for health care and quality of life, should be encouraged. Does the elder want measures to be taken to prolong life at all costs or wish for a natural death if the alternative may mean prolonged maintenance on machines? Are there any persons the elder feels comfortable with who can act as a proxy to insure that the elder's wishes will be carried out? Answers to these questions are helpful when discussing the elder's wishes. The discussion should include the family and perhaps the clergy and friends, before a directive is completed, to identify if those who are to be involved are comfortable with the decisions and will adhere to the directive. For elders without family, the nurse may become a sounding board.

Box 26-9   Barriers to Completion of Advance Directives for the Elderly

- Inability to speak English
- Religious/ethnic affiliation
- Memory
- Inability to concentrate
- Eyesight
- Hearing
- Print size of document/reading material
- Family structure and support
- Procrastination, or wait to do later
- Dependence on family to make decisions
- Lack of knowledge about directives
- Difficult topic to discuss
- Waiting for physician to initiate discussion
- Physician waiting for patient to initiate discussion
- Believe a lawyer is needed for completion of forms
- Fatalism or the acceptance of "will of God"
- Fear of signing away life
- Fear of being untreated

Modified from Mezey M: Advance directives protocol: nurse's helping to protect patient's rights, *Geriatr Nurs* 17(5), 1996; Berrio MW, Levesque ME: Advance directives: most patients don't have one. Do yours? *Am J Nurs* 96(8):25, 1996.

No one can think of all the possible contingencies that might require decisions with serious illness or a current condition. The nurse can help the elder understand treatments that are available to sustain life and the implications of such interventions as resuscitation efforts (cardiopulmonary resuscitation), intubation, and artificial nutrition, as well as the technical terms associated with them.

Suicide

Suicide by the elderly, per se, is mentioned here because it is an alternative way of dying that the aged may choose. Suicide no longer holds the societal stigma it once did. In 1994 the suicide rate was 2.6% in the aged population and is thought to be rising (U.S. Bureau of Census, 1995). The number of successful suicides increases with age, particularly with aged males, who have a suicide rate twice that of the population as a whole. The motive of the aged who attempt suicide is not to attract attention or to gain sympathy but rather a genuine desire to end life.

The aged, as mentioned earlier in this chapter, often would rather die than experience the indignities of severe illness, dependency, rejection, and isolation. In their own way, whether in an overt act of suicide or the insidious culmination of excessive or predetermined drug use (such as alcohol or mixing medications), refusal to eat, or the willing of oneself to die, the suicide presents a final statement, an effort to retain control of life and life decisions. Interestingly enough, if the terminally ill aged have needs met in a hospice or other care environment and are kept in the mainstream of life, suicide, although an option, is rarely considered.

Physician-Assisted Death. Physician-assisted death, physician-assisted suicide, physician-aid in dying, and active euthanasia are interchangeable terms. Changes in dying in the latter half of the twentieth century have resulted in the patient's right to refuse life-sustaining medical measures and the hospice movement. They have also spurred growing debate over physician-assisted suicide and active euthanasia. Reasons for the debate arise from advances in high-tech support systems that maintain cardiac and respiratory function, the increasing aged population, the changing trajectory of illness with large numbers of patients alive for months and years with cancer or other incurable illnesses, limits on health care resources and misconceptions about the rising cost of care of the dying, and greater emphasis on patient autonomy with policy shifts from societal to individual rights (Foley, 1996).

The following definitions are presented to help with understanding key terms used in the discussion of assisted dying. *Active euthanasia* is "the commission of any act that directly leads to the death of a patient. The intent of the act is to mercifully cause the death of the patient" (Minogue, 1996, p. 64). *Physician-assisted suicide* occurs "when the physician facilitates a patient's death by providing the necessary means and/or information to enable the patient to end his or her life" (Minogue, 1996, p. 80). An example of this might be the physician providing the patient with sleeping pills and instructions about the lethal dose. This is considered passive euthanasia because the physician has not withheld or withdrawn life-sustaining treatment. The physician who would inject lethal poison into a patient who voluntarily requested to be euthanized would be considered to be practicing active euthanasia. At this time both active and passive euthanasia are considered criminal acts by law.

In May 1992 the *Journal of the American Medical Association* reported that 73% of the general public in a large sample approved of some form of euthanasia.

The Netherlands is held up as the example of the only nation that permits physician-assisted death and active euthanasia. Though it is not legal, it is tolerated (Morrison and Meier, 1994; O'Keefe, 1995; DeSpelder and Strickland, 1996; Hendin, 1996). The comparison between the Netherlands, a more homogeneous population with almost all possessing medical insurance, to the United State with great heterogeneity of races, cultures, religions, languages, and lifestyles makes it extremely difficult to arrive at consensus on this issue.

Limited knowledge is available about the circumstances under which physician-assisted death is requested and whether an actual or potential demand really exists. One major question asked is, Why does one request euthanasia? Some answers have indicated it is because those who are dying fear the loss of dignity, pain, and being dependent on others and are tired of life (Morrison and Meier, 1994).

Passage of Measure 16, the Death with Dignity Act, by the State of Oregon in 1994, makes Oregon the first in the world to pass legislation in favor of physician-assisted dying. However, implementation has been stalled by judicial review (DeSpelder and Strickland, 1996; Hendin, 1996).

If deemed legally acceptable by the court, the Death with Dignity Act would allow a terminally ill Oregon resident with fewer than 6 months to live to obtain a lethal prescription from a physician to end his or her life. Before a patient could receive a physician's help, he or she must be mentally competent, give informed consent, obtain a second opinion, and be a legal resident of Oregon. If those criteria are met, the patient requesting the prescription takes the drug without the assistance of the physician (passive euthanasia). The law prohibits lethal injection (active euthanasia). Nurses have had strong opinions pro and con on the topic.

The American Nurses' Association position statement on assisted suicide was developed to provide nurses with a point of reference for discussion and understanding of the many difficulties involved in the issue of a patient's request to terminate his or her life. The American Nurses' Association advises nurses not to participate in assisted suicide, citing such action a "violation of the *Code for Nurses with Interpretive Statements* and the ethical traditions of the profession" (Ana, 1985; Canavan, 1996, p. 8). The nurse is involved in many end-of-life care situations because she or he is the primary care provider who implements decisions of others around end-of-life care. It should not mean patients who want their life terminated should be abandoned.

Considerable confusion exists regarding terminology and interpretation of what effects the nurse's role may have. Many nurses believe that turning off the ventilator, turning off tube feedings, stopping intravenous fluids, or giving as much pain medication as is needed, even if the side effect is death, constitutes assisted suicide. It is important for the nurse to understand that withdrawal of such measures as feeding tubes and ventilators is allowing natural death to occur, which is very different than actively doing something to cause death (Murphy, 1996).

The general trend in American law is toward greater freedom for the individual to choose when and how to die. Many believe that patient-assisted suicide could be a reality soon based on constitutional grounds of the right to privacy (Messinger, 1993) or the due process clause of the Fourteenth Amendment to the U.S. Constitution (Sedler, 1993; Wilkes, 1996; Carter, 1996).

As a means of stimulating thoughtful discussion on this topic, Table 26-9 includes some pros and cons from Morrison and Meier (1994). Murphy (1996) suggests *now* is the time for nurses individually, among themselves, and collectively, in professional organizations, to consider the implications of physician-assisted suicide and what their role will be while it is still a topic of social debate, rather than be caught unprepared without professional consensus as to their position if it should be legalized, as it could be (Murphy, 1996).

It is clear that continuing discussion and new perspectives are needed to resolve this supremely important question. *California Nurse* (Liaschenko and Drought, 1993)

Table 26-9	Arguments for and against Physician-Assisted Suicide

For	Against
Physicians have a duty to alleviate uncontrollable pain and suffering, including the obligation to provide an assisted death at a competent patient's request.	Society runs the risk of sliding into a practice of involuntary euthanasia and subtle coercion of vulnerable and disenfranchised patients.
Patients have the right to autonomy, which presently includes the right to forego or have withdrawn life-sustaining therapy.	There is a potential for abuse. Involuntary euthanasia has a higher priority in permissive environments where euthanasia is legal.
It allows the terminally ill to preserve their autonomy and exert final control.	The healing ethos of medical practice may be adversely affected, and public trust in physicians may be eroded.

Data from Morrison S, Meier DE: Physician-assisted dying: fashioning public policy with an absence of data, *Generations* 18 (4):48, 1994.

Nursing Diagnoses

The following potential diagnoses must be considered as well as diagnoses unique to the particular individual:

Coping, ineffective
Family processes, altered
Grieving, anticipatory
Grieving, dysfunctional
Hopelessness
Pain

Personal identity disturbance
Powerlessness
Role performance, altered
Social isolation
Spiritual distress

NURSING PROCESS AND NURSING DIAGNOSIS
Grieving: Anticipatory—Loss of Self through Terminal Illness

Etiologies and Related Factors
Terminal diagnosis

Defining Characteristics
Verbal expression of distress
Sadness
Crying
Altered eating patterns
Altered sleep patterns
Altered dreams
Reminiscence
Lability
Withdrawal
Exacerbation of psychopathology

Knowledge
Grief process
Theories of loss and grief
The dying process
Interpersonal relationships
Role of caregiver in facilitating grief expression
Ritual and rites that are important
Therapeutic communication
Legalities: advance directives, organ donations
Own mortality feelings
Community resources

Clinical Judgment and Related Skills
Utilization of communication skills
Listening
Share perceptions
Provide for privacy
Reinforce self-worth
Encourage (as or when appropriate) family, friends, and client opportunities for closure
Provision of control in decision making
Physical comfort measures to maintain independence for as long as possible
Share concerns
Help client plan and get important business in order
Nonjudgmental acceptance
Facilitate religious/spiritual/social needs as needed
Assist family as well as client to cope with impending loss
Ability to separate own feelings and philosophy of death and dying from those of client
Make necessary referrals

Evaluation
Client completes task(s) that he/she identified or defined
Expresses some philosophy related to living and dying
Achieves the security to die in own way

NEEDS ADDRESSED AND TASK STRENGTHS

Need to maintain family continuity; need for spiritual expression and awareness of meaning; need for comfort and choices in dying
Awareness and acceptance of life cycles

Expression of own life experience
Universality
Sensitivity to meanings
Cultivation of spirituality
Sense of humor

introduced some cogent questions regarding this issue; these are included at the end of the chapter for student discussion.

Planning for the Care of Survivors

As with grief discussed earlier in this chapter, outliving those one loves may create an emptiness that can never be fully assuaged. Table 26-3 is again cited as an aid to facilitating the needs of survivors. The nurse must be prepared for this most difficult of all tasks.

• • •

This chapter has dealt with the apogee and perigee of human experience. The highest levels of nursing function and the deepest feelings are uncovered in the nurse who is privileged to accompany the aged through the processes of fully living the last days before dying.

KEY CONCEPTS

- Grief is an emotional and behavioral response to loss.
- There are many theories or frameworks that outline grief responses; however, grief responses are individual. What is appropriate for one societal group may be considered aberrant by another group.
- One never completely resolves grief. Instead, the individual incorporates the grief as a part of his or her life.
- Dying is a multifaceted active process. It affects all involved, the one who is dying, the family, the professional caregivers.
- The stages or phases of dying and the type of coping are not obligatory or prescriptive of the way one should die. Such expectations place an added burden on the one who is dying.
- An individual is living until he or she has died.
- The dying older adult is a living person with all the same needs for good and natural relationships with people as the rest of us.
- Hope is empowering. It generates courage and motivates action and achievement. The degree of hope that a dying individual possesses depends on a caring relationship with others.
- The health professional who cares for the dying must have outside interests and support systems before considering care of the dying.
- Living can be more painful than dying.
- Hospice is a process or unique ideology that links the needs of terminally ill, the family, and staff to fulfill the remainder of a dying individual's life by enabling or returning control to the dying person.
- Advance directives allow an individual control over life and death decisions by written communication and allows an appointed person (a proxy) to be his or her advocate when he or she are not able to communicate desires personally.
- Most medical and nursing organizations do not support physician-aid in dying and suicide. These issues will continue to generate controversy within the health professions into the next century.

▲ CASE STUDY

Jesse simply could not believe his wife was dying. The doctor told him she was in the early stages of multiple myeloma, and she could die in less than a year or she might have remissions and live another decade. They had worked hard all their lives and raised two sons. Now that they were both retired and financially well fixed, even though they were not yet 65, they had thought the best years of their lives were ahead. But, both Jesse and Jeannette were the type to approach a problem head on, and they gathered all the relevant material they could find and assiduously studied all they could find about multiple myeloma. Jeannette said she did not want to mention her problem to others because she didn't think she could deal with "their piteous cancer looks." She also stressed that she expected to have long remissions and to live to be 75 years old, at least, so why trouble friends and family. So Jesse could not share his fear and grief because he had promised to respect Jeannette's wishes in that regard. She began a series of chemotherapeutic drugs, and friends began to notice her lethargy. They began to worry about her, but she insisted, "I'm just fine." Six months passed with a steady downward course in Jeannette's condition. Her sons began to suspect she had a malignancy, and one son, Rob, asked outright, "Are you hiding a serious illness from us?" She denied it, but Rob also noticed that Jesse was withdrawing into himself and frequently retreated into the booze bottle. He knew something was wrong but was at a loss. When Rob went to the family physician for his annual checkup, the office nurse said, "Oh, Rob, how is your mother doing now?" At Rob's insistence the nurse told him of his mother's diagnosis. Discuss your rationale and feelings as the office nurse, and determine a plan of action that seems appropriate at this time. Develop a long-range plan of care for this family.

Based upon the case study, develop a nursing care plan using the following procedure*:

List comments of client that provide *subjective data*.

List information that provides *objective data*.

From these data identify and state, using accepted format, two *nursing diagnoses* you determine are most significant to this client at this time.

---

*Students are advised to refer to their nursing diagnosis text and identify possible or potential problems.

Determine and state *outcome criteria* for each diagnosis. These must reflect some alleviation of the problem identified in the nursing diagnosis and must be stated in concrete and measurable terms.

Plan and state one or more interventions for each diagnosed problem. Provide specific documentation of source used to determine appropriate intervention.

Evaluate success of intervention. Interventions must correlate directly with the stated outcome criteria in order to measure the outcome success.

STUDY QUESTIONS/ACTIVITIES

Explore your responses to being given a terminal diagnosis: what coping mechanisms work for you? With which awareness approach would you be comfortable?

How would you recognize spiritual distress? Relate particular interventions you think would be helpful to an individual who was feeling spiritually distressed.

Discuss what you believe are the significant aspects of "religion" or "spirituality" in your life. Do not feel you must do so if it is an uncomfortable topic for you to share.

If you feel able, discuss your grief process when you dealt with the loss of someone special in your life.

Practice with a partner several methods you will use to introduce the topic of dying with a client who is critically ill and not expected to live.

Describe how you would deal with a dying person and his or her family when they are especially protective of each other.

Discuss and strategize how you would bring up the topic of advance directives.

What advance directive is legally recognized in your state?

Explore with family and friends their thoughts on completing an advance directive.

Complete your own advance directive.

STUDENT DISCUSSION QUESTIONS RELATED TO ASSISTED SUICIDE

What is the cultural and historic meaning of "killing"?

In Biblical times was it believed that God killed?

Is there a general denial of the responsibility that accompanies the enormous technologic power we have developed over life and death?

Are we afraid we are "playing God"?

Is loss of dignity and loss of self as significant in the desire to die as unbearable pain?

For those in favor of euthanasia, is it related to an inability to tolerate or witness the suffering of others?

Is the Hippocratic Oath, grounded in allegiance to Greek gods and selectively practiced, relevant to decisions about euthanasia?

What would be appropriate safeguards from misuse, neither too restrictive nor too liberal?

What nursing actions do you consider assisted suicide?

RESEARCH QUESTIONS

How does religiosity influence coping and grief resolution?

What are the phenomenologic aspects of dying at various ages: 65, 75, 85, etc.? What is the significance of the variations? Similar studies are needed related to the particular type of death.

Do patterns of grief of elders differ depending upon whether the person is spouse, sibling, or child?

What are the variables that influence elders to die at home?

What percentage of hospice patients are over age 65, and what are the conditions of their terminal illness?

When do elders usually complete an advance directive?

What are the nurses' interpretation of assisted dying versus euthanasia?

How do long-term care facilities cope with the dying elder?

How do nurses foresee their role if assisted suicide is legalized?

RESOURCES

Films and Videos

Walk Me to the Water is available from Box 258, Mountain Road, New Lebanon, NY 12125, (518) 794-9622. "*Walk Me to the Water* clearly and powerfully portrays the needs of the dying. It is an excellent and loving contribution to the field of death education. For those facing a terminal illness, their family members, and the health care professionals involved—this film is a must!" (Elisabeth Kübler-Ross, MD)

A Woman's Tale is a film by Paul Cox that is available in video outlets and presents the details of a life as it nears an end. "Beauty in life may come from makeup or clothing, but for beauty in death you have to fall back on character," Martha says at one point. In its better moments, *A Woman's Tale* is indeed what Mr. Cox must have intended: a vivid embodiment of that thought.

A Home Alone, J. Rowe, Filmakers Library, New York, NY (30 minutes). From the "Saying Goodbye" series on bereavement, this program shows the special problems that men have in dealing with feelings of loss.

To Dance with the White Dog, Republic Pictures Corporation, 12636 Beatrice Street, Los Angeles, CA 90066-0930. This Hallmark Hall of Fame television presentation is available in stores for video rental. It is based on the book by Terry Kay. Alone and struggling with his own ailing health after the sudden death of his wife, Sam's spirit begins to fade until the sudden appearance of a mysterious white dog who awakens in him the joy of life and the undying love of his wife.

The Way We Die, Fanlight Productions, 47 Halifax Street, Boston, MA 02130, (800) 937-4113. Purchase or rental available. Through interviews with doctors, patients, and family members and through intimate interactions between medical personnel and their terminally ill patients, the video encourages health professionals to work with their patients to devise treatment plans in accord with their needs, values, and wishes and to pay attention to the larger issue of what illness means for a particular patient and family.

Organizations

Institute of Noetic Sciences
PO Box 909
Sausalito, CA 94966-0909
Apollo 14 Astronaut Edgar Mitchell founded the Institute of Noetic Sciences in 1973 to expand knowledge of the nature and potentials of the mind and spirit and to apply that knowledge to advance health and well-being for humankind and our planet.

Parapsychology
Parapsychological Association
PO Box 7503
Alexandria, VA 22307

Hospices
National Hospice Organization
Suite 402
1901 N Fort Myer Drive
Arlington, VA 22209
(703) 243-5900
Toll-free hospice referral number: (800) 658-8898

Advocates for hospice patients; provides education and workshops to professionals.

Legal Assistance
American Bar Association
1155 E 69th Street
Chicago, IL 60637

The Widowed
National Association for Widowed People, Inc
PO Box 3564
Springfield, IL 62708

Parents Without Partners
7910 Woodmont Avenue
Washington, DC 20014

Society of Military Widows
PO Box 1714
La Mesa, CA 92041

The Compassionate Friends
PO Box 1347
Oak Brook, IL 60521

Widowed Persons Service (WPS)
NRTA-AARP
1909 K Street, NW
Washington, DC 20049

Euthanasia
American Euthanasia Foundation
95 N Birch Road, Suite 301
Ft Lauderdale, FL 33304

Choice in Dying, Inc., The National Council
for the Right to Die
200 Varick Street
New York, NY 10014

General Organizations

Ars Moriendi
7301 Huron Lane
Philadelphia, PA 19119

Center for Death Education and Research
1167 Social Science Building
University of Minnesota
267 19th Ave, South
Minneapolis, MN 55455

Foundation of Thanatology
630 West 168th Street
New York, NY 10032

Association for Death Education and Counseling
638 Prospect Avenue
Hartford, CT 06105-4298
(203) 232-4825

International, interdisciplinary organization offering seminars, workshops, and conferences.

National Institute for the Seriously Ill and Dying
Henry Avenue & Abbottsford Road
Philadelphia, PA 19129

Information about Advance Directives

Alzheimer's Disease and Related Disorders Association
(312) 335-8700

American Association of Critical-Care Nurses
(800) 899-2226

American Association of Retired Persons
(202) 434-2277

American Bar Association
Commission on Legal Problems of the Elderly
(202) 662-8690

American Hospital Association
(312) 422-3000

American Nurses' Association
(202) 651-7000

Center for Healthcare Ethics
St Louis University Health Sciences Center
(314) 577-8195

Choice in Dying
(800) 989-WILL (9455)

National Hospice Organization
(703) 243-5900

Publications

The National Interfaith Coalition on Aging (NICA) is comprised of national-level representatives concerned with the future of older adults in America. It holds an annual conference and publishes *Reform*, a newsletter. Address: 298 South Hull Street, Athens, GA 30605.

REFERENCES

American Nurses' Association, *Code for nurses with interpretative statements,* Kansas City, Mo, 1985.

American Nurses' Association: *Standards and scope of hospice nursing practice,* Kansas City, Mo, 1987, The Association.

American Nurses' Association: *Position statement on nursing care and do-not-resuscitate decisions,* Washington, DC, 1992, The Association.

Arbuckle NW, DeVries B: The long-term effects of late life spousal and parental bereavement on personal functioning, *Gerontologist* 35(5):637, 1995.

Berrio MW, Levesque ME: Advance directives: most patients don't have one. Do yours? *Am J Nurs* 96(8):25,1996.

Botwinick J et al: Predicting death from behavioral test performance, *J Gerontol* 33:(6)755, 1978.

Bowlby J: Process of mourning, *Int J Psychoanal* 42:317, 1961.

Bowling A: Who dies after widow(er)hood? A discriminate analysis, *Omega: Journal of Death and Dying* 19:135, 1989.

Brabant S, Forsyth CJ, Melanon C: Grieving men: thoughts, feelings and behaviors following deaths of wives, *Hospice Journal Physical, Psychosocial, and Pastoral Care of the Dying* 8(4):33, 1992.

Canavan K: ANA advises nurses not to participate in assisted suicide, *Am Nurs,* p 8, June 1996.

Carr AC, Schoenberg B, Peretz D, et al: Object-loss and somatic symptom formation. In Schoenberg B et al, editors: *Loss and grief: psychological management in medical practice,* New York, 1970, Columbia University Press.

Carter SL: Rush to a lethal judgement, New York, *Time Magazine,* July 2, 1996.

Cartwright A: Is religion a help around the time of death? *Public Health* 105(1):79, 1991.

Caserta MS, Lund DA: Intrapersonal resources and the effectiveness of self-help groups for bereaved older adults, *Gerontologist* 33(5):619, 1993.

Cleeland D: Pain and its treatment in outpatients with metastatic cancer, *N Engl J Med* 330:592, 1994.

Cohen E: Durable powers of attorney: an overview, *Aging Connection* 8(2):8, 1987.

Coolican MB, Stark J, Doka KJ, Corr CA: Education about death, dying, and bereavement in nursing programs, *Nurs Educa* 19(6):38, 1994.

Corr CA: Coping with dying: lessons that we should and should not learn from the work of Elisabeth Kübler-Ross, *Death Studies* 17(1):69, 1993.

Corr CA: A task-based approach to coping with dying. In DeSpelder LA, Strickland AL: *The pathway ahead,* Mountainview, Calif, 1995, Mayfield Publishing Company.

Danis M; Southerland LI, Garrett JM et al: A prospective study of advance directives for life-sustaining care, *N Engl J Med* 324:882,1991.

Delong MF: Caring for the elderly. V. Managing end of life issues, *NURSEweek* 8(9), 1995.

Depaola SJ, Neimeyer RA, Lupfer MB et al: Death concern and attitudes toward the elderly in nursing home personnel, *Death Studies* 16(6):537, 1992.

DeSpelder LA, Strickland AL: *The pathway ahead: readings in death and dying,* Mountainview, Calif, 1995, Mayfield Publishing Company.

DeSpelder LA, Strickland AL: *The last dance: encountering death and dying,* ed 4, Mountainview, Calif, Mayfield Publishing Company, 1996

Dessonville CL, Thompson LW, Gallagher D: The role of anticipatory bereavement in the adjustment to widowhood in the elderly, *Gerontologist* 23:309 (special issue), 1983.

Doka KJ: The spiritual crisis of bereavement. In Doka KJ, Morgan JD, editors: *Death and spirituality,* Amityville, NY, 1993, Baywood Publishing Company.

Emanuel LL, Barry MJ, Stoeckle JD et al: Advance directives for medical care: a case of greater use, *N Engl J Med* 324:889,1991.

Emanual LL, Emanual EJ: The medical directive: a new comprehensive advance care document, *JAMA* 261:3288, 1989.

Engel G : Grief and grieving, *Am J Nurs* 64:93, 1967.

Erikson E: *Childhood and society,* New York, 1963, WW Norton.

Foley KM: Death in America: a new dynamic for an old reality—the national debate, *Aging Today* 17 (1):7, 1996.

Forbes SB: Hope: an essential human need in the elderly, *J Gerontol Nurs* 20(6):5, 1994.

Futterman EH, Hoffman I, Sabshin M: Parental anticipatory mourning. In Schoenberg B, Carr AC, Peretz D et al, editors: *Psychosocial aspects of terminal care,* New York, 1970, Columbia University Press.

Gass K: Coping strategies of widows, *J Gerontol Nurs* 13(8):29, 1987.

Gilfix M: Legal planning is essential for Alzheimer's victims, *Senior Spectrum* 6(12):5, 1987

Glaser B, Strauss A: *Awareness of dying,* Chicago, 1963, AVC, Inc.

Godow S: Death and dying: a natural connection? *Generations* 11:15, 1987.

Goodman M, Rubinstein RL, Alexander BB, Luborsky M: Cultural differences among elderly women in coping with the death of an adult child, *J Gerontol* 46(6):S321, 1991.

Gorer G: *Death, grief, mourning,* London, 1965, Cressett Press.

Gray VR: Dealing with dying, *Nursing '73* 3:27, 1976.

Harper BC: *Death: the coping mechanisms of the health professional,* Greenville, SC, 1977, Southeastern University Press.

Hendin H: The psychiatrist. In Wilkes P: The next pro-lifers, *New York Times Magazine,* p. 25, July 21, 1996.

Herth K: Relationship of hope, coping styles, concurrent losses and setting of grief resolution in the elderly widow(er), *Res Nurs Health* 13:109, 1990.

Hess PA: Loss, grief, and dying. In Beare P, Myers J: *Adult health nursing,* ed 3, St Louis, 1998, Mosby.

Hooyman N, Kiyak H: *Social gerontology,* Boston, 1988, Allyn and Bacon Co.

Horacek BJ: Toward a more viable model of grieving and consequences for older persons, *Death Studies* 15(5):459, 1991.

Keleman S: Stages of dying, *Voices* 10:46,1974.

Kelly JD: Grief: Re-forming life's story, *J Palliat Care* 8(2):33, 1992.

Krohn B: When death is near, *Geriatr Nurs* (in press).

Kübler-Ross E: *On death and dying,* New York, 1969, MacMillan.

Lentzner HR, Pamuk ER, Rhodenhiser EP et al: The quality of life in the year before death, *Am J Public Health* 82(8):1093, 1992.

Liaschenko J, Drought T: Euthanasia: pro and con, *Calif Nurse* 89(1):1, 1993.

Lindeman E: Symptomatology and management of acute grief, *Am J Psychiatr* 101:141,1944.

Lindley DB: Process of dying: defining characteristics, *Cancer Nurs* 14(6):328, 1991.

Lund DA, Caserta MD, Dimond MF: Gender differences through two years of bereavement among the elderly, *Gerontologist* 26(3):314,1986.

MacKay S: Durable power of attorney for health care: is DPAHC the best advance directive for patients residing in long-term care facilities? *Geriatr Nurs* 13(2):99,1992.

Martocchio BC: *Living while dying,* Bowie, Md, 1982, RJ Brady Co.

McCaffery M, Bebee A: *Pain: clinical manual for nursing practice,* St Louis, 1989, Mosby.

Meier DE, Fuss BR, O'Rourke D et al: Marked improvement in recognition and completion of health care proxies: a randomized controlled trial of counseling by hospital patient representatives, *Arch Intern Med* 156(11):1227, 1996.

Messinger TJ: A gentle and easy death: from ancient Greece to beyond Cruzan—toward a reasoned legal response to the societal dilemma of euthanasia, *Denver University Law Review* 71(1):229, 1993.

Mezey M, Ramsey GC, Mitty E: Making the PSDA work for the elderly, *Generations* 18 (4):13, 1994.

Mezey M: Geriatric nursing standard of practice protocol: advance directives—nurses helping to protect patient rights, *Geriatr Nurs* 17(5) 1996.

Mickley JR, Soeken K, Belcher A: Spiritual well-being, religiousness and hope among women with breast cancer, *Image J Nurs Sch* 24(4):267, 1992.

Minogue B: *Bioethics: a committee approach,* Boston, 1996, Jones and Bartlett Publishers.

Mittleman M: Taking grief to heart, *Harvard Health Letter* 21(8):8, 1996.

Morrison RS, Meier DE: Physician-assisted dying: fashioning public policy with an absence of data, *Generations* 18(4):48, 1994.

Moyers W: *Healing and the mind,* WNET public television, February, 1992.

Murphy P: In Canavan K: ANA advises nurses not to participate in assisted suicide, *Am Nurs,* p 8, June 1996.

O'Hara PA, Harper DW, Lyne D et al: Patient death in a long-term care hospital: a study of the effect on nursing staff, *J Gerontol Nurs* 22(8):27,1996.

O'Keefe M: The Dutch way of dying, *San Francisco Sunday Examiner,* p A8, Feb 19, 1995.

Parkman C: Using advance directives: part 2, *NURSEweek* 9(12):10,1996.

Parks CM: *Bereavement,* New York, 1972, Tavistock.

Parks CM, Weiss RS: *Recovery from bereavement,* New York, 1983, Basic Books.

Pattison EM: The experience of dying, *Am J Psychother* 21:32, 1967.

Pietruszka FM: Management of bereavement in the elderly, *Physician Assistant* 16(4):31, 1992.

Rando TA: *Grief, dying and death,* Champaign, Ill, 1984, Research Press.

Raphael B: *Anatomy of bereavement,* New York, 1983, Basic Books.

Rees WD, Lukin SG: The mortality of bereavement, *Br Med J* 4:13, 1967.

Retsinas J: A theoretical reassessment of the applicability of Kübler-Ross's stages of dying, *Death Studies* 12:207, 1988.

Richter J: Support: a resource during crisis of mate loss, *J Gerontol Nurs* 13(11):18, 1987.

Rigdon I, Clayton B, Dimond M: Toward a theory of helplessness for the elderly bereaved: an invitation to a new life, *Adv Nurs Sci* 9(2):32, 1987.

Schmitt L: *The right to choose: capacity study of demented residents in nursing homes* (executive summary), Franciscan Sisters of the Poor, Hospital Systems Inc, 1996.

Schreck IR: Commentary on grieving men: thoughts, feelings, and behavior following death of wives, *ONS Nursing Scan Oncol* 2(4):1, 1993.

Schuman J: Palliative care in a Catholic institution (abstract), *Proceedings of the Third Congress of the International Psychogeriatric Association,* 1987.

Sedler RA: The constitution and hastening inevitable death, *Hasting Cent Rep* 23(5): 20, 1993.

Siegel JM, Kuykendall DH: Loss, widowhood, and psychological distress among the elderly, *J Consult Clin Psychol* 58(5):519, 1990.

Sisneros J: *Language change as a function of growth after loss,* compiled for N112, San Francisco State University School of Nursing, 1994.

Solari-Twadell PA, Schmidt-Bunkers S, Wang CE, Snyder D: The pinwheel model of bereavement, *Image J Nurs Sch* 27(4):323, 1995.

Steele L: Risk factor profile for bereaved spouses, *Death Studies* 16(5):387, 1992.

Stroebe M, Gergen MM, Gergen KJ, Stroebe W: Broken hearts or broken bonds: love and death in historical perspective, *Am Psychol* 47(10)1205,1992.

Thomas V: Hospice nursing: reaping the rewards, dealing with the stress, *Geriatr Nurs* 4:22, 1983.

Ulrich LK: The challenge of hospice care, *Bull Am Protestant Hosp Assoc* 21:6, 1978.

US Bureau of the Census: *Statistical abstract of the United States: 1995,* ed 115, Washington, DC, 1995.

US Department of Health and Human Services: *Vital Statistics report to vital and health statistics,* Public Health Service, Center for Disease Control and Prevention, National Center for Health Statistics, Series 10, #193, December, 1995.

Watson W, Maxwell RJ: Elements of the social structure of dying. In Watson W, Maxwell RJ, editors: *Human aging and dying: study in sociocultural gerontology,* New York, 1977, St Martin's Press.

Weenolsen P: *The art of dying,* New York, 1996, St Martin's Press.

White N, Cunningham WR: Is terminal drop pervasive or specific? *J Gerontol* 43(6):141, 1988.

Wilkes P: The next pro-lifers, *New York Times Magazine,* July 21, 1996.

Worden JW: *Grief counseling and grief therapy: a handbook for mental health practitioners,* ed 2, New York, 1991, Springer.

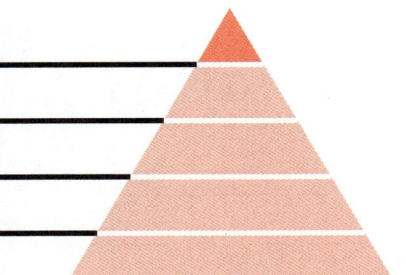

The Medical Directive

INTRODUCTION

As part of a person's right to self-determination, every adult may accept or refuse any recommended medical treatment. This is relatively easy when people are well and can speak. Unfortunately, during serious illness they are often unconscious or otherwise unable to communicate their wishes—at the very time when many critical decisions need to be made.

The Medical Directive allows you to record your wishes regarding various types of medical treatments in several representative situations so that your desires can be respected. It also lets you appoint a proxy, someone to make medical decisions in your place if you should become unable to make them on your own.

The Medical Directive comes into effect only if you become incompetent (unable to make decisions and too sick to have wishes). You can change it at any time until then. As long as you are competent, you should discuss your care with your physician.

COMPLETING THE FORM

You should, if possible, complete the form in the context of a discussion with your physician. Ideally, this should occur in the presence of your proxy. This lets your physician and your proxy know how you think about these decisions, and it provides you and your physician with the opportunity to give or clarify relevant personal or medical information. You may also wish to discuss the issues with your family, friends, or religious mentor.

The Medical Directive contains six illness situations that include incompetence. For each one, you consider possible interventions and goals of medical care. Situation A is permanent coma; B is near death; C is with weeks to live in and out of consciousness; D is extreme dementia; E is a situation you describe; and F is temporary inability to make decisions.

For each scenario you identify your general goals for care and specific intervention choices. The interventions are divided into six groups: (1) cardiopulmonary resuscitation or major surgery; (2) mechanical breathing or dialysis; (3) blood transfusions or blood products; (4) artificial nutrition and hydration; (5) simple diagnostic tests or antibiotics; and (6) pain medications, even if they dull consciousness and indirectly shorten life. Most of these treatments are described briefly. If you have further questions, consult your physician.

Your wishes for treatment options (I want this treatment; I want this treatment tried, but stopped if there is no clear improvement; I am undecided; I do not want this treatment) should be indicated. If you choose a trial of treatment, you should understand that this indicates you want the treatment *withdrawn* if your physician and proxy believe that it has become futile.

The Personal Statement section allows you to explain your choices and say anything you wish to those who may make decisions for you concerning the limits of your life and the goals of intervention. For example, in situation B, if you wish to define "uncertain chance" with numerical probability, you may do so here.

Next you may express your preferences concerning organ donation. Do you wish to donate your body or some or all of your organs after your death? If so, for what purpose(s) and to which physician or institution? If not, this should also be indicated in the appropriate box.

In the final section you may designate one or more proxies, who would be asked to make choices under circumstances in which your wishes are unclear. You can indicate whether or not the decisions of the proxy should override your wishes if there are differences. And, should you name more than one proxy, you can state who is to have the final say if there is disagreement. Your proxy must understand that this role usually involves making judgments that you would have made for yourself, had you been able—and making them by the criteria you have outlined. Proxy decisions should ideally be made in discussion with your family, friends, and physician.

WHAT TO DO WITH THE FORM

Once you have completed the form, you and two adult witnesses (other than your proxy) who have no interest in your estate need to sign and date it.

Many states have legislation covering documents of this sort. To determine the laws in your state, you should call the state attorney general's office or consult a lawyer. If your state has a statutory document, you may wish to use the Medical Directive and append it to this form.

You should give a copy of the completed document to your physician. His or her signature is desirable but not mandatory. The Directive should be placed in your medical records and flagged so that anyone who might be involved in your care can be aware of its presence. Your proxy, a family member, and/or a friend should also have a copy. In addition, you may want to carry a wallet card noting that you have such a document and where it can be found.

MY MEDICAL DIRECTIVE

This Medical Directive shall stand as a guide to my wishes regarding medical treatments in the event that illness should make me unable to communicate them directly. I make this Directive, being 18 years or more of age, of sound mind, and appreciating the consequences of my decisions.

SITUATION A

If I am in a coma or a persistent vegetative state and, in the opinion of my physician and two consultants, have no known hope of regaining awareness and higher mental functions no matter what is done, then my goals and specific wishes—if medically reasonable—for this and any additional illnesses would be:

- ☐ Prolong life; treat everything
- ☐ Attempt to cure, but reevaluate often
- ☐ Limit to less invasive and less burdensome interventions
- ☐ Provide comfort care only
- ☐ Other (please specify):

SITUATION B

If I am near death and in a coma, and, in the opinion of my physician and two consultants, have a small but uncertain chance of regaining higher mental functions, a somewhat greater chance of surviving with permanent mental and physical disability, and a much greater chance of not recovering at all, then my goals and specific wishes—if medically reasonable—for this and any additional illness would be:

- ☐ Prolong life; treat everything
- ☐ Attempt to cure, but reevaluate often
- ☐ Limit to less invasive and less burdensome interventions
- ☐ Provide comfort care only
- ☐ Other (please specify):

SITUATION C

If I have a terminal illness with weeks to live, and my mind is not working well enough to make decisions for myself, but I am sometimes awake and seem to have feelings, then my goals and specific wishes—if medically reasonable—for this and any additional illness would be:

*In this state, prior wishes need to be balanced with a best guess about your current feelings. The proxy and physician have to make this judgment for you.

- ☐ Prolong life; treat everything
- ☐ Attempt to cure, but reevaluate often
- ☐ Limit to less invasive and less burdensome interventions
- ☐ Provide comfort care only
- ☐ Other (please specify):

SITUATION D

If I have brain damage or some brain disease that in the opinion of my physician and two consultants cannot be reversed and that makes me unable to think or have feelings, but I have no terminal illness, then my goals and specific wishes—if medically reasonable—for this and any additional illness would be:

- ☐ Prolong life; treat everything
- ☐ Attempt to cure, but reevaluate often
- ☐ Limit to less invasive and less burdensome interventions
- ☐ Provide comfort care only
- ☐ Other (please specify):

SITUATION E

If I ... (Describe a situation that is important to you and/or your doctor believes you should consider in view of your current medical situation):

- ☐ Prolong life; treat everything
- ☐ Attempt to cure, but reevaluate often
- ☐ Limit to less invasive and less burdensome interventions
- ☐ Provide comfort care only
- ☐ Other (please specify):

SITUATION F

If I am in my current state of health (describe briefly: _____)
and then have an illness that, in the opinion of my physician and two consultants, is life threatening but reversible, and I am temporarily unable to make decisions, then my goals and specific wishes—if medically reasonable— would be:

- ☐ Prolong life; treat everything
- ☐ Attempt to cure, but reevaluate often
- ☐ Limit to less invasive and less burdensome interventions
- ☐ Provide comfort care only
- ☐ Other (please specify):

Please check appropriate boxes:

Each situation (A–F) has the following response columns:
I want. | I want treatment tried. If no clear improvement, stop. | I am undecided. | I do not want.

1. **Cardiopulmonary resuscitation** (chest compressions, drugs, electric shocks, and artificial breathing aimed at reviving a person who is on the point of dying). — *Not applicable*

2. **Major surgery** (for example, removing the gallbladder or part of the colon). — *Not applicable*

3. **Mechanical breathing** (respiration by machine, through a tube in the throat).

4. **Dialysis** (cleaning the blood by machine or by fluid passed through the belly).

5. **Blood transfusions or blood products.** — *Not applicable*

6. **Artificial nutrition and hydration** (given through a tube in a vein or in the stomach). — *Not applicable*

7. **Simple diagnostic tests** (for example, blood tests or x-rays). — *Not applicable*

8. **Antibiotics** (drugs used to fight infection). — *Not applicable*

9. **Pain medications,** even if they dull consciousness and indirectly shorten my life. — *Not applicable*

HEALTH CARE PROXY

I appoint as my proxy decision-maker(s):

_____
Name and Address

and *(optional)*

_____
Name and Address

I direct my proxy to make health-care decisions based on his/her assessment of my personal wishes. If my personal desires are unknown, my proxy is to make health-care decisions based on his/her best guess as to my wishes. My proxy shall have the authority to make all health-care decisions for me, including decisions about life-sustaining treatment, if I am unable to make them myself. My proxy's authority becomes effective if my attending physician determines in writing that I lack the capacity to make or to communicate health-care decisions. My proxy is then to have the same authority to make health-care decisions as I would if I had the capacity to make them, EXCEPT *(list the limitations, if any, you wish to place on your proxy's authority):*

I wish my written preference to be applied as exactly as possible/with flexibility according to my proxy's judgement. *(Delete as appropriate.)*

Should there be any disagreement between the wishes I have indicated in this document and the decisions favored by my above-named proxy, I wish my proxy to have authority over my written statements/I wish my written statements to bind my proxy. *(Delete as appropriate.)*

If I have appointed more than one proxy and there is disagreement between their wishes, _____
shall have final authority.

Signed: _____
         Signature   Printed Name

        _____
         Address   Date

Witness: _____
         Signature   Printed Name

        _____
         Address   Date

Witness: _____
         Signature   Printed Name

        _____
         Address   Date

Physician *(optional):*

I am _____'s physician. I have seen this advance care document and have had an opportunity to discuss his/her preferences regarding medical interventions at the end of life. If _____ becomes incompetent, I understand that it is my duty to interpret and implement the preferences contained in this document in order to fulfill his/her wishes.

Signed: _____
         Signature   Printed Name

        _____
         Address   Date

ORGAN DONATION

☐ I hereby make this anatomical gift to take effect after my death:

I give   ☐ my body
         ☐ any needed organs or parts
         ☐ the following parts_____

to   ☐ the following person or institution _____
         ☐ the physician in attendance at my death
         ☐ the hospital in which I die
         ☐ the following physician, hospital storage bank, or other medical institution: _____

for
☐ any purpose authorized by law   ☐ transplantation
☐ therapy of another person   ☐ research
☐ medical education

☐ I do not wish to make any anatomical gift from my body.

MY PERSONAL STATEMENT *(use another page if necessary)*

Please mention anything that would be important for your physician and your proxy to know. In particular, try to answer the following questions: (1) What medical conditions, if any, would make living so unpleasant that you would want life-sustaining treatment *withheld*? (Intractable pain? Irreversible mental damage? Inability to share love? Dependence on others? Another condition you would regard as intolerable?). (2) Under what medical circumstances would you want to stop interventions that might already have been started? (3) Why do you choose what you choose?

If there is any difference between my preferences detailed in the illness situations and those understood from my goals or from my personal statement, I wish my treatment selections/my goals/my personal statement *(please delete as appropriate)* to be given greater weight.

When I am dying, I would like—if my proxy and my health-care team think it is reasonable—to be cared for:
☐ At home or in a hospice   ☐ In a hospital
☐ In a nursing home   ☐ Other *(please specify)*

Signed _____   Date _____

Witness _____   Date _____

Witness _____   Date _____

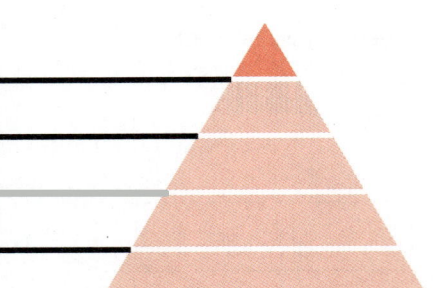

Durable Power of Attorney

California Medical Association
DURABLE POWER OF ATTORNEY FOR HEALTH CARE DECISIONS
(California Probate Code Sections 4600-4753)

WARNING TO PERSON EXECUTING THIS DOCUMENT

This is an important legal document. Before executing this document, you should know these important facts:

This document gives the person you designate as your agent (the attorney-in-fact) the power to make health care decisions for you. Your agent must act consistently with your desires as stated in this document or otherwise made known.

Except as you otherwise specify in this document, this document gives your agent power to consent to your doctor not giving treatment or stopping treatment necessary to keep you alive.

Notwithstanding this document, you have the right to make medical and other health care decisions for yourself so long as you can give informed consent with respect to the particular decision. In addition, no treatment may be given to you over your objection, and health care necessary to keep you alive may not be stopped or withheld if you object at the time.

This document gives your agent authority to consent, to refuse to consent, or to withdraw consent to any care, treatment, service, or procedure to maintain, diagnose, or treat a physical or mental condition. This power is subject to any statement of your desires and any limitations that you include in this document. You may state in this document any types of treatment that you do not desire. In addition, a court can take away the power of your agent to make health care decisions for you if your agent (1) authorizes anything that is illegal, (2) acts contrary to your known desires or (3) where your desires are not known, does anything that is clearly contrary to your best interests.

This power will exist for an indefinite period of time unless you limit its duration in this document.

You have the right to revoke the authority of your agent by notifying your agent or your treating doctor, hospital, or other health care provider orally or in writing of the revocation.

Your agent has the right to examine your medical records and to consent to their disclosure unless you limit this right in this document.

Unless you otherwise specify in this document, this document gives your agent the power after you die to (1) authorize an autopsy, (2) donate your body or parts thereof for transplant or therapeutic or educational or scientific purposes, and (3) direct the disposition of your remains.

If there is anything in this document that you do not understand, you should ask a lawyer to explain it to you.

1. CREATION OF DURABLE POWER OF ATTORNEY FOR HEALTH CARE

By this document I intend to create a durable power of attorney by appointing the person designated below to make health care decisions for me as allowed by Sections 4600 to 4753, inclusive, of the California Probate Code. This power of attorney shall not be affected by my subsequent incapacity. I hereby revoke any prior durable power of attorney for health care. I am a California resident who is at least 18 years old, of sound mind, and acting of my own free will.

2. APPOINTMENT OF HEALTH CARE AGENT

(Fill in below the name, address and telephone number of the person you wish to make health care decisions for you if you become incapacitated. You should made sure that this person agrees to accept this responsibility. The following may not serve as your agent: (1) your treating health care provider; (2) an operator of a community care facility or residential care facility for the elderly; or (3) an employee of your treating health care provider, a community care facility, or a residential care facility for the elderly, unless that employee is related to you by blood, marriage or adoption. If you are a conservatee under the Lanterman-Petris-Short Act (the law governing involuntary commitment to a mental health facility) and you wish to appoint your conservator as your agent, you must consult a lawyer, who must sign and attach a special declaration for this document to be valid.)

I, _____ , hereby appoint:
(insert your name)

Name _____

Address _____

Work Telephone (_____) _____ Home Telephone (_____) _____

as my agent (attorney-in-fact) to make health care decisions for me as authorized in this document. I understand that this power of attorney will be effective for an indefinite period of time unless I revoke it or limit its duration below.

(Optional) This power of attorney shall expire on the following date: _____

3. AUTHORITY OF AGENT

If I become incapable of giving informed consent to health care decisions, I grant my agent full power and authority to make those decisions for me, subject to any statements of desires or limitations set forth below. Unless I have limited my agent's authority in this document, that authority shall include the right to consent, refuse consent, or withdraw consent to any medical care, treatment, service, or procedure; to receive and to consent to the release of medical information; to authorize an autopsy to determine the cause of my death; to make a gift of all or part of my body; and to direct the disposition of my remains, subject to any instructions I have given in a written contract for funeral services, my will or by some other method. I understand that, by law, my agent may <u>not</u> consent to any of the following: commitment to a mental health treatment facility, convulsive treatment, psychosurgery, sterilization or abortion.

4. MEDICAL TREATMENT DESIRES AND LIMITATIONS (OPTIONAL)

(Your agent must make health care decisions that are consistent with your known desires. You may, but are not required to, state your desires about the kinds of medical care you do or do not want to receive, including your desires concerning life support if you are seriously ill. If you do not want your agent to have the authority to make certain decisions, you must write a statement to that effect in the space provided below; otherwise, your agent will have the broad powers to make health care decisions for you that are outlined in paragraph 3 above. In either case, <u>it is important that you discuss your health care desires with the person you appoint as your agent and with your doctor(s).</u>

(Following is a general statement about withholding and removal of life-sustaining treatment. If the statement accurately reflects your desires, you may initial it. If you wish to add to it or to write your own statement instead, you may do so in the space provided.)

> I do **not** want efforts made to prolong my life and I do **not** want life-sustaining treatment to be provided or continued: (1) if I am in an irreversible coma or persistent vegetative state; or (2) if I am terminally ill and the use of life-sustaining procedures would serve only to artificially delay the moment of my death; or (3) under any other circumstances where the burdens of the treatment outweigh the expected benefits. In making decisions about life-sustaining treatment under provision (3) above, I want my agent to consider the relief of suffering and the quality of my life, as well as the extent of the possible prolongation of my life.
>
> *If this statement reflects your desires, initial here:* _____

Other or additional statements of medical treatment desires and limitations: _____
_____
_____
_____

(You may attach additional pages if you need more space to complete your statements. Each additional page must be dated and signed at the same time you date and sign this document.)

5. APPOINTMENT OF ALTERNATE AGENTS (OPTIONAL)

(You may appoint alternate agents to make health care decisions for you in case the person you appointed in Paragraph 2 is unable or unwilling to do so.)

If the person named as my agent in Paragraph 2 is not available or willing to make health care decisions for me as authorized in this document, I appoint the following persons to do so, listed in the order they should be asked:

First Alternate Agent: Name _____
Address _____
Work Telephone (_____) _____ Home Telephone (_____) _____

Second Alternate Agent: Name _____
Address _____
Work Telephone (_____) _____ Home Telephone (_____) _____

6. USE OF COPIES

I hereby authorize that photocopies of this document can be relied upon by my agent and others as though they were originals.

DATE AND SIGNATURE OF PRINCIPAL
(You must date and sign this power of attorney)

I sign my name to this Durable Power of Attorney for Health Care at _____, _____
(City)   *(State)*

on _____ . _____
(Date)   *(Signature of Principal)*

STATEMENT OF WITNESSES

(This power of attorney will not be valid for making health care decisions unless it is either (1) signed by two qualified adult witnesses who are present when you sign or acknowledge your signature <u>or</u> (2) acknowledged before a notary public in California. If you elect to use witnesses rather than a notary public, the law provides that none of the following may be used as witnesses: (1) the persons you have appointed as your agent and alternate agents; (2) your health care provider or an employee of your health care provider; or (3) an operator or employee of an operator of a community care facility or residential care facility for the elderly. Additionally, at least one of the witnesses cannot be related to you by blood, marriage or adoption, or be named in your will. IF YOU ARE A PATIENT IN A SKILLED NURSING FACILITY, YOU <u>MUST</u> HAVE A PATIENT ADVOCATE OR OMBUDSMAN SIGN BOTH THE STATEMENT OF WITNESSES AND THE DECLARATION ON THE FOLLOWING PAGE.)

I declare under penalty of perjury under the laws of California that the person who signed or acknowledged this document is personally known to me to be the principal, or that the identity of the principal was proved to me by convincing evidence;* that the principal signed or acknowledged this durable power of attorney in my presence, that the principal appears to be of sound mind and under no duress, fraud, or undue influence; that I am not the person appointed as attorney in fact by this document; and that I am not the principal's health care provider, an employee of the principal's health care provider, the operator of a community care facility or a residential care facility for the elderly, nor an employee of an operator of a community care facility or residential care facility for the elderly.

First Witness: Signature _____

Print name _____

Date _____

Residence Address _____

Second Witness: Signature _____

Print name _____

Date _____

Residence Address _____

(AT LEAST ONE OF THE ABOVE WITNESSES MUST ALSO SIGN THE FOLLOWING DECLARATION)

I further declare under penalty of perjury under the laws of California that I am not related to the principal by blood, marriage, or adoption, and, to the best of my knowledge I am not entitled to any part of the estate of the principal upon the death of the principal under a will now existing or by operation of law.

Signature: _____

*The law allows one or more of the following forms of identification as convincing evidence of identity: a California driver's license or identification card or U.S. passport that is current or has been issued within five years, or any of the following if the document is current or has been issued within five years, contains a photograph and description of the person named on it, is signed by the person, and bears a serial or other identifying number: a foreign passport that has been stamped by the U.S. Immigration and Naturalization Service; a driver's license issued by another state or by an authorized Canadian or Mexican agency; or an identification card issued by another state or by any branch of the U.S. Armed Forces. If the principal is a patient in a skilled nursing facility, a patient advocate or ombudsman may rely on the respresentations of family members or the administrator or staff of the facility as convincing evidence of identity if the patient advocate or ombudsman believes that the representations provide a reasonable basis for determining the identity of the principal.

SPECIAL REQUIREMENT: STATEMENT OF PATIENT ADVOCATE OR OMBUDSMAN

(If you are a patient in a skilled nursing facility, a patient advocate or ombudsman must sign the Statement of Witnesses above <u>and</u> must also sign the following declaration.)

I further declare under penalty of perjury under the laws of California that I am a patient advocate or ombudsman as designated by the State Department of Aging and am serving as a witness as required by subdivision (e) of Probate Code Section 4701.

Signature: _____   Address: _____

Print Name: _____

Date: _____

CERTIFICATE OF ACKNOWLEDGMENT OF NOTARY PUBLIC

(Acknowledgement before a notary public is <u>not</u> required if you have elected to have two qualified witnesses sign above. If you are a patient in a skilled nursing facility, you <u>must</u> have a patient advocate or ombudsman sign the Statement of Witnesses on page 3 <u>and</u> the Statement of Patient Advocate or Ombudsman above)

State of California   )

)ss.

County of _____   )

On this _____ day of _____ , in the year _____ ,

before me, _____ ,
                                             (here insert name and title of the officer)

personally appeared _____
                                                   (here insert name of principal)

personally known to me (or proved to me on the basis of satisfactory evidence) to be the person(s) whose name(s) is/are sub-scribed to this instrument and acknowledged to me that he/she/they executed the same in his/her/their authorized capacity(ies), and that by his/her/their signature(s) on the instrument the person(s), or the entity upon behalf of which the person(s) acted, executed the instrument.

WITNESS my hand and official seal.

_____

        (Signature of Notary Public)

                                                                                                    NOTARY SEAL

COPIES

YOUR AGENT MAY NEED THIS DOCUMENT IMMEDIATELY IN CASE OF AN EMERGENCY. YOU SHOULD KEEP THE COMPLETED ORIGINAL AND GIVE PHOTOCOPIES OF THE COMPLETED ORIGINAL TO (1) YOUR AGENT AND ALTERNATE AGENTS, (2) YOUR PERSONAL PHYSICIAN, AND (3) MEMBERS OF YOUR FAMILY AND ANY OTHER PERSONS WHO MIGHT BE CALLED IN THE EVENT OF A MEDICAL EMERGENCY. THE LAW PERMITS THAT PHOTOCOPIES OF THE COMPLETED DOCUMENT CAN BE RELIED UPON AS THOUGH THEY WERE ORIGINALS.

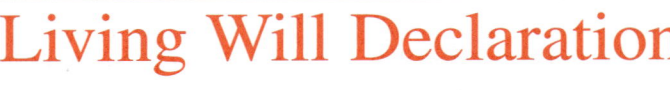

Living Will Declaration

FLORIDA LIVING WILL

INSTRUCTIONS

PRINT THE DATE

PRINT YOUR NAME

Declaration made this _____ day of _____ , 19 ___.

I, _____ , willfully and voluntarily make known my desire that my dying not be artificially prolonged under the circumstances set forth below, and I do hereby declare:

If at any time I have a terminal condition and if my attending or treating physician and another consulting physician have determined that there is no medical probability of my recovery from such condition, I direct that life-prolonging procedures be witheld or withdrawn when the application of such procedures would serve only to prolong artificially the process of dying, and that I be permitted to die naturally with only the administration of medication or the performance of any medical procedure deemed necessary to provide me with comfort care or to alleviate pain.

It is my intention that this declaration be honored by my family and physician as the final expression of my legal right to refuse medical or surgical treatment and to accept the consequences for such refusal.

In the event that I have been determined to be unable to provide express and informed consent regarding the witholding, withdrawal, or continuation of life-prolonging procedures, I wish to designate, as my surrogate to carry out the provisions of this declaration:

PRINT THE NAME, HOME ADDRESS AND TELEPHONE NUMBER OF YOUR SURROGATE

Name: _____

Address: _____

Zip code: _____

Phone: _____

I wish to designate the following person as my alternate surrogate, to carry out the provisions of this declaration should my surrogate be unwilling or unable to act on my behalf:

PRINT NAME, HOME ADDRESS AND TELEPHONE NUMBER OF YOUR ALTERNATE SURROGATE

Name: _____

Address: _____

Zip code: _____

Phone: _____

ADD PERSONAL INSTRUCTIONS (IF ANY)

Additional instructions (optional):

I understand the full import of this declaration, and I am emotionally and mentally competent to make this declaration.

SIGN THE DOCUMENT

WITNESSING PROCEDURE

Signed: _____

Witness 1: _____

Signed: _____

Address: _____

TWO WITNESSES MUST SIGN AND PRINT THEIR ADDRESSES

Witness 2: _____

Signed: _____

Address: _____

Courtesy Choice in Dying, Inc.

SAMPLE

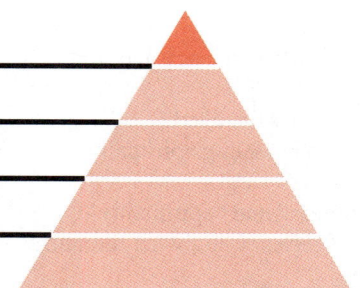

CHAPTER 27

Transcendence, Spirituality, and Legacies

Students learn

I will become a model of morality for younger persons who look up to me and expect me to teach them about my experience of life. Most important, aging means that it is time for me to start living for my soul, or to prepare myself for another life after death.

Mai, age 23

Aging is neither a disease nor a villain that robs one of life's dreams; dreams become more real, fantasies develop into realities, and life is transformed beyond the mundane. I am learning to be slower about saying, "He is confused."

Jerry, age 30

Elders speak

I was raised to believe that some things happen to you only because God felt you could handle them, and that He would not give you more than you could handle. I do believe to this day that one must have a sense or feeling of a higher power or greater power in order to cope with certain changes physically and mentally as we get older.

Dorothy, age 72

What is the advice I would give to others about aging? Keep on learning from nature, art, books, study, and society. It's a life-long project. Most important is to have loving relationships and never to be vindictive no matter how put-upon one may feel. Family harmony has always been important to us, and I hope and pray that their love for one another will prevail when I am gone.

Alice, over 70

I would like everyone I've ever met or known to be glad that I was in their world, even if just for a moment.

Aveline, over 70

In my dream Charlie and I were walking together again. I knew he would disappear because he was dead. He kept reassuring me but insisted I call him by another name as he had assumed another. Even in the dream I felt doubt.

Jennie, age 69

My thoughts are different now, with a major shift but no detectable passage, preoccupied with meanings rather than the next task of the day. I drift around at times hunting for my glasses or forgetting the rolls in the oven and the coffee in the micro while I ponder the various cycles of my life. They are becoming bound together; concatenations that achieve wholeness. Age-associated memory impairment? Someday, each will understand that the old materialistic mental monologue of "facts" is insignificant, no longer capturing attention in the face of the deepest mysteries.

Virginia, ageless

Upon completion of this chapter, the student will be able to:

1. Identify several mechanisms by which individuals achieve transcendence and find meaning in illness and death.
2. Describe several evidences of transcendence as experienced by the aged.
3. Relate particular interventions geared to the individual who is feeling spiritually distressed.
4. Discuss the commonalities and differences between "religion" and "spirituality."
5. Define the concept of "legacy" and name several types of legacies and what the nurse can do to facilitate their expression.
6. Compare changes in life views likely to be evident in elders to those of young adults.

The purpose of this chapter is to bring the reader in touch with the less visible aspects of aging; the meanings that are fundamental to the preparation to depart this life. This last portion of the cycle of life is potentially as orderly and as fulfilling as birth. We believe it is possible to transcend the limitations of the body through a focus on spirituality. A strong sense of values and ethics, significant relationships, enduring hope, and motivation are linked together to form the foundation for reaching one's highest fulfillment. Transcendence is the high-level emotional response to religious and spiritual life and finds expression in numerous rituals and modes of cosmic consciousness. Rituals provide a means of connecting with all others through the ages who have observed like rituals. These modes of thinking and feeling are sometimes unfamiliar to individuals immersed in the necessary materialistic concerns of young adulthood, yet there are moments throughout life when one is deeply aware of being part of a larger scheme. Though some of this chapter may be obscure, it is the springboard for learning to appreciate the full life cycle. The privilege of briefly walking alongside an elder on the last great journey can be truly inspiring.

TRANSCENDENCE

Transcending is inspired by the desire to go beyond the self as delimited by the material and the concrete aspects of living, to expand self-boundaries and life perspectives. It embodies aspects of belonging, connecting, giving life, holding commitments, struggling and surrendering ego, turning inward and becoming free (Forbes, 1994). Creative thought and actions are vehicles of both self-actualization and self-transcendence; the bridge to universal expression and existence. Self-transcendence is generally expressed in five modes: creative work, religious beliefs, children, identification with nature, and mystical experiences (Reed, 1991). Chapter 25 considered the creative spirit and its myriad expressions. This chapter deals with the meanings of life: the culmination of life experience and various mechanisms by which one transcends the purely physical limitations of existence. The way one perceives time, experiences extensions

of the self, and copes with the sure knowledge that death is inevitable may be the ultimate victory or defeat.

Asceticism, self-denial, and rigorous rituals may be used by some to reach the peaks of human experience; many others find more prosaic approaches just as effective. The thesis of Maslow's writings is that mystic, sacred, and transcendent experiences frequently arise from the ordinary elements of one's life (Maslow, 1970). Planting and harvesting, one of the most persistent interests of elders, is the "substance of things hoped for, the evidence of things not seen" (Hebrews 11:1). Gardening, reading, holding an infant, dealing with loss, and numerous other normal events have elements of mystery.

With each death of a loved one, throughout life, one is reborn to a slightly altered state. When deaths of significant others abound in the later years, it is imperative that elders be given opportunity to express how they personally have been altered by the loss. We could speculate that with each personal loss one moves slightly closer to the universal and away from the individual until toward the end one feels an affiliation with all living things, animal, plant, and mineral. Some of the old have achieved a state of existence that transcends the limits of the failing body.

An 86-year-old widow seemed to blend with her world of plants, birds, and flowers. Each new blossom or bird call excited her as she mused in her small apartment and garden. Her conversation was sprinkled with minute discoveries, each of which thrilled her. She became so close to nature that some thought her eccentric. In her last years of life her interest in the living and growing things consumed her. Hours were spent gazing at leaves, grass, ants, and twigs. The cycles of nature seemed to become a part of her being as she experienced her own limited existence. She was found dead in her apartment one morning. It was then learned that her breasts were eroded with cancer. She had not gone to a physician and had never given evidence of pain; rather a sense of mild euphoria filled her last months.

Chidester (1990), a professor of religion, organized transcendence into segments that resemble anthropologic studies: the primal, the Eastern, and the Western. All evolved out of the human necessity to make meaning of the major events in life and to develop rituals by which to support the transitions: birth and death being the central issues. Symbolic death and rebirth form the essence of transcendent rituals and in one form or another are common to all transcendent mechanisms.

Primal Transcendence

In primal transcendence native peoples achieved meaning and structure primarily through natural phenomena. They interpreted the elements, the natural occurrences, as the source of help or harm. Dreams and animals were deified and became the channels to the supernatural.

In some groups the spirits of the dead were thought to reside in animals, or to return to earth through the birth of a child. Natural objects, animals or birds were the emblems of particular groups, containing their spirits and distinguishing features. This is beautifully expressed in the poem of Birago Diop of Mali (Taylor, 1990, p. 160) (Box 27-1).

Eastern Transcendence

Eastern transcendence in the overall sense, with many variations, embodies reverence for life, ancestors, balance, and order. Liberation from passions, disorder, and lack of discipline form the foundations of spiritual growth and transcendence of the purely physical. Many mechanisms are used to achieve this state of peace and enlightenment. Westerners have observed and employed some of these and are in awe of those who have achieved mastery. The Eastern respect for the aged and ancestors is often cited by gerontologists who view it as a cultural phenomenon more than a spiritual necessity.

Western Transcendence

Western modes of transcendence have been fraught with the struggle between good and evil, the separation of mind and body, the Cartesian duality of which Benner (1994) writes. Each life event is judged as it is integrated; personal responsibility is highly valued, and one can expect no help from ancestors or atavistic aids to achieve a transcendent state of universal love. Cause and effect are in linear motion. Transcending evil to reach eternal bliss or attain rewards after death is an overriding expectation of many.

As the world continually shrinks and peoples of the world intermingle, there are few purely classic examples of any one transcendent system. As jeans, colas, and T-shirts have infiltrated the world, so have the predominant ways of dealing with the exigencies of life. Among the enlightened elders with whom we have worked it often seems as if elements of primitive animism, Eastern cyclic death/rebirth, and Western universal love have all been observed.

Gerotranscendence

Tornstam (1994, 1996) theorizes that human aging brings about a general potential for what he terms *gerotranscen-*

dence, a shift in perspective from the material world to the cosmic and concurrent with it an increasing life satisfaction. He found, in a survey of 912 Danish elders, that shifts in cosmic awareness and ego transcendence were accompanied by satisfaction and a lesser need for social activity. The higher the level of transcendence, the more internal were the sources of satisfaction.

This satisfaction is qualitatively different than disengagement (Cumming and Henry, 1961) or the achievement of ego integrity (Erikson, 1950). Disengagement or activity is of little significance in this transformation. There is not an either/or duality but a more profound, all-pervasive change in perspective. Gerotranscendence is conceptualized as a metamorphosis, an alteration in conception of time, space, life, death, and self.

This theory leaves little room for the concept of the ageless self (Kaufman, 1986) or identity continuity throughout adult life because Tornstam's theory assumes that one's orientation to existence undergoes profound changes in the process of aging. Continuity theory contends there is little change in perspective throughout life but only various shifts in emphasis and that one's middle-aged propensities are in some basic way present throughout later life. Tornstam says, "Simply put, gerotranscendence is a shift in metaperspective, from a midlife materialistic and rational vision to a more cosmic and transcendent one, accompanied by an increase in life satisfaction" (Tornstam, 1996, p. 38).

Indices of gerotranscendence are summarized in Box 27-2. It is thought to be a gradual and ongoing shift generated by the normal processes of living, sometimes hastened by serious personal disruptions. Time for reflection becomes

---

Box 27-1   African Ancestors

Those who are dead are never gone:
they are there in the thickening shadow.
The dead are not under the earth:
they are in the tree that rustles,
they are in the wood that groans,
they are in the water that runs,
they are in the water that sleeps,
they are in the hut, they are in the crowd,
the dead are not dead.
Those who are dead are never gone:
they are in the breast of the woman,
they are in the child who is wailing
and in the firebrand that flames.
The dead are not under the earth:
they are in the fire that is dying,
they are in the grasses that weep,
they are in the whimpering rocks,
they are in the forest, they are in the house,
the dead are not dead.

<table>
<tr><td>

Box 27-2   **Characteristics of Individuals with a High Degree of Gerotranscendence**

Have high degrees of life satisfaction
Engage in self-controlled social activity
Experience satisfaction with self-selected social activities
Social activities not essential to their well-being
Midlife patterns and ideals no longer prime motivators
Demonstrate complex and active coping patterns
Greater need for solitary philosophizing
May appear withdrawn when engaged in inner development
Accelerated development of gerotranscendence fomented by life crises
Feel shifts in perception of reality

</td></tr>
</table>

Data from gerotranscendence theory development of Lars Tornstam.

of overriding importance and, we should be cautious about coercing elders into activity. In prior studies Tornstam found, when studying Swedish citizens between ages 15 and 80, that loneliness decreased with every consecutive age group, and time alone became more valued.

Tornstam believes that many theories of what aging is about arise from the personal values of rather young gerontologists and their wishes about what reality ought to be. These imposed expectations and other elements in our culture may inhibit/prohibit the full possibilities of old age. We would agree.

Peak Experiences

A peak experience is when one momentarily transcends self in love, wisdom, insight, worship, commitment, or creativity. It is the time when restricting boundaries seem to vanish, and one feels more aware, more complete, more ecstatic, or more concerned for others. Peak experiences include many modes of transcending one's ordinary limitations. Spiritual and paranormal experiences, creative acts, courage, and humor may all potentiate peak experiences. They are the extraordinary events in one's life that clearly demonstrate self-actualization and personal authenticity (see Chapter 25 for additional discussion).

Levin (1993) defines these mystical experiences as including déjà vu, clairvoyance, and other occurrences in which the self-perceptions reach beyond the ordinary limits. These mechanisms move humans beyond the boundaries of visible, concrete reality and toward a wholly integrated "self." The *self,* as used by Jung, means the supreme oneness of being: integration of aspects of self that are generative and destructive, light and dark, conscious and unconscious, male and female. The ability to embrace the possibility of every potential behavior as native to self instills compassion and a sense of oneness with the world. Keeping oneself open to transcendence involves finding the places where such ex-

periences can break through: soul-stirring concerts, sunrises, sunsets, or raging storms on mountaintops (Kimble, 1993). Each individual seeks states of being in which they feel part of a larger whole.

Compassion, Love, and Caring

Love in its most universal sense is transcendent. *Love* suffers numerous definitions, but transcendent love goes beyond attachment. Attachment is the most common and egocentric love; a necessary aspect of being fully human. The step beyond is to love that which ties all together in appreciation and caring. Wayne, a chaplain of our acquaintance, was driving home on a crowded freeway when he was overcome with emotion. He pulled to the side and began sobbing. He later explained that he suddenly had an overwhelming sense of being connected to everyone and everything he saw. That extraordinary brief cosmic experience changed his entire orientation to life and its meaning.

One may transcend the self in caring for others. "Informed caring for the well-being of others" (Swanson, 1993) is the essence of the best in nursing. In all the great religions there has been evidence of compassion for the suffering of mankind, and some say that compassion is the quality that makes us most human. To our discredit as humans, we seem to be regressing in these capacities.

Empathy is the quality responsible for creating a caring environment, and without experiential understanding there is little possibility of empathy (Watson, 1985; 1987). Wheeler and Barrett (1994) contend that empathy is a skill that can be taught. Swanson (1993) suggests informed caring for the well-being of others requires the following:

- A basic belief in people
- Apprehension of another's reality
- Being with another
- Doing for another when necessary
- Enabling the other

Transcendent Sex. Sublimation, or reaching the sublime realization of sexuality, requires a connection with the spiritual beginnings of sexual acts. "In both sex and religion there is the common mystic element which is the essence of both ecstasies" (Goldberg, 1958, p. 8). For thousands of years procreation, fertility, and sex were celebrated as integral to religious rites (Goldberg, 1958). Sex and sexuality can be expressions of great spirituality, the great mystery of the universe and continuous replenishment. Sex is the source of life itself, but on an individual level it can be as mechanical or mystical as one believes it to be.

As relevant to aging, one might inquire, "What are your thoughts about sexuality at this stage of your life?" Most elders dismiss the topic rather quickly, "Oh, that is no longer important" or "It is physically too taxing." However, one lady whom I consider enlightened said, "It is a definite presence in all of life, even in later life." She understands it is much more than a mechanical act, it is the supreme mystery. Further discussion of sexuality is found in Chapter 16.

Time Transcendence

Life as experienced ordinarily involves the chronologic passage of time. Some types of conscious experience alter our time perception, but the subconscious destroys time. Therefore the release of the subconscious transcends the limitations of time that conscious life experience generally imposes on us. If we conquer time, we conquer annihilation and the dimensions of time that lie within the mind. Recognizing the importance of time perception, particularly in old age, is a fertile field to explore more fully.

Influences on time perception include age, imminent death, level of activity, emotional state, outlook on the future, and the value attached to time. Conclusions from studies of the aged generally support the view that they perceive time as passing quickly and favor the past over the present or the future. Community-dwelling elderly studied by Strumpf (1982) were present oriented and valued past, present, and future equally, although they viewed the past as the most important time of their lives and derived most enjoyment out of reviewing the past.

Newman (1987) has studied changes in time perception that occur in the process of aging and found that as one grows older there is an expanded sense of time in relation to one's quality of life. The emphasis is on the inner experience as crucial to expanding consciousness. The implications of this study are profound and reinforce the necessity of providing elders with validation of the need to rock, meditate, fantasize, and perform many other "passive" activities that may, in fact, be consciousness expanders.

Transcendence of time through dreams is a most wonderful compensatory capacity of humans. The dream of my infant daughter is embedded in my psyche forever though she is no longer an infant; now in her forty-fifth year I can hardly remember her as an infant, but in a vivid dream she was there again, and I was holding and rocking her. She will never leave me nor I her.

Universal Linkages

Elders who link their lives with their participation in historic events may seek a secure place in the stream of generations that will transcend the limitations of the brief mortal existence. Even the events one would think devastating often leave one with a sense of participation in a grander plan. Settersen and Holup (1996) found that the majority of combat veterans thought the events had important positive effects on their later development.

Historic events rated most significant included wars, space exploration, changes in transportation, the civil rights movement, assassinations, and the development of the nuclear age. Martin and colleagues (1996) were able to categorize these significant events as recent micro events (personal and present occurrences), distant micro events (personal childhood events that left an emotional residual), recent macro events (world economic, political, and environmental occurrences), and distant macro events (major markers of world events, such as wars, depressions, etc.). Those considered most potent by the very old were distant macro events and recent micro events. These findings stir questions regarding effects of early events on adult identity formation and constriction of concerns as energy is depleted in advanced old age.

Thorsheim and Roberts (1995) found that shared reminiscing enhanced the capacity of elders to see the uniqueness of others while simultaneously seeing unknown aspects of self. This strengthened cohort linkages with others.

Seeking One's Roots. Seeking one's roots is going beyond the self to reach preceding generations. In a graveyard in New England a simple hand-cut marker has held a message for 200 years, "Vishna Miller, 1782-1797." Who were you, Vishna? Where did your mystical name originate? How did you die when just beginning to live? My ancestor begins to breathe life. The search for me begins anew. Genealogy is more than a hobby of the old. It is the means to reach back to those who have gone before. Journals, old letters, autobiographies, photos, cemeteries, and treasured objects carry me back to communicate with my forbears. I hear and see myself in them. I more clearly see my charge to the future.

Margery Kemp, born in 1373, an illiterate healer, dictated her memoirs to a priest near the end of her life. Though married and the mother of 14 children, she left them and traveled alone from England, throughout Europe, and to the Holy Land (Collis, 1964). Would this not stir the longings of anyone named Kemp? Much of genealogy is carried on to seek one's connections in the stream of time as well as to preserve the legacy of the past.

Hope as a Transcendent Mechanism

A definition of hope, based upon extensive study and analysis, is provided by Morse and Doberneck (1995): "Hope is a response to a threat that results in the setting of a desired goal; the awareness of the cost of not achieving the goal; the planning to make the goal a reality; the assessment, selection and use of all internal and external resources and supports that will assist in achieving the goal; and the reevaluation and revision of the plan while enduring, working and striving to reach the desired goal" (p. 284). Hope is the belief in the future and the expectation of fulfillment. Hope is the anchor that sustains life in the most difficult times and in the face of doubts and ennui. Some level of hope must be maintained in order to survive and to die in peace. Hope embodies desires and expectations and the limitless possibilities of humans in all times and places: present, past, and future.

For an elder, hope is a major means of coping, and those who lose hope lose the capacity and desire for survival. O'Conner (1996) enumerates the critical aspects of hope: (1) the presence of an inner human energy, (2) positive expectations for the future, (3) motivation for action, and (4) formulations of meaningful, realistic goals. She further states that a person without hope has no goals or expectations for the future. All practicing nurses have observed how a small goal or hope for the future can sustain an elder. The grandson's graduation from college, the daughter's return from her travels, even a birthday may keep an elder alive until the event is safely fulfilled.

Nurses seldom recognize the small things they may do, routinely and preconsciously, to impart hope. Grooming conveys a quiet belief that it matters; pain relief and comfort measures reinforce the recognition of an individual's needs and reinforce the value of that individual. Hickey (1986) supplies several approaches that may assist nurses to more clearly foster and sustain hope in the physically failing elder: (1) confirm the value of life, (2) identify a reason for staying alive, (3) establish a support system, (4) incorporate humor, (5) incorporate religion, and (6) set realistic goals. The nurse is not able to "do" these things for the elder. The nurse becomes a sounding board as the elder sorts through these important elements of survival.

Hope is much more than magical thinking. Components of hope as delineated by Morse and Doberneck (1995) include the following:

- Recognition of a predicament or threat
- Realistic assessment of the severity and implications
- Determining various methods of resolution or ways out of dilemma
- Recognizing negative outcomes that may occur and preparing to deal with them
- Remaining realistically optimistic about outcomes
- Assessing conditions and resources that may influence outcomes
- Seeking supportive relationships and realistic tangible supports
- Evaluation of progress toward goals and revision as necessary
- Determination to endure

These components resemble any problem-solving process with the added element of the deep belief that problems can be solved and that one can endure and learn from the outcome if it is less perfect than hoped for.

Transcendence in Illness

Serious illnesses influence how one perceives the meaning of life. There is often a distinct shift in goals, relationships, and values among those who have survived life-threatening episodes. There may be a heightened awareness of beauty and of caring relationships, but a long period of emotional "splinting" may be necessary while recovering from the psychic wound of body betrayal. Newman (1994) contends that disease can be a manifestation of health as one confronts the crisis and as it reveals special meanings.

Steeves and Kahn (1987) found from their work in hospice care that certain conditions facilitate the search for meaning in illness. They noted the following:

- Suffering must be bearable and not all-consuming if one is to find meaning in the experience.

- A person must have access to and be capable of perceiving objects in the environment. Even a small window on the world may be sufficient to match the energy one has to attend.
- One must have time free of interruption and a place of solitude to experience meaning.
- Clean, comfortable surroundings and freedom from constant responsibility and decision making free the soul to search for meaning.
- An open, accepting atmosphere in which to discuss meanings with others is important.

The following nursing actions may facilitate the search for meaning in suffering:

1. Make opportunities for the person to talk.
2. Ask how they have experienced the changes.
3. Accept the process as it unfolds, including anger and bitterness that may accompany the search.
4. Listen and facilitate expression of feelings about life and death.
5. Recognize and confirm any evidence of a rebirth of a sense of beauty. Often there has been a "peak experience" the patient may share if made comfortable enough to do so.
6. Lead discussion groups for recovering patients, knowing that for many enlightenment is a lonely process.
7. Seek the meaning to self while learning from the elders with whom we are privileged to walk for however brief the time.

Sister Rosemary Donley (1991) defines the nursing role in the spiritual search of suffering persons as compassionate accompaniment; meaning entering into another's reality and quietly, attentively sharing the experience. "Nurses need to be with people who suffer, to give meaning to the reality of suffering, and, in so far as possible, to remove suffering and its causes. Here lies the spiritual dimensions of health care" (Donley, 1991, p. 180). Young (1993) felt that nurses are in an ideal position to assist by making opportunities for the sharing of spiritual feelings. Nightingale (Macrae, 1995; Davis and Hale, 1995) believed that all creativity, insight, and sense of higher purpose were evidences of divine intelligence and a potent resource for healing; that physical laws were evidence of the divine; and that carrying out the natural laws and taking responsibility for them brought healing. She did not seek miracles but thought prayer could bring one in tune with universal law and the spiritual energy of the divine.

Chronic Illness. Chronic illnesses, those slow, insidious, unpredictable disorders that wear down the soul, must be examined separately from acute illness when searching for meanings. The chronically ill individual is frequently judged; expected to "get better," shunned, punished, or rejected by well-intentioned people with very subtle, "health-oriented" expectations that can't be met. Stephenson and Murphy (1986) have termed the experience of chronic illness, "existential grief."

The challenge is to find meaning and some purpose in the affliction that, unchallenged, entwines and chokes identity. Holstein and Cole (1996) say, "Thus, part of the 'work' of chronic illness is to tell a new story about the self that integrates the illness into the ongoing story" (p. 18).

The pain that often accompanies chronic illness adds another dimension to the self that must be addressed and given meaning. We do not concur with those who say "you must learn to live with it." We believe pain relief to the greatest extent possible is necessary to release the mind and soul from the grip of intractable pain. Additional discussion of pain can be found in Chapters 8 and 9.

Meaning is derived from cultural ideals, images, and metaphors (Holstein and Cole, 1996). There is little tolerance in the Eurocentric culture for dependency, help-seeking, inactivity, and indecision. For the most part, aspects of a declining life are "culturally construed as personal and medical failures, devoid of social or cosmic meaning" (Cole, 1994, pp. 4-5).

Cartesian duality and linear time are two deeply embedded thought frameworks that do injustice to the person with a chronic disability. The individual embodies the whole of his or her life story at any given time. There is no former self and present self, and there is no cause-effect model that explains the totality of the individual. Wholeness involves the total life history.

Healing. The evolution of the word *heal* from the Old Norse usage, through Old and Medieval English and its German derivations (Partridge, 1959), gives a fuller sense of the meaning of the word that has largely been lost in present-day tendencies to equate heal with cure and cure with eradication of physical disease. This sometimes inexplicably occurs but it is not our emphasis. The words *hail, heil,* be *whole,* be *healthy* and *be well* all underlie the word *heal.* Originally these were used in greeting another and to convey blessings and the desire for communion (intimate fellowship and rapport). Clearly, the desire for interaction was integral to hailing (healing). Likewise, in departures, "Good-bye" was a contraction of the original "God be with you." My old friend, Catherine, always said, "Go with God" when I would leave her.

This somewhat esoteric examination of word origins is meant only to convey the larger meaning of the word *heal.* Underpinning this whole text is our conviction that wholeness in person, holiness, and healing are possibilities regardless of tissue and organ disturbances or the wear and tear of living. "Going with God," in whatever sense one conceives of God, is our meaning when we talk of healing.

Healing often occurs in the search for the meaning of untoward events and most particularly when in true communion with another. Healing emanating from the mind/soul is an ancient method that has been neglected and even denigrated by the scientific community. Recently, medicine and nursing have been receptive to the idea that prayer may heal and restore well-being (American Association of Critical Care Nurses, 1995; MacLennan and Tsai, 1995). Finally, the amazing power of the mind is being recognized as essential to the healing process.

Nurses may introduce the discussion with elders and explore experiences they have had with extraordinary events that stirred the subconscious or paranormal powers within themselves. The nurse's receptivity and caring are essential components of the healing process. This releases the forces of self-healing.

Healing may be experienced in many ways. The result may or may not be the eradication of a disease but always brings about the integration of a condition or situation into a sense of wholeness, wellness, and greater understanding. To do so, "we will need a rapprochement between ancient wisdom and modern science, between mystery and mastery" (Cole, 1992, p. 17). Stoll (1979) espouses the interrelatedness of forgiveness, love, and trust in achieving health and wholeness (Figure 27-1). We would emphasize the importance of self-forgiveness and hope.

Suicide as Transcendence

Buchanan et al (1995) found that among elders they surveyed the notion of death as a means to rise beyond morbid life conditions was seen as an option. The wish to die may be a transcendent phenomenon at certain times with some elders. Long ago Robert Murphy, in a Pendle Hill (the Friends' publishing house) pamphlet, wrote about transcendent suicide although he didn't classify it as such. Simply, he saw suicide as a declaration of hope and an affirmation of personal strength, an individual acting out the statement, "I simply refuse to live in this way. There must be more to life."

There can be great strength and protest in suicidal thoughts and gestures, and these qualities must become the focus of therapeutic efforts. The individual may be seeking to transcend the limits experienced by the present self. As always, the nurse may learn much by truly listening and providing affirmation of an individual's strength and courage. The desire for assisted suicide and the topic of suicide in general is discussed in Chapters 14, 21, and 24. Our point here is to affirm that suicide can be a search for transcendence through death.

SPIRITUALITY

Spirituality is difficult to define, though many have tried. Moberg (1979), one of the major contributors to our understanding of spirituality and aging, defines spirituality as the "totality of man's inner resources, the ultimate concerns around which all other values are focused, the central philosophy of life that guides conduct, and the meaning-giving center of human life which influences all individual and social behavior" (p. 2). Thibault et al (1991) state, "Spirituality refers to the manner in which a person integrates three domains—knowledge or belief system, inner life experiences, and exterior life and institutional activities in support of these beliefs" (p. 29).

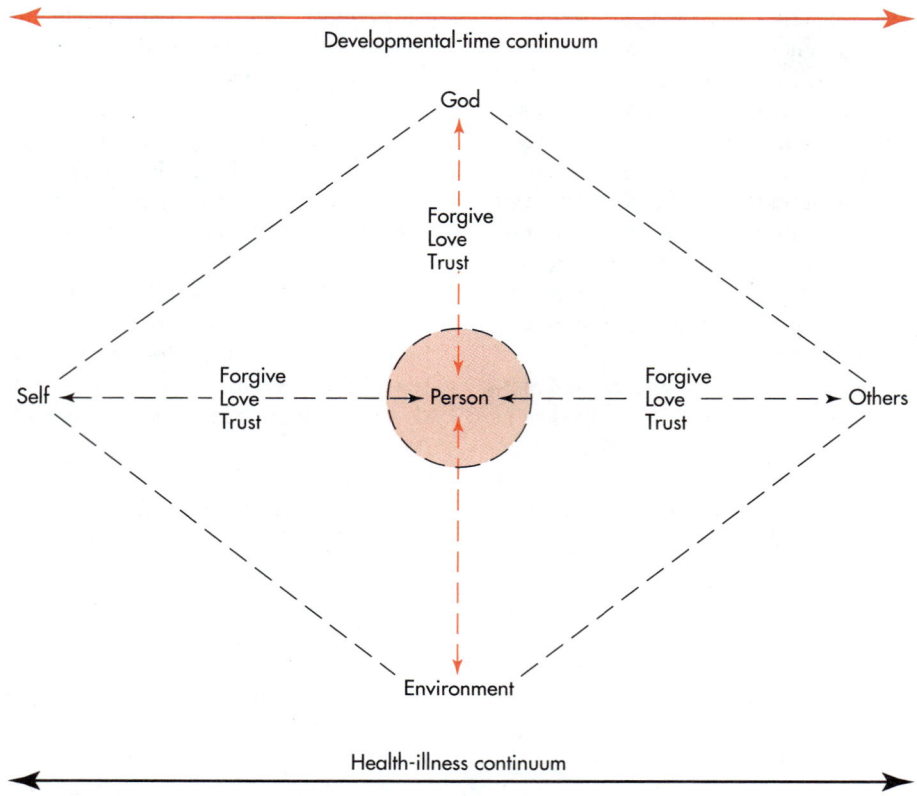

Figure 27-1. Stoll's model of spiritual interrelatedness via forgiveness, love, and trust, resulting in meaning purpose, and hope in life. (Redrawn from Frisch NC, Kelley J: *Healing life's crises: a guide for nurses,* Albany, NY, 1996, Delmar.)

Spiritual well-being is defined as "the affirmation of life in a relationship with God, self, community, and environment that nurtures and celebrates wholeness" (National Interfaith Coalition on Aging, 1975).The spiritual path leads one into self-discovery, self-acceptance, affirmation of self-love, and a connection with all others that is brought about by loving the most unlovable aspects of self and of others. When on a spiritual path, we find our own unique way to contribute love to the world.

Some see the essence of aging as a spiritual journey in which one connects with the transcendent self and the route of spiritual growth (Berggren-Thomas and Griggs, 1995). The nursing role is not to intervene but to accompany along the path and be fully present with the individual. Reflection, feedback, comfort, and affirmation are all a part of being with the elder and providing the supports that release energy for spiritual seeking. The importance of the spiritual to an individual's well-being, hopeful attitudes, and will to live are of increasing interest to nurses and other professionals (Ross, 1996).

Nurses may interpret a patient's spiritual needs in terms of religious affiliation, rites, and rituals. Religion is only one aspect of spirituality, and it may or may not fill an individ-

ual's spiritual needs. Spiritual needs are much broader and more personal than any particular religious persuasion. The spiritual aspect transcends the physical and psychosocial to reach the deepest individual capacity for love, hope, and meaning. The spiritual person can rise above that which is humanly expected in a situation. For example, a dying elder in great pain whom I was attending said to me, "This is so hard for you." I could scarcely believe he was able to see beyond himself.

The last few years have seen a "revival" of interest in philosophy, religion, and spirituality. It is more than a "New Age" fad. The phenomenon seems to be the insistent emergence of a need long sacrificed to the God of Science. Henderson (1996) calls it a spiritual renaissance that has captured the interest of professionals.

Benner (1994) discusses the emergence of interest among nurses in interpretive phenomenology that opens the possibility of new meanings, individually defined. Interpretive phenomenology is a way of looking at human experience through the interpretation of the individual experiencing the events. It is looking at the whole of it and how it makes sense to that person. Meanings, commitments, and concerns cannot be encompassed in ordinary scientific research cal-

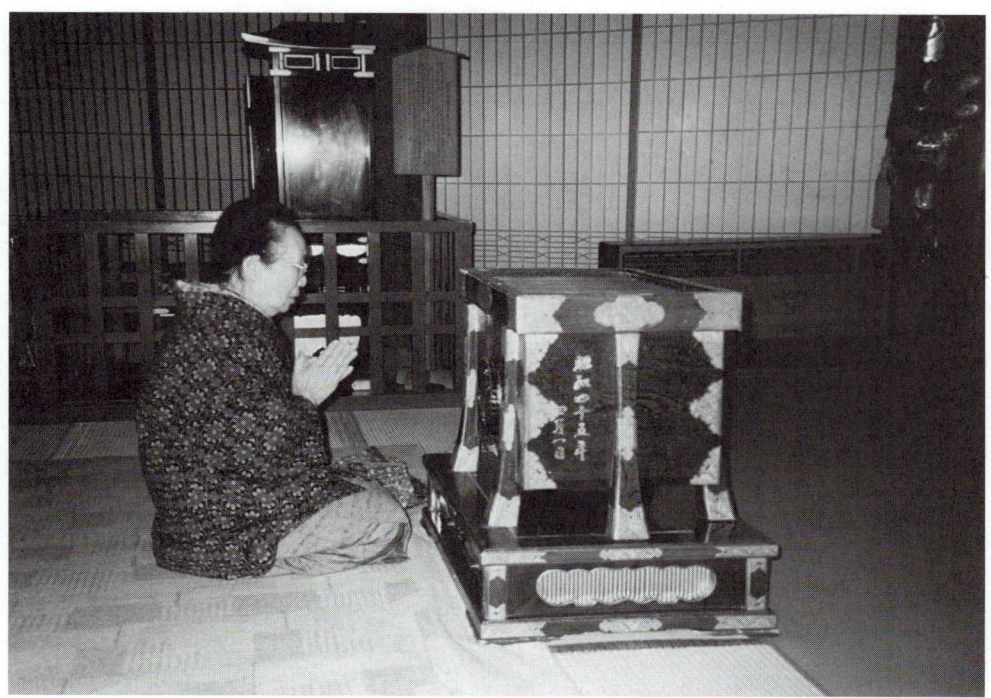

Prayer. (Courtesy Priscilla Ebersole.)

culations. The particular science of interpretation is dubbed *hermeneutics;* thus one reads of hermeneutic phenomenology, the method by which experience is interpreted and then analyzed. From an accumulation of many interpretations from numerous individuals new understanding of the human experience can emerge. This is the essence of what this chapter is about.

van Manen (1990) suggests research guidelines for hermeneutic phenomenologic research:

- Commit to an area of serious interest.
- Investigate experience as it is lived rather than through a conceptualized pattern.
- Reflect on the essential themes that characterize the phenomena.
- Describe the phenomena through writing and rewriting.
- Examine the parts and the whole.

One might say historical research at its best or biography at its best displays evidence of hermeneutic phenomenologic examination. The principles for evaluation are seen in Box 27-3.

Spiritual healing has been neglected for so long we have almost forgotten that in antiquity priests and healers wore the same hat. Two nurses in Toronto, Canada, thought it time to again look at spiritual healing (MacLennan and Tsai, 1995). They began with questions about whether nurses were concerned about spiritual needs, and if so were they applying concepts related to spirituality in nursing practice.

Box 27-3	**Evaluation of Phenomenologic Hermeneutic Reports**

A coherent linkage makes sense of contradictions.
The whole context and comprehensiveness of the account are appropriate.
It attempts to solve a central issue
The account deals with all the questions posed.
Questions arise from the text itself.
Historic and contextual sense are preserved.
The account critiques previous interpretations and leaves room for reinterpretation.
It raises questions that will stimulate further interpretive research.
Its insights and critical discussion can generate future possibilities.

Data from Madison GB: *The hermeneutics of postmodernity,* Indianapolis, 1988, Indiana University Press.

They found that nurses tended to avoid dealing with spiritual needs because they felt they were too personal. How can one begin to discuss spiritual matters?

- Ask the individual his or her source of strength and hope.
- Ask if the individual sees any connection between physical health and spiritual beliefs.
- Discuss sources of spiritual strength throughout life.

Box 27-4	Assessing and Intervening in Spiritual Distress

Assessment

Brief history
  Losses
  Challenged belief/value system
  Separation from religious and cultural ties
  Death
  Personal and family disasters
Symptoms (defining characteristics) such as:
  Unmet needs
  Threats to self
  Change in environment, health status, self concept, etc.
  Seeking spiritual assistance
  Questioning meaning of own existence
  Depression
  Feelings of hopelessness, abandonment, fear
Assessment of etiology of spiritual distress:
  Depletion anxiety
  Helplessness/hopelessness
  Perceived powerlessness
  Medication reactions
  Hormonal imbalances

Interventions

Create a therapeutic environment.
Assess support system.
Assess past methods of decreasing distress, i.e., prayer, imagery, healing, memories/reminiscence therapy, medication, relaxation.
Determine environmental changes needed to enhance functioning.
Assess and assist implementation of coping mechanisms.
Refer to clergy.
Evaluate effects of nursing interventions.
Evaluate medications and their interactions.
Activate and evaluate appropriate community referrals.
Use techniques to assist client and family in reducing spiritual distress.

- Signs of spiritual distress include doubt, despair, guilt, boredom, ennui, and anger at God (Box 27-4). Interventions may involve calling clergy; sharing spiritual readings, poems, and music; obtaining religious articles such as the Bible or a rosary; or praying.

Interestingly, old women who have taken and are taking care of their developmentally disabled adult children say prayer and belief in God have sustained them through the great difficulties they have faced (Forbes, 1994). Humans are spiritual animals who need love and meaning no less than food, clothing, shelter, and health care.

Religion

The religious impulse, as conceptualized by Maslow, resides within each person and in its highest fulfillment integrates the life experience rather than splitting life into the sacred and the profane. Maslow believes the organizational and ritual aspects of religion can be expressions of meaning and become empty gestures only when one separates self from the source of spirituality. Davis (1995) makes the discrimination between religion as an organized practice of beliefs and the spiritual, which embodies deeply held beliefs encompassing love, compassion, and respect for life; ritual practice may or may not be present in the spiritual.

Throughout history and in all cultures, sacraments, symbols, and metaphor have been used to recognize, organize, and understand human experience (Table 27-1). Even the cognitively impaired have been found to respond positively to faith rituals and symbols (Richards, 1990). Shared purpose and shared preparation using appropriate materials bring individuals into contact with others and with the transcendental. Krause (1995) found that religiosity, as measured by involvement in church activities, tended to increase self-esteem among older adults and particularly among blacks. Silverman (1990) contends that in addition to the comfort and security of these rituals our sense of connectedness with others is enhanced by ceremonies. "Religious beliefs and practices are regarded by some as reflections of even more basic realities, such as psychological need for economic and political power" (Cole, 1992, p. 17). Kennedy et al (1996) found that religious preference and practice were inversely related to depressive symptomatology for those religious persons who were able to attend services of their faith. Those who were unable to attend services, particularly Catholic and Jewish persons, had a greater prevalence of depression.

Jung proposed the presence in humans of a natural religious energy. He believed religion can unite the inner and outer man in equal degree (Fordham, 1966). No completely rational approach can do this, but art, dreams, fantasies, and other intuitive expressions may assist the person, steeped in logic, to reach into the soul and become whole. There are many ways one can touch religious energies within and outside of formalized religion. We have seen evidence of this embedded desire for religious expression in the eagerness with which many people grasp cults and "isms" of all kinds, some with destructive rather than constructive beliefs and outcomes.

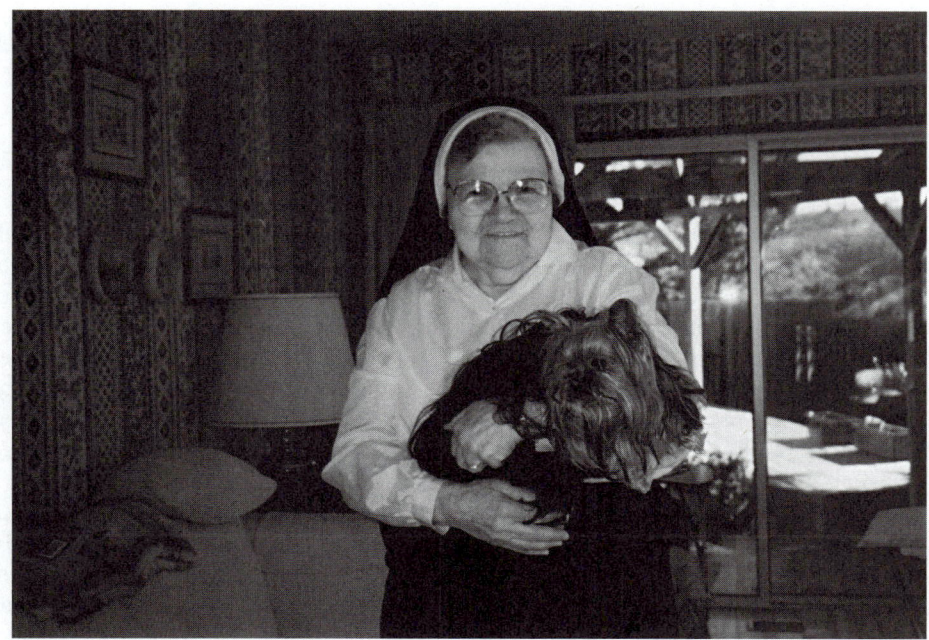

The religious life. (Courtesy Irene M. Bobak.)

Table 27-1   Religious Population of the World: 1994

[In thousands, except percent. Refers to adherents of all religions as defined and enumerated for each of the countries in *World Encyclopedia (1982),* projected to mid 1994, adjusted for recent data]

Religion	Total	Percent distri-bution	Africa	Asia	Latin America	Northern America	Europe	Eurasia*	Oceania
Total population	**5,661,525**	**100.0**	**722,814**	**3,345,498**	**474,240**	**288,788**	**514,655**	**287,164**	**28,365**
Christians	1,901,148	33.6	351,682	304,887	442,140	247,293	422,159	109,747	23,240
Roman Catholics	1,058,069	18.7	132,102	132,053	411,514	100,386	267,972	5,615	8,427
Protestants	391,143	6.9	93,865	87,051	17,513	99,652	75,441	9,903	7,718
Orthodox	174,184	3.1	30,685	3,904	1,789	6,217	36,869	94,129	591
Anglicans	78,038	1.4	28,873	755	1,319	7,593	33,625	1	5,872
Other Christians	199,707	3.5	66,158	81,125	0,004	33,445	8,252	100	623
Muslims	1,033,453	18.3	293,993	675,297	1,395	5,500	13,194	43,967	107
Nonreligious†	923,104	16.3	2,936	733,740	19,327	22,910	58,199	82,236	3,758
Hindus	764,000	13.5	1,608	759,059	912	1,315	725	2	379
Buddhists	338,621	6.0	23	336,755	559	578	279	401	26
Atheists	239,111	4.2	344	167,739	3,329	1,367	16,362	49,407	563
Chinese folk-religionists‡	149,336	2.6	14	149,037	76	126	61	1	21
New-religionists§	128,975	2.3	23	126,869	548	1,473	51	1	10
Tribal religionists	99,150	1.8	69,872	28,197	967	42	1	—	71
Sikhs	20,204	0.4	29	19,557	8	363	237	1	9
Jews	13,451	0.2	128	4,289	458	5,907	1,761	813	95
Shamanists	11,010	0.2	1	10,754	1	1	2	250	1
Confucians	6,334	0.1	1	6,300	2	26	2	2	1
Baha'is	5,835	0.1	1,631	2,817	827	379	93	7	81
Jains	3,987	0.1	57	3,906	4	4	15	—	1
Shintoists	3,387	0.1	—	3,383	1	1	1	—	1
Other religionists	20,419	0.4	472	12,912	3,686	1,503	1,513	329	4

From U.S. Bureau of the Census: *Statistical abstract of the United States: 1995,* ed 115, Washington, DC, 1995.
—Represents zero. *Source's term for the former Soviet Union. †Persons professing no religion, nonbelievers, agnostics, freethinkers, and dereligionized secularists indifferent to all religion. ‡Followers of traditional Chinese religion (local deities, ancestor veneration, Confucian ethics, Taoism, etc.) §Followers of Asiatic 20th-century New Religions, New Religions movements, radical new crisis religions, and non-Christian syncretistic mass religions.
Source Encyclopaedia Britannica, Inc, Chicago, IL, *Britannica Book of the Year,* (Reprinted with permission. Copyright 1994).

The prevalence and importance of religious beliefs and activities in later life have been investigated with various conclusions. Koenig (1987) studied more than 1000 individuals between 55 and 94 years of age who lived in and around Springfield, Illinois. From this large, although geographically limited, population he came to the following conclusions:

- Religious activities and attitudes are very common among older adults (Table 27-2).
- A large proportion of older persons claim that religion helps them to cope, both when asked directly about religion as a source of strength in difficult times and when asked indirectly how they coped with or survived stressful life events.
- There is a strong correlation between well-being and religion even when controlling for health, wealth, and social support. This is particularly true for women 75 years old and over.
- Black women tend to be significantly more religious than black men and whites of both genders (Levin and Taylor, 1993).
- Correlations between well-being or adjustment and religion tend to increase over time, suggesting that as other sources of well-being decline religion may become even more important.

Nine of every ten older Americans say religion is important in their lives and three fourths of those say it is very important (Moore, 1995). Moberg (1996) suggests that religion and spirituality are important independent variables in health and well-being that gerontologists routinely fail to consider. Levin (1994) attributes this to an antipathy to religion that is inherent in the modern scientific world view and stereotypical barriers to religious research among funding agencies and publishers. Recently the highly respected Mayo Clinic stated in their newsletter, "Could spiritual beliefs and practices enhance your health and well being as well? More and more, the medical profession is considering that possibility. As a result, spirituality's role in today's high-tech medical world is increasingly being explored" (Mayo Clinic Health Letter, 1996).

In many early societies religion and health care were tightly interwoven, and the priesthood controlled both. As scientific method changed the practice of medicine, health and spirituality grew apart, though the residue of the priesthood remains in the practice of medicine.

Courtney et al (1992) studied the correlation between religiosity and adaptation in a group of centenarians. They found a significant relationship between religiosity and physical health and successful coping. The very old are more likely to be interested in the nonorganizational aspects of religion than in active participation (Table 27-3).

The church is the social institution with the greatest potential for reaching the aged with needed service. Typically, 40% to 60% of congregations are composed of retired persons. The major reason they are not better served is for lack of gerontologic training in the seminaries (Seeber, 1988). There are several movements afoot to remedy this. There is an increase in aging ministry courses across the United States, and many denominations are sponsoring conferences or seminars on aging issues. The *Journal of Religion and Aging* has emerged, and several organizations of aging are forming committees.

Nurses who are involved in religious organizations can be advocates for increasing the attention given to the needs of the aged. They may even spearhead particular services to the aged such as peer counseling, health screening activities,

---

Table 27-2   Religious Preference, Church Membership, and Attendance: 1967 to 1993

[In percent. Covers civilian noninstitutional population, 18 years old and over. Data represent averages of the combined results of several surveys during year or period indicated. Data are subject to sampling variability, see source]

Year	Religious preference					Church/ synagogue members	Persons attending church/ synagogue[a]	Age and region	Church/ synagogue members, 1992-93
	Protestant	Catholic	Jewish	Other	None				
1967	67	25	3	3	2	[b]73	43	18-29 years old	59
1975	62	27	2	4	6	71	41	30-49 years old	68
1980	61	28	2	2	7	69	40	50 years and over ...	76
1985	57	28	2	4	9	71	42	East[c]	69
1990	56	25	2	6	11	65	40	Midwest[d]	72
1991	56	25	2	6	11	68	42	South[e]	76
1992-93	56	26	2	7	9	69	40	West[f]	55

From U.S. Bureau of the Census: *Statistical abstract of the United States: 1995,* ed 115, Washington, DC, 1995.
[a]Persons who attended a church or synagogue in the last seven days. [b] 1965 data. [c]ME, NH, RI, NY, CT, VT, MA, NJ, PA, WV, DE, MD, and DC. [d]OH, IN, IL, MI, MN, WI, IA, ND, SD, KS, NE, and MO. [e]KY, TN, VA, NC, SC, GA, FL, AL, MS, TX, AR, OK, and LA. [f]AZ, NM, CO, NV, MT, ID, WY, UT, CA, WA, OR, AK, and HI.
Source Princeton Religion Research Center, Princeton, NJ, *Emerging Trends,* periodical. Based on surveys conducted by The Gallup Organization.

day care, home visitation programs, and respite for families. "Parish nurses" are becoming visible nationwide as churches and hospitals join forces to provide health maintenance and monitoring activities for parishioners (Schank et al, 1996). Hoag Memorial Hospital in Newport Beach, California, has pioneered the development of these programs in alliance with several churches (Hammers, 1992).

When religion is important to an elder, every effort should be made to make it accessible or find available alternatives. The nurse must often introduce the topic of religion or spirituality. The spiritual dimension of life, in whatever way interpreted by the elder, is a significant force for adaptation and perceived meanings. Decontextualization of social and psychologic phenomena in order to objectify data and make generalizations robs experience of meaning.

Homebound Elders and Religious Connections. Powers (1996) notes that at the time elders need spiritual connections the most they may break down. The spiritual nourishment that comes from being an integral part of a congregation of like-minded individuals is diminished when an elder becomes homebound and can no longer attend services or observe comforting rituals. Some individuals

deeply need the connection with others and to participate in meaningful ways in the activities of the church.

According to Rev Elwood Spackman, interviewed by Powers, roles can be devised that meet these needs for the elders unable to attend services. He suggests they be given names of parishioners with particular prayer requests and those needing telephone reassurance. Parish newsletters and tapes of sermons can be provided to isolated elders, as well as visits from youthful members of the church. He also suggests that family members may be encouraged to create meaningful rituals that can be observed at home.

Some parishioners find televised church services comforting, including participating in the singing. Singing is seldom considered as a transcendent mechanism, though participating in song and dance renew the spirit and take one beyond self into the higher human attributes.

Wesley Woods Geriatric Center in Atlanta, Georgia, reports a program designed to maintain a sense of spiritual community for homebound elders who are no longer able to attend services (Powers, 1996). For those elders who throughout their life maintained strong ties with a church community the sense of loss when unable to attend services

Table 27-3 Religious Congregations—Summary: 1991

[Excludes Alaska and Hawaii. A religious congregation is a community of people who meet together for worship, for fellowship, and for service to their members and the larger communities in which they live. Excludes informal congregational groups that did not have an official meeting place, denominational organizations, religious charities, and religiously-owned or -affiliated institutions. Based on a sample survey of 1,003 congregations with telephones conducted by the source; for details, see source]

Size of congregation	Number of congregations	Areas of activity	Percent of all congregations providing support or service[d]	Source of revenue or type of expenditure	Amount (mil. dol.)
Total	[a]**257,648**	Human services	91.7	**Revenues, total**[i]	**48,412**
Fewer than 100 members[b]	[b]52,065	Recreation[e]	72.6	Individual giving	39,223
100-199 members	[c]70,464	Marriage counseling	70.5	Fees, charges for services	1,851
200-299 members	39,553	Family counseling	61.8	School tuition	1,352
300-399 members	23,521	Meal services[f]	50.1		
400-499 members	16,051	Single adults programs	46.5	**Expenditures, total**	**47,648**
500-999 members	31,826	Health	89.5	Current operating[i]	34,183
1,000-1,999 members	15,451	Visitation and support[g]	87.4	Wages, salaries	16,532
2,000 or more members	8,717	Alcohol/drug prevention	47.3	Fringe benefits	3,696
		International	73.9	Supplies services	10,400
Fewer than 100 nonmembers	136,513	Relief abroad	61.5	Donations[i]	6,626
100-199 nonmembers	63,956	Education &/or health	39.0	Within denomination	4,655
200-299 nonmembers	20,883	Public benefit	62.2	To other organizations	1,317
300-499 nonmembers	12,150	Abortion activities[h]	41.8	Construction, capital improvements[j]	5,051
500 or more nonmembers	19,804	Education	53.3	Savings	1,788

From U.S. Bureau of the Census: *Statistical abstract of the United States: 1995,* ed 115, Washington, DC, 1995.
[a]Includes those which don't know or did not answer. [b]Includes churches with fewer than 100 nonmembers. [c]Includes churches with fewer than 100 members but with 100 or more nonmembers. [d]Congregations could give multiple responses. [e]Includes camp programs and other youth programs. [f]Includes food kitchens. [g]Programs for sick and shut-ins. [h]Pro-life or pro-choice. [i]Includes other items, not shown separately. [j]Includes acquisition of real property.
Source INDEPENDENT SECTOR, Washington, DC, *From Belief to Commitment: The Community Service Activities and Finances of Religious Congregations in the United States,* 1993 Edition (copyright).

can be acute. It is not only the ritual but the fellowship that is lost. Some of the suggestions for maintaining ties are to provide tapes of services, involve youth groups in home visitations, develop prayer circles in which homebound members not only are included in the prayers of others but also have several individuals to pray for, thus keeping spiritual linkages strong. Family members can be encouraged to set aside a special time where all join in hymns, Bible reading, and watching a televised sermon. Important rituals may also be included as the individuals desire. These ideas are actually resurrections of those practiced several generations ago when families lived in isolated areas.

Wesley Woods undoubtedly has a predominantly protestant, Methodist approach to religious needs even though it is interdenominational in practice. It is extremely important that elders be connected with their preferred spiritual roots and rituals whether Protestant, Jewish, Buddhist, Shinto or any of the numerous religions in our multicultural society. Additional discussions of cultural differences are found in Chapter 24.

Striepe, a parish nurse coordinator in Spencer, Iowa, gives these suggestions for approaching spirituality with a homebound elder (Powers, 1996, p. 13):

"How do you feel spiritually?"
"How satisfied are you with your spiritual health?"
"When do you feel most connected to God?"
"What helps you feel connected?"
"Have you had an intense spiritual experience that dramatically changed your relationship with God?
"What gives you joy?"
"Would you be interested in visits with young people from your congregation?"

Spiritual Needs and Resources

Life satisfaction, happiness, morale, and health have all been studied in relation to religion and spiritual expression. Gerontologists are cognizant of the significance of religion and spirituality in the adaptational capacity of elders. However, spirituality has not achieved the central focus it merits in the study of aging. At the 1971 White House Conference on Aging, spiritual well-being was an aspect of aging deemed significant enough for a section focus. At the 1995 White House Conference on Aging, 45 conference resolutions were adopted; none addressed spirituality directly, but all supported the fundamental needs of elders that form the foundation for health, economic security, and life satisfaction.

Nursing Assessment and Intervention to Encourage Spiritual Well-Being

Hungelmann et al (1996) have developed an assessment tool that provides a way of establishing the diagnosis of spirituality that emphasizes strengths, as well as possible spiritual distress Figure 27-2 and Appendix 27-A). The scale is multidimensional, including factors that affect psychologic and physical welfare. The authors identify four areas of nursing intervention: affirmation through listening and discovering the gift and

identifying need; therapeutic communication as a vehicle for identifying strengths, as well as pain; reminiscing that encourages the emergence of the life story; and referral to clergy or another health professional when desire or need is indicated.

What is this to gerontic nurses? First, the awareness of one's own spirit; then, knowing that caring for an aging body is the least of work with the elderly. Recognizing the primacy of the spirit is necessary. Some very spiritual individuals are unable to articulate their knowing; do not negate that aspect of an individual's experience because it is not expressed verbally. Realization that biopsychosocial aspects of aging are all shards of the spirit will integrate every aspect of your work in gerontic nursing. Haase et al (1992) have developed a conceptual model useful in understanding spirituality (Figure 27-3). This model clarifies the components of spirituality.

ALTERED MIND STATES

In every society and every age humans have sought spiritual enlightenment through altered mind states by the use of substances, rituals, and deprivations. There seems an inherent need in almost every culture to incorporate methods of seeking some enlightenment outside the common daily experience. Some of these exceptional experiences are treasured, and some are feared. The ritual use of peyote by the Southwest Indians, sake by the Japanese, isolation and deprivation by some of the Northwest tribes, withdrawal into nirvana by East Indians, and LSD by the flower children are only a few of the most obvious of these. These examples simply exemplify some of the routes individuals take to move out of the common thought modes that may keep them trapped in the mundane levels of existence.

For some, mind states are altered without the use of a particular substance or mechanism. These altered mind states may be frightening. Professionals may validate the experiences and assist the person to achieve a coping style that bal-

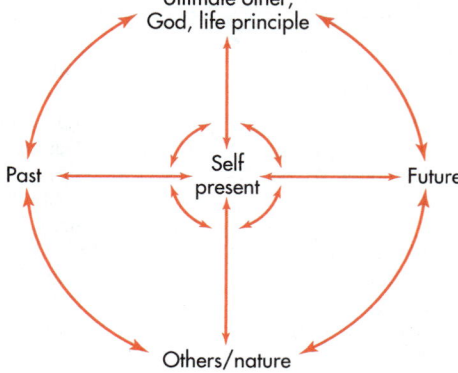

Figure 27-2. Model of spiritual well-being, reflecting harmonious interconnectedness of the major themes of time and relationships. (Reprinted with permission of *Journal of Religion and Health* from Hunglemann J, Kenkel-Rossi E, Klassen L et al: Spiritual well-being in older adults: Harmonious interconnectedness, *J Religion Health* 24(2):52, 1985.)

ances the internal reality with the demands of daily living. In the following discussion of some of these situations, examples and suggestions are given for facilitating acceptance and valuing these extraordinary occurrences.

Confusion and Transcendence

Nursing literature and gerontologic studies approach the issue of confusion in the elderly as a problem. It often becomes a problem for the individual in negotiating the milieu and for health care providers who have certain expectations of the realities of effective functioning. However, we propose another way of assessing and dealing with confusion. What is the human need addressed by the confusion? A better time? A more comfortable place? More loving persons? Attention? In our observations we have noted the following positive effects of confusion in certain persons:

1. Individuals are largely unaware of biologic disturbances and the betrayal of their bodies as they mentally roam in spiritual territories.
2. Some find security and safety in imagining they are in a familiar place. We encountered a specific example of this in an elderly man who thought he

was in a bordello and spent much of his time searching for "the girls." This was indicative of a need for safety and sexual expression.
3. Often we find those who augment their need for belonging when they imagine nurses to be cousins, granddaughters, or other significant persons from their past. Some talk at length to invisible companions.
4. The attempts to order others about and the insistence on obscure demands or enigmatic activities are a means of compensating for an erosion of self-esteem and power.

However, we have been most impressed by the value of delirium when one is dying. The snatches of reality (as consensually defined) are often interspersed with extended periods of otherworldliness in which the individual is clearly in a transcendent level of consciousness. Distortions become symbols of meaning, ceremonies occur, and dream consciousness invades the wakeful states, producing occult meanings. Conversations occur with persons long gone as the individual makes peace with those he or she loved. Often there is a feeling of persons beckoning and waiting "on the other side."

One ordinarily thinks of transcendent experiences as accompanied by a supreme mind state or a moment of

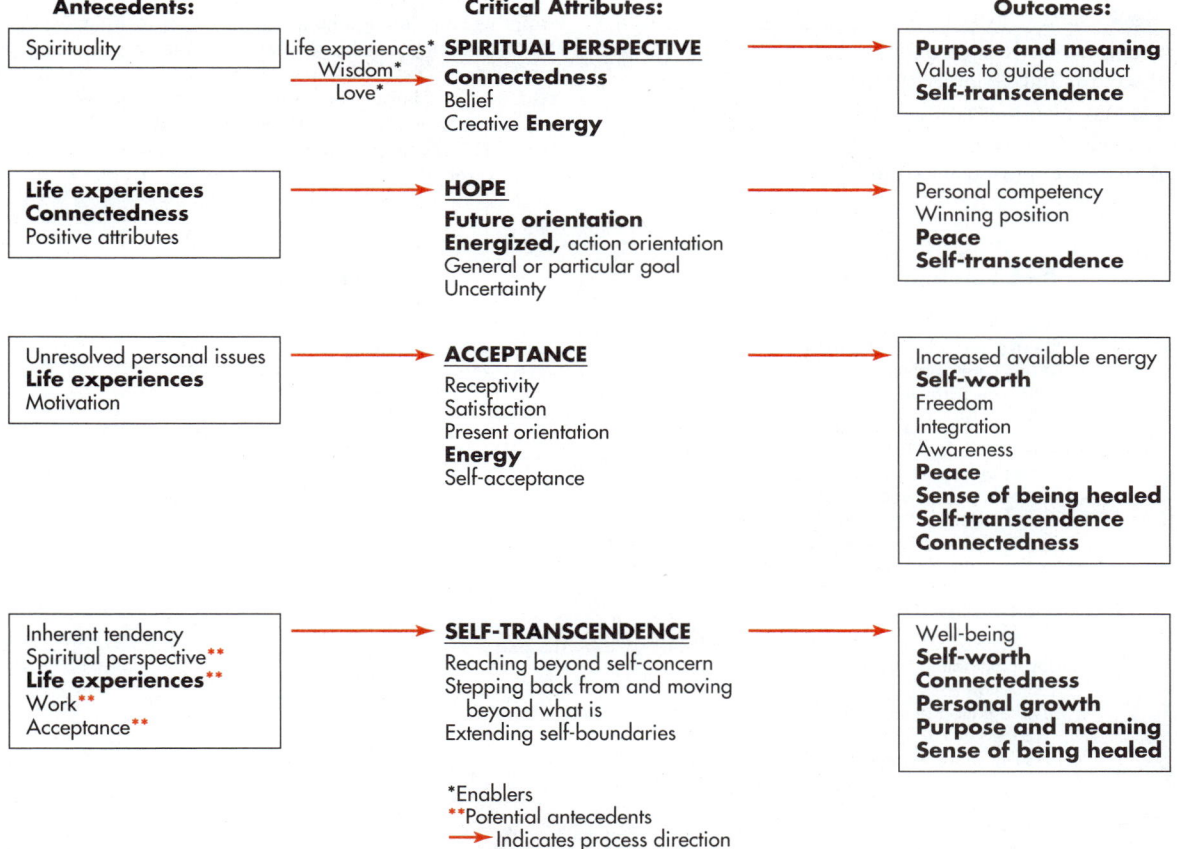

Figure 27-3. Components of spirituality: a process model. (From Haase JE, Britt T, Coward DD et al: Simultaneous concept analysis of spiritual perspective, hope, acceptance and self-transcendence, *Image J Nurs Sch* 24(2):142, 1992.)

extreme clarity. The following is an example of a "confused" elder in a transcendent state:

J was lingering on earth, strongly willing himself to "whip the cancer." Each day he struggled slowly, with assistance, to his chair in the living room where he kept up the pretense of ordinary living, joking and chatting with visiting friends and family. When he returned to his bedroom and the rented hospital bed, he would intermittently lapse into delirious states. In those altered states of consciousness his mind would leave the mundane affairs of the household, and he would be mentally inaccessible to those with him. He carried on long conversations with persons from the past—challenging, answering, forgiving, and setting things right. He often spoke in symbols and enigmatic phrases. His mind seemed to leap with equal ease to the distant past and the unknown future. He spoke with those family members who had preceded him in death and discussed his coming. Most interestingly, he participated in death ceremonies with the Cheyenne Indians and went through the litany of Christ on the cross. In his lucid periods, as judged by his awareness of daily events, he still spoke of beating the cancer. Within 6 weeks he died.

From this and similar experiences we suggest nurses begin to assess more astutely the meaning of confusion and the need that it may be satisfying. It seems clear that in many instances certain episodes of confusion may be the individual's manner of meeting a felt need (Figure 27-4).

There is much we do not yet understand about the dynamics of confusion. It is frequently thought to arise from brain dysfunction and certainly often does in the mechanistic sense. It may also be that the mind is indeed an essence of itself that moves toward the resolution of psychosocial needs and cosmic consciousness during confusional states.

Parapsychologic Phenomena

Some older persons may have experienced unusual events such as telepathic messages, predictive dreams, premonitions, out-of-body experiences, or poltergeist activity. They may be reluctant to share them unless the listener maintains an accepting attitude. For some persons it will be important that they can share these paranormal experiences that may have made them feel abnormal or bizarre. Some persons who do not appear to be psychotic experience such events. If they have sought professional help, they may have become frustrated, since our present understanding of these events is limited. They are most often thought to be psychotic. Even persons with lifelong psychotic disorders may experience valid parapsychologic events. Therapists open to the limits of their knowledge will offer validation, support, and reassurance and refer the individual to organizations studying such phenomena. They are interested in the patterning of such events and the relationships to stresses, illness, accidents, and personality components. Many persons who experience such events develop a great sense of alienation or attempt to deny the experiences.

George had the sense that he was floating above the scene of the accident. He heard a commotion and even moaning that emanated from his body, though he had no sense of making a sound. He saw his body being carefully lifted onto the stretcher and put in the ambulance. There was no pain or distress. Slowly, it seemed, he reentered his body, and by the time they arrived at the hospital he was very aware of being in considerable pain. He didn't mention this strange experience even though, in afterthought, it was quite frightening.

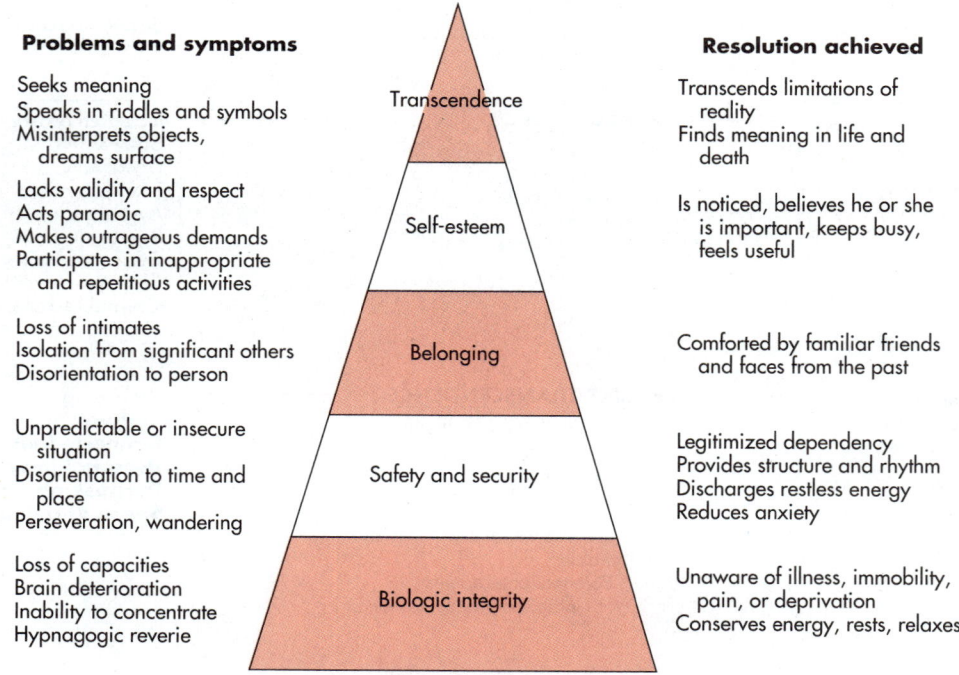

Problems and symptoms

Seeks meaning
Speaks in riddles and symbols
Misinterprets objects,
    dreams surface

Lacks validity and respect
Acts paranoic
Makes outrageous demands
Participates in inappropriate
    and repetitive activities

Loss of intimates
Isolation from significant others
Disorientation to person

Unpredictable or insecure
    situation
Disorientation to time and
    place
Perseveration, wandering

Loss of capacities
Brain deterioration
Inability to concentrate
Hypnagogic reverie

Transcendence
Self-esteem
Belonging
Safety and security
Biologic integrity

Resolution achieved

Transcends limitations of
    reality
Finds meaning in life and
    death

Is noticed, believes he or she
    is important, keeps busy,
    feels useful

Comforted by familiar friends
    and faces from the past

Legitimized dependency
Provides structure and rhythm
Discharges restless energy
Reduces anxiety

Unaware of illness, immobility,
    pain, or deprivation
Conserves energy, rests, relaxes

Figure 27-4. Needs met through confusional states. (Developed by Priscilla Ebersole.)

Harriet had a prophetic dream about her son-in-law, so vivid she couldn't go back to sleep. She "knew" he would be crushed by a falling tree the following day and begged him not to go into the woods. There was no doubt in her mind. It was as if the event had occurred for her before it occurred in reality, as it did, the next afternoon.

Freida "knew" the moment her grandmother died, though the family was not notified until the next day.

These are only some of the examples we have heard of extraordinary occurrences for which we have no explanation. However, nurses must become aware that many elders have experienced some of these phenomena.

A nurse may initiate a revealing conversation by saying, "There are many things going on in this universe that we do not understand. Have you ever experienced something that there was no logical explanation for, such as a premonition?" "Were you frightened by it?" "Did you tell anyone?" "How did you explain it to yourself?" Such conversations can be enlightening and also renew an individual's awareness of the unknown possibilities existing in all situations.

Near-Death Experience

From antiquity to the present, near-death experiences have been reported that have given insight into the experience of death itself. Persons who have survived tell us what it is like to ostensibly return from the dead. They describe feelings of peace, tranquility, and unconditional love. Some do not wish to return but feel they must. Serdahely et al (1988) have examined some of these experiences and suggest ways nurses may encourage individuals to share them. The urge to express these transcendental experiences is often strong but mixed with fears of being considered crazy. It is particularly difficult to express the out-of-body experiences that commonly occur. It seems as if one's essence disengages from the body and, psychiatrically, this would be labeled as an episode of depersonalization. The health care provider must realize these may have profound significance and lasting impact on the individual who has experienced them.

Katherine Anne Porter (1965) had a near-death experience when she contracted influenza during the 1918 pandemic. The experience is shared in her short story, "Pale Horse, Pale Rider." An excerpt follows:

Miranda sighed and lay back on the pillow and thought, I must give up, I can't hold on any longer. There was only that pain, only that room, and only Adam. There were no longer any multiple planes of living, no touch filaments of memory and hope pulling taut backwards and forwards holding her upright between them (p. 304).

That was a child's dream of the heavenly meadow, the vision of repose that comes to a tired body in sleep, she thought, but I have seen it when I did not know it was a dream. Closing her eyes she would rest for a moment remembering that bliss which had repaid all the pain of the journey to reach it; opening them again she saw with a new anguish the dull world to which she was condemned, where the light seemed filmed over with cobwebs, all the bright surfaces corroded, the sharp planes melted and formless, all objects and beings meaningless, ah, dead and withered things that believed themselves alive (p. 314)!

Miranda wondered again at the time and trouble the living took to be helpful to the dead. But not quite dead now, she reassured herself, one foot in either world now; soon I shall cross back and be at home again (p. 316).

To elicit a discussion of a near-death experience you might ask, "Do you recall any unusual feelings or perceptions during any critical episode you survived?" Suggestions for dealing with persons experiencing these remarkable events include the following:

1. Speak as if the patient can hear you even though he or she appears totally nonresponsive. Patients frequently later report hearing comments about them that either anger or disturb them.
2. Be receptive and nonjudgmental when listening later to an account of the event.
3. Reassure the individual that these experiences are quite commonly reported and that they are not evidences of psychoses.
4. Recognize the emotional impact this may have on the individual and explore the meaning attached to it.
5. Anticipate anger from some persons who felt compelled to come back from the near-death experience.
6. Explore your own biases and keep an open mind to the unknown aspects of our universe.

We know so little of human potential and of the mystical. Let us keep ourselves open to the unknown and immeasurable.

Hallucinations and Visions

Hallucinations and visions have great meaning for some people. These differ from ordinary fantasies in that the individual believes their origin is external. History has given us many examples of such events: Saint Paul's confrontation with God, the voices heard by Joan of Arc, and the vision of the Virgin at Lourdes. Sometimes these are collectively witnessed. Most of them seem to have some religious or ethereal motif. These are mentioned because they are poorly understood and often judged a psychotic symptom or a miracle. Religious old people sometimes report visions of angels or other heavenly emissaries. Most often they see a person who has died and may feel comforted.

Meditation

Many types and rituals of meditation have flourished in Western societies in the past two decades. Some have been used for thousands of years in Eastern cultures. Whatever the method, the goal is to quiet the mind and center oneself. When the mind slows, the body relaxes, and less oxygen and nutrients are needed. In addition, meditation has been found to yield the following benefits (Bloomfield, 1975):

- Increased measured intelligence
- Increased short-term and long-term recall
- Decreased anxiety, depression, and irritability

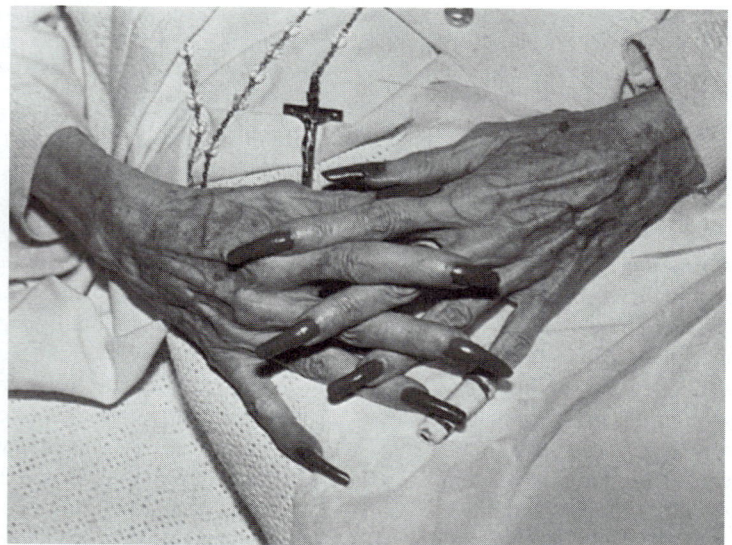

Expression of the inner and outer woman. (Courtesy American Society on Aging.)

- Greater perceived self-actualization (realization of potential)
- Better mind-body coordination
- Increased perceptual awareness
- Normalization of blood pressure
- Relief from insomnia
- Normalization of weight

These are all significant to aged people; the fact that we see the polar opposites of these benefits so frequently attests to the stress level of many older citizens, which might be reduced through meditation.

Effective meditation requires about 20 minutes of focusing on a sound, a thought, or an image. Practicing 2 or more times daily will bring calmness, better health, and higher energy levels in its wake. It can be accomplished in any setting, but a place with few distractions is helpful. People who meditate with consistency often begin to be aware of a transcendent state of being. Although meditation has unique meanings for each person, some common dynamics that tend toward self-actualization exist:

- It is noncompetitive.
- It integrates body-mind function.
- It is not dependent on others.
- It taps into beliefs about oneself.
- There is always room for improvement.
- You are in control.
- You cannot fail.

Nurses may introduce the values of meditation to the aged and serve as guides in the beginnings of such activities. Chanting psalms, reciting poetry by rote, praying, practicing yoga, keeping a dream diary, and playing a musical instrument are all mechanisms of release and renewal that may bring one into higher states of awareness.

Dreams—Personal and Collective

Jung's view of the work of dreams is most appropriate in a gerontology text. He saw the goal of the last half of life as reconciliation of one's various repressions by the use of dreams, myths, and symbols to become a whole person. To discover the hidden and embrace the unconscious is the process of individuation and transcendence, which may occupy one intensely after midlife. To explore the hidden, one may analyze dreams. They are the window of the unconscious.

To fully use dream material for self-transcendence, the concept of collective unconscious must be explored. Jung (1961) views the collective unconscious as composed of archetypal images or symbols. They include powerful, collectively carried, instinctual reactions:

Anima: feminine principle

Animus: masculine principle

Wise old man: king, hero, medicine man, savior

Great mother: infinite love, understanding, help, protection, tyranny over the dependent

In dreams for a brief time we possess qualities "beyond ourselves"—we are phenomenally courageous, infinitely wise and forgiving, not ego centered but intimately aware of all life and feel oneness with life (Fordham, 1966).

Jung believed each person could best analyze and interpret his or her own dreams by meditating on them and examining them in great detail. To understand the meaning, several steps are employed. Establish the context of the present life situation, then examine each image or symbol carefully for all the possible meanings. He suggests a series of dreams may be a most satisfactory basis for interpretation, since important images occur repeatedly in dreams.

Following is an example of a dream an old woman had following the death of her roommate. "I have dreamed of her every night since she died. She sometimes sings to me, and she is waiting for me on an island and says she won't go on without me. She's holding a big bowl of soup." We talked about the dream, about death, and about the fear of dying alone. She spoke of how her roommate knew she loved soup and also mentioned that her roommate was deaf. The dream seemed to give her assurance that she would not be alone in death (a compensatory aspect of the dream because so many do die alone) and that physical limitations were conquered through death (the singing of her deaf roommate). In a symbolic sense the soup could mean nourishment, love, a blending, an offering, or it could be from the present context of her life, in which she seldom got the soup she enjoyed. The old woman died 2 weeks after her roommate. Jung might call this a "prospective" dream because it prepared her for a future place and time.

Dreams provide access to the unconscious of the individual or the collective unconscious. The individual may express desires, conflicts, fears, prophecies, hidden aspects of personality, compensation, or modifications of recent or distant experiences. Dreams that connect one with the collective unconscious may be very vivid, seem highly significant, and include surprising or incomprehensible symbols that seem to have no relationship to the dreamer's life. Jung believes these dreams are especially significant in transcending the personal and deepening one's experience by connection with remote people through symbols significant to many. Jung believed that dreams function to promote growth and individuation and that they are sources of information and creative power.

We believe nurses should express interest in the dreams of their aged clients and explore meanings with them. Sharing a dream is a revealing and intimate gesture.

Henry and Stephens (1977) speculated that dreams and fantasies are the ties between the two brain hemispheres, the creative and the logical. They are the synthesizers. Jung, Faraday (who discovered the benzene ring through the symbolism of a dream in 1825), and many other theorists have made important discoveries through dreams that connected the creative and logical parts of the brain. Significantly, Faraday's dream was an example of continuity rather than linearity of thought, another attribute of the nondominant hemisphere.

Dombeck (1995) reports a dream sharing group in which "dream telling" is a mechanism for increasing spiritual awareness. It has been found to be a healing experience for victims of abuse, disadvantaged youths, and prisoners. There were no efforts at dream interpretation but only to explore feelings, commonalities with others, and speculations about personal meanings.

We did not find reports of such activity with elders but believe it might be very illuminating. We would be particu-

larly interested in recurring dreams and the meaning for the elder. Dream research seems a fruitful area of study with elders.

Fantasies and Daydreams

Most studies indicate a decreasing importance and intensity of daydreams and fantasies in old age. However, we must remember cohort effects and realize that those born 75 years ago were culturally conditioned in a way that put little importance on dreams and fantasies. We might assist the aged to value their self-exploratory activities by giving credence to them.

Memories could well be included with dreams and fantasies because they become so intertwined in the later years. The conscious and unconscious seem to merge in a more holistic manner when the very old move back and forward in time with ease, weaving recurrent dreams, hopes, and fantasies into their memories. Often we mistakenly label this fluidity as confusion or inaccuracy if we hold strict boundaries and a segmented personal reality. We might take lessons from the old who have learned to make peace with their multiple realities.

Hypnosis

Throughout the history of medicine, hypnosis has appeared again and again as a means of healing, yet it has not gained a respected status. The eclectic psychiatrists today have largely abandoned hypnosis and free association, but most are aware that the mind has more power over illness and health than the physician. The ingredient of interpersonal trust enhances hypnotic responsiveness. The aged subjected to minimum stimulation over long periods are thought to be susceptible to hypnotic suggestion. Some drugs also increase suggestibility.

NURSING INTERVENTIONS

When focusing on the supreme needs of an individual, those for transcending the usual limits of life experience, nursing interventions may become obscure. Finding meaning in life is a uniquely individual task and does not occur quickly or through the efforts of another. Young, attentive nurses often find the aged leading the way toward development of the spirit. We can provide a milieu of acceptance, openness, and validation. These attitudes come from our own awareness of the importance of the inner person and our willingness to accede to its supremacy. This means we cannot always measure coping by visible evidence nor can we be the arbiter of meaning.

LEGACIES

The search for meaning seems to be the basic motivation for leaving a legacy (Birren and Deutchman, 1991) (Box 27-5). Extending one's meaning to others can be an important and

<table>
<tr><td>

Box 27-5

Special Characteristics of Older Adults

1. Desire to leave a legacy provides a sense of continuity.
2. "Elder" function is a natural propensity of the old to share with the young accumulated knowledge and experience.
3. Attachment to familiar objects gives a sense of continuity, aids the memory, and provides comfort, security, and satisfaction.
4. Change in the sense of time experienced as a sense of immediacy, of here and now, of living in the moment.
5. Personal sense of the entire life cycle.
6. Creativity, curiosity, and surprise may promote active and productive lives in the absence of disease and social problems.
7. Feeling of consummation or fulfillment in life that brings "serenity" and "wisdom."

</td><td>

Box 27-6

Example of Legacies

Oral histories
Autobiographies
Shared memories
Taught skills
Works of art and music
Publications
Human organ donations
Endowments
Objects of significance
Written histories
Tangible or intangible assets
Personal characteristics such as courage or integrity
Bestowed talents
Traditions and myths perpetuated
Philanthropic causes
Progeny: children and grandchildren
Methods of coping
Unique thought: Darwin, Einstein, Freud, and others

</td></tr>
</table>

gratifying activity in the last years. Throughout life, shared experiences provide satisfaction, but in the last years this exchange allows one to gain a clearer perspective on how his or her movement on earth has had impact.

A legacy is one's tangible and intangible assets that are transferred to another and may be treasured as a symbol of the bequeathor's immortality. Courage, wisdom, and insights that we perceive in our elders also become part of their legacy (Wyatt-Brown, 1996). Not only the giver but the receiver is essential to the concept of legacy; reciprocity is essential (Kivnick, 1996).

Old people must be encouraged to identify that which they would like to leave and whom they wish the recipients to be. This process has interpersonal significance and prepares one to leave the world with a sense of meaning. It can provide a transcendent feeling of continuation and tangible or intangible ties with survivors.

Interestingly, *Generations*, the publication of the American Society on Aging, devoted an entire issue to the consideration of legacies (vol 20, no. 3, 1996). Most of the issue was focused on the legacy of health and economic policies and the transmission of wealth and burden. This is certainly significant, and many elders and others now wonder what legacy of debt and conflict we are leaving for the generations to follow.

Legacies are diverse and may range from memories that will live on in the mind of others to bequeathed fortunes. Box 27-6 is a partial list of legacies. The list in Box 27-6 is as diverse as individual contributions to humanity. Erikson's seventh stage of man identifies the generative function as the main concern of the adult years and the last stage (eighth) as that of reviewing with integrity or despair what one has ac-

complished. We propose that legacies are generative and are identified and shared best as one approaches the end of life. This activity reinforces integrity.

Autobiographies/Life Histories

Oral histories are an approach to immortality. As long as one's story is told, one remains alive in the minds of others. Doers leave their products and live through them. Powerful figures are remembered in fame and infamy. The quiet, unobtrusive person survives in the memory of intimates and in family anecdotes. Everyone has a life story. The quest for immortality grew out of words, the human ability to articulate meaning and personality to others. Without words, experience would contain no past or future. The short span of one's days would amount to only a series of sensory impressions, not even rising to the perceptual level, since percepts are formed through internalized concepts and words spoken to the self.

Autobiographies and recorded memoirs can serve a transcendent purpose for those who are alone—and for many who are not. Nurses can encourage older people to write, talk, or express in other ways the meaning of their lives. The human experience and the poignant anecdotes bind people together and validate the uniqueness of each brief journey in this level of awareness and the assurance that one will not be forgotten. Dying patients can express and order their memories through audiotapes that are then bequeathed to families if the aged person desires. Sharing one's personal story creates bonds of empathy, illustrates a point, conveys some of the deep wisdom that we all contain, and connects us with our deepest human consciousness.

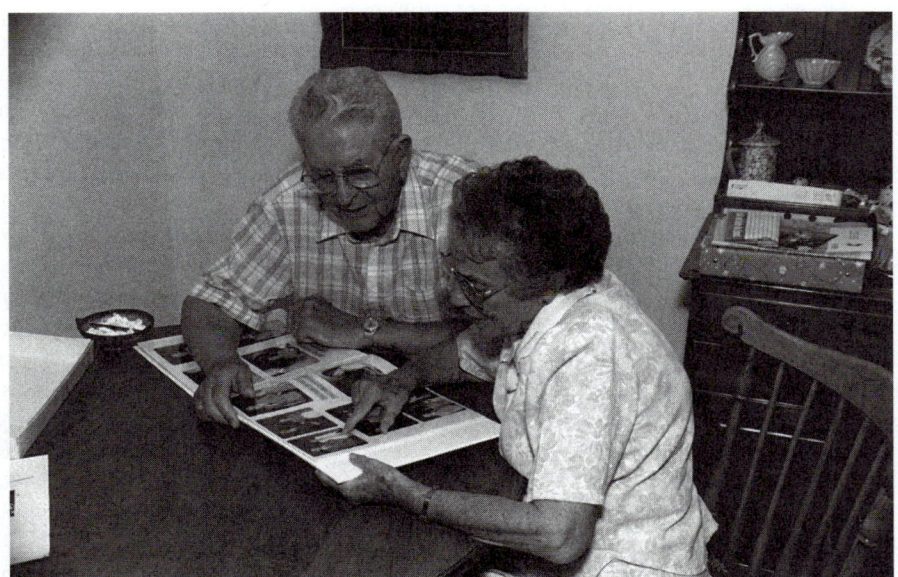

Generational continuity. (Courtesy Rod Schmall.)

These stories are influenced by gender, culture, history, social class and context, race and ethnicity (Schuster, 1996; Harrienger, 1996). All come together to form a unique, never-to-be-reproduced individual legend. In addition, stories from a grandparent will bring to life historical periods that have previously seemed sterile (Kivnick, 1996). Reaching across generations in this way decreases self-absorption and releases "grand-generativity" that incorporates care for the present and concern for the future (Kivnick, 1993).

A real story touches not only the mind, but also the imagination and the unconscious depths in a person, and it may remain with him or her through many years, coming to the surface of consciousness now and then to yield new insights (Luke, 1982).

Collective Legacies

Each person is a link in the chain of generations (Erikson, 1963) and as such may identify with generational accomplishments. An old man may feel himself a significant part of a generation that survived the Great Depression. A middle-aged man may identify with the generation that walked on the moon. Those years of youthful idealism are impressed in one's memory by the political or ideologic climate of the time. That is the stage when one searches for a fit in the larger society.

The importance of this to nurses lies in how they use this knowledge. For instance, the nurse may ask, "Who were the great men of your time? Which ones were important to you? What events of your generation changed the world? What were the most important events you experienced?" Sometimes it is helpful to mention certain historic events and ask about individual reactions.

Childless individuals are becoming more prevalent with each passing generation, and they must find a way to outlive the self through a legacy. Many choose a "social" legacy (Rubinstein, 1996). Florence Nightingale would be one such person, with the legacy left to nurses.

Legacies Expressed through Others

There are many ways that one's legacy is expressed through the development of others: in a teaching/learning situation or through mentorships, patronage, shared talents, and organ donations. Some creative works and research are legacies left to successive generations for continued modification and growth (Philip, 1995). In other words, one's legacy may be a product of his or her own brought to fruition through someone else who may also become an intermediary. Thus people and generations are tied in sequential development. Some examples may illustrate this type of legacy.

An aged man cried as he talked of his grandson's talent as a violinist. They shared their love for violin, and the grandfather believed he had genetically and personally contributed to his grandson's development as a musician.

A professor emeritus spoke of visiting his son in a distant state and hearing him expound ideas that had been partially developed by the professor and his father before him.

Great-aunt Laura worried about preserving the environment for future generations, so she took young children on nature walks to stimulate their interest in birds, plants, and animals. She also donated land for a natural park.

People who amass a fortune and allocate certain funds for endowment of artists, scientific projects, and intellectual exploration are counting on others to complete their legacy.

The following are suggestions for assisting elders to identify and develop their legacy:

1. Find out lifelong interests.
2. Establish a method of recording.

3. Identify recipients—either generally or specifically.
4. Record legacy.
5. Distribute as planned.
6. Provide for systematic feedback of results to older person.

It is gratifying to the old if a legacy can be converted into some tangible form, ensuring that it will not be readily dismissed or forgotten. The poem by Kivnick (Box 27-7) is a tangible legacy. The following vehicles can convey legacies:

Summation of life work
Photograph albums, scrapbooks
Written memoir
Taped memoirs (video or audio)
Artistic representations
Memory gardens
Mementos
Genealogies
Recorded pilgrimages
See Resources for detailed information.

Living Legacies. Many old people wish to donate their bodies to science or donate body parts for transplant. This is one mechanism to transcend death. Parts of the body keep another alive, or, in the case of certain diseases, the deceased body may provide important information leading to preven-tive or restorative techniques in the future. Donation of body parts in old age may not be encouraged because they are often less viable than those from younger people. Persons interested in providing such a legacy should be encouraged to call the nearest university biomedical center and obtain more information. The nurse then has a postmortem obligation to the client to assist in carrying out his or her wishes.

Keating (1996) identifies the generational transfer of a farm as a living legacy. Though not an organ donation, it is certainly a living donation. In the days of primogeniture this was a simple affair though not necessarily satisfactory. Now it is more complex. A study conducted in Canada, New Zealand, and the United States showed that keeping the farm intact and in the family was a high priority (Keating, 1996). A successful resolution included keeping all family members content and maintaining a viable farm operation (Stalker et al, 1996). This was done successfully when all family members were involved in the planning early on and various aspects of the farm management were turned over to the children who best could manage them. In other cases encumbrances on the farm or fluctuating market values imposed inequities on various siblings. Most parents attempted to compensate nonsuccessor children in some way.

Box 27-7	**Hang On**

Chorus:

Hang on to the work that you do every day,
Hang on to the love every step of the way.
Hang on to the memories, hang on to tomorrow,
Hang on to the hope and the joy and the sorrow,
Each day is a victory still to be won,
So hang on with dignity, proudly hang on.

Verses:

When Lily retired she played tennis each day,
And she tutored the children who lived out her way.
Twice a week in her car she delivered hot meals,
To the old folks who treasured the gift of her wheels.
And though nightly exhausted she fell into bed,
"Keeping busy prevents feeling old," Lily said.

(Chorus)

At 75 John McNeal lost his wife.
She died in the cabin where they'd spent their life.
After long months of raging and praying and crying
A new life emerged from the pain of her dying.
Now John puts up berries as she used to do,
And in the glass jars feels her love shining through.

(Chorus)

Mother was 90 the year that she died;
Her strength long since gone, she stayed mostly inside.
But she planted a tree in the last warmth of Fall,
Little more than a stick with no branches at all.
"It will bloom in the Spring," Mother said,
"And my dear,
I believe we will have to pick apples next year!"

(Chorus)

Today I write letters where I'd march before,
Against all injustice and nuclear war.
Now I can't go to jail as I once used to do,
But I still have this message; I'll leave it with you.
If we do all we can, giving what we can give,
And we work side by side for as long as we live.
Black and white, man and woman, the young and the old,
Then a future of justice and peace will unfold.

(Chorus)

©1996 Helen Kivnick

From Kivnick HQ: Remembering and being remembered: the reciprocity of psychosocial legacy, *Generations* 20(3):49, 1996.

Property and Assets. Wealth may be viewed as a means toward power more often than transcendence; therefore old people are often reluctant to disperse material goods before their death and frequently never make out a will (Table 27-4). Some elders use the future legacy as a means to exert power and control over offspring. One man said, "So long as I have that bankroll, they've got to treat me with respect" (Lustbader, 1996). The power to exert in-fluence, to punish and reward is often bound up in an anticipated estate distribution (Lustbader, 1996).

Many people have considerable assets to leave to their families, philanthropic foundations, or on occasion to friends, pets, or strangers, yet many old people die each year leaving inheritances with no specified beneficiaries. Many of these are retained in county and state treasuries until someone successfully substantiates a claim to them.

| *Table 27-4* | Characteristics of Americans over 70 with Wills, 1994 |

Demographic characteristics	Total (N = 20,985,637)		
	Number	Percent in category	Percent with a will
Age			
70 to 75	9,378,603	45.2	69.0
76 to 80	5,535,085	26.7	69.4
81 to 85	3,601,910	17.4	69.8
Over 86	2,227,069	10.7	67.5
Household annual income			
1 to 9,000	4,233,067	20.4	49.4
9,001 to 16,000	5,143,461	24.8	67.1
16,001 to 28,650	5,538,312	26.7	73.5
Over 28,651	5,827,827	28.1	80.9
Household assets*			
0 to 15,437	4,094,753	19.7	34.2
15,438 to 73,475	4,866,556	23.5	63.8
73,476 to 174,425	5,561,756	26.8	79.1
Over 174,425	6,219,604	30.0	87.2
Gender			
Male	7,878,890	38.0	72.2
Female	12,863,777	62.0	67.2
Religious preference			
Protestant	13,140,646	63.4	69.8
Catholic	5,466,421	26.4	67.4
Jewish	836,390	4.0	76.9
No preference	989,966	4.8	64.1
Other	300,461	1.4	65.7
Race			
White	17,649,063	85.1	76.4
Black	2,171,214	10.5	29.1
Hispanic	782,575	3.8	24.1
Other	139,817	0.7	16.0
Education			
Less than high school	11,514,125	55.5	61.6
High school diploma	6,467,750	31.2	75.7
College degree	2,760,792	13.3	84.7
Marital/family status			
Married, spouse present	9,960,669	48.0	75.9
Married, spouse absent	315,959	1.5	66.7
Living with someone	133,850	0.6	57.9
Divorced or separated	1,020,959	4.9	52.5
Widowed	8,626,674	41.6	64.8
Never married	684,555	3.3	51.6
Total	20,985,637	100	69.0

From O'Connor C: Empirical research on how the elderly handle their estates, *Generations* 20(3):13, 1996.
NOTE: Based on 8,223 respondents and 5,694 households. Data are weighted to represent the over-70 U.S. population in 1994. One age-eligible person was selected at random from each household; however, if that person was married, information about the entire household was obtained only once.
*Assets include home value, real estate, transportation, business, IRA, stocks, bonds, CDs, checking, and savings.
SOURCE: AHEAD survey.

Freud contended that, in the unconscious, everyone is convinced of his own immortality (O'Connor, 1996). Families often consider wills a taboo subject and refuse to discuss them but upon distribution may be sorely disappointed. When older people leave large gifts to "unnatural" or "unworthy" legatees, the will is often challenged by children or other relatives (Frolik, 1996).

There are certain ways to plan estates that are decidedly advantageous for the planner, as well as the recipient, in terms of control, avoidance of lengthy probate proceedings, and taxation. Since the laws are complex and everchanging, it would be advisable to use the services of an estate planner (see Chapter 14). The nurse's responsibility regarding wills may be limited to advising older people to obtain legal counsel while they are healthy and competent and plan how they would like to distribute their worldly goods.

Knowledge. We carry the thought legacies, without conscious awareness, of individuals such as Ban Zhao*, Sappho†, Lao-Tzu‡, Hippocrates§, St. Augustine‖, James Madison¶, Nightingale#, Helen Hunt Jackson** and others who underlie many of our thoughts and actions. Erik Homberg Erikson, one of the respected thinkers of our time, is just one of many formulators of human thought constructs who left numerous published works for future generations and has markedly influenced the understanding of life span development in our era. His legacy will continue with modifications and reinterpretations. As has been said in many ways before, we build on the thought and works of those who have preceded us. In a sense all creative thinkers and teachers leave their legacy in their students and devotees.

Personal Possessions. Possessions carry more meaning as time passes; individuals change, but the possession remains much the same. A possession is a way of symbolically hanging onto individuals who are gone or times that are past. For some it is a means of hanging onto the self that is changing with time. Cherished possessions passed on through several generations may have achieved meaning through the close family member to whom they belonged (Tobin, 1996). One's personally significant items become highly charged with memories and meaning, and transferring them to friends and kin can be a tender experience. They should never be dispersed without the individual's knowledge.

*Ban Zhao, Chinese astronomer, mathmetician, and poet, circa 115 AD.
†Sappho, Greek educator and priestess of the feminine love cult, circa 610 BC.
‡Lao-Tzu, Chinese founder of Taoism, circa 575 BC.
§Hippocrates, Greek father of medicine, circa 425 BC.
‖St Augustine, Christian theologian, circa 400 AD.
¶James Madison, father of the US Constitution, circa 1775 AD.
#Florence Nightingale, mother of organized nursing, circa 1860 AD.
**Helen Hunt Jackson, author, defender of Native Americans, their rights, and intermarriage, circa 1884 AD.

It is vital that people approaching death be given the opportunity to appropriately distribute their important belongings to those whom they feel will also cherish them. Nurses may encourage them to plan the distribution of their significant items carefully because it is often very difficult to decide when and how best they should be given. Some choose to distribute them before dying, and in those cases nurses often need to help family members accept these gifts, appreciating the meaning and recognizing the significance.

TRANSCENDENT NURSING AND LEGACIES

"The responsibility of the nurse is not to make people well, or to prevent their getting sick, but to assist people to recognize the power that is within them to move to higher levels of consciousness" (Newman, 1994, p. xv). We have dealt with transcendence, spirituality and several mechanisms used to establish a legacy, methods of expanding one's limited existence. Often this becomes a major concern before one's death, and the nurse will find it an absorbing task. It is well to remember that some persons may avoid any such interest or concern, particularly when angry, in pain, or denying their own mortality. Nurses need not push the individual to accomplish this task but should be available to assist the person and family members. Certain questions allow the aged person to consider a legacy if he or she is ready to do so, for example:

What is the meaning to you of your life experience right now?

Have you ever thought of writing an autobiography?

If you could leave something to the younger generation, what would it be?

Have you ever thought of the impact your generation has had on the world?

What has been most meaningful in your life?

These suggestions should stimulate ideas for spontaneous statements, which are revealing in an interpersonal context. When discussing meanings of life, it is possible a client will become despairing and find no meaning. In those cases we would suggest that life-review may be in process, and the nurse can assist with this (see Chapter 21).

The basic mysteries of life elude scientific researchers, yet they are the essence of existence with meaning. Remembering, feeling, dreaming, worshiping, and grasping one's connection to the universe are the realities of the human spirit. "Temporal transcendence" (Brewer, 1986), the blending of past-present-future, may guard the inner self from being old unless the spirit is crushed. Being old is not the centrality of the self—spirit is. Spirit synthesizes the total personality, provides integration, energizing force, and immortality.

Nursing Diagnoses

The following potential diagnoses must be considered
   as well as diagnoses unique to the particular
   individual.
   Coping, ineffective
   Grieving, anticipatory
   Grieving, dysfunctional
   Hopelessness
   Pain

Personal identity disturbance
Powerlessness
Social isolation

NURSING PROCESS AND NURSING DIAGNOSIS
Spiritual Distress (*Distress* of the Human Spirit)

Etiologies and Related Factors
Separation from religious and cultural ties
Intrinsic challenges to beliefs and value system

Defining Characteristics
Verbal expression of distress/disgust/disillusionment
Sadness/depression
Anger at God and religion
Verbalizes inner conflict regarding beliefs
Altered sleep patterns/distressing dreams
Questions meaning of existence
Self-blaming
Withdrawal
Regards illness as punishment by God

Knowledge
Depression
Spiritual assessment
Concept of anomie
Interpersonal relationships
Ritual and rites that are important in various religions
   and cultures
Therapeutic communication
Own spiritual needs
Community resources

Clinical Judgment and Related Skills
Utilization of communication skills
Listening
Assess level of depression
Share perceptions
Provide for privacy
Reinforce self-worth
Provision of control in decision making
Share concerns regarding client's distress
Nonjudgmental acceptance
Facilitate expression of religious/spiritual/social needs
Recognition of cultural variations
Ability to separate own beliefs, values, and spiritual
   philosophy from those of client
Make necessary referrals

Evaluation
Client completes task(s) that he/she identified or defined
Expresses some philosophy related to living and dying
Achieves the desired sense of spiritual peace
Client expresses meaning in current situation.

NEEDS ADDRESSED AND TASK STRENGTHS

Need for spiritual expression and awareness of
   meaning; need for philosophy that is sustaining
Awareness and acceptance of life cycles and universal
   connections

Expression of own life experience
Universality
Sensitivity to meanings
Cultivation of spirituality
Sense of humor
Rituals that provide meaning and comfort

KEY CONCEPTS

- Transcending the material and physical limitations of existence through ritual and spiritual means is an especially important aspect of aging.
- Gerotranscendence is a theory, proposed by Tornstam, that implies a natural shift in concerns that occurs in the aging process. Elders are thought to spend more time in reflection, less on materialistic concerns and to find more satisfaction in life. This is an attempt to define aging not by the standards of young and middle aduthood but as having distinctive characteristics of its own.
- Peak experiences are those times when one seems to have risen above the ordinary and participated in the mystical.
- Illnesses that occur have the potential for altering one's fundamental beliefs and hopes. It is important for nurses to give elders the opportunity to discuss the meanings of an illness. Some find these experiences bring new insights, others are angry. Empathic nurses will provide a sounding board while the elder makes sense of an illness within a satisfactory framework.
- Spiritual healing has ancient religious roots, but scientists are now recognizing and accepting the power of the mind in restoring health and, if not restoring health, enhancing one's ability to cope.
- Though many do not attend churches, elders have a high level of interest in the spiritual and religious elements of life.
- Nurses need not neglect to discuss spirituality with elders. They will only respond if it has significance for them.
- Life satisfaction, happiness, morale, and health are all related in some ways to beliefs, hope, and motivation that may be derived from a spiritual awareness.
- Dreams and fantasies are avenues to the subliminal life and often yield insights to the elder in search of meanings.
- Near-death experiences are remarkably consistant in producing a sense of profound peace. These studies indicate that the experience of death may indeed be a culmination.

▲ CASE STUDY

Melba had no children but numerous nieces and nephews, though she did not feel particularly close to any of them. She had been a nursing instructor at a community college and had enjoyed her students but had not developed a sustained relationship with any of them after they had completed her courses. At the level of nursing education there seemed to be little opportunity for mentorship, though she had occasionally taken a student under her wing and arranged special experiences that they particularly desired. Because she had taught several courses each year, she never really developed a strong affiliation to a specialty but considered herself a pediatric nurse. She had not made any major contributions to the field in terms of research or publications; a few reviews, CE workshops, and some nursing newsletters had really been the extent of her work outside that required. Her husband died in 1988, and she had felt very much alone since that time, especially after her retirement 3 years ago. Prior to that time she had been too busy to think about the ultimate meaning of all her years of teaching and wifely activities. With time on her hands she began to wonder what it all meant. Had she done anything meaningful? Had she really made a difference in anything or in anyone's life? Was anyone going to remember her in any special way? So many questions were making her morose. She had never been a religious person, though her husband had been a devoted Catholic. He had felt that God had a purpose for him in life, and though he wasn't always able to understand what it might be, he seemed to feel satisfied. She began to wonder if she should go to church . . . would that make her feel less depressed? One Sunday morning she had decided to attend her neighborhood Catholic church, but on her way out she slipped on the icy walkway and sustained Colle's fractures on both wrists. After a brief emergency room visit for assessment, immobilization of the wrists, and medications, she was sent back home with an order for home health and social service assessment on the following day. Of course, she had extreme difficulty managing the most basic self-care while keeping her wrists immobilized and was very dejected. When the home health nurse arrived the next morning, to her amazement, it was a former student who had graduated 4 years previously. Melba was more chagrined than pleased and greeted her with, "Oh, I hate to have you see me so helpless. I've been feeling so useless and, now with these wrists, I am totally useless." If you were the home health nurse, how would you begin working with Melba, knowing that your visits would be limited to just a few?

Based upon the case study, develop a nursing care plan using the following procedure*

List comments of client that provide *subjective data*.

List information that provides *objective data*.

From these data identify and state, using accepted format, two *nursing diagnoses* you determine are most significant to this client at this time.

Determine and state *outcome criteria* for each diagnosis. These must reflect some alleviation of the problem identified in the nursing diagnosis and must be stated in concrete and measurable terms.

Plan and state one or more *interventions* for each diagnosed problem. Provide specific documentation of source used to determine appropriate intervention.

---

*Students are advised to refer to their nursing diagnosis text and identify possible or potential problems.

Plan at least one intervention that incorporates the client's existing strengths.

Evaluate success of intervention. Interventions must correlate directly with the stated outcome criteria in order to measure the outcome success.

STUDY QUESTIONS/ACTIVITIES

Discuss the meanings and the thoughts triggered by the student's and elder's viewpoints as expressed at the beginning of the chapter. How do these vary from your own experience?

RESEARCH QUESTIONS

Kane (1996) suggests the following aspects of legacies need to be studied:

How do elders balance their own present needs against estate planning?

Who makes out wills and when?

How do bequests relate to gifts given during one's lifetime?

Is the perpetuation of one's name an important aspect of a legacy?

What are the motivating differences between gifts during life and those after one's death?

How do recipients view the adequacy of their legacy?

These are important questions that we might suggest for nursing research.

RESOURCES

Consciousness Research and Training Project, Inc.
Dr. Joyce Goodrich
315 E 68th St, Box 96
New York, NY 10021-5692

Dr. Lawrence LeShan's approach to paranormal healing is taught in focused 5-day residential seminars; includes elements of holistic health, wellness, and consciousness theory.

Saybrook Institute Graduate School and Research Center
450 Pacific, 3rd Floor
San Francisco, California 94133
(800) 825-4480

Focused on understanding and enhancing the human experience; offers an innovative, individualized, and rigorous distance learning experience in humanistic psychology and human science.

Openway
Route 10, Box 105
Charlottesville, VA 22903
(804) 293-3245

4-year certificate training center for healers; healing energy systems, inner work, and hands-on healing.

American Society on Aging
Forum on Religion, Spirituality and Aging
833 Market Street, Suite 511
San Francisco, California 94103-1824
(415) 974-9600

Membership in organization provides newsletter, conferences, educational programming, networking opportunities, information clearinghouse, and access to leaders in the field.

Center for Aging, Religion and Spirituality
Dr. Mel Kimble
2481 Como Ave
St Paul, MN 55108
(612) 641-3581

Center established in 1994 to strengthen the field of religion, spirituality, and aging, to provide educational materials, and research and to foster interdisciplinary work. Sponsored by the College of Chaplains and the American Association of Homes and Services for the Aging.

Center for the Study of Health, Faith, and Ethics
211 E. Ontario, Suite 800
Chicago, IL 60611-3215

REFERENCES

American Association of Critical Care Nurses (AACN): Prayer and medicine: do they mix? *AACN News,* p 1, Feb 1995.

Benner P: *Interpretive phenomenology: embodiment, caring and ethics in health and illness,* Thousand Oaks, Calif, 1994, Sage.

Berggren-Thomas P, Griggs MJ: Spirituality in aging: spiritual need or spiritual journey, *J Gerontol Nurs* 21(3):5, 1995.

Birren JE, Deutchman DE: *Guiding autobiography groups for older adults: exploring the fabric of life,* Baltimore, 1991, Johns Hopkins University Press.

Bloomfield H: *Discovering inner energy and overcoming stress,* New York, 1975, Dell.

Brewer EDC: Researching religion and aging: an unlikely scenario. In Oliver DB, editor: *New directions in religion and aging,* New York, 1986, Haworth Press.

Buchanan D, Farran C, Clark D: Suicidal thought and self-transcendence in older adults, *J Psychosoc Nurs* 33(10):31, 1995.

Chidester D: *Patterns of transcendence: religion, death and dying,* Belmont, Calif, 1990, Wadsworth Publishing.

Cole T: The humanities and aging: an overview. In Cole T, Van Tassel D, Kastenbaum R, editors: *Handbook of aging and the humanities,* New York, 1994, Springer.

Cole TR: The aging spirit: agism and the journey of life in America, *Aging Today* 13(4):17, 1992.

Cole TR: What have we made of aging? *J Gerontol* 50B(6):S341, 1995.

Collis L: *Memoirs of a medieval woman: the life and times of Margery Kemp,* New York, 1964, Harper & Row.

Courtney BC, Poon LW, Martin P et al: Religiosity and adaptation in the oldest-old. In Poon LW, editor: *The Georgia centenarian study,* Amityville, NY, 1992, Baywood.

Cumming E, Henry WE: *Growing old: the process of disengagement,* New York, 1961, Basic Books.

Davis J: A ball player's approach to spirituality, *Innovator,* p 2, Spring/Summer 1995.

Davis J, Hale K: Spirituality and the caregiver, p 7, *Innovator,* Spring/Summer 1995.

Dombeck M-TB: Dream telling: a means of spiritual awareness, *Holistic Nursing Practice* 9(2):37, 1995.

Donley R: Spiritual dimensions of health care: nursing's mission, *Nurs Health Care* 12(4):178, 1991.

Erikson EH: *Childhood and society,* New York, 1950, WW Norton.

Erikson EH: *Childhood and society,* ed 2, New York, 1963, WW Norton.

Forbes EJ: Spirituality, aging, and the community-dwelling caregiver and care recipient, *Geriatr Nurs* 16(6):297, 1994.

Fordham F: *An introduction to Jung's psychology,* New York, 1966, Penguin Books.

Frolik LA: Legacies of possessions: passing property at death, *Generations* 20(3):9, 1996.

Goldberg BZ: *The sacred fire: the story of sex in religion,* New York, 1958, University Books.

Haase JE, Britt T, Coward DD et al: Simultaneous concept analysis of spiritual perspective, hope, acceptance and self-transcendence, *Image J Nurs Sch* 24(2):141, 1992.

Hammers M: Parish nurses give new meaning to Sunday services, *Nurseweek* 5(14):8, 1992.

Harrienger M: *Writing a life: the composing of grace.* Paper presented at the meeting of the Gerontological Society of America, Washington, DC, November 19, 1996.

Hebrews 11:1, *Holy Bible,* Chicago, 1964, John A Dickson.

Henderson R: The spirituality 'renaissance': professional interest grows, *Aging Today* 17(2):11, 1996.

Henry JP, Stephens PM: *Stress, health and the social environment,* New York, 1977, Springer-Verlag.

Hickey SS: Enabling hope, *Cancer Nurs* 9(3):133, 1986.

Holstein MB, Cole TR: Reflections on age, meaning, and chronic illness, *J Identity Health* 1(1):7, 1996.

Hungelmann J, Kenkel-Rossi E, Klassen L et al: Focus on spiritual well-being: harmonious interconnectedness of mind-body-spirit—use of the Jarel spiritual well-being scale, *Geriatr Nurs* 17(6):262, 1996.

Jung C: *Memories, dreams, reflections,* translated by Jaffe A, editor, New York, 1961, Random House.

Kane RA: Toward understanding legacy: a wish list, *Generations* 20(3):92, 1996.

Kaufman SR: *The ageless self: sources of meaning in later life,* Madison, 1986, University of Wisconsin Press.

Keating NC: Legacy, aging and succession in farm families, *Generations* 20(3):61, 1996.

Kennedy GJ, Kelman HR, Thomas C, Chen J: The relation of religious preference and practice to depressive symptoms among 1,855, *J Gerontol* 51B(6):P301, 1996.

Kimble M: A personal journey of aging: the spiritual dimension, *Generations* 17(2):27, 1993.

Kivnick HQ: Everyday mental health: a guide to assessing life strengths, *Generations* 17(1):13, 1993.

Kivnick HQ: Remembering and being remembered: the reciprocity of psychosocial legacy, *Generations* 20(3):49, 1996.

Koenig H: Religion and well-being in later life (abstract). *Proceedings of the Third Congress of the International Psychogeriatric Association, Chicago,* 3:1, 1987.

Krause N: Religiosity and self-esteem among older adults, *J Gerontol* 50B(5):P236, 1995.

Levin JS: *Religion in aging and health: theoretical foundations and methodological frontiers,* Thousand Oaks, Calif, 1994, Sage.

Levin JS: Age differences in mystical experience, *Gerontologist* 33(4):507, 1993.

Levin JS, Taylor RJ: Gender and age differences in religiosity among black Americans, *Gerontologist* 33(1):16, 1993.

Luke H: *The inner story,* New York, 1982, Crossroad.

Lustbader W: Conflict, emotion and power surrounding legacy, *Generations* 20(3):54, 1996.

MacLennan S, Tsai S: A nursing perspective on spiritual healing, *Perspectives* 19(1):9, 1995.

Macrae J: Nightingale's spiritual philosophy and its significance for modern nursing, *Image J Nurs Sch* 27(1):8, 1995.

Martin P, Raiser MV, Poon LW, Johnson MA, Bramlett M: *Significant events in the lives of the oldest old.* Paper presented at the meeting of the Gerontological Society of America, Washington, DC, Nov 20, 1996.

Maslow A: *Religions, values and peak-experiences,* New York, 1970, Viking Press.

Mayo Clinic Health Letter: Health and spirituality: medicine ponders how the two may interact, *Mayo Clinic Health Letter* 14(11):4, 1996.

Moberg DO: Religion in gerontology: from benign neglect to belated respect, *Gerontologist* 36(2): 264, 1996.

Moore DW: Most Americans say religion is important to them, *Gallup Poll Monthly,* No 353, p 16, Feb 1995.

Morse JM, Doberneck B: Delineating the concept of hope, *Image J Nurs Sch* 27(4):277, 1995.

Moyers W: *Healing and the mind,* WNET public television, February 1992.

National Interfaith Coalition on Aging: *Spiritual well being,* Washington, DC, 1975, National Interfaith Coalition on Aging.

Newman M: Aging as increasing complexity, *J Gerontol Nurs* 13:16, 1987.

Newman MA: *Health as expanding consciousness,* ed 2, New York, 1994, National League for Nursing Press.

O'Connor C: Empirical research on how the elderly handle their estates, *Generations* 20(3):13, 1996.

O'Connor P: Hope: a concept for home care nursing, *Home Care Provider* 1(4):175, 1996.

Partridge E: *Origins: a short etymological dictionary of modern English,* New York, 1959, Macmillan.

Philip CE: "Lifelines," *J Aging Studies* 9(4):265, 1995.

Porter KA: *The collected stories of Katherine Anne Porter,* New York, 1965, Harcourt Brace.

Powers M: Homebound elders still need spiritual connections, *Aging Today* 17(5):13, 1996.

Reed PG: Toward a nursing theory of self-transcendence: deductive reformulation using developmental theories, *Advances Nurs Sci* 13(4):64, 1991.

Richards M: Meeting the spiritual needs of the cognitively impaired, *Generations* 14(4):63, 1990.

Ross L: The spiritual dimension: its importance to patients' health, well-being and quality of life and its implications for nursing practice, *Capsules Comments Psychiatr Nurs* 3(1):54, 1996.

Rubinstein RL: Childlessness, legacy and generativity. *Generations* 20(3):58-61, 1996.

Schank MJ, Weis D, Matheus R: Parish nursing: ministry of healing, *Geriatr Nurs* 17(1):11, 1996.

Schuster E: *Transformative functions of life writing.* Paper presented at the meeting of the Gerontological Society of America, Washington, DC, Nov 19, 1996.

Seeber J: Needed: a ministry trained in aging, *Aging Connection* 9(4):3, 1988.

Serdahely W, Drenk A, Serdahely J: What care givers need to understand about the near-death experience, *Geriatr Nurs* 9(4):238, 1988.

Settersten RA, Holup J: *Linking lives and history: cohort differences in the personal meanings of historical events and changes.* Paper presented at the meeting of the Gerontological Society of America, Washington, DC, Nov 20, 1996.

Silverman H: Ceremonies and aging, *Generations* 14(4):51, 1990.

Stalker N, McGregor J, Rock G: *From one generation to the next: successful farm transfer from the perspectives of retiring and successor farm family members.* Report to the Rural Education Development Association. Edmonton, Alberta, Canada, 1996.

Steeves R, Kahn D: Experience of meaning in suffering, *Image J Nurs Sch* 19(3):114, 1987.

Stephenson J, Murphy D: Existential grief: the special case of the chronically ill and disabled, *Death Studies* 10:135, 1986.

Stoll R: Guidelines for spiritual assesment, *AJN* 79(9): 1574, 1979.

Strumpf N: *The relationship of life satisfaction and self-concept to time experience in older women,* doctoral dissertation, New York, 1982, New York University.

Swanson KM: Nursing as informed caring for the well-being of others, *Image J Nurs Sch* 25(4):352, 1993.

Taylor S: African ancestors. In Chidester D: *Patterns of transcendence: religion, death and dying,* Belmont, Calif, 1990, Wadsworth Publishing.

Thibault JM, Ellor JW, Netting FE: Conceptual framework for assessing the spiritual functioning and fulfillment of older adults in long-term care settings, *J Religious Gerontol* 7(4):29, 1991.

Thorsheim HI, Roberts B: Finding common ground and mutual social support through reminiscing and telling one's story. In Haight BK, Webster JD: *The art and science of reminiscing: theory, research, methods and applications,* Washington, DC, 1995, Taylor and Francis.

Tobin S: Cherished possessions: the meaning of things, *Generations* 20(3):46, 1996.

Tornstam L: Gerotranscendence: a theoretical and empirical exploration. In Thomas LE, Eisenhandler SA, editors: *Aging and the religious dimension,* Westport, 1994, Greenwood Publishing Group.

Tornstam L: Gerotranscendence: a theory about maturing into old age, *J Aging Identity* 1(1):37, 1996.

Trager J: *The women's chronology,* New York, 1994, Henry Holt.

United States Bureau of the Census: *Statistical abstract of the United States: 1995,* ed 115, Washington, DC, 1995, US Government Printing Office.

van Manen M: *Researching lived experience: human science for an action sensitive pedagogy,* Ontario, Canada, 1990, Althouse.

Watson J: Nursing on the caring edge: metaphorical vignettes, *Advances Nurs Sci* 10(1):10, 1987.

Watson J: *Nursing: human science and human care,* Norwalk, Conn, 1985, Appleton-Century-Crofts.

Wheeler K, Barrett EAM: Review and synthesis of selected nursing studies on teaching empathy and implications for nursing research and education, *Nurs Outlook* 42(5):230, 1994.

Wyatt-Brown AM: The literary legacies: continuity and change, *Generations* 20(3):65, 1996.

Young C: Spirituality and the chronically ill Christian, *Geriatr Nurs* 14(6):298, 1993.

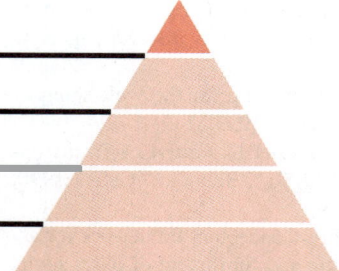

Jarel Spiritual Well-Being Scale

DIRECTIONS: Please circle the choice that <u>best</u> describes how much you agree with each statement. Circle only <u>one</u> answer for each statement. There is no right or wrong answer.

	Strongly Agree	Moderately Agree	Agree	Disagree	Moderately Disagree	Strongly Disagree
1. Prayer is an important part of my life.	SA	MA	A	D	MD	SD
2. I believe I have spiritual well-being.	SA	MA	A	D	MD	SD
3. As I grow older, I find myself more tolerant of others' beliefs.	SA	MA	A	D	MD	SD
4. I find meaning and purpose in my life.	SA	MA	A	D	MD	SD
5. I feel there is a close relationship between my spiritual beliefs and what I do.	SA	MA	A	D	MD	SD
6. I believe in an afterlife.	SA	MA	A	D	MD	SD
7. When I am sick I have less spiritual well-being.	SA	MA	A	D	MD	SD
8. I believe in a supreme power.	SA	MA	A	D	MD	SD
9. I am able to receive and give love to others.	SA	MA	A	D	MD	SD
10. I am satisfied with my life.	SA	MA	A	D	MD	SD
11. I set goals for myself.	SA	MA	A	D	MD	SD
12. God has little meaning in my life.	SA	MA	A	D	MD	SD
13. I am satisfied with the way I am using my abilities.	SA	MA	A	D	MD	SD
14. Prayer does not help me in making decisions.	SA	MA	A	D	MD	SD
15. I am able to appreciate differences in others.	SA	MA	A	D	MD	SD
16. I am pretty well put together.	SA	MA	A	D	MD	SD
17. I prefer that others make decisions for me.	SA	MA	A	D	MD	SD
18. I find it hard to forgive others.	SA	MA	A	D	MD	SD
19. I accept my life situations.	SA	MA	A	D	MD	SD
20. Belief in a supreme being has no part in my life.	SA	MA	A	D	MD	SD
21. I cannot accept change in my life.	SA	MA	A	D	MD	SD

From Hungelmann J, Kenkel-Rossi E, Klassen L, Stollenwerk R, Marquette University College of Nursing, 1987, Milwaukee, Wisconsin (Copyright).

JAREL SPIRITUAL WELL-BEING SCALE
Factor I Faith/Belief Dimension

(Scoring: SA = 6   SD = 1)

Item 1 _____
Item 2 _____
Item 3 _____
Item 4 _____
Item 5 _____
Item 6 _____
Item 8 _____   SubScore _____

Factor II Life/Self Responsibility

(Reverse Scoring: SA 1   SD6)

Item 7 _____
Item 12 _____
Item 14 _____
Item 17 _____
Item 18 _____
Item 20 _____
Item 21 _____   SubScore _____

Factor III Life Satisfaction/Self Actualization

(Scoring SA 6   SD 1)

Item 9 _____
Item 10 _____
Item 11 _____
Item 13 _____
Item 15 _____
Item 16 _____
Item 19 _____   Subscore _____   Total score _____

FURTHER STATISTICAL DATA: RELIABILITY AND VALIDITY
Validity

Concerns the ability of an instrument to measure what it purports to measure and the degree to which it accomplishes this objective (*Anastasi*, 1988).

Content Validity

Items developed from Phase I (grounded approach methodology). Review of scale by panel of experts in spiritual well-being/gerontology.

Construct Validity

Convergent (Criterion-related)
deCran's study (n = 114) of rural elderly, using JAREL scale and Paloutzian & Ellison Spiritual Well-Being scale, reports a correlation of .8175 (p = .000) between the two scales (1990).

Discriminate
Brophy, Stollenwerk, Hungelmann & Binder's study of depression, spiritual well-being and residence among older adults (n = 446), using JAREL scale, report statistically significant differences between the scores of Catholic, Protestant, Other Christians, and Non-Christian subjects and those of Agnostic/skeptic and Atheist subjects.

Factor Analysis
Reported by Hungelmann et al (1987)

Reliability

Stability
Test-Retest (2-week interval) Pearson Product Moment Correlation r = 0.88 (Hungelmann et al (1987).

Internal Consistency (Homogeneity)
Hungelmann et al (1987) (n = 294) Cronbach Alpha r = 0.85.

Fulton (1992) (n = 266) Cronbach Alpha r = 0.89

deCran's (1990) (n = 114) Cronbach Alpha r = 0.91.

Hungelmann & Stollenwerk (1992) (n = 420) Cronbach Alpha r = 0.79.

(6/93)

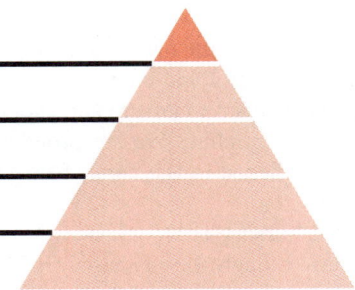

CHAPTER 28

The Professionalization
of Gerontic Nursing

A student speaks	**I met this old nurse, and she told of the old days when everything but the patients was dipped in Lysol solution. Bedpans were carried down a long hall to be emptied and patients might be in the hospital for weeks or months. I asked why she chose to be a nurse, and she said it was because she knew that she was up to the challenge.**

Gerri, nursing student, 34 years old

A faculty member speaks	**Nursing care of the aged brings one in touch with the most basic and profound questions of human existence: the meanings of life and death; sources of strength and survival skills; beginnings, ending, and reasons for being. It is a commitment to discovery of the self—and of the self I am becoming as I age.**

Stephanie Nagley

A geriatric nurse pioneer speaks	**The twentieth century in history and the first century in organized American nursing probably share the most creative time in history since the Creation. I should make a point of organized nursing, for while nursing is a one-to-one action, its ramifications into economics, politics, health, and numerous other areas lead me to the conclusion that professional nursing has taken place only within the many-faceted world in which we now live.**

Mary Opal Wolanin, elder-nurse pioneer

An elder speaks	**Those who deal with the aged must let them know that they are loved, respected, and important in this existence of ours. They must be treated with respect and not as "throwaways." After all, God makes no junk.**

Aveline, over 70

LEARNING OBJECTIVES

Upon completion of this chapter, the reader will be able to:

1. Identify certification mechanisms of professional nursing that can inform and assure the public of an individual's qualifications for safe gerontic nursing practice.
2. Compare various gerontic nursing roles and requirements.
3. Specify several ethical issues that are currently of importance to gerontic nursing.
4. Discuss nursing research studies and the role of nurses in their development.
5. Identify the key elements of the most recent American Nurses' Association Standards of Practice for Gerontological Nursing
6. Discuss several formal geriatric organizations and their significance to the practicing nurse.
7. Compare the roles of the advanced practice nurse in acute care, home health, and the community.
8. Identify several factors that have influenced the progress of gerontologic nursing as a specialty practice.
9. Explain components of gerontic nursing care that are fundamental regardless of role and the setting where nursing care is provided.

SCOPE AND PURPOSE OF GERONTIC NURSING

The numerous needs of the aged and the special nature of their care requires the most devoted and sophisticated nurses. Gerontic nursing is limited only by the expertise and understanding of the nurse and the desires and needs of the client. The logic of gerontic care is based on comprehensive understanding and a holistic approach to care, inclusive of the medical aspects of geriatric care and the scientifically based understanding of gerontologic care. Gerontic nursing care includes all of these elements.

This chapter will examine the foundations of gerontic nursing, the educational needs of gerontic nurses, the developing roles, and the future expectations. Historically, nurses have been in the front lines caring for the aged. They have provided hands-on care, supervision, administration, program development, teaching, and research and are to a great extent responsible for the rapid advance of gerontology as a profession in the last 25 years. Nursing is the first of the professions to develop standards of gerontologic care and the first to provide a certification mechanism to ensure specific professional expertise through credentialing. We are proud to be the standard-bearers of excellence in the care of the aged (Box 28-1).

The purpose of gerontologic nursing is to enhance the quality of life for aged persons through the promotion of health, supports for maximum levels of independence and least restrictive lifestyles, opportunities for continued development throughout the life span, and peaceful death. Physical and emotional problems of aging that impinge on these goals are the special concern of gerontic nurses.

This chapter is designed to highlight the history and current scope of gerontic nursing practice, certification, education, and practice roles. The major focus will be to explore

---

Box 28-1	**Professionalization of Gerontic Nursing**

1904	First article published in *American Journal of Nursing* (AJN) on care of the aged
1925	AJN considers geriatric nursing as a possible specialty in nursing
1950	Newton and Anderson publish first geriatric nursing textbook
	Geriatrics becomes a specialization in nursing
1962	ANA forms a national geriatric nursing group
1966	ANA creates the Division of Geriatric Nursing
1970	ANA establishes Standards of Practice for Geriatric Nursing committee, chaired by Dorothy Moses, included Lois Knowles and Mary Shaunnessey
1973	ANA Defined Standards of Practice for Geriatric Nursing
1974	Certification in geriatric nursing practice offered through ANA, process implemented by Laurie Gunter and Virginia Stone
1975	*Journal of Gerontological Nursing* published by Slack, first editor, Edna Stilwell
1976	ANA renames Geriatric Division; "Gerontological"
	ANA publishes Standards for Gerontological Nursing Practice, committee chaired by Barbara Allen Davis
	ANA begins certifying geriatric nurse practitioners
	Nursing and the Aged edited by Burnside and published by McGraw-Hill
1977	First gerontological nursing track funded by Division of Nursing and established by Sr. Rose Therese Bahr at University of Kansas School of Nursing
1979	*Education for Gerontic Nursing* written by Gunter and Estes; suggested curricula for all levels of nursing education
	ANA Council of Long Term Care Nurses established, group first chaired by Ella Kick
1980	*Geriatric Nursing* first published by AJN, Cynthia Kelly, editor
1981	ANA Division of Gerontological Nursing issues statement regarding scope of practice (see below)
1983	Florence Cellar Endowed Gerontological Nursing Chair established at Case Western Reserve University, first in the nation; Doreen Norton first scholar to occupy chair
1984	National Gerontological Nurses Association established
	Division of Gerontological Nursing Practice becomes Council on Gerontological Nursing (councils established for all practice specialties)
1986	ANA publishes survey of gerontological nurses in clinical practice
1987	ANA revises and issues Standards and Scope of Gerontological Nursing Practice
1989	ANA certifies gerontological clinical nurse specialists
1990	ANA establishes a Division of Long Term Care within the Council of Gerontological Nursing
1992	ANA redefines long term care to include life-span approach
1993	National Institute of Nursing Research established as separate entity
1994	ANA redefines Standards and Scope of Gerontological Nursing Practice

the various roles in gerontic nursing and to describe the function of nurses occupying these roles, but the overriding role of gerontic nurses is in advocating for the needs of the vulnerable aged. We will also explore issues and trends of concern to gerontic nurses in the present and the future, orienting nurses to the challenges, the aspects of the setting, practice issues, and information related to the job market. There are continuing ageist attitudes among some health care professionals, but we have found this to be changing, and we expect they will be considerably reduced by the entrée of the baby boomers into the ranks of the old, both as professionals and as recipients of care. The special emphases in current gerontic nursing that must be addressed by those in the field are the brief contacts with elders within the acute care setting and the need to monitor the increasing number of assistive personnel, as well as coordinating interdisciplinary care and multidisciplinary teams. These have added to the complexity and the challenges experienced by nurses in the field.

In 1973 the American Nurses' Association (ANA) first defined standards of geriatric care. In 1976 and 1987 these were redefined as standards of gerontologic nursing practice. In 1994 the ANA updated the scope of gerontologic nursing practice, which now focuses on "assessing the health and functional status of aging adults, planning and providing appropriate nursing and other health care services, and evaluating the effectiveness of such care" (American Nurses' Association, 1995c). They further emphasize health, dignity, and comfort as the undergirding goals of all care of the elderly.

Current standards of practice focus on the following:
- The ramifications of the aging process
- The different rates at which people age
- The multiplicity and collectiveness of an older person's losses
- The grief work necessary in accepting losses
- The interrelationship between the social, economic, psychologic, and biologic factors

- The frequently atypical response of the aged to disease and to the treatment of disease
- The accumulated disabling effects of multiple chronic illness and/or degenerative processes

(See Resources at the end of the chapter to order copies of the standards of practice.)

DEVELOPMENT OF GERONTIC NURSING

Historically, nurses have been in the front lines caring for the aged. They have provided hands-on care, supervision, administration, program development, teaching, and research and are to a great extent responsible for the rapid advance of gerontology as a profession in the last 30 years. Nursing is the first of the professions to develop standards of gerontologic care and the first to provide a certification mechanism to assure the public of their expertise.

Certification

ANA certification in gerontologic nursing is one evidence of professional competency and a sign to health care administrators of a commitment by nurses to the care of older adults (Gaines, 1994). The certification program for gerontic nurses began in 1975. The original protocol has since been expanded to include nurse practitioners, clinical specialists, geriatric consultants, researchers, administrators, and educators.

In October 1989 the first ANA examination for certification of gerontologic nurse clinical specialists was given. This is a major step toward recognition of this specialized practice arena. Presently there are 13,381 geriatric generalists certified; 2,655 gerontologic nurse practitioners; and 816 geriatric clinical nurse specialists (Gropper, 1997).

For additional information on certification and specialty practice contact:

American Nurses' Credentialing Center
600 Maryland Avenue, SW, Suite 100 West
Washington, DC 20024-2571
(800) 284-CERT

Graduate nursing programs prepare nurses to be credentialed as the following:
1. Geriatric nurse practitioners
2. Community health nurses
3. Gerontologic nurse clinical specialists
4. Geriatric case managers for acute and long-term care
5. Nurse administrators in acute and long-term care
6. Gerontologic faculty and staff development roles
7. Geropsychiatric specialists

Accreditation

The National League for Nursing (NLN) accreditation process for nursing curricula is very general and does not include a specific requirement or evidence of gerontologic care in a curriculum, though recently there is more emphasis on it. Without licensing and NLN accreditation that

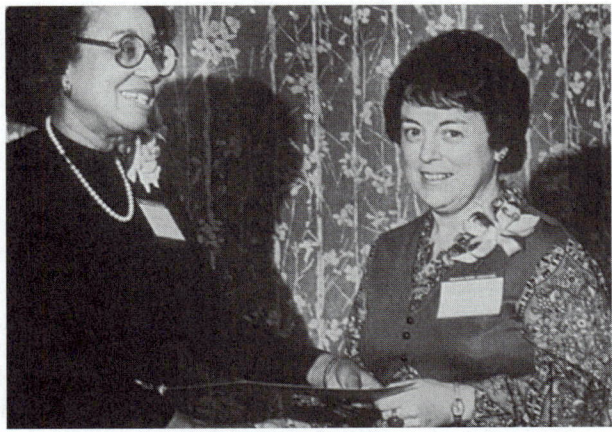

Laurie Gunter issuing first ANA certificate in Geriatric Nursing.

require gerontologic nursing content, the strength in a program will continue to be influenced mainly by the strength of the faculty in the topic. It is recommended that a 3-credit course should be mandated in every undergraduate program, and this should include a clinical component (Fulmer and Matzo, 1995).

The development of an integrated, nationally distributed test for nurse licensure (National Council Licensing Examination, [NCLEX]) was implemented for the first time in 1982. In response to this there are more fully integrated curricula and more attention to the preparation of nurses to care for a broad range of client needs, but as yet there is not a proportionate emphasis on gerontic nursing preparation. Since 70% of the working nurses are engaged in the care of the aged the majority of the time, this is a glaring deficiency.

Gerontic Nursing Organizations

The National Gerontological Nursing Association (NGNA), organized in 1984, is the first and only national association created specifically for all levels of nurses specializing in the delivery of health care to the elderly. This nonprofit association is comprised of registered nurses (RNs), licensed practical nurses (LPNs), and certified nurse assistants (CNAs); however, the great majority of the nearly 2000 members are RNs. The functions of the NGNA are listed in Box 28-2.

The NGNA was conceived by a group of four nurses in the Washington, DC, area. This small local group evolved into a national organization with members in all 50 states and the District of Columbia. Today, NGNA membership totals over 1860 RNs, LPNs, and interested others committed to caring for older persons. It is the only nursing organization that welcomes nurses at every educational level and in every type of practice setting (Braun, 1993).

Box 28-2 NGNA Functions

- Provide a forum for identifying and exploring gerontologic nursing issues
- Sponsor and conduct lectures, seminars, debates, and similar educational programs for gerontologic nurses, health care providers, and the general public
- Disseminate information and research results related to gerontologic nursing
- Promote activities designed to educate and inform the general public about health care issues with emphasis on those issues affecting the elderly
- Formulate programs designed to demonstrate innovative techniques and approaches in gerontologic health care to enable nurses and others to better meet the needs of America's aging population
- Advocate for elders for gerontologic health care through public policy and governmental involvement

---

NGNA has recently demonstrated its commitment to gerontologic nursing growth and elder care by completing a Delphi study that encompassed critical issues, problems, future directions, and priorities of gerontologic nursing. The results are discussed in this chapter in the section on nursing research (Luggen, 1997).

The National Conference of Gerontological Nurse Practitioners (NCGNP) began in 1976 with a group of a dozen gerontologic nurse practitioners (GNPs) in the northwestern states who convened annually to share their concerns and expertise. It developed, with the support and assistance of Mountain States Health Corporation, the W.K. Kellogg Foundation, and Ross Laboratories, into a strong national organization devoted to advancing and updating the knowledge necessary for the practice of gerontologic nurse practitioners. The purpose of NCGNP is to promote high standards of health care for older persons through advanced gerontologic nursing practice, education, and research. (For the address of the organization see Resources.) At present there are over 500 members nationwide.

Another group, one that specifically addresses the needs of directors of nursing (DONs) in long-term care, is the National Association of Directors of Nursing Administration in Long-Term Care (NADONA/LTC). From their president, Joan Worden, we learned that the original 40 founding members held their first conference in St Louis in 1986. They now have 4200 members in 50 states, with 32 chapters. Their mission statement states their intention of promulgating a network of DONs and assistant DONs through education, communication, and service to the members. These activities are conducted within the parameters of the code of ethics, constitution, and charter of the organization with the ultimate goal of providing quality care for those individuals receiving long-term care and concern for the morale and satisfaction of those delivering long-term care. The address for NADONA/LTC can be found in the Resource section at the end of this chapter.

Our neighbors, the Canadian gerontologic nurses, have grown enormously in strength and purpose in recent years. Although the percentage of their elder population in most provinces is somewhat less than ours, the social services and functional aids provided (at no cost to those more than 65 years of age) are a model toward which we may strive.

In general, they have provided a full range of supports for the maintenance of elders in their homes and have had a holistic approach to gerontic care through their national health system. In 1986 the Canadian Gerontological Nursing Association (CGNA) developed a philosophy, conceptual framework, and standards for gerontologic nursing practice. Philosophically, the goal is to enhance life and maximize independence while fully recognizing the individual's uniqueness. The conceptual framework is based on the interrelatedness of health and environment as it relates to application of nursing knowledge and process.

The seven standards and criteria of CGNA include (a) respect for the uniqueness of each older person, (2) promotion of function and maximum independence, (3) assistance toward environmental mastery, (4) practice based on the specific and evolving knowledge of aging, (5) emphasis on sustaining interpersonal relationships, (6) advocacy on behalf of the rights and responsibilities of elders, and (7) the application of nursing process (Canadian Gerontological Nursing Association, 1987). The specific and detailed guidelines are available from the Canadian Gerontological Nursing Association, PO Box 368, Postal Station K, Toronto, Ontario M4P 2GT.

Their professional development of standards of practice and educational requirements in Canada are somewhat behind those of U.S. nursing (Hirst et al, 1996). As recently as 1990 there was only one graduate program (University of Manitoba) that identified gerontologic nursing as a program emphasis (Hirst et al, 1996). Recent advances in public awareness of the population needs and pressures upon policy makers has resulted in significantly increased geriatric criterion-referenced licensure examination content. In this respect, they have advanced beyond the gerontologic competencies included in the United States NCLEX examination.

The Gerontological Society of America (GSA) and the American Society on Aging (ASA) are interdisciplinary organizations devoted to the development and promotion of progress in research and service to the aged. Both of these organizations have large contingents of nurse members. Nurses form the largest group of professionals belonging to GSA.

Long-term care nurses are particularly active in two other national organizations, the American Association of Homes and Services for the Aging (AAHSA) and the American Health Care Association (AHCA) (see Resources for addresses). These organizations are highly visible in promoting legislation to strengthen the stature and practice opportunities in long-term care in numerous venues.

Worldwide, nursing organizations devoted to upgrading the care of the aged are emerging as each of the developed and developing countries confront the needs of the frail aged and find that there are no longer sufficient supports within the family to maintain them. Even in very remote places the young find it necessary to migrate to the cities for work and the elders are left behind in the village.

Gerontologic Nursing Research

In 1981, the ANA Commission on Nursing Research determined that priority should be given to nursing research that would generate knowledge and guide practice toward promotion of wellness and competency to manage personal health, prevent health problems and their negative impact on daily life, protect and assist the vulnerable, and contribute to cost-effective, accessible health care. These goals are more relevant today than when originally articulated.

The great increase in doctorally prepared nurses in the last decade is reflected in numerous research endeavors that are qualitatively impressive. Geriatric nursing research is generally conducted by doctorally prepared nursing faculty, though faculty without specific credentials in gerontology also conduct studies (Maddox, 1995). Although nursing research is vital and necessary to nursing care, clinicians may feel inadequate or uninterested, believing that the process is too difficult, they are not qualified, or time constraints preclude research. These situations can be remedied by using research consultants from university nursing faculty or the teaching/research hospital staff. Since baccalaureate- and master's-prepared nurses are trained in various levels of the research process, obtaining their participation may only need encouragement and support by their teams and administration. The gerontic nurse is in a field in which many clinical areas have not been explored in depth, and she or he can make a significant contribution.

Support for Nursing Research. The Research Act of 1974 provided training and instruction in research through the establishment of traineeships and fellowships in the National Institute on Aging (NIA) or elsewhere to conduct research on aging. Another federal agency, the Center for Nursing Research of the U.S. Department of Health and Human Services, helps to foster research. The American Nurses Foundation, another supporter of nursing research, awards small research grants each year. Some private foundations have been generous in supporting nursing research; most notably, the W.K. Kellogg Foundation and Robert Wood Johnson Foundation.

The National Center for Nursing Research became the National Institute of Nursing Research in 1993 when President Bill Clinton signed the act establishing it as a separate entity. This action added status to the recognition of nurses as health researchers (Gaines and Martin, 1994).

Two of the priorities for nursing research funding are strategies for management of cognitive impairment (1997) and chronic illness (1997). Dr Ada Sue Hinshaw, first director of the Institute, was especially concerned about the use of restraints in hospitals and nursing homes in the United States. Though much has been accomplished to reduce their use, more research is needed to find out why some other countries are able to manage their elderly in a more humane way than we do (Gaines and Martin, 1994). Currently the Institute supports research that includes the development of mental stimulation exercises for Alzheimer's patients and a variety of other programs to promote healthier lifestyles for rural and impoverished Americans. The Institute awards eligible schools of nursing predoctoral and postdoctoral research training grants and fellowships for individual research training (see Resources) (Gaines and Martin, 1994).

Nurses need to be aware of trends in research funding. At present grants and funds are directed heavily toward studies of the aged in institutions, women's issues, and minority aging.

The NIA is currently focused on research into retirement; health institutions; social support; health behaviors and attitudes, "disease-prone" personality types, nutrition, exercise, and sleep; family and household patterns; and conditions under which informal care systems sustain frail elders in their homes. There is intense interest in prevention of illness and institutionalization with the hope of ultimately reducing the costly Medicaid and Medicare expenditures. Ethics in research are discussed later in this chapter and in Chapter 14.

Retrieval of Gerontological Information. The informatics age has initiated access to the internet for gerontologic information. There are numerous resources, but GSA publishes updates of Web addresses in each issue for those interested in pursuing this avenue of information. The complexity of gerontologic information retrieval and management is affected by the multidisciplinary nature of the subject. Solutions are appearing in large computerized databases for retrieval of gerontologic information and in the establishment of permanent committees of information specialists within the gerontologic organizations.

There are problems with these large data banks, stemming from the sometimes spurious use by researchers. More and more "secondary" research is emerging because investigators crunch computerized statistics to arrive at conclusions for which the original research was never intended. At this point no one seems particularly concerned by the ethics of this practice.

At present the American Association of Retired Persons (AARP) in conjunction with the Library of Congress is serving as the National Information and Resource Clearinghouse on Aging. However, this source is weak in information about foreign sources and international studies.

Several reference tools have been developed that can be used in searching gerontologic literature, particularly acquisition lists that are available from most gerontologic centers and in new reference books in gerontology. The Virginia Henderson Library for nurses, the archives of nursing history at the University of Virginia and the University of Wisconsin are useful. In addition, special collections can be found in places such as the University of Pennsylvania, where the Doris Schwartz papers and considerable information on the development of public health nursing are housed.

Nurses will find librarians helpful in locating desired information or instituting computerized subject searches through Medical Literature Analysis and Retrieval System (MEDLARS) or MEDLARS On-Line (MEDLINE), National Institute of Medicine. There is a small fee for data retrieval. The *International Nursing Index, Cumulative Nursing Index, Psychological Abstracts,* and *Dissertation Abstracts* are additional sources of specific information.

Examples of Gerontologic Nursing Research. Research studies contribute to the knowledge of gerontologic nursing from geriatric nursing organizations, clinicians, faculty, and students.

Example of organizational research. The NGNA sponsored a Delphi survey to plan future directions for growth and development in gerontologic nursing and care of the elderly. Based on five questions, 100 respondents participated. The questions included future directions in practice, education, and research; impact of national health care trends/issues on gerontologic nursing practice; critical issues/problems of gerontologic nurses; and elder care (Luggen, 1997). The last question addressed the priorities for gerontologic nursing research (see Appendix 28-A for the results).

Example of faculty/clinical case manager core search. A research study of interest was conducted by a nurse case manager and a university clinical director of research at the University of Arizona College of Nursing. They interviewed case managers and clients regarding affective, cognitive, and behavioral nursing interventions that facilitated higher levels of self-care, fewer hospitalizations, and increased quality of life. More specific discussion of this study may be found in the case management section of this chapter.

Example of graduate student research. A student developed a study of the implementation of an influenza immunization program for homebound elders. The conclusions were that Medicare funding for the home visit, as well as the vaccine, would increase elder participation, and cost savings would increase participation. This study demonstrates that students can improve the quality of life for homebound elders and that students can develop innovative methods to impact health services.

ETHICAL CONSIDERATIONS IN GERONTIC NURSING

The Code of Medical Ethics of the American Medical Association (AMA) states:

The primary bond between medical practice and nursing is mutual ethical concern for the patients . . . Where orders appear to the nurse to be in error or contrary to customary medical and nursing practice, the physician has an ethical obligation to explain those orders to the nurse involved. Whenever a nurse recognizes or suspects error or discrepancy in a physician's orders, the nurse has an obligation to call this to the attention of the physician . . . In emergencies, when prompt action is necessary and the physician is not immediately available, in the performance of reasonable care a nurse may be justified in acting contrary to the physician's standing orders for the safety of the patient (American Medical Association, 1992).

Although this position is of importance to nurses, there are many other considerations particular to nursing practice. Ethics produces many dilemmas for nurses who attempt to follow personal value dictates and maintain professional integrity. Commonly held misconceptions are the source of some of the dilemmas, and confusion about the real issues at stake contribute to the difficulties. As has been pointed out all too often, legalities are not necessarily ethical, and ethical decisions are not necessarily legal. Some of the major ethical issues in the care of the elderly that nurses are concerned about include those in Box 28-3.

New areas of risk liability are evolving as the health care delivery system continues to change. At the same time, traditional areas remain. Nurses continue to be professionally accountable for their own actions, but there are increasingly higher levels of liability exposure because of advanced technologic requirements in care, potential of miscommunication, and lack of precise documentation. A major liability risk is failure to communicate and to access chain of command (Fiesta, 1995).

Developing skills in ethical decision making must begin early in the experience of student nurses while they learn the concepts, principles, and decision-making process involved in clinical case studies involving ethical issues. Standards of professional organizations guide nurses in decisions regarding responsibilities, obligations, and rights of members. An example is that of the ANA Code for Nurses of 1994, which opposes active euthanasia by the nursing profession.

Reigle (1996) gives an example of the variations in the level of ethical responsibilities. The novice advanced practice nurse (APN) is expected to recognize an ethical issue, communicate concern, and seek clarification. If the issue remains a problem after discussing with others, the APN can pursue additional assistance.

An example cited by Reigle (1996) is that of an elderly woman admitted to an in-patient psychiatric unit for depression. Her declared incompetence prevents her from refusing electroconvulsive treatments. A psychiatric, clinical nurse specialist (CNS) might identify this situation as an ethical dilemma and can seek further clarification, such as the functional capacity of the patient and the process of how incompetence was determined. Further avenues for information would be the psychiatrist and the patient.

Ethics rounds, case reviews, and strong collegial relationships facilitate the process of ethical decisions. An open system of communication and respectful environment facilitate ethical decisions as opposed to a closed system or authoritative environment.

Special Legal and Ethical Considerations

Organ Donation. In several states professionals are required by law to discuss organ donation with dying individuals or their family members, and documents must reflect that the discussion has taken place. Because this is a recent requirement and one of which many professionals are

---

Box 28-3	**Ethical Issues**

- When and how to die; currently the issue of assisted suicide is at the forefront and is not supported by the ANA
- Restraints—chemical and physical
- Generational equity in distribution of resources
- Competency judgments
- Sustained artificial feeding and fluids for the nonresponsive individual
- Elder abuse—identification, reporting, and management
- Neglect versus individual rights
- Human rights in long-term care institutions
- Care of the psychiatric client in nursing homes
- Appropriate psychogeriatric care
- Iatrogenic disorders
- Burdens of spousal caregivers
- Burdens of family caregivers
- Economic inequities of old women
- Numerous demonstration projects that are not sustained and leave the aged stranded; finances of agencies that limit the number of visits (for instance, Visiting Nurses Association limited to small number of visits; physicians limited to one visit per month to boarding care patients)
- Burgeoning expense of medical care and the need to deplete personal resources before assistance can be obtained
- Untrained and unqualified personnel caring for the ill aged in some settings
- Abuse of conservatorships and guardianships
    The following are inhibitions to ethical behavior:
- Organizational constraints such as administrative dictates and inadequate staffing
- Trust in others' intelligence and judgment
- Self-deception or inability to perceive correctly the ethics of a situation
- Lack of clear-cut supports for taking an ethical stand
- Fear of reprisal or job loss
- Uncertainty about rights of others and of ourselves
- Ambiguous legal power for enforcing rights

unaware, nurses are often in a dilemma. Educational efforts about organ procurement have traditionally been aimed at nurses, and the extraordinarily high levels of support among nurses implies the considerable success of these efforts. In many settings there are organ procurement specialists available who are specially trained to discuss the issues with individuals and families. When this is done with respect and sensitivity, families often feel some comfort in knowing something of their loved one will go on and that there is some small gain in their loss.

OBRA and OSHA. Since 1987, as a follow-up to the 1986 Institute of Medicine report on long-term care, there have been continued revisions and updates of long-term care requirements intended to protect clients and staff, more accurate qualitative (to comply with the Office of Budget Reconciliation Act [OBRA]) and comprehensive assessment of clients through the use of the federally constructed Minimum Data Set (MDS), more exacting diagnoses and care plans, and emphasis on routine and periodic training of the hands-on providers (largely nurse aides). In addition, and perhaps most importantly, there has been an emphasis on patients' rights and freedom from chemical and physical restraints. Clearly, state and federal requirements are moving in the direction of more humane and holistic care of the elders in long-term care. Increasing requirements through the Occupational Safety and Health Agency (OSHA) for protection from tuberculosis, hepatitis, and AIDS benefit staff and patients. All of these improvements have added to the quality, cost, and necessity of nursing expertise in long-term care settings. There are similar efforts to institute these protections in acute care settings. Recently, there have been some efforts to reduce the requirements that are particularly cumbersome.

Nursing Roles Related to Ethics and Legalities

New areas of concern are rising in the wake of myriad bioethical dilemmas and health care system restructuring.

Box 28-4	**Legal Reforms Affecting Nursing**

Increased peer review requirements, protection from lawsuits
Increased powers of disciplinary boards
Increased reporting requirements
Requirements for continuing education
Caps on malpractice awards
Punitive damage limits
Expert witness requirements
Informed consent limits
Professional standards of care reasserted
Extension of "Good Samaritan" statutes

Modified from Bovbjerg RR: Legislation on medical malpractice: further developments and a preliminary report card, *UC Davis Law Review* 22(4):499, 1989.

Legal reforms affecting nursing care delivery can be seen in Box 28-4. Nursing advocacy for vulnerable clients is more critical than ever. Nurses are essential to the adequate function of institutional ethics committees. Nursing representation on ethics committees emphasizes the position of nurses as the professionals most frequently involved on a daily basis with the implementation of ethical decisions. Advocacy is inherent in that position.

Advocacy is generally seen as necessary for those who cannot recognize or articulate their own needs. Situations that commonly require advocacy by nurses include: interdisciplinary communication, issues in dying, and individual preferences of the aged individual. Perhaps the most powerful function of the nurse advocate is as ombudsman and spokesman for the aged to state and federal legislators. Further discussions of advocacy can be found in Chapters 14, 15, and 26. These provide additional discussion of ethics and legalities of care.

A relatively new role as legal nurse consultant began emerging in the 1980s. In the past 5 to 7 years it has developed considerably. The American Association of Legal Nurse Consultants (AALNC) was organized in 1989 and has grown to include 1400 members with 23 local chapters. The organization supports, provides education, and markets the role. National conferences include current legal issues and updates on medical research, practice, and procedures (Mason, 1994).

Legal nurse consultants function in a variety of ways in independent consulting practice or hired as expert witnesses

---

Box 28-5	**Nurse's Role as Court Examiner**

1. Functional, cognitive assessment, social and medical history.
2. Written recommendations for judge and other members of team.
3. Testify/attend hearing as expert witness.
   a. Two weeks to prepare.
   b. Give broad recommendations, no medical diagnosis (example: "assessment consistent with a dementing illness," NOT "subject has dementia").
4. Reimbursement: Hourly consultant basis. Two to three hours includes time writing report plus court time.
5. Nurse's reactions to the role of court examiner.
   a. Most satisfying: Protecting rights of older people.
   b. Least satisfying: Bureaucracy paperwork. Waiting 2 to 3 months for payment.
   c. Most challenging: Finding subjects who are not at address and making recommendations that may place limitations of older person's rights.

Extrapolated from Fletcher K, Small N: Evolving roles of GNPs, *NCGNP Newsletter* 43:1,2, 1994; presented by Fiona C. Druy, Court appointed examiner, District of Columbia, Office on Aging.

in their clinical specialty. They may provide summaries related to allegations, identify standards of care in issues related to causation and damage, collaborate with an attorney in preparing legal pleadings, trial briefs, depositions, and support at trials. The practicing legal nurse consultant is self-regulated as defined within the AALNC Scope of Practice, the ANA Standards of Practice and Code of Ethics, and the American Bar Association Code of Ethics.

Educational requirements are established by the state's Board of Registered Nursing (BRNs), and sometimes supplemental education is required (Mason, 1994). Workshops train interested nurses in the role and methods to gain access to the legal world. An example of the components of the role of nursing court examiners is provided in Box 28-5.

EDUCATION FOR GERONTIC NURSING

Mezey (1995) discusses two methods of geriatric curriculum development that have failed to adequately impact nursing education. The first model regards gerontologic study as a graduate nursing specialty without a need to include any geriatrics in basic nursing programs (associate and baccalaureate), and the second model, for BSN and AD programs, focuses on minimal content with the expectation that the nurse acts to refer to the advanced nurse practitioner or physician specialist.

An other problem that has prevented adequate curricula is the lack of consideration of the diversity of the aged. Those from 65 to 95 years old, the well elderly, the frail elderly, and those of various ethnic origins are all lumped together as "the aged." Further, neglect of the intergenerational issues of grandparenting and elder care that impact the young family are not integrated into maternal/child and community care.

A national effort was made to identify issues in gerontologic education by the Department of Health and Human Services, Public Health Service (Klein, 1995). A forum on geriatric education and training was assembled to develop a national agenda for action in geriatric education. The results and recommendations are published in *A National Agenda for Geriatric Education: White Papers* (Klein, 1995). A model nursing curriculum at both undergraduate and graduate levels is recommended.

In the model for nursing curricula 17 recommendations were given. It is recommended that by the year 2000 all undergraduate nursing programs should have a separate geriatric nursing course, all basic nursing programs should contain core content in gerontologic nursing, and accreditation should be contingent on meeting this requirement. A specialty in geriatrics in master's programs and a geriatric minor in other advanced programs should also be available. Content issues that are sorely neglected and need to be included are mental health, elder abuse, acute care, long-term care, and minority and rural aging.

The NGNA members, guided by Ann Luggen, have produced an extensive and detailed core curriculum for gerontologic nursing (Luggen, 1996). This provides sufficient information for the development of nursing courses at any level and in any program.

We believe those in the field of nursing must seriously consider specific minimum requirements at each level of education to fulfill the responsibility of nurses to the public

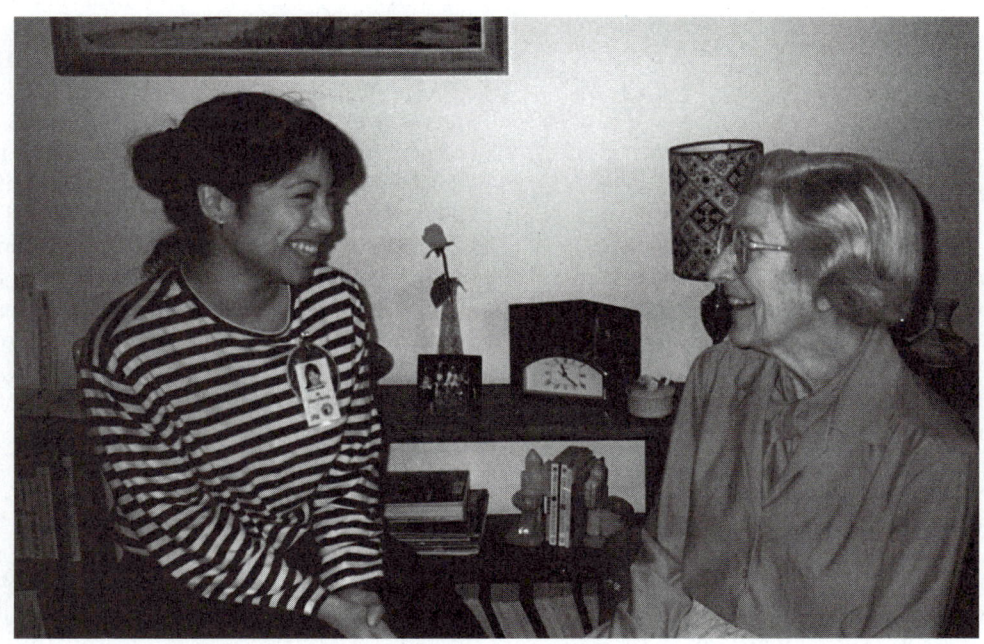

A student learns from an elder. (Courtesy Priscilla Ebersole.)

Table 28-1   Gerontologic Nursing Profile of Baccalaureate Faculty Members

Characteristic	Full-time	Clinical Part-time	adjunct	n
Specific preparation (formal, continuing education, or both) in gerontological nursing	83%	7%	10%	217
Conducting research in gerontological nursing or aging	97%	1%	2%	98
Published books or articles on gerontological topics	93%	2%	5%	95
Certified by American Nurses' Association as gerontological nurse, gerontological nurse practitioner, or clinical specialist in gerontological nursing	76%	32%	21%	63
Master's degree with major emphasis in gerontological nursing	67%	7%	26%	58
Master's degree in nursing with minor emphasis in gerontological nursing	86%	11%	3%	35
Master's degree or graduate certificate in gerontology	88%	0	12%	33
Completed doctoral dissertation in gerontological nursing or aging	100%	0	0	29
Licensed as a gerontological nurse practitioner	75%	4%	21%	217
Completed doctoral dissertation in gerontology (non-nursing)	89%	0	11%	9

From Yurchuck ER, Brower T: Faculty preparation for gerontological nursing, *J Gerontol Nurs* 20(1):17, 1994.

Table 28-2   Undergraduate Faculty Members with Work Experience in Selected Practice Areas

Practice area	Associate degree	Baccalaureate degree	Number of institutions
Home health care			
None	86%	14%	35
1% to 3%	56%	44%	64
4% to 6%	49%	51%	39
11% to 15%	56%	44%	36
Nursing home			
None	69%	31%	45
1% to 3%	54%	46%	65
4% to 6%	47%	53%	17
11% to 15%	59%	41%	34
Health screening			
None	69%	31%	45
1% to 3%	54%	46%	65
4% to 6%	47%	53%	17
11% to 15%	59%	41%	34

From Yurchuck ER, Brower T: Faculty preparation for gerontological nursing, *J Gerontol Nurs* 20(1):17, 1994.

and the profession. Nurses choosing a gerontic specialty will need, in addition to content about aging individuals, special attention to the following:

Family services and counseling
Agency referral mechanisms
Politics of aging
Economics of aging
Physical and psychologic changes of aging
Professional collaboration
Political strategies
Institutional change
Strategies of paraprofessional education

A model project, funded by the W.K. Kellogg Foundation and headed by Verle Waters of Ohlone College in Fremont, California, has had an amazing impact. Nearly 400 community college programs nationwide in affiliation with as many nursing homes are educating their nursing students in geriatric care (Carnigan, 1992). Learning opportunities for students are numerous in those settings.

One is not limited in gerontic education to the acute care setting or the nursing home. Creative faculty consider sites such as retirement homes, private practice with families, nutrition centers, home-care agencies, day-care centers, and housing complexes. The acute care hospitals and nursing homes are integral to the total picture but might be included later in the students' learning experience after they have worked with elders who have less acute or complex conditions. In addition, nursing homes provide opportunities for leadership training and research application for more advanced students (Matzo, 1994; Sears and Wilson, 1996).

Importance of Faculty

The profile of faculty members and their preparation and preferences are seen in Tables 28-1 and 28-2. The direction of gerontic nursing now and in the future relies heavily on the nursing faculty that may or may not stimulate a student's interest in the aged. Numerous educational resources in the form of journals, texts, audiovisual, and curriculum outlines have become readily available. In addition, faculty members have begun to publish teaching strategies and learning modules that have been successful in their particular programs and that may assist other programs in solidifying their geriatric content. However, without faculty interest this information will lie fallow.

ROLES IN GERONTIC NURSING CARE

A gerontic nurse may be a generalist or a specialist. The generalist functions in a variety of settings: hospital, home, and community, providing nursing care to individuals and their families. The generalist draws on the expertise of the specialist in planning and evaluating care. The gerontic spe-

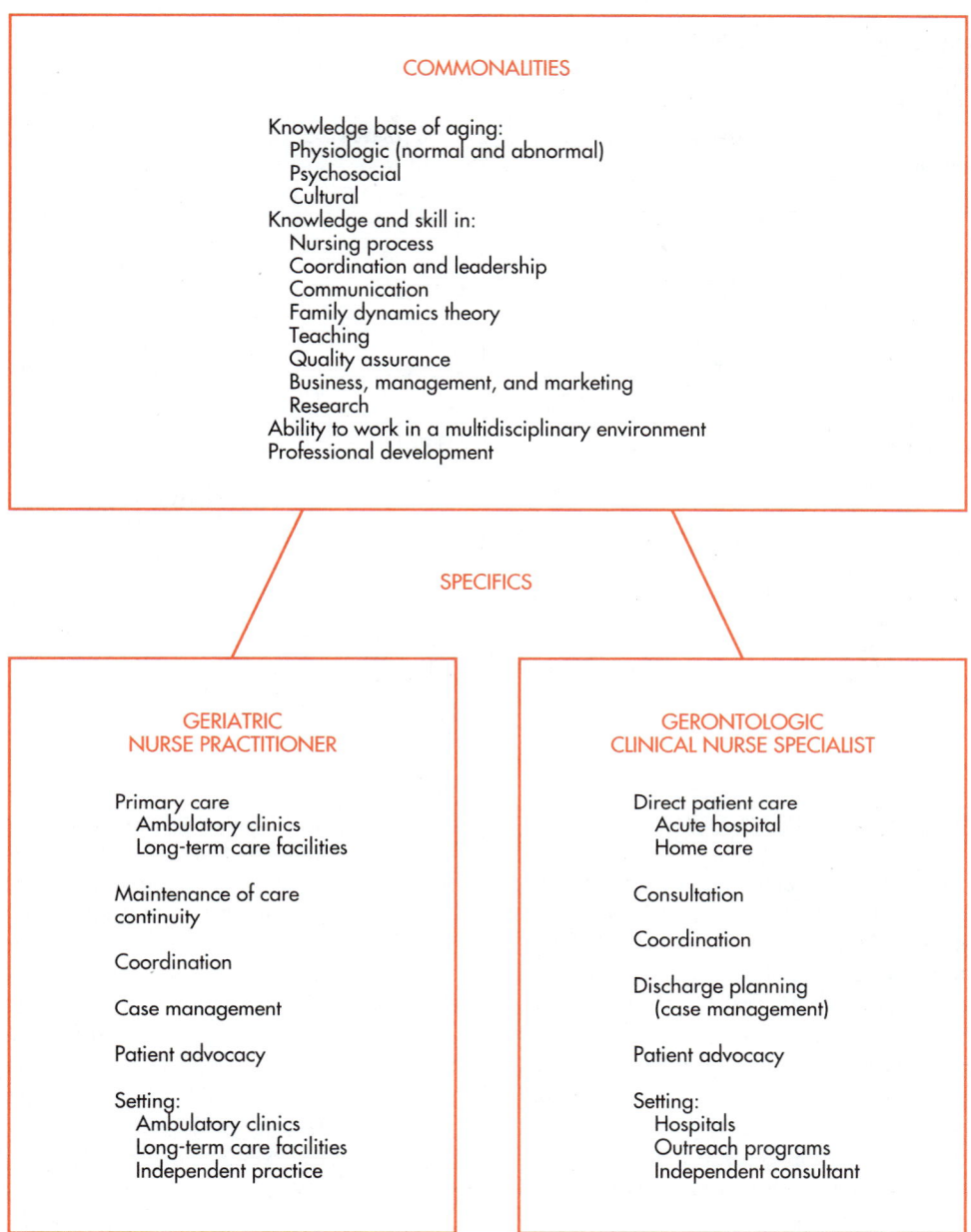

Figure 28-1. Established roles: commonalities and specifics. (Developed by P. Hess and H. Monea.)

cialist has advanced preparation and performs all of the functions of the generalist but has developed additional clinical expertise, understanding of health and social policy; and proficiency in planning, implementing, and evaluating health programs. To understand the variations of these categories and the progression of specialization see Figure 28-1. Table 28-3 shows the organization of nursing relating to care of the elderly (Mezey and Fulmer, 1995).

Geriatric Nurse Practitioner

Originally the development of the gerontologic or geriatric nurse practitioner (GNP) emerged to meet the need for con-

sistent, accessible, quality care for persons in underserved areas such as nursing homes or remote rural areas. Today, GNPs practice in nursing homes, acute care, subacute facilities, retirement complexes, health maintenance organizations (HMOs), day-care settings, community clinics, physicians' offices, independent practices, and in any situation requiring expert nursing in combination with midlevel medical practitioner skills.

Education and certification prepare the GNP for midlevel medical management of groups of clients/patients: to take health histories; perform physical examinations; institute and evaluate many laboratory tests; monitor and manage the

Table 28-3   Organization of Nursing Relating to Care of the Elderly

Title	No. years education	Degree	Responsibilities related to care of the elderly
Professors of geriatric nursing	8 plus	PhD, Ed D, or DNS	Research Teaching
Geriatric nurse practitioners	6	MS	Both medical and nursing functions in ambulatory and institutional settings Case managers
Gerontological nurse specialists	6	MS	Specialized nursing care of elderly clients Teachers and role models Case managers
Registered nurse— baccalaureate level	4-5	BS	Community health, hospital, home health agencies, nursing homes Case managers
Registered nurse—associate level	2-3	ADN or	Hospital and nursing home staff nurses
Licensed practical nurses	1-1½		Nursing home staff Home nursing staff
Nursing aides and orderlies	0-6 mo.		Nursing home staff Hospital staff

From Mezey MD, Fulmer TT: Nursing. In Maddox, GL, editor: *The encyclopedia of aging,* ed 2, New York, 1995, Springer.
Sources U.S. Bureau of the Census. *Statistical Abstract of the United States,* 1988, ed 10, Washington, DC, US Government Printing Office; American Nurses' Association. *Facts about nursing,* Kansas City, Mo, 1992-1993, ANA, pp 1-4.

common acute, episodic, and chronic health problems of the aged; and prescribe medications in states that include prescribing as part of the expanded practice act. Many activities overlap physician medical management, and in those cases decisions are guided by protocols developed by both the GNP and the physician. First and foremost the GNP is a nurse and is acutely aware of and involved in teaching, counseling, health education, health screening, and preventive care.

A GNP is educated in one of the many graduate programs around the country that offer a master's degree in nursing along with practitioner knowledge and skills and that meet the qualifications for certification. Certification can be obtained through the ANA, and the individual must comply with regulations for advanced practice, which vary from state to state.

A growing number of persons associated with long-term care and HMOs believe that GNPs are best qualified to act as primary care managers of the health problems of the aged. The role and function of the GNP in the community is also diverse and may include that of the primary case manager to the aged. A vital function is coordination and collaboration with other professionals, paraprofessionals, families or surrogates to facilitate and promote health care planning and chronic care management.

The need for nurse practitioners in rural communities is great. Nurse practitioner clinics have been established in small communities that can rarely attract physicians and are notoriously underserved medically, even when there is generally an oversupply of physicians elsewhere. Functions of the GNP include performing physical examinations and assessments, electrocardiograms, inhalation therapy, radiologic examinations, suturing, nutrition counseling, education in dental care, first aid, and alcoholism care. GNPs are involved in preventive, primary, and tertiary health care.

Mobile screening units that travel to rural areas are a way to reach the many elderly who need services but who are too threatened by interference in their lifestyle. Many of these older people distrust agencies and fear the loss of independence if they seek help. GNP mobile outreach programs are a way of identifying and monitoring the health of elders who are unknown to any health care agency.

GNPs have developed distinctive roles in a variety of settings. Terri Goheen functions as a primary care practitioner in Appalachia in nursing homes and in a cardiology clinic. Kathy Fletcher teaches on inpatient units, psychogeriatric units, and has an independent clinical practice (Fletcher and Small, 1994). This example shows how an enterprising GNP can negotiate for two part-time positions. Nurses interested in this type of work are encouraged to peruse the article. Beth Landis, a nurse practitioner (NP) with a degree in adult primary care and a minor in gerontology, holds a locum tenens position, which means she is offered short-time positions in a variety of places to meet special needs (Landis, 1997). See Box 28-6 for a summary of her role activities.

Gerontologic Clinical Nurse Specialist

The gerontologic clinical nurse specialist (GCNS) is prepared at the master's level and is a specialist prepared as a caregiver, educator, and advocate of and for the aged. The

With a degree in adult primary care with a minor in gerontology and experience in women's health and internal medicine, Beth Landis expanded her horizons from burnout to travel. Aspects of locum employment included the following:

1. Average assignments of 6 to 8 weeks or varying from 2 to 30 weeks
2. Housing and utilities paid for, with the company handling all details
3. Travel expenses to the site reimbursed
4. Health care, disability, and continuing education
5. Option to choose location, job description, length of contract
6. Orientation from 1 to 8 hours
7. Carries own texts for resource
8. Broad range of specialty experiences: HMOs, occupational health facilities, extended care facilities—women's health, student health, ambulatory surgery, and emergency department
9. Options open for any length of unpaid vacation time between assignments

   Her latest assignment is in a community clinic operated by the Cherokee Nation in Oklahoma, where she is maximizing her practitioner skills and integrating hypertension and diabetes caregiving.

Compiled from *Nurse Practitioner World News* 2:1, Jan/Feb 1997.

GCNS initiates wellness interventions in care plans for elders in both institutional and community settings, provides health education programs for older consumers, and provides informal and formal programs for caregivers of the aged. The GCNS educates others to dispel myths and stereotypes held by the public, health care providers, and the elderly themselves. In agencies that are used for teaching and research, the GCNS functions as a role model for students.

As an advocate, the GCNS is involved in legislation to promote health promotion programs to decrease cost and to increase life satisfaction. The GCNS ensures that hospitalized elders receive quality care and assistance in making major decisions about care and placement options for discharge. As a researcher, the GCNS is in a position to develop original and applied research on nursing care of the aged and to conduct research to determine the outcomes of nursing interventions designed to promote wellness in all settings.

The GCNS is most effective as a consultant to those who plan care for the elderly, such as social service, staff, and discharge planners in the acute setting. Although case management is common to both the GNP and the GCNS, the GCNS is more often in place to direct the complex-

ities of discharge planning that require extensive knowledge not only of aging but also of the community resources, the family situation, and the aged's choice and level of independence.

Possessing multidisciplinary management skills is significant to this role. Monitoring health and social needs of the aged client requires the ability to communicate with and understand other professional and paraprofessional roles. Traditionally, the GCNS provides indirect patient care in hospitals as educators, quality improvement, and consultant.

Advanced Practice Nursing

The ANA describes APN as an "umbrella" term for RNs with 2 to 4 years of education beyond that of basic nursing. Four ANA titles fall under this rubric: clinical nurse specialist (CNS), nurse practitioner (NP), certified nurse-midwife (CNM), and certified registered nurse anesthetist (CRNA) (American Nurses' Association, 1995a). Only the CNS and NP are relevant to the gerontologic nurse. Geriatric advanced practice nurses (GAPNs) are in a combined role with more breadth, depth, and versatility in practice than is usually found in either of the separate roles. They are typically involved in providing comprehensive care that includes health screening, counseling, crisis intervention, and education of clients, families, and professionals. They also initiate and collaborate in research to promote health status and develop innovative APN models for acute, community, long-term, and ambulatory care.

Although GAPNs have demonstrated their value and expertise, their utilization is restricted by barriers in reimbursement and "turf" issues. Some states are more conducive to practice than others. The common barriers are the following:

1. Restrictive state nurse practice acts
2. Limited prescriptive authority
3. Lower reimbursement
4. Malpractice insurance limitations
5. Limitations of institutional privileges

These barriers are chiefly influenced by the medical professional. (Ruiz et al, 1995). The GAPNs are often found in the community arena providing direct patient care and assessing both acute and chronic illnesses (Ruiz et al, 1995). As previously discussed, NPs (Callender-Price, 1996) are part of a new role in hospitals. To compare the similarities of expertise and roles see Box 28-7.

The journal *Nurse Practitioner* provides an annual summary of legislation and policies in each state that affect the practice of APNs (Pearson, 1997). It is important to keep apprised of these, because the situations for NP practice are rapidly changing. There is an NP statutory prescribing authority; this also is changing rapidly.

Martin and Hutchinson (1997) studied the work world of 23 NPs in Florida and found their practice concerns focused on status and restricted opportunities. They tried to cope with these issues by confronting, bargaining, and

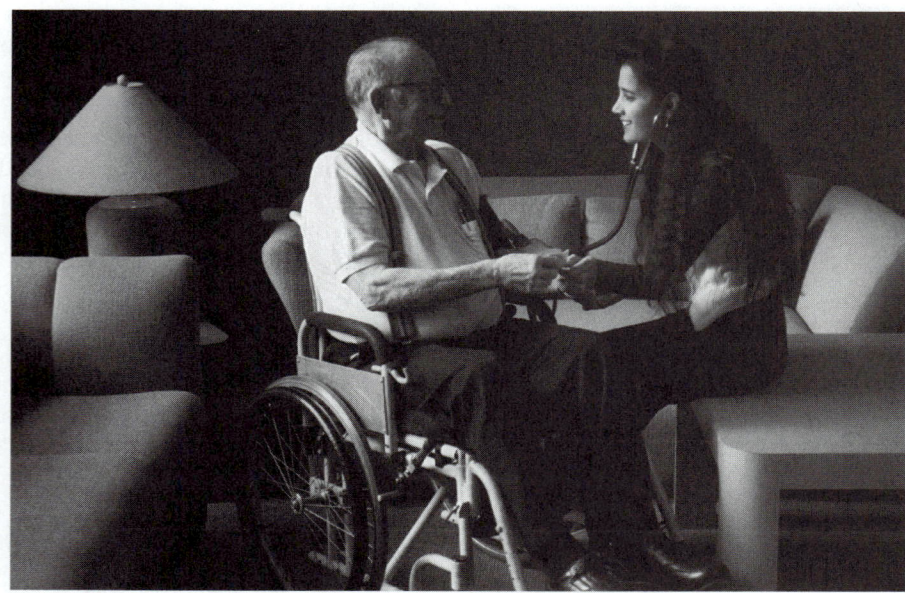

Advanced nurse practitioner at work. (Courtesy Mary Duffy/O'Keefe Duffy, San Jose University School of Nursing.)

Box 28-7 **Roles of GNPs and GCNSs**

Gerontological Nurse Practitioners (GNPs)
  Traditionally community based
  Unique role focus
    Provision of direct patient care
    Physical and psychosocial assessment
    Treatment of acute/chronic illness
    Prescriptive authority
Gerontological Clinical Nurse Specialists (GCNSs)
  Traditionally acute care based
  Unique role focus
    Indirect patient care activities
      Quality improvement
      Change agent
      Consultant
      Educator
Common priorities for both GNPs and GCNSs
  Improvement of functional ability of older persons
  Emphasis on diagnosis and treatment of human
    responses to health and illness
  Patient and family education and interaction
  Interdisciplinary collaboration

From Ruiz BA, Tabloski PA, Frazier SM: The role of the gerontological advanced practice nurse in geriatric care, *J Am Geriatr Soc* 43(9):1061, 1995.

disengaging when the situation was demeaning or uncomfortable. Some NPs were very frustrated by their work situation and sought other positions that provided more autonomy in decision making. The researchers recommend replication of this study in different states to determine the commonalities and variances of practice concerns. The reader is urged to read this very informative research.

The merging of CNS and NP roles began when curriculum changes occurred in the 1980s. In 1992, the idea was introduced to merge the two advanced roles into a case management model to follow clients into various settings. Issues debated include curriculum overload, weakening reimbursement policies, certification problems, and increasing/decreasing independence (Page and Arena, 1994). Shuren (1996) notes that blending the expertise of the NPs (primary skills) and the CNS (specialty knowledge) will expand the role of the APN to a higher level of care with complex health problems. Current issues of concern are related to cost-effectiveness affecting the role of medicine in health care, restructuring medical training to produce more primary care physicians, and replacing anticipated residency shortages in acute care. Some advantages and disadvantages of merging the roles are outlined in Box 28-8. A CNS, Betsy Kelley (1995), voices her feelings about the trend toward merging of the roles in advanced practice (Box 28-9).

The US Department of Health and Human Services Division of Nursing announced they have agreed to merge the APN roles by the year 2010 (Redding, 1994). Nurses planning to return to school should review clinical offerings, inquire about the combined role, and seek clarification. If not sure, you are not alone—faculty are struggling to foresee the role, settings, and title (Redding, 1994). Change is here, climb on board! With the various opportunities and positive outlook for advanced practitioners, both traditional and innovative opportunities exist. Michalek (1994) gives guidelines to consider for either the new or established nurse. Included is the process of the search, from networking, search, resume, interviews, and adjusting to a new job with use of a mentor.

Box
28-8
Advantages and Disadvantages of CNS and NP Merger

Advantages	Disadvantages
Increased cost-effectiveness	No in-depth discussion of the effect on patients, families
Increased independence of advanced practice nurse	NP reimbursement policies may be weakened
Defining role increase while health care reform continuing	Graduate education issues:
More prescriptive privileges for CNS, depending upon pharmacology requisites.	a. Lengthen role content
Powerful lobbying force with more professionals	b. Role strain/role confusion
	c. Limited market place

Compiled from Page NE, Arena, DM: Rethinking the merger of the clinical nurse specialist and the nurse practitioner roles, *Image J Nurs Sch* 26(4):315, 1994.

Box
28-9
Kudos to Page and Arena

Kudos to Page and Arena for their article "Rethinking the Merger of the Clinical Nurse Specialist and the Nurse Practitioner Roles" (*Image,* Winter. 1994). As a practicing CNS this is an issue that is near and dear to my heart.

Over the last couple years I have seen some disturbing trends. One is the increasing conversion of CNS positions to case manager positions. Although I feel CNSs are eminently qualified to be case managers, I grieve for my colleagues that did not want this role change. I regret too, the loss of CNS expertise in many of the systems and education endeavors for which CNSs take the lead.

As an adjunct faculty member I have seen an increasing tendency in academia to downplay the CNS role by offering a blended track, rather than two distinct tracks; as well as a marked decrease in the number of students enrolled in a "pure" CNS track. I see this as clearly due to an aggressive marketing campaign by these schools for their nurse practitioner programs, to the exclusion of the CNS programs. I have seen the frenzy of colleagues who are returning to school in droves for an NP postmaster's certificate. Yet they cannot articulate why or how this will be of use to them.

Many people have expressed fear that the CNS role is dead or suffering from a terminal illness, and that this explains why so many are jumping on the NP bandwagon. I maintain that the role is very much alive and needed now more than ever. We need the expertise of *both* nurse practitioners and CNSs, but as two distinct entities, not as a hybrid of both. I agree with the point made in the article regarding the likelihood of the "imposter phenomenon" in the blended role.

It is incumbent upon those of us who believe in the CNS role to lobby for the preservation of it in our practice settings and our colleges of nursing. We need to be much better at explaining the work of the CNS, providing examples of cost savings and revenue generation due to the role, marketing our services, and becoming visionaries regarding expanding role possibilities. If you believe in the role, fight for it. Nursing as a profession cannot afford to lose us!

Betsy Kelley, RN, MS, CCRN, CS, *Beta Epsilon*
Clinical Nurse Specialist
Critical Care/Emergency Services
Rex Hospital
Raleigh, NC

From Kelley B: Kudos to Page and Arena, *Image J Nurs Sch* 27(2):89, 1995.

Lambert and Lambert (1996) have written an excellent chapter about the intricacies of establishing an independent practice that includes valuable information and guidelines with consideration of community need, location of business, partnership, corporation or sole practice, state laws, legal considerations, scope of practice, insurance, marketing, potential clientele, referrals, and detailed information on reimbursement. Although APNs have selected to be in independent practice for the past 30 years, new aspects have emerged, and the reader will find this material valuable, interesting and thought provoking (Gross, Morrow, 1993). Refer to the example of private practice in home health care described by Sweeney (1996).

With the changing health care scene, it is vital for the survival of ANPs to be knowledgeable and use strategic marketing expertise. Components of a marketing portfolio are included in Table 28-4 (Davis Doughty, 1996). Buchanan (1994) developed a tool that describes characteristics of various roles of the advanced practice nurse: practitioner, educator, researcher, and leader/manager.

Cardiovascular Nurse Interventionist: A Role for the Advanced Nurse Practitioner. We know that cardiovascular disease (CVD) is the number one cause of death. Engler and Engler (1994) propose a role for APNs in the community to prevent CVD. They recommend a master's degree program for APNs in prevention of risk factors for "cardiovascular nurse interventionists" (CVIs). There seem to be no specialized training programs in schools of nursing that have a CVD prevention program with formal coursework and clinical residency. Some responsibilities of the

| Table 28-4 | Components of a Marketing Portfolio for APNs |
| | | | | |

	Scope	Focus	Length	Purpose
Biography	Credentials and experience	Prepares for presentation	One page only	Introduction for presentation
Resume	Work history	Work results	One to two pages (bullets)	Listing how APN made a difference in work setting
Curriculum vitae	• Credentials • Scholarly works • Honors • Publications	Academic communications	Three to five plus pages	Listing of academic accomplishments
Portfolio	Supporting documents of accomplishments	Determined by outcome sought, e.g., grant or position	Varies, multiple documents	Marketing the APN
Video tapes*	Demonstration of skills, expertise	Determined by position sought	30 to 60 minutes	Marketing APN skills to potential partners, employers

From Davis Doughty SE: Developing markets for advanced nursing practice. In Hamrick AB, Spross JA, Hanson CM: *Advanced nursing practice: an integrative approach,* Philadelphia, 1996, WB Saunders.

cardiovascular nurse interventionist would include evaluation of risk factors for CVD, health, laboratory, and medication assessment, patient education and counseling, diagnostic testing (exercise, electrocardiogram [ECG], etc.) and magnetic resonance imaging (MRI). They could practice in acute care, physicians' offices, occupational health, homes, and cardiac rehabilitation settings. As a direct provider, the CNI could be in private practice or collaborating with cardiologists or internal medicine physicians (Engler and Engler, 1994).

Nurse Case Managers

The emergence of nurse case managers as gatekeepers and brokers of health care may well benefit community-residing patients who need long-term health care. Increasingly, case management begins in acute care as a means of best integrating and utilizing resources for prompt and safe discharge planning. Case management involves planning, coordinating, and monitoring services to meet the needs of elderly clients with emotional, functional, and physical problems who find it difficult to maintain themselves independently in the community. Case managers pull together the available resources and coordinate them to provide the client the best help. Nurses, who are most likely to view the holistic needs of individuals, are actively involved in case management and will undoubtedly develop the role more fully. In industry, occupational health nurses have filled the case management role effectively for years.

Nurses are uniquely prepared to be case managers. They have knowledge of the biologic and social sciences, the humanities, health maintenance, disease processes, and medications. Nurses also have extensive experience in collaboration with other care professionals. The tasks of a case manager differ depending on the organizational setting, the type of geriatric clientele served, and the nature of the practice (whether it is solely the coordination or the delivery of

primary care). Minimum preparation for a nurse case manager (NCM) is a baccalaureate degree and 3 years of appropriate clinical experience. However, many existing management programs prefer a nurse with a master's degree who has experience as a clinical specialist or nurse practitioner in areas related to the aged and experience in the type of service setting the case manager is likely to use.

It is well known that case management is based on a compilation of services that contains costs and improves quality of care while reducing fragmentation and duplication of services. Historically, case management in nursing developed in acute care but today crosses all areas of health care including community, clinics, mental health day care, and outreach programs.

Case management is alive and thriving, but there is no generic definition. The term encompasses many different models of care depending on what agency or setting you view. "The term, 'case management' has become as generic as the use of the word 'senility'" (Quinn, 1994). Public health nurses have used the model since 1890s, when Lillian Wald, the champion of public health services, established American Public Health Nursing and later pioneered the concept of using visiting nurses as case managers for a life insurance company, successfully saving lives and reducing costs. In the 1980s, DRGs and HMOs developed their own case management programs to contain costs of health care (Kersbergen, 1996). Box 28-10 presents compilation of historical development. Stahl (1996) provides a summary of the components of case management (Box 28-11).

The National Academy of Certified Care Managers (NACCM) is completing a certification process. They expect 3,000 to 4,000 for the first examination, with a potential of 70% passing rate (Klein, 1995). Since 1993, case managers can be certified nationally and credentialed as a certified case manager by passing a test for certification for case

Box 28-10	**Brief History of Case Management in the United States**
1860s	Providing health care to poor and immigrants; growth and coordination problems
1877	First interagency cooperative coordination of services to the poor and immigrants to prevent duplicate of services
1890s	Lillian Wald founded American Public Health Nursing based on philosophy of self-help (health choices), coordinated and developed New York City's private and public health human services that previously were nonfunctional.
1909-1925	Wald pioneered the concept to Metropolitan Life Insurance Company for case management with visiting nurses during period of illness; successful in saving millions of dollars

Human Service Agencies

1940s	World War II; provision of care by Veterans' Administration for returning veterans in Los Angeles for all services in one place
1960-70	Civil Rights movement impacted case management; facilitated client to be active instead of passive, resulting in provider becoming accountable for quality of service
1970s	Programs for Mentally Disabled
	Poorly coordinated community services for support when institutionalized mentally disabled discharged into community as state hospitals closed
	Evolution of legislation requiring case management services—viewed as the "keystone" to care of deinstitutionalized people

Health Care System Changes

1980s	Expansion of case management through various changes in health care system:
	1. DRG's focus to prevent lengthy hospitalization
	2. Insurance companies controlling high cost of clients with catastrophic illnesses
	3. Development of case management health maintenance programs to control costs
1990s	Multiple settings with predominantly case load evaluators.

Compiled from Kersbergen AL: Case management: a rich history of coordinating care to control costs, *Nursing Outlook* 44(4):169, 1996

managers (CCM). The test is broad and includes interdisciplinary knowledge. For nurses, there are three categories for eligibility depending on range of case management experience (full/part time) and licensure (RN). Initial certification is valid for 5 years. To renew certification without reexamination requires 80 contact hours of continuing education every 5 years (Certification for case managers, 1992).

Certification guards the quality of case management for protection from individuals who are not qualified and safeguards the vulnerable older consumer who trusts professionals. There are cautions against "institutionalizing" a definition so that future changes in the role can be incorporated (Klein, 1995). At this time there are a few nursing certifications for NCMs. Mahn and Spross (1996) discuss the NCM in an advanced practice role and believe the potential for certification as an NCM "will become a reality" since the competency of APNs includes in-depth aspects of case management.

Case management research reveals that clients with NCMs use fewer days in hospitals, intensive care, and emergency rooms and have fewer hospital admissions (Lamb and Stempel, 1994). In one study, results indicated positive changes in client behavior because of the case manager's approach to care (Newman et al, 1991). Lamb and Stempel (1994) implemented a small but significant study to discover

the difference. They selected 16 clients who had been served by NCMs and encouraged them to share their "stories" about working with an NCM by asking questions such as "What was happening to you when you met your nurse case manager?" "How do you think it might have been different if the nurse case manager had not been there?" (Lamb and Stempel, 1994). Three stages were identified:

- Bonding: the nurse case manager develops trust, elder clients know they are cared about and the nurse has the expertise to help them.
- Working: the major factor was the demonstration of *concern* while the nurse motivates elders to explore options and patterns and to rethink their situation regarding changing how they care for themselves and accepting care from others.
- Changing: the elder and nurse share a role of being an "insider-expert" until the client is confident of being responsible. When the elder becomes the "insider-expert," dramatic growth occurs; one elder expressed it as "being pulled out of a pit or deep hole."

It was found that clients tended to bond with NCMs through developing trust and confidence in their expertise. They also felt motivated to rethink their own ability to solve problems, as well as to accept appropriate care from others. Finally, they felt

---

Box 28-11	**Steps in Case Management**

Stahl (1996) recommends the following seven steps:

1. Case finding: Identify cases from managed care organizations (MCO) case managers that would meet patient's needs at much lower cost than acute care setting.
2. Screening/intake: Screen potential patients who could be served.
3. Assessment: Assess level of patient's acuity related to appropriate price services, including total assessment of physical, mental, functional, social, and financial status, to fit and influence quality of care and financial objectives.
4. Care planning: Plan strategies to meet need of patient. Lead interdisciplinary team care planning and act as liason with MCO's case manager so outcomes are mutually agreed upon.
5. Service arrangements: Work with patient and family to access publicly funded programs for continuity of care after discharge.
6. Ongoing monitoring and follow-up: Support patient goals by involving the MCO's case manager with interdisciplinary team. Build positive business relations by sharing relevant clinical data and compliance by patient.
7. Evaluation: Plan strategy of determining various clinical quality outcome measures and financial measures.

Adapted with permission from Stahl DA: Case management in subacute care, *Nurs Manag* 27(8):20, 1996. Copyright Springhouse Corporation.

---

there was an equality when they shared with the NCM their own self-knowledge and became the "insider-expert."

From these findings, Lamb and Stemple (1994) recommend that case managers need increased time with clients in order to develop and maintain the critical therapeutic relationships. Through teaching, coordinating, and monitoring care of their clients, they enable the elderly to be their own "inside-experts" in self-care. We applaud the researchers for demonstrating a nursing process that can make a valuable difference in nursing case management for the elderly. We need contemporary pioneers like Lillian Wald who have the drive, the courage, and the vision to engage insurance conglomerates in establishing a demonstration project with NCMs as she did in 1909 with visiting nurses. NCMs could save millions and give excellent case management services, . . . Where are you, Lillian?

Another study in nursing case management demonstrated how the caring relationship between the chronically ill older adult and the NCM can be significant in improving the quality of life. Community-based NCMs were cost-effective (decreased emergency department visits, hospital admissions, length of hospital stay, and primary care physician visits). The key to success was the caring relationship that the case manager established with the clients and families (Boyd et al, 1996).

The future of case management will continue to be changed, refined, and altered as the epic of health care reform impacts the United States health care system. Aside from being cost-effective, the case manager can increase patient compliance with discharge follow-up and/or monitoring. Tables 28-5 and 28-6 (Klein, 1995) provide information on case management models in the institution and community.

Institutional Nursing Roles

Gerontic nursing within institutions may involve intensive, acute, subacute, and long-term care. Nurses' role as defined by institutional expectations include numerous levels of function and opportunities for creative practice.

Long-Term Care Administrator. Ballard (1995) studied the role of long-term care nurse administrators and found the need for nurse administrators to increase educational preparation in management, economics, and corporate issues. The survey of 94 DONs and 94 nursing home administrators specifically identified necessary skills as those of human resource management, negotiation, nursing expertise, and finances. It is critical that nursing education respond to these identified educational needs because long-term care is an expanding field in which many nurses will find themselves and find satisfaction only if adequately educated.

Roles in Acute Care. The number of elderly now requiring medical and surgical treatment in the acute care setting has increased significantly. Fifty percent of the elderly age 75 and over account for 21% of all inpatient days (Fulmer and Walker, 1992). The implication is clear: the role of the nurse in the acute care setting—to promote the health status or wellness of the elderly despite medical diagnosis or surgical procedures—will be a critical one. Studies reveal that older patients are at greater risk of experiencing unfavorable incidents—41% of medical patients over age 70 have experienced adverse incidents related to hospitalization. The interventions implicated most frequently are psychotropic medications, physical restraints, and urinary catheters (NICHE, 1994). The challenge for critical care nurses is to differentiate between iatrogenic problems, changes that occur secondary to the disease process, and those that reflect the normal aging process. Thus it is essential that each nurse determine priorities, use the multidisciplinary team judiciously, and coordinate patient care accordingly. Coordination is critical in our highly specialized health care delivery system. Nurses are in an ideal position to coordinate all aspects of care and assess

Table 28-5   Case Management Models

	Institution based			Community based		Private case management	Physician office
	Hospital	Health maintenance organization	Area agency on aging	Health department	Home health care and visiting nurse association		
Services provided	In-depth geriatric assessment; some follow through with identified problems (fewer than 3% of hospitals provide traditional case management)	Depends on plan; full spectrum of long-term care services for beneficiaries in some instances	Mostly non-service providing; information and resource linkage; limited purchase of services for low-income clients in some areas	Identification of clients at risk; referral and resource linkage	Occasional long-term client assessment, service, service plan, service provision, and resource allocation; some family counseling	Assessment, service plan, resource linkage, follow-up, and monitoring; some service provision and family counseling	Assessment, screening, referral; authorization of home health, hospice, nursing home care and certificates of medical necessity for equipment and supplies; patient & family counseling
Client eligibility	Guidelines set up according to specific program	Can be restricted to Medicare enrollees with disabilities and/or long-term care needs	Usually frail elders over 60	All ages served; focus often on services for children—some programs for elderly with health care needs	Anyone with health/personal care needs; age neutral; large percentage of elders	Majority of clients are elderly; all accepted (also focus on adult children of elders)	All ages served, generally patient/clients who are elderly
Cost	Some third-party reimbursement from Medicare/Medicaid; much variation depending on hospital and services provided	Medicare/Medicaid reimbursement; typical monthly premium range: $36 to $135 and/or co-payment; some annual cost caps	Mostly federal tax supported; some volunteer contributions and Medicaid waiver funds; occasional fee for service	State/county tax supported; no direct out-of-pocket fees	Third-party payment for home care segment; long-term case management either folded into visit charge or extra $40 to $60 per hour	Out-of-pocket $200 to $400 per assessment; typically $50 per hour for follow-up service	Grant demonstrations; part of overhead; Medicare reimbursement for home health and hospice "care plan oversight": $58 for 30 minutes aggregated over 1 month
Referral turnover time	Varies—can be 1- to 2-month wait for initial appointment	Screening time varies for new enrollees, members sooner	Varies—often 2 to 3 weeks	Varies—1 week to 2 months	Usually 1 to 2 days for acutely ill clients, less than 1 week for others	Often 1 to 3 days	1 to 2 days; office case management meetings often held weekly or bimonthly
Professional availability	Usually an interdisciplinary team; nurse, physician, and social worker common	Varies—usually nurse, social worker, or other social service professional	Usually nurse and social worker	Nurse (occasionally nutritionist)	Nurse/social worker provide long-term care management; interdisciplinary team approach during acute care phase	Usually nurse or social worker; long-term professional relationship; 7 days a week availability	Interdisciplinary team; physician, office nurse, home health nurse, social worker; sometimes pharmacists, therapists and DME vendors
Geographic access	May be increased access in urban areas	Limited availability; few programs at the present time	Operational throughout country; services may vary within states	Services to elders may be geographically limited	Spotty throughout country	Increased access in large urban areas	Available through individual physician practices

From Klein S: *A national agenda for geriatric education: white papers*, Washington, DC, 1995, US Department of Health and Human Services, Public Health Service, Health Resources and Services Administration, Bureau of Health Professions.

Table 28-6   Nursing Function in Caring for the Aged in the Institutions and in the Community

	Long-term care	Acute care	Community care
	Provide a milieu for living and holistic support in illness and dying	Support patient in achieving highest level of autonomy possible in situation	Make clients and families aware of options and resources Involve clients in citizens' councils and political action groups Support legislation affecting opportunities for the aged
	Teach resident and families Counsel resident and families Learn about and use community resources, advise family and patient of same Establish short-term and long-term goals: evaluate progress toward both periodically Secure and maintain health, recreation, and social history	Provide appropriate information to patient and families about treatment plan, medications, and diagnosis in collaboration with physician	Teach clients and families Consult and collaborate with agencies and multiprofessional representatives Educate clients to self-responsibility for health
	Plan and coordinate care Teach ancillary personnel Communicate resident's needs in written and verbal form	Collaborate with multiprofessionals, patient, and family to develop a comprehensive care plan Supervise ancillary personnel	Promote health through clinic and home contact. Provide appropriate resources Identify health, social, or economic needs Counsel clients and family members
	Give treatments, medications, and rehabilitative exercises Observe and evaluate patient response to treatment, medication, and care plan Teach health care maintenance to staff and residents	Recognize implications of syndromes for patient care (e.g., renal failure, coronary disease, emphysema) Protect patient from injury or iatrogenic disease Perform physical and psychologic assessment and integrate in nursing care plan Initiate action as outlined in nursing protocols regarding various conditions	Report care finding and make appropriate referral Assess environmental safety Assess response to illness and compliance with treatment Provide information about medications and treatments
	Keep physician aware of changes in residents' conditions Institute life-saving measures in the absence of a physician Perform physical assessment of residents Ensure adequate medical, dental, and podiatric care for residents Maintain hydration, nutrition, aeration, and comfort	Provide emergency treatment as needed for cardiopulmonary crisis, amelioration of shock, hemorrhage, convulsions, poisoning Alert physician to changes in patient status and abnormal findings of tests Maintain hydration, nutrition, aeration, and comfort	Provide health surveillance Identify health, social, and economic need Assist client and family to modify patterns detrimental to health Evaluate deviations from normal and advise clients of appropriate action Identify existing or impending illness

Box 28-12	**Acute Care Model 1—Geriatric Consultation Team**

Strumpf discusses models of care for acutely ill elders. The first model, the geriatric consultation team, has been used for more than 10 years. Team members from nursing, medicine, social work, and psychiatry respond to problems about functional and mental status, drug therapy, rehabilitation possibilities, and discharge planning.

Data from Strumpf NE: Innovative gerontological practices as models for health care delivery, *Nurs Health Care* 15(10):522, 1994.

the influence of microsystems and macrosystems on the patient and the patient's relationship to the system.

Strumpf (1994) discusses three models of care for acutely ill elders in hospitals. Three boxes (28-12, 28-13 and 28-14) summarize the original model of geriatric consultation team, the five models of the Hartford Hope project, and an innovative nurse-managed day care hospital.

Subacute Care Nursing Roles. Subacute units are new, and nursing staff roles include myriad functions as around-the-clock specialists and medical/surgical experts and in discharge planning for critical home care, pulmonary rehabilitation, and oncology. The nurse clinician coordinates services (Gill and Balsano, 1994). The issue of lack of appropriately trained staff often arises.

Acute care nurses who are hired often have some difficult adjustment. They need to be prepared for the adjustment, as well as functioning as providers of teaching and technologic expertise in the new setting. Being in transition and relied upon as the expert in the situation is a difficult role to negotiate.

Gray (1994) quotes Dave Kyllo of AHCA: "The milieu of a subacute is such that although it looks like a med/surg unit, it is more family focused, flexible, and laid-back than hospitals . . . they're more adaptable. If a physical therapist comes in for a treatment and the patient is napping, they're more likely to let (him/her) rest and come back later."

At this time, variations in quality of care and in staffing are apparent. One successful model of subacute geriatric practice for frail older adults is that provided by a large managed care organization in which dedicated subacute units are served by a multidisciplinary staff (von Sternberg et al, 1997). The units are called transitional care centers (TCCs) and are housed in five nursing homes. A board-certified geriatrician and a GNP work with the nursing, therapy, and social work staff to form a consistent team at each nursing home. Full-time nurse practitioners are assigned to remain in a specific TCC facility while other team members rotate through.

The patient's progress is followed closely by the TCC team from admission until discharge. Some of the conditions of clients in this service involve orthopedic problems, musculoskeletal injuries, cerebrovascular accidents (CVAs), postsurgical patients with tissue wounds, and uncomplicated infections. Patients are holistically assessed each week, including advance directives, for status change and discharge planning. After weekly meetings, the geriatrician and the GNP are available to meet with families. The GNP reviews new admissions and monitors the patient's status 2 or 3 times each week.

This model demonstrates that high-quality, cost-effective subacute care can be provided by a large managed care organization when a GNP is available on an ongoing basis (von Sternberg et al, 1997).

Case manager in subacute care. Implementing the role of the case manager has been difficult in subacute care for a variety of reasons: a new role, poorly understood in the industry, not knowing or understanding the role, expecting the case manager to develop referrals, and lack of planned goals for the manager. The basic tenet of case management is to meet the needs of the client and support caregivers while coordinating access to cost-effective services. Expectations of "sales and marketing" in the job description can be overwhelming. Both the employer and the employee need to be clear about job responsibilities and have the expectations detailed in a contract (Stahl, 1996). Because of the newness of the role, there are often basic conflicts of role expectations in a subacute care program, including territoriality, politics, and a push for marketing. The official definition of subacute care can be found in Chapter 13.

The services of an APN with case management skills may be critical to the success of newly developing subacute care units. Table 28-7 gives an example of the range of abilities of these specialists.

Certified Geriatric Rehabilitation Nurse. Professionals associated with rehabilitation are increasingly finding the need to specialize; some teams limit their practice to a specific disorder or body system. Indeed, some nurses have become specialists in the management of decubiti, contractures, diabetes, and other chronic disorders of the aged. Rehabilitation nurses in institutional and community settings diagnose and treat human responses of individuals and groups to an actual or potential disability that interrupts or alters function and life satisfaction. The goal is to assist the individual or group in the restoration and maintenance of maximum health. Rehabilitation nurses assist individuals to make the most of their abilities rather than focusing on their losses. These nurses are finding it increasingly difficult, because of understaffing, to find time for therapeutic teaching and family orientation.

New roles and functions for the rehabilitation nurse are evolving in subacute care units. Ideal acute rehabilitative care involves a certified rehabilitation registered nurse (CRRN) as case manager in an expanded practice role. This role entails the following:

- A primary care concept
- Option to delegate to rehabilitation technicians

Box 28-13 **Acute Care Model 2—HOPE (Hospital Outcomes Project for the Elderly)**

A cluster of five models that focus primarily on nursing care.

Geriatric Resource Nurse (GRN)—Integrating Expertise

A team composed of primary nurses, trained geriatric resource nurse, gerontologic nurse specialist, and geriatric physicians helps staff with specific problems of the elderly, such as delirium, physical functioning, incontinence, etc. Implemented nationally. Originated in New England area, 1980s.

Acute Care of the Elderly (ACE)—Designed Environments

A 29-bed specialty unit designed for acutely ill older patients with attention to physical needs of older patients; appropriate colors, carpeting, art, music, activity room, and recliners in patient rooms.

Team of nurses, gerontologic nurse specialist, social workers, nutritionists, and physical therapist to prevent functional decline and multiple clinical problems.

Developed by University Hospitals of Cleveland conjointly with Frances Payne Bolton School of Nursing at Case Western Reserve University. An innovative though expensive model that has demonstrated rapid implementation, which is accomplished easily because of the interdisciplinary team.

Geriatric Nurse Specialist (GNS)—Targeting Common Problems

Clinical specialist who consults and educates staff about specific problems of the aged. NICHE project used this inexpensive way to focus on nursing care and issues of delirium.

Developed by University of Chicago hospitals. Disadvantage: immediate access to GNS not available.

Comprehensive Discharge Planning (CDP)—Planning Ahead

Focus of GNS is on high-risk older patients and caregivers. Assessment occurs at admission and every 48 hours thereafter. Available to family members and patients 7 days a week. Continuity of care continues after discharge. Developed by University of Pennsylvania Hospital for continuity of care while minimizing readmissions. Findings concur success; extended time between discharge and readmission.

Case Management: Multidisciplinary Approach

A multidisciplinary case management model for patients with complex conditions, high acuity, and increased potential for complications, noncompliance, and absence of a support system. Developed at Beth Israel Medical Center, New York.

Compiled from Strumpf NE: Innovative gerontological practices as models for health care delivery, *Nurs Health Care* 15(10):522, 1994; NICHE Project Faculty: Geriatric models of care: which one's right for your institution? *Am J Nurs* 94(7):21, 1994.

- Supplementation of physical therapy, occupational therapy, and speech therapy on a continuing basis
- Patient and family education

CRRN is the designation for RNs who have successfully completed special education and attained national certification in rehabilitation nursing. The Rehabilitation Nursing Foundation (RNF) is sponsored by the Association of Rehabilitation Nurses, an international organization of professional nurses dedicated to providing expert care for individuals (and groups) with actual or potential disabilities. The RNF is engaged in developing educational opportunities and scientific research to further the specialty of rehabilitation nursing and thus the health care provided to all disabled individuals. The RNF provides educational and research opportunities to nurses in all practice settings.

The Association of Rehabilitation Nurses provides opportunities for subspecialization in pediatrics, pain management, and geriatrics with foci on the roles of educator, manager, consultant, liaison, administrator, and researcher. Certification as a gerontological rehabilitation nurse pre-

pares one to serve the young-old, the old, and the frail elderly. These specialists practice in the full range of institutional and community settings and for governmental agencies, insurance companies, and private service companies. There are 8900 members of the International Rehabilitation Association; however, over 13,000 nurses have been certified as rehabilitation nurses by the organization, and 1700 have declared geriatric rehabilitation as their specialty (Association of Rehabilitation Nurses, 1997).

Hospital-Based Community Outreach Nurse. A nurse gerontologist was hired by a hospital in Wisconsin to make home visits to medically isolated elderly (those without a physician or satisfactory health care linkages) in a community with high-density elderly population to reduce inappropriate reliance on the hospital's emergency department. Outreach mechanisms used to contact unserved elders were distribution of pamphlets, publication in hospital news, and communicating with apartment managers, social service providers, community agency workers, and other related community businesses frequented by the elderly for possible referrals. Contacts were made with those identified to deter-

Box 28-14	**Acute Care Model 3—Community Care**

Strumpf discusses alternatives for institutional care and models that successfully care for frail elders at home and those early discharges from hospitals.

A pioneer project developed by the School of Nursing at the University of Pennsylvania implemented a nurse-managed day hospital reimbursed by Medicare: Collaborative Assessment & Rehabilitation for Elders program (CARE).

The design is based on the British geriatric care model of "maximizing independence, promoting health and function, and enhancing quality of life for chronically ill elders living in the community."

After a comprehensive evaluation, the patient receives an individualized plan of care for short-term, intensive interventions that can include any or all of the out-patient basis services, such as nursing or medical management, physical, or occupational therapy, mental health, nutrition, coping strategies, and family/caregiver support. A study outcome is in progress.

Data from Strumpf NE: Innovative gerontological practices as models for health care delivery, *Nurs Health Care* 15(10):522, 1994.

Table 28-7   Advanced Nursing Practice (ANP) Competencies and Nurse Case Management (NCM) Skills and Functions

ANP competency	NCM knowledge/skill	NCM function
Direct care	*In-depth, specialized assessment skills *Expert, clinically relevant technical skills *Establishment of patient outcomes	*Find and screen cases *Conduct health assessments *Develop and review critical pathways *Coordinate interventions of other providers *Link patient with appropriate resources *Monitor patient's progress toward goals *Evaluate effects of interventions
Expert guidance and coaching	*Education of patient, family, and other providers	*Educate staff nurses and other providers about clinical, fiscal, and system processes *Coach patients and families through developmental, health, and illness transitions
Consultation	*Provision of case consultation *Securing of consultation to enhance care and NCM	*Participate in work redesign *Initiate systemwide process improvements (e.g., documentation tools)
Research interpretation and use	*Collection, analysis, and synthesis of data	*Evaluate program outcomes such as quality and costs of care
Collaboration	*Communication, coordination, and negotiation	*Monitor service plan regarding quality, timeliness, quantity, costs of services, and effectiveness *Develop critical pathways and other clinical guidelines
Change agency	*Assessment of systems and organizations	*Initiate systemwide improvements *Identify needs for new services/programs
Ethical decision making	*Recognition and raising of ethical dilemmas	*Meet both system/fiscal and client goals

Mahn VA, Spross JA: Nurse case management as an advanced practice role. In Hamrick AB, Spross JA, Hanson CM: *Advanced nursing practice: an integrative approach,* Philadelphia, 1997, WB Saunders.

mine if they were in touch with a physician or if they were agreeable to participate in St. Mary's hospital outreach program.

The home visit was made within 24 hours to all those identified and included completion of assessment, development of a nursing care plan, and establishment of linkage to a primary care physician. Three situations were encountered upon assessment: (1) identification of an acute care health problem with immediate transport by ambulance to the hospital's emergency department with follow-up by a physician, (2) an untreated chronic health care problem with as-

sistance to the elder to select a physician, or (3) an infrequent health care problem with the need to establish linkage to a primary care physician. After 6 years this program showed that 750 elderly persons were provided with satisfactory health care linkages. The majority were able to remain independent in the community. The study did not state the reduction in emergency room use by elders in the area (Haworth, 1993).

In-Service Educator and Staff Developer. The in-service educator position or staff development role is most effectively filled by a nurse with a master's degree in education and a sound base in teaching/learning strategies. In smaller institutions this position may not formally exist. In such situations the professional nurse is responsible for training paraprofessionals and seeking education for herself appropriate to continued professional development.

Many nurses in long-term care have been schooled in programs that provided little theoretic understanding of normal aging or the special needs of the aged. It then becomes incumbent on the nurse to design an appropriate supplemental program. As the training person for paraprofessionals, the nurse may need additional training in teaching/learning and communication skills. Given the Omnibus Budget Reconciliation Act (OBRA) requirements for long-term care, staff development is best accomplished by nurses who are optimistic and self-confident enough to instill confidence in others. Ferreting out the strengths of paraprofessionals and building on them requires tact and understanding.

Emerging Roles in the Community

Nurses' roles have changed and evolved over the years yet are returning to the earlier emphasis on providing care in the home. Although there is a continued need for specialization in the acute care setting, shorter hospital stays and earlier discharge have created a need for more nurses in community health services with equally specialized abilities and comprehensive knowledge of older adult care. Individuals are frequently discharged from the hospital while requiring highly specialized care that families must supply with the support of professionals. Nurses are increasingly confronted with the need to design the management of complex illnesses in the home. Teaching and counseling the family are significant aspects of the geriatric specialist's nursing role.

Nurses entering home care from acute care think their qualifications and skills will transfer directly and qualify them to work in the home. These nurses who are new to community health report feelings of being adrift? Working in the community requires additional skills beyond handson and technical care. The hospital nurse comes from a structured environment where collegial support and supplies are readily available, but in the home, "what to do when you contaminate a piece of equipment or run out of sterile saline solution and the nearest supplies are 10 miles away?" (Hanner, 1994). Hanner notes the components of home nursing require creativity, autonomy, and accountability in a first home visit. There is a growing concern about the lack of information and support for nurses making the transition from hospital to home health nursing (Hanner, 1994).

Working in a home sets up different parameters and dynamics. The nurse has to be prepared for everything and anything when knocking on that door. Dealing with the home environment requires sensitivity, flexibility, ingenuity, adaptability, intuitiveness, skillful communication, and the ability to quickly problem solve. Psychosocial skills are imperative. The environment is out of the nurse's control—

control belongs to the client. In the home, there are other family members, friends, neighbors, pets, ringing phones, and unexpected interferences or crises.

With some families the nurse becomes the saviour, friend, chauffeur, financial adviser, counselor, educator, and advocate. The priority is not always the "treatment" of a disorder but rather assistance in the resolution of a family issue that is problematic. Stulginsky (1993a) shares experiences of a first home visit (Box 28-15).

The experienced home health nurse can quickly assess and reduce some of the burnout of elderly caregivers. For example, a 75-year-old man, taking care of his 70-year-old wife dying of cancer was getting up at 5 AM, not getting to sleep until midnight, and literally living at her bedside because of 4-hourly scheduled feedings and a complex schedule of medications. The nurse, consulting with the pharmacist, arranged to have medications mixed to simplify the schedule.

Home health nurses also experience frustration in not being able to give quality care because of business ramifications; for example, nurses do not get paid for many of the things they do (Box 28-16).

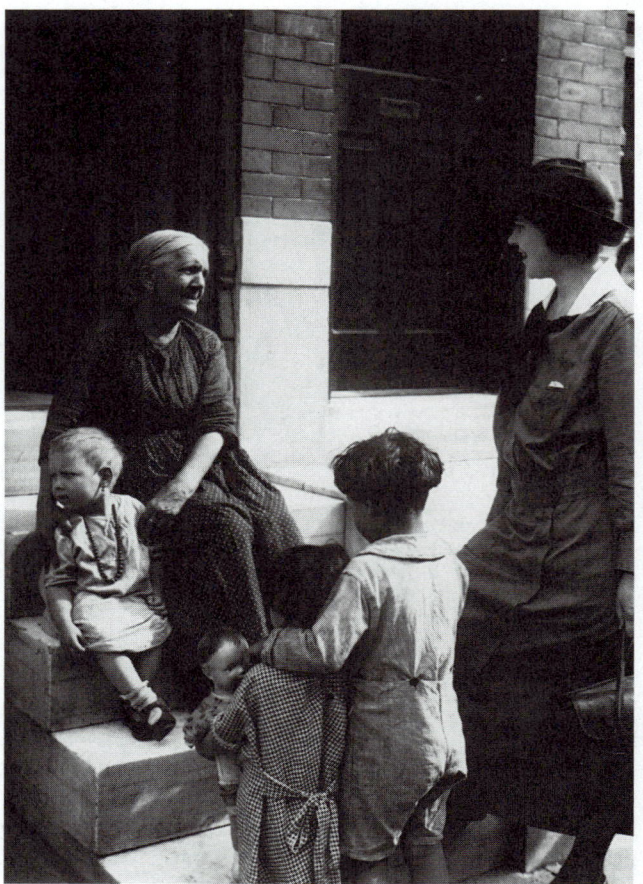

The public health nurse served the family. (Courtesy Center for the Study of the History of Nursing, School of Nursing, University of Pennsylvania.)

A concern about home care nursing has been the quality control issue. The Joint Commission on Accreditation of Healthcare Organizations (1994) has developed an initial framework for potential inclusion of performance measurements in the accreditation process (Box 28-17). Their focus will increasingly include clinical care issues relevant to the health care professional. The standards and written policies and procedures are outlined in Table 28-8 (Joint Commission on Accreditation of Healthcare Organizations, 1996). This may act as an impetus to more fully address the special needs of the aged in home care.

Home Care Nursing: Private Practice. Sweeney (1996) describes the process and experiences of setting up a private geriatric nursing practice with a colleague, Reidy: Community Nursing Service for the Elderly. The practice was established in a community in upstate New York with a population of 50,000. They encountered the usual problems of private practice nurses: the public and the health care system did not understand their goals. They overcame barriers in referral sources, financial issues, and legal implications. By surveying the community, they found more than 15% of the population was 65 and over. Initially they began in an office but soon learned that elders preferred home visits.

Their business thrived, and they now have 80 employees and are licensed by the New York State Health Department as a home health agency. They train all of their own workers and certify home health aides for others as well. Educational programs are offered to keep personnel updated. In 1993 another building was purchased that is used as a training and educational center.

Sweeney believes their success is due to the quality of their services, dependable staff, and low fees. Their nursing activities are presented in Table 28-9. Sweeney believes that similar community-based nursing practices could improve the quality of life of elders and reduce health care costs.

Home Care Agency Nurse-Administrator. Schank, Weis, and Matheus (1996) note that nurse-owned community health care agencies are proliferating and assuming an ever-larger share of this $31 billion industry. According to the National Independent Nursing Network (NINN), nurses are now driving home health care and controlling the business side. This has been the nurses's realm for decades, but only recently have nurses actually reaped the fiscal benefits. It is estimated that nearly 7.1 million Americans received medical care at home in 1995, primarily because of advances in home medical technology and the effectiveness

---

Box 28-15	**Nurses' Home Health Experience: The Practice Setting**

It was my first visit, I was nervous. I was covering the weekend and was told this would be easy and quick. The 80-year-old woman living with her daughter had just been discharged after several days in the hospital for recurring congestive heart failure. All I needed to do was physical assessment and check the effectiveness of her meds. Her multiple admissions were starting to get to the daughter, a single working parent . . . I was met at the door by an overwrought daughter who told me her mother was bleeding, she had called the doctor, her young son was upstairs sleeping, and she had to show up at work or be fired. Please, wouldn't I come in and take care of her mom? She would return within an hour, once she had negotiated with her boss for more time off, but it had to be done face-to-face. "I just can't call in one more time over the phone," she told me. I wasn't sure what to do., she seemed so beside herself. I don't think I was even party to the decision, she was gone so fast. I went looking for the patient's room. After introducing myself and performing a quick physical assessment, I noted the presence of blood at the rectum and on the sheets and wondered about how much had been lost. "That smell" led me to the bathroom where a trash can filled with soaked sanitary pads gave me the answer. I knew I was looking at a massive GI bleed. The phone rang, it was the doctor. I reported my findings and he said he would meet the family at the ER. What family? I returned to the patient and spoke to her about the urgent need to

rehospitalize her. She was shaking visibly as she flatly refused. I fantasized for a moment about how things would be different if I'd found her like this in a hospital. We would have already started fluids and she'd probably be on the way to the ICU and a host of people would be with me. But here we were, the two of us, blood oozing from her rectum. I wasn't sure what to do. I needed to call 911 but she was refusing treatment. I was with someone else's mother, in someone else's house. I couldn't remove her against her will, and what was I supposed to do with the youngster sleeping upstairs? I had little power here. My advice, which typically carried weight, meant nothing. Although my insides screamed treatment, I found myself quietly sitting on the edge of her bed talking. We held hands. I felt her pain as she told me she had just discovered that her two best friends had died, how she was sure that she'd never return home, how she felt like such a burden to her daughter; how becoming old was one loss after another. I know I blinked back tears. I'll never know what it was that we did or said that made her change her mind. All I know is that the daughter came back as the EMTs arrived. As the daughter and her child got into her car to follow the ambulance, I wondered whether I should be going to the hospital too, should I ride along with this frightened old woman so afraid of dying? We never covered this in orientation. As I drove home from my "simple" first visit, all I could think of was how different this type of nursing was going to be.

From Stulginsky MM: Nurses' home health experience. I. The practice setting, *Nurs Health Care* 14(8):402, 1993

Box 28-16   **Nurses' Home Health Experience: Home Visits**

Home care nurses don't get paid for what they do, neither do agencies—they get reimbursed for some kind of a thing that goes along the medical model, and that's the least of what you do. The most wonderful visit I ever had was down in Baltimore in a row home. He was a brand new diabetic, new to insulin, and I went into the house to teach. There was no heat, hot water, or electricity, and he didn't know what to do. He gave me the business card of the landlord who was a slum lord, I had heard his name in connection with scandals . . . and there was no phone number on the card, just a post office box . . . the guy had paid his rent . . . so I made a few phone calls to some public agencies, it took about 15 minutes. The next day I came back he had heat, hot water, and electricity.

(Obviously Medicare would not have reimbursed your agency for what you did on that visit, it wasn't skilled nursing, how did you handle that?) To get reimbursement? I documented that I gave him a list of his medications and instructed the patient regarding frequency and dosage. (Does that bother you in any way?) No, it doesn't bother me at all. What I did was much more valuable than teaching him about diabetes . . . although I probably gave him the list but no teaching occurred, he was too distracted. (What you're saying is that you couldn't have walked out of the home without addressing that issue). No, and we have many situations like that . . . (You mean the way the regs are written we're forced into certain situations out of ethical need?) Exactly right.

From Stulginsky MM: Nurses' home health experience. II. The unique demands of home visits, *Nurs Health Care* 14(9):477, 1993.

Box 28-17   **Definitions of Dimensions of Performance**

Doing the right thing
- The efficacy of the procedure or treatment in relation to the patient's condition
- The degree to which the care or service for the patient has been shown to accomplish the desired or projected outcome(s)
- The appropriateness of a specific test, procedure, or service to meet the patient's needs
- The degree to which the care provided is relevant to the patient's clinical needs, given the current state of knowledge

Doing the right thing well
- The availability of a needed test, procedure, treatment, or service to the patient who needs it
- The degree to which appropriate care is available to meet the patient's needs
- The timeliness with which a needed test, procedure, treatment, or service is provided to the patient
- The degree to which the care is provided to the patient at the most beneficial or necessary time
- The effectiveness with which tests, procedures, treatments, and services are provided
- The degree to which the care is provided in the correct manner, given the current state of knowledge, to achieve the desired or projected outcome for the patient
- The continuity of the services provided over time to the patient with respect to other services, clinicians, and providers
- The degree to which the care of the patient is coordinated among services, among organizations, and across time
- The safety of the patient (and others) to whom the services are provided
- The degree to which the risk of an intervention and risk in the care environment are reduced for the patient and others, including the staff members
- The efficacy with which services are provided
- The relationship between the outcomes (results of care) and the resources used to deliver patient care
- The respect and caring with which services are provided
- The degree to which the patient or a designee is involved in his or her own care decisions and to which those providing services do so with sensitivity and respect for the patient's needs, expectations, and individual differences

Source Joint Commission on Accreditation of Healthcare Organizations: *1995 Accreditation manual for home care,* vol 1, *Standards,* Oakbrook Terrace, Ill, 1994, The Commission. Reprinted with permission.

---

and reduced cost of care in the home. However, caution is necessary because this lucrative market is being entered by individuals without adequate nursing or medical qualifications. NINN nurse-administrators encourage nurses to join them for support and guidance in establishing such a business (see Resources for information).

Home Care Case Management Nurse. Home health care providers have become much more than the traditional agency overseers of multiproblem, poverty-stricken families. Home care is now an extension of the acute hospital and involves complex equipment, treatments, and extensive teaching to provide even the minimal supports needed in the home

Table 28-8	Home Care Standards and Written Policies and Procedures	
	Standard	**Policy or procedure**
RI.1.3.1	The organization has a functioning process in place to address and respect patient rights. The process is supported by a framework that includes the following mechanisms: Approved mechanisms that address the participation of the patient in all aspects of care, including formulation of advance directives.	Advance directives policy.
PE.1.6	The initial assessment of each patient admitted is conducted within a certain time frame preceding or following admission, as specified by policy.	Policy on time frame for conducting the initial assessment.
PE.2	Each patient is reassessed periodically during the course of care.	Policy on reassessments—content and intervals.
TX.3.1.1	As appropriate to the scope of care, reports of the patient's condition, the outcome of current treatment, and his or her response are periodically provided to the responsible physician.	Policy on written reports to the physician.
TX.4	Care planning includes a review and revision process as necessary.	Policy for care plan review and revision.
CC.2.4.1.1	As appropriate and according to organizational policy, the orientation to assigned responsibilities occurs on-site.	Policy for orientation of staff to assigned responsibilities and new cases.
EC.2.2.2	Environmental management processes are implemented for hazardous materials and wastes.	Policies and procedures for hazardous materials and waste identification, handling, transportation, and disposal.
HR.3.3.2	In-service education or other continuing education programs provided for staff are appropriate to their responsibilities and to the maintenance of skills necessary for the care of patients.	Policy and procedure on educating staff concerning advance directives.
HR.4	An individual's demonstrated ability to achieve expectations stated in a job description is assessed.	Policy for performance evaluation.
IM.2.1	The organization determines the need for appropriate levels of security and confidentiality of data and information.	Policy on confidentiality and release of information.
IM.3.3.1	Qualified individuals review the completeness, accuracy, and timely completion of information in home care records to determine compliance with the organization's policies.	Policies regarding completion, timeliness, and accuracy of home care records.
IM.5	The communication of data and information is timely and accurate as required by law and regulation.	Policies regarding completion, timeliness and accuracy of information and communication.
IM.7.1.2	Authentication is done by written signatures, initials, or a computer key.	Policy on authentication of entries.
IM.7.3.1	The home care record of a patient discharged from home health, hospice, clinical respiratory, and/or pharmaceutical service is completed within a time period specified in the organization's policy.	Policy on time frame for completion of the home care record for discharged patients.
IM.7.3.3	When the patient is transferred within the organization or to another organization, relevant information is provided to the organization and, as appropriate, to the patient's physician.	Transfer policy defining relevant information to be shared.

From Joint Commission on Accreditation of Healthcare Organizations: Home care standards and written policies and procedures, *Joint Commission Perspectives* 16(1):19, 1996, Oakbrook Terrace, Ill. Reprinted with permission.

(Michela, 1995). High-tech home care presents a myriad of problems never before dealt with in the home or by families. Careful monitoring, documentation, and teaching are the triad of care in the home. Home health care is booming in this age of shortened hospital stays caused by diagnostic-related groups' (DRGs) reimbursement limitations and increasing numbers of frail aged. The trend in health care is away from the institution and toward the community.

As appears evident, RNs play a pivotal role in the provision of quality home care, particularly since the drastic change in intensity of home care that has occurred. Some ventilator-dependent patients are at home with their families, as are other patients requiring sophisticated and intense care. Highly expert nurses are needed to assist in the management of such cases. Nurses must be able to think independently and holistically and be highly skilled. Physicians must rely on the nurse's judgment in making medical decisions; thus the home care nurse-manager must possess high-level nursing and managerial skills, judgment, and tact, and the ability to communicate with many levels of professionals and all types of families. Although home care is provided by many of the disciplines, nursing is the key; it is necessary that nurses be given a primary care role to organize and coordinate care.

The role of the Visiting Nurse Association and community health nurse has been significant but poorly recognized in regard to case management. Although they have historically acted as primary care agents and case managers, these nurses have not organized to promote this role. Private insurance companies are investigating coverage for home health services but need to be assured that the cost will not be overwhelming. Case managers will be needed to monitor

Table 28-9   Nursing Activities

Category	Outcome	Nursing function
Advocacy	Helping elders and families "work the system"; familarize family with responsible options	Independent judgment; technical, interpersonal, and critical thinking skills, using integrated thoughtful process*
Assessment	Identify needs with nursing process	Assess physical, mental, and emotional needs; communicate with physician and others as needed
Crisis intervention	Monitor unstable health conditions and relieve anxiety	Nurses available 24 hours a day to answer calls and meet the health needs of clients
Education and counseling	Maintain health and reduce complications	Clients/families are provided handouts on medications in easy-to-read format; counseling provided regarding disease process
Consultation	Recognize conditions that require additional treatment	Referrals to physicians and professionals after thorough assessment
Referrals	Contact others who will help to normalize client's condition	Communicate appropriate information to professionals and agencies as needed with interdisciplinary collaboration
Screening tests	Increase awareness and knowledge of client problem, while reducing duplication and cost	Perform, interpret, and report test results as needed (e.g., urine and blood tests)
Treatments	Recognize critical conditions that require immediate attention and reduce discomfort and cost	Contact medical personnel and perform the required treatment (e.g., medication preparation, enema, catheterization)
Training	Provide qualified persons to prepare home care workers	Instruct and train persons to work in the home through organized classes
Continuing education	Educate regular employees on an ongoing basis regarding home care	Provide 12 hours of education to home care workers on a monthly basis
Community education	Educate the community regarding home care needs of elders and availability of services	Prepare and be available to provide caregivers with information requested
Case management	Ensure client is being properly cared for in the home and emphasize the value of the nurse's home visit; provide continuous care between home and institution	Ensure billing for visit is separate; supervise and instruct caregiver; assess and identify client home care needs; follow up and plan with discharge planner and report to physician

*Deihl DH. *Private practice: out on a limb and loving it.*
From Sweeney JM: Nurses in home care: a success story, *Geriatr Nurs* 17(4):187, 1996.

quality and cost, providing an open opportunity for nurses to declare their expertise and efficiency and to approach the market with a widespread case management plan.

Particular issues of concern to the nurse, necessary to maximize home care services, include (1) knowledge of the extent of insurance coverage, (2) ability to precisely describe clients' service needs, (3) familiarity with the professional health care practice acts and home care licensure standards, both state and federal, (4) establishment of links and coordination of efforts of a multidisciplinary team, and (5) pursuit of legal leverage when needed to adequately provide for clients (Michela, 1995).

Acceptable standards of care are also needed to ensure the quality of home care. The skyrocketing demand and the prospective payment system of Medicare (DRGs) have spawned hundreds of home care agencies of varying quality and capacities. Only the provider and the customer know what goes on in the home, and the consumer may not recognize inadequate care.

The Parish Nurse.   Churches have been involved in health care delivery for more than 2000 years. The contemporary model was developed by a Lutheran minister and former hospital chaplain, Granger Westburg. His vision in the 1980s was of nurses promoting health and preventing disease within congregations (Schank et al, 1996). Thousands of parish nurses have now found gratifying roles in urban and rural settings and serve all ages and faiths. Their roles include the following:

Education (CPR, advance directives, selecting a nursing home, medications)

Case managers and advocates in obtaining health care

Counselors for grieving and psychosocial issues

Providing referrals

Training volunteers as peer counselors and developing support groups

Parish nurses are usually employed by health care institutions, which contract with the congregation for services or a church-sponsored nurse. A workweek can be from 10 to 20 hours or full time. Educational recommendations are being developed by the Health Ministries Association.

A successful educational program has been established at Marquette University Parish Nurse Preparation Institute of Wisconsin. The training has two phases. During the first phase, the content includes assessment skills, roles, spiritual caregiving, legal issues, and on-site observational experience with a practicing nurse. The second phase involves a 9-month fellowship/mentoring experience in a congregation. Funding, doctrinal issues, and perception of the nursing role may sometimes present problems. This program received the 1995 Global Visio-Community Outreach Award from the Wisconsin Hospital Association and the Marshall Iisley Trust Foundation.

Armmer and Humbles (1995) established a parish nursing model, the Christian Nurses Preventive Health Project (CNPHP) with funding from a community foundation to provide health promotion services to African-American church congregations in underserved areas of Peoria, Illinois. The activities of the program included health promotion, blood pressure monitoring, health counseling, breast self-examination, health education, and a monthly health newsletter. Medications and blood pressure screening were the most-used services. Teaching aids adapted to African-Americans were found useful. The church environment instilled trust and interest in health care.

The role of the parish nurse will continue to offer valuable services that fit the national trend to maintain elderly in their homes, reduce costs of institutionalization, promote self-care, and prevent disease. Bringing healing and spiritual beliefs into a whole approach to health has been sorely neglected in the modernist era; postmodernism is again realizing the power of this approach.

Counselor and Health Educator for Elders and Their Family Members.

Throughout this text, information to assist nurses in the role of counselor and health educator has been included. Often the nurse is in direct contact with clients as a counselor or health educator, but with the present shortage of adequately prepared gerontic nurses, his or her function is often indirect, educating those who have direct contact with the aged. The nurse prepared in gerontics may provide counseling and education to social service agency personnel, who are often overwhelmed by aged clients' crises or talk of dying. Long-term care staff members need education about the independence potential of their aged patients. Police officers need education regarding their contacts with aged persons.

Nurses in the community are often teachers. It is important to expand the concept of teaching beyond that of skills and direct information. As early as 1978, Monea (1985) educated older persons to become peer counselors: she taught peer counseling strategies to older adults through experiential learning sessions. They learned to use touch, listening ability, sensory awareness, and reminiscence and to deal with anger, pride, and ruffled feelings. These abilities helped them serve as counselors for peers who were lonely, disabled, and distressed. In this way one nurse was able to indirectly affect the quality of life for many elderly persons. See Chapter 17 for more discussion of caregivers and their provision for elder family members.

Nurse-Managed Elder Health Care Centers.

Nurse-managed centers for the health care of older adults are flourishing and proving to provide quality care, to generate client enthusiasm, and to be cost effective. Given the emphasis on cost, we expect more of these to appear throughout the United States. In 1990, there were approximately 250 centers, both rural and urban, providing services to the underserved at affordable cost to aged clients. Half of these care centers were free standing, whereas the others were associated with hospitals, public health or home care agencies, retirement communities, or senior centers. Many were managed and staffed by faculty and students of schools of nursing (American Nurses' Association, 1992).

The nurse-managed health care centers furnish services such as assessment and screening, education and counseling, consultation, and home care. An interdisciplinary team of nurse, physician, and social worker usually assesses each client entering the system. Nurses occupy chief management positions. Emphasis is placed on determining how well the activities of daily living and instrumental activities of daily living are performed and what supports are used or needed. Specific abilities evaluated include dressing, bathing, mobility, toileting, preparing meals, taking medications, and handling finances. The nurse also identifies problems in behavioral management of persons with congnitive impairment and assists the client and family to handle the situation better. Caregiver assistance is provided through individual counseling, family conferences, and formalized educational programs.

A free-standing clinic in southern California, the Older Women's Health Care Clinic, is a model, staffed entirely by geriatric nurse practitioners, and is designed to serve the health and wellness needs of females over the age of 50 (Magit, 1980). The major aspect of the nurse's role in this setting is as educator, need assessor, and resource coordinator. Physicians are used appropriately for referral, but it has been found that approximately 80% of the problems older women bring can be dealt with effectively by nurse practitioners in the clinic.

Morgan (1996) reports on a successful nurse-managed clinic in California and attributes much of the success to the demographic analysis, preliminary needs assessment, accessible site location, and the sharing of space and resources with affiliated agencies and groups.

Nurses are now increasingly serving senior centers, retirement communities, environmental planning agencies, engineering and architectural firms, nutrition sites, and storefront multiservice centers, where they function as primary care providers. The critical issue in these nurse-managed centers is the relatively autonomous function and the direct reimbursement available to the nurse providers. Functions can be seen in Figure 28-2.

The Wellness Nurse.

Continuing care retirement communities (CCRCs) offer nursing opportunities for an autonomous role as a wellness nurse. The role of the nurse is

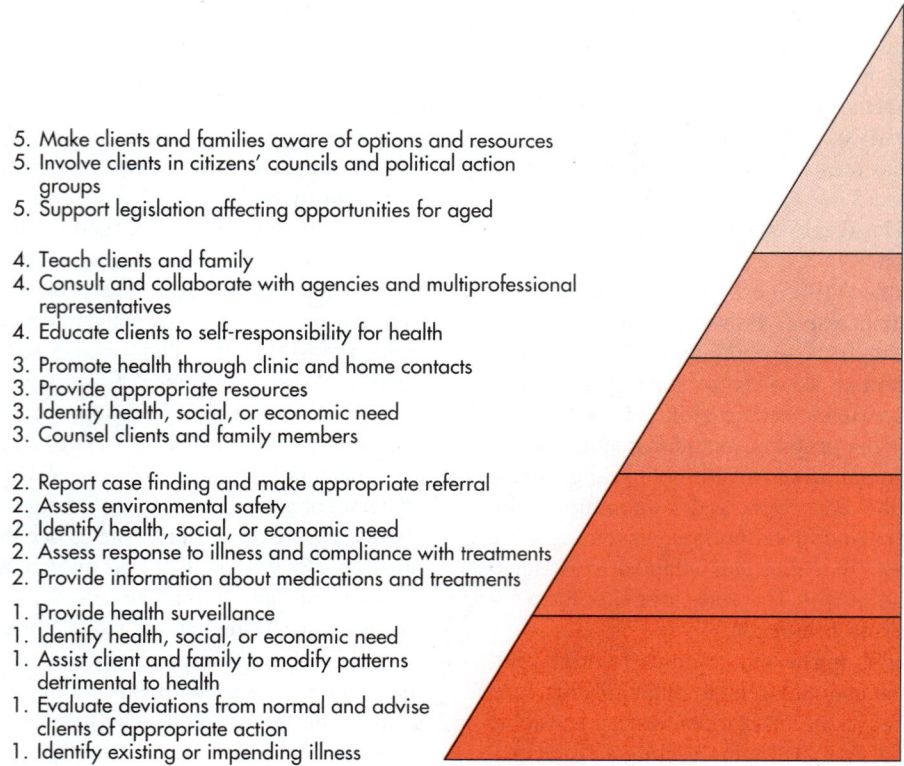

5. Make clients and families aware of options and resources
5. Involve clients in citizens' councils and political action groups
5. Support legislation affecting opportunities for aged

4. Teach clients and family
4. Consult and collaborate with agencies and multiprofessional representatives
4. Educate clients to self-responsibility for health

3. Promote health through clinic and home contacts
3. Provide appropriate resources
3. Identify health, social, or economic need
3. Counsel clients and family members

2. Report case finding and make appropriate referral
2. Assess environmental safety
2. Identify health, social, or economic need
2. Assess response to illness and compliance with treatments
2. Provide information about medications and treatments

1. Provide health surveillance
1. Identify health, social, or economic need
1. Assist client and family to modify patterns detrimental to health
1. Evaluate deviations from normal and advise clients of appropriate action
1. Identify existing or impending illness

Figure 28-2. Nursing functions in community health clinics.

essentially to sustain the residents in their independent setting. They work with the higher functioning residents and provide a range of nursing services, including assessment, monitoring of changes in chronic conditions, wellness educational programs, triage, and consultation. They keep the resident at the most appropriate level of care (Petit, 1994). Emotional support by the wellness nurse is especially significant during the resident's transition into the retirement community. They may help prevent relocation trauma (see Chapter 13). The wellness nurse also assesses new residents who may have moved because of pressure from their children and are at risk of great dissatisfaction (Petit, 1994).

Administrators in CCRCs view the wellness nurse in terms of costs versus benefits; that is, reducing the need for use of the expensive nursing care center. The wellness nurse attempts to keep elders healthy at the least cost. Petit advises that nurses considering employment in CCRCs gain a "clear understanding of organization's expectations." The opportunities for developing wellness nursing in CCRCs continues to grow as life care centers become ever more popular (Garland, 1992). They provide an excellent learning opportunity for nursing students and the possibility for significant nursing research to contribute knowledge of healthy elders to the growing field of gerontology.

Well Elder Clinics and Outreach Nurses. Well elder clinics are often located in low-rent housing developments, retirement complexes, life care centers, and senior centers

and sometimes in shopping malls—anyplace where seniors are likely to congregate. The role of these outreach nurses is to develop rapport with administrators of these facilities and be available to seek out those elders who may be frail and need monitoring, to teach staff and residents signs of increasing vulnerability, to monitor general health of any elders who come to them, and to make referrals as indicated. This role with well elders is one that can provide gratifying and enriching experiences for nursing students.

Christensen (1996) had dreaded the geriatric component of her nursing school requirements until placed in a well elder clinic sponsored by a local hospital. In this experience she performed physical and psychosocial assessments, performed venipunctures and learned to properly handle laboratory specimens off site, monitored vital signs, and referred individuals for further testing and examination when any irregularities were encountered. Most importantly, she began to know some elders, their concerns, and life histories. She said in summarizing her experience, "I now realize that growing old is much more than pressure ulcers and cataracts. My experience has shown me firsthand the need we have as nurses and as students to dispel the stereotypes of old age" (p. 92).

Informatics Nursing. The ever-expanding use of electronic networks has made it possible to disseminate information, to provide health care services to individuals in their homes via computer linkages, and to develop distance learning programs and client support networks. Patricia Brennan (1989), the pioneer in nursing informatics, has developed ComputerLink, an electronic network designed to provide nursing support, information, and advocacy to individuals 24 hours a day to be used at the convenience of caregivers and the aged when they feel a need. This and similar programs are being developed by nurse-entrepreneurs throughout the nation. Brennan's research demonstrated the effectiveness of such linkages in the management of chronic and complex illnesses and in fostering self-care techniques in home-based patients. She predicts nursing informatics will develop into a strong domain of nursing and that in the future much nursing will not be delivered face to face. Most importantly, she and Turley (1996) caution nurses to keep the *nurse* in nursing informatics and not lose sight of the primary role of nursing as patient advocates and supporters.

Telephone Advice Nurse. Similar to the informatics nurse, and a forerunner of this type of care delivery, is telephone advice nurse. The telephone allows community-residing elders and their families to initiate nursing assistance, support, and counseling at their discretion and thus increases their self-reliance. This provides a vital link between the health care system and elderly persons in their homes and has become especially important in the era of managed health care.

The initial function is as a triage manager, requiring great expertise in making cursory assessments through phone contact. Initial assessment and ongoing support are provided through the phone contact between the nurse and the elderly individual or members of his or her support system. To perform a good, brief assessment without being perfunctory, the nurse needs to develop a complete picture of the elderly person's situation based on information gathered in the phone conversation. The nurse must focus on specific areas to determine (1) the immediate concern that triggered seeking help, (2) the ability of the person to exercise safe judgments, and (3) the health history, with emphasis on essential and instrumental self-care abilities.

Nursing care through telephone contact requires that the nurse have crisis intervention skills, a method of systematic assessment, a creative approach to intervention, and the ability to listen to what is verbalized and to hear what is not stated. This role requires a great deal of knowledge and experience. Most importantly, the telephone advice nurse has the opportunity to ensure that the individual has sufficient information to make wise care decisions. The nurse must frequently advocate for the client when adequate or sufficient care does not seem to be forthcoming from a particular health care system. This has become a significant issue in the last few years because we see clients being viewed as dollar-consuming end products rather than individuals. Rural, isolated individuals are particularly vulnerable and will likely need this service.

Gerontic Nurses as Alternative Healers. Engebretson (1996) proposes that the concepts underlying health and healing are fundamentally similar for nurses and alternative healers. The shared domains of health care include activities such as attitudinal and relationship strengthening; spiritual, physical and mental, wellness; and promotion of self-care and appropriate help seeking. After decades of enchantment with technology, nurses are increasingly blending the holistic mode into caregiving activities of all kinds. The mature nurse can be of any chronologic age but has gone through the developmental phases of nursing, which we believe involve nurse identity, technical expert, skillful assessor, master interventionist, and finally, strategic holistic planner. A method employed by alternative healers is that of linkage between novices and experts in practice. Nurses seldom have that luxury, but we recognize the value of seeking expertise and mentorship whenever possible.

Whatever nursing role one occupies, the challenge in caring for the aged is exciting and takes one on a path of self-discovery that requires maximum sensitivity, maturity, and self-awareness. Nursing the aged is an exhilarating journey into oneself and the meanings of life. The field is open; unending opportunities and challenges await the nurse of today and the future in working with the aged to achieve the most positive closure on the lived experience. Organized nursing celebrated its centennial in 1996, and throughout the celebration it was noted that we must look at our past to plan well for the future. Nurse-elders are our guides in this venture, representatives of our past and portenders of our future. Mary Opal Wolanin (1996) brings it into perspective very quickly, "Florence Nightingale was born in 1820 and died in 1910. I was born in 1910 and began nursing in 1931. In the span of two lives we have seen the whole of organized nursing. What is so different about this past century of nursing? What is different about this whole world in which we live? I believe the difference is organization and use of each other's strength. We are within the context of our time and technology" (American Nurse, 1996, p. 29).

THE FUTURE OF GERONTIC NURSING

Opportunities abound for role development and refinement for nurses caring for the aged. The major specialties and components of the role are presented in Box 28-18. Alert and creative nurses can design their own practices and develop a range of services to sustain elders in the least restrictive settings that will add satisfaction and joy to the extended years of life that so many elders are now experiencing. In addition, the whole group of late middle-aged baby boomers will be seeking services while they age, of a nature we can scarcely imagine. Already, many elders and almost-elders seek the information they need for self-care on the Web pages of the internet. The vastly better informed populace and the erosion of physicians' status and control of elders' lives will make profound differences in the care available and in nursing opportunities.

> **Box 28-18**
> **Major Specialties and Components of Gerontic Nursing**
>
> A. Practitioner
> ___ 1. Completes care plan for individuals and families during the clinical time
> ___ 2. Implements plan of care as prescribed and planned
> ___ 3. Utilizes critical thinking during implementation
> ___ 4. Applies theory, science, and art in practice
> ___ 5. Relates nursing actions, interactions as influencing factors on individual, family outcomes.
> ___ 6. Utilizes research in actions and interactions
> ___ 7. Implements standardized protocols and monitors responses
> ___ 8. Compares actual to predicted responses
> ___ 9. Communicates and collaborates with other professions
> B. Educator
> ___ 1. Implements teaching intervention for knowledge deficits
> ___ 2. Utilizes nursing science and theory base in teaching
> ___ 3. Implements individualized approach to care
> ___ 4. Demonstrates the art of nursing in teaching individual, families, and staff
> ___ 5. Participates in discharge planning teaching and community-based workshops for individual and family nursing diagnoses or problems
> C. Researcher
> ___ 1. Utilizes research findings to solve clinical problems
> ___ 2. Critiques research for applicability
> ___ 3. Identifies research questions and communicates them to nurse researchers or managers
> ___ 4. Utilizes nursing theory to explain phenomenon in practice
> ___ 5. Identifies research questions and implements primary studies in the hospital and community
> D. Leader/Manager
> ___ 1. Participates in group conferences
> ___ 2. Implements appropriate style relative to the organizational structure of the nursing care delivery system
> ___ 3. Functions as an advocate for the individual and family
> ___ 4. Functions effectively within the organizational structure
> ___ 5. Functions to develop a positive nursing care delivery system within the organization to support therapeutic intervention
> ___ 6. Supports implementation of clinical research studies in the hospital and community.

From Buchanan LM: Therapeutic nursing intervention knowledge and outcome measures for advanced practice, *Nurs Health Care* 15(4):190, 1994.

We have presented background issues and a range of interesting roles in gerontic nursing. The real attraction to gerontic nursing, however, is based on the awareness of the individual nurse that life's greatest meanings and insights tend to emerge in the later years. Depth, breadth, and sensitivity are required of nurses who care for the aged. Continuous personal growth and learning are some of the ongoing rewards for nurses who elect to work with the aged. We have presented brief summaries of numerous roles and opportunities in gerontic nursing. The themes of change, challenge, stress, and success have been obvious in the continuing professionalization of gerontic nursing summarized in this chapter. We wish you energy, power, and peace in your nursing career toward healthy and humanistic aging care. To capture the in-depth essence of the various roles reviewed the reader is encouraged to select and read the references listed—an exciting and enriching experience.

KEY CONCEPTS

- The development of gerontic nursing as a specialty began nearly 25 years ago when the ANA first formulated standards of geriatric nursing care.
- Certification assures the public of nurses' committment to specialized education and qualification for the care of the aged.
- Requirements for accreditation of nursing programs should require solid evidence of special study in the care of the aged.
- The major U.S. organizations devoted exclusively to nurses caring for the aged are the National Gerontological Nursing Association, the National Conference of Gerontological Nurse Practitioners, and the National Association of Directors of Nursing Administration in Long Term Care.
- Clinical research in gerontic nursing is becoming more prevalent because nurses are better prepared and more confident in conducting research.
- Nurses caring for the aged are increasingly concerned about ethical and legal issues that are arising. Their responsibility for outcomes is also increasing. Nurse attorneys, legal consultants, and court examiners are contributing their expertise to clarifying these issues.
- The major changes in health care delivery have resulted in numerous revised, refined, and emergent roles for nurses in the field of gerontology.
- Advanced practice nurses have either nurse practitioner qualifications or clinical nurse specialist education. Advanced practice role opportunities for nurses are numerous and are seen as potentially saving money in health care delivery while facilitating more holistic health care.
- Gerontic nurses who desire to do so have found many opportunities for independent practice.
- Gerontic nursing at its best requires specialized education, maturity, commitment, and sensitivity.

▲ **Needs Addressed and Task Strengths**	
Student nurses' need for recognition, for intellectual stimulation, and achievement (to meet need for belonging, self-esteem, and individual and collective sell-actualization); interpersonal involvement Need for relevant education adapted to goals and personal past Need to be heard Need for adequate resources and opportunities Need for personal responsibility in pursuing learning needs	Perceptive Appreciation of faculty experience Ability to take risks Ability to appreciate learning role Motivated by personal experience Compassionate Assertive Seeking excellence

▲ CASE STUDY

Janice had achieved a Master's Degree in English literature and was simply thrilled to have completed her graduate studies. She began searching for a job that would use her talents and her great love for literature, particularly women's literature. After several months of fruitless searching there seemed to be no position available in which she could capitalize on her expertise. However, as fate sometimes decrees, her grandmother became unable to care for herself and needed a live-in caretaker. As her parents were both working it seemed she was the only one available as a caregiver. Reluctantly, but somewhat relieved at having something to do, she agreed to move in with Grandmother Winnie as a temporary measure until someone suitable could be found. Neither she nor her parents had any idea where to begin to get help or resources to aid them. Janice tried to do what she thought her grandmother needed but wasn't sure about the schedule for her numerous medications and at times her grandmother was not sure either. One night her grandmother began moaning and mumbling, and Janice couldn't understand what she needed or wanted. The more she tried to get her grandmother to speak clearly, the more agitated Winnie became. Finally she called her parents, and they took Winnie to the emergency room of the nearby community hospital. It was several hours before Winnie was seen by a doctor, assessed, admitted, and settled into a hospital room. It had been a difficult night for the whole family but was most unsettling for Janice because she learned that her grandmother's medications had been improperly given and also that she was dreadfully dehydrated. This was not something Janice was accustomed to. She had always done a careful and thorough job of anything she attempted and seldom felt she had not been successful in accomplishing her goal. She realized her care of grandmother had been inadequate because she had no knowledge of the best ways to care for her. At dawn, finally on their way home, she broke down crying and said to her parents, "It will be my fault if grandmother dies. I wish I had known how to take care of her better." Her grandmother recovered after several days of monitoring and intravenous fluid and electrolyte replenishment. The hospital arranged for a home health nurse to monitor Winnie's progress and assist Janice in finding the resources needed to augment her care.

Following that episode, Janice became impressed with the skill of the home health nurse and decided to enter an accelerated nursing program designed for individuals who had already achieved a degree in another field. She found her studies fascinating and clinical practice interesting and gratifying but was amazed that so little time was spent in the curriculum on studying the complexity of medication interactions and hardly anything was said about caring for elders in the home. She continually asked questions, but faculty had little or no actual experience in home care and thus were unable to meet her particular needs. One day, in disgust she commented loud enough for those around her to hear, "I thought this program would be just what I need, but they don't teach me what I need to know." Toward the end of her studies she requested and was granted a precepted experience in a home care agency.

Based up on the case study of the student nurse, Janice, develop an intervention plan for the remainder of her studies:

List her comments that provide *subjective data.*

List information that provides *objective data.*

From these data identify the student nurse's present needs.

Develop a plan for the remainder of her education that you would consider ideal.

State the *outcome criteria* that you would expect.

How would you *evaluate* the success of her nursing education, considering her needs.

STUDY QUESTIONS/ACTIVITIES

Discuss how an individual's personal needs should influence the direction of their studies.

Discuss your thoughts about the relevance of the nursing educational system to the actual care of the aged.

Discuss your expectations of and obligations toward professional organizations that relate to nursing and gerontology.

Discuss the ethical questions related to nursing that are most troubling to you at present.

Survey your community for available positions in nursing and summarize the areas of need and those that are being neglected.

Interview a supervising nurse in each of the following settings: hospital, emergency room, home care, hospice, and nursing home and ask what they consider to be the greatest needs in the care of the aged within their settings. Ask what they consider the advantages of their setting in the care of the aged.

Describe several gerontic nursing roles and the characteristics that distinguish each. Determine which of the gerontic nursing roles would be most fitting for you given your particular personality and nursing goals.

Discuss several major factors that have influenced or hindered the progress of gerontologic nursing as a specialty practice.

Discuss various methods in which you have obtained expertise in gerontic nursing. Identify those most effective and the reasons this was so.

Compare variations in institutional and community roles in gerontic nursing and discuss some of the underlying differences.

Prioritize some of the immediate needs in the field of gerontic nursing and how best these might be addressed.

Explain components of gerontic nursing care that remain fundamental regardless of role and setting where nursing care is provided.

Discuss some of the pioneers in gerontic nursing and how their contributions and thoughts have affected your feelings about gerontic nursing.

Develop a statement of your feelings related to the care of the aged

Select a partner and discuss in the most realistic manner possible what you expect you and your life will be like when you are 75 years old.

Write a short essay (2 or 3 pages) about the old person you have enjoyed or respected most in your life time.

RESEARCH QUESTIONS

What are the range of activities of a nurse in acute care during an 8-hour shift and how much time is spent in caring for needs related specifically to those of aged patients?

What aspects of gerontic nursing roles do nurses find most gratifying?

Women studies have been done on the pros and cons of nursing home nursing but we need broader and more specific information on what attracts nurses to the field.

Why do nursing home nurses stay and why do they leave?

What is the actual time spent in baccalaureate nursing programs on clinical experiences caring for the aged?

What is the actual time in the curriculum of baccalaureate nursing schools spent on content related only to the care of the aged?

The field of historic investigation is ripe for further studies, and there are pioneering gerontic nurses that need to be interviewed regarding their perceptions of the specialty. Others who need to be studied: Doreen Norton. Irene Burnside, Margaret Dimond, Neville Strumpf, Lois Evans, Lois Knowles, Barabara Lee, and Loretta Ford. What are the perspectives of gerontic nurse pioneers on the future of nursing the aged?

RESOURCES

American Association of Homes and Services
for the Aging
901 E Street, NW, Suite 500
Washington, DC 20004-2037
(301) 490-0677

National League for Nursing (NLN)
Accreditation Board
10 Columbus Circle
New York, NY 10019

American Health Care Association
1201 L Street NW
Washington, DC 20005
(202) 842-8444

American Nurses' Association (ANA)
Accreditation Board
600 Maryland Ave SW
Suite 100 W
Washington DC 20024-2571
(202) 554-4444

American Society on Aging
833 Market Street, Suite 511
San Francisco, CA 94103-1824
(415) 974-9600

Gerontological Society of America
1275 K Street, NW, Suite 350
Washington, DC 20005-4006
(202) 842-1275

Association for Gerontology in Higher Education (AGHE)
600 Maryland Ave, SW, West Wing 204
Washington, DC 20024
(202) 484-7505

Gerontic Nursing Education Programs

Because of the rapid development of numerous graduate, undergraduate, and certificate programs in gerontic nursing throughout the United States, it is advisable to contact the accrediting bodies directly for current information. Information regarding certificate and degree programs (undergraduate and graduate) in gerontology, standards, guidelines, and program directories are available.

Films and Videos

Code Gray: Ethical Dilemmas in Nursing, Jamaica Plains, Mass, 1984. Fanlight Productions (motion picture videorecording). One 16 mm film or videocassette; 28 min; sound; color.

Ethics, Values, and Health Care, Irvine, Calif, 1980, Concept Media (film-strip). Eight rolls; color; 34 mm and 8 cassettes (two-track, monaural, approximately 20 min/each); including guide.

Ethics, Law, and Nursing, Chicago, Nursing Management FIlms (video recording). One videotape cassette divided into three units; 60 min; sound; color; includes study guide and bibliography.

Ethics in Nursing, Fairfax, Va, 1986. School of Nursing, George Mason University (videorecording). Nine videocassettes in five units (4 hr); sound; color; includes study guide with bibliography. (The five units are Concept of morality; Ethical theories; Ethical principles; Allocation of scarce resources, theory; Allocation of scarce resources, application.)

No Heroic Measures, Urbana, Ill, Carle Medical Communications (videotape). Color: 22 min. Free 3-day previews are available in 1/4 inch video to media libraries and previous CMC customers on written request. For others the preview fee is $15.00, which must accompany preview request and is applicable to purchase or rental within 90 days. Preview tapes may not be used for classroom or inservice instruction.

In addition, an extensive list of audiovisual titles in bioethics can be generated through BIOETHICSLINE and AVLINE, National Library of Medicine.

Organizations

American Nurses' Association, 600 Maryland Avenue, SW, Suite 100 West, Washington, D.C. 20024-2571

National Conference of Gerontological Nurse Practitioners. Inc. officers and committee chairpersons: NCGNP Central Office. P.O. Box 270101, Fort Collins, CO 80527-0101, (303)493-7793.

National Gerontological Nurses Association (NGNA), 7250 Parkway Drive, Hanover, MD 21076

The National Association of Directors of Nursing Administration in Long-Term Care (NADONA/LTC) is the only national organization for directors, assistant directors, and former DONs in long-term care facilities. NADONA/LTC. Membership, 10999 Reed Hartman Hwy #229, Cincinnati, OH 45242-8331, 1-800-222-0539.

Publications

Codes and Guidelines

American Nurses' Association: *Code for nurses with interpretive statements.* Kansas City, MO, 1985. The Association. This pamphlet identifies the 11 statements of the code, with interpretive comments about each one.

American Nurses' Association: *Human rights guidelines for nurses in clinical and other research,* Kansas City, MO. 1985. The Author. The guidelines focus on protection of human rights in research, with emphasis on right to anonymity, right to privacy and dignity, and right to freedom from intrinsic risk of injury. The guidelines also focus on mechanisms for protection of human subjects in research.

The Council on Gerontologic Nursing Practice, American Nurses' Association, 600 Maryland Avenue, S. W., Suite 100 West, Washington, D.C. 20024-2571.

Hastings Center, Institute of Society, Ethics and the Life Sciences. Publishes the *Hastings Center Report,* leading journal in bioethics, plus case studies, bibliographics, books, and monographs. Guidelines on the termination of life-sustaining treatment and the care of the dying. New York, 1987. The Center, Department T, 255 Elm Rd, Briarcliff Manor, NY 10510 and 360 Broadway, Hastings-on-Hudson, NY 10706.

Kennedy Institute of Ethics, Bioethics Library, Georgetown University, maintains *Bioethics-line*, the only computerized database on the subject of bioethics, Georgetown University, 37th & P Sts, Washington, DC 20057, (202)625-2383.

Legal and Ethical Aspects of Health Care for the Elderly. Kapp M, Pies HE, Doudera AE, editors. Ann Arbor, MI 48109, (313)764-1380.

Compiled Bibliography

Pence T: *Ethics in Nursing: AN Annotated Bibliography,* ed 2. New York, 1986, National League for Nursing. This bibliography contains more than 1200 annotated references related to ethics in nursing. Reference data from 1901 to 1986 arranged by topic, alphabetically by annotated citations, and also by secondary author index.

REFERENCES

American Medical Association: Opinions on interprofessional relations, 3.02, p 17, *Code of medical ethics: current opinion,* Chicago, 1992, The Association.

American Nurse's Association: Community nursing centers gaining ground as solution to health issues, *Am J Nurs* 92(7):71, 1992.

American Nurses' Association: Advanced practice nursing: a new age in health care. In American Nurses' Association: *Nursing facts,* Washington, DC, 1995a, The Association.

American Nurses' Association: *Nursing facts,* Washington, DC, 1995b, The Association.

American Nurses' Association: *Scope and standards of gerontological nursing practice,* Washington, DC, 1995c, The Association.

Armmer FA, Humbles P: Extending health care to urban African-Americans via parish nursing, *Nurs Health Care* 16(2):64, 1995.

Association of Rehabilitation Nurses: *The gerontological rehabilitation nurse,* Glenview, Ill, 1997, The Association.

Ballard TM: The need for well-prepared nurse administrators in long-term care, *Image J Nurs Sch* 27(2):153, 1995.

Boyd ML, Fischer B, Davidson AW, Neilsen CA: Community-based case management for chronically ill older adults, *Nurs Manage* 27(11):31, 1996.

Braun J: Editorial, *Geriatr Nurs* 14(2):62, 1993.

Brennan P: Keep the nurse in nursing informatics! A comment on guidelines for reporting innovations in computer-based informatics systems for nursing. *Computers Nurs* 7(5):239, 1989.

Buchanan LM: Therapeutic nursing intervention knowledge and outcome measures for advanced practice, *Nurs Health Care* 15(4):190, 1994.

Callender-Price N: Nurse practitioners move into acute care, *Nurseweek* 9(15):1, 1996.

Canadian Gerontological Nursing Association: *Gerontological Nursing Guidelines,* GNA, PO Box 368, Postal Station K, Toronto, Ontario, M4P2GT, Canada.

Carnignan AM: Community college-nursing home partnership: impact on nursing care, *Geriatr Nurs* 13(3):139, 1992.

Certification for case managers: CCM certification guide, Rolling Meadows, Ill, 1992, Certification of Insurance Rehabilitation Specialists Commission.

Christensen JC: Well elder clinics: changing a student's views on aging, *Geriatr Nurs* 17(2):91, 1996.

Davis Doughty SE: Developing markets for advanced nursing practice. In Hamrick AB, Spross JA, Hanson CM: *Advanced nursing practice: an integrative approach,* Philadelphia, 1996, WB Saunders.

Engebretson J: Comparison of nurses and alternate healers, *Image J Nurs Sch* 28(2):95, 1996.

Engler MB, Engler MM: An emerging new role: cardiovascular nurse interventionist, *Nurs Health Care* 15(4):199, 1994.

Fiesta J: *Law for the nurse manager, legal update,* part 1, 27(5):22, 1995.

Fletcher K, Small N: Evolving roles of GNPs, *NCGNP Newsletter* 33:3, 1994.

Fulmer TT, Matzo M: *Strengthening geriatric nursing education,* New York, 1995, Springer.

Fulmer TT, Walker MK: Overview: goals of critical care nursing of the elderly. In Fulmer TT, Walker MK, editors: *Critical care nursing of the elderly,* New York, 1992, Springer.

Gaines JE: Here comes everybody in APN, *Advanced Practice Nurse,* p 42, Spring/Summer, 1994.

Gaines JE, Martin AR: A new scientific star, *Advanced Practice Nurse,* p 39, Spring/Summer 1994.

Garland S: Homes with nursing that aren't nursing homes, *Bus Week* May 4:182, 1992.

Gill HS, Balsano AE: The move toward subacute care: key considerations for any nursing home wanting to make a go of it, *Nurs Homes* (5):7, 1994.

Gray BB: Subacute care market creates RN opportunities, *Nurseweek* 7(12):1, 1994.

Gropper R: Personal communication, American Nurses' Association Credentialing Division, Washington, DC, March 5, 1997.

Gross S, Morrow J: Going solo: NP entrepreneurs, part I, *CCNP Newsletter* 6(6):3, 1993.

Hanner MB, Home health nursing: understanding the practice, *Geriatr Nurs* 15(6):328, 1994.

Haworth MJ: Hospital-based community outreach to medically isolated elderly, *Geriatr Nurs* 14(1):23, 1993.

Hirst SP, King T, Church J: The emergence of gerontological nursing education in Canada, *Geriatr Nurs* 17(3):120-122, 1996.

Joint Commission on Accreditation of Healthcare Organizations: Home care standards and written policies and procedures, *Joint Commission Perspectives* 16(1):19, 1996.

Joint Commission on Accreditation of Healthcare Organizations: *1995 accreditation manual for home care,* vol 1, *Standards,* Oakbrook Terrace, Ill, 1994, Joint Commission on Accreditation of Healthcare Organizations.

Kelley B: Kudos to Page and Arena, *Image J Nurs Sch* 27(2):89, 1995.

Kersbergen AL: Case management: a rich history of coordinating care to control costs, *Nurs Outlook* 44(4):19, 1996.

Klein S: *A national agenda for geriatric education: white papers,* Washington, DC, 1995, US Department of Health and Human Services, Public Health Service, Health Resources and Services Administration, Bureau of Health Professions.

Lamb GS, Stempel JE: Nurse case management from the client's view: growing as insider-expert, *Nurs Outlook* 42(1):7, 1994.

Lambert VA, Lambert CE: Advanced practice nurses: starting an independent practice, *Nurs Forum* 31(1):11, 1996.

Landis B: A locum tenens position: how it works for one NP, *Nurs Practitioner World News* 2(1):5, 1997.

Luggen AS: NGNA's strategic plan, *Geriatr Nurs* 18(1):33, 1997.

Luggen AS, editor: *Core curriculum for gerontologic nursing,* St Louis, 1996, Mosby.

Maddox G, editor: *Encyclopedia of aging,* New York, 1995, Springer.

Magit J: Personal communication, Senior Health and Peer Counseling Center, Santa Monica, Calif, 1980.

Mahn VA, Spross JA: Nurse case management as an advanced practice role. In Hamrick AB, Spross JA, Hason CM: *Advanced nursing practice: an integrative approach,* Philadelphia, 1996, WB Saunders.

Martin PD, Hutchinson SA: Negotiating symbolic space: strategies to increase NP status and value, *Nurs Pract* 22(1):89, 1997.

Mason M: Nurse on the case, *Advanced Practice Nurse,* p 2, Spring/Summer, 1994.

Matzo M: Baccalaureate nursing students as research clinicians in long term care, *Geriatr Nurs* 15:250, 1994.

Mezey MD, Fulmer TT: Nursing. In Maddox GI, editor: *The encylcopedia of aging,* New York, 1995, Springer.

Michela NJ: Jumping the hurdles of high-tech home care, 16(6):249, 1995.

Michalek MR: The advanced practice job search, *Advanced Practice Nurse,* p 12, Spring/Summer, 1994.

Monea H: *Peer counseling: perspectives in learning with the older adult,* San Francisco, 1985, Commission on Aging.

Morgan L: Nurse-run clinic lightens the load for crowded ED, *Nurseweek* 9(21):6, 1996.

Newman M, Lamb G, Michaels C: Nursing case management: the coming together of theory and practice, *Nurs Health Care* 12:404, 1991.

NICHE Project Faculty: Geriatric models of care: which one's right for your institution? *Am J Nurs* 94(7):21, 1994.

Page NE, Arena DM: Rethinking the merger of the clinical nurse specialist and the nurse practitioner roles, *Image J Nurs Sch* 26(4):315, 1994.

Pearson LJ: Annual update of how each state stands on legislative issues affecting advanced nursing practice, *Nurs Pract* 22(1):18, 1997.

Petit JM: Continuing care retirement communities and the role of the wellness nurse, *Geriatr Nurs* 15(1):28, 1994.

Quinn J: *National committee issues guidelines for case management of long term care,* news release, Connecticut Community Care, Inc, Dec 13, 1994.

Redding BA: Titling and the advanced practice nurse, *Advanced Practice Nurse,* p 7, Spring/Summer, 1994.

Reigle J: Ethical decision-making skills. In Hamrick AB, Spross JA, Hason CM: *Advanced nursing practice: an integrative approach,* Philadelphia, 1996, WB Saunders.

Ruiz BA, Tabloski PA, Frazier SM: The role of gerontological advanced practice nurses in geriatric care, *J Am Geriatr Soc* 43(9):1061, 1995.

Schank MJ, Weis D, Matheus R: Parish nursing: ministry of healing, *Geriatr Nurs* 17(1):11, 1996.

Sears LE, Wilson CS: Leadership experience in gerontological nursing for associate degree students in long term care, *Geriatr Nurs* 17:128, 1996.

Shuren AW: The blended role of the clinical nurse specialist and the nurse practitioner. In Hamrick AB, Spross JA, Hason CM: *Advanced nursing practice: an integrative approach,* Philadelphia, 1996, WB Saunders.

Stahl DA: Case management in subacute care, *Nurs Manage* 27(8):20, 1996.

Strumpf NE: Innovative gerontological practices as models for health care delivery, *Nurs Health Care* 15(10):522, 1994.

Stulginsky MM: Nurses' home health experience. Part I. The practice setting, *Nurs Health Care* 14(8):402, 1993a.

Stulginsky MM: Nurses' home health experience. Part II: The unique demands of home visits, *Nurs Health Care* 14(9):477, 1993b.

Sweeney JM: Nurses in home care: a success story, *Geriatr Nurs* 17(4):187, 1996.

Turley JP: Toward a model for nursing informatics, *Image J Nurs Sch* 28(2):95, 1996.

von Sternberg T: Post-hospital sub-acute care: an example of a managed care model, *J Am Geriatr Soc* 45(1):87, 1997.

Wolanin MO: Ceremony spotlights legendary nurses, *Am Nurs* 28(5):26, 1996.

Wolanin MO: Good old days? *Am Nurs* 28(4): 29, 1996.

Yurchuck ER, Brower T: Faculty preparation for gerontological nursing, *J Gerontol Nurs* 20(1):17, 1994.

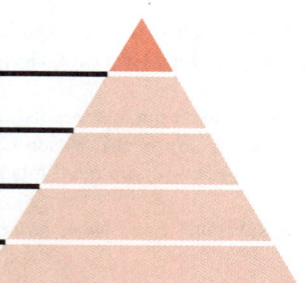

NGNA Strategic Plan Derived from the DELPHI Survey: Results

General Results of DELPHI

Question	Results	N	Mean	Mode	Median
What is the future direction of gerontologic nursing?	1. Focus on the education of nursing students and caregivers about normal aging, assessment and management skill; gerontology questions on NCLEX.	15	1.0	1	2.0
	2. Provide managed care in the outpatient setting; increase emphasis on wellness and home care; increase skills to keep elders at home and out of the hospital.	11	1.7	1	1.0
	3. Conduct clinically based gerontology research	9	2.0	1	1.5
What are major issues and trends affecting gerontology nursing?	1. The changes in the health care system and reform in all settings	21	1.9	1	1.0
	2. Federal regulations related to (a) decreases in Medicare and Medicaid funding; (b) more third-party payment directly to nurses; (c) federal budget reduction proposed impact on long-term care; (d) proposed changes in Social Security benefits	22	2.3	2	2.0
	3. Increasing numbers of aging individuals, especially older women and the old-old; increased numbers of baby boomers; more healthy young people	20	2.5	2	2.0
What are the critical issues and problems of gerontologic nurses?	1. Changes need to be effected in the health care system to provide safe care to elderly clients	19	2.1	1	1.5
	2. The poor gerontologic knowledge/skills in basic nursing programs need to be addressed	10	2.3	1	2.0
	3. The lack of educationally and experientially prepared gerontologic nurses in the workplace needs to be addressed	13	2.5	1	2.0
What are the critical issues and problems of older adults?	1. Fear and the loss of insurance/Medicare or Social Security	11	2.3	1	2.0
	2. Economics, money, decreasing resources, poverty	14	2.6	1	2.5
	3. Refusal of insurance companies to pay for needed services	10	2.7	2	2.5
What should be the future focus of research conducted by gerontology nurses?	1. Provide methods of promoting and maintaining health and independence of older adults	20	2.1	1	2.0
	2. Measure the efficacy of interventions	13	2.5	1,2	2.0
	3. Discern nursing actions to motivate older adults to change lifestyles and behaviors	13	2.8	1	3.0
What are advanced practice issues?	1. Clear definition of roles and titles: NP, CNS, APN, GN	13	1.9	2	2.0
	2. Adequate opportunities for clinical practice in educational programs in terms of preceptors and role models.	17	2.3	1,2,3	2.0
	3. Faculty prepared to teach advanced practice	17	2.5	1	2.0
Does replacing nurses with nonprofessionals affect care?	1. Replacement results in substandard, compromised quality of care for those patients with complex health and socioeconomic problems and emotional problems	22	1.8	1	1.0
	2. It depends on who leads the team—a good gerontology NP can direct activities, and ancillary personnel can provide good care	21	2.7	2	2.0
	3. A change in quality will affect nursing's professional image	14	2.9	2	3.0
What are the problems of an aging workforce?	1. Institutions must enforce geriatrics as an important nursing specialty to recruit new nurses into the field	9	1.8	1	1.0
	2. School of nursing must promote gerontology as a practice area that all students need and must require a gerontology course	23	2.1	1	2.0
	3. Role models and mentors must be found for nursing students so the new nurses will want to work with older adults after graduation	15	2.1	1	2.0

From Luggen AS: NGNA's strategic plan, *Geriatr Nurs* 18(1):33, 1997.

Question	Results	N	Mean	Mode	Median
With the population aging, can nursing meet care needs?	1. Faculty in nursing school need to encourage gerontology nursing practice and involve new nurses in clinical care of older adults	22	2.1	1	2.0
	2. Courses in gerontology need to be required in nursing schools	23	2.4	1	2.0
	3. Gerontologic nursing can be portrayed as an exciting practice; the uniqueness of the specialty can be shown; scholarships, fellowships, and internship can be given	20	2.5	1	2.0
Is gerontology content adequately represented in the curriculum?	(ADN)				
	1. AD programs have inadequate content	10	1.7	1	1.5
	2. AD programs have little content about elders except in the clinical practicum; content is integrated and has an illness focus	16	1.8	1	2.0
	3. Content is improving but needs to be stronger	16	1	1	2.0
	(BSN)				
	1. Gerontology content is usually integrated but difficult to find	13	1.3	1	1.0
	2. Faculty do not value gerontology content	21	1.3	1	1.0
	3. Content is found in assessment and community health courses.	10	1.7	2	2.0
	(MSN)				
	1. Unless the student's major is gerontology, content is not clearly delineated	19	1.1	1	1.0
	2. Students in adult health specialties should be getting this content	16	1.5	1,2	1.5
	3. It depends on the program administration and number of faculty prepared to address issues of older adults	16	1.9	2	2.0
What strategies should be used to teach gerontology nursing?	1. Begin with well elders in community settings; learn elder life history and coping patterns. Student should monitor elder throughout curriculum to experience changing needs	22	2.1	1	1.0
	2. Conduct projects with healthy elders, such as health screening. Visit long-term care facilities and adopt an older person for the semester or the year. Interview older adults throughout all courses	24	2.5	2	2.0
	3. Use active models of education that foster thinking, problem solving, communication, team building, and multidisciplinary skills	19	3.0	3	3.0
What should be the educational preparation of nurses and other health care professionals who care for older adults?	1. Include gerontology in the curriculum, with the same emphasis as other specialty areas	25	1.5	1	1.0
	2. Provide gerontology education and consultation for nurses who care for this population. Maintain continuing education for those without formal preparation	21	2.2	1	2.0
	3. Design a core curriculum of gerontology nursing base. NGNA could assume responsibility for development and dissemination of this document	21	2.6	2	2.0
What are other significant areas of importance to gerontologic nurses in caring for older adults?	1. Federal regulations and paperwork: the nurse has become the regulations police. Survey teams do not assess patients' quality of care/life. They focus on unpredictable, arbitrary parameters. This inhibits creativity in caring and takes nurses from the bedside	18	2.2	1	2.0
	2. Our image: gerontologic nursing needs respect and needs to improve its image nationally	16	2.7	1,2	2.5
	3. Advocacy: political advocacy is needed for passage of legislation to benefit older adults and gerontology nurses	20	2.3	1	3.0
	4. Chronic health disease and long-term care	11	2.8	2,4	3.0

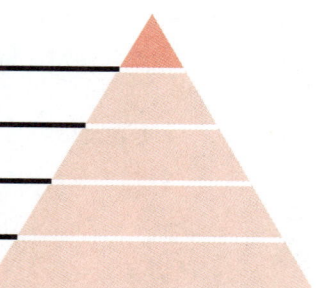

NANDA-Approved Nursing Diagnoses: 1997-1998

Activity intolerance
Activity intolerance, risk for
Adaptive capacity, decreased: intracranial
Adjustment, impaired
Airway clearance, ineffective
Anxiety
Aspiration, risk for
Body image disturbance
Body temperature, altered, risk for
Bowel incontinence
Breastfeeding, effective
Breastfeeding, ineffective
Breastfeeding, interrupted
Breathing pattern, ineffective
Cardiac output, decreased
Caregiver role strain
Caregiver role strain, risk for
Communication, impaired verbal
Community coping, potential for enhanced
Community coping, ineffective
Confusion, acute
Confusion, chronic
Constipation
Constipation, colonic
Constipation, perceived
Coping, defensive
Coping, family: potential for growth
Coping, ineffective family: compromised
Coping, ineffective family: disabling
Coping, ineffective individual
Decisional conflict (specify)
Denial, ineffective
Diarrhea
Disuse syndrome, risk for
Diversional activity deficit
Dysreflexia
Energy field disturbance
Environmental interpretation syndrome, impaired
Family processes, altered: alcoholism
Family processes, altered
Fatigue
Fear

Fluid volume deficit
Fluid volume deficit, risk for
Fluid volume excess
Gas exchange, impaired
Grieving, anticipatory
Grieving, dysfunctional
Growth and development, altered
Health maintenance, altered
Health-seeking behaviors (specify)
Home maintenance management, impaired
Hopelessness
Hyperthermia
Hypothermia
Incontinence, functional
Incontinence, reflex
Incontinence, stress
Incontinence, total
Incontinence, urge
Infant behavior, disorganized
Infant behavior, disorganized: risk for
Infant behavior, organized: potential for enhanced
Infant feeding pattern, ineffective
Infection, risk for
Injury, perioperative positioning: risk for
Injury, risk for
Knowledge deficit (specify)
Loneliness, risk for
Management of therapeutic regimen, community: ineffective
Management of therapeutic regimen, families: ineffective
Management of therapeutic regimen, individual: effective
Management of therapeutic regimen, individuals: ineffective
Memory, impaired
Mobility, impaired physical
Noncompliance (specify)
Nutrition, altered: less than body requirements
Nutrition, altered: more than body requirements
Nutrition, altered: risk for more than body requirements
Oral mucous membrane, altered
Pain
Pain, chronic

Parent/infant/child attachment, altered: risk for
Parental role conflict
Parenting, altered
Parenting, altered, risk for
Peripheral neurovascular dysfunction, risk for
Personal identity disturbance
Poisoning, risk for
Post-trauma response
Powerlessness
Protection, altered
Rape-trauma syndrome
Rape-trauma syndrome: compound reaction
Rape-trauma syndrome: silent reaction
Relocation stress syndrome
Role performance, altered
Self-care deficit, bathing/hygiene
Self-care deficit, dressing/grooming
Self-care deficit, feeding
Self-care deficit, toileting
Self-esteem disturbance
Self-esteem, chronic low
Self-esteem, situational low
Self-mutilation, risk for
Sensory/perceptual alterations (specify) (visual, auditory, kinesthetic, gustatory, tactile, olfactory)

Sexual dysfunction
Sexuality patterns, altered
Skin integrity, impaired
Skin integrity, impaired, risk for
Sleep pattern disturbance
Social interaction, impaired
Social isolation
Spiritual distress (distress of the human spirit)
Spiritual well-being, potential for enhanced
Suffocation, risk for
Swallowing, impaired
Thermoregulation, ineffective
Thought processes, altered
Tissue integrity, impaired
Tissue perfusion, altered (specify type) (renal, cerebral, cardiopulmonary, gastrointestinal, peripheral)
Trauma, risk for
Unilateral neglect
Urinary elimination, altered
Urinary retention
Ventilation, inability to sustain spontaneous
Ventilatory weaning response, dysfunction (DVWR)
Violence, risk for: directed at others
Violence, risk for: self-directed

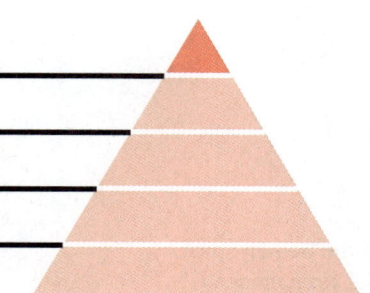

Geriatric Research, Education, and Clinical Centers (GRECCs)

DEPARTMENT OF VETERANS AFFAIRS
VETERANS HEALTH ADMINISTRATION

THOMAS T. YOSHIKAWA, M.D.
Assistant Chief Medical Director for Geriatrics and
    Extended Care (114)
VA Central Office
810 Vermont Ave, N.W.
Washington, DC 20420
(202) 535-7165
FTS 535-7165

MARSHA E. GOODWIN, R.N.-C., M.A., M.S.N.
Director, Geriatrics and Grants Management Service (114B)
VA Central Office
810 Vermont Ave, N.W.
Washington, DC 20420
(202) 535-7531
(FTS) 535-7531

GRECC Directors

Ann Arbor GRECC
VA Medical Center
Ann Arbor, MI 48105
(313) 761-7686
FTS 700/373-7493

Baltimore GRECC
VA Medical Center
Baltimore, MD 21201
(410) 605-7185
FTS 700/580-5410

Boston GRECC: Bedford Division
VA Medical Center
Bedford, MA 01730
(617) 275-7500
FTS 700/840-0631

Boston GRECC Brockton/West Roxbury Division
VA Medical Center
West Roxbury, MA 02132
(617) 323-7700, Ex. 5992
FTS 700/885-5992

Durham GRECC
VA Medical Center
Durham, NC 27705
(919) 286-6932
FTS 700/671-6932

Gainesville GRECC
VA Medical Center
Gainesville, FL 32602
(904) 374-6077
FTS 700/947-6077

Little Rock GRECC
VA Medical Center
Little Rock, AR 72206
(501) 660-2031
FTS 700/742-2031

Madison GRECC
VA Medical Center
Madison, WI 53705
(608) 262-7089
FTS 700/364-7089

Miami GRECC
VA Medical Center
Miami, FL 33125
(305) 324-3388
FTS 700/351-3388

Minneapolis GRECC
VA Medical Center
Minneapolis, MN 55417
(612) 725-2051
FTS 700/780-2051

Palo Alto GRECC
VA Medical Center
Palo Alto, CA 94304
(415) 858-3933
FTS 700/463-4146

St. Louis GRECC
VA Medical Center
St. Louis, MO 63125
(314) 894-6510
FTS 700/280-6510

Salt Lake City GRECC
VA Medical Center
Salt Lake City, UT 84148
(801) 582-1565 Ex. 2475
FTS 700/588-2475

San Antonio GRECC
VA Medical Center
San Antonio, TX 78284
(210) 617-5197
FTS 700/779-5197

Seattle/American Lake GRECC: Seattle Division
VA Medical Center
Seattle, WA 91808
(206) 764-2308
FTS 700/396-2308

American Lake Division
VA Medical Center
Tacoma, WA 98483
(206) 582-8440, Ex. 6930
FTS 700/396-6930

Sepulveda GRECC
VA Medical Center
Sepulveda, CA 91343
(818) 895-9311
FTS 700/966-9311

West Los Angeles GRECC
VA Medical Center
Los Angeles, CA 90073
(310) 824-4301
FTS 700/748-6105

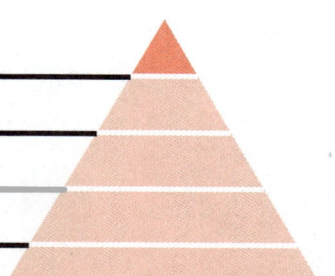

Note: Extensive federal, national, state, and university organizations can be found in the *Directory of Aging Resources* published by *Business Publishers,* Directory Division, 951 Pershing Dr., Silver Spring, MD 20910-9973.

Administration on Aging
330 Independence Ave. SW
Cohen Bldg, Room 4760
Washington, DC 20201
(202) 619-0556

Alzheimer's Association
919 N. Michigan Ave.
Suite 1000
Chicago, IL 60657-1676
(312) 335-8870

Alzheimer's Disease Education and Referral Center
P.O. Box 8250
Silver Spring, MD 20907-8250

American Academy of Home Care Physicians
10480 Little Patuxeny Parkway
Suite 760A
Columbia, MD 21044
(410) 730-1623

American Academy of Physical Medicine and Rehabilitation
122 S. Michigan Ave.
Suite 1300
Chicago, IL 60603-6107
(312) 922-9366

American Association for Continuity of Care
1730 N. Lynn St.
Suite 502
Arlington, VA 22209
(703) 525-1191

American Association of Diabetes Educators
444 N. Michigan Avenue, Suite 1240
Chicago, IL 60611-3901

American Association for Geriatric Psychiatry
P.O. Box 376A
Greenbelt, MD 20768
(301) 220-0952

American Association for International Aging
1133 20th St. NW
Suite 333
Washington, DC 20036
(202) 822-8893

American Association of Homes and Services for the Aging
901 E Street NW
Suite 500
Washington, DC 20004

American Association of Public Health Dentistry (AAPHD)
10619 Jousting Lane
Richmond, VA 23235-3838
(804) 272-8344

American Association of Retired Persons (AARP)
601 E Street NW
Washington, DC 20049
(202) 434-2277

American Bar Association Commission on Legal Problems of the Elderly
1800 M St. NW
Washington, DC 20036
(202) 331-2297

American Cancer Society National Office
1599 Clifton Rd. NE
Atlanta, GA 30329
(404) 320-3333

American College of General Practitioners
330 East Algonquin Road
Arlington Heights, IL 60005
(800) 323-0794

American College of Healthcare Administrators
325 S. Patrick St.
Alexandria, VA 22314
(703) 549-5822

American College of Nursing Home Administrators
4650 East-West Freeway
Washington, DC 20014

American Congress of Rehabilitation Medicine
5700 Old Orchard Rd.
Skokie, IL 60077
(708) 966-0095

American Council of the Blind
1155 15th St. NW
Suite 720
Washington, DC 20005
(202) 467-5081

American Dental Association
211 East Chicago Ave.
Chicago, IL 60611-2678
(312) 440-2500

American Dietetic Association
216 W. Jackson Blvd.
Suite 800
Chicago, IL 60605-6995
(312) 899-0040

American Federation for Aging Research (AFAR)
1414 Avenue of the Americas
18th Floor
New York, NY 10019
(212) 752-AFAR
FAX: (212) 832-2298

American Foundation for the Blind, Inc.
National Services on Aging
15th West 16th St.
New York, NY 10011
(212) 620-2000

American Geriatric Society
770 Lexington Ave.
Suite 400
New York, NY 10021
(212) 308-1414

American Health Care Apparel
327 Northhampton St.
Easton, PA 18042

American Health Care Association
1201 L St. NW
Washington, DC 20005-4014
(202) 842-4444

American Heart Association
7320 Greenville Ave.
Dallas, TX 75231
(214) 373-6300

American Hospital Association (AHA)
840 Lakeshore Dr.
Chicago, IL 60611
(312) 280-6357

American Lung Association
1740 Broadway
New York, NY 10019-4373
(212) 315-8700

American Medical Association (AMA)
515 N. State St.
Chicago, IL 60610
(312) 464-5000

American Medical Directors Association (AMDA)
10480 Little Patuxeny Parkway
Suite 760
Columbia, MD 21044
(800) 876-2632

American Nurses' Association
600 Maryland Ave. SW
Washington, DC 20024-2571
(202) 544-4444
FAX: (202) 544-2262

American Nursing Home Association
(see American Health Care Association)

American Occupational Therapy Association
1383 Piccard Dr.
P.O. Box 1725
Rockville, MD 20849-1725
(301) 948-9626

American Optometric Association
1505 Prince Street, Suite 300
Alexandria, VA 22314
(703) 739-9200

American Parkinson's Disease Association
60 Bay St.
Suite 401
Staten Island, NY 10301
(800) 223-ADPA or (718) 981-8001

American Psychiatric Association
1400 K St. NW
Washington, DC 20005
(202) 682-6000
FAX: (202) 682-6114

American Psychiatric Nurses' Association
6900 Grove Road
Thorofare, NJ 08086

American Psychological Association
Division of Adult Development
750 First St. NE
Washington, DC 20002-4242
(202) 336-5500

American Public Health Association
1015 15th St. NW
Washington, DC 20005
(202) 789-5600

American Public Welfare Association
810 1st St. NE
Suite 500
Washington, DC 20002-4267
(202) 682-0100

American Red Cross
National Headquarters
430 17th St. NW
Washington, DC 20006
(202) 737-8300

American Society for Geriatric Dentistry
211 East Chicago Ave.
17th Floor
Chicago, IL 60611
(312) 440-2500 x 2660

American Society for Parenteral and Enteral Nutrition
8630 Fenton St.
Suite 412
Silver Spring, MD 20910-3805
(301) 587-6315

American Society of Consultant Pharmacists
1321 Duke St.
Alexandria, VA 22314-3563
(703) 739-1300
FAX: (703) 739-1321

American Society on Aging
833 Market St.
Suite 511
San Francisco, CA 94103-1824
(415) 882-2910

American Speech-Language-Hearing Association
10801 Rockville Pike
Rockville, MD 20852
(301) 897-5700
(800) 638-8255

Arthritis Foundation
P.O. Box 19000
Atlanta, GA 30326
(404) 872-7100

Association for Gerontology in Higher Education
1001 Connecticut Ave. NW
Suite 410
Washington, DC 20036-5504
(202) 429-9277

Association of Hospital-Based Nursing Facilities
Suite 501A
3500 Masons Hill Business Park
Huntington Valley, PA 19006
(215) 657-9992

Association of Humanistic Gerontology
1711 Solano Ave.
Berkeley, CA 94707

Association of University Programs in Health Administration
Office of Long-term Care and Aging
1911 North Fort Meyer Dr.
Suite 503
Arlington, VA 22209
(703) 524-5500

Children of Aging Parents
1609 Woodbourne Rd.
Suite 302-A
Levittown, PA 19057
(215) 945-6900

Commission on Legal Problems of the Elderly
1800 M St. NW
Washington, DC 20036
(202) 331-2297

Concern in Care of the Aging
(See American Association of Homes for the Aging)

Consultant Dietitians in Healthcare Facilities
P.O. Box 60
Armada, MI 48005
(313) 784-9766

Consumer Nutrition Hotline
(800) 366-1655

Consumer Product Safety Commission
5401 Westbound Ave.
Washington, DC 20207
(301) 492-6580

Council of Nursing Home Services
(See American Nurses Association)

Department of Veterans Affairs
Veterans Health Administration
Nursing Service Program (118c)
810 Vermont Ave. NW
Washington, DC 20420
(202) 299-4000

Design for Aging/Architecture for Health
American Institute of Architects
1735 New York Ave. NW
Washington, DC 20006
(202) 626-7361

Dietary Managers Association
One Pierce Place
Suite 1220W
Itasca, IL 60143-3111
(708) 775-9200

Dietitians and Health Care Facilities Consultant
P.O. Box 2067
Pensacola, FL 32513
(414) 432-9224

Directory of Aging Resources
Business Publishers, Inc.
951 Pershing Drive
Silver Springs, MD 20910-4464
Updated periodically, Cost approx $100
(800) BPI-6737
FAX: (301) 585-9075

Drug Enforcement Administration
Washington, DC 20537
(202) 307-1000

Family Caregiver Alliance
425 Bush Street, Suite 500
San Francisco, CA 94108

Federal Council on Aging
330 Independence Ave. SW
Room 4280 HHS-N
Washington, DC 20201

Food and Drug Administration (FDA)
Professional and Consumer Programs
5600 Fishers Lane
Suite 1685
Parklawn Bldg.
Rockville, MD 20857
(301) 443-5006

Foundation for Hospice and Home Care
519 C St. NE
Washington, DC 20002
(202) 547-6586

Gerontological Nutritionists
4103 44th St.
Sacramento, CA 95820
(916) 451-7149

Gerontological Society of America
1275 K St. NW
Suite 350
Washington, DC 20005-4006
(202) 842-1275

Gray Panthers
1424 16th St. NW
Suite 602
Washington, DC 20036
(202) 387-3111

Healthcare Financial Management Association
1050 17th Street N.W., Suite 700
Washington, DC 20036
(202) 296-2920

Healthcare Financing Administration
200 Independence Avenue S.W.,
Suite 314G
HHH Building
Washington, DC 20201
(202) 690-6113

Health Care Organization
Division of Long Term Care
Room 2F5, Oak Meadows Bldg.
Baltimore, MD 21207
(410) 966-6049

Health Resources and Services Administration
Room 1405, HRSA
5600 Fisher Lane
Rockville, MD 20857
(301) 443-2216

House Select Committee on Aging
House Office Bldg.
Annex 1, Room 712
Washington, DC 20515

Huntington's Disease Society of America
140 W. 22nd St.
New York, NY 10011-2420
(212) 242-1968

Institute for Retired Professionals
New School of Social Research
60 W. 12th St.
New York, NY 10011

International Federation on Aging
Secretariat - Canada
380 St. Antoine St. W.
Suite 3200
Montreal, Quebec
H24 3X7
(514) 987-8191
FAX: (514) 987-1948

International Senior Citizens Association
537 S. Commonwealth Ave.
Suite 4
Los Angeles, CA 90020
(213) 380-0135

**Joint Commission on Accreditation
of Healthcare Organizations**
1 Renaissance Blvd.
Oakbrook Terrace, IL 60181
(708) 916-5600

Lighthouse National Center for Vision and Aging
800 Second Ave.
New York, NY 10017
(212) 808-0077

Managed Care and Aging Network
American Society on Aging
833 Market Street, Suite 511
San Francisco, CA 94103-1824

Managed Care: An AARP Guide
American Association of Retired Persons
611 E Street, NW
Washington, DC 20049

Managed Care Information Center
3100 Highway 138
PO Box 1442
Wall Township, NJ 07719-1442

Mental Disorders of the Aging
Research Branch DCR
Room 11 C-03
5600 Fishers Lane
Rockville, MD 20857

National Alliance of Senior Citizens
2525 Wilson Blvd.
Arlington, VA 22201

National Arthritis Foundation
P.O. Box 19000
Atlanta, GA 30326
(800) 283-7800

National Asian-Pacific Center on Aging
Melbourne Tower
1511 Third Ave.
Suite 914
Seattle, WA 98101
(206) 624-1221

National Association for Hispanic Elderly
3325 Wilshire Blvd.
Suite 800
Los Angeles, CA 90010-1724
(213) 487-1922

National Association for Home Care
519 C St. NE
Washington, DC 20002-5809
(202) 547-7424

National Association for Senior Living Industries
184 Duke of Gloucester St.
Annapolis, MD 21401-2523
(410) 263-0991

National Association of Area Agencies on Aging
1112 16th St. NW
Suite 100
Washington, DC 20036
(202) 296-8130

National Association of Directors of Nursing Administration in Long-Term Care (NADONA-LTC)
10999 Reed Hartman Highway
Suite 229
Cincinnati, OH 45242
(800) 222-0539

National Association of Home Care
519 C Street N.E.
Washington, DC 20002-5809
(202) 547-7424

National Association of Meal Programs
206 E St. NE
Washington, DC 20002
(202) 547-6157

National Association of Medical Equipment Suppliers (NAMES)
625 Slaters Lane
Suite 200
Alexandria, VA 22314
(703) 836-6263

National Association of Nutrition and Aging Services Programs
2675 44th St. SW
Suite 305
Grand Rapids, MI 49509
(616) 531-9909
(800) 999-6262

National Association of Psychiatric Health Systems
1319 F St. NW
Suite 1000
Washington, DC 20004
(202) 393-6700

National Association of Rehabilitation Facilities
1730 N. Lynn St.
Suite 502
Arlington, VA 22209
(703) 525-1191

National Association of Social Workers
750 First Street N.E.
Washington, DC 20002
(202) 408-8600

National Association of Spanish Speaking Elderly
2025 I St. NW
Suite 219
Washington, DC 20006

National Association of State Units on Aging
2033 K St. NW
Suite 304
Washington, DC 20006
(202) 785-0707

National Association of the Deaf
814 Thayer Ave.
Silver Spring, MD 20910-4500
(301) 587-1788
TTY: (301) 587-1789

National Cancer Institute
Office of Communications
Room 10A24
9000 Rockville Pike
Rockville, MD 20892
(800) 4-CANCER

National Caucus and Center on Black Aged
1424 K St. NW
Suite 500
Washington, DC 20005
(202) 637-8400

National Center for Nutrition and Dietetics
(see American Dietetic Association)

National Citizens Coalition for Nursing Home Reform
1224 M. St. NW
Suite 301
Washington, DC 20005
(202) 393-2018

National Clearinghouse on Technology and Aging
College of Health and Human Services
Ohio University
Athens, OH 45701
(614) 593-2133
FAX: (614) 593-0555

National Committee for Prevention of Elder Abuse
(see Institute on Aging)

National Conference on Geriatric Nurse Practitioners
P.O. Box 270101
Fort Collins, CO 80527-0101
(303) 493-7793

National Consumers League
815 15th St. NW
Suite 928
Washington, DC 20005
(202) 639-8140

National Council of Senior Citizens
1311 F St. NW
Washington, DC 20004-1171
(202) 347-8800
FAX: (202) 624-9595

National Council on the Aging
(Includes National Institute of Senior Citizens and
National Institute on Adult Day Care)
409 3rd St. SW
Suite 200
Washington, DC 20024
(202) 479-1200

National Eye Institute
Bldg. 21, Room 6A-32
9000 Rockville Pike
Bethesda, MD 20852
(800) 638-8255

National Gerontological Nursing Association
c/o Mosby
Suite 510
7250 Parkway Dr.
Hanover, MD 21076
(800) 723-0560

National Hospice Organization (NHO)
1901 North Moore St.
Suite 901
Arlington, VA 22202
(703) 243-5900

National Indian Council on Aging
6400 Uptown Blvd. NE
Suite 510W
Albuquerque, NM 87110
(505) 242-9505

National Institute of Mental Health
Public Inquiries
Room 15C-05
5600 Fishers Lane
Rockville, MD 20857
(301) 443-4513

National Institute of Nursing Research
1341 G Street, NW, Suite 600
Washington, DC 20005

National Institute on Aging
Public Information Office
Federal Bldg. 31-C, Room 5C27
9000 Rockville Pike
Bethesda, MD 20892

National Interfaith Coalition on Aging
(see National Council on the Aging)

National Institute of Diabetes and Digestive and Kidney Diseases
National Institutes of Health
3 Information Way
Bethesda, MD 20892-3580

National League for Nursing
350 Hudson St.
New York, NY 10014
(212) 989-9393

National Library Service for the Blind and Physically Handicapped
Library of Congress
1291 Taylor St. NW
Washington, DC 20542

National Meals on Wheels Foundation
1133 20th St. NW
Suite 321
Washington, DC 20036
(202) 463-6039

National Osteoporosis Foundation
1150 17th Street N.W., Suite 500
Washington, DC 20036
(202) 223-2226

National Parkinson's Foundation
Bob Hope Rd.
1501 NW 9th Ave.
Miami, FL 33136
(305) 547-6660

National Policy Center on Housing and Living Arrangements for the Older Americans
University of Michigan
2000 Bonisteel Blvd.
Ann Arbor, MI 48109

National Rehabilitation Association
633 S. Washington St.
Alexandria, VA 22314
(703) 836-0850

National Rehabilitation Information Center
4407 Eighth St. NE
Washington, DC 20017-2277
(202) 635-5822

National Senior Citizens Law Center
1815 H St. NW
Suite 700
Washington, DC 20006
(202) 887-5280

National Stroke Association

8480 East Orchard Rd.
Suite 1000
Englewood, CO 80111-5015
(303) 771-1700

National Student Nurses Association

555 W. 57th St.
Suite 137
New York, NY 10019
(212) 581-2211

Non-Prescription Drug Manufacturer Association

1150 Connecticut Ave. NW
Washington, DC 20036
(202) 429-9260

**Occupational Safety and Health Administration
Information and Consumer Affairs**

200 Constitution Ave. NW
Washington, DC 20210
(202) 523-8151

Older Women's League (OWL)

666 11th St. NW
Suite 700
Washington, DC 20001
(202) 783-6686

Oncology Nursing Society

501 Holiday Dr.
Pittsburgh, PA 15220-2749
(412) 921-7373

Public Health Service

Room 721H
200 Independence Ave. SW
Washington, DC 20201
(202) 245-6867

Senate Special Committee on Aging

Dirksen Senate Office Bldg.
Room 623
Washington, DC 20510

Senior Care Centers of America, Inc.

26 E. Second St., A-1
Moorestown, NJ 08057
(609) 778-0624

Social Security Administration

6401 Security Boulevard
Baltimore, MD 21235

Society for Ambulatory Care Professionals (SACP)

(see American Hospital Association)

U.S. Department of Health and Human Services

Superintendent of Documents
P.O. Box 371954
Pittsburgh, PA 15250-7954

Veterans Administration

(see Department of Veterans Affairs)

Video Respite™

Innovative Caregiving Resources
P.O. Box 17332
Salt Lake City, UT 84117
(801) 272-9446

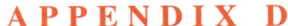

Resources on the Internet

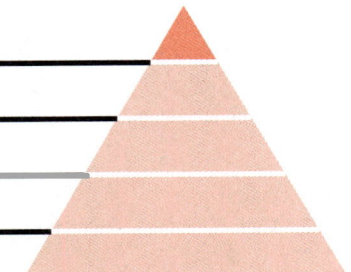

Name/Type	Location
Beginning Note	
Internet and E-Mail Resources on Aging	http://www.aoa.dhhs.gov/aoa/pages/jpostlst.html
Directory of WEB and Gopher Aging Sites	http://www.aoa.dhhs.gov/aoa/webres/craig.htm
Aging in general	
Universities	
Case Western Reserve University	
University Center on Aging and Health	http://www.cwru/edu/CWRU/Bulletin/ArtsSciences/gerontology.html
University of California at San Francisco	
Institute for Health and Aging	http://nurseweb.ucsf.edu/www/iha.htm
University of Maryland	
Baltimore Veterans Administration Center GREEC	http://www.gl.umbc.edu/˙abbott/geri.html
Worldwide	
University of Melbourne (Australia)	
National Ageing Research Institute	http://hermes.its.unimelb.edu.au/U5533827/narihome.html
Simon Fraser University (Canada)	
Gerontology Research Centre	http://biblio.ucs.sfu.ca/gero/
Free University of Berlin (Germany)	
Research Group on Aging and the Life Course	http://fub46.zedat.fu-berlin.de:8080/˙ifs/fall/falleol.htm (English)
	http://fub46.zedat.fu-berlin.de:8080/˙ifs/fall/falldl.htm (German)
TNO Centre for Ageing Research (Netherlands)	http://www.tno.ml/instit/cvo.html
Moscow State University (Russia)	
Institute for Longevity Research	http://alpha.genebee.msu.su/
Alzheimer's disease, dementia, and related disorders	
General	
Alzheimer's Disease Education and Referral Center (ADEAR)	http://www.alzheimers.org/adear
Alzheimer's Disease Research Centers	http://www.biostat.wustl.edu/ADCnet
Genetics	
Genline	http://www.hslib.washington.edu/genline/alzheimer.html
Alzheimer's Disease Genetics Initiative (NIMH)	http://nimh.sratech.com/adann.html
Government (U.S.)	
Experimental Therapeutics Branch (NIH)	http://www.nih.gov/ninds/neurosci/clinical/etb/etbproto.htm
Grant information	
Research on Aging search engine	http://cos.gdb.org/best/fedfund/nih-select/aging.html
Research on Alzheimer's search engine	http://cos.gdb.org/best/fedfund/nih-select/alzheimer.html

Continued

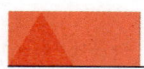

Name/Type	Location
Grant Information—cont'd	
NIH Guide to Grants and Contracts	
NIHGDE-L	NIHGDE-L@list.nih.gov (see article for details)
NIHTOC-L	NIHTOC-L@list.nih.gov (see article for details)
back files	gopher.nih.gov
	http://www.nih.gov/grants/
Claude D. Pepper Older Americans Independence Center	http://www.gl.umbc.edu/˙abbott/pepp2.html
anonymous FTP	ftp.cu.nih.gov
NIH Grant Line bulletin board system	call 301-594-7270 for information
Libraries	
Benjamin B. Green-Field National Alzheimer's Library and Resource Center	(312) 335-9602 (voice)
919 North Michigan Avenue, Suite 1000	(312) 335-0214 (fax)
Chicago, IL 60611-1676	Call the telephone number above for technical information for logging on.
Bulletin boards (direct dial-up access)	
AGE-NET—A bulletin board maintained by the National Association of State Units on Aging and available free to national organizations, federal agencies, advocates, service providers.	For further information by telephone call: 1-800-989-6537.
American Association of Homes and Services for the Aging (AAHSA)—AAHSA maintains an on-line bulletin board for its members which are non-profit nursing homes. Members pay $9.95 for the SpaceWorks software that runs this bulletin board and is installed on a member's personal computer. There is an additional charge of $9.95 per hour to use the service.	Call 1-202-783-2242 for information.
American College of Health Care Administrators—The members of this association are administrators and executives affiliated with both for-profit and not-for-profit facilities. The association has a "LTC On-Line Bulletin Board" for its members. The SpaceWorks bulletin board software which is installed on a member's personal computer is free. There is an hourly charge of $9.95 to use the service.	Call 1-703-739-7900 for information.
National Aging Information Center—Their dial-in bulletin board system accommodates modem speeds between 2400 and 28800.	To connect call 1-202-554-9800.
The Rural Resource—Developed for the rural aging network and funded by the Administration on Aging and the National Association of Area Agencies on Aging.	For further information call the system operator at 1-913-588-1424.
Discussion groups/listservs	
GERINET—The most general of all the discussion groups in aging. It is a very active listserv whose subscribers discuss a wide range of topics in aging and gerontology.	A Web site is at: http://tile.net/tile/cgi-bin/gerinet.html
Supersites for links	
Directory of WEB and Gopher Aging Sites. Compiled by Bruce M. Craig	http://www.aoa/dhhs.gov/aoa/webres/craig.htm
This home page is produced by the U.S. Administration on Aging	
EldercareWeb	
See the full description of this site at #216. It has links to hundreds of full-text documents and direct links to approximately 35 websites.	http://www.ice.net/ ~ kstevens/ELDERWEB.HTM
American Association of Retired Persons—Internet Resource Guide to Aging	gopher://cwis.usc.edu:70/00/Library/Research/Researchby.subject/ SocSci/Gerontology/internet_aarp.txt
Yahoo—Health: Geriatrics and Aging	http://www.yahoo.com/Health/Geriatrics_and_Aging
Yahoo—Society and Culture: Death	http://www.yahoo.com/Society_and_Culture/Death/
Yahoo—Society and Culture: Seniors	http://www.yahoo.com/Society_and_Culture/Seniors/

Continued

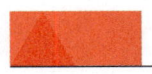

Name/Type	Location
Government agencies and organizations	
United States	
Administration on Aging	http://www.aoa.dhhs.gov or
	gopher://gopher.os.dhhs.gov/11/dhhs/aoa/aoa
Census, Bureau of the	http://www.census.gov/
Health Care Financing Administration	
Administers the Medicare and Medicaid programs	http://www.ssa.gov/hcfa/hcfahp2.html
National Center for Health Statistics	
Includes information about	http://www.cdc.gov/nchswww/nchshome.htm
Social Security Administration (SSA)	http://www.ssa.gov/
Senate Special Committee on Aging	http://www.destek.net/cybermkt/govemail.htm or
	gopher://ftp.senate.gov:70/11/committee/aging
Veteran's Administration	http://www.va.gov/
Australia	
Department of Human Services and Health	http://www.health.gov.au/hsh/struct/aged&cc.htm
Canada	
Health, Canada. Seniors Directorate	http://hpbl.hwc.ca/links/english.html
Available in English and French	http://www.hwc.ca/datahpsb/seniors/senpage.html (English)
	http://www.hwc.ca/datahpsb/seniors/frpage.htm (French)
Community Services and Agencies United States	
Southern California, University of Ethel Percy Andrus	http://www.usc.edu/Univ/entries/gerontology.html
Gerontology Center	http://www.usc.edu/dept/gero/lds/index.html
Leonard Davis School of Gerontology	gopher://cwis.usc.edu/11/University_Information/
	Academic_Departments/
Alzheimer's disease and dementia	
Caregiving	
Alzheimer's Association (U.S.)	http://www.alz.org/
Alzheimer's Association (Victoria, Australia)	http://www.vicnet.net.au/vicnet/community/alzheim/index.html
Yahoo—Health: Disease and Conditions—Alzheimer's Disease	http://www.yahoo.com/Health/Diseases_and_Conditions/
	Alzheimer_s Disease/
Research (Alzheimer's disease and dementia)	
National Institutes of Health (U.S.)—funded research on	for a list of Alzheimer's research locations with grants from NIH:
Alzheimer's disease	gopher://gopher.nih.gov/77/gopherlib/indices/crisp/
	index?alzheimer
	for a list of funded grants in Alzheimer's disease use the Community
	of Science's search engine:
	http://cos.gdb.org/best/fedfund/nih-select/alzheimer.html
Consumer topics	
General	
Health care	http://www.noah.cuny.edu/aging/aging.html
Ask NOAH about: Aging	
Organizations	
Canadian Association of Retired Persons	http://www.mbnet.mb.ca/crm/lifestyl/advoc/carp.html
	Link from #50, section on Long Term Care
National Association for Home Care	http://www.nahc.org/
National Center on Elder Abuse	http://www.cyber.nl/ageingresearch/dutch/pub2.html
National Senior Service Corps	http://www.senior.com/npo/nssc.html
A network of 3 federally-supported programs (foster	
grandparents, senior companions, and retired and senior	
volunteers) that helps people 55 and older find service	
opportunities.	
Service Corps of Retired Executives (SCORE)	http://www.senior.com/score.html
	gopher://www.sbaonline.sba.gov:70/11/Local-Information

Continued

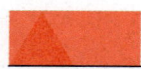

Name/Type	Location
Research (General)	
National Institute on Aging (U.S.) Laboratory of Neurosciences	http://adobe.nia.nih.gov/
National Institutes of Health (U.S.)	http://gos.gdb.org/best/fedfund/nih-select/aging.html
Libraries, information centers, databases	
Alzheimer's Disease Education and Referral Center (ADEAR)	Requests to search their database may be sent to their e-mail address at: adear@alzheimers.org (See also #272)
Andrus Gerontology Center Library (University of Southern California) Includes many links to other Web sites	http://www.usc.edu/Library/Gero/
MEDLINE database search (1986-1995) on search terms "aging" and "theory" Prepared for the National Center for Biotechnology Information (NCBI) GenBank	http://ncbi.nlm.nih.gob/cgi-bin/medline?aging+%26+theory
National Aging Information Center (U.S.) (NAIC) Makes available a "Bibliographic Database of Documents in Aging," "Statistical Tables on Aging"	http://www.ageinfo.org

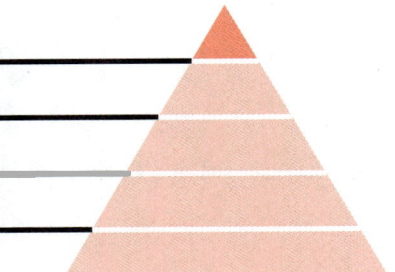

Journals on Aging

AARP News Bulletin
American Association of Retired Persons
601 E. St. NW
Richmond, VA 23235-3838

Age and Aging
Bailliere Tindall
7-8 Henrietta St.
Convent Garden
London, England
WCZE 8QE

Age Page
National Institute of Aging
USDHHS
US Government Printing Office
Washington, DC 20402

Aging International
International Federation on Aging
380 St. Antoine St. W.
Suite 3200
Montreal, Quebec H24 3X7

Aging
Raven Press
1185 Ave. of the Americas
New York, NY 10036

American Journal of Alzheimer's Care and Related
Disorders and Research
Prime National Publishing Corp.
470 Boston Post Rd.
Weston, MA 02193

Answers: For Adult Children of Aging Parents
Publication Consultants
5725 Paradise Drive, Suite 400
Corte Madera, CA 94925-9800

Clinical Gerontologist
Haworth Press
10 Alice St.
Binghamton, NY 13904-1580

Educational Gerontology
Hemisphere Publishing Corp.
1900 Frost Rd.
Suite 101
Briston, PA 19007

Elderly Care
Viking House
17-19 Peterborough Road
Harrow, Middlesex HA1
UK

Experimental Aging Research
Taylor and Francis Publishing
1900 Frost Road, Suite 101
Bristol, PA 19007-1598

Experimental Gerontology
Pergamon Press, Inc.
660 White Plains Rd.
Tarrytown, NY 10591

Generations
American Society on Aging
833 Market St.
Suite 511
San Francisco, CA 94103-1824

Geriatric Nursing
Mosby
11830 Westline Industrial Dr.
St. Louis, MO 63146

Journal of Geriatric Psychiatry and Neurology
Decker Periodicals, Inc.
One James Street South
PO Box 620, L.C.D. 1
Hamilton, Ontario
Canada L8N 3K7

Geriatrics
Avanstar Communications, Inc.
Cleveland, OH 44130

Gerontologist
Gerontological Society of America
1275 K St. NW
Suite 350
Washington, DC 20005-4006

Gerontology and Geriatrics Education
Haworth Press, Inc.
10 Alice St.
Binghamton, NY 13904

Gray Panther Network
Gray Panthers
1424 18th St. NW
Washington, DC 20036

Home Care Provider
Mosby

International Journal of Aging and Human Development
Baywood Publishing Co., Inc.
26 Austin Ave., Box 337
Amityville, NY 11701

Journal of Adult Development
Plenum Publishing Corp
233 Spring Street
New York, NY 10013

Journal of Aging and Health
Sage Publications
2455 Telber Rd.
Newbury Park, CA 91320

Journal of Aging and Social Policy
Haworth Press, Inc.
10 Alice St.
Binghamton, NY 13904

Journal of Case Management
Springer Publishing Company
536 Broadway
New York, NY 10012-3955

Journal of Clinical Geropsychology
Plenum Publishing Corp.
233 Spring Street
New York, NY 10013

Journal of Geriatric Psychiatry
International Universities Press, Inc.
59 Boston Rd.
Madison, CT 06443-1542

Journal of Gerontological Nursing
Slack, Inc.
6900 Grove Rd.
Thorofare, NJ 08086-9447

Journal of Long Term Care Administration
American College of Health Care Administrators
325 S. Patrick Ave.
Alexandria, VA 22314

Journal of Nutrition for the Elderly
Haworth Press, Inc.
10 Alice St.
Binghamton, NY 13904

Journal of Women's Health
Mary Ann Leibert, Inc.
1651 Third Avenue
New York, NY 10128

Modern Maturity
American Association of Retired Persons (Long Beach)
3200 E. Carson St.
Lakewood, CA 90712

New Horizons
NGNA
7250 Parkway Drive
Hanover, MD 21076

Nurse Practitioner
Vernon Publications, Inc.
3000 Northrup Way
Suite 200
Bellevue, WA 98004

Perspectives
Journal of the Gerontological Nursing Association
PO Box 368
Station K
Toronto, Ontario
Canada M4P 2G7

Perspective on Aging
National Council on the Aging
409 3rd St. SW
Washington, DC 20024

Psychology and Aging
American Psychological Association
750 First Street, NE
Washington, DC 20002-4242

Senior Citizens News
National Council of Senior Citizens
1311 F St. NW
Washington, DC 20004-1171

Urologic Nursing
Mosby
11830 Westline Industrial Dr.
St Louis, MO 63146

WOCN
Mosby
11830 Westline Industrial Dr.
St Louis, MO 63146

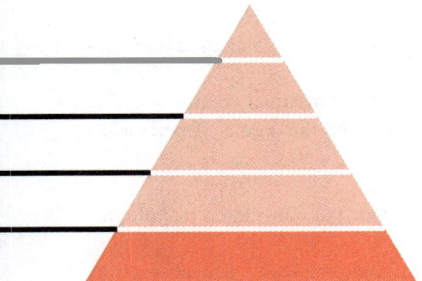

Glossary

accoutrement Implement, appliance, or equipment needed to augment the failing functional capacities of aged persons.

achieved roles Roles that are earned by fulfilling certain expectations; for example, nurse.

actinic keratosis Localized reddish, scaly thickening of the skin that may become cancerous.

activities of daily living Fundamental tasks and demands of daily life.

acupuncture Stimulation of small nerve fibers by twirling needles inserted at acupuncture points identified on body charts developed primarily by the Chinese (and others); meant to relieve pain and illness.

addiction Physiologic dependence on a substance.

advance directives Legally affirm the right of competent adult patients to declare in advance their wishes regarding refusal of aggressive treatment in the face of terminal illness when death is imminent or when unable to express their wishes concerning treatment.

advanced practice nurse (APN) A category of nurse with qualifications that meet the criteria in the nurse's state of residence for legally carrying out advanced practices beyond those of a registered nurse. An advanced practice nurse may be a nurse practitioner, a clinical specialist, a nurse anesthetist, or a midwife; sometimes various combinations of these.

advocacy Representing the interest of others by acting in their behalf or by attempting to influence policies that affect them.

age-integrated Social situations, particularly housing, in which all ages are involved.

ageism Tendency to impose limitations or expectations related soley to chronologic age.

aging Process of growing old, which begins at conception and ends at death.

ancillary General term used to refer to a body of accessory or auxiliary personnel.

anomie Feeling of alienation and meaninglessness related to a breakdown of social norms and values.

anthropometric measurement Measurement of individual muscle mass and body fat; human body size and proportions.

anxiety Vague sense of impending doom characterized by uneasiness and physiologic changes. Usually results from a real or perceived threat to the self.

aphasia Condition usually resulting from a cerebrovascular accident, in which a person has lost the ability to use or understand spoken or written words.

apnea Temporary cessation of respiration.

arcus senilis White rim that forms around the iris of the eye and is particularly common with advancing years.

ascetic One who practices self-denial or self-mortification in the pursuit of ideals and religion.

ascribed roles Roles that are socially defined and occupied by virtue of position; for example, mother.

assisted living Situation in which an elderly person is housed in a separate apartment in a retirement or similar complex and is provided meals and assistance with functional activities, as needed, to remain as independent as possible.

biofeedback Method of learning, by machine feedback, to control autonomic (sympathetic and parasympathetic) functions. Used for stress reduction, symptom control, and awareness of mind/body interrelation.

biorhythm General term applied to the rhythmic cycles of body processes related to internal and external forces.

capitation Method of payment whereby a provider is paid a fixed amount for each enrollee, regardless of the type or amount of services required.

catastrophic reaction Disintegration of behaviors and thoughts, bordering on panic; induced when demands exceed one's coping capacity. Reaction is characteristic of persons with organic mental disorders when exposed to taxing situations.

chore services Regular assistance with personal care and housekeeping.

chronic pain Pain lasting longer than 6 months, may be continuous or intermittent.

chronic illness Irreversible presence, accumulation, or latency of disease states or impairments that involve the total human environment for supportive care and self care, maintenance of function, and prevention of further disability (Lubkin IM: *Chronic illness, impact and interventions,* Boston, 1986, Jones and Bartlett).

chronobiology Scientific study of the effects of time on living systems and biological rhythms.

chronopharmacology The study of interactions of biological rhythms with medicine.

chronotherapy The administration or adjustment of medication to coincide with the biological rhythms of the body.

circadian rhythm Undulation of rhythmic biologic processes, which recur at approximately 24-hour intervals.

cognition Act or process of perceiving or knowing; cerebral functioning.

cohort Persons born in a given year or period of years (usually a decade), aging together, and experiencing sociohistoric events that influence development in a certain way; for example, what influence did the Great Depression have on the cohort born between 1900 and 1910?

comfort State of ease and satisfaction of the bodily wants and freedom from pain and anxiety.

companion Person who gives in-home help, fellowship, information and referral, and limited health aide services to potentially isolated adults.

confidant One with whom intimate thoughts are shared.

confidante Female confidant.

congregate dining Hot meals served in congregate style 5 days per week at community centers.

conservatorship Legal arrangement whereby one person or institution assumes responsibility for an adult individual. When a conservator of person is appointed, it has been determined by the court that the individual is unable to provide for food, clothing, shelter, and health care. When a conservator of estate is appointed, the court has determined that the individual is substantially unable to manage financial affairs. The individual is known as a conservatee, and there is no finding of incompetency. Term used interchangeably with guardianship.

continuing care retirement communities (CCRCs) Retirement communities that offer several levels of living and health care ranging from total independence to total dependence and until death. There are numerous types of plans but most require a large cash outlay up front and a monthly maintenance fee. They are available only to the relatively affluent and provide what amounts to insurance care until death.

court investigator Person appointed by the court, without personal interest in the proceedings, to perform investigations on cases pertaining to adult guardianships and conservatorships in the state of California.

crisis That period of time during which usual patterns of coping are ineffective and result in disorganization of the life of an individual and/or family.

cross-sectional Term used in surveys to describe comparative data of two groups of persons at one point in time.

cross-sequential Data that compare several cohorts at different points in time.

crystallized intelligence Dominant brain activity that encompasses orderly and scientific problem solving, rote memory, vocabulary, facts, and formulas.

culture An aggregate of values, beliefs, and customs that form a collectively shared identity.

defense mechanism Unconscious psychologically protective behaviors used by the individual to maintain psychic equilibrium.

dementia Severe impairment or loss of intellectual capacity and personality integration.

dependency Falling below the established self-sufficiency level physically, mentally, socially, and or economically.

depersonalization Psychiatric term meaning estrangement from oneself, accompanied by a sense of unreality and loss of control of one's body and identity.

deviance Behavior that is contrary to the accepted norms.

dilemma Situation requiring a choice between two equally desirable or undesirable alternatives.

disengagement Term used by Cumming and Henry to describe the mutually desirable withdrawal of society and aged individuals from dynamic interchange.

disorientation Condition in which an individual cannot correctly state where he is, the time or date, and the names of persons he should know.

dysphagia Difficulty in swallowing.

eccentricity Odd or peculiar behavior not considered pathologic.

edentulous Having no teeth.

egocentricity Qualities of self-centeredness, self-absorption, showing little regard or awareness of others' needs.

Elderhostel Adult education program providing low-cost room and board and specially designed classes for elders on college campuses.

elite aged Those elderly, nonagenarians, centenarians, and beyond, who remain alert and functional.

entropic Concept of a limited amount of energy tending toward inertness or "running down."

environmental press Concept that explains negative, maladaptive behaviors as the result of too much or too little environmental stimulation, thus taxing an individual's adaptive capacity.

ethics Moral principles and values held by groups, individuals, and cultures.

eustress Balance of selfishness and altruism, which facilitates self-care and through which an individual has the desire and energy to care about others.

euthanasia Painless death for sufferers of incurable disease who are not close to death; helping those who are dying to exit from life with as little anguish as possible.

euthenic Environment of maximum pleasure, comfort, and safety.

extended care Term covering several types of care beyond hospitalization for acute illness, which includes residential care, intermediate care, and skilled nursing provided in a nursing home.

extrapyramidal reaction Disturbances in the functional unit of the nervous sytsem that regulates motor activities such as muscle control and coordination.

extravert One who is interested in and responsive to others and concerned with the physical and social environment.

fluid intelligence Nondominant brain activity that encompasses spatial awareness, intuitive thought, creative thought, poetry, music, and esthetic appreciation.

forensic Legal or rhetorical issues prepared for argumentation.

foster family care Families trained and reimbursed for care of health-impaired adults in their own homes.

frail aged Elderly who need considerable assistance to manage their lives, and are generally in precarious health and living situations.

functional In psychiatry, a term used to discriminate mental illnesses that have no physiologic base. When generally applied to the aged, it connotes the ability to carry out the activities of daily living.

Ganzfeld effect Completely patternless visual field such as a whitewashed surface, which produces a sensation of inability to see.

generative Actions that promote new growth, creative problem solving, and actualization of another's adaptive capacity.

geron Word of Greek origin meaning an old man.

gerontic nursing Care of the well and ill elderly, based on nursing and gerontologic principles, to develop high-level wellness through nurturant, protective, and generative interventions.

gerontocracy Governing body consisting of old men (and women); the aristocracy of old age.

geropsychiatry Term applied to services for the mentally ill aged.

guardianship Legal arrangement whereby one person or institution assumes responsibility for an adult individual. The individual is known as a ward, and there is a finding of legal incompetency. The person is labeled incompetent and may not enter into contracts; for example, marry or buy items on installment plans. When a guardian of person is appointed, it has been determined by the court that the individual is unable to provide for food, clothing, shelter, and health care. When a guardian of estate is appointed, the court has determined that the individual is substantially unable to manage financial affairs.

hardy aged Those who are able to endure with courage, characterized by a combination of control, competence, and compassion. The hallmark is maintenance of control in one's own life.

health The integration of physical, mental, and social well-being oriented to maximizing one's internal and external environment to experience a balance of harmonious and satisfactory living.

hearty aged Those who are enthusiastic, warmhearted, affectionate, and sincere or any combination of these personality characteristics.

hemiplegia Paralysis of one side of the body resulting from brain or spinal cord trauma; in old age it is usually the result of cerebrovascular accidents.

heuristic Questions that stimulate interest as a means of further investigation.

hierarchy Ascendance in order of importance.

holistic Integration of all needs and interdependence of all functions.

holistic health Shift in emphasis from knowledge of disease to knowledge of human beings and their integrated function; states of disease and health are seen as related to shifts in energy systems.

home health care Intermittent skilled services (medical, rehabilitative, or therapeutic services) provided in the home by registered nurses, licensed practical nurses, nurses' aides, and physical therapists, etc., as prescribed by a physician.

homemaker services Limited personal care of client and light housekeeping for a short period of time.

hospice Concept that combines an alternative to traditional care of the terminally ill, offering a combination of home and, if necessary, institutional care, with a focus on pain control, family involvement, and living to one's fullest until death. Survivors' support services are also a part of hospice care.

humanist Person concerned with human welfare, values, dignity, and a belief in human potential for betterment.

hyperkalemia Abnormally high levels of potassium in blood.

hyperthermia Much higher than normal body temperature.

hypnagogic Vivid images that occur in the period going from wakefulness into sleep.

hypnapompic Dream images that remain as one emerges from sleep into wakefulness.

hypnosis Intense concentration on one thought induced by self or other; characterized by heightened susceptibility to suggestion.

hypokalemia Abnormally low levels of potassium in blood.

hypothermia Abnormal condition in which body temperature is much below normal.

hypothyroidism Decreased secretions of thyroid hormones.

iatrogenic Disorder caused by the manner in which a physician or surgeon diagnoses or treats an illness.

idiosyncratic Individualized, unique, unusual, or peculiar reaction.

impaction Tightly packed, large amount of feces that cannot be evacuated without assistance.

incontinence Inability to control the evacuation of urine or feces.

infraradian rhythm Rhythmic bioprocesses occurring in longer than 24-hour intervals.

interactionist Philosophy of care that emphasizes the effects of interpersonal influence and the alteration of self and other perceptions in a reciprocal manner.

interdisciplinary health care Two or more disciplines that may be involved in the care of one individual.

interiority Development of self-awareness through reflective activity.

introvert Person concerned primarily with his own thoughts and feelings.

kinkeeper Individual within a family who maintains contacts and cultivates relationships in the kin network.

legacy Anything handed down from the past or anticipated to bestow on future generations.

lentigenes Large brown spots (often called liver spots) similar to freckles that appear as one ages on exposed skin areas, particularly the hands. They are the result of erratic pigmentation produced by melanocytes.

life-care See continuing care retirement communities.

life review Process, as defined by Butler, by which individuals integrate and accept the conflicted aspects of their lives; characteristically occurs in old age.

longitudinal Term describing studies of persons over time.

managed care System of providing medical care in which individuals enrolled in a health plan are provided medical care, regardless of the intensity needed or length of time needed, by a select group of providers according to strict guidelines established by the profit or nonprofit adminstrative group. Vertically integrated managed care organizations provide numerous levels of service within one parent or organization, whereas horizontally integrated systems subcontract with a range of providers to provide various levels and types of services. Vertically integrated systems are presently the most common. Average adjusted per capita cost are paid monthly by each enrollee, or, most commonly by Medicare or Medicaid. In 1996 there were almost 5 million Medicare beneficiaries enrolled in 234 risk-based managed care plans across the United States. Risk-based programs must accept all eligible individuals regardless of their health status and are compensated at higher per capita rates. It is to their ultimate economic advantage to keep all members as healthy and functional as possible.

mastery Being in command or control of a situation; intrinsic ego motivation toward learning and accomplishment.

Meals on Wheels Home-delivered hot meals for people unable to prepare own hot meal at noon.

Medicaid Title XIX of the Social Security Act, established in 1965, to make health care available to those persons who had less than the minimum income and did not qualify for Medicare services.

Medicare Title XVIII of the Social Security Act, establishd in 1965, to provide a measure of health coverage to all Social Security recipients.

meditation A form of relaxation and coping with stress that uses a wide variety of techniques to clear the mind of stressful outside interferences.

mentor Wise and trusted advisor or counselor who paves the way for younger colleagues.

metaphors Words or phrases used to comparatively illustrate objects or concepts.

milieu Environmental description that incorporates surroundings, conditions, and ambiance.

morality A personally defined set of values that guide one's behaviors and decisions.

multidisciplinary Team efforts toward planning and interventions formulated and carried out by two or more disciplines.

myth Traditional or legendary story that attempts to convey a basic truth.

napping Periods of sleep, generally during the day, which last from 15 to 60 minutes and do not attain the level of deep sleep.

network System of interrelated supportive structures of persons.

nursing care plan The outcome of a process of nurse and client input which includes assessment, problem identification, goal setting, planning, intervention, and evaluation.

nurturant Qualities of one who provides nourishment, support, encouragement, and education to facilitate the growth and development of another.

oldest-old Those 85 years and older; enduring beyond average life span.

ombudsman Nursing home advocate prepared to represent objectively and sensitively with concerns for resident's realities.

organic Refers to illnesses that have a physiologic base.

pain Whatever the person says it is, existing whenever he or she says it does (McCaffery M, Beebe A: *Pain: clinical manual for nursing practice,* St Louis, 1989, Mosby).

paradoxic agitation Unexpected excitability following administration of analeptic medications.

peer Person who is equal to another in abilities, qualifications, or rank; often used in relation to age or status.

percepts Integrated product or mental set resulting from sensory input, beliefs, and expectations.

personal space Area surrounding an individual (up to 1 m) that is perceived as private and invasion of which is viewed as personally intrusive.

pharmacodynamics The study of the mechanisms of action of drugs and their biochemical and physiologic effects.

pharmacokinetics Absorption, distribution, metabolism, and excretion of drugs.

point of-service-program (POS) Option offered by an HMO in which enrollees may engage doctors not in the provider's cadre, but the costs to the recipient will be higher for selecting this type of plan.

polypharmacy Dispensing of multiple drugs for one individual who has one or several health problems.

power of attorney Authority to act, which one person gives to another, to authorize the donee to perform actions on the donor's behalf. This authority may not be legally valid if the donor can be found to be mentally incompetent at the time of designation or thereafter. There is no action or supervision by the court in these situations.

preretirement The 5 years before retirement when one ordinarily begins making specific retirement plans and may gradually withdraw from the work force.

presbycardia Limited cardiac reserve as a result of old age.

presbycusis Normal decrements in hearing acuity, speech intelligibility, auditory threshold, and pitch discrimination that occur in aging.

presbyopia Decreased ability of the eyes to accommodate for close and detail work as one advances in age.

preventive care giving That which alters the environment or enhances function to prevent or forestall deterioration or illness.

primary care Prevention of disease and promotion of health.

primary relationships Relationships with intimates, close friends, and family.

prolongevity Extension of the life span beyond the present achievable maximum.

protective Qualities of one who guards another from injury or danger and provides a safe environment.

protocol Customs, regulations, and basic expectations that guide actions and decisions in various situations.

pseudodementia Condition in which an individual displays the characteristics of dementia without a physiologic basis; usually induced by profound depression.

psychoactive General term applied to any substance that alters mentation and/or emotion.

psychotropic Substances or activities that alter mind functions.

reality of orientation Term used to designate specific approaches used to assist confused or disoriented persons toward awareness of reality.

reciprocity Mutually satisfying exchange of power and resources.

relocation stress Term used to describe a transitional stressful state experienced by some individuals when moving from one place to another. Though it has been thought to have a negative health impact on the elderly, it appears that adequate preparation and orientation to the move mitigate the negative effects for most.

reminiscence Recollection of past personal experiences and significant events.

remotivation Term used to describe techniques used to stimulate persons to become motivated to learn and interact.

respite Temporary taking in of or providing care to a frail or impaired person in order to give regular caretakers a vacation.

sandwich generation Generation between the old and young who are care givers to both; usually a middle-aged couple.

secondary care Retardation of existing illness or pathologic conditions of physical, mental, social, or environmental origin.

secondary relationships Relationships with those who provide or accept services; acquaintances and friends.

self-actualization Process of most fully developing one's unique capacities.

senile Term pertaining to the supposed characteristics of old age, particularly mental infirmity; often used in a pejorative manner.

sensory deprivation Condition in which there is insufficient stimuli to sensory apparatus to allow integrative percepts to develop.

sensory overload Bombardment of the sensory apparatus by environmental stimuli that reaches levels physically and psychologically overwhelming.

single room occupant (SRO) Designation used in gerontologic literature to describe those older persons who dwell in one room of central-city, low-cost hotels.

Social Security Program established in 1935 as a means of providing income in old age through work life contributions.

social time clock Term used by Neugarten to describe the role expectations that dictate socially appropriate behavior at a given age.

somatotherapies Treatment aimed at curing the ills of the body.

soul food Food that possesses emotional significance and provides personal satisfaction; often has some cultural or traditional origins.

stress Any biopsychosocial stimulus that alters the equilibrium of the body.

substance abuse Overindulgence in and dependence on any substance to an extent that is detrimental to health.

sundowner Term describing one who habitually becomes confused or disoriented in the evening.

Supplemental Security Income Program established in 1972 to provide limited assistance to persons who are aged or disabled and have insufficient income to survive.

surrogate One who substitutes for or takes on the role of another.

tardive dyskinesia Descriptive term for abnormal movements of mouth, tongue, maxilla, and mandible as a result of long-term use of certain drugs, particularly of some major tranquilizers.

telehealth care Form of health care delivery in which telephone and electronic networks of services are available to participants for the management of health problems. These are particularly important for rural and underserved areas.

terminal drop Rapid decline in cognitive function and coping ability that occurs 1 to 5 years before death.

territoriality Emotional attachment to and defense of certain areas related to one's existence.

tertiary care Restorative measures that return the dysfunctional individual to a level of health and well-being.

topographic Freudian conceptualization of the layers of human consciousness.

transcendence Ability to step beyond one's usual human limitations.

transcutaneous nerve stimulation Use of mild electric impulses, which activate large nerve fibers to transmit impulses that prevent pain signals from reaching the brain.

translocation Relocation of an individual, with or without belongings; process of adjusting to new surroundings following displacement or dislocation.

ultradian Biorhythms that occur in cycles of less than 24 hours.

visualization Mode of mind activity that is meant to increase tranquility or promote healing by the imagining of specific situations or scenes.

well-being Achievement of a good and satisfactory existence as defined by the individual.

wellness Balance between one's internal and external environment and one's emotional, social, cultural, and physical processes.

will Legal expression or declaration of a person's mind or wishes as to the disposition of property, to be performed or take effect after death.

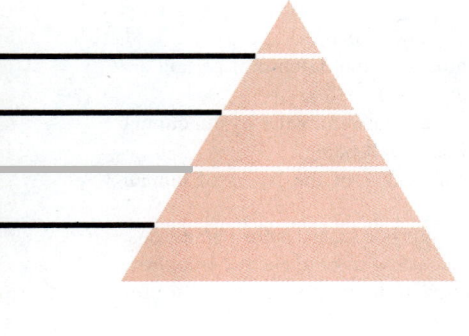

Name Index

Aasen, N, 694
Abel, E, 615
Aber, CS, 729
Abraham, IL, 764
Abrams, WB, 256, 275
Abrass, I, 149
Ackerman, D, 583, 584, 585
Adamchak, DJ, 10
Adams, PF, 269
Adams, RG, 614
Adams, S, 664
Adams, WL, 721
Adelman, M, 593
Adelmann, PK, 707
Adsit, J, 279, 280
Agarwal, S, 35
Aizenstein, S, 390
Akiyama, H, 608, 614
Albert, MS, 793
Albert, SG, 278
Aldwin, C, 692
Alessi, CA, 192
Alexopoulos, GS, 756, 848
Algase, D, 501
Ali, N, 394
Allen, CK, 810
Allen, RE, 810
Allen, SM, 621, 628
Allison, M, 180, 182
Almeida, OP, 755
Altman, DF, 96
Ancoli-Israel, S, 186, 189, 190, 853
Anderson, B, 904
Anderson, CJ, 589
Anderson, JC, 665
Anderson, JW, 171, 186
Anderson, LM, 141
Anderson, MA, 143, 145, 146, 147, 280
Anderson, PB, 45
Anderson, R, 279
Anderson, SJ, 555
Anderson, TB, 610
Anderson, WF, 98
Andres, R, 86, 144
Andrews, JF, 456, 459
Andrews, VH, 687
Anetzberger, G, 564

Angel, JL, 870
Anson, K, 644
Antonovsky, A, 707
Antonucci, T, 614
Antonucci, TC, 608
Applegate, J, 869
Aravanis, SC, 562
Arbore, P, 770
Arbuckle, NW, 614, 730, 945
Arena, DM, 1030
Armmer, FA, 1045
Armstrong, CH, 926
Arras, JD, 269, 492
Ascione, FJ, 364, 367, 369
Ashley, I, 565
Asmuth, MV, 923
Aspland, K, 278
Atchley, RC, 18, 719, 720
Atkinson, P, 752
Avioli, R, 611
Avison, WR, 687
Avorn, J, 832
Back, AP, 447
Back, C, 917
Back, K, 52
Bahr, RT, 23, 24
Bailey, BJ, 276
Bailis, S, 536, 540
Baker, F, 558, 593, 594, 823
Balazs, EA, 37
Baldessarini, RJ, 839, 844, 847
Baldwin, L, 548
Ballard, TM, 1034
Balsano, AE, 1037
Baltazar, B, 925
Baltes, P, 793
Baltes, PB, 56
Baly, A, 503
Ban, T, 842
Banaski, JL, 91
Bandura, A, 45
Banks, JT, 45
Banting, DW, 223
Banzinger, G, 502, 904
Barder, L, 760
Barer, BM, 707
Barer, D, 439
Barker, S, 757
Barnard, RJ, 91

Barnes, RF, 845
Barnett, K, 583, 584
Barrett, CJ, 593
Barrett, EAM, 988
Barry, HC, 194, 196, 198
Barry, R, 256
Barsky, A, 65
Barsky, AJ, 759
Bartashuk, LM, 97
Barth, JT, 822
Bartlett, JG, 94
Bartley, SK, 718
Bartol, M, 815, 817, 818
Bartz, B, 87, 95
Basch, A, 297, 298
Bass, E, 448
Bassen, S, 925
Basu, JL, 794
Bates, MS, 330, 334
Bates-Jensen, BM, 281, 282
Battegay, R, 679
Bauer, DC, 391
Bay, MK, 96
Beale, CL, 648
Beard, BB, 4
Beare, P, 91
Beck, A, 763
Beck, AT, 758, 790
Beebe, A, 329, 335, 337, 341, 954
Beehr, TA, 717
Beel-Bates, CA, 190
Beers, M, 596, 597, 832
Beffert, U, 802
Begley, S, 54
Beizer, JL, 841, 851, 853, 855
Belanger, AJ, 301
Belgrave, L, 822, 881
Bell, J, 13
Bellecci, P, 57
Belvin, DB, 96
Benary-Isbert, M, 587
Bender, BS, 42
Benedict, A, 197
Benet, S, 56
Benezra, EE, 679, 684
Bengston, VL, 609
Bengtson, VL, 524, 721
Benison, B, 204

Benner, P, 31, 103, 263, 267, 987, 992
Bennett, D, 840
Bennett, M, 41
Bentley, DW, 94
Beregi, E, 134
Beresford, JM, 593
Bergener, SC, 815, 816
Berger, R, 592
Berger, RM, 657
Berggren-Thomas, P, 992
Bergman, G, 496
Bergstrom, N, 280, 281, 282
Berkman, LF, 642, 666
Berkow, R, 256, 801
Berlin, H, 587
Berman, HJ, 871, 916
Berman, RU, 631
Bernstein, A, 925
Berrio, MW, 965, 966
Berry, W, 793
Beverly, L, 181
Bhatt, A, 424
Billhorn, DR, 587
Binney, E, 20, 21
Biordi, D, 644, 645, 708, 719
Birnbaum, B, 38
Birren, B, 43, 45
Birren, J, 32, 43, 45, 51
Birren, JE, 75, 765, 1003
Bixler, EO, 184
Black, JS, 910
Black, KJ, 758
Blair, G, 657
Blakeney, B, 657
Blanchard-Fields, F, 692
Blaney, P, 691
Blatter, CW, 658
Blazer, 752
Blazer, DG, 750, 751, 753, 757, 762
Bleathman, C, 819
Bliwise, DL, 185
Blum, N, 589
Blumenthal, JA, 197
Blumenthal, SJ, 262
Boaz, RF, 626
Boczkowski, JA, 337
Boerner, RJ, 750

Subject Index

Addington v. Texas, 543
ADEA; *see* Age Discrimination in
Employment Act
ADH; *see* Antidiuretic hormone
Adherence, 309-310, 363-366, 371, 749
Adjustment disorders, 749-750
Adjuvant medications, 335
ADLs; *see* Activities of daily living
Administration on Aging (AOA), 18, 200,
926, 1060
Adrenal corticoids, stress and, 74
Adrenal gland, age-related changes in, 95
Adrenergic agents, sexual response and,
595
Adrenergic decongestants, side effects of,
385
Adrenocorticosteroids, malnutrition and,
370
Adrenocorticotropic hormone (ACTH),
95, 243
Adrenogenic hormones, age-related
changes in, 95
Adult education, self-actualization and,
905-910
Adult foster care, 497, 498
Adult nurse practitioners, 22
Adult Protective Services, 558-559
Advance directives, 543, 965-968,
973-974, 977-979
Advanced nursing practice (ANP), 1030,
1031, 1039
Advanced practice nurse (APN), 1023,
1029-1032
Adverse drug interactions, 358-359, 360,
361, 366
Advil; *see* Ibuprofen
Advocacy, 544-545, 967-968, 983, 1024
drug interactions and, 360-361
legal protection and, 562
national issues in, 545
principles of, 545
sexuality and, 600-601
Advocates Senior Alert Process (ASAP),
548
Aeration, assessment of, 104
Aerobic exercise, 72, 199
Aerophylline; *see* Theophylline
AFAR; *see* American Federation for Aging
Research
Affectual disturbance, cognitive
impairment and, 811-812
African Ancestors, 987
African-Americans, 33, 879-881, 1045
caregiving by, 622-623
widowhood and, 731
AFTER Rehabilitation and Training
Center for Limb
Deficiencies/Amputations, 316
Afternoon, sensory deprivation and, 441,
443
Agar, cross-link theory and, 36
Age
biologic, 32
chronologic, 2, 3, 32, 51
metabolic, 32
psychologic, 32

Age—cont'd
social, 32
subjective, 2
Age Discrimination in Employment Act
(ADEA), 714
Age norms, 51, 52
Age spots, 243
Age-associated memory impairment
(AAMI), 796
Aged; *see* Elders
Age-grading, sociologic aging and, 51
Ageism, 642-644, 744
compassionate, 21
contributors to, 643
of scientists, 643
"Ageism in Advertising: A Study of
Advertising Agency Attitudes
Towards Maturing and Mature
Consumers," 643
Ageist attitudes, 12
Ageist discrimination, 940
Ageless self, 987
Agencies, communities and, 631
Agency for Health Care Policy and
Research (AHCPR), 17, 275, 282,
284, 288, 333, 344
Agenda behaviors, 423
Age-related changes, 85-132
assessment of, 104-107, 114-117,
118-132
auditory, 100, 101
biochemical, 101
body composition, 89
cardiovascular, 90-91, 114
case study, 109-110
endocrine, 95-96, 117
facial, 88
functional assessment of, 105-106
gastrointestinal, 96-97, 115
genetic, 101
hair and, 87-88
health assessment and, 102-103, 104
immunologic, 100-101
integrated assessment of, 106-107
loss of tissue elasticity and, 88-89
mental assessment of, 106
nails and, 87-88
nervous system, 97, 116
nursing diagnosis and, 108-109
peripheral vascular, 91-92
physical assessment of, 104-105,
114-117, 118-132
physiologic, 85-101
posture and, 86-87, 88
recording of data in, 107
renal, 94-95
resources for, 110-111
respiratory, 92-94
sensory, 97-98
sexuality and, 590-591
skin and, 87-88, 115
in sleep, 187, 188
vision, 98-100
Age-related macular degeneration
(ARMD), 450

Aggression
cognitive impairment and, 810
passive, 749
AGHE; *see* Association for Gerontology
in Higher Education
Aging, 1-29
abuse and neglect in, 562-568
age-related changes and; *see* Age-
related changes
almost-old and, 3
already-old and, 3-4, 5
anthropology and, 33
area agency on, 1035
assessment of, 561
attitudes toward, 12-16
biomedicalization of, 18-21, 31
brain in, 794-796
business of, 18
case study and, 26-27, 58, 569-571
centenarians and, 4-6, 57
chronic illness and; *see* Chronic illness
chronologic age and, 2, 3
creativity and, 914-931
crises and, 679-682
definition of, 2, 3
demographics of, 6-11
depression and, 757
development of gerontology and, 16-22
disease versus, 20
elders and; *see* Elders
elite-old and, 4-6
ethnography of, 33
evolutionary basis for, 33
family life contributions in, 626-627
forensics and, 20-21
frailty in, 558-562
future of, 24-25, 568-569
global, 10-11, 12, 13, 14
healthy, 20, 65, 67; *see also* Health
immunologic theory and, 40-41
intimacy and sexuality and, 583-605
journals on, 1071-1072
legal concerns of; *see* Legal concerns
of aging
longevity and, 54-57
medications contraindicated in, 380
nursing diagnoses and, 570
oldest-old and; *see* Oldest-old
pain in, 332-333
perspectives on, 33
physiologic, 85
politics of, 17-18, 19
primary, 54
professionalization of care for; *see*
Gerontic nursing
psychologic aspects of, 43-50
research and, 16-17
resources for, 27, 59
respect for, 13-16
sociologic, 51-54
special drug considerations in, 381-383
study of, 16
successful, 32, 85-86, 905-911
theories of; *see* Theories of aging
in United States, 6-10
usual, 31-32, 85-86

Center
 on Aging, 896
 for Aging, Religion and Spirituality,
  1011
 for Death Education and Research, 973
 of Design for an Ageing Society, 505
 for Healthcare Ethics, 974
 for Nursing Research, 1021
 for the Partially Sighted, 473
 for the Study of Health, Faith and
  Ethics, 1011
 for Women's Health Research, 869
Centers for Disease Control and Prevention
  (CDC), 198, 308, 309, 593
Central anticholinergic effects of
  antipsychotics, 837
Central apnea, 189
Central nervous system (CNS)
 drug toxicity and, 361
 effects of drugs on, 335
Central nervous system stimulants, 850
Cephalosporins, 352, 359
Cerebral oxygenation, interruption of, falls
  and, 411-412
Cerebrovascular accident (CVA), 273,
  278, 598
Ceremonies, religious, 994
Certificate in Added Qualifications in
  Geriatrics, 21-22
Certification
 for case managers (CCM), 1032-1033
 gerontic nursing and, 21-22, 1018,
  1019
Certified geriatric rehabilitation nurse,
  1037-1038
Certified nurse assistants (CNAs), 1020
Certified nurse-midwife (CNM), 1029
Certified registered nurse anesthetist
  (CRNA), 1029
Certified rehabilitation registered nurse
  (CRRN), 1037-1038
Cerumen impaction, 457
CFUs; *see* Colony-forming units
CGNA; *see* Canadian Gerontological
  Nursing Association
Chair confinement, interventions for, 285
Challenge
 crisis as, 67
 hardiness and, 45
Changes, age-related; *see* Age-related
  changes
Charcoal, drug interactions and, 359
Charity contributions, 903
Chelating agents, malnutrition and, 370
Chemistry
 blood, laboratory values and, 136-138,
  141-145
 serum, laboratory values and, 135-136,
  140-141
Chemosensation, 443
Chemosensory center, 445
Chest wall, age-related changes in, 93
CHF; *see* Congestive heart failure
Childless individuals, legacies of, 1005
Childproof containers, compliance with
  medications and, 371-372

Children
 of Aging Parents (CAPS), 635, 1062
 attitudes of, toward aging, 16
 boomerang, 721
 death of, coping with, 949
Chin, double, 88
Chinese, 505, 878, 879, 888-889, 891
Chloral hydrate, 383, 849, 853
 drug interactions and, 360
 side effects of, 385
Chloramphenicol
 blood glucose levels and, 276
 drug interactions and, 359
 vitamin deficiencies and, 386
Chlordiazepoxide, 355, 380, 383, 849,
  852, 853
Chlorhexidine, 226
Chloroquine, 359
Chlorothiazide, 355
Chlorpheniramine, 383, 448
Chlorphenoxamine, 448
Chlorpromazine, 354, 355, 380, 448, 834,
  835, 837, 838, 843, 848
 effects of, on sexual function, 595
 relative potency of, 835
 side effects of, 836
Chlorpropamide, 355
 drug interactions and, 359, 360
 toxicity and, 362
Chlorprothixene, 448, 843
Chlor-Trimeton; *see* Chlorpheniramine
Choice in Dying, Inc., 973, 974
Cholecystitis, 96
Cholelithiasis, 96
Cholesterol
 in diet, 171
 laboratory values and, 137, 139, 144
Cholestyramine, 353, 360
 drug interactions and, 359
 malnutrition and, 370
 vitamin deficiencies and, 386, 387
Cholinergic system, age-related changes
  in, 97
Cholinesterase inhibitors, 844
Cholinomimetic agents, 844
Choral reading of poetry, 923
Christian Affirmation of Life, 966
Christian Nurses Preventive Health Project
  (CNPHP), 1045
Chromatin, 101
Chromosome, major
  histocompatibility, 42
Chronic airflow limitation (CAL), 222
Chronic care, 68
Chronic grief, 943, 944-945
Chronic illness, 255-328, 310
 activities of daily living and, 264-265,
  266
 adaptive devices and, 269, 270, 315
 aging and, 258-259
 assessment of, 264-267
 assistive devices and, 269-271
 caring and, 267-268
 case study, 313, 314
 chronotherapeutics and, 265-267
 compliance in, 309-310

Chronic illness—cont'd
 definition of, 256
 disorders of, 275-309
  coronary problems, 299-308
  diabetes mellitus, 275-278
  incontinence, 284-299
  musculoskeletal impairments, 309
  pressure sores, 280-284, 285, 286,
   287, 321-323, 324-325
  pressure ulcers, 280-284, 285, 286,
   287, 321-323, 324-325
  stroke, 278-280
  tuberculosis, 308-309
 exercise and, 205
 fatigue and, 262
 gender and, 262
 grief and, 263
 health beliefs in, 309-310
 home care and, 311-313
 interventions in, 267-271
 long-term care and, 310-311
 moral dimensions of, 263-264
 nursing diagnosis for, 312
 pain and, 262, 991
 prevention of iatrogenic disturbances in,
  271, 272
 rehabilitation and, 271-275
 research on, 1021
 resources for, 314-316
 self-care and, 268
 sexuality and, 263, 597, 598-599
 small-group approaches to, 268-269
 substance abuse and, 262-263
 trajectory of, 260-261, 311
 wellness and, 78-80, 258
 work of, 991
Chronic insomnia, 187
Chronic lung disease, exercise and, 205
Chronic obstructive pulmonary disease
  (COPD), 94, 222, 303-308, 599,
  758
 interventions for, 307
 sleep alterations and, 188
Chronic pain; *see* Pain, chronic
Chronic stressors, 686-687
Chronicity, 78, 256-264
Chronicle Publishing Company, 710
Chronobiologic terms, 357
Chronobiology
 definition of, 357
 pharmacologic, 355-358
Chronologic age, 2, 3, 32, 51
Chronopharmacology, 357, 358
Chronotherapeutics
 chronic illness and, 265-267
 definition of, 357
Chronothesy, 357
Chronotolerance, 357
Chronotoxicity, 357
Church volunteers, caregiving and, 620
CI; *see* Cognitive impairment
Cigarette smoking, 98
Cilia, age-related changes in, 92
Cimetidine, 352, 354, 380, 844
 anticholinergic drug levels in, 837
 drug interactions and, 359

Being a Nursing Assistant

EIGHTH EDITION

Francie Wolgin

MSN, RN, C
System Leader for Education and Employee Development
St. Joseph Mercy Hospital (SJMH)
Ann Arbor, Michigan

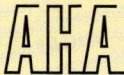
American Hospital Association

Prentice Hall Health ■ Upper Saddle River, New Jersey 07458

Library of Congress Cataloging-in-Publication Data

Wolgin, Francie.
    Being a nursing assistant. — 8th ed. / Francie Wolgin.
        p.   cm.
    Includes index.
    ISBN 0-13-084083-1
    1. Nurses' aides.   2. Care of the sick.   I. American Hospital
Association.
    [DNLM: 1. Nurses' Aides.   2. Nursing Care—methods.
WY 193 W861b 2000]
RT84.S35   2000
610.73'06'98—DC21
DNLM/DLC
for Library of Congress   99–31931
                                                                       CIP

Publisher: *Julie Alexander*
Editor-in-Chief: *Cheryl Mehalik*
Director of Marketing: *Leslie Cavaliere*
Marketing Manager: *Tiffany Price*
Acquisitions Editor: *Barbara Krawiec*
Managing Editor Development: *Marilyn Meserve*
Advertising Coordinator: *Cindy Frederick*
Director of Manufacturing & Production: *Bruce Johnson*
Managing Editor: *Patrick Walsh*
Senior Production Editor: *Janet Bolton*
Composition: *TSI Graphics*
Senior Production Manager: *Ilene Sanford*
Creative Director: *Marianne Frasco*
Cover Design: *Wanda España*
Cover Image: *Laina Leckie*
Interior Design: *Seventeenth Street Studio*
Managing Photography Editor: *Michal Heron*
Photographers: *George Dodson, Michal Heron, Michael Gallitelli*
Printing and Binding: *Press of Ohio*

Published for The Hospital Research and Education Trust by Prentice-Hall Inc., Upper Saddle River, New Jersey 07458

Printed in the United States of America
10 9 8 7 6 5 4 3

ISBN 0-13-084083-1

PRENTICE HALL INTERNATIONAL (UK) LIMITED, *London*
PRENTICE HALL OF AUSTRALIA PTY. LIMITED, *Sydney*
PRENTICE HALL OF CANADA INC., *Toronto*
PRENTICE HALL OF HISPANOAMERICANA, S.A., *Mexico*
PRENTICE HALL OF INDIA PRIVATE LIMITED, *New Delhi*
PRENTICE HALL OF JAPAN, INC., *Tokyo*
PRENTICE HALL (SINGAPORE) PTE., LTD.
EDITORA PRENTICE HALL DO BRASIL, LTDA., *Rio de Janeiro*

Dedication

I would like to dedicate this book to my daughter, Rebecca, and to my colleagues, committed to empowering and developing others.

NOTICE

The procedures described in this textbook are based on consultation with nursing authorities. The author and publisher have taken care to make certain that these procedures reflect currently accepted clinical practice; however, they cannot be considered absolute recommendations.

The material in this textbook contains the most current information available at the time of publication. However, federal, state and local guidelines concerning clinical practices, including without limitation, those governing infection control and universal precautions, change rapidly. The reader should note, therefore, that new regulations may require changes in some procedures.

It is the responsibility of the reader to familiarize himself or herself with the policies and procedures set by federal, state and local agencies, as well as the institution or agency where the reader is employed. The authors and the publishers of this textbook, and the supplements written to accompany it, disclaim any liability, loss or risk resulting directly or indirectly from the suggested procedures and theory, from any undetected errors, or from the reader's misunderstanding of the text. It is the reader's responsibility to stay informed of any new changes or recommendations made by any federal, state and local agency as well as by his or her employing health care institution or agency.

Note on Gender Usage

The English language has historically given preference to the male gender. Among many words, the pronouns, "he" and "his" are commonly used to describe both genders. The male pronouns still predominate our speech, however, in this text "he" and "she" have been used interchangeably when referring to the Nursing Assistant and/or the patient. The repeated use of "he or she" is not proper in long manuscript, and the use of "he or she" is not correct in all cases. The author has made great effort to treat the two genders equally. Throughout the text, solely for the purpose of brevity, male pronouns and female pronouns are often used to describe both males and females. This is not intended to offend any reader of the female or male gender.

Notice Re "The Nursing Assistant in Action"

The names used in the case studies throughout this text are fictitious.

To the Student

A self-instructional workbook for this text is available through a college bookstore under the title, *Workbook for Being a Nursing Assistant, 8th edition* [ISBN # 0-13-086676-8]. If not in stock, ask the bookstore manager to order a copy for you. If your course is being offered off-campus, ask your instructor where to obtain a copy. The workbook can help you with course material by acting as a tutorial review and study aid.

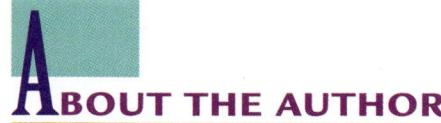

ABOUT THE AUTHOR

■ Francie Wolgin, MSN, RN, C

Francie Wolgin, System Leader for Education and Employee Development, St. Joseph Mercy Hospital (SJMH), Ann Arbor, Michigan, served four years as Director of Operations Support and Practice Development at SJMH, and as president of the National Nursing Staff Development Organization. Her St. Joseph Mercy Hospital department is responsible for the training and development of all Patient Care Associates, including the orientation and ongoing competency assessment of Nurses and Patient Care Assistants. Her department is also responsible for the training programs of the Patient Care Technicians. In addition, Ms. Wolgin serves as an adjunct faculty member at the University of Michigan School of Nursing, serves on the advisory board of Cross Country University, and serves on the editorial board of *Nursing Management.*

Ms. Wolgin's previous positions include Director of Nursing Practice Development and Clinical Associate at the School of Nursing, Duke University Medical Center; several management, staff development, and administrative positions at the University of Cincinnati Hospital; and a faculty appointment at the University of Cincinnati College of Nursing and Health. She served on the *Journal of Nursing Staff Development* editorial board for several years. She is the author of *Advanced Skills and Competency Assessment for Caregivers, Volumes I and II, Being a Nursing Assistant, 7th edition,* as well as many articles. She contributes to books on staff development, competency, and training of advanced nursing assistants. Extensive experience as a direct care giver in a variety of positions gives her both perspective and firsthand knowledge of the challenges and opportunities available throughout the health care continuum.

GUIDELINES AND PROCEDURES

Guidelines

Important principles of care are highlighted throughout the text to guide your care of the patient.

Key Idea

Important points are highlighted with a Key Idea icon.

Age-Specific Considerations

This feature points out age-specific considerations to take into account when performing a task or skill.

Procedures

Preparation and Follow-up steps are included with procedures when appropriate, so you have everything you need to successfully complete each procedure in one easy-to-find place.

OBRA Designation

This icon identifies mandatory OBRA content.

Marginal Glossary

Key Terms are presented in the margin with each term printed in color and followed by the definition.

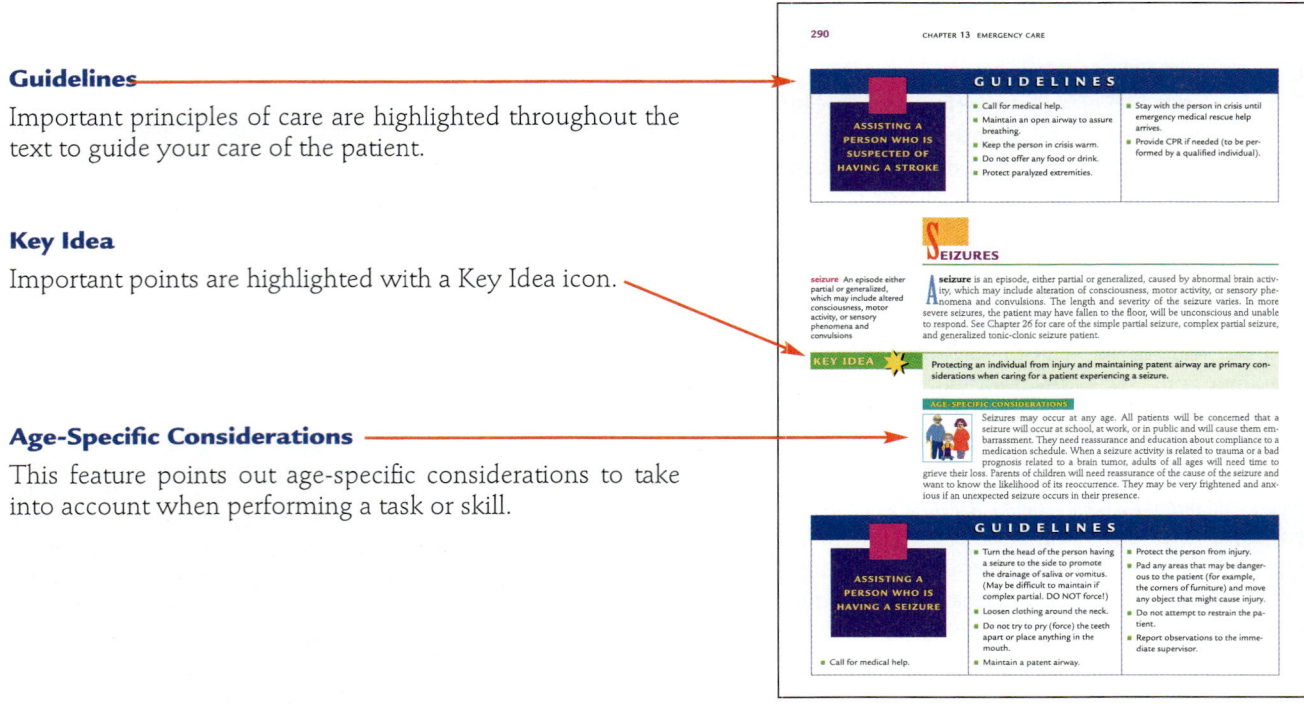

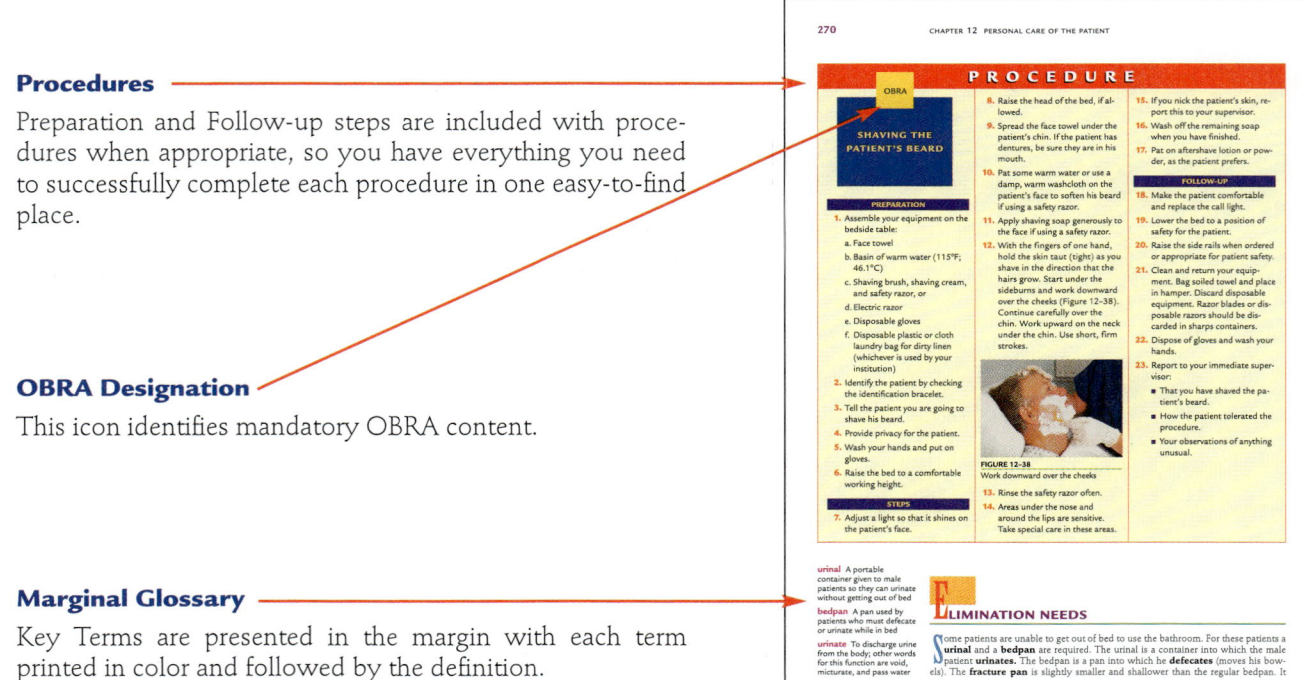

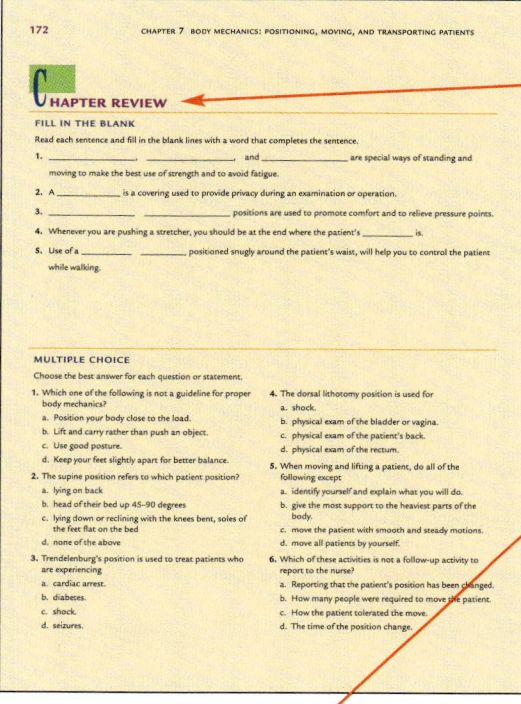

ᴇND-OF-CHAPTER MATERIAL

Chapter Review

Fill-in-the-blank and multiple-choice questions test your understanding of chapter content and help you prepare for the certification exam.

Getting Connected

These multimedia activities include something for every type of learner. Log on to our free Companion Website for helpful hints, an interactive study guide, and links to websites that feature additional information about chapter topics. Our free audio glossary CD helps you learn key terms. See how procedures are performed and get helpful advice on developing a professional image with our *Care Provider Skills Series* and *Focus on Professionalism* videos.

Critical Thinking

These questions will challenge you to apply what you have learned.

Time Out/Tips for Time Management

Designed to promote your personal and career growth and development, these tips appear at the end of each chapter and help you develop communication, planning and organizational skills, as well as self-discipline.

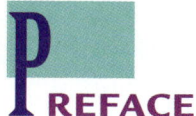

PREFACE

You are entering a challenging and ever-changing health care environment. Being a nursing assistant isn't just another job, but a serious occupation where you are an important part of a team providing health care services. Nursing assistants work in a variety of settings, ranging from within the home, to an office or a clinic, or to an extended care or acute care hospital setting. *Being A Nursing Assistant, 8th Edition* and all the accompanying supplements have been significantly revised, redesigned, and expanded to provide practical core material which makes up the foundation of your practice. As you may know, nursing programs are frequently requiring students to enter the program with nursing assistant certification or training evidence. What you learn as a nursing assistant will become your basic foundation of health care knowledge if you choose to enter a nursing program.

Some of the chapters will be more important to you than others, depending on your practice area or workplace setting. Material that may not seem necessary to know today can become vital if you find yourself being cross-trained to work in a different position, or to accept a job in a different health care setting.

Continuing developments in care technology and increased use of computers to document patient care will necessitate changes or, perhaps, the elimination of certain procedures and tasks. There are, however, core aspects of caring that will be ongoing. Examples include communicating effectively and providing compassionate care that takes into consideration the patient's physical, emotional, and spiritual needs, as well as cultural and age-specific considerations.

This book has been revised and rewritten following an extensive assessment process. The ideas and expressed needs of instructors and students across the country were given serious consideration. Colleagues and educators who have both experience and practical expertise in a variety of practice settings and specialties have contributed as chapter authors and reviewers. Their varied areas of expertise, knowledge, and competency assessment have been skillfully edited and integrated into this book. As a result, *Being a Nursing Assistant, 8th Edition* has been completely updated to prepare you for today's health care environment with new content and technology that includes:

- **Free CD** will help you master key terminology with an audio glossary. It can be used in either a computer or a CD player.
- **Age-Specific Considerations** are integrated throughout the book.
- **Expanded end-of-chapter exercises** will help you prepare for the certification exam with fill-in-the-blank and multiple-choice questions. Critical thinking questions will challenge you to apply what you have learned, while time management tips will help you develop communication, organizational, and planning skills. The *Getting Connected* section brings it all together with multimedia activities using our companion Website, CD, and videos.
- **Career-related topics** include a section on computer skills as well as information on accepting, keeping, and resigning from a job.
- **Updated infection control chapter** includes Hepatitis C, revised Contact Precautions, and an introduction to aseptic and sterile technique for nursing assistants who will be working in areas where this information is needed.
- **New material** has been added to keep you up-to-date with the latest developments and trends in health care, including noninvasive blood pressure monitoring; restorative care; skin care; communication skills; computer skills; GI system and ostomy care; adults >75 to 100+; care of patient following a total hip or total knee

replacement; restraint care and protective device information; cancer; AIDS care; sun downing; home health care; mental health care; substance abuse; and depression.

- **New procedures and guidelines** cover care of patients with stroke, burns, hemorrhage, shock and seizures, and feeding a patient with dysphagia.
- **Nursing Assistant in Action feature** provides scenarios based on actual, real-life issues and challenges which you may encounter on the job. This feature appears for each chapter, and is located either in the text or on the Website.

Your instructor will modify content or steps of procedures when necessary to comply with the standards of your community or state. Because there are significant differences and state variations as to which skills may be performed by nursing assistants, your instructor offers the most current information that applies to your role. You are responsible for knowing what the scope of your role is, as well as the particular policies, protocols and procedures of your employer. Your instructor or employer may provide you with this information, if not, it is important that you ask where you can obtain such information. Only perform those procedures you have been educated or validated to do.

Being a Nursing Assistant, 8th Edition will prepare you to be a successful nursing assistant by providing the core content and procedures you will need to function in a wide variety of practice settings. Welcome to the continuously challenging and learning environment that is health care!

■ The Teaching/Learning Package

Instructors and students who have used previous editions of *Being a Nursing Assistant* will notice that we've created a new interior and exterior design to be more appealing to today's students. While we've changed our look, we didn't change the basics that have helped students successfully master material, such as exceptional readability, clear, easy-to-follow procedures, and a complete supplements package. Our supplements package includes all the traditional components such as an instructor's guide and student workbook and, in addition, has been updated to take advantage of new technology:

- **New Companion Website** (www.prenhall.com/wolgin), tied chapter-by-chapter to the text, gives students an on-line study guide that provides immediate feedback, helps bolster their self-confidence with Student Success Profiles, gives them a forum for posting questions and discussion topics related to the text, and provides links to interesting and relevant sites on the World Wide Web. The Companion Website also enables instructors to create a customized syllabus and download Powerpoint slides and transparency masters.
- **Free CD** helps students master key terminology with an audio glossary.
- **Instructor's Guide** makes managing and preparing for class a snap with teaching suggestions, chapter overviews, objectives and key terms, student assignments, answers to end-of-chapter questions, as well as full page reproductions of student workbook pages with answers.
- **Student Workbook** features a variety of activities, including multiple-choice questions, labeling, fill-in-the-blank, and matching. We've also included competency checklists where appropriate for self-assessment.
- **Computerized Test Manager** will help you prepare tests with a large bank of test questions. Available in Windows, DOS, and Macintosh versions.
- **Body Systems Overhead Transparencies** showing 25 color illustrations of major body systems. (Available on-line.)
- **Care Provider Skills Video Series** allow students to see how procedures are actually performed. Videos are available individually or in a ten-video set.
- **Focus on Professionalism Video** teaches students how to develop a professional image by demonstrating what professionalism is—and isn't.

BRIEF CONTENTS

DETAILED CONTENTS

PROCEDURES

■ Indicates mandatory OBRA content. The page number follows the procedure title.

GUIDELINES

■ Indicates mandatory OBRA content. The page number follows the guideline title.

ACKNOWLEDGMENTS

This Eighth Edition of *Being a Nursing Assistant* has been prepared by Francie Wolgin, MSN, RN, CNA and her dedicated team of professionals. Individually, they each worked with extraordinary commitment on this revision. Together, they formed a team of highly dedicated professionals who have upheld the highest standards of current instruction for Nursing Assistants.

The **Hospital Research Education Trust** (**HRET**) of **American Hospital Association** gratefully acknowledges the author, **Francie Wolgin**, and her team for their expertise, perseverance, and above all their dedication in the development of this textbook.

For their contributions to individual chapters and to the overall enhancement of the Eighth Edition, we gratefully thank:

Phylis Brandon-Root, BSN, RN   Infusion Specialist, St. Joseph Mercy Home Care, Ann Arbor, MI (Chapter 11). Also, contributor to *Advanced Skills and Competency Assessment for Caregivers, Vol II.*

Barb Boylan Lewis, BSN, MA, CETN   Enterostomy Therapy Nurse, St. Joseph Mercy Hospital, Ann Arbor, MI. Member of the Wound, Ostomy, and Continence Nurses' Society (WOCN). Chapter Contributor to *Being a Nursing Assistant, 7th Edition.* (Chapter 20)

Marti A. Burton, RN, BS   Former Practical Nursing Instructor at Metrotech Technology Center, Oklahoma City, OK. Custom Designer of Health Education Curriculum and Author of the new State of Oklahoma Practical Nursing textbook. (Chapter 16)

Jane M. Campbell, MSN, RN, CS   Gerontology Clinical Nurse Specialist, UNC Memorial Hospital, Chapel Hill, N.C. (Chapter 32)

Ruth Churly-Strohm MSN, RN, PNP   Education Specialist, Education and Employee Development SJMHS, Ann Arbor, MI. Also, trained as a Pediatric Nurse Practitioner. Former faculty member at the University of Michigan School of Nursing, Ann Arbor, MI (Chapter 3)

Lisa F. Friedman, MS, RN   Education Specialist, Education and Employee Development, SJMHS, Ann Arbor, MI and Coordinator Policies and Procedures. Former Education Coordinator, Urology and Neurology, St. Joseph Mercy Hospital, Ann Arbor, MI. Previous Nursing Instructor, Madonna University, Livonia, MI and Coordinator Patient Care Assistant Consortium Class and PCT Program, Ann Arbor, MI. Chapter Contributor to *Being A Nursing Assistant, 7th Edition,* and *Advanced Skills and Competency Assessment for Caregivers, Volume I and II.* Co-authored the Instructor's Guides for *Being a Nursing Assistant, 7th Edition,* and *Advanced Skills and Competency Assessment for Caregivers, Volume I and II.* (End-of-Chapter Questions; Chapter 6 and 8)

Julee Huss, RN   Supervisor and Nurse Educator, The Shook Home, Chambersburg, PA. Dysphasia and Validation Therapy, (Chapter 21 and 32)

Christeen Conlin Holdwick, MA, RN, CNAA   System Leader Organization Development, SJMHS, Ann Arbor, MI. Formerly Director of Women and Children, St. Joseph Mercy Hospital, Ann Arbor, MI. Formerly held administrative and faculty positions in areas of chemical dependency, pediatrics, and psychiatry. Chapter contributor to *Being A Nursing Assistant, 7th Edition.* (Chapter 30)

Gloria Sveller, MSN, RN   Education Coordinator, Education and Employee Development, SJMHS, Ann Arbor, MI. Coordinator of the Patient Care Assistant Education and PCT Program. Former Director of Staff Development, Orchard Hills-Mercy Living Center, Pontiac, MI. Former Faculty Member, Mercy School of Nursing. (Chapter 6)

Kathy Wickman, BSN, MA, CETN   Wound, Ostomy and Continence Specialist, St. Joseph Mercy Hospital, Ann Arbor, MI. (Chapter 20)

Jan Treston-Aurand, MS, RN, CIC   Infection Control Practitioner, St. Joseph Mercy Health System, Ann Arbor, MI. Received 1995 AORN Research Award; Chapter Contributor to *Being A Nursing Assistant, 7th Edition* and *Advanced Skills and Competency Assessment for Caregivers, Volume I.* (Chapter 5)

Thanks to the following Seventh Edition contributors:

Terry Ainsworth, MS, RN, NP   Duke University Medical Center. (Chapter 14 and 15)

Barb Boylan Lewis, BSN, MA, CETN   St. Joseph Mercy Hospital, Ann Arbor, MI (Chapter 20)

Christeen Conlin Holdwick, MA, RN, CNAA   St. Joseph Mercy Hospital, Ann Arbor, MI (Chapter 30)

Martha Dawson, MSN, RN, VP   University of Louisville Hospital. (Chapter 22)

Lou Ebrite, PhD, MS, BS, RN   University of Central Oklahoma, Edmond, OK (Chapters 10, 12, 27, 28, 29, 34)

Cinda Fluke, MEd, RN, CNAA   Director of Medical Nursing, Parkland Hospital, Dallas Texas. (Chapter 9 and 32)

Lisa F. Friedman, MS, RN   St. Joseph Mercy Hospital, Ann Arbor, MI. (Chapter 8)

Geraldine Heneghan, MS, RN, CETN, CRN   EKA-Division Medical, Capital Heights, MD. (Chapter 17 and 20)

Amy F. Larson, MS, RN, CNRN   St. Joseph Mercy Hospital, Ann Arbor, MI. (Chapter 20)

Melodee J. Leimnetzer, MSM, RN   Lifelink Corporation, Bensenville, IL. (Chapter 11)

Lisa McDowell, MS, RD, CNSD   Coordinator of Clinical Nutrition, St Joseph Mercy Hospital, Ann Arbor, MI. (Chapter 21)

Jerene Maune, MS, RN, CETN, CVN   Johns Hopkins Wound Healing Center, Baltimore, MD. (Chapters 17 and 20)

Mary Morochnick, BA, RN   Nurse Manager Rehabilitation, DUMC. (Chapter 23)

Glenda Pavia, RN, CRRN   Rivergate Terrace, Riverview, MI. (Chapters 6, 33, and 35)

JoLynn Pulliam, MS, RN, CPHQ   St. Joseph Hospital and Supervisor at St. Mary Hospital in Livonia, MI. (Chapters 16, 18, 24, 25, and 31)

Caroline Schultz, MS, OTR   Work Capacity Services, St. Joseph Mercy Hospital, Ann Arbor, MI. (Chapter 7)

T. Jane Swain, MS, RN, VP   St. Elizabeth Medical Center, Covington, KY. (Chapter 13)

Jan Treston-Aurand, MS, RN, CIC   St. Joseph Mercy Hospital, Ann Arbor, MI. (Chapter 5)

Kelly M. Warnock, RN   Duke University Medical Center, Durham, NC. (Chapter 19)

In addition, the author would like to acknowledge and thank the following organizations and individuals for contributing immeasurably to this edition.

Prentice Hall Health
Julie Alexander, publisher, Prentice Hall Health, for the implementation of her visionary approach and creative ideas.

Cheryl Mehalik, editor-in-chief, nursing/health related professions/health occupations, for guidance in making the text user friendly and a pleasure to use.

Barbara Krawiec, acquisitions editor, health related professions, for her intuition and understanding of the task; for supporting the author in assembling a contributing group of professionals with the expertise and the knowledge needed for this ambitious project.

Marilyn C. Meserve, senior managing editor, development, health related professions, for providing hands-on commitment, zealous energy, and unique coordinating skills from the beginning of the project through its completion.

Stephanie Camangian, editorial assistant, Prentice Hall Health, for providing critical editorial support and assistance in various stages of the project.

Leslie Cavaliere, marketing director, special thanks for her contributions to the cover design, and to the overall marketing plan for the program.

Tiffany Price, marketing manager, Prentice Hall Health, for the development and the implementation of the marketing strategies, the outreach, and the promotions for all components of the program.

Cindy Frederick, marketing coordinator, Prentice Hall Health, for her dynamic and lively advertising and marketing coordination and support for the program.

Judy Stamm, sales manager, and the sales team for their support, suggestions, and resources.

Pat Walsh, managing editor, production, Prentice Hall Health, for providing production leadership and guidance to meet the needs of the project, including the text, the multi-media components, and the additional supplemental parts of the program.

Janet Bolton, project manager, production, for her management, coordination of materials, cross-checking all phases of production, the control and mastery of technical details, and communication with all involved on the project.

Ilene Sanford, senior production manager, for her planning and management of the many details and schedules behind the printing and binding process.

Marianne Frasco, design director, Prentice Hall Health, for her patience and creative contributions in bringing together the design of the book, including both the interior and the cover.

TSI Graphics staff for their work on composition.

Michal Heron, managing photography editor, evidenced special skill and dedication in capturing nuances in photographic expression. She worked tirelessly to complete the extensive photo program on time. Consensus as to which pictures were best from among hundreds Michal shot is amazing evidence of her skill and creativity. It is always a pleasure to work with Michal. In addition, Gloria Sveller and Lisa Friedman were particularly helpful in securing items needed for many photographs taken on site in Ann Arbor, MI and they arranged to have other items sent to Michal's other shooting sites.

Organizations

Special thanks to Garry Faja, President and CEO, Saint Joseph Mercy Health System, and Julie MacDonald, Senior VP, St. Joseph Mercy Hospital, Ann Arbor, MI, for their support throughout the project and for granting permission to reprint or adapt, within this book and its supplements, materials and forms from Saint Joseph Mercy Health System, St. Joseph Mercy Hospital and Home Care. Appreciation is also extended to Kathleen Rhine, VP, Human Resources, SJMHS.

I would also like to thank and acknowledge the assistance of Charles P. Craig, MD; Russell Olmsted, MPH, CIC; and Kathy Allen Bridson, RN, CTC of SJMHS Department of Infection Control Services for their review and contributions to Chapter 5. Thanks also to Judy Meyers, MS, RN for her contributions to the Restraint Policy appearing in Chapter 6. Special thanks to everyone who facilitated and participated in the photo shoot, and especially to my team and Volunteer Services, for their support.

Supplement Teams

In order to ensure an integrated and complementary supplements package, a team who currently educate Nurse Assistants and Patient Care Technicians was assembled. Working in collaboration with Francie Wolgin, JoLynn Pulliam authored the Student Workbook. Lisa Friedman updated and expanded the complementary Instructor's Guide and the Test Item File. Sherry Simpson developed additional questions for the Website. The new Nursing Assistant in Action Features appearing on the Website were written by Francie Wolgin, Marti Burton, and Jane Campbell. The supplements evidence their dedication to providing quality products to support student learning exercises and experiences. Mirada Slater and Amy Way deserve special thanks for their support.

Technical Advisors

The publisher wishes to acknowledge the cooperation of organizations and individuals who assisted in the photography program for Edition 7 and 8. For their invaluable contribution to the accuracy of these photographs, the technical advisors who supervised the procedures portrayed in these photographs were:

Lisa Friedman, MS, RN	Education Specialist
David Micham, BS, RRT	RT Education Coordinator
Gloria Sveller, MSN, RN	Education Coordinator
Dolores McAdoo, RN	Instructor
Susan Reddel, RN	Instructor

For assistance in the photography shoots by providing space, technical assistance, materials, and a pool of extremely competent CNAs to model in our photographs, our very special thanks to:

Mary Lou Proch, Director of Education
Sara Anthony, Education Department
Nurses and Staff of Eight Tower East
Sarasota Memorial Hospital
Sarasota, FL

Victoria Haines, Staff Services Assistant
Sarasota Memorial Hospital Staff Services
Sarasota, FL

Paul Farineau, Education Director
Home Health Services of Sarasota
Sarasota, FL

Elizabeth Bess, Director
Cindi Aun, RN, Director of Nursing
Joyce Stobbs, BS Director of Social Services
Heartland Health Care and Rehabilitation Center
Sarasota, FL

Deborah Metheny, RN, MS, Assistant Director SCTI
Pamela Bull LaGasse, RN, EdD, Department Chairperson, Allied Health
Sarasota County Technical Institute
Sarasota, FL

David Bobish, Director of Nursing
Physicians Dialysis Center
Sarasota, FL

Photography Models: For their gracious assistance in finding models to portray the patients in our photographs:
Cynthia Clements, Jan Wright and members of the following organizations:
The New Sarasotans Club
Sarasota, FL

First Congregational United Church of Christ
Sarasota, FL

St. Andrew United Church of Christ
Sarasota, FL

Broadway Theatre Academy
Susan Swanson, Director
Sarasota, FL

◼ Credits

ACE is the registered trademark of Peg Bandage, Inc.
Acetest is the registered trademark of Miles, Inc., Diagnostics Div.
Band-Aid is the registered trademark of Johnson & Johnson Medical, Inc. and Johnson
  & Johnson Consumer Products, Inc.
Clinitest is the registered trademark of Miles, Inc., Diagnostics Div.
K-Pad is the registered trademark of Katecho, Inc.
T.E.D. is the registered trademark of The Kendall Co.
Velcro is the registered trademark of Velcro USA, Inc.

◼ Reviewers

The following reviewers provided invaluable feedback and suggestions. We wish to thank each of these professionals for their contributions.

Reviewers for the Eighth Edition

Patti Biro
Director of Healthcare Programs
Del Mar College
Corpus Christi, TX

Marie Boucher RN
Director
Helping Hands Trade School
Waterville, ME

Judith T. Kautz MS, RN
Education Director
Pima Medical Institute
Tucson, AZ

Catherine Mainville RN, BS
Rhode Island Central Directory for Nurses
Providence, RI

Nancy Pimentel RN
Life-Stream/Cognosco
New Bedford, MA

Diane Weeks RN
Onondaga Cortland Madison Boces
Cortland, NY

Kathy Williford RN, MSN
Department Chair - Nursing
Edgecomb Community College
Tarboro, NC

Reviewers for the Seventh Edition

Judith Ann Avie, RN, BSN, MEd IT
Vice President
United Training Services
Professional Services Department
Southfield, MI

Also: Instructor
        Instructional Design and
          Development
        Wayne State University

Also: Instructor
        College of Health Science
        University of Detroit Mercy

John Bennett, RN, BSN, MSN
Instructor
Education and Training
South Hills Home Health Agency
Homestead, PA

Gloria J. Bizjak
Curriculum Specialist
Maryland Fire and Rescue Institute
University of Maryland
College Park, MD

Susan J. Bormolini, BSN, MA
Director
Human Resources Department
Rutland Regional Medical Center
Rutland, VT

Former: Project Coordinator
      Vermont Nursing Initiative
      Rutland Regional Medical Center
      Rutland, VT

Marie L. Boucher, RN
Senior Instructor
CNA Program
Helping Hands Trade School
Waterville, ME

Judy Bravin, RN, BSHA
Coordinator/Instructor
Nurse Assistant/Ward Clerk Department
Belleville Area College
Granite City, IL

Brenda Chamberlin, RN, MHSA
Coordinator Nursing Assistant Education
State of Vermont
Montpelier, VT

Lydia R. Chavana, CLS, MT, (ASCP)
Director of Allied Health Careers
Medical-Administration Department
South Texas Vo-Tech
McAllen, TX

Martha Cox, MSN, RN
Clinical Nurse Educator
Hospital Education Department
Duke University Medical Center
Durham, NC

Diane Cunningham, MS, RNc, FHCE
Nurse Educator
Research, Education, Quality Division
University Hospital
Salt Lake City, Utah

Laura Duprat, RN, MS, MPH
Former: Project Coordinator
      Integrated Clinical Practice
      Beth Israel Hospital
      Boston, MA

Kathryn Gahl, BS, BSN
Head Nurse
The Genesis Center and Women's Health
St. Nicholas Hospital
Sheboygan, WI

Kathleen Geran, RN, MS
Educator/Consultant
Quality, Education and Development
Fletcher Allen Health Care
Burlington, VT

Eva B. Gifford, RN
Health Occupations Department
Cumberland County Technical Education
  Center
Bridgeton, NJ

Catherine Glennon, RN, MHS, OCN
Oncology and Neurology Department
Georgetown University Hospital
Washington, DC

Josephine Hookway, RN, CNN, NP
Continuing Education Department
Beaufort County Community College
Washington, NC

Mary Jubeck, RN, MSN
Director
Education and Training
South Hills Home Health Agency
Homestead, PA

Fran LaMonica, RN, MS
Director
Cardiac Care Units
Mercy Hospital and Medical Center
Chicago, IL

Jill K. Mason, MS, RN, CNA
Vice President - Acute Care Services
Nursing Administration Department
Blessing Hospital
Quincy, IL

Mary Jo Pacifico, RN, BS
Piñellas Technical Education Center
Clearwater Campus
Clearwater, FL

Sue Ellen Pikula, BSN, RN, ETN
Nurse Educator
Educational Services Department
Cape Coral Hospital
Cape Coral, FL

Ellen Reed Riley, RNC
Director
Advantage Health Education
Riverside, CA

Connie Scott, MS, RN
Vice President Specialty Services
Blessing Hospital
Quincy, IL

Sharon Showalter, RN, BSN
Green Hills Center
West Liberty, OH

Catherine Smith, RN, BS
Allied Health Coordinator
Continuing Education Department
Sand Hills Community College
Pinehurst, NC

Jane P. Suder, RN
Educator/Consultant
Fletcher Allen Health Care
Burlington, VT

Gloria Sveller, BSN, MA, C
Director of Staff Development
Orchard Hills - Mercy Living Center
Pontiac, MI

Kristi Vander Hyde, BS, BSN, RN, CIC
Staff Specialist
Infection Control Services Department
University of Michigan Medical Center
Ann Arbor, MI

Judith Walker, MS, RN
Director of Birthing Services
Butterworth Hospital
Grand Rapids, MI

Leslie Williams, RN, MN
Education Facilitator, Education
  Department
Centura Health Education
Denver, CO

Kristina R. Wenzel, RN, MBA
Project Coordinator
School of Nursing
University of Colorado Health Sciences
  Center
Denver, CO

Lauren Zelmiker, RN
Lead CNA Instructor
Nursing Education
Beacon Career Institute
Miami, FL

Terry Zeman, RN, BSN, MSEd
Clark State Community College -BEC
Springfield, OH

INTRODUCTION

Welcome to the diverse and challenging field of health care. You are, or will be, working in the health care system where the delivery of patient care services is the focus of employer and employee alike. Whether you work in a large metropolitan hospital, a suburban nursing home, an inner-city or rural outpatient clinic, or the patient's home, *the patient* is the most important person. All personnel are there to provide care or to treat the sick and injured.

Being a Nursing Assistant offers you an extensive resource to help you as you study—learn and train—and as you are on the job. Your instructor will guide your learning/training during class, lectures, practice sessions, and clinical experiences, and will teach you the procedures and policies that are required in your state and in the institution, agency, or delivery site where you will be working because methods and policies vary from state to state and from one health care setting to another.

Health care delivery systems are continually changing to meet the ever-growing demands for health care services. Institutions, agencies, and their personnel must respond rapidly to make use of new research findings, insights, techniques, or equipment changes. If this text, or any other source, takes one approach to a situation and your instructor takes a different approach, follow your instructor. Your instructor is an expert in health care delivery and is the authority for your course.

On the job, you will be supervised by the nurse manager, supervisor, or team leader. They may not necessarily be the same person, although they might be. We use the term immediate supervisor throughout this book to refer to the person who supervises you and keeps a record of your performance. During your training, if you do not understand a procedure, ask your instructor for help. On the job, ask your nurse manager or team leader. It is far better to get help if you are not sure, than to do something wrong.

The more you know about how *Being a Nursing Assistant, 8th Edition* is organized the more help you will gain from using it. Take the time now to read the next few pages to find out what's in *Being a Nursing Assistant, 8th Edition*—where it is and how to find it.

■ Contents

All chapters and main headings, as well as procedures, guidelines, and "Nursing Assistant in Action" features that appear in the chapters are listed in the Contents.

■ Introduction

A paragraph at the beginning of each chapter highlights the content, issues, or concepts presented in the chapter. You may find it helpful to consider what you already know about the chapter content and to develop a list of questions you hope to answer as you read the chapter. Such efforts at focusing on the content are very helpful. Other techniques for studying are provided in *Using This Textbook* which follows the Glossary description.

■ Objectives

Each chapter begins with a list of objectives that tells you what you should be able to do by the end of the chapter. The objectives describe measurable or reachable goals—procedures or tasks to be performed, guidelines to be followed, information to be recalled and used. Use the Chapter Review at the end of the chapter to help you review the content and assess how well you have understood the content and met the objectives.

■Key Terms

Listed at the beginning of each chapter are key terms that are used in the chapter. Learning the meaning of the key terms before reading the chapter will greatly improve your ability to understand and remember what you learn. Key Terms are printed in bold where they are introduced in the text, appear with definitions in the side margins, and are printed alphabetically in an end-of-book glossary.

■Alert

In chapters dealing with procedures or tasks involving exposure to body fluids, blood, or airborne pathogens, a warning is given to adhere to *Standard Precautions* and wear protective equipment as indicated.

■Key Ideas

Throughout the book, Key Ideas address the most important aspects or focus of the content. Concepts discussed in the text are highlighted by the use of Key Ideas.

■Age-Specific Considerations

Identified with a specific icon and located throughout the text, this information points out "age-related/age-specific" issues that should be considered by the nursing assistant when performing a task or a skill.

■Procedures

In this text, a *procedure* consists of nursing tasks that are divided into a logical, orderly series (sequence) of actions or *Steps*. When appropriate, the procedure also includes *Preparation* steps and *Follow-up* steps. In health care institutions, procedures are done according to a standard method. Procedures may vary slightly from institution to institution in wording, sequence, or style, but the underlying principles or ideas are always the same. The procedures presented in this text will be the same or similar to procedures you will follow in the institutions and agencies where you are employed. Be sure you know the methods, policies, and procedures of the institution where you are working.

■Guidelines

There are basic principles, ideas, and methods that must be remembered for the overall total care of a patient. As an example, you will always treat the patient with courtesy, kindness, and empathy. Such a principle or guideline does not make up a full procedure. In some situations, the order in which the tasks are done does not matter. For example, you will check the patient unit (the room) to make sure that everything needed is there. Tasks like this do not follow definite numerical order. Therefore, they are not true procedures. They are called Guidelines.

■Summary

A paragraph at the end of each chapter recaps the content, issues, or concepts presented in the chapter. You may find it helpful to consider what additional information you recall about the content, issues, or concepts mentioned in the summary and to see how many of your own questions you were able to answer as you read the chapter. Such efforts at focusing on the content are very helpful. Other techniques for studying—learning and remembering—are provided in *Using This Textbook* which follows the Glossary description.

■ The Nursing Assistant in Action

These scenarios are based on actual, real-life issues and challenges you may encounter on the job. The statement of each situation is followed by probing questions. These questions address your response to the situation, including actions you might take to safeguard the health of your patient and your patient's right to confidentiality. Use these situations and the questions accompanying them to explore your moral, ethical, or legal obligations in the situation described. Also, take advantage of actual situations as they present themselves to develop questions of your own to assist you as you seek solutions or appropriate responses.

■ Chapter Review

Each chapter presents a *Chapter Review* in the form of fill-in-the-blank and multiple choice questions. These questions will help you review the chapter's main ideas. The questions also will remind you of the things you have learned and the objectives you have met. The questions are not intended to be a test or quiz. You may wish to discuss the answers to the questions with classmates and/or your instructor. This type of discussion will help you to remember what you have learned. Reread and study any parts of the chapter that deal with a question you could not answer.

■ Getting Connected

In this section you will find suggestions and help through the use of multimedia extension activities. First, there is the free, interactive Companion Website. This Website, designed specifically for this book, gives hints, instant feedback, and textbook references to chapter-related multiple choice questions. You will also find the *Nursing Assistant in Action* feature on the Website. Tied into the content of each chapter, you will find a real-life issue scenario followed by probing questions. These questions will help you explore what your actions should be when you encounter a similar scenario. Secondly, you will be directed to use the *Audio Glossary CD-ROM disk* enclosed with your textbook to hear the pronunciation of the key terms in the chapter. Thirdly, a recommended video is suggested for your use to extend and enhance the chapter content.

■ Critical Thinking

You will be able to expand your understanding by applying your critical-thinking skills to the key questions presented in this section. For each of the questions presented, you are asked to think of what you might do to solve the problem.

■ Time Out

In this section you will find *Tips for Time Management.* These tips will help you develop communication, planning, and organizational skills.

■ Preparing for the Competency Evaluation Exam

Expanded end-of-chapter exercises will help you prepare for the certification exam with fill-in-the-blank and multiple-choice questions. In addition, in Chapter 35 you will find a sample test with an answer key containing questions similar to those that appear on the Nurse Assistant Competency test. General information you will need to know to help you prepare/qualify for the Competency Evaluation Exam is also provided. For example, there is information about OBRA regulations regarding course requirements, explanations of the clinical skills exam and written/oral exam, test fees and time requirements. Be sure to ask your instructor about specific state requirements that apply to you.

■ Employment Opportunities

The health care field, like any other, offers options to the Nursing Assistant who is pursuing that "first job" as well as the one who is seeking "opportunities for advancement." Chapter 35 provides information about where to look for work, how to interview, accepting a job, and making career moves along the employment continuum. Continuing education that supports cross-training and career path planning that encourages multi-skilling are also presented. Take the opportunity to discuss your short-term and long-term goals with your instructor or supervisor.

■ Medical Terms and Abbreviations

The Appendix provides an extensive list of medical terms, abbreviations, and specialties. You should learn as many medical terms and abbreviations as you can. Understanding terminology and abbreviations used in the health care field will make you more confident, help you understand instructions you are given, and assist you in reporting accurately. Knowledge of the "words" used will greatly improve your ability to communicate effectively.

■ Glossary

The end-of-book Glossary provides a complete alphabetical listing of all the Key Terms used in the text. Following the definition of each term, the number(s) of the chapter(s) in which the term is used appears in parentheses. For example, "**seizure** An episode, either partial or generalized, which may include altered consciousness, motor activity, or sensory phenomena and convulsions (13, 26)."

■ Using This Textbook

After you purchase *Being a Nursing Assistant, 8th Edition,* or when your instructor gives you your first assignment, take a little time to get to know this textbook. Make a quick survey of the text. Look at the *Detailed Contents* and find out what's listed there. As you read the chapter titles, you will get a sense of how the content is organized.

Chapter 1 introduces the "big picture" of the health care system. In Chapter 2 you learn about the role of the nursing assistant. The importance of good communication skills in caring for patients is presented in Chapter 3. Chapter 4 discusses patients, residents, and clients and you learn that individuals in need of care are referred to differently in different settings. Continue going through the entire *Detailed Contents* on your own, noting what's in each chapter. You may want to star or highlight chapter content that is of special interest or importance to you.

Be sure to find the *Appendix: Medical Terms, Abbreviations, and Specialties, Glossary,* and *Index* listed at the end. Turn to each section and find out what's there. You will probably find that you refer to these sections often. That's good. Make the book work for you!

■ Preview Before You Read

As you read or study each chapter in this book, you will find it helpful to preview the chapter first. Whenever you are reading and learning new material you wish to remember, take the time to focus your energies and to set up the proper internal environment for learning. Preview first.

Preview the chapter by reading the Introduction, Objectives, Key Terms, Main Headings, and Summary. Notice that you have not read the chapter itself, just the skeleton or bare bones. Examine photographs, illustrations, drawings, charts, and tables.

Always be sure to:

- Take notes (write words or phrases, or perhaps make drawings or sketches).
- Make connections with what you already know about the topic.
- Make a list of questions (no more than three or four) about what you want to learn.

Read the chapter carefully, paying particular attention to the Objectives, Key Terms, Key Ideas, and Age-Specific Considerations. They will help you identify key concepts, ideas, and issues in the chapter. Follow your instructor's directions, and note information about policies and practices that relate to your institution.

Always be sure to:

- Keep in mind the Objectives for the chapter.
- Note words or phrases that are **bold** or seem important to you.
- Take a closer look at tables, charts, photographs, and illustrations.
- Jot down information that answers your preview questions.
- Use the Chapter Review to help you recall and meet the objectives.
- Ask your instructor for help with concepts, procedures, or guidelines you find difficult.
- Re-read sections related to questions you are unable to answer.

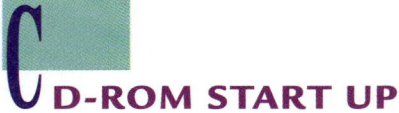

CD-ROM START UP

- From the START menu select RUN
- Type your CD-ROM drive letter, then type :\setup.exe (CLICK OK)
- Follow the on screen instructions
- See read me file for additional information

For support call 1-800-677-0337; 8-5; M-F CST or email: media.support@pearsoned.com.

Being a Nursing Assistant

The Health Care System

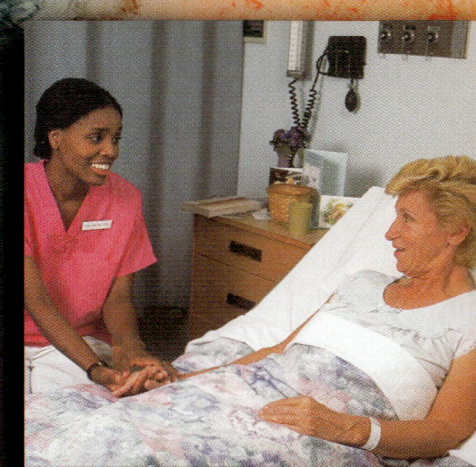

1

INTRODUCTION

This chapter introduces you to the health care system. It is a challenging, ever changing environment that embraces the delivery of health care services to individuals in need of care, the facilities in which these services are provided, and the health care providers who deliver these services. Some factors affecting the health care environment include: an aging population, advances in medicine, new possibilities for delivering care, governmental legislation, managed care plans, and insurance companies. Patient care is delivered in a variety of ways on an inpatient and outpatient basis in a variety of long-term and short-term care settings, including the patient's home. In all situations, health care providers are expected to provide quality compassionate care in a cost effective manner.

Different types of facilities and services are presented along with several nursing models. One of the newest models, patient-focused care, is a multidisciplinary team approach that places the patient and the patient's needs first—at the center, prompting and directing the delivery of services. It is important for you as a nursing assistant to understand the environment of the health care system, the organizational structure of your particular setting or facility, and the nursing model, or structure, on which your health care team is based.

OBJECTIVES

When you have completed this chapter, you will be able to:

- Explain the purpose and organization of the health care delivery system.

- Explain how managed care influences the health care delivery system.

- Describe the effects of DRGs on the American health care system.

- Describe three ways of organizing the patient care services/nursing health care team.

- Identify the members of the patient care services/nursing health care team.

- Explain the purpose and function of a multidisciplinary team approach to patient care.

- Explain the difference between the qualifications of the registered nurse and the licensed practical nurse, and between the jobs of the patient/nursing assistant and the unit clerk/secretary.

KEY TERMS

diagnosis

DRGs

functional nursing

health care institution

hospice

hospital

immediate supervisor

multidisciplinary team

nurse

nurse manager

nursing assistant

patient-focused care

primary nursing

task oriented

team leader

team nursing

THE HEALTH CARE ENVIRONMENT

health care institution (facility) Hospital, hospice, nursing home, convalescent home, or clinic where health care services are provided both on an inpatient and outpatient basis

The health care environment is a continually changing and challenging place to work. Health care organizations and the people who work in them strive to improve their roles and work. Even as they provide compassionate, quality patient care and contribute to society at large, **health care institutions (facilities)** and their care providers study to improve their knowledge and develop in their roles as caregivers. These efforts to learn new skills are important as change in the health care system is happening faster than ever.

The health care delivery system is designed to meet the health care needs of all individuals. It has five functions.

The five basic functions of a *health care delivery system* are to:

1. Provide care for ill and/or injured people

2. Prevent disease

3. Promote individual and community health

4. Provide facilities for the education of health workers

5. Promote research in the sciences of medicine and nursing

To give more people access to health care, to get the best possible results, and to keep costs down, health providers are constantly reviewing agency, institution, and patient needs and hospitalization requirements. Health providers continually ask questions like these.

- What do they do or what is their mission?

- Where do they do it?

- Who can do the work?

- How can they get the best results at the lowest cost?

- What does the individual patient or family desire from the health care providers?

- Is this treatment needed, necessary, or in the patient's best interests?

Efforts to answer these questions makes providers:

- Think about or focus on the bigger issues of disease prevention and the health status of entire communities, not just about medical care for the sick and injured who come to an institution for help.

- Rethink the roles of hospitals and the ways different institutions and providers can cooperate. For example, people might go to walk-in or same-day surgery clinics rather than to hospitals, and many services might be provided in people's homes.

- Rethink what must be handled by a doctor or nurse and what can be done by others, including helping patients and their families assume an active role in self-care.

- Look for the best ways to meet the goals of those who seek health services.

- Listen to what patients and their families say they want in addition to the actual services and treatments people seek out.

- Discuss with patients various treatments, goals, costs, and/or alternatives to treatment in order to provide the best care for the patient.

■ Health Care Reimbursement

Trying to reduce or control the ever increasing cost of health care has been a big challenge. Most health care administrators struggle to reduce their expenses yet provide the quality of care expected by patients, families, and accreditation bodies. Managed care or managed lives contracts are negotiated with major employers. Price, access, outcomes, satisfaction, and quality all influence the decision. Unless individuals covered in the contracts chose to pay themselves, they have limited or minimal choice to use facilities or providers not part of their system.

■ Medicare and Medicaid

Medicare and Medicaid are two different government programs that greatly influence health care. Medicare is a federal U.S. government program funded by Social Security and available to all individuals over age 65, regardless of income. It also covers the health care of some disabled or handicapped persons of all ages.

Medicaid is a separate program, funded by each state to help meet the medical and health care needs of low-income individuals or families. Medicaid programs and eligibility vary from state to state. Children of single mothers who have minimal income or who are unemployed would receive medical coverage through Medicaid. Some individuals may qualify for coverage under both Medicare and Medicaid, for example an 80-year-old woman who has very limited income.

Many of the questions providers ask relate to insurance companies, managed care plans, and government legislation. For example, the federal Medicare program and other insurers look at services used by patients who fall into **diagnosis-related groups (DRGs).** A **diagnosis** is a physician's determination of a patient's disease or condition. Researchers look at groups of patients with related or similar diagnoses (a DRG) and develop statistics on the average length of hospital stay and average cost.

DRGs Diagnostically related groups of patients; a DRG includes patients whose diagnoses are related, usually by body system or broad disease type, such as heart disease

diagnosis Finding out what kind of disease or medical condition a patient has; a diagnosis is always made by a physician

■ Diagnosis-Related Groups (DRGs)

DRGs were developed at Yale University and in 1983 they became a basis for payment for Medicare patients as well as a method for doctors to assess patients for the provision of quality care. There are over 400 DRGs. Age, comorbidities (more than one disease or chronic illness; for example a person with diabetes and hypertension), and complications will influence the assigned DRG coding number. Payments are set fees based on the DRG assigned.

Current Procedural Terminology (CPT-4)

CPTs are currently in their 4th edition. These are groups of five numbers used to classify procedures or medical services performed for billing purposes.

■ Managed Care

Managed care is a term used to describe a wide variety of prepayment agreements, negotiated contracts and discounts, agreements for prior service authorization or approval, and performance audits. In managed care there is a standard benefit package, open enrollment, information or data on quality of care and payments or contributions paid to a benchmark plan. A benchmark is a comparison or reference point, for example, the comparison of an organization's costs to the regional or national averages of similar providers. Physicians are encouraged to, and rewarded for, practicing efficiently through fixed payments. In essence, managed care is a business strategy whereby health care financing and delivery are combined into one organization for the purposes of balancing costs, quality of care, and access. There has not been evidence of a decline in quality of care in patients covered by managed care.

HEALTH CARE DELIVERY SITES

Health care delivery sites, professional, and nonprofessional workers depend on the revenue received in exchange for services provided to patients based on standard systems, contracted, or negotiated prices. The amount of money received by providers is frequently predetermined by national standards or based on statistics such as the average length of hospital stay and average cost. Health care professionals also use DRGs to group patients and determine the best answers to the questions outlined earlier in this chapter. These answers will change with advances in patient care techniques and technology.

Health care is delivered in an ever expanding variety of settings, facilities, and sites. Examples include:

- Acute care facility

- Adult day care

- Adult group living center

- Birthing center

- Community care home

- Free-standing surgical center

- Home health agency (home care)

- **Hospice** inpatient center

- Long-term care nursing facility

- Mental health facility or Partial treatment units

- Outpatient clinic

- Physician offices

- Rehabilitation facility

- Residential care home

- Respite care

- Skilled nursing facility

- Subacute care facilities

hospice An extended, or long-term, care facility that provides health care services to terminally ill patients and their families

Each facility or health care delivery site requires an organizational structure that supports the purpose and functions of the delivery site. Figure 1–1 provides an organizational plan for a **hospital** organizational chart identifying the various departments required in such a facility. It highlights the nursing branch and indicates the line of communication and responsibility—chain of command—within the facility. There is a flatter management in a skilled nursing facility (Figure 1–2).

hospital A short-term, or emergency, care facility that provides health care services to patients

As prevention becomes increasingly important, health care screening and assessment sites will be found at shopping malls, fairs, senior citizen centers, schools, churches, or other places where people gather. Patients are staying fewer days in the hospital and in many cases are receiving the majority of their health care, including surgical procedures, in outpatient or ambulatory settings. This means there are sicker, more critically ill patients in the hospital settings and a higher demand for health care workers in the variety of sites and places where health care is given to people.

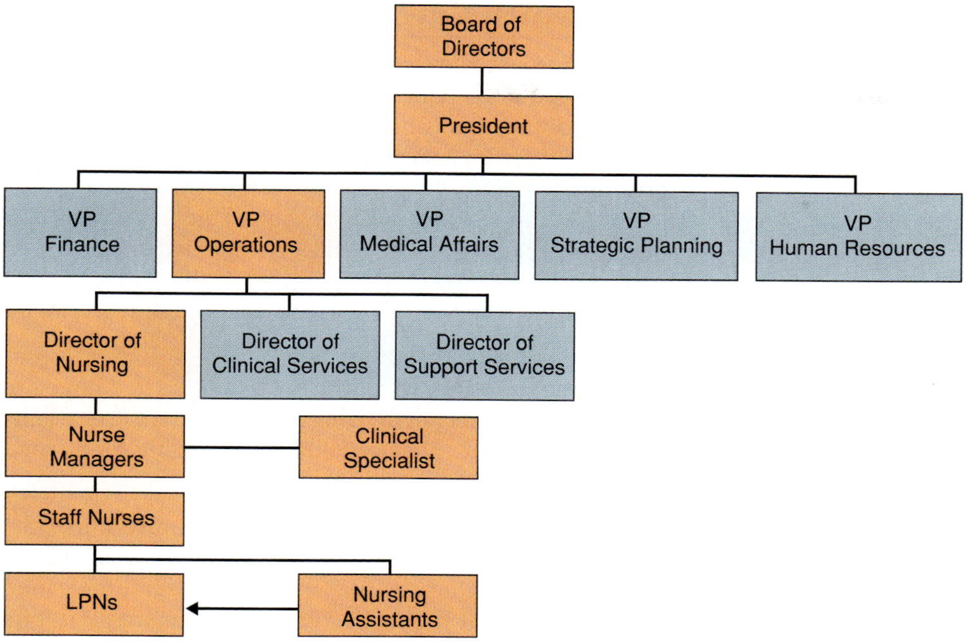

```
                    ┌─────────────┐
                    │   Board of  │
                    │  Directors  │
                    └─────────────┘
                    ┌─────────────┐
                    │  President  │
                    └─────────────┘
```

| VP Finance | VP Operations | VP Medical Affairs | VP Strategic Planning | VP Human Resources |

```
┌──────────────┐   ┌──────────────┐   ┌──────────────┐
│ Director of  │   │ Director of  │   │ Director of  │
│   Nursing    │   │  Clinical    │   │   Support    │
│              │   │  Services    │   │  Services    │
└──────────────┘   └──────────────┘   └──────────────┘

┌──────────────┐   ┌──────────────┐
│    Nurse     │   │   Clinical   │
│   Managers   │   │  Specialist  │
└──────────────┘   └──────────────┘

┌──────────────┐
│ Staff Nurses │
└──────────────┘

┌──────────────┐   ┌──────────────┐
│     LPNs     │ ← │   Nursing    │
│              │   │  Assistants  │
└──────────────┘   └──────────────┘
```

FIGURE 1–1

The nursing branch of a hospital organizational chart

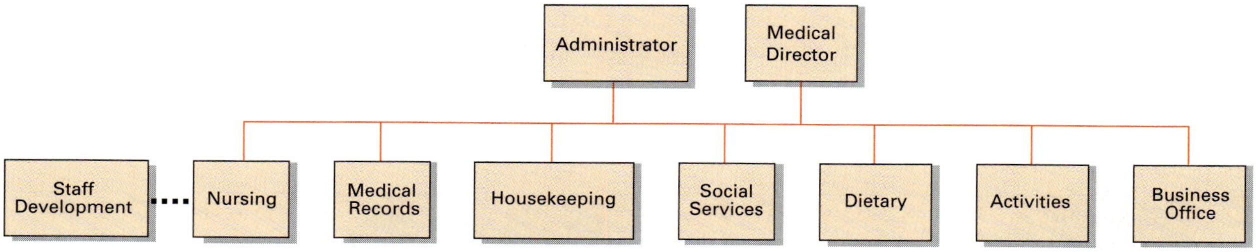

```
        ┌──────────────┐   ┌──────────────┐
        │Administrator │   │   Medical    │
        │              │   │  Director    │
        └──────────────┘   └──────────────┘
```

| Staff Development | Nursing | Medical Records | Housekeeping | Social Services | Dietary | Activities | Business Office |

FIGURE 1–2

Organization of a long-term care facility

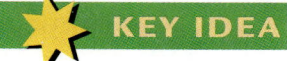

You will learn new terms and see many changes as you work in the health care field. Remember: The goal of all health care professionals is to improve patient care and the health of the community. If you stay focused on that important aim, you'll accept change as a necessary step to achieve that goal.

KEY IDEA

THE PATIENT/HEALTH CARE TEAM

The structure, or organization, of each health care team is unique. The size, complexity, and scope of services will determine the need for administration and/or layers of management. The current trend is to flatten the levels of administration and have decision making as close to the patient or at the lowest level as it can reasonably occur within the organization. The health care team model fits within the larger organizational structure of the facility. Refer to Figure 1–1 to identify the nursing branch of a health care facility.

■ Organization of the Health Care Team

Some models will work better in some settings than others. The nature of the patient care required, function, size, and location of a patient care facility affect staffing needs. What works best in a major metropolitan area is not necessarily the best option for a rural location. Also, the needs of the patients or residents in a hospice, nursing home, hospital, or home care setting differ greatly. Several models of patient/health care teams are described here. Each model indicates the relationship of the members of the nursing staff to each other and directs the interaction of staff with patients. Become familiar with the health care team models discussed here and realize that wherever you work the organization of the team may vary. Each one's role is important to the patient's care.

■ **Functional Nursing:** The **nurse manager** or charge nurse assigns and directs all patient care responsibilities for the nursing staff. This system is sometimes called *direct assignment*. In this organization, one nurse would be responsible for all medications; another for taking all vital signs.

■ **Team Nursing:** The nurse manager is sometimes called the resource nurse. She or he divides the staff into teams. Each team has a leader. The nurse manager assigns a group of patients to each team. The team leader then makes out the patient care assignments for all the members of the team. Team members may be registered nurses (RN), licensed practical nurses (LPN), or **nursing assistants** (NA) or patient care assistants (PCA) (Figure 1–3). The **team leader** is teacher, adviser, and helper to all the team members. This system is **task oriented.** This means that nursing care is arranged according to what must be done for a group of patients.

functional nursing A method of organizing the health care team in which the head nurse assigns and directs all patient care responsibilities for the nursing staff; this is sometimes called direct assignment

nurse manager The RN leader responsible for the care delivery, personnel supervision, and operating budget of a unit, area, or facility

team nursing A task-oriented method of organizing the health care team in which the team leader gives patient care assignments to each team member

FIGURE 1–3

The nursing care health team

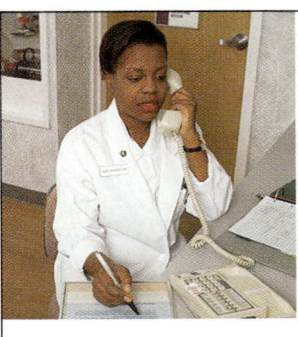

PROFESSIONAL REGISTERED NURSE
Four-year university education with a bachelor's degree
or
Two-year junior or community college education with an associate degree
or
Three-year diploma from a hospital nursing school
and
Passed state board examinations

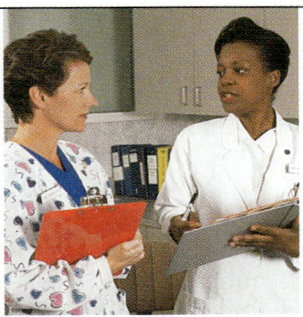

LICENSED PRACTICAL NURSE (LPN)
or
LICENSED VOCATIONAL NURSE (LVN)
One-year training program
Passed state board examinations
PLPN/MLPN—Pharmaceutical Licensed Practical Nurse is one who administers drugs or medications after taking a special course and passing a special examination

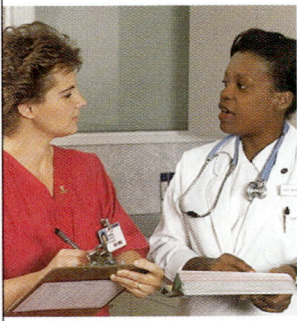

PERSONAL CARE ATTENDANT
PERSONAL CARE ASSISTANT
HOMEMAKER
NURSING ASSISTANT
NURSING AIDE
NURSE'S AIDE
NURSE'S ASSISTANT
HOME HEALTH AIDE
HOME HEALTH ASSISTANT
GERIATRIC AIDE
GERIATRIC ASSISTANT
ORDERLY
NURSING ATTENDANT
All are names used for the nonprofessional worker, who, under the direction and supervision of the registered nurses, carries out basic bedside nursing functions

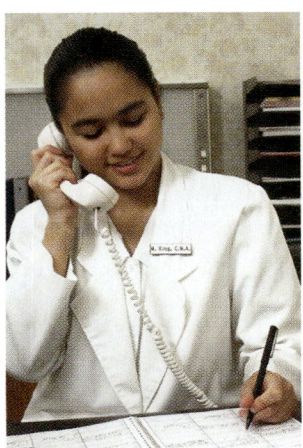

WARD CLERK
HEALTH UNIT SECRETARY
HEALTH UNIT CLERK
HEALTH UNIT COORDINATOR
Works at the desk of the nurses' station
—Does clerical work
—Answers the telephone at the nurses' station
—Helps to direct traffic on the floor
—Fills out requisition slips
—Transcribes physician's orders

- **Primary Nursing:** Primary nursing is a method of patient care delivery in which the professional **nurse** is responsible and accountable for the entire nursing care of the patient 24 hours a day. The nurse is responsible for assessing the patient's needs and for planning, implementing, and evaluating the patient's nursing care. The purpose is to ensure that the professional nurse works directly with the patient. In addition, responsibilities include family teaching, patient education, discharge planning, and coordinating discharge plans with community agencies to assist the patient after discharge. This system is patient oriented. This means that the nursing care is arranged according to the total needs of the individual patient; it is sometimes called *patient oriented* or total nursing care. The primary nurse will be assisted by associate nurses who provide care when the primary nurse is not scheduled on duty.

- **Partners in Practice:** Patient care is delivered with a combination of a nurse or primary care nurse working in partnership with a patient care assistant as a team. An assigned patient group is shared between these two partners who work closely to meet the care needs of their patients. In some settings, this model schedules both the nurse and NA to work the same schedule as much as possible to enable them to deliver care more effectively. Depending on the needs of the unit, other partner examples could include: nurse and LPN or RN and respiratory therapist.

Patient-focused Care

Along with the nursing models just described, there is an increasing trend in health care to use a **patient-focused care** delivery model. This model may involve a small team of cross-trained caregivers assigned to deliver patient care in a specific unit or area. In this case, the members are cross-trained to draw blood samples, run EKG strips, and provide other skilled care as needed. The patient receives more personalized care as there are fewer personnel in direct contact with each patient.

Figure 1–4 represents a patient-focused care delivery model involving a **multidisciplinary team** used in a health care facility. The team plans, makes decisions, and delivers

nursing assistant A person who helps the registered nurse to care for patients; nursing assistants work in hospitals, long-term care or other health care facilities, or in the patient's home

team leader The nurse responsible for one area of a nursing unit, including patient care assignments

task oriented Nursing care that is arranged according to what must be done

primary nursing A patient-oriented method of organizing the health care team in which the professional registered nurses are responsible for the total nursing care of the patient

nurse A person educated and trained to provide health care for people and to help physicians and surgeons; nurses are licensed as registered nurses (RNs) and licensed practical nurses (LPNs)

patient-focused care A care delivery model in which multidisciplinary teams plan, make decisions, and deliver care with the patient's needs a focus rather than the needs or convenience of various departments or caregivers

multidisciplinary team A team of professionals and nonprofessionals from different disciplines that plans, makes decisions, and implements the delivery of patient care that is focused, or centered, on the patient's needs rather than any particular discipline's (department's) needs

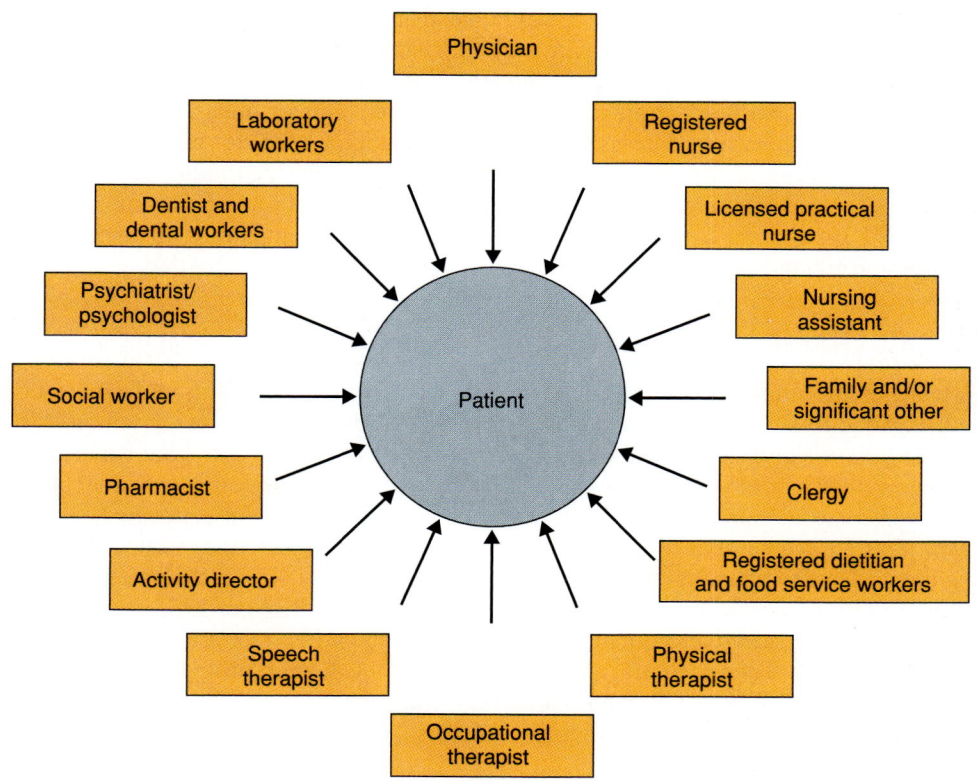

FIGURE 1–4

A multidisciplinary team provides patient-focused/ patient-centered care; when possible the team includes the patient and the patient's family

care with the patient as the central point of focus, rather than the needs of various departments and services. This design intends to provide seamless care across the continuum or episode of health care. The managers are more like coaches in this model, and the health care team workers are all working toward the common goal of delivering personalized, cost effective care focused or centered on patient needs. A multidisciplinary team involves as many or as few departments (members) as the patient's needs require.

AGE-SPECIFIC CONSIDERATIONS

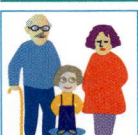 Health care institutions not only provide care based on different models, but also according to the age of the patient. This is called age specific care. This means that health care institutions recognize that patients are not all the same and need to be treated and cared for in ways that are appropriate for the stage of life in which they are. While the goals of care may be the same for all patients, how the caregivers interact with the patient, how the patient is taught, the equipment used for various ages, and safety measures needed for different age groups may vary widely. Age specific care recognizes that as patients grow, mature, and age, they need different approaches to care in order to best meet their care needs.

THE NURSING ASSISTANT: PART OF THE TEAM

As a nursing assistant, you are a member of a health care team (Figure 1–3). Everyone on the team must understand teamwork and know what they are supposed to do and then to do it to the best of their abilities with a spirit of cooperation. You will be working under the supervision of a professional nurse and cooperatively with other members of the nursing service staff. The figure provides a list of the many names used when referring to a health care worker who carries out the basic bedside nursing functions. Remember that the nurse recognizes the nursing assistant as a valuable worker, as a member of the team. Look at your head nurse, team leader, or **immediate supervisor** as someone who will help you to learn and understand your job.

It is not uncommon to see a variety of care delivery systems even within the same facility. Some models work more effectively in a given unit or area. As different ideas evolve, and the realities of decreasing reimbursement or payment for health care services continues, you can count on being exposed to different delivery models in your career. There will also be significant differences in the role expectations of nursing assistants. Figure 2–1 in Chapter 2 provides an example of the different duties and roles of the PA/NA, the advanced NA, and the Patient Care Technician.

Relationship of Nurse and NA/PCA

You are an important member of the health care team. Your assignments and expectations will vary in different facilities and on different units. A key to your success in your role is to discuss your assignment, duties, and any questions you may have with your supervisor or the nurse with whom you are working. Review the photos and information in Figure 1–3 for specific information about the credentials and responsibilities of the nursing health care team. This figure identifies the health care team members and describes some of the training they receive to function or be licensed in the role of RN, LPN, and clerk/secretary.

As a result of the Omnibus Budget Reconciliation Act (OBRA) of 1987, nursing assistants working in skilled and nursing care facilities are required to complete an approved training program. Then they must pass a competency evaluation program consisting of a written test and a skills test. Refer to Chapter 35 for more information about competency requirements and evaluation for nursing assistants.

immediate supervisor
An individual responsible for providing direction, critiquing performance, and giving feedback related to that performance

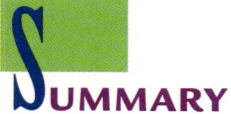 SUMMARY

The health care environment is continually changing. Members of the health care team work in a variety of inpatient and outpatient settings or in the home. These health care workers are expected to provide quality, compassionate care using a variety of patient care models, but always in a cost effective manner. Medicare, managed care companies, networks, insurers, and others set their payments to, or negotiate contracts with, health care institutions in exchange for the services provided to patients. Your employer will explain your responsibilities for patient care charges as they relate to your particular setting. Examples are charting or accounting for supplies used. Patient-focused or patient-centered care, wherein multidisciplinary teams plan, make decisions, and place the patient at the center of their care delivery, is a current trend. Understanding the organizational structure of your particular setting or facility will help you understand how and where your nursing team fits in the overall structure of your facility or agency and appreciate the specific function your team and you in particular serve in the delivery of patient services.

Notes

_____

_____

_____

_____

_____

_____

_____

_____

_____

_____

_____

_____

_____

_____

Your Role as a Nursing Assistant

INTRODUCTION

The nursing assistant is an important member of the health care team. Depending on where you work and the role you play on the team, your duties may include a range of direct and indirect patient care tasks. Job descriptions identify specific expectations, roles, and duties. Job descriptions will vary among institutions and agencies, but they reflect the institution's mission, patient care service philosophy, objectives, and/or policies. In addition to performing the required job duties, each caregiver is expected to demonstrate good interpersonal skills in interacting with other members of the health care team and with patients. Good organizational skills—time management and goal setting—along with the ability to relieve personal stress, are real assets in nursing assistants. A personal code of ethics and an awareness of the legal aspects of being a nursing assistant are essential in order to function as a caregiver.

OBJECTIVES

When you have completed this chapter, you will be able to:

- Display qualities that are desirable in a good patient/nursing assistant.
- Identify duties and role functions of nursing assistants.
- Practice good personal hygiene.
- Behave ethically.
- Keep confidences to yourself.
- Work accurately.
- Be dependable.
- Follow rules and instructions.
- Develop cooperative staff relationships.
- Show respect for patients' rights.
- Explain how laws affect you and the patients you care for.
- Report incidents.

KEY TERMS

accountable

accuracy

competency

cooperation

dependability

ethical behavior

hazard

hygiene

incident

informed consent

interpersonal skills

malpractice

negligence

stress

THE NURSING ASSISTANT: AN IMPORTANT CAREGIVER

accountable To be answerable for one's behavior; legally or ethically responsible for the care of another

competency A demonstrable skill or ability

Being a nursing assistant is not just another job—it is a serious occupation. There are many new things to learn and so many things to do as a caregiver. The fundamental patient care tasks and procedures for which you will be **accountable** can be found on the health care institution's or agency's job description. Your instructor can review any state licensing or certification **competency** requirements that apply to you.

KEY IDEA

Remain sensitive to what you would want if you or one of your loved ones were the patient. *Empathy* and *understanding* from those caring for a patient are part of the treatment. Frequently, they are as important as medicine or therapy in helping the patient to get well.

■ Role of the Nursing Assistant

Whether you are called nursing assistant, patient care assistant, patient care associate, certified nurse assistant, or some other title to reflect these roles, you will be working under the supervision of the nurse manager or team leader. We will use the terms *nursing assistant* and *immediate supervisor* to refer to you and the person who supervises you. Your immediate supervisor usually makes your assignments, provides feedback on how well you are doing, and keeps track of your overall performance. Ask your immediate supervisor for help when you do not know how to do an assigned procedure or when you are unsure of yourself. It is better to get help than to do something wrong.

If you think you are being asked to do more than you were taught to do, remember that everything you do as a nursing assistant will be supervised by a registered professional nurse. That professional nurse can either provide any additional instruction you may need or will direct you to the proper person or department for such education. Everyone in health care is expected to be continually learning new and updated information on how to best care for patients and their loved ones.

■ Duties and Functions of the Nursing Assistant

A general summary of a job description will state that the nursing assistant works under the direct or general supervision of a registered nurse, contributing to the delivery of patient care through performance of selected day-to-day activities; maintenance of a functional and aesthetic environment conducive to patient well-being; demonstration of unit/area designated competencies; and interaction with patients considering their developmental, age-specific, cultural, and spiritual preferences. Refer to Table 2–1 to review an example of the specific duties and functions expected of three different levels of nonlicensed caregivers. Special education is provided for each level.

KEY IDEA

Caregivers are expected to have good interpersonal skills that enable them to get along well with others, approach and resolve conflicts constructively, problem solve, and maintain confidentiality of information acquired in their role as caregivers.

TABLE 2–1

Patient Care Team—Nonlicensed Caregivers' Duties/Functions

PATIENT CARE TECHNICIAN	PATIENT CARE ASSOCIATE II	PATIENT CARE ASSOCIATE I
TREATMENT/PROCEDURES AS FOLLOWS:	BASIC HYGIENE/ADLS:	PREPARE AND MAINTAIN CLEAN ENVIRONMENT FOR PATIENTS:
<ul><li>Venipuncture</li><li>Blood cultures</li><li>Start, prime, discontinue IV (not to include regulating rate)</li><li>Suctioning—Tracheal, Oral</li><li>NMT's—Routine</li><li>Routine oxygen therapy</li><li>Pulse oximetry</li><li>Intermittent clean caths</li><li>Insert/d/c of urinary cath</li><li>Sterile/clean dressing changes (may use thirds solution chlorpactin, NS, bacitracin), No blind packing</li><li>PCIS documentation</li><li>Peripheral vascular checks</li><li>ROM/splints</li><li>Emergency equipment check</li><li>Assist patient with C & DB</li><li>Flush heplocks with NS</li><li>Trach care</li><li>Blood glucose monitoring</li><li>Remove NG tubes</li><li>Respond to call lights</li></ul>Unit Specific Tasks:<ul><li>Obtain blood specimens (arterial lines, heplock, CVC)</li><li>Flush A-lines, heplocks, and CVCs (as a function of blood drawing)</li><li>Hold pressure post PTCA sheath removal and/or intra-aortic balloon pump cath</li></ul>	<ul><li>Bathing/showering patients</li><li>Vital signs</li><li>Blood glucose monitoring</li><li>Obtain body weights</li><li>Strip/make beds</li><li>Oral hygiene, skin care</li><li>Shampooing, shaving</li><li>Foley care</li><li>Toileting</li><li>Transfer, turn, ambulate patients</li><li>Set up for meals</li><li>Pass trays and nourishment</li><li>Document calorie counts</li><li>Record I & Os (oral intake)</li><li>H. S. care</li><li>Transport functions</li><li>Body fluid cleaning</li><li>Respond to call lights</li><li>PCIS documentation</li><li>Assist w/menu selecting</li><li>Prepare body postmortem</li><li>Orient patient/family to room</li><li>Collect/dispose of soiled linen</li><li>Order late trays</li><li>Collect meal trays</li><li>Deliver soiled tray cart to soiled sending room</li><li>Drain IV bags; d/c IVs</li><li>D/C foley catheters</li><li>Assist with minor treatments/procedures</li><li>ROM</li><li>Unit tests per unit policy (i.e., guaiac stool, obtain sterile urine specimen from indwelling catheter)</li><li>Assist patient with C & DB</li><li>Use of equipment such as K-pad, Hoyer lift, bed scale, cardiac chair safely</li><li>Enemas</li><li>Simple clean dressing change</li></ul>	<ul><li>Mop floors in rooms/halls/spot mop</li><li>Clean toilets/sinks in patient rooms</li><li>Clean nursing stations</li><li>Clean soiled utility room</li><li>Clean med room</li><li>Clean supply room</li><li>Dusting furniture, ceiling, and windows</li><li>D/C cleaning of patient rooms</li><li>Empty trash in patient rooms*</li><li>Strip beds*</li><li>Make beds—unoccupied/occupied w/assistance</li><li>Prepare room for patient arrival</li><li>Replenish soaps, toilet papers, towels, etc. in patient rooms*</li><li>Disinfect showers/tub between use/daily general clean*</li><li>Body fluid cleaning*</li><li>Needlebox exchanges*</li><li>Stock/clean pantry area</li><li>Stocking of other supplies</li><li>Minor maintenance duties</li><li>Monitor level of linen</li><li>Assist w/stocking and replenishing of unit supply carts/medication carts</li><li>Check/restock emergency equipment/supplies housed in patient rooms</li><li>Answer phones and communicate messages*</li><li>Assure working condition of selected equipment</li></ul>Under the direction of the RN:<ul><li>Respond to call lights</li><li>Assist other nursing associates with making occupied beds and assisting with patient ADLs</li><li>Assist with meal set up, delivery of trays and return of food cart</li><li>Escort patients in a wheelchair for procedures or discharge</li></ul>
All Basic Hygiene/ADLs as listed under PCA II Prepare and maintain clean environment for patients (responsible for * items under PCA I) **Not all-inclusive lists**	Prepare and maintain clean environment for patients (responsible for * items under PCA I)	

SOURCE: Chart courtesy of St. Joseph Mercy Hospital, Ann Arbor, Michigan.

PERSONAL QUALITIES

You have decided that you want to be the best nursing assistant you can be and do the best possible job. What kind of person makes a good nursing assistant? Certain traits, attitudes, and habits are often observed in people who are successful in their work in health care institutions, especially on the nursing team. **Interpersonal skills**, such as courtesy and **cooperation**, enable people to interact or work together in a productive and satisfying manner. Some of these traits are built into your personality—you have had them all along. Others can be learned through practice. Refer to Chapter 3 for more information about interpersonal skills and communicating with patients and coworkers.

Use the Traits and Attitudes checklist to see where you stand. Put a check mark in the "yes" column to indicate qualities you already have or in the "can learn" column next to those you think you can work on to make them a part of your personality.

interpersonal skills Skills used in interacting with other persons, such as courtesy; good interpersonal skills enable people to interact or work together in a productive and satisfying manner

cooperation Working or acting together; uniting to produce an effect or to share an activity for mutual benefit

Traits and Attitudes Checklist

	Yes	Can Learn
1. I am trustworthy, dependable, and honest.	_____	_____
2. I relate easily to new people.	_____	_____
3. I make friends quickly.	_____	_____
4. I enjoy working with people.	_____	_____
5. I get along well with others.	_____	_____
6. I am sensitive to the feelings of others.	_____	_____
7. I am considerate and tactful.	_____	_____
8. I want to help people.	_____	_____
9. I try to be gracious and polite at all times.	_____	_____
10. I get satisfaction when serving others.	_____	_____
11. I show sympathy and patience with others.	_____	_____
12. I try to control my temper.	_____	_____
13. I believe the work I do is important.	_____	_____
14. I want to improve my performance.	_____	_____
15. I like to learn new things.	_____	_____
16. I rarely let my private life interfere with my work.	_____	_____
17. When the work is heavy and everyone is tense, I try a little harder.	_____	_____
18. I have a sense of humor.	_____	_____
19. I exercise regularly and/or have a way to reduce stress in my life.	_____	_____
20. I feel comfortable helping those who are less able to help themselves.	_____	_____

Personal Hygiene and Appearance

All members of the nursing team are teachers by the example they set. They influence each other to become better in their jobs. The practice of good personal **hygiene**, as used in a health care environment, becomes a teaching tool. Here are things to remember about personal cleanliness and your appearance:

- Dress properly and neatly. Follow the dress code of the health care institution where you work.

- Use good personal hygiene, bathing or showering daily.

- Keep your mouth and teeth clean and in good condition.

- Keep your hair clean and neatly combed. Long hair should be braided, pulled back, or pinned up.

- Keep your nails short and clean. Wear only clear nail polish, if any.

- Wear no or very little makeup.

- Try to be completely free of odor. Do not use heavy perfume, scented sprays, or heavy shaving lotion. Use an unscented deodorant.

- Have a physical checkup every year.

- Eat a well-balanced diet every day.

- Get plenty of sleep. Be alert when you come to work.

- Keep your body fit; do daily exercises.

- Wear clean clothes every day.

- Wear comfortable, low-heeled, enclosed shoes with nonskid soles and heels.

- Keep your shoes polished and the laces clean.

- Repair rips and hems and replace missing buttons on your clothing.

- Never wear jewelry, such as large, dangling earrings, bracelets, or pendants.

- Wear a white sweater if you are cold.

- Always wear your name pin and institutional badge.

- Always wear a wristwatch with a second hand.

- Always carry a pen and a pad of paper.

Patients believe a health care environment is, or should be, one of the cleanest places in the world. You will want, therefore, to be especially clean and fresh looking yourself.

hygiene The science that deals with the preservation of health; when used to describe an object or a person, it means clean and sanitary

ORGANIZING YOUR WORK

Most people working in health care today find the demands of their jobs very hard to meet. Along with your patient assignment, you will be given a list of other duties to complete. Some information you need will be given in a report or written on the patient's care plan or care map. It is helpful to plan how you will complete your assignment and begin immediately. Avoid putting off or delaying completion of your work.

■ Time Management

Time management is planning, prioritizing, and organizing your work or tasks to be completed in a given period of time, usually measured in hours and minutes. You will need to *prioritize* your work, meaning you do the most important things first. You decide which things are most important by reviewing your assignment, noting what needs attention first, second, and so on. Decisions you make will be influenced by doctors' orders, nurses' instructions, scheduled tests or appointments, and immediate physical, safety, or welfare needs of your patients.

Patient needs take priority over housekeeping or cleaning needs. Your supervisor will help you determine when you need to change your priorities. Frequently, new needs and unexpected situations arise in the workplace that require you to adjust your priorities, for example, requests to assist with other patients' needs or unforeseen emergencies. If you use your time to complete assigned tasks, including cleaning and returning equipment and supplies and charting sooner than the last part of your scheduled shift, you will be less hurried and feel more satisfied in your work. It is helpful to make and carry a written list to remind you of your assignments. This list can be checked as you complete assigned duties and provide patient care, and it serves as a reminder of what you need to do.

■ Goal Setting

Goal setting means identifying a target or desired end and developing an action plan to move toward it. You set a goal when you decided to become a nursing assistant. For example, you identified the educational program and applied for acceptance, or you secured a position where the education was provided as part of your orientation. Attending classes, studying, practicing your new skills, and preparing for your final tests and/or examination are the action steps to accomplish this goal.

■ Stress Reduction

stress A physical, mental, or emotional tension or strain triggered by a stimulus that requires some response or type of adjustment

Stress is a physical, mental, or emotional tension triggered by a stimulus that requires some response or type of adjustment. Everyday sources of stress are loss, fear, threat, frustration, uncertainty, and conflict. The demands you experience in your personal life and in your role as a nursing assistant can cause you to feel an uncomfortable level of stress or anxiety.

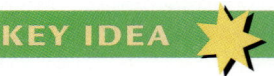

KEY IDEA

When there is too little *stress*, nothing much happens or gets done. Too much stress can leave one feeling overwhelmed, even immobilized.

Stress can come from inside or outside. Internal (inside) stresses are self-imposed by what a person thinks or does. External (outside) stresses are caused by demands posed by other people, things, circumstances, or events.

There are many things you can do to relieve stress. It is best to try several ways to see what works for you. The means one person uses to relieve stress may not relieve stress for another person. It may even cause additional stress.

Avoid people, situations, or things that can increase your stress. Some people drink alcohol to excess, use street or recreational drugs, or gamble to have fun or "relax." For many, these activities lead to serious addiction and/or dependency, become serious personal or money problems, and interfere with the ability to work, causing attendance problems. If you or your loved ones are having problems, there are numerous confidential community resources available for individuals desiring help or support to change.

GUIDELINES

WAYS TO REDUCE STRESS

- Exercising physically at least three times a week for 20–30 minutes.

The activity can be the same each time or any combination of the following: running, walking briskly, swimming, dancing, playing basketball or soccer, or aerobic exercises—activities that get your heart rate higher.

- Gardening, yard work, house cleaning, or hobbies.
- Listening to music that is soothing and relaxing to you.

- Talking with understanding friends or family members who can help you put things in perspective.
- Using humor, watching comedy movies, or listening to funny people.
- Reading, meditation, or prayer.
- Soaking in a hot bath or swimming.

ETHICAL BEHAVIOR

Ethical behavior means doing what you ought to do because it is right and consistent with good and moral conduct. As a member of the nursing team, a patient/nursing assistant will be expected to subscribe to the same high standard that professional nurses and health care providers do. Nursing has a Code for Nurses that outlines the values, norms, and ideals of the profession. It provides guidance for conduct and a framework within which to look at and evaluate nursing actions. As a nursing assistant, you should observe this code for ethical behavior.

Patients derive their images of the nursing service primarily from the behavior of the individuals with whom they come in contact. All members of the nursing team must adhere to standards of personal ethics that reflect credit on the nursing profession. Members of the nursing team are responsible for their individual conduct in accord with the professional standards of care. Each member of the health care team has the ability to positively or negatively influence the individuals with whom they come in contact.

ethical behavior To keep promises and do what you should do; to act in accordance with the rules or standards for right conduct or practice

GUIDELINES

OBRA

CODE OF ETHICS

- Be conscientious in the performance of your duties. This means do the best you can.
- Be generous and sensitive in helping your patients and your fellow workers.

- Carry out faithfully the instructions you are given by your immediate supervisor.
- Perform *only* procedures that you have been educated to do or that are on (or below) the level of duties/responsibilities listed in your job description.
- Respect the right of all patients to beliefs and opinions that might be different from yours.
- Let the patient know that it is your pleasure, not just your job, to assist him or her.

- Try to demonstrate that you are sincere in your involvement in the care of a human being. Always show that the patient's well-being is of the utmost importance to you.
- Do not accept tips from patients. You are expected to do a good job for the salary paid by your employer. Graciously decline any tips offered and reassure patients they do not need to offer tips to receive or reward good care.

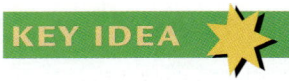

KEY IDEA   Ethical behavior means doing what you ought to do because it is right and consistent with good and moral conduct.

Practicing high ethical behavior does more than reflect well on the patient's opinion of the nursing profession. It will help you personally improve the status of the nursing assistant. A patient or visitor who observes a conscientious, willing, and honest nursing assistant will think well of that person and the entire nursing staff. All members of the nursing team must adhere to standards of personal ethics that will reflect credit on the nursing profession.

- **Ethics of Confidentiality:** Figure 2–1 outlines patient confidentiality considerations.

accuracy The quality of being exact or correct; exact conformity to truth and rules; free from errors or defects

- **Ethics of Accuracy:** Accuracy is a part of being dependable (Figure 2–2). In a health care institution, you are concerned with human lives. What might appear to you to be a tiny mistake or oversight could delay the recovery of a patient. It is vitally important for you to follow your nurse's or team leader's instructions exactly. Be accurate when you are recording a temperature. Be alert when you answer the patient's call light. Should a mistake occur, report it to your immediate supervisor at once. If you do not understand something, ask again. Always remember: There is a reason for every step in the policies of the health care institution.

- **Ethics of Dependability:** Your health care institution is organized to function efficiently when a certain number of people are on the job. If you are not there, patients could be deprived of the care they need. Also, your absence may cause your

FIGURE 2–1
The ethics of confidentiality

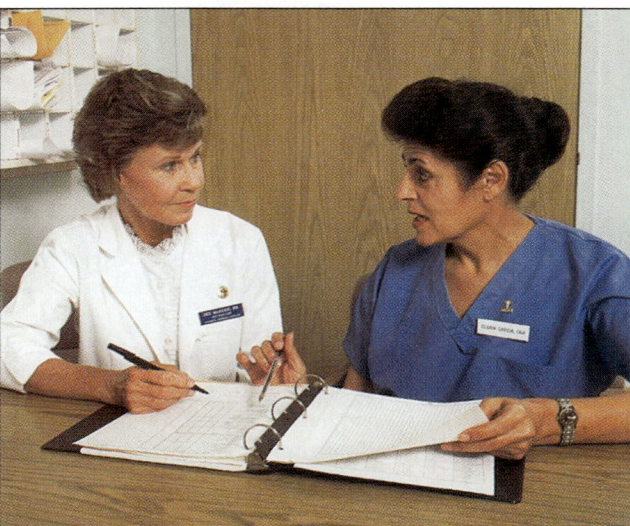

Discuss patient information only with the doctor, the R.N., your team leader, or your supervisor.

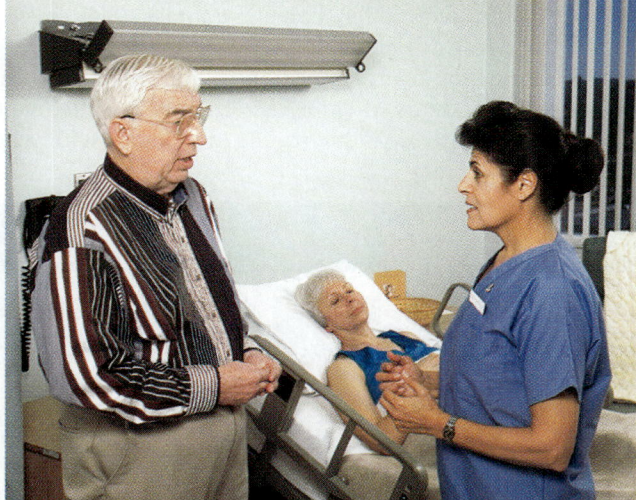

Do not discuss patient information with:
- Another patient
- Relatives and friends of the patient
- Visitors to the hospital
- Representatives of news media
- Fellow workers, except when in conference
- Your own relatives and friends

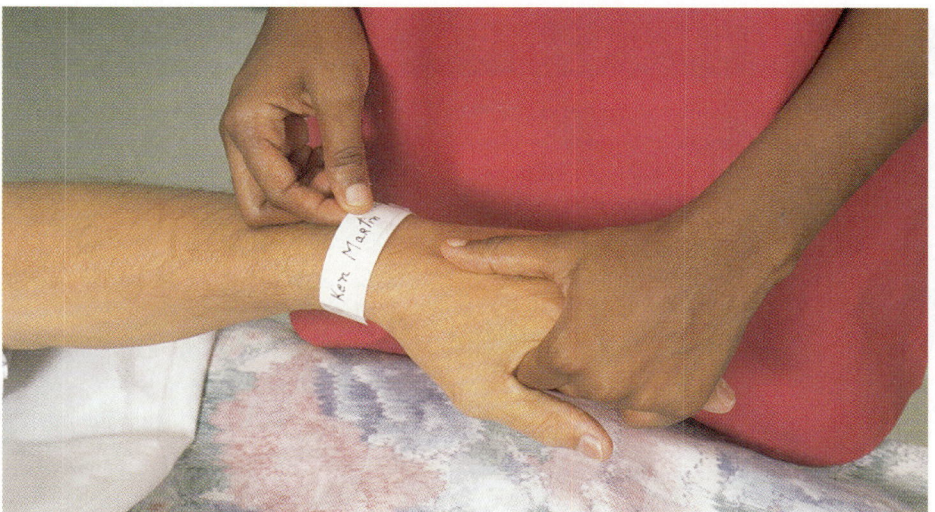

fellow workers to have an overload of work. It is essential that you arrive promptly every day unless you are ill. If you are sick, call the nursing office at the appropriate time. **Dependability** means more than coming to work on time every day. It means that the immediate supervisor who asks you to do something can rely on you to do it at the proper time and in the proper way (Figure 2–3).

Everybody follows instructions and goes by rules. Otherwise, the job would never get done. Even the top people in the health care institution have to follow rules. On page 24 are some useful guidelines to remember in your work. They can help to make you a better nursing assistant.

dependability A quality shown by coming to work every day on time and doing what is asked at the proper time and in the proper way

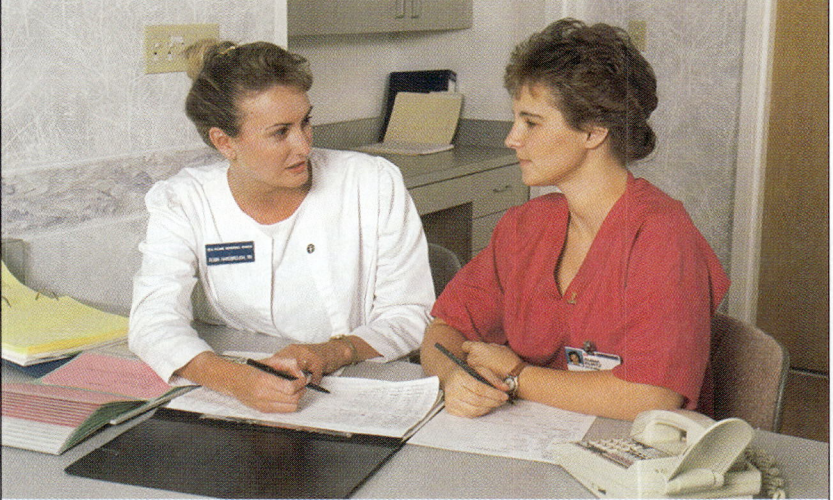

FIGURE 2–3

Be dependable

- Report to work on time.
- Keep absences to a minimum.
- Keep promises.
- Do an assigned task as well as you can: finish it quickly, quietly, and efficiently.
- Perform a task you know should be done, without having to be told.

GUIDELINES

OBRA

WORK RULES AND INSTRUCTIONS

- In your written or verbal communication, be *accurate* to the best of your ability.
- Follow carefully the instructions of your immediate supervisor.

- If you do not understand something, ask your immediate supervisor for more information or to explain the reason why.
- There are good reasons for every work rule and every procedure in the health care institution. Be aware of them all or at least know where you can look them up.
- Report accidents or errors immediately to the immediate supervisor.
- Keep confidences to yourself, except when it might be dangerous to a patient. For example, a patient

tells you she is not taking her medicine. Report this to your immediate supervisor.
- Do not waste or destroy supplies or equipment.
- Be ready to adjust quickly to new situations.
- Try to get things done on time. Use a systematic work schedule.
- Work to be a good team member.

Staff Relationships

You will find your fellow workers and other health care personnel more agreeable and helpful if you treat them properly (Figure 2–4). Some good practices are:

- Report to the immediate supervisor whenever you leave the unit for any purpose and at the end of your shift. Report to the supervisor again when you return.

- Volunteer to assist coworkers as time allows or when you recognize your help is needed.

- Direct all questions you may have about patients and their care to your immediate supervisor.

- Tell your nurse manager or team leader about personal problems that you feel might be interfering with your work. There may be confidential employee assistance programs to help you.

- Avoid talking about your personal problems with other staff members; never discuss your personal problems with patients.

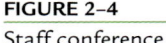

FIGURE 2–4

Staff conference

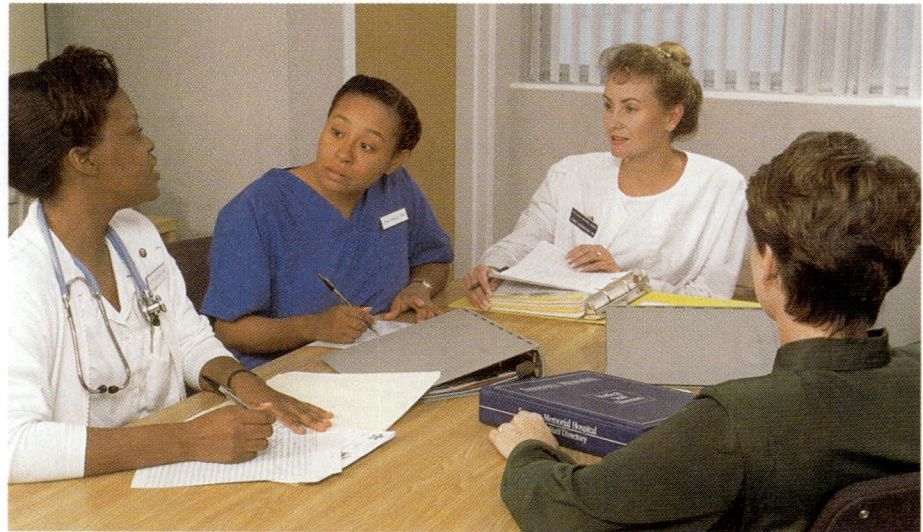

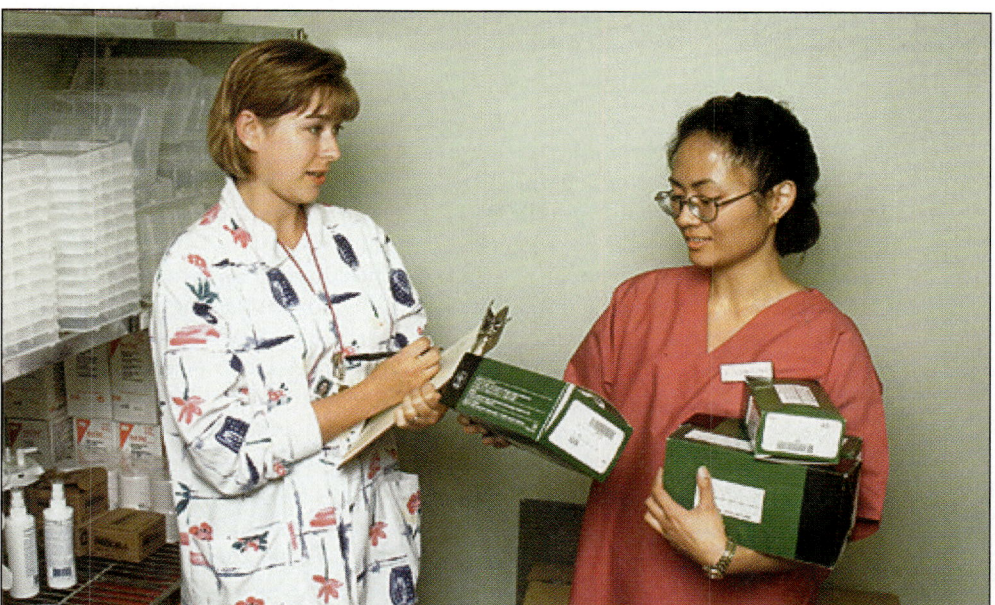

FIGURE 2–5
Cooperate with your fellow workers

"I'll do my best to get the job done right."
- Accept jobs assigned to you without complaint.
- Follow the advice of your supervisors.
- Show a willingness to learn.

- Follow all instructions given to you by your immediate supervisor. If you are confused about any of your assignments, discuss them with the immediate supervisor.

- Report all complaints from patients and visitors to the immediate supervisor. Never ignore complaints, no matter how silly or unreasonable they may seem to you.

- Perform all your duties in a spirit of cooperation and follow orders willingly (Figure 2–5).

- Be courteous and express your appreciation in interacting with team members. Of course, always remember to say *please* and *thank you*.

LEGAL ASPECTS OF PATIENT CARE

Laws concerning patients and workers in health care institutions are written to protect both the patients and the workers. As nursing assistants, you need to understand how the law affects you and the patients you care for. One important legal aspect you will learn about is incident or occurrence reporting. This plays an important role in responsible patient care and the safety program of your institution. It is advisable that you know the laws of your particular state.

The Patient's Bill of Rights

The American Hospital Association has written a *Patient's Bill Of Rights* to be used as a guide for doctors, health care providers and employees in hospitals, and patients. This document describes the basic rights to which the patient is entitled. See Figure 2–6 for

A PATIENT'S BILL OF RIGHTS

MANAGEMENT ADVISORY

PATIENT AND COMMUNITY RELATIONS

INTRODUCTION

Effective health care requires collaboration between patients and physicians and other health care professionals. Open and honest communication, respect for personal and professional values, and sensitivity to differences are integral to optimal patient care. As the setting for the provision of health services, hospitals must provide a foundation for understanding and respecting the rights and responsibilities of patients, their families, physicians, and other caregivers. Hospitals must ensure a health care ethic that respects the role of patients in decision making about treatment choices and other aspects of their care. Hospitals must be sensitive to cultural, racial, linguistic, religious, age, gender, and other differences, as well as the needs of persons with disabilities.

The American Hospital Association presents *A Patient's Bill of Rights* with the expectation that it will contribute to more effective patient care and be supported by the hospital on behalf of the institution, its medical staff, employees, and patients. The American Hospital Association encourages health care institutions to tailor this bill of rights to their patient community by translating and/or simplifying the language of this bill of rights as may be necessary to ensure that patients and their families understand their rights and responsibilities.

BILL OF RIGHTS*

1. The patient has the right to considerate and respectful care.

2. The patient has the right to and is encouraged to obtain from physicians and other direct caregivers relevant, current, and understandable information concerning diagnosis, treatment, and prognosis.

   Except in emergencies when the patient lacks decision-making capacity and the need for treatment is urgent, the patient is entitled to the opportunity to discuss and request information related to the specific procedures and/or treatments, the risks involved, the possible length of recuperation, and the medically reasonable alternatives and their accompanying risks and benefits.

   Patients have the right to know the identity of physicians, nurses, and others involved in their care, as well as when those involved are students, residents, or other trainees. The patient also has the right to know the immediate and long-term financial implications of treatment choices, insofar as they are known.

3. The patient has the right to make decisions about the plan of care prior to and during the course of treatment and to refuse a recommended treatment or plan of care to the extent permitted by law and hospital policy and to be informed of the medical consequences of this action. In case of such refusal, the patient is entitled to other appropriate care and services that the hospital provides or transfer to another hospital. The hospital should notify patients of any policy that might affect patient choice within the institution.

4. The patient has the right to have an advance directive (such as a living will, health care proxy, or durable power of attorney for health care) concerning treatment or designating a surrogate decision maker with the expectation that the hospital will honor the intent of that directive to the extent permitted by law and hospital policy.

   Health care institutions must advise patients of their rights under state law and hospital policy to make informed medical choices, ask if the patient has an advance directive, and include that information in patient records. The patient has the right to timely information about hospital policy that may limit its ability to implement fully a legally valid advance directive.

5. The patient has the right to every consideration of privacy. Case discussion, consultation, examination, and treatment should be conducted so as to protect each patient's privacy.

6. The patient has the right to expect that all communication and records pertaining to his/her care will be treated as confidential by the hospital, except in cases such as suspected abuse and public health hazards when reporting is permitted or required by law. The patient has the right to expect that the hospital will emphasize the confidentiality of this information when it releases it to any other parties entitled to review information in these records.

*These rights can be exercised on the patient's behalf by a designated surrogate or proxy decision maker if the patient lacks decision-making capacity, is legally incompetent, or is a minor.

FIGURE 2–6

Patient's Bill of Rights (Reprinted with permission from the American Hospital Association, Copyright 1992.)

7. The patient has the right to review the records pertaining to his/her medical care and to have the information explained or interpreted as necessary, except when restricted by law.

8. The patient has the right to expect that, within its capacity and policies, a hospital will make reasonable response to the request of a patient for appropriate and medically indicated care and services. The hospital must provide evaluation, service, and/or referral as indicated by the urgency of the case. When medically appropriate and legally permissible, or when a patient has so requested, a patient may be transferred to another facility. The institution to which the patient is to be transferred must first have accepted the patient for transfer. The patient must also have the benefit of complete information and explanation concerning the need for, risks, benefits, and alternatives to such a transfer.

9. The patient has the right to ask and be informed of the existence of business relationships among the hospital, educational institutions, other health care providers, or payers that may influence the patient's treatment and care.

10. The patient has the right to consent to or decline to participate in proposed research studies or human experimentation affecting care and treatment or requiring direct patient involvement, and to have those studies fully explained prior to consent. A patient who declines to participate in research or experimentation is entitled to the most effective care that the hospital can otherwise provide.

11. The patient has the right to expect reasonable continuity of care when appropriate and to be informed by physicians and other caregivers of available and realistic patient care options when hospital care is no longer appropriate.

12. The patient has the right to be informed of hospital policies and practices that relate to patient care, treatment, and responsibilities. The patient has the right to be informed of available resources for resolving disputes, grievances, and conflicts, such as ethics committees, patient representatives, or other mechanisms available in the institution. The patient has the right to be informed of the hospital's charges for services and available payment methods.

The collaborative nature of health care requires that patients, or their families/surrogates, participate in their care. The effectiveness of care and patient satisfaction with the course of treatment depend, in part, on the patient fulfilling certain responsibilities. Patients are responsible for providing information about past illnesses, hospitalizations, medications, and other matters related to health status. To participate effectively in decision making, patients must be encouraged to take responsibility for requesting additional information or clarification about their health status or treatment when they do not fully understand information and instructions. Patients are also responsible for ensuring that the health care institution has a copy of their written advance directive if they have one. Patients are responsible for informing their physicians and other caregivers if they anticipate problems in following prescribed treatment.

Patients should also be aware of the hospital's obligation to be reasonably efficient and equitable in providing care to other patients and the community. The hospital's rules and regulations are designed to help the hospital meet this obligation. Patients and their families are responsible for making reasonable accommodations to the needs of the hospital, other patients, medical staff, and hospital employees. Patients are responsible for providing necessary information for insurance claims and for working with the hospital to make payment arrangements, when necessary.

A person's health depends on much more than health care services. Patients are responsible for recognizing the impact of their lifestyle on their personal health.

CONCLUSION

Hospitals have many functions to perform, including the enhancement of health status, health promotion, and the prevention and treatment of injury and disease; the immediate and ongoing care and rehabilitation of patients; the education of health professionals, patients, and the community; and research. All these activities must be conducted with an overriding concern for the values and dignity of patients.

FIGURE 2–6 *(continued)*

Patient's Bill of Rights

the complete twelve provisions. Patients are responsible for knowing and exercising their rights in accordance with the laws of their state.

The words negligence and malpractice are often used interchangeably, as if they were the same thing. Officially, **negligence** is the commission of an act or failure to perform an act where the respective performance or nonperformance *deviates* from the act that should have been done by a reasonably prudent person under the same or similar conditions. **Malpractice** is negligence when applied to the performance of a professional. When a nursing assistant does not follow the directions of an immediate supervisor, and such failure causes or results in injury to the patient, then the nursing assistant has committed a negligent act. Examples of negligent acts nursing assistants might commit follow.

- Failure to raise the side rails on a patient's bed and the patient falls

- Failure to open the bottom of the mechanical lift to its widest position before use and the patient falls

- Failure to follow instructions to turn the patient every two hours, and to document same, and the patient develops decubitus ulcers

- Failure to place the patient's feet on the provided footrests of the wheelchair and as a result the wheels of the wheelchair run over and injure the patient's feet

Standards of care are based on laws, administrative policy, and guidelines published for nursing assistants. The professional standards of care are usually defined with respect to community, state, or national standards. These standards of care permit you to be judged based on what is expected of someone with your education and experience. All health care institutions and home health agencies have their standards of care, which you must follow.

Good Samaritan laws have been developed to protect individuals trying to give assistance to people requiring emergency care outside the health care institution. In the states that have Good Samaritan laws, you will be granted immunity if you act in good faith to provide care to the level of your education, to the best of your ability, as a reasonable and prudent person.

negligence The commission of an act or failure to perform an act, where the respective performance or nonperformance deviates from the act that should have been done by a reasonably prudent person under the same or similar conditions

malpractice Negligence when applied to the performance of a professional

TABLE 2–2

Additional Legal Terms and Definitions

TERM	DEFINITION
Accident/incident	An unforeseen event that occurs without intent.
Accountability	The act of being liable or legally responsible.
Advanced directive (living will)	Instructions given in advance that life-support systems shall not be used in the event that the patient's death will occur soon and a physician has determined that there can be no recovery and the application of life-support systems would only artificially prolong the dying process.
Assault	An unsuccessful attempt or threat to commit bodily harm.
Battery	An assault that is actually carried out where the person is injured.
Civil law	Concerned with the legal rights and duties of private persons.
Crime	A violation against a citizen or society.
Invasion of privacy	Invasion of the right to live in seclusion without being subjected to undesired publicity.
Liability	An obligation incurred or that might be incurred through any act or failure to act.
Wills	A statement for the distribution of personal belongings and property following death.

Consent is the right to refuse your care when an adult is conscious and clear of mind. Whatever their reasons, adults have this right. A parent or legal guardian can refuse to let you care for their child. You, the nursing assistant, must report to your immediate supervisor if any adult refuses to permit you to care for him or a significant other. **Informed consent** is a voluntary act by which a conscious and mentally competent person gives permission for someone else to do something for him.

Civil rights must be guaranteed to all citizens. This includes freedom from discrimination because of *religion, ethnic origin, sex, race, physical handicap,* and *age.*

For example:

- An employer cannot discriminate in hiring practices.

- A nursing assistant cannot discriminate in care for patients.

Defamation of character means making false or damaging statements or misrepresentations about another person that defame or injure his reputation. There are two types of defamation of character:

Slander: A spoken statement (gossip)

Libel: A written statement

Abandonment is the act of leaving, walking off the premises, deserting, or neglecting a patient. If the nursing assistant is unable to care for his patient, suitable and qualified substitutes must be made with consent of the patient; otherwise, a breach of duty could occur. An example would be leaving a patient care unit/area at the end of your shift when there was no one else there to care for the patients.

Criminal law applies to felonies against society. The elements of crime and punishment are usually part of each state's legislation and judicial opinions.

False imprisonment refers to a situation in which a person is restrained or detained without proper consent. Restraints cannot be applied to any patient without a written order from the physician. It is important to review the restraint policy and procedures and follow them as outlined.

Incidents

An **incident,** or occurrence, is an event that is outside or does not fit the routine operation of the health care institution or the routine care of the patients. It may be an accident or something that might cause one. For example, a staff person stumbles into a patient in a wheelchair because someone spilled liquid and failed to wipe it up. Such incidents can affect the patients, visitors, and members of the institution's staff. Prevent accidents. Report **hazards**. Be alert for potential dangers, such as spilled liquids and trash.

Types of incidents are:

- Patient, visitor, or employee accidents

- Thefts from patients, visitors, or employees

- Thefts of facility property

- Accidents occurring on outlying hospital property, such as sidewalks, parking lots, or entrances

informed consent A voluntary act by which a conscious and mentally competent person gives permission for someone else to do something for him

incident An unforeseen event that occurs without intent

hazard A source of danger; a possible cause of an accident

Prevent accidents. Report hazards. Be alert for potential dangers, such as spilled liquids and trash.

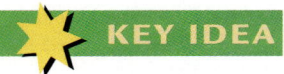 **KEY IDEA**

Whenever an incident occurs, a report must be made. Each agency will have a special form to use. Your supervisor or instructor will review the specific accident/incident

form with you (Figure 2–7). Report any incident you observe immediately. Also report any unsafe conditions you think might lead to an incident. Reporting is very important to the safety program of the health care institution and for the protection of all health care workers. For the institution to have adequate records and be prepared for possible liability suits or damage claims, all the facts related to the incidents must be known. Incident reports are filed with the hospital's administration and are not part of the patient's chart.

FIGURE 2–7
Accident/Incident Report

MEMORIAL HOSPITAL
ACCIDENT/INCIDENT REPORT — Medical Record # ________

1. Patient ☒ Visitor ☐ Employee ☐ Other ☐
2. Date of this report 12/25 19xx — Date of incident 12/25/xx
3. Name Johnson, Henry A. Age 43 Sex Male Marital Status ________
   Department ________ Position ________
4. Location incident occurred at Room 407 — Time 1:00 a.m. p.m.
5. Reported to ________ — Patient seen by Dr. Ralph A. Jones
   ________ Time ____ a.m. p.m. — ________ Time 1:05 a.m. p.m.
6. Statement of doctor or resident (diagnosis, parts of body affected and treatment)
   Patient examined—no injuries sustained—left elbow slightly
   abraded.
   ________ Attending Physician ________ M.D.
7. Describe incident and how accident occurred. (Statement of nurse or person in charge.)
   Patient found on floor—stated he attempted to get out of bed, slipped off and fell to floor.
   Slight abrasion of left elbow. No hospital property damaged.
   Signed ________ Title ________
8. Witness name Fred R. Smith Address 33 Yale St., New Brunswick, N.J.
   Witness name ________ Address ________
9. Name of machine involved ________
10. Kind of work performed by machine ________
11. Part of machine causing injury ________
12. Any protective device on machine ________
13. Action taken to prevent recurrence ________
    ________ Signed ________ Title ________
14. Did employee lose time? Yes ☐ No ☐ If yes, give last day worked mo ☐ day ☐ yr ☐
    If unable to resume work, give probable date of return mo ☐ day ☐ yr ☐ if already returned mo ☐ day ☐ yr ☐
15. If patient accident, signed ________ Date ________
    Ass't. Adm. Nursing Service
    Reported to administration on ________ at ________ a.m p.m. Signed ________ Adm.

Department director must complete necessary information in duplicate. Duplicate must be forwarded immediately to chairman of the safety committee.

Reviewed by safety committee on ________ Signed ________ Chairman.

(FILL OUT IN DUPLICATE)

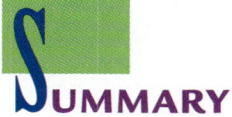

SUMMARY

The nursing assistant is an important member of the health care team. In your role as caregiver, you will be ensuring that patients do not suffer any extra pain and will be making a patient's stay in the health care institution easier. Good interpersonal skills and hygiene are expected in a nursing assistant. Good organizational skills can help make the many duties and responsibilities of the job more manageable and less stressful. As a member of the nursing team, a nursing assistant will be expected to subscribe to the high standard that professional nurses and health care providers set for themselves. Always remember that patients are entitled to respect for their human rights. They must be kept safe and properly cared for at all times. Laws concerning patients and workers in health care institutions protect both the patients and the workers. Be aware of the legal aspects of your job and understand the importance of reporting incidents in your institution's overall safety program.

Notes

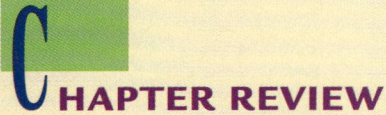

CHAPTER REVIEW

FILL IN THE BLANK

Read each sentence and fill in the blank line with a word that completes the sentence.

1. When you are legally or ethically responsible for the care of another, you are said to be _____.

2. Working or acting together for mutual benefit is called _____.

3. Good _____ includes good personal cleanliness and appearance.

4. You demonstrate good _____ when you plan, prioritize, and organize your work in order to get it done in a given time period.

5. _____ behavior includes keeping promises, doing what you should do, and acting in accordance with the rules and standards for right conduct and practice.

MULTIPLE CHOICE

Choose the best answer for each question or statement.

1. Caregivers are expected to have good communication skills to allow them to understand their patients and to work as a team.
   a. True
   b. False

2. Positive traits in a nursing assistant are all of the following except
   a. being trustworthy.
   b. enjoying working with others.
   c. liking things only a certain way.
   d. liking to learn new things.

3. The code of ethics includes following all of these standards except
   a. carrying out faithfully the instructions you are given.
   b. respecting the right of all patients to beliefs that are different from yours.
   c. letting the patient know it is your pleasure to do your job.
   d. All of the above.

4. Do not discuss patient information with
   a. other patients.
   b. relatives and friends of the patient.
   c. your family.
   d. All of the above.

5. Negligence is doing something or not doing something when a reasonably prudent nursing assistant would have done it under the same conditions.
   a. True
   b. False

6. Whenever an incident happens, remember that it is an unforeseen event that occurs without intent and so does not need to be reported.
   a. True
   b. False

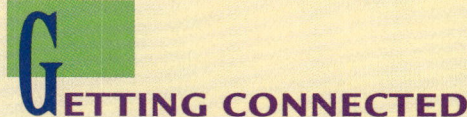

GETTING CONNECTED

MULTIMEDIA EXTENSION ACTIVITIES

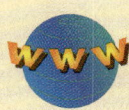

www.prenhall.com/wolgin

Use the above address to access the free, interactive Companion Website created for this textbook. Get hints, instant feedback, and textbook references to chapter-related multiple choice questions. Read and react to the "Nursing Assistants in Action." Link to other interesting sites.

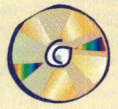

Audio Glossary

Use the CD-ROM disk enclosed with your textbook to hear the pronunciation of the key terms in the chapter.

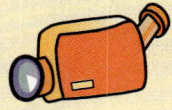

Video

Watch the "Patient Rights" video from the Care Provider Skills series and the "Focus on Professionalism" video.

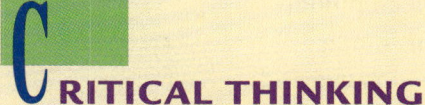

CRITICAL THINKING

USING KEY QUESTIONS

Read each question and think of what you might do in each situation.

1. What can you do to practice good hygiene?
2. Why is it so important to be accurate in everything you do, say, or write as a nursing assistant?
3. You are a new nursing assistant. How can you show that you are dependable?
4. You are a new nursing assistant. How can you show that you are cooperative?
5. What types of incidents should be reported?

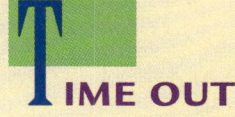

TIME OUT

TIPS FOR TIME MANAGEMENT

COMMUNICATION TIP You may be treated unfairly by a supervisor at work. This can cause you to feel hurt or angry. Take time to cool down before you react to the situation. Think through the causes of the supervisor's behavior. Avoid wasting time by discussing the unfairness with other staff members. Approach the supervisor at a later time and ask to calmly discuss what occurred. Clear the air by hearing both sides of the situation.

Communication Skills

3

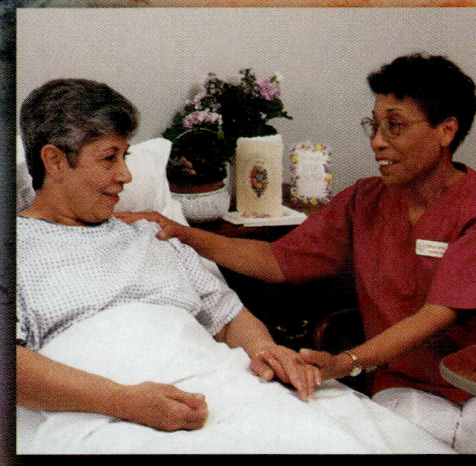

INTRODUCTION

This chapter describes how communication occurs through words and actions. As a nursing assistant, you will communicate with patients, their families or significant others, and other health care staff. It is important that you be positive and effective as a communicator. Personal qualities that promote positive communication and that you will use in communicating with patients, their families, and other health care staff are discussed. Some barriers to effective communication are also presented. Special consideration will be needed when communicating with visually- or hearing-impaired individuals as well as the pediatric patient. Information on how to communicate and document objectively or report your observations of patients is also presented.

When you have completed this chapter, you will be able to:

- Demonstrate a courteous and professional manner toward patients, families, visitors, and coworkers.
- Keep your emotions under control while on the job.
- Deal with patients and visitors in an empathetic and tactful manner.
- Show interest and concern about the patient's welfare.
- Communicate effectively with pediatric patients and their parents.
- Use communication skills effectively when relating to patients and their visitors.
- List seven barriers to effective communication.
- Answer the patient's call light signal promptly.
- Meet the patient's physical and psychological needs.
- Teach a visually or hearing impaired patient how to use the call light.
- Take complete and accurate telephone messages.
- Use your senses of sight, touch, hearing, and smell to observe your patients.
- List the behaviors to observe in a patient.
- List the behaviors to report when they are observed in infants or children.
- Differentiate between objective and subjective reporting.
- Report observations promptly, accurately, and objectively.
- Identify the basic parts and functions of a computer used to document and communicate patient information.

body language

boot up

central processing unit (CPU)

communication

courtesy

cursor

cyanosis

data

edema

empathy

feedback

hardware

keyboard

light pen

log on

memory

monitor

mouse

network

objective observations

objective reporting

observation

password

pediatric patient

PIN

printer

prompt

retrieval

screen

secretions

software

subjective observations

subjective reporting

tact

terminal

COMMUNICATION SKILLS

communication The exchange of thoughts, messages, or ideas by speech, signals, gestures, or writing between two or more people

Communication refers to the exchange of information with others. This information can be about facts, feelings, opinions, or ideas. Communication may be verbal or nonverbal. Verbal communication may be spoken or written. Greetings like "Hello" and "Good morning," phone conversations, and letters and greeting cards are examples of verbal communication. Nonverbal communication involves body language. It may be as simple as a wave of the hand or a wink, or it may involve the entire body. All communication, whether verbal or nonverbal, involves these three important elements:

- a sender: the one sending the message
- a receiver: the one receiving the message
- a message: the information shared or emotion expressed

Even if all three elements are present, the communication may not be understood, or it may be misinterpreted. For example, the sender may speak too quickly, the receiver may be busy or preoccupied and not listening, or the message may include difficult or unknown terms. Any one of these factors may affect the communication. There are certain responsibilities or criteria attached to each element in the communication. Only when these criteria are met will the communication be understood and less subject to misinterpretation.

- The sender must obtain the receiver's attention, be organized, speak clearly, and make sure the message is understood
- The receiver must listen carefully, respond appropriately, and ask for clarification, if needed
- The message must be organized, simple, and clear

Verbal Communication (Communicating through Words)

Verbal communication occurs through the exchange of spoken words. Ideas, facts, or information is transferred from the sender to the receiver. For example, when you arrive at your workplace and greet a coworker, you are communicating verbally. You are the sender, your coworker is the receiver, and your greeting is the message. Likewise, your coworker who receives your message then responds to your greeting. This response to the message, which actually may repeat the message, is called **feedback**. The exchange of greetings between you and a coworker can express very different meanings, depending upon the tone of your voice, the speed or quickness of your spoken words, your inflection, and the actual words you use. If your greeting is warm and lighthearted, you convey the idea that you are having a good day and are pleased to be there. Such a greeting may (but not necessarily) draw a similar positive response from your coworker even if he or she is not having an equally pleasant day.

feedback Response of the receiver to the sender's message; the response, or feedback, lets the sender know if the message is acknowledged and clearly understood

Written Communication

Written communication occurs when you use handwritten or printed words, photographs, or drawings to communicate. The patient's record or chart is a form of written communication. Your assignment, too, may be written on a sheet of paper or posted on the unit bulletin board. Other examples of written communication are the patient's ID bracelet, NPO and OXYGEN IN USE signs, and the different color stripes and arrows the hospital may utilize in main corridors to help you get from place to place within the facility.

■ Nonverbal Communication and Body Language

Spoken and written words are used for most communications. But there are other ways that are sometimes more effective to get a message across. Hand movements (gestures), expressions on your face, and body movements may tell the story better than words. Although no words are spoken, a powerful message can be sent. Often, one can look at a person and see that the person is happy, sad, angry, willing, or unwilling to perform a requested task. For example, if someone is slamming charts or refusing to answer a question by turning his or her body away from you, the nonverbal message is negative, but you do get a message. A very different message is communicated when you see someone hugging another, smiling, or making eye contact with another person.

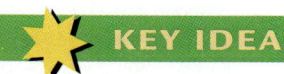

> **KEY IDEA**
>
> The three key elements in all communication are the sender, the receiver, and the message. The same message can have different meanings depending on how quickly or slowly you speak, your tone of voice, your facial expression, or gestures you make.

■ Barriers to Effective Communication

Good or effective communication is communication in which the "sender" conveys (sends) the intended message and draws an appropriate response (feedback) from the "receiver." Communication is good or effective when it is respectful, honest, clear, and appropriate. Bad, negative, or ineffective communication fails to convey the intended message or draws an inappropriate response. Communication can fail or break down for many reasons. It will be helpful to learn what ways of speaking, topics, issues, or situations may be barriers to communications. Some barriers to effective communication are:

1. Clichés, familiar, or overused phrases said with little or no thought, such as "Don't worry" or "It was meant to be"

2. Questions that can be answered with "Yes" or "No" responses, tending to end the communication

3. Language misunderstandings or misinterpretations of meaning

4. Cultural differences, including beliefs and practices

5. Sensitive topics

6. Judgmental attitudes on the part of the sender or receiver

7. Failure to listen to feedback (response to your message) or giving the receiver only partial attention

COMMUNICATION AND RELATING TO PEOPLE

Relating to people means making a connection between yourself and another person. The relations between yourself and patients, visitors, parents, and fellow workers depend on your approach and response to them. If you have a kind, courteous, sensitive, tactful, empathetic, and open manner, you will find it easier to form positive connections (Figure 3–1). Relationships depend on receiving as well as giving information, so listening attentively is as important as what you say. Communication skills are necessary to be successful as a nursing assistant.

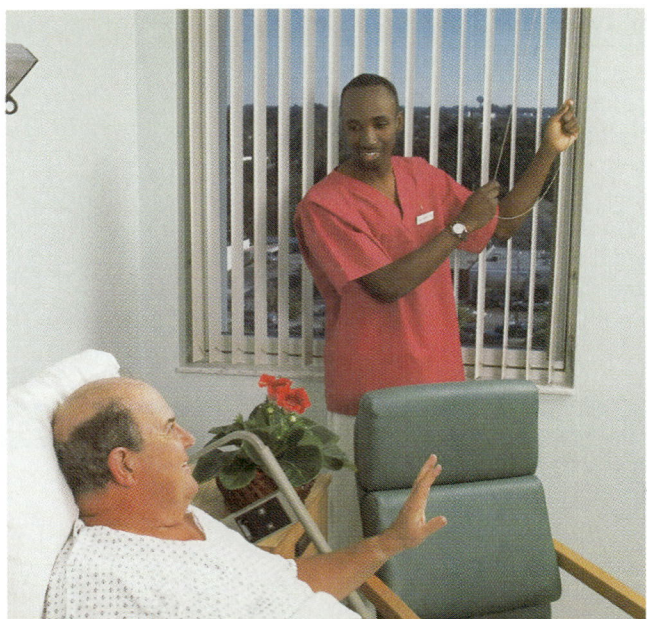 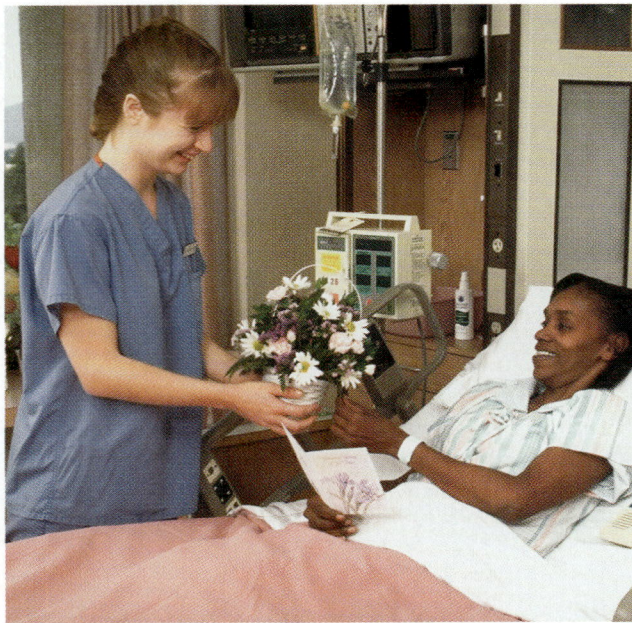

FIGURE 3–1

Helpful personal qualities include courtesy, emotional control, empathy, and tact

Taking care to be nonjudgmental when you listen and observe others will help to improve your communication with them. Maintaining emotional control by not allowing others to easily upset you with their words and actions is an essential skill for health care providers. When people are worried, anxious, or sick, their ability to control their fear and stress is reduced. Patients, coworkers, or your supervisor may share that they do not like the way you are doing a particular task or assisting them. Try to focus on the suggestion or constructive criticism being offered, rather than becoming angry or upset with the person sending the message to you.

Remember that courtesy, empathy, tact, and emotional control do much to enhance positive communication. Consider them here and think of ways to make them part of your personality.

courtesy Being polite and considerate

- **Courtesy:** consideration and respect shown for another person's needs. It means cooperating, sharing, and giving. Being polite and considerate of others shows that you care about them. Think how you would feel if you were in their place, and you will understand how far a cheerful word and a smile can go.

empathy The ability to put yourself in another's place and to see things as they see them

tact Doing or saying the right things at the right time

- **Empathy:** feelings, thoughts, and motives of one person are understood and/or felt by another person without pity. A nursing assistant should use empathy or empathize with the patient, visitor, and coworkers.

- **Tact:** doing and saying the right things at the right time. Tact also includes knowing when it is best to say nothing.

- **Emotional Control:** calm and self-control in the presence of a patient, another staff member, or a visitor who may upset or anger you. You may feel like making a rude or nasty remark or reply. Don't do it. Stop and realize that the patient may be worried, nervous, or tense. This may also be the case for family and friends who visit the patient. Fellow workers may be under stress because of a problem at home or on the job. Try to be understanding and learn to control anger and cope with all situations.

Learning to accept constructive criticism and suggestions without feeling you are being personally attacked is an essential part of your job. Try to avoid becoming defensive. If your supervisor criticizes you or tells you to do something, you may feel like saying, "That is not my job" or "Why do you pick on me?" Stop and examine your attitude. Calm down and then perform the right or correct action. It can be helpful to discuss the situation at a later time after you and your supervisor/coworker are better able to hear each other and consider a different point of view. Try to focus on the work or skill being discussed. It is easy to personalize criticisms or suggestions. Consider that your supervisor may be wanting to help you modify or improve your skills or interactions, while still valuing you as a person.

Relationships with Patients

Many things make a difference in a patient's behavior and attitude during an illness. The patient may become frightened, angry, or sad. Some factors or influences are the diagnosis, seriousness of the illness, age, previous illnesses, past experience in hospitals, and mental condition. Other things that might make a difference are the patient's personality, disposition, and financial condition.

Each patient's reaction to pain, treatment, annoyances, and even kindness is different. Always treat each patient as an individual, a person who needs your help. Respect confidences the patient shares with you, recognizing that giving the patient the opportunity to speak about physical problems or other concerns is a real kindness. Refer to Chapter 2 for more information regarding confidentiality and a code of ethics for health care staff.

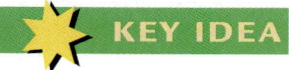
KEY IDEA

Keep confidences. Never talk to anyone except your immediate supervisor about a patient's condition. Take care to see that you are out of earshot from others when you are discussing a patient's problem. Discussing one patient's medical condition with another patient is an invasion of privacy. Never discuss your patients with family members or friends.

Always try to give the patient confidence in the hospital, the doctors, and the nursing staff. Never discuss or criticize any of your fellow staff members in front of a patient.

Remember that the patient's behavior is the result of things that worry or bother him (Figure 3–2). The patient may be hostile, mean, and nasty. You may simply be the nearest person to talk to or to lash out against. Try not to take what is said to you personally and respond in kind.

Whatever problems a patient has, you can be sure one person considers them very important—the patient. Try to be understanding. Be a good listener, even when you would rather leave.

Patients and visitors often relieve their feelings of helplessness and hopelessness through words and behavior. It may sometimes appear that they are trying to take it out on you. Be patient with them as much as possible. Remember that the patient may be suffering emotionally as well as physically; talking may relieve the emotional suffering.

Try to be as tactful as you can. When a patient begins to recover, give praise and encouragement. Do not hold a patient's behavior against them. Remember some behaviors are difficult but the individual is not a bad person because they are unkind or focused on themselves.

Always listen when a patient makes a complaint or brings up a problem. Patients' questions about the doctor or the time and plans for discharge should be referred to your immediate supervisor.

While these considerations apply to adult and pediatric patients alike, the following is particularly important to remember as you relate to children, or pediatric patients.

Sometimes a child cries when his parents are getting ready to leave the hospital. You can show empathy to both the child and parents by making the separation easier for them. Pick up the child (if permitted) and pat and soothe him. Turn the child's attention to something other than the anxiety, fear, and pain of being separated from the parents.

FIGURE 3–2
A patient worries about many things

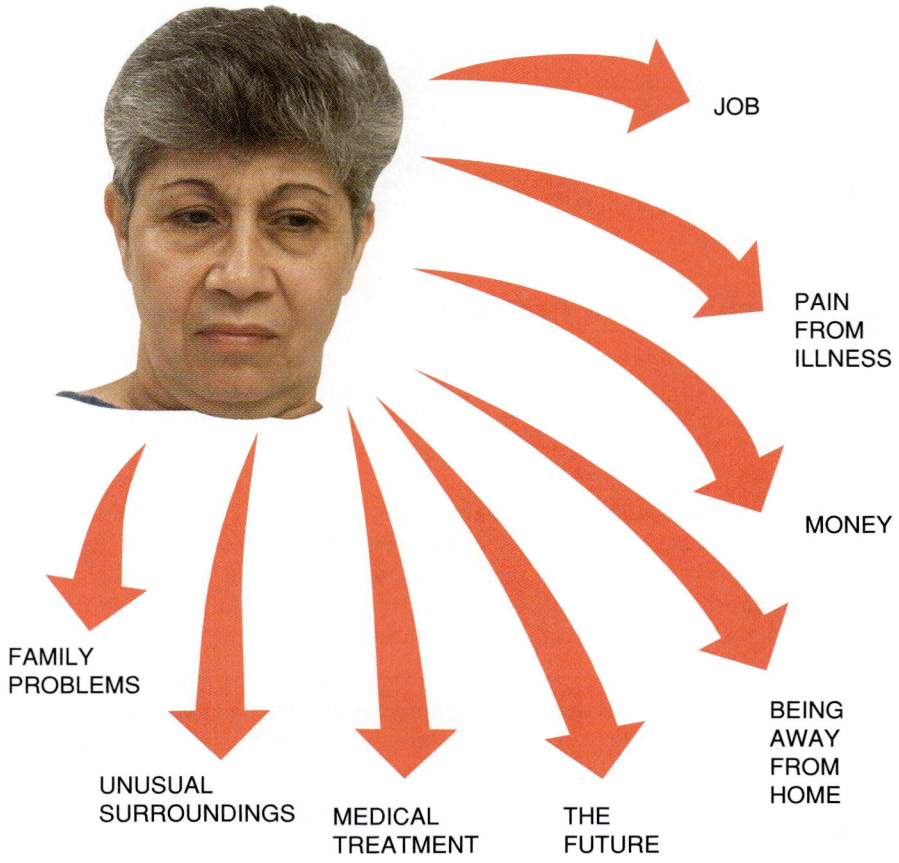

JOB

PAIN
FROM
ILLNESS

MONEY

BEING
AWAY
FROM
HOME

FAMILY
PROBLEMS

UNUSUAL
SURROUNDINGS

MEDICAL
TREATMENT

THE
FUTURE

Crying is the normal, natural way for children to express their feelings and fears. Try to understand why a child is crying excessively. Do not let it irritate you.

Never tell a child that you are going to take his temperature or blood pressure. The child may think you are going to take something away. Say you are going to measure his temperature or blood pressure instead. Explain the procedure; let the child examine the stethoscope or such to gain confidence and trust.

■ Communicating with Patients

As a nursing assistant, you are close to patients during their stay in the hospital. Often they tell you about their needs, pains, and worries. As you listen, you are both in close communication. Every time you touch a person's body, whether you speak any words or not, you are communicating something. How you assist a person in any action that involves touching the body says something. If you are careful, firm, and gentle, it tells the person something far different than if you are rough.

Pay attention to your posture. The way you move when you enter a patient's room or how you stand by the bed are ways of communicating through **body language**. Try to make these movements communicate energy, a sense of interest, and a willingness to help. A frown, an impatient body movement, or a shrug may give the patient the message, "Do not bother me." Also, a certain way of standing or walking may send the message "I am lazy" or "I don't want to be bothered."

When you feel rushed, take a moment to collect yourself and focus on the patient. Look at the patient when you speak to him (Figure 3–3). This tells the patient that he has your attention. If you are looking away when talking, the patient gets the impression that your attention is elsewhere. Speak clearly and distinctly in a normal tone of voice.

body language
Communication through hand movements (gestures), facial expressions, body movements, and touch

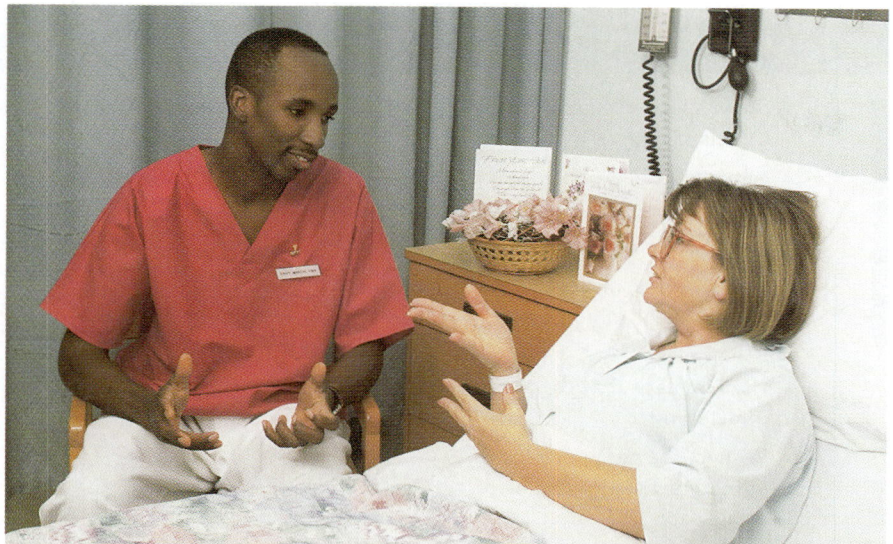

FIGURE 3–3
Explaining and clarifying information is part of the nursing assistant's job

Talk with the patient, not just to or at him. Ask the patient what he likes or dislikes, thinks, or wants. Wait for the response and listen to the responses in an interested manner. If you are particularly busy, let a patient know when you will have some time to be able to sit and talk with him. If you think there will be a delay in your return with something the patient requested, be sure to let him know.

Vulgar words or slang are not appropriate or necessary. Also, do not use medical terms or abbreviations when talking to patients and their visitors. If you use medical language and the patient does not understand, you might give the wrong idea about what is happening to the patient (Figure 3–4).

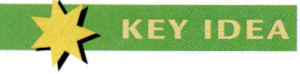

Keep your voice pleasant, not too loud or too high pitched. Speak clearly and slowly enough to be easily understood. Never whisper or mumble, even when you think the patient is asleep or cannot hear you. This is annoying to the patient.

KEY IDEA

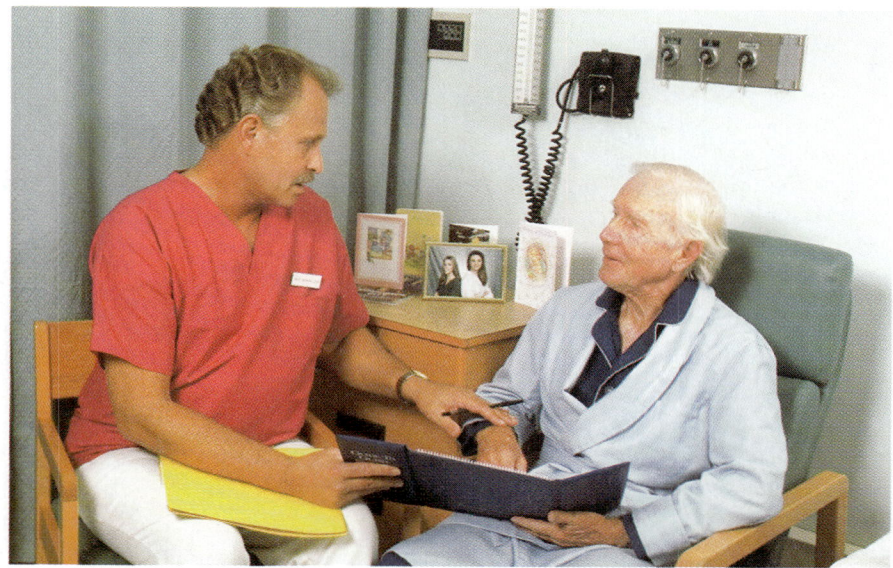

FIGURE 3–4
Communicating with patients is an important part of the nursing assistant's job

GUIDELINES

OBRA

COMMUNICATING WITH PATIENTS

- Address adults using Mr., Ms., or Mrs. and their last name unless they request otherwise.

- Show an interest in what the patient is saying.
- Let your facial expressions show that you are interested (Figure 3–4).
- Use good manners.
- Speak clearly, distinctly, and slowly. Speak in a normal, pleasant tone.
- Use language that the patient can understand.
- Respect the patient's moods. Sometimes silence can help.

- Make your body movements look pleasing and energetic.
- When someone in need asks you for assistance, whether to bathe or turn her or to get something that is out of reach, you should give your assistance willingly and graciously, no matter whose assigned patient it is. Avoid communicating a rushed or unhelpful response.

Remember that, although some patients seem to be semicomatose, comatose, or unconscious, they may be fully aware of what is happening around them and can often hear what is happening. Therefore, always speak and behave as if the patient can hear every word. They may hear more than you think. Patients frequently report conversations that occurred when they were seemingly comatose or unconscious.

Be sensitive to those times when the patient does not want to talk. Respect changes in the patient's mood or behavior. Saying nothing may have more meaning than any words or facial expressions. Sometimes a pat on the shoulder or holding a hand means more to a patient than anything you might say. Simply being near the stretcher or bed at the moment of trouble may be the most comforting message of all. It may help to silently sit near the patient for a few minutes when you know the patient is upset, afraid, or lonely. Use these guidelines when interacting with your patients.

■ Communicating with the Pediatric Patient

pediatric patient Any patient under the age of 16 years

In most hospitals, anyone under age 16 is called a **pediatric patient** (Figure 3–5). These patients may be grouped in several ways. For example, pediatric patients are sometimes

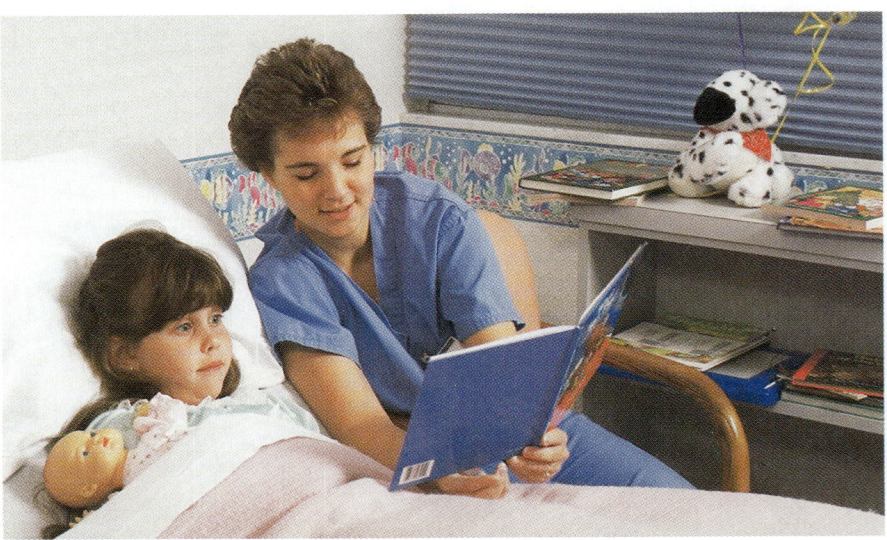

FIGURE 3–5
Pediatric patients have special needs

grouped according to age because children of different ages need different kinds and amounts of care. Children also may be grouped according to their medical or surgical condition. Refer to Chapter 15 for information on chronological-age considerations and nursing assistant behaviors in communicating with the pediatric patient. Also, see Chapter 31 for information about communicating with pediatric patients and medical and surgical conditions that necessitate hospitalizing pediatric patients.

Call a child by his first name or nickname. Using his name tells the child that you know who he is. It shows respect for the child as a person and is a mark of courtesy.

Do not use commands (Figure 3–6). Do not call any child "stupid" or "dumb." Using such words can be very harmful to a child, because if they are repeated often enough children may begin to think of themselves as stupid or dumb. Then they may begin to behave as if they were stupid, because they think this is what is expected of them.

Very small children simply cannot tell you in words what they want. It is hard for them to communicate with you. Children will try to tell you things by the sounds they make, through the use of gestures or pointing, and by the way they move. You should try to understand what their sounds and movements mean.

Try to learn the reason for their crying and then try to comfort them. Reasons for crying, of course, depend on how old the child is and perhaps on what happened before they started crying.

When you are giving children personal care, use every chance you have to show your interest in them and your affection for them. This is done in different ways with children of different ages. Although children may not complain or seem to feel sorry for themselves, they may be uncomfortable or unhappy. They need your kindness and empathy. Your smile, a tender touch, or affectionate words can tell the child that you are interested in and care about him or her. Refer to Chapter 15 for age-specific considerations and recommendations.

Importance of the Child's Family

A child is still a member of a family, even when in the hospital. The person or persons who care for the child at home represent the family. Many hospitals and pediatric patient care units have a policy of allowing a family member to stay with the child and even encourage them to do so.

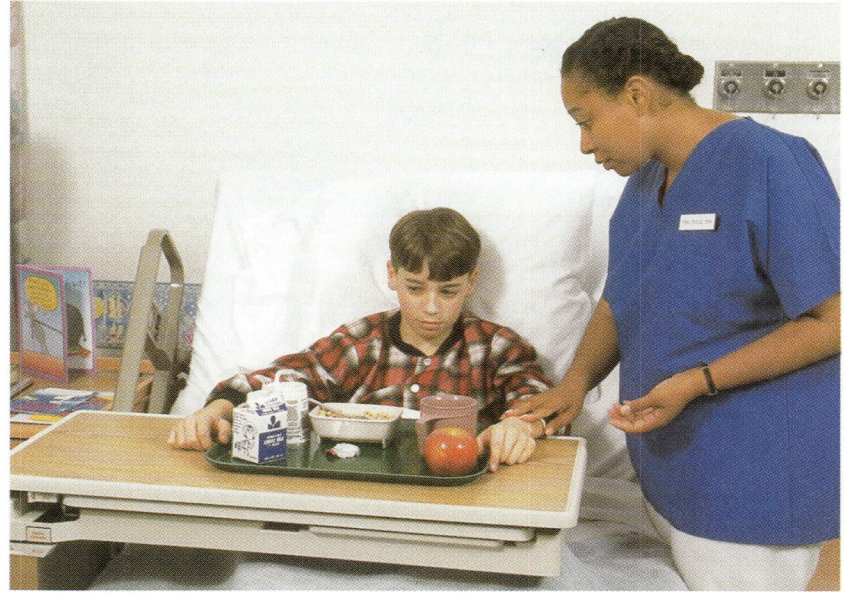

FIGURE 3–6

Do not say "Don't play with your food"; you could say "Aren't you hungry?"

KEY IDEA

This may be the first time the child has been away from home. The child may be frightened or may view hospitalization as punishment. Such a patient needs to be held, touched, and talked to in order to be comforted and reassured.

Several important things need to be considered and remembered with the pediatric patient:

- Family members need to be with their children, and children need their families.

- Family members are normally concerned and often are worried and frightened.

- Most children first learn about the world from their families.

- The younger the child, the more important the family is in helping to ease the child's fears.

Things you can do to help are:

- Do the best possible job of caring for the child. This is usually reassuring to the family members.

- Show interest and concern about the family members' welfare. Ask, "Is there something we can do?"

- Do not make judgments about the family members' attitudes or behavior, even if they seem strange to you.

- Encourage and allow family members to help take part in the child's care when possible and if permitted.

- Sometimes family members seem to be worried about something concerning their child in the hospital and are afraid to talk about it. If you suspect this, tell your immediate supervisor.

Communicating with Older Adults

Most older adults are able to easily communicate. Changes in vision or reduced hearing occur with many elderly persons. However, communicating with patients who have Alzheimer's disease, can be challenging because they are confused and disoriented. Refer to Chapter 32 for guidelines and more detailed information.

Communicating with Family and Visitors

Visiting hours are often the highlight of the day for patients. Knowing that family and friends are interested and concerned can do a lot to relax a patient's tensions, ease feelings of loneliness or isolation, relieve fears, and cheer the spirit.

Visitors may be worried and upset over the illness of a member of the family. They need your kindness and patience. Pleasant comments about flowers or gifts brought by visitors for the patient may be helpful (Figure 3–7).

If it appears that visitors are upsetting or tiring the patient, notify your immediate supervisor, who can caution the visitors or ask them to leave.

In some situations, visiting hours may be longer or shorter. Sometimes there are special circumstances where exceptions need to be made to meet the needs of particular families or visitors. Usually a note is put in the patient's chart or plan of care to alert

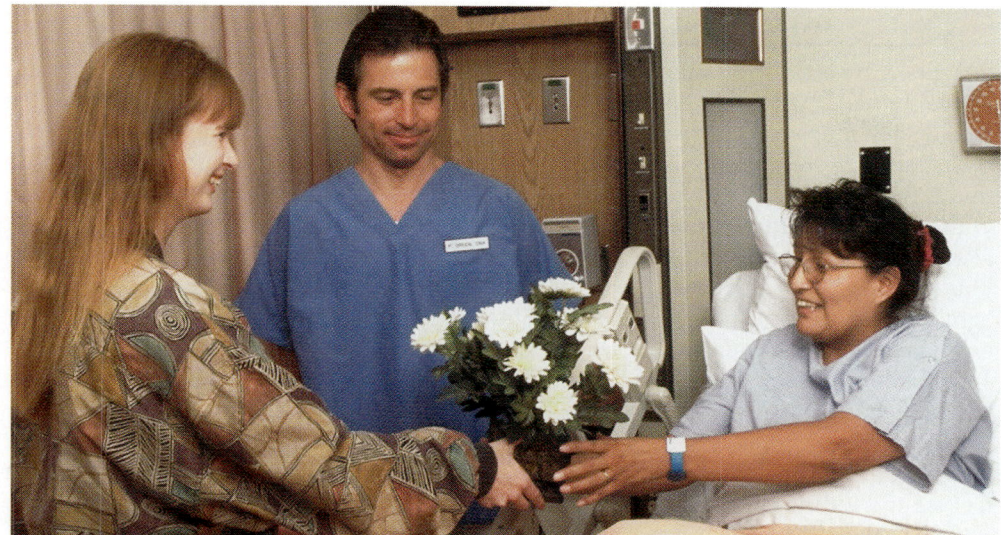

FIGURE 3–7
The nursing assistant should make visitors feel welcome

staff that a particular exception has been made. Your instructor will tell you about the visiting hours and any rules for visitors in your health care institution. These rules, of course, must be followed. Two main rules usually apply to visitors in any health care institution:

- Visitors are not allowed to take institutional property away with them.
- Visitors cannot bring food or drink to the patient unless permission has been given by the nurse or doctor.

Certain actions are helpful in your contacts with visitors. Follow these guidelines when interacting and communicating with visitors.

GUIDELINES

OBRA

COMMUNICATING WITH VISITORS

- Listen to the visitor. Whether it is a suggestion, a complaint, or "passing the time of day," listen to the person. Some suggestions by visitors can be very helpful. Some complaints may be valid. When a complaint is presented, tell the person, "Thank you for bringing this matter to my attention. I will tell my supervisor about this," and then report it to your immediate supervisor.

- Do not get involved in the family's private affairs and feelings. Never take sides in family quarrels.

Never give information or opinions to someone about other family members.

- Be prepared to give information regarding the hospital to visitors. Tell them what facilities are available for coffee, snacks, or meals, and the hours of operation. Tell them where to find a public telephone. Direct them to other places in the institution, for example, the business office or the gift shop.

■ Communication: Patients with Sensory Impairments

Patients with sensory loss present special challenges. Your patients who are visually impaired, or blind, will have the same personal care needs as your other patients. Providing care will be much easier if you explain what you wish to do and encourage the patient's cooperation. Your patient has probably accepted his visual disability and learned to do things for himself quite well. Assume your patient has normal intelligence and treat him with the respect and courtesy you would any other patient. The patient's care plan should identify how the patient can best see or hear. If this information is not available to you, then ask your patient if he has any vision at all and determine if the patient sees light, dark, shadows, and so on. Discuss things that might be helpful to the patient. For example, where his cane should be placed if the patient has one or describing the size and shape of the room, the location of the bathroom, the bedside chair, overbed table, and nightstand.

For patients who have serious vision losses, the call light is used differently. Blind or visually-impaired patients must be shown and taught how to use the signal. Have them feel around for the cord and practice using it while you are there.

If the call light is the kind that you push to turn on, you can call it a "push" button. If it works like a light switch, you can compare it to that. When working with patients who have serious visual losses, you should not expect them to turn off the signal. You can do that routinely when you respond to the signal call.

Communicating with the deaf or hearing-impaired patient who is able to read and write will be easier if you remember to carry a small pad and a pen. You can communicate with your patient in writing. Print short questions that are easy for the patient to read. The patient can respond by writing the answers. Use questions that can have either "yes" or "no" answers, if possible. Pictures or drawings can be used with patients who cannot read.

Also, if the patient wears a hearing aid, be sure it is operating and assist the patient if he has difficulty manipulating it. Refer to Chapter 26 for care of hearing aids.

Some patients can read lips. If this is true for your patient, always position yourself so that the patient is able to see your lips. Speak slowly and distinctly. Don't shout!

Many facilities have staff available to communicate with patients who present particular challenges to any staff members who do not have the training to sign, for example. Take advantage of this support staff and encourage your patient to do so. You may find it particularly helpful to learn to sign words and simple phrases.

Patients with serious hearing losses can easily learn how to pull or push the call light if you show them how to do it instead of telling them. Remember, they cannot hear you.

■ Communicating with Non-English-Speaking Patients

Sometimes patients come to the hospital who do not speak English or for whom English is a second language. It would be ideal if your facility employed workers who speak languages other than English or if you could learn certain medical terms or phrases in several languages to assist you in communicating with your patients. There may be a list of personnel or volunteers who can be called to translate when it is necessary to communicate with non-English-speaking patients. Also, communication boards with pictures or drawings of equipment, such as a bedpan, TV, phone, water pitcher, and so on, are helpful tools to use in communicating with patients. In the absence of these options, a family member or friend can be very helpful.

■ Communicating with Other Staff Members

Communication is essential in providing patients with the coordinated care they need. Staff communicate through the patient record, in report or team meetings, in conversations or consultations about particular patient needs or problems, and verbally.

■ Answering the Patient Call Signal

Every patient has a way of sending a signal to the nursing staff when something is needed. It is important to answer the patient's call for service or help without delay (Figure 3–8).

All patients have a call light or signaling device. It is important to show the patient and family how to use the call light system at the time of admission. When the patient presses the button on the end of the cord, a light flashes near the nurses' station and over the patient's door. This device may be called a call light or call bell. A hand bell system can be used if no electronic system is available. You should always keep alert for such signals. Answer the signal as soon as it flashes. Every minute seems forever to the patient who is waiting. When the patient signals:

- Go to the patient at once, quietly and in a friendly way.

- Turn off the call signal, and address the patient by name.

- Say, "Mr. Jones, what can I do for you?"

- Do whatever the patient asks, but be sure it is correct and safe for this patient. If you are in doubt, ask your immediate supervisor. Relate what the patient wants and then follow your supervisor's directions.

- Take patient and visitor concerns seriously (Figure 3–9). If you are unable to do something to correct the situation, refer the matter or problem to your supervisor.

- When necessary, use the emergency signal to get qualified personnel to assist you. Emergency signals are usually in one or more convenient locations: at the bedside, in the bathroom, shower, or tub room.

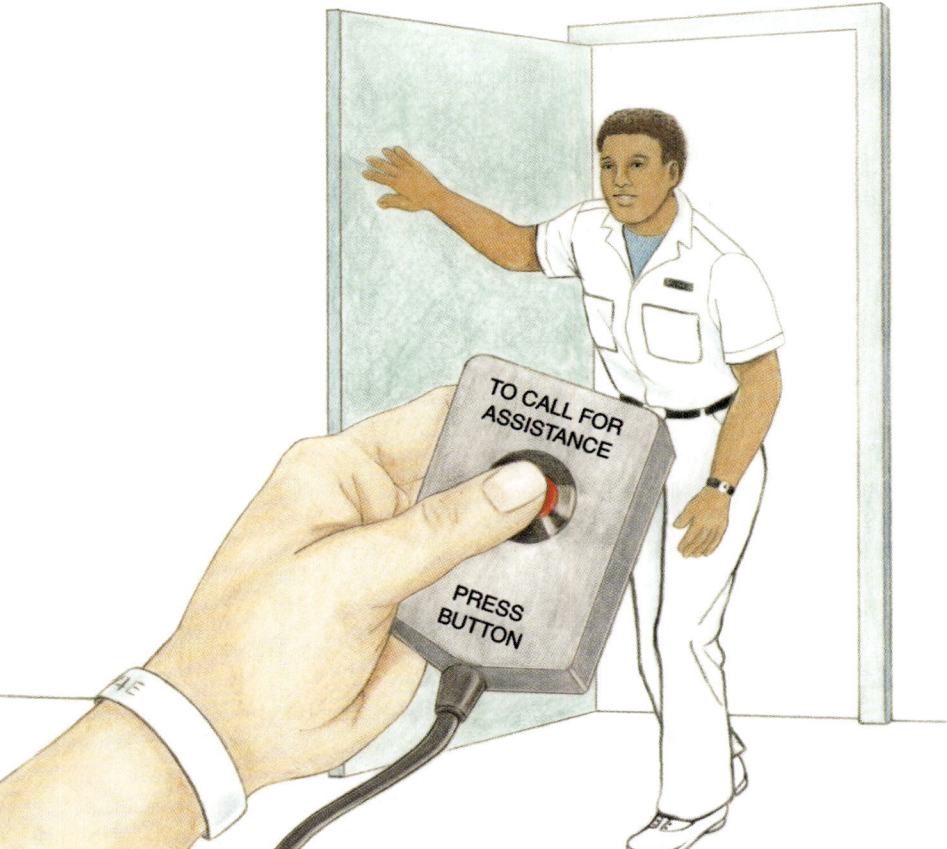

FIGURE 3–8
Answer the patient's call as quickly as possible

TO CALL FOR ASSISTANCE

PRESS BUTTON

FIGURE 3–9
Take patients' family
concerns seriously

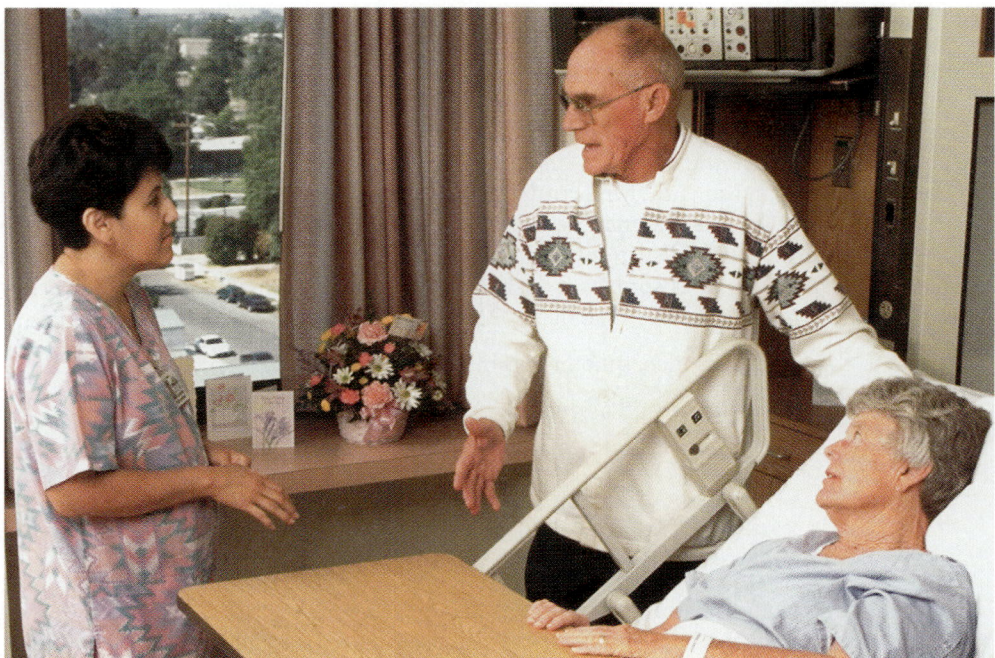

- Place the call light where the patient can reach it easily.

- Caution: A young child or an incapacitated adult may not be able to use the call light. Listen for calls for help from these patients and go quickly to see what they need. Check these patients often to see if they need something. Often, special call lights are available for patients with handicaps.

Using the Telephone

When you use the telephone or an intercommunication system (intercom), speak clearly and slowly. When you answer the telephone, for example, say, "Third floor, west. Mrs. Brown, nursing assistant, speaking." When you take a message for someone else, write it down immediately. Then repeat it to the person calling to make sure it is correct. Verify the spelling of the caller's name so you are sure you have it right. Record the following:

- The person being called

- The date and time the call was received

- The caller's name and phone number

- The message

- Your name and title

Reporting Incidents

Incidents can occur at any time, and no incident should be viewed as too insignificant to report. When you are unsure if a situation warrants an incident report, discuss the matter with your supervisor. A simple notation on the patient's chart may be adequate. Always ask for help when you are unsure. Your concern indicates that you care and that you are responsible. Remember: The patient's safety and well-being are your first responsibility. Refer to Chapter 2 for more detailed information on reporting incidents.

Complaints and Grievance Procedures

There are times when employees, patients, or families have concerns or issues that they want to bring to the attention of supervisors or administration. This communication occurs in the form of a verbal or written letter of complaint. There are some facilities that have formal grievance procedures for employees to use when they have been unable to resolve an issue with their coworkers or supervisor. If there is such a procedure in your facility, it will be mentioned in your orientation. The human resources staff or individual can review this process with you should you need more information.

OBSERVING THE PATIENT

Get into the habit of observing the patient during all your contacts. These contacts include the bed bath, bed making, meal times, visiting hours, and any other time you are with the patient (Figure 3–10). **Observation** of the patient is a continuous process. Observing begins the first time you see a patient and ends when he is discharged from the hospital.

Observation means more than just careful watching. It includes listening and talking to the patient and asking questions. It means being aware of a situation and interpreting it. Be alert to changes in a patient's condition or anything unusual that occurs whenever you are with a patient. Report any changes in the patient's condition or appearance. Also watch for changes in the patient's attitude, moods, and emotional condition. Pay attention to any complaints. For example, report to your immediate supervisor if:

- A patient who had an abdominal operation two or three days ago says, "The calf of my leg is sore."

- A patient who is being given a blood transfusion says, "I feel itchy."

observation Gathering information about the patient by noticing any change

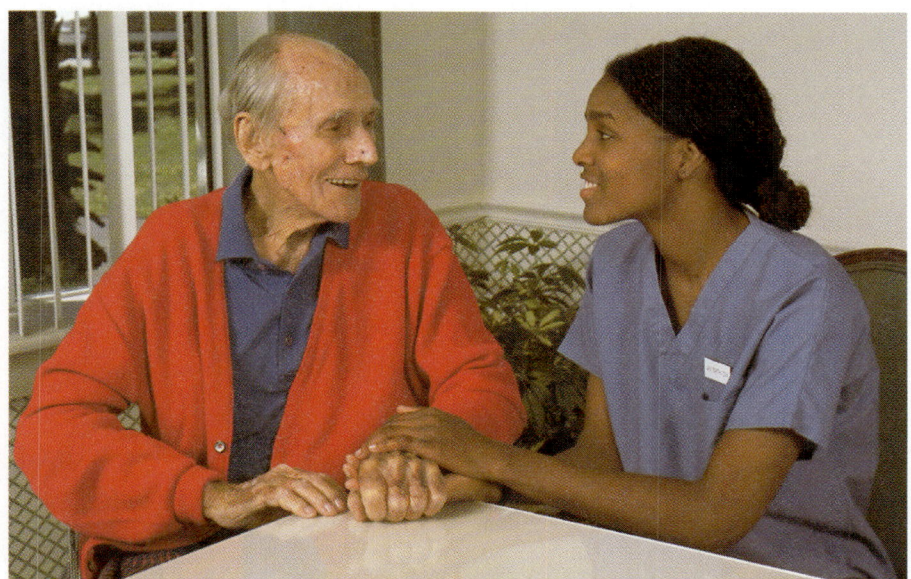

FIGURE 3–10
Observation of the patient includes listening and talking

METHODS OF OBSERVATION

Learning how to make useful observations is one of the most important things you will do in your work and will give you satisfaction and a feeling of achievement (Figure 3–11). The process of observation never ends, and you learn by doing. Because observations are so important in the total care of all patients, doctors, nurses, and all health care givers never stop learning.

Objective Observations: Signs

objective observations Signs that can be observed and reported exactly as they are seen

Use all your senses (looking, listening, touching, smelling) when making **objective observations**:

- You can see some signs of change in a patient's condition. By using your eyes, you can observe a skin rash, reddened areas, or swelling (**edema**).

edema Abnormal swelling of a part of the body caused by fluid collecting in that area; usually the swelling is in the ankles, legs, hands, or abdomen

- You can feel some signs with your fingers: a change in the patient's pulse rate, puffiness in the skin, dampness (perspiration).

- You can hear some signs, such as a cough or wheezing sounds, when the patient breathes.

- You can smell some signs, such as an odor on a patient's breath.

- Listen to the patient talking for other changes in his condition.

Subjective Observations: Symptoms

subjective observations Symptoms that can be felt and described only by the patient himself, such as pain, nausea, dizziness, ringing in the ears, and headache

Subjective observations are symptoms that can be felt and described only by the patient. Examples are pain, nausea, dizziness, ringing in the ears, or headache. Table 3–1 provides a list of things to observe in the patient.

FIGURE 3–11
Be alert when making observations. Touching, listening, and looking help you gather information about the patient

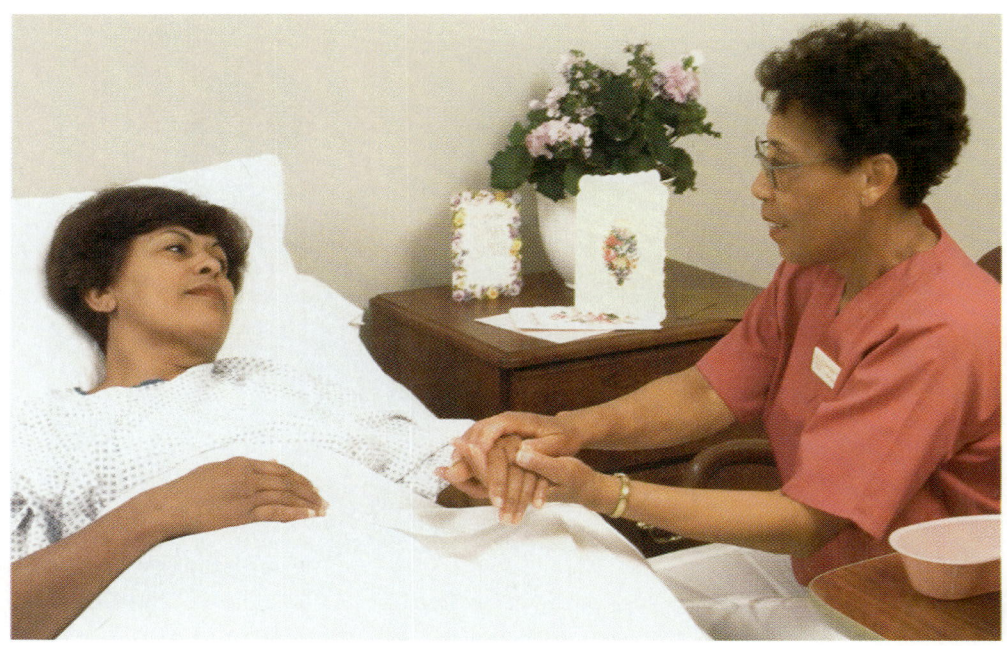

TABLE 3–1

Things to Observe in a Patient

WHAT TO OBSERVE	QUESTIONS TO ASK YOURSELF
General Appearance	Has this changed? If so, in what way? Is there a noticeable odor (smell)?
Mental Condition or Mood	Does the patient talk a lot? Very little? Does he talk about the future or the past? Does he talk about where he hurts? Is the patient anxious and worried? Is he calm? Or is he very excited? Is he talking sensibly? Or not making sense? Is he confused or disoriented? Is he speaking rapidly? Slowly? Is he cooperative? Uncooperative? Is he belligerent or aggravated?
Position	Does the patient lie still, or does he toss around? Does he like to lie in one position better than others? Does he prefer being on his back? On his side? Is he able to move easily?
Eating and Drinking Habits	Does the patient complain that he has no appetite? Does he dislike his diet? How much does he eat? Does he eat some of each kind of food? Is he always thirsty, or does he very seldom drink water? Does he eat all the food on his tray? Does he eat half the food on his tray? Does he refuse to eat?
Sleeping Habits	Is the patient able to sleep? Is she restless? Does she complain about not being able to sleep? Do these complaints agree with your observations? Does she sleep more than is normal? Is she constantly asleep?
Skin	Is the patient's skin unusually pale (pallor)? Is it flushed (red)? Is the skin dry or moist? Are his lips and fingernails turning blue (cyanotic)? Is any swelling (edema) noticeable? Are there reddened areas? Are these at the end of the spine, or on the heels, or at other pressure points? Is the skin shiny? Is there any puffiness? Is there puffiness in the legs and feet? Is his skin cold and clammy? Is it hot? Are there bruises or unusual markings?
Eyes, Ears, Nose, and Mouth	Does the patient complain that he sees spots or flashes before his eyes? Does bright light bother him? Are his eyes red (inflamed)? Is it hard for him to breathe through his nose? Does he seem to have large amounts of mucus discharge from the nose? Does he complain that he has a bad taste in his mouth? Is there an odor on his breath? Is the patient able to hear you?
Breathing	Does the patient wheeze? Does she make other noises when she breathes? Does she cough? Does she cough up sputum and how much? What is the color? Is it bloody? Does she have difficulty breathing (dyspnea) or shortness of breath?
Abdomen, Bowels, and Bladder	Does the patient's stomach appear to be distended (puffed up)? Does he complain of gas, belching, or nausea? Is he vomiting (having emesis)? What is the appearance of the vomitus? Does it contain red blood? Does it look like coffee grounds? Is the patient constipated? How often does he have a bowel movement? What is the color and consistency (hard or soft) of feces (stool)? Is there any blood, or clumps of mucus, or pieces of white material in the feces? How often does the patient void (urinate)? How much does he void each time? Does he say that he has pain during urination or that it is difficult to start to urinate? Is there sediment (cloudiness) or blood in the urine? Is it concentrated? Does the urine have a peculiar odor or color? Is the patient unable to control his bowels or urine (incontinent)?
Pain	Where is the pain? How long does the patient say she has had it? How does she describe the pain? Is it constant? Does it come and go? Does she say that it is sharp, dull, aching, or knifelike? Has she had medicine for the pain? Does the patient say that the medicine relieved the pain?
Daily Activities	Does the patient dress himself? Does he walk without help? Does he walk with help? Does he avoid walking altogether?
Personal Care	Without help, does the patient brush his teeth? Comb his hair? Go to the bathroom? Wash his face? Does he ask for assistance?
Movements	Is the patient shaking (having tremors or spasms)? Is she limp? Are her movements uncontrollable?

◾ Observation of an Infant or Child

secretions The substances that flow out of or are produced by glandular organs; the process of producing this substance; for example: sweat, bile, lymph, saliva, or urine

Observing an infant or a child means looking at her appearance and physical condition, bodily functions and **secretions**, and movements and behavior. When you observe changes in any of these, it is very important that you report them to your immediate supervisor right away. Report things that can be measured, such as a high temperature. Also report the things you see in a pattern of change, such as the child's behavior. Your careful observation and quick reporting could save a baby's life. The following are things to report when you observe them in infants or children:

Appearance and Physical Condition

- The child's temperature is high or very low

- The pulse is unusually fast, slow, or irregular

- The child is breathing rapidly or is having trouble breathing

- The abdomen seems to be swollen

- The child's skin does not look normal; it may be yellow, show purplish patches, appear unusually pale, or have a blue cast

cyanosis When the skin looks blue or gray, especially on the lips, nailbeds, and under the fingernails; in a black patient, it may appear as a darkening of color: This occurs when there is not enough oxygen in the blood

- There may be blueness **(cyanosis)** in the fingernails or lips

- There are secretions, bleeding, or odor coming from the baby's navel (umbilicus)

Bodily Functions and Secretions

- The child has not urinated during your hours of work or has voided very little

- The child has diarrhea

- A large amount of mucus is being secreted from the mouth or nose

- The child is producing a large amount of saliva

- The child is having trouble swallowing

- The child is coughing or choking

- The child is vomiting

Movement and Behavior

- The child is lying in an abnormal position

- The muscles are twitching

- There is no movement in the legs or arms

- The child is lying very quietly or seems unusually still

- The child is crying or is excessively irritable

Reporting and Recording Observations

Reporting and recording observations involves care and accuracy. You will have to sort out and report appropriately objective and subjective information. Forms you will use and charting techniques will vary from facility to facility. Some records will be handwritten; others will be computerized. You will be taught whatever system is in use in your facility or agency.

◼Subjective and Objective Reporting

It is very important for you to understand the difference between **objective reporting** and **subjective reporting**. Reporting subjective information must be done accurately by repeating what the patient tells you regarding herself. Remember, only the patient can describe or make a judgment about what she feels. Examples are pain, nausea, dizziness, ringing in the ears, and headaches.

Objective reporting means reporting exactly what you measure or observe, that is, what you see, hear, feel, or smell. Examples of measurements include: temperatures, vital signs, blood pressures, weights, size or actual amounts. The nursing assistant must always use objective reporting (see Figure 3–12).

Here are some examples of objective reporting:

- Mrs. Barbary in Room 110, window bed, is perspiring profusely

- Mr. Ellis in Room 432, door bed, had a bowel movement that was white; a specimen was collected

- Mrs. Delcara, Room 510, A bed, has an area on her left heel that is hard, red, and it measures the size of a quarter

- Mrs. Walker in Room 330, A bed, lips are dark blue

- Mrs. Carlin in Room 101, window bed, right ankle is much larger than her left ankle

- Mr. Joseph in Room 404 is clenching his teeth together and is talking very differently than he was talking at breakfast

- When Mr. Roberts in Room 581, B bed, breathes he makes loud wheezing sounds, which he was not doing when I made his bed an hour ago

objective reporting
Reporting exactly what you observe

subjective reporting
Giving your opinion about what you have observed; the nursing assistant should never use subjective reporting

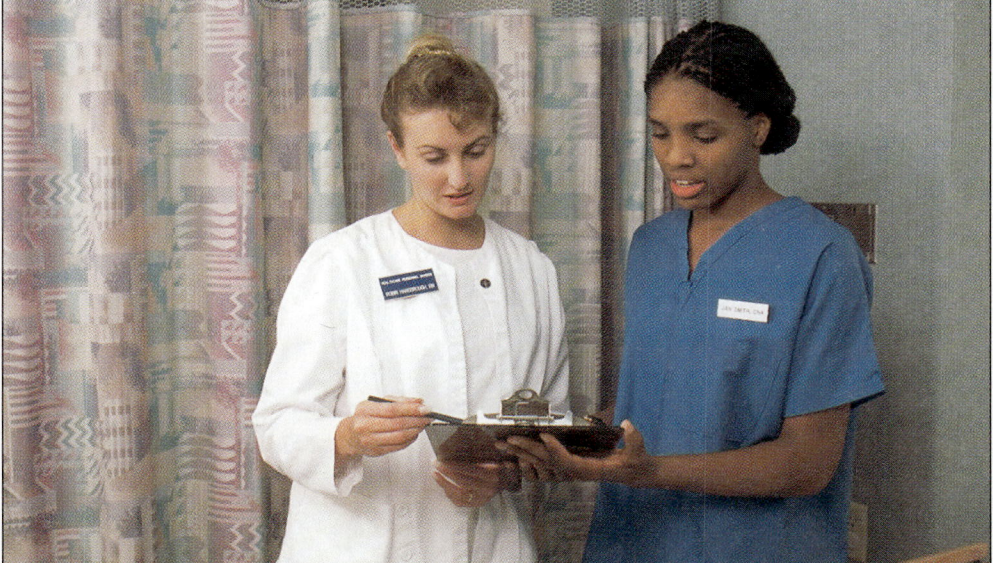

FIGURE 3–12
Guidelines to follow when reporting observations

Guidelines to Follow When Reporting Your Observations
- Write down the patient's name, room number, and bed number.
- Write or report your observations to the head nurse or team leader as soon as possible.
- Report the time you made the observation.
- Report the location of the observation.
- Report exactly, but report only what you observe, that is, report objectively.

- Mrs. Smith, Room 8031, is breathing rapidly, and the breaths appear to be shallow

- Mr. Williams, Room 204, B bed, urine looks red tinged; a urine specimen was collected

- Cindy Jones, Room 107, A bed, has a red area the size of a dollar bill on her upper right back

- Mr. Jones, Room 101, A bed, urine was bright red; left in urinal in his bathroom for you to see

Figure 3–13 gives examples of the right way and the wrong way of reporting.

■ Forms and Records Used in Documentation

Every facility has its own forms and record keeping or documentation system. Some facilities' records are written down in long hand while other facilities have computerized their documentation system (Figure 3–14). Your instructor or staff development educator will explain the particular way you are expected to chart the care you have given to patients. Refer to Figure 12–2 in Chapter 12 for an example of a form you may be asked to use to chart daily care of patients.

Recording the date and time of your observations accurately is a very important part of documentation. Some facilities/agencies use a 24-hour "clock," or military time, for recording rather than the standard, or conventional, 12-hour clock with A.M. and P.M. Table 3–2 is a conversion table that gives the 12-hour clock for the A.M. and P.M. hours (conventional time) on the left and the corresponding 24-hour clock hours (military time) on the right. If you are using military time, the hours from midnight to noon are referred

FIGURE 3–13

Subjective versus objective reporting

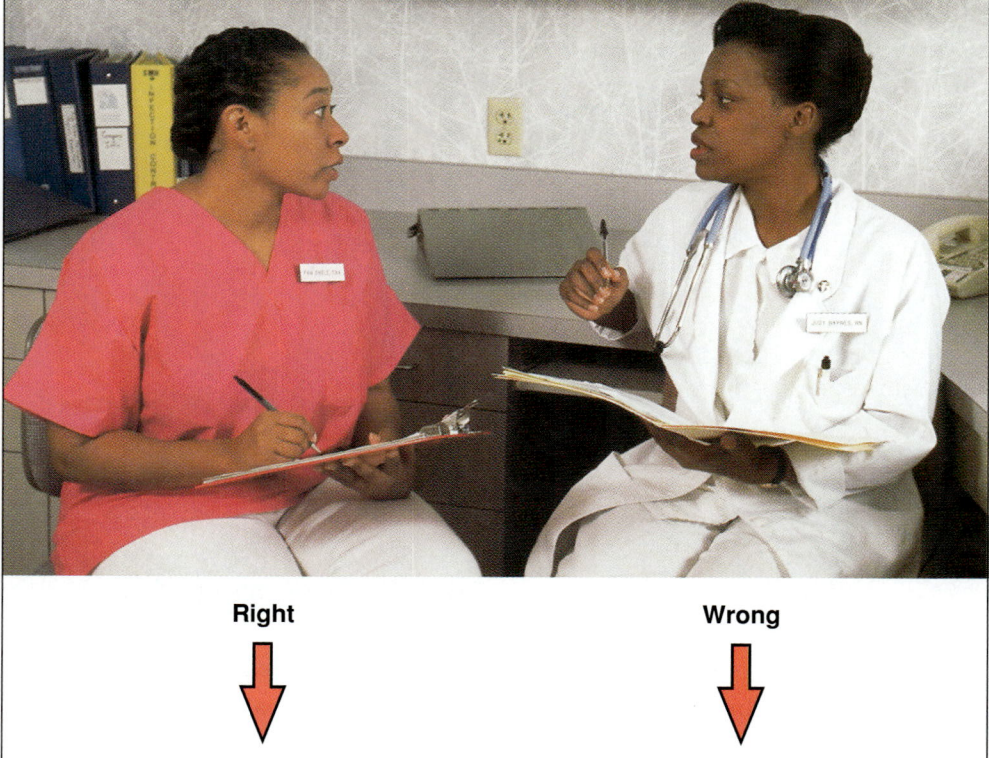

Right

Objective Reporting: "Mr. Jones, 402, B bed, the patient's lips are blue. They didn't look that way at 10 A.M."

Wrong

Subjective Reporting: "There was a draft in the room. He was cold so his lips looked blue."

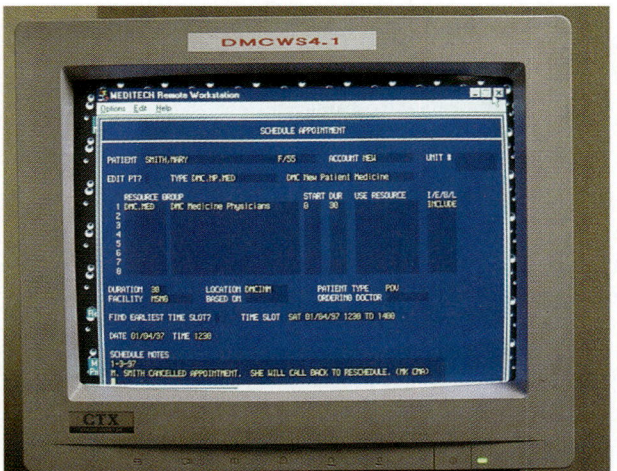

FIGURE 3–14

Computerized charting

to as "____ hundred hours." For example, 2:00 A.M. is "0200" (two hundred hours). The P.M. hours (after noon to midnight) on the 12-hour clock can easily be converted to military time by adding the time on the 12-hour clock to 12. Therefore, if it is 4:00 P.M., military time would be 12 + 4 or 1600 hours.

Computerization of Medical Records

Health care facilities are increasingly computerizing their records. It is necessary for all health care givers to be trained to document on the computerized record (Figure 3–14). This training usually lasts for several days, especially if the caregiver has had little or no computer training or **keyboard** (typing) experience. Even those employees or students who do have some computer experience will need to learn how to use the system—computer equipment and **software** programs—in use in their facility. A **password** is given or chosen by each person to give them access to the system. A particular advantage of a computerized record keeping or charting system is that a particular patient's chart or record can be pulled up in multiple places. For example, a physician can chart, check lab results, or write orders from another location in the facility or from an office outside the facility.

keyboard An input device similar to a typewriter keyboard; has additional keys that allow the user to make selections to direct computer activity

software Set or sets of instructions that direct computer operations; computer programs

password A word or phrase that identifies a person and allows access to or entry to a program or record

TABLE 3–2

24-Hour Clock Conversion

12-HOUR CLOCK (CONVENTIONAL TIME)	24-HOUR CLOCK (MILITARY TIME)	12-HOUR CLOCK (CONVENTIONAL TIME)	24-HOUR CLOCK (MILITARY TIME)
1:00 A.M.	0100	1:00 P.M.	1300
2:00 A.M.	0200	2:00 P.M.	1400
3:00 A.M.	0300	3:00 P.M.	1500
4:00 A.M.	0400	4:00 P.M.	1600
5:00 A.M.	0500	5:00 P.M.	1700
6:00 A.M.	0600	6:00 P.M.	1800
7:00 A.M.	0700	7:00 P.M.	1900
8:00 A.M.	0800	8:00 P.M.	2000
9:00 A.M.	0900	9:00 P.M.	2100
10:00 A.M.	1000	10:00 P.M.	2200
11:00 A.M.	1100	11:00 P.M.	2300
12:00 (Noon)	1200	12:00 (Midnight)	2400 (0000)

Advantages of computerized records are:

- Many caregivers can access the record with ease.

- The problem with reading handwriting is avoided as the record is clearly printed.

- Eventually record storage will be kept on disks rather than on volumes of paper.

- Patients can be issued cards with computer chips that contain pertinent medical history. These cards can be presented to emergency departments, health care providers, and/or clinics, as needed. The possibility of errors and delays in treatment can be reduced.

- There will be fewer questions about services provided and payments can be processed sooner.

Computer Documentation

The use of computers has become commonplace in health care over the past decade. Many organizations have expanded the technology used in ordering, reporting, and documenting patient care to include electronic or computer as well as handwritten systems. Computers are used for many different reasons—from ordering laboratory tests and food service to recording information about the patient's progress and activities of daily living. Health care workers are expected to have basic familiarity with computers and how computers function. For some, the thought of using a computer is unnerving while others consider it a fact of life. The basic function of a computer is to break knowledge down into a simple form, store it, then rapidly move it from one place to another in a very efficient and rapid fashion. Computers are tools to assist in communicating information and getting work done.

Basic Parts, or Components, of a Computer

Computers are made up of two key components: a **central processing unit (CPU)**, or "brain," and a data storage device, or **memory**. The central processing unit performs several functions and moves pieces of data, one at a time, to and from data storage or memory. There are several other pieces of equipment or hardware that are necessary to know about in order to become comfortable using a computer.

Hardware

Hardware includes all of the parts that physically make up the computer, the electronic and mechanical parts of the computer that can be touched or manipulated. Hardware includes the keyboard, **mouse**, **monitor**, or terminal, and the **printer**. The hardware is used to enter **data** into the central processing unit (CPU), the brain of the computer, where it is processed for storage or for output and printing. The central processing unit and memory are contained in a box or tower that can be found near the computer monitor, which is also called a **terminal**.

Similar to a television, the terminal or computer monitor displays data or information on a **screen**, usually in color. The **cursor** is a blinking or flashing line or box that indicates the user's location on the computer screen. A message that appears on the computer screen is called a **prompt**. A prompt is a signal that the user needs to either make a selection on the screen or to enter data in order for the computer program to continue.

Data can be entered by way of a keyboard or by making selections with a mouse or light pen. The computer keyboard is similar to a typewriter, with additional keys that allow the user to make selections to direct computer activities. The arrow keys on the keyboard allow a user to move the cursor up or down and to the right or left on the computer monitor. There are also special *function keys* on a computer keyboard. The function

---

central processing unit (CPU) Central processing unit, the "computer brain" where information is stored or directed to appropriate pathways

memory The capacity of the computer to store data

hardware The actual physical equipment that is used by a computer to process data

mouse A pointing and selecting device to input data; a small tabletop electronic pointing device used to make selections on a computer screen

monitor A screen, similar to a television screen, that allows the user to see input and output

printer An output device for creating a hard copy

data Information that a user enters into a computer

terminal A computer monitor that allows the computer operator to see input and output on a screen

screen A portion of data that is displayed at one time within the confined area of the computer monitor

cursor Flashing bar, or symbol, that indicates where the next character is to be placed or location on the computer screen

prompt A reminder that the user must take some action so further processing of the data can continue

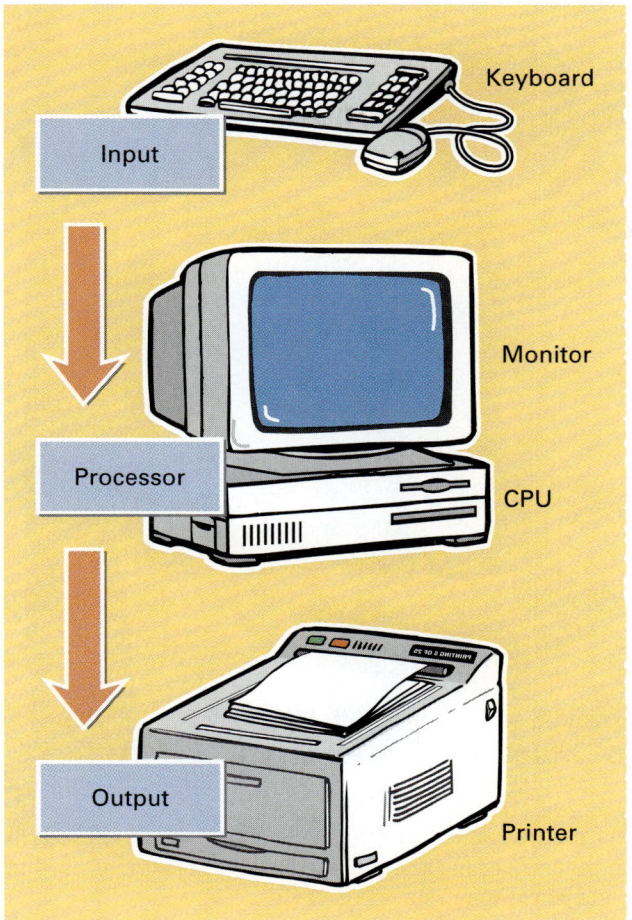

FIGURE 3–15

Computer system components

keys are spare keys, which operate differently depending on the *software,* or *program,* being used. On the right of the keyboard, there is a number pad, similar to a calculator, which is used for entering numerical data for calculations. As a computer user, you will need to be familiar with the placement of letters, numbers, and function keys on the keyboard so you can record data or execute other computer functions. In addition, you will need to know how to use a mouse or light pen.

A mouse is one type of electronic pointing device used to make selections on a computer monitor. To become comfortable using a mouse requires eye–hand coordination and a bit of practice. The mouse has a roller ball in the base and two buttons on the surface. The user lightly rests his/her hand on the mouse and gently moves it on a desk or tabletop. When the mouse is moved on the top of the table or desk, the cursor moves on the monitor. Once the cursor is in the desired position on the screen, the user presses or "clicks" the left button to make a selection. The right button is used less frequently and is similar to the spare keys on the keyboard; it offers options for additional functions with specific software.

Another electronic pointing device is the **light pen**, which looks exactly like its name implies, an oversized pen. A wire connects the light pen to the CPU on one end and emits a small light signal to which the computer can respond at the other end. Sometimes there is a button on the side of the light pen that the user pushes to make the selection on the screen. The light pen can be held as a pen when designed to make selections by scanning the data, such as bar codes. Otherwise, the light pen can be held across the palm of the hand, like a knife handle, using the index finger to push the button for making selections. The latter method for making selections is the "point and click"

light pen A hand-held device shaped like a pen that has an electronic sensor for making selections on a computer screen

FIGURE 3–16

Caregiver enters data using a keyboard

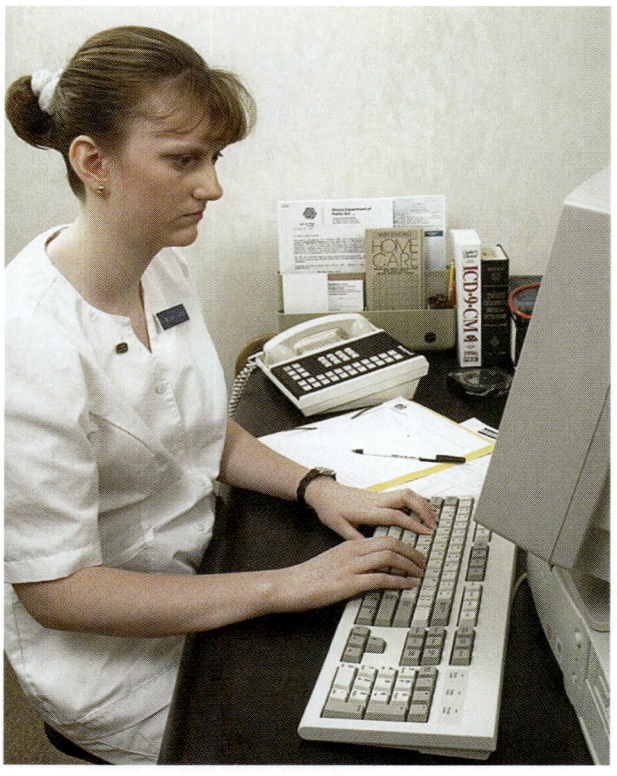

method. With either method, the user requires practice to refine the skill. Portable wireless pen-based computers, or laptop computers, are increasingly used in office settings, outpatient clinics, and home care.

A printer is used to transfer data from memory into information on paper. There are different types of printers available. A laser printer burns the ink into the paper while an ink jet printer sprays tiny dots of ink onto the page. Both laser and ink jet printers feed paper through the rollers one page at a time. A dot matrix printer has small metal pins that press ink from a ribbon on the page and feeds perforated paper on tractor pins through the printer. With the continuous feed paper, users sometimes experience problems with paper jams or inappropriately torn paper resulting in misalignment of the next page. It is important to tear the paper only at the perforated end of the page or feed the

FIGURE 3–17

Portable wireless pen-based computer

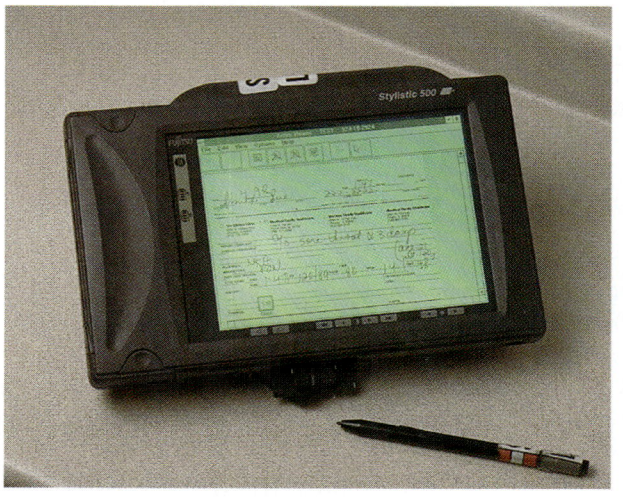

paper through to the end of the page. A printer may be found next to the other hardware at an individual work station or in a central location where several work stations have access to it.

Hardware is connected to the CPU by cables. Occasionally, the cables become loose and create problems with the hardware. Simple problem solving can be done by tracing wires to their ports and checking the connections. Hardware varies from one manufacturer to another. Once you are comfortable with one type of hardware, you often can figure out what to do with a similar piece of hardware from a different manufacturer.

Software

Software is a term used to describe the programs or set of instructions that make the computer work. Software, or the computer program, contains instructions that direct computer activity. Without software the computer would not function. Software is loaded, or installed, on the computer by computer analysts or programmers who are familiar with information systems (IS).

Computer programs exist for a number of activities. The most common types of software seen in patient care areas are used for:

1. Ordering patient care activities

2. Recording patient care information

3. Interfacing with other departments to obtain information or reports

Organizations usually provide training to prepare employees to use new software. The training is often done directly on the computer and is known as computer-based training (CBT). Learning to use new software takes time, practice, and patience.

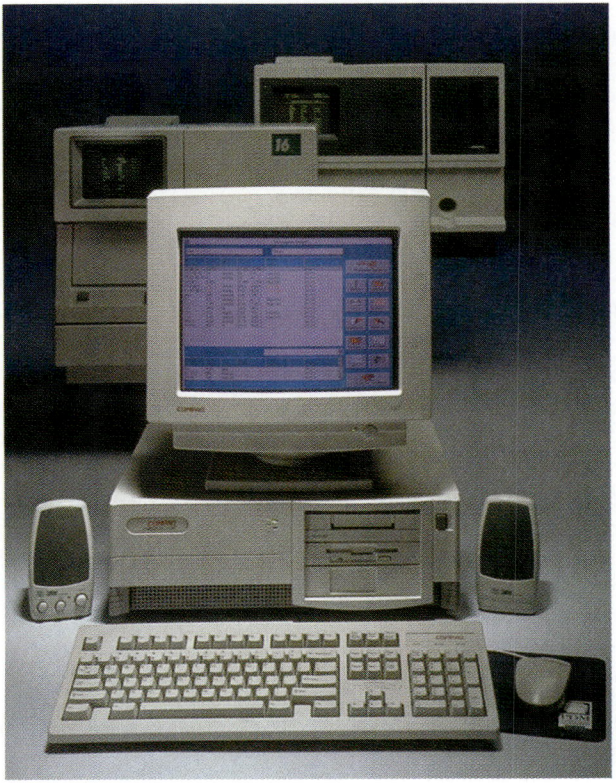

FIGURE 3–18

Windows software on a patient management system

■ Network

When working in a large organization, several computers may be connected to each other by wires, cables, or telephone lines to create a **network**. If a work station is connected to a network, the user can have access to any of the software or hardware that is part of the network. In fact, a user could go to any work station in the organization, *log on* to the network, and use that computer to enter data.

Computers hooked to a network are often left on and ready to use. The monitor may be blank or have a *screen saver* of some nature. The user simply needs to touch any key to get to the log-in screen. A user will **log on** when he enters his user identification (ID) and password, which is a confidential code allowing network access. The user ID and password are listed in the computer for security purposes. This is the same concept as a **personal identification number (PIN)** used at an electronic bank teller machine. If the ID is in the list of people identified as valid and legitimate users and the password matches the ID, then the user will have access to the network. If the ID or password does not match those on the list, access will be denied. Security is important to eliminate inappropriate users.

Individual, or stand-alone, work stations may need to be turned on and off daily. Turning a computer on is called **booting up**. When a user wants to turn off the computer, he must exit the programs that are running and log out. The user must always log off the computer appropriately or the ID and password will continue to be in operation. This means that another person wanting to use the computer may actually be doing so under the previous user's name rather than her own. Be sure to log off or sign off each time you complete recording patient information so your electronic signature and the patient data are removed from the screen. The terminal will then be ready for the next user. Table 3–3 contains additional definitions for frequently used computer terms.

■ Confidentiality

All patient centered computer information is considered confidential because it deals with the private and personal information about patients and their conditions. Most computer systems have a method of protecting patient confidentiality, such as tracking the number of entries or excursions made into the patient's data base. If anyone other than the designated caregiver is looking at the patient data in the computer, there is a breach of patient confidentiality. Only those delivering care to the patient at a given time are permitted access to patient data.

Most computer systems have the capacity to track the number of entries or excursions into the system. If a person not actually involved with patient care explores data, the system manager will be able to detect it. Staff members who breach patient confidentiality may be subject to disciplinary action up to termination of employment.

Computers are expensive and a large investment for organizations. Many organizations have limited numbers of computers in given patient care areas. In some areas, such as intensive care, a computer may be at each patient's bedside, whereas in other areas there may be one work station for every four patients. Computers make it efficient to record and store information for **retrieval** or recall. The patient medical record can be available for others to access when necessary. It is especially useful for large hospital systems to have a computerized patient record so information from across the patient's continuum of care can be retrieved. Although data is stored in the computer, a hard, or printed, copy of the patient's record is also available. In the future, employers will expect most caregivers to be computer literate.

■ Medical Terminology

Refer to the Appendix for a listing of medical terms and abbreviations commonly used in health care facilities. The Appendix also provides an extensive listing of medical specialties, with title of the physician delivering each specialty and a brief description of the specialty itself. Learn where the general medical reference materials are kept in your facility and in the unit(s) or area(s) to which you are assigned.

---

network Several computers that are connected or wired together, having access to central computer programs; can interface to obtain information; located at different work stations

log on To sign on to the computer using a password or personal identification number

PIN Personal identification number; password

boot up To start up the computer

retrieval To recall data stored in computer memory

TABLE 3–3

Frequently Used Computer Terms

TERMS	DEFINITIONS
Boot	To start up the computer.
Downtime	Time a computer cannot be used because of maintenance or mechanical failure.
Drive	Pathway that sends signals to the right place at the right time.
Hard copy	A printed copy of data in a file; printout; output.
Information systems	Refers to managing data through the use of computers; a unit or department in an organization deals with computers.
Input	Entering data into the computer system.
Interface	Technology that allows two or more computers to exchange programs and data. Also referred to as a network.
Log on	To sign on to use the computer.
Memory	The capacity of the computer to store data.
Main memory	The part of the central processing unit that stores data and program instructions. It does not perform any of the logical operations, for example, computations or sorting.
Output	Processed data translated into final form information.
Program	A set or sets of instructions that tell the computer hardware what to do in order to complete the required data processing. Also called software.
Report	Structured information provided upon request or at selected intervals.
Retrieve	Recall data from computer memory.
Security code	A group of characters that allows an authorized computer user access to certain programs or features. Password.
Screen	A portion of data that is displayed at one time within the confined area of the computer monitor.
Sign on code	Secure password to prevent unauthorized persons from using the system.
Work station	A location that contains a CPU, computer monitor, keyboard, and mouse or light pen; may be an individual unit or part of a network.

SUMMARY

Communication occurs through the exchange of gestures and words and the observation of actions. This chapter has identified ways to communicate effectively with patients, their families, and other health care providers using your actions, words, and observation skills. Both your verbal and written communication skills are important. Subjective reporting includes what you learn directly from a patient. Objective reporting refers to what you are able to hear, see, feel, or smell. In your work, you will be educated (taught/trained) and expected to chart or document on a variety of forms and systems.

Notes

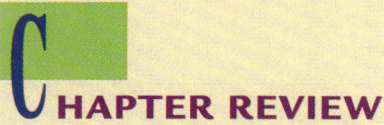

CHAPTER REVIEW

FILL IN THE BLANK

Read each sentence and fill in the blank line with a word that completes the sentence.

1. Signs that can be observed and reported exactly as they are seen are called _____ _____.

2. _____ _____ is a type of communication through movements (gestures), facial expressions, body movements, and touch.

3. For the pediatric patient, _____ is extremely important in helping calm the fears of the patient.

4. It is very important to answer the _____ _____ when the patient signals so that they can receive help without delay.

5. _____ are an electronic medical record that make it easy for institutions to record and store information for retrieval or recall.

MULTIPLE CHOICE

Choose the best answer for each question or statement.

1. Communication
   a. may be written.
   b. may be spoken.
   c. is an exchange of information with others.
   d. All of the above.

2. Which of the following is not a key element of communication?
   a. The sender must obtain the receiver's attention and make sure the message is understood.
   b. The sender must speak loudly.
   c. The receiver must listen carefully and respond appropriately.
   d. The message must be organized, simple, and clear.

3. The patient's medical record is an example of
   a. verbal communication.
   b. written communication.
   c. nonverbal communication.
   d. body language.

4. Which of the following is not a barrier to effective communication?
   a. Clichés
   b. Language misunderstandings
   c. Simple, well-organized messages
   d. Judgmental attitudes

5. In order to maintain patient confidentiality, you should do all of the following except
   a. discuss one patient's problems with another patient.
   b. keep confidences.
   c. keep out of earshot of others when discussing a patient's concerns.
   d. only discuss the patient's problems with your supervisor.

6. Which of the following guidelines does not promote good communication?
   a. Showing an interest in the patient
   b. Speaking loudly at all times
   c. Using good manners
   d. Using language the patient can understand

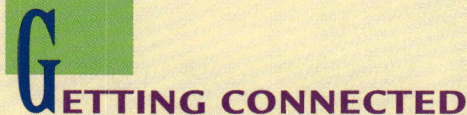

GETTING CONNECTED

MULTIMEDIA EXTENSION ACTIVITIES

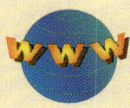

www.prenhall.com/wolgin

Use the above address to access the free, interactive Companion Website created for this textbook. Get hints, instant feedback, and textbook references to chapter-related multiple choice questions. Read and react to the "Nursing Assistants in Action." Link to other interesting sites.

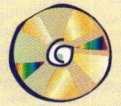

Audio Glossary

Use the CD-ROM disk enclosed with your textbook to hear the pronunciation of the key terms in the chapter.

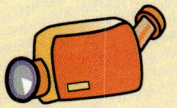

Video

Watch the "Age-Specific Competencies" video from the Care Provider Skills series to learn about communicating with different age groups.

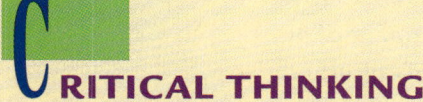

CRITICAL THINKING

USING KEY QUESTIONS

Read each question and think of what you might do in each situation.

1. Your patient expects professional behavior. What does this mean?

2. Your patient has a complaint about the food. What should you do?

3. Your patient is blind. How will you show him how to use the call bell?

4. You notice that your pediatric patient is looking a little blue (cyanotic). What should you do?

5. One of your patients asks about another very ill patient across the hall. What can you tell her?

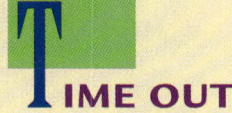

TIME OUT

TIPS FOR TIME MANAGEMENT

COMMUNICATION TIP   Write information on a pocket note pad for reporting or recording later. Do not depend on your memory. You will deal with a great many numbers, and you will confuse one patient's vital signs and another patient's intake if you do not write it down. If you don't write out the information, you will waste time repeating the task to get the correct numbers.

Patients, Residents, and Clients

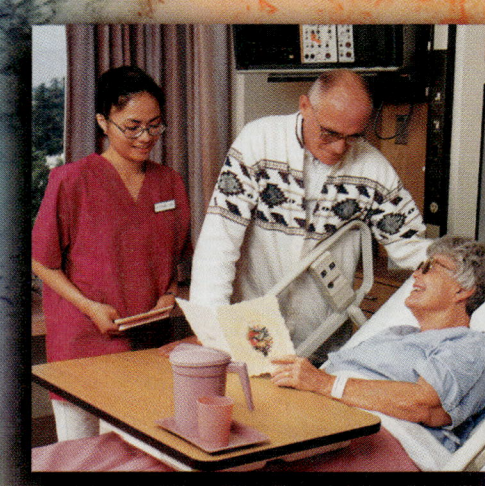

4

INTRODUCTION

All individuals are influenced by the values and beliefs of their cultures. Cultures share similarities as well as differences when it comes to dealing with pain, the causes and treatment of illness, and death. This chapter offers an overview of cultural diversity and suggests some strategies to enable you to provide customer focused service and to meet the physical and psychological needs of your patients, residents, or clients. The importance of rest is presented along with approaches or actions you can take to promote sleep. The chapter also reviews approaches to dealing with difficult behaviors.

When you have completed this chapter, you will be able to:

- Describe seven goals of customer focused care.

- Demonstrate an understanding of cultural differences among patients, residents, and clients.

- Provide service that meets the basic human needs of those who are in your care.

- Identify actions you can take to promote rest and sleep for your patients.

- Use methods to deal with disruptive behavior.

- Describe how unmet needs can influence patient behavior.

client

culture

customer-focused care

ethnic diversity

need

patient

physical crisis management

resident

service

UNDERSTANDING AND RELATING TO PATIENTS, RESIDENTS, AND CLIENTS

In various health care settings or facilities, you will hear the individuals to whom you are providing care referred to as patients, clients, or residents. **Patients** usually refers to those admitted to inpatient or outpatient hospitals, physician offices, or clinics. Individuals in nursing homes, long term care or extended care facilities are frequently referred to as **residents.** (Residents usually live at a facility for an extended period of time.) Individuals cared for by home health agencies or providers are generally referred to as **clients.** While your place of employment may refer differently to those you provide care for, the most important thing to remember is to treat all individuals within your care with respect and courtesy, keeping in mind any cultural differences.

CUSTOMER-FOCUSED CARE

Chapter 1 reviewed the various ways care is delivered or provided to individuals. See Chapter 1 for more information about customer-focused care.

> The common aspect of all care is that it should be directed to meet the needs of the individual and his family. You are providing care for, and service to, those who are unable to care for themselves.

Service is an important part of patient care. Patients, families, and visitors will judge the care given to their loved ones based on attentiveness, quality of food, cleanliness of the environment, and employee behavior. Most important are personal interactions, attention, and perceived helpfulness of the staff. Many studies have been done to determine the degree of customer satisfaction with health care. Leebov (1990)[1] found that employee behavior toward customers is the most powerful marketing and customer satisfaction tool available to an organization or facility. It is important to know that dissatisfied customers or patients usually do not complain. Instead, nine out of ten will go to another health care provider rather than return. They will also tell an average of 20 other relatives, friends, or acquaintances about their experience. A negative experience hurts the overall reputation of the facility.

When you care for others, treat them and their families the way you would like to be treated (Figure 4–1). Provide the service and care you would expect if they were your loved ones.

◼ Seven Goals of Customer-Focused Care

There are seven goals of **customer-focused care,** which is designed to meet the needs of patients, residents, and clients (customers). While all of them are important, the care needs of your patients should be your primary concern.

---

[1] Leebov, W. *Customer Service in Healthcare,* Chicago: American Hospital Publishing, 1990, p. 3.

Sidebar:

patient An individual admitted to an inpatient or outpatient hospital, physician office, or clinic

resident An individual cared for in a nursing home or other long term/extended care facility

KEY IDEA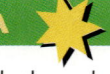

client An individual cared for by a home health agency or provider

service Factors such as attentiveness, quality of food, and cleanliness of environment, which affect the care and comfort of the individual receiving health care

customer-focused care Care designed to meet the needs of patients, residents, and clients (customers)

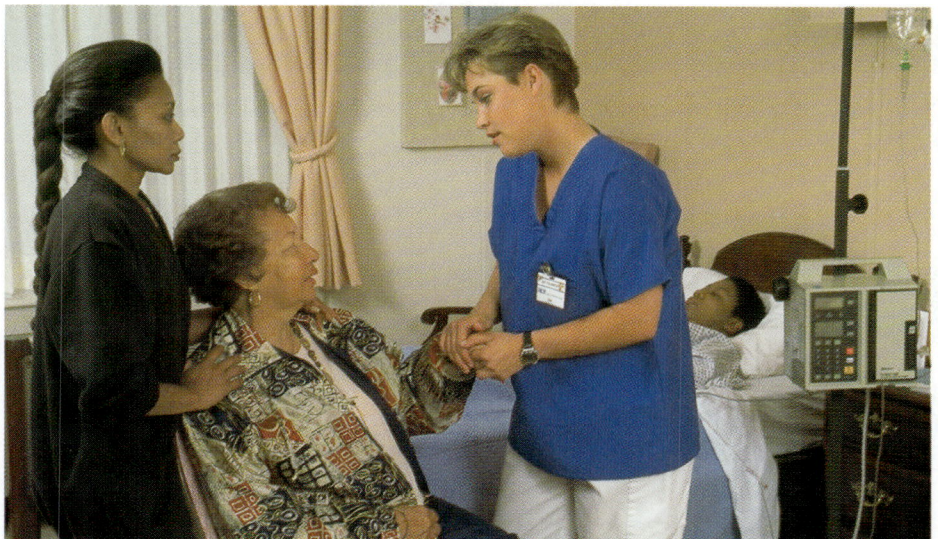

FIGURE 4–1
Treat individuals who are in your care, as well as their families, the way you would like to be treated

1. Care provided reflects respect for the individual.

2. Caregivers are working together in a planned way, so that care is coordinated.

3. Information is communicated.

4. The patient's physical comfort and care needs are met.

5. The patient is relieved of fear when possible.

6. Family and/or friends are involved.

7. Care is considered over the continuum, rather than a discrete episode or time period. Many conditions or illnesses, such as pregnancy, cancer, AIDS, and diabetes, will require medical care and services from a variety of providers.

CULTURAL DIFFERENCES AND DIVERSITY

Ethnic diversity refers to the variety of races, religions, and cultures in the world. A **culture** is the thoughts, beliefs, and values of a social group. Ethnic diversity is increasing in the United States. Currently, one in every four Americans is Hispanic, African American, or Asian. By the year 2000, Latin Americans will comprise the largest ethnic minority group in the United States, and one-third of children attending schools will be nonwhite.

Thus, as part of a nursing care team, it will be very important to increase your knowledge of the various cultural differences and similarities in views of pain, the causes of illness, treatment, and death. Your supervisor can provide more specific information regarding cultural differences and similarities.

ethnic diversity The variety of races, religions, and cultures in the world

culture The thoughts, beliefs, and values of a social group

The more you can learn about an individual's cultural beliefs and differences, the better you can provide sensitive care and services to your patients, residents, or clients.

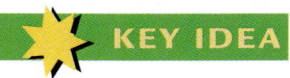

KEY IDEA

GUIDELINES

APPRECIATING CULTURAL DIVERSITY

- Learn as much as you can about other cultures, especially those cultures of patients in your care or those of your coworkers.
- Treat everyone with respect.
- Develop understanding for differences.
- Appreciate the talents and contributions of others.
- Be open, flexible, and adaptable.
- Practice effective communication skills.
- Be quick to apologize if you see you have offended someone.
- Thank others who help you better understand or teach you more about their culture.

■ Transcultural Nursing

Since you have chosen to be a nursing assistant, we assume that you enjoy working with and helping people. For sick people to feel well again, they must first be helped to feel relaxed, comfortable, accepted, and safe, regardless of their ethnic background (Table 4–1).

As part of the nursing care team, you will assist with the delivery of nursing care to people from many different countries and backgrounds (Figure 4–2). People may adhere to religious beliefs, values, traditions, practices, or rituals that are very different from your own. They may have very different food habits, manners, lifestyles, social roles, family systems, birth and death practices, or perceptions of privacy, territoriality, and touch. They may use languages, customs, or behavior patterns completely foreign to you. You must learn to be tolerant, accepting, and understanding of these differences. Behave in ways that show respect for the patient's customs and beliefs.

TABLE 4–1

Cross-Cultural Communication Guidelines

- Establishing and building relationships is the core and aim of all effective communication in a cross-cultural setting.
- Recognize your own cultural filters, including the values (and stereotypes) that shaped them. Work at understanding your own cultural preferences.
- Speak at a comfortable pace for your foreign associates. Repeat what was said. Summarize often; confirm and clarify.
- Be respectful of (cultural) differences. Listen, observe, and describe, rather than evaluate.
- Don't settle for surface meaning. Patiently search for what is really being communicated.
- Respect the appropriate level of formality in other cultures.
- Avoid taboos; pay particular attention to your nonverbal behavior.
- Beware of jokes; they cannot readily be translated into another language, culture, or value system.
- Check yourself constantly for cultural assumptions.
- Be very conscious of the context in which the communication takes place.

SOURCE: Reprinted with permission from Gottfried Oosterwal, Ph.D., *Community in Diversity: A Participant Workbook*, 1995, p. iii–21.

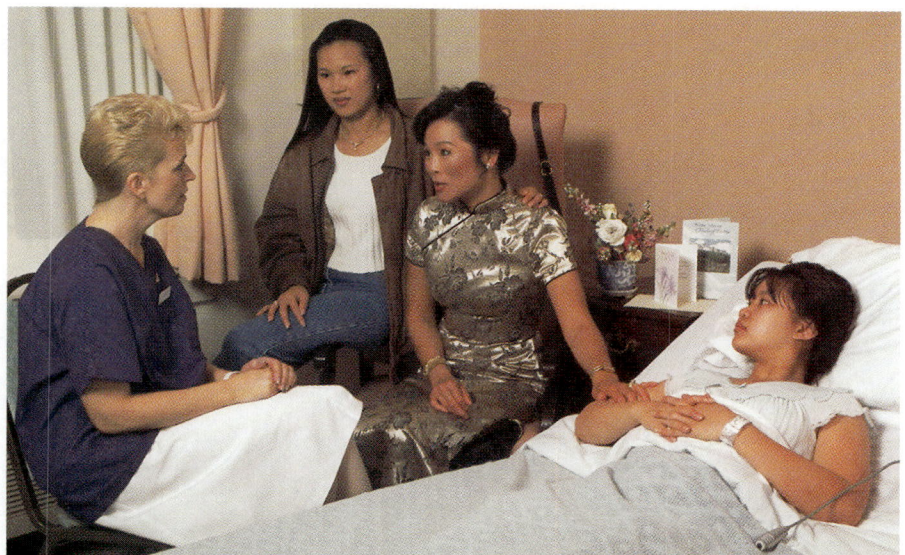

FIGURE 4–2

As a nursing assistant, you will help deliver care to people from different countries and backgrounds

Different does not mean better or worse, only another way of doing or seeing things. Because your own ways are familiar to you, they seem like the right ways, and other languages, values, lifestyles, traditions, or diets may seem strange. Your customs may seem just as strange to the patient as her customs seem to you. This can lead to misunderstandings. Remember, there is no right or wrong in these matters.

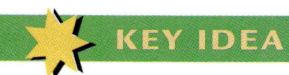 **KEY IDEA**

Many patients are frightened by illness and the hospital or health care setting. Part of your job is to show the patient that the health care institution is a friendly place and that your major concern is for her well-being.

Patients born in other countries may be fearful because of problems in understanding our language and culture. Be sure to discuss these problems with your immediate supervisor, who can suggest ways of dealing with these patients effectively, for example:

- If the patient speaks and understands little or no English, your nurse manager or team leader may suggest the use of flash cards, pictures, nonverbal communication, a translator, or materials written in the patient's language to communicate with the patient and thereby reduce stress and anxiety (Figure 4–3).

- There are no universal gestures. For example, the American "thumbs up" or "OK" sign may be a terrible insult to Turkish, Greek, or Brazilian individuals. Unless you know and understand the meanings of gestures in another culture, avoid using them.

- Space has different meanings to different people. It is better to ask before approaching or touching someone. Each culture has its own comfort zone in which communication takes place. It may be 18 inches or arm's length in the United States or Canada, but the range in other countries can be 5 inches to 50 inches. Caregivers may have patients or visitors who unknowingly intrude upon each other's space or comfort zones.

- A patient from another culture may answer "yes" to all questions asked because in his culture it is rude to say no. Your nurse manager or team leader may suggest that you phrase your questions so that a "yes" or "no" answer is not required. For

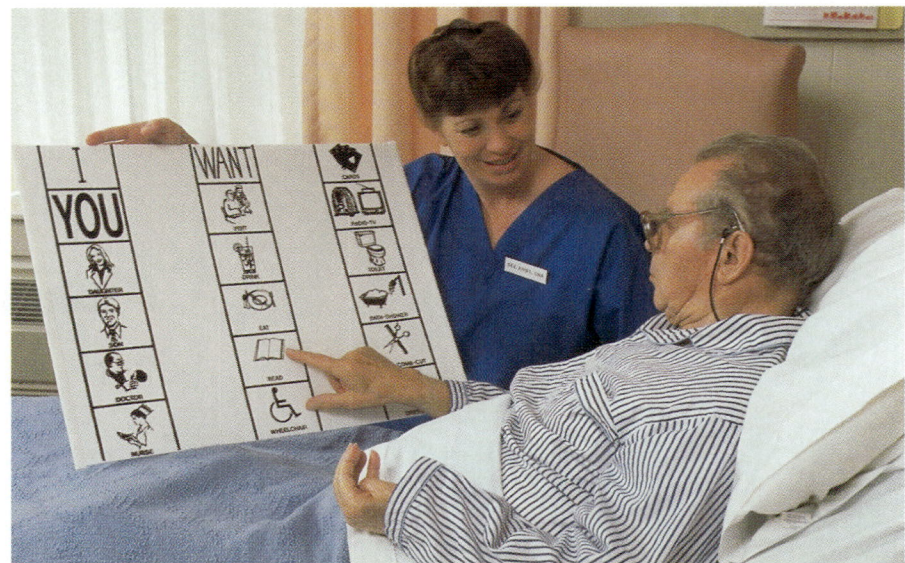

example, instead of asking, "Do you want the lights out now?" you could say, "What time would you like me to turn off the lights?"

- A patient may refuse to eat hospital food because of religious or cultural dietary laws or beliefs. In many Latin American cultures, for instance, the concept of keeping the body in balance involves the use of foods identified as "hot" foods or "cold" foods. Depending on the illness, which is also considered "hot" or "cold," a patient may prefer to eat a particular food in order to bring the body into balance. An example of a "hot" food among Puerto Ricans might be corn meal or peas, while a "cold" food would be bananas or lima beans. There are also hot and cold medicines and herbs. Similar beliefs are found among Asian cultures, which believe in the philosophy of Tao. According to Taoism, harmony is maintained through a balance of yin and yang. Yin represents cold, darkness, and female, while yang represents hot, light, and male. Certain conditions or illnesses are considered either yin or yang and require the opposite types of food or herbs for treatment. A yin food would include mostly fruits and vegetables, while yang foods include meat, chicken, and most, but not all, kinds of fish.

  Some groups avoid certain types of food altogether. A patient may be a strict vegetarian, avoiding not only meat, fish, and poultry, but also all dairy products. Other patients may avoid certain foods on certain religious occasions. Some may fast on religious holidays. Patients have the right to decide what they will eat and when they eat it. Your nurse manager or team leader may be able to make special arrangements for this patient's food. If the facility cannot provide the requested foods, arrangements can be made for the family or friends to bring food.

- People from many cultures place more importance on modesty than Americans. They may want to keep certain parts of the body, such as the head, the face, arms, or legs, covered at all times. Your nurse manager or team leader may suggest ways of draping the patient so necessary care can be given without violating the patient's sense of modesty, dignity, and privacy.

- People have different ideas about death and the hereafter. Adherents of some religions believe that the body should not be touched or moved after death until the proper religious authority arrives. Your nurse manager or team leader may suggest that you straighten the patient's limbs before death occurs.

BASIC HUMAN NEEDS

Every person has basic physical and psychological needs that must be met. A **need** is a requirement for survival. Most people can satisfy their own needs; however, sometimes they need help. As a nursing assistant, you will help your patients meet some of their most basic needs until they no longer need your assistance. Your knowledge of these needs and your objective observations, when reported promptly, will help your supervisor, nurse manager, or team leader to determine if all the patient's needs are being met by the plan of care.

need A requirement for survival

Basic Physical and Psychological Needs

All human beings have basic physical needs that must be met in order to live. These needs do not all have to be met completely every day. But the more each person's needs are fulfilled, the better the quality of life.

Psychological needs must be satisfied to have a healthy emotional and social outlook. These, also, do not have to be met completely every day. However, the more completely each need is met, the better the emotional state of the individual.

Some psychologists divide human needs into five categories, arranged into a hierarchy, or order of priority, developed by Abraham Maslow (Figure 4–4). Maslow's idea is that human beings work on meeting lower-level, physical needs (food, water, shelter) first, then move on toward meeting higher-level needs (security, belonging, and so on).

Rest and Sleep

Your body requires rest and sleep. One must first be in a state of rest to fall asleep. Rest is a state wherein one feels comfortable, calm, and free of stress and anxiety. Certain

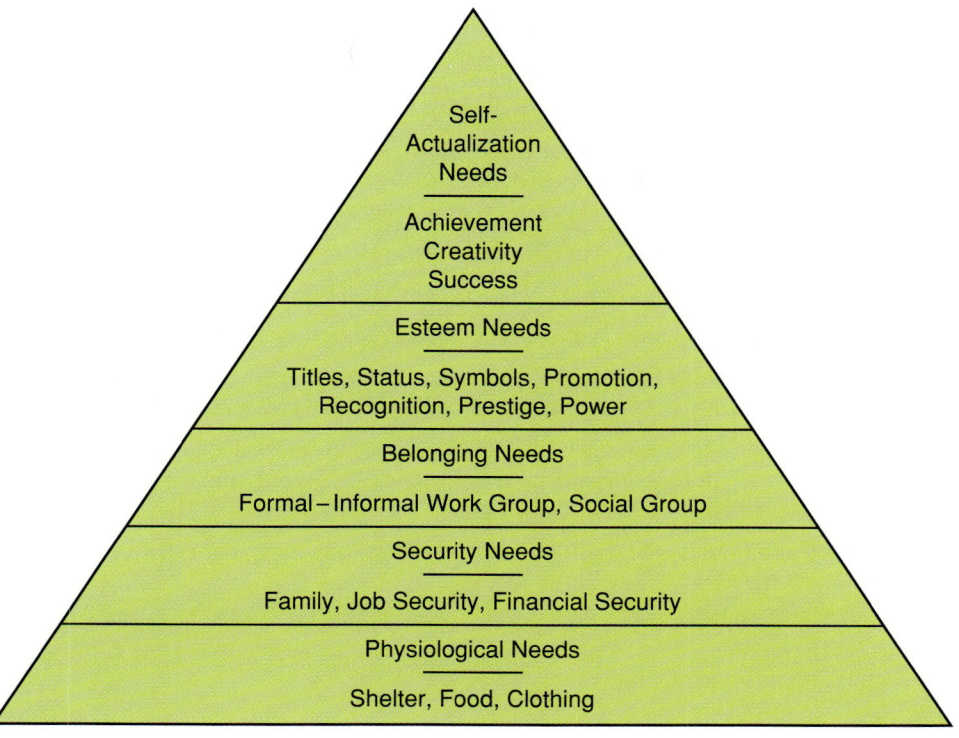

FIGURE 4–4
Maslow's hierarchy of needs

activities may be restful to one individual, but not so for others. Examples are listening to music, reading, watching TV, swimming, walking, sewing, golfing, drawing, or gardening. Determining those activities that are restful for each individual is important as it will help you to promote rest. Basic needs for water, food, and comfort must be met for a person to rest (Table 4–2).

Sleep is a natural periodic suspension of consciousness during which the natural restorative powers of the body occur. In this state of unconsciousness, there is reduced voluntary muscle activity and lowered metabolism as the body requires less energy during sleep. In sleep, the body is at rest. The blood pressure, temperature, pulse, and respirations are lower than when awake. While there is a general unawareness of the environment and people around you while asleep, most individuals are easily awakened by noise, alarms, the sound of a baby crying, etc.

Sleep is an essential and distinctive aspect of human behavior. Each person's body has individual requirements regarding their basic needs for sleep and rest. Nearly one-third of the average adult lifespan is spent sleeping. Sleep requirements decrease with age. Newborns average 20 hours of sleep per day, while elderly persons require 5–6 hours per day. Infants and children sleep more soundly and have a harder time awakening than older adults.

It is during sleep that tissues heal and the body is restored or refreshed. One's mental alertness and energy levels are restored during sleep. Stress, tension, and anxiety are reduced. Following sleep, one can usually think more clearly and function more effectively.

Individuals have different sleep/wake patterns or rhythms during a 24-hour period. You are probably aware of your preferred biological clock or pattern. Some individuals require only a few hours of sleep while others need 8–10 hours to feel refreshed. Your body may or may not require brief nap periods. You may be alert in the early morning, awaking before your alarm rings, but ready to go to sleep early in the evening. There are other people who

TABLE 4–2

Rest and Sleep

FACTORS AFFECTING SLEEP	APPROACHES/ACTIONS
Age	Be aware that older persons awaken easily and children tend to sleep more soundly.
Anxiety/Stress/Emotional Problems	Listen and offer emotional support. Encourage the patient to talk about what is bothering him. There may be resource persons available for consultation/support or medications ordered to reduce anxiety. Check with your supervisor.
Environment/Strange Sounds/Noise	Keep the door closed at night to reduce noise. A child may want a toy or blanket from home to comfort him. Reduce noise: Try not to use the intercom system at night, speak in low voices to prevent awakening patients unnecessarily.
Light	Keep bathroom light on or off, per patient's preference.
Strange Bed/Pillow	Patient may be allowed to have her preferred pillow brought in from home.
Exercise	Avoid exerting patients less than two hours prior to sleeping time.
Caffeine/Nutrition	Cheese and milk can promote rest and sleep. Offer decaffeinated drinks, water, or juices rather than tea, coffee, or cola drinks at bedtime or in the evening.
Illness Symptoms: Pain	Need for sleep is increased. Try repositioning or pain medication as ordered. Report if it does not help. Distractions such as TV, reading, and humor may promote rest.
Vomiting, Diarrhea, Other	Medications usually are ordered to treat the symptoms; offer skin care and mouth care as needed.
Lifestyle Changes	The patient may not be comfortable with his roommate—a change may be needed. The recent death of a close relative or friend may be causing depression. Encourage the patient to talk about her grief/loss.

TABLE 4-3

The Sleep Cycle

Presleep	NonREM Stage 4
NonREM Stage 1	Deepest stage of sleep
Lightest sleep state	Hard to awaken
Easily aroused	Body rests and restores
NonREM Stage 2	Lower vital signs
Sound sleep	Lasts 15–30 minutes
Increased relaxation	REM Sleep (Rapid Eye Movement)
Lasts 10–20 minutes	Vivid dreaming
NonREM Stage 3	Mental restoration occurs
Begin deep sleep	Review problems and events of the
Muscles completely relax	prior day
Slow and regular respiratory and	Hard to arouse
heart rates	Starts 50–90 minutes after sleep begins
Lasts 15–30 minutes	

SOURCE: Material adapted from J. Fry, "Sleep Disorders," *Merritt's Textbook of Neurology*, Baltimore, MD: Williams & Wilkins, 1995.

prefer to sleep in the early morning, but have no trouble staying up late at night. Health care facilities routinely interfere with the sleep cycles of both the health care providers and the patients. Caregivers are needed around the clock, and various aspects of patient care occur at times that are unwelcome to the patients. Whenever possible, it is important to consider each individual's preferences and needs when you plan their care needs. For example, you may have a patient who prefers to sleep in the morning and have their bath in the early afternoon. It is possible to plan your assignment to accommodate their preference.

There are two phases of sleep, REM (rapid eye movement) and NonREM (nonrapid eye movement). REM sleep accounts for 25 percent of the time spent sleeping, while NREM sleep makes up 75 percent of the time.

The sleep cycle lasts about 85–100 minutes and repeats itself three to five times over a 6–8 hour period of sleep (see Table 4–3 on the sleep cycle). An adult will usually fall asleep within 10–15 minutes, and go through a sequence of stages 1, 2, 3, and 4, followed by the reverse (stages 4, 3, and 2). Next, the first REM sleep period occurs. The cycles of sleep will continue three to five times. Deep sleep occurs more often during the first half of the total time spent in sleep. Vivid dreaming in the REM sleep episodes increases in intensity and duration during the second half of sleep. When people are ill or hospitalized, they frequently do not experience prolonged blocks of sleep time and thus experience less time in REM sleep, leaving them feeling less restored or rested.[2]

■ Influences on Patient Behavior: Unmet Needs

When basic needs are not met, most people show some reaction or change in behavior. If a physical need is not met, the person might become irritable or weak. When an emotional need is not met, the person's reactions may include anxiety, depression, aggression, anger, or a physical ailment without apparent cause. An unwanted diagnosis, a serious illness, age, and previous experience, along with personality, financial situation, and family relationships can all be the source of unmet needs, thus affecting a patient's behavior.

Report these reactions to your immediate supervisor. By reviewing a patient's actions, your supervisor will be able to determine if a need is unmet and evaluate the plan of care to attempt to fulfill the need and thus change the patient's behavior.

---

[2] Material adapted from J. Fry, "Sleep Disorders," *Merritt's Textbook of Neurology*, Baltimore, MD: Williams & Wilkins, 1995.

Remember, too, that each person has a different reaction to pain, treatment, and even attempted kindness, so when you try to make adjustments to fulfill needs, you should consider him as an individual. If you observe the patient's behavior carefully, you will be better able to report it and make changes to fulfill needs.

DEALING WITH DIFFICULT BEHAVIOR

Patients, their families, and friends are usually experiencing varying amounts of stress and anxiety. An illness can be very frightening and can reduce a person's ability to cope with a stressful situation. Some patients or their significant others may have a particularly hard time dealing with or accepting an illness or injury. An individual may be overcome by stress, grief, or guilt. An individual may be suffering from a mental problem or other illness and may not be able to understand or recognize her own behavior. Some medications can also cause side effects that leave a person disoriented, combative, or hallucinating.

KEY IDEA Your challenge as a nursing assistant is to deal with a patient's disruptive behavior in such a way that keeps you, the patient, and others in the environment safe from harm.

Below are some causes of disruptive behavior, along with appropriate actions.

Causes or Reasons	Appropriate Actions
1. Illness or injury (insulin shock, head injury, respiratory problems)	Keep safe from injury. Reassure. Make minimal attempts to reason with the individual.
2. Mental illness/emotional problems	Reduce stimuli. Give short, concrete directions. Do not ask "why" questions. Do not argue or correct grandiose delusions. Ignore strange behaviors, focus on safety. Acknowledge the person's difficulty.
3. Medication reactions; confused/ disoriented, "feel bugs crawling on them"	Focus on safety. Report to your supervisor.
4. Stress	Be supportive. Acknowledge the stressor, if you know it.
5. Anger	Remain calm.
6. Misbehavior	Don't focus on negative behavior. Be clear about limits.

PHYSICAL CRISIS MANAGEMENT

physical crisis management Methods for dealing with a dangerous situation involving a patient, resident, or client

Physical crisis management refers to how you deal with a dangerous situation. Many facilities have training programs or courses for employees who work in high-risk areas, such as psychiatry or the emergency department. There is a high probability that

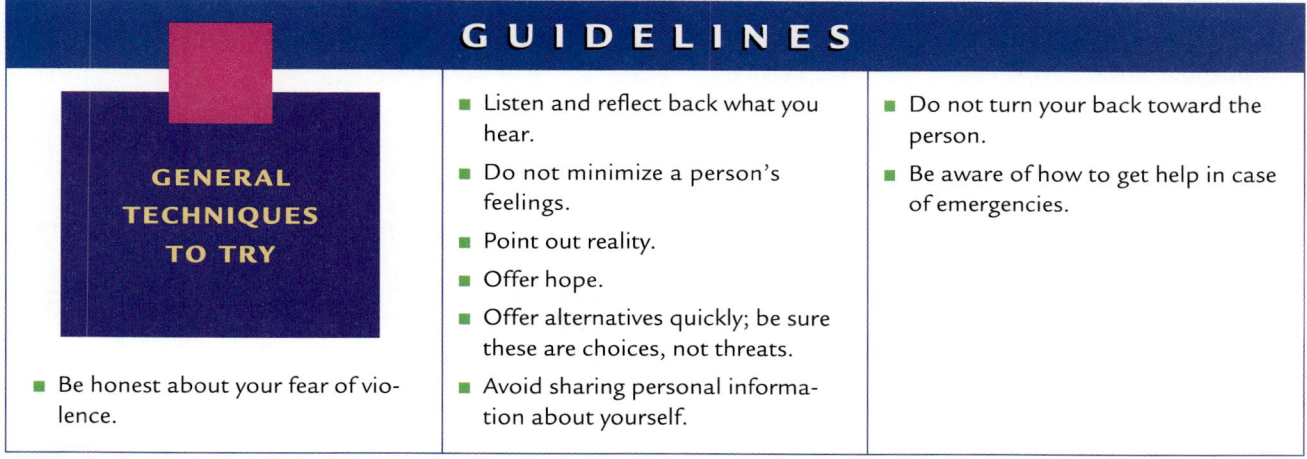

GUIDELINES

DEALING WITH THE DISRUPTIVE INDIVIDUAL — OBRA

- Be objective.
- Remain calm, but firm and controlled.

- Act appropriately and do not raise your voice or yell back.
- Do not display your own anger or threaten the person.
- Respect personal space, stay at least an arm's length away from the person.
- Be alert.
- Take time to determine the facts, whenever possible.
- Watch body positioning and non-verbal body language.

- Do not stare or avoid eye contact.
- Remember many people want their "say," not their "way."
- Call for help or assistance if you cannot defuse the situation.

GUIDELINES

GENERAL TECHNIQUES TO TRY

- Be honest about your fear of violence.

- Listen and reflect back what you hear.
- Do not minimize a person's feelings.
- Point out reality.
- Offer hope.
- Offer alternatives quickly; be sure these are choices, not threats.
- Avoid sharing personal information about yourself.

- Do not turn your back toward the person.
- Be aware of how to get help in case of emergencies.

you will encounter someone who is unable to control his behavior or emotions because he has a physical or mental illness or is under the influence of drugs or alcohol. When patients or visitors are very stressed, they may not be in control of their feelings or emotions. Sometimes they yell and become insulting or verbally abusive to health care givers in any setting. It is helpful to anticipate this and review some basic guidelines to assist you in coping with these kinds of problems.

SUMMARY

Seven goals of customer-focused care, which is designed to meet the needs of patients, residents, and clients, help you provide service to those who are in your care. It is important to keep cultural variations in the way people view illness and treatment in mind when you communicate with and provide care for patients whose ethnic backgrounds differ from your own. When you encounter a patient whose behavior is disruptive, you can use a number of techniques to try to defuse the situation.

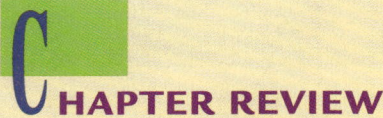

CHAPTER REVIEW

FILL IN THE BLANK

Read each sentence and fill in the blank line with a word that completes the sentence.

1. A _____ is an individual cared for by a home health agency or provider.

2. A _____ is an individual cared for in a long term/extended care facility.

3. The more you learn about an individual's _____ and differences, the better you can provide sensitive care and services to your patients, residents, or clients.

4. A _____ is a requirement for survival.

5. Every person has basic _____ and _____ needs.

MULTIPLE CHOICE

Choose the best answer for each question or statement.

1. Which of the following is not a goal for customer-focused care?
   a. Care provided reflects respect for the individual.
   b. Information is communicated.
   c. The patient is relieved of fear whenever possible.
   d. The food is always warm and comforting.

2. Which of the following actions do not promote sleep and rest?
   a. Being aware of the noise around you.
   b. Always turning off all the lights.
   c. If possible, allow the patient to use their own pillow.
   d. Offer skin and mouth care as needed.

3. Which of the following is not a good technique to try when dealing with a disruptive patient?
   a. Yell back at the patient.
   b. Be objective.
   c. Be alert.
   d. Remain calm, but firm.

4. Which of the following is considered a physiologic need?
   a. social groups
   b. status, titles
   c. shelter
   d. family

5. Which of the following is not a guideline for appreciating cultural diversity?
   a. Treat everyone with respect.
   b. Take what the patient says literally.
   c. Be open, flexible, and adaptable.
   d. Thank others who help you to better understand about their culture.

6. Which of the following is true?
   a. Using flash cards and pictures with patients who do not speak English helps to reduce stress and anxiety.
   b. Use the universal "OK" sign to communicate with people of all cultures.
   c. Hold the patient's hand and look directly in their eyes when talking with people of all cultures.
   d. All of the above.

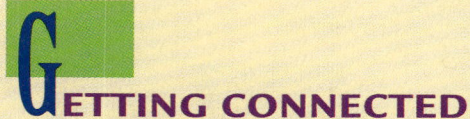

GETTING CONNECTED

MULTIMEDIA EXTENSION ACTIVITIES

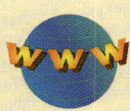

www.prenhall.com/wolgin

Use the above address to access the free, interactive Companion Website created for this textbook. Get hints, instant feedback, and textbook references to chapter-related multiple choice questions. Read and react to the "Nursing Assistants in Action." Link to other interesting sites.

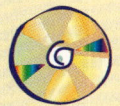

Audio Glossary

Use the CD-ROM disk enclosed with your textbook to hear the pronunciation of the key terms in the chapter.

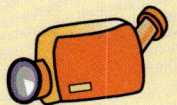

Video

Watch the video "Dealing with Dementia" from the Care Provider Skills series and the video "Professionalism: Dealing with Anger."

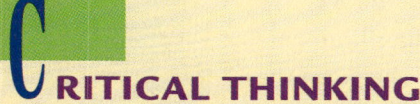

CRITICAL THINKING

USING KEY QUESTIONS

Read each question and think of what you might do in each situation.

1. Imagine you are assigned to care for a patient who speaks little or no English. What methods might you use to help communication?

2. What gestures or communication aides might you use to bridge the language gap with your patient?

3. What kind of behavior might you see in a patient who has unmet physical needs?

4. Imagine you encounter a patient who is unable to control his behavior because of injury and intoxication. What guidelines and techniques would you use to help diffuse the situation?

5. Think of an encounter where you have received good customer-focused care. Which of the seven goals were satisfied to make you feel like you received good care?

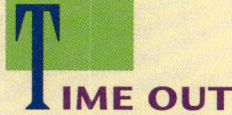

TIME OUT

TIPS FOR TIME MANAGEMENT

SELF-DISCIPLINE TIP   Avoid the temptation to do more talking than working. Save social chit-chat for break time. Make your conversations patient-centered, not self-centered. Keep your conversations with coworkers professional and positive.

Infection Control

5

The health care environment is an area that requires the people who work there to have a basic knowledge and understanding of disease and disease transmission. This chapter introduces the nursing assistant to the history of the germ theory and its evolution into today's practice. Health care workers and patients alike have benefited from knowledge about disease transmission. An example of this is the recently updated guideline from the Centers for Disease Control and Prevention (CDC) for the protection of health care workers (HCW) in health care institutions. CDC's expanded guideline consists of two tiers of precautions: Standard Precautions and Transmission-based Precautions. In this chapter, the relationship between Universal Precautions and the new CDC guideline, particularly Standard Precautions, is presented. With the information and examples provided on infection control, nursing assistants will be able to protect themselves more fully, as well as their patients, from acquiring one of the most serious and dreaded complications of hospitalization—a *nosocomial* infection. The importance of asepsis and sterile technique is introduced. Guidelines for maintaining a sterile field and procedures to put on sterile gloves and open sterile packages are included.

When you have completed this chapter, you will be able to:

- Differentiate between helpful and harmful microorganisms.
- List four conditions affecting the growth of bacteria.
- Summarize the history of infection control.
- List five ways microorganisms are spread.
- Explain how microorganisms are destroyed.
- Identify what precautions are used for all patients.
- List the three elements necessary for transmission of infection.
- Describe the three main purposes of asepsis.
- Demonstrate the procedure for handwashing.
- Identify OSHA standards for occupational exposure to bloodborne pathogens.
- Identify recommendations for prevention and control of Hepatitis C.

KEY TERMS

asepsis

aseptic

autoclave

bacteria

disinfection

friction

hepatitis B

hepatitis C

infection

infection control

isolation

microorganism

normal flora

nosocomial infection

pathogen

Rickettsiae

spores

sterile field

sterilization

transmission

virus

HISTORY OF INFECTION CONTROL

People once believed that sickness was caused by evil spirits. About 500 years ago, scientists began to suspect that some diseases were caused by very small living things they called germs. The germ theory of disease was not actually *proven* until about 100 years ago. A French scientist named Louis Pasteur made two important discoveries about bacteria. First, he discovered that many diseases are caused by **bacteria**. Second, he discovered that bacteria could be killed by excess heat.

bacteria Unicellular microorganism

Pasteur's name has been used to refer to the heat method of killing germs. For example, pasteurization is the process of heating milk to 140°F (60°C) and keeping it at that temperature for one-half hour. Pasteurization kills harmful bacteria and makes milk safe for us to drink.

A few years after Pasteur's discoveries, a British surgeon, Joseph Lister, found that germs could also be killed by carbolic acid. Lister recognized that many deaths in hospitals seemed to be connected with unclean conditions. He was the first to *demand* that surgical wounds were to be kept clean and the air in the operating room kept pure. His success was demonstrated by a reduction in deaths in people undergoing amputation, which decreased from 45 percent to 15 percent.

aseptic Germ free, without disease-producing organisms

Lister's theories led to changes in hospitals by introducing the principles and methods of aseptic surgery. **Aseptic** means germ free, or without disease-producing organisms. Lister developed a technique to keep germs out of open wounds as well as identifying a method to destroy germs. His method was to spray the skin around the wound with carbolic acid. Also, surgical instruments were made aseptic by being dipped in a carbolic acid solution. This technique was a major advance in the battle against disease.

Nosocomial Infections

People working in hospitals began to realize that some disease-producing germs were everywhere. Scientists learned that germs multiply very rapidly—every 12 minutes. They also found that if germs are not controlled, they may spread infection and disease from one person to another. Therefore, it was necessary to apply the principles of asepsis to the health care practice in order to prevent **nosocomial infections** (infections acquired while a person/patient is in the hospital). Nosocomial infections can range from simple and uncomplicated to major and life-threatening. Patients often have weakened immune systems and are prone to exposure from the people, equipment, and environment within a health care facility. Additionally, patients are at risk for iatrogenic infection, which can occur following surgery, medication, or a treatment. *Iatrogenic* means *caused by medical treatment*. Bacteria causes two common nosocomial infections: Methicillin-resistant Staphlococcus aureus (MRSA) and Psuedomonas aeruginosa. They are both resistant to antibiotic treatment and difficult to control. Vancomycin-resistant enterococci (VRE) is another difficult to control infection that has been seen in both hospitals and long-term care facilities.

nosocomial infection Hospital acquired infection

The success of modern medicine in controlling and preventing infection is due to the focus, or emphasis, on the individual health care worker as the primary source, or means, of spreading infection and thus the means of preventing infection.

NATURE OF MICROORGANISMS

microorganism A living thing that is so small it cannot be seen with the naked eye but only through a microscope

A germ is a microorganism. Micro means very small. Organism means living thing. So a **microorganism** is a living thing that is so small it cannot be seen with the naked eye, only through a microscope. Different kinds of microorganisms (also called microbes)

are bacteria (**Rickettsiae**), fungi, protozoa, and viruses. Microorganisms occur nearly everywhere in nature. They occur most abundantly where they find food, moisture, and a temperature suitable for their growth and multiplication. Since conditions that are favorable for microorganisms are those under which people normally live, it is inevitable that we live among numerous microbes.

Microorganisms are best known to the average person by the diseases they cause in human beings. The disease-producing microorganisms or *germs* are called **pathogens**. Figure 5–1 demonstrates the role different pathogens can play in disease causation. They grow best at body temperature, 98.6°F; 37°C. Pathogens destroy human tissue by using it as food. They may also give off waste products called toxins that are absorbed into and poison the body.

Rickettsiae An example of bacteria found in the tissues of fleas, lice, ticks, and other insects; Rickettsiae are transmitted to humans by insect bites

pathogen Disease producing microorganism

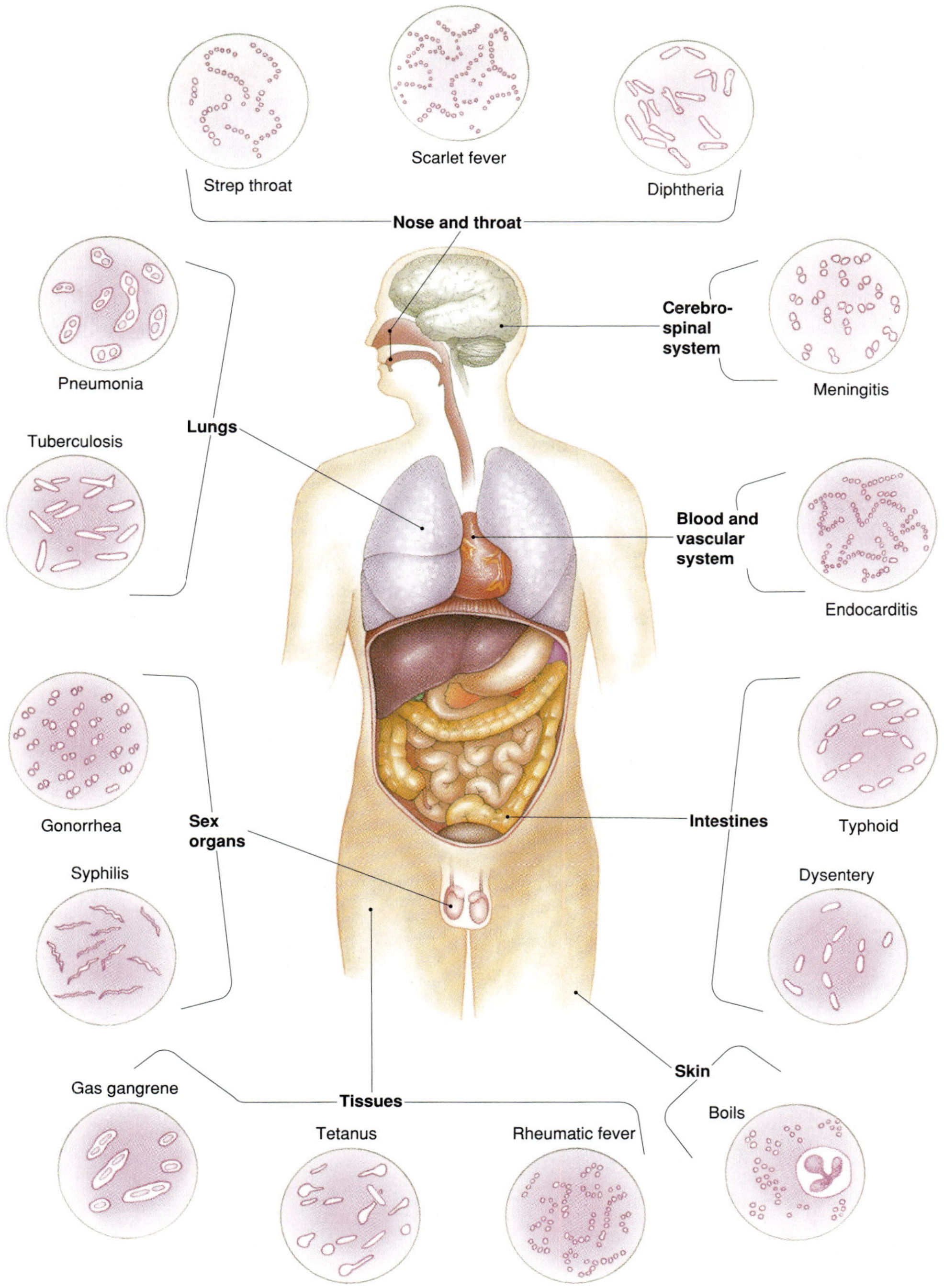

FIGURE 5–1

Pathogens cause disease in the human body

Strep throat

Scarlet fever

Diphtheria

Nose and throat

Pneumonia

Tuberculosis

Lungs

Cerebro-spinal system

Meningitis

Blood and vascular system

Endocarditis

Gonorrhea

Syphilis

Sex organs

Intestines

Typhoid

Dysentery

Gas gangrene

Tissues

Tetanus

Rheumatic fever

Skin

Boils

normal flora
Microorganisms that are necessary for health, and usually live and grow in specific locations; they are nonpathogenic when in or on a natural reservoir

Some microorganisms, particularly bacteria and fungi, are helpful and necessary for healthy functioning of a person and are referred to as normal flora. **Normal flora** in the human digestive system breaks down the foods not used by the body and turns them into waste products. Also, certain microbes cause a chemical change in food called fermentation. Fermentation is the change that produces cottage cheese from milk, beer from grains, and cider from apples.

Microbes each have their own normal environment, or home, called their natural habitat. When organisms gain access to areas of the body in which they do not belong (Figure 5–2), they become pathogens. For example, Escherichia coli belongs in the colon where it helps to digest food. When it gets into the bladder or into the bloodstream, it can cause a urinary infection, or a *bloodstream* infection.

Bacteria grow well in moist, warm, dark areas. For example, meat must be stored at extremely cold temperatures and then cooked to extremely high temperatures in order to eliminate the risk of potential bacterial contamination that has occurred through improper handling or cooking. Some bacterial microbes require oxygen to live. Figure 5–3 describes four conditions that affect the growth of bacteria.

In the hospital you will often hear the words staph, or staphylococcus, and strep, or streptococcus. Staphylococcus and streptococcus are examples of two types of bacteria that may become pathogens if given the right opportunity. They are commonly found on the human skin and may enter the body through a portal of entry. Portal of entry is an area where the primary defense to an organism is violated and there is now a direct access to the inside of the body. Our primary defense is the skin, and it is violated every time the skin is cut, such as when there is a surgical incision or when a tube/drain is placed. When staphylococci get inside the skin, they may produce a local infection. There may be soreness, tenderness, redness, and/or pus (infection). Sometimes staphylococcus infections can affect the whole body.

virus A type of microorganism; much smaller than bacteria and can survive only in other living cells

A virus is another type of microorganism. **Viruses** are much smaller than bacteria, and cause many of our diseases. Examples are measles, AIDS (acquired immunodeficiency syndrome), and influenza. Viruses can survive only in other living cells.

Figures 5–4a and 5–4b show ways that microorganisms are NOT spread. Touching a patient does not require use of gloves or other protective equipment, provided the patient's skin is intact and not draining or weeping. Visiting with a patient and adjusting the bed sheets also does not require protective equipment unless the linen is soiled. Examples of situations with the potential for spreading microorganisms and for which protective equipment such as gowns, gloves, and masks may be indicated are the emptying of a urinary bag, starting an IV, and doing a dressing change.

FIGURE 5–2
Bacteria may enter the body through invasive points of entry such as IV sites, indwelling catheters, and surgical sites. Bacteria may also enter the body through cuts or through the nose and mouth

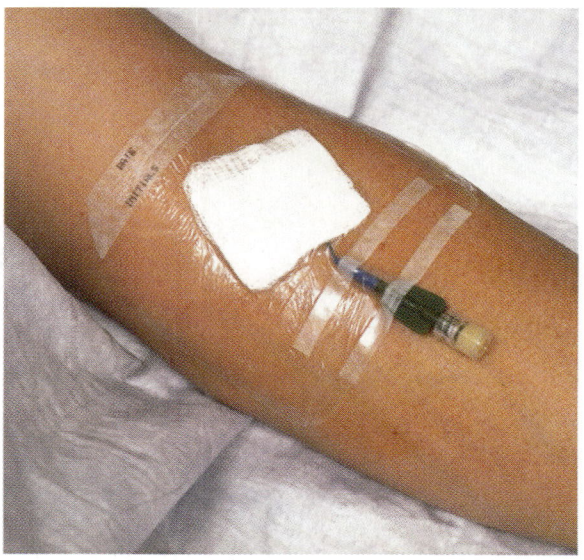

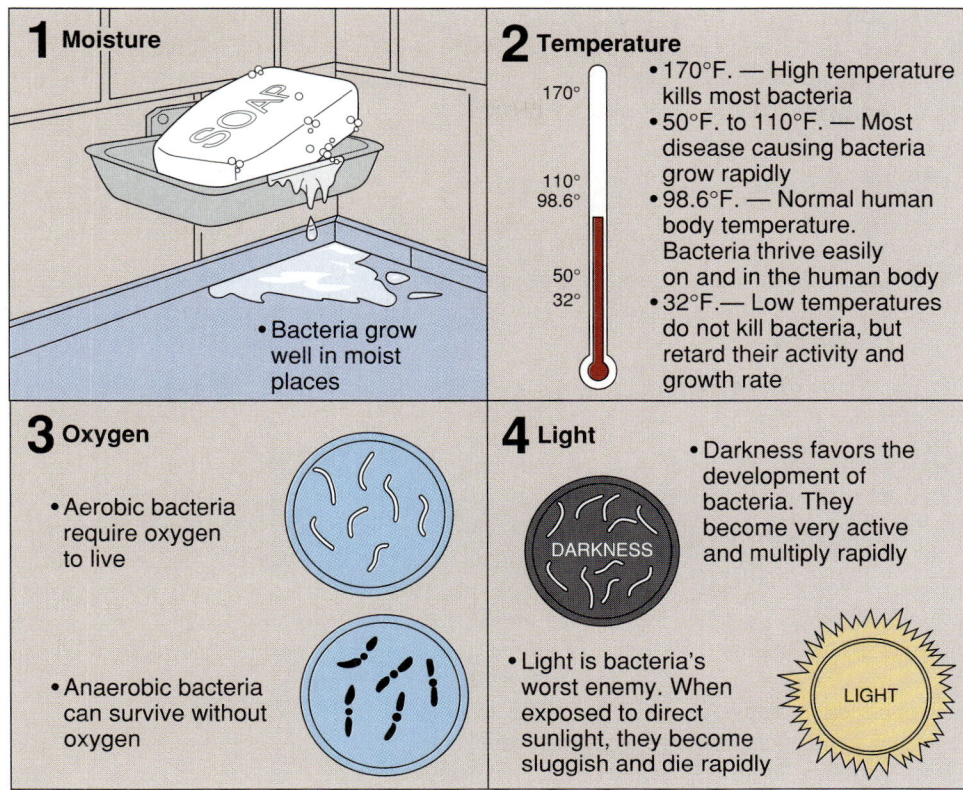

FIGURE 5–3
Four conditions affecting the growth of bacteria

1 Moisture

SOAP

• Bacteria grow well in moist places

2 Temperature

170°
110°
98.6°
50°
32°

• 170°F. — High temperature kills most bacteria
• 50°F. to 110°F. — Most disease causing bacteria grow rapidly
• 98.6°F. — Normal human body temperature. Bacteria thrive easily on and in the human body
• 32°F.— Low temperatures do not kill bacteria, but retard their activity and growth rate

3 Oxygen

• Aerobic bacteria require oxygen to live

• Anaerobic bacteria can survive without oxygen

4 Light

• Darkness favors the development of bacteria. They become very active and multiply rapidly

DARKNESS

• Light is bacteria's worst enemy. When exposed to direct sunlight, they become sluggish and die rapidly

LIGHT

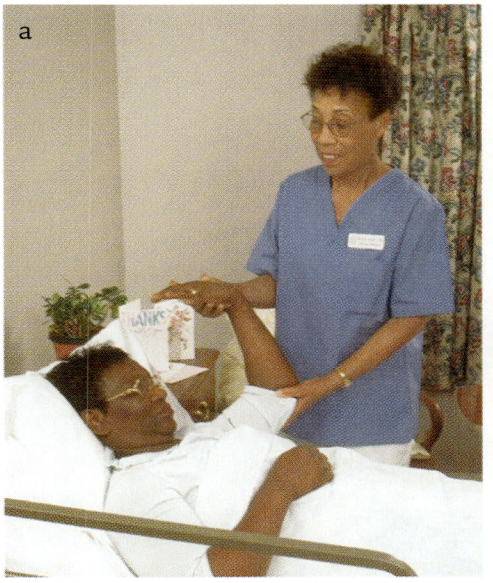

a

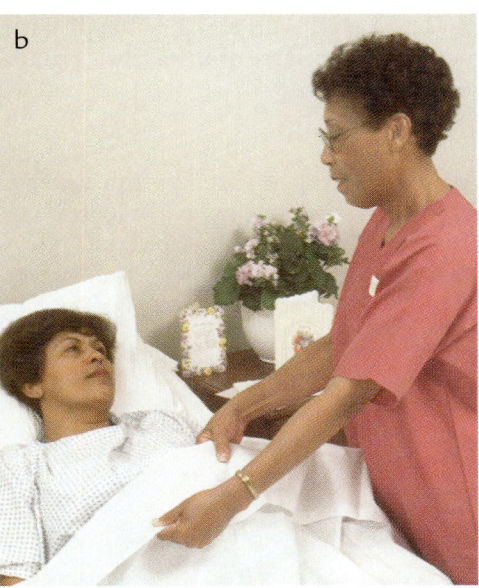

b

FIGURE 5–4a
Gloves are not required when touching a patient, provided the skin is not draining or weeping

FIGURE 5–4b
Gloves are not required when adjusting sheets of a patient, provided the linen is not soiled

PREVENTING THE SPREAD OF INFECTION

It is a major goal of health care institutions to prevent the spread of pathogens. This battle is called **infection control**. In spite of the best efforts of health care personnel, there are always some harmful microorganisms around us. We can reduce the number

infection control The effort to prevent the spread of pathogens

of organisms, however, by maintaining simple cleanliness procedures. We can keep ourselves clean by bathing and frequent handwashing. We can keep the institution and its equipment clean with soap, water, and special solutions that assist in the removal of bacteria, as well as keeping down bacterial growth.

◼ Disinfection and Sterilization

Two very important methods for killing microorganisms or keeping them under control are

1. **Disinfection**—the process of destroying as many harmful organisms as possible. It also means slowing down the growth and activity of the organisms that cannot be destroyed.

2. **Sterilization**—the process of killing all microorganisms, including spores, in a certain area.

Spores are bacteria that have formed hard shells around themselves as a defense. These shells are like a protective suit of armor. Spores are very difficult to kill; some can even live in boiling water. Spores can be destroyed by being exposed to pressurized steam at a high temperature. Machines called **autoclaves** can produce this high-temperature, pressurized steam (Figure 5–5). Autoclaves are used to kill spores and other disease-producing bacteria. Another method of sterilization uses a chemical gas instead of heat to destroy microorganisms. This method can be used to sterilize equipment made of plastics without melting it. When an object is free of all microorganisms, it is called sterile. These are both effective ways of sterilizing objects used in a health care institution.

Sterilization is necessary if the article comes in direct contact with an open wound or the bloodstream, as in the case of surgical instruments, and is referred to as a critical item. Noncritical items are supplies and equipment that are used in the care of patients, but do not come in contact with an open or draining area. Therefore, noncritical items can be cleaned with a hospital-approved disinfectant, between patient use, to prevent the spread of disease or **infection** (Figure 5–6).

◼ Asepsis

Asepsis means the absence of microorganisms. Asepsis can be achieved by preventing the conditions that allow pathogens to live, multiply, and spread. As a nursing assistant, you will share the responsibility for preventing the spread of disease and infection by using aseptic techniques. The main purposes for asepsis in caring for patients are

- Protecting the patient against becoming infected a second time by the same microorganism. This is called reinfection.

disinfection The process of destroying as many harmful organisms as possible

sterilization The process of killing all microorganisms, including spores

spores Bacteria that have formed hard shells around themselves as a defense

autoclave Device used to achieve sterility of an item through heat, pressure, and steam

infection Due to a pathogen producing a reaction that may cause soreness, tenderness, redness, and/or pus, fever, change in drainage, and so on

asepsis The absence of microorganisms (germs)

FIGURE 5–5

Autoclaves are used to kill spores and other disease-producing bacteria

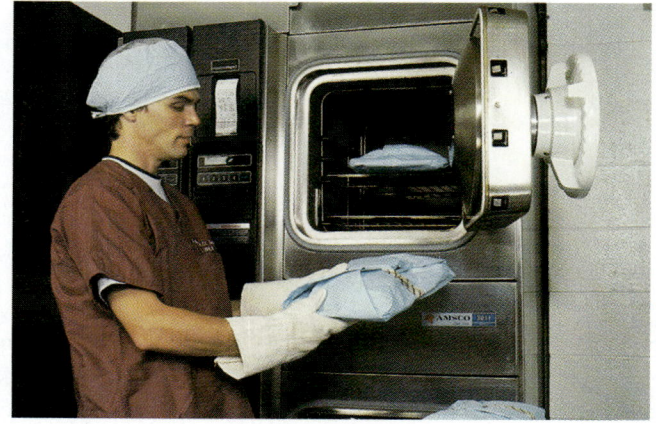

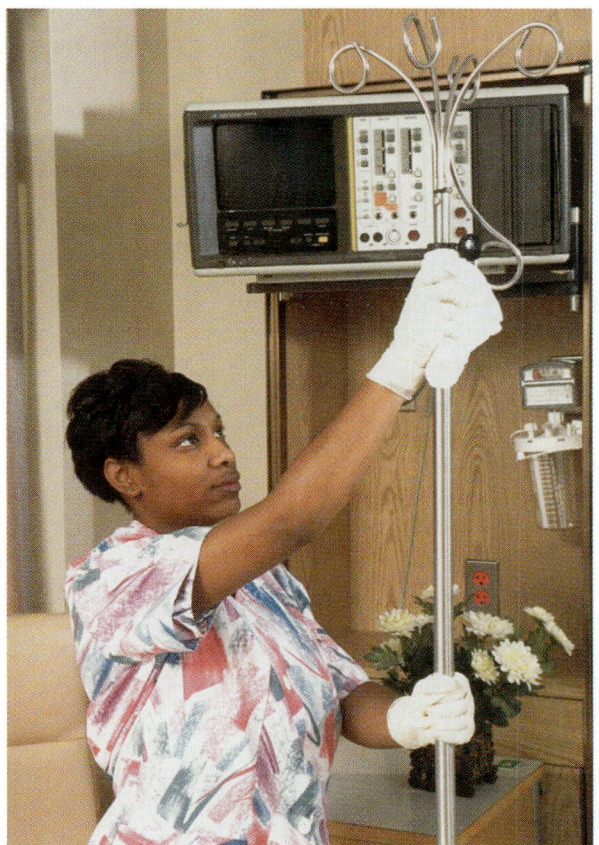

FIGURE 5–6
The IV pole is cleaned with
approved disinfectant

- Protecting the patient against becoming infected by a new or different type of microorganism from equipment, another patient, or a member of the hospital staff. This is called cross contamination.

- Protecting the patient from becoming infected with the patient's own organisms.

When the patient acquires an infection that was not present prior to or at the time of admission to the hospital, it is called a nosocomial, or hospital, acquired infection. For the transmission of any infection within a hospital, three things are necessary:

- a source of the infecting microorganisms

- a patient or susceptible host

- a means of transmission for the microorganism

The presence of these three factors, or components, is also referred to as the chain of infection. Infection control strategies are aimed at interrupting this chain of infection.

The source of the microorganisms may be the patient, the health care worker, or basically anyone, as well as the inanimate environment, for example, equipment. The patient becomes a susceptible host (one who can catch the disease or become infected) as the ability to resist an infection varies with different people. Certain criteria, such as age, underlying disease, current medication, or treatments, can greatly affect an individual's ability to "resist" infection. The final component that is necessary for an infection to develop is a route of transmission. You must understand the concept of **transmission**, or how the disease is spread, in order to protect yourself as well as your patient. There are three main routes of transmission that need to be focused on within a hospital: contact, droplet, and airborne.

transmission The spread
of microorganisms

KEY IDEA

Most diseases are spread through body fluids. Some diseases are spread through the air. Hospitals have isolation policies designed to protect health care workers from exposure to infectious diseases.

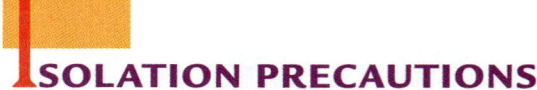

isolation To separate or set apart

ISOLATION PRECAUTIONS

The Centers for Disease Control and Prevention (CDC) have updated their guideline for protecting health care workers (HCW) and patients from exposure to infectious diseases. The guideline consists of two tiers of precautions.

The first and most important tier contains those precautions designed to decrease the risk of transmission of disease to the HCW through exposure to body fluids. This tier is called "Standard Precautions" and is used when caring for all patients, regardless of the patient's diagnosis and whether or not the patient is known to have an infectious disease.

The second tier of the CDC guideline is designed for patients documented or suspected to be carrying or infected with pathogens that require extra precautions in addition to the "Standard Precautions." This second tier of precautions, known as "Transmission-based Precautions" includes: 1) Airborne Precautions, 2) Droplet Precautions, and 3) Contact Precautions.

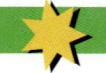

KEY IDEA

The CDC's expanded guideline is presented in order to provide an example of safe practice and precautions. It is your responsibility to learn and to follow the isolation policies used at your health care institution.

Not all hospitals will choose to follow the CDC guidelines exactly. Most hospitals will have isolation policies that are similar in underlying principal but may be different in detail. All hospitals that comply with regulatory rules, for example, OSHA, will have at least the following:

1. A barrier-based isolation policy that applies to all patients and is designed to reduce the risk of transmission of microorganisms from blood or other blood-containing body fluids. These policies may be referred to as Universal Precautions.

   Many health care institutions have chosen to expand on these required precautions to include not only blood and blood-containing body fluids, but any moist body substance. These expanded precautions are often called Body Substance Isolation or Body Substance Precautions.

2. An isolation policy to prevent the transmission of infectious diseases that are spread on air currents. These policies are often called Airborne Precautions (like the CDC's) or Respiratory Isolation.

3. Policy standards for the safe handling of "sharps" to prevent injuries and deep exposure to body fluids. In some cases, standards for sharps handling are included in the institution's barrier-based policies (see #1).

Most institutions follow basic precautions like those just outlined; others will have expanded and adopted more detailed practices they felt were warranted. Since health care institutions choose to adopt and implement guidelines differently, it is important that you be familiar with the isolation policies used at your institution.

Many institutions will choose to use the new terminology and implement the precautions as they are described in this chapter. In those health care facilities where CDC guidelines are not followed, staff training will provide information regarding changes in policy and practice. Your immediate supervisor will provide direction and clarification, as needed.

Standard Precautions

All health care institutions have isolation precautions that are designed to reduce the risk of exposure to microorganisms and prevent the spread of infectious diseases. Typically, the main system of precautions used by health care institutions applies to all patients, since many diseases, such as **hepatitis B** virus (HBV), **hepatitis C** virus (HCV) and human immunodeficiency virus (HIV), the virus that causes AIDS, can be spread before the patient even develops symptoms of the disease. Therefore, Standard Precautions must be used when caring for all patients.

Both HBV and HIV are spread through several routes:

1. parenteral (direct inoculation of blood on a needle through the skin)

2. mucous membranes (blood contamination of the eye or mouth)

3. sexual

4. perinatal (from infected mother to newborn infant)

Standard Precautions, CDC's first tier of precautions, is designed to provide safety to health care workers and patients and to assist in controlling the spread of nosocomial infections.

hepatitis B Bloodborne disease that affects the liver and is easily transmitted within the health care setting following parenteral exposure

hepatitis C Prior to 1988 known as nonA-nonB hepatitis. Transmitted best through needle sticks and may result in chronic liver disease

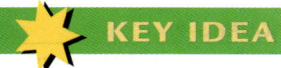 **KEY IDEA**

Remember: The CDC's Standard Precautions are similar to Universal Precautions in that both are directed at body fluids that are blood or blood serum derived or fluids that contain blood, but Standard Precautions are broader in that they also include precautions for any moist body substance. Examples are: tears, eye drainage, saliva, ear drainage, vaginal secretions, semen, urine, stool, sputum, nasal drainage, drainage from open wounds or incisions.

Standard Precautions apply to:

1. Blood

2. All body fluids-secretions and excretions—except sweat, regardless of whether or not they contain visible blood

3. Nonintact skin

4. Mucous membranes

To comply with these precautions the following practice on page 88 is expected.

GUIDELINES

CARE AND CLEANING OF NONCRITICAL ITEMS

Following use of a noncritical item, check for visible contamination, such as blood or other body substances.

■ If the item is not visibly soiled, carefully wipe the item clean with alcohol or the cleaning solution recommended by the manufacturer and /or the current hospital cleaner.

■ If the item is visibly soiled with blood or body fluids, the item should first be wiped, cleaned, and then disinfected.

Recommended cleaning, or disinfecting, solutions and methods must be effective against microbes while not harming the device in any way,

for example, corroding the metal or cracking the plastic. The solution may include:

a. 70 percent to 90 percent ethyl or isopropyl alcohol

b. Sodium hypochlorite (household bleach) 1 part bleach to 10 parts water

c. Phenolic germicidal detergent

d. Iodophor germicidal detergent

e. Quaternary ammonium germicidal detergent

PROCEDURE

OBRA

APPLICATION OF A GOWN

STEPS

1. Wash your hands. If you are wearing a long-sleeve uniform, roll your sleeves above your elbows (Figure 5–15a).

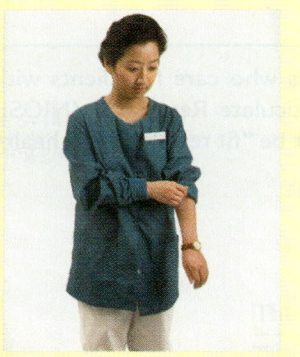

FIGURE 5–15a
Roll up sleeves

2. Unfold the isolation gown so the opening is at the back (Figure 5–15b).

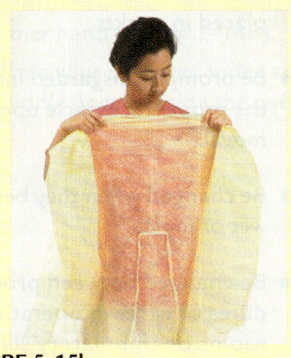

FIGURE 5–15b
Unfold gown so the opening faces you

3. Put your arms into the sleeves of the isolation gown (Figure 5–15c).

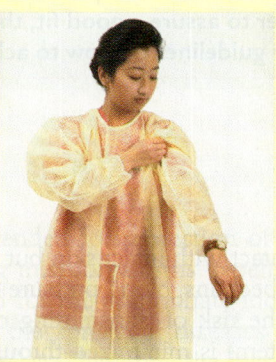

FIGURE 5–15c
Put your arms into the sleeves

4. Fit the gown at the neck, making sure your uniform is covered (Figure 5–15d).

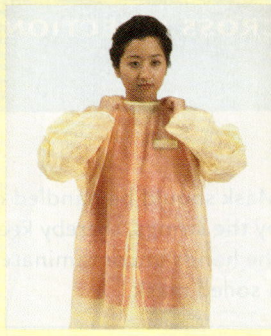

FIGURE 5–15d
Fit gown at your neck

5. Reach behind and tie the neck back with a simple shoelace bow or fasten an adhesive strip (Figure 5–15e).

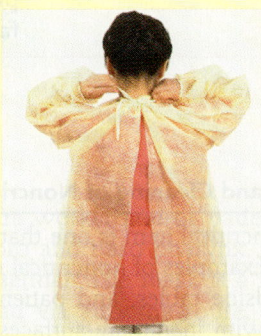

FIGURE 5–15e
Tie neck back with simple bow

PROCEDURE (CONTINUED)

6. Grasp the edges of the gown and pull to the back (Figure 5–15f).

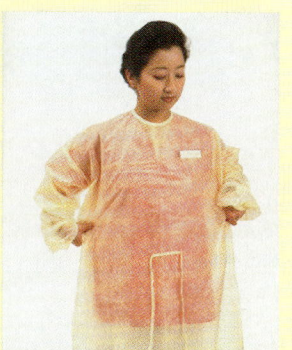

FIGURE 5–15f

Grasp gown edges and pull them back

7. Overlap the edges of the gown, completely closing the opening and covering your uniform completely (Figure 5–15g).

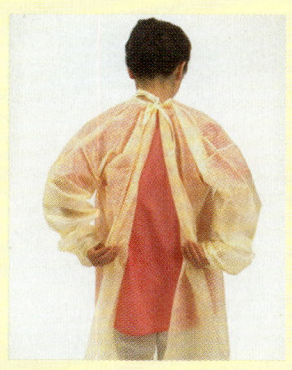

FIGURE 5–15g

Completely cover back of your uniform

8. Tie the waist ties in a bow or fasten the adhesive strip (Figure 5–15h).

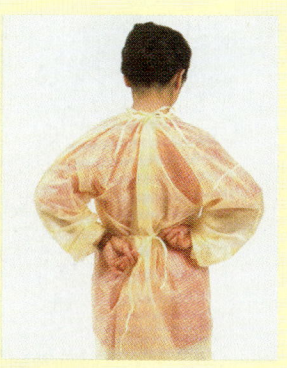

FIGURE 5–15h

Tie waist ties in a bow

PROCEDURE

OBRA

REMOVING A GOWN

STEPS

1. Keep gloves on, then untie the waist belt or ties (Figure 5–16a).[1]

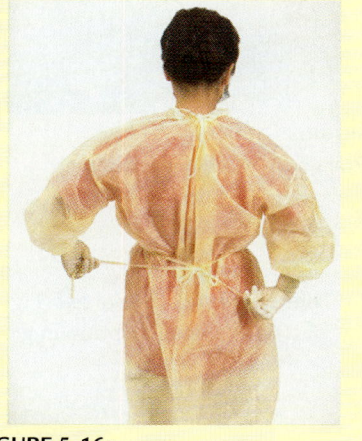

FIGURE 5–16a

Untie waist ties

2. Untie the neck ties, being cautious not to come in contact with neck, or have someone else untie the gown for you (Figure 5–16b).

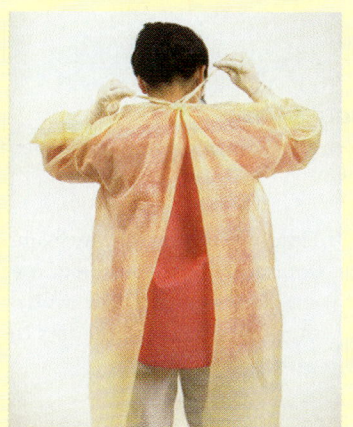

FIGURE 5–16b

Carefully untie neck ties

[1] This procedure is based on AORN standards. In practice there are two acceptable approaches regarding removing gloves and gown. The most important point is to avoid contamination or contact exposure to blood and body fluids. In the case where there is blood on your gown and gloves, it is most important to remove your gloves last after you have touched the contaminated gown. Follow your instructor's direction and always wash your hands after removing and discarding gowns, masks, and/or gloves.

PROCEDURE (CONTINUED)

3. Pull the sleeve off by grasping each shoulder at the neck line (Figure 5–16c).

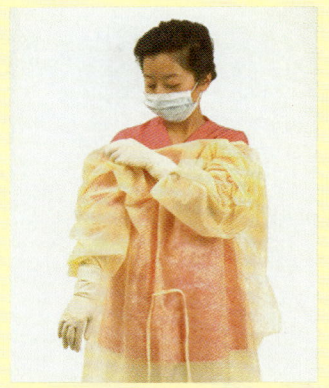

FIGURE 5–16c
Grasp gown at shoulder to pull sleeve off

4. Turn the sleeves inside out as you remove them from your arms (Figure 5–16d).

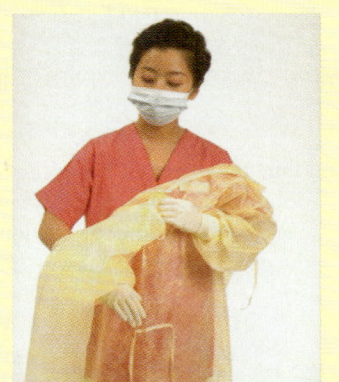

FIGURE 5–16d
Turn sleeves inside out as you remove them

5. Holding the gown away from your body by the inside of the shoulder seams, fold it inside out, bringing the shoulders together (Figure 5–16e).

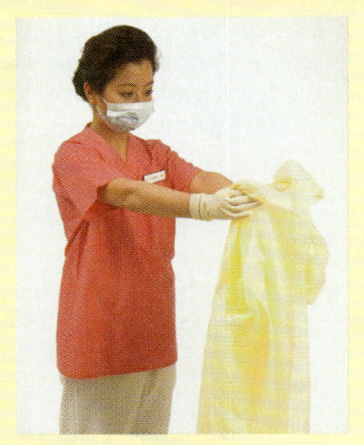

FIGURE 5–16e
Hold gown away from you as you fold it inside out

6. Roll the gown up with the inside out and discard (Figure 5–16f).

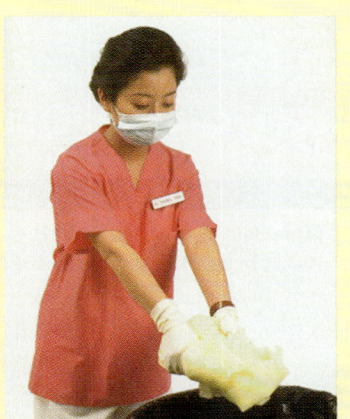

FIGURE 5–16f
Roll gown inside out and discard

7. Remove gloves being careful to not contaminate yourself (Figure 5–16g). (See description in glove removal.)

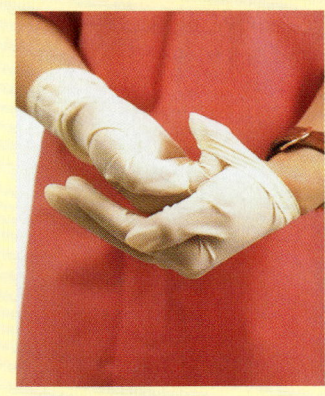

FIGURE 5–16g
Remove gloves

8. Remove mask touching only the strings and discard (Figure 5–16h).

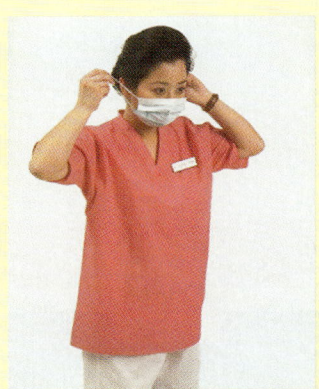

FIGURE 5–16h
Remove mask

FOLLOW-UP

9. Wash hands (Figure 5–16i).

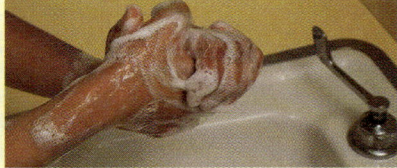

FIGURE 5–16i
Wash hands

▪ Changes in Isolation Strategies

As information on disease transmission becomes more available and more scientific, certain isolation strategies of the past are being eliminated. The practices that have no longer been found necessary consist of the following: double bagging of linen, meltaway bags, special precautions for cleaning dishware and utensils used by patients in isolation, and protective or reverse isolation. The rationale for the change in each isolation strategy follows:

1. Double bagging of linen is unnecessary since all linen is considered infectious and therefore needs to be handled in such a manner as to avoid dispersal of microorganisms. This includes using a plastic bag if the linen is soiled or wet in order to prevent contamination of floors, linen chutes, or bins. The practice of double bagging is not necessary, however.

2. Meltaway bags are unnecessary since all linen is handled as infectious.

3. No additional special precautions are needed for dishes, glasses, cups, or eating utensils for the patient in isolation. Dishes should be handled according to standard hospital procedure or in the home setting may be washed with hot, soapy water or in the dishwasher. Disposable dishes and utensils are not necessary for patients in isolation precautions.

4. Protective or reverse isolation was shown to be ineffective in preventing infection in immunosuppressed patients, as the patient's own flora was primarily responsible for their infection. Good handwashing, limiting visitors, and not allowing fresh fruits, vegetables, or flowers is the most effective prevention method for this population. Some hospitals have more specific precautions for immune compromised patients.

OSHA STANDARDS FOR OCCUPATIONAL EXPOSURE TO BLOODBORNE PATHOGENS

Who is at risk? All facilities will identify all job classifications that have occupational exposure to blood and other potentially dangerous body fluids and materials. Since July 6, 1992, OSHA (Occupational Safety and Health Administration, U.S. Department of Labor) standards mandate that training and immunization must be provided to all employees within ten days of initial assignment to a job that puts the employee at occupational risk. This training must be updated annually. All employees must be given the choice to elect or refuse immunization. If refused, the employee has the right to change his or her mind at a later date and receive immunization at no charge.

Employers are required to provide a means of protecting their employees from potential exposure to hepatitis B. Employees must use standard precautions, protective clothing, protective eye wear or face shields, and equipment to prevent exposure to potentially infectious materials. However, the best defense against infection by hepatitis B is vaccination.

Hepatitis B vaccine (grown on yeast) became available in 1987 and is now the only type produced in this country. There are minimal adverse reactions and no possibility of infection from this vaccine. The hepatitis B vaccine is contraindicated for individuals who are hypersensitive to yeast or any component of the vaccine. Employees with a history of cardiopulmonary disease should consult their physician prior to accepting this vaccination. Hepatitis B vaccination is not recommended for use by pregnant women or nursing mothers.

Immunization is accomplished in a three-injection series. Any employee with a potential for occupational exposure qualifies to receive the vaccine. All costs associated with this immunization must be provided by the employer.

Hepatitis C virus (HCV) is now the most common chronic bloodborne infection in the United States. Most people with HCV are chronically infected and might not be aware of their infection because they do not have any clinical symptoms. Infected persons serve as a source of transmission to others and are at risk of developing chronic liver disease. HCV is transmitted primarily through large or repeated percutaneous exposures to blood. Prior to ten years ago, HCV was transmitted in blood transfusions; however, today, blood is screened for this virus. Injecting drug use consistently has accounted for a substantial proportion of HCV infections.

Another bloodborne pathogen that puts health care workers at potential risk is human immunodeficiency virus (HIV). The acquired immunodeficiency syndrome (AIDS) caused by HIV is a severe viral disease that affects the immune system and is characterized by opportunistic infections. The risk is due to exposure by semen, vaginal secretions, cerebrospinal fluid, synovial fluid, pleural fluid, pericardial fluid, peritoneal fluid, amniotic fluid, saliva, blood, blood products, and other body fluids and waste. Annual reeducation and the enforced use of standard precautions is the best means of preventing exposure. (Refer to Chapter 30 for AIDS.)

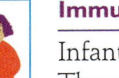

AGE SPECIFIC CONSIDERATIONS

Immunization

Infants less than three months of age have an immature immune system. They rely on passive immunity from their mothers. This makes them more prone to infections. The elderly also are more prone to infections. As the body ages, changes in the pulmonary system, such as decreased muscle strength, decreased vital capacity, and decreased cough, make the elderly more prone to infection.

KEY IDEA

There are times you may be asked to assist a nurse performing a procedure using aseptic or sterile technique. Do not perform sterile procedures independently unless you have been instructed to do so. Your instructor will be familiar with any practice rules or restrictions.

ASEPSIS AND STERILE TECHNIQUE

When working in a health care environment, it is important to assist patients to maintain their best possible physical state. To do so, caregivers might be required to practice the principles of asepsis (aseptic technique). When practiced correctly, these standards protect the patient from exposure to germs and help prevent infections.

Asepsis means the absence of microorganisms. Asepsis can be achieved by preventing the conditions that allow pathogens to live, multiply, and spread. As a caregiver, you share the responsibility to prevent the spread of infection by using aseptic, or sterile, technique. (*Aseptic technique* and *sterile technique* are terms that can be used interchangeably. For the rest of this chapter, we will use the term *sterile technique*.)

Sterile technique encompasses the steps followed to prevent contamination by germs. By following these steps very carefully, you will be able to maintain a sterile, or aseptic (germ-free), environment in which to do certain tasks.

When practicing sterile technique, keep the following in mind:

GUIDELINES

MAINTAINING A STERILE FIELD

- A **sterile field** is an area that you can create to work from when you are doing a sterile procedure. This area must remain dry in order to remain sterile. You can use a sterile wrap from a package to create this field, or you can use sterile towels supplied as part of a supply kit.

- Only sterile items can be on a sterile field. Sterile items have gone through the process of sterilization, which can destroy all living microorganisms. If an unsterile item is placed on the field, the field becomes unsterile.

If an unsterile item touches a sterile item, the sterile item becomes unsterile.

- Only the top of a table or counter of a sterile field is considered to be sterile. Anything hanging over the edge of a sterile field is unsterile. The edges of a sterile field itself (approximately 1 inch into the field) are considered unsterile, so be careful that you do not touch these areas with sterile items.

- Do not cross over your sterile field—that is, unless you are wearing sterile gown and gloves, do not reach over a sterile field. Microbes may drop from your arms or hands onto the sterile field, making it unsterile.

- Do not turn your back on your sterile field. You do not know what is happening when you cannot see your field. Place the sterile field in a location that will allow

you to keep it in sight and do your work efficiently.

- You may not touch the sterile field unless you have sterile gloves on.

- When you have sterile gloves on, your hands must be kept above your waist, in front of your body, and in your sight at all times. You may not touch anything that is not sterile. If you touch an unsterile item, your gloves become contaminated and must be replaced.

- You may drop sterile items onto a sterile field, but if they touch any unsterile items or the unsterile edge of the field, the sterile item becomes contaminated.

- Anything on your sterile field that absorbs moisture from an unsterile item becomes unsterile. For example, if there is wetness on the table on which you open your sterile package and this wetness soaks into your sterile field, the field becomes contaminated.

sterile field An area created to work from when you are doing a sterile procedure

Surgical conscience is a term used to describe the way you must act and think when you are working with sterile technique. It is your responsibility to be aware of and maintain your own sterile technique. For example, if no one is around and you contaminate your sterile field, you must be aware of this and start over. This protects the patient from microorganisms and germs that could cause an infection.

It is important to know the difference between clean technique and sterile technique. Some procedures are performed with clean technique. For example, clean technique might be used to change a dressing over a closed surgical wound or to reinforce a dressing. Clean technique involves using clean gloves and clean supplies (they do not need to be sterile, but they may be). You do not need to use sterile technique when doing something "cleanly," but you must still avoid contaminating your clean supplies and clean gloves. Clean items become contaminated if you drop them on the floor; clean gloves become contaminated if you use them to touch something dirty. The RN will tell you what type of technique (clean or sterile) to use during a procedure.

PROCEDURE

PUTTING ON STERILE GLOVES

STEPS

1. Wash hands.
2. Select a pair of wrapped gloves in a size that will fit your hands snugly.
3. Check to be certain that the gloves are sterile.
   a. Package intact with no signs of dampness?
   b. Seal of sterility?
4. Place package on a clean, dry, flat surface.
5. Open the wrapper, handling only the outside (Figure 5–17a and b).

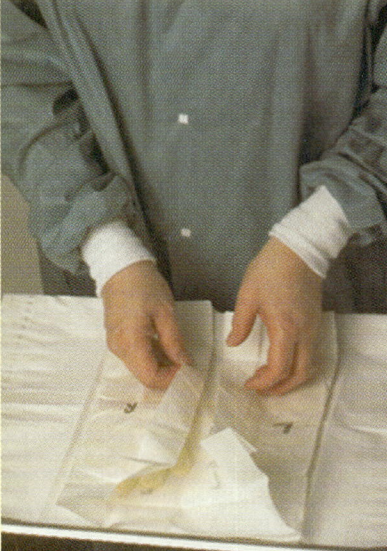

FIGURE 5–17b
Handle only outside of wrapper

6. Use your left hand to pick up the right glove. Touch only the inside folded cuff (Figure 5–18) *Do not touch the outside of the glove!*

7. Put the glove on your right hand (Figure 5–19).

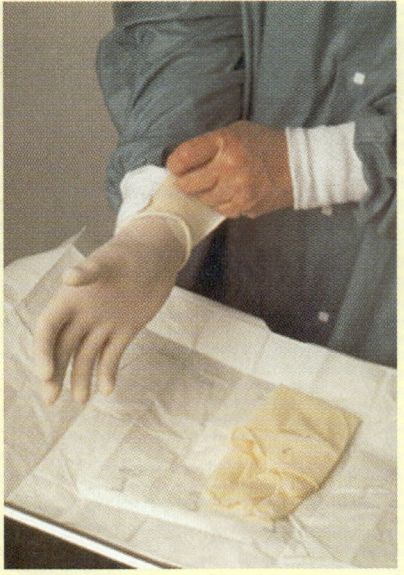

FIGURE 5–19
Put glove on your right hand

8. Use your gloved right hand to pick up the left glove:
   a. Place the finger of your gloved right hand under the cuff of the left glove (Figure 5–20).

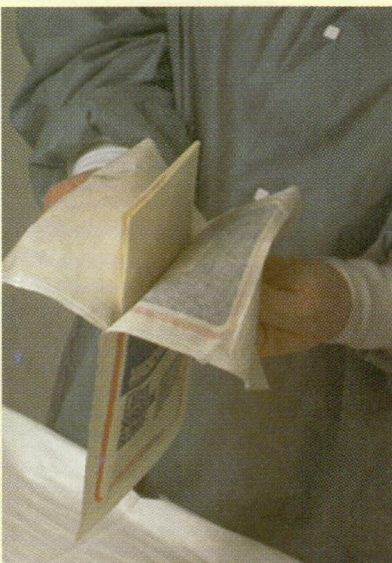

FIGURE 5–17a
Open wrapper

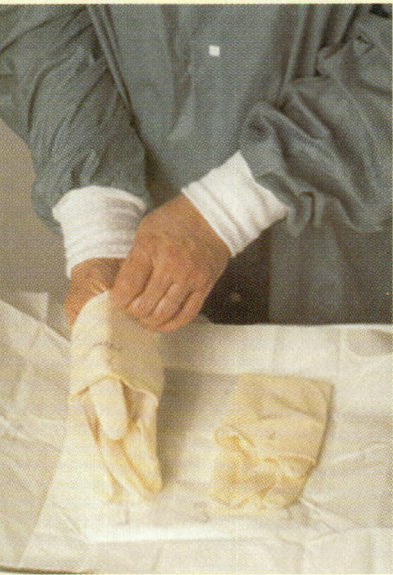

FIGURE 5–18
Touch only the inside of glove

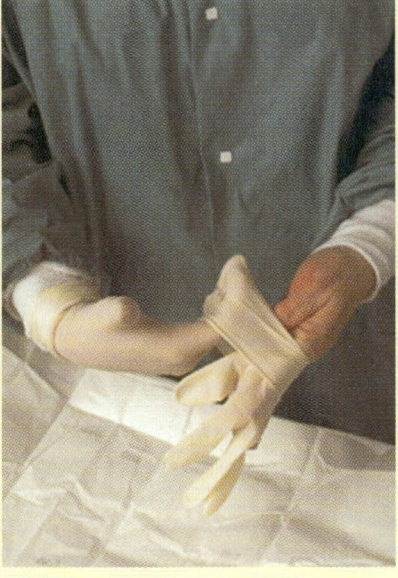

FIGURE 5–20
Place fingers of gloved hand inside left-hand glove cuff

PROCEDURE (CONTINUED)

b. Lift the glove up and away from the wrapper, and pull it onto your left hand.

c. Continue pulling left glove up to wrist. Be certain that the gloved right thumb does not touch your skin or clothing (Figure 5–21).

9. With your gloved left hand, place fingers under the cuff of the right glove and pull it up over your right wrist.

10. Adjust the fingers of the glove as necessary.

11. If either glove tears, remove them both and begin the procedure again with another pair.

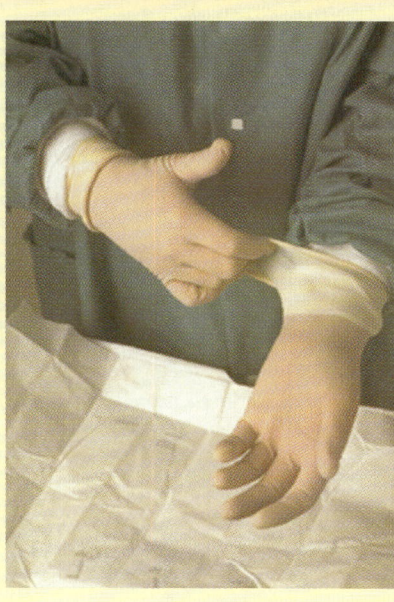

FIGURE 5–21

Pull glove on hand up to wrist

PROCEDURE

OPENING A STERILE PACKAGE

STEPS

1. Wash hands.

2. Assemble the equipment and supplies

   a. Sterile gloves

   b. Sterile package

3. Check to be certain all supplies are sterile:

   a. Package intact, with no signs of dampness?

   b. Seal of sterility?

4. Place the package on dry, flat, clean work surface (an over-bed table, for example). Position the package so that the first edge to be unfolded will be pulled away from you. (By opening the package away form you with the first motion, you will not have to reach across your sterile area again.) The outer wrap of the package will serve as a sterile field to work on (Figure 5–22a).

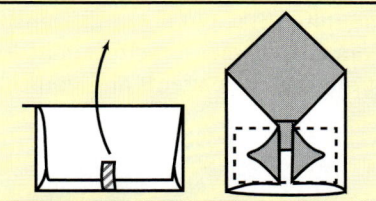

FIGURE 5–22a

Open first edge of package away from you

5. Slowly pull the corners at the right and left of the package (Figure 5–22b). This exposes the inside of the package.

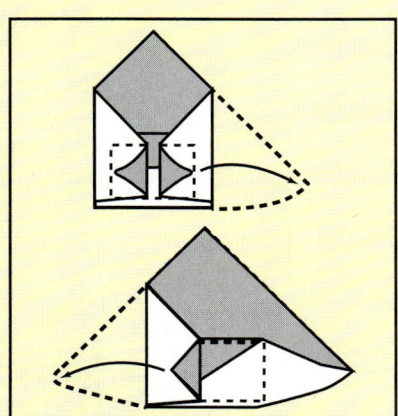

FIGURE 5–22b

Pull right and left corners of package to expose inside

6. Carefully pull back the corner pointing toward you (Figure 5–22c).

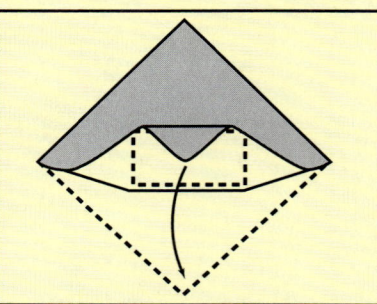

FIGURE 5–22c
Pull the last edge of package toward you

7. If you are going to add sterile items to your field, do so now (Figure 5–23). Remember that the edge (1 inch around) of your sterile field, and anything hanging over the edge of your work area, is contaminated.

8. Do not touch anything inside your sterile package or sterile field until you have put your sterile gloves on.

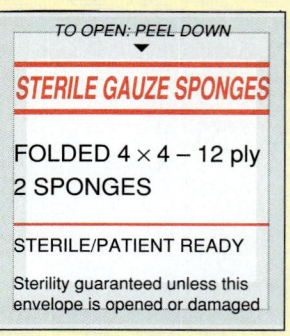

FIGURE 5–23a
Check that sterile package is clean and dry

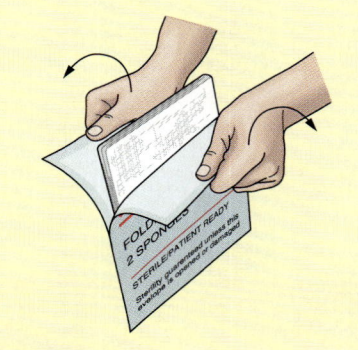

FIGURE 5–23b
Grasp each side of package at the top

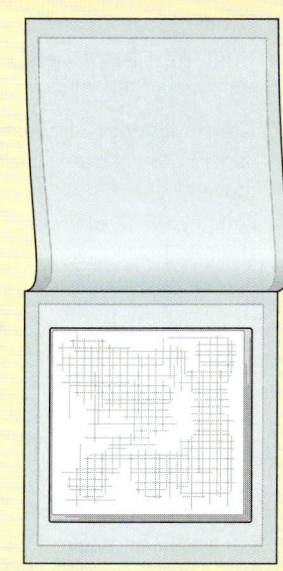

FIGURE 5–23c
Peel down the sides of package and lay flat

Aseptic and sterile technique are particularly important in any area where surgical procedures are performed or in an operating environment. An instructor will review objectives and performance expectations specific to the procedures that are performed.

Summary

The work of being a nursing assistant is not without risk. However, these risks are greatly minimized or eliminated by following the recommendations in this chapter, such as when to wear protective items, handwashing, and having the hepatitis B vaccine. Handwashing is the most important measure you can take to prevent the spread of microorganisms. Knowing how disease or infection is transmitted is the first step, but you then must utilize the Standard and Transmission-based Precautions necessary to interrupt the chain of transmission effectively. It is your responsibility to do all you can to prevent infections in your patients and yourself by following the described practices.

Notes

Patient Withholds Information

THE NURSING ASSISTANT IN ACTION

Mr. Joles was admitted to your unit yesterday. He has been coughing vigorously since he was admitted. You hear the physician ask him if he has been doing any traveling lately and if he has been out of the country. He responds no. Later that night he motions for you to come into his room. He tells you that he was not honest with the doctor when they talked that afternoon. Mr. Joles says that he is worried now. The fact is, he was out of the country for a week while in Mexico on business. He didn't want his wife to know about the trip so he didn't tell the doctor. Mr. Joles shares with you that he now wonders if his coughing is related to the trip. He also shares that he frequently needs to go for a walk in the hall to clear his head.

What Is Your Response/Action?

1. What are the important pieces of information from this situation?

2. What would be your first step in reacting to this situation?

3. What, if anything, would you do on your own in this situation?

4. What, if anything, would you report to your supervisor?

5. How can you protect yourself against infection in this situation?

6. How important is your action in this situation?

7. What might happen to the patient if you take no action?

8. What did you learn from this situation that you will apply in future situations?

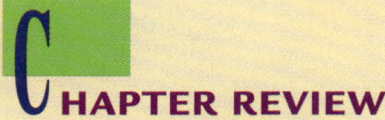

CHAPTER REVIEW

FILL IN THE BLANK

Read each sentence and fill in the blank line with a word that completes the sentence.

1. If you wear contaminated gloves in public places, you risk spreading _____.

2. A noncritical care item, such as a blood pressure cuff, can generally be _____versus disinfected.

3. _____ is the process of rubbing two surfaces together, such as skin.

4. Use _____ precautions when caring for a patient with TB.

5. When a patient is in contact precautions, you should always wear_____ when caring for the patient.

MULTIPLE CHOICE

Choose the best answer for each question or statement.

1. Aseptic means
   a. germ free.
   b. disease free.
   c. bacteria free.
   d. All of the above.

2. Normal flora means
   a. the normal plants seen around the hospital.
   b. the nonpathogenic microorganisms that live in our bodies.
   c. the pathogenic microorganisms that live in our bodies.
   d. All of the above.

3. Bacteria grows best in
   a. warm, moist, dark places.
   b. temperatures that are at less than 76 degrees.
   c. dry, bright, surfaces.
   d. All of the above.

4. Sterilization means
   a. process of killing all microorganisms.
   b. process of destroying as many microorganisms as possible.
   c. process of removing half of the microorganisms.
   d. All of the above.

5. In order for an infection to spread, all of the following factors need to be present except
   a. a source.
   b. a susceptible host.
   c. a means of transmission.
   d. a wet environment.

6. Which of the following types of precautions should be used for all patients?
   a. standard precautions.
   b. airborne precautions.
   c. contact precautions.
   d. droplet precautions.

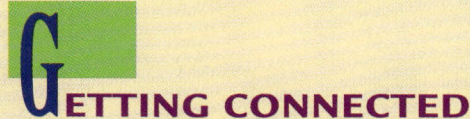

GETTING CONNECTED

MULTIMEDIA EXTENSION ACTIVITIES

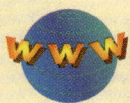

www.prenhall.com/wolgin
Use the above address to access the free, interactive Companion Website created for this textbook. Get hints, instant feedback, and textbook references to chapter-related multiple choice questions. Read and react to the "Nursing Assistants in Action." Link to other interesting sites.

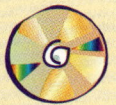

Audio Glossary
Use the CD-ROM disk enclosed with your textbook to hear the pronunciation of the key terms in the chapter.

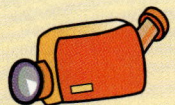

Video
Watch the video "Infection Control" from the Care Provider Skills series.

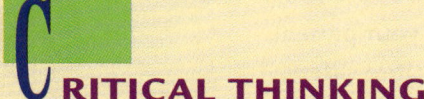

CRITICAL THINKING

USING KEY QUESTIONS

Read each question and think of what you might do in each situation.

1. You see another health care worker enter the room of a patient with airborne precautions without a mask. What do you do?

2. You hear the patient say she might have been exposed to chicken pox and is worried she might have them. What do you do?

3. You are really rushed for time. You wonder if you really need to wash the commode chair between patients. What do you do?

4. A patient's family member is afraid he might catch HIV from being in the same room with the patient. Can this happen?

5. Your patient has hepatitis C. What kind of personal protective equipment might you need?

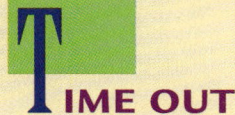

TIME OUT

TIPS FOR TIME MANAGEMENT

PLANNING TIP When you are assigned to care for an isolation patient, plan to do as many tasks as possible while you are in the room. Think through the tasks you plan to do so you can gather all your supplies before entering the isolation room. You can save the time and supplies you would use if you had to put on a mask, gown, and gloves several times to perform different tasks or to go get additional supplies.

Safety

6

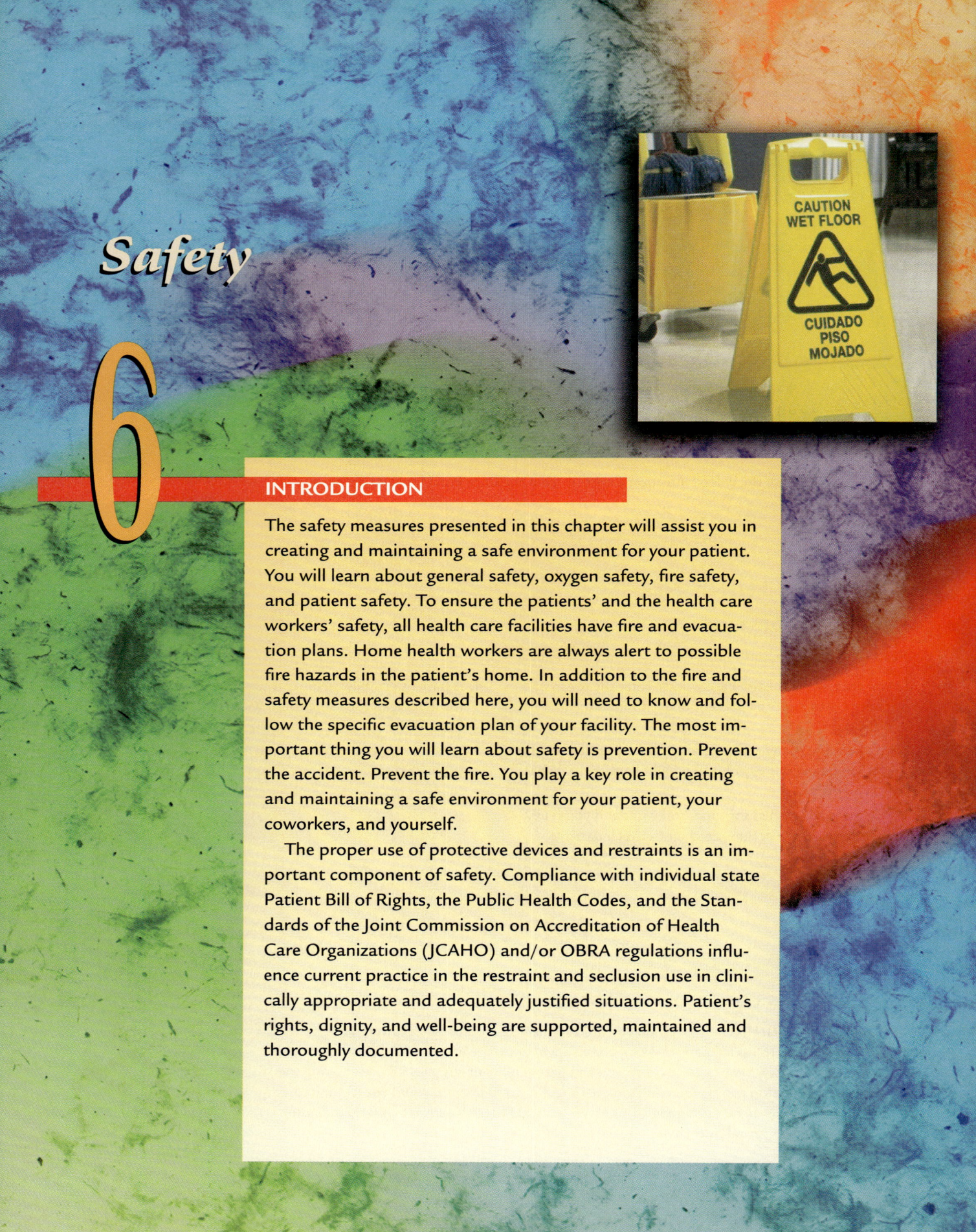

INTRODUCTION

The safety measures presented in this chapter will assist you in creating and maintaining a safe environment for your patient. You will learn about general safety, oxygen safety, fire safety, and patient safety. To ensure the patients' and the health care workers' safety, all health care facilities have fire and evacuation plans. Home health workers are always alert to possible fire hazards in the patient's home. In addition to the fire and safety measures described here, you will need to know and follow the specific evacuation plan of your facility. The most important thing you will learn about safety is prevention. Prevent the accident. Prevent the fire. You play a key role in creating and maintaining a safe environment for your patient, your coworkers, and yourself.

The proper use of protective devices and restraints is an important component of safety. Compliance with individual state Patient Bill of Rights, the Public Health Codes, and the Standards of the Joint Commission on Accreditation of Health Care Organizations (JCAHO) and/or OBRA regulations influence current practice in the restraint and seclusion use in clinically appropriate and adequately justified situations. Patient's rights, dignity, and well-being are supported, maintained and thoroughly documented.

OBJECTIVES

When you have completed this chapter, you will be able to:

- List the general rules of safety in a health care setting.
- List safety precautions in caring for children.
- Describe the special safety precautions necessary when oxygen is being used.
- Explain what you can do to prevent fires and what to do in case of a fire.
- Understand the basics of emergency care.
- Identify OBRA regulations regarding the use of restraints.
- Discuss restraint alternatives.
- List the safety rules for patient ambulation.

KEY TERMS

ambulate

ambulation

cannula

clove hitch

flowmeter

gait training

nasal

OBRA regulations

oxygen

protective devices

restraint alternative

restraints

GENERAL SAFETY MEASURES

People with health-care needs are challenged by illness, disability, concerns, and medications. Many of them cannot care for themselves in an emergency and rely on health care personnel for protection. As a member of the care team you must make every effort to guard against accidents, prevent fires and other kinds of emergencies, and know what to do in case of emergency. Follow the guidelines for safety measures.

In some settings, bed rails are less commonly used and may be considered a form of unnecessary restraint. Be sure you know the policy of your employer with regard to side rails.

AGE-SPECIFIC CONSIDERATIONS

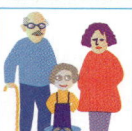

For all restraint procedures: Patients of all ages must be treated with respect. Children and the elderly might feel as though they are being punished for doing something wrong. If the patient is confused, being restrained often increases anxiety and attempts to "escape." Talk frequently and reassuringly to all patients in restraints. Explain that the devices are being used to prevent them from accidentally pulling on lines, tubes, drains or from falling. Check on the patient frequently and advocate for the removal of the restraint as soon as the patient's mental capacity has improved or when the medical device is no longer needed.

In addition to the safety measures followed for adult patients, the care of young children in the hospital or home setting requires additional safeguards to prevent accidents and ensure a safe environment. The guidelines that follow are based on the chronological-age characteristics and needs of young children. Refer to Chapter 15 for information on chronological-age development.

GUIDELINES

OBRA

SAFETY MEASURES

- Use handrails on stairways (Figure 6–1). In hallways and stairs, keep to the right and avoid collisions. Take special care at intersections (Figure 6–2).
- Use care when opening doors that open into busy areas (Figure 6–3).
- Be sure to lock the brakes on the wheels on beds, stretchers, examining tables, wheelchairs, bedside commodes, and shower chairs. Use care in transferring patients from them.

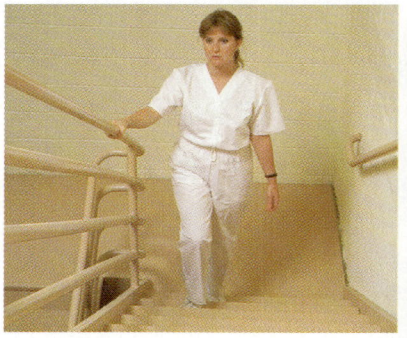

FIGURE 6–1
Be safety conscious at all times

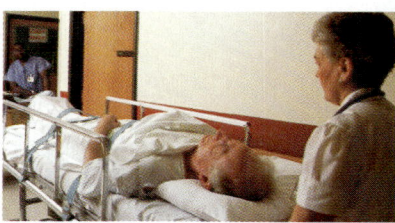

FIGURE 6–2
Use caution at intersections

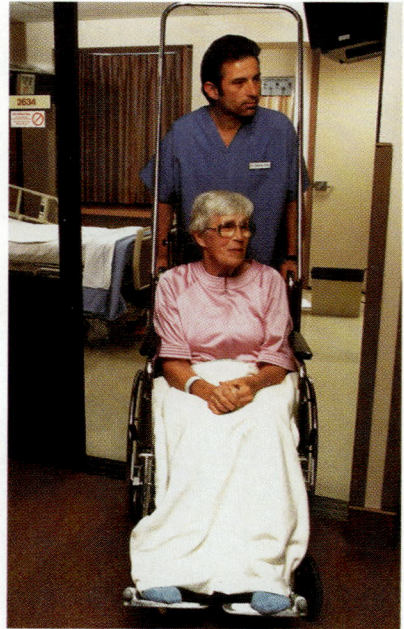

FIGURE 6–3
Be careful going through doorways

GUIDELINES (CONTINUED)

- Be very careful of the position of the patient's feet during wheelchair transport. Keep hands and feet in view while transporting by stretcher.

- When you see something on the floor that doesn't belong there, pick it up. Spilled liquids can be very dangerous (Figure 6–4). Remember that the housekeeping or environmental department may clean a room or area only once a day. Incidental spills in patient areas are the responsibility of all health care workers.

- Follow the instructions of your supervisor in giving care and be aware of special instructions for a patient, such as:
  - No weight bearing.
  - Keep head (or foot) of bed elevated at all times.
  - Do not position patient on right side.
  - May be out of bed with assistance only.

- Never use the contents of an unlabeled container; take it to your supervisor at once (Figure 6–5). Store cleaning fluids only in assigned areas which should be locked.

- Check meal trays for dentures and check soiled linen for overlooked items such as misplaced instruments, needles, or other articles, and dispose of them properly.

- Place used disposable razors in approved containers, never in a waste basket.

- Use disposable gloves when the possibility of coming in contact with blood or body fluids is present.

- If ordered, keep bed side rails up and in the locked position (Figure 6–6).

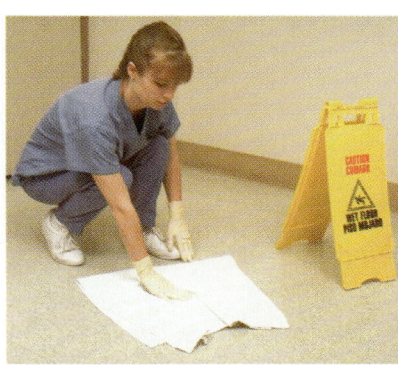

FIGURE 6–4
Clean up spills immediately

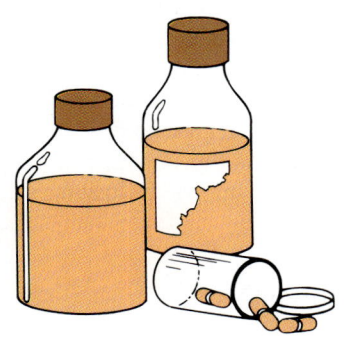

FIGURE 6–5
Never use the contents of an unlabeled container; take the container to your supervisor immediately

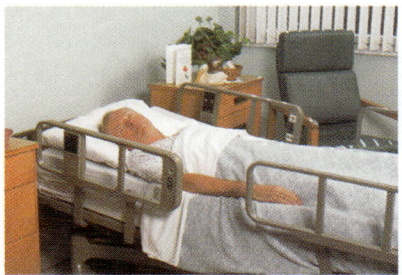

FIGURE 6–6
Keep the side rails up and in the locked position for patients who are confused, restless, or coming out of anesthesia

GUIDELINES

SAFETY MEASURES FOR YOUNG CHILDREN

Use care to remove items that could be harmful to young children. Children must be watched closely to prevent injuries.

- Never leave small children unattended unless they are in a protective crib.

- Frequently check a child in a protective device.

- Keep out of the child's reach all articles used in the child's care.

- Clean up spills and messes immediately.

- Keep crib railings up and locked. Bed rails for toddlers and older children should be used according to physician's order.

- Keep exit doors, stairway doors, and linen chutes closed when not in use and locked if possible.

- Keep drapery and window blind cords out of child's reach.

- Examine all toys for small or loose parts that can cause choking.

- Remove from the bed or floor large objects the child can stand on, increasing the risk of falls.

- Be sure windows are closed and locked.

- Lock the wheels on beds and cribs.

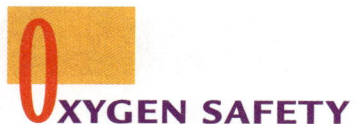

OXYGEN SAFETY

flowmeter A device used to control and regulate the flow of oxygen

oxygen A colorless, odorless, tasteless gaseous element that is essential for respiration; air is 21 percent oxygen

A special device called a regulator or **flowmeter** is needed when **oxygen** is used (Figure 6–7). It controls and regulates the rate or flow of oxygen that is being administered to the patient. If your patient is being given oxygen be sure that you know the policies of your employer regarding its use and care of the equipment. The amount of oxygen given to a patient is expressed in liters and is given according to the order of a physician or respiratory specialist. As the nursing assistant, you may be instructed to set up and monitor liter flow in some institutions. *The physician's or respiratory therapist's order must be followed exactly.*

Respiratory therapy departments take care of administration of oxygen and of the equipment used in most hospitals. In some settings, the nursing assistant may be expected to transport oxygen tanks and must know the facility's policies regarding safety in handling and storage of the tanks.

Room air is 21 percent oxygen. Oxygen, by itself, does not burn. However, it is one of the elements needed to cause fire, along with heat and fuel. Special precautions must be taken when more than the normal amount of oxygen is present, such as in a patient's room where oxygen is being administered. Extra oxygen supports combustion and can make things catch fire and burn more rapidly than in normal room air. Since patients may also be given oxygen therapy in the home, it is important that you advise the patient and/or the patient's caregiver of the caution they must take when oxygen is in use. Observing the following safety rules for oxygen use can help to prevent fires.

FIGURE 6–7

Although some oxygen delivery systems look different, they all have the same parts and function

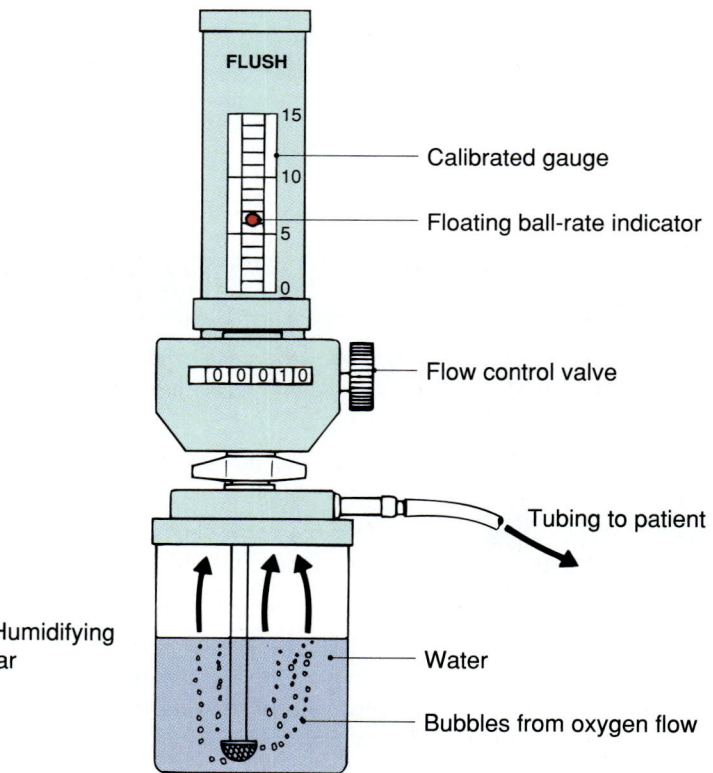

GUIDELINES

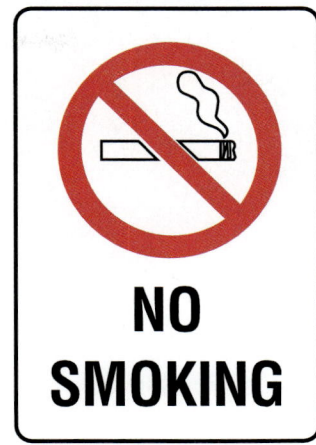

OBRA

OXYGEN SAFETY

- Place a NO SMOKING—OXYGEN IN USE sign on the door of the room and over the patient's bed (Figure 6–8).
- Keep the oxygen tubing free of kinks (see Figure 6–7).

FIGURE 6–8

No Smoking sign should be used when oxygen is in use

- Monitor any electrical appliance or device in the patient's room that could potentially create a spark, including items such as electric razors, hairdryers, and heating pads.
- Be observant for any lighters, matches, or smoking materials the patient or visitors may have and report them to your supervisor at once.
- If a humidifying jar is used, the correct level of distilled water must be maintained in the jar and the water in the jar should "bubble" as the oxygen passes through it (see Figure 6–7).

■ Oxygen Therapy

Use of an oxygen mask or **nasal cannula** is determined by the physician or respiratory therapist, depending on the needs of the patient. Both devices are made of plastic and come in direct contact with the patient's skin during use. Any area—behind the ears, on the cheeks, and at the nostrils—where there is contact combined with perspiration and moisture must be checked frequently for breakdown and protected if necessary.

The oxygen mask, used most often for a patient who cannot be relied on to consistently breathe through his nose, covers the mouth and nose (Figure 6–9). Keep the inside of the mask clean at all times.

nasal Pertaining to the nose and nasal cavity

cannula A flexible tube that can be inserted into a body cavity and used to draw fluids out or give oxygen or fluids

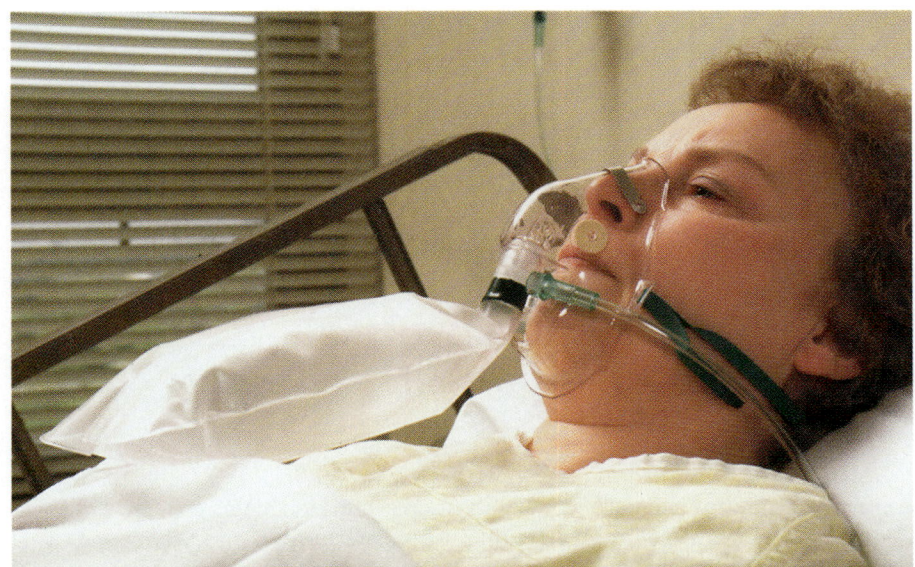

FIGURE 6–9

Oxygen is administered by an oxygen mask

FIGURE 6–10
The tubing of cannulas is flexible

FIGURE 6–10
The tubing of cannulas is flexible

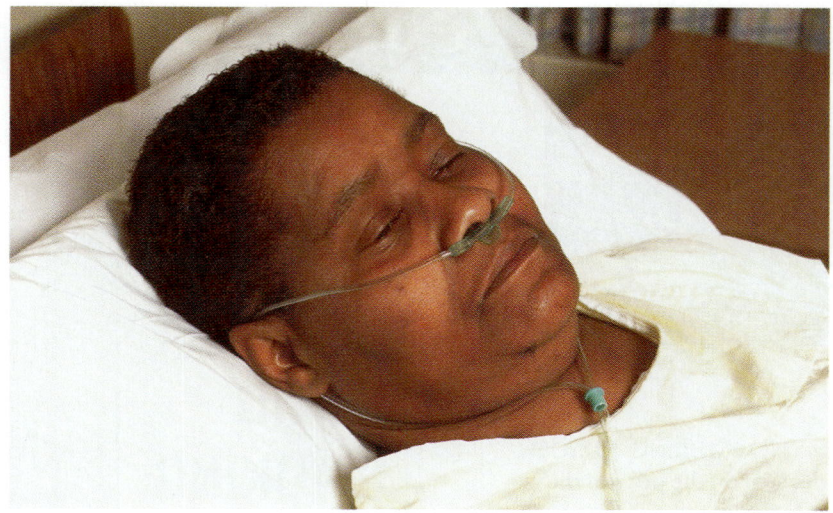

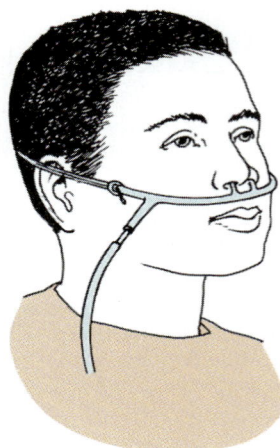

FIGURE 6–11
Nasal cannulas move easily, so check their placement frequently

The oxygen cannula is placed inside the patient's nostrils, extending upward about 1/2 inch. Two small holes in the tubing provide the patient with oxygen. The tubing of cannulas is flexible (Figure 6–10). In one type, the tubing wraps around the patient's ears and is secured under the chin; in another, the tubing extends from the nostrils across the cheeks and wraps around the patient's head. Nasal cannulas move easily, so their placement should be checked frequently (Figure 6–11).

FIRE SAFETY AND PREVENTION

Fire can start at any time in any setting. It may come as the aftermath of a disaster or a single incident. All health facilities have fire and disaster plans to provide safe transport and evacuation of patients and health care workers to a safe environment within the facility or outside the facility. If you work in a home setting you will develop an evacuation plan with your client and/or the client's caregiver. The best plan, however, is prevention, and preventing fires is everyone's job—be sure you know and observe all fire safety rules.

If a fire breaks out, you must:

1. Know what to do

2. Remain calm

3. Carry out what you have learned

KEY IDEA

Elevators are not to be used without approval of the Fire Department.

Be sure you are familiar with your institution's fire plan (Figure 6–12) and disaster plan. Know where your facility's fire extinguishers are located and what type of rating they have. Fire extinguishers may be rated A, B, or C according to the type of fire they may be used on.

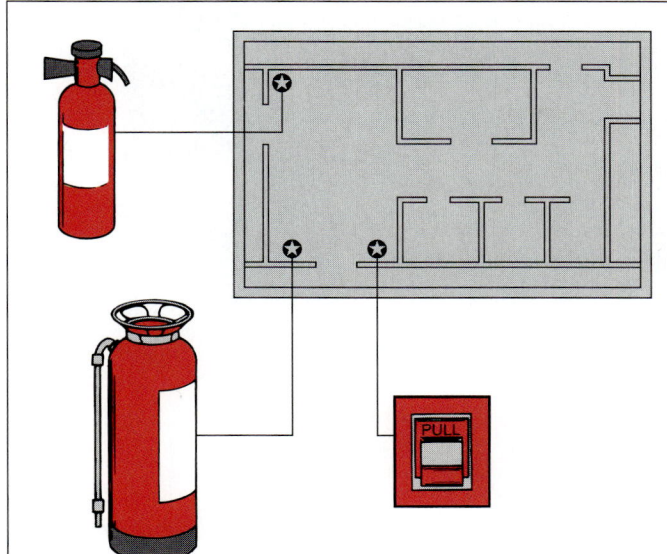

• Know the floor plan of your department and the hospital as a whole

• Pay particular attention to exit routes

• Know the exact location of fire alarms and fire extinguishing devices

• Know how to report a fire

• Know the emergency plan of your hospital and what you should do

• Know how to use fire extinguishers

FIGURE 6–12

Fire safety planning

A for paper, wood, and trash

B for burnable liquids such as oil or grease

C for electrical fires

ABC for use on any type of fire

If a situation does require the actual use and discharge of a fire extinguisher, remember the word **PASS.**

P   Pull the PIN on the upper handle (Figure 6-13a).

A   Aim low. Point the nozzle at the base of the fire (Figure 6-13b).

S   Squeeze the handles releasing the extinguisher's agent.

S   Sweep from side to side aiming at the base of the fire (Figure 6-13c).

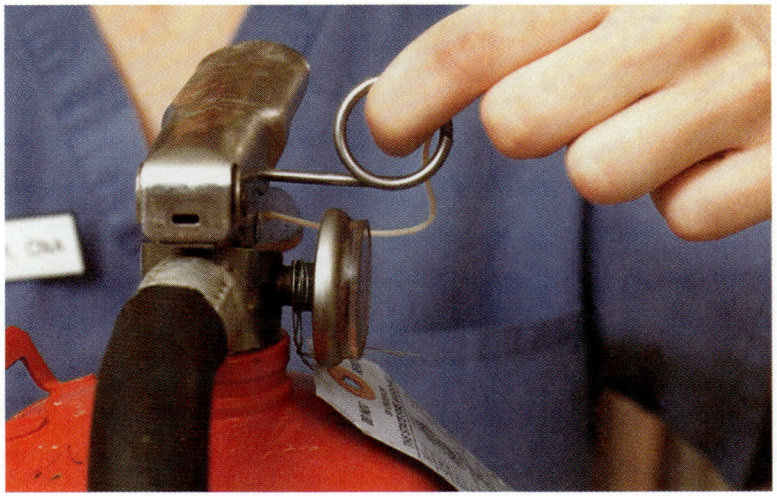

FIGURE 6–13a

Pull the pin on the upper handle of the fire extinguisher

FIGURE 6–13b

Aim low toward the base of the fire

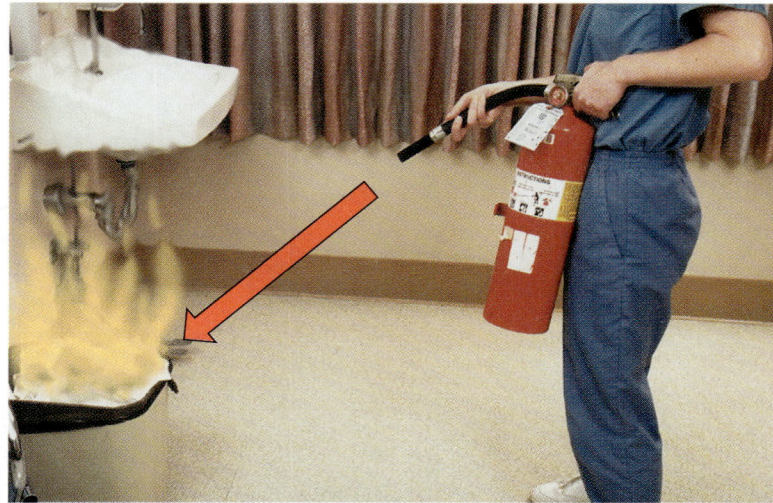

FIGURE 6–13c

Sweep the area from side to side

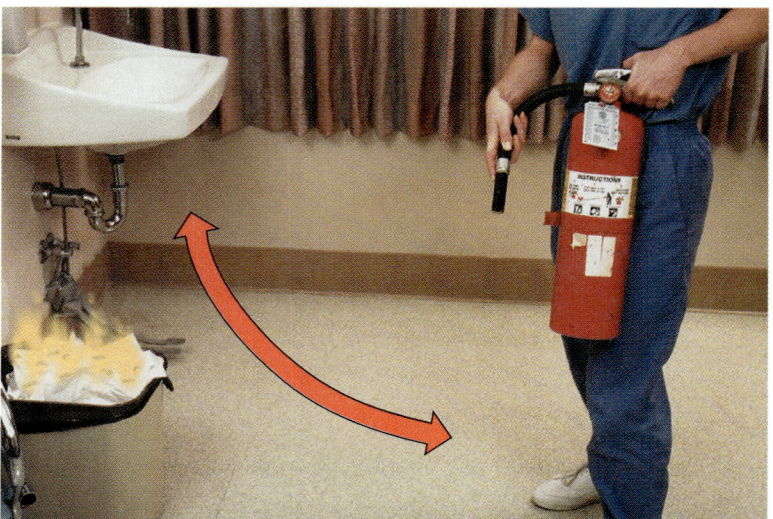

■ Major Causes of Fire

- ■ Smoking and matches
- ■ Misuse of electricity
- ■ Defects in heating systems
- ■ Spontaneous ignition
- ■ Improper rubbish disposal

Remember that it takes three things to start a fire (Figure 6–14):

- ■ HEAT, in the form of sparks or flame
- ■ FUEL, any burnable material
- ■ OXYGEN, present in the air we breathe

Smoking

Smoking is the number one cause of fires in health care institutions. Many facilities have adopted a nonsmoking policy (Figure 6–15). Some have identified areas

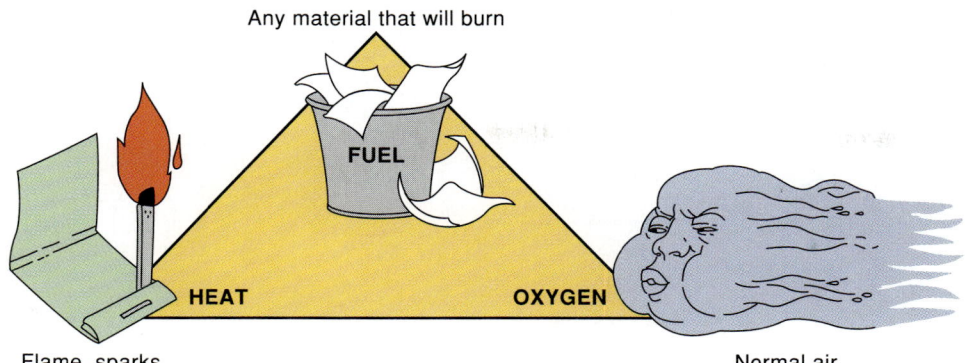

Any material that will burn

FUEL

HEAT

OXYGEN

Flame, sparks

Normal air

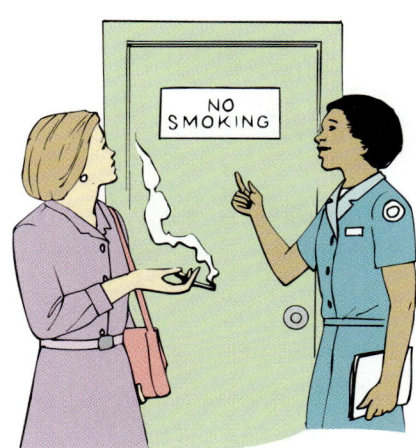

FIGURE 6–15
Smoking and nonsmoking areas are clearly identified

NO SMOKING

where smoking is permitted. It is important that employees, visitors, and patients smoke only in approved areas and observe the following rules:

- Provide ashtrays for those who smoke. Never use or allow anyone else to use disposable cups or dishes as ashtrays.

- Be sure that ashtrays are not emptied into trash containers until all smoking materials are safely extinguished.

- Provide supervision for any patient who wishes to smoke if the patient is confused or weak. Sedated patients should not smoke.

- Report any violation of your employer's smoking policy to your supervisor at once.

Misuses of Electricity

- Use care to be sure electrical equipment does not come in contact with water.

- Limit use of extension cords; if used, make sure they are in accordance with your faculty's policies.

- Many electrical devices are equipped with three-pronged grounding plugs. Do not use any such device if the rounded middle pin on the plug has been broken or cut off.

- Check cords and plugs for fraying or cracking prior to use. Report all electrical hazards at once.

FIGURE 6–16

Misuses of electricity

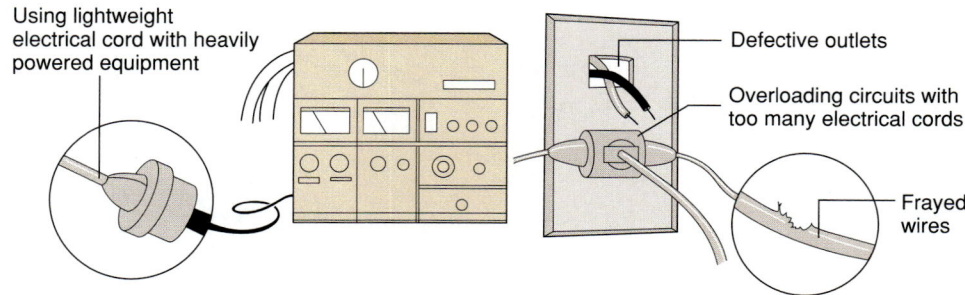

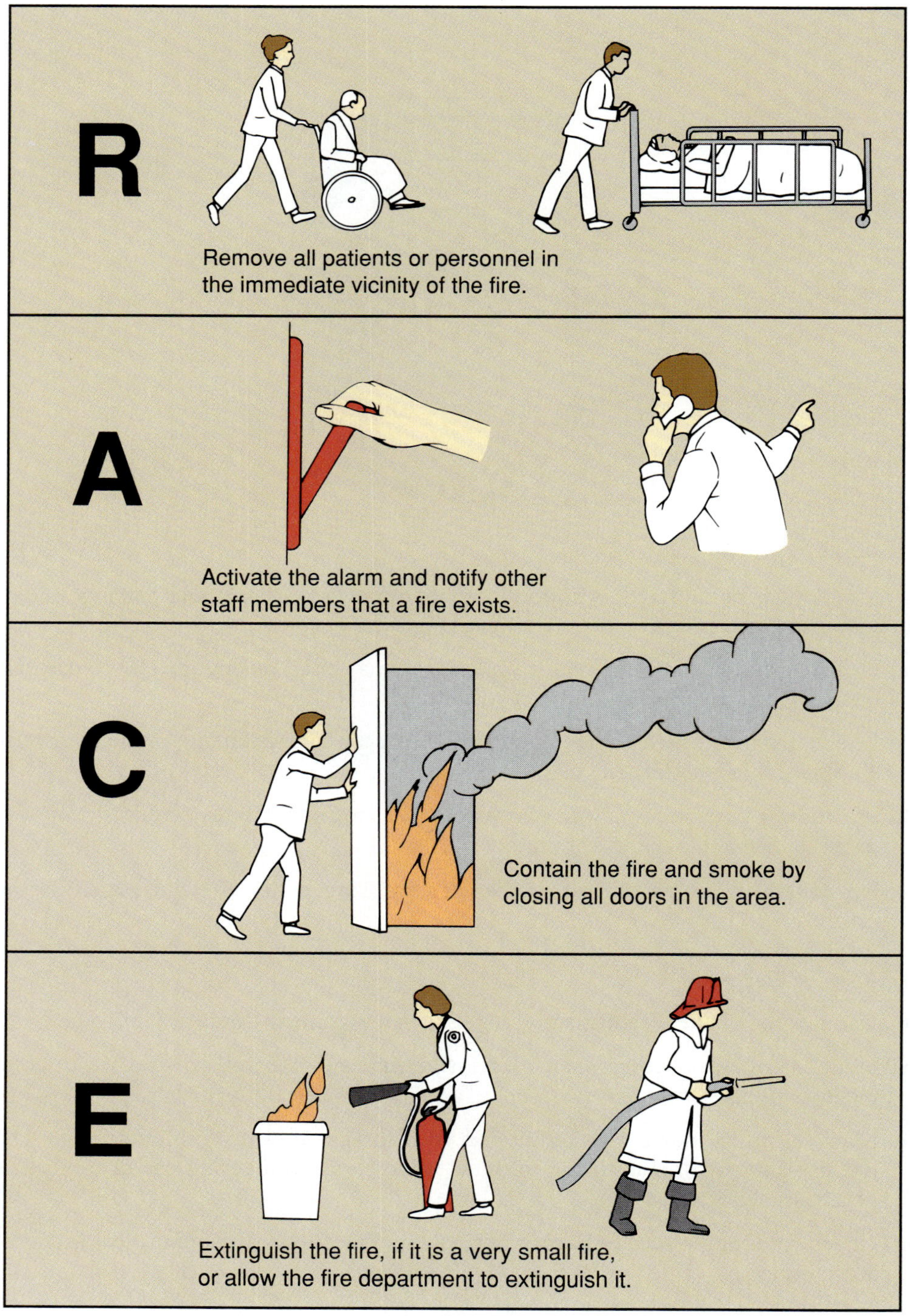

Using lightweight electrical cord with heavily powered equipment

Defective outlets

Overloading circuits with too many electrical cords

Frayed wires

FIGURE 6–17

In case of a fire, remember the word **R A C E**

R Remove all patients or personnel in the immediate vicinity of the fire.

A Activate the alarm and notify other staff members that a fire exists.

C Contain the fire and smoke by closing all doors in the area.

E Extinguish the fire, if it is a very small fire, or allow the fire department to extinguish it.

▌In Case of a Fire

If a fire occurs, remain calm and remember that many lives can depend on your actions. Keeping in mind the word **R A C E** can assist you in remembering what to do (see Figure 6–17 on page 122):

- **R**emove the patient from the immediate vicinity of the fire

- **A**ctivate the alarm and alert other staff members that a fire exists, following the policy of your employer

- **C**ontain or confine the fire by closing all the doors in the area

- **E**xtinguish the fire if it is safe to do so

Know and follow your employer's evacuation plan. Your institution will hold scheduled fire "drills" to assist staff in knowing exactly what to do in case of fire, including specific rescue techniques. Be sure that you dispose of all rubbish in the manner and place designated by your facility.

If you are working in a home setting, have fire drills regularly. In case of a fire, be sure to follow the evacuation plan that you developed earlier with the patient and/or the caregiver or other family members if they are present. Having an evacuation plan in advance of such a situation will help you to remain calm and facilitate the removal of your client to a safe environment.

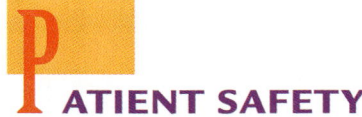

PATIENT SAFETY

Falls in health care facilities account for a large percentage of patient-related accidents. You can help prevent falls by:

- Anticipating the patients' needs

- Placing call light and personal items within easy reach

- Correctly positioning patients in beds and chairs

- Keeping personal items within easy reach of the patient

- Maintaining a clutter-free environment

- Answering call lights promptly

- Cleaning up spills at once

- Knowing and following your employer's fire emergency plan

▌Protective Devices

Physical **restraints** are used as **protective devices** to prevent a patient from harming himself or someone else or to protect him during a medical procedure. Restraints are applied only with the recommendation of a nurse or therapist and *only* with a physician's order (Figure 6–18). The nurse or therapist will decide what type of restraint is to be used and the length of time it is to be left in place. Hospitals follow the Joint Commission on Accreditation of Health Care Organizations (JCAHO) regulations regarding the use of restraints. Never tie or secure a restraint to any movable part of a bed or chair.

restraints Protective measures ordered by a physician to prevent patients from harming themselves or others

protective devices Measures taken to keep a patient safe or to prevent injury

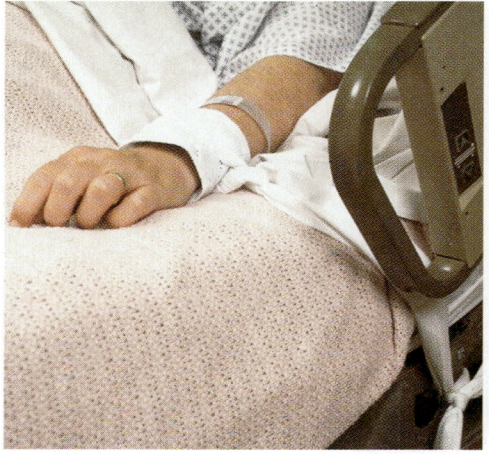

FIGURE 6–18a

Soft protective devices: A soft limb tie

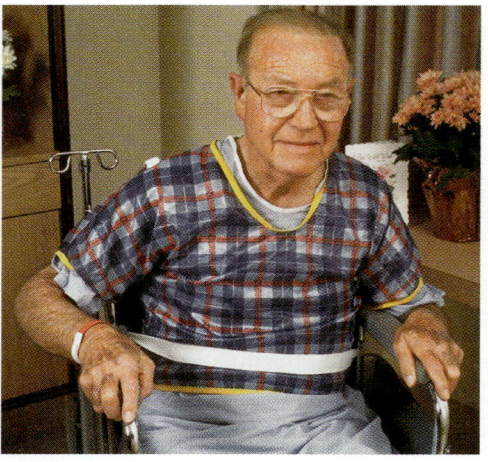

FIGURE 6–18b

Safety vest

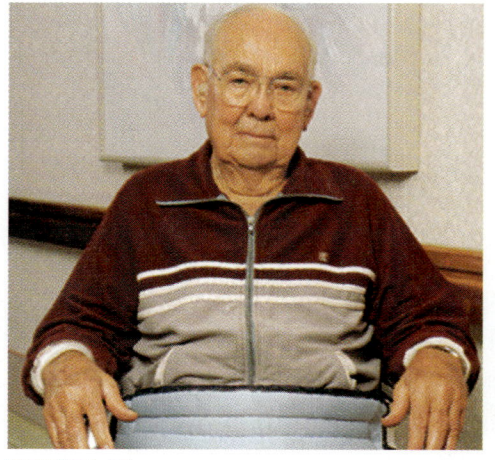

FIGURE 6–18c

Pelvic support

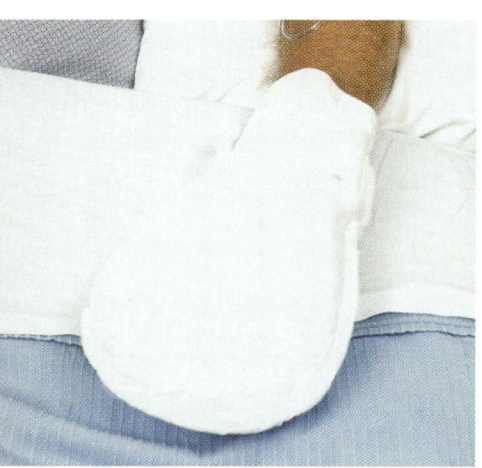

FIGURE 6–18d

Soft cloth mitten

KEY IDEA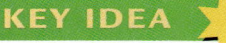

Proper documentation is needed to ensure protection of patient's rights and to record the observation and care of the patient. Care is documented on the restraint flowsheet or unit/division specific documentation form. Depending on the facility, the frequency of checks and documentation standards will vary. Psychiatric patients are checked every 15 minutes while others are 30 minutes or per facility policy.

PROCEDURE

OBRA

APPLYING A WAIST RESTRAINT

PREPARATION

1. Select the appropriate restraint.

2. Wash your hands.

3. Introduce yourself, identify the patient, and explain what you will do.

4. Provide privacy for the patient.

STEPS

5. Lock the wheels on the chair, commode, or toilet.

6. Wrap the waist restraint or belt around the patient's abdomen and cross the straps behind her back. Follow your institution's guidelines for wrist and ankle restraints.

PROCEDURE (CONTINUED)

7. Bring the crossed straps out to the sides and pull through the loops at the sides of the restraints.

8. Secure the restraint and make sure it is not too tight by inserting two fingers between the restraint and the patient's abdomen.

9. Wrap the straps of the restraint once around the metal part of the chair arm near the chair back before securing the straps, out of the resident's reach at the back of the chair.

10. Your instructor will demonstrate a **clove hitch** tie which maintains the restraint securely while making sure it can be readily untied in case of emergency.

FOLLOW-UP

11. Make the patient comfortable. Place the call light and personal items within easy reach of the patient before you leave the room, assuring him that you will be available if he needs assistance.

12. Document repeated checks per policy.

Check the patient *every 15–30 minutes* while restrained, carefully checking pressure points on the skin each time. **Release the restraint every two hours to offer food and liquids, toilet, exercise, and to reposition the patient.**

clove hitch A type of knot that can be easily released in case of emergency

PROCEDURE

OBRA

APPLYING A VEST RESTRAINT

PREPARATION

1. Select the appropriate restraint.
2. Wash your hands.
3. Introduce yourself, identify the patient, and explain what you will do.
4. Provide privacy for the patient.

STEPS

5. Lock the wheels on the bed or chair.

6. APPLY THE VEST RESTRAINT AS YOU WOULD ANY VEST, THAT OPENS DOWN THE FRONT. MAKE SURE ANY SEAMS OR ROUGH EDGES ARE NOT IN CONTACT WITH THE PATIENT'S SKIN.

7. Wrap the ties around the patient's waist crossing them behind his back pulling them through the loops at the sides.

8. Secure the restraint with a clove hitch or single loop knot out of the patient's reach.

9. Make the patient comfortable. Place the call light and personal items within easy reach of the patient.

10. Check to make sure the restraint is not too tight before you leave the room, assuring the patient that you will be available if he needs assistance.

FOLLOW-UP

11. Document repeated checks per policy.

Check the patient *every 15–30 minutes* while restrained, carefully checking pressure points on the skin each time. **Release the restraint every two hours to offer food and liquids, toilet, exercise, and to reposition the patient.**

PATIENT RESTRAINT POLICY EXAMPLE

Compliance with individual state Patient Bill of Rights, the Public Health Codes, and the Standards of the Joint Commission on Accreditation of Health Care Organizations (JCAHO) and/or OBRA regulations influence current practice in the restraint and seclusion use in clinically appropriate and adequately justified situations. Patient's rights, dignity, and well-being are supported and maintained. The least restrictive method of restraint and/or seclusion that meets the patient's assessed need is applied. Restraints are the *last resort* of a physical management after a thorough assessment of the patient. It should be noted that the restraints can have strong, negative psychological and physical effects such as:

- increased disorganized behavior
- confused behavior
- social isolation
- discomfort
- demoralization
- humiliation

- sense of being punished
- increased risk of injury or death
- increased risk of pressure ulcers
- increased risk of pneumonia
- increased cardiac load
- increased risk of disconditioning

Restraint or seclusion may be initiated by a nurse in an emergency situation in response to dangerous patient behavior. Use of restraint as a part of a facility, department or unit specific approved protocol does not require a doctor's written order. A physician's order is required for use of restraint or seclusion in behavior health areas when a patient's assessed need requires the use of restraint outside a defined, approved protocol.

Definitions

Physical Restraint

Involuntary use of any method physically restricting a person's freedom of movement, physical activity, or normal access to his or her body, as either part of an approved protocol or use of individual orders.

Seclusion

Involuntary confinement of a person alone in a room where the person is physically prevented from leaving.

Performance Improvement

Use of restraint is documented and monitored. Data is collected and reviewed for the purpose of identifying problems with use of restraint and seclusion, care of patients, and the role of participants in restraining/secluding patients. Charts are routinely reviewed when the institution or agency has accreditation site visits.

Alternatives to Restraints

Alternatives are based on respecting the patient's dignity, understanding behavior as a symptom of an unmet need, freedom of choice, and optimum patient outcomes. Alternatives include:

- If possible, collaboration with patient and family to try to make sense of agitation or worrisome behavior

- Careful assessment and collaboration with the treatment team to attempt to make sense of the patient's behavior

- Individualized care planning which attempts to correlate behavior with the unmet need

- On the restraint record, document alternatives used prior to the application of restraints

Types of Restraints Used

Leather (hard) limb, cloth limb, vest, waist, pelvic, mitts, and net bed.

Restraint and Seclusion Standards Do Not Apply in the Following Situations

Restraint devices may be used for a patient *without a doctor's order* under the below conditions. Individual needs are assessed by appropriate professional staff (where indicated). The assessment is documented and use of the device is added to the patient plan of care.

- A restraint device used during transportation via wheelchair or cart.

- Children (six months to four years) wear vests while in high chairs, wheelchairs, or any transportation vehicle.

- Medical immobilization is customarily employed during medical, diagnostic, or surgical procedures or tests, and is considered a regular part of such procedures or tests, including body restraint during surgery.

- Individual patient needs are assessed for adaptive support mechanisms intended to permit a patient to achieve maximum normative bodily functioning, such as orthopedic appliances, braces, wheelchairs, geri chairs, other appliances, or devices used to posturally support the patient.

- Individual patient needs are assessed for protective devices intended to compensate for a specific physical deficit or to prevent safety incidents not related to cognitive dysfunction, such as bedrails, tabletop chairs, protective helmets, or at times, halter-type devices (i.e., to prevent a cognitively intact patient from falling out of a chair due to a physical inability to support his or her own body).

- A time out of 15 minutes or less is used with children.

- Forensic and correction officer restriction used for security purposes.

- In home care, if applied by a family member.

- Patient seizure precautions will have four side rails, up with protective seizure pads in place.

- The institution's standard of care for patients who are sedated, recovering from anesthesia, or post operative/post-procedure may have soft restraints applied to maintain safety for the patient tubes, wounds, and dressings using the following criteria for application and removal of restraints. A nursing assessment determines the individual patient's needs. See table below regarding criteria for exemption.

Customary patient care and regular hourly observation is performed and documented on the Division Specific Flow Sheet or the Restraint Flow Sheet to ensure safe use (Figure 6–19).

Criteria for Exemption from Policy with Sedated/Anesthetized Patients

APPLICATION CRITERIA	RELEASE CRITERIA
Low level of consciousness. Can be aroused but unable to maintain wakefulness.	Maintain wakefulness.
Exhibits confusion and/or disorientation.	No confusion and/or disorientation.
Unable to remember instructions.	Remembers and repeats instructions.
Grabs at tubes, dressing, etc.	Doesn't grab at tubes, dressing, etc.
Likelihood of falling out of bed or rolling onto an operative site.	Little likelihood of falling out of bed or onto operative site.

proper application and care of patients in leather restraints).

PROCEDURE

OBRA

APPLICATION AND CARE OF THE PATIENT IN LEATHER RESTRAINTS

PREPARATION

1. Select the appropriate restraint.
2. Wash your hands.
3. Introduce yourself, identify the patient, and explain what you will do.
4. Provide privacy for the patient.

STEPS

5. Lock the wheels on the bed or stretcher.
6. Leather restraints are applied in the following manner:
   a. Apply cuffs with smooth edge towards the patient, snugly to the wrists and ankles.
   b. Draw straps through the slots of the cuff.
   c. Secure straps to the metal portion of bed frame (Do not secure straps to side rails) and lock. Allow 2–3 inches slack to allow for movement.
   d. The key will be placed near the patient and within easy reach of the staff (tape to outside of the foot of the bed).

CARE OF THE PATIENT

- The circulatory status of the restrained limb(s) will be evaluated at least every 15 minutes.
- In the event there is a change in the circulatory condition, the limb will be released immediately and measures taken to improve circulation.
- Wrist and ankle leather restraints are padded, whenever possible, using unsterile ABD pads and tape to prevent abrasions and tensions from occurring.
- Restraints are applied allowing for some patient movement when opposite or all extremities are restrained.
- Restraints are released individually to provide skin care and active or passive range of motion exercises at least every 2 hours and prn while the patient is awake.
- When locked restraints are used, the key must be accessible to remove restraints in an emergency situation (keep taped to the outside of the foot of the bed).
- Make sure the patient is as comfortable as possible.
- Assure patient that you or someone else will check on him every 15 minutes and will be available should he need assistance (fluids, blanket, urinal, etc.)

FOLLOW-UP

7. Document repeated checks per policy. Proper documentation is needed to ensure protection of patient's rights and to record the observation and care of the patient. Care is documented on the restraint flowsheet or unit/division specific documentation form.
8. Wash hands.

Patient and Family Discussion and Involvement

The staff discusses the use, or possible use, of restraint with the patient and family whenever possible. Provide patient and family with a copy of the Restraints Information sheet. (Table 6–1).

Patient Care Documentation

The nurse or authorized staff member is responsible for completing the Restraint Flow Sheet (Figure 6–19) or Appropriate Division Specific Flow Sheet.

Reporting Change of Condition

The physician is notified when there is a change in the patient's behavior or physical condition which affects the need for a more restrictive type of restraint device or other medical intervention.

Early Release

Monitoring and reassessment may permit the reduction (to a less restrictive device) or early termination of restraint and/or seclusion. Staff may release/reduce restraint or seclusion

TABLE 6–1

Restraints: Patient and Family Information Sheet

I. What is a restraint?

A restraint is any object or device which is used to limit movement or decreases the patient's ability to reach a part of their body. Restraints are used to protect the patient from injuring themselves or others.

II. Why are restraints used?

Restraints are applied only when needed to protect a patient or others from injury.

III. When are restraints used?

Restraints are used to protect a patient only after many other methods have been tried. These may include:

- taking the patient to the bathroom,
- changing the patient's position,
- having someone spend time with the patient (perhaps family),
- moving the patient closer to the nurses station,
- addressing the patient's pain level.

IV. What to expect while a patient is restrained:

- Restraints will be removed as soon as possible.
- Restraints can sometimes be removed while family is present. It is very important to discuss this with the nurse before the restraint can be removed.
- A caregiver will check the patient every hour. Every two hours, the patient in restraints will be offered something to drink, and asked if he/she needs to use the restroom.

V. How family can help?

- Send time with your family member.
- Talk calmly and provide reassurance.
- Help caregivers understand the patient's needs and gestures.
- Help communicate information to the patient.
- Bring personal reminders/items from home.

SOURCE: Courtesy St. Joseph Mercy Hospital, Ann Arbor, Michigan. Used with permission.

before the time limit based on reassessment. The original order can be reapplied if alternatives remain ineffective, when restraint or seclusion is terminated early and the same behavior(s) become evident.

Physician Responsibilities: Patient Assessment and Orders

Patient Assessment

The physician (or designee) assesses the individual patient's need for restraint and/or seclusion. Reassessment associated with time limited orders is used primarily to determine the continuing need for the restraint and/or seclusion. The physician provides clinical oversight or qualified, trained staff to apply or remove restraint and/or seclusion in emergent situations or under written protocols.

Orders

- Orders are to be obtained from the patient's physician within two hours of the application of restraint. If an order is not received in the two hour time frame, the restraints must be discontinued.

- **No PRN orders.**

- Order must include type of restraint, reason for restraint, and maximum duration of use not to exceed 24 hours.

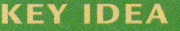 **KEY IDEA**   Any protective device that the patient/resident cannot release on his own is considered a restraint.

Restraint Alternatives

restraint alternative
Protective measures such as a saddle or wedge cushion, self-releasing belt or lap tray that are used to help prevent falls but do not physically restrain an individual

A **restraint alternative** is a protective device or technique that prevents the patient or resident from harming himself or others but does not physically restrain the individual. A thorough assessment of each patient by the members of the care team will determine which restraint alternative is appropriate. Documentation of the type of restraint used, why it was used, when it was applied, and when it was removed is important.

Some of the choices are:

- A wedge or saddle cushion, which helps to prevent sliding forward and possibly falling while seated in chair (Figure 6–20a)

- A self-releasing belt, sometimes preferred by patients who are aware and able to make appropriate choices for themselves (Figure 6–20b)

- A lap tray, which can help prevent falling out of a chair

- A lap pillow, which helps to prevent the patient from falling forward and ease the pressure the patient might otherwise experience (Figure 6–21)

- Seat belt style lap belt with latch (Figure 6–22)

- Using Posey grip or a similar product to keep patient from slipping in chair (Figure 6–23a and Figure 6–23b)

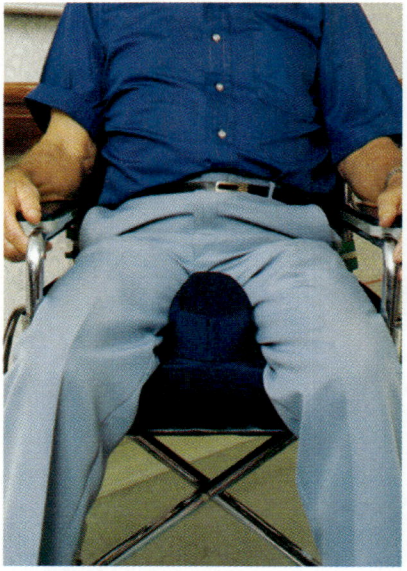

FIGURE 6–20a
Restraint alternatives: A saddle cushion, which prevents sliding forward

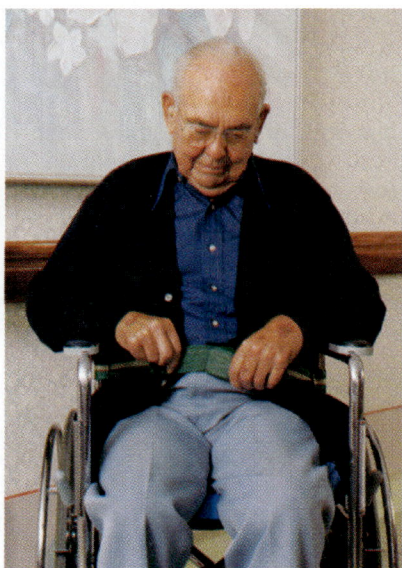

FIGURE 6–20b
Self-releasing safety belt

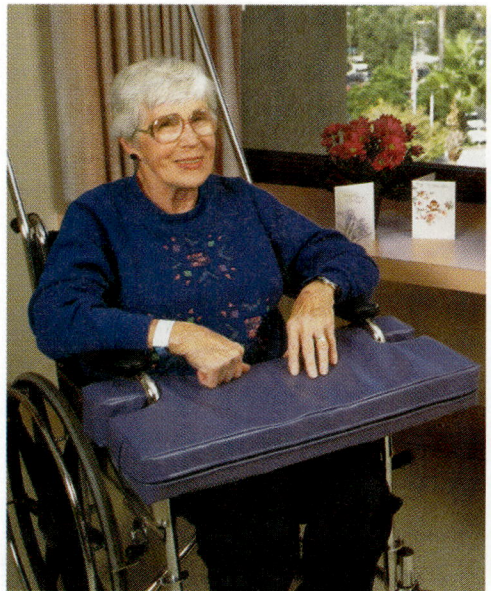

FIGURE 6–21
Lap pillow

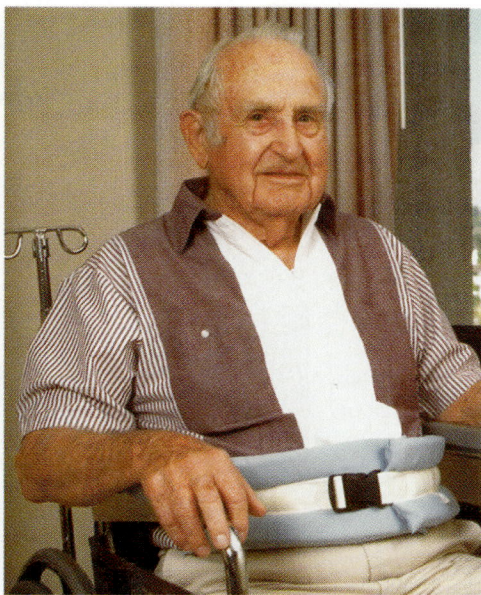

FIGURE 6–22
Seat-belt–style lap belt with latch

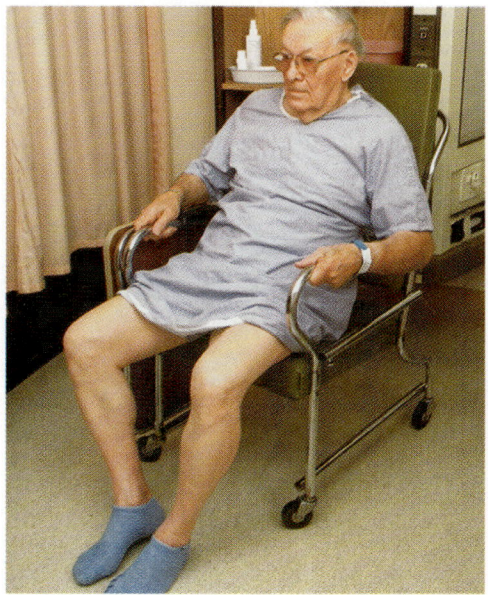

FIGURE 6–23a
Patient slipping in chair

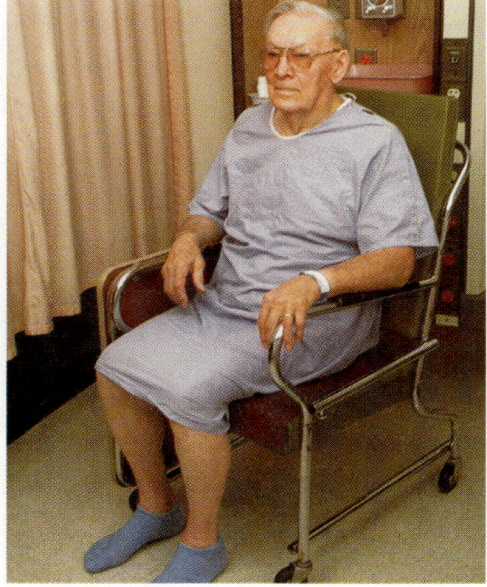

FIGURE 6–23b
Using Posey grip to keep patient from slipping in chair

- A chair alarm safety device alerts staff to a problem (Figure 6–24).

- Patient positioning devices for wheelchair provides support (Figure 6–25a and Figure 6–25b).

- A diversion, something of interest to the patient, which can help to take his mind off wandering behavior.

- Any device used as a restraint (including side rails) is to be used only with the order of a physician and only to ensure the physical safety of the patient. (Figure 6–26a and Figure 6–26b).

FIGURE 6–24

Chair alarm safety device

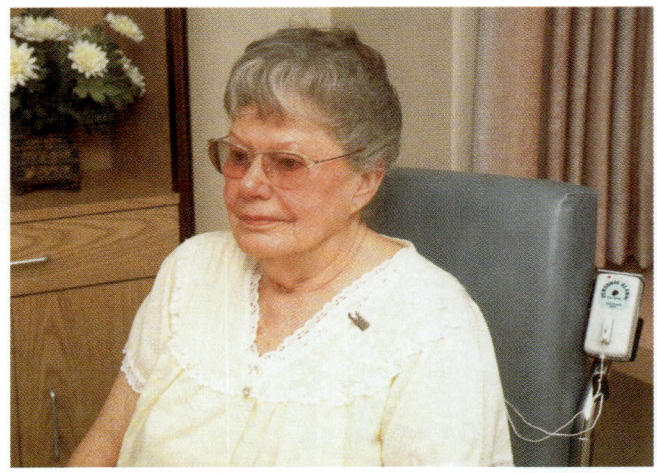

FIGURE 6–25

Patient positioning devices for wheelchair

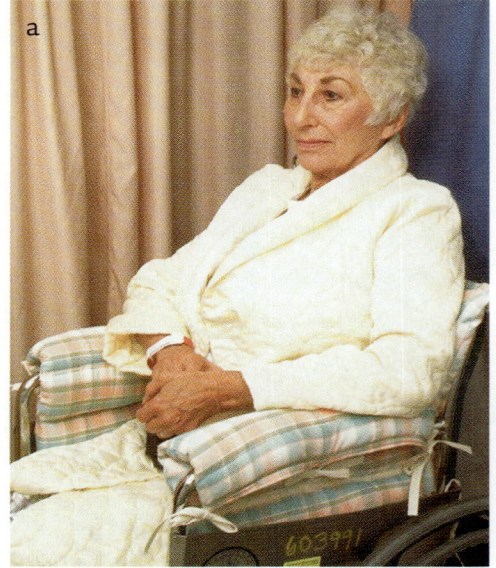

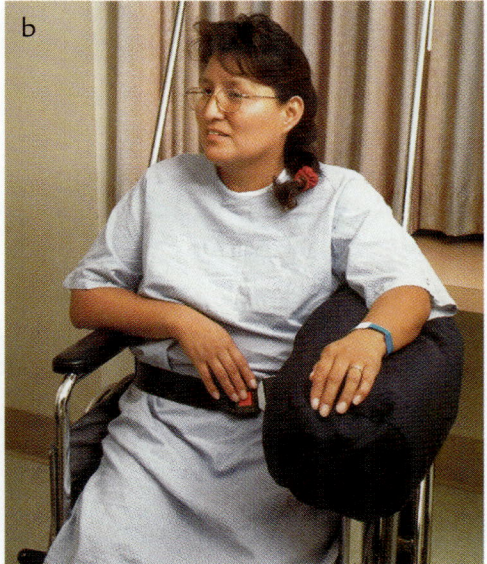

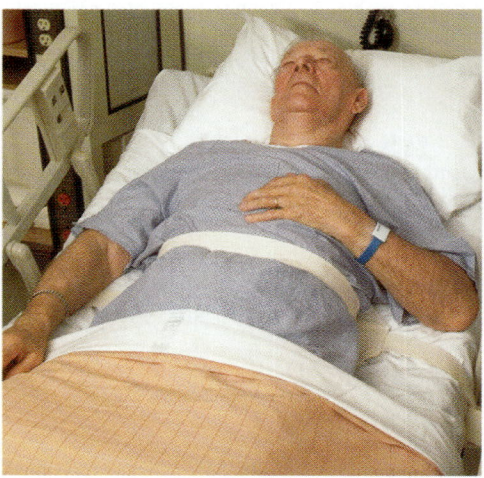

FIGURE 6–26a

Roll belt in bed restraint front

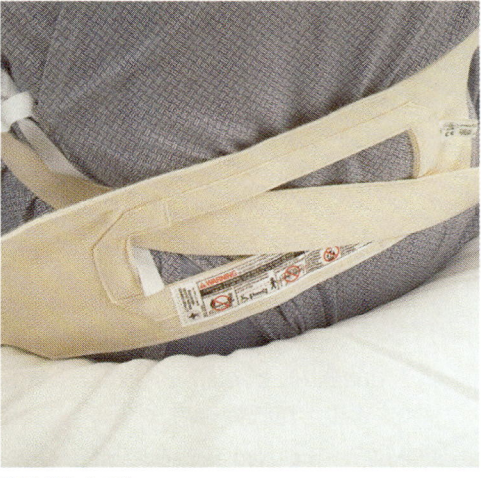

FIGURE 6–26b

Roll belt in bed restraint back

- Restraining devices are to be applied correctly and used only according to the policy of the institution.

- Explain the purpose of the restraining device to the patient and family members prior to its use even if the patient is not fully able to understand.

- Check the restrained patient *every 30 minutes* to be certain the restraint is not too tight and that the resident's needs are being met.

- Release the restraint every two hours, reposition or exercise the patient, offer food and fluids, toilet the patient, and check the patient's skin for redness or irritation. Document all findings including the responses of the patient to the use of the restraint.

- Know the federal (OBRA) guidelines for the use of restraints.

- Use a clove hitch so that the restraint can be easily released in an emergency.

Restraining the Pediatric Patient

To restrain means to keep someone from doing something or to prevent an action from happening. As with adults, all restraints used for pediatric patients are applied only on the instruction of the nurse or physician. The kind of restraint used for a child depends on why she is being restrained, age, and level of understanding.

- Elbow restraints (Figure 6–27) may be applied to a child who has eczema to keep him from scratching himself, to a child who has had surgery on his mouth or eyes, or has an IV, to keep his hands away from those areas. Elbow restraints prevent a child from bending his elbows and, therefore, from reaching or scratching his face.

- Mitten restraints are also used to prevent scratching.

Remember, restraints can cause injury and must be used with extreme care.

Applying Elbow Restraints

- Elbow restraints are made of canvas and tongue depressors or a padded arm-board. They are tied firmly around the child's arm so that they will not slide below the elbow. The child can move the arm but cannot bend the elbow to reach his or her face.

- Such restraints should be removed frequently to prevent muscle cramp and to access the skin. One restraint should be removed at a time, and someone should be present to control the child's arm movements for the time it is off.

- A child may often be frustrated emotionally because of the restraints. His satisfaction must be provided in new ways. Ask your immediate supervisor for guidance in caring for a restrained child.

FIGURE 6–27
Elbow restraint

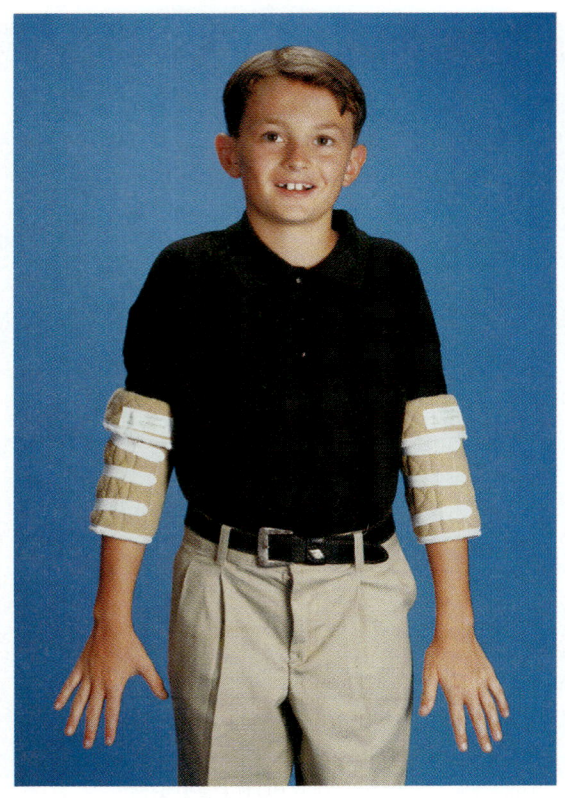

OBRA Regulations

OBRA, the Omnibus Budget Reconciliation Act of 1987, includes a regulation regarding physical restraints which states, in part, that "any device that limits movement or restricts normal access to one's body" may be used only in circumstances in which a patient may harm himself or someone else or to protect a patient during a medical procedure and only with a physician's order. This regulation applies to nursing facilities that provide long-term care to elderly and disabled patients. Even when a physician writes an order for a physical restraint, the care team is obligated by law to seek the least restrictive method of maintaining the resident's safety, carefully documenting each step of the process.

The nursing assistant is the care team member who has the greatest amount of contact with the resident and will be more aware of the resident's needs and preferences. A resident who is confused and unable to understand or express his own needs may become restless, agitated, or even aggressive when he is hungry, frightened, or simply needs to go to the bathroom. Long-term care residents cannot be restrained for the staff's convenience—to prevent wandering or getting out of the bed or chair—and all possible causes for unusual or agitated behavior must be investigated prior to considering a restraint for that person. It is very frustrating to be unable to move as you wish; consequently, there is great danger that a restrained person may become injured attempting to do nothing more than gain someone's attention.

Ambulation Safety with a Cane, Walker, or Crutches

Various pieces of equipment may be ordered by the physician to assist the patient to ambulate safely. These pieces of equipment include *canes, crutches,* and *walkers.*

They support the patient while walking. Each of these pieces of equipment must be adjusted for each individual patient. The hand piece must be level with the patient's hip to accommodate a slight bend of the elbow while the patient is standing and holding the cane, crutches, or walker. The patient must never use these pieces of equipment to help get to a standing position. They are only something to assist the patient to walk.

- *Cane:* Usually used on the patient's stronger side to balance his weight between the cane and the weaker side (Figure 6–28).

- *Walker:* Ordered when the patient requires some support when walking due to imbalance or weakness. The walker is safe to push down upon only when all four legs of the walker are on the ground in a level position. When the walker is being moved the patient's feet should be stationary. When the walker is stationary, the patient can move his feet. The walker must be picked up and moved and never slid along the ground unless the walker has wheels. Make sure the walker is the correct size for the patient (Figure 6–29).

- *Crutches:* Ordered to decrease weight borne by one or both feet and legs or to provide stability (Figure 6–30). Instructions will permit full weight bearing, partial weight bearing, weight bearing to tolerance, or non-weight bearing. Make sure that all pads and grips are securely in place. Check the screws to make sure all hardware is tight. Inspect the rubber tips for wear and make sure they are dry, and free of dirt and/or stones. If the patient is weak, unsteady, or unable to maintain balance, help him to a position of safety and report this to your immediate supervisor.

Ambulation is the action of walking. Gait is the rhythm and movement of the feet and the speed of walking. **Gait training** is done by the physical therapist as the first step toward helping the patient to **ambulate** independently. A gait belt is a device used to hold the patient securely while ambulating him.

ambulation To walk or move about in an upright position

gait training Rehabilitative exercise to help the patient improve his walking ability

ambulate To walk or move about

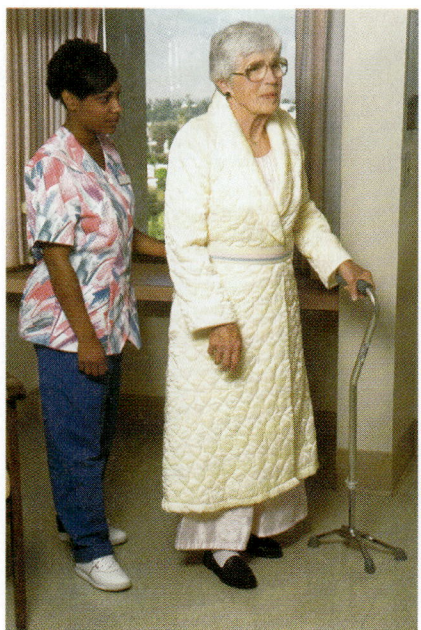

FIGURE 6–28

CNA assists patient using a cane

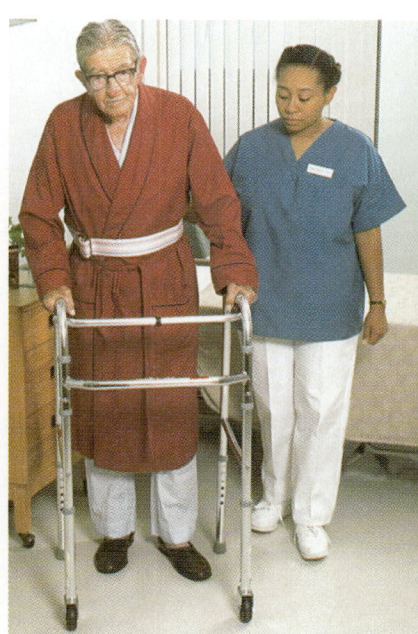

FIGURE 6–29

Walker

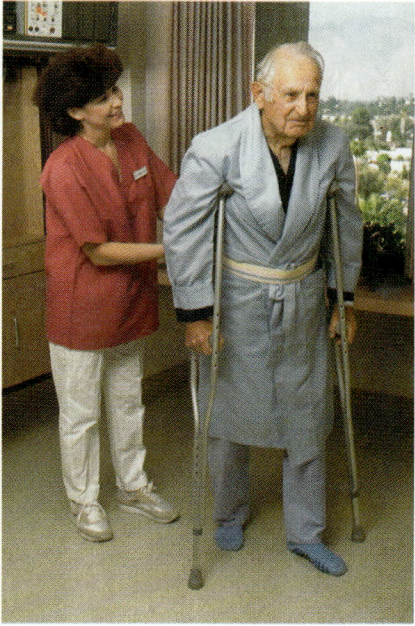

FIGURE 6–30

Crutches

GUIDELINES

OBRA

PATIENT AMBULATION SAFETY

- Apply good body mechanics at all times (see Chapter 7).
- Be sure of the patient's ability to ambulate before you attempt to assist him.
- If you need help or if you are in doubt, ask your immediate supervisor for assistance.

- Communicate with the patient by explaining the procedure and telling the patient what you expect of him.

Summary

Safety is a most important consideration. This chapter has reviewed safety measurement precautions to take when caring for patients, listed special considerations and guidelines to follow when oxygen is used, and covered electrical and fire safety. The care and safety of patients requiring protective devices or restraints was also outlined. You are the team member who probably interacts most with the patient, or client. Therefore, your observations and actions are essential to the safety of the patient.

Notes

_____

_____

_____

_____

_____

_____

_____

_____

_____

_____

Restraint Alternatives

Mrs. Cox is an elderly woman who easily becomes confused, gets up out of her bed and walks around every few minutes. You are concerned that she is frail and weak and afraid she may accidentally fall and hurt herself. As a nursing assistant you are aware that patient safety is important.

What Is Your Response/Action?

1. What decision do you have to make?

2. What possible actions might you consider?

3. Which action will you take?

4. What are your responsibilities if Mrs. Cox falls?

5. What did you learn that you can apply to other situations?

CHAPTER REVIEW

FILL IN THE BLANK

Read each sentence and fill in the blank line with a word that completes the sentence.

1. Be sure to lock the _____ on wheelchairs, stretchers, and commode chairs.

2. The special device used with oxygen that controls and regulates the amount of oxygen is called the _____.

3. An _____ extinguisher can be used on all types of fires.

4. _____ is the number one cause of fires in health care institutions.

5. Never tie or secure a restraint device to a _____ part of a bed or chair.

MULTIPLE CHOICE

Choose the best answer for each question or statement.

1. All of the following are general safety measures except

   a. Use care when opening doors into busy areas.

   b. Be careful going through intersections.

   c. Be careful when cutting up food for patients.

   d. Be careful taking patients through doorways.

2. All of the following is true about oxygen except

   a. it is a colorless, odorless, tasteless gas.

   b. the more oxygen a patient has the better.

   c. oxygen is one of the key elements needed for fire.

   d. room air is 21% oxygen.

3. If you need to use a fire extinguisher, remember Pass: pull the Pin, Aim low, Squeeze the handle, and Sweep from side to side aiming at the fire.

   a. True

   b. False

4. All of the following are misuses of electricity except one.

   a. Electrical equipment in contact with water.

   b. Use of numerous extension cords.

   c. Use of frayed cords and plugs.

   d. Use of three pronged plugs.

5. When a patient is in a restraint device, he or she needs to be released at least every four hours to offer food and liquids, toilet, exercise and to reposition the patient.

   a. True

   b. False

6. When ambulating a patient,

   a. apply good body mechanics.

   b. be sure of the patient's ability to ambulate before you attempt to move him.

   c. always communicate to the patient what you expect of him.

   d. All of the above.

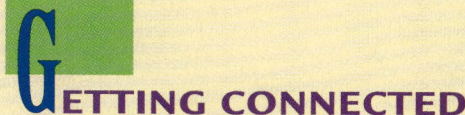ETTING CONNECTED

MULTIMEDIA EXTENSION ACTIVITIES

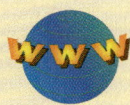

www.prenhall.com/wolgin

Use the above address to access the free, interactive Companion Website created for this textbook. Get hints, instant feedback, and textbook references to chapter-related multiple choice questions. Read and react to the "Nursing Assistants in Action." Link to other interesting sites.

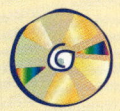

Audio Glossary

Use the CD-ROM disk enclosed with your textbook to hear the pronunciation of the key terms in the chapter.

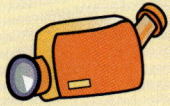

Video

Watch the "Complying with Legal Standards" and the "Being Reliable" sections of the "Focus on Professionalism" video and the "Patient's Right to Refuse Care" section of the "Patient's Rights" video from the Care Provider Skills series.

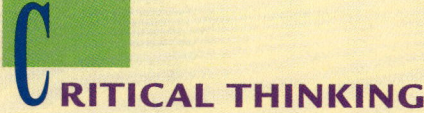RITICAL THINKING

USING KEY QUESTIONS

Read each question and think of what you might do in each situation.

1. You are taking care of a small child today. What kind of safety precautions should you take?

2. Suddenly you smell smoke. What should you do?

3. The nurse/physician determines a waist restraint device is needed for your patient. How will you apply it?

4. Your patient is on oxygen. What are some safety precautions you will take?

5. What are some alternatives to restraint?

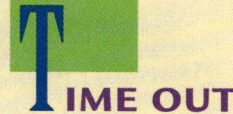IME OUT

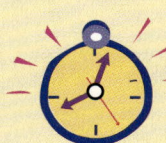

TIPS FOR TIME MANAGEMENT

ORGANIZATION TIP Allow extra time for tasks that slow you down. For example, if you like to take your time, organize your day so that you have the time you need to read assignments and write on charts.

Body Mechanics: Positioning, Moving, and Transporting Patients

7

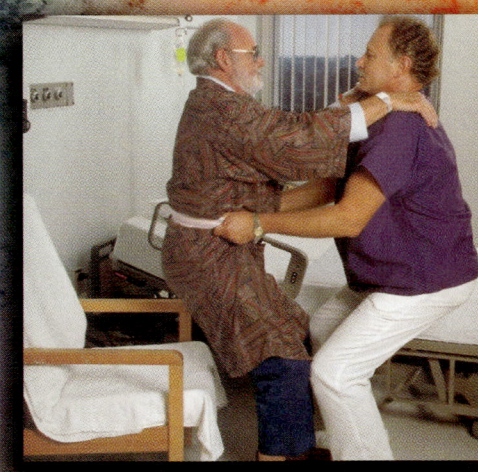

INTRODUCTION

The use of proper/protective body mechanics during the positioning, moving, and transporting of patients will help you avoid fatigue and injury as a health care worker. Learning how to apply the techniques correctly will improve safety for you and for the patient.

When you have completed this chapter, you will be able to:

- Describe techniques for proper/protective body mechanics.
- Lift, hold, or move an object or patient using techniques for proper/protective body mechanics.
- List the different positions for patients, assist patients into those positions, and drape for privacy.
- List the guidelines for moving and lifting patients.
- Move a helpless patient up in bed.
- Move a patient up in bed with the patient's help.
- Move the mattress to the head of the bed with the patient's help.
- Move a helpless patient to one side of the bed on the patient's back.
- Log roll the patient.
- Turn a patient on either side.
- Transport and reposition a patient in a wheelchair, move the patient from the bed to a wheelchair and back into bed.
- Move the helpless patient using a portable mechanical patient lift.
- Transport a patient by stretcher, and move the patient from the bed to a stretcher and back into bed.
- Assist a patient to ambulate.
- Assist a falling patient.

KEY TERMS

bedridden

body alignment

dorsal lithotomy position

dorsal recumbent position

drape

draping

Fowler's position

incontinent

knee-chest position

left lateral position

nonambulatory

prone position

proper/protective body mechanics

semi-Fowler's position

side-lying positions

Sims's position

stretcher

supine position

transporting

Trendelenburg's position

PROPER/PROTECTIVE BODY MECHANICS

The term **proper** or **protective body mechanics** refers to the techniques of standing and moving one's body, using the strongest muscles to avoid fatigue or injury. You should understand the techniques of proper/protective body mechanics and learn to apply them to work tasks. As a result, you will feel less tired at the end of the day.

GUIDELINES

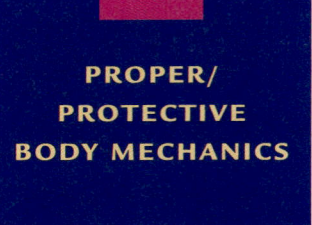

OBRA

PROPER/ PROTECTIVE BODY MECHANICS

- When an action requires physical effort, try to use the largest muscles or groups of muscles possible. For example, use both hands rather than one hand to pick up an object.

- Use good posture. Keep your body aligned in front of your work.

Maintain the natural curves in your back, keeping ears, shoulders, and hips in vertical alignment. Bend your knees. Keep your weight balanced evenly on both feet.

- Keep your feet slightly more than hip width apart to give you a broad base of support and good balance.

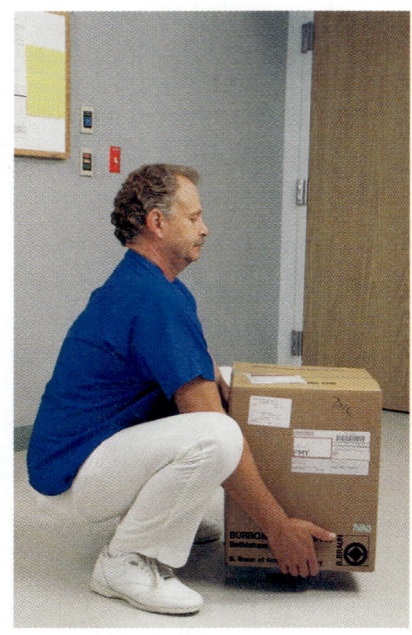

FIGURE 7–1a
Squat close to the load

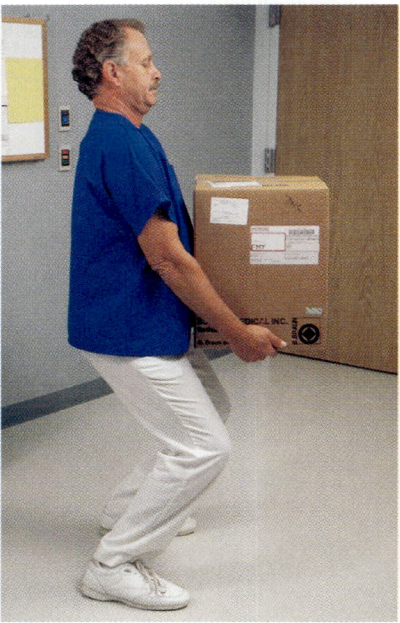

FIGURE 7–1b
With arms fixed close to your sides, lift by pushing up with your strong leg muscles

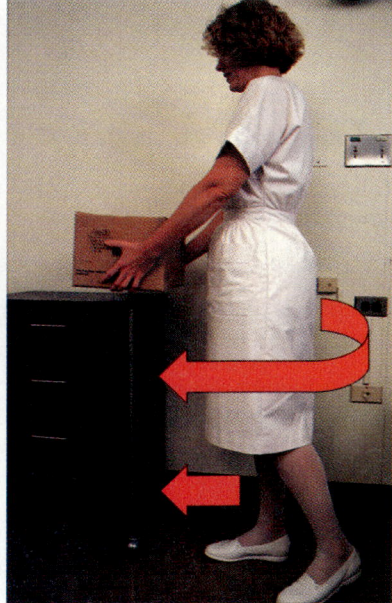

FIGURE 7–2
Pivot feet

- Position your body close to the load being lifted.

- When you have to move a heavy object, push it or roll it rather than lift and carry.

- Use your arms to support the object. Keep your arms in a fixed position with elbows close to your sides. The muscles of your legs, not the muscles of your back and arms, should do the job of lifting.

- When you are doing work such as giving a back rub, making a corner on a bed, or moving the patient, align your body in the direction of your work. Avoid twisting at the waist. Always turn or pivot with your feet, or shift your weight from one foot to the other.

- When you lift an object (Figure 7–1a):
  - Squat close to the load.
  - Maintain the natural curves in your back.
  - Grip the object firmly.
  - Hold the load close to your body.
  - Keep your arms fixed and close to your sides.
  - Lift by pushing up with your strong leg muscles (avoid lifting load with arms to chest and then standing) (Figure 7–1b).

- Ask for assistance if you think you may not be able to lift the load yourself.

- Lift smoothly; don't jerk. Always count "one, two, three" when working with another person, or say "ready" and "go" so that you work in unison. Do this with both the patient and with other health care workers.

- When you want to change the direction of movement:
  - Pivot (turn) feet (Figure 7–2).
  - Use short steps.
  - Turn your whole body using your feet to avoid twisting your back and neck.

POSITIONING AND DRAPING THE PATIENT

Draping covers a patient's entire body or parts of the body with a sheet, blanket, bath blanket, or other material. Draping is usually done during the physical examination of the patient and during surgery. A **drape** is the actual cover used to provide privacy during an examination or an operation,

Horizontal Recumbent Position (Supine Position)

In the **supine position,** the draping covers the entire body. The patient lies on his or her back with the legs together and extended or with the knees bent slightly to relax the muscles of the abdomen. A pillow is placed under the patient's head; the drape is spread loosely over the patient's body (Figure 7–3).

Dorsal Recumbent Position

In the **dorsal recumbent position,** the patient's legs are separated, the knees are bent, and the soles of the feet are flat on the bed. Drape the female patient by putting a sheet,

proper/protective body mechanics Special ways of standing and moving one's body to make the best use of strength and to avoid fatigue

draping Covering a patient or parts of a patient's body with a sheet, blanket, bath blanket, or other material during a physical examination or prior to surgery

drape A covering used to provide privacy during an examination or operation

supine position Lying on one's back

dorsal recumbent position Lying down or reclining; refers to the back or the back part of an organ

FIGURE 7–3

Horizontal recumbent position (supine position)

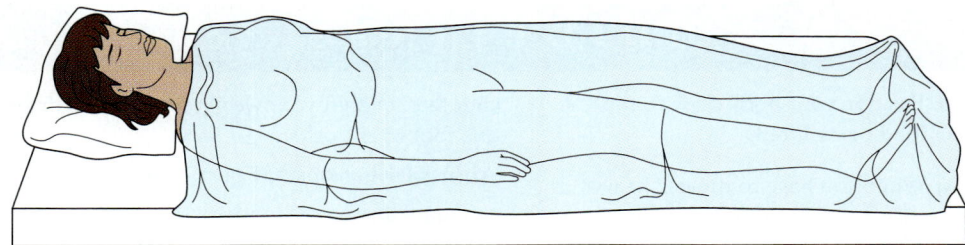

FIGURE 7–3

Horizontal recumbent position (supine position)

folded once, across her chest. Put a second sheet crosswise over her legs loosely so that the perineal region (the area of the body between the thighs) can be exposed for examination (Figure 7–4).

FIGURE 7–4

Dorsal recumbent position

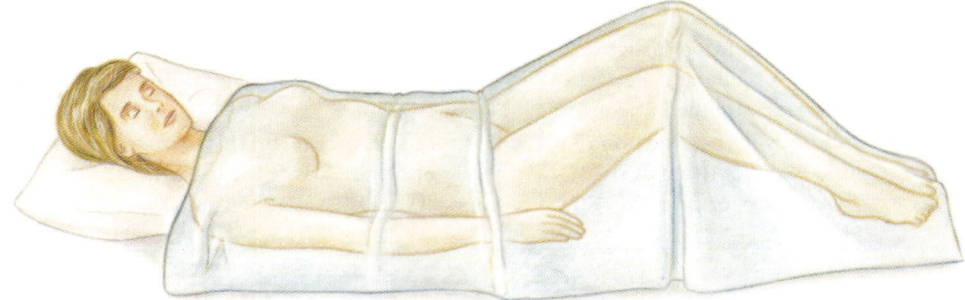

Fowler's position The position in which the head of the patient's bed is at a 45°–90° angle

semi-Fowler's position The position in which the head of patient's bed is at a 30°–45° angle

Fowler's Position

Fowler's position is also called the *high Fowler's position.* The patient is partly sitting, with the back rest of the bed at a 45°–90° angle. The knees are slightly bent. For the **semi-Fowler's position**, the incline is less than the Fowler's position. The head of the bed is raised 30°–45° and the patient's knees are slightly bent (Figure 7–5).

FIGURE 7–5

Fowler's position

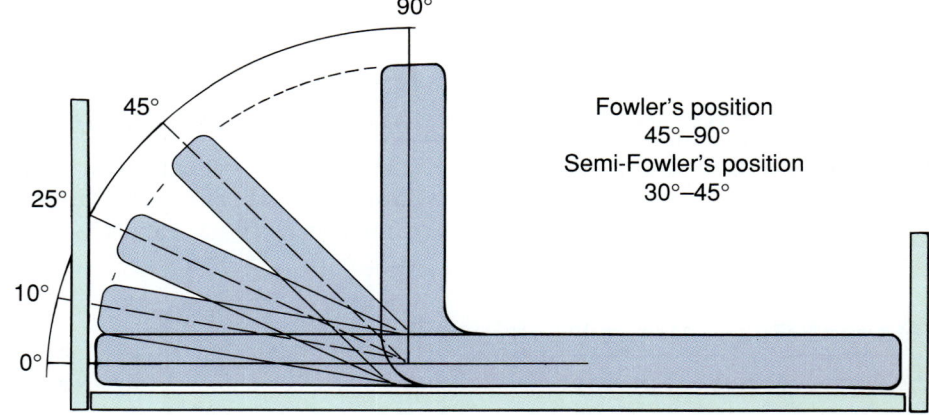

90°

45°

25°

10°

0°

Fowler's position
45°–90°
Semi-Fowler's position
30°–45°

knee-chest position A bent posture with the knees and chest touching the examining table, sometimes used for examining the rectum or for women who have recently given birth, to allow the uterus to fall forward into its natural position

Knee-Chest Position

In the **knee-chest position**, the patient rests on the knees and chest. The head is turned to one side with the cheek on a pillow. The patient's arms are extended slightly, bent at the elbows. Although the arms help support the patient, the main body weight is supported by the knees and chest. The knees are bent so that they are at right angles to the thighs. Draping is done with two sheets, one for the upper part of the body and one for the lower part (Figure 7–6). This position is used in rectal and vaginal examinations.

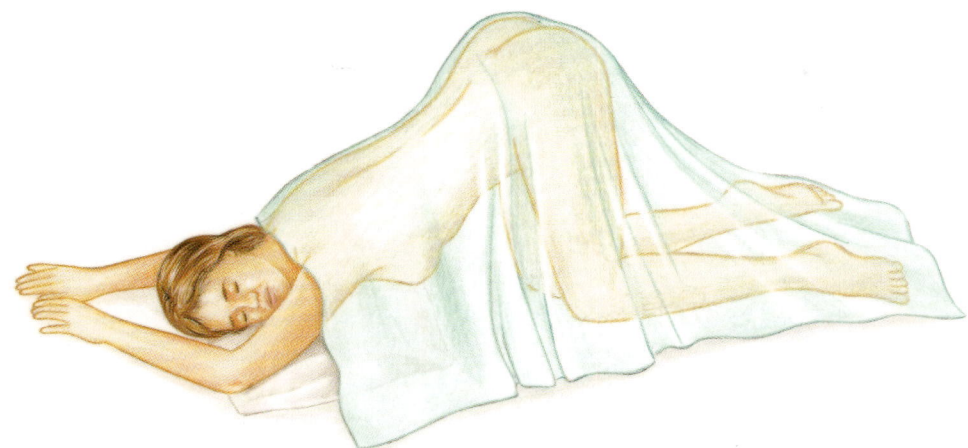

FIGURE 7–6
Knee-chest position

■ Side-Lying Positions

Side-lying positions are positions of comfort to relieve pressure points. Pillows are used to provide support and prevent skin breakdown (Figure 7–7).

side-lying positions
Lying on one's side

FIGURE 7–7
Side-lying position

TOP VIEW

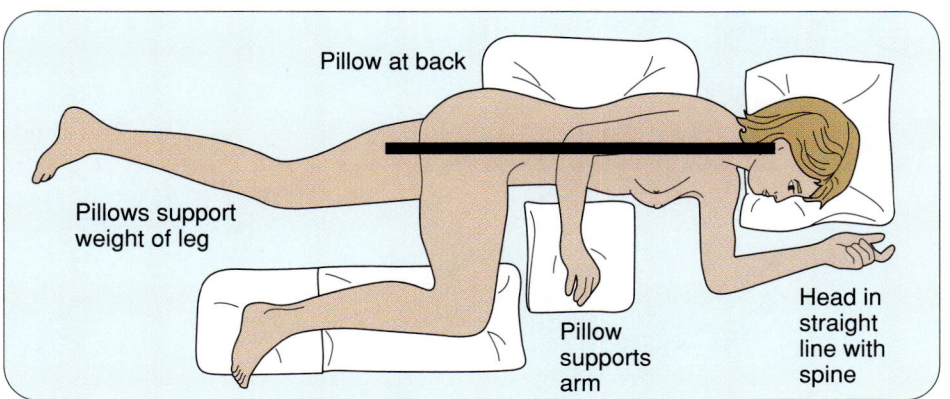

Pillow at back

Pillows support
weight of leg

Pillow
supports
arm

Head in
straight
line with
spine

FRONT VIEW

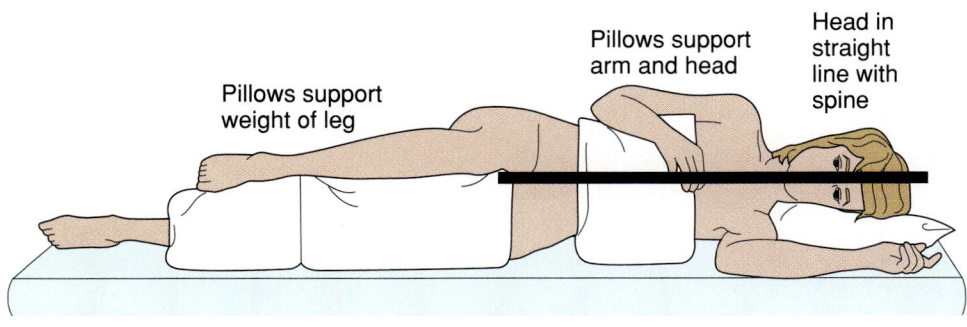

Pillows support
weight of leg

Pillows support
arm and head

Head in
straight
line with
spine

■Trendelenburg's Position

In **Trendelenburg's position**, the draping covers the entire body. The patient's head is low; the body is on an incline, carefully supported to prevent the patient from slipping out of position or being injured (Figure 7–8). This position is used for postural drainage, prolapsed cord situations, and so on.

Trendelenburg position
Position in which the bed or operating table on which a patient is lying is tilted so that the patient's head is about one foot below the level of his or her knees to allow more blood flow to the head and prevent shock; also called *shock position*

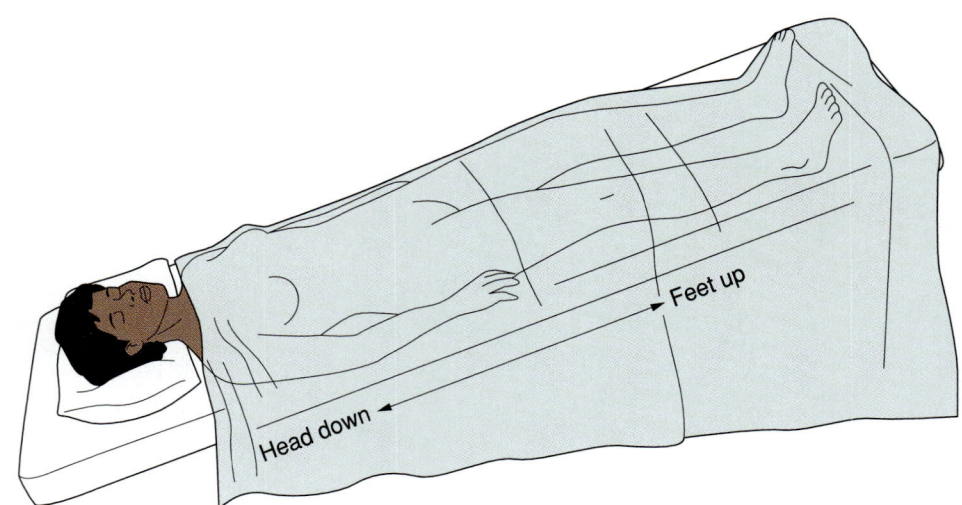

FIGURE 7–8
Trendelenburg position

■Reverse Trendelenburg

In reverse Trendelenburg position, the patient's body is on an incline so that the feet are lower than the head. Again, the body is completely draped (Figure 7–9).

FIGURE 7–9
Reverse Trendelenburg position

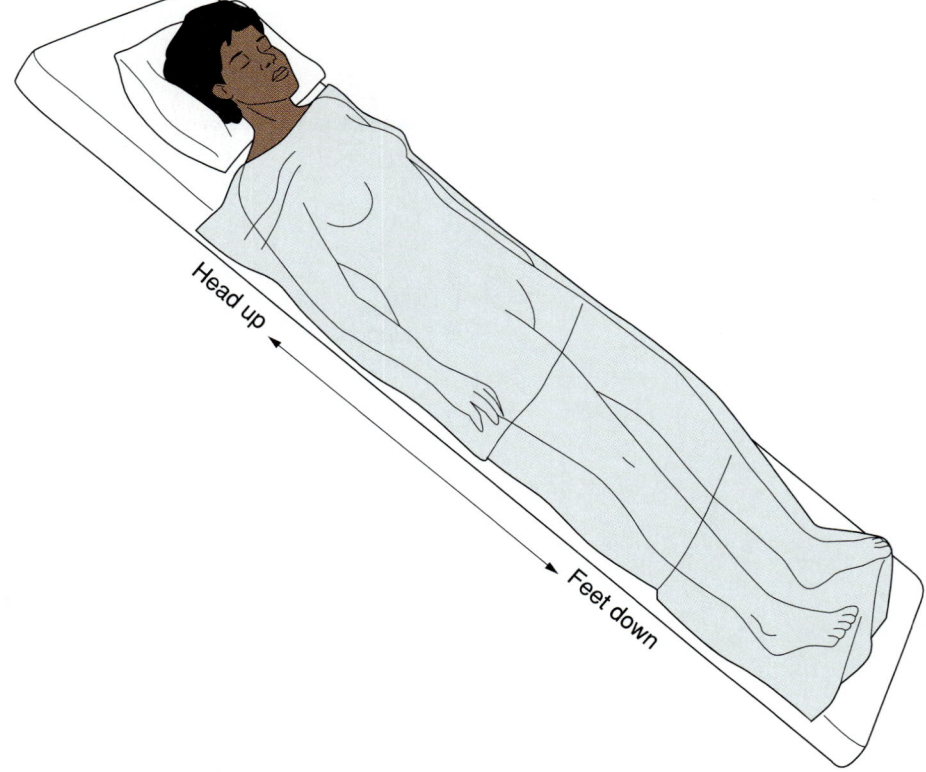

◼ Dorsal Lithotomy Position

The **dorsal lithotomy position** is the same as the dorsal recumbent position, except that the patient's legs are well separated and the knees are bent more (Figure 7–10). This position is used often for examination of the bladder, vagina, rectum, and perineum. If an examination table is being used, the patient's feet are sometimes placed in stirrups.

dorsal lithotomy position The position in which a patient lies on the back, with legs spread apart and knees bent

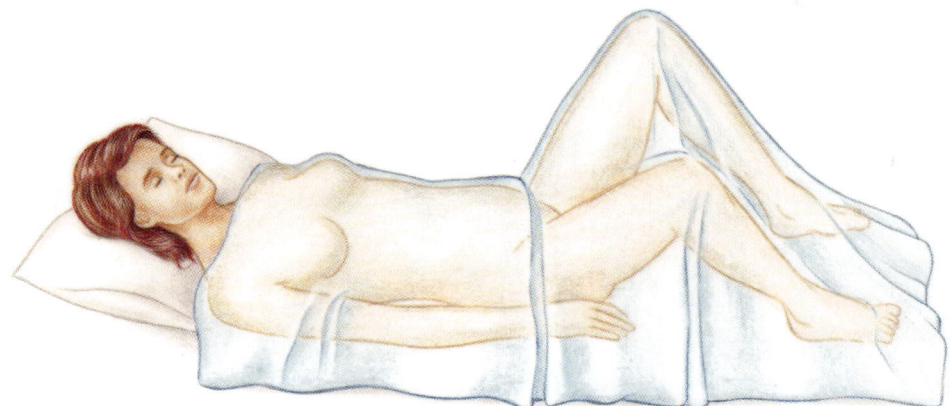

FIGURE 7–10
Dorsal lithotomy position

◼ Prone Position

In the **prone position**, the patient lies on the abdomen with the arms at the sides or bent at the elbows. The patient's head is turned to the side (Figure 7–11).

prone position Lying on one's stomach

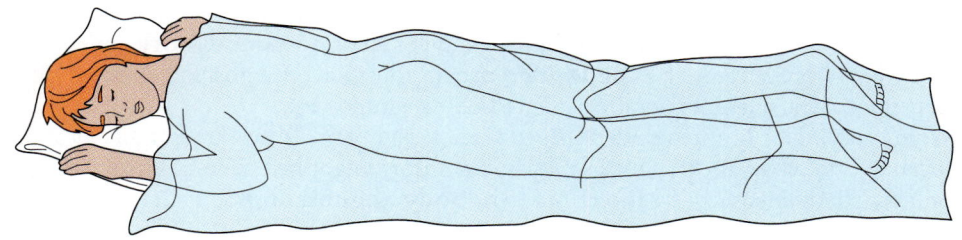

FIGURE 7–11
Prone position

◼ Left Sims's Position

Sims's position is also called the *semiprone position.* The patient lies on the left side. The patient's cheek is resting on a small pillow that is placed under the head. The right knee is bent against the patient's abdomen. The left knee is also bent, but not as much. The left arm is placed behind the body; the right arm rests in a way that is comfortable for the patient (Figure 7–12). This position is used for rectal examinations and enemas. Draping covers the entire body.

Sims's position Position in which the patient lies on the left side with the right knee and thigh drawn up, often used for a rectal examination

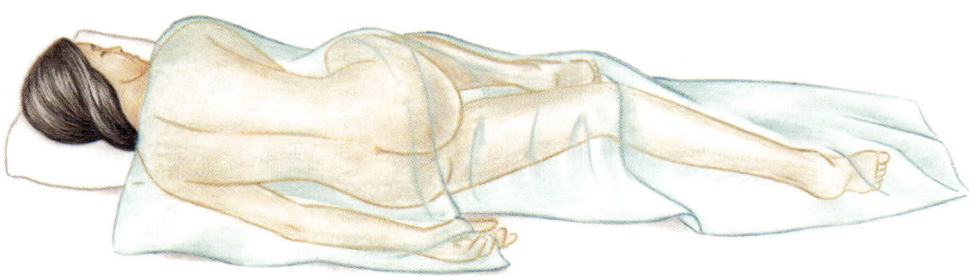

FIGURE 7–12
Left Sims's position

■ Left Lateral Position

left lateral position Lying on the left side

In the **left lateral position**, the patient lies on the left side. The hips are closer to the edge of the bed than the shoulders. The knees are bent, one more than the other (Figure 7–13).

FIGURE 7–13
Left lateral position

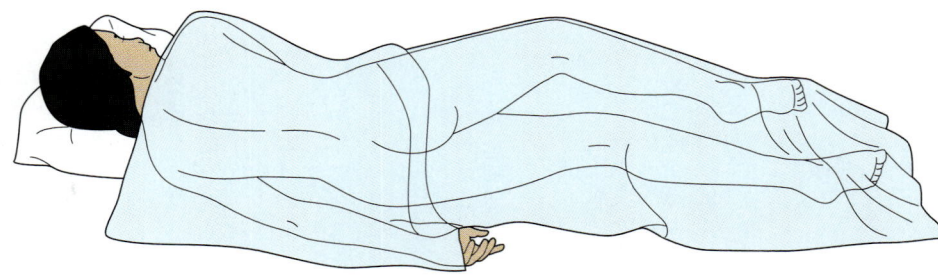

MOVING AND LIFTING PATIENTS

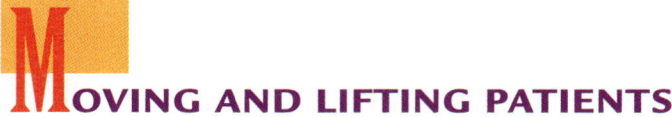

KEY IDEA

Moving and lifting patients who cannot assist you can be difficult. For this reason, you must take special care to support and align the patient's body properly.

nonambulatory Unable to walk

bedridden Unable to get out of bed

body alignment The correct, or anatomical, positioning of a patient's body; also the arrangement of the body in a straight line

Many of your tasks require lifting and moving a helpless or **nonambulatory** patient who cannot walk or move himself. A **bedridden** patient must have his position changed often. Proper support and alignment of the patient's body are important.

When moving or lifting a patient, the patient's body should be straight and properly supported; otherwise, the patient's safety and comfort might be affected. The correct positioning of the patient's body is referred to as **body alignment**. Body alignment means the arrangement or adjustment of the patient's body so that all parts of the body are in their proper positions in relation to each other.

Many conditions and injuries, as well as special patient care treatments, make it difficult or even dangerous for a patient to be in a certain position. As a member of the nursing team, you will be responsible for making sure that the patient you are caring for is in the position ordered by the doctor.

GUIDELINES

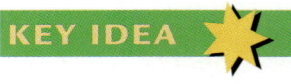

OBRA

MOVING AND LIFTING PATIENTS

- Before you begin each procedure, identify yourself and explain what you are going to do and encourage the patient to participate and help as much as possible.
- Before moving the patient, place tubing from catheters and IVs where they won't be pulled.

- Give the most support to the heaviest parts of the patient's body.
- Hold the patient close to your body for the most support.
- Move the patient with smooth and steady motions. Avoid sudden jerking movements.

A pull or lift sheet can help you move the patient in bed more easily. A regular extra sheet folded over many times and placed under the patient can be used as a pull sheet. The cotton draw sheet can also be used as a pull sheet. When moving the patient, roll and pull the sheet up tightly on each side next to the patient's body. Grip the rolled portion to slide the patient into the desired position. By using the pull sheet, friction and irritation to the patient's skin are avoided.

AGE-SPECIFIC CONSIDERATIONS

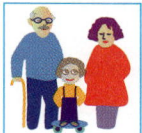

Moving and Lifting Patients

For all lifting and moving procedures: Patients of all ages must be treated with respect. In adolescence, patients are experiencing rapid change in their bodies and in their emotions. Avoid the use of medical jargon to gain their trust and respect. Guard their privacy as you move and transfer these patients. Adults often fear losing control when ill and are prone to feelings of helplessness. Explain clearly what you are doing and encourage them in areas where they may have some control. The older adult experiences numerous physiological changes as the aging process progresses. However, getting older is not a disease process. Allow for a longer response time when giving directions, speak clearly and in lower tones, and make sure the patient is wearing glasses/hearing aides (if applicable) to aide in communication.

PROCEDURE

OBRA

MOVING THE HELPLESS PATIENT UP IN BED

PREPARATION

1. Ask another nursing assistant to work with you.
2. Wash your hands.
3. Identify the patient by checking the identification bracelet.
4. Ask visitors to step out of the room, if this is your hospital's policy.
5. Tell the patient that you and your partner are going to move her up in the bed, even if she appears to be unconscious.
6. Provide privacy for the patient.

STEPS

7. Place the pillow from under the patient's head up against the headboard. This will protect the patient's head.
8. Lock the wheels on the bed.
9. Raise the height of the bed to a comfortable working position.
10. Lower the backrest and footrest, if this is allowed.
11. Stand on one side of the bed. The other nursing assistant will stand on the opposite side.
12. Both nursing assistants should stand straight, pivoting with feet slightly toward the head of the bed and hip width apart. The foot closest to the head of the bed should be pointed in that direction. Both should bend their knees and maintain the natural curves in the back.
13. The use of a draw, pull, or turning sheet is always preferred for mov-

ing a helpless patient up in bed. This is to avoid friction between the patient's skin and bedding. Roll the sides of the sheet to be used as a pull sheet close to the patient. Each nursing assistant then grasps one side of the rolled portion of the sheet firmly so that, when the patient is moved up, the sheet will stay in place under the patient (Figure 7–14).

14. You will be sliding the patient's body when you move her up in bed. Slightly bend your knees as you start to slide the patient shifting your weight from one foot to the other.
15. When you say "one, two, three" in unison, you and your partner will move together to slide the patient gently toward the head of the bed or to the desired position.
16. Make the patient comfortable.
17. Replace the pillow, as per the patient's request.

PROCEDURE (CONTINUED)

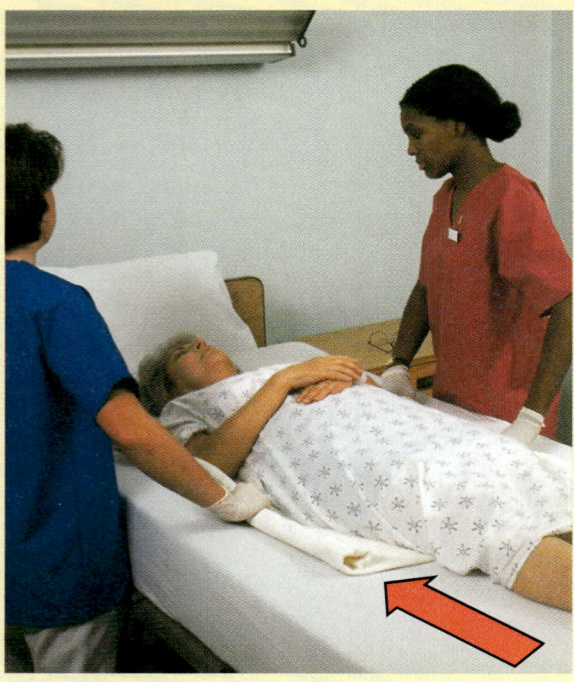

FIGURE 7–14
Use draw sheet to move helpless patient up in bed

FOLLOW-UP

18. Lower the bed to a position of safety for the patient.

19. Raise the side rails where ordered, indicated, and appropriate for patient safety.

20. Place the call light within easy reach of the patient.

21. Wash your hands.

22. Report to your immediate supervisor:

- That the patient's position has been changed.
- The time the patient's position was changed.
- How the patient tolerated the procedure.
- Your observations of anything unusual.

PROCEDURE

OBRA

MOVING A PATIENT UP IN BED WITH THE PATIENT'S HELP

PREPARATION

1. Wash your hands.

2. Identify the patient by checking the identification bracelet.

3. Ask visitors to step out of the room, if this is your hospital's policy.

4. Tell the patient that you are going to move him up in bed. Before you begin, ask your head nurse or team leader if the patient is a car-

diac patient and is allowed the necessary exertion for this move.

5. Provide privacy for the patient.

6. Lock the wheels on the bed.

7. Raise the height of the bed to a comfortable working position.

8. Lower the backrest and footrest if this is allowed.

STEPS

9. Remove the pillow from under the patient's head. Put the pillow at the top of the bed against the headboard. This will protect the patient's head from hitting the headboard.

10. Put the side rails in the up position on the far side of the bed.

11. Put one hand under the patient's shoulder. Put your other hand under the patient's hip. Provide

assistance to the weaker side of the patient.

12. Ask the patient to bend his knees and brace his feet firmly on the mattress.

13. Have your feet hip width apart. The foot closest to the head of the bed should be pointed in that direction.

14. Bend your knees. Maintain the natural curves in your back.

15. Bend your body from your hips and pivot slightly toward the head of the bed.

16. At the signal, "one, two, three," have the patient push toward head of bed with his hands and feet.

17. At the same time, help the patient to move toward the head of

P R O C E D U R E   (CONTINUED)

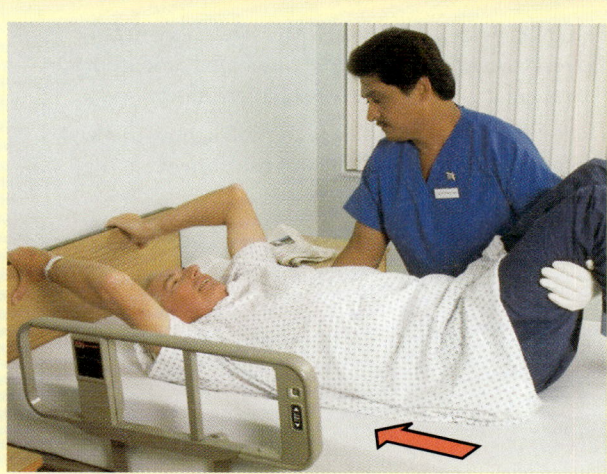

FIGURE 7–15
Helping slide the patient toward the head of the bed

the bed by sliding the patient with your hands and arms, as you shift weight from back foot to foot closest to head of bed (Figure 7–15).

18. Replace the pillow under the patient's head and shoulders.

FOLLOW-UP

19. Make the patient comfortable.

20. Lower the bed to a position of safety for the patient.

21. Raise the side rails where ordered, indicated, and appropriate for patient safety.

22. Place the call light within easy reach of the patient.

23. Wash your hands.

24. Report to your immediate supervisor:

   - That the patient's position has been changed.
   - The time the patient's position was changed.
   - How the patient tolerated the procedure.
   - Your observations of anything unusual.

P R O C E D U R E

OBRA

MOVING THE MATTRESS TO THE HEAD OF THE BED WITH THE PATIENT'S HELP

PREPARATION

1. Wash your hands.

2. Ask another nursing assistant to work with you.

3. Identify the patient by checking the identification bracelet.

4. Ask visitors to step out of the room, if this is your hospital's policy.

5. Tell the patient that you are going to move her mattress to the head of the bed.

6. Provide privacy for the patient.

7. Lock the wheels on the bed.

8. Raise the bed to a comfortable working position.

9. Lower the backrest, if allowed.

STEPS

10. If you are working alone, put the side rail in the up position on the far side of the bed.

11. If you are working with a partner, each of you should stand at opposite sides of the bed and loosen the sheets.

12. Lock arms with the patient and remove the pillow (Figure 7–16). Put the pillow on the chair.

13. Ask the patient to grasp the headboard with both hands.

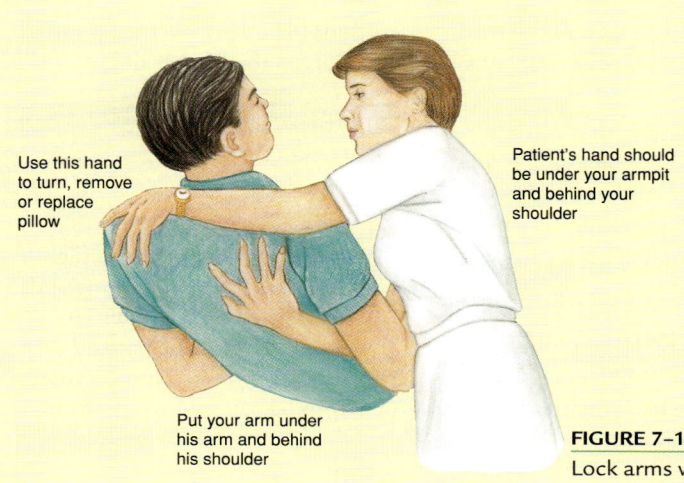

Use this hand to turn, remove or replace pillow

Patient's hand should be under your armpit and behind your shoulder

Put your arm under his arm and behind his shoulder

FIGURE 7–16
Lock arms with patient

PROCEDURE (CONTINUED)

14. Ask the patient to bend her knees and brace her feet firmly on the mattress.

15. Grasp the mattress loops, or grasp the sides of the mattress if there are no loops.

16. At the signal, "one, two, three," have the patient pull with her hands toward the head of the bed and push with her feet against the mattress (Figure 7–17).

17. At the same time, both nursing assistants slide the mattress toward the head of the bed, keeping the knees bent and the backs straight.

18. Lock arms with the patient and put the pillow back in place.

FOLLOW-UP

19. Make the patient comfortable.

20. Lower the bed to a position of safety for the patient.

21. Raise the side rails where ordered, indicated, and appropriate for patient safety.

22. Place the call light within easy reach of the patient.

23. Wash your hands.

24. Report to your immediate supervisor:

- That the mattress was moved to the head of the bed with the patient's help.
- The time the mattress was moved to the head of the bed.
- How the patient tolerated the procedure.
- Your observations of anything unusual.

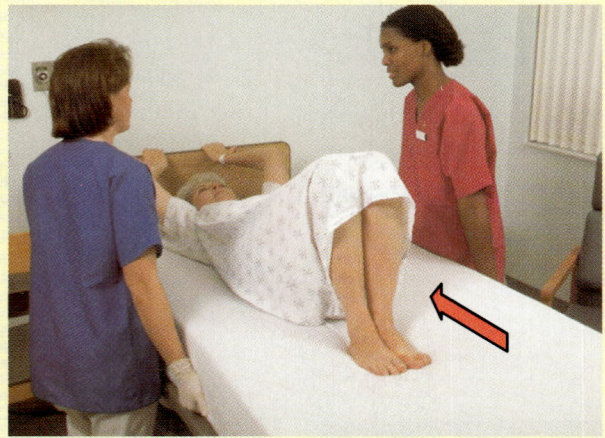

FIGURE 7–17

On your signal, have patient push with her feet

PROCEDURE

OBRA

MOVING A HELPLESS PATIENT TO ONE SIDE OF THE BED ON THE PATIENT'S BACK

PREPARATION

1. Wash your hands.

2. Identify the patient by checking the identification bracelet.

3. Ask visitors to step out of the room, if this is your hospital's policy.

4. Tell the patient that you are going to move him to one side of the bed on his back without turning the patient.

5. Provide privacy for the patient.

6. Lock the wheels on the bed.

7. Raise the bed to a comfortable working position.

8. Lower the backrest and footrest, if this is allowed.

9. Put the side rail in the up position on the far side of the bed.

STEPS

10. Loosen the top sheets, but don't expose the patient.

11. With one leg slightly in front of the other and front knee slightly bent, slide both your arms under the patient's back to his far shoulder. Slide the patient's shoulders toward you on your arms as you shift weight from the front leg to the back leg

PROCEDURE (CONTINUED)

while straightening the front leg (Figure 7–18).

12. Slide both your arms as far as you can under the patient's hips and slide his hips toward you, again shifting weight from front leg to back leg. Use a pull (turning) sheet whenever possible.

13. Place both your arms under the patient's lower legs and slide them toward you on your arms, again shifting your weight from one leg to the other (Figure 7–19).

14. Adjust the pillow, if necessary.

15. Remake the top of the bed.

FOLLOW-UP

16. Make the patient comfortable.

17. Lower the bed to a position of safety for the patient.

18. Raise the side rails where ordered, indicated, and appropriate for patient safety.

19. Place the call light within easy reach of the patient.

20. Wash your hands.

21. Report to your immediate supervisor:
    - That the patient has been moved to one side of the bed on his back.
    - The time the patient's position was changed.
    - How the patient tolerated the procedure.
    - Your observations of anything unusual.

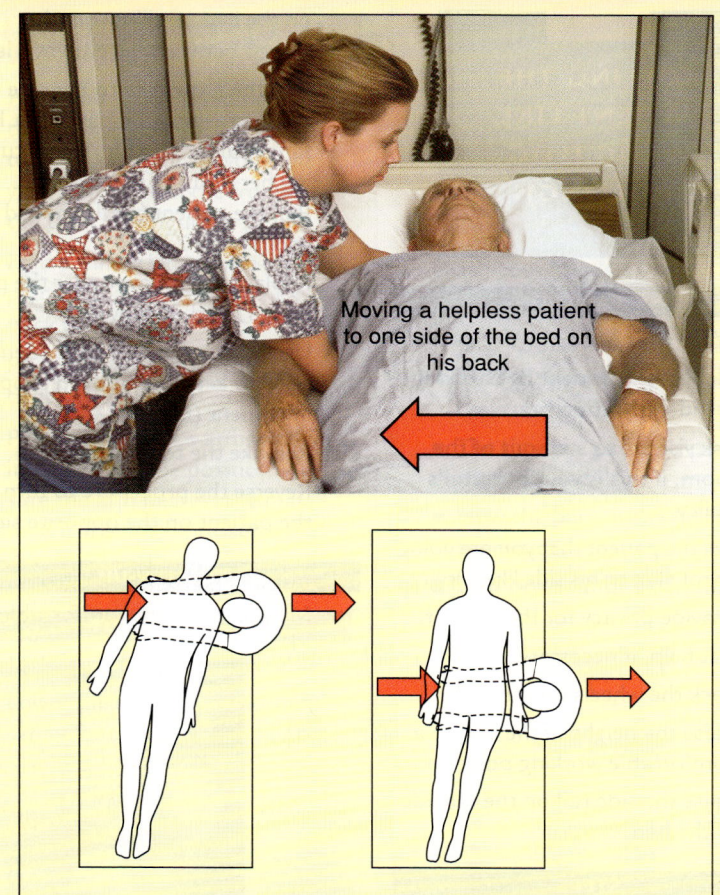

FIGURE 7–18

Moving a helpless patient to one side of the bed on his back. As a safety measure, this procedure must be done before turning a patient onto his side. It insures that the patient, when turned, is located in the center of the mattress.

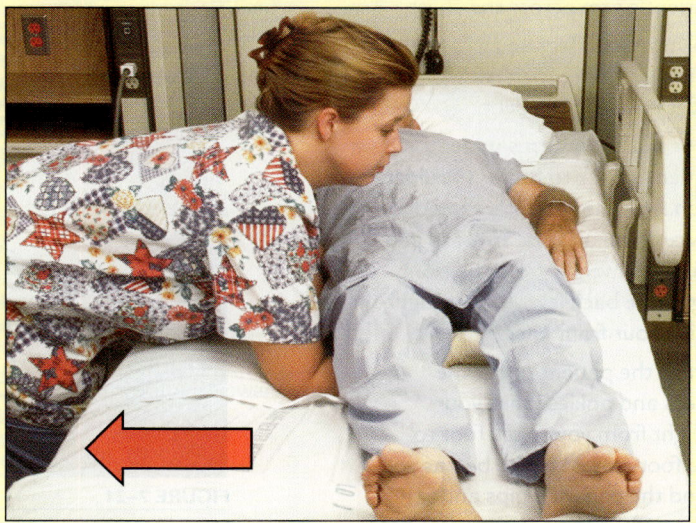

FIGURE 7–19

Using both your arms, slide patient's lower legs toward you

PROCEDURE

OBRA

TURNING A PATIENT ONTO THE PATIENT'S SIDE AWAY FROM YOU

PREPARATION

1. Wash your hands.
2. Identify the patient by checking the identification bracelet.
3. Ask visitors to step out of the room, if this is your hospital's policy.
4. Tell the patient you are going to turn him on the other side.
5. Provide privacy for the patient.
6. Lock the wheels on the bed.
7. Raise the height of the bed to a comfortable working position.
8. Lower the backrest and footrest.
9. Put the side rail in the up position on the far side of the bed.

STEPS

10. Loosen the top sheets, but don't expose the patient.
11. With one leg positioned in front of the other, slide both your arms under the patient's back to the far shoulder as you shift your weight from the back leg to the front leg. Slide the patient's shoulders toward you on your arms as you shift your weight from the front leg to the back leg.
12. Slide both your arms as far as you can under the patient's hips and slide the hips toward you again as you shift your weight from the back leg to the front leg. Use a pull (turning) sheet whenever possible.

13. Place both your arms under the patient's lower legs and slide them toward you on your arms as you shift your weight from the front leg to the back leg.
14. Cross the patient's arms over the chest, and bend the patient's knees, placing the feet on the bed.
15. Place one hand on the patient's shoulder near you.
16. Put your other hand along the hip/thigh nearest you.
17. Turn the patient gently on his side, facing away from you (Figure 7–23).
18. Fold a pillow lengthwise. Place it against the patient's back for support.
19. Place a pillow under the patient's head.
20. Make sure the patient's arms and legs are in a comfortable position. Put a pillow between the knees if this helps to make the patient comfortable. Be sure the arm nearest the mattress is free from pressure.

21. Remake the top of the bed.
22. Lower the bed to its lowest horizontal position.

FOLLOW-UP

23. Make the patient comfortable.
24. Lower the bed to a position of safety for the patient.
25. Raise the side rails where ordered, indicated, and appropriate for patient safety.
26. Place the call light within easy reach of the patient.
27. Wash your hands.
28. Report to your immediate supervisor:
    - That the patient's position has been changed.
    - The time the patient's position was changed.
    - How the patient tolerated the procedure.
    - Your observations of anything unusual.

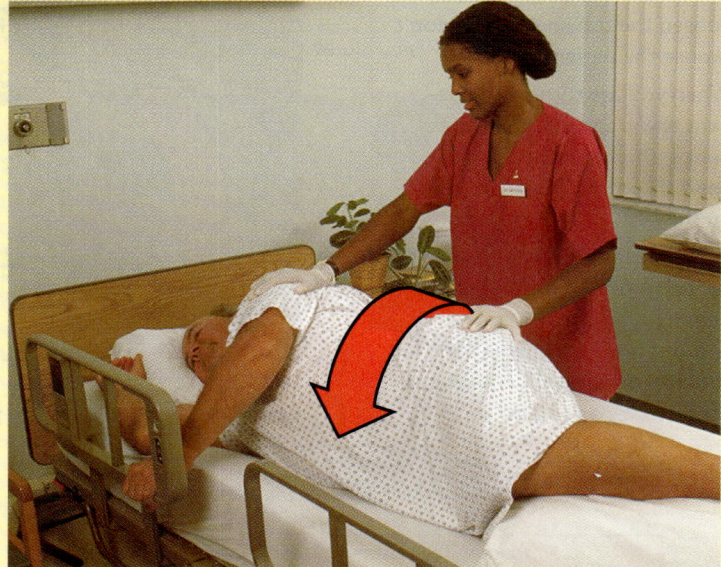

FIGURE 7–23

Gently turn the patient on his side, facing away from you

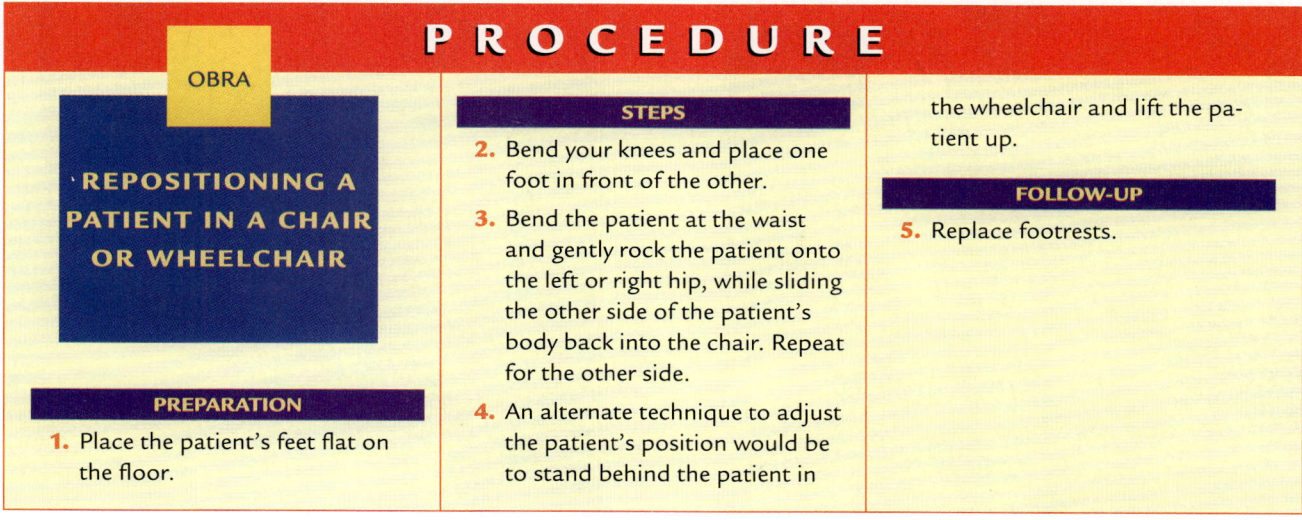

PROCEDURE

OBRA

REPOSITIONING A PATIENT IN A CHAIR OR WHEELCHAIR

PREPARATION

1. Place the patient's feet flat on the floor.

STEPS

2. Bend your knees and place one foot in front of the other.

3. Bend the patient at the waist and gently rock the patient onto the left or right hip, while sliding the other side of the patient's body back into the chair. Repeat for the other side.

4. An alternate technique to adjust the patient's position would be to stand behind the patient in the wheelchair and lift the patient up.

FOLLOW-UP

5. Replace footrests.

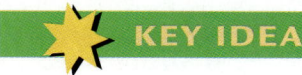

KEY IDEA

When repositioning a patient in a wheelchair, it is important to remember always to apply techniques for protective body mechanics.

TRANSPORTING A PATIENT BY WHEELCHAIR

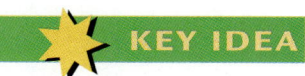

KEY IDEA

The patient in a wheelchair should be well covered if not dressed in a robe and slippers.

When **transporting** a patient by wheelchair, you may cover the feet as well as the shoulders with a sheet or a blanket, making sure it does not get caught in the wheels. In some institutions the seat of the wheelchair is covered with a piece of linen or with a disposable bed protector if the patient is **incontinent** (unable to control the bowels or bladder). The wheelchair must be wiped off with a disinfectant solution after it has been used by each patient.

When you are transporting a patient in a wheelchair, you should push the wheelchair from behind keeping your body close to the chair, except when entering or leaving elevators (Figure 7–24). When you are entering an elevator, pull the wheelchair into the elevator backward (Figure 7–25). When you are leaving an elevator, ask everyone else to step out first. Push the button marked "open." Turn the chair around, and pull it out of the elevator backward. This may not be necessary with very wide elevators. Take caution not to make contact with other individuals as you push the wheelchair out. Don't move the wheelchair while the elevator is in motion.

When you are moving a patient down a steep incline or ramp, you should take the chair down backward (Figure 7–26). To do this, stand behind the chair with your back facing the direction you want to go. Walk backward, holding the chair and moving it carefully down the ramp. Glance back now and then to make sure of your direction and to avoid collisions, as if you were driving a car in reverse.

transporting Moving something or someone from one place to another

incontinent Unable to control the bowels or bladder

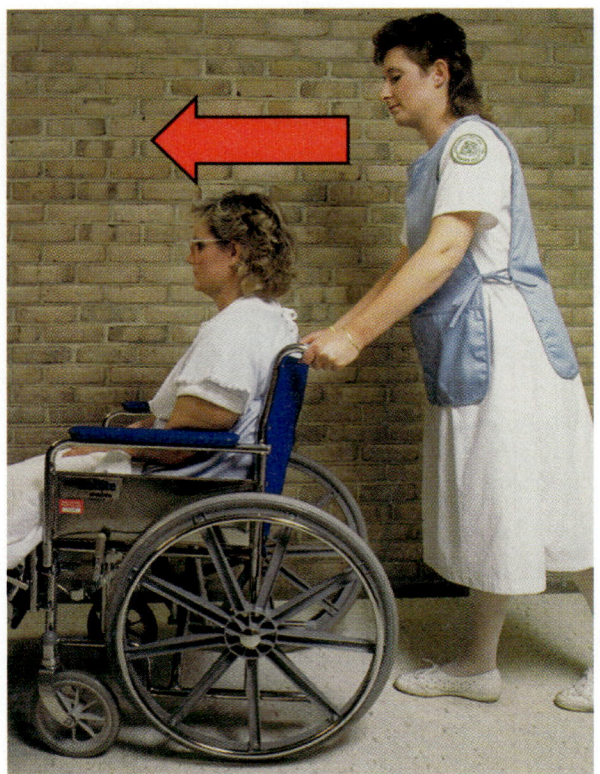

FIGURE 7–24
Transporting the patient by wheelchair

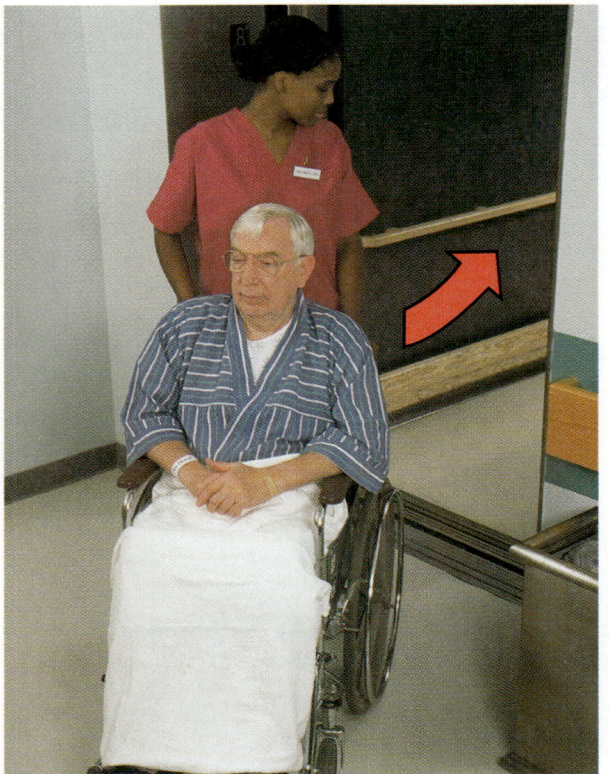

FIGURE 7–25
Entering an elevator with a patient in a wheelchair

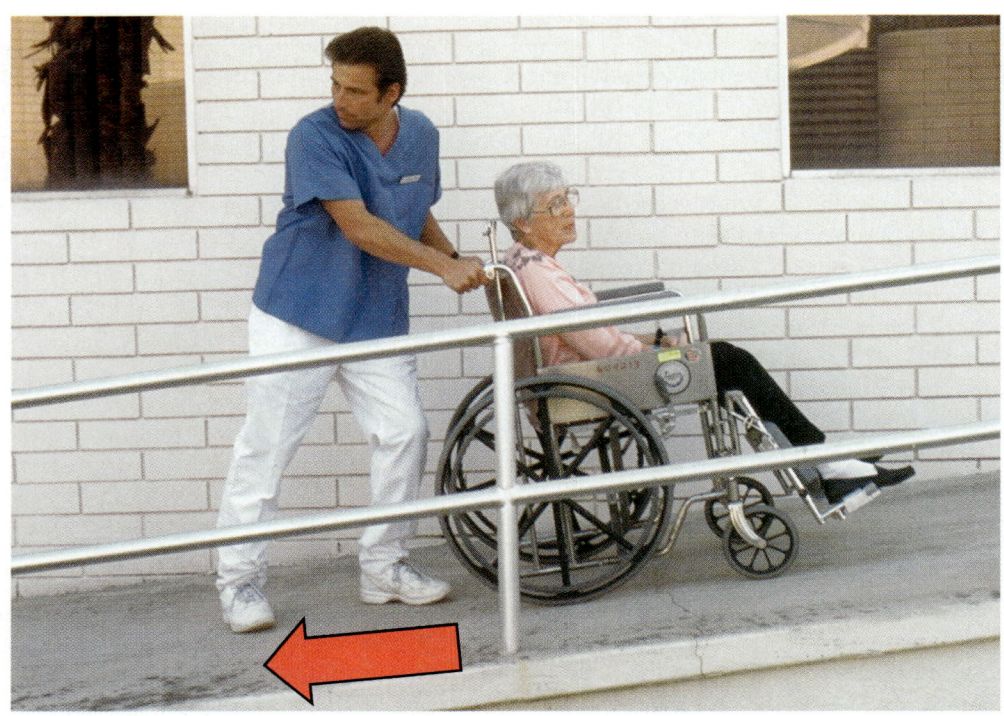

FIGURE 7–26
Moving down a ramp with a patient in a wheelchair

PROCEDURE

OBRA

MOVING THE NONAMBULATORY PATIENT INTO A WHEELCHAIR OR ARM CHAIR FROM THE BED

PREPARATION

1. Assemble your equipment:
   a. Wheelchair or arm chair
   b. Blanket or sheet
   c. Gait belt, if needed or required.
   d. Robe, if desired or needed.
2. Wash your hands.
3. Identify the patient by checking the identification bracelet.
4. Ask visitors to step out of the room, if this is your hospital's policy.
5. Tell the patient you are going to help her into a wheelchair.
6. Provide privacy for the patient.
7. Lock the wheels on the bed.
8. Spread a blanket or sheet on the chair. Have the corner of the blanket between the handles over the back so the opposite corner will be at the patient's feet.
9. Ask another nursing assistant to help you (Figure 7–27a-b).

STEPS

10. Put the patient's robe and non-skid rubber sole shoes or slippers on while she is in bed.
11. Move the patient to the edge of the bed.
    a. Slide both your arms under the patient's back to the shoulder; then slide the patient's shoulders toward you on your arms.
    b. Slide both your arms as far as you can under the patient's

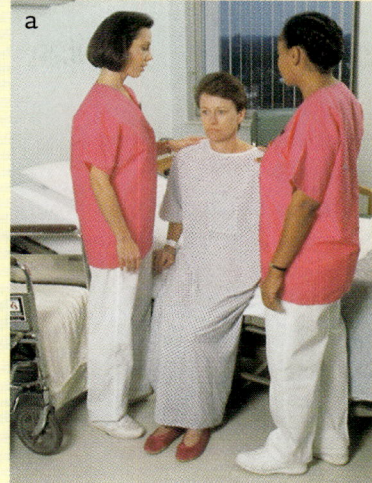

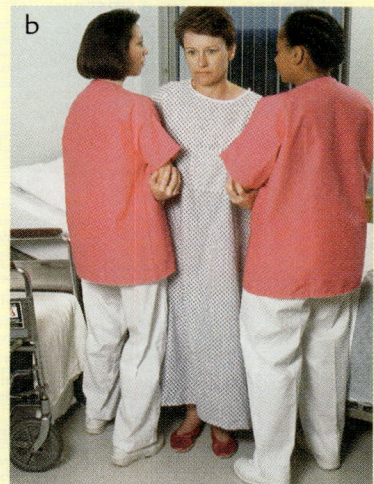

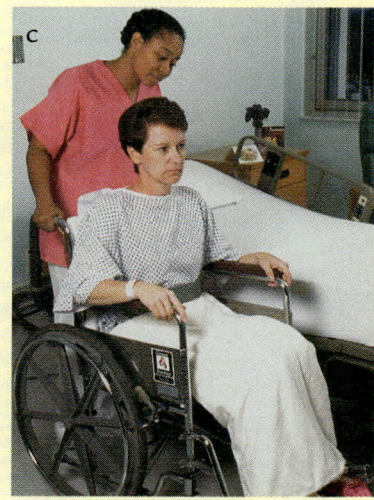

FIGURE 7–27
Assisting patient to a wheelchair

hips and slide the hips toward you. Use a pull (turning) sheet whenever possible.
    c. Place both your arms under the patient's lower legs and slide them toward you on your arms.
12. Raise the side rail.
13. Lower the bed to its lowest horizontal position so that when you dangle the patient, the feet will touch the floor when he sits up.
14. Raise the back rest so the patient is in a sitting position in bed.
15. Lower the side rail on the side where you and the other nursing assistant will be working.
16. Place both hands under the patient's legs and turn them to the dangling position. The patient's feet should be firmly on the floor. One nursing assistant supports the patient's back and head and raises them at the same time. The other nursing assistant places her arm around the patient's shoulders to support the patient's back while the patient is in the dangling position. Give the patient a minute to adjust. Observe the patient's color.
17. Place a gait belt around the patient's waist.
18. Scoot the patient forward to the side of the bed. Place the patient's feet flat on the floor. Support the patient behind the shoulder so that the patient is sitting upright.
19. Place the wheelchair at the bedside with the back of the chair in line with the middle of the bed. Lock the wheels on the chair.
20. Fold up the footrests of the wheelchair so they are out of the way. If the wheelchair has leg rests, adjust them to hang straight down, or remove the footrests/leg rests.

PROCEDURE (CONTINUED)

21. Lock the brakes on the wheel-chair.

22. Ask patient to hug you in front, around your waist. Then block the patient's knees between your knees and grasp the gait belt at the patient's sides.

23. The second nursing assistant should be positioned with one knee on the bed.

24. The first assistant, in front, should gently pull the patient forward into the wheelchair while the second assistant guides the patient's hips onto the chair.

25. Fasten the safety straps around the patient to keep him from falling out of the chair.

26. Arrange the blanket snugly but firmly around the patient. Make sure that no part of the blanket can possibly get caught in the wheels.

27. Adjust the footrests so that the patient's feet are resting comfortably on them.

28. Use the signal cord to call your immediate supervisor and take the patient's pulse and blood pressure if you observe any of the following:

   a. The patient becomes very pale.

   b. The patient seems to be perspiring a lot.

   c. The patient says something like, "I feel weak," "I feel dizzy," or "I feel faint."

29. Adjust the chair to a comfortable angle (Figure 7-27c).

30. Put a pillow behind the patient's back or shoulders, if needed.

FOLLOW-UP

31. Wash your hands.

32. Report to your immediate supervisor:

   ■ That the patient has been moved out of bed into a chair or wheelchair.

   ■ The time the patient's position was changed.

   ■ How the patient tolerated the procedure.

   ■ Your observations of anything unusual.

PROCEDURE

OBRA

HELPING A NONAMBULATORY PATIENT BACK INTO BED FROM A WHEELCHAIR OR ARM CHAIR

PREPARATION

1. Wash your hands.

2. Identify the patient by checking the identification bracelet.

3. Ask visitors to step out of the room, if this is your hospital's policy.

4. Tell the patient you are getting her back into bed.

5. Ask another nursing assistant to help you.

6. Place a pull sheet on the bottom sheets; fan-fold from the top of the bed to the foot.

7. Lock the wheels on the bed.

8. Raise the head of the bed as high as it will go to a sitting position.

9. Lower the bed to its lowest horizontal position.

10. Raise the side rail on the far side of the bed.

STEPS

11. Bring the wheelchair with the patient to the bedside.

12. Position the wheelchair so that the seat of the chair is in line with the middle of the bed. The chair should be positioned so the patient is transferred from the patient's strongest side.

13. Lock the brakes on the wheelchair.

14. Raise the footrests of the wheelchair, lifting the patient's feet off them and onto the floor at the same time. Remove the footrests if possible.

15. Open up the blanket and safety straps that are on the patient in the wheelchair.

16. Scoot the patient forward in the seat. Place the patient's feet flat on the floor. Support the patient behind the shoulder so that the patient is sitting upright.

17. Place a gait belt around the patient's waist.

18. Ask the patient to hug you in front, around your waist. Then block the patient's knees between your knees and grasp the gait belt at the patient's sides.

19. The second nursing assistant should be positioned with one knee on the bed behind the wheelchair.

20. The first assistant, in front, should gently pull the patient forward and up while the second

PROCEDURE (CONTINUED)

assistant guides the patient's hips onto the bed.

21. Raise that side rail.

22. Raise the bed to waist height.

23. One nursing assistant goes to the far side of the bed.

24. Lower that side rail.

25. Slide both your arms under the patient's back to the shoulder; then slide the patient's shoulders toward you on your arms.

26. Slide both your arms as far as you can under the patient's hips and slide the hips toward you. Use a pull (turning) sheet whenever possible.

27. Keep your knees bent and your back straight as you slide the patient.

28. Place both your arms under the patient's lower legs and slide them toward you on your arms.

29. Both nursing assistants then roll the pull sheet toward the patient and slide the patient up in bed using the pull sheet, using side to side weight shift.

30. Put a pillow under the patient's head.

31. Remake the top of the bed.

FOLLOW-UP

32. Make the patient comfortable.

33. Lower the bed to a position of safety for the patient.

34. Raise the side rails where ordered, indicated, and appropriate for patient safety.

35. Place the call light within easy reach of the patient.

36. Wipe the wheelchair with disinfectant solution and return the chair to its proper place.

37. Wash your hands.

38. Report to your immediate supervisor:

- That the patient has been put back into bed.
- The time the patient was put back into bed.
- How the patient tolerated the procedure.
- Your observations of anything unusual.

PROCEDURE

OBRA

HELPING AN AMBULATORY PATIENT WHO CAN STAND, BACK INTO BED FROM A CHAIR OR A WHEELCHAIR

PREPARATION

1. Wash your hands.

2. Identify the patient by checking the identification bracelet.

3. Ask visitors to step out of the room, if this is your hospital's policy.

4. Tell the patient you are getting him back into bed.

5. Provide privacy for the patient.

6. Lock the wheels on the bed.

7. Bring the wheelchair very close to the bed so that the patient's strongest side is closest to bed.

8. Lock the brakes on the wheelchair.

9. Raise the head of the bed to a sitting position.

10. Lower the bed to its lowest horizontal position.

STEPS

11. Raise the footrests of the wheelchair, or remove them. Place the patient's feet on the floor.

12. Open up the safety straps on the wheelchair.

13. Help the patient out of the wheelchair to stand, pivot (turn), and sit on the side of the bed. The patient's feet should be resting firmly on the floor.

14. Lean the patient against the backrest.

15. Put one arm around the patient's shoulders for support. Put your other arm under the patient's knees.

16. Swing the patient's body slowly around, helping the patient lift the legs onto the bed.

17. Raise the side rail.

18. Lower the head of the bed.

19. Help the patient move to the center of the bed.

20. Place a pillow under the patient's head.

21. Remove the patient's robe and nonskid shoes or slippers.

22. Remake the top of the bed.

FOLLOW-UP

23. Make the patient comfortable.

PROCEDURE (CONTINUED)

24. Lower the bed to a position of safety for the patient.

25. Raise the side rails where ordered, indicated, and appropriate for patient safety.

26. Place the call light within easy reach of the patient.

27. Fold the blanket from the wheelchair and put it in its proper place.

28. Wash the wheelchair with an antiseptic or disinfectant solution and return it to its proper place.

29. Wash your hands.

30. Report to your immediate supervisor:

- That you have helped the patient back into bed.

- The time you helped the patient back into bed.

- How the patient tolerated the procedure.

- Your observations of anything unusual.

PROCEDURE

OBRA

USING A PORTABLE MECHANICAL PATIENT LIFT TO MOVE THE HELPLESS PATIENT

PREPARATION

1. Assemble your equipment Mechanical patient lift and sling. (Figure 7–28a-b):

2. Wash your hands.

3. Identify the patient by checking the identification bracelet.

4. Ask visitors to step out of the room, if this is your hospital's policy.

5. Tell the patient you are going to get him out of bed by using the portable mechanical patient lift. This kind of lift is sometimes referred to as a Hoyer Lift (Figure 7-29). (You may need the help of a second nursing assistant as a partner.)

FIGURE 7–28a
(Photo courtesy of Guardian Products, a division of Sunrise Medical)

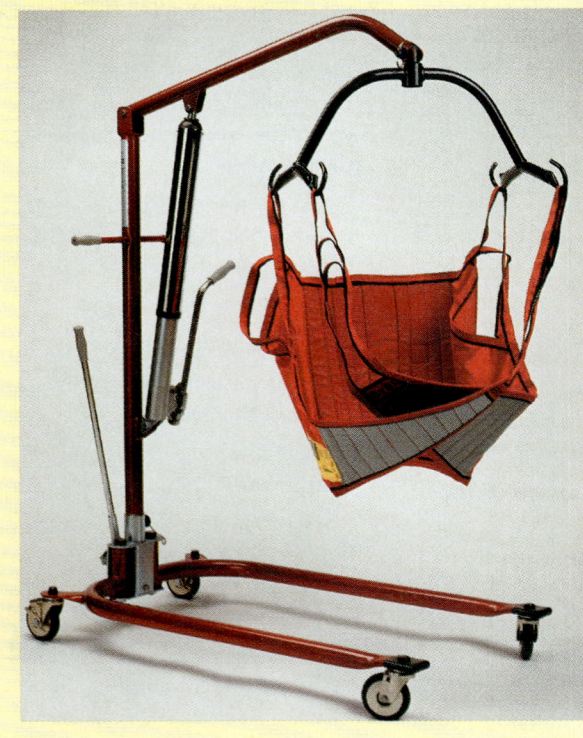

FIGURE 7–28b
Components of a mechanical lift

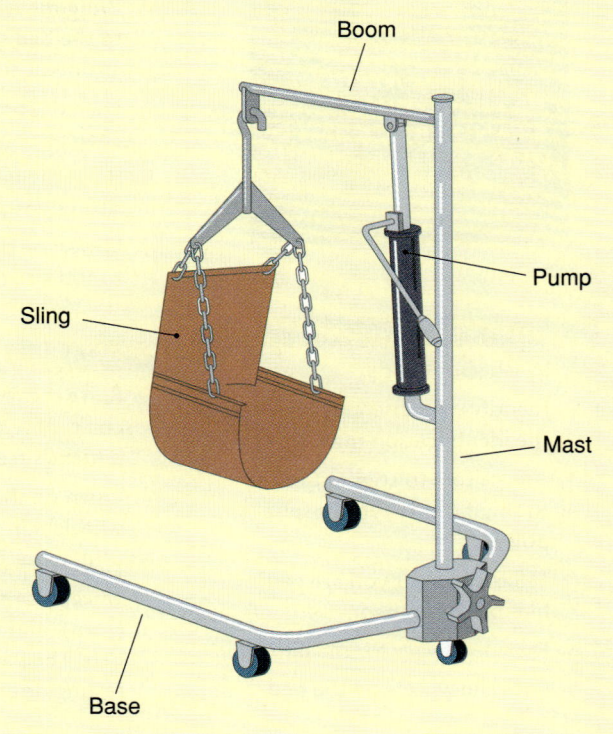

Boom

Pump

Sling

Mast

Base

PROCEDURE (CONTINUED)

6. Provide privacy for the patient.

7. Position the chair next to the bed with the back of the chair in line with the headboard of the bed. Lock the wheels of the bed and the mechanical lift.

8. Cover the chair with a blanket or sheet.

STEPS

9. By turning the patient from side to side on the bed, slide the sling under the patient.

10. Attach the sling to the mechanical lift with the hooks in place through the metal frame. Be sure to apply hooks with open, sharp ends away from the patient.

11. Have the patient fold both arms across his chest, if possible.

12. Using the crank, lift the patient from the bed.

13. Have your partner, a second nursing assistant, guide the patient's legs.

14. Lower the patient into the chair.

15. Remove the hooks from the frame of the portable mechanical patient lift.

16. Wrap the patient with the blanket.

17. Secure the patient to the chair with safety straps, if necessary.

18. Leave the patient safe and comfortable in the chair for the proper amount of time, according to your instructions.

19. To get the patient back to bed, put the hooks through the metal frame of the sling, which is still under the patient.

20. Raise the patient by using the crank on the mechanical patient lift. Lift him from the chair into the bed. Have your partner guide the patient's legs.

21. Lower the patient into the center of the bed.

22. Remove the hooks from the frame.

23. Remove the sling from under the patient by having the patient turn from side to side on the bed.

24. Put a pillow under the patient's head.

25. Remake the top of the bed.

FOLLOW-UP

26. Make the patient comfortable.

27. Lower the bed to a position of safety for the patient.

28. Raise the side rails where ordered, indicated, and appropriate for patient safety.

29. Place the call light within easy reach of the patient.

30. Wash the mechanical patient lift with an antiseptic or disinfectant solution and return it to its proper place.

31. Wash your hands.

32. Report to your immediate supervisor:

- That the patient was taken out of bed by means of the portable mechanical patient lift.

- The time the patient was taken out of bed.

- The prescribed length of time that the patient sat in a chair.

- That the patient was put back into bed by means of the portable mechanical patient lift.

- The time the patient was put back into bed.

- How the patient tolerated the procedure.

- Your observations of anything unusual.

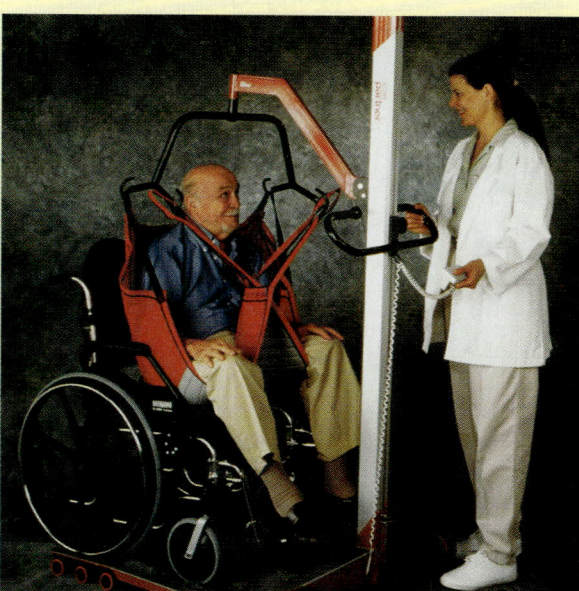

FIGURE 7–29

Hoyer Lift (Photo courtesy of Guardian Products, a division of Sunrise Medical)

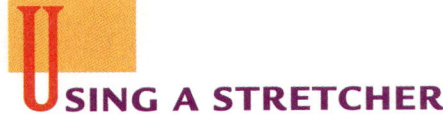

USING A STRETCHER

stretcher A wheeled cart on which patients are moved from one place to another

A hospital **stretcher** is a wheeled cart on which patients are moved from one place to another. When moving a helpless patient from the patient's bed to a stretcher, you will need a second nursing assistant working as your partner.

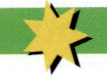 **KEY IDEA**

Whenever you are moving a stretcher, you should stand at the end where the patient's head is and push the stretcher so the patient's feet are moving first. Keep your body close to the stretcher. Be careful to protect the patient's head at all times.

When entering an elevator, push the stop button so the doors of the elevator will not close until you are ready. Pull the stretcher into the elevator with the head end first (Figure 7–30). Stand at the patient's head while the elevator is in motion. When you leave the elevator, press the stop button and push the stretcher out foot-end first.

Use side rails or restraining straps whenever you move a patient on a stretcher. Check the straps before you move the stretcher. Guide the stretcher from the foot-end when going down a ramp (Figure 7–31).

FIGURE 7–30

Entering an elevator with a stretcher

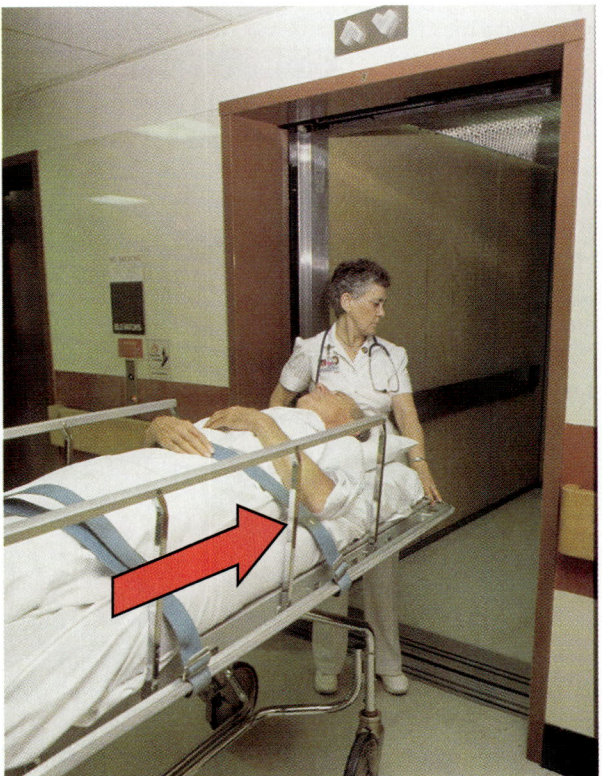

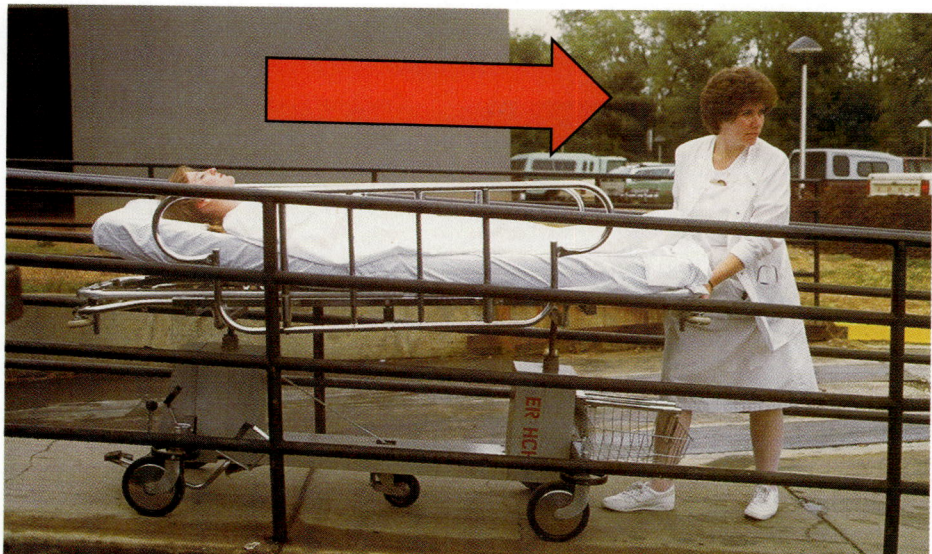

FIGURE 7–31
Moving down a ramp with a stretcher

PROCEDURE

OBRA

MOVING A PATIENT FROM THE BED TO A STRETCHER

PREPARATION

1. Assemble your equipment:
   a. Stretcher
   b. Sheet or blanket
2. Ask another nursing assistant to help you. The two of you should work in unison to move the patient from the bed to a stretcher.
3. Wash your hands.
4. Identify the patient by checking the identification bracelet.
5. Tell the patient you are going to move him from the bed to a stretcher.
6. Ask visitors to step out of the room, if this is your hospital's policy.
7. Provide privacy for the patient.

STEPS

8. Loosen the top sheets.
9. Cover the patient with a blanket or sheet. Remove the top sheets without exposing the patient.
10. Move the stretcher next to the bed.
11. Raise the bed so that it is the same height as the stretcher. Lock the wheels on the bed.
12. Lock the wheels on the stretcher.
13. You will stand on the far side of the bed, using your body to hold the bed in place.
14. Your partner will stand on the far side of the stretcher, using her body to hold the stretcher in place.
15. Position your legs so that one is in front of the other, bend your knees, and maintain the natural curves in your back.
16. At the signal, "one, two, three," push, pull, and slide the patient from the bed to the stretcher, while shifting your weight from the front leg to the back leg (if you are the assistant positioned on stretcher side) or from the back leg to the front leg (if you are the assistant positioned on bed side). Use a pull (turning) sheet whenever possible (Figure 7–32).
17. Support the patient's head and feet, keeping the body covered with a loose blanket or sheet.
18. Fasten the stretcher straps around the patient at the hips and shoulders.
19. Put the side rails of the stretcher in the up position for the patient's safety.

FOLLOW-UP

20. Wash your hands.
21. Report to your immediate supervisor:
    - That you have moved the patient from the bed to a stretcher.
    - The time you moved the patient to the stretcher.
    - How the patient tolerated the procedure.
    - Your observations of anything unusual.

PROCEDURE (CONTINUED)

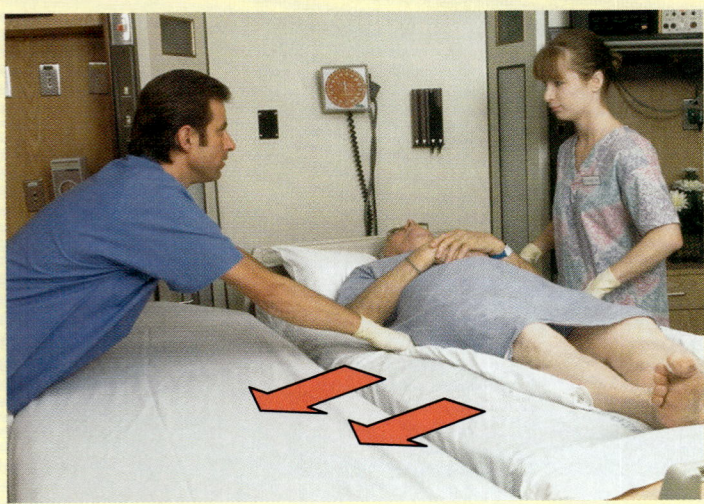

FIGURE 7–32
Moving the patient from the bed to the stretcher

PROCEDURE

OBRA

MOVING A PATIENT FROM A STRETCHER TO THE BED

PREPARATION

1. Assemble your equipment:
   a. Stretcher
   b. Sheet or blanket
2. Ask three other nursing assistants to help you. You should work in unison to move the patient from the bed to a stretcher.
3. Wash your hands.
4. Identify the patient by checking the identification bracelet.
5. Tell the patient you are going to move him from the stretcher to the bed.
6. Ask visitors to step out of the room, if this is your hospital's policy.

7. Provide privacy for the patient.
8. Lock the wheels on the bed.
9. Fan-fold the top sheet to the bottom of the bed.
10. Bring the stretcher next to the bed.
11. Raise the bed so that it is level with the stretcher.
12. Lock the wheels on the stretcher.

STEPS

13. Two nursing assistants stand by the far side of the bed, using their bodies to hold the bed in place.
14. The other two nursing assistants stand by the far side of the stretcher, using their bodies to hold the stretcher in place.
15. Open the stretcher straps.
16. Bend your knees, maintaining the natural curves in your back, and position your legs so that one is in front of the other.
17. At the signal, "one, two, three," slide the patient from the stretcher to the bed. Use a pull (turning) sheet whenever possible.
18. Keep the patient covered with a loose blanket or sheet and support the head and feet.

FOLLOW-UP

19. Make the patient as comfortable as possible.
20. Replace the top sheets, removing the blanket without exposing the patient.
21. Lower the bed to a position of safety for the patient.
22. Raise the side rails where ordered, indicated, and appropriate for patient safety.
23. Place the call light within easy reach of the patient.
24. Wash your hands.
25. Report to your immediate supervisor:
    - That you have moved the patient from the stretcher to the bed.
    - The time you moved the patient from the stretcher to the bed.

ASSISTING THE PATIENT TO AMBULATE

■ Using a Gait Belt

Use of a gait belt positioned snugly around the patient's waist will help to control the patient while walking. Position yourself slightly behind the weaker side of the patient. Have the patient's stronger side close to a wall if available. Keep one hand on the gait belt at all times (see Chapters 6 and 32).

■ Using a Cane, Walker, or Crutches

Canes, crutches, and walkers (Figure 7–33) are pieces of equipment that may be used by the patient to ambulate safely. These pieces of equipment help support the patient while walking and may be ordered by the physician. (See Chapters 6, 16, and 32.)

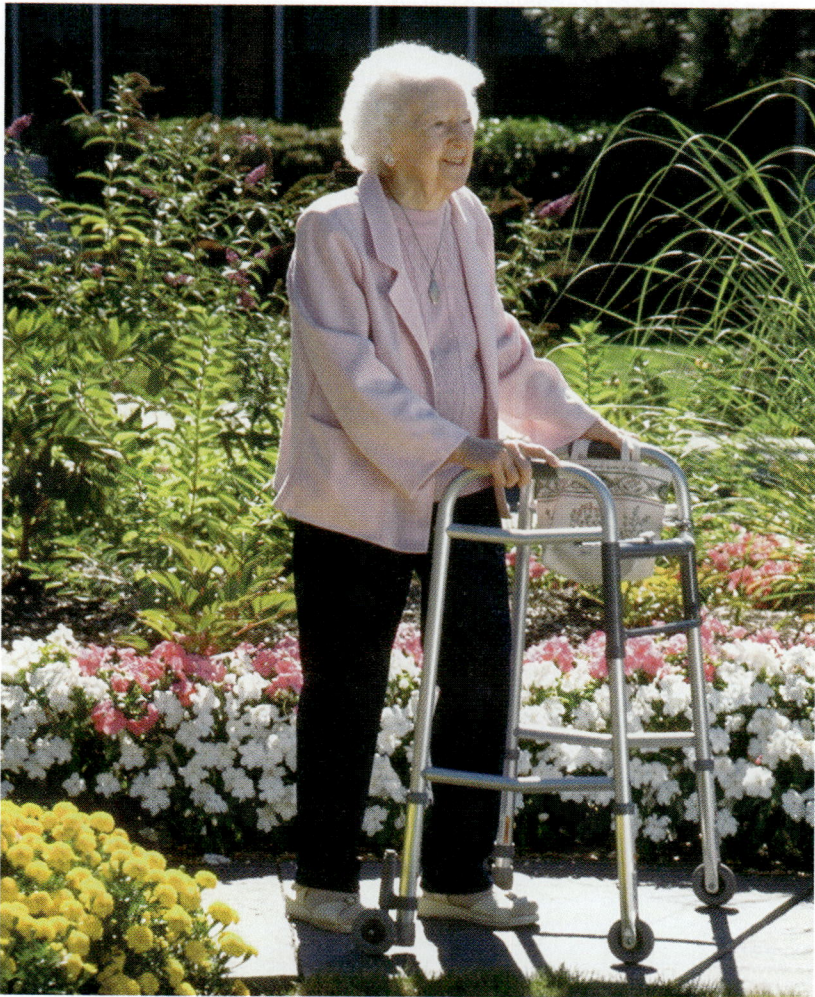

FIGURE 7–33

A walker may be used when the patient requires some support due to imbalance or weakness

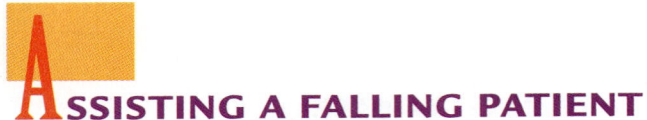

ASSISTING A FALLING PATIENT

GUIDELINES

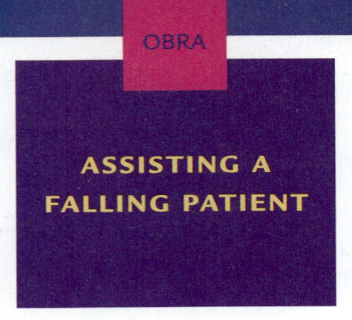

OBRA

ASSISTING A FALLING PATIENT

- If a patient begins to fall, move your feet apart to increase your stability, bend your knees, and lower your body to the floor with

the patient. Keep the patient's body close to you.

- Hold onto the patient from behind, placing your arms under the patient's arms and placing your hands on their transfer or gait belt to help ease them to the floor.

- Maintain the natural curves in your back.

- If the patient is next to a wall when he begins to fall, use the wall to assist in easing the patient to the floor.

- Protect the patient's head from injury.

- Stay with the patient, call for help, and do not move the patient until you are instructed to do so.

- Always ask for assistance to help patient back to a standing position.

- Report the details to your supervisor or charge nurse and complete an incident report.

SUMMARY

The use of proper/protective body mechanics during daily work tasks such as positioning, moving, and lifting patients will help you avoid back and shoulder injuries and leave you with more energy at the end of the day. Always ask for assistance when you feel you are unable to perform a task safely on your own.

Notes

THE NURSING ASSISTANT IN ACTION

Should a Policy Be a Guideline For You?

Your employer has a policy that employees are to use mechanical lifts when lifting patients. You are a male nursing assistant in excellent physical condition. Mr. Chapman is a frail, confused, elderly man who weighs about 130 pounds. You know you can easily pick Mr. Chapman up and place him in his bedside chair. Since he is confused he would not know if you used the lift or not.

What Is Your Response/Action?

1. What decision do you have to make?

2. What possible alternatives to following the policy might you have?

3. Would you consider documenting that you used the lift simply to satisfy policy, even though you did not use it? Why or why not?

4. What action will you take?

5. What did you learn about yourself in this situation?

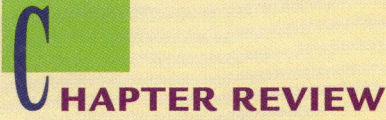

CHAPTER REVIEW

FILL IN THE BLANK

Read each sentence and fill in the blank lines with a word that completes the sentence.

1. _____ _____ _____ are special ways of standing and moving to make the best use of strength and to avoid fatigue.

2. A _____ is a covering used to provide privacy during an examination or operation.

3. _____ _____ positions are used to promote comfort and to relieve pressure points.

4. Whenever you are pushing a stretcher, you should be at the end where the patient's _____ is.

5. Use of a _____ _____ positioned snugly around the patient's waist will help you to control the patient while walking.

MULTIPLE CHOICE

Choose the best answer for each question or statement.

1. Which one of the following is not a guideline for proper body mechanics?
   a. Position your body close to the load.
   b. Lift and carry rather than push an object.
   c. Use good posture.
   d. Keep your feet slightly apart for better balance.

2. The supine position refers to which patient position?
   a. lying on back
   b. head of their bed up 45–90 degrees
   c. lying down or reclining with the knees bent, soles of the feet flat on the bed
   d. none of the above

3. Trendelenburg's position is used to treat patients who are experiencing
   a. cardiac arrest.
   b. diabetes.
   c. shock.
   d. seizures.

4. The dorsal lithotomy position is used for
   a. shock.
   b. physical exam of the bladder or vagina.
   c. physical exam of the patient's back.
   d. physical exam of the rectum.

5. When moving and lifting a patient, do all of the following except
   a. identify yourself and explain what you will do.
   b. give the most support to the heaviest parts of the body.
   c. move the patient with smooth and steady motions.
   d. move all patients by yourself.

6. Which of these activities is not a follow-up activity to report to the nurse?
   a. Reporting that the patient's position has been changed.
   b. How many people were required to move the patient.
   c. How the patient tolerated the move.
   d. The time of the position change.

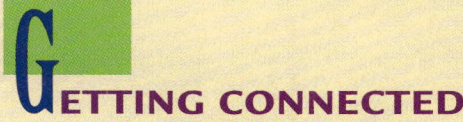

GETTING CONNECTED

MULTIMEDIA EXTENSION ACTIVITIES

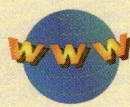

www.prenhall.com/wolgin

Use the above address to access the free, interactive Companion Website created for this textbook. Get hints, instant feedback, and textbook references to chapter-related multiple choice questions. Read and react to the "Nursing Assistants in Action." Link to other interesting sites.

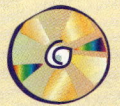

Audio Glossary

Use the CD-ROM disk enclosed with your textbook to hear the pronunciation of the key terms in the chapter.

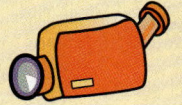

Video

Watch the "Body Mechanics" video and the "Transfer and Ambulation" video from the Care Provider Skills series.

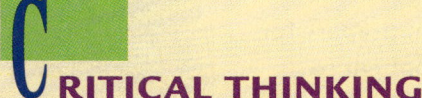

CRITICAL THINKING

USING KEY QUESTIONS

Read each question and think of what you might do in each situation.

1. You are walking down the hall with your patient, who suddenly says she feels faint and thinks she may fall. What do you do?

2. The nurse tells you that your patient is to have a vaginal exam. What position would you place her in?

3. What is the difference between an ambulatory and nonambulatory patient? How does this difference affect your procedures for moving a patient?

4. You are pushing your patient in a wheelchair and come upon a steep ramp. How should you proceed with your patient?

5. Why is draping important when examining a patient?

TIME OUT

TIPS FOR TIME MANAGEMENT

SELF-DISCIPLINE TIP   Ask for help when you need it. It is safer for you and for the patients if you have assistance with procedures that you cannot handle alone. Others with more experience may not require the same amount of help for the same things, but everyone needs help sometimes.

Admitting, Transferring, and Discharging a Patient

8

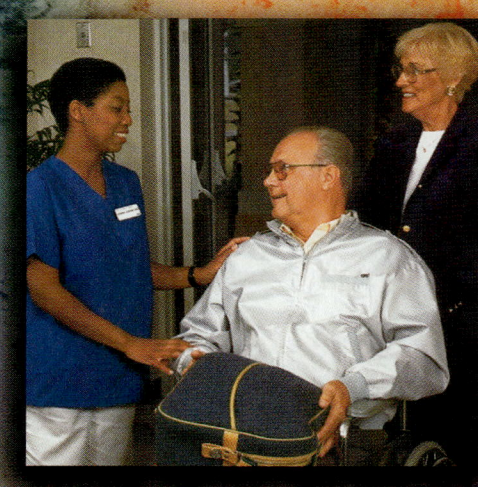

INTRODUCTION

The admission process is a patient's first glimpse of the individuals who will be providing health care. Nursing assistants can ease the patient's anxiety and help the patient prepare for whatever is ahead. Often, it is necessary for the patient to move from one room in an institution to another. Performing this procedure smoothly will ease anxiety and promote comfort for the patient in the new room. Finally, an expertly performed discharge procedure will increase the patient's confidence at home.

OBJECTIVES

When you have completed this chapter, you will be able to:

- Explain your role in following the patient plan of care.
- Admit a patient to the nursing unit by following the correct procedure.
- Weigh and measure a patient.
- Follow the correct procedure to transfer a patient to another room or unit within the institution.
- Describe the components of a discharge and patient health education plan and explain the importance of the plan.
- List the discharge planning activities.
- Discharge a patient from the institution following the correct procedure.
- Help make the patient feel comfortable and secure during all activities.

KEY TERMS

admission

assessing

convalescence

discharge

evaluating

holistic

implementing

patient plan of care

physiological

planning

psychological

sociocultural

spiritual

transfer

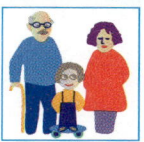

AGE-SPECIFIC CONSIDERATIONS

Admitting, Transferring, and Discharging a Patient

Being admitted to a health care facility or being transferred to a new place in a health care institution is a nervous time for patients of all ages. Children wonder what might happen to them and may be frightened of the equipment and noises of the environment. Allow parents to stay with the child as much as possible. Explain things to the child in simple language. Let the child touch and explore as much equipment as possible. For the adolescent, avoid the use of medical jargon. Maintain privacy, but let them know their parents are available if they want them. For adults and the elderly, give them as much decision making as possible. Explain things in terms that they can understand and allow time for questions and concerns.

At the time of discharge, prepare the patient to go home. For children, this might mean explaining in simple terms the healing process at home and any instructions. Most care needs will be handled by their parents. Adolescents will want to know more about what to do at home and about restrictions. Avoid the use of medical jargon. Answer questions directly with the adolescent and not just with the parents. When discharging the adult and the elderly patient, consider their lifestyles and learning preferences. Emphasize how the information will help them and allow time for questions.

ADMITTING THE PATIENT

admission The administrative process that covers the period from the time the patient enters the institution door to the time the patient is settled

A patient coming into a health care institution may be frightened and uncomfortable. The patient may or may not be seriously ill or in pain, but this is a time when you, as a member of the nursing team, are very important to the patient. Being pleasant and courteous from the time the patient enters the institution door until he is settled will make the patient's **admission** process easier.

KEY IDEA

A nice, relaxed environment and welcome will create a favorable first impression of the health care facility for the patient.

Introduce yourself (Figure 8–1). Learn the patient's name and use it often. Do not call an adult patient by the first name unless given permission to do so. Remember that the way you speak and behave will have a lot to do with the patient's impression of the institution. Smile and be friendly. Do not appear to be rushed or busy with other things. Do your work quietly and efficiently.

When admitting a patient to your institution, keep in mind the purpose for the patient's admission. A patient might be having surgery, undergoing a procedure, seeking treatment for an illness, or require long-term assistance with living.

Each institution will have its own policies and procedures for admitting a patient. The nursing team will provide the patient (and the patient's family) with general information to help them to become more familiar with the institution. This information includes a description of the unit's usual activities, usual meal times, information about any tests or procedures the patient is to have, and information about the visiting hours of the unit.

■ Patient Plan of Care

patient plan of care A written plan stating the nursing diagnosis, the patient goals or expected outcomes, and the nursing orders, interventions, or actions to be taken

Upon admission or shortly thereafter, an individualized **patient plan of care** is written by the registered nurse. This plan serves as a course of action to assist the patient to achieve optimum wellness (Figure 8–2). Patient plans of care are one way for the nursing

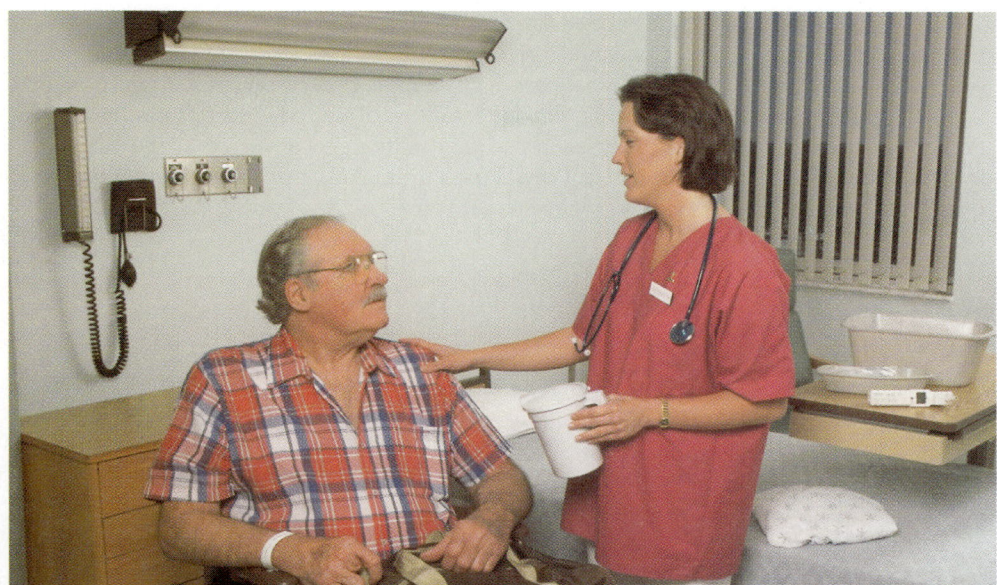

FIGURE 8–1

Help to make the admission of the patient as pleasant as possible

team to communicate. They provide a structure for **assessing**, **planning**, **implementing**, and **evaluating** individualized care. The assessing and planning stages involve gathering information to identify needs and problems and deciding what to do and how to do it; the implementing and evaluating stages involve carrying out the plan and then determining whether or not the plan worked. Each plan is written to meet the individual needs of the patient. One reason for the written care plan is to ensure that continuous and consistent care is provided for each patient. The registered nurse will review and discuss the patient's choices and decisions related to the patient's care. These choices and decisions will be reflected in the patient's plan of care.

The admitting registered nurse begins the plan by collecting information for a health history and completing a physical examination. Patient problems and nursing diagnoses are identified, long- and short-term goals are determined, and nursing interventions or actions are planned to help the patient reach these goals. The registered nurse reevaluates the plan of care daily to meet the changing needs of the patient. This reevaluation is continued until discharge and includes patient health education and a discharge plan. All members of the multidisciplinary health care team collaborate on the plan of care and assist the patient to reach the goals by carrying out the interventions written into the plan.

assessing Gathering facts to identify needs and problems

planning Deciding what to do and how to do it

implementing Carrying out or accomplishing a given plan

evaluating Determining whether a plan (such as the patient care plan) has been effective

NURSING CARE PLAN

DATE IDENTIFIED	NURSING DIAGNOSIS	DATE RESOLVED	PATIENT GOAL EXPECTED OUTCOME	NURSING ORDERS INTERVENTIONS/ ACTIONS

FIGURE 8–2

A sample care plan form

The parts of the plan of care most directly involving the nursing assistant are the activities of daily living, direct bedside care, and making and reporting objective, factual observations. Nursing assistants can observe and report patient progress toward meeting goals. (See Chapter 12 for a checklist of the activities of daily living.) The nursing assistant may read the plan of care for each assigned patient to ensure that the plan is followed. When the plan of care is well developed and used appropriately, it is the single most important tool in providing quality patient care.

PROCEDURE

OBRA

ADMITTING THE PATIENT

PREPARATION

1. Assemble your equipment on the bedside table:

   a. Admission checklist, if used in your institution

   b. Urine specimen container and laboratory requisition slip

   c. Institution gown or pajamas (if part of institutional policy)

   d. Clothing list

   e. Portable scale

   f. Blood pressure cuff and stethoscope

   g. Admission pack (contents vary in each health care institution)

   h. Thermometer

   i. Bedpan and/or urinal, emesis basin, and wash basin (may be in admission pack in some health care institutions)

2. Wash your hands.

3. Fan-fold the bed covers down to the foot of the bed to open the bed.

4. Place the hospital gown or pajamas at the foot of the bed.

5. Put the bedpan, urinal, emesis basin, wash basin, and admission pack in the proper place in the bedside table drawer or stand.

STEPS

6. When the patient arrives on the floor, introduce yourself to the patient and to any visitors. Smile, be friendly. Call the patient by his name. Offer to shake hands and tell the patient your name and job title.

7. Escort the patient to his room. The patient may be escorted to the room by an auxiliary worker. Introduce the patient to any roommates.

8. Ask the visitors to leave the room while you finish admitting the patient, if this is your hospital's policy.

9. Close the door in a private room, or draw the curtain around the bed for privacy.

10. Ask the patient to change into the hospital gown or his own pajamas. If necessary, help the patient get undressed and into the gown. Weigh the patient (see Procedure: Weighing and Measuring the Patient).

11. Help the patient to get into the bed or allow him to sit in a chair if he is not ordered on bedrest.

12. Raise the side rails on the bed, if necessary.

13. Complete the admission checklist of your institution (Figure 8–3).

14. Have the patient place any personal toilet articles and small belongings into or on top of the bedside table. If the patient is unable to do this, you may do it yourself.

15. Ask your immediate supervisor if the patient is NPO or is allowed to have drinking water. If drinking water is allowed, fill the water pitcher.

16. To familiarize the patient with his new surroundings, point out the signal cord or call bell (Figure 8–4). Attach the signal cord to the bed where the patient can reach it easily. Test the signal cord, demonstrating and explaining how the intercom system works. Permit the patient to try the signal cord light.

17. Explain the health care institution's policy on radios, television, newspapers, and mail. Tell the patient at what times his meals will be served. Help the patient to fill out the dietary slip for the next meal, if this is part of your institution's procedure.

18. Make the patient comfortable. Adjust the lights to the patient's preference. Be sure the top sheets and blankets are arranged properly.

19. If the patient is allowed to have the head of the bed elevated and the knee gatch adjusted as high or low as is comfortable, adjust these to a position of comfort. (Check before gatching the bed as a specific order may be required.) If the bed is self-adjustable, explain how the bed works and show the patient how to adjust it. Lower the bed to a position of safety for the patient.

20. Pull the curtains back to the open position.

PROCEDURE (CONTINUED)

ADMISSION CHECKLIST
(Fill in every statement and check every appropriate item)

Patient's name _____   Room Number _____

Time of admission _____ a.m./p.m.   Date of admission _____

Admitted by stretcher _____ wheelchair _____ walking _____

Check identification bracelet? Yes ☐ No ☐   Bed tag in place? Yes ☐ No ☐

Side rails up? Yes ☐ No ☐

Bruises, marks, rashes, or broken skin noted? Yes ☐ No ☐

    If yes, describe _____

Weight _____   Height _____   Scale used? Yes ☐ No ☐

Temperature _____   Pulse _____   Respirations _____   Blood Pressure _____

Admission urine specimen collected? Yes ☐ No ☐   Sent to lab? Yes ☐ No ☐

Is the patient allergic to food? Yes ☐ No ☐   Allergic to drugs? Yes ☐ No ☐

Reason for admission _____

Complaints _____

What are your concerns about this hospitalization (Circle all that apply)

    Illness   Test/procedures   Family   Job   Financial

    Surgery   Insurance   Other   None

Have you felt downhearted and blue or see things as hopeless? Yes ☐ No ☐

Do you know why? _____

_____

What is your source of hope and strength?

_____

Is there anything else we should know about in order to take care of you? (Dietary, cultural, religious needs or requests?) _____

_____

Highest grade in school completed: _____

How do you learn best? (Check all that apply)

    Reading   Videos

    Verbal instructions   Hands on   With Family Present   Interpreter needed:

Do you have difficulty with reading? Yes ☐ No ☐

Language spoken if not English: _____

Do you have education needs in any of these areas? (Circle all that apply)   Ability to learn or barriers to learning:

Activity/exercise   Coping/stress   Diet   Disease process

Wound/Incision care   Treatments   Medications   Self Care

Dentures? Yes ☐ No ☐   Partial? Yes ☐ No ☐   Full? Yes ☐ No ☐

    Denture Cup? Yes ☐ No ☐

Vision problems? Yes ☐ No ☐   Does the patient wear glasses? Yes ☐ No ☐   Contacts? Yes ☐ No ☐

Valuables: Money? Yes ☐ No ☐   Describe _____

    Jewelry? Yes ☐ No ☐   Describe _____

Is the patient hard of hearing? Yes ☐ No ☐   Hearing aid? Yes ☐ No ☐

    Artificial limb? Yes ☐ No ☐   Brace? Yes ☐ No ☐

Has the patient been admitted to this hospital before? Yes ☐ No ☐

Is the clothing list complete? Yes ☐ No ☐   Signed by _____

Is the signal cord attached to the bed? Yes ☐ No ☐

Have drugs brought into the hospital by the patient been given to the charge nurse? Yes ☐ No ☐

Name of the nurse drugs were given to _____

Was the patient told not to eat or drink anything until the doctor's visit? Yes ☐ No ☐

Admitted by _____

FIGURE 8–3

Admission checklist

PROCEDURE (CONTINUED)

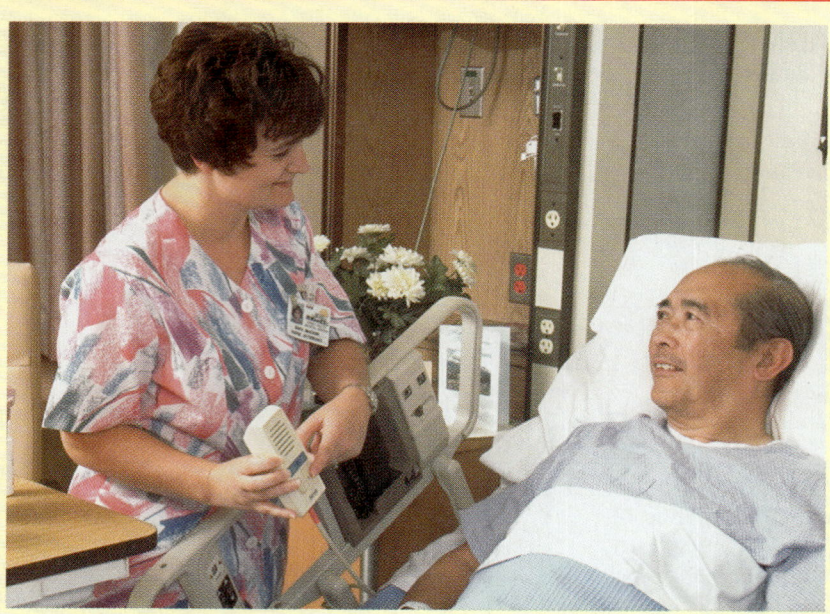

FIGURE 8–4
Point out the call button to the patient

21. Raise the side rails where ordered, indicated, and appropriate for patient safety.

FOLLOW-UP

22. Wash your hands.

23. Report to your immediate supervisor:

- That you have completed the admission.
- That the patient is in bed or sitting in a chair.
- That you have completed the admission checklist.
- That the side rails are in the up or down position.
- How the patient tolerated the procedure.
- Your observations of anything unusual.

There are several ways that the patient plan of care can help the nursing assistant provide quality care on a daily basis. The plan of care provides:

- Specific instructions regarding care to be given
- Information needed prior to giving care
- Guidelines for continuity of care
- Information essential for organizing and planning work or special duties

Each health care institution has its own policies and procedures related to the patient's plan of care. Be sure you understand and follow your employer's policies.

◼ Weighing and Measuring

Weights and heights are recorded to provide an important database. Accuracy is important because some medications are ordered based on weight. Nutrition problems are another area where weights are very important and used for comparison and progress evaluation.

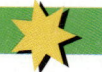

KEY IDEA

Many health care institutions have special equipment such as the scale with a mechanical lift for weighing the patient who is unable to stand. Some institutions have special scales with bars on them to assist the patient in standing straight and to keep the patient from falling. For example, a bed scale is used for the patient on complete bedrest. Follow your institution's procedures for these different types of scales. (Figure 8–5a-d)

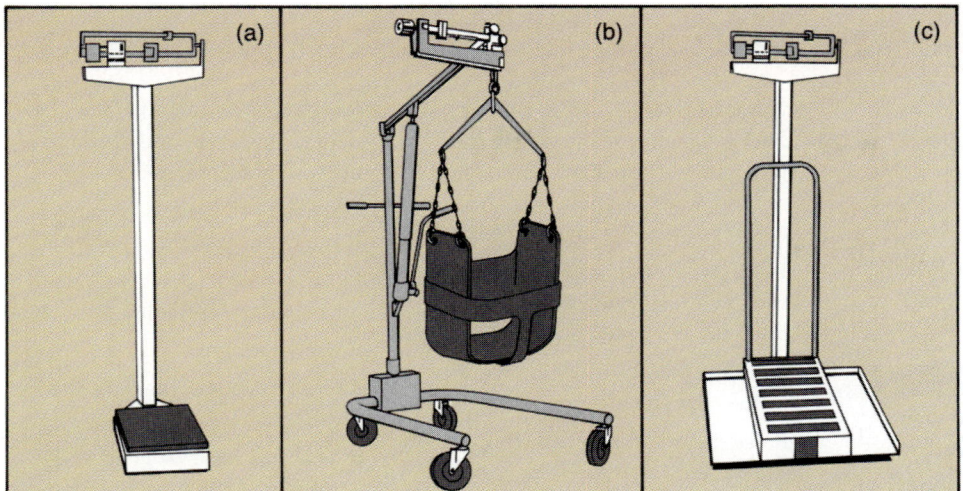

FIGURE 8–5

Types of scales: (a) Standing scale, (b) Scale with a mechanical lift, (c) Wheelchair scale, (d) Bed scale

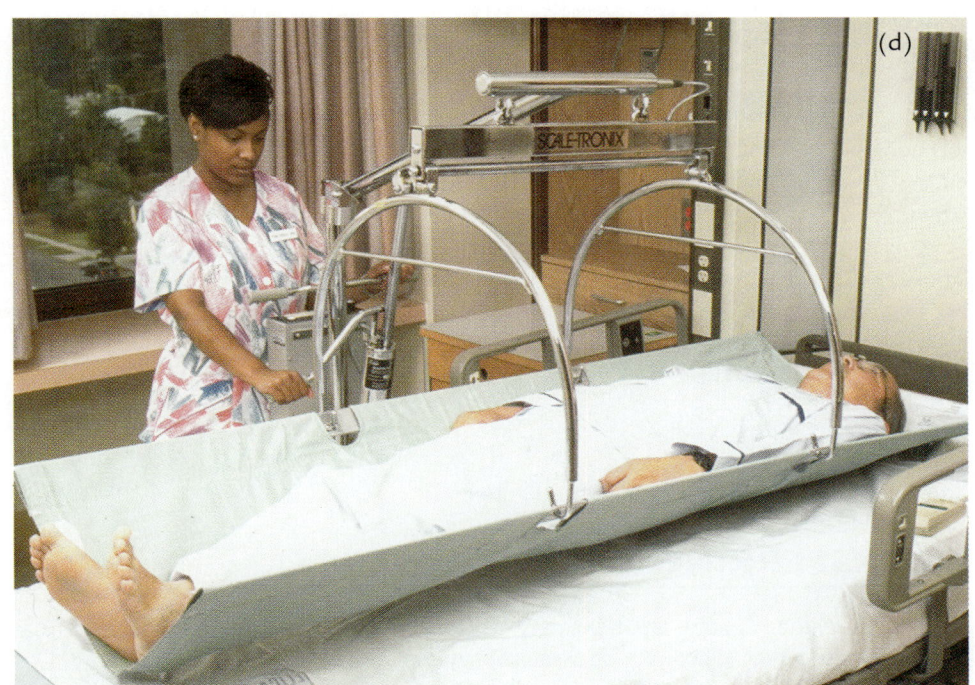

PROCEDURE

OBRA

WEIGHING AND MEASURING THE HEIGHT OF A PATIENT WHO IS ABLE TO STAND

PREPARATION

1. Assemble your equipment:

   a. Portable balance scale

   b. Paper towel

   c. Notepaper

   d. Pen or pencil

2. Wash your hands.

3. Identify the patient by checking the identification bracelet.

4. Ask visitors to step out of the room, if this is your hospital's policy.

5. Tell the patient that you are going to weigh her.

6. Pull the curtain around the bed for privacy.

PROCEDURE (CONTINUED)

7. Balance the scale. To do this, make sure the scale is standing level. Both weights (poises) must point to zero (0). If they do not, turn the balance screw until the pointer of the balance beam stays steadily in the middle of the balance area. The scale is now balanced.

STEPS

8. Help the patient to stand with both feet firmly on the scale.

9. Ask the patient to place both hands at her side.

10. Adjust the weights (poises) until the balance pointer is again in the middle of the balance area.

11. Note the patient's weight by adding together the numbers on both the large balance and the small balance. Write it down on the notepaper.

12. Raise the measuring rod above the patient's head.

13. Have the patient turn so that her back is against the measuring rod. Be sure that the patient is standing as straight as possible, with her heels touching the measuring bar.

14. Bring the measuring rod down so that it rests horizontally on the patient's head.

15. Note the patient's height. Write it down on the notepaper.

16. Raise the measuring rod. Help the patient to step off the scale.

17. Assist the patient back into bed or help the patient to put on her robe and slippers.

FOLLOW-UP

18. Make the patient as comfortable as possible.

19. Lower the bed to a position of safety for the patient.

20. Pull the curtains back to the open position.

21. Raise the side rails where ordered, indicated, and appropriate for patient safety.

22. Place the call light within easy reach of the patient.

23. Put the scale back where it belongs. Clean if soiled.

24. Wash your hands.

25. Report to your immediate supervisor:

   - That you have weighed and measured the height of the patient.

   - Note if the patient has dressings or braces, as this must be considered for the correct weight.

   - The patients's weight and height.

   - How the patient tolerated the procedure.

   - Your observations of anything unusual.

TRANSFERRING THE PATIENT

During the patient's stay, a patient may be transferred from one unit or facility to another (Figure 8–6). This may be done for several reasons:

- The patient may have requested a private room, but none was available at the time of admission

- The patient may ask to be transferred from a private room to a semiprivate room

- The patient may be moved to another unit because of a change in the patient's medical condition

transfer Moving a hospital patient from one room, unit, or facility to another

The patient may become alarmed if a doctor orders a **transfer**. In this case, try to calm the patient. Explain that the change is being made for the patient's benefit. Before you help in transferring the patient, be sure his new unit is ready.

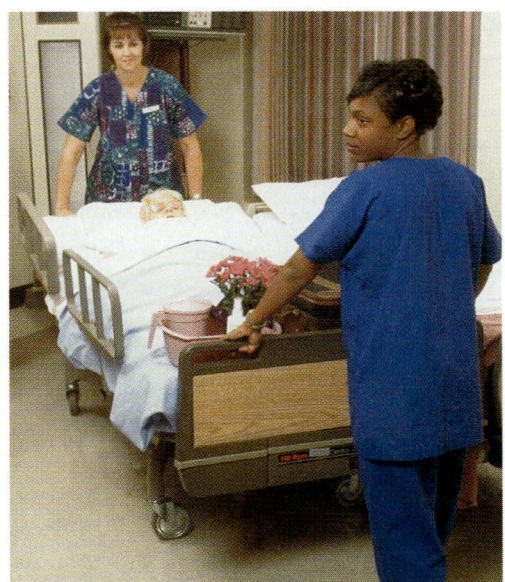

FIGURE 8–6
Transferring a patient

PROCEDURE

OBRA

TRANSFERRING THE PATIENT

PREPARATION

1. Assemble your equipment, according to the needs of the patient:
   a. Wheelchair
   b. Stretcher or the patient's bed
   c. Cart

2. Check to be sure the new unit is ready to receive the patient.

3. Wash your hands.

4. Identify the patient by checking the identification bracelet.

5. Ask visitors to step out of the room, if this is your hospital's policy.

6. Tell the patient you are going to transfer her to her new room.

7. Collect the patient's personal belongings, patient's record, and equipment that are to be moved with her.

STEPS

8. Transport the patient to the new unit:
   a. The patient can be moved in her own bed from one room to another. Personal belongings can be placed on the bed and moved with the patient. Or, if she has many personal articles, you may use a cart to move them.
   b. You may have to transport the patient by stretcher or wheelchair to her new room. Here you will help the patient from the stretcher or wheelchair into her new bed. In these cases, put the patient's belongings and equipment on a cart. Move them after the patient is settled and safe in the new unit.

9. Follow all safety precautions when wheeling the patient to her new unit. (Some institutions have a transportation service that does this for you.)

10. Give the patient both physical and emotional support (Figure 8–7). For example, she may need to be reassured that her family and visitors will be given her new room number.

11. Introduce the patient to her new roommate.

12. Make the patient comfortable in her new room.

13. Introduce her to the nursing staff who will be caring for her. Hand the patient's record to the clerk or nursing caregiver accepting the patient.

14. Arrange the room. Help the patient to put away her personal items or possessions.

15. Lower the bed to a position of safety for the patient.

16. Pull the curtains back to the open position.

PROCEDURE (CONTINUED)

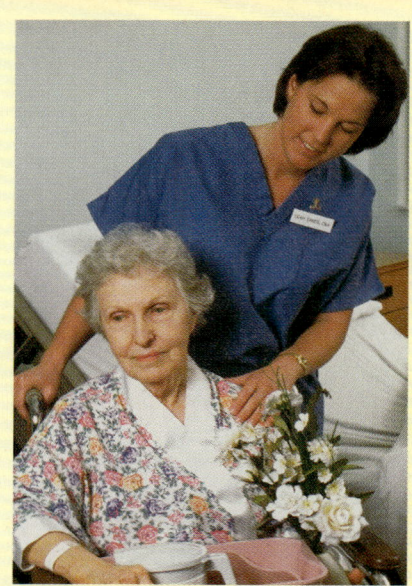

FIGURE 8–7
Give both physical and emotional support

17. Raise the side rails where ordered, indicated, and appropriate for patient safety.

18. Place the call light within easy reach of the patient.

FOLLOW-UP

19. Wash your hands.

20. Report to the nurse manager or team leader in the new nursing unit that the patient is now in the new unit. Describe how the patient reacted to the transfer.

21. Return to your own floor. Strip the bed and take the equipment that was not transferred to the dirty utility room, or follow the procedure used in your institution.

22. Wash your hands.

23. Report to your immediate supervisor:
    - That the patient has been transferred to the new unit.
    - The time of the transfer.
    - The patient's reaction to the transfer.
    - Your observations of anything unusual.

discharge The official procedure for helping patients to leave the health care institution, including teaching them how to care for themselves at home

DISCHARGING THE PATIENT

Written permission from a doctor is required for the patient to be **discharged**, or officially processed out of the health care institution. Your supervisor will tell you when the doctor has ordered that the patient is to be discharged.

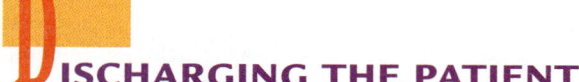
KEY IDEA

If the patient wants to leave and you have not been told that the discharge order has been written by the physician, report this to your immediate supervisor immediately.

In many institutions, the patient must be taken to the business office, cashier, or discharge desk before the patient leaves the facility. (In certain instances a member of the patient's family may do this.)

A patient is sometimes discharged from one health care institution to another, for example, from a hospital to a nursing home. This patient may leave the facility in an ambulance. Your immediate supervisor will give you special instructions for the care of this patient. Some patients may require a caregiver or nurse to accompany them in transfer.

Normally, there is a certain hour by which most patients are discharged. This is so that the room can be cleaned and made ready for new patients, who are often admitted early in the afternoon.

■ Discharge and Health Teaching

As a result of the DRGs (diagnosis-related groups) system of Medicare payment to health care institutions, patients are staying in health care institutions for shorter periods of time. This means the patients may have a longer **convalescence,** or recovery period, at home.

convalescence The period of recovery after illness or surgery

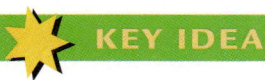

Teaching patients how to care for themselves at home is the responsibility of the entire nursing team.

The nurse will instruct you as to your part in the patient's health teaching as written in the policies of your health care institution. The patient's family should be included in the education process whenever possible. The plan for discharge and health education is of vital importance to the well-being of the patient following discharge from the health care institution.

Four important factors must be included in the discharge and health teaching plan to meet the needs of the whole patient. This is often referred to as the **holistic** approach. It must reflect the four dimensions of the whole "person" who is the patient. They are:

holistic An approach that reflects the four dimensions of a "whole" person: physiological, psychological, sociocultural, and spiritual

- **Physiological:** as seen in a person's biological response (physical changes) to alterations in the body's structures and functions

- **Psychological:** as seen in a person's cognitive (level of knowledge) and emotional responses to himself and the surrounding environment

- **Sociocultural:** as seen in a person's noninherited intra- and interpersonal responses to socialization practices learned and transmitted from families and communities

- **Spiritual:** as seen in a person's personal response to inspirational forces

physiological Referring to a person's biological response to alterations in the body's structures and functions

psychological Referring to a person's cognitive and emotional responses to the self and the surrounding environment

Your immediate supervisor will include the following topics in the discharge instructions and patient health education plan.

Explanation of the patient's disease/disorder:

- History and/or explanation of disease or disorder

- Signs and symptoms expected and those not expected

- What to report to the physician

sociocultural Referring to a person's interpersonal responses to socialization practices in the family and community

Explanation of medications as ordered by the physician:

- Name of medication

- Dose: how much the patient is to take

- The correct times to take the medication

- The purpose and expected effects of the medication

- Signs and symptoms of side effects of the medication

- What to report to the physician

spiritual Referring to an individual's personal response to inspirational forces

Explanation of treatments ordered by the physician:

- Purpose of treatments

- Time of treatments

- How to perform treatments

- Return demonstrations of treatments

- What to report to the physician

Explanation of nutrition and diet:

- Type of diet ordered by physician
- Foods allowed and disallowed on this diet
- Amounts of food to be consumed
- Available home health agencies for help; name, phone number, and address

Explanation of care in the home environment:

- Elimination of hazards in the home environment
- Available transportation to the physician's office or clinic
- Available housekeeping services
- Available economic support agencies; name, phone number, and address

Explanation of progression of activities of daily living:

- Outline activities of daily living for the first two weeks following hospitalization, with progressive activities
- Signs and symptoms of inability to perform activities
- What to report to the physician

Explanation of future appointments that have been made with the physician or clinic:

- Time and date of appointment
- Name of physician and/or clinic
- Phone number and address of physician or clinic
- The reason why these future appointments are necessary for follow-up care

Explanation of referral agencies:

- Names of agencies
- Address of agencies
- Phone number of agencies
- Name of contact person at the agency

Discharge Planning

Your immediate supervisor is responsible for the following discharge planning activities. You will be instructed on what you should do as your part of this discharge plan. Be sure to follow your immediate supervisor's instructions.

Your immediate supervisor will:

- Start discharge planning at the time of admission.
- Work with the physician, health care team members, case manager, social worker, dietitian, family, and significant others.
- Contact the necessary community agencies for referral, if necessary. Include the discharge plan in patient education with family members and/or significant others present when possible.
- Assess the patient's ability for self-care in the home setting.
- Give the patient and/or family members a written plan for all medications (stating time and amount), exercises, and any other pertinent data.

- Make future appointments in the physician's office, clinic, health agency, outpatient department, physical therapy, and social services, as indicated.

- Give the patient and/or family members a written schedule of appointments (date and time). Discuss activities of daily living with the patient and interested family members.

- Give the patient and family members a written outline for any exercises or special activities.

- Advise proper time for continuance of normal activities and lifestyle. Advise patient and/or family members to call, giving the phone number and extension, if they have any questions after they get home.

- Document the entire discharge plan and the patient's reaction to the plan on the permanent record.

- If permitted by your institution's policies, give the patient a copy of the discharge checklist.

PROCEDURE

OBRA

DISCHARGING THE PATIENT

PREPARATION

1. Assemble your equipment, according to the needs of the patient:
   a. Wheelchair
   b. Stretcher
   c. Discharge slip, if used in your institution
   d. Cart
2. Wash your hands.
3. Identify the patient by checking the identification bracelet.

STEPS

4. Help the patient collect and pack personal possessions (Figure 8–8).
5. Be sure all valuables and medications are returned to the patient.
6. Help the patient get dressed, if necessary.

7. Check that the written instructions are given to the patient by your immediate supervisor, such as:
   a. Doctor's orders to follow at home
   b. Prescriptions
   c. Follow-up schedule of appointments with the doctor or clinic

8. Bring the wheelchair to the patient's bedside and help the patient into it.

9. Before wheeling the patient off the floor, get the discharge slip from your immediate supervisor.

10. Take the patient in the wheelchair to the discharge desk,

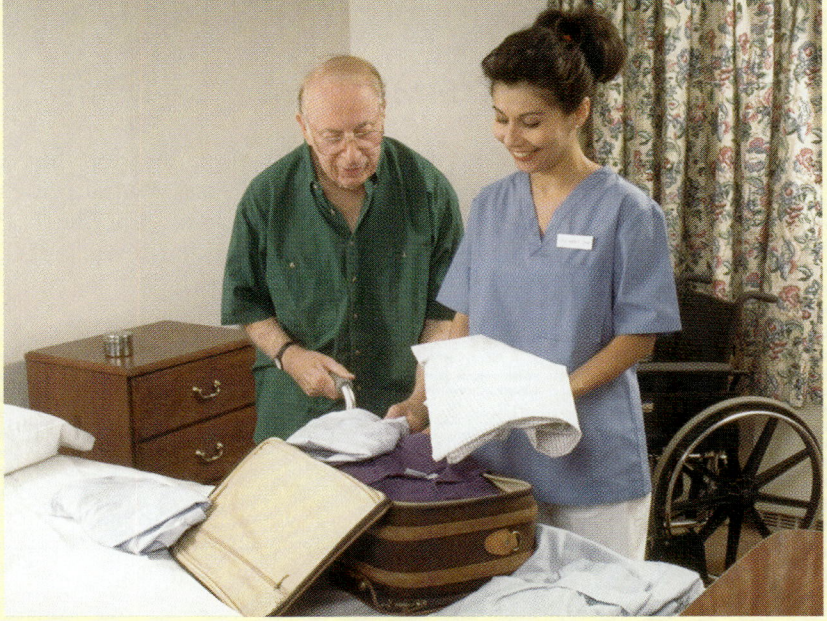

FIGURE 8–8
Help the patient collect and pack personal possessions

PROCEDURE (CONTINUED)

cashier, or business office, if the patient's family has not already done so. Give the clerk the discharge slip. Get a release form in return.

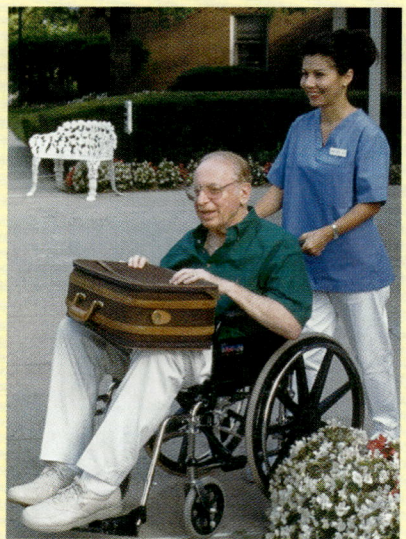

FIGURE 8–9
Wheel the patient to the door

11. Wheel the patient to the front door. Help the patient out of the wheelchair and into his car (Figure 8–9).

12. Say goodbye to the patient.

13. Take the wheelchair and release form back to the floor.

FOLLOW-UP

14. Strip the linen from the bed unless this is done by the environmental services department in your institution. Place it in the dirty linen hamper.

15. Notify the environmental service or housekeeping department that the discharge has taken place and the unit is ready to be cleaned.

16. Wash your hands.

17. Give your supervisor the release form from the business office, cashier, or discharge desk. Then report to your immediate supervisor:

- That the patient has been discharged.
- The time of the discharge.
- The type of transportation used for the discharge.
- Who accompanied the patient: husband, wife, daughter, friend.
- That patient was given a copy of the discharge.
- Patient's reaction to the discharge.
- That environmental service has been notified that the unit is ready to be cleaned.
- Your observations of anything unusual.

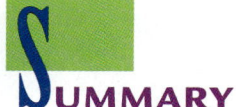

SUMMARY

Nursing assistants can significantly affect the way the patient experiences the admission, transfer, and discharge processes. By following the patient plan of care as well as proper admitting, transfer, and discharge procedures, the nursing assistant can help the patient to feel comfortable, cared for, and secure in the health care environment.

Notes

Patient Plans to Leave Without Medical Approval

THE NURSING ASSISTANT IN ACTION

You are talking with Melissa B., a 17-year-old patient in the medical unit. Melissa tells you, "Don't tell anyone but I'm going to get out of here tonight. When my boyfriend comes to visit we are going to ask to go downstairs for a Coke. But then we are going to go right on out the door. I don't want my parents to know where I am. I just have to be alone with my boyfriend for awhile." Melissa does not have a discharge order in her chart, and in fact, is scheduled for more tests the next day.

What Is Your Response/Action?

1. What are the important pieces of information in this situation?

2. What possible responses could you make to Melissa?

3. What action will you take?

4. Where does patient confidentiality fit into this situation?

5. What did you learn that you can apply in other situations?

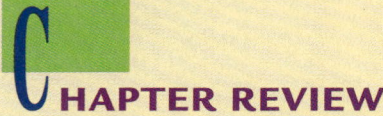HAPTER REVIEW

FILL IN THE BLANK

Read each sentence and fill in the blank line with a word that completes the sentence.

1. The process that covers the time when the patient enters the institution until they are settled in is called

   _____.

2. Do not use an adult's first name without first being given _____.

3. Using a _____ lift is often a good idea for patients who cannot stand by themselves.

4. _____ permission is needed from a physician prior to a patient being discharged.

5. The _____ approach to care includes the physiological, psychological, sociocultural, and spiritual aspects of the patient.

MULTIPLE CHOICE

Choose the best answer for each question or statement.

1. A nice, relaxed environment and a warm welcome will create a favorable first impression of the institution for the patient.
   a. True
   b. False

2. The patient plan of care is written by the registered nurse and serves as a guide or suggestion for the care the patient is to receive.
   a. True
   b. False

3. The weight of the patient is very important because
   a. it will determine the final cost of care.
   b. it will determine who is treated first.
   c. it will be used to determine the dose of some medications.
   d. All of the above.

4. Patients may be transferred to any of the following except
   a. to another hospital.
   b. to another room.
   c. to another unit.
   d. to a school.

5. When discharging a patient, do all of the following except
   a. wash your hands.
   b. help the patient collect and pack her belongings.
   c. have the patient take his dirty linen home.
   d. make sure the patient takes home all his written instructions.

6. Written discharge instructions often include the medications the patient is to take at home, activity restrictions, diet instructions, and dates of return appointments.
   a. True
   b. False

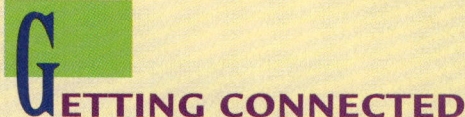

GETTING CONNECTED

MULTIMEDIA EXTENSION ACTIVITIES

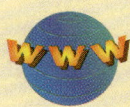

www.prenhall.com/wolgin

Use the above address to access the free, interactive Companion Website created for this textbook. Get hints, instant feedback, and textbook references to chapter-related multiple choice questions. Read and react to the "Nursing Assistants in Action." Link to other interesting sites.

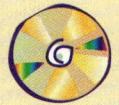

Audio Glossary

Use the CD-ROM disk enclosed with your textbook to hear the pronunciation of the key terms in the chapter.

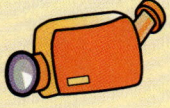

Video

Watch the "Lifting Techniques" section of the "Body Mechanics" video and the "Transfer and Ambulation" video from the Care Provider Skills series.

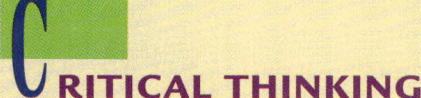

CRITICAL THINKING

USING KEY QUESTIONS

Read each question and think of what you might do in each situation.

1. As a nursing assistant, how can you use the nursing care plan?

2. Describe things that you can do to welcome a patient and his or her family to your institution?

3. What types of equipment are necessary to admit a patient to your institution?

4. What are the different types of scales available to weigh a patient in your institution?

5. What can you do to help a patient settle into a new room after a transfer?

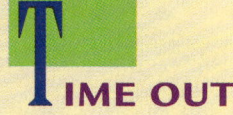

TIME OUT

TIPS FOR TIME MANAGEMENT

ORGANIZING TIP When you help with the discharge or transfer of a patient, use a methodical approach, such as beginning at the top drawer of the night stand and emptying all belongings into a bag or suitcase. Progress down the night stand, then empty the closet. Remove the patient's belongings from the trays in the overbed table. Then check the bathroom and under the bed. This will prevent spending time later looking for a belonging that was left behind.

The Patient's Environment

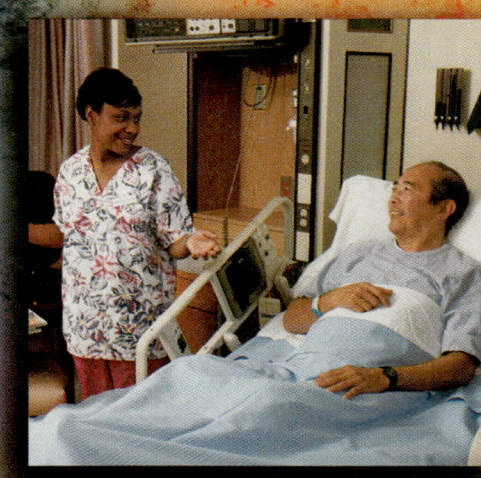

9

INTRODUCTION

One of the responsibilities of a nursing assistant is to maintain the patient's room and general environment in a tidy and organized manner. The environment must be convenient for the patient, while affording the space needed for the nursing assistant and others to perform their work. This chapter addresses the needs of the patient's environment, including various supplies and equipment, along with ideas for maintaining the space. You will review the typical room arrangement as well as safety tips to assist you in avoiding accidents while providing a safer environment for the patient. Some health care facilities or agencies refer to the person receiving care as patient, resident, or client depending on the setting in which care is provided. These references are made from time to time within this chapter when referring to a patient in a hospital, long-term care facility, or home setting.

When you have completed this chapter, you will be able to:

- Describe the typical patient's unit and list the equipment it contains.
- Check the unit for convenience to the patient, organization, and safety.
- Describe the purpose of each piece of equipment.
- Create an appropriate environment in the home in which to provide care for the patient.
- Provide a safe environment for the patient by eliminating safety hazards and anticipating safety needs.

KEY TERMS

alternating-pressure mattress

bed cradle

bedpan

Central Supply Department

disposable equipment

emesis basin

equipment

flammable

intravenous pole

lamb's wool

patient lift

patient unit

specialty bed

stretcher

urinal

walker

wheelchair

THE PATIENT'S UNIT

The **patient unit** consists of all the room space, furniture, and **equipment** provided by the hospital for one patient. Each unit can be screened off for privacy by draw curtains (Figure 9–1).

After a patient has been assigned to the unit for which you are responsible, make sure everything that belongs in the unit is there and in its proper place. If the patient is left handed, put the bedside stand and call light near the left hand; if the patient is right handed, place them near the right hand.

A hospital unit designed for children may be different from an adult unit (Figure 9–2). A child's age and the reason for the hospitalization will determine how the unit is arranged and the equipment that will be needed.

The unit should be arranged for the convenience of the patient. The call light system must be easily accessible for the patient, along with items of importance such as eyeglasses and the telephone (Figure 9–3). Depending on the patient's needs, other items may need to be close also (such as a urinal or emesis basin). When you straighten the room throughout your shift, consider how it should be arranged in anticipation of what will be happening. For example, the over bed table should be cleared prior to a meal tray being delivered. If a procedure is to be done, space will need to be prepared for the supplies used in that procedure. Keeping the room tidy and organized is a priority so that the patient and family are comfortable and care can be provided without clutter or obstacles in the way.

patient unit The space for one patient, including the hospital bed, bedside table, chair, and other equipment

equipment Materials, tools, devices, supplies, furnishings, necessary things used to perform a task

FIGURE 9–1

Adjust curtain for the patient's privacy

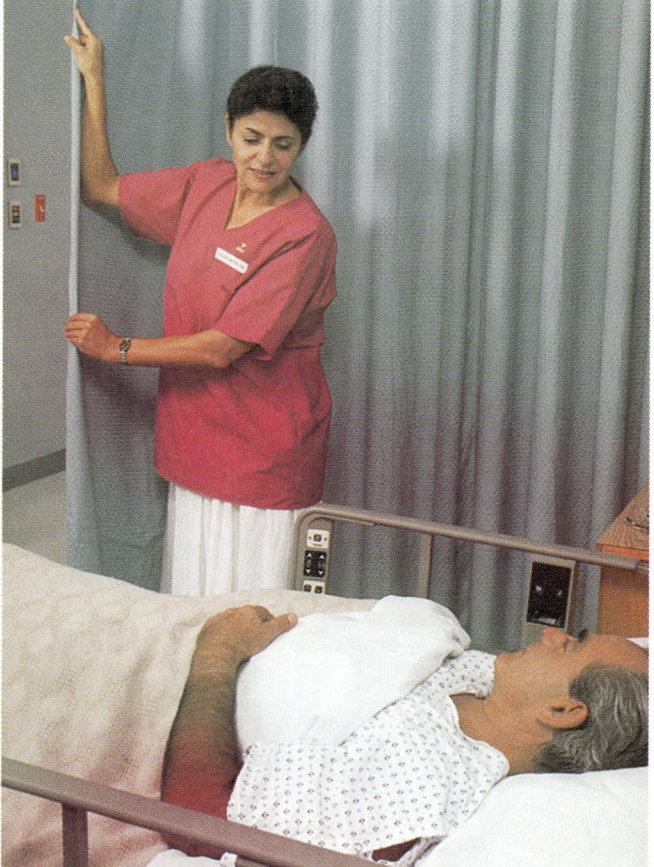

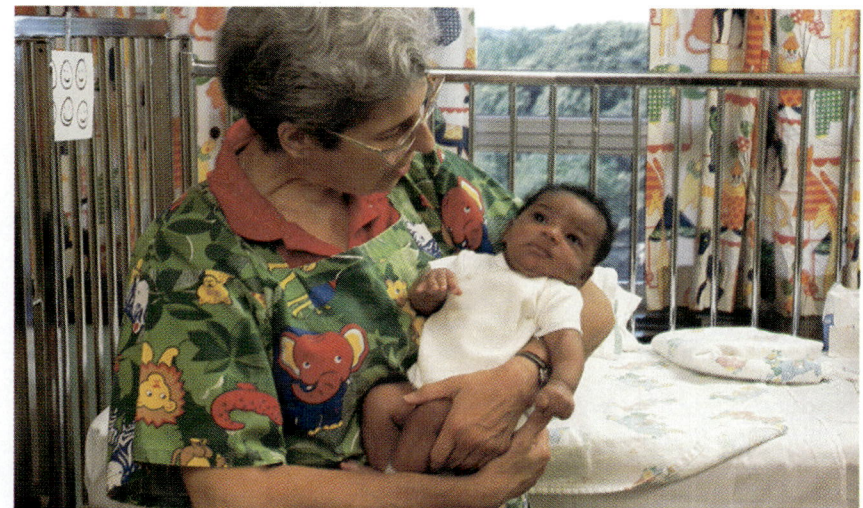

FIGURE 9–2
The pediatric unit

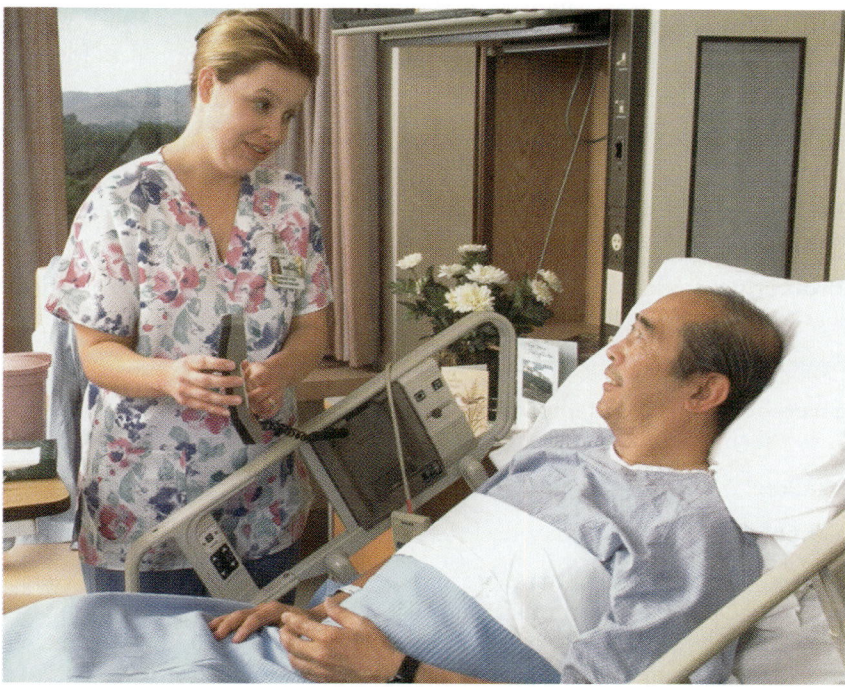

FIGURE 9–3
Check the patient's unit; place the call light and the patient's personal items within easy reach

■ Equipment

The modern health care facility has many pieces of equipment needed for patient care and treatment. This equipment might include:

- **Alternating-pressure (A-P) mattress:** A device like an air mattress placed beneath a bedridden or elderly patient or a patient at risk for pressure ulcers. It reduces pressure on the head, shoulders, back, heels, elbows, and bony or prominent surfaces.

- **Bed board:** A large board placed beneath the mattress to provide additional support for patients with back, muscle, or bone problems.

- **Bed cradle:** This cradle looks like a half-barrel cut the long way (Figure 9–4). It is used to cover a part of the patient's body where she is having great pain, to eliminate pressure and to support the weight of the top linen, to eliminate additional pain in the area, or when you do not want anything to touch that area.

alternating-pressure mattress A pad similar to an air mattress that can be placed beneath the patient to reduce pressure on the head, shoulders, back, heels, elbows, and bony prominences

bed cradle A frame shaped like a barrel cut in half lengthwise used to keep bed linens off a part of the patient's body

FIGURE 9–4

The bed cradle is used to keep bed linens off a part of the patient's body

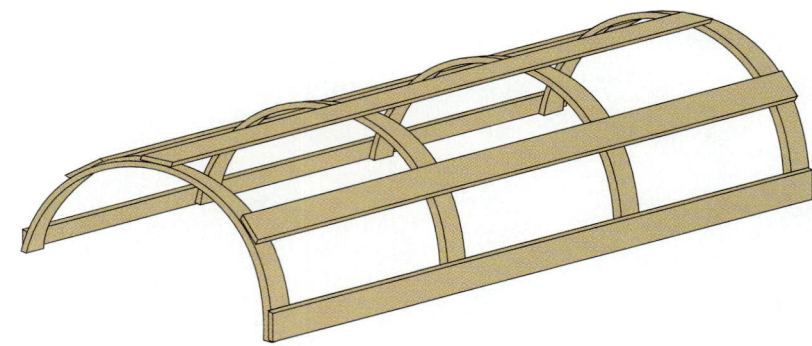

intravenous pole A tall pole, also called IV pole, which attaches to a bed or is on rollers or casters; this pole is used to hold the containers or tubes needed, for example, during a blood transfusion

lamb's wool A wide strip of lamb's hide with the fleece attached or an imitation material used to increase patient comfort

patient lift A mechanical device with a sling seat used for lifting a patient into and out of such equipment as the hospital bed, bathtub, or wheelchair

specialty bed A bed that constantly changes pressure under the patient. Used to minimize pressure points in the treatment or prevention of pressure ulcers

stretcher A narrow rolling table with or without a mattress or simply a canvas stretched over a frame used to transport patients; the latter may also be called a litter or a gurney

walker A stable frame made of metal tubing used to support the unsteady patient while walking; the patient holds the walker while taking a step, moves it forward, and takes another step

wheelchair A chair on wheels used to transport patients

disposable equipment Equipment that is used one time only or for one patient only and then thrown away

Central Supply Department A central place for storing supplies and equipment, also called special purchasing department or central supply department

- **Binders:** Strips of heavy cotton cloth with Velcro fasteners. Binders are wrapped securely around the patient's body over the abdomen to give support and comfort following abdominal surgery.

- **Foot board:** A small board placed upright at the foot of the bed and used to keep the patient's feet aligned properly to prevent foot drop.

- **Intravenous poles:** These are called IV poles. They support the bags and tubes used in various treatments. Some IV poles are on casters or rollers for easy movement. Other IV poles fit into the bed frame.

- **Lamb's wool:** Wide strips of lamb's wool cloth (or soft synthetic materials) used to increase patient comfort.

- **Portable patient lift:** A mechanical device used to move the patient from bed to chair and back again when the patient needs full assistance.

- **Protective devices:** Devices, usually of cotton, used to restrain a patient's arms, legs, or body to prevent him from self-injury.

- **Specialty bed:** Used to eliminate pressure points and prevent pressure ulcers.

- **Stretcher:** A narrow table with a mattress on wheels used to transport patients. Also called a litter, gurney, or cart.

- **Walker:** A supportive device used by the patient for help in walking.

- **Wheelchair:** A chair with wheels used to transport patients.

A number of the preceding items are shown in Figure 9–5. Other equipment may be used at a particular hospital or health care facility. The nursing assistant will be expected to be familiar with many pieces of equipment and know how to operate, maintain, and clean it. When unfamiliar with the equipment, the nursing assistant must ask for an in-service or review instructions prior to working with the item.

Disposable Equipment

Today, in many health care facilities, reusable equipment has been replaced by **disposable equipment** (Figure 9–6). Reusable equipment requires washing and disinfecting. Disposable equipment needs almost no care and is usually prepackaged. It may be made of plastic or paper. Some of this equipment is used only one time and then thrown away. Other disposable equipment may be used several times for one patient only, being cleaned between uses and thrown away when the patient is discharged, or sent home with the patient.

Nursing assistants usually get disposable equipment from the **Central Supply Department** as needed. Central Supply may also be called Supply Processing and Distribution. This is a central place for storing supplies and equipment. You may need a written or computer generated requisition slip to get equipment from Central Supply. In some facilities, disposable equipment is stored in a clean utility room in each area, which is kept stocked by the Central Supply Department.

FIGURE 9–5
Health care equipment

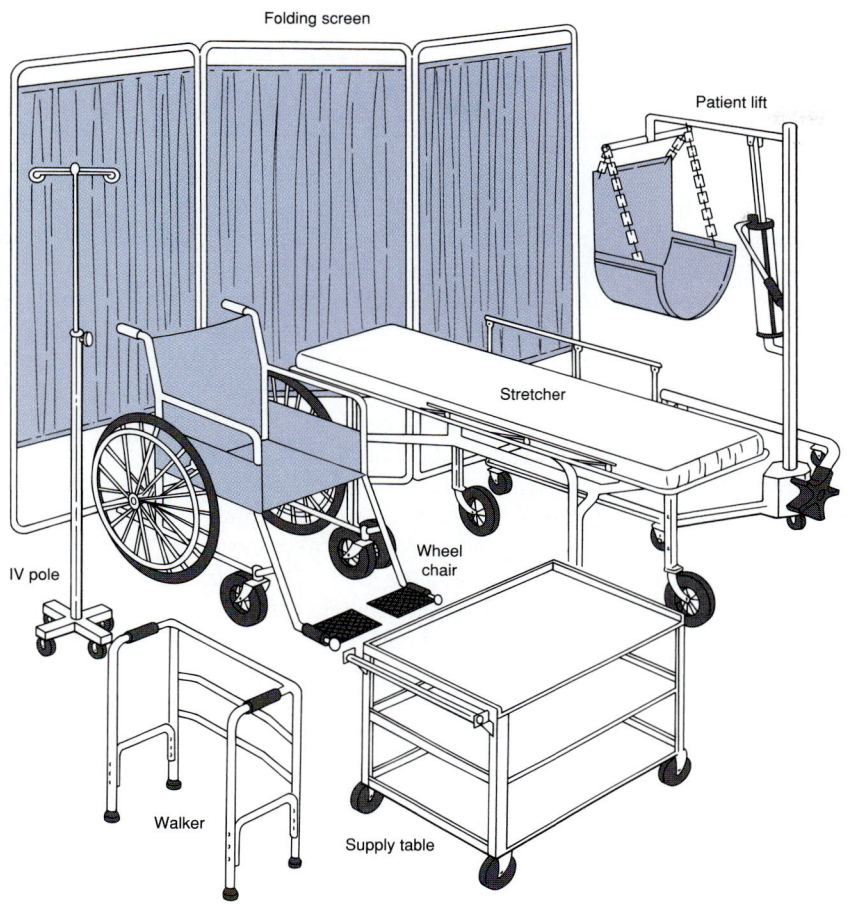

Folding screen

Patient lift

Stretcher

IV pole

Wheel chair

Walker

Supply table

FIGURE 9–6
Disposable equipment

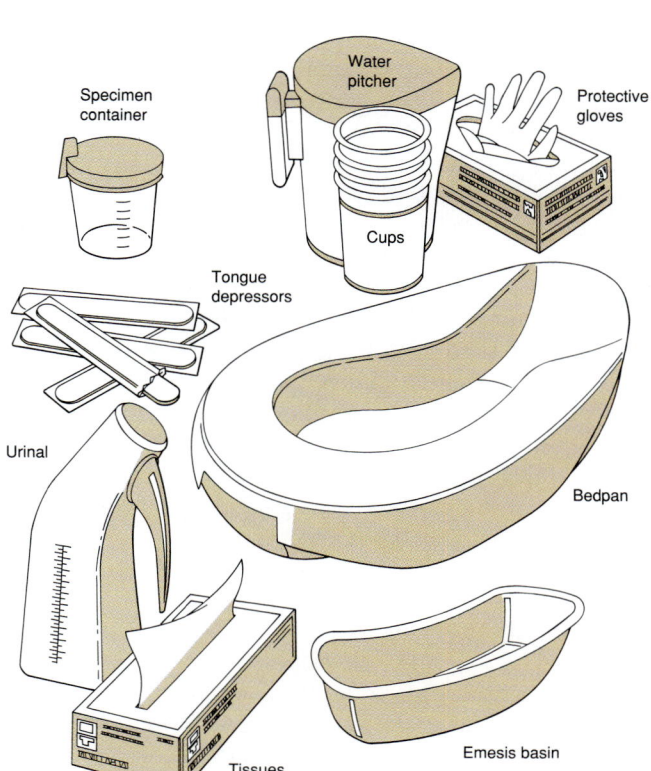

Specimen container

Water pitcher

Protective gloves

Cups

Tongue depressors

Urinal

Bedpan

Tissues

Emesis basin

bedpan A pan used by patients who must defecate or urinate while in bed

emesis basin A pan used for catching material that a patient spits out, vomits, or expectorates

urinal A portable container given to male patients in bed so they can urinate without getting out of bed

CREATING A COMFORTABLE ENVIRONMENT

Patients must be made to feel comfortable in their environment. The hospital room is the patient's environment during a stay in the hospital. The room temperature, lighting, position of the bed, and the volume of the TV and telephone should be adjusted to suit the patient, unless conditions do not allow it or it interferes with another patient. Always respect the privacy of the patient, realizing that the room is the *patient's* while they are hospitalized. Knock on the patient's door before entering and wait for acknowledgment from the patient (if the patient is able to respond). Provide privacy for the patient by drawing the curtain or closing the door when activity or procedures might expose the patient. Provide comfort for the patient in any way possible such as repositioning, providing extra blankets, refilling the water pitcher, or meeting other needs.

In addition to these considerations, when caring for a patient in a long-term care environment, the nursing assistant will find other ways in which a patient may be made more comfortable. Long-term care patients, referred to as residents, bring furniture and personal belongings to the facility to decorate their rooms and make them more like home. As a nursing assistant, you will be responsible for protecting these items on behalf of the resident. To make a resident more comfortable, you may seat him in a favorite chair, play the resident's favorite music on the stereo, or utilize other personal items to aid the resident. In each situation, you will demonstrate respect for the resident's belongings. As in the hospital setting, knock before entering a resident's room.

CARING FOR A PATIENT IN A HOME SETTING

Working in the home environment presents slightly different challenges. The atmosphere and life style will be different in every home in which you work. You must respect the rights of your patient (client) and his family to have beliefs and opinions, culture, and customs that might be different from your own. People of different backgrounds may eat foods you have never seen or tasted; they may behave differently toward their family members than you would; their religious beliefs may seem unusual to you; and their standards of cleanliness or general life style may be different from yours. Accept these differences with respect and understanding, without judging or criticizing. Let your patient, the client, know it is your pleasure, not just your job, to assist him. Recognize you are a guest in your patient's home.

Be careful in the home not to disturb the patient's personal belongings, letters, pictures, and the like. You may suggest they be moved, however, to another place so that you can give better care. It is also important that you not perform heavy cleaning chores, such as moving heavy furniture, waxing floors, shampooing carpets, washing windows, and carrying firewood. You are there to provide care and comfort measures, as you would if the patient were in the hospital. The patient may need equipment or supplies similar to those used in the hospital. If you determine a need for these items, they can be provided in the home to facilitate the patient's care.

■ Safety

You can create a safe environment for your patient and yourself by eliminating, preventing, or correcting conditions that could cause accidents. Safety includes proper infection control, electrical and fire safety, and accident prevention.

As you go about your work, be alert and look for the hazards listed below. Make a note of these things and bring them to the attention of the patient, family member, or your supervisor, whichever is appropriate. Some of the most common safety hazards in the home are:

- Damaged electrical wiring on large and small appliances or equipment

- Faulty or uneven stairs or loose debris on stairs

- Loose rugs that slip, or those without a non-skid backing

- Poisons (such as cleaning solutions)

- **Flammable** cleaning rags, mops, and brooms (these should be cleaned after each use and stored in a well-ventilated place)

- Sharp objects such as knives, razors, and hypodermic needles

- Wet floor (spills should be wiped up immediately)

- Cluttered hallways or walkways

- Unstable furniture

- Electrical cords that cross a walkway

- Liquids spilled onto equipment

- Wheels on equipment that roll unevenly

- Dimly lit hallways and walkways

flammable Capable of burning quickly and easily

Refer to Chapter 6 for more information on fire safety measures and Chapter 11 for overall safety awareness and accident prevention guidelines to follow while caring for a patient in the home.

Fire Safety and Burn Prevention

- Avoid using flammable liquids.

- Use flame-resistant clothing for the patient and follow the washing instructions on the label inside the clothing to keep them flame resistant.

- Caution the patient against smoking while seated on upholstered furniture or the bed, especially when sleepy.

- If the patient is a smoker, use a deep, wide-rimmed ashtray and set it on a table. Extinguish smoldering butts when the patient is finished smoking.

- Do not use an extension cord or electric cord and plug unless it is in excellent condition. Many facilities have a tag or require maintenance approval.

- Arrange furniture with fire safety in mind. Place furniture well away from stoves, space heaters, fireplaces, doorways, and stairs.

- If a fire occurs, get the patient out of the area. Know the exit route.

- Have a fire extinguisher available and a smoke alarm in the home.

- Follow the safety rules of your local fire department; they can train you as to how to use an extinguisher.

- Keep matches away from children and confused adults.

- Check the temperature of water before using it on the patient.

▪ Reporting an Accident or Emergency by Telephone

If an accident or emergency does occur, you must be ready to handle the situation calmly and wisely. Report every accident to your supervisor immediately. It is important to know emergency phone numbers. In the home, keep emergency numbers next to the phone. The list should include:

- Emergency Medical Service (often *911*)
- Police department
- Fire department
- Responsible family member at work
- Your home care supervisor or agency
- Patient's physician
- Nearest hospital
- Ambulance service
- Poison control center

If there is no phone in the home, arrange in advance to use a neighbor's phone in case of an emergency. Some home care agencies provide cellular phones for employees to use in these situations.

In the hospital or long term care facility, you should know the emergency numbers for fire and medical emergencies. Refer to Chapters 6 and 13 for more information on fire safety and medical emergencies.

▪ Calling for Help

No matter who you call, you must be clear when reporting the accident or emergency. Be sure to:

1. Give your name.

2. Give the name of the patient and identify your location, room number, or address.

3. Clearly state the problem; objectively state exactly what has happened or what help you need. If calling a city emergency number, give the above information, as well as the phone number of the patient's physician to the person who answers the phone call.

4. If you have a phone number for a member of the family, give that number, also.

By being prepared, you will be better able to handle emergency situations when they arise. Even more important, by observing safety hazards and taking preventive steps you may be able to avert an emergency totally. You should always strive for a safe, accident-free environment for every patient.

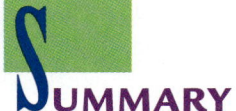

SUMMARY

The patient's environment is important to the recovery or care of the patient in numerous ways. It must provide comfort in order for the patient to rest. It must be perceived as safe for the patient to have peace of mind. For the family, the environment should be presentable and inviting; however, it must also afford staff a clean, safe, adequate space in which to work. Considering all of these needs, it is easy to understand how vital the nursing assistant is in maintaining the patient's environment. In reviewing the equipment and supplies necessary for patient care, the arrangement of the furniture and equipment, and safety concerns listed, the nursing assistant is able to prepare an efficient, organized, and safe patient environment. Regardless of which setting the patient is in, the nursing assistant, by maintaining the environment as such, enhances the quality of care for each patient.

Patient Lives in Clutter

THE NURSING ASSISTANT IN ACTION

You are working in a home care setting caring for Mr. Monroe. There is clutter everywhere in his home. He keeps old newspapers and magazines stacked in every corner. Boxes of old papers and magazines are stacked in spare rooms. One day while Mr. Monroe is resting, a recycling group calls asking for donations. You tell them that Mr. Monroe has many boxes of donations. When you ask Mr. Monroe which boxes he wants to donate he becomes very upset. He says he does not want to donate any of his belongings and that he will report you to your supervisor for trying to take away his things.

What Is Your Response/Action?

1. What are the important pieces of information in this situation?

2. What possible actions could you take?

3. Was your original action (offering to donate the papers and magazines) appropriate? Why or why not?

4. What action will you take now?

5. What will you say to your supervisor, if anything, about this situation.

6. What did you learn that you can apply to other situations?

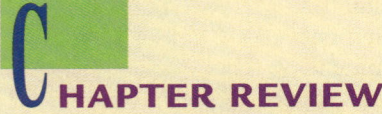

CHAPTER REVIEW

FILL IN THE BLANK

Read each sentence and fill in the blank line with a word that completes the sentence.

1. An _____ _____ mattress is a device placed beneath a bedridden patient to decrease the risk for pressure ulcers.

2. Equipment that is used for one patient only is called _____ equipment.

3. A _____ _____ is a frame shaped device used to keep linens off the bed.

4. Lamb's wool is a piece of material used to increase the patient's _____.

5. When working in the home, you must respect the patient's beliefs and attitudes even if they are _____ from yours.

MULTIPLE CHOICE

Choose the best answer for each question or statement.

1. The unit should be arranged for the convenience of the patient.
   a. True
   b. False

2. All of the following are pieces of patient equipment except
   a. binders.
   b. foot board.
   c. walkers.
   d. covers.

3. When caring for the patient, arrange her personal items, call light, and water where she will need to get up and get them. This will assure that she will get exercise.
   a. True
   b. False

4. All of the following is an example of a piece of disposable equipment except
   a. cups.
   b. foot board.
   c. bed pan.
   d. tissues.

5. To create a comfortable environment for the patient, do all of the following except
   a. put the TV on the channel the patient likes.
   b. keep the lights and heat at a level comfortable for the patient.
   c. keep the side rails up at all times.
   d. provide privacy for the patient.

6. Provide a safe environment for your patient by
   a. removing loose rugs that slip.
   b. keeping hallways uncluttered.
   c. cleaning up spills.
   d. All of the above.

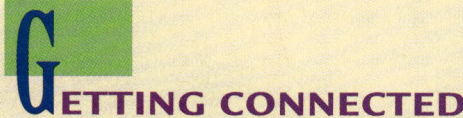

GETTING CONNECTED

MULTIMEDIA EXTENSION ACTIVITIES

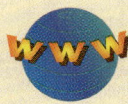

www.prenhall.com/wolgin

Use the above address to access the free, interactive Companion Website created for this textbook. Get hints, instant feedback, and textbook references to chapter-related multiple choice questions. Read and react to the "Nursing Assistants in Action." Link to other interesting sites.

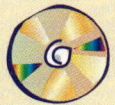

Audio Glossary

Use the CD-ROM disk enclosed with your textbook to hear the pronunciation of the key terms in the chapter.

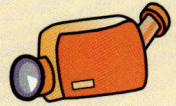

Video

Watch the "Patient's Rights" video from the Care Provider Skills series.

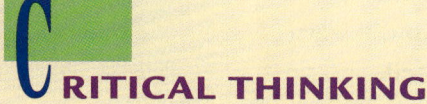

CRITICAL THINKING

USING KEY QUESTIONS

Read each question and think of what you might do in each situation.

1. You are getting a new patient to your institution. What kind of equipment will be needed?

2. Your patient has a history of falling. What kinds of things will you do to make the patient's environment safe?

3. What types of disposable equipment is used in your unit/institution?

4. What types of nondisposable equipment is used in your unit/institution?

5. You are caring for a patient in their home who has had an accident. How would you call for help?

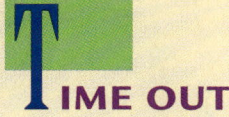

TIME OUT

TIPS FOR TIME MANAGEMENT

PLANNING TIP Make any routine appointments for dentists, eye doctors, teacher conferences, etc. for times when you are not normally at work. It is very difficult to "catch-up" after coming in late, or to leave in the middle of a shift.

Bedmaking

10

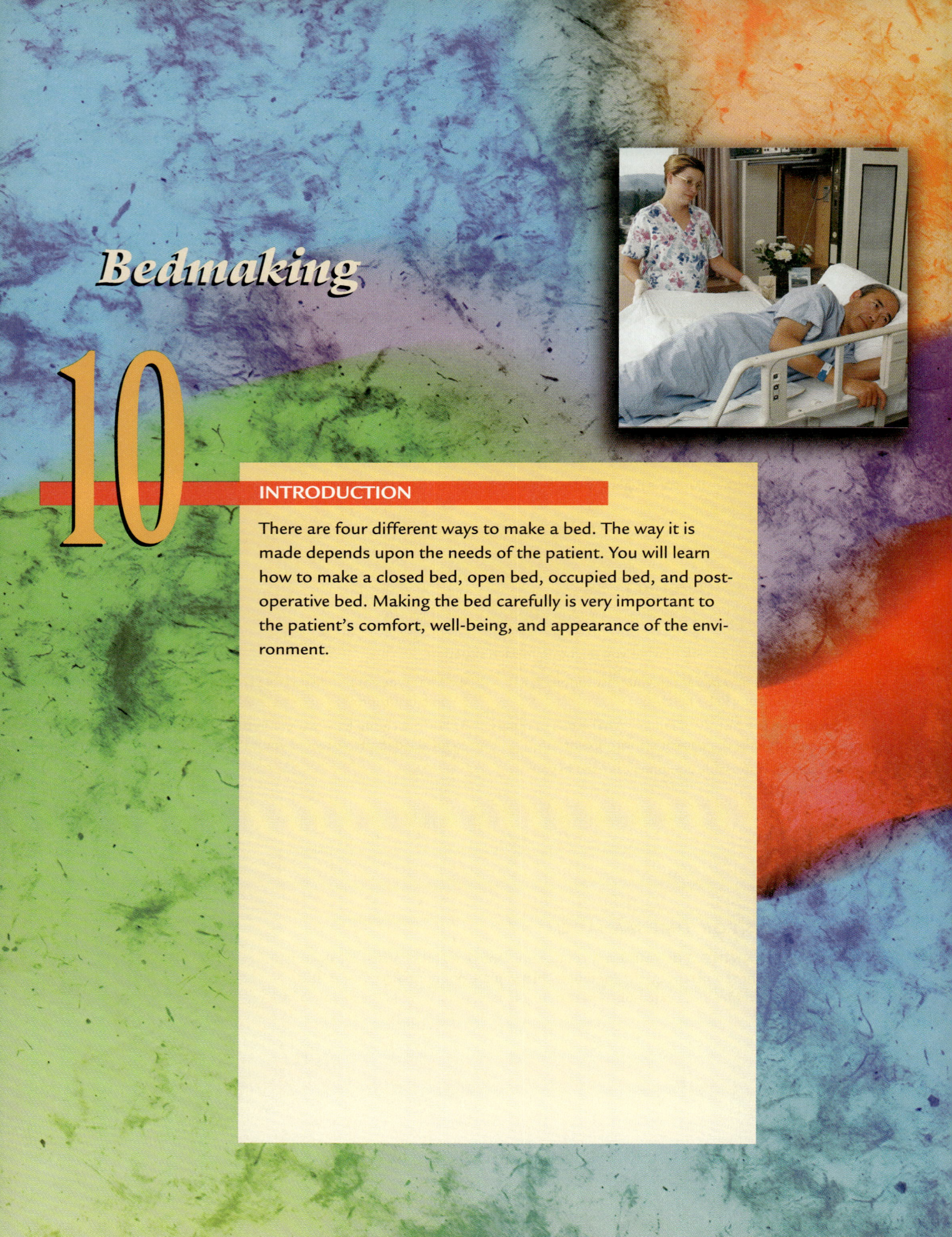

INTRODUCTION

There are four different ways to make a bed. The way it is made depends upon the needs of the patient. You will learn how to make a closed bed, open bed, occupied bed, and post-operative bed. Making the bed carefully is very important to the patient's comfort, well-being, and appearance of the environment.

When you have completed this chapter, you will be able to:

- Explain the reason for making the patient's bed with great care.
- Identify and describe the four basic methods of making a bed.
- List the guidelines to follow for bedmaking.
- Make the closed bed.
- Make the open, fanfolded bed.
- Make the occupied bed.
- Make the postoperative bed (surgical, OR [operating room], stretcher, recovery room bed).

KEY TERMS

closed bed

decubitus ulcers

draw sheet

fanfold

occupied bed

open bed

postoperative bed

decubitus ulcers Tissue breakdown resulting from pressure or reduced blood flow (often called pressure sores or bed sores)

closed bed Bed made with bedspread in place

open bed Bed made with top sheet folded so as to give patient easy entrance

occupied bed One with a patient in it

postoperative bed Bed made with top sheet folded lengthwise and positioned to one side, allowing transfer of the patient from the surgical stretcher to the bed without unnecessary movement

BEDMAKING

Some patients are unable or are not permitted to get out of bed. As a result of this, many patients eat, bathe, and use a bedpan in bed. Therefore, it is important to make the patient's bed with great care and to straighten sheets from time to time and adjust the pillow for the patient's comfort.

Whether the patient is in a health care facility or at home, the bed needs to be made without any wrinkles in the sheets. Wrinkles are not only uncomfortable but restrict the patient's circulation and can cause skin breakdown **(decubitus ulcers)**.

FOUR BASIC BEDS

The **closed bed** is made after environmental service personnel have cleaned the unit following a patient's discharge. The bed is made up closed. The top covers are pulled up to the head of the bed so it will stay clean until a new patient is assigned to it. When a patient is assigned to a unit, the closed bed is made into an **open bed** by fanfolding the top sheets down to the foot of the bed. The **occupied bed** is made with the patient in the bed. The **postoperative bed** may also be called the surgical, OR (operating room), recovery, or stretcher bed. The top sheets are folded lengthwise and positioned on one side of the bed. The postoperative bed allows transfer of the patient from the surgical stretcher to the bed without unnecessary movement.

KEY IDEA

A guideline that protects the patient and the patient's visitors as well as the nursing assistant from germs is to never shake linen and to always hold it away from the uniform.

GUIDELINES

OBRA

BEDMAKING

- Do not shake the bed linen. Shaking spreads germs to everything and everyone in the room, including you.

- Do not allow any linen to touch your uniform.

- Dirty, used linen should never be put on the floor. Place in a laundry bag.

- Fold linen in on itself as you remove it from the bed.

- Do not take extra linen into a patient unit. It is considered contaminated (or dirty) and cannot be used elsewhere.

- Set aside torn linen to send for repair.

- Never use a pin on any item of linen as it may come unfastened and injure the patient.

- Report to your immediate supervisor if you see patients or visitors trying to remove articles of linen from the unit for any reason.

Some health care institutions use melt-away plastic bags for laundry bags. These bags dissolve during the washing process.

- The bottom sheet must be firm, tight, and smooth under the patient.

GUIDELINES (CONTINUED)

This is very important for the patient's comfort.

- Plastic should never touch a patient's skin. If using a plastic draw sheet, be sure to cover it entirely with a cotton draw sheet. Small disposable bed protectors may be used with the draw sheet or in place of it.

- By fanfolding the top of the bed, you make it easy for the patient to get back into the bed.

- The cotton **draw sheet** is about half the size of a regular sheet. When cotton draw sheets are not available, a large sheet can be folded in half widthwise (with small and large hems together).

The fold must always be placed toward the head of the bed and the hems toward the foot of the bed.

Remember that you save time and energy by first making as much of the bed as possible on one side before going to the other side. Practice good body mechanics and follow standard precautions when making any bed.

■ Closed Bed

As a nursing assistant, you will have occasion to make many beds. It is important to remember that a clean, comfortable bed has a positive effect on the patient's physical and mental well-being.

draw sheet Small sheet made of plastic, rubber, or cotton placed across the middle of the bed to cover and protect the bottom sheet and assist in moving the patient

PROCEDURE

OBRA

MAKING THE CLOSED, EMPTY BED

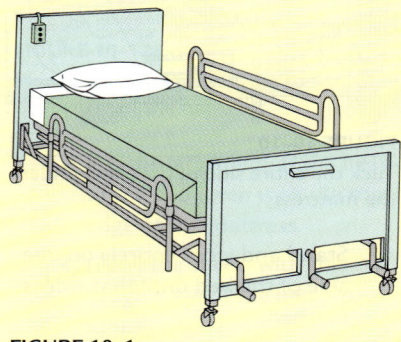

FIGURE 10–1
The closed, empty bed

PREPARATION

1. Assemble your equipment on a chair near the bed:

   a. Mattress cover, if used

   b. Bottom sheet

   c. Cotton and plastic draw sheets (or disposable bed protector)

   d. Top sheet

   e. Blanket

   f. Bedspread

   g. Pillowcase

   h. Pillow

   i. Pillow protector, if used

2. Place a chair near the bed.

STEPS

3. Wash your hands.

4. Put the pillow on the chair.

5. Stack the bed linen on the chair in the order in which you will use them: first things to be used on top, last things to be used on the bottom.

6. Adjust the bed to the highest horizontal position for comfort while you work (Figure 10–2).

7. Push the mattress to the head of the bed until it touches the headboard.

8. If mattress pads are used in your facility, place the pad on the

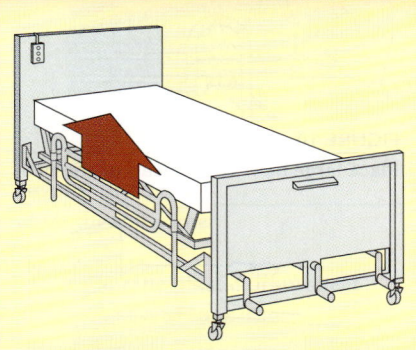

FIGURE 10–2
Adjust bed to highest horizontal position for comfort

mattress even with the head edge of the mattress.

9. Fold the bottom sheet lengthwise and place it on the bed:

   a. Place the center fold of the sheet in the center of the mattress from head to foot (Figure 10–3).

   b. Place the large hem to the head of the bed (Figure 10–4).

   c. Put the small hem at the foot of the bed, even with the edge of the mattress (Figure 10–5).

10. Open the sheet. It should now hang evenly the same distance over each side of the bed. The

P R O C E D U R E (CONTINUED)

e. One bath blanket

f. Pillowcase

g. One blanket (optional per patient preference and room temperature)

h. One bedspread

i. One plastic laundry bag

2. Identify the patient by checking the identification bracelet.

3. Tell the patient you are going to make the bed.

4. Provide privacy for the patient.

STEPS

5. Wash your hands and put on gloves.

6. Lower the backrest and knee rest until the bed is flat, if that is allowed. Raise the bed to a comfortable working height and lock in place. Keep side rails up to provide safety for the patient.

7. Loosen all the sheets around the entire bed.

8. Take the bedspread and blanket off the bed and fold them over the back of the chair, leaving the patient covered only with the top sheet.

9. Cover the patient with the bath blanket by placing it over the top sheet. Ask the patient to hold the bath blanket. If the patient is unable to do this, tuck the top edges of the bath blanket under the patient's shoulders. Without exposing the patient, remove the top sheet from under the bath blanket (Figure 10–34).

10. If the mattress has slipped out of place, move it to its proper position touching the headboard. Ask another nursing assistant to help.

11. Raise the bedside rail on the opposite side from where you will be working and lock in place (Figure 10–35).

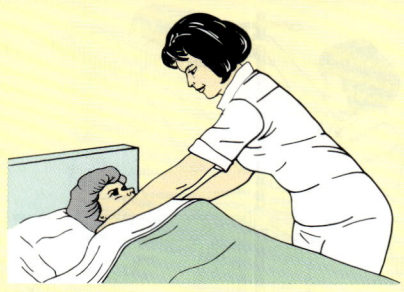

FIGURE 10–34
Tuck top of bath blanket under patient's shoulders

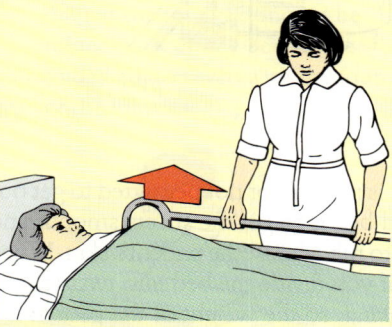

FIGURE 10–35
Raise and lock side rails

12. Ask the patient to turn onto her side toward the side rail. Help the patient to turn, if necessary. The patient is now on the far side of the bed (Figure 10–36).

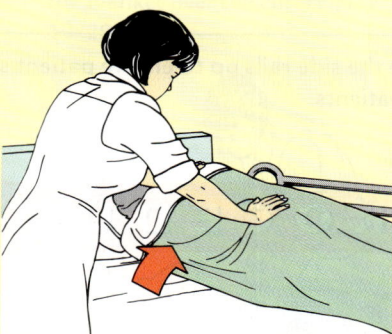

FIGURE 10–36
Help patient turn toward side rail

13. Adjust the pillow for the patient according to instructions. If the patient cannot sit up, lock arms with her and raise her to remove the pillow. If you are leaving the pillow under the patient's head,

then move it over to the side of the bed, adjusting it so that it is comfortable.

14. Fold the cotton draw sheet toward the patient and tuck it against her back.

15. Raise the plastic draw sheet (if it is clean) over the bath blanket and the patient. If the plastic draw sheet is dirty, also fold it toward the patient.

16. Fold the bottom sheet toward the patient and tuck it against her back. This strips your side of the bed down to the mattress (Figure 10–37).

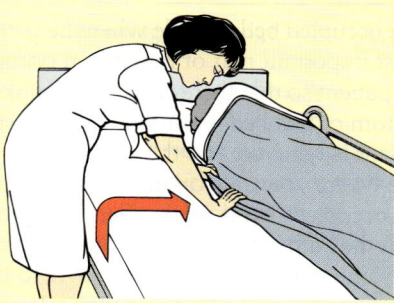

FIGURE 10–37
Fold and tuck bottom sheet against the patient's back

17. Take the large clean sheet and fold it in half lengthwise. Do not permit the sheet to touch the floor or your uniform.

18. Place the sheet on the bed, still folded, with the fold running along the middle of the mattress. The small hem end of the sheet should be even with the foot edge of the mattress. Fold the top half of the sheet toward the patient. Tuck the folds against her back, below the plastic draw sheet (Figure 10–38).

19. Miter the corner at the head of the mattress. Tuck in the clean bottom sheet on your side from head to foot of the mattress (Figure 10–39).

PROCEDURE (CONTINUED)

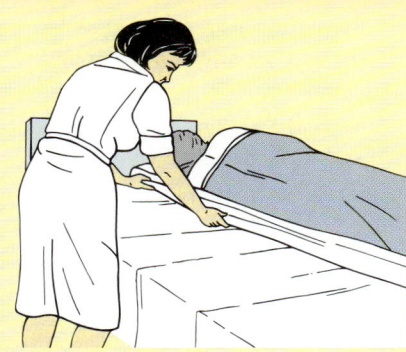

FIGURE 10–38
Tuck folds of clean sheet against the patient's back below the plastic draw sheet

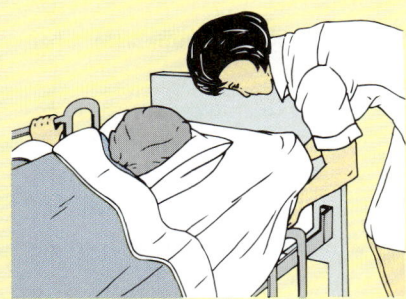

FIGURE 10–39
Miter the corner

20. Pull the plastic draw sheet toward you, over the clean bottom sheet, and tuck in.

21. Place the clean cotton draw sheet over the plastic sheet, folded in half. Fold the top half toward the patient, tucking the folds under her back, as you did with the bottom sheet. Tuck the draw sheet under the mattress.

22. Raise the bedside rail on your side of the bed and lock in place (Figure 10–40).

23. Go to the opposite side of the bed.

24. Lower the bedside rail. Ask the patient, or help her, to roll over the "hump" onto the clean sheets away from you. Be careful not to let the patient become wrapped up in the bath blanket while turning (Figure 10–41).

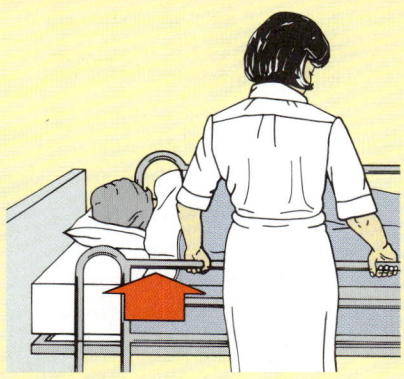

FIGURE 10–40
Raise and lock side rail on your side of bed

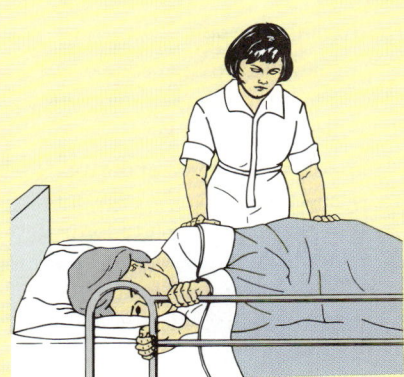

FIGURE 10–41
Roll or assist patient over hump onto clean sheets

25. Remove the old bottom sheet and cotton draw sheet from the bed. Pull the fresh bottom sheet toward the edge of the bed. Tuck it under the mattress at the head of the bed and make a mitered corner. Then tuck the bottom sheet under the mattress from the head to the foot, pulling firmly to remove any wrinkles (Figure 10–42).

26. Pull the plastic draw sheet and clean cotton draw sheet toward you.

27. Then, one at a time, tuck the draw sheets under the mattress along the side.

28. Be sure to pull all the sheets tight as you tuck them in for a tight foundation.

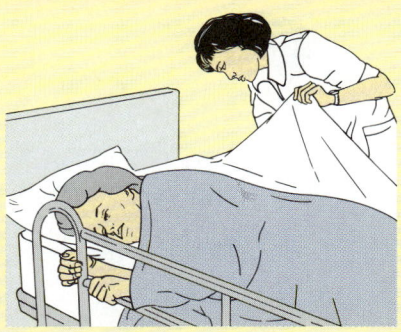

FIGURE 10–42
Pull bottom sheet tight and miter the corner

29. Have the patient turn on her back, or turn her yourself, loosening the bath blanket as she turns.

30. Change the pillowcase and place the pillow under the patient's head (Figure 10–43).

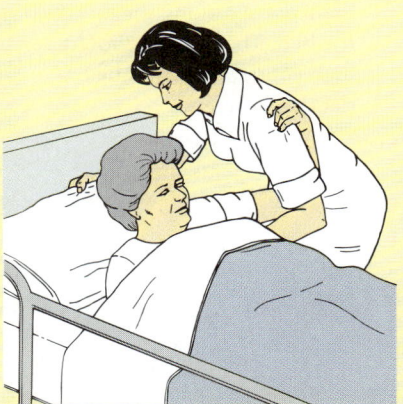

FIGURE 10–43
Place pillow under patient's head

31. Spread the clean top sheet over the bath blanket with the wide hem to the top. The middle of the sheet should run along the middle of the bed. The wide hem should be even with the head edge of the mattress. Remove the bath blanket, moving toward the foot of the bed, without exposing the patient (Figure 10–44).

PROCEDURE (CONTINUED)

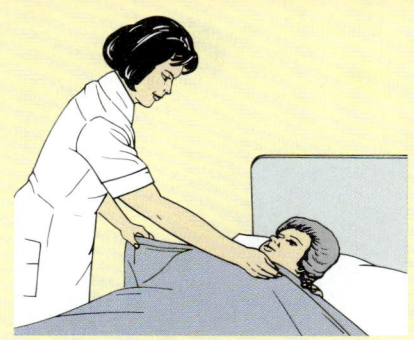

FIGURE 10–44

Remove bath blanket without exposing patient

32. Tuck the clean top sheet under the mattress at the foot of the bed. Make sure you leave enough room for the patient to move her feet freely. Miter the corners of the sheet.

33. Spread the blanket over the top sheet. Be sure the middle of the blanket runs along the middle of the bed. The blanket should be high enough to cover the patient's shoulders.

34. Tuck the blanket in at the foot of the bed. Make a mitered corner with the blanket.

35. Place the spread on the bed in the same way. Make a mitered corner with the spread.

36. Go to the other side of the bed and pull the top sheet, blanket, and spread over and straighten. Remove bath blanket. Turn the top covers back and miter the top sheet; then miter the blanket, and then miter the spread. Be sure the top covers are loose enough for the patient to move her feet.

37. To make the cuff:

  a. Fold the top hem edge of the spread over and under the top hem of the blanket.

  b. Fold the top hem of the top sheet back over the edge of the spread and blanket to form a cuff. The rough edge of the hem of the sheet must be turned down so the patient does not come in contact with it.

38. Raise the backrest and knee rest to suit the patient, if this is allowed.

39. Make the patient comfortable and replace the call light.

40. Lower the bed to a position of safety for the patient.

41. Raise the side rails when ordered or appropriate for patient safety.

42. Bag and dispose of used linen in the laundry hamper.

FOLLOW-UP

43. Dispose of gloves and wash your hands.

44. Report to your immediate supervisor:

- That you have made the occupied bed.
- How the patient tolerated the procedure.
- Your observations of anything unusual.

SUMMARY

A wrinkle-free bed is very important to the patient's comfort and well-being. There are four basic ways to make a bed. Each serves a special purpose. The closed bed is made with the top covers pulled to the head of the bed. An open bed, which has the top covers fanfolded to the foot of the bed, is made when a patient can be out of the bed. When a patient is bedridden, the occupied bed is made. A postoperative bed is made so the sheets are folded to one side for ease in moving a patient from the recovery stretcher to the bed. One of the guidelines in bedmaking is to never use a safety pin on the linen as it could open and injure the patient.

Notes

Covering Up the Evidence

THE NURSING ASSISTANT IN ACTION

You are working in a long-term care facility. When you turn Mrs. Herrera, you notice some small urine stains on the bottom sheet. The nursing assistant who is helping you turn the patient says, "Let's just change the draw sheet. It will cover the stains and keep them from coming in contact with Mrs. Herrera's skin. It sure would be a lot easier than trying to change the whole bottom sheet. We can change the bottom sheet tomorrow when she is in the whirlpool." Mrs. Herrera weighs about 225 pounds and is difficult to turn.

What Is Your Response/Action?

1. What decision do you have to make?

2. What possible responses could you make to the nursing assistant?

3. Which action will you take?

4. If you found a bed that had urine stains covered by a draw sheet, what would you do?

5. What did you learn that you can apply in other situations?

Home Health Care

11

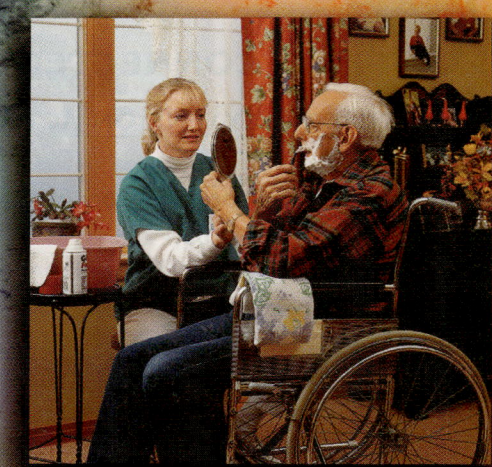

INTRODUCTION

Home health care is a rapidly expanding industry. As health care providers strive to reduce health care costs by decreasing the length of stay, patients are being discharged sooner or receiving services and surgery as outpatients. This chapter will help you discover the uniqueness of home health care and the special role that the nursing assistant or home health aide plays as part of the home care team. Working with patients and their families in their natural home environment presents a different set of challenges and opportunities than may be present in an institutional setting. One noticeable difference is that many agencies refer to individuals receiving care as clients rather than patients. Also, nursing assistants who are trained to work in the home are referred to as home health aides.

The area of home health offers many different types of situations in which you may choose to work. The types and ages of clients served, the hours worked, and the role responsibilities of the home health aide vary from agency to agency across the country. However, all home health aides through the type of personal care they render have an opportunity to significantly influence the quality of life of their clients. In this chapter, the qualities and attributes required of someone working in the home care field are discussed. Although the home health aide may be assigned many responsibilities and procedures that are the same as those performed in other settings, such as hospitals, some are unique to the home health care setting and are covered in detail in this chapter.

When you have completed this chapter, you will be able to:

- Differentiate between working in the home and in the health care institution.

- Describe the four categories of home health care providers.

- Define the role of the home health aide.

- Show respect for the beliefs, opinions, culture, and customs of patients and their families.

- List 26 basic tasks and procedures you may be assigned to perform in the home.

- Assist in the implementation of the discharge plan by communicating with the home care team.

- List nine procedures the home health aide may *not* do in the home.

- Describe 21 potential safety hazards in the home.

- Write a list of the phone numbers that should always be kept next to the phone for use in reporting an accident or emergency.

- List six rules to follow for storing infant formula.

- List three types of infant formula.

- Sterilize water, bottles, nipples, and caps.

- Demonstrate an infant sponge bath in the home.

- Demonstrate an infant tub bath in the home.

- List at least four safety precautions when caring for infants.

- Identify eight housekeeping responsibilities the home health aide may be assigned to perform in the home.

- Discuss how to apply at least five principles of infection control to the home setting.

- Discuss nutrition and food service as it applies to the home setting.

- Record your activities and those of the patient during your scheduled home visit.

- Describe the types of patient information that should be reported to the supervisor immediately.

KEY TERMS

bed-bound

caregiver

efficiency

family unit

flammable

formula

hospice care

infection control

long-term supportive care

microorganism

punctuality

responsibility

short-term intermittent skilled nursing care

sterilize

time/travel record

WORKING IN THE HOME HEALTH CARE FIELD

Home health care allows the patient to remain in his home while receiving an array of services that can encompass short-term intermittent skilled nursing, rehabilitative care, **long-term supportive care**, or hospice care depending upon his needs (Figure 11–1). Services can be provided on an intermittent basis, such as once a month, or up to 24 hours a day, 7 days a week. The primary purpose of intermittent skilled care is to educate acutely ill patients and their families on how to best meet the patients' specific needs. The goal is to promote maximum independence in self-care and functional ability, encouraging patients' active participation in their own health care. Throughout this chapter the words *client* and *patient* are used interchangeably.

Long-term supportive care is available for chronically ill patients who are unable to care for themselves and live alone or have limited family support. Hospice care is available for patients with terminal conditions who choose to remain at home until their death.

Federal government regulations require home health aides to complete a training program and competency evaluation check to verify skills prior to the time of hire. Additional hours of continuing education are also required yearly. See Chapter 35 for more information about skills competency and continuing education.

For Medicare and Medicaid reimbursed agencies, an assessment tool called OASIS is now being utilized at the start of care for each client. OASIS stands for *Outcome and Assessment Information Set* and is used to clearly describe clients' needs, provide data for assessment and care planning, and facilitate information sharing with all care givers. The OASIS and any other assessment information will be used to determine the home health aide care plan and frequency of visits.

■ Home Health Care Agencies and Other Employees

Substantial differences can exist among the variety of agencies providing home health care. The four main categories of home health care providers include privately owned, for-profit or not-for-profit agencies; publicly operated health departments; hospital-based home health services; and national networks of investor owned or not-for-profit agencies. There are state-by-state differences concerning license requirements for home health care agencies. Some agencies may be certified to provide Medicare and Medicaid

---

ALERT

For all patient contact, adhere to Standard Precautions (see Chapter 5, pages 78-108). Wear protective equipment as indicated.

long-term supportive care The care of chronically ill patients who are unable to care for themselves and live alone or have limited family support

---

FIGURE 11–1

The nursing assistant cares for patients in the home

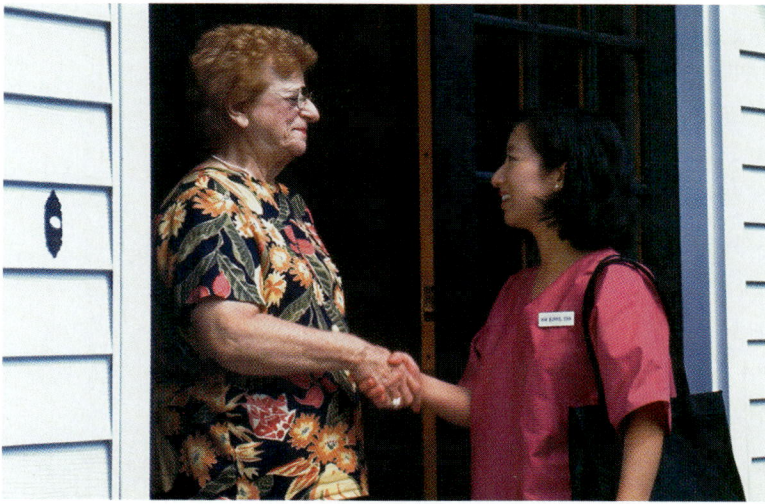

reimbursed services and others may only provide services for patients on a private fee-for-service or insurance reimbursed basis. The type of services that may be provided are often dependent on the client's health insurance coverage. Medicare and Medicaid typically will pay for home health aides only if the client has a need for a skilled nurse. While the types of home care services provided by agencies vary, all offer basic nursing services. Staffing patterns are determined by the types of services provided. Some agencies offer various levels of home services, including those that do not provide hands-on care. These assistants may be called homemakers or companions, and their duties do not include the personal care that home health aides give. Homemaker and companion's tasks are focused on housekeeping, meal preparing, errands, and providing company for the client or someone to assist in obtaining further assistance when needed. In most cases, however, the home care nursing staff will consist of registered nurses, licensed practical/vocational nurses, and home health aides.

The Home Health Aide

With *professional supervision*, the home health aide is able to assist the patient with the activities of daily living and maintain a safe, clean, and comfortable environment. The patient in the home should receive high-quality nursing care. All the nursing skills and principles explained in this textbook must be applied by the home health aide. Adhere to the same high standards of ethical professional behavior outlined in Chapter 2.

Just as the nursing assistant in the health care institution works under the direct supervision of a registered nurse or physician, so does the home health aide in the home. The main difference between working in the home and in the health care institution is that in the home the home health aide may be alone while working. It is essential that the home care aide keep the supervisor and home care nurse informed about any changes observed in the patient's condition.

HELPFUL PERSONAL QUALITIES OF THE HOME HEALTH AIDE

As a member of the health care team, you are expected to maintain a professional attitude in the home. The same qualities that will make you a successful nursing assistant in a health care institution will be necessary if you are to be successful as a home health aide. The best home health aides are those who are dependable, trustworthy, considerate, tactful, ethical, courteous, self-starters, sympathetic, energetic, polite, careful, observant, sensitive, and good listeners. Communication skills are an essential part of your job. You will be in close contact with the patient, family members, and visitors. Since you will be spending more time in the home than any other team member, patients and families may share important information with you that they may not tell the nurse or therapist.

It is important to respect the privacy and confidentiality of your patient. Do not discuss the patient's condition with visitors in the home. All observations and information obtained from the patient should be shared only with the members of the home care team. You should never discuss your personal problems with the patient.

Demonstrate honesty and accuracy when handling the patient's money and valuables. Show respect by treating the patient's possessions carefully. Display dependability by never leaving before an assignment is completed. Self-discipline, time management, and the motivation to do a good job are especially important qualities, since you are working alone in the home.

- Sharp objects such as knives, razors, and lawn tools
- Wet floors (spills should be wiped up immediately)
- Cluttered walkways
- Unstable furniture
- Ambulatory devices that need repair; for example, replacement of rubber tips on walkers, canes, or crutches

■ Fire Safety and Burn Prevention

flammable Capable of burning quickly and easily

- Avoid using **flammable** liquids. Use flame-resistant clothing for the patient and follow the washing instructions on the label inside the clothing to keep them flame resistant (Figure 11–5).
- Caution the patient against smoking while seated on upholstered furniture or the bed, especially when sleepy.
- Caution the patient and/or family to refrain from smoking when oxygen is being used in the home.
- If the patient is a smoker, use a deep, wide-rimmed ashtray and set it on a table. Extinguish smoldering butts when the patient is finished smoking.
- Do not use an extension cord or electric cord and plug unless it is in excellent condition.
- Arrange furniture with fire safety in mind. Place furniture well away from stoves, space heaters, and fireplaces, and out of walkways.
- If a fire occurs, get the patient out of the house. If the patient is bedridden, follow your agency's policy regarding fire emergencies. Know the exit route. If the apartment is above the first floor, know where the stairs are.

FIGURE 11–5

Many garment-related fires cause injuries when a loose-fitting portion of a garment, such as a sleeve or skirt hem, comes in contact with a stove burner, lighted candle, space heater, or fireplace fire; flaming liquids also cause serious injuries when they splash on to a garment and ignite its fabric or when the textile is wet with a flammable liquid (such as lighter fluid), which is then ignited by a nearby spark or flame

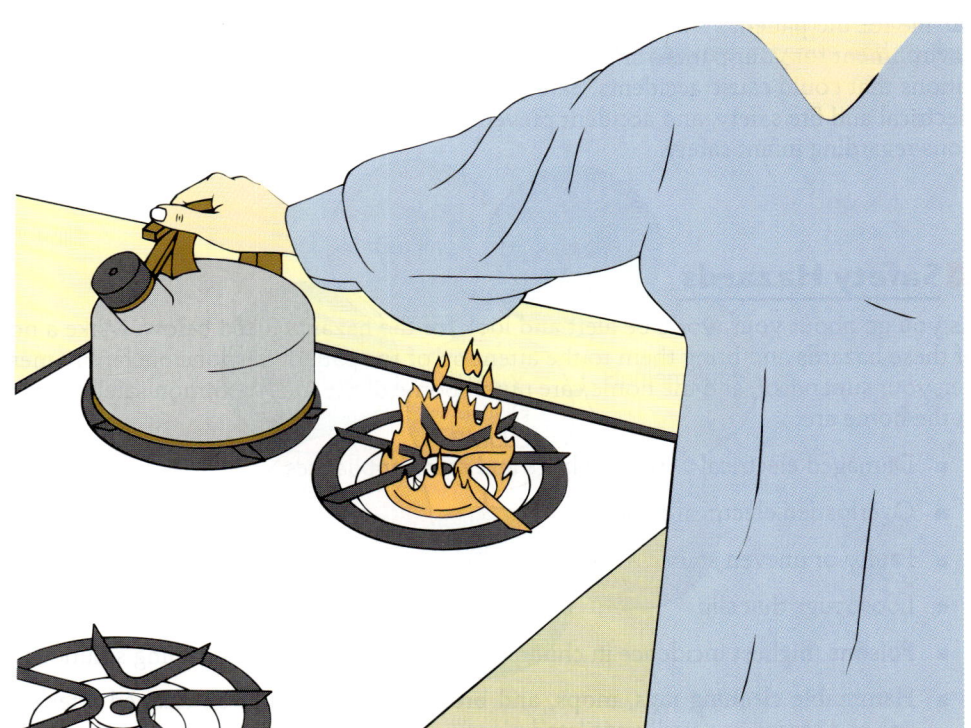

- To provide a safe quick exit, make sure the key remains in the lock of any door(s) that lock on the inside with a key.
- Encourage the family to have a fire extinguisher and smoke detector in the home. Make sure smoke detectors are working and batteries are tested monthly.
- Follow the safety rules of your local fire department.
- Keep matches away from children and confused adults.
- Check the temperature of water before using it on the patient.

REPORTING AN ACCIDENT OR EMERGENCY BY TELEPHONE

If an accident or emergency does occur, you must be ready to handle the situation calmly and wisely. Report every accident to your supervisor immediately.

Phone Numbers to Keep Handy

It is important to have emergency phone numbers written next to the phone. The list should include:

- Emergency Medical Service (often *911*) if available
- Police department
- Fire department
- Responsible family member at work
- Your home care supervisor or agency
- Patient's physician
- Nearest hospital
- Ambulance service
- Poison control center
- Pharmacy

If there is no phone in the home, arrange in advance to use a neighbor's phone in case of an emergency.

Calling for Help

Most states have laws regarding a patient's right to execute an Advance Directive. Make sure you are aware of your agency's policy regarding the types of medical emergencies that are affected by an Advance Directive and how you are to handle them. Many areas have a special phone number to call when an accident or emergency occurs in the home. You may call that number or the physician phone number that you have been given by the family or agency. No matter whom you call, you must be clear in reporting the accident or emergency. Be sure to:

- Give your name and title
- Give the name of the patient

- Clearly state the problem; objectively state exactly what has happened

- Give the address and phone number of where you are

- Clearly state the condition of the patient or person who has had the accident or is in a crisis

- If calling a city emergency number, give the phone number of the patient's physician to the person who answers the phone call

- If you have a phone number for a member of the family, give that number to the emergency answering service

- Remain with the patient until help arrives

CARE OF THE INFANT IN THE HOME

Home care services to infants may include normal newborn follow-up as well as care of the sick infant. Agencies throughout the country will vary in their policies regarding the types of staff who are assigned to do infant care in the home. If you are employed by an agency that includes infant care in the home health aide job description, refer to Chapter 31 of this textbook regarding the care of infants and pediatric patients. Infant care procedures you may be asked to perform *in the home* are given here in Chapter 11.

If for any reason the mother is unable to feed or care for the baby, you may be asked to do it. Refer to Chapter 31 regarding breastfeeding, burping, bathing, care of the circumcision, and diapering. This is an opportunity to demonstrate to a new mother the newborn's need for handling, affection, and security.

Preparing Formula

formula A liquid food prescribed for an infant containing most required nutrients

If the mother is breastfeeding her baby, you may bring the baby to her when it is time for a feeding. If the baby is being bottle-fed, you may need to prepare the **formula**. The home care nurse will obtain orders from the infant's physician as to the type of formula needed to meet the infant's special needs. There are several types of milk-based and milk-free formulas available. The nurse will provide instructions on the dilution of the formula, number of ounces per feeding, and the number of feedings per day. Be sure to read directions on the label.

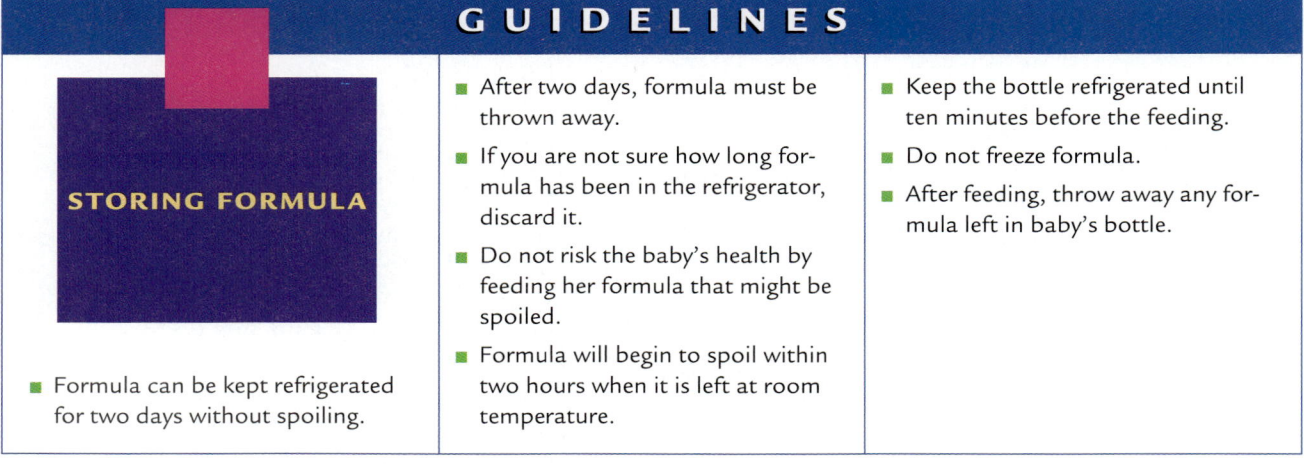

GUIDELINES

STORING FORMULA

- Formula can be kept refrigerated for two days without spoiling.

- After two days, formula must be thrown away.
- If you are not sure how long formula has been in the refrigerator, discard it.
- Do not risk the baby's health by feeding her formula that might be spoiled.
- Formula will begin to spoil within two hours when it is left at room temperature.

- Keep the bottle refrigerated until ten minutes before the feeding.
- Do not freeze formula.
- After feeding, throw away any formula left in baby's bottle.

■ Different Types of Formula

- Ready-to-feed
- Powder
- Concentrated liquid

Unopened cans and bottles do not have to be refrigerated. Wash all cans and bottles before opening. Remember to shake all cans of liquid and concentrated formulas before opening them. Use a *clean, sterile can opener* to open all cans. After assembling all needed equipment, wash hands before and after preparation of the formula or sterilization of bottles. Dishwashers provide an easy way to clean baby bottles and nipples. Check with the nurse or the parents to see if special precautions or sterilization is necessary.

Ready-to-feed (Prepared) Formula

While expensive to buy, this type of formula needs no preparation. Shake and open the can and pour the contents into sterile (clean) bottles. Some ready-to-feed formulas come in disposable bottles, to which you attach a sterile nipple and ring, and it is ready to feed the baby. DO NOT ADD WATER.

Powdered Formula

Follow the instructions provided by the nurse regarding the amounts of powder and sterile water to mix together. Be sure to mix the powder with water that you have boiled and allowed to cool. Mix the powder and sterile water in sterile bottles. Once mixed, this formula must be kept refrigerated.

Note: Powder mixes best when you use boiled water which has cooled to a warm temperature. Shake for five seconds.

Concentrated Liquid Formula

Follow the instructions provided by the nurse regarding the dilution of the concentrate. You must boil the water before you mix the formula. As with the powdered formula, this must be mixed in sterile bottles or a sterile pitcher. Once mixed, this formula must also be kept refrigerated.

In certain areas, you will not be instructed to boil water to **sterilize** bottles and nipples. Ask your supervisor or the home care nurse for instructions for your area.

sterilize Destroying all microorganisms

PROCEDURE

STERILIZING TAP WATER

PREPARATION

1. Wash your hands.
2. Assemble your equipment:
   a. Saucepan
   b. Water
   c. Timer, watch, or clock

STEPS

3. Fill the saucepan two-thirds full with water and place on burner.

4. When the water comes to a full boil, begin timing. Allow the water to remain at a full boil for 20 minutes in covered pan.

5. Allow the water to cool before using it to mix the formula.

PROCEDURE

STERILIZING BOTTLES

PREPARATION

1. Wash your hands.
2. Assemble your equipment:
   a. Bottles
   b. Nipples, caps, and jar
   c. Bottle brush
   d. Dishwashing detergent
   e. Hot water from the tap
   f. Large pot with cover or a special sterilizing pot for baby bottles
   g. Small towel
   h. Tap water
   i. Timer, watch, or clock
   j. Tongs

STEPS

3. Scrub bottles, nipples, and caps with hot soapy water. Use the bottle brush to clean inside the bottles. Always squirt hot, soapy water through the holes in the nipples to clean out any dried-on formula.
4. Rinse thoroughly with hot water.
5. Fold the small towel to fit the bottom of the pot and lay it in the pot to prevent the bottles from breaking (this is not necessary when using a bottle rack).
6. Stand the washed bottles on the towel in a circle around the inside of the pot (Figure 11–6).

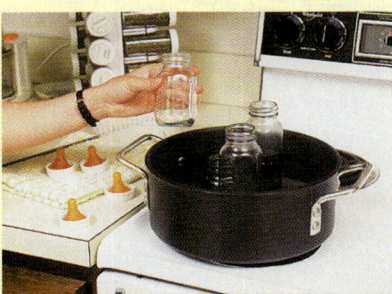

FIGURE 11–6
Sterilizing bottles

7. Place the caps and nipples into the clean, empty jar and place it into the pot at the center of the bottles.

8. Pour water into and around the bottles and into the jar with the nipples until two-thirds of each bottle is under water. Place the tongs upright in the pot to sterilize them.
9. Cover the pot and place on the stove.
10. When the water comes to a full boil, begin timing. Allow the water to remain at a full boil for 25 minutes.
11. Using the sterile tongs, remove the nipples and caps in the jar 10 to 15 minutes after the full boil began. With the nipples still inside the jar, stand the jar on the table to cool.
12. Take the cover off the pot and allow it to cool.
13. Remove the sterile bottles from the pot with sterile tongs.

FOLLOW-UP

14. Empty the water out of the pot. The pot is now sterilized and can be used for mixing the formula, if needed.

HOUSEKEEPING RESPONSIBILITIES IN THE HOME

The tasks expected of you will vary from home to home depending on the availability and ability of family members. If the home care nurse asks you to do the shopping for the patient, keep an accurate written account of the amount of money given to you by the patient. Be sure to save the register receipts for the total amount spent. Return the correct amount of change. Include this information, along with the date and time, in your written report.

It is best to clarify any questions with your supervisor as to what will be expected of you before you make your first visit to the home. This will avoid future misunderstandings. Patients and their family members will sometimes request you to do tasks that are not appropriate or allowed by your agency. It is helpful to be open and honest when communicating with the patient and family members. Refusal of these tasks should be done in a firm but tactful manner. If problems arise, notify your supervisor and request that she or the nurse explain your role to the family.

■ Cleaning Responsibilities May Include:

- Washing linens and clothing used by the patient only

- Sweeping the floor or vacuuming the carpet in the patient's immediate area of use

- Straightening up and dusting the patient's immediate area

- Cleaning the bathroom, including tub, toilet, sink, floor, and mirror after assisting the patient with his bath

- Returning used items to their proper places

- Disposing of soiled, disposable items, following your agency's policy on the handling and disposal of waste materials; refer to Chapter 5 for information on waste management

- Cleaning spills and crumbs from the stove, counters, sink, and floor following preparation of meals for the patient

- Washing dishes used by the patient only

■ Infection Control in the Home

It is your **responsibility** to assist in preventing the spread of **microorganisms** in the home by using proper handwashing techniques, standard precautions, and maintaining a clean environment for the patient. Refer to Chapter 5 for detailed instructions on handwashing and standard precautions. Wash fruits and vegetables before cooking or serving. Refrigerate or freeze all perishable foods as appropriate. You should use hot water and detergent when washing dishes. Wash dishes and cooking vessels immediately after using. Be sure to rinse well. Dispose of garbage and soiled supplies promptly.

Cleaning the tub and commode with a disinfectant will help to eliminate odors and will cut down on the growth of bacteria. If there is more than one person using the bathroom, encourage them to use their own towels. Never place soiled linen or clothing on furniture or carpets. Place them in a plastic bag until the family can wash them, unless the nurse has asked you to do the laundry. Laundry bleach is an inexpensive and effective disinfectant that can be found in most homes. Be careful not to allow bleach to come in contact with carpets and materials that could become damaged by the bleaching action.

If there are no cleaning supplies available, discuss this with your supervisor or the home care nurse. In some homes, cleaning supplies and even patient care supplies may be limited. You will have to be flexible and improvise with what is available. For example, you may substitute baking soda on a wet toothbrush or a solution of mouthwash and water if there is no toothpaste.

■ Nutrition and Food Service

Prior to mealtime, assist the patient to wash his face and hands. Some patients, especially those with dentures, will find the meal more appetizing if they rinse their mouth out with mouthwash and water. Assist with oral hygiene as desired by the patient. Position the patient for maximum comfort and to reduce risk of choking or aspiration.

Some patients may have prepared meals delivered to their homes if they live alone and are unable to prepare their own meals. The delivered meals usually consist of one warm meal and one cold meal. The nurse may ask you to set up the meal and assist the patient as needed. In some cases, you may have to prepare a light meal or snack for the patient. The kind of written instructions left in the home by the nurse will vary from agency to agency; however, most will leave basic instructions or a home health aide assignment sheet in the home.

If the patient's special diet needs are not included on the instruction sheet, check with your supervisor or the nurse before preparing the meals. When preparing foods, consider

infection control
Restraining or curbing the spread of microorganisms

responsibility A duty or obligation; that for which one is accountable

microorganism A living thing so small it cannot be seen with the naked eye but only through a microscope

the patient's likes and dislikes, including cultural preferences and religious practices, allergies to foods, and ability to chew and swallow. Some patients have difficulty in chewing because dentures do not fit well, their own teeth are in poor condition, or because they have mouth sores. If you notice this, report it to your supervisor or the nurse and try to provide softer, more easily chewed foods. The food should always be prepared and arranged in an attractive manner and served on a clean surface. Check all foods for spoilage before serving.

If you are assigned to stay with the patient for a full 8-hour shift, inquire as to when the patient prefers to have his meals. If you will be in the home for a shorter period of time to render care and are to prepare a meal for the patient, schedule your visit so you will be in the home during the meal time. If you have to leave the home before the meal is to be served, a cold meal may be prepared and left in the refrigerator or within reach of the patient.

bed-bound Unable to get out of bed

The **bed-bound** patient's appetite may be small. Even if the meals are small, they must be well balanced and contain enough fluids.

Refer to Chapter 21 for nutritional information. When purchasing and preparing food, it is important to read the food product labels to be certain that the food is allowed on the patient's prescribed diet (Figure 11–7).

Nutrition Facts

Serving Size 1 cup (49g)
Servings Per Container about 10

Amount Per Serving	Cereal	Cereal with 1/2 cup Skim Milk
Calories	170	210
Calories from Fat	5	5
	% Daily Value**	
Total Fat 0.5g*	1%	1%
Saturated Fat 0g	0%	0%
Polyunsaturated Fat 0g		
Monounsaturated Fat 0g		
Cholesterol 0mg	0%	0%
Sodium 0mg	0%	3%
Potassium 200mg	6%	11%
Total Carbohydrate 41g	14%	16%
Dietary Fiber 5g	21%	21%
Insoluble Fiber 5g		
Sugars 0g		
Other Carbohydrate 36g		
Protein 5g		
Vitamin A	0%	4%
Vitamin C	0%	2%
Calcium	2%	15%
Iron	8%	8%
Thiamin	8%	10%
Riboflavin	2%	10%

FIGURE 11–7

Reading labels will help you select foods suited to the patient's diet

REPORTING AND RECORDING

A carefully written record of your activities and those of the patient must be kept. These notes help you and other team members monitor any changes in the client's status. The format of written home health aide assignments will vary from agency to agency. Some agencies combine the assignment sheet and the patient's daily record on the same form.

Regardless of the type of record form, it is very important that you document everything you do while in the home, including how the patient tolerated activities and procedures. It is important to record the patient's orientation to time, place, and person. Record the patient's food intake, activity level, vital signs, and urine sugar and acetone results.

Be sure your handwriting is neat and legible. It is best to write each activity down as soon as it is completed, while you are still in the home. Do not rely on your memory. If you are to report to your supervisor before you leave the home or after you have completed all of your patient home visits for the day, be sure this is done. However, observations of any problems or changes in the patient's condition should be reported to the supervisor or home care nurse immediately.

Figure 11–8 shows a sample of a home health aide daily progress record. To document the activities of daily living on a flow sheet see Chapter 12.

AGE-SPECIFIC CONSIDERATIONS

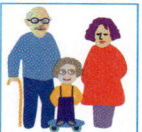

Caring for patients in the home requires the same attention to the age-specific care needs of the patient as in a health care institution. The ages of the family members also become important, as they provide physical and emotional care for the patient. Keep in mind safety features for all age groups, such as choking hazards for small children, gun safety for older children, and tripping hazards and oxygen safety for the elderly (Figure 11–9). Elderly patients will often require reinforcement of the proper use of new adaptive equipment (Figure 11–10). Infection control issues include proper mixing of formula for infants and proper food preparation and storage of leftovers.

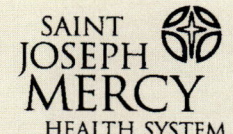

SAINT JOSEPH MERCY HEALTH SYSTEM
A Member of Mercy Health Services

St. Joseph Mercy Home Care
Ann Arbor, Michigan

Home Health Aide Note
Level II

Month _____ Year _____

Client Name _____

Client ID# _____

	Sun	Mon	Tue	Wed	Thu	Fri	Sat
Date							
Shift							
Time							

PERSONAL CARE

Assist: ☐ Shower
☐ Tub
☐ Bed
☐ Sponge
Hair Care
Shampoo
Skin Care
Shave
Peri Care
Foot & Nail Care
Oral Hygiene
Denture Cleaning
Maint. clean, safe environ.
Linen Change
Laundry
Dress
Non-Sterile Dressing
TED Hose Applied
Other _____
_____
_____

VITAL SIGNS

	Sun	Mon	Tue	Wed	Thu	Fri	Sat
T _____							
P _____							
R _____							
BP _____							
WT _____							
Medication Assistance							

ELIMINATION

	Sun	Mon	Tue	Wed	Thu	Fri	Sat
Bed Pan							
Bathroom							
Empty drainage/ostomy bag							
Catheter Care							
Commode							
Date last BM							
Consistency							
Incontinent Care							

OTHER

_____
_____
_____
_____
_____

6901-009 R3/97 (PC) D

	Sun	Mon	Tue	Wed	Thu	Fri	Sat
Date							
Shift							
Time							

ACTIVITY

Total Bedrest
Bed Rails Up
Reposition
Up in Chair
Dangle
Assist w/ROM Exercise
Ambulate with assistance
Ambulate w/o assistance
Walker
Crutches
Cane
Wheelchair
Use of transfer belt
No wt. bearing
☐ R ☐ L

DIETARY

	Sun	Mon	Tue	Wed	Thu	Fri	Sat
Nothing by mouth							
Diet _____							
Encourage Fluids							
Restrict Fluids							
Assist w/ meal preparation							
Feed Client							

SAFETY CONSIDERATIONS/MEASURES

	Sun	Mon	Tue	Wed	Thu	Fri	Sat
Seizure Precautions							
Bleeding Precautions							
O_2 Precautions							
O_2 at ____L/min____hrs/day							
Hypo/hyperglycemic Prec							
_____							
_____							

REPORTING

Are there client changes that need to be reported? ☐ Yes ☐ No

Office Staff Notified	Date	Time

_____   _____
Home Health Aide Signature   Date/Time

FIGURE 11–8

The home health aide daily progress note. Courtesy St. Joseph Mercy Hospital, Ann Arbor, MI. Reprinted with permission.

FIGURE 11–9

Practice oxygen safety with an elderly patient with COPD

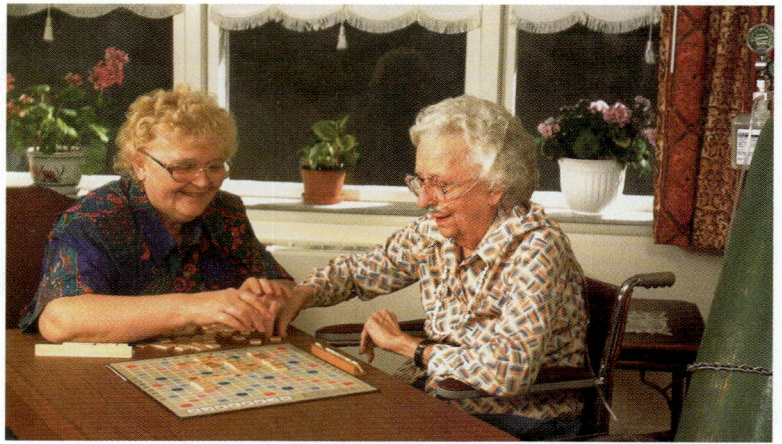

FIGURE 11–10

CNA reinforcing the proper use of adaptive equipment

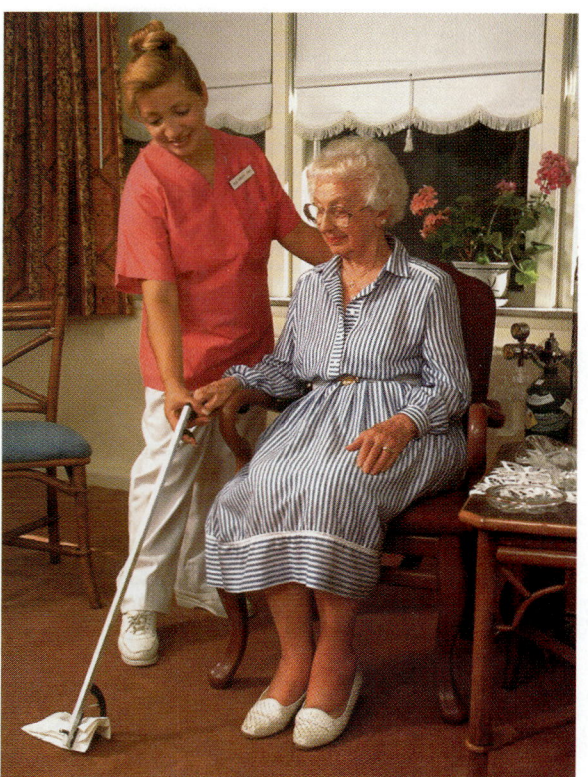

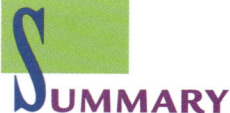UMMARY

The primary purpose of home health care is to allow the patient to remain in his natural environment while being restored to his maximum level of independence in self-care and functional ability. The frequency and duration of services may vary from once a month to 24-hour care. The role of the home health aide is to assist the patient with activities of daily living and maintenance of a clean, safe, and comfortable environment. The home health aide must be able to work independently and effectively with patients and families regardless of age, ethnicity, cultural or religious beliefs, and medical problems.

Patient Wants More Help Than You Can Give

You are a nursing assistant assigned to give personal care to Mrs. Sondheim in home health. She is 78 years old and lives alone. When you arrive today, Mrs. Sondheim tells you that the guest room needs to be readied for her grandchildren who are coming to visit. She asks you to move the boxes in the guest room to the garage, then rearrange some of the furniture. She tells you to vacuum and dust the guest room and to change the linens on the beds. When you remind Mrs. Sondheim that your duties are limited to her personal care and needs, she becomes upset. She says, "Then don't give me a bath and shampoo today; do the guest room instead. That's what I *really* need."

What Is Your Response/Action?

1. What are the important pieces of information in this situation?

2. What possible actions might you consider?

3. What action will you take?

4. What justification do you have for your decision?

5. What did you learn that you can apply in other situations with clients?

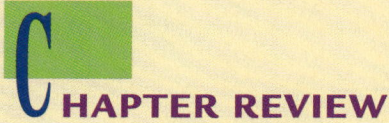

CHAPTER REVIEW

FILL IN THE BLANK

Read each sentence and fill in the blank line with a word that completes the sentence.

1. A group of people brought together by shared needs, interests, and mutual concerns for the well-being of all its members is a _____.

2. _____ _____ involves the restraining or curbing the spread of microorganisms.

3. A patient who is unable to get out of bed is _____ _____.

4. If an accident or medical emergency occurs in the home, call _____.

5. One of the principle concerns of the home health aide is patient _____.

MULTIPLE CHOICE

Choose the best answer for each question or statement.

1. When caring for a person in his or her home, home health aides generally refer to that person as a client.
   a. True
   b. False

2. Which of the following is not a helpful characteristic of a home health aide?
   a. Polite
   b. Trustworthy
   c. Inconsiderate
   d. Careful

3. Efficiency refers to
   a. getting all of one's duties done in an organized fashion.
   b. getting all of one's duties done in a short amount of time.
   c. arriving on time.
   d. arriving early.

4. Which of the following is not a reason why a person may need home health assistance?
   a. Family works outside the home.
   b. Patient does not want help.
   c. The client cannot shop and prepare meals.
   d. The client cannot provide transportation.

5. Which of the following is not a duty of the home health aide?
   a. Preparing bottles.
   b. Shopping for food for the client.
   c. Changing sterile dressings.
   d. Collecting specimen samples.

6. Which of the following phone numbers does not need to be kept handy?
   a. Fire station
   b. Police station
   c. Pizza delivery
   d. Pharmacy delivery

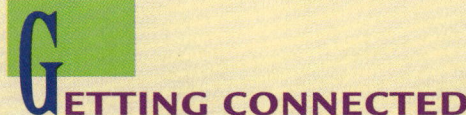

GETTING CONNECTED

MULTIMEDIA EXTENSION ACTIVITIES

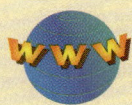

www.prenhall.com/wolgin

Use the above address to access the free, interactive Companion Website created for this textbook. Get hints, instant feedback, and textbook references to chapter-related multiple choice questions. Read and react to the "Nursing Assistants in Action." Link to other interesting sites.

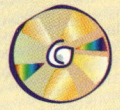

Audio Glossary

Use the CD-ROM disk enclosed with your textbook to hear the pronunciation of the key terms in the chapter.

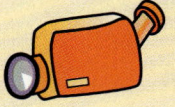

Video

Watch the "Communication" section from the "Dealing with Dementia" video and the "Patient's Rights" video from the Care Provider Skills series.

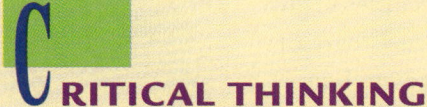

CRITICAL THINKING

USING KEY QUESTIONS

Read each question and think of what you might do in each situation.

1. Where can you find the necessary instructions regarding the patient's care that is to be provided in the home?

2. What kind of things should you *not* do in a patient's home?

3. What should you do if you notice a safety hazard in the patient's home?

4. A new mother asks you to show her how to sterilize a bottle. What do you tell her?

5. What kind of observations about your patients should you report to your supervisor immediately?

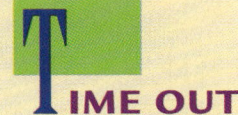

TIME OUT

TIPS FOR TIME MANAGEMENT

COMMUNICATION TIP   Take time to see, hear, and appropriately touch a patient when you are giving care. You may observe or detect a problem in the early stages, so it can be prevented from becoming worse. Avoid becoming so task oriented that you forget the whole person who is your patient.

Personal Care of the Patient

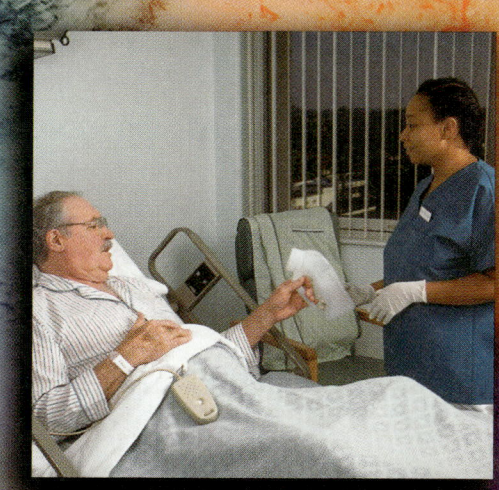

12

INTRODUCTION

This chapter provides you with the knowledge and skills needed to provide daily care for patients. This includes giving or assisting with oral hygiene, bathing, perineal care, care of nails and feet, back rub, changing the patient's gown, hair care, shaving, and elimination. Special care for patients who are incontinent is also presented.

When you have completed this chapter, you will be able to:

- Establish a schedule of personal care.
- Record what you have done for the patient on the activities of daily living (ADL) flow sheet (or other appropriate form).
- Care for the patient's mouth using good oral hygiene techniques.
- Bathe the patient.
- Give perineal care.
- Care for the patient's nails and feet as instructed.
- Give a back rub.
- Change the patient's gown.
- Care for the patient's hair.
- Shave the patient's beard; remove facial hair.
- Help the patient use a bedpan, a urinal, or a bedside commode.
- Care for the incontinent patient.

KEY TERMS

activities of daily living (ADL)

bedpan

commode

dentures

eliminate (defecate)

flow sheet

fracture pan

incontinence

oral hygiene

perineum (perineal area)

self-care

urinal

urinate

Daily Care of the Patient

Each patient is an individual with a special set of needs. Care must be unhurried and personalized to meet each patient's special needs. The tasks that are listed here may seem very routine, but the nursing assistant can greatly increase the comfort of patients by performing them.

KEY IDEA

One example of a special need would be a patient who is going to surgery. Patients scheduled for surgery are usually NPO (nothing by mouth). You would not give any drinking water but you would provide oral hygiene to increase comfort.

AGE-SPECIFIC CONSIDERATIONS

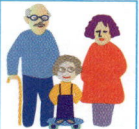 When performing personal care for small children, keep in mind that they may experience stranger anxiety. Try to have the parent assist or remain close by to comfort the child. Babies lose body heat more quickly than adults, so dry their skin quickly. Adolescents value privacy and are generally very modest. Allow them as many choices as possible when assisting with or providing personal care. Adults and geriatric patients may have concerns over loss of control and feelings of helplessness if they cannot perform their own care. Try and maintain as many personal habits and practices as possible.

Early Morning Care: Before Breakfast (Sometimes called Early A.M. Care)

- Offer the bedpan or urinal or assist ambulatory patient to bathroom or commode
- Wash the patient's hands and face
- Help with oral hygiene
- Pass fresh drinking water, if permitted
- Clean the overbed table and position it to receive food tray
- Raise the head of the bed, if permitted
- Reposition patient as needed, if permitted

Morning Care: After Breakfast (Sometimes called A.M. Care)

- Before giving personal care, provide privacy for the patient
- Offer the bedpan or urinal
- Assist with oral hygiene
- Help the patient to bathe—follow instructions from your immediate supervisor
- Give the patient a complete bed bath, partial bed bath, shower, or tub bath
- Change the patient's gown
- Help the male patient to shave his face, if allowed
- Make the bed

- Straighten the unit
- Reposition patient as needed, if permitted

Afternoon Care: After Lunch

- Offer the bedpan or urinal
- Wash the patient's hands and face
- Assist with oral hygiene
- Change the patient's gown, if necessary
- Straighten the unit
- Pass fresh drinking water

Evening Care: After Supper, Before Bedtime (Sometimes called P.M. Care)

- Offer the bedpan or urinal
- Wash the patient's hands and face
- Assist with oral hygiene
- Give a back rub, if allowed
- Change the draw sheet, if necessary or at patient's request
- Smooth and tighten the sheets
- Offer the patient an extra blanket
- Pass fresh drinking water

Activities of Daily Living: The Flow Sheet

In many health care facilities, the nursing assistant is required to record—check off (√) or initial—what has been done for the patient on an **activities of daily living (ADL) flow sheet** (Figure 12–1) or a *patient care flow sheet* (Figure 12–2). Follow the nurse's instructions regarding this documentation.

activities of daily living (ADL) The activities or tasks usually performed every day, such as toileting, washing, eating, or dressing

flow sheet A checklist or chart for recording the activities of daily living

O RAL HYGIENE

Care of a person's mouth and teeth is called **oral hygiene**. A sick person's mouth often has a bad taste because of medications or the illness. The tongue may be covered with a grayish coating that spoils the appetite. With good care, the patient's mouth will feel fresh and clean and may increase the desire to eat. Giving oral hygiene is an essential part of daily patient care (Figure 12–3). Teeth should be brushed every morning, every evening, and after eating (Figure 12–4a). Flossing teeth once a day is desirable to promote healthy gums (Figure 12–4b and Figure 12–4c). In your work, you will be giving oral hygiene to conscious and unconscious patients. When necessary, you will be cleaning their **dentures** (false teeth).

Oral hygiene is given to unconscious patients and patients who are NPO (nothing by mouth) every two hours. The purpose is to keep the lips and oral tissues moist. Unless this is done, the lips and oral tissues tend to dry out, split, and bleed, and may develop a mucus coating much more rapidly.

oral hygiene Cleanliness of the mouth

dentures Artificial teeth. Dentures may replace some or all of a person's teeth; they are described as being partial or complete and upper or lower

ACTIVITIES OF DAILY LIVING CHECKLIST

SELF   —Done by patient
ASSIST —Patient assisted by nursing staff
TOTAL   —Done by nursing staff
✔   —Check procedure performed.
         Include time if appropriate.

DATE															
DIET	B'fast	Dinner	Supper	B'fast	Dinner	Supper	B'fast	Dinner	Supper	B'fast	Dinner	Supper	B'fast	Dinner	Supper
Ate all food served															
Ate approx. 1/2 food served															
Refused to eat															
PROCEDURE	11-7	7-3	3-11	11-7	7-3	3-11	11-7	7-3	3-11	11-7	7-3	3-11	11-7	7-3	3-11
A.M. or H.S. Care															
Oral Hygiene															
Bath–Bed bath complete															
Bed bath partial															
Shower															
Tub															
Self Care															
Back Care															
Bed Made															
ELIMINATION															
Bowel movement															
Involuntary B.M.															
Voided															
Incontinent															
Foley cath.															
Sitz Bath @															
ACTIVITY															
Bed rest complete															
Dangle															
Bed rest–B.R.P.															
Up in chair															
Up in room															
Walk in hall															
Ambulatory															
POSITION CHANGED															
Flat in bed															
Semi–Fowler's															
Deep breathe, cough															
Range of motion															
Turn from side to side															
Side Rails–Up															
Down															
Fresh Water @															
SIGNATURE & TITLE															

FIGURE 12–1

The activities of daily living checklist

Catherine McAuley Health System

8765-004 N 4/93

St. Joseph Mercy Hospital
5301 East Huron River Drive
P.O. Box 995
Ann Arbor, Michigan 48106

Patient Care Flow Sheet

Admission Date	OP Date	POD

Date		MIDNIGHTS							DAYS								AFTERNOONS							
		24	01	02	03	04	05	06	07	08	09	10	11	12	13	14	15	16	17	18	19	20	21	22	23
VITAL SIGNS	Temperature																								
	Pulse																								
	Respiratory Rate																								
	Blood Pressure																								
	CVP																								
FLUID INTAKE	Oral																								
	Feeding/NG						CREDITS					CREDITS					CREDITS								
	IV/IVPB																								
	Hyperal/Lipids																								
	Blood																								
	Total 8°																	24° Total							
FLUID OUTPUT	Urine																								
	Emesis																								
	Nasogastric Tube																								
	Total 8°																	24° Total							

ACTIVITY	Safety Code						EVENING SHIFT
	Progression Weight						
	SCDs / TEDs						

SAFETY / RESTRAINT	Type of restraint and						DAY SHIFT
	Location of restraint						
	Observation q1°						
	Turn/ROM q2°						
	Fluids offered						MIDNIGHT SHIFT
	Toilet patient q2°						
	Skin status under restraint checked						
	Circulation checked						

FIGURE 12–2

The patient care flow sheet (Chart adapted with permission of St. Joseph Mercy Hospital, Ann Arbor, Michigan)

Date		24	01	02	03	04	05	06	07	08	09	10	11	12	13	14	15	16	17	18	19	20	21	22	23
	Diet and Amount	BREAKFAST								LUNCH								SUPPER							
	Weight																								
GI / GU	Stool character and number																								
	Guaiac and date of last stool																								
	Bowel sounds																								
	Bladder																								
RESPIRATORY	Assessment																								
	Cough / Deep Breathe																								
INTEGUMENT	Surgical incision / Dressing																								
	Drains / characteristics																								
	Wound Care																								
TESTS AND SPECIMENS	Test results (mg/dL)																								
	Treatment/Medications																								
BLOOD GLUCOSE	Patient response																								
	ACCU-CHECK Instrument No.																								
	Date of last quality check																								
	CHEMSTRIP Lot No.																								
	Same as Calibration Lot (Yes, No)																								
	Sample type (cap, venous)																								
	Initials																								
NEUROLOGICAL	Assessment																								
	Best Eye Opening																								
	Best Verbal Response																								
	Best Motor Response																								
	Total Score																								
	Grasp																								
	Leg Lift / Foot Presses																								
	Pupils R																								
	L																								
HYGIENE	AM Care / HS Care																								
	Foley Care / Perineal Care																								
	Oral Care																								

KEY

Bowel Sounds:
✓ = Present in all 4 quadrants

Bladder:
✓ = Able to empty bladder Urine clear and yellow
F = Foley to DD
F✓ = Foley to DD, urine clear and yellow

Respiratory Assessment:
✓ = Bilateral breath sounds clear and respirations quiet and regular
☆ = See description

Surgical Incision:
I✓ = incision well approximated no drainage
D✓ = dressing dry / intact
★ = See description

Best Motor Response:
6 = Obeys commands
5 = Localizes pain
4 = Flexion withdrawal
3 = Flexion abnormal
2 = Extension abnormal
1 = No response

Grasp and Leg Lift
R = L, R> L, or R < L
and
W = Weak
S = Strong

Pupils
Record size in mm and
R = reactive to light
NR = nonreactive to light

Neurological Assessment:
✓ = Alert and oriented X3
☆ = See description

Best Eye Opening:
4 = spontaneous
3 = to speech
2 = to pain
1 = no response

Best Verbal Response
5 = Oriented to time, person, place
4 = Confused
3 = Inappropriate words
2 = Incomprehensible sounds
1 = no response

FIGURE 12–2 (continued)

The patient care flow sheet

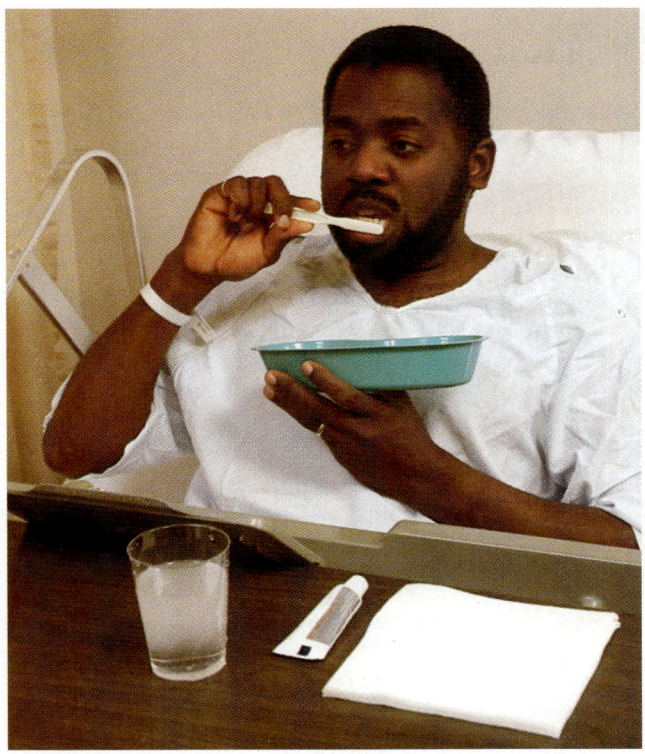

FIGURE 12–3

Oral hygiene is an essential part of daily patient care

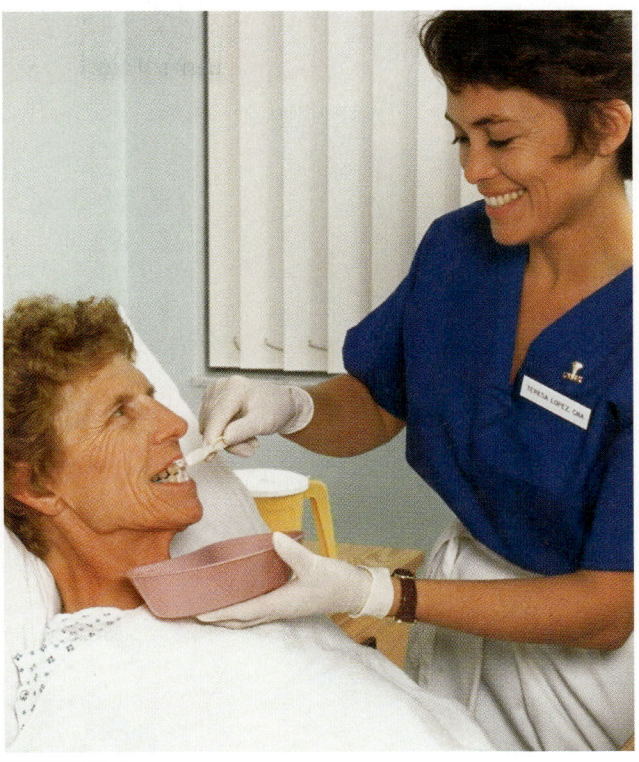

FIGURE 12–4a

In your work as a nursing assistant, you will be giving oral hygiene to patients

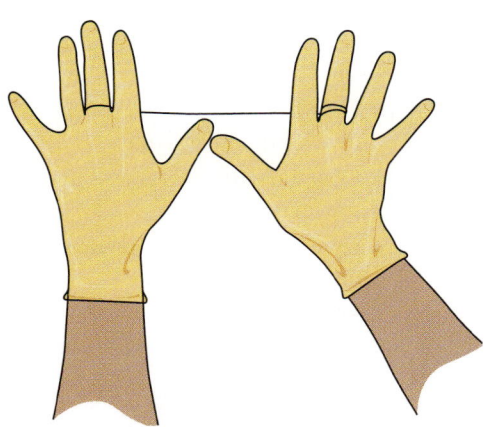

FIGURE 12–4b

Wrap dental floss around middle fingers

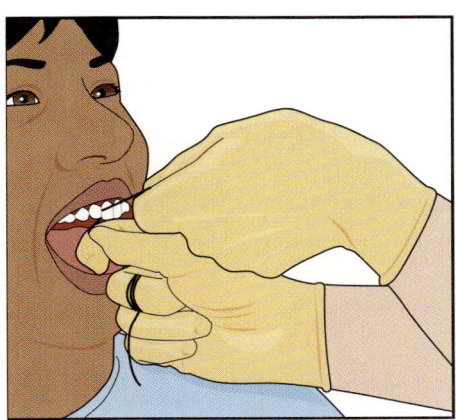

FIGURE 12–4c

Hold dental floss firmly between each thumb and forefinger to properly floss around each tooth

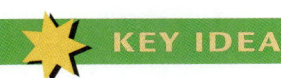

KEY IDEA

A person's mouth and teeth need more care when a person is ill than when he or she is well. Always wear gloves when performing oral hygiene. Oral hygiene can be performed at the bedside or in the bathroom. Look at the mouth and gums for redness or skin breakdown.

PROCEDURE

OBRA

ORAL HYGIENE

PREPARATION

1. Assemble your equipment on the bedside table:
   a. Mouthwash
   b. Fresh water
   c. Disposable cup
   d. Straw (optional)
   e. Toothbrush
   f. Toothpaste
   g. Emesis basin
   h. Face towel
   i. Disposable gloves
   j. Dental floss and disposable face mask
2. Identify the patient by checking the identification bracelet.
3. Tell the patient you will help her clean her teeth and mouth.
4. Provide privacy for the patient.
5. Wash your hands and put on gloves.
6. Raise bed to a comfortable working height.

STEPS

7. Position patient to a sitting position, if possible.
8. Spread the towel across the patient's chest to protect the gown and top sheets.
9. Mix one-half cup of water with one-half cup of mouthwash in the disposable cup.
10. Let the patient take a mouthful of the mixture if allowed and rinse her mouth.
11. Hold the emesis basin under the patient's chin so she can spit out the mouthwash solution.
12. Put toothpaste on the wet toothbrush.
13. If the patient can do it, let her brush her teeth. If she cannot, brush her teeth for her. Brush the tongue to freshen breath and remove bacteria.
14. Help the patient rinse the toothpaste out of her mouth, using the mouthwash solution or fresh water.
15. Floss the patient's teeth using a 12–14 inch piece of dental floss. Wear a disposable face mask while flossing a patient's teeth as there is potential for gum bleeding and your face will be in close proximity when flossing teeth.

    Wrap ends of the dental floss around your middle fingers. (See Figure 12–4b) Ask the patient to open her mouth. As you hold the dental floss between your thumb and forefingers, gently insert the floss between each tooth, down to but not into the gum (See Figure 12–4c). When finished, offer water or mouthwash to have the patient rinse her mouth.
16. Clean and put your equipment in its proper place. Discard disposable equipment.

FOLLOW-UP

17. Make the patient comfortable and replace call light.
18. Dispose of your gloves and wash your hands.
19. Lower the bed to a position of safety for the patient.
20. Raise the side rails when ordered or appropriate for patient safety.
21. Report to your immediate supervisor:
    - That you have assisted the patient with oral hygiene.
    - How the patient tolerated the procedure.
    - Your observations of anything unusual.

PROCEDURE

OBRA

CLEANING DENTURES (FALSE TEETH)

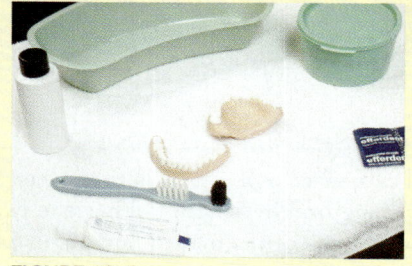

FIGURE 12–5
Preparation for cleaning dentures

PREPARATION

1. Assemble your equipment on the bedside table (Figure 12–5):
   a. Paper towel
   b. Mouthwash
   c. Disposable denture cup
   d. Emesis basin
   e. Toothbrush or denture brush
   f. Towel

PROCEDURE (CONTINUED)

g. Denture toothpaste

h. Disposable gloves

2. Identify the patient by checking the identification bracelet.

3. Tell the patient you wish to clean his dentures.

4. Provide privacy for the patient.

5. Wash your hands and put on gloves.

6. Raise bed to a comfortable working height.

STEPS

7. Position patient to a sitting position, if possible.

8. Spread the towel across the patient's chest to protect the gown and top sheets.

9. Ask the patient to remove his dentures. (Have paper towel in the emesis basin ready to receive them.) Assist the patient who is unable to remove his own dentures.

10. Take the dentures to the sink in the lined emesis basin (Figure 12–6).

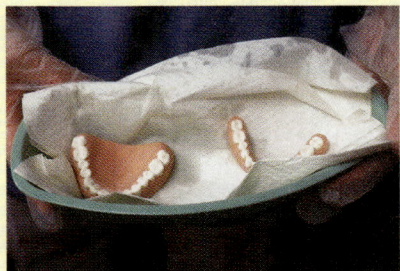

FIGURE 12–6
Place dentures in a lined emesis basin

11. Place a paper towel or washcloth in the bottom of the sink to guard against breaking dentures if you drop them accidentally. Fill the sink with water.

12. Apply toothpaste or denture cleanser to the dentures. With the dentures in the palm of your hand, brush all surfaces until they are clean (Figure 12–7).

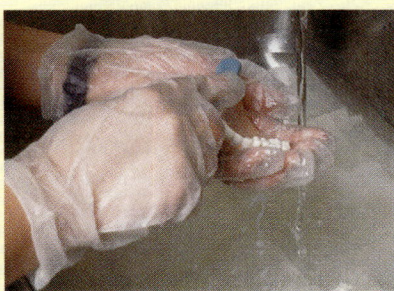

FIGURE 12–7
Brush all surfaces of the dentures

13. Rinse dentures thoroughly under cool running water (Figure 12–8).

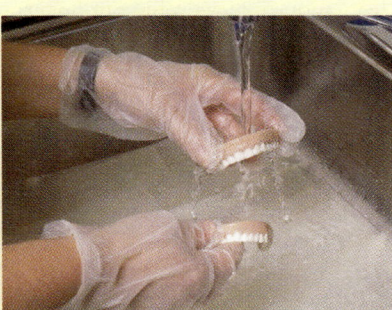

FIGURE 12–8
Rinse dentures thoroughly

14. Fill the clean denture cup with cool water, some mouthwash and water, or dental solution. Place the dentures in the cup and close the lid.

15. Help the patient rinse his mouth with water and/or mouthwash.

16. Have the patient replace the dentures in his mouth if this is what he wants. Be sure dentures are moist before replacing them.

17. Leave the labeled denture cup with the clean solution on the bedside table where the patient can reach it easily. Some patients remove dentures between cleanings.

18. Clean and replace all your equipment. Discard disposable equipment in the proper container.

FOLLOW-UP

19. Make the patient comfortable.

20. Dispose of your gloves and wash your hands.

21. Lower the bed to a position of safety.

22. Raise the side rails when ordered or appropriate for patient safety.

23. Place the call light within easy reach of the patient.

24. Report to your immediate supervisor:

- That you have cleaned the patient's dentures.

- Your observations of anything unusual.

PROCEDURE

OBRA

ORAL HYGIENE FOR THE UNCONSCIOUS PATIENT (SPECIAL MOUTH CARE)

PREPARATION

1. Assemble your equipment on the bedside table:

a. Towel

b. Emesis basin

c. Special disposable mouth care kit of commercially prepared swabs. Or if such a kit is not available:

- Tongue depressor to hold mouth open or teeth apart, if necessary

- Applicators or gauze sponges

- Lubricant such as glycerin, petroleum jelly, or a solution of lemon juice and glycerin

d. Disposable gloves

PROCEDURE (CONTINUED)

2. Identify the patient by checking the identification bracelet.

3. Tell the patient what you are going to do. Even though a patient seems to be unconscious, he still may be able to hear you.

4. Provide privacy for the patient.

5. Wash your hands and put on gloves.

6. Raise the bed to a comfortable working height.

STEPS

7. Stand at the side of the bed. Turn the patient's head to the side facing you.

8. Put a towel on the pillow under the patient's head and partly under the face.

9. Lower head of bed, if possible. Gravity causes saliva to automatically run out of the mouth and prevents drainage into lungs.

10. Put the emesis basin on the towel under the patient's chin.

11. Tell the unconscious patient you are going to open his mouth. Press on his cheeks or open the mouth using gentle pressure with hand on chin. **Never** put your fingers into the mouth of an unconscious or uncooperative patient.

12. Open the commercial package of swabs, if available. Wipe the patient's entire mouth to remove debris and dried mucus (roof, tongue, and inside the cheeks and lips) with the prepared swab (Figure 12–9).

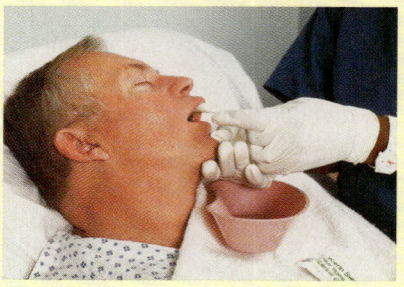

FIGURE 12–9
Wipe the entire inside of the patient's mouth, including the inside of the cheeks and lips

13. Put used swabs into the emesis basin. Some commercial swabs leave a coating of glycerin solution on the entire inside of the mouth, tongue, and teeth.

14. If a disposable mouth care kit of commercially prepared swabs is not available:

   a. Moisten the applicators with mouthwash solution.

   b. Use your free hand to insert the applicator in the patient's mouth. **Never** put your fingers in the unconscious patient's mouth.

   c. Thoroughly wipe the roof of the mouth, the teeth, and the tongue.

   d. Change applicators when soiled.

   e. Place the used applicators and other supplies in the emesis basin.

   f. Use clear water on more applicators to rinse out the patient's mouth.

15. Dry the patient's face with the towel.

16. Using an applicator, put a small amount of water-soluble lubricant on the patient's lips and tongue.

17. Clean and return your equipment to its proper place. Discard disposable equipment.

FOLLOW-UP

18. Raise head of the bed if it was lowered. Make the patient comfortable.

19. Dispose of your gloves and wash your hands.

20. Lower the bed when ordered or appropriate for patient safety.

21. Raise the side rails when ordered or appropriate for patient safety.

22. Place the call light within easy reach of the patient.

23. Report to your immediate supervisor:

   ■ That you have given the patient oral hygiene.

   ■ How the patient tolerated the procedure.

   ■ Your observations of anything unusual.

HELPING THE PATIENT TO BATHE

Patients who are able to manage their own daily personal care—oral hygiene and bathing—should be encouraged to do so. There are several important reasons for bathing the patient. Bathing gets rid of dirt on the patient's body. It eliminates body odors and cools and refreshes the patient. The bath stimulates circulation, helps to prevent skin breakdown, and can be relaxing.

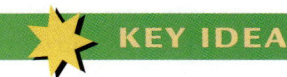

> Patients who are ordered to be on **self-care** should be encouraged to do as much as possible for themselves.

self-care Activities or care tasks performed by the patient

The physician may order one of four types of baths, based on the patient's condition. The patient may be given a complete bed bath, a partial bed bath, a tub bath, or a shower.

Bathing requires movements of certain parts of the body; the patient's legs and arms are lifted and the head and torso are turned. This activity exercises muscles that might otherwise remain unused. (Range of motion exercises are covered in Chapter 33: Rehabilitation and Return to Self-Care.) At this time, the nursing assistant has the opportunity to observe the patient for any unusual body changes such as skin rashes, pressure ulcers, or reddened areas. (Refer to Chapter 17: Integumentary System and Related Care for a discussion of skin disorders associated with confinement to bed.)

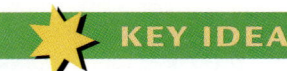

> Change the bath water from time to time as it appears soapy or gets cool.

Types of Baths

Complete bed bath	The patient who is too weak or ill is given a complete bed bath. When you are giving this bath, you will get little or no help from the patient. Sometimes the doctor will write an order placing the patient on complete bed rest. In this case, the patient is not permitted to do anything.
Partial bed bath	Patients may be able to take care of most of their own bathing needs. In this case you bathe only the areas that are hard for the patient to reach, such as the back or feet.
Tub bath	The tub bath might be ordered by the doctor for therapeutic reasons.
Shower	Showers may be permitted for patients who are recovering from their illness (convalescent patients). These patients have been judged by their doctor to be strong enough to get out of bed and walk around.

GUIDELINES

OBRA

BATHING THE PATIENT

- Usually the complete bed bath is given as part of morning care. After the bath, the hair is combed, the gown changed, and the occupied bed is made.

- Use good body mechanics. Keep your feet separated, stand firmly, bend your knees, and keep your back straight.

- Raise the patient's bed to a comfortable working position with the side rails up on the far side of the bed.

- Change the water during the bed bath as necessary. For example, change the water whenever it becomes soapy, dirty, or cold.

- Only one part of the body is washed at a time. Wash, rinse, and dry each part or area very well. Then cover it right away with the bath blanket.

- Soap has a drying effect on the patient's skin. Be sure to rinse off all the soap.

GUIDELINES (CONTINUED)

- When you are not using the soap, keep it in the soap dish instead of the basin. In this way, the water will not dissolve the soap and get too soapy.
- Putting the patient's hands and feet into the water makes the patient feel relaxed.
- Observe the condition of the patient's skin when you are giving the bath. Report any redness, rashes, broken skin, or tender places you see on the patient's body.
- Never trim or cut fingernails or toenails without special instructions from the nurse.
- At the beginning of the bath, put the patient's bottle of lotion for the back rub in the basin of water to keep it warm or put lotion on your hands and rub your hands together to warm it up.
- Deodorant should be used if the patient asks for it. It should be applied after the bath has been completed and before the clean gown is put on.
- Check the patient's gown and bed linens for personal items or valuables and return them to the patient before putting the gown in the laundry hamper.

PROCEDURE

OBRA

THE COMPLETE BED BATH

PREPARATION

1. Assemble your equipment on the bedside table (Figure 12–10):

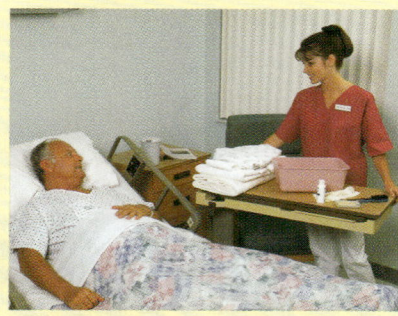

FIGURE 12–10
Preparation for the complete bed bath

   a. Soap and soap dish

   b. Washcloths

   c. Wash basin

   d. Bath thermometer, if available

   e. Face and bath towels

   f. Talcum powder or corn starch (optional)

   g. Clean gown

   h. Bath blanket

   i. Orange stick for nail care, if used by your institution

   j. Lotion

   k. Comb or hair brush

   l. Disposable plastic or cloth laundry bag for dirty linen (whichever is used by your institution)

   m. Clean bed linen, stacked on the chair in order of use, if the bed is to be made following the bed bath

   n. Disposable gloves

2. Identify the patient by checking the identification bracelet (Figure 12–11).

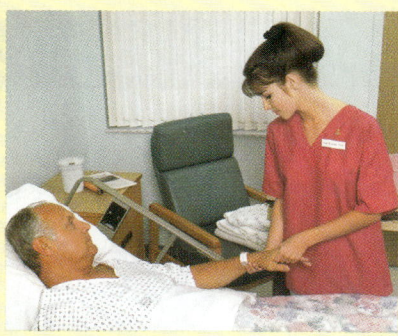

FIGURE 12–11
Identify the patient

3. Wash your hands (Figure 12–12) and put on gloves.

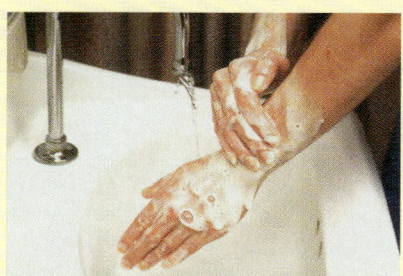

FIGURE 12–12
Wash hands and forearms

4. Tell the patient you are going to give him a bed bath.

5. Provide privacy for the patient (Figure 12–13).

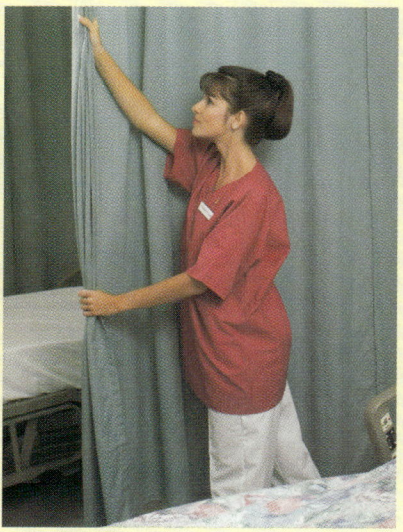

FIGURE 12–13
Provide privacy for the patient

PROCEDURE (CONTINUED)

STEPS

6. Assist the patient with oral hygiene.

7. Offer the bedpan or urinal.

8. Place the laundry bag on a chair near the bed.

9. Raise the bed to a comfortable working position and lock it in place (Figure 12–14).

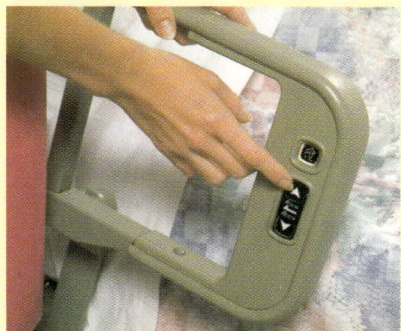

FIGURE 12–14
Raise bed to a comfortable working position

10. Pull out all the bedding from under the mattress. Leave it hanging loosely at all four sides of the bed (Figure 12–15).

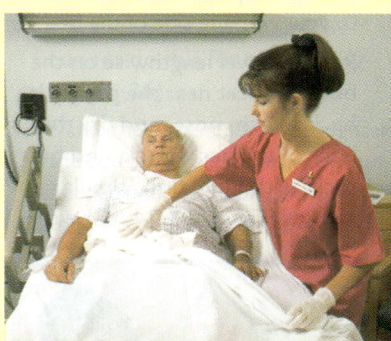

FIGURE 12–15
Pull out all bedding from under the mattress

11. Take the bedspread and regular blanket off the bed. Fold them loosely over the back of the chair, leaving the patient covered with the top sheet.

12. Place the bath blanket over the top sheet.

13. Remove the top sheet from underneath without uncovering (exposing) the patient. Fold the sheet loosely over the back of the chair if it is to be used again; if not, put it in the laundry bag.

14. Lower the headrest and knee rest of the bed, if permitted. The patient should be in a flat position, as flat as is comfortable and as is permitted.

15. Remove the patient's gown and ornamental jewelry. (It is not necessary to remove wedding rings.) Keep the patient covered with the bath blanket. If the gown belongs to the patient, put it away as requested. Place the hospital gown in the laundry bag. Put the jewelry into the drawer of the bedside table.

16. Fill the wash basin two-thirds full of warm water (115°F; 46.1°C).

17. Help the patient to move to the side of the bed closest to you. Use good body mechanics.

18. Put a towel across the patient's chest and make a mitten with the washcloth (Figure 12–16). Wash the patient's eyes from the nose to the outside of the face. Ask the patient if he wants soap used on his face. Wash the face, ears, and neck. Be careful not to get soap in his eyes. Rinse and dry by patting gently with the bath towel (Figure 12–17).

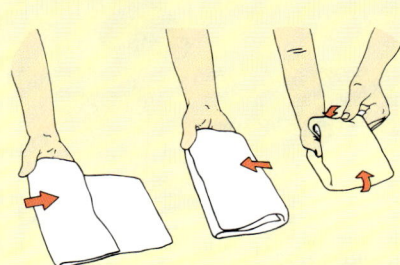

FIGURE 12–16
Make a mitten with the washcloth

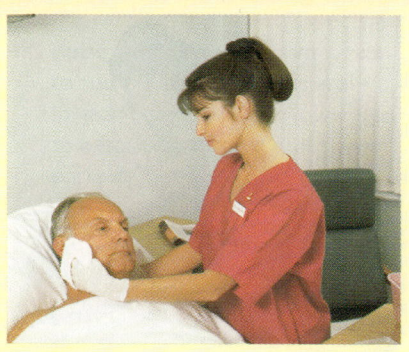

FIGURE 12–17
Wash face, ears, and neck

19. Put a towel lengthwise under the patient's arm farthest from you. This will keep the bed from getting wet. Support the patient's arm with the palm of your hand under his elbow. Then wash his shoulder, armpit (axilla), and arm. Use long, firm, circular strokes. Rinse and dry the area well (Figures 12–18 a and b and 12–19).

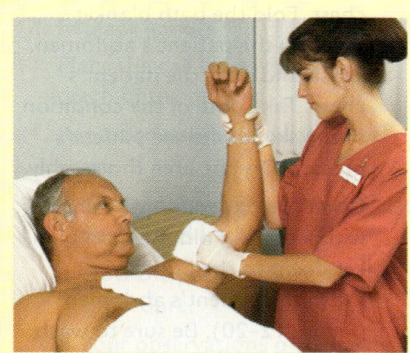

FIGURE 12–18a
Wash his shoulder

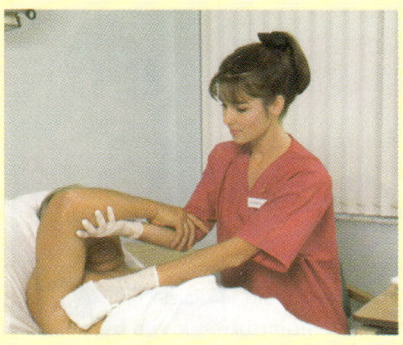

FIGURE 12–18b
Wash his armpit

PROCEDURE

OBRA

PERINEAL CARE FOR THE FEMALE PATIENT

PREPARATION

1. Assemble your equipment:
   a. Bath blanket
   b. Bedpan and cover
   c. Soap
   d. Basin with warm water (115°F; 46.1°C)
   e. Bath thermometer
   f. Disposable gloves
   g. Disposable bed protector
   h. Washcloth and towel
   i. Disposable plastic or cloth laundry bag for dirty linen (whichever is used by your institution)

2. Identify the patient by checking the identification bracelet.

3. Tell the patient that you are going to provide perineal care.

4. Provide privacy for the patient.

5. Provide safety with the side rail up on the opposite side of the bed.

6. Lower the side rail on the side nearest you.

STEPS

7. Position the patient on her back (a side-laying position is also used with some patients).

8. Remove the bedspread and blankets and place on a nearby chair or table for use after the bath.

9. Cover the patient with the bath blanket.

10. Being careful not to expose the patient, slide the sheet out from under the bath blanket and leave fanfolded at the foot of the bed.

11. Ask the patient to raise her hips, and then slide the bed protector under her.

12. Put on gloves. Offer the patient a bedpan. If used, raise the side rail, measure output if necessary, discard the contents in the toilet, and clean the bedpan. Remove gloves. Wash your hands.

13. Ask patient to flex her knees and separate her legs. If the patient is on her side, use a pillow or folded bath blanket between the knees to separate the legs comfortably and to allow easier access to the perineal area.

14. Slide down the bath blanket to expose the perineal area only, keeping the legs covered.

15. Put on gloves.

16. Wet the washcloth in the basin, form it into a mitt, add a small amount of soap. Too much soap will be difficult to rinse off, and may be drying or irritating to the skin.

17. Separate the vulva with one hand.

18. To wash gently:
    - Using the mitt, stroke the outer labia *once* from top downward to the perineum.
    - Rinse the washcloth, and repeat this *one* stroke to rinse the area.
    - Using the soaped mitt, stroke the other outer labia *once* from top, downward to the perineum.
    - Rinse the washcloth, and repeat this *one* stroke.
    - Repeat the above steps for both inner labia.
    - Separate the labia with one hand.
    - Wash and rinse with the same *one* downward stroke.

19. Rinse the washcloth, using the mitt to rinse the area washed.

20. More than one rinse, or wash, may be necessary to clean the area thoroughly.

21. Dry the area with the towel.

22. Turn the patient on her side away from you, and flex the knee of her upper leg slightly, if this is permitted depending on her restrictions.

23. Wet washcloth, form into a mitt, and apply soap.

24. Wash the anal area, using gentle front (perineum) to back (coccyx) strokes.

25. Rinse carefully as before. Repeat the wash and rinse if necessary.

26. Dry gently.

27. Reposition patient on her back or her side.

28. Remove the protective pad from the bed and dispose of it.

29. Dispose of gloves and wash your hands. Apply clean disposable gloves.

30. Pull the sheet over the top of the bath blanket. Slide the bath blanket out from under the sheet. Bag and discard in laundry hamper.

31. Place the spread and blanket back on the patient. Tuck in as required.

FOLLOW-UP

32. Empty the basin of water, clean according to policy, place in proper storage, dispose of washcloths and towel. Dispose of gloves and wash your hands.

33. Document the procedure (and output if appropriate). Remember to document any redness, sores, rashes, swelling, bleeding, discharge, or discomfort the patient may have in that area.

CARE OF NAILS AND FEET

Follow your health care facility's policy regarding care of nails and feet, specifically that of cutting nails. Always receive specific instructions from your supervisor before cutting a patient's nails. Routine and proper nail and foot care can help prevent infections and foot odor. For the elderly, those with poor circulation, and patients with diabetes, the lack of nail and foot care could result in an infection and even cause the patient to have a foot amputated.

For toenails and feet, follow the same procedure as for a partial bath. Allow the feet to soak for ten minutes in the warm water. Using the washcloth, rub the dry skin from the heels of the feet and wash well between the toes. Dry the feet thoroughly, especially between the toes. An orange stick can be used to gently remove any dirt from under the nails. If you have permission to do so, trim the nails straight across. Many institutions will not allow you to use an emery board or file as it may damage the soft tissue around the nails. Fingernails can be soaked in the emesis basin and then trimmed if needed. Be very careful not to trim any nail too short. Report any redness or problems noted.

The best time to observe the nails and feet is during the bath. If the nails are dirty or need trimming, this is a good time to do it. Nails should be trimmed at least weekly.

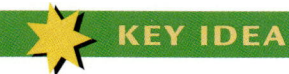 **KEY IDEA**

THE BACK RUB

Back rubs are usually given during morning care, right after the patient's bath. They also are given (1) as part of evening care, (2) when changing the position of a bedridden patient, (3) for very restless patients who need relaxing, and (4) on a doctor's orders for "special back care. (Figure 12–33a-c)"

A back rub relaxes the muscles, stimulates circulation, and refreshes the patient. Because of pressure caused by the bedclothes and the lack of movement to stimulate circulation, the skin of a bedridden patient needs special care to prevent skin breakdown.

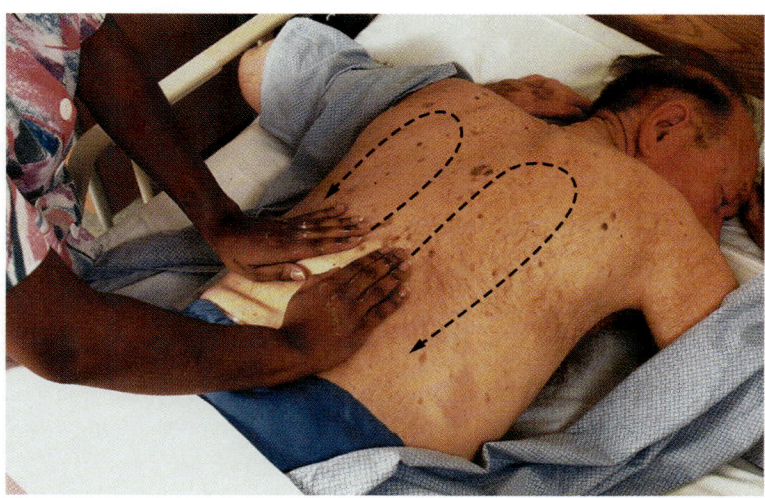

FIGURE 12–33a

Back rubs are usually given during morning care, right after the patient's bath

FIGURE 12–33b
Use firm circular motions with hands and fingertips over each bony area

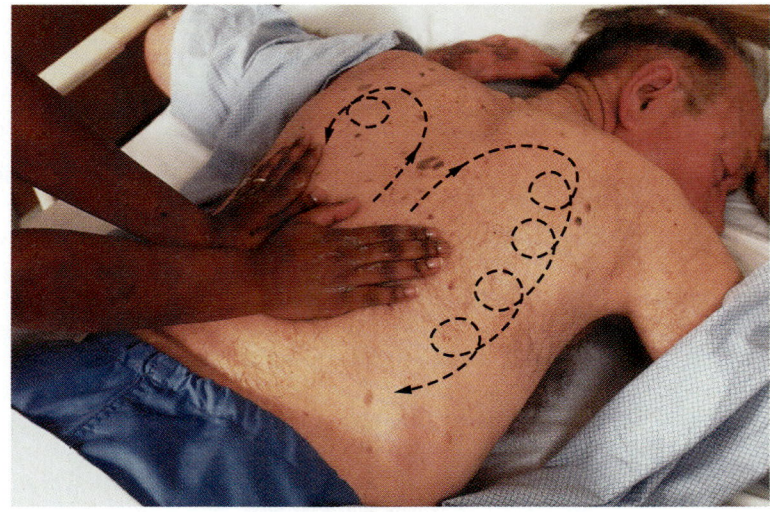

FIGURE 12–33c
Repeat firm circular motions covering the entire back

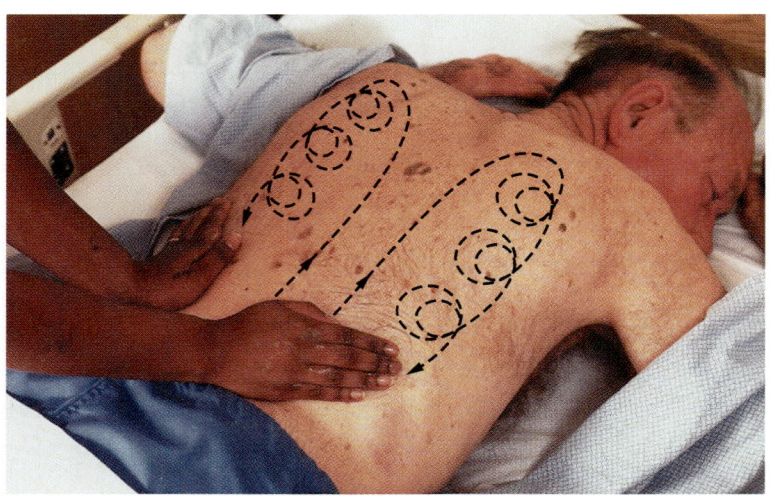

PROCEDURE

OBRA

GIVING THE PATIENT A BACK RUB

PREPARATION

1. Assemble your equipment on the bedside table:

   a. Towels

   b. Lotion

   c. Basin of warm water (115°F; 46.1°C)

2. Identify the patient by checking the identification bracelet.

3. Tell the patient you are going to give him a back rub.

4. Provide privacy for the patient.

5. Wash your hands.

6. Raise the bed to a comfortable working position.

STEPS

7. Ask the patient to turn on his side or abdomen so his back is toward you. Use the position that is most comfortable for the patient and for yourself.

8. The side rail should be in the up position on the far side of the bed.

9. Lotion may be warmed by placing the container in a basin of warm water (Figure 12–34).

PROCEDURE (CONTINUED)

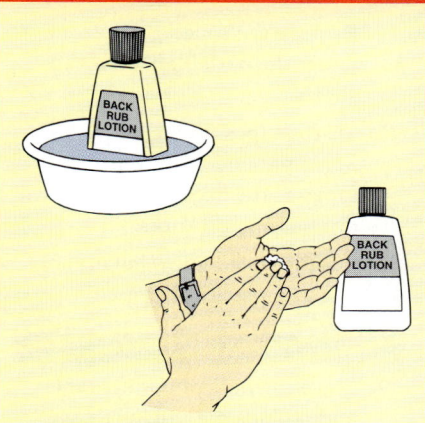

FIGURE 12–34
Apply warm lotion to your hands

10. Open the ties on the patient's gown or remove pajama top.

11. Pour a small amount of lotion into the palm of your hand.

12. Rub your hands together using friction to warm the lotion.

13. Keep your knees slightly bent and your back straight.

14. Apply lotion to the entire back with the palms of your hands. Use firm, long strokes from the buttocks to the shoulders and back of the neck.

15. Exert firm pressure as you stroke upward from the buttocks toward the shoulders. Use gentle pressure as you stroke downward from shoulders to buttocks (Figure 12–33a).

16. Use a circular motion on each bony area (Figure 12–33b).

17. This rhythmic rubbing motion should be continued from one and one-half minutes to three minutes (Figure 12–33c).

18. Dry the patient's back by patting gently with a towel.

19. Close and retie the gown.

20. Assist the patient in turning back to a comfortable position and replace the call light.

FOLLOW-UP

21. Arrange the top sheets of the bed neatly.

22. Lower the bed to a position of safety for the patient.

23. Raise the side rails when ordered or appropriate for patient safety.

24. Put your equipment back in its proper place. Discard disposable equipment.

25. Wash your hands.

26. Report to your immediate supervisor:

- That you have given the patient a back rub.
- The time it was given.
- How the patient tolerated the procedure.
- Your observations of anything unusual.

CHANGING THE PATIENT'S GOWN

When you change a patient's gown be careful not to expose the patient's body unnecessarily. It is important to prevent the patient from feeling any embarrassment or sudden chill from exposure to cool air.

PROCEDURE

OBRA

CHANGING THE PATIENT'S GOWN

PREPARATION

1. Assemble your equipment on the bedside table:

a. A clean gown

b. Disposable gloves

c. Disposable plastic or cloth laundry bag for dirty linen (whichever is used in your institution)

2. Identify the patient by checking the identification bracelet.

3. Tell the patient you are going to change his gown.

4. Provide privacy for the patient.

5. Wash your hands and put on gloves.

6. Adjust the bed to a comfortable working height.

STEPS

7. Ask the patient to turn on his side with his back toward you so you can untie the tapes.

8. If the patient cannot be turned, you will have to reach under his neck to untie the tapes.

PROCEDURE (CONTINUED)

9. Loosen the soiled gown around the patient's body.

10. Get the clean gown ready to put on the patient. Unfold it and lay it across the patient's chest on top of the bath blanket or top sheets.

11. Take off one sleeve at a time, leaving the old gown in place on the patient.

12. Slide each arm through one sleeve of the clean gown (Figure 12–35).

13. If the patient cannot hold his arm up, put your hand through the sleeve. Take his hand in yours and slip the sleeve up the patient's wrist and arm. Do this for both arms. Then pull the gown down over the patient's chest. If the patient has a sore arm, remove the sleeve on the unaffected arm first. Then remove the sleeve on the sore (affected) arm. To put the clean gown on, put the sleeve on the sore (affected) arm first. Then slide the unaffected arm through the second sleeve.

14. Remove the soiled gown from under the bath blanket or top sheets.

15. Tie the tapes on the clean gown. Some patients want only the tapes at the neck tied so they will not be lying on knots.

16. Put the soiled gown in laundry bag and place in hamper.

FOLLOW-UP

17. Make the patient comfortable and replace the call light.

18. Lower the bed to a position of safety for the patient.

19. Raise the side rails when ordered or appropriate for patient safety.

20. Remove the gloves and wash your hands.

21. Report to your immediate supervisor:
    - That you have replaced the patient's soiled gown with a clean one.
    - Your observations of anything unusual.

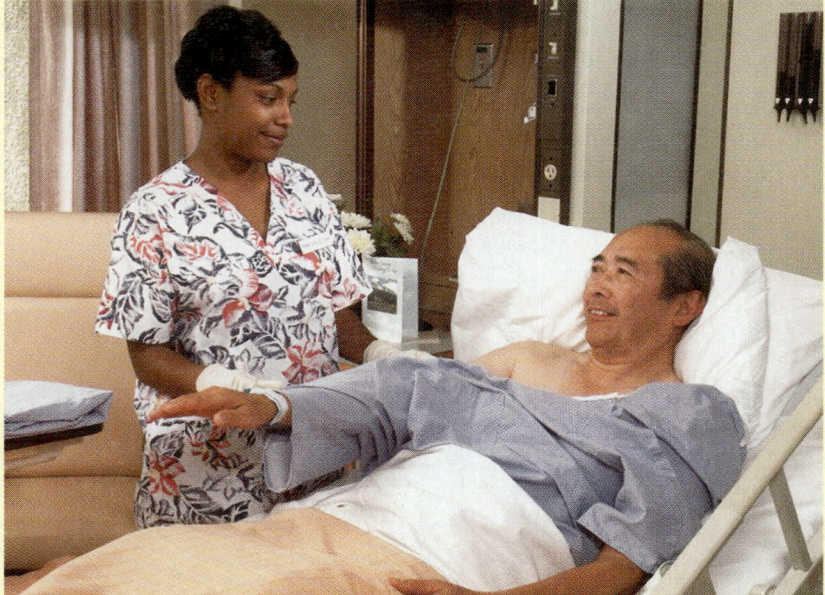

FIGURE 12–35
Slide each arm through one sleeve of the patient's clean gown

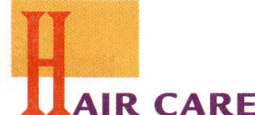

HAIR CARE

Patients who will be in the health care institution for a long time may occasionally need to have their hair shampooed. Often the doctor must write the order for a shampoo. The nurse must give you instructions for giving the shampoo. For patients on bed rest, the patient must be in bed when the shampoo is given. Other patients may be allowed to shampoo in the tub or shower.

PROCEDURE

OBRA

SHAMPOOING THE PATIENT'S HAIR

PREPARATION

1. Assemble your equipment on the bedside table:

   a. Basin of warm water (105°F; 40.5°C)

   b. Pitcher of warm water (115°F; 46.1°C)

   c. Bath thermometer

   d. Large basin

   e. Water trough (shampoo tray) or plastic sheet

   f. Disposable bed protector

   g. Pillow with waterproof case

   h. Face and bath towels

   i. Washcloth, to cover the patient's eyes

   j. Paper cup

   k. Bath blanket

   l. Cotton

   m. Disposable gloves

   n. Disposable plastic or cloth laundry bag for dirty linen (whichever is used in your institution)

2. Identify the patient by checking the identification bracelet.

3. Tell the patient you are going to give her a shampoo.

4. Provide privacy for the patient.

5. Wash your hands and put on gloves.

6. Raise the bed to its highest horizontal position.

STEPS

7. Brush the patient's hair. Have her turn her head from side to side so the hair can be brushed one exposed side at a time.

8. Place a chair at the side of the bed near the patient's head. The chair should be lower than the mattress. The back of the chair should be touching the mattress.

9. Place the small towel on the chair. Put the large basin on the chair.

10. Put small amounts of cotton in the patient's ears for protection.

11. Ask the patient to move across the bed so that her head is close to where you are standing.

12. Remove the pillow from under the patient's head. Cover the pillow with the waterproof case. Place the pillow between the shoulder blades, so that the head tilts back when the patient lies down.

13. Put the bath blanket on the bed. From underneath, fanfold the top sheets to the foot of the bed without exposing the patient.

14. Place the disposable bed protector on the mattress under the patient's head.

15. Place the shampoo trough under the patient's head. A trough can be made by rolling over the three sides of the plastic sheet three times. This makes a channel for the water to run off. Put the end of the channel under the patient's head. Have the other open end hanging over the side of the bed. This free end of the plastic sheet should be put into the large basin on the chair.

16. Loosen the patient's gown at the neck.

17. Dampen the washcloth and ask the patient to hold the damp washcloth over her eyes (Figure 12–36).

18. Fill the basin with warm water. Put the basin on the bedside table with the paper cup.

19. Fill the pitcher with warm water. Have the pitcher on the bedside table, for extra water, if needed.

20. Fill the paper cup with water from the basin. Pour it over the hair; repeat until completely wet.

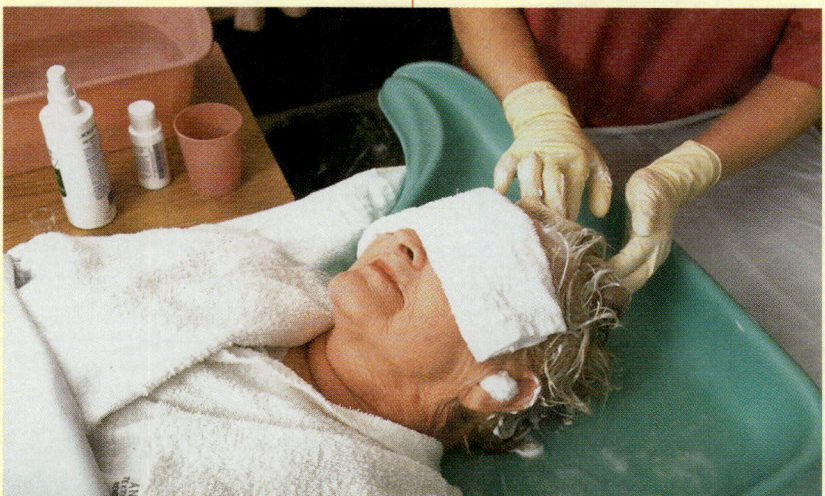

FIGURE 12–36

Apply a damp wash cloth over patient's eyes. Use both hands to carefully shampoo hair

PROCEDURE (CONTINUED)

21. Apply a small amount of shampoo and, using both hands, wash the hair and massage the patient's scalp with your fingertips. Avoid using fingernails as they could scratch the scalp.

22. Rinse the soap off the hair by pouring water from the cup over the hair. Have the patient turn her head from side to side. Repeat this until the hair is free of shampoo.

23. Dry the patient's forehead and ears with the face towel.

24. Remove the cotton from the ears.

25. Raise the patient's head and wrap the head with a bath towel.

26. Rub the patient's hair with the towel to dry it as much as possible.

27. Remove your equipment from the bed. Change the patient's gown, if necessary.

28. Comb the patient's hair. Leave a towel wrapped around the head or spread a towel out over the pillow under the head until the hair is completely dry. If a dryer is available, use it to dry the patient's hair. Use low or warm setting and move dryer to avoid burning the scalp.

29. Remove the bath blanket and at the same time bring the top sheets back up to cover the patient.

FOLLOW-UP

30. Make the patient comfortable and replace the call light.

31. Lower the bed to a position of safety for the patient.

32. Raise the side rails when ordered or appropriate for patient safety.

33. Clean and return your equipment. Discard disposable equipment.

34. Remove the gloves and wash your hands.

35. Report to your immediate supervisor:

- That you have given the patient a shampoo.
- How the patient tolerated the procedure.
- Your observations of anything unusual.

KEY IDEA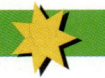

As with other types of personal care, a patient may be too weak or ill to take care of her own hair. It may be difficult for her to raise her arms. Combing and brushing a patient's hair almost always leaves the patient looking and feeling better.

PROCEDURE

OBRA

COMBING THE PATIENT'S HAIR

PREPARATION

1. Assemble your equipment on the bedside table:
   a. Towel
   b. Comb or brush
   c. Hand mirror, if available
   d. Disposable gloves
   e. Disposable plastic or cloth laundry bag for dirty linen (whichever is used by your institution)

2. Wash your hands and put on gloves.

3. Identify the patient by checking the identification bracelet.

4. Provide privacy for the patient.

5. Tell the patient you are going to brush or comb her hair.

6. Raise the bed to a comfortable working height.

STEPS

7. If possible, comb the patient's hair after the bath and before you make the bed.

8. Lay a towel across the pillow under the patient's head. If the patient can sit up in bed, drape the towel around her shoulders.

PROCEDURE (CONTINUED)

9. If wearing glasses, ask the patient to remove them before you begin. Be sure to put the glasses in a safe place.

10. Part the hair down the middle to make it easier to comb.

11. Brush or comb the patient's hair carefully, gently, and thoroughly, combing small amounts of hair at a time.

12. For the patient who cannot sit up, separate the hair into small sections. Comb each section separately, using a downward motion. Ask the patient to turn her head from side to side or turn it for her so you can reach the entire head (Figure 12–37).

13. Comb the patient's hair into the style the patient requests.

14. If the patient has very long hair, suggest braiding it to keep it from getting tangled.

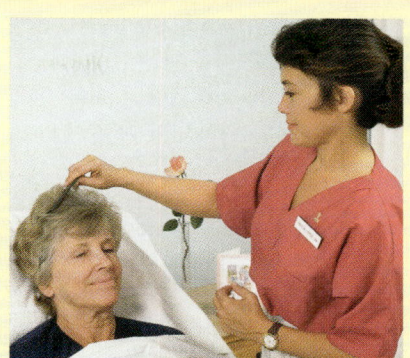

FIGURE 12–37
Comb each section of hair separately

15. Be sure you brush the back of the head. Observe any breaks in skin or abnormal findings.

16. Remove the towel when you are finished.

FOLLOW-UP

17. Let the patient use the mirror.

18. Make the patient comfortable and replace the call light.

19. Lower the bed to a position of safety for the patient.

20. Raise the side rails when ordered or appropriate for patient safety.

21. Clean and return your equipment to its proper place.

22. Remove the gloves and wash your hands.

23. Report to your immediate supervisor:

- That you have combed the patient's hair.
- How the patient tolerated the procedure.
- Your observations of anything unusual.

SHAVING THE PATIENT'S BEARD

A regular morning activity for most men is shaving their beard. A patient is often well enough to shave himself. In this case, you will give him only the help that is necessary, such as being sure he has the equipment he needs. Sometimes patients are too ill or weak to shave themselves. In such cases, you will do it. Before shaving any patient's face, be sure to get permission from your immediate supervisor. Certain patients may not be permitted to shave or be shaved.

Shaving can be done with an electric razor or a safety razor. Often, the patient will have his own electric razor which you will be able to use.

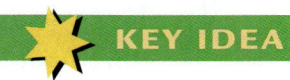

KEY IDEA

Many hospitals have special rules and policies regarding electrical equipment being brought into the hospital. Follow the nurse's instructions regarding electric razors. Due to bleeding precautions certain patients should not be shaved with a safety razor.

PROCEDURE

OBRA

SHAVING THE PATIENT'S BEARD

PREPARATION

1. Assemble your equipment on the bedside table:
   a. Face towel
   b. Basin of warm water (115°F; 46.1°C)
   c. Shaving brush, shaving cream, and safety razor, or
   d. Electric razor
   e. Disposable gloves
   f. Disposable plastic or cloth laundry bag for dirty linen (whichever is used by your institution)

2. Identify the patient by checking the identification bracelet.

3. Tell the patient you are going to shave his beard.

4. Provide privacy for the patient.

5. Wash your hands and put on gloves.

6. Raise the bed to a comfortable working height.

STEPS

7. Adjust a light so that it shines on the patient's face.

8. Raise the head of the bed, if allowed.

9. Spread the face towel under the patient's chin. If the patient has dentures, be sure they are in his mouth.

10. Pat some warm water or use a damp, warm washcloth on the patient's face to soften his beard if using a safety razor.

11. Apply shaving soap generously to the face if using a safety razor.

12. With the fingers of one hand, hold the skin taut (tight) as you shave in the direction that the hairs grow. Start under the sideburns and work downward over the cheeks (Figure 12–38). Continue carefully over the chin. Work upward on the neck under the chin. Use short, firm strokes.

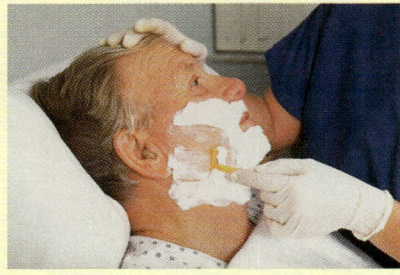

FIGURE 12–38
Work downward over the cheeks

13. Rinse the safety razor often.

14. Areas under the nose and around the lips are sensitive. Take special care in these areas.

15. If you nick the patient's skin, report this to your supervisor.

16. Wash off the remaining soap when you have finished.

17. Pat on aftershave lotion or powder, as the patient prefers.

FOLLOW-UP

18. Make the patient comfortable and replace the call light.

19. Lower the bed to a position of safety for the patient.

20. Raise the side rails when ordered or appropriate for patient safety.

21. Clean and return your equipment. Bag soiled towel and place in hamper. Discard disposable equipment. Razor blades or disposable razors should be discarded in sharps containers.

22. Dispose of gloves and wash your hands.

23. Report to your immediate supervisor:
    - That you have shaved the patient's beard.
    - How the patient tolerated the procedure.
    - Your observations of anything unusual.

urinal A portable container given to male patients so they can urinate without getting out of bed

bedpan A pan used by patients who must defecate or urinate while in bed

urinate To discharge urine from the body; other words for this function are void, micturate, and pass water

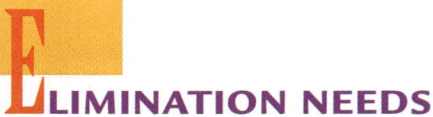

ELIMINATION NEEDS

Some patients are unable to get out of bed to use the bathroom. For these patients a **urinal** and a **bedpan** are required. The urinal is a container into which the male patient **urinates**. The bedpan is a pan into which he **defecates** (moves his bowels). The **fracture pan** is slightly smaller and shallower than the regular bedpan. It is used by the patient whose illness or injuries don't allow the patient sufficient movement to utilize a bedpan. The female patient uses the bedpan for urination and defecation.

Wear gloves whenever handling a bedpan or urinal after use. You should always cover the bedpan and remove it from the patient's bedside to the bathroom as quickly as possible after use. At this time you would collect a specimen if required. You would also measure the urine if the patient is on intake and output.

eliminate (defecate) To rid the body of waste products; to excrete, expel, remove, put out; (To have a bowel movement; to excrete waste matter from the bowels)

fracture pan A bedpan with a flat end that goes under the patient

PROCEDURE

OBRA

OFFERING THE BEDPAN

PREPARATION

1. Assemble your equipment on the bedside table (Figure 12–39):

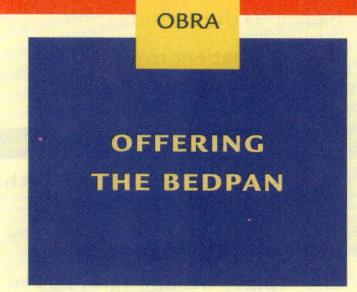

FIGURE 12–39
Assemble equipment

   a. Bedpan and cover, or fracture pan and cover (may be placed on chair) (Figure 12–40)

   b. Toilet tissue

   c. Wash basin with warm water (115°F; 46.1°C)

   d. Soap

   e. Hand towel

   f. Powder

   g. Disposable bed protector

   h. Disposable gloves

2. Identify the patient by checking the identification bracelet.

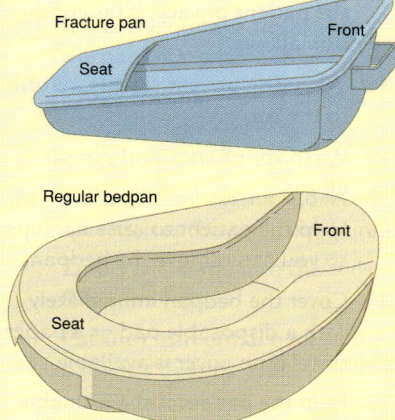

FIGURE 12–40
Choose appropriate type of bedpan and cover

3. Ask the patient if she would like to use the bedpan.

4. Provide privacy for the patient.

5. Wash your hands and put on gloves.

6. Raise the bed to a comfortable working position.

STEPS

7. Take the bedpan out of the bedside table. Warm the bedpan if necessary by running warm water inside it and along the rim. Dry the outside of the bedpan with paper towels. Put powder on the bedpan to decrease friction.

8. Fold back the top sheets so that they are out of the way.

9. Raise the patient's gown, but keep the lower part of her body covered.

10. Ask the patient to bend her knees and put her feet flat on the mattress if she is able. Then ask the patient to raise her hips. If necessary, help the patient to raise her buttocks by slipping your hand under the lower part of her back. Place the protective pad and then the bedpan in position with the seat of the bedpan (smooth round rim) under the buttocks (Figure 12–41 a). (Place the fracture pan with the flat end under the patient's buttocks.)

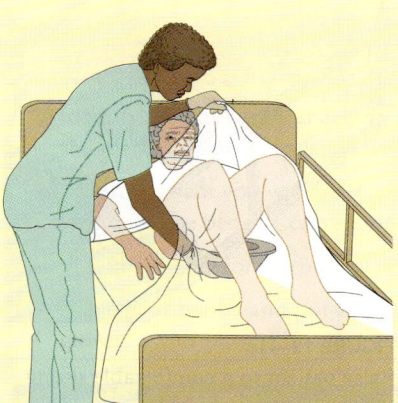

FIGURE 12–41a
Position bedpan under the buttocks

11. Sometimes the patient is unable to lift her buttocks to get on or off the bedpan. In this case, turn the patient on her side with her back to you. Put the bedpan against the buttocks. Then turn the patient onto the bedpan (Figure 12–41 b).

12. Replace the covers over the patient.

PROCEDURE (CONTINUED)

9. Ask the patient to signal when he is finished.

10. Dispose of your gloves and wash your hands. Leave the room to give the patient privacy, if his condition allows.

11. When the patient signals, return to the room. Wash your hands.

12. Put on gloves and help the patient clean himself.

13. Assist the patient back to bed.

14. Close the cover on the commode.

15. Help the patient to wash his hands in the basin of water.

16. Make the patient comfortable.

17. Remove the bedpan from under the commode. Cover it and carry it to the patient's bathroom.

18. Check the excreta (feces or urine) for abnormal (unusual) appearance.

19. Measure output if patient is on intake and output. If a specimen is required, collect it at this time.

20. Empty the bedpan into the toilet.

21. Health care institutions have different equipment in the bathroom for cleaning the bedpan. Follow your institution's instructions for cleaning the bedpan.

22. Dispose of your gloves and wash your hands.

23. Put the clean bedpan back in the bedside table. Put the commode in its proper place.

FOLLOW-UP

24. Lower the bed to a position of safety for the patient.

25. Raise the side rails when ordered or appropriate for patient safety.

26. Place the call light within easy reach of the patient.

27. Report to your immediate supervisor:
    - That the patient has voided or defecated.
    - If a specimen was collected.
    - How the patient tolerated the procedure.
    - Your observations of anything unusual.

THE INCONTINENT PATIENT

incontinence The inability to control the bowels or bladder

Some patients are not able to control their bladder or bowels. This condition is called **incontinence.** A draw sheet and a reusable or disposable bed protector are used on the bed. These patients should be checked frequently to make sure they are clean and dry. Follow the procedure for a partial bed bath each time the patient is soiled. (See perineal care earlier in this chapter.) For urinary incontinence in some patients, the physician may order an indwelling catheter. Due to the increased risk of a urinary infection with an indwelling catheter, an external condom catheter may be ordered for males. For some patients, bowel and bladder retraining will be ordered. Your supervisor will instruct you on the procedures for retraining each individual patient.

KEY IDEA ⭐ Washing and drying the patient thoroughly will decrease the probability of the patient getting decubitus ulcers and infections.

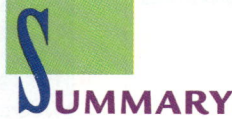

SUMMARY

Meeting the needs of your patients in regard to their activities of daily living is a major responsibility. Assisting patients with oral hygiene, bathing, perineal care, care of nails, feet, and hair, and elimination in a skillful manner will increase their comfort and well-being. Following each procedure correctly will provide for safety for you and the patient. Each patient is to be treated as an individual. Your observations while helping patients are important to other members of the health care team as they evaluate care needed.

THE NURSING ASSISTANT IN ACTION

Doctors Overheard Discussing Patient

You are in the elevator at work along with a couple of doctors and three visitors. The doctors start a conversation about one of the patients you are assigned to care for today. You notice the visitors paying attention to the doctors' conversation about treatment options for Mr. Chu, your patient.

What Is Your Response/Action?

1. In your own words, describe how you would feel in this situation.

2. What are your concerns?

3. What are your options in this situation?

4. Which of these options would you follow? Explain why.

5. What did you learn from this situation that you will apply in future situations?

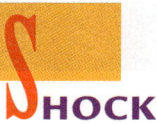HOCK

Shock may accompany many emergency situations. **Shock** is the failure of the **cardio-vascular system** to provide sufficient blood circulation to every part of the body. Diagnostic signs of shock are

- Eyes are dull and lack luster
- Pupils may be dilated
- Face is pale and cyanotic (blue)
- Respirations are shallow, irregular, or labored
- Pulse is rapid and weak
- Skin is cold, clammy (moist), and pale

The shock patient may be:

- Nauseated
- Anxious and restless
- Thirsty

The shock patient may:

- Collapse
- Vomit

■ Types of Shock

Shock may be caused by many factors, such as

- Excessive blood loss
- Any severe injury
- Insufficient oxygen
- Spinal cord damage
- Reaction of nervous system to fear, the sight of blood, and so on
- Inadequate heart function
- Infection
- Loss of body fluid or changes in body chemistry
- Extreme allergic reaction

Hemorrhagic shock is caused by blood loss. The reduction of blood volume means that circulation is impaired; this may occur for several reasons.

- External bleeding
- Internal bleeding
- Loss of plasma (the straw-colored liquid component of blood) due to burns or crushed tissues

shock The failure of the cardiovascular system to provide sufficient blood circulation to every part of the body

cardiovascular system Circulatory system which includes heart, arteries, veins, and capillaries

Respiratory shock is caused by insufficient oxygen in the blood. The inability to fill the lungs completely is the result of impaired breathing. This may happen because of

- A chest wound
- Broken ribs
- A collapsed lung
- Airway obstruction
- Spinal cord damage that has paralyzed the muscles of the chest

Neurogenic shock is caused by loss of control of the nervous system. This may occur because of

- Trauma to the spinal cord
- Infection

Psychogenic shock or fainting is caused by a reaction of the nervous system to fear, bad news, the sight of blood, or a minor injury. Sudden dilation of the blood vessels occurs and the blood flow to the brain is reduced. The person faints, and unless other problems are present, fainting is usually self-correcting. When the head is lowered, blood circulates to the brain and normal function is restored. However, injury due to fainting, such as falling and injuring a body part, can occur.

Cardiogenic shock is caused by inadequate functioning of the heart. When the heart does not continuously operate due to disorders that weaken the heart muscle, the heart may no longer have the strength to pump blood to all parts of the body.

Septic shock is caused by infection. Toxins released into the bloodstream have a harmful effect on the blood vessels, causing them to dilate (get larger), which results in incomplete filling of the circulatory system.

Metabolic shock is caused by loss of body fluids and changes in body chemistry. This happens because of

- Loss of body fluids through diarrhea, vomiting, or urination
- Severe disturbance of body salts or the acid-base balance in diseases

GUIDELINES

ASSISTING THE PATIENT IN SHOCK

- Call for medical help.
- Maintain an open airway to assure breathing.
- Keep the person quiet and lying down with the feet and legs slightly higher than the body and head unless contraindicated

(Figure 13–2). Maintain normal body temperature.

- If a broken bone is suspected, keep the person in crisis flat. Do not move.
- Control bleeding.
- Do not offer any food or drink.
- Talk to the person in crisis and offer reassurance.
- Stay with the person in crisis until emergency medical rescue help arrives.

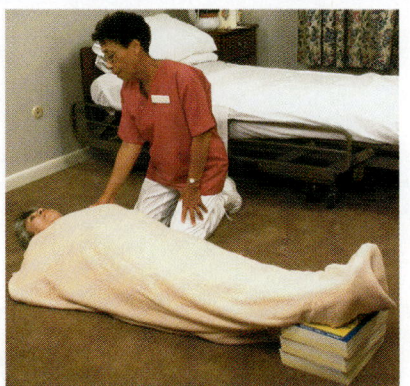

FIGURE 13–2
Keep the person quiet and lying down with the feet and legs slightly higher than the body and head; maintain normal body temperature

Anaphylactic shock or allergic reaction occurs when a person comes in contact with something to which he or she is extremely sensitive or allergic. This may be caused by

- Insect stings (bees, yellow jackets, wasps, and hornets)
- Inhaled substances (dust, pollen)
- Injected substances (drugs such as penicillin)
- Ingested substances (foods, medications)

HEART ATTACK, CHEST PAIN, AND CARDIAC ARREST

heart attack Interruption or damage to the blood supply to the heart muscle; myocardial infarction

The heart muscle has its own blood supply. Interruption or damage to this blood supply is a **heart attack**, or myocardial infarction, which may cause damage to the heart muscle. Since it is difficult to determine if chest pain is really a heart attack, all chest pain is treated as if it could be a heart attack.

Signs and symptoms of a heart attack include

- Chest pain or discomfort, with lightheadedness
- Shortness of breath
- Lowered blood pressure
- Shallow and difficult respirations
- Profuse perspiration or sweating
- Wet, clammy, cold skin
- Rapid, weak, irregular pulse or lack of a pulse
- Pale color
- Nausea and vomiting
- Loss of consciousness or fainting

If there is chest pain, it is severe and crushing and may radiate to the inner left arm, the jaw, or the neck; the person in crisis may refer to the chest pain as a belt around his chest or heaviness in his chest. Sharp, stabbing, or short twinges of chest pain are usually not signs of a heart attack.

cardiac arrest The unexpected stopping of the heartbeat and circulation

Cardiac arrest is the unexpected stopping of the heartbeat and circulation (loss of heart function). This situation calls for immediate emergency care.

Signs and symptoms of cardiac arrest include

- Loss of consciousness
- Absence of pulse
- Absence of heart sounds
- Absence of breath sounds
- Enlargement of the pupils of the eye
- Ashen gray color of the skin
- Lips and nailbeds may turn blue

GUIDELINES

OBRA

ASSISTING THE PERSON HAVING A HEART ATTACK, CHEST PAIN, OR MYOCARDIAL INFARCTION

- Call for medical help or activate the EMS system.
- Help the person in crisis into a comfortable position that allows the easiest breathing.
- Loosen clothing if it is tight.
- Encourage the person in crisis to remain quiet.

- Measure respiration and pulse at frequent intervals.
- Talk to the person in crisis; offer reassurance to him.
- Do not offer any food or drink.
- Stay with the person in crisis until emergency medical rescue help arrives.

CARDIOPULMONARY RESUSCITATION (CPR)

Cardiopulmonary resuscitation (CPR) is a basic, life-saving procedure for sudden cardiac or respiratory arrest. The technique of CPR provides basic emergency life support until emergency medical help arrives. CPR keeps oxygenated blood flowing to the brain and other vital body organs until medical treatment can be given to restore normal heart function.

cardiopulmonary resuscitation (CPR) An emergency procedure used to reestablish effective circulation and respiration in order to prevent irreversible brain damage

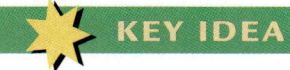

KEY IDEA

Only a person who has been trained in CPR can safely perform the rescue techniques. The only way of learning CPR is to enroll in an approved, supervised program.

Note: The following material is not intended to be a CPR course. An authorized CPR course includes practice on mannequins supervised by a certified trained instructor to direct you in CPR with written and performance examinations. The American Heart Association and the American Red Cross, as well as other community service organizations, offer classes in CPR. Most health care institutions require all employees to be certified in CPR and to complete periodic recertification. Only a person who has been trained in CPR should perform the rescue techniques. Different techniques are required for adults versus pediatric patients and must be learned.

There are three basic rescue skills to CPR. These are referred to as the ABCs of CPR.

- A, airway
- B, breathing
- C, circulation

Airway

The first action to take is to check the person for unresponsiveness. Tap or gently shake the person and shout "Are you O.K.?" If there is no response, call for assistance now (call for another individual or 911) so you can proceed to start CPR.

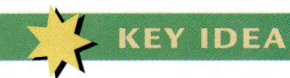

KEY IDEA

The most important factor in successful resuscitation is the immediate opening of the airway. There are many possible causes of an obstructed airway. The most common cause in an unconscious person is the tongue.

The recommended technique for opening the airway must be simple, safe, easily learned, and effective. Since the head-tilt/chin-lift method meets these criteria, it is considered the method of choice. (Appropriate training should be obtained in an approved course before applying in practice. You may also be taught the jaw-thrust technique.)

To accomplish the head-tilt maneuver, one hand is placed on the victim's forehead and firm backward pressure is applied with the palm to tilt the head back. To complete the head-tilt/chin-lift maneuver, the fingers of the other hand are placed under the bony part of the lower jaw near the chin to gently lift the chin up (Figure 13–3). This supports the jaw and helps to tilt the head back. Do not use this technique if there is a possibility of injuries to the head, neck, or spine as to not do further damage.

Look to see if there is any chest movement.

Listen for any breath sounds.

Feel for the victim's breath on your cheek (Figure 13–4).

If the victim does not spontaneously begin breathing after you have opened the airway, then begin rescue breathing.

■ Breathing

Mouth-to-mouth rescue breathing is the most effective way of getting oxygen into the lungs of the victim. The American Heart Association teaches mouth-to-mouth, mouth-to-nose, mouth-to-stoma, and mouth-to-barrier device breathing. The mouth-to-barrier method is preferred to reduce the risk of contact exposure.

The barrier device or mask should have a one way valve so that exhaled air does not enter the rescuer's mouth (Figure 13–5). If rescue breathing is deemed necessary, the barrier device is positioned over the victim's mouth and nose, ensuring an adequate seal. Mouth-to-barrier device breathing is then initiated using slow inspiratory breaths (1½ to 2 seconds), as described following.

Keeping the airway open by the head-tilt/chin-lift maneuver, you should gently pinch the nose closed with the thumb and index finger of the hand on the forehead. Open your mouth wide and place it tightly over the victim's mouth, creating a tight seal. Blow two slow breaths lasting 1½ to 2 seconds and then remove your mouth. Turn your head to the side with your ear close to the victim's mouth and listen for a return of air. If there is no return of air, or if you met resistance while trying to blow air into the patient, you must recheck the head and neck position. If the airway is obstructed, no air can flow to the lungs.

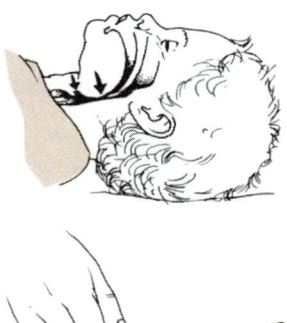
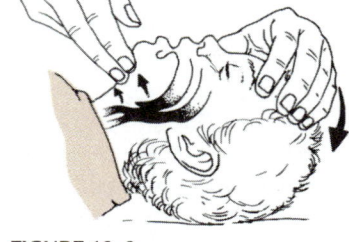

FIGURE 13–3
The head-tilt/chin-lift maneuver

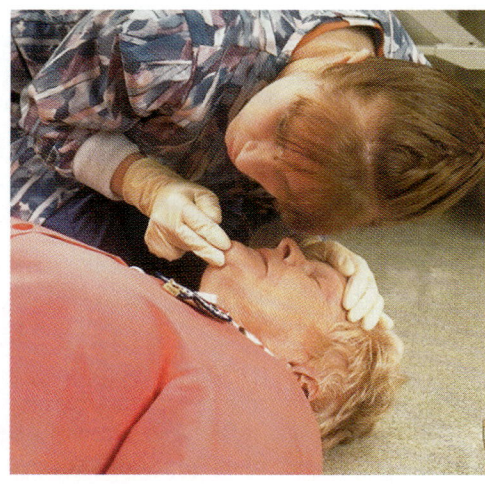

FIGURE 13–4
Open the airway and look, listen, and feel

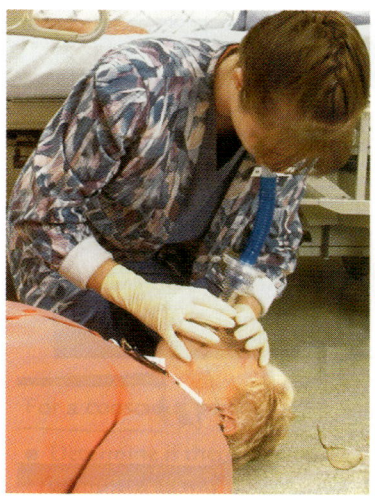

FIGURE 13–5
One-way valve protective device

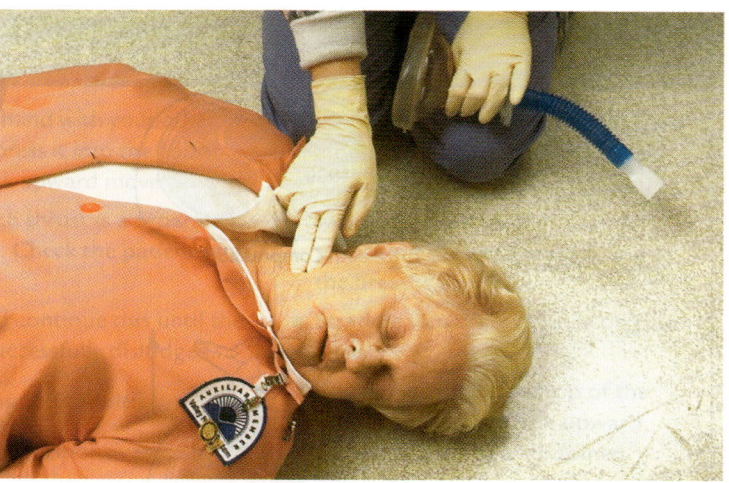

FIGURE 13–6
With the tips of your fingers find the groove next to the Adam's apple and feel for a pulse

After you have given the victim two breaths, check to see if the heart is beating. To feel the carotid pulse, use your hand that has been lifting the chin. With the tips of your fingers, find the groove next to the Adam's apple and feel for a pulse for 5–10 seconds (Figure 13–6). Check the pulse after the first minute and then every few minutes thereafter. If the heart is beating, you must breathe for the victim at a rate of 12 breaths per minute (one breath every 5 seconds) for an adult while maintaining the open airway. If the heart is not beating (no pulse), you will then have to artificially pump the heart and circulate the victim's blood using external chest compressions.

For both one-rescuer and two-rescuer CPR, deliver 10–12 breaths per minute. In one-rescuer CPR, pause after every 15th chest compression for two ventilations. In two-rescuer CPR, pause after every 5th chest compression for one ventilation.

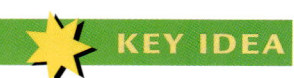

KEY IDEA

Note: To protect both the victim and yourself when performing CPR, a pocket face mask or other protective device must be used as a barrier. The barrier will protect the victim and yourself from transferring any communicable diseases either individual may be carrying.

There are many types of protective barrier devices; your instructor and the facility where you are working will determine which device you will use. No device, however, can guarantee 100 percent protection from transmission of germs.

■ Circulation

External chest compression along with mouth-to-mouth resuscitation will allow oxygenated blood to circulate to the brain and other organs. To perform external chest compression, kneel next to the victim's chest. Place the heel of one hand on the lower third (1/3) of the sternum, place your other hand on top; the fingers may be either interlaced or extended but should be kept off the chest wall (Figure 13–7). As you compress downward, your shoulders should be directly over the victim's midline and your arms kept straight (Figure 13–8). For an adult victim you will depress 1 1/2 to 2 inches. When you release this pressure, do not remove your hands from the sternum. These compressions should be rhythmic so that compression and release are of equal duration. Deliver 15 compressions for every 2 breaths when you are providing mouth-to-mouth rescue breathing. Deliver a rate of 80–100 compressions per minute.

TABLE 13-1

Common Poisons

POISON	SYMPTOMS AND SIGNS
Acetaminophen	Nausea, vomiting, heavy perspiration. The victim is usually a child.
Acids	Burns on or around the lips. Burning in mouth, throat, and stomach, often followed by heavy vomiting.
Alkalis (ammonia, bleaches, detergents, lye, washing soda, certain fertilizers)	Check to see if mouth membranes appear white and swollen. There may be a "soapy" appearance in the mouth. Abdominal pain is usually present. Vomiting may occur, often full of blood and mucus.
Arsenic (rat poisons)	"Garlic breath," with burning in the mouth, throat, and stomach. Abdominal pain can be severe. Vomiting is common.
Aspirin	Delayed reactions, including ringing in the ears, rapid and deep breathing, dry skin, and restlessness.
Corrosive Agents (disinfectants, drain cleaners, household acids, iodine, pine oil, turpentine, toilet bowl cleaners, styptic pencil, water softeners, strong acids)	(See Acids)
Food Poisoning	Difficult to detect since symptoms and signs vary greatly. Usually you will note abdominal pain, nausea and vomiting, gas, loud, frequent bowel sounds, and diarrhea.
Iodine	Upset stomach and vomiting. If a starchy meal has been eaten, the vomitus may appear blue.
Metals (copper, lead, mercury, zinc)	Metallic taste in mouth, with nausea and abdominal pains. Vomiting may occur. Stools may be bloody or dark.
Petroleum Products (some deodorizers, heating fuel, diesel fuels, gasoline, kerosene, lighter fluid, lubricating oil, naphtha, rust remover, transmission fluid)	Note characteristic odors on patient's breath, on clothing, or in vomitus.
Plants—Contact (poison ivy, poison oak, poison sumac)	Swollen, itchy areas on the skin, with quickly forming "blister-like" lesions.
Plants—Ingested (azalea, castor bean, elderberry, foxglove, holly berries, lily of the valley, mistletoe berries, mountain laurel, mushrooms and toadstools, nightshade, oleander, rhododendron, rhubarb, rubber plant, some wild cherries)	Difficult to detect, ranging from nausea to coma. Always question in cases of apparent child poisoning.
Strychnine (rat poisons)	The face, jaw, and neck will stiffen. Strong convulsions occur quickly after ingesting.

AGE-SPECIFIC CONSIDERATIONS

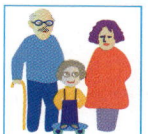

Babies, toddlers, and small children are prone to put things in their mouths and have no fear. Parents need to install childproof locks on cabinets containing medications, toxic cleaning products, or other poisonous substances. Teens may experiment with toxic substances such as sniffing glue or get high or binge drink alcohol, which can result in alcohol poisoning or death. Parents need to caution teens and young adults that they should be cautious at parties or on dates to avoid leaving their drinks unattended or consuming punches as there has been an increase in use of "date-rape" drugs, which can be lethal in large doses. Adults may ignore warning labels and use cleaning or toxic chemicals in inadequately ventilated places. Elderly persons with poor eyesight may accidentally inject a toxic substance or, in confusion, overdose on prescribed medications.

GUIDELINES

ASSISTING THE PERSON WHO HAS BEEN POISONED

- Observe the person in crisis.
- Check the mouth for signs of burns.
- Check the breath for a significant odor.
- Ask questions of the person in crisis and other persons present to gather as many facts as possible before you act. Look for a medication container or bottle that may have been holding the poison.

- Call the regional poison control center immediately. The number is always found on the inside cover or on the first page of the telephone book.
- Call for medical help.
- Follow the directions given to you from the poison control center. If you have been instructed to induce vomiting, save any vomitus from the person in crisis.
- If the person in crisis is unconscious:
  - Do not give anything by mouth.
  - Position the person on his or her back with the head facing you.
  - Maintain a clear airway.
- If the person stops breathing, perform artificial respiration, using a pocket face mask or other barrier device to protect yourself.

Note: This should be done only on the directions from the poison control center. There are times when you should not perform mouth to mouth resuscitation due to the type of poison ingested.

- If it is necessary to move the person in crisis to a safe area, do so, but remember not to injure yourself while you are doing this.
- Keep the person in crisis warm and comfortable.
- Do not leave until emergency medical rescue help arrives.

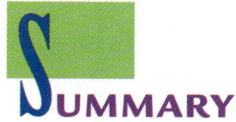

SUMMARY

This chapter has provided an overview of common emergencies and guidelines to follow for situations requiring immediate action. These situations include shock, heart attack (myocardial infarction), chest pain, cardiopulmonary resuscitation, stroke, seizures, hemorrhage, burns, and poisoning. The Chapter Review will help you evaluate what you have learned from the contents of this chapter.

Notes

Responding in an Emergency

THE NURSING ASSISTANT IN ACTION

You are working in a long-term care facility on the evening shift. A tornado touches down near the facility and causes wind damage. As soon as the winds calm, you find several residents are injured. One has fallen, but is conscious and complains of left leg pain. Several have cuts from broken glass, but none of them are bleeding badly. One resident is unconscious and may not be breathing.

What Is Your Response/Action?

1. What are the important pieces of information in this situation?

2. Which resident is your first concern?

3. What action will you take and why?

4. Other nursing assistants ask you what they should do. What will you tell them?

5. What did you learn about handling an emergency with multiple injuries?

The Human Body

14

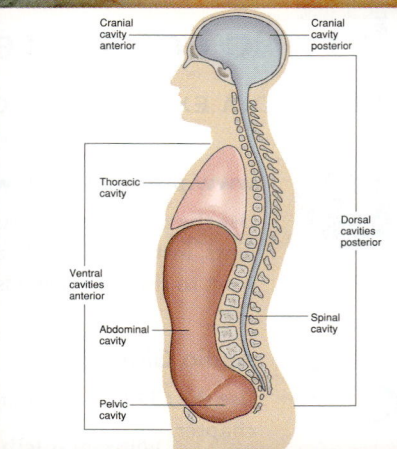

INTRODUCTION

This chapter presents a basic review of the structures and functions of the human body. An explanation of the reproduction and structure of cells and the grouping and organization of cells, tissues, and organs is given. Understanding of the functions and relationships among the many organs and systems in the human body is essential for the nursing assistant. One such system is the respiratory system—nose, pharynx, larynx, trachea, bronchi, and lungs. The respiratory system gives the body air to supply oxygen to the cells through the blood and eliminates carbon dioxide. A table lists all the body systems, the functions of each system, and the organs that comprise each system. Anatomical position is discussed in relationship to care of the patient.

When you have completed this chapter, you will be able to:

- List the things all living cells have in common.
- Relate the parts of a cell to their functions.
- Explain the process of cellular division.
- List the basic groupings of cells that build a human body.
- Name the primary kinds of tissues, their functions, and examples of their location in the human body.
- Identify the organs and basic functions of each body system.
- Describe the body in anatomical position.

anatomy

anterior

blood and lymph tissue

cardiac muscle tissue

cell

connective tissue

deep

dorsal

epithelial tissue

inferior

muscle tissue

nerve tissue

organ

physiology

posterior

superficial

superior

system

tissue

ventral

ANATOMY AND PHYSIOLOGY

anatomy The study of the structure of an organism

physiology The study of the functions of the body dealing with the physical and chemical processes of cells, tissues, and organs of living organisms

Anatomy is the study of the body structure and the relation of its parts. **Physiology** is the science that deals with the physical and chemical processes of cells, tissues, and organs of living organisms. The study of anatomy and physiology is the basis for understanding the clinical procedures that you will perform as a nursing assistant.

CELLS, TISSUES, AND ORGANS

This section provides descriptions of the structure and relationship of cells, tissues, and organs in the human body. *Cells* describes the structure of the cell and the process of cell division. *Tissues* identifies the various type and function of tissues found in the body. *Organs* explains the relationship of various tissues to specific organs and organs to specific body systems.

Cells

cell The basic unit of living matter

The **cell** is the fundamental building block of all living matter. Cells are microscopic in size. They are the living parts of organisms. The human body is made up of millions of cells. There are many kinds of cells and each has a special task within the body. Living cells have many things in common:

- They come from preexisting cells
- They use food for energy
- They use oxygen to break down food
- They use water to transport various substances
- They grow and repair themselves
- Most reproduce themselves (Only mature neural cells do not reproduce themselves.)

Structure of the Cell

Cells consist of three main parts: the nucleus, the cytoplasm, and the cell membrane (Figure 14–1).

FIGURE 14–1

The cell

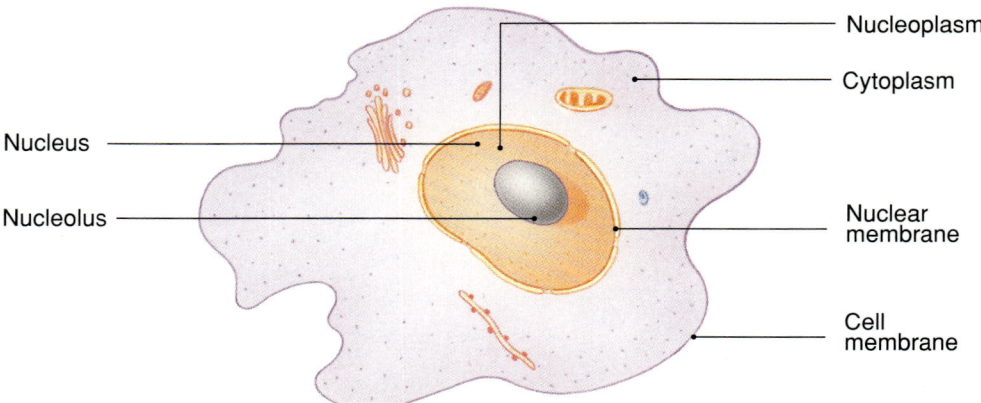

Nucleoplasm

Cytoplasm

Nucleus

Nucleolus

Nuclear membrane

Cell membrane

The nucleus is important to the process of heredity, growth, and cell reproduction. It contains chromosomes which control cell activity. Chromosomes are threadlike structures that contain deoxyribonucleic acid (DNA) and control heredity factors. They control physical and chemical traits a person inherits, for example eye color, skin color, and height.

The cytoplasm is the substance surrounding the nucleus and is where the activities of the cell take place. Messenger RNA molecules pass from the nucleus into the cytoplasm and direct the formation of the protein molecules necessary to maintain life. Through messenger RNA, the nucleus controls the kinds of chemical reactions carried out by the cell. The cell membrane keeps the cytoplasm within cell bounds and allows certain substances to pass in and out of the cell.

Cell Division

Cells reproduce by division. In any cell preparing for division, the nucleus initially duplicates its chromosomes exactly. As the cell continues to divide, the duplicate chromosomes, or chromosome pairs, divide and move to opposite sides of the nucleus. Then the rest of the cell contents divide and go with one or the other pair of chromosomes. After a new cell membrane forms between the two sides division is complete. The new cells are identical.

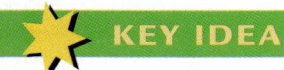

Current research to discover the causes of many diseases involves studying the cell and its immediate environment. With today's explosion of scientific knowledge about the cell, it is hoped that scientists will more readily find ways to cure or prevent many diseases.

■ Tissues

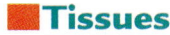

Individual cells usually do not work alone. Groups of cells of the same type that work together to perform a particular function are called **tissues** (Figure 14–2). Some of the primary kinds of tissues (Table 14–1) in the human body are:

tissue A group of cells of the same type

epithelial tissue Tissue that lines, protects, secretes, absorbs, and receives sensations

connective tissue Tissue that connects, supports, covers, lines, pads, or protects other body structures

- **Epithelial tissue:** The function of this tissue is to protect, secrete, absorb, and receive sensations. Examples are skin, linings of the intestines, and linings of the glands and organs.

- **Connective tissue:** The function of this tissue is to connect, support, cover or line, and pad or protect. Examples are bone, blood, ligaments, and tendons.

TABLE 14–1

Primary Kinds of Tissue

TYPE OF TISSUE	FUNCTION	LOCATION IN THE BODY
Epithelial tissue	Protect, secrete, absorb, receive sensations	Lining of mouth and nose, skin, lining of stomach
Connective tissue	Connect, support, cover	Tendons, bones, layer of fatty tissue under skin
Muscle tissues (a) striated (b) smooth (c) cardiac	Movement—stretch, contract	Muscle groups in arms, legs, abdomen, back and internal organs
Nerve tissue	Transmit impulses to and from the central nervous system and to and from the body systems	Throughout the body
Blood and lymph tissue	Circulate nutrients, oxygen, and antibodies throughout the body; remove waste products	Circulatory system

FIGURE 14–2

Types of body tissue

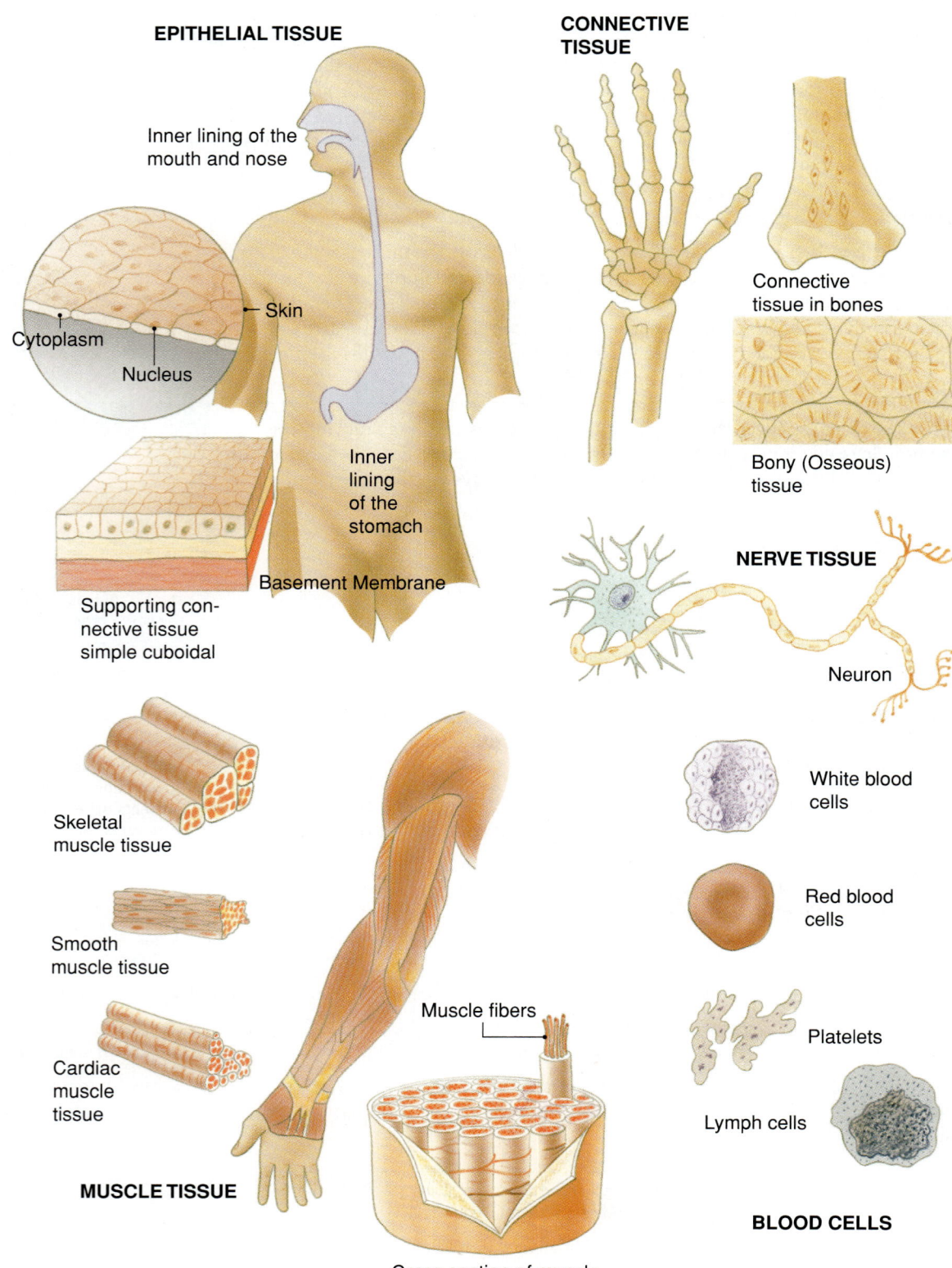

EPITHELIAL TISSUE

Inner lining of the mouth and nose

Skin

Cytoplasm

Nucleus

Supporting con-
nective tissue
simple cuboidal

Inner
lining
of the
stomach

Basement Membrane

CONNECTIVE
TISSUE

Connective
tissue in bones

Bony (Osseous)
tissue

NERVE TISSUE

Neuron

White blood
cells

Red blood
cells

Platelets

Lymph cells

BLOOD CELLS

Skeletal
muscle tissue

Smooth
muscle tissue

Cardiac
muscle
tissue

MUSCLE TISSUE

Muscle fibers

Cross section of muscle

- **Muscle tissue:** The function of this tissue is movement. Striated tissue is found in voluntary muscles, those you can move consciously. Smooth tissue is found in the involuntary muscles, such as those that push food and water through the gastrointestinal tract or those that allow actions such as dilation (making opening larger) or contraction (making opening smaller) of the pupil of your eye and blood vessels. **Cardiac tissue** is specific smooth muscle tissue found only in the involuntary muscles of the heart.

- **Nerve tissue:** The function of this tissue is to carry nervous impulses from a portion of the brain or spinal cord to all parts of the body and vice versa. The body cannot renew nerve tissue.

- **Blood and lymph tissue:** In this type of tissue the cells are singular and move within a fluid to every part of the body (technically these are in the family of connective tissue).

■Organs

Tissues are grouped together to form **organs**, such as the heart, lungs, and liver. Each organ has a specific function. Figure 14–3 shows the organs of the body and their

muscle tissue Tissue that ensures movement; it is capable of stretching and contracting

cardiac muscle tissue Involuntary muscle tissue found only in the heart

nerve tissue Tissue that carries nervous impulses between the brain, the spinal cord, and all parts of the body

blood and lymph tissue Tissue composed of singular cells that move within a fluid to every part of the body, circulating nutrients, oxygen, and antibodies and removing waste products

organ A part of the body made of several types of tissue grouped together to perform a certain function; examples are the heart, stomach, and lungs

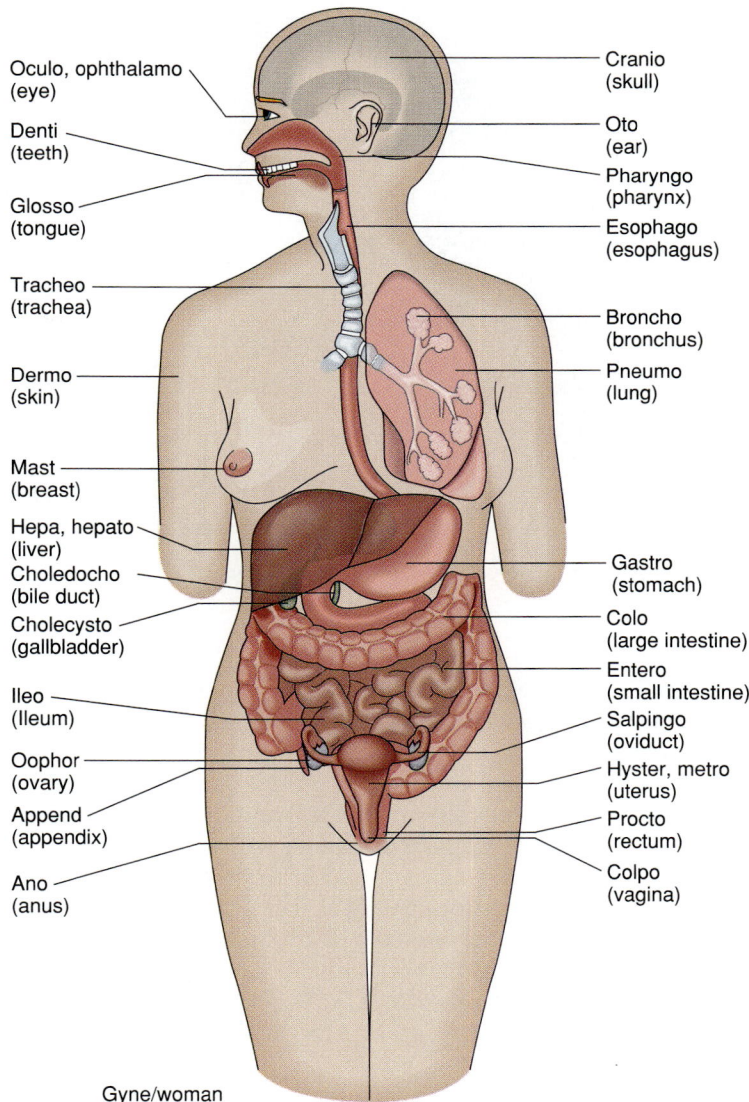

Oculo, ophthalamo (eye)
Denti (teeth)
Glosso (tongue)
Tracheo (trachea)
Dermo (skin)
Mast (breast)
Hepa, hepato (liver)
Choledocho (bile duct)
Cholecysto (gallbladder)
Ileo (Ileum)
Oophor (ovary)
Append (appendix)
Ano (anus)

Cranio (skull)
Oto (ear)
Pharyngo (pharynx)
Esophago (esophagus)
Broncho (bronchus)
Pneumo (lung)
Gastro (stomach)
Colo (large intestine)
Entero (small intestine)
Salpingo (oviduct)
Hyster, metro (uterus)
Procto (rectum)
Colpo (vagina)

Gyne/woman

FIGURE 14–3

Organs of the body

FIGURE 14–3 *(continued)*
Organs of the body

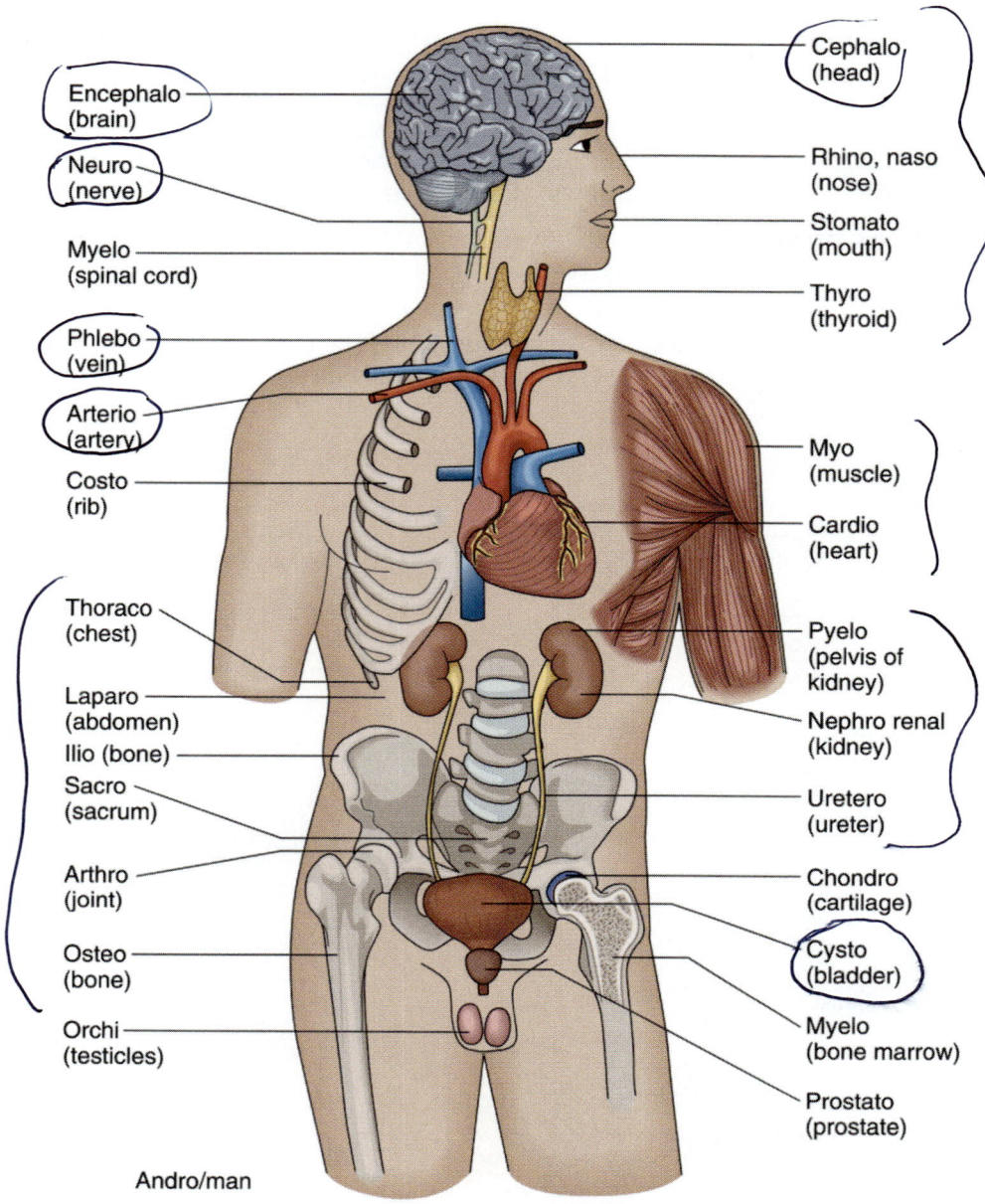

Encephalo (brain)
Neuro (nerve)
Myelo (spinal cord)
Phlebo (vein)
Arterio (artery)
Costo (rib)
Thoraco (chest)
Laparo (abdomen)
Ilio (bone)
Sacro (sacrum)
Arthro (joint)
Osteo (bone)
Orchi (testicles)

Cephalo (head)
Rhino, naso (nose)
Stomato (mouth)
Thyro (thyroid)
Myo (muscle)
Cardio (heart)
Pyelo (pelvis of kidney)
Nephro renal (kidney)
Uretero (ureter)
Chondro (cartilage)
Cysto (bladder)
Myelo (bone marrow)
Prostato (prostate)

Andro/man

approximate locations. The prefixes associated with the organs (cardio, pneumo, gastro, and so on) are combined with roots and suffixes to form the medical terminology discussed in the Appendix.

The body has two major cavities, the dorsal cavity and the ventral cavity (Figure 14–4). The dorsal cavity is divided into the cranial and the spinal cavities. The ventral cavity is divided into the thoracic and abdominal cavities. Some organs are located in body cavities. For example, the brain is found in the cranial cavity in the head. The heart and lungs are found in the thoracic cavity. The stomach, spleen, liver, pancreas, kidneys, small and large intestines, urinary bladder, and, in the female, the ovaries and uterus are located in the abdominal cavity. The abdominal cavity is lined with a membrane called the peritoneum which protects organs from rubbing together when they move. This membrane also keeps organs in place within the abdominal cavity.

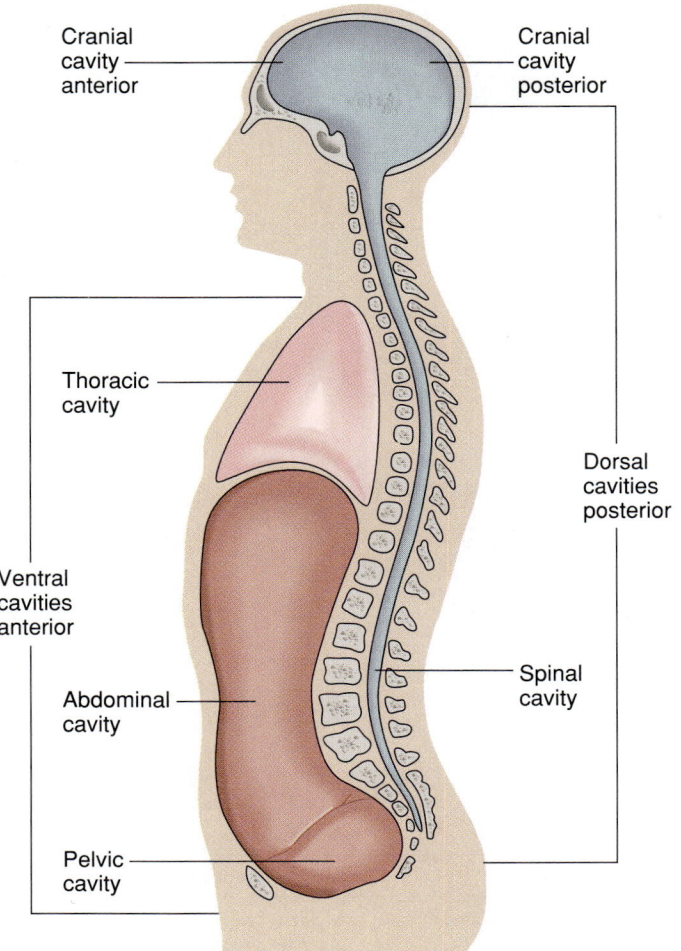

FIGURE 14–4

Body cavities

Cranial cavity anterior

Cranial cavity posterior

Thoracic cavity

Dorsal cavities posterior

Ventral cavities anterior

Spinal cavity

Abdominal cavity

Pelvic cavity

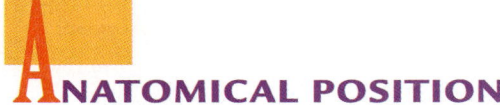

BODY SYSTEMS

Cells, tissues, and organs make up the body systems that keep the human body healthy and functioning normally. Figure 14–5 shows an example of three types of tissue combining to form an artery. Arteries are organs found in the circulatory system. Organs that work together to perform similar tasks make up body **systems**. It is easier to study anatomy and physiology by body systems (Table 14–2). Always remember that systems cannot work by themselves but are dependent upon each other.

system A group of organs acting together to carry out one or more body functions

ANATOMICAL POSITION

As part of the study of each system, it is helpful to take an overall look at the body and to become familiar with the names given to body areas. In any demonstration or diagram, the body or body part shown is in the anatomical position (Figure 14–6). The

FIGURE 14–5

Three types of tissue combine to form an artery

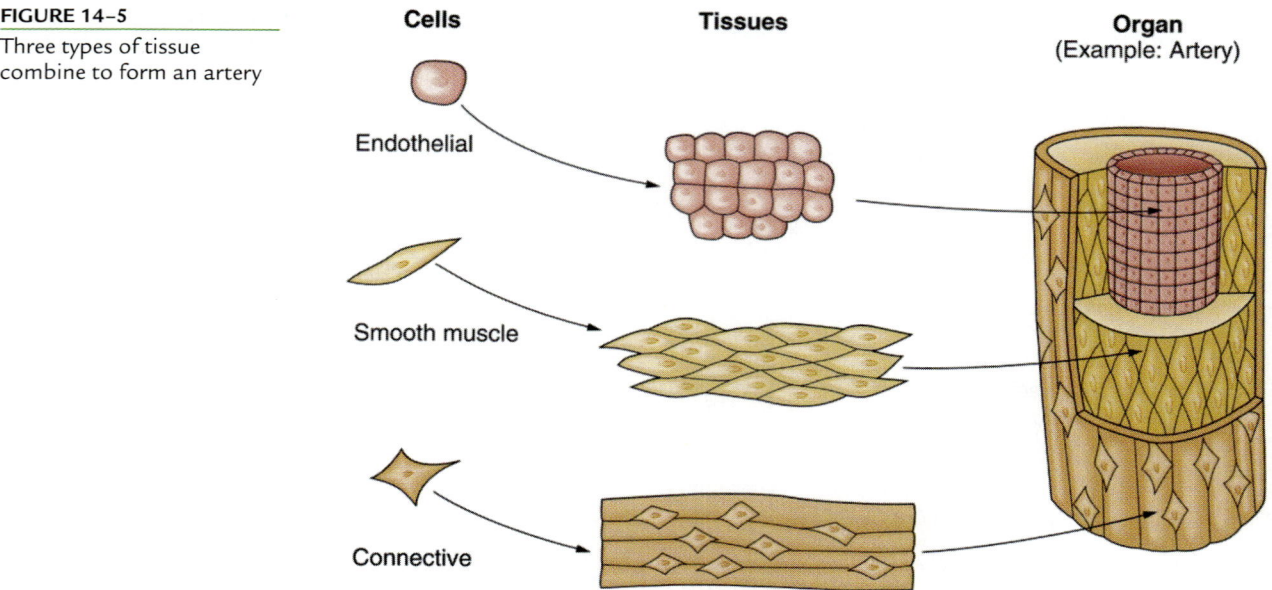

TABLE 14–2

Body Systems

SYSTEM	FUNCTION	ORGANS
Skeletal	Supports and protects the body	Bones; joints
Muscular	Gives movement to the body	Muscles; tendons; ligaments
Digestive (gastrointestinal)	Takes in and absorbs nutrients and eliminates wastes	Mouth; teeth; tongue; esophagus; salivary glands; stomach; duodenum; small and large intestines; liver; gallbladder; ascending, transverse, and descending colon; rectum; anus; appendix
Nervous	Controls activities of the body	Brain; spinal cord; nerves
Urinary (excretory)	Removes wastes from the blood, produces urine, and eliminates urine	Kidneys; ureters; bladder; urethra
Reproductive	To reproduce; allows a new human being to be born; for sexual fulfillment and expression of sexuality	**Male:** testes, scrotum, penis, prostate glands **Female:** ovaries, uterus, fallopian tubes, vagina
Respiratory	Gives the body air to supply oxygen to the cells through the blood and eliminates carbon dioxide	Nose; pharynx; larynx; trachea; bronchi; lungs
Circulatory	Carries food, oxygen, and water to the body cells and removes wastes	Heart; blood; arteries; veins; capillaries; spleen; lymph nodes; lymph vessels
Endocrine	Secretes hormones directly into the blood to regulate body functions	Thyroid and parathyroid glands; pineal gland; adrenal glands; testes; ovaries; breasts; thymus; pancreas; and pituitary gland
Integumentary	Provides first line of defense against infection, maintains body temperature, provides fluids, and eliminates waste	Skin; hair; nails; sweat and oil glands

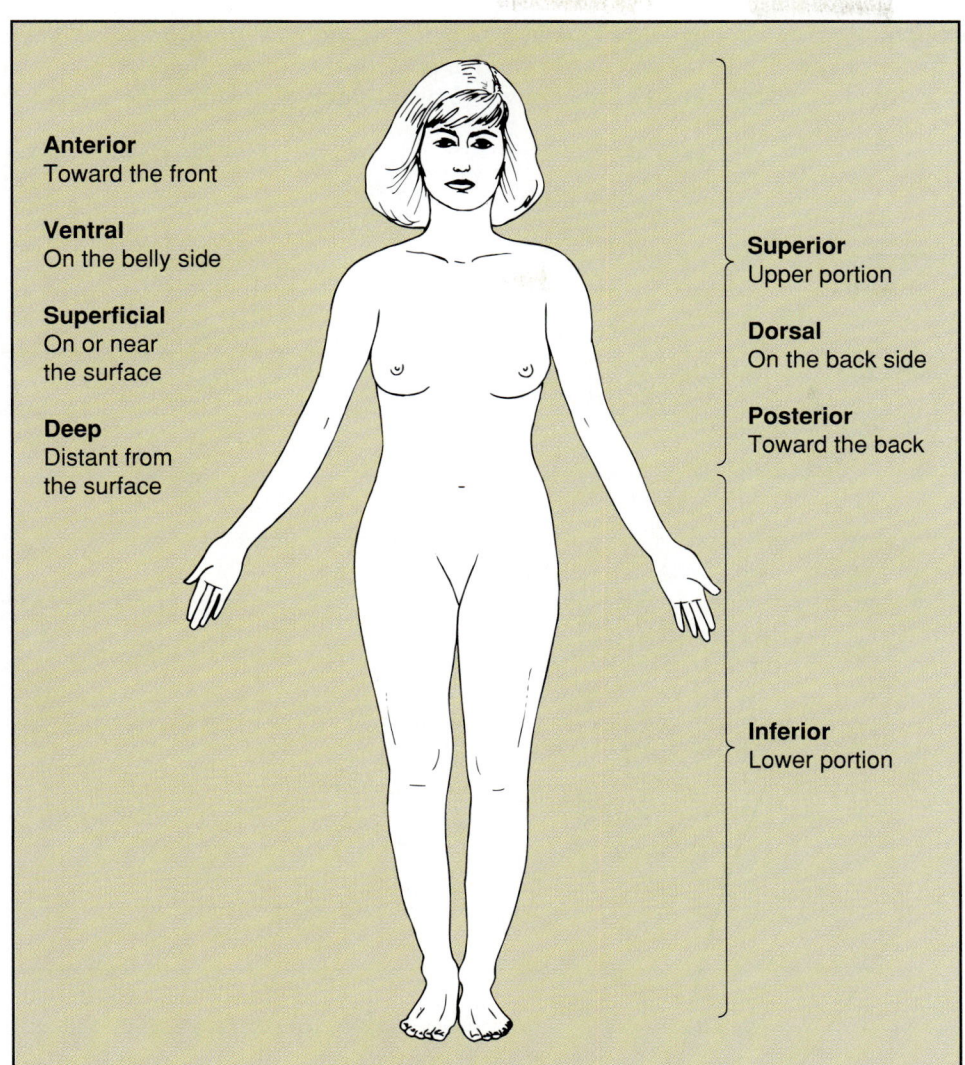

FIGURE 14–6
The body in anatomical position

Anterior
Toward the front

Ventral
On the belly side

Superficial
On or near
the surface

Deep
Distant from
the surface

Superior
Upper portion

Dorsal
On the back side

Posterior
Toward the back

Inferior
Lower portion

superficial On or near the surface of the body

deep Distant from the surface of the body

person is standing up straight, facing you, palms out and feet together. When you look at a person in the anatomical position, remember that the left side is always on your right side. This is especially important in studying diagrams. The front of a person is referred to as the **anterior** or **ventral** side. The back, containing the spine (backbone), is called the **posterior** or **dorsal** side. The areas of the body closer to the head are called **superior.** Those closer to the feet are called **inferior.** These terms may also be used to describe the position of an organ in the body.

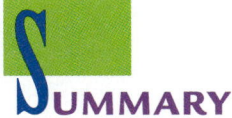

SUMMARY

The study of anatomy and physiology forms the basis for understanding the clinical procedures performed by nursing assistants. The cell is the basic building block of the human body. Cells combine to form tissues, and tissues combine to form organs. Organs that perform similar tasks work together as systems. When a person becomes ill or is involved in an accident, body structures may be damaged and their functions

anterior Located in the front; opposite of posterior

ventral On the abdominal, anterior, or front side of the body

posterior Located in the back or toward the rear

dorsal Refers to the back or to the back part of an organ

superior The upper portion of the body

inferior The lower portion of the body

disrupted. Remember when you look at a patient in anatomical position your right is the patient's left. The terms anterior or ventral, posterior or dorsal, superior, and inferior are used to describe areas of the body and the position of organs.

Notes

THE NURSING ASSISTANT IN ACTION

Are Abnormal Cells Always Cancer Cells?

You are working on the medical unit in an acute care hospital. When you walk into Ms. Melvin's room she is crying. She replies to your concerned question about what is wrong by saying, "I heard the doctor and the nurse talking outside my door. They said the lab found abnormal cells in the specimen they sent. That means cancer, doesn't it? Cells that aren't normal are cancer cells. Oh, no, have I got cancer? Have I? Tell me!" You heard in report this morning that Mrs. Melvin's tests were positive for cancer.

What Is Your Response/Action?

1. What are the important pieces of information in this situation?

2. What possible responses might you consider?

3. What response will you make and why?

4. What other action, if any, will you take?

5. What did you learn that you can apply to other situations?

■ Development

cognitive The mental processes by which knowledge is acquired

As noted earlier in this chapter, development refers to the accomplishment of and the increase in the ability to use motor, language, cognitive, and social skills that people acquire over their life span. **Cognitive**, language, social, **fine motor**, and **gross motor** skills are necessary for performance of the tasks that all humans must master. Newborns have few of these skills at birth. However, they seem to be born with the uncanny ability to capture the hearts of their parents—the initial caregivers. Parents move instinctively toward their newborn infant at the slightest signal that the infant is in distress. As humans age chronologically from infant to toddler, then from toddler to preschooler, and so on, they learn to think, to "coo" or talk, to socialize, to pick up small objects, and to walk. Human beings develop skills in each of these areas in a particular pattern, or sequence. Most people, as the old saying reminds us, learn to crawl before they learn to walk. Humans build on skills they have developed at a previous stage of development (Table 15–2).

fine motor Refers to the movement of small muscles, such as those in the hands and fingers

gross motor Refers to the movement of large muscles, such as those used in walking or hitting a ball

TABLE 15–2

Developmental Tasks and Chronological Age

SKILL AREA	INFANT: BIRTH–1 YEAR	TODDLER: 1–2 YEARS	PRESCHOOL: 2–5 YEARS	SCHOOL AGE: 5–12 YEARS
Cognitive	Learns about new things by feeling and working with objects encountered in the immediate environment and by placing or trying to place those objects in the mouth	Expands knowledge of things by learning words associated with objects in the environment	Comprehends tired, hungry, and other bodily experiences Recognizes colors	Learns relationship of objects to other objects and to self Learns relationship between objects and feelings
Social	Attaches to primary caregiver(s) Infant begins by recognizing faces and smiling; at about 6 months the infant begins to recognize primary caregiver(s) and expresses fear of strangers Plays simple interactive games like peek-a-boo and pat-a-cake	Learns self and primary caregiver(s) are different or separate from each other Undresses self Imitates and performs tasks seen in environment Expresses needs or indicates wants without crying	Begins to separate easily from caregiver(s) Dresses with supervision Washes and dries hands Plays interactive games (tag)	Acts independently, but emotionally close to caregiver Performs work and gets rewarded for it Dresses without supervision Forms same-sex play groups and clubs
Language	Vocalizes, squeals, and imitates sounds Says "dada" and "mama"	Says three words other than dada and mama Follows simple instructions	Names one picture Follows directions Combines words to make simple sentences of two or three words; uses plurals Gives first and last names	Defines words Knows and describes what things are made of
Gross Motor	Lifts head first, then chest Rolls over, pulls to sit, crawls, and stands alone	Walks well, kicks, stoops and jumps in place Throws balls	Runs well, hops, pedals tricycle Balances on one foot	Skips, balances on one foot for 10 seconds Overestimates physical abilities
Fine Motor	Reaches for objects and rakes up small items Grasps rattles Feeds self crackers	Unbuttons clothes Builds tower of 4 cubes Scribbles Uses spoon Picks up very small objects	Buttons clothes Builds tower of 8 cubes Copies simple figures or letters, for example "o" Begins to use scissors	Draws man with 6 parts Copies detailed figures and objects

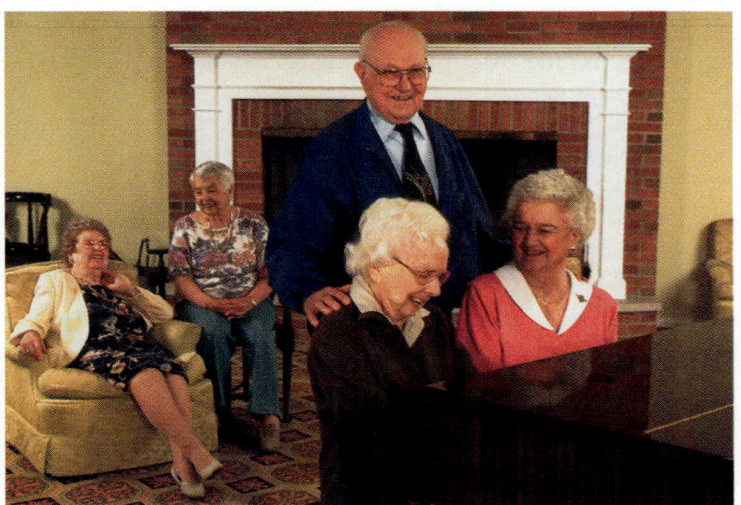

FIGURE 15–2
Socialization with others is important for older adults

ADOLESCENT: 12–18 YEARS	YOUNG ADULT: 18–40 YEARS	MIDDLE ADULT: 40–64 YEARS	OLDER ADULT: 65–75 YEARS	OLD AGE: 76–100+
Understands abstract concepts like illness and death	Fully developed; continues to develop knowledge-base related to school or job	Fully developed	Fully developed	Fully developed May be impaired
Experiences turmoil with rapidly changing moods and behavior Demonstrates interest in peer group almost exclusively Distances from parents emotionally Expresses concern with body image Experiences falling in and out of love	Establishes independence from parents Forms an individual lifestyle Adjusts to companions Selects a career Copes with career, social and economic constraints Chooses a mate Learns to live cooperatively with mate Becomes a parent	Builds socioeconomic status Assists younger and older to cope Fulfilled by work, family, or by giving or caring for others Copes with physical changes of aging Relates to grown children and the empty nest Deals with aging parents Copes with the death of parents	Develops mutually supportive relationships with grown children Adjusts to loss of friends and relatives Copes with loss of spouse Adjusts to retirement Forms new friends Adjusts to new role in the family Copes with dying	Develops mutually supportive relationships with grown children and grandchildren Copes with loss of spouse, friends, and sometimes children Forms new friends/withdraws Adjusts to new role in the family Copes with dying
Vocabulary increases Understands more abstract concepts, for example grief	Fully developed	Fully developed	Fully developed	Fully developed
Awkwardness may be apparent as individuals learn to deal with rapid increases in size due to growth spurts	Fully developed	Beginning physical changes of aging such as decreased energy and endurance	Physical changes associated with the aging process are more significant	Pronounced physical changes associated with the aging process Stamina, sight, and hearing diminished
Fully developed	Fully developed	Fully developed	Physical changes associated with the aging process begin to appear	Physical changes associated with the aging process present

Chronological Age

Chronological age is linked to developmental skill acquisition, but not exactly in a lock-step fashion. For example, most children start walking by their first birthday. However, some start to walk as early as eight months, and still others wait until they are 16 months old. The normal chronological-age range given (for walking) is from 8 months to 16 months, so the children cited in this example have all developed the ability to walk within the usual chronological-age range. Once development skills are mastered, the person is able to perform them most of the time.

Illness

Illness can have a profound effect on a person's ability to use skills that are already developed. When people are ill, they often behave at a lower developmental stage than their chronological age would suggest. For example, parents of a hospitalized 4-year-old may express concern that their child, who is toilet-trained, is once again wetting the bed. The nursing assistant's role is to reassure the parents that such a behavioral change is not unusual. Sometimes children cope with the anxiety and pain often accompanying hospitalization by reverting to behaviors that kept them anxiety- and pain-free at an earlier age. Support the child, parents, and other family members by addressing their anxieties and fears, and the temporary setback will usually resolve itself.

Injuries

Injuries such as head injuries or a stroke can necessitate the re-learning of skills from earlier stages of development. For example, a stroke could mean that a person would have to re-learn how to walk or talk. Frustration limits one's ability to cope with such difficult situations and may cause them to revert back to an earlier developmental level as well. Instead of thinking logically and realizing that with rehabilitation their walking may improve, they throw something across the room in exasperation at their inability to walk as they had before.

CHRONOLOGICAL-AGE CONSIDERATIONS

Knowledge of developmental-task masteries associated with chronological age is key to your ability to relate appropriately with patients and to provide needed nursing care. You must also be aware that illness and injury may sometimes impact negatively on a person's performance. The approach, or technique, you will use in delivering care to patients in the Infant: Birth–1 year range will be different from the approach you will use with patients in the School-age: 5–12 year range. Your behavior will be based on chronological-age considerations of the patient (Figure 15–3). Table 15–3 lists typical nursing assistant behaviors that correspond to or are based on the patient's chronological age and typical task masteries or competencies to be considered as you provide care. Chapter 32 addresses many specific age considerations for older adults.

TABLE 15–3

Appropriate Nursing Assistant Behaviors for Various Age Groups

INFANT: BIRTH–1 YEAR	TODDLER: 1–2 YEARS	PRESCHOOL: 2–5 YEARS	SCHOOL-AGE CHILD: 5–12 YEARS
Keep child with parent(s). Use parents to comfort rather than restrain child during hurtful or scary experiences. Explain procedures to parents so they can calm patient. Keep small objects (such as IV tube caps and safety pins) out of child's reach. Ensure that the side of the bed is up. Place visually interesting objects where child can observe them. Provide age- and disease-appropriate toys.	Keep child with parent(s). Use parents to comfort rather than restrain child during hurtful or scary experiences. Explain procedures to parents so they can calm patient. Keep small objects (such as IV tube caps) out of child's reach. Ensure that the side of the bed is up. Toddlers are accustomed to being "on the go." Efforts to interfere with their movements may provoke negative displays, obstinacy, even temper tantrums. Interact with children on their terms, which may mean moving about with them.	Keep child with parent(s). Use parents to comfort rather than restrain child during hurtful or scary experiences. Explain procedures in simple words, describing only what patients will see, what things will look like outside the body. For example, if child will have an IV, demonstrate the tubing and IV needle hub. Don't show or talk about things that will not be visible to the child, such as the needle. Provide activities that engage the child and lessen anxiety when appropriate.	Allow independent movement as appropriate. Explain procedures in greater detail. Offer choices, when possible, to allow children to experience some control over their bodies and environment. For example, ask if patient would like you to make the bed now or after breakfast. Explain how long a painful procedure will take. This will avoid or shorten the child's attempts to stall the experience. When possible, give a tour before hospitalization to acquaint child with the environment.

ADOLESCENT: 12–18 YEARS	YOUNG ADULT: 18–40 YEARS	MIDDLE ADULT: 40–65 YEARS	OLDER ADULT: 65–75 YEARS AND OLD AGE: 76–100+
Show interest in visits by the patient's peers, supporting and complimenting positive behavior. Involve adolescents fully in decisions about their health care. Express interest in and support adolescents who exhibit concern about scars or imperfections, even if they are minor. Body image is very important at this age.	Involve patient in decision making about all aspects of health care. Review with patient what treatments are scheduled, including when they will take place, and so on. Knowing what to expect next helps the patient adapt to unfamiliar surroundings and routines. Listen to patient's concerns about the effect illness will have on progress toward lifelong goals like meaningful relationships, offspring, and employment.	Involve patient in decision making about all aspects of health care. Ask if patient would like a family member or other person present to provide support, help with hearing and clarifying information when needed, or making a health care decision. Provide information when the family member or other person arrives. Review with patient what treatments are scheduled, including when they will take place, and so on. Knowing what to expect next helps the patient adapt to unfamiliar surroundings and routines.	Ask patient about the routine followed at home, and adapt the hospital routine as much as possible to the patient's at-home routine. Review with patient what treatments are scheduled, including when they will take place, and so on. Knowing what to expect next helps the patient adapt to unfamiliar surroundings and routines. Ask if patient would like a family member present to provide support in making a health care decision. Provide information needed when the family member arrives.

FIGURE 15–3

Involve adolescents in their care

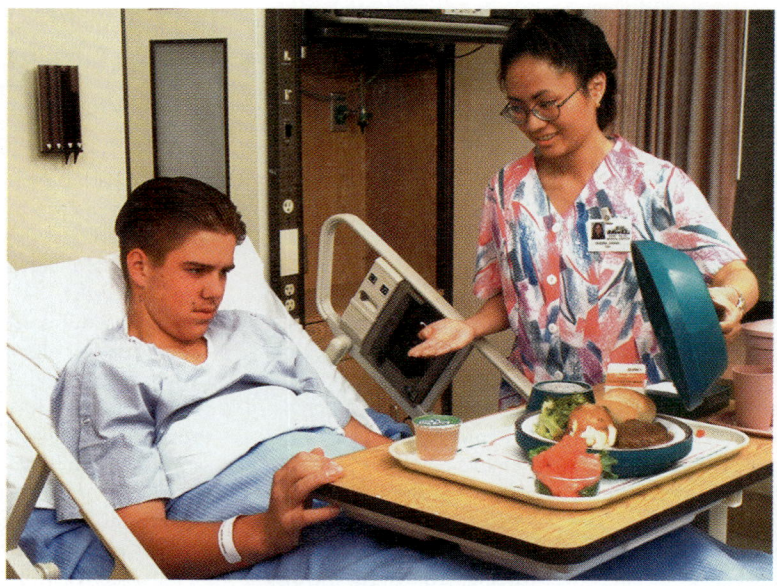

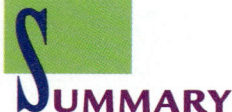 **S**UMMARY

Growth and development refers to the physical, intellectual, emotional, and social changes that occur over the life span of every human being. Although both may occur at different rates for different individuals, there are general principles and characteristics that describe the typical person within each stage of development. Illness and injury impact individual's ability to use their developed skills; however, human beings continue to adapt to triumphs and adversities throughout their entire lives. Consideration of specific developmental capabilities based on chronological age of patients is key to determining your role. Basic knowledge and understanding of the general principles of normal growth and development, including chronological-age differences, provide nursing assistants with a sound basis for delivering informed patient-centered care.

Notes

Baby Talk

You are working in a long-term care facility. One of the nursing assistants, Shawndel, talks "baby talk" to the residents. She asks the residents if they need to "go potty" or if they have a "tummy ache." One day you ask Shawndel why she talks that way. She responds, "Well, old people are in their second childhood. They're just like children, so why not talk to them the way I talk to my kids? Besides, I'm not mean or anything."

What Is Your Response/Action?

1. What are the important pieces of information in this situation?

2. From your understanding of growth and development, how would you respond to Shawndel?

3. How might Shawndel's treatment affect the residents?

4. What action could you take to ensure that you treat patients appropriately for their age?

5. What did you learn that you can apply to other situations involving co-workers?

The Musculoskeletal System and Related Care

16

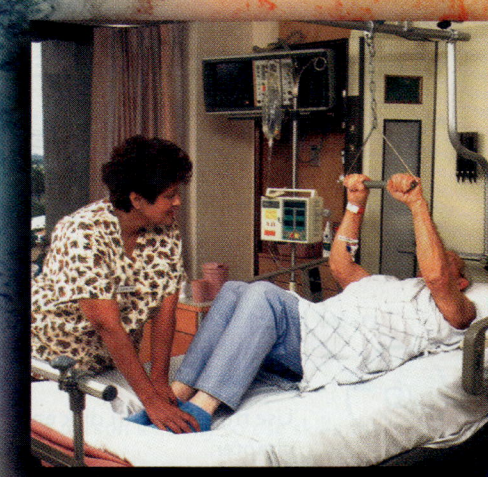

INTRODUCTION

The human body works most efficiently when a person is physically active. Thus, proper care of the musculoskeletal system plays an important role in maintaining overall good health. The nursing assistant can have a positive impact by helping patients care for themselves and encouraging them to be as active as possible. This chapter provides the background necessary for carrying out these responsibilities. It describes the musculoskeletal system, common diseases and disorders affecting it, and the nursing assistant's role in orthopedic nursing care.

OBJECTIVES

When you have completed this chapter, you will be able to:

- Identify the functions of the muscular system.

- Explain how groups of muscles work together to perform body motion.

- List the functions of the skeletal system.

- List the four general types of bones and give examples of each.

- Name three major types of joints and give examples of each.

- Label a diagram of the skeletal and surface muscles.

- Describe how aging affects the musculoskeletal system.

- List common diseases and disorders of the musculoskeletal systems.

- Describe the scope of orthopedic nursing care and the purposes of orthopedic equipment.

- Describe and explain the reasons for special skin care for the orthopedic patient.

- List important points to observe while performing any nursing task involving patients in traction.

- List important points to observe while performing any nursing task involving patients in plaster casts.

- Identify several types of supportive devices and the nursing assistant's role in caring for patients who use such devices.

KEY TERMS

abduction

adduction

atrophy

contract

contracture

extension

flex

flexion

fracture

joint

ligament

orthopedics

relax

traction

trapeze

walker

flex To bend; the act of bending a body part

relax To place in a resting position, in which muscle tension decreases and fibers lengthen

flexion Bending of a joint (elbow, wrist, knee)

extension Straightening or lengthening a muscle, thereby making the angle formed by bones and muscles greater

abduction Movement of an arm or leg away from the center of the body

THE MUSCULAR SYSTEM

The muscular system makes possible all the body's motion: that of the whole body and that which occurs inside the body. Besides moving the body, muscles help to keep the body warm, especially during activity. Muscles have an exceptionally rich blood supply, so they are the most infection-free of all the body's basic tissues (see Figure 16–1).

Groups of muscles work together to perform a body motion. Other groups perform the opposite motion. These pairs of muscle groups are called *antagonistic groups*. For example, when you **flex** your arm (bring it toward your shoulder), your biceps muscle contracts and the triceps muscle **relaxes**. When you extend your arm (straighten it), the biceps relax while the triceps contract.

You should know the terms for the basic ways in which muscles can move parts of the body. **Flexion** is bending at a joint, such as the elbow (Figure 16–2b and Figure 16–2d), wrist, or knee. Its opposite is **extension**, or straightening (Figure 16–2a and Figure 16–2c). **Abduction** means moving a part away from the body midline. Conversely, **adduction** means moving it toward the body (Figure 16–2e and Figure 16–3).

If a muscle is kept inactive for too long, it tends to shrink and waste away. This is called **atrophy**. In addition, immobility (remaining perfectly still) can lead to **contracture**, a permanent muscle shortening. Preventing these conditions is among the reasons

FIGURE 16–1

The musculoskeletal system

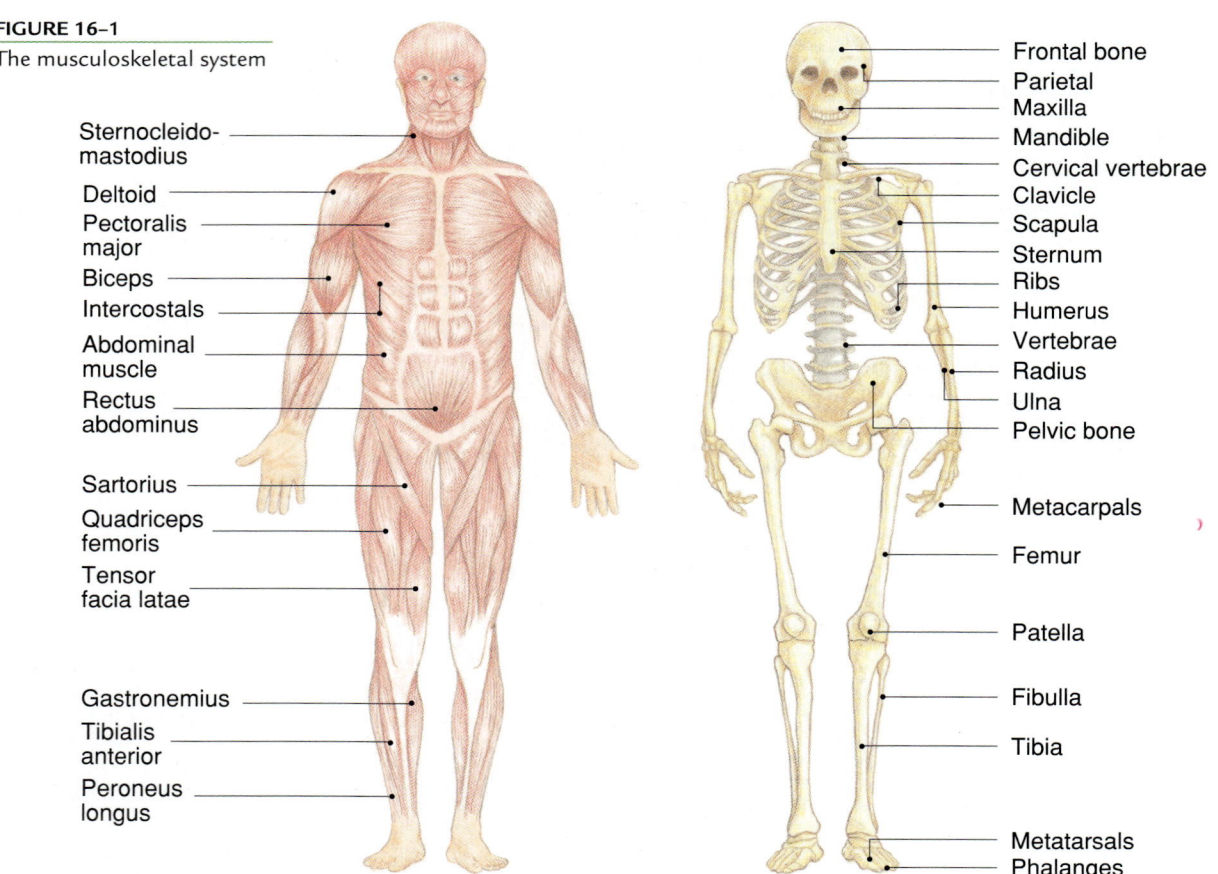

Sternocleido-mastodius
Deltoid
Pectoralis major
Biceps
Intercostals
Abdominal muscle
Rectus abdominus
Sartorius
Quadriceps femoris
Tensor facia latae
Gastronemius
Tibialis anterior
Peroneus longus

Frontal bone
Parietal
Maxilla
Mandible
Cervical vertebrae
Clavicle
Scapula
Sternum
Ribs
Humerus
Vertebrae
Radius
Ulna
Pelvic bone
Metacarpals
Femur
Patella
Fibulla
Tibia
Metatarsals
Phalanges

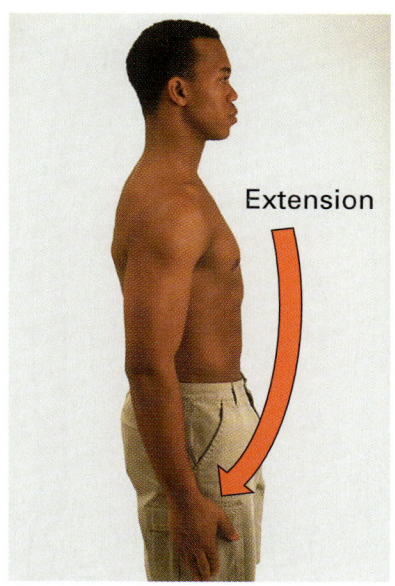

FIGURE 16–2a
Extension

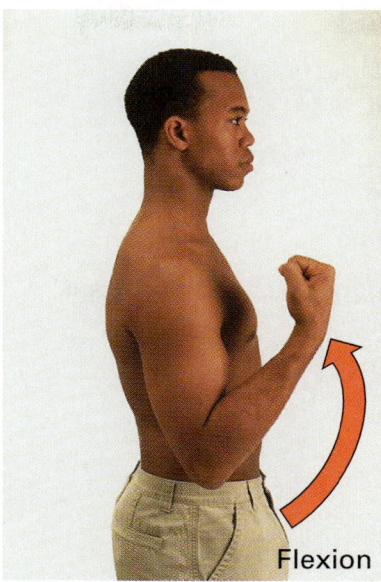

FIGURE 16–2b
Flexion

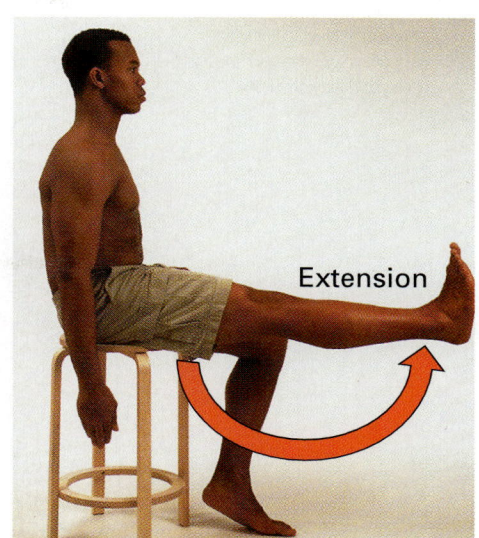

FIGURE 16–2c
Extension

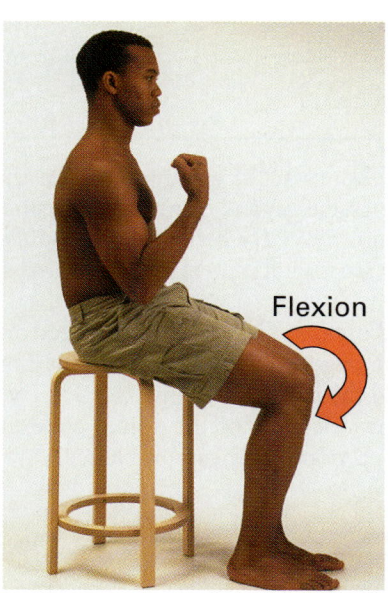

FIGURE 16–2d
Flexion

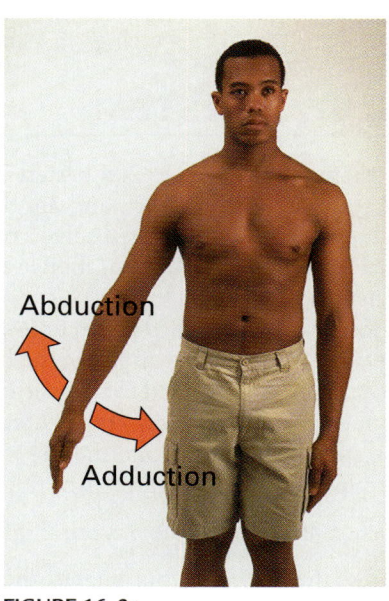

FIGURE 16–2e
Abduction and Adduction

why regular exercise is important to good health. Patients who cannot be physically active may be given range-of-motion exercises to prevent these problems.

The largest muscle groups are the strongest ones. Using your large muscle groups for heavy tasks can help you avoid straining your other muscles and hurting yourself. For example, when helping to lift a patient or making a bed, remember to use the strong muscles of your legs rather than those of your back. (For more information on moving and lifting patients, see Chapter 7.)

adduction Movement of an arm or leg toward the center of the body

atrophy Wasting away of muscles; decrease in muscle size

contracture An abnormal shortening of a muscle

FIGURE 16–3
(a) Adduction and
(b) abduction, moving a
body part toward and away
from the body midline

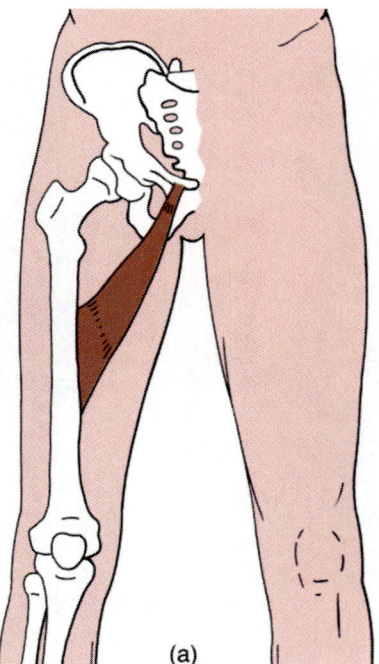

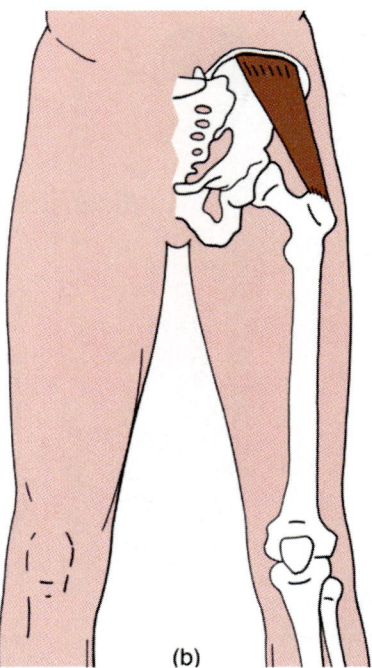

(a)   (b)

THE SKELETAL SYSTEM

The skeletal system is made up of 206 bones. The bones act as a framework for the body, give it structure and support, and are the passive organs of motion. In other words, bones do not move by themselves but are moved when a nerve impulse stimulates a muscle to **contract** (shorten). Bones also store vital minerals that are necessary for many other body activities.

Another function of the bones is to protect the vital organs. The bones of the head are designed to protect the very delicate tissue of the brain (Figure 16–4). They are joined by *sutures,* similar to a zigzag pattern, and totally surround the brain and cranial nerves. Two other kinds of bones that protect vital organs are the vertebrae of the spinal column, which protect the spinal nerve cord, and the ribs, which guard the heart and lungs.

There are four types of bones (Figure 16–5):

1. *Long bones,* such as the big bone in your thigh, the femur

2. *Short bones,* like the bones in your fingers, the phalanges

3. *Irregular bones,* such as the vertebrae that make up the spinal column

4. *Flat bones,* like the bones of the rib cage

Bone cells grow and reproduce slowly. Therefore, **fractures** (broken bones) can mend, but the process is slow and gradual. The new bone hardens gradually as calcium is deposited. Blood supply to bone tissue is poor in comparison to other areas of the body. Therefore, bone has relatively low resistance to infection.

contract Get smaller; shortening the length of muscle, thereby making the angle formed by bones and muscles smaller

fracture A break in a bone

■ Joints (Motion)

In a healthy human body, all the systems of the body work together. No one system can stand alone. During each body movement, the skeletal system, muscular system, nervous

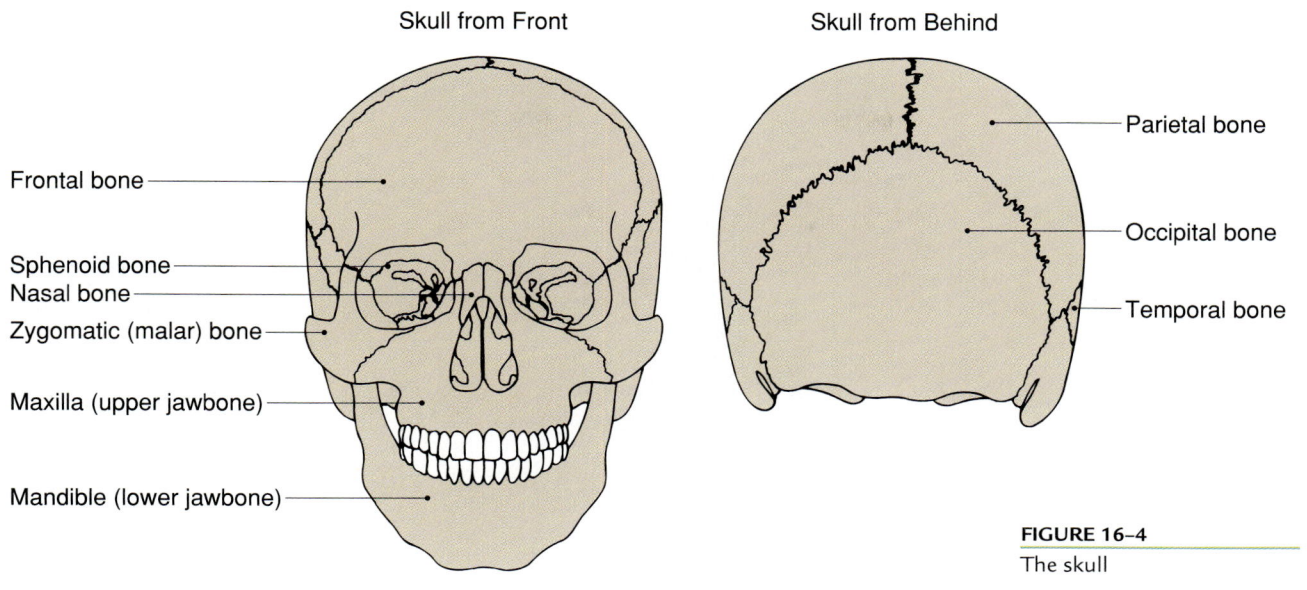

Skull from Front

Frontal bone

Sphenoid bone
Nasal bone
Zygomatic (malar) bone

Maxilla (upper jawbone)

Mandible (lower jawbone)

Skull from Behind

Parietal bone

Occipital bone

Temporal bone

FIGURE 16–4
The skull

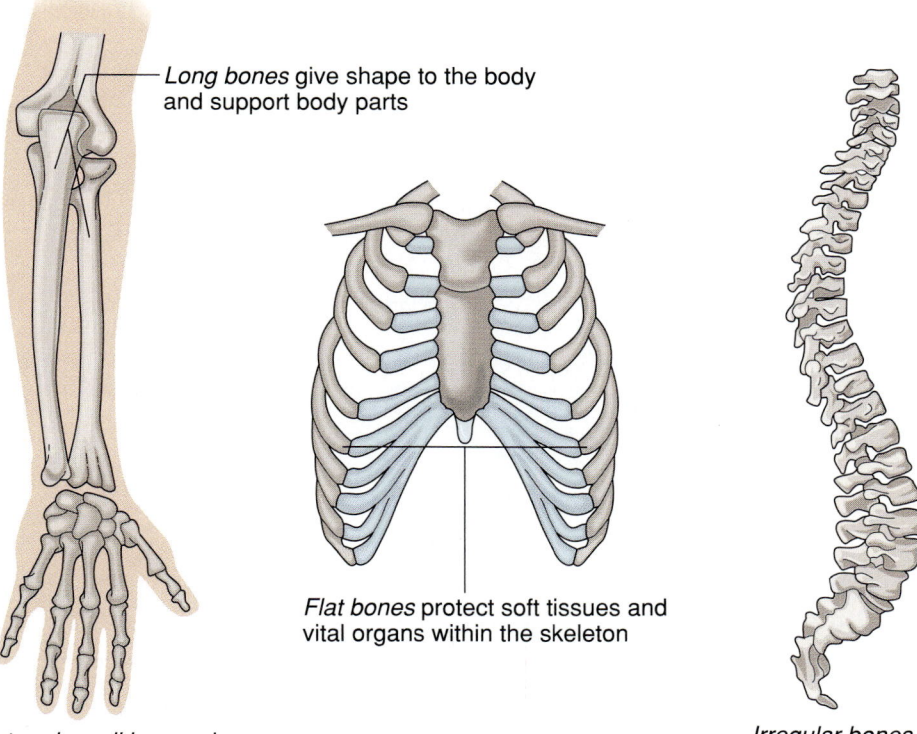

Long bones give shape to the body and support body parts

Flat bones protect soft tissues and vital organs within the skeleton

Short and small bones give flexibility to the body

Irregular bones

FIGURE 16–5
Types of bones

system, and circulatory system are all interacting. This body movement occurs at the joints, a perfect example of how several systems must work together.

   Joints are the meeting place where one bone connects with one or more other bones. They are the necessary levers for all motion. Joints are made up of many structures. The tough, white fibrous cord, the **ligament**, connects bone to bone. The _tendons_ connect muscle to bone. Joints—especially those in the shoulder, hip, and knee—are enclosed in a strong capsule lined by a membrane that secretes a fluid called _synovial fluid._ This fluid

joint A part of the body where two bones come together

ligament Tough, white fibrous cord that connects bone to bone

FIGURE 16–6

Types of joints

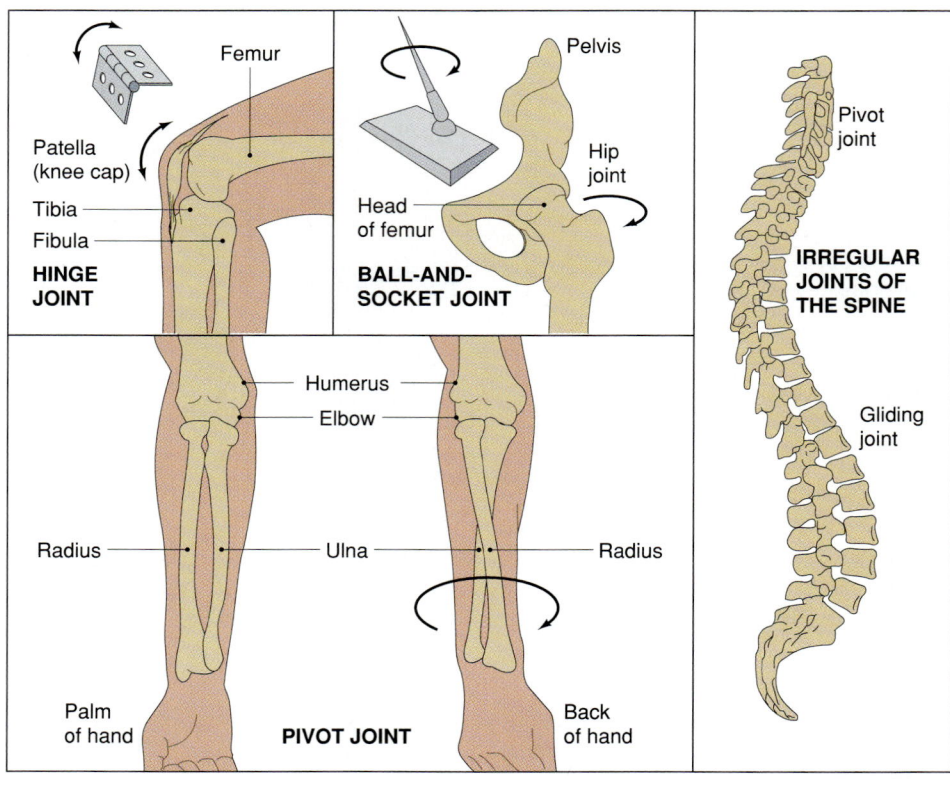

acts as a buffer, very much like a waterbed, so that the ends of the bones do not get worn out from too much motion. Other structures that protect the bone include the pad of cartilage at the end of the bone, a sac of synovial fluid (which is known as a bursa), and a disk of cartilage called the meniscus. Many such safeguards are built into the body. The human body has several kinds of joints (Figure 16–6). The hinge joint, such as in the knee, is freely movable. There are also fewer movable joints, such as those between the vertebrae. Some joints do not move at all, such as the joints between the bones of the head, which protect the brain.

THE MUSCULOSKELETAL SYSTEM AND THE NORMAL AGING PROCESS

The musculoskeletal system undergoes changes as a person gets older. Unless the person remains physically active, muscles become weaker and lose their tone. The body therefore loses strength and endurance. Such changes affect many parts of the body, including the organs. For example, weakening muscles may cause heart function to decrease and breathing to become more difficult.

Cartilage deteriorates with age, and tissue hardens. As a result, joints become stiff, making movement more difficult. A person may react to this difficulty by being less active. If so, the reduced activity can bring about further loss of muscle tone.

Bones become porous and brittle with age; they do not remain as hard as they once were. The body's absorption of calcium decreases. Some older people lose calcium, especially if they do not bear weight (stand). This makes the bones even weaker. Therefore, bones in an older person break more easily.

The spinal column (bones of the spine) may also change, bringing about a stooped posture and loss of height. Some people become as much as two inches shorter than they were as a young adult.

COMMON DISEASES AND DISORDERS OF THE MUSCULOSKELETAL SYSTEM

The changes of aging can make a person more likely to be injured as one gets older, but diseases and disorders of the musculoskeletal system can occur at any age. Following are the most common conditions:

- *Bursitis:* inflammation of the bursa (sac of synovial fluid)

- *Contusion:* injury to soft tissue

- *Sprain:* strain of a ligament or tendon surrounding a joint; ligaments may be partially torn

- *Joint dislocation:* injury in which a bone end that forms part of a joint is displaced (pulled out so that it is no longer in anatomic position)

- *Fracture:* break in a bone (Figure 16–7)

    - *Simple fracture:* broken bone with no external wound

    - *Compound fracture:* broken bone with an external wound or fragment of bone protruding through the skin

- *Surgical amputation:* removal of a portion of a limb

FIGURE 16–7

Types of bone fractures

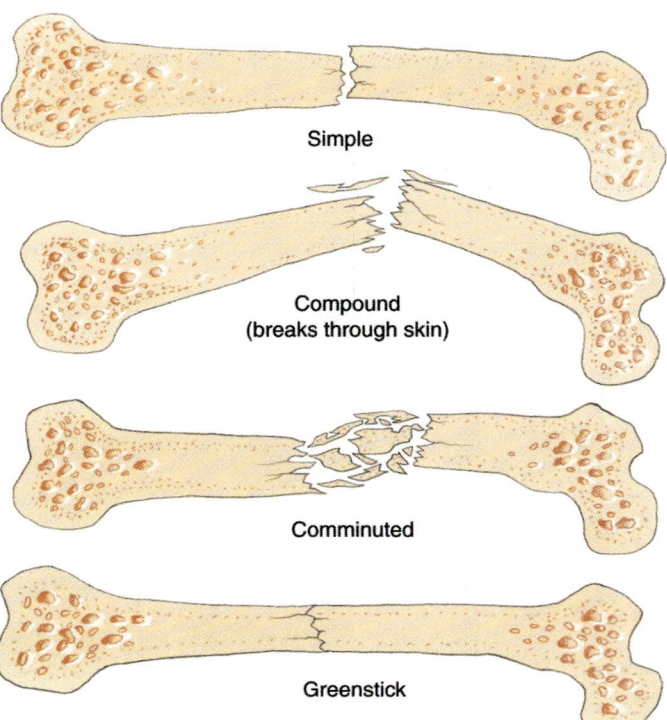

Simple

Compound
(breaks through skin)

Comminuted

Greenstick

- *Low back pain:* pain that often is accompanied by muscle spasms

- *Rheumatoid arthritis:* inflammation of the lining of the joints

- *Osteoarthritis:* degeneration of the cartilage of the joints

- *Osteogenic sarcoma (cancer):* malignant bone tumor

- *Osteoporosis:* reduced amount of normal bone tissue, resulting in softening

- *Muscular dystrophy:* a condition characterized by a progressive atrophy of muscular tissue

- *Osteomyelitis:* inflammation of or an infection in the bone caused by bacteria introduced by trauma or surgery

- *Tuberculosis:* an infectious disease that usually affects the lungs, but can affect bone tissue. TB can invade the spinal vertebrae destroying the disks and resulting in the collapse and wedging of the vertebrae and shortening the spine. If pressure in the spinal cord occurs, paralysis may result. The patient may require some of the same orthopedic care discussed in this chapter.

- *Poliomyelitis:* (not seen often) viral infection causing an inflammation of the grey matter of the spinal cord, resulting in partial or complete paralysis

- *Trauma to spinal cord:* accidental injury damaging the spinal cord and resulting in paralysis of some area of the body. Trauma to the spinal cord may result in paralysis of the arms, legs, and body below the level of the injury. This immobility causes the patient to require a lot of supportive care.

- *Guillain-Barré syndrome:* a disease of the nervous system resulting in ascending paralysis

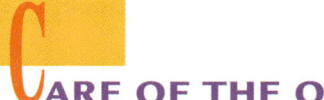

CARE OF THE ORTHOPEDIC PATIENT

orthopedics The medical specialty that covers the treatment of broken bones, deformities, or diseases that attack the bones, joints, and muscles

Orthopedics (also spelled *orthopaedics*) is the science of the prevention and correction of deformities and the treatment of diseases of the bones, muscles, joints, and fasciae (supporting membranes) either by manipulation, special apparatus, or surgery. Orthopedic nursing requires special knowledge and skills in addition to routine patient care. To care for the orthopedic patient, the nursing assistant needs knowledge of body mechanics and specialized procedures related to the treatment of this type of patient. Nursing assistants will need to be familiar with special equipment such as splints, casts, traction devices, and walkers.

Modern science is constantly developing new ways and means to help the orthopedic patient. In the past, traction and bed rest were the method of treatment for most patients with orthopedic problems. Today, improved methods of surgery, lighter casting materials, shortened hospital stays, and the identified physiologic benefits of early ambulation (walking or moving about while standing) have led to changes in the care of orthopedic patients. A patient who is put in traction remains there for a shorter period of time than in past years. Early ambulation using assistive devices such as canes and walkers promotes faster healing with fewer circulatory side effects such as blood clots.

The emphasis on early ambulation requires the nursing assistant to provide both ambulatory and non-ambulatory orthopedic care. Both types of orthopedic care pose special challenges:

- Routine nursing care is difficult to give when a patient is in a cast or traction. It will often be necessary to carry out some procedures with the least possible disturbance to these orthopedic devices.

■ Especially if the patient must endure a long period of restricted mobility, he may become unduly discouraged. Encouraging independence through the use of special devices for walking or retrieving objects out of reach promotes muscle tone and a positive mental outlook for the patient.

Orthopedic Equipment

Orthopedic care may involve the use of special equipment. These orthopedic devices are used for several purposes:

1. To provide support for the injured part until it heals

2. To prevent deformity and weakness in the injured muscles and joints

3. To help the patient to ambulate with safety as early as possible in the healing process

Support for the injured part may be provided by bandages, adhesive strapping, splints, or plaster casts applied externally. Support may also be applied directly to a bone by using pins, metal plates, or prosthetic devices (for example, the replacement of a joint). These specialized *prostheses* (artificial aids) are applied in the operating room, using specialized surgical procedures. To prevent stiffness or deformity, the patient will be asked to use the affected part within limits ordered by the doctor. Frequently, the patient needs the support of a brace, crutches, or a walker.

When a patient must wear a brace, there are often specific restrictions. Some braces must be worn continually, while others must be applied before getting out of bed. It is important to check the patient's plan of care to see if any specific instructions are included.

To promote early ambulation, the physician often prescribes a **walker** for the patient to use. A walker is a metal frame device with handgrips and four legs. It is open on one side. This device provides stability and security for a patient who is weak on one side or restricted in the amount of weight he can put on one foot. The use of the walker will depend on what kind of surgery or injury the patient had. Always check with your supervisor before assisting a patient to use a walker (Figure 16–8).

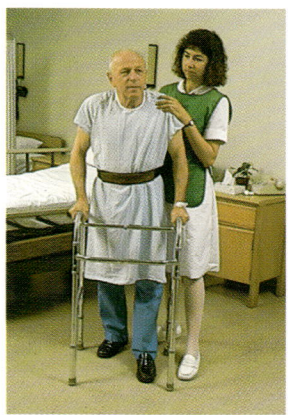

FIGURE 16–8

Assisting a patient to use a walker

walker A metal frame device with handgrips and four legs that is open on one side; provides stability and security for the patient who is weak on one side or restricted in the amount of weight he can put on one foot

Special Skin Care for the Orthopedic Patient

Besides routine nursing care, the orthopedic patient may need special skin care. In the early stages of an injury or after surgery, the patient may be confined to bed because of traction. Even a casted patient will have restricted mobility. This type of patient is particularly susceptible to pressure ulcers.

The nursing assistant should change the patient's position every two hours following the doctor's instructions, give special back care, and change the area of pressure as often as is possible to prevent pressure ulcers. Providing a smooth, clean, dry bed and keeping the cast clean can promote patient comfort and prevent pressure ulcers. A **trapeze**, suspended from an over-the-bed frame, allows the patient to move or lift himself, to aid in back care, and to use the bedpan.

trapeze A triangle-shaped bar attached to the overbed frame of a traction setup which enables the patient to pull himself up in bed

Care of the Patient in Traction

Traction means the exertion of pull by means of weights and pulleys. Countertraction (exertion of pull in the opposite direction) must be present to maintain body alignment. Traction is used to promote and maintain the alignment of broken (fractured) bones and for other orthopedic conditions and treatment. It may be applied to the skin externally or to the bone internally through surgery. It is maintained by the use of a special frame on the bed (Figure 16–9).

traction Exertion of pull by means of weights or pulleys, often used for realignment of bones or other limb tissues

THE SKIN (INTEGUMENTARY SYSTEM)

integumentary system
The body system that includes the skin, hair, nails, and sweat and oil glands, that provides the first line of defense against infection, maintains body temperature, provides fluids, and eliminates wastes

The components of the **integumentary system** include the skin, hair, nails, and sweat and oil glands. The skin provides the first line of defense against infection, the maintenance of body temperature, the balance of body fluids, and the elimination of wastes.

Skin covers and protects underlying structures from injury or bacterial invasion. Skin also contains nerve endings from the nervous system. A cross section of the skin is shown in Figure 17–1.

The skin helps regulate the body temperature by controlling the loss of heat from the body. To promote heat loss, the blood vessels near the skin dilate, and the increased blood flow brings more heat to the skin's surface. Then the skin temperature rises and more heat is lost from the hot skin to the cooler environment. Even more important in heat loss is the evaporation of sweat (perspiration) that carries heat away from the skin.

Perspiration is released from the body through *sweat glands,* which are distributed over the entire skin surface. The glands open through ducts or pores. The body also disposes of certain waste products through perspiration.

Conversely, when the body must conserve heat, sweating stops and blood vessels constrict. This prevents the blood from carrying heat to the skin. The skin temperature falls, decreasing heat loss. In this way, the body temperature is kept almost constant.

Oil glands below the skin's surface secrete a thick, oily substance through the ducts that lead to the skin surface. In this way, the skin is lubricated and kept soft and pliable. The oil also provides a protective film for the skin, which limits the absorption and evaporation of water from the surface. During the aging process, these oil glands sometimes fail to function properly, and the skin becomes dry, scaly, and delicate.

■ Appendages of the Skin

In addition to the skin and the sweat and oil glands, other parts of the integumentary system include the hair and the nails. Each hair has a root embedded in the skin into which the oil glands of the skin open. Fingernails and toenails grow from the nail bed at the base underneath. If the nail bed is destroyed, the nail stops growing.

FIGURE 17–1

A cross section of the skin

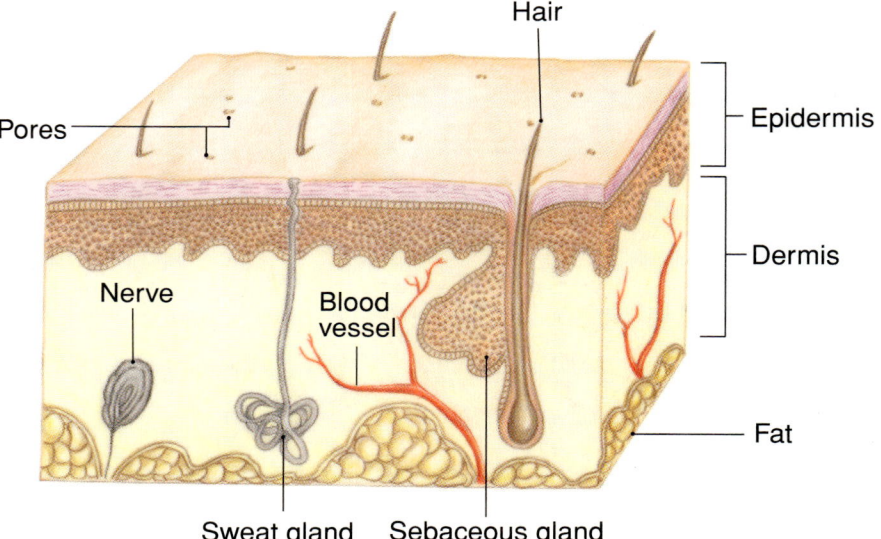

The skin covers the entire body. The outer layer of the skin (the layer you can see) is called the **epidermis**. Cells are constantly flaking off or being rubbed off this outer layer of skin. Beneath the epidermis is the **dermis**. In this layer of skin are the new cells that will replace the cells that are lost from the epidermis. *Pigment* is found in the epidermis and is responsible for the color of the skin. In sunlight, through a chemical reaction, the amount of pigment increases and a suntan results. Fairskinned people have less pigment and are more easily sunburned.

Moisture on the skin can pick up dust and dirt from the air. This moisture can also mix with the skin particles being flaked off the epidermis. This process causes a condition that promotes the growth and spread of bacteria, which is the main reason for keeping the skin clean. The skin is where the battle against infection begins.

epidermis The outer layer or surface of the skin

dermis The inner layer of skin

◼ Primary Functions of the Skin

The primary functions of the skin are to:

- Cover and protect underlying body structures from injury and invasion by micro-organisms
- Help regulate body temperature by controlling loss of heat from the body
- Provide a first line of defense against infection
- Store energy in the form of fat and vitamins
- Eliminate wastes through perspiration
- Allow sensory perception, that is, the sense of touch (the nerves in the skin can sense heat, cold, pain, and pressure)

◼ Inspecting the Skin

Patients who are totally immobile, are incontinent, and have limited sensation are at greatest risk for skin breakdown.

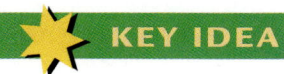
KEY IDEA

Caregivers are often the first to notice subtle changes in a patient's skin or appearance which may signal serious health problems. When examining a person's skin, be sure to note the following:

- Skin color
- Skin temperature
- Excessive moisture or dryness
- Darkened or reddened areas, especially over bony prominences
- Rashes
- Swelling
- Bruising
- Skin tears
- Wounds/ulcers
- Other abnormalities

■ Common Disorders of the Skin

The common disorders of the skin are:

lesion An abnormality, either benign or cancerous, of the tissues of the body, such as a wound, sore, rash, boil, tumors, or growths

- Skin lesions: a **lesion** is an abnormality of body tissues, either benign or cancerous, such as a wound, sore, rash, boil, tumors (lumps), or growths

- Scales: layers of dead skin found on the skin surface

- Excoriations: reddened, scratched, or broken areas caused by the wearing away of the skin's surface

pressure ulcers Also called bedsores; areas of the skin that become broken and painful; caused by continuous pressure on a body part and usually occur when a patient is kept in one position for a long period of time

- **Pressure ulcer:** area of tissue destruction or a lesion resulting from prolonged, unrelieved, pressure

- Vascular ulcer: area of skin breakdown related to abnormalities of the vascular system

- Diabetic ulcer: an ulcer that occurs in people with diabetes resulting from dysfunction of the nerve

- Furuncle: acute inflammation that starts in a hair follicle

- Impetigo: superficial infection caused by streptococci staphylococci, or other bacteria

- Fungus: caused by plantlike organisms, which includes Athlete's foot

- Infestations
    - Pediculosis capitus (scabies/head lice)
    - Pediculosis corporis (body lice)
    - Pediculosis pubis (crab lice)

- Herpes zoster (shingles): inflammatory condition caused by the chicken pox virus that produces painful eruptions

- Dermatitis: reaction to irritating or allergenic materials

- Psoriasis: chronic condition of crusty circular patches for which the cause is unknown

- Burns: excessive exposure to heat or fire

- Maceration: skin breakdown (reddened area) caused by excessive moisture usually in skin folds of perineum of incontinent patients

atrophic skin Thin, fragile, less elastic skin frequently associated with aging

- **Atrophic skin:** fragile, thin skin, often associated with aging

friction injuries Injuries resulting from the patient sliding against hard surfaces

- **Friction injuries:** result from the patient sliding against hard surfaces

shear injuries Result from the skin remaining in place on top of a surface while the underlying structures, such as the bone, slide downward

- **Shear injuries:** result from skin remaining in place on top of a surface and the underlying structures, such as the bone, sliding downward without the skin moving

AGE-SPECIFIC CONSIDERATIONS

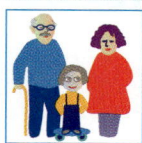

Changes in the Skin

As people age, they develop atrophic skin, which can become thin, fragile, and less elastic (like tissue paper). Atrophic skin can be injured more easily. Elderly people need gentle cleansing and moisturizing (applying lotion) to keep their skin as healthy as possible and prevent skin tears and scrapes, which can lead to infection.

An elderly person's skin may also develop brown spots, particularly on the hands and arms. Fingernails and toenails may thicken and become abnormally shaped.

Always report any changes in skin condition to your immediate supervisor, particularly:

- Redness of skin *(erythema),* which can mean increased body temperature, prolonged pressure, infection, or injury

- A blue or gray color *(cyanosis),* which can mean decreased circulation, a life-threatening condition

- A black or "scablike" skin area *(eschar),* which can disguise a more serious skin problem underneath. A scab does not necessarily mean that a wound is healing well

- A very pale or white color can mean circulatory problems related to anemia, impaired circulation to body parts, or shock

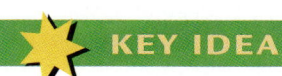

KEY IDEA

An elderly person usually experiences loss of fat under the skin, which makes sitting or lying on hard surfaces even more uncomfortable. In addition, loss of fat makes a person feel cold even when room temperatures feel warm to others. For this reason, it is important to keep elderly patients dressed warmly or well covered in bed or when you are giving nursing care.

CARE OF THE PATIENT WITH POTENTIAL SKIN PROBLEMS

Pressure Ulcers

Pressure ulcers, also called decubitus ulcers or bedsores, are areas where the skin has broken down because of prolonged underlying pressure (Figure 17–2). Injury to the skin comes from pressure on a part of the body where there is loss of circulation (blood flow), which destroys tissues. The pressure cuts off circulation and nourishment to skin areas over the **bony prominences**. These are places where bones are close to the surface of the skin. The pressure can come from the weight of the body lying in one position for too long or from splints, casts, or bandages. If pressure ulcers are not treated, they quickly get larger and become very painful. Even wrinkles in the bed linen can be a cause of pressure sores.

bony prominences
Places where bones are close to the surface of the skin

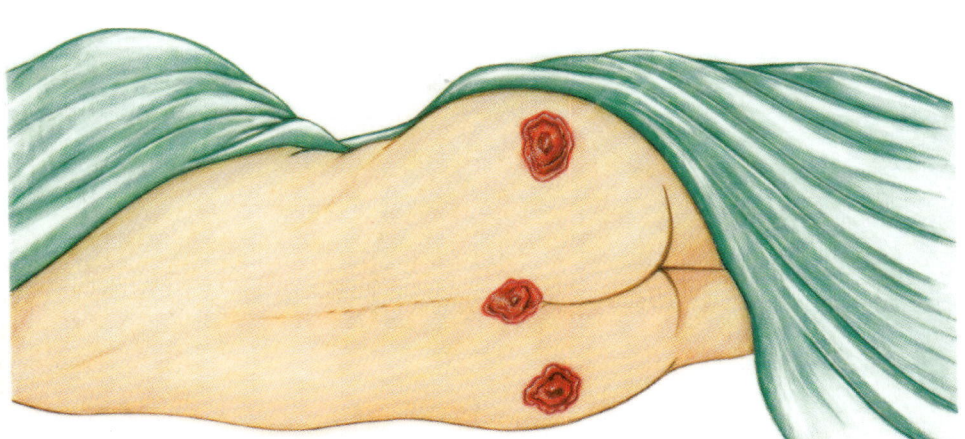

FIGURE 17–2
Pressure ulcers are broken areas of the skin caused by the loss of circulation to that area; ulcers are the result of continual pressure when a patient remains in the same position too long

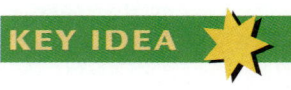

KEY IDEA   Injury to the skin comes from pressure on a part of the body where there is loss of circulation (blood flow), which destroys tissues.

Pressure ulcers are often made worse by continued pressure, moisture, and lack of cleanliness. Irritating substances on the skin such as perspiration, urine, feces, material from wound discharges, or soap that has been left on the skin after a bath all tend to make skin conditions worse.

Risk Factors for Pressure Ulcer Development

Certain conditions are associated with pressure ulcer breakdown. Patients with even one of these risk factors is at risk for skin breakdown. The patient with more than one risk factor is at even greater risk. These patients need considerable assistance from the nurses to prevent pressure ulcers. The conditions for risk include:

- Loss of sensory perception: patients who are unresponsive and have a limited ability to feel pain over large parts of their bodies

- Moist skin: skin that is almost constantly moist from perspiration, urine, or loose stools can break down

- Limited activity: patients who are bedfast and chairfast

- Immobility: patients who do not move on their own while in bed or in the chair

- Friction and shear: frequent sliding down and pulling up in bed can cause the patient to slide over the sheets

- Poor nutrition or poor hydration: patients who do not eat all their food and are not on tube feedings can be vulnerable to skin breakdown

Notify your supervisor if a patient starts to decrease activity and stops eating regular meals and snacks. Early small areas of skin breakdown also need to be reported immediately. They can signal much larger problems.

Signs of a Pressure Ulcer

The signs of a pressure ulcer on the skin are heat, redness, tenderness, discomfort, and a feeling of burning. When there is a darkened or reddened area that doesn't fade after 20 minutes, a pressure ulcer has formed (Figure 17–3). If pressure is not relieved, the skin

FIGURE 17–3

Tissue under pressure; the ulcer visible on the surface is often much smaller than the skin damage below the skin surface

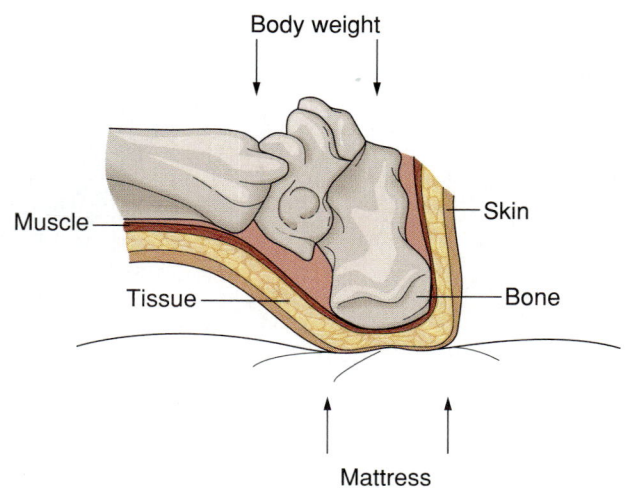

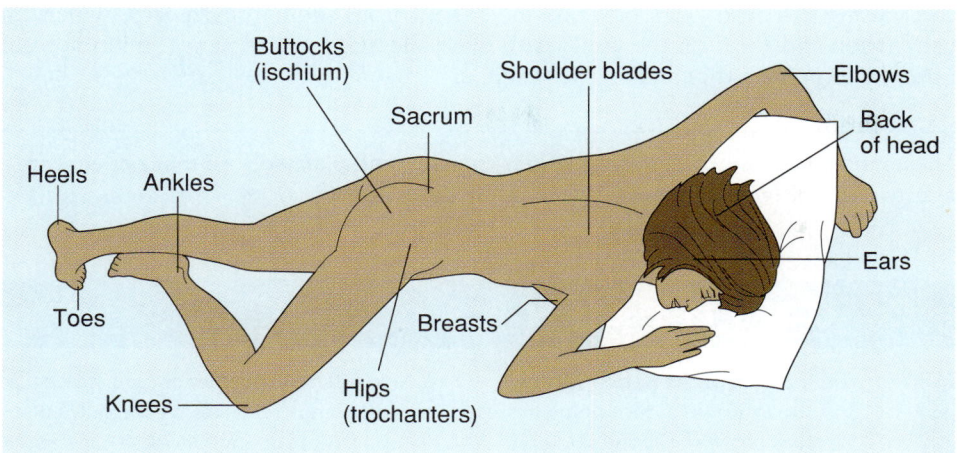

FIGURE 17–4

Check for signs of pressure ulcers over bony prominences

may break open. Specific treatment for pressure sores are prescribed by a doctor or nurse specialist. The wound must be kept clean. As you have already learned, the skin is the body's first line of defense against infection.

Places to check on the body for signs of pressure are the bony areas (prominences) (Figure 17–4). These include the shoulder blades, elbows, knees, heels, hips, sides of ankles, back of the head, above the ears, and the lower tip of the spine (sacrum). Sitting in any type of chair for too long can cause pressure over the bones in the buttocks (ischium). Usually these areas are covered only by a thin layer of skin.

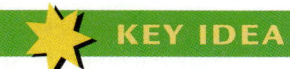

Bony prominences are the areas where pressure sores are most likely to occur when patients lie or sit on them continually.

KEY IDEA

Preventing Pressure Ulcers

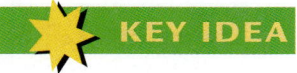

Preventing pressure ulcers is the responsibility of the entire healthcare team. We now know that nearly all pressure sores *can* be prevented.

KEY IDEA

Once a mild ulcer has formed, it can be very hard to cure. It is critical that nursing assistants report the first sign of a pressure sore to their immediate supervisor so that steps can be taken to prevent further damage.

Immobile patients and bedridden patients are at risk for developing friction and shear injury from sliding over rough surfaces. When the head of the bed is elevated too high, the patient slides down in bed causing a *friction/shear injury*. Position the head of the bed below 30 degrees (Figure 17–5) unless there is a medical reason to have it elevated. Patients on tube feedings and who have difficulty breathing will need to have the head of the bed elevated. If the head of the bed needs to be elevated, raise the knees slightly

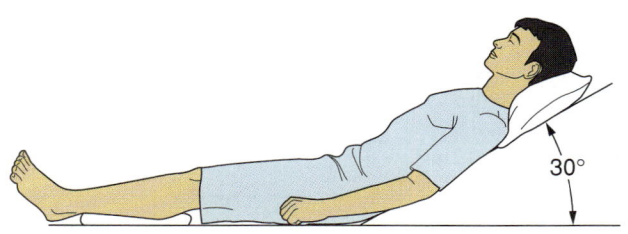

FIGURE 17–5

Example of head of bed raised 30 degrees; heels are raised off the bed before raising the head. This prevents the patient from sliding downward, which can cause friction and shear on the skin. Use a draw sheet to pull the patient up in bed and for turning to prevent friction and shear injuries.

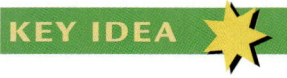 **KEY IDEA**

The nursing assistant can group activities together and plan work so that patients are assisted into different positions within a safe time frame.

obese Very overweight

GUIDELINES

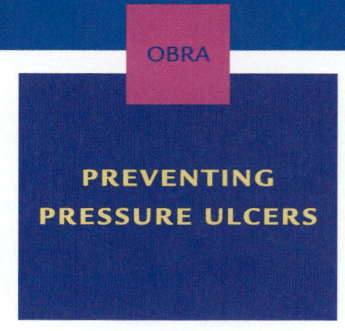

OBRA

PREVENTING PRESSURE ULCERS

The nursing assistant can help to prevent bedsores by doing the following:

■ Change the patient's position every two hours. A turning schedule at the bedside is helpful when there are multiple caregivers (Figure 17–6).

■ Be careful when using bedpans. Pressure from sitting on the rim and friction when moving the patient on and off the bedpan can create or worsen ulcers. Never leave the patient on the bedpan longer than necessary. Use care when removing the bedpan to avoid spilling urine on the skin. Urine is irritating to the skin and can cause further damage to a reddened or tender area. Powdering the rim of the bedpan can minimize friction when removed.

■ Keep the patient's body as clean and dry as possible. Change the patient's gown or clothing if it is damp. Wash the patient's skin with mild soap or use special incontinent cleansers to remove urine or feces. Rinse well with clean warm water. Use moisture barriers on the skin to prevent contact with discharged materials from wounds, which can cause irritation.

■ If a part of the patient's body shows signs of developing a pressure ulcer, notify the skin care nurse or health care provider and do not position the patient on that area until the redness or ulcer has disappeared. Position the patient on the turning surfaces that do not have ulcers.

■ Use powder or corn starch sparingly where skin surfaces come together and form creases. Examples are under the breasts of women patients, between buttocks, and in the folds of skin on the abdomen or groin. Do not apply powder in areas of open sores or surgical incisions. When bathing the patient, be sure

to wash the powder or corn starch off completely. This is especially important in caring for obese patients. Corn starch is less caking when in contact with moisture and is preferred over powders. To help prevent caking, the corn starch or powder should be rubbed into the skin, much like when applying lotion.

■ **Obese** (very overweight) patients tend to develop sores where body parts rub against each other, causing friction. Places to check on obese patients are the folds of the body where skin touches skin, such as under the breasts, between the folds of the buttocks, and between the thighs. Pillows are used to pro-

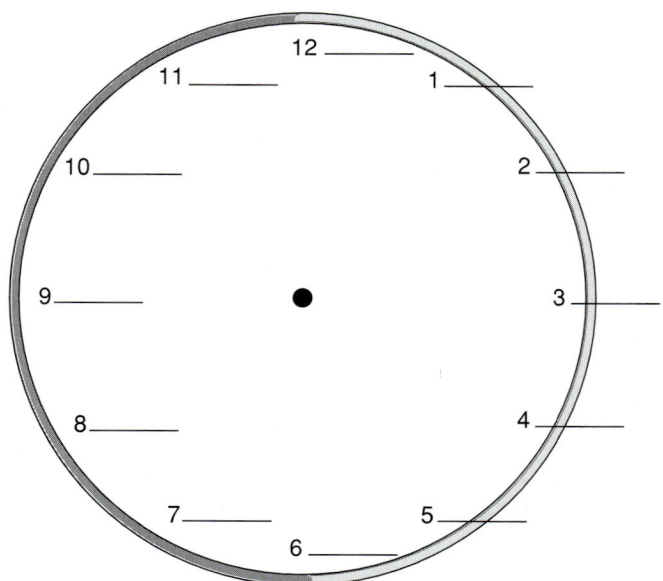

Turning schedule: Indicate position change on the lines above.
R = right side; L = left side; B = back; S = stomach; C = chair.

FIGURE 17–6

A sample turning schedule

GUIDELINES (CONTINUED)

vide support, separate skin surfaces, and prevent skin breakdown. It is necessary to avoid all skin-to-skin contact. Use pillows between the knees.

- Keep linens wrinkle free and dry at all times.

- Remove crumbs, hair pins, and any other hard objects from the bed promptly.

- If the patient is **incontinent** (unable to control urine or feces), use incontinent pads. These can be disposable or reusable. Never use more than two layers of incontinent pads. If more than two layers of incontinent pads are used, the patient will be at greater risk of pressure sore development. To be sure that plastic never touches the patient's skin, place a sheet between the patient and the plastic

disposable pads (Figure 17–7). Change the incontinent pads immediately when they become wet.

- Disposable plastic diapers can be used when the incontinent patient is out of bed. However, they must

be removed when the patient is returned to bed. The closed, wet plastic environment can result in maceration of the skin and skin breakdown.

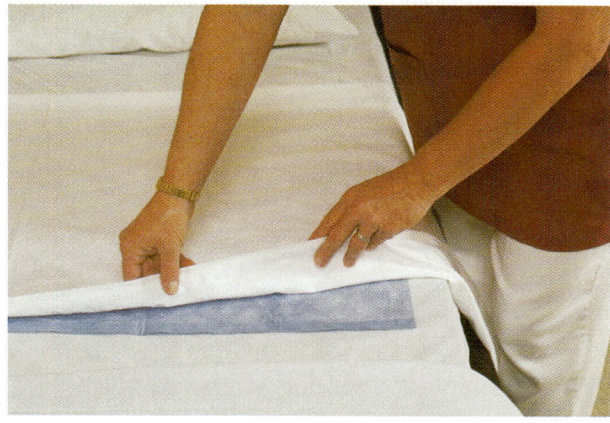

FIGURE 17–7

Place a sheet between disposable plastic incontinent pads and the patient

Foot Care

incontinent Unable to control urine or feces

Preventing pressure ulcers on the feet requires special attention and knowledge.

Pressure sores on the feet can be serious, sometimes leading to amputation and even death.

KEY IDEA

GUIDELINES

OBRA

FOOT CARE

- Never soak a patient's feet without a doctor's order.
- Wash a patient's feet daily with mild soap and water.

- Rinse well and dry the feet thoroughly. Do not pull towels through toes as this can cut the skin.
- Apply lotion to the feet except for the area between toes.
- Notify the nurse or podiatrist for nail care. Do not attempt to trim a patient's nails unless you have been trained to do so.
- Use pillows to dangle heels (Figure 17–8). Place each pillow lengthwise under the calf and tuck in to prevent heel from touching.

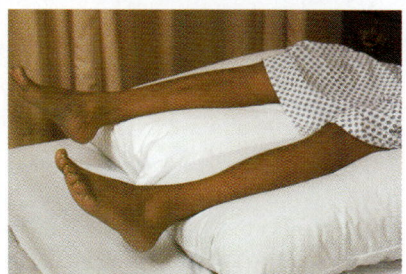

FIGURE 17–8

Use pillows to dangle the heels to prevent pressure areas

EQUIPMENT AND DEVICES THAT REDUCE PRESSURE ON THE SKIN

Special equipment may be ordered to reduce the pressure on the skin. Devices are available to protect patients while they are in bed or sitting in chairs. Bed and chair cushions are made from a variety of materials. Foam mattresses and overlays can be used for patients at low risk. Air and gel mattresses provide greater pressure reduction for people at high risk for breakdown.

■ Mattresses, Overlays, and Beds

Foam Mattresses

- *Purpose:* A softer mattress prevents pressure ulcers.

- *Precautions:* Turn patients every two hours and elevate the heels of immobile patients. Ask if your institution has this type of mattress.

Four-Inch High Density Foam

- *Purpose:* An overlay for assisting in the prevention of pressure ulcers.

- *Precautions:* Place foam in plastic covering to prevent soiling. Use for one patient only, then discard.

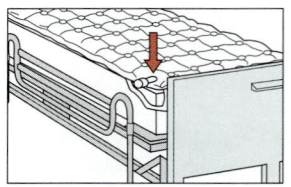

Static Air Mattress

- *Purpose:* An overlay for preventing pressure ulcers.

- *Precautions:* Follow the manufacturer's operating instructions. Do not puncture. Turn the patient every two hours and elevate the heels of immobile patients. Use for one patient only, then discard (Figure 17–9).

Alternating Air Mattress

- *Purpose:* Redistributes the pressure on a timed, automatic basis.

- *Precautions:* Be sure the motor and mattress are working correctly. Do not puncture. Use only one loosely applied sheet between the patient and the mattress.

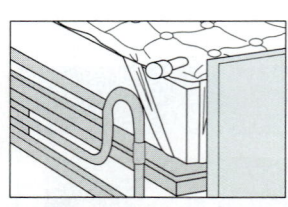

FIGURE 17–9

Static air mattress overlay

Specialty Bed

- *Purpose:* Provides pressure relief over most of the body and is an excellent device to promote wound healing.

- *Precautions:* Patients still need to be turned while on a specialty bed and their heels and the back of the head still need to be elevated off the bed surface while the patient is immobile. Use the manufacturer's recommended incontinent pads (Figure 17–10).

Eggcrate Mattress

- *Purpose:* Provides comfort.

- *Precautions:* These mattresses do not protect patient from pressure ulcers.

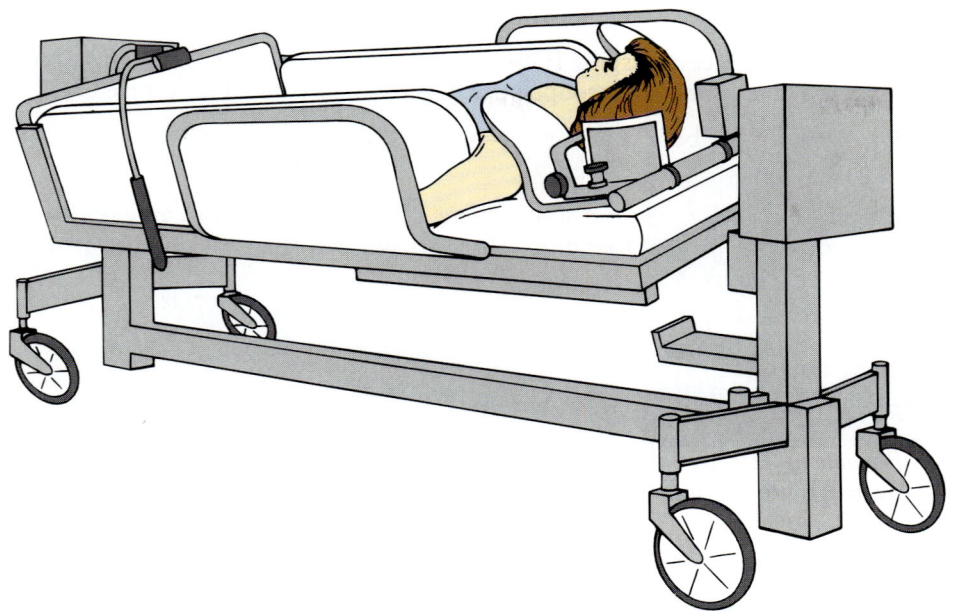

FIGURE 17–10
Specialty bed; immobile patients will continue to develop heel ulcers on most types of specialty beds and will need the heels elevated

■ Chair Cushions

Special pressure reduction devices can be used in chairs. Patients at risk for pressure ulcers need therapeutic foam (four-inch, high-density foam, gel pads or air pads) in their chairs (Figure 17–11). Do not allow patients to sit on *round doughnuts* without a doctor's order as this can cause poor circulation.

Wheelchair cushions conform to the body when a patient is sitting. Place the cushion properly in the chair and cover with a cloth.

■ Extremities: Foot, Heel, Arms

A pillow placed lengthwise under the calf with the heel dangling is the best device for protecting the heels. Many other products do not stay in place or the straps for attachment cause pressure ulcers.

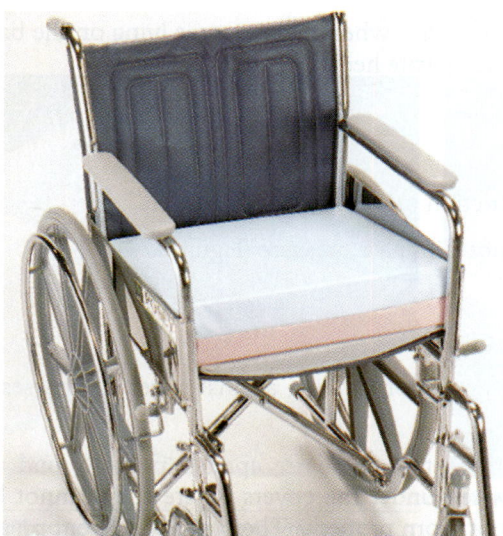

FIGURE 17–11
Foam cushion in wheelchair

circulatory system The heart, blood vessels, blood, and all organs that pump and carry blood and other fluids throughout the body

heart A four-chambered, hollow, muscular organ that lies in the chest cavity and pumps the blood through the lungs and into all parts of the body

THE CIRCULATORY SYSTEM: ANATOMY AND PHYSIOLOGY

The **circulatory system** (Figure 18–1) is made up of the blood, the heart, and the blood vessels (arteries, veins, and capillaries). The **heart** acts as a pump for the blood, which carries the nutrients, oxygen, and other elements needed by the cells. The blood vessels are the pathways through which the blood travels.

The Blood

The blood is a kind of transportation system that transports needed elements to the cells of the body and removes waste products.

- The blood carries oxygen from the lungs to the cells

- The blood carries carbon dioxide from the cells to the lungs

- The blood absorbs (picks up) nutrients from the duodenum (small intestine) and carries them to the cells

- The blood carries waste products from the cells to the kidneys to be eliminated in urine

FIGURE 18–1

The circulatory system

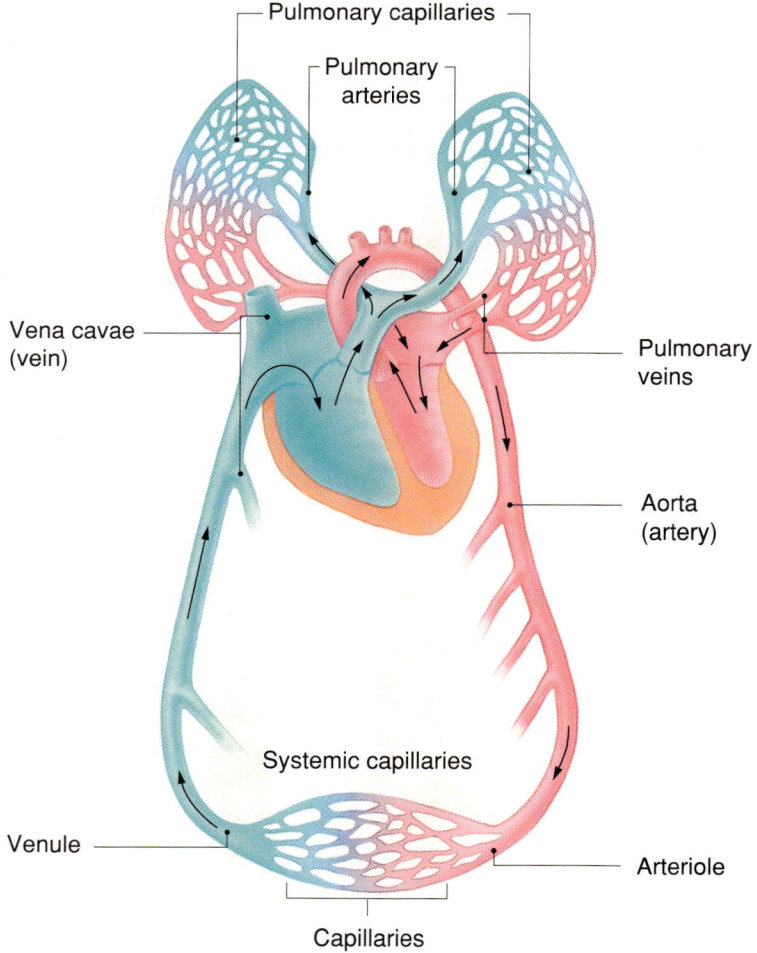

To carry out this function, the blood must move continuously throughout the body. This continuous movement is called **circulation**.

The blood and blood vessels perform other functions as well:

- The blood transports hormones from the endocrine glands.

- The blood vessels help regulate body temperatures through dilation (enlargement) and constriction (narrowing). To bring more blood and warm up a body part, the blood vessels dilate. Constriction reduces the blood supply and lowers body temperature.

- The blood helps maintain the fluid balance of the body by helping to move sodium and potassium into and out of body cells. These elements affect how much water the body will either retain or excrete.

- The white cells of the blood defend the body against disease. They do so by destroying microorganisms they identify as a threat to the body. The white cells are sent into the blood and carried to the site of infection. There they engulf the microorganisms, and the blood carries them away to be excreted out of the body.

The liquid portion of the blood is called **plasma**. It contains red blood cells, white blood cells, and platelets. Platelets help to stop bleeding when the body is injured by forming clots at the site of the injury.

The red blood cells carry oxygen. People who have too few red blood cells have a type of **anemia**.

The white blood cells fight infection. People who have too few white blood cells have a lowered resistance to disease. An increase in white blood cells in the blood can mean that an infection is present somewhere in the body. If a patient has an inflammation in some area of the body, a physician often prescribes warm, moist compresses. These are applied to dilate the blood vessels in the area and to bring more of the important white blood cells to the place of infection to help fight it.

circulation The continuous movement of blood through the heart and blood vessels to all parts of the body

plasma The liquid portion of the blood

anemia A shortage of red blood cells

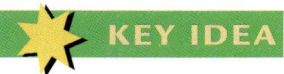

The blood carries oxygen and nutrients to the cells of the body. It carries away carbon dioxide (to be eliminated through the lungs) and waste products (to be eliminated through the kidneys).

The Heart

The heart (Figure 18–2) is located in the chest cavity, pointing slightly to the left. It is the pump that circulates the blood through the lungs and into all parts of the body. It is a muscular organ made up of four chambers: two atria and two ventricles.

The two larger chambers are called ventricles. The right ventricle sends the blood only as far as the lungs. Here, in the **pulmonary** circulation, the blood picks up oxygen and gets rid of carbon dioxide. This blood then returns to the heart, carrying its load of oxygen on the surface of the red blood cells. The left ventricle then pushes the blood into systemic circulation (circulation throughout the rest of the body).

pulmonary Pertaining to the lungs

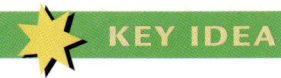

The ventricles have thick walls of muscle. When they contract, the left ventricle pushes the blood through the largest blood vessel, the aorta, to all parts of the body.

FIGURE 18–2
The heart

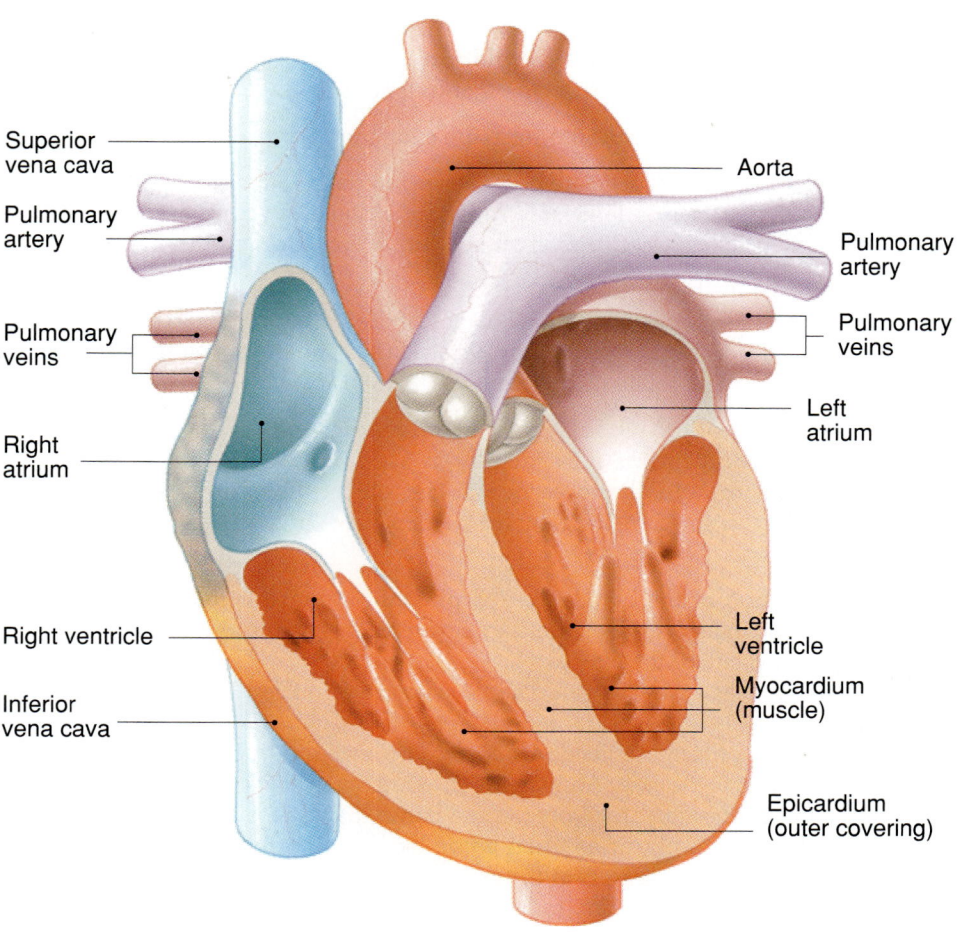

Superior vena cava

Pulmonary artery

Pulmonary veins

Right atrium

Right ventricle

Inferior vena cava

Aorta

Pulmonary artery

Pulmonary veins

Left atrium

Left ventricle

Myocardium (muscle)

Epicardium (outer covering)

The Blood Vessels

The blood vessels carrying blood that is oxygenated (having a lot of oxygen) are called **arteries**. An exception is the pulmonary artery, which carries the blood to the lungs. Arteries branch into a vast network throughout the body (Figure 18–3). As they branch out, the blood vessels become smaller and smaller until finally they are so thin they become capillaries.

The walls of the capillaries are only one cell layer thick. Through these walls, gases, nutrients, waste products, and other substances are exchanged among the blood in the capillaries, the tissue fluid, and the individual cell.

After the RBCs in the blood have given up their oxygen, it returns to the heart through the **veins** (Figure 18–4).

The heart muscle must be supplied with blood carrying oxygen. The first branches of the aorta, the coronary arteries, come from the heart's left ventricle. These arteries surround the heart and carry needed oxygen to **cardiac** (heart muscle) tissue. If one of these coronary branches is blocked by a blood clot (thrombus), the patient has a heart attack, which can result in the death of some heart tissue. The event is called a myocardial infarction (MI).

artery Blood vessel that carries oxygenated blood away from the heart

vein Blood vessel that carries blood from parts of the body back to the heart

cardiac Pertaining to the heart

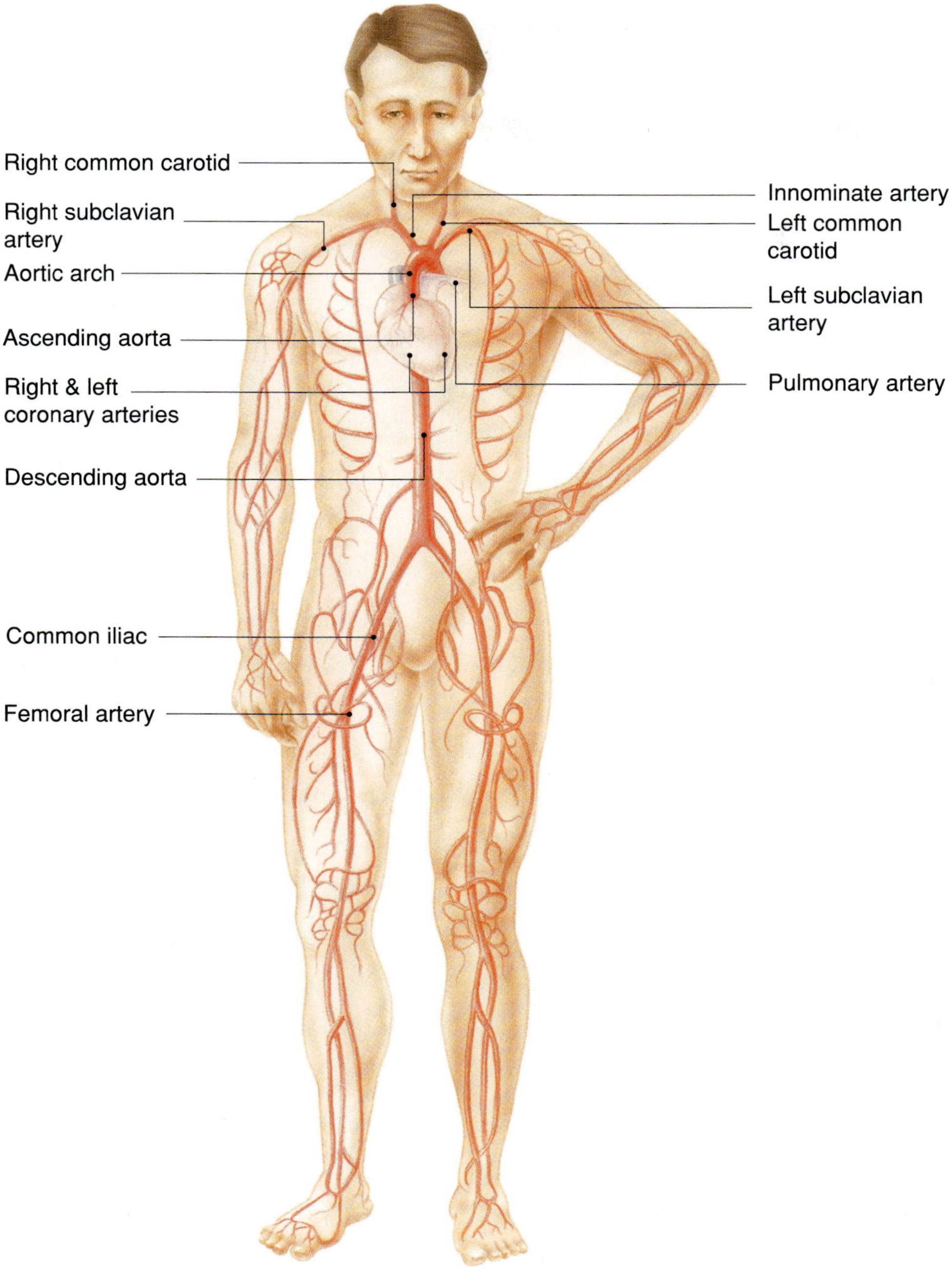

FIGURE 18–3
The system of arteries

Right common carotid

Right subclavian artery

Aortic arch

Ascending aorta

Right & left coronary arteries

Descending aorta

Common iliac

Femoral artery

Innominate artery

Left common carotid

Left subclavian artery

Pulmonary artery

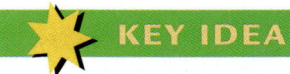

The following points summarize the basic differences between the arteries and veins:

- All arteries carry blood away from the heart.

- All veins carry blood back to the heart.

- All arteries (except the pulmonary artery) carry oxygenated blood.

- All veins (except the four pulmonary veins) carry deoxygenated blood.

KEY IDEA

FIGURE 18–4
The system of veins

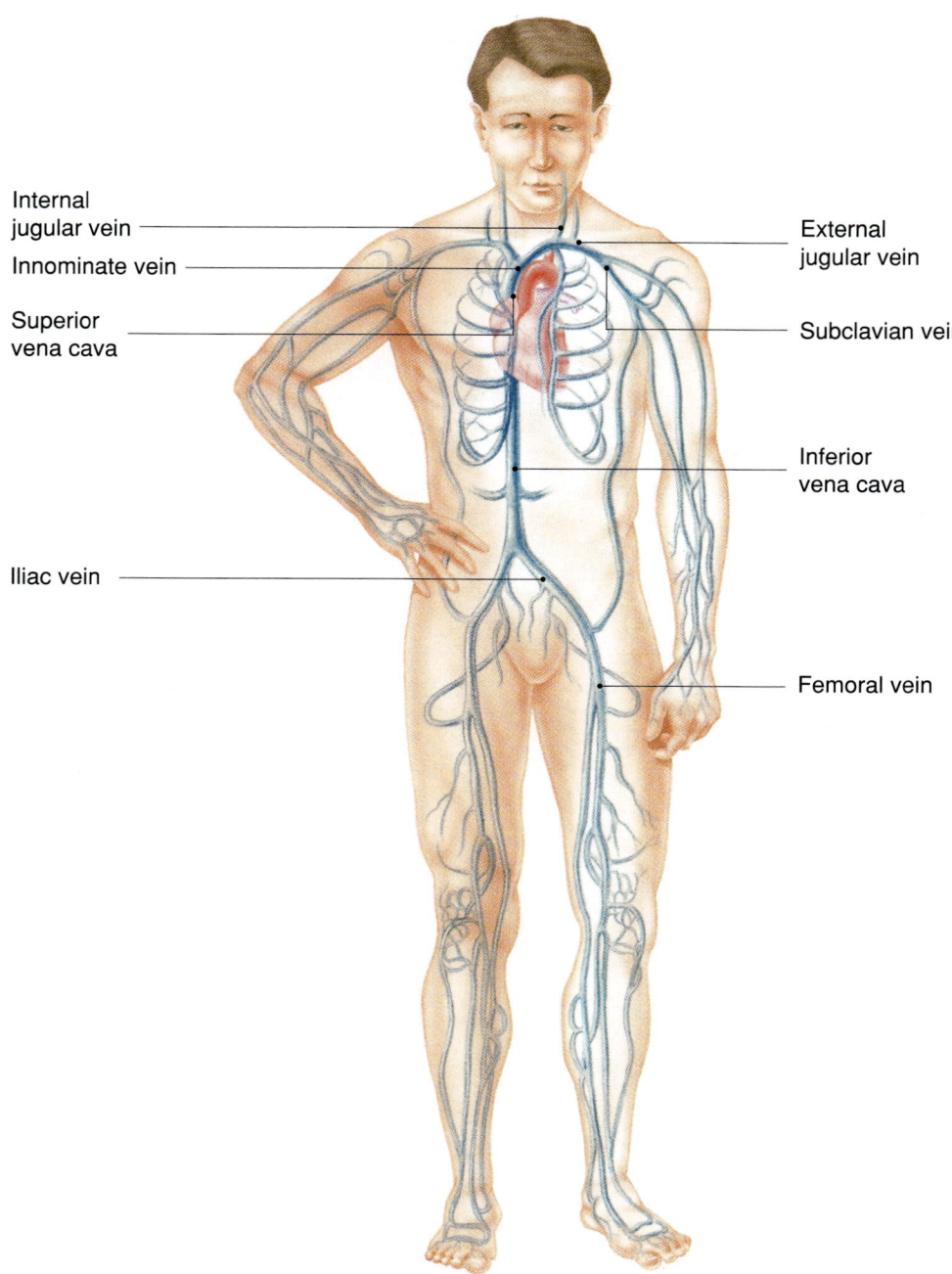

Internal jugular vein

Innominate vein

Superior vena cava

Iliac vein

External jugular vein

Subclavian vein

Inferior vena cava

Femoral vein

Inactivity and Blood Circulation

When a patient is inactive, the blood circulation tends to slow down. The patient may also have a lower **blood pressure** (force of the blood pushing against the walls of the blood vessels). Sometimes this can cause the blood to form clots. Blood clots are dangerous. Sometimes a clot flows with the blood and becomes lodged in the blood vessels of the lungs. This condition, called a pulmonary embolism, is life-threatening.

If you have orders to help a patient out of bed for the first time after an illness or after surgery, remember that the patient's circulation is slower and the blood pressure may be lower. Therefore, be sure the patient moves carefully and slowly. Allow the patient to sit at the edge of the bed and dangle the legs until the circulation stabilizes (comes back to normal). Then carefully help the patient to a standing position.

blood pressure The force of the blood pushing against the walls of the blood vessels

Sometimes this procedure will cause the blood to leave the brain suddenly, and the patient may be dizzy or feel faint. You may need more than one person to help you with the patient. Be sure to check the patient's activity restrictions with the supervisor.

THE CIRCULATORY SYSTEM AND THE NORMAL AGING PROCESS

As a person grows older, the movement of blood through the body tends to slow down. The heart muscle weakens, so the heart pumps with less force. It must work harder to keep the blood moving, yet it works less effectively. Thus, the blood flow decreases. The reduced output of the heart is one reason older people tend to tire more easily and have less reserve energy than younger people.

The heart may change in size. If it works harder to circulate the blood through the vessels, the greater work causes this muscle to grow larger. (In general, muscles get larger when they perform more work.) When some people age, they drastically reduce their physical activity. For such people, the heart may become smaller because it does not work as hard.

The blood vessels change as well. With age, they may harden and lose their ability to stretch. This causes them to become narrow. Fatty deposits and other substances may clog these narrowed vessels. Such changes further diminish blood flow and increase blood pressure. They also increase the risk of a blood vessel rupturing or becoming blocked. Thus, changes in the blood vessels can bring about physical and mental problems.

COMMON DISEASES AND DISORDERS OF THE CIRCULATORY SYSTEM

Among the diseases and disorders that most often affect the circulatory system are the following:

- Arteriosclerosis: The walls of the arteries become thicker with fatty deposits and less elastic than they should be for the normal regulation of blood flow and blood pressure.

- Angina pectoris: Heart pain that results from insufficient blood flow and oxygen to the heart muscle.

- Myocardial infarction (MI): Obstruction of a blood vessel in the heart muscle results in death of heart tissue due to lack of oxygen.

- Endocarditis: The inner lining of the heart becomes inflamed.

- Rheumatic heart disease: The organism that causes rheumatic fever damages the valves of the heart.

- Congestive heart failure: The heart is unable to pump enough blood, and fluid builds up in the lungs.

- Hypertension: The blood pressure in the arteries is elevated (high).

- Leukemia: This is the term for cancer of the blood.

GUIDELINES

OBRA

PROVIDING CARE FOR PATIENTS WITH PERIPHERAL VASCULAR DISEASE

- Carefully inspect the feet when bathing the patient's feet or in

response to patient complaint of foot discomfort. Report broken or cracked skin, color changes to red, white, black, or blue; swelling, pain, loss of function; corns or calluses, or loss of function.

- After washing, thoroughly dry the feet and between the toes, then apply lotion if the skin is dry.
- Avoid cutting toenails unless instructed to do so by a nurse or doctor.

- Elevate feet when patient is sitting up in a chair for more than a few minutes or support them with a foot stool.
- Discourage habits that hinder circulation (wearing tight garters or socks, crossing legs at the knees, smoking).
- Avoid heating pads, unprotected exposure to heat or cold, as sensation is reduced.

GUIDELINES

PROVIDING CARE FOR PATIENTS WITH HYPERTENSIVE DISEASE

- Treatment usually includes drugs that lower the blood pressure, a low sodium diet, and encouragement of regular exercise. Encourage patient to follow the treatment and continue to take their medications even when they are feeling they do not need to do so.

- Avoid, decrease, or quit smoking.
- Observe and report the following signs and symptoms: Flushed face, dizziness, nosebleeds, sudden headaches, changes in speech patterns, or blurred vision.

- Anemia: The quantity and quality of red blood cells decreases.

- Cerebrovascular accident (CVA): A blockage in or rupturing of arteries in the brain causes a stroke (death of brain tissue).

- Peripheral Vascular Disease: Conditions resulting from restricted or poor functioning of the valves in the veins.

THE RESPIRATORY SYSTEM: ANATOMY AND PHYSIOLOGY

respiratory system The group of body organs that carries on the body function of respiration; the system brings oxygen into the body and eliminates carbon dioxide

The **respiratory system** (Figure 18–5) provides a route or pathway for oxygen to get from the air into the lungs, where it can be picked up by the blood. The organs that make up this system include the nose and mouth, pharynx (throat), trachea (windpipe), larynx (voice box), lungs, and bronchi.

Because we must have oxygen to live, it is necessary to keep this pathway open. The structures themselves help to do this. The trachea and bronchi are kept open by incomplete cartilage rings.

On the top of the trachea, opening from the pharynx (the throat), is a structure known as the larynx. In addition to being the opening to the trachea, it also contains the vocal cords, which make it possible for us to talk.

FIGURE 18–5
The respiratory system

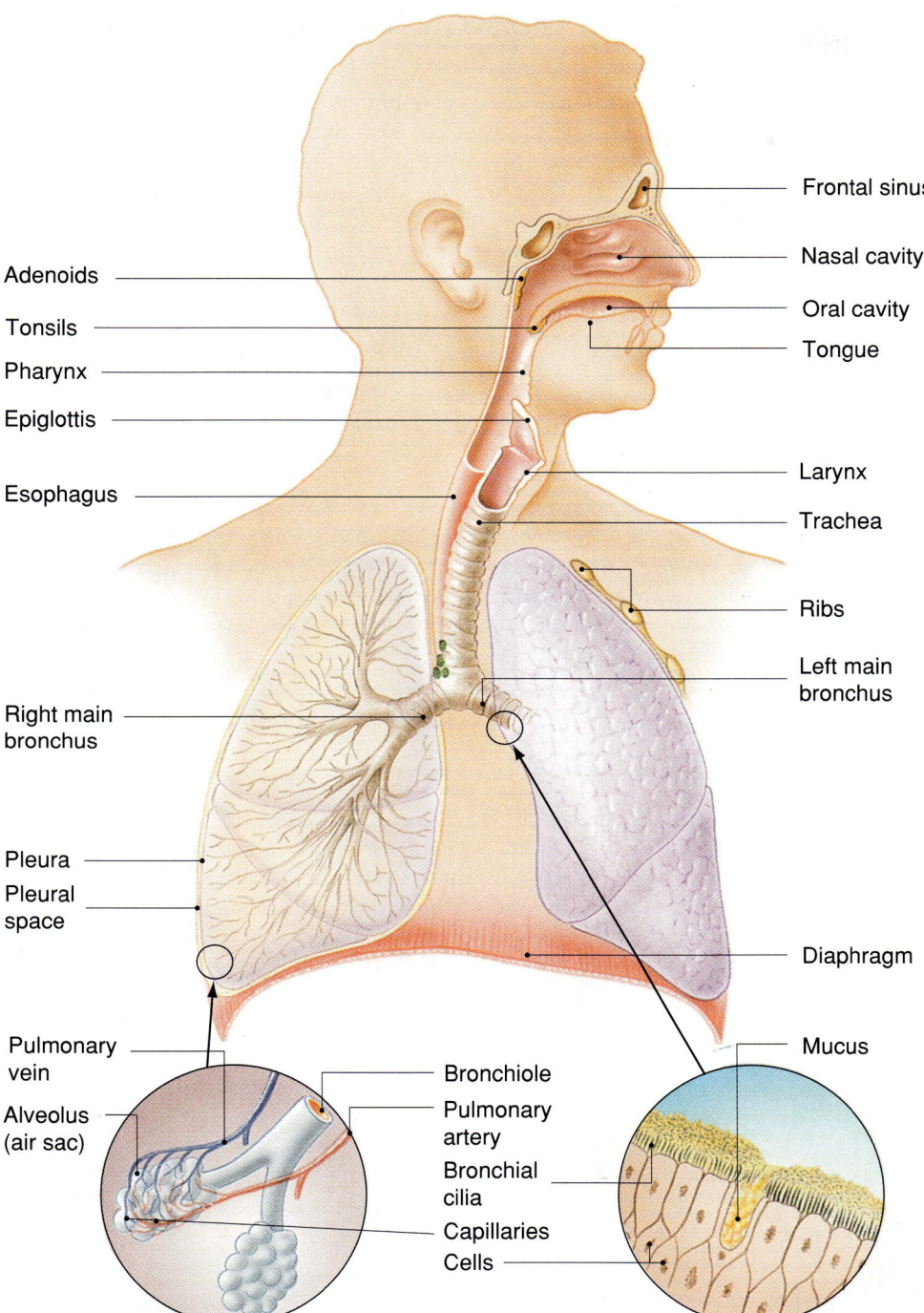

Frontal sinus

Nasal cavity

Oral cavity

Tongue

Adenoids

Tonsils

Pharynx

Epiglottis

Esophagus

Larynx

Trachea

Ribs

Left main bronchus

Right main bronchus

Pleura

Pleural space

Diaphragm

Mucus

Pulmonary vein

Alveolus (air sac)

Bronchiole

Pulmonary artery

Bronchial cilia

Capillaries

Cells

An important piece of cartilage, the epiglottis, covers the opening to the trachea when food is swallowed, preventing the food from going into the lungs. A very weak patient or one who is having trouble breathing must be watched carefully during feeding so that food does not get into the trachea. This is known as aspiration of food. An unconscious patient who vomits may also be in danger of aspirating vomitus. If an unconscious patient vomits, turn the patient's head to one side immediately. You must watch the patient with great care, because if the pathway for oxygen is blocked, the patient will die without immediate treatment.

Oxygen and Carbon Dioxide Exchange

As in the body's other systems, the important work of the respiratory system is done at the level of the cell. The exchange of oxygen and carbon dioxide occurs in an area of the lungs that is so small you would have to use a microscope to see it. At the end of the last branch of the bronchus—the alveolar duct—is a small sac, the alveolus. Many oxygen molecules fill this sac after the body breathes in. The blood has less oxygen, so it can pick up a large amount of oxygen from the alveolar sac and release the CO_2 it is carrying. The blood is then returned to the heart to transport the oxygen around the body.

The respiratory system then is responsible for getting oxygen to the blood. Internal respiration occurs when cells that need the oxygen receive it in exchange for carbon dioxide, which is the cells' gas waste product. Both functions—the exchanges of oxygen in the lungs and at the cellular level—are equally important.

Breathing is regulated in the medulla, a part of the brain.

KEY IDEA

The circulatory and respiratory systems are tightly linked. The respiratory system delivers oxygen from the air to the blood to be transported through the circulatory system. The circulatory system delivers carbon dioxide from the body to the lungs, where the respiratory system removes it from the body. Thus, neither system can complete its work without the other.

Respiratory Care after Surgery

Often, especially after surgery, a patient must be encouraged to breathe deeply in order to keep all the air sacs open and inflated. Sometimes a nursing assistant is asked to encourage the patient to cough, especially if there is inflammation of the lung tissue. In many of the larger health care institutions, the Pulmonary Medicine Department (Respiratory Therapy) will, by a doctor's order, institute a treatment that will encourage the patient to breathe deeply and cough. An incentive spirometer is used postoperatively for this in most hospitals.

After a patient has had some kind of abdominal surgery, he may, fearing pain, resist coughing. One way to make the patient more comfortable is to place a pillow over the patient's abdomen and instruct the patient to hold it firmly against the abdomen when he coughs.

The patient is usually instructed to breathe in and out slowly and deeply twice. After breathing in deeply a third time, the patient should cough twice instead of letting the air out slowly. Make sure he covers his mouth with a tissue and turns his head away from you.

THE RESPIRATORY SYSTEM AND THE NORMAL AGING PROCESS

As adults age, the elasticity of the lung tissue can decrease. Also, the airways can become obstructed due to repeated infections or irritants, such as smoking or air pollution. This is known as chronic obstructive pulmonary disease (COPD), which refers to a group of disorders, such as bronchitis, asthma, and emphysema.

As the body ages, the circulatory system becomes less responsive. Cardiac output decreases and the structures of the heart become more rigid. The respiratory system ages as well. Geriatric adults often have less muscular strength, less lung capacity, and weaker cough.

Infants and small children have little ability to maintain a reserve of energy and are more apt to become severely ill quickly. Crying can elevate vital signs. The intercostal muscles of infants are not fully developed and therefore may have a difficult time clearing secretions.

COMMON DISEASES AND DISORDERS OF THE RESPIRATORY SYSTEM

The following diseases and disorders are among the most common ones affecting the respiratory system:

- Infection of the upper respiratory tract: the common cold

- Sinusitis: inflammation of the sinuses

- Pharyngitis: inflammation of the throat

- Cancer of the larynx (voice box): the growth of cancer in the larynx

- Pneumonia: infection of the lung

- Lung cancer: the growth of cancer in the lungs

- Chest trauma: injury to the chest

- **Tuberculosis (TB):** infection caused by a microorganism that is easily transmitted from one person to another through the air

- Chronic obstructive pulmonary disease (COPD): obstruction of the airways caused by repeated infections or exposure to irritants

- Bronchitis: inflammation of the bronchi

- Emphysema: obstruction of airflow in the lungs

- Asthma: allergy with wheezing and dyspnea (difficulty breathing)

tuberculosis (TB) A highly infectious disease that usually affects the lungs

Tuberculosis (TB) has been increasing over the last few years. This disease is spread through the air by droplets produced from an infected person's coughing, sneezing, or talking. If you care for a patient who has tuberculosis, you must wear a special mask at all times and adhere to Standard Precautions. Be sure to check with the supervisor to identify any other special precautions to be taken.

A patient with COPD has several needs. He will find it difficult to breathe and will get short of breath with common activities like walking. He has a great deal of fear that he will not be able to breathe and may have a reduced appetite. Mouth care becomes very important as this patient will often breathe deeply through the mouth. Mouth breathing dries up the saliva normally present in the mouth. Saliva provides moisture that assists in cleansing the mouth. The patient may be receiving oxygen therapy (Figure 18–6). It is very important to permit a COPD patient to do as much as he comfortably can for himself. This helps to maintain his sense of independence and ability to function. Expect that frequent rest periods may be needed for the patient to perform the routine activities of daily living.

FIGURE 18–6

A patient with COPD
requiring oxygen

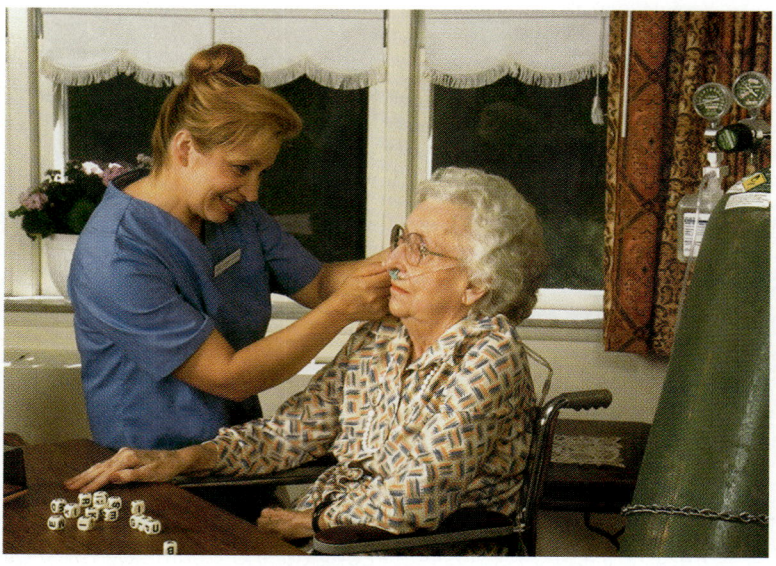

◼ Indications a Patient May Require Supplemental Oxygen

When caring for a patient there are signs that the patient may need extra or supplemental oxygen. Consider the following questions and report if you observe any to be occurring:

- Are their respirations labored?

- Has the respiration rate increased?

- Does the patient report feeling short of breath?

- Is the patient using accessory muscles (neck or intercostal muscles) to assist their ventilation?

- Is the patient wheezing?

- Are there signs of cyanosis—bluish nail beds or bluish hue—to the lips or mucous membranes?

◼ Therapies Related to Respiratory Disease

A patient who has a respiratory disease may be receiving oxygen or special breathing treatments (Figure 18–7). A patient using oxygen must never smoke or come near an open flame because the oxygen will burn or explode. When a patient is receiving a breathing treatment, oxygen may also be used, so remember to avoid any situation involving smoking or being around an open flame. It may be important to remind visitors or family members of these precautions (Figure 18–8).

The oxygen orders must be followed carefully. Some patients must keep the oxygen on at all times. A patient who is receiving breathing treatments will have them ordered to be done at specific times. Check with the supervisor for specific instructions for the patient.

Try to give patient care at times that fit well with the ordered treatments. For example, after a breathing treatment, a patient generally feels better and can breathe more easily. Giving a bath or ambulating a patient after receiving treatment will enable the patient to be more active and less likely to tire.

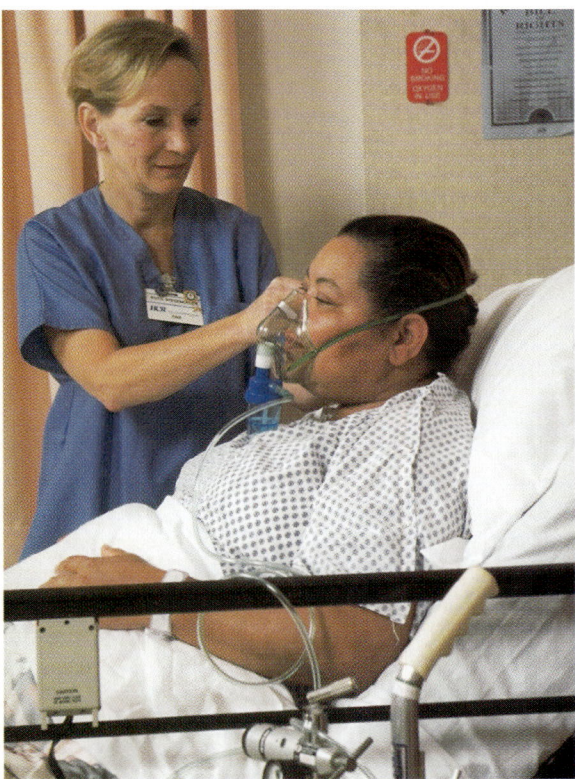

FIGURE 18–7
Patients with respiratory disease often require treatments that involve the use of oxygen

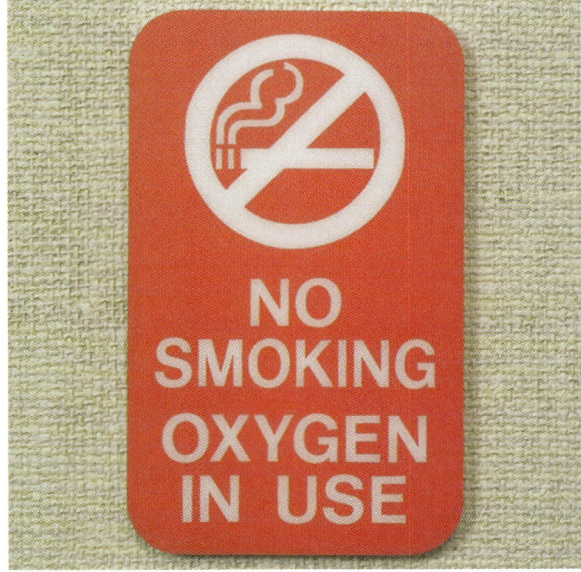

NO SMOKING OXYGEN IN USE

FIGURE 18–8
Visitors may need reminders not to smoke near a patient when oxygen is in use

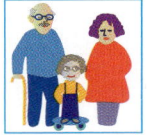

AGE-SPECIFIC CONSIDERATIONS

The use of nasal cannulas can cause irritation to the skin of the ears in the geriatric population. The nasal cannula is looped over the ears and tightened under the chin. This constant pressure of the tubing on the ears is the source of irritation and can be relieved by placing cotton or other soft material between the skin and the tubing.

Many patients, both young and old, feel claustrophobic wearing a face mask. It is often difficult to convince these patients to wear such a device and other alternatives to oxygen delivery must be considered. Another important consideration is the elderly patient with sensitive skin. If the mask is used for an extended period of time, skin break-down may be a problem. For this reason it is important to clean the area under the mask where there is skin and mask contact. Secondly, do not overtighten the mask straps. A secure fit to the face is desired, but not so tight as to impede circulation.

KEY IDEA

> The chronic obstructive pulmonary diseases (COPD) and tuberculosis (TB) are two of many conditions that require special instructions for care and safety. Be sure to check with the supervisor for what the doctor's current orders are.

Summary

The circulatory and respiratory systems affect the flow of blood and the exchange of oxygen between the blood and the cells of the body. The primary exchange takes place in the lungs in the alveoli. A secondary exchange is at the cellular level. The circulatory and respiratory systems work closely together. A condition that affects one system may affect the other. Patients with conditions affecting either or both systems will be limited in their activities of daily living.

Notes

THE NURSING ASSISTANT IN ACTION

Heart Patient Wants to Smoke

Miss Dupay is a patient who was admitted to your unit for medical tests to determine why her heart frequently races and skips beats. Her doctor, Dr. Cheryl Coates, has told Miss Dupay that her heart problems may be related to her habit of smoking a pack of cigarettes a day. Miss Dupay knows about the hospital's No Smoking policy. Even so, she smokes in her bathroom and frequently asks to leave the floor to go to some other place to smoke. She has not been given off-floor privileges. Today, she asks you to let her leave the floor in a wheelchair so she can go outside "for a breath of fresh air."

What is Your Response/Action?

1. What are the important pieces of information in this situation?

2. What are your options in this situation?

3. What are your concerns?

4. What are your ethical boundaries?

5. What, if anything, would you do on your own in this situation?

6. What, if anything, would you report to your supervisor?

7. What did you learn from this situation that you will apply in future situations?

Measuring Vital Signs

19

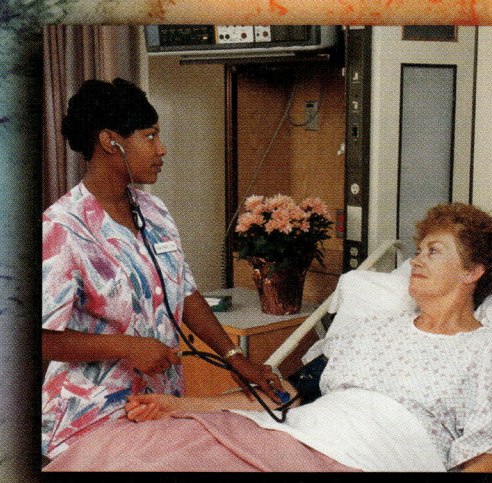

INTRODUCTION

By measuring or "taking" a person's vital signs, you are recording measurements that reflect the physical well-being of a person. Everyone has a normal vital sign range. The vital signs are often the first key indicators that something adverse (wrong or abnormal) is going on with the patient. Vital signs which are routinely measured on every patient include temperature, respirations, blood pressure, and pulse rate.

OBJECTIVES

When you have completed this chapter, you will be able to:

- List and describe the different types of thermometers.
- Read a Fahrenheit and centigrade (Celsius) thermometer accurately.
- Demonstrate the procedure for measuring oral temperatures.
- Demonstrate the procedure for measuring rectal temperatures.
- Demonstrate the procedure for measuring axillary temperatures.
- Demonstrate the proper use of a battery-operated electronic thermometer.
- Count the radial and apical pulse.
- Report the rate and rhythm of the pulse accurately.
- Count a patient's respirations accurately.
- Determine if the patient's breathing is labored or abnormal.
- Explain systolic pressure.
- Explain diastolic pressure.
- Demonstrate the use of aneroid and mercury types of blood pressure equipment accurately and efficiently.
- Measure a patient's blood pressure accurately.

KEY TERMS

abdominal respiration

aneroid sphygmomanometer

apical pulse

apnea

axillary

blood pressure

centigrade

Cheyne-Stokes respiration

diastolic blood pressure

dyspnea

exhaling

Fahrenheit

force

inhaling

irregular respiration

labored respiration

mercury sphygmomanometer

oral

pulse

pulse deficit

radial pulse

rate

rectal

rhythm

shallow respiration

sphygmomanometer

stertorous respiration

stethoscope

systolic blood pressure

thermometer

Fahrenheit A system for measuring temperature. In the Fahrenheit system, the temperature of water at boiling is 212°. At freezing, it is 32°. These temperatures are usually written 212°F and 32°F.

centigrade A system for measurement of temperature using a scale divided into 100 units or degrees; in this system, the freezing temperature of water is 0°C and water boils at 100°C; often referred to as Celsius

thermometer An instrument used for measuring temperature

oral Anything to do with the mouth; examples are eating and speaking

axillary The area under the arms; the armpits

rectal Pertaining to the rectum

BODY TEMPERATURE

Body temperature is a measurement of the amount of heat in the body. The body creates heat in the process of changing food into energy. The body can also lose heat through perspiration (sweating), respiration (breathing), and excretion. The balance between the heat produced and the heat lost is the body temperature. The normal adult body temperature is 98.6° **Fahrenheit (F)** or 37° **centigrade** or **Celsius (C)**. There is a normal range in which a person's body temperature may vary and still be considered normal.

◼ Types of Thermometers

The body temperature is measured with an instrument called a **thermometer**. There are several different types of thermometers.

- Glass
  - Oral
  - Rectal
  - Security
- Battery-operated electronic
- Chemically treated

The *glass thermometer* is a delicate, hollow glass tube with a liquid metal called mercury, an element that is very sensitive to temperature, sealed inside it. Mercury expands (gets larger) when the temperature goes up and contracts (gets smaller) when the temperature goes down. Even if the temperature rises only slightly, the mercury will expand and travel up the tube, reflecting the change. The outside of the glass thermometer is marked with lines, or calibrations, and numbers. These markings help us measure exactly the temperature readings displayed by the level of the mercury. There are three types of glass thermometers (Figure 19–1):

- **Oral** thermometers are used to measure the patient's temperature by mouth and also by the **axillary** method.

- **Rectal** thermometers are used to measure temperature by inserting the thermometer into the patient's rectum.

FIGURE 19–1

Types of glass thermometers

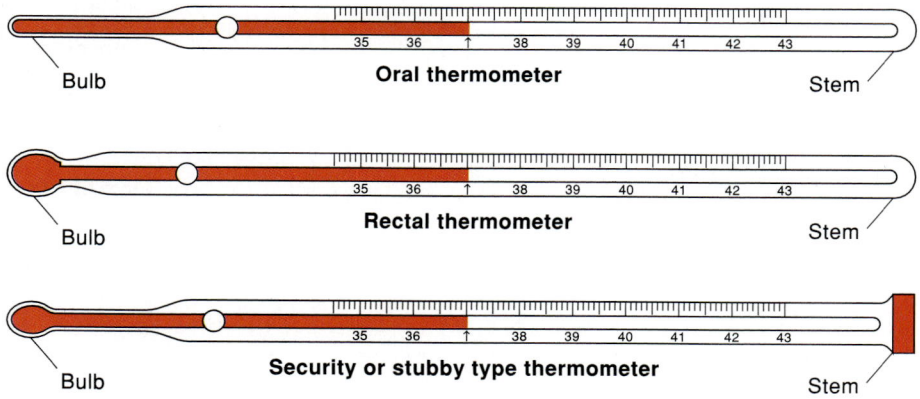

Bulb   **Oral thermometer**   Stem

Bulb   **Rectal thermometer**   Stem

Bulb   **Security or stubby type thermometer**   Stem

■ Security thermometers are used for taking an infant's rectal temperature. Many institutions use the security or stubby type with a red knob at the stem for rectal temperatures and those with a green or blue knob at the stem for oral temperatures. Follow your institution's policy.

Battery-operated electronic thermometers eliminate human error and variations that can occur in reading a glass thermometer. An electronic thermometer is used with a disposable sheath (plastic cover) over the probe. The sheath is discarded after each use. The ear (aural) thermometer is an electronic thermometer that measures the temperature by inserting the probe gently in the ear canal. This device is capable of converting and displaying the temperature as an oral or rectal temperature. Be sure to indicate whether your thermometer converts to an oral or rectal temperature. Figure 19–2 is an example of an electronic thermometer that measures the temperature of the tympanic membrane or eardrum.

The latest electronic thermometers instantly calculate the body temperature when a sheath-covered probe is inserted into the opening of the outer ear canal. This type of thermometer is available for industrial and home use.

Chemically treated paper or plastic thermometers are now used by some health care institutions. These change color to indicate the patient's temperature.

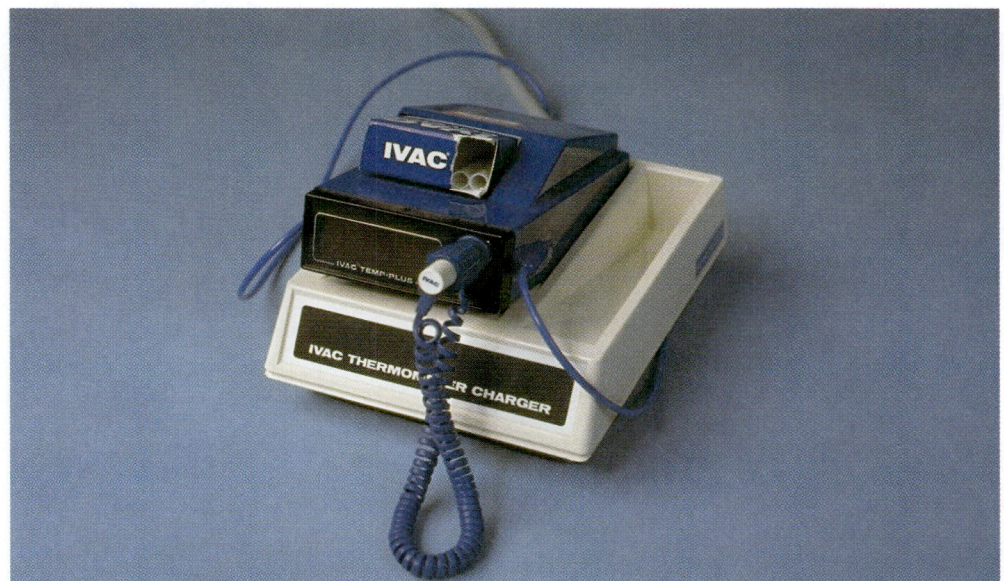

FIGURE 19–2

A type of electronic thermometer that measures the temperature by inserting the probe in the ear canal

GUIDELINES

OBRA

CARE OF GLASS THERMOMETERS

■ Because glass thermometers break and shatter easily, they must be handled with care. Be especially careful to avoid breaking a thermometer while it is in a patient's mouth or rectum.

■ The liquid metal, mercury, inside the thermometer is a poison; that is, it may be harmful if it is ingested (taken into the body by mouth) or if it has contact with the skin for a prolonged period of time.

■ Check the containers in which the thermometers are kept. Follow your instructions for cleaning these containers.

■ Never clean a glass thermometer with hot water as it will cause the mercury to expand so much that the thermometer will break.

PROCEDURE

OBRA

SHAKING DOWN THE GLASS THERMOMETER

PREPARATION

1. Assemble your equipment on the bedside table:

    Thermometer in container

2. Wash your hands.

3. Before using the thermometer, check to make sure that it is not cracked or that the bulb is not chipped. The bulb is the end that is inserted into the patient's body. Never touch the bulb end of the thermometer.

STEPS

4. Hold the thermometer firmly between your fingers and your thumb at the stem, farthest from the bulb.

5. Stand clear of any hard surfaces such as counters and tables to avoid striking and breaking the thermometer while you are shaking it. For practice, you might stand with your arm over a pillow or mattress in case you accidentally drop the thermometer.

6. When you are sure that you have a good hold on the thermometer, shake your hand loosely at the wrist. Do it as if you were shaking water from your fingers (Figure 19–3).

    Note: Shake the mercury down to the lowest point below the numbers and lines.

7. Snap your wrist again and again. This will shake down the mercury to the lowest possible point, below the numbers and lines (calibrations).

FOLLOW-UP

8. Always shake down the mercury before and after using a glass thermometer.

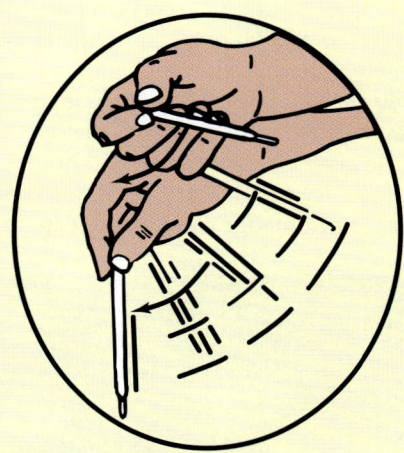

FIGURE 19–3
Shake down a glass thermometer by holding the thermometer stem firmly between your thumb and index finger as you snap your wrist

PROCEDURE

OBRA

READING A FAHRENHEIT THERMOMETER

STEPS

1. With your thumb and first two fingers, hold the thermometer at the stem. Never touch the bulb end.

2. Hold the thermometer at eye level. Turn the thermometer back and forth between your fingers until you can clearly see the column of mercury.

3. Notice the scale or calibrations. Each long line stands for 1 degree.

4. There are 4 short lines between each of the long lines. Each short line stands for two-tenths (or 0.2) of a degree.

5. Between the long lines that represent 98° and 99°, look for a longer line with an arrow directly beneath it. This special line points out normal body temperature (98.6°F).

6. Look at the end of the mercury. Notice the first line or number where the mercury ends (Figure 19–4). If it is one of the short lines, notice the previous longer line toward the silver tip that goes into the patient's mouth. The temperature reading is the degree marked by that long line plus 2, 4, 6, or 8 tenths of a degree. For example, if the mercury ends after the 99 line, but on the second short line, the temperature is 99.4°F. If the mercury ends between the two lines, take the line it is closer to.

    Note: Accuracy is extremely important. Look at the mercury carefully when reading a thermometer.

7. Write down the patient's temperature right away. If you are using a vital sign book, check to find the right column next to the patient's name and the right

P R O C E D U R E (CONTINUED)

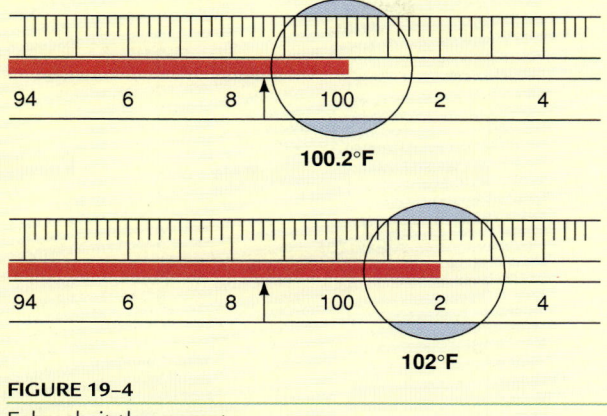

100.2°F

102°F

FIGURE 19–4
Fahrenheit thermometer

time of day. Write the patient's temperature using the figure you read on the thermometer. Some institutions will write 99.4°F. Others will write 99⁴. Follow the method used in your institution.

P R O C E D U R E

OBRA

READING A CENTIGRADE (CELSIUS) THERMOMETER

STEPS

1. With your thumb and first two fingers, hold the thermometer at the stem.

2. Hold the thermometer at eye level. Turn the thermometer back and forth between your fingers until you can clearly see the column of mercury.

3. Notice the scale or calibrations. Each long line shows 1 degree.

4. There are 9 short lines between each number. These short lines are 1, 2, 3, 4, 5, 6, 7, 8, and 9 tenths of a degree. If the mercury ended after the 36 and on the third short line, the temperature

would read 36.3°C (Figure 19–5). If the mercury ended after the long line 37 and on the eighth short line, the temperature would read 37.8°C. If the mercury ends after line 37 on the fifth short line, the temperature would be referred to as 37.5°C.

Note: Accuracy is extremely important. Look at the mercury carefully when reading a thermometer.

5. Write down the patient's temperature right away. If you are using a vital sign book, check to find the right column next to the patient's name and the right time of day. Write the patient's temperature using the figure you read on the thermometer. Some hospitals write 37°C. Others will write 37. Follow the method used in your hospital.

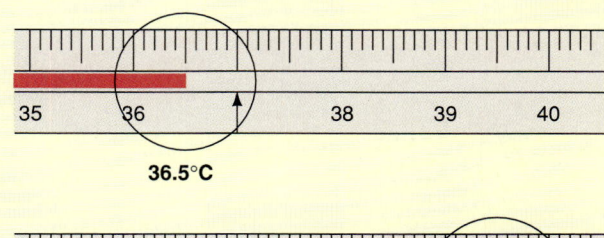

36.5°C

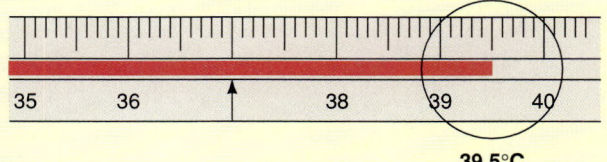

39.5°C

FIGURE 19–5
Centigrade thermometer

▪ Recording the Patient's Temperature

For recording the patient's temperature, three symbols are used:

° = degrees   F = Fahrenheit   C = Centigrade or Celsius

You will record the patient's temperatures according to the method used in your institution (Figures 19–6 and 19–7).

FIGURE 19–6

The two major scales used in the United States for measuring temperature

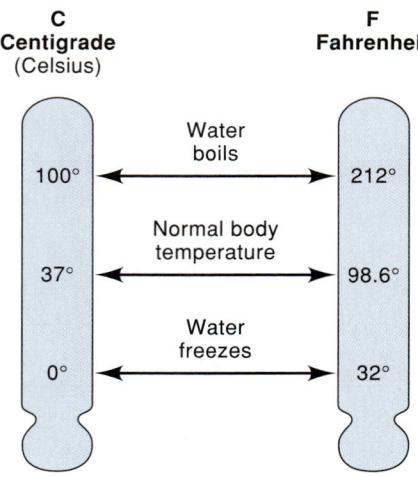

FIGURE 19–7

Temperature conversion

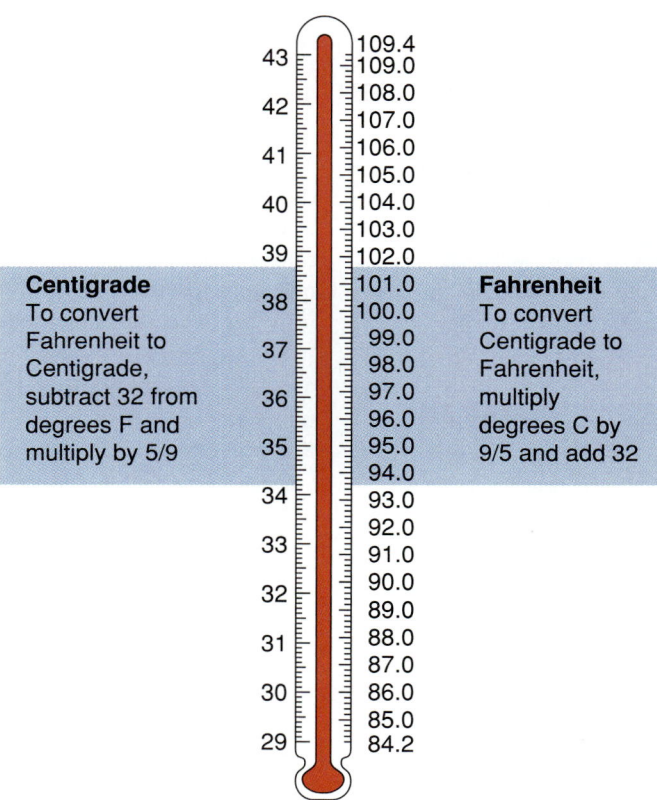

Fahrenheit temperature can be written in two ways:

$$98.6°F \quad \text{or} \quad 98\underline{^6} \, F$$

If you are using a centigrade (Celsius) thermometer, the temperature would be written

$$37°C \quad \text{or} \quad 37.3°C \quad \text{or} \quad 37\underline{^3}°C$$

Write an R in front of the temperature reading if a rectal temperature was taken. Write an A if an axillary temperature was taken. Write an O if an oral temperature was taken. See Table 19–1 for normal temperature readings.

TABLE 19–1

Normal Temperature Readings

METHOD	CENTIGRADE	FAHRENHEIT
Oral	37.0	98.6
Axillary	36.4	97.6
Rectal	37.5	99.6

PROCEDURE

OBRA

MEASURING AN ORAL TEMPERATURE

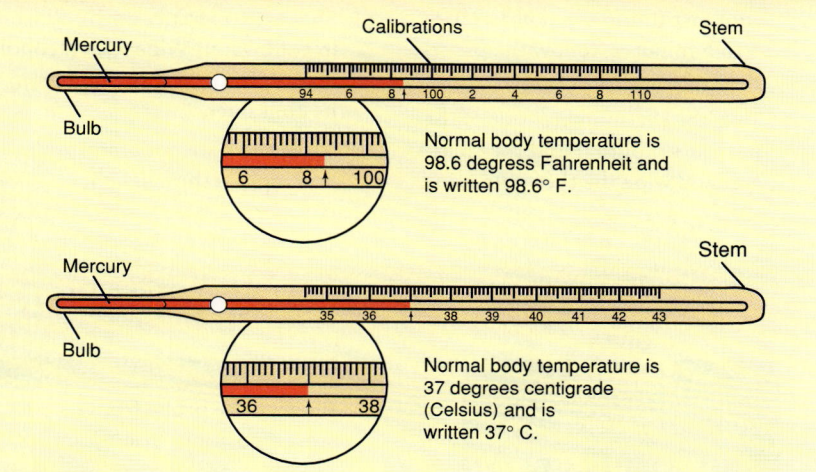

Normal body temperature is 98.6 degress Fahrenheit and is written 98.6° F.

Normal body temperature is 37 degrees centigrade (Celsius) and is written 37° C.

FIGURE 19–8
Normal body temperatures

PREPARATION

1. Assemble your equipment:

   a. Oral thermometer (Figure 19–8)

   b. Tissue or paper towel

   c. Vital sign form used in your institution

   d. Pen or pencil

2. Identify the patient by checking the identification bracelet.

3. Wash your hands.

4. Tell the patient you are going to take his temperature.

5. Ask the patient if he has recently had hot or cold fluids or been smoking. If the answer is yes, wait 10 minutes before taking an oral temperature.

6. Provide privacy for the patient.

7. The patient should be in bed or sitting in a chair.

8. Take the thermometer out of its container. Dry with a paper towel.

9. Shake the mercury down.

STEPS

10. Gently put the bulb end in the patient's mouth under the tongue (Figure 19–9).

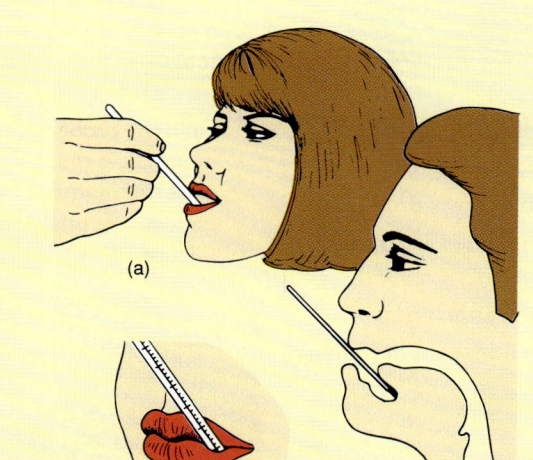

FIGURE 19–9
Gently place bulb end into patient's mouth under the tongue

a. Insert the thermometer gently into the patient's mouth under the tongue.

b. Position the thermometer to the side of the mouth.

c. Instruct the patient to keep the thermometer under the tongue by gently closing the lips around the thermometer. Ask him to keep his mouth

PROCEDURE (CONTINUED)

and lips closed around the thermometer.

11. Leave the thermometer in the patient's mouth for 8 minutes. (*Note:* The latest research states that oral temperature is more accurate when the oral thermometer remains in the mouth for 8 minutes. However, if in your institution the policy is for 3 to 5 minutes, follow the procedure of your institution.)

12. Take the thermometer out of the patient's mouth. Hold the stem end and wipe the thermometer with a tissue. Wipe the stem of the thermometer toward the bulb end.

13. Read the thermometer.

14. Record the temperature according to your institution's policy.

FOLLOW-UP

15. Shake the mercury down. Rinse in cold water. Wipe with alcohol and replace the thermometer in its container.

16. Make the patient comfortable and replace the call light.

17. Lower the bed to a position of safety.

18. Raise the side rails when ordered or appropriate for patient safety.

19. Wash your hands.

20. Report to your immediate supervisor:
    - If the oral temperature was above 100°F or 37.5°C or below 97°F.
    - Your observations of anything unusual.

PROCEDURE

OBRA

USING A BATTERY-OPERATED ELECTRONIC ORAL THERMOMETER

PREPARATION

1. Assemble your equipment:
   a. Disposable plastic probe cover
   b. Battery-operated electronic thermometer
   c. Oral (blue) attachment
   d. Vital sign form used in your institution
   e. Pen or pencil

2. Identify the patient by checking the identification bracelet.

3. Tell the patient you are going to take her temperature.

4. Wash your hands.

5. Provide privacy for the patient.

6. Check to be sure that the oral (blue top) probe connector is properly placed in its receptacle on the base of the unit.

STEPS

7. Remove the probe from its stored position. Insert it into a sheath or probe cover.

8. Insert the covered probe into the patient's mouth slowly until the metal tip is at the base under the tongue to the back of the patient's mouth.

9. Hold the probe in the patient's mouth. It is much heavier than a glass thermometer and some patients are unable to hold it. (Figure 19–10).

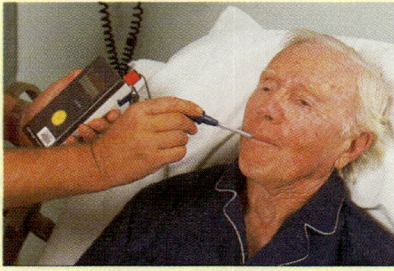

FIGURE 19–10
Hold the probe in the patient's mouth

10. Wait about 15 seconds for the buzzer to ring for a computed temperature reading, then remove the probe from the patient's mouth.

11. Record the temperature on the vital sign form used in your institution. This is very important because when you return the probe to its stored position the reading automatically returns to zero.

12. Without touching it, discard the used probe cover (sheath) immediately into a waste receptacle.

FOLLOW-UP

13. Return the probe to its stored position in the face of the thermometer.

14. Store the thermometer in its charging stand whenever it is not in use.

15. Make the patient comfortable and replace the call light.

16. Lower the bed to a position of safety.

17. Raise the side rails when ordered or appropriate for patient safety.

18. Wash your hands.

19. Report to your immediate supervisor:
    - If the oral temperature was over 100°F; 37.5°C.
    - Your observations of anything unusual.

PROCEDURE

USING A BATTERY-OPERATED ELECTRONIC TYMPANIC OR AURAL (EAR) THERMOMETER

PREPARATION

1. Assemble your equipment:

   a. Disposable plastic probe cover

   b. Battery-operated electronic thermometer

   c. Vital sign form used in your institution

   d. Pen or pencil

2. Identify the patient by checking the identification bracelet.

3. Tell the patient you are going to take her temperature.

4. Wash your hands.

5. Provide privacy for the patient.

STEPS

6. Make sure the probe is connected to the unit.

7. Remove the probe from its stored position. Insert the cone-shaped end of the thermometer into a probe cover or attach a disposable probe.

8. Position the patient's head so one ear is directly in front of you.

9. For an adult or child, pull the outer ear up and back to open the ear canal. For an infant, pull the ear straight back.

10. Gently insert the covered probe into the patient's ear; slowly use a slight rocking motion if needed to insert the probe as far as possible and seal the ear canal. (Figure 19–11).

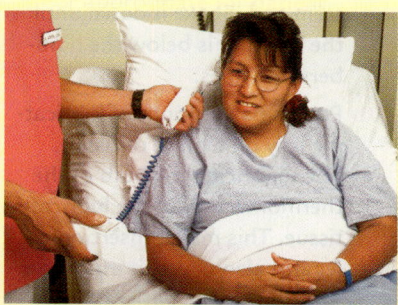

FIGURE 19–11
Gently insert covered probe into patient's ear

11. Watch and wait for about 10–15 seconds for a flashing light or buzzer to ring indicating a computed temperature reading, then remove the probe from the patient's ear.

12. Read and record the digitally displayed temperature on the vital sign form used in your institution. This is very important because when you return the probe to its stored position the reading automatically returns to zero. Some units have built in convertors so the temperature may be displayed as an equivalent oral or rectal value in centigrade or Fahrenheit.

13. Without touching it, eject and discard the used probe cover (sheath) immediately into a waste receptacle.

FOLLOW-UP

14. Return the probe to its stored position in the face of the thermometer.

15. Store the thermometer in its charging stand whenever it is not in use.

16. Make the patient comfortable and replace the call light.

17. Lower the bed to a position of safety.

18. Raise the side rails when ordered or appropriate for patient safety.

19. Wash your hands.

20. Report to your immediate supervisor:

    ■ If the tympanic temperature was over 100°F; 37.5°C.

    ■ Your observations of anything unusual.

■ Measuring Rectal Temperature

Remember that you will always use a rectal thermometer for taking rectal temperatures. Notice that the glass rectal thermometer has a small round bulb on one end. This bulb prevents the thermometer from injuring the sensitive lining of the patient's rectum. Under the following conditions you might take a rectal temperature. Ask your supervisor for verification.

■ When the patient is an infant or child; follow the policies of your health care institution for pediatric patients

■ When the patient is having warm or cold applications on the face or neck

■ When the patient cannot keep her mouth closed around the thermometer

■ When the patient finds it hard to breathe through the nose

■ When the patient has sneezing or coughing spells

PROCEDURE (CONTINUED)

FOLLOW-UP

11. Make the patient comfortable and replace the call light.

12. Lower the bed to a position of safety.

13. Raise the side rails when ordered or appropriate for patient safety.

14. Wash your hands.

15. Report to your immediate supervisor:

   ■ If the pulse rate was under 60 or over 100 for an adult. If the pulse was irregular, circle in red the number on the vital

sign form used by your institution. Sometimes "irr." is written near the number.

■ Your observations of anything unusual.

■ The Apical Pulse and Pulse Deficit

The pulse rate should be the same as the heart rate. However, in some patients the heartbeats are not strong enough to be transmitted along the arteries to be felt with a radial pulse. This may be due to some forms of heart disease. For these patients, an apical pulse would be taken. An **apical pulse** is a measurement of the heartbeats at the apex of the heart, located just under the left breast (Figure 19–19).

Sometimes the patient has a **pulse deficit**, a difference between the apical heartbeat and the radial pulse rate. To determine this, the apical pulse (heart rate) is counted with a stethoscope over the apex of the heart. At the same time, the pulse rate is counted at the radial pulse. The two figures are compared. The difference between the apical heartbeat and the radial pulse beat is the pulse deficit. This is called the *apical pulse deficit*. For maximum accuracy, both pulses should be taken at the same time by two nursing assistants. A different method can be used with one nursing assistant who takes the apical pulse first and then takes the radial pulse. This second method is not considered as accurate as the first method.

apical pulse A measurement of the heartbeats at the apex of the heart, located just under the left breast

pulse deficit A difference between the apical heartbeat and the radial pulse rate

FIGURE 19–19
Measuring the apical pulse

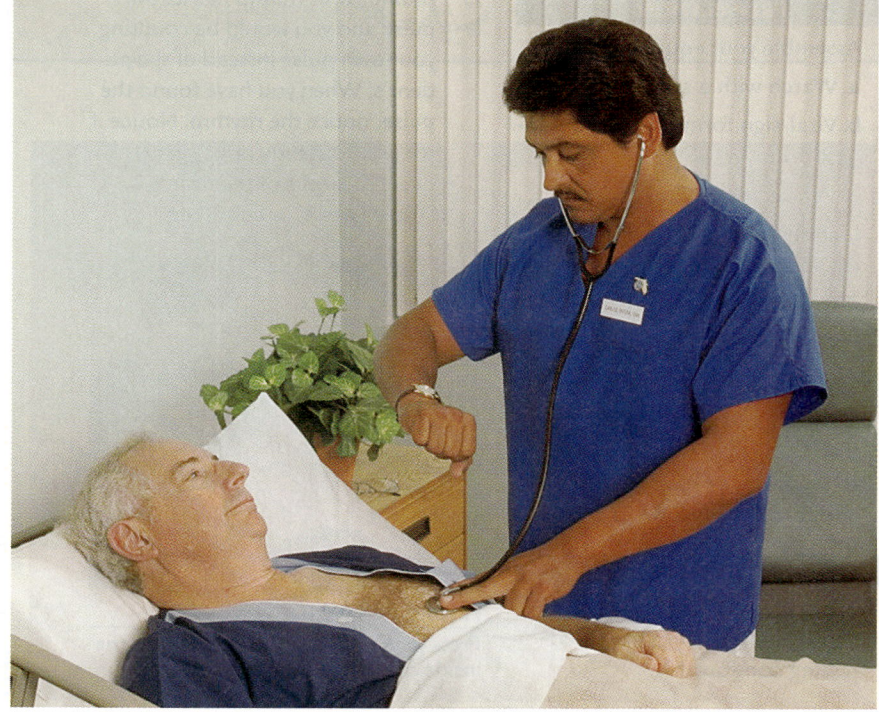

PROCEDURE

OBRA

MEASURING THE APICAL PULSE

PREPARATION

1. Assemble your equipment:
   a. Stethoscope and antiseptic swabs
   b. Watch with a second hand
   c. Vital sign form used in your institution (*Note:* In many institutions, this reading is reported directly to your immediate supervisor rather than writing it on the form used)
   d. Pen or pencil and note paper
2. Identify the patient by checking the identification bracelet.
3. Explain to the patient that you are going to take her apical pulse.
4. Wash your hands.
5. Provide privacy for the patient.
6. Clean the earplugs on the stethoscope with antiseptic swabs. Put the earplugs in your ears. Warm the bell or diaphragm of the stethoscope by holding it tightly for a few seconds.

STEPS

7. Uncover the left side of the patient's chest. Avoid overexposing the patient.
8. Locate the apex of the patient's heart by placing the bell or diaphragm of the stethoscope under the patient's left breast. Listen for the heart sounds.
9. Count the heart sounds for a full minute.
10. Write the full minute count on the note paper.

FOLLOW-UP

11. Cover and make the patient comfortable.
12. Replace the call light.
13. Lower the bed to a position of safety.
14. Raise the side rails when ordered or appropriate for patient safety.
15. Clean the earplugs of the stethoscope with antiseptic swabs. Return the equipment to its proper place.
16. Wash your hands.
17. Report to your immediate supervisor:
    - That you have taken the patient's apical pulse.
    - What the apical pulse rate was.
    - Your observations of anything unusual.

PROCEDURE

MEASURING THE APICAL PULSE DEFICIT

PREPARATION

1. Assemble your equipment:
   a. Stethoscope and antiseptic swabs
   b. Watch with a second hand
   c. Vital sign form used in your institution (*Note:* In many situations, this reading is reported directly to your immediate supervisor rather than writing it on the form used)
   d. Note paper, pen, or pencil
2. Identify the patient by checking the identification bracelet.
3. Explain to the patient that you are going to take his pulse.
4. Wash your hands.
5. Provide privacy for the patient.

STEPS

6. There are two methods of taking the apical pulse deficit.
   - *Method A:* Two nursing assistants do this procedure together at the same time. One counts the radial pulse and the other counts the apical pulse for one full minute each. The difference between the two pulses is known as the apical pulse deficit. This method is used for maximum accuracy.
   - *Method B:* The nursing assistant first takes the apical pulse, and then the radial pulse. The difference between the two pulses is known as the apical pulse deficit. However, since the readings are not taken at the same time, it is not considered as accurate as the first method.
7. Count the apical pulse and the radial pulse for one full minute and record both figures.

PROCEDURE (CONTINUED)

8. Record the difference between the figures as the pulse deficit.

FOLLOW-UP

9. Make the patient comfortable and replace the call light.

10. Lower the bed to a position of safety.

11. Raise the side rails when ordered or appropriate for patient safety.

12. Clean the equipment and return it to its proper place.

13. Wash your hands.

14. Report to your immediate supervisor:

- That you have taken the patient's apical pulse deficit.
- The apical pulse rate.
- The radial pulse rate.
- The pulse deficit.
- Your observations of anything unusual.

RESPIRATIONS

inhaling The process of breathing in air in respiration

exhaling The process of breathing out air in respiration

labored respiration Working hard to breathe

stertorous respiration The patient makes abnormal noises like snoring sounds when breathing

abdominal respiration Breathing in which the patient is using mostly the abdominal muscles

The human body must have a steady supply of air. The body needs oxygen from the air in order to change food into heat and energy. When you breathe in, air is drawn into the lungs. In the lungs, oxygen is taken out of the air and absorbed into the blood stream. The blood then carries the oxygen to the body cells. In the body cells, the oxygen is used to produce energy for the body (oxidation).

Respiration is the process of **inhaling** (breathing in) and **exhaling** (breathing out). One respiration includes breathing in and breathing out once. When a person breathes in, the chest gets larger (expands). When a person breathes out, the chest gets smaller (contracts). When you count respirations, the patient should be lying on his back. You watch the chest rise and fall as the patient breathes, or you feel the chest rise and fall with your hand. Either way, you should count respirations without the patient knowing it (Figure 19–20). If the patient thinks that breathing is being counted, he will not breathe naturally. You want to count natural breathing. Besides counting respirations, you will be noticing whether the patient seems to breathe easily or seems to be working hard to get his breath. When a person is working hard to get breath, it is called **labored respiration**. You must also notice whether the breathing is noisy.

FIGURE 19–20
The patient must be unaware that you are counting respirations

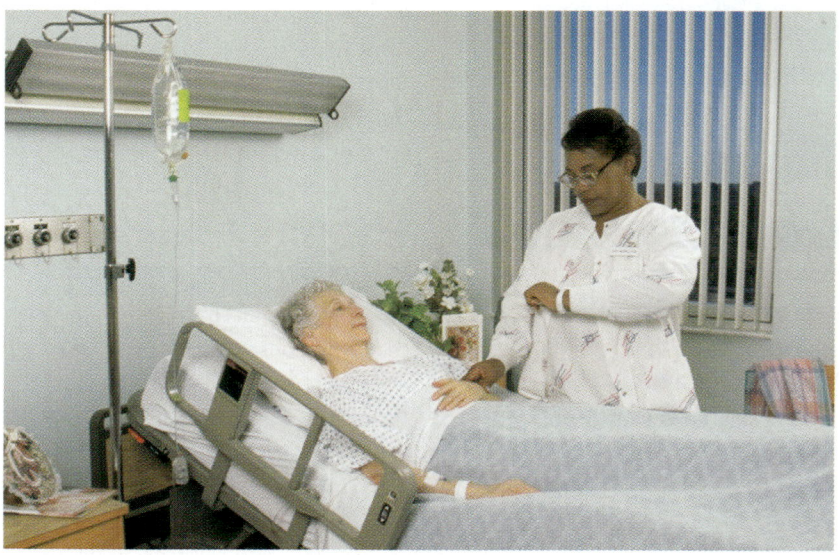

Normally, adults breathe at a rate of from 16 to 20 times a minute. Children breathe more rapidly. The elderly breathe more slowly. Exercise, digestion, emotional stress, disease conditions, some drugs, stimulants, heat, and cold can all affect the number of times per minute that a person breathes.

■ Abnormal Respiration

While you are counting the patient's respirations, it is important to observe and make note of anything about his breathing that appears to be abnormal. Different types of abnormal respiration that you should be familiar with are:

1. **Stertorous respiration:** The patient makes abnormal noises like snoring or snorting sounds when breathing.

2. **Abdominal respiration:** The patient is using mostly the abdominal muscles to breathe.

3. **Shallow respiration:** Breathing with only the upper part of the lungs.

4. **Irregular respiration:** The depth of breathing changes and the rate of the rise and fall of the chest is not steady or regular.

5. **Cheyne-Stokes respiration:** One kind of irregular breathing. At first the breathing is slow and shallow; then the respiration becomes faster and deeper until it reaches a peak. The respiration then slows down and becomes shallow again. The breathing may then stop completely for 10 seconds and then begin the pattern again. This type of respiration may be caused by certain cerebral (brain), cardiac (heart), or pulmonary (chest) diseases or conditions.

6. **Dyspnea:** Insufficient oxygenation of the blood resulting in labored or difficult breathing.

7. **Apnea:** Periods of not breathing.

shallow respiration Breathing with only the upper part of the lungs

irregular respiration The depth of breathing changes and the rate of the rise and fall of the chest is not steady

Cheyne-Stokes respiration One kind of irregular breathing. At first the breathing is slow and shallow; then the respiration becomes faster and deeper until it reaches a peak. The respiration then slows down and becomes shallow again. The breathing may then stop completely for 10 seconds and then begin the pattern again; this type of respiration may be caused by certain cerebral (brain), cardiac (heart), or pulmonary (lung) diseases or conditions

dyspnea Insufficient oxygenation of the blood resulting in labored or difficult breathing

apnea Periods of not breathing

PROCEDURE

OBRA

MEASURING RESPIRATION

PREPARATION

1. Assemble your equipment:
   a. Watch with a second hand
   b. Vital sign form used in your institution
   c. Pen or pencil
2. Identify the patient by checking the identification bracelet.

3. Wash your hands.
4. Provide privacy for the patient.

STEPS

5. Hold the patient's wrist just as if you were taking his pulse. This way he will not know you are watching his breathing. Count the patient's respirations, without him knowing it, immediately after counting his pulse rate.

6. If the patient is a child who has been crying or is restless, wait until he is quiet before counting respirations. If a child is asleep, count his respirations before he wakes up. Always count a child's pulse and respirations before

you measure his temperature. (Most children get upset when you measure their temperature which would abnormally elevate their pulse and respirations.)

7. One rise and one fall of the patient's chest counts as one respiration.

8. If you cannot clearly see the chest rise and fall, fold the patient's arms across his chest. You can feel his breathing as you hold his wrist.

9. Check the position of the second hand on the watch. Count "one" when you see the patient's chest rising as he breathes in. The next time his chest rises, count "two."

PROCEDURE (CONTINUED)

Keep doing this for a full minute. Report the number of respirations you count within that minute.

10. You may be permitted to count for 30 seconds. Count the respirations for one-half minute and then multiply the number you counted by 2. For example, if you count 8 respirations in 30 seconds (a half-minute), your number for a full minute is 16.

11. If the patient's breathing rhythm is irregular, always count for a full minute. Observe the depth of the breathing while counting the respirations.

12. Write down the number you counted immediately on the vital sign form used by your institution. Be sure you write it in the proper column, opposite the correct patient's name.

13. Note whether the respirations were noisy or labored.

FOLLOW-UP

14. Make the patient comfortable and replace the call light.

15. Lower the bed to a position of safety.

16. Raise the side rails when ordered or appropriate for patient safety.

17. Wash your hands.

18. Report to your immediate supervisor:
   - Whether the respirations were noisy or labored.
   - Whether the respirations were irregular.
   - The time they were measured.
   - If the respirations were less than 14 or more than 28 a minute.
   - Your observations of anything unusual.

BLOOD PRESSURE

blood pressure The force of the blood exerted on the inner walls of the arteries, veins, and chambers of the heart as blood flows or circulates through the structures

Blood pressure is the force of the blood pushing against the walls of the blood vessels. When you take a patient's blood pressure, you are measuring this force of the blood flowing through the arteries.

There is always a certain amount of pressure in the arteries. This is because the heart, by pumping blood, is constantly forcing it to circulate through the body. The blood goes first into the arteries. It then circulates throughout the whole body. The amount of pressure in the arteries depends on two things:

1. The rate of heartbeat

2. How easily the blood flows through the blood vessels

systolic blood pressure The force with which blood is pumped when the heart muscle is contracting; when taking a patient's blood pressure, the systolic blood pressure is recorded as the top number

The heart contracts as it pumps the blood into the arteries. When the heart is contracting, the pressure is highest. This pressure is called the **systolic pressure**. As the heart relaxes between each contraction, the pressure goes down. When the heart is most relaxed, the pressure is lowest. This pressure is called the **diastolic pressure**. When you take a patient's blood pressure, you are measuring both.

In young, healthy adults, the normal blood pressure range is between 100 and 140 millimeters (mm) mercury (Hg) for systolic pressure. Normal diastolic pressure is between 60 and 90 millimeters (mm) mercury (Hg). The way these figures are written is:

diastolic blood pressure In taking a patient's blood pressure, one records the bottom number as the reading for the diastolic pressure; this is the relaxing phase of the heartbeat

$$120/80 \text{ or } \frac{120 = \text{Systolic}}{80 = \text{Diastolic}}$$

When a patient's blood pressure is higher than the normal range for her age and condition, it is referred to as high blood pressure or hypertension. When a patient's blood pressure is lower than the normal range for her age or condition, it is referred to as low blood pressure or hypotension.

■ Instruments for Measuring Blood Pressure

When you take a patient's blood pressure, you will be using an instrument called a **sphygmomanometer**, which is a combination of three Greek words:

- sphygmo, meaning pulse

- mano, meaning pressure

- meter, meaning measure

This instrument, however, is usually referred to as the blood pressure cuff. The four main parts of this instrument are the manometer, valve, cuff, and bulb.

Two kinds of instruments are used for taking blood pressure. One is the **mercury** type. The other is the **aneroid (dial)** type. Both kinds have an inflatable, cloth-covered rubber bag or cuff that is wrapped around the patient's arm. Both kinds also have a rubber bulb for pumping air into the cuff. The procedure for measuring blood pressure is the same, except for measuring the reading. When you use the mercury type, you will be watching the level of a column of mercury on a measuring scale (Figure 19–21). When you use the dial (aneroid) type, you will be watching a pointer on a dial (Figure 19–22).

When you measure a patient's blood pressure, you will be doing two things at the same time. You will listen to the brachial pulse as it sounds in the brachial artery in the patient's arm. You also will watch an indicator (either a column of mercury or a dial) in order to take a reading.

You will use a stethoscope (Figure 19–23) to listen to the brachial pulse. The **stethoscope** is an instrument that makes it possible to listen to various sounds in the patient's body, such as the heartbeat or breathing sounds in the chest. The stethoscope is a tube with one end that picks up sound when it is placed against a part of the body. This end is either bell shaped (called a bell) or it is round and flat (called a diaphragm). The other end of the tube splits into two parts. These parts have tips on the ends and fit into the listener's ears.

In many institutions, the blood pressure equipment hangs on the wall over the bed. A smaller-sized cuff must be used for children and a larger-sized for obese (overweight)

sphygmomanometer An apparatus for measuring blood pressure

mercury sphygmomanometer Blood pressure equipment containing a column of mercury

aneroid sphygmomanometer Dial-type blood pressure equipment

stethoscope An instrument that allows one to listen to various sounds in the patient's body, such as the heartbeat or breathing sounds

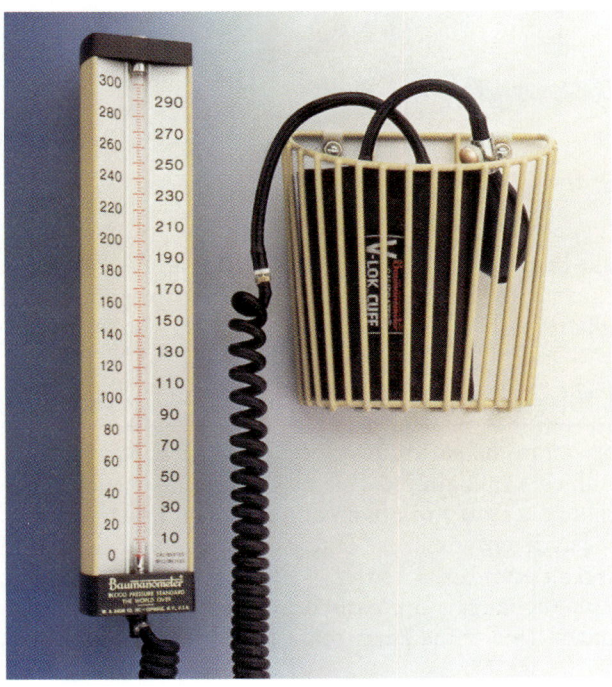

FIGURE 19–21
Mercury sphygmomanometer (Photo courtesy of W. A. Baum Co., Inc.)

FIGURE 19–22

Aneroid
sphygmomanometer

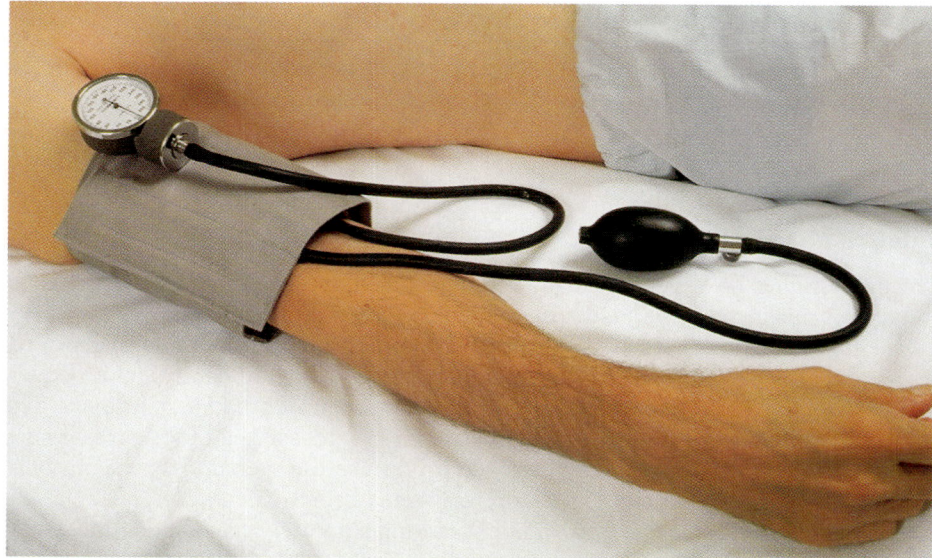

FIGURE 19–23

Stethoscope

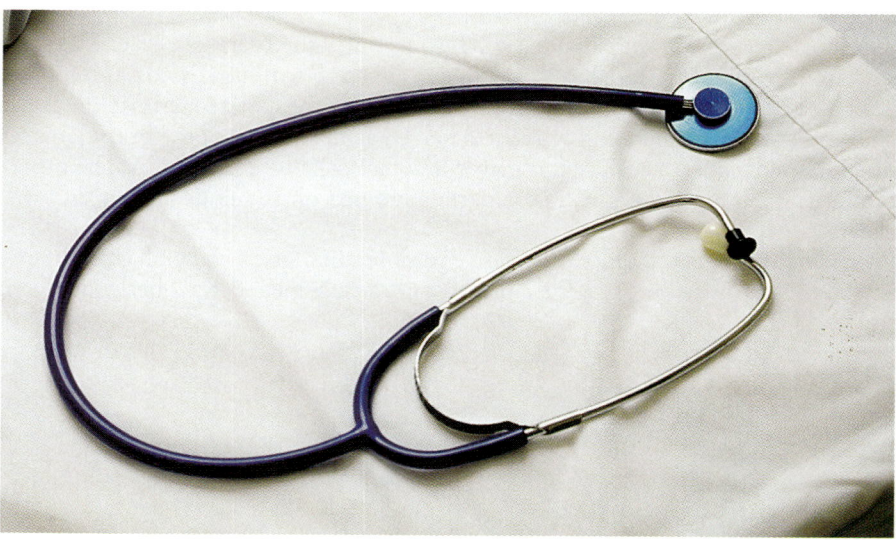

patients. Do not take blood pressure on an arm that has an IV (intravenous) setup in it, or surgical site on it (example: post-mastectomy), or from a patient with an A.V. shunt (catheter used for dialysis).

◼ Electronic Blood Pressure Monitoring Apparatus

The latest development in the electronic blood pressure apparatus is an infrared photoelectric system in which a miniature cuff is placed around the left index finger, inflating to the correct pressure necessary to obtain a proper reading and then deflating once the measurement has been determined. Use of this type of equipment eliminates the use of a stethoscope and human error.

With an automatic digital blood pressure monitor a cuff is placed around the wrist. The arm must be at the level of the heart, and no stethoscope is needed.

GUIDELINES

NONINVASIVE BLOOD PRESSURE MONITORING (NIBP)

- Patient selection: No exclusion based on age—with appropriately sized cuffs and hoses, NIBP monitors can be used on patients of all ages.

- Do **not** use NIBP in patients with the following:
  - Highly irregular or rapid cardiac rhythms.
  - Excessive bodily movement or excessive external movement.
  - Extreme hypotension or hypertension.

- Do not place an NIBP cuff on the following:
  - The same extremity with an IV infusion line.
  - The same extremity where SpO_2 is being monitored.
  - An extremity with impaired circulation.

- NIBP monitors have performance limits; in rare circumstances, they cannot determine extremes in blood pressure.

- Inflation of the cuff will impede IV flow.

- Identified patients for whom NIBP monitoring is not acceptable should be communicated to all caregivers. These include those with atrial dysrhythmias and tremors.

- Application of device and initial monitoring:
  - Upper arm is preferred site for cuff placement.
  - Forearm and ankle can also be used.

- Select proper cuff size. Cuff width should equal 40% of arm circumference. Too loose or too small a cuff will lead to falsely high readings. Too large a cuff can lead to falsely low readings.

- Obtain at least one BP reading through auscultation to use as baseline reading.

PROCEDURE

OBRA

MEASURING BLOOD PRESSURE USING A SPHYGMOMANOMETER

PREPARATION

1. Assemble your equipment:
   a. Sphygmomanometer (blood pressure cuff)
   b. Stethoscope
   c. Antiseptic swabs
   d. Vital sign form used in your institution
   e. Pen or pencil

2. Identify the patient by checking the identification bracelet.

3. Tell the patient that you are going to measure his blood pressure.

4. Wash your hands.

5. Provide privacy for the patient.

6. Wipe the earplugs of the stethoscope with antiseptic swabs.

STEPS

7. Have the patient resting quietly. He should be either lying down or sitting in a chair.

8. If you are using the mercury apparatus, the measuring scale should be level with your eyes.

9. The patient's arm should be bare up to the shoulder, or the patient's sleeve should be well above the elbow without limiting or constricting circulation.

10. The patient's arm from the elbow down should be resting fully extended on the bed. Or it might be resting on the arm of the chair or your hip, well supported, with the palm upward.

11. Unroll the blood pressure cuff and loosen the valve on the bulb. Squeeze the compression bag to deflate it completely.

12. Snugly and smoothly, wrap the cuff around the patient's arm 1/2" to 1" above the elbow. Do not wrap it so tightly that the patient is uncomfortable from the pressure. You may need to use a different-size cuff for a

P R O C E D U R E (CONTINUED)

patient with very thin arms (a child, for example) or very large arms. (Figure 19–24).

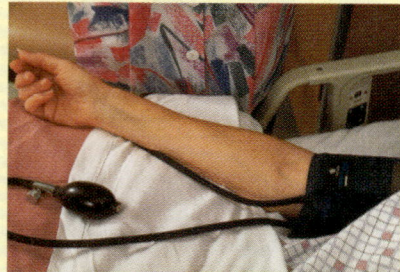

FIGURE 19–24

Placement of blood pressure cuff

13. Leave the area clear where you will place the bell or diaphragm of the stethoscope.

14. Be sure the manometer is in position so you can read the numbers easily.

15. Put the earplugs of the stethoscope into your ears.

16. With your fingertips, find the patient's brachial pulse at the inner aspect of the arm above the elbow (brachial artery) (Figure 19–25). This is where you will place the diaphragm or bell of the stethoscope. The diaphragm should be held firmly against the patient's skin, but it should not touch the cuff of the apparatus (Figure 19–26).

17. Tighten the thumbscrew of the valve to close it by turning it clockwise. Be careful not to turn it too tightly. If you do, you will have trouble opening it.

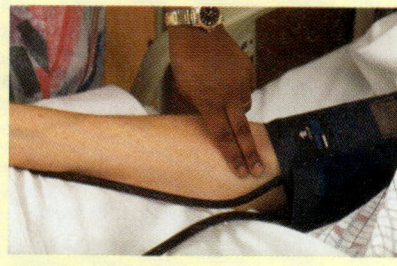

FIGURE 19–25

Checking for the brachial pulse

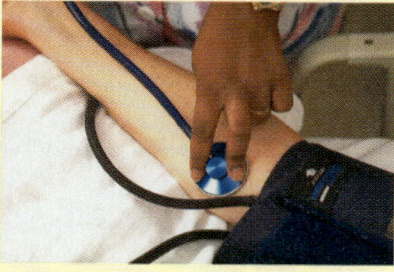

FIGURE 19–26

Place diaphragm over the brachial artery

18. Hold the stethoscope in place. Inflate the cuff quickly. When the radial pulse is no longer felt, inflate the cuff an additional 30 mm Hg. (Inflating the cuff to an unnecessarily high pressure is painful to the patient.)

19. Open the valve counterclockwise. This allows the air to escape. Let it out slowly until the sound of the pulse comes back. A few seconds must go by with-

out sounds. If you do hear pulse sounds immediately, you must stop the procedure and completely deflate the cuff. (Repeat number 18, this time inflating the cuff slightly higher.) Again, slowly loosen the thumbscrew to let the air out. Listen for a repeated pulse sound. At the same time, watch the indicator.

20. Note the calibration (number) that the pointer passes as you hear the first sound (Figure 19–27). This point indicates the systolic pressure (or the top number).

21. Continue releasing the air from the cuff. When you hear the last beat, note the calibration. This is the diastolic pressure (or bottom number).

22. Deflate the cuff completely and remove it from the patient's arm.

23. Record your reading on the vital sign form used in your institution.

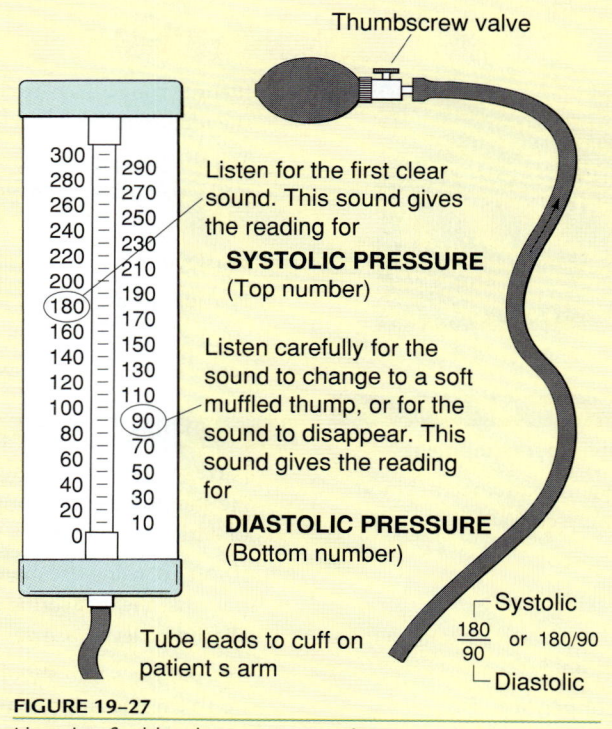

FIGURE 19–27

Listening for blood pressure sounds

PROCEDURE (CONTINUED)

FOLLOW-UP

24. After using the blood pressure cuff, roll it up over the manometer and replace it in the case.

25. Wipe the earplugs and diaphragm of the stethoscope again with an antiseptic swab. Put the stethoscope back in its proper place.

26. Make the patient comfortable and replace the call light.

27. Lower the bed to a position of safety.

28. Raise the side rails when ordered or appropriate for patient safety.

29. Wash your hands.

30. Report to your immediate supervisor:
    - That you have measured the patient's blood pressure.
    - The time that you measured the blood pressure.
    - Your observations of anything unusual.

AGE-SPECIFIC CONSIDERATIONS

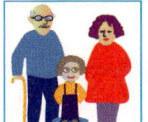

Vital Signs

Age specific care for vital signs is very important. Be sure to use the appropriate size equipment for your patient. Use the appropriate size cuff and the most appropriate type of thermometer. If this is not followed, inaccurate vital signs will be obtained. When using glass thermometers, be sure to follow your institution's policy for the use of glass thermometers, especially with children. Glass thermometers can break easily, and mercury exposures are dangerous for patients of all ages. If you will care for patients in several age groups, be sure to know the "normal" vital signs for each group.

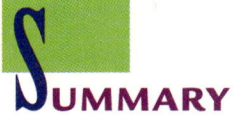

SUMMARY

In this chapter you learned how to measure the patient's vital signs—temperature, pulse, respirations, and blood pressure. You learned the normal reading or normal range for each type of measurement using the various types of equipment available or appropriate. For example, the normal reading for a temperature measured rectally is 99.6°F; 37.5°C while the reading for a normal temperature measured orally is 98.6°F; 37.0°C. There are also several different types of rectal and oral thermometers available. Procedures presented here demonstrate how to use many types of equipment and the facilities you will work in will have similar equipment. Over the years as you continue to work in the health care field, you will see the development of and will be trained to use new equipment. What is most important is that you know and understand the criteria for normal readings and that you know what equipment to use and how to use it when you are measuring a patient's vital signs.

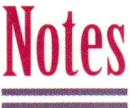

Notes

FIGURE 20–3
Large intestine

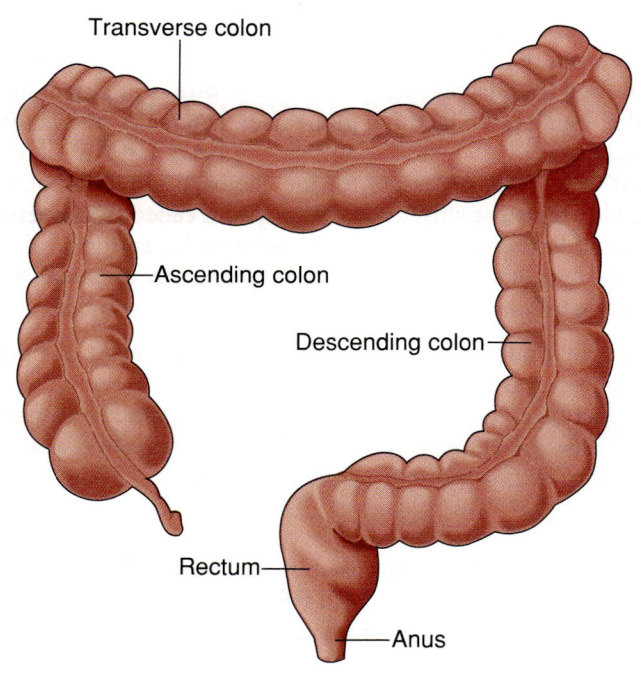

FIGURE 20–3
Large intestine

rectum The lowest portion of the large intestine, which curves in an *S*-shape and stores fecal material

sphincter Ring-shaped muscle that surrounds and controls a natural opening in the body, such as the anus

The lowest portion of the large intestine curves in an S-shape into the **rectum** (Figure 20–3). The rectum is made of very delicate tissue. It has an internal sphincter muscle and an external sphincter muscle. A **sphincter** is a ring-shaped muscle that surrounds and controls a natural opening in the body, such as the anus. Sometimes blood vessels that supply this area become enlarged and filled with blood clots, causing hemorrhoids.

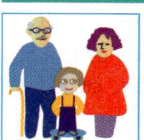

AGE-SPECIFIC CONSIDERATIONS

Age-Related Changes in the Gastrointestinal System

As a person ages, changes occur in the gastrointestinal system that cause the process of digestion to be less efficient. The flow of saliva decreases, as does the number of taste buds, so a person's appetite is likely to decrease as well. In addition, an older person may experience difficulty chewing and swallowing. A weakened gag reflex means an increased risk of choking. Reduced digestive juices make food more difficult to digest, and the absorption of vitamins and minerals is also reduced.

Due to the changes in the gastrointestinal system as a patient ages, care needs of the elderly patient need to be adapted. Decreases in saliva as well as an increased difficulty with chewing and swallowing may result in the need for longer meal times for the elderly. They benefit from sitting up while eating to aid digestion and prevent choking. Due to decreases in peristalsis, the elderly may need more fiber and fluids in their diets. The muscular contractions that move food through the digestive system, slows down.

■ Common Disorders and Diseases of the Gastrointestinal System

- *Malignancy:* cancerous tumor that can occur anywhere and in any organ of the gastrointestinal system

- *Ulcers:* gastric (stomach) ulcers, duodenal ulcers, and ulcerative colitis; lesions of mucous membrane exposed to digestive juices

- *Hernias:* occur when there is a weakness in the walls of the muscle, and the underlying tissue pushes through

- *Cholecystitis:* inflammation of the gallbladder

- *Cholelithiasis:* stones in the gallbladder

- *Constipation:* difficult, infrequent defecation with passage of unduly hard and dry fecal material

- *Diarrhea:* abnormally frequent discharge of fluid fecal material from the bowel

- *C. Diff (Clostridium Difficile):* an infectious bacterial disease that causes severe gastrointestinal discomfort and diarrhea; treated with antibiotics

- *Appendicitis:* inflammation of the appendix

- *Peritonitis:* inflammation of the peritoneal cavity

- *Intestinal obstruction:* interruption in the normal flow of intestinal contents along the gastrointestinal tract

- *Hemorrhoids:* varicose veins of the anal canal or outside the external sphincter of the rectum and anus

- *Hepatitis:* inflammation of the liver caused by viruses

- *Hepatic cirrhosis:* chronic disease of the liver caused by viruses

- *Jaundice:* abnormally high concentration of bilirubin in the blood causing a yellow discoloration of the skin and sclerae of the eyes

- *Polyps:* growths on the lining of the intestines that can become cancerous if not treated

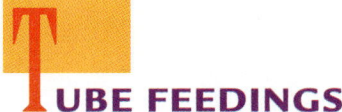

TUBE FEEDINGS

Often times nursing assistants care for patients who have tubes in the body for the purpose of putting food into the body (or for draining fluids from the body). Frequently, a patient cannot eat or drink because of an illness, surgery, or an injury. In these cases, other methods are used to meet the patient's food and fluid needs. The use of feeding tubes is ordered by the doctor, and the nurse carries out the order. One of the main roles of the nursing assistant caring for a patient with a feeding tube is to protect the patient and keep the patient safe. Think about how uncomfortable it is to have tubing inserted into your body. Provide comfort for the patient and always be careful when you work around feeding tubes. Remember to check and follow the policy of your particular institution or agency regarding your role in caring for a patient with a feeding tube.

Nasogastric Tubes

A **nasogastric tube** (NG tube) is inserted by a skilled nurse or a physician through one of the patient's nostrils, down the back of the throat, and through the esophagus into the patient's stomach. These tubes are used for suctioning the stomach and short-term tube feedings. In such feedings, a nutrition formula is given to a patient through the tube at regular times. Nasogastric feeding is also called **gavage** (Figure 20–4).

Fluids are removed from the patient's body through tubes by gravity or **suction**. When fluids are removed by gravity, the collecting container is placed near the patient at a level that is lower than the patient's body. The fluid drips into the container. Suction is used to remove thick secretions that cannot be drawn out easily by gravity. Low-level or intermittent suction is most often used. A suction canister will be connected to a suction machine (Figure 20–5a) or to a wall mounted suction unit (Figure 20–5b).

nasogastric tube A tube placed through one of the patient's nostrils (naso-), down the back of the throat, and through the esophagus into the patient's stomach (-gastric)

gavage Feeding through a nasogastric tube

suction Using negative pressure to remove material, usually fluid

FIGURE 20–4

Nasogastric tubes (stomach tubes)

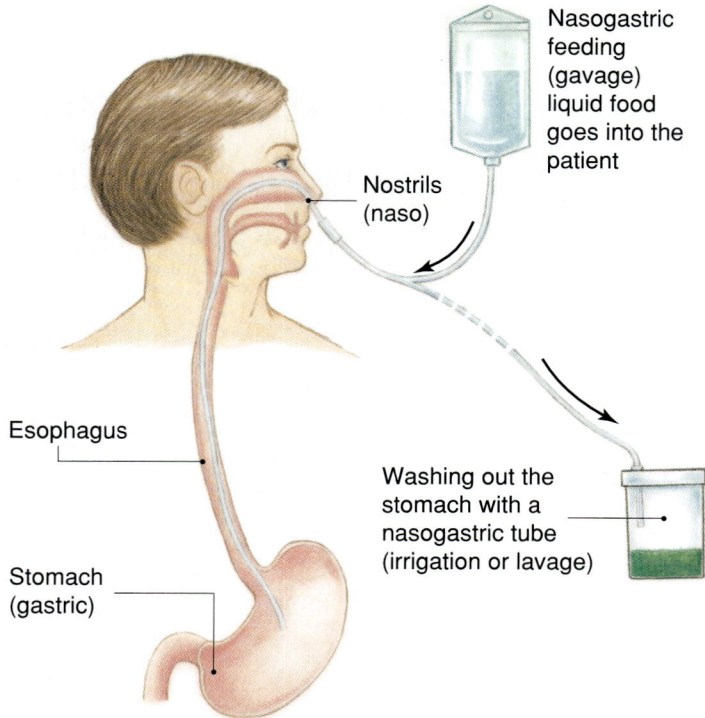

Nasogastric feeding (gavage) liquid food goes into the patient

Nostrils (naso)

Esophagus

Washing out the stomach with a nasogastric tube (irrigation or lavage)

Stomach (gastric)

FIGURE 20–5a

Patient with portable suction (vacuum) apparatus with a nasogastric tube

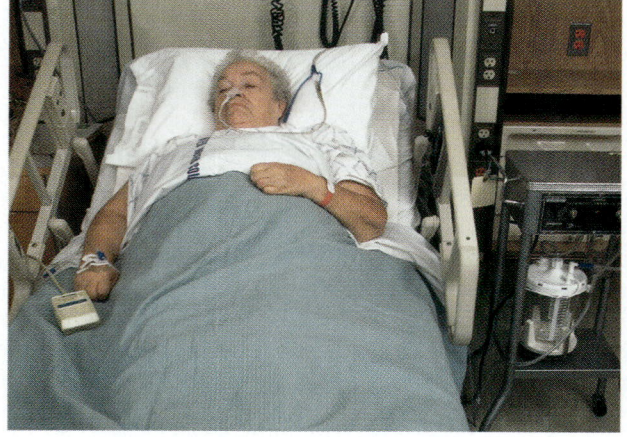

FIGURE 20–5b

Patient connected to wall mounted suction unit

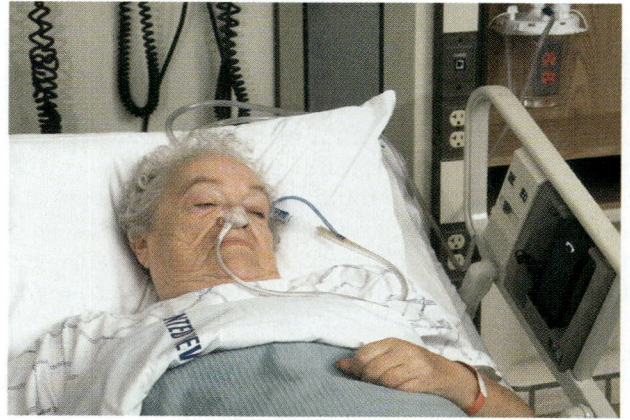

The nasogastric tube can be used to withdraw a specimen of the stomach contents for testing. When a nasogastric tube is being used to drain substances out of the stomach or to collect a specimen, the patient is given nothing by mouth (NPO). The food would only be drawn back out through the tube. Another procedure called a **lavage** refers to the washing out of the stomach through a nasogastric tube, usually with normal saline.

lavage The washing out of the stomach through a nasogastric tube, usually with normal saline

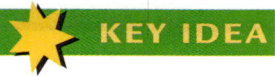

> **KEY IDEA**
>
> When a nasogastric tube is used to drain substances from the stomach or to collect a specimen, the patient is given nothing by mouth (NPO).

GUIDELINES

CARING FOR THE PATIENT WITH A NASOGASTRIC TUBE (NG)

- Before giving any fluid through an NG tube, be sure to check to see that the tube is in the stomach by inserting air through a syringe while listening with a stethoscope over the stomach

- Confirm that a doctor has checked the x-ray and approved use of the tube.

- Never pull on the tube when moving the patient or changing the patient's position.

- Remember to fasten the connecting tubing to the patient's clean gown after you have finished bathing the patient. This eases the strain on the tube and prevents accidental withdrawal. The NG tube may be taped to the bridge of the patient's nose. Notify the nurse if tape becomes loose.

- Keep the tube clean and free from mucous deposits at the entrance to the nostril.

- Observe the patient's nostrils for any signs of pressure damage from the tube and report them to the nurse for retaping of the tube.

- If the patient begins to gag or vomit while the tube is in place, report this immediately.

- Report immediately to your supervisor if you see what appears to be leakage from the tube or suction system. Never open the collecting containers to empty the drainage without instructions to do so.

- Report if the level of fluid in the container stops rising. The tubing may be blocked or drainage may be complete.

- The drainage collected through the tube is measured at regular intervals. Note the color, kind, and amount of material and record on the output side of the intake and output sheet.

- If a specimen of the drainage is needed, collect the amount at the time specified.

- If there is a rapid increase in the amount of material being drained or any change in the material itself, report to your supervisor.

■ Gastrostomy Tubes

A **gastrostomy** is an opening made through the abdomen to the stomach for the purpose of feeding (Figure 20–6). Children and adults who are unable to eat by mouth, (typically with disorders of the gastrointestinal or central nervous system) are likely to have a gastrostomy. There are three main types of gastrostomy tubes: a long-term surgical gastrostomy tube; a percutaneous endoscopic gastrostomy (PEG) tube; and a percutaneous endoscopic gastrostomy with a jejunal extension (PEG-J) tube. A surgical gastrostomy, in which a **gastrostomy tube (GT)** is inserted into the stomach, is done in an operating room with the patient under general anesthesia. After a surgical gastrostomy, patients are usually fitted with a "replacement tube" made of silicone. The PEG technique is simple to perform and safer than the standard surgical procedure for elderly or weak patients. A PEG-J is used to feed patients who are at risk for aspiration. The tube has an extension that feeds into the jejunum (Figure 20–7).

The tubes usually have a balloon to keep the tube in the stomach and a retainer device to keep the tube stabilized at its exit site. It is very important that the tube site is cleaned

gastrostomy An opening made through the abdomen to the stomach for the purpose of feeding

gastrostomy tube (GT) Tube inserted into the abdomen for the introduction of fluids

---

from a refrigerator without warm-   ing the tube feeding to prevent

PROCEDURE (CONTINUED)

8. Place the disposable bed protector under the patient's hips and buttocks.

9. Turn the patient on the left side. Bend the right knee toward the chest. (This is the left Sims's position.)

10. Put the bedpan at the foot of the bed within easy reach.

11. Close the clamp on the enema tubing.

12. Fill the graduated pitcher with 500 cc of water, 105°F (40.5°C). Measure the temperature of the water with the bath thermometer.

13. Pour the water from the graduated pitcher into the enema container.

14. Open the clamp on the enema tubing to let water run through the tubing into the bedpan. This will get rid of any air that may be in the tubing to avoid giving the patient flatus and will also warm the tube. Close the clamp.

15. Put the lubricating jelly on a piece of toilet tissue. Lubricate the enema tip by rubbing the jelly on it with the tissue. Be sure the tip is well lubricated and the opening is not plugged.

16. Expose the patient's buttocks by raising the blanket in a triangle over the anal area. Put gloves on now.

17. Raise the upper buttocks so you can see the anal area.

18. Gently insert the enema tip 2 inches through the anus into the rectum.

19. Open the clamp. Hold the enema container 12 inches above the anus. Allow about 200 cc of water to enter the rectum.

20. Lower the enema bag below the bed frame. Let the water run back into the enema bag without removing the tube from the patient's rectum.

21. Hold the enema bag 12 inches above the anus. Let 200 cc of water run into the patient's rectum; then lower the bag. Allow the water to run back into the enema bag. Keep the tube in the patient's rectum.

22. Continue letting water in and out of the rectum for 10 to 20 minutes, as you are instructed.

23. Tell the patient to take slow deep breaths. Explain that this kind of breathing will help relieve the pressure and cramps caused by the enema. It will also help her to relax.

24. Observe the amounts (large or small) of flatus the patient expels as the water runs out of the patient into the enema bag.

25. Remove the tubing when the treatment is finished. Wrap the enema tip in the paper towel. This is to avoid contamination. Place it in the disposable enema container.

26. Help the patient onto the bedpan. Raise the back of the bed, if allowed. Put the toilet tissue where the patient can reach it easily. Give the patient the signal cord. Check on the patient every few minutes.

27. The patient may be allowed by the nurse to go to the bathroom to expel more flatus. If so, assist the patient to the bathroom. Tell the patient to notice the amount of flatus (large or small amounts) that is expelled.

28. Discard the disposable enema equipment while the patient is on the bedpan or in the bathroom.

29. Return to the patient when she is finished using the bedpan or bathroom. Check the contents for bowel movement, color of stool, consistency, amount, unusual material, or anything abnormal. If you observe anything unusual, collect a specimen. Ask the patient if flatus was expelled.

30. Empty the bedpan, clean it, and put it in its proper place.

31. Remove the disposable bed protector and discard it.

32. Remove the bath blanket. At the same time, raise the top sheets to cover the patient.

33. Wash the patient's hands, or have the patient wash them.

FOLLOW-UP

34. Make the patient comfortable.

35. Lower the bed to a position of safety for the patient.

36. Raise the side rails where ordered, indicated, and appropriate for patient safety.

37. Place the call light within easy reach of the patient.

38. Wash your hands.

39. Report to your immediate supervisor:

- That you have given the patient a Harris flush.
- The time the Harris flush was given and how long it was continued.
- The results, amount of flatus expelled, and unusual material noted.
- Whether or not a specimen was obtained.
- How the patient tolerated the procedure.
- Your observations of anything unusual.

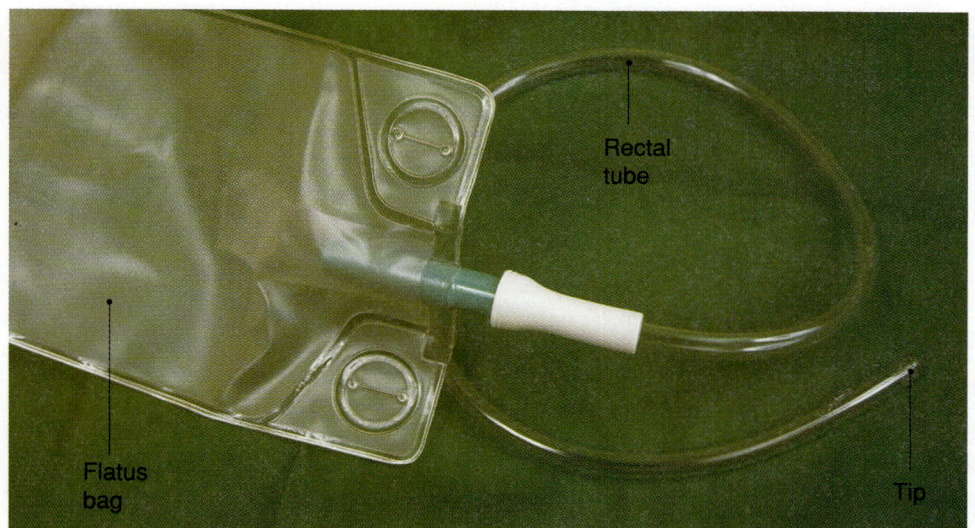

FIGURE 20–16
Disposable flatus bag and rectal tube

Rectal tube

Flatus bag

Tip

Disposable Rectal Tube with Connected Flatus Bag

A rectal tube with connected bag is used to relieve intestinal gas (flatus) that often accumulates in the patient's lower bowel (Figure 20–16). You will use the rectal tube only once a day for 20 minutes, unless otherwise instructed. The whole kit—tube and bag—is discarded after one use.

PROCEDURE

USING THE DISPOSABLE RECTAL TUBE WITH CONNECTED FLATUS BAG

PREPARATION

1. Assemble your equipment:
   a. Disposable rectal tube with connected flatus bag
   b. Small piece of adhesive tape
   c. Tissue
   d. Lubricating jelly
   e. Disposable gloves
2. Wash your hands.
3. Identify the patient by checking the identification bracelet.
4. Ask visitors to step out of the room, if this is your hospital's policy.

5. Tell the patient that you are going to insert a rectal tube for the purpose of relieving him of gas (flatus).
6. Provide privacy for the patient.

STEPS

7. Turn the patient on the left side. Bend the right knee toward the chest. (This is the left Sims's position.)
8. Expose the patient's buttocks by raising the blanket in a triangle over the anal area. Put on the disposable plastic gloves.
9. Lubricate the tip of the rectal tube. Do this by squeezing lubricating jelly onto the tissue and rubbing the jelly on the tip. Be sure the opening at the end of the tube is not clogged. (If the rectal tube is prelubricated, this step is not necessary.)

10. Raise the upper buttocks so you can see the anal area.
11. Gently insert the rectal tube 2 to 4 inches through the anus into the rectum.
12. Use a small piece of adhesive tape to attach the tube to the patient's buttocks in order to hold the tube in place.
13. Let the tube remain in place for 20 minutes. Then remove and discard the equipment. (Usually this procedure is done once in a 24-hour period.)

FOLLOW-UP

14. Make the patient comfortable.
15. Lower the bed to a position of safety for the patient.
16. Raise the side rails where ordered, indicated, and appropriate for patient safety.
17. Place the call light within easy reach of the patient.

PROCEDURE (CONTINUED)

18. Wash your hands.

19. Report to your immediate supervisor:

- The time the rectal tube was inserted and the time it was removed.

- The patient's comments about the amount (small or large) of flatus that was expelled through the tube.

- How the patient tolerated the procedure.

- Your observations of anything unusual.

■ Rectal Suppositories

Rectal suppositories are inserted into the rectum to aid in elimination, to promote healing, to relieve pain, or to re-toilet train an incontinent patient. Adults use a single or double-cone shaped suppository; children use a long, thin suppository. Simple, nonmedicinal suppositories are made of soap, glycerine, or cocoa butter, and may be administered by nursing assistants. Medicinal suppositories, which contain drugs, are not administered by nursing assistants.

ostomy A surgical procedure (operation) in which a new opening, called a stoma, is created in the abdomen, usually for the discharge of wastes (urine or feces) from the body

stoma A surgically made opening connecting the urinary or intestinal tract with the outside, such as in a urostomy or colostomy

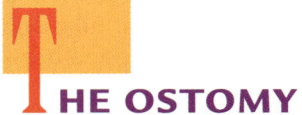

THE OSTOMY

An **ostomy** is a surgical procedure in which a new opening, called a **stoma**, is created, usually in the abdomen, for the discharge of wastes (urine or feces) from the body. A stoma created surgically may be used to divert the path of the patient's feces from the rectum. This is done when the colon is diseased or injured. The ostomy is often performed to remove tumors. Sometimes the surgery is done to permit repair of bowel injuries. An ostomy may be created to treat Inflammatory Bowel Disease (IBD) like ulcerative colitis and Crohn's disease.

KEY IDEA

An ostomy is a surgical procedure that provides the patient with an artificial opening connecting a body passage with outside, such as in a tracheotomy or colostomy. An ostomy may be temporary or permanent.

Figures 20–17 through 20–21 describe types of ostomies and show the position of the stoma in each case.

FIGURE 20–17

Following surgery, the type of discharge from a sigmoid or descending colostomy may be semiliquid until, through management of diet, the stool begins to resemble a normal bowel movement

Sigmoid colostomy   Descending colostomy

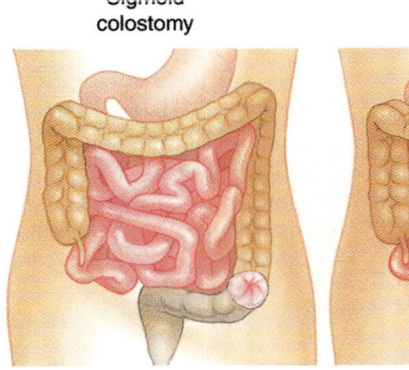
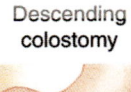
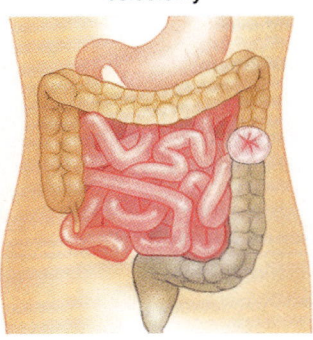

Transverse
(double barrel)   Transverse-
loop colostomy

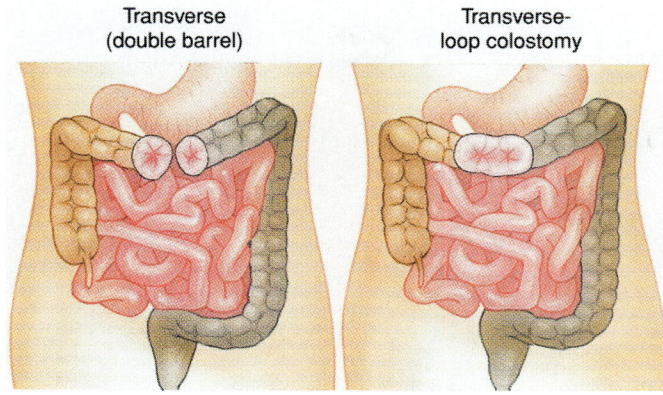

FIGURE 20–18

Frequently, the transverse double barrel and the transverse loop colostomy are temporary; common patient problems with these types of ostomies include skin irritation and leakage from the appliance

Bilateral
cutaneous
ureterostomy

Ileal conduit

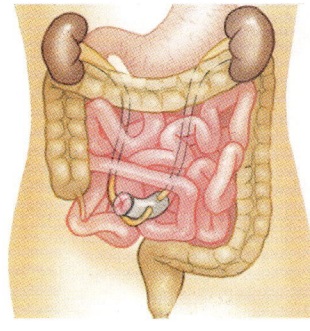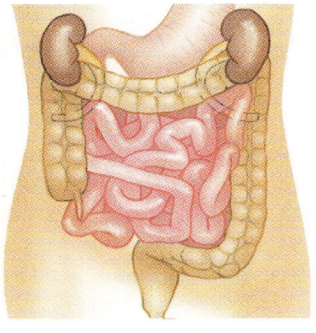

FIGURE 20–19

Urinary diversion is performed for malfunction of the urinary bladder. When the patient has a bilateral cutaneous ureterostomy or an ileal conduit, prevention of leakage and skin protection are of utmost importance

Ascending colostomy

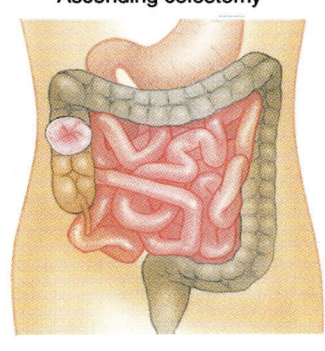

FIGURE 20–20

The ascending colostomy is essentially the same as the transverse colostomy. Common patient problems include skin irritation, leakage from the appliance and odor control

Ileostomy

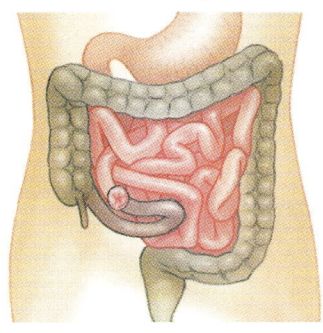

FIGURE 20–21

The ileostomy; a common patient problem with the ileostomy is skin irritation

FIGURE 20–22

Ostomy appliance in place over the stoma

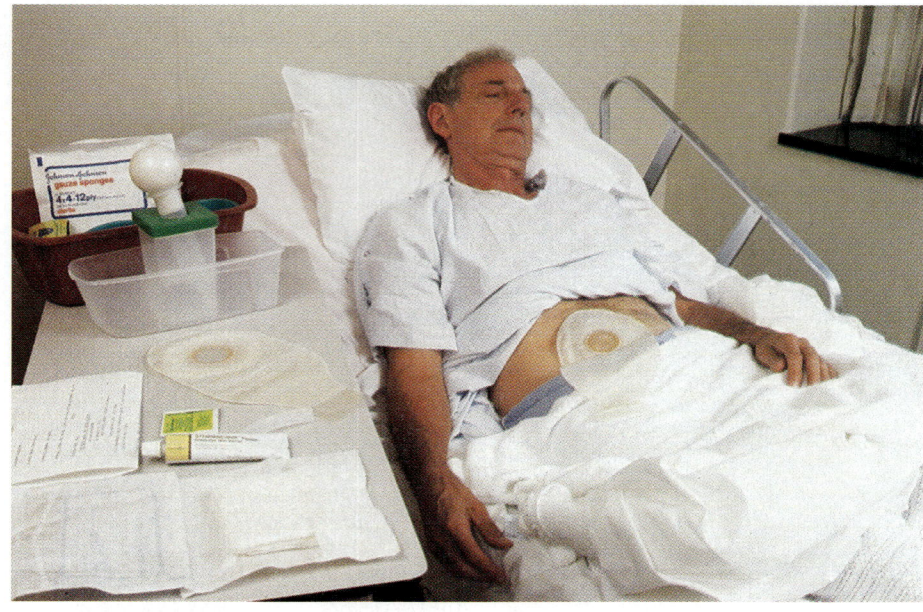

ostomy appliance
Collecting pouch usually attached to the skin around the stoma with adhesive

A person with a stoma must wear an **ostomy appliance** to collect waste from the stoma (Figure 20–22). This is a collecting pouch usually adhered to the skin around the stoma with an adhesive barrier. The stoma is red due to its abundant blood supply. It may bleed slightly during care. This is normal and is not something that should worry the patient. However, bleeding that does not stop should be reported.

As a nursing assistant, you may be taking care of a patient who has had the surgery for some time and already has been fitted with an ostomy appliance. Sometimes the patient is able and wants to care for the ostomy himself. In this case, assist the patient as he needs. Ask the patient how you can assist, as each patient develops a routine in doing self-care and will appreciate your interest and concern. A new surgical patient with a new ostomy is cared for by a registered nurse who teaches self-care and does a frequent assessment of the stoma.

Psychological Aspects of Ostomies

The psychological reaction of the patient to an ostomy will vary with each patient. Dealing with the ostomy may at first be a bit overwhelming to the patient. Faced with an altered body image, the patient may feel a keen sense of loss, become quiet and withdrawn, or very angry, hostile, noisy, and disruptive. The patient may develop mood changes, appearing very anxious or depressed. Anxiety is a natural and common response; fear is another. Either emotion can cause the patient to develop feelings of doom or panic. Family members and significant others who provide emotional support are very important. Allow the patient time to express his feelings during your contact with him.

The nurse or Enterostomal Therapy Nurse (a nurse specializing in Ostomy care) should be contacted to arrange for an Ostomy Visitor if the patient desires. An Ostomy Visitor is someone who has had ostomy surgery and has had special training. The shared experience of someone who has had an ostomy and is living with a stoma can help the patient see that positive adjustment is possible. As the caregiver it is important not to convey either verbally or nonverbally a negative reaction to the patient. Your patient needs encouragement and support.

Caring for an Ostomy

It is desirable for the patient to be moving toward independence in ostomy self care prior to discharge. It is important for the patient to know and demonstrate how to empty the appliance, clean the tail and replace the clamp prior to discharge. To get to that point, you can assist by practicing with the patient how to empty the ostomy pouch.

Shortly after surgery and until the patient is up without assistance, it is easier for the patient to have the pouch emptied while in bed. Ideally, in the future, the patient will be able to empty the pouch while sitting on the toilet, with the pouch between the legs. It is often difficult for the patient to do this during the post-op stay, but you should inform the patient that the toilet method is the best and most natural (especially away from home, for example, in a public restroom). With this method, no extra equipment (containers) is needed.

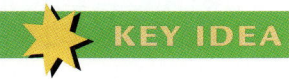

KEY IDEA

It is easier to empty the ostomy pouch when it is about 1/3 filled. Hot water destroys the pouch's odor proofing.

PROCEDURE

OBRA

EMPTYING THE OSTOMY POUCH

PREPARATION

1. Assemble your equipment:
   a. Plastic container (for contents of pouch)
   b. Toilet tissue
   c. Disposable bed protector
   d. Basin with warm water
   e. Soap
   f. Wet washcloth
   g. Hand towel
   h. Disposable gloves
   i. Container of water, if pouch is to be rinsed (optional)

2. Identify the patient by checking the identification bracelet.

3. Tell the patient you will empty the ostomy pouch. If the patient is able, assist them.

4. Provide privacy for the patient.

5. Raise the bed to a comfortable working position. Raise the head of the bed. This helps the stool settle into the bottom of the pouch and also allows the patient to see what you are doing.

6. Put on gloves.

7. Encourage the patient to watch. Ask, "Would you like to empty the pouch?"

STEPS

8. Cover the patient with the bath blanket. Without exposing the patient, fanfold the top sheet and the bedspread to the bottom of the bed.

9. Place the disposable bed protector under the patient's hips and put container and roll of toilet tissue on the bed where it is easily accessible to you.

10. Holding the bottom of the pouch up, remove the clamp from the pouch and set the clamp aside.

11. Drain the pouch into the container. If the stool is thick, slide fingers down the outside of the pouch, squeezing out the contents into the container.

12. After emptying the pouch, measure the contents, if necessary, and then flush.

13. *Optional:* Rinse pouch with container of water, if patient wishes. Empty rinse water in plastic container. (Some patients like to rinse out the pouch. The pouch is odor proof whether it is clean or full of stool as long as the pouch is intact.)

14. Wipe the end of the pouch off with the tissue on the outside and also on the inside of the narrow opening.

15. Wipe off the clamp with tissue and place the clamp back on the bottom of the pouch.

16. If the patient has helped, give him a wet washcloth with soap and water to wash his hands.

FOLLOW-UP

17. Cover the patient. Lower the head of the bed if required or patient's preference.

18. Make the patient comfortable and replace the call light.

19. Lower the bed to a position of safety.

20. Raise the side rails when ordered or appropriate for patient safety.

21. Clean basin with soapy water, rinse, dry, and replace in its proper place. Discard disposable equipment. Bag and dispose of soiled linen in the laundry hamper.

22. Dispose of gloves and wash your hands.

23. Report to your immediate supervisor:
    - That the ostomy pouch was emptied.
    - Record as output on I + O records.

PROCEDURE

OBRA

CHANGING THE OSTOMY APPLIANCE

PREPARATION

1. Assemble your equipment:

   a. Disposable bed protector

   b. Bath blanket

   c. New pouch (may be 1 or 2 pieces

   d. Toilet tissue

   e. Basin of warm water (115°F; 46°C)

   f. Non cream-based soap or cleanser as ordered by your immediate supervisor

   g. Washcloth

   h. Disposable gloves

   i. Towels

2. Identify the patient by checking the identification bracelet.

3. Tell the patient that you will assist them in changing the ostomy appliance.

4. Wash your hands and put on gloves.

5. Provide privacy for the patient.

6. Raise the bed to a comfortable working position.

STEPS

7. Place a towel over the patient's abdomen, exposing only the appliance.

8. Place the disposable bed protector under the patient's hips. This is to keep the bed from getting wet or dirty.

9. Gently remove the soiled pouch. Use a push-pull method to remove barrier.

10. Dispose of the pouch in the appropriate container. Wipe the area around the ostomy with a warm wet wash cloth. This is to remove any stool from the skin.

11. Rinse the entire area well. Be careful not to leave any soap on the skin. (Soap has a drying effect and may irritate the skin.)

12. Dry the area gently with a bath towel.

13. Prepare the new barrier (Figure 20–23). A colostomy stoma needs a barrier ⅛″ larger than the stoma measurement. It may need to be sized and cut out. For urostomy and ileostomy stomas, no skin should show between the wafer and the stoma. The opening of the wafer should fit around the stoma at the area where the skin meets the stoma. Use stoma

adhesive paste if necessary. Note: There are 1- and 2-piece appliances. Become familiar with the supplies available to you.

14. Apply new wafer to skin; hold in place for 30 seconds with your hand to help adhesive stick well (Figure 20–23c). Apply clamp to bottom of pouch.

15. Remove the disposable bed protector. Change any damp linen. Bag and dispose of soiled linen in the laundry hamper.

FOLLOW-UP

16. Make the patient comfortable and replace the call light.

17. Lower the bed to a position of safety.

18. Raise the side rails when ordered or appropriate for patient safety.

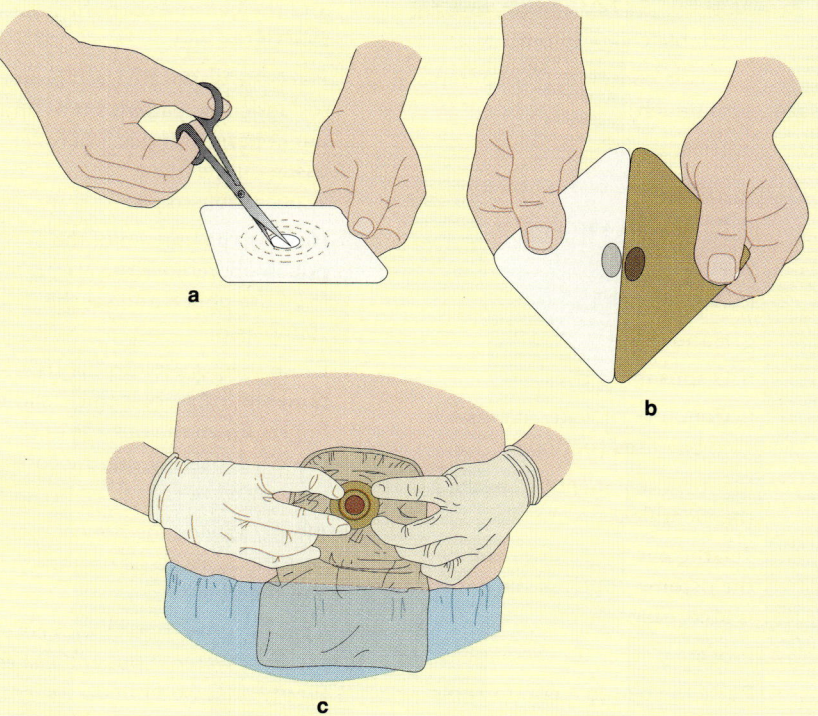

FIGURE 20–23

Replacing an ostomy appliance. (a) Use a measuring guide to size and cut opening in the barrier. (b) Remove covering if wafer is self adhesive, or apply stoma adhesive paste. (c) Hold in place for 30 seconds.

PROCEDURE (CONTINUED)

19. Remove all used equipment.

20. Wash your hands.

21. Report to your immediate supervisor:

- That the ostomy wafer and pouch were changed.

- The amount of drainage.

- The consistency of the stool.

- The color and appearance of the stoma and skin around stoma.

- How the patient tolerated the procedure.

- Your observations of anything unusual.

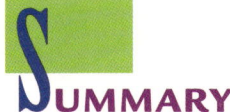

SUMMARY

Caring for patients with digestive-related problems requires a knowledge of the gastrointestinal system itself as well as the common disorders and diseases of the system. It is also important to be familiar with the types of age-related changes that can occur in the gastrointestinal system. Tube feeding is a common procedure and it is important to understand the guidelines for care of a patient on tube feedings. Causes of diarrhea and constipation have been discussed to enable the nursing assistant to make changes to prevent and remedy problems. Learning how to recognize and manage diarrhea and constipation also contribute to a patient's comfort and health. The nursing assistant is relied upon to understand the proper technique for safe administration of the procedures given in this chapter and to have knowledge of the patient care guidelines. The nursing assistant is also responsible for reviewing and following the policies and procedures of the institution or agency where the nursing assistant is employed regarding each of these procedures and their administration and the nursing assistant's role.

Notes

malnutrition Poor
nutrition status

The prevalence of malnutrition in the hospital is very high. **Malnutrition** means poor nutrition status. Patients with a poor appetite need encouragement to meet their nutritional needs. The patient's surroundings should be cheerful and attractive. The sight and aroma of food should be as appetizing as possible. You often can increase patients' appetites by showing them what they will be eating and providing some positive comments about the food. Obtaining patients' food preferences is one important way you may be able to increase their intake. In some settings, it is possible for patients to eat with others. The companionship and socialization can also encourage or promote the desire to eat—thereby improving the patient's appetite.

ASSISTING PATIENTS WITH FOODS

Mealtime is a break in the often boring hospital routine and gives the patient something to look forward to. Many patients also enjoy making food selections from the menu. This is another time when you can encourage the patient to select a well-balanced meal.

When the food tray is delivered, do everything you can to make the patient's meal as pleasant and comfortable as possible. Make sure the room is clean, quiet, free of unpleasant odors, and not too warm or cold. Take away things that might spoil the patient's appetite—items such as an emesis basin, urinal, or bedpan.

AGE-SPECIFIC CONSIDERATIONS

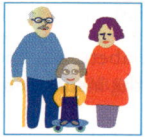

Patients of all ages enjoy social contact while eating. Children have food preferences just like adults. Encourage children to eat, but do not force them. Offer small amounts frequently. For adolescents, try to obtain foods that are familiar, and favorites too. Emphasize healthy choices, but in a way that is typical for the age group, i.e., pizza. For the elderly, perform and encourage oral care prior to meals to improve the preceptor of taste and the flavor of food. Encourage the patient to sit up in the chair for meals and to wait 30–60 minutes after meals for food to digest.

PROCEDURE

OBRA

PREPARING THE PATIENT FOR A MEAL

PREPARATION

1. Assemble your equipment:
   a. Bedpan or urinal
   b. Basin of warm water (115°F; 46.1°C)
   c. Washcloth
   d. Towel
   e. Robe and slippers

2. Identify the patient by checking the identification bracelet.

3. Wash your hands.

STEPS

4. Tell the patient you are getting her ready for her next meal.

5. Provide privacy for the patient.

6. Offer the bedpan or urinal or assist the patient to the bathroom.

7. Have the patient wash her hands or offer the patient assistance.

8. Raise the backrest so the patient is in a sitting position, if this is allowed. If not, you might prop up her head by using several pillows.

9. Clear the overbed table. Put it in a convenient position for the patient's meal.

10. If the patient wants to sit in a chair to eat and this is allowed, assist her with her robe and slippers. Help the patient out of bed and to the chair.

P R O C E D U R E (CONTINUED)

FOLLOW-UP

11. Make the patient comfortable and replace the call light.

12. Check that the telephone is still within reach.

13. Lower the bed to a position of safety for the patient.

14. Raise the side rails when ordered or appropriate for patient safety.

15. Wash your hands.

16. Report the following to your immediate supervisor:

- The patient is ready for the next meal.

- How the patient tolerated the procedure.

- Your observations of anything unusual.

P R O C E D U R E

OBRA

SERVING THE FOOD

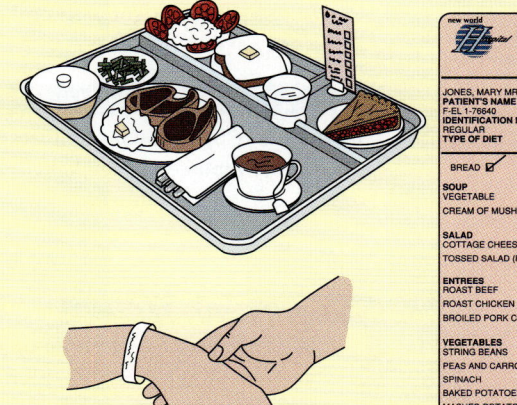

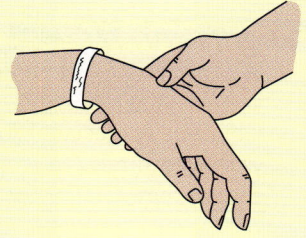

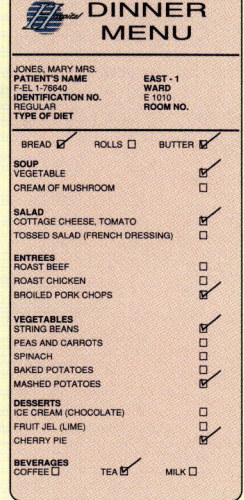

FIGURE 21–2

Check to be sure the name on the menu card matches the patient's identification band

PREPARATION

1. Wash your hands.

2. Check the tray before you give it to the patient. Make sure the tray looks appetizing and nothing is missing (including silverware). Make sure nothing has spilled. Correct anything that is wrong.

3. Be sure you are giving the right tray to the right patient. Check the menu card, which will have the patient's name on it, against the identification band to be sure they match (Figure 21–2).

STEPS

4. Put the tray on the overbed table. Adjust it to a height comfortable for the patient.

5. Arrange the dishes and silverware so the patient can reach everything easily. Be sure drinking water is handy.

6. Help any patient who needs it (Figure 21–3). For example, if a patient seems to be weak or asks for help, you might offer to spread the napkin on his lap or tuck it under his chin. Spread butter on the bread. Cut up whatever

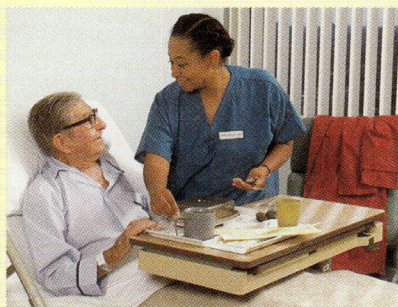

FIGURE 21–3

Help any patient requiring assistance to eat

needs cutting. Pour tea or coffee. Do not give any more help than is really needed. The more a patient can do for himself, the better.

7. A patient may discover that he cannot eat when the food is served. Report this to your supervisor. If permitted, you may take the tray away and keep the hot food warm until the patient wants to eat.

8. When you are sure the patient can go on with his meal by himself, leave the room.

9. Go back for the food tray when the patient has finished eating.

PROCEDURE (CONTINUED)

10. Note how much the patient has eaten and how much he has had to drink.

11. Record the intake for those patients who are on calorie counts or intake and output records.

12. Record how the patient has eaten his meal on the daily activity flow sheet. Record this information separately for breakfast, lunch, and supper:

    a. Did the patient eat all the food served?

    b. Did the patient eat about half the food served?

    c. Did the patient eat very little food?

    d. Did the patient decline to eat anything?

13. Take the tray away and put it in its proper place.

14. If the patient ate sitting in a chair, help him back into bed.

15. Put personal articles back where the patient wants them.

16. If the patient ate in bed, brush crumbs from the bed, smooth out the sheets, and straighten the bedding.

17. Assist the patient with oral care as needed.

FOLLOW-UP

18. Make the patient comfortable and replace the call light.

19. Lower the bed to a position of safety for the patient.

20. Raise the side rails when ordered or appropriate for patient safety.

21. Wash your hands.

22. Report the following to your immediate supervisor:

    - That you have served the patient his food.

    - The amount of food eaten (all, half, or refused to eat).

    - Your observations of anything unusual.

AGE-SPECIFIC CONSIDERATIONS

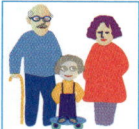

When caring for patients of all ages, try to find out food preferences and favorites. When possible, give them some choice in when and what they eat. Children appreciate what is familiar, therefore encourage family to assist with mealtimes. To assist the elderly, make sure there is adequate lighting so that they can see the food. Have them wear their glasses as well.

Patients Requiring Assistance to Eat

Some patients are incapable of feeding themselves and, therefore, will have to be fed. The reason might be

- The patient cannot use his hands

- The doctor wants the patient to save his strength and to be on "complete bed rest"

- The patient may be too weak to feed himself

- The patient may have difficulties with swallowing (for example, due to a stroke or cleft palate) and may need assistance

- The patient may have dysphasia, which is difficulty in chewing or swallowing due to damage to the nerves and muscles involved in swallowing (from head and neck cancer, multiple sclerosis, Parkinson's or Alzheimer's disease)

Usually, it is hard for adults to accept the idea of not being able to eat independently. Because he may be physically challenged or handicapped, the patient may experience feelings of resentment or even depression. Be friendly and natural. Encourage the patient to do as much as he can for himself. Also, remember that because of medical reasons a patient may not always be allowed to help. You will learn how to judge the amount of help the patient can give you when he is being fed. For example, if the patient is strong enough, you might let him hold his own bread.

When feeding a challenged patient, the most important thing is not to rush him through his meal. The time it takes to chew food, for example, may seem long to you, but the patient is probably very weak; otherwise, he would be able to eat without your help.

Remember that you should not bring the food tray or have it delivered until you have prepared the patient for the meal and are ready to feed him. Again, make sure you are serving the correct tray to the patient. Preparations before mealtime are the same for the challenged patient who cannot feed himself. Be observant throughout. Watch for signs of choking, coughing, or anything unusual.

Signs and symptoms of dysphasia include pocketing of food in the mouth, drooling, coughing, especially following sips of liquids, choking on food, frequent clearing of the throat, and speaking in a wet, gargly voice.

GUIDELINES

FEEDING A PATIENT WITH DYSPHASIA

- Positioning the patient with a 90° flexion of hips and a 45° neck flexion is recommended. Pillows can be used behind the back and neck if needed to maintain this position. If the patient is in bed, the knees can be cranked up to prevent the patient from slipping down.

- Feeding liquids can be easier using a cut-out cup and reminding the patient to keep his head down, suck in a small amount of liquid, swallow, then rest.

- Place solid food on the tongue with a spoon. Wait and be sure the mouth is empty before offering more food. Very cold foods or Italian ices between every 5–6 bites can make it easier for some patients to eat. Avoid offering dry foods, for example, bread, waffles, and pancakes. Extra honey, syrup, butter, or applesauce can help make these foods easier to swallow for patients who desire them.

- Encourage the patient to swallow twice after each bite.

- Present food from the midline and below.

- Be patient and offer verbal cues as needed.

- Check that the mouth is empty after the feeding and have the patient remain sitting up for 30 minutes.

PROCEDURE

OBRA

FEEDING THE PHYSICALLY CHALLENGED PATIENT OR THE PATIENT WHO IS UNABLE TO FEED HIMSELF

PREPARATION

1. Assemble your equipment on the overbed table:

   a. Patient's tray

2. Check the name on the card on the tray against the patient's identification bracelet.

3. Tell the patient you are going to feed him or assist with the meal.

STEPS

4. Wash your hands.

5. If allowed the patient should be in high Fowler's position.

6. If you plan to be seated while you feed the patient, bring a chair to a convenient position beside the bed.

7. Check the tray to make sure everything is there. If anything is missing, have it brought in or get it yourself.

8. Tuck a napkin under the patient's chin.

9. Season the food the way the patient likes it. However, do this only if his request agrees with the prescribed diet.

10. For most patients unable to feed themselves you will use a spoon. Fill the spoon only half-full. Give the food to the patient from the tip of the spoon, not the side. Put the food in one side of the patient's mouth so he can chew it more easily. If a patient is paralyzed on one side of his body, make sure you feed him on the side of his mouth that is not paralyzed.

11. If the patient cannot see the tray, name each mouthful of food as

PROCEDURE (CONTINUED)

you offer it. Offer the different foods in a logical order, soup or juice before the main course. Alternate between liquids and solid foods throughout the meal. Feed the patient as you yourself would want to eat. Or follow the patient's suggestions about how he wants to alternate between various kinds of foods and a beverage.

12. If the patient is unable to see and would like to feed himself, you can describe the position of the food on the tray. For example, cold liquids are in the left corner, hot liquids in the right corner. Describe the food on the plate in terms of a clock face (Figure 21–4). For example, "Baked potato at 2 o'clock, peas at 4 o'clock, carrots at 5 o'clock, roast beef at 8 o'clock, and bread at 11 o'clock."

13. Try to maintain the patient's independence as much as possible.

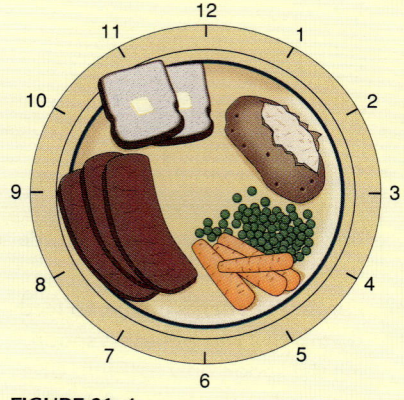

FIGURE 21–4
Describe the food on the plate and its placement in terms of a clock face

14. Warn the patient if you are offering something hot. Never offer extremely hot liquids; allow them to cool. Use a straw for giving liquids (Figure 21–5). Use a new straw for each beverage.

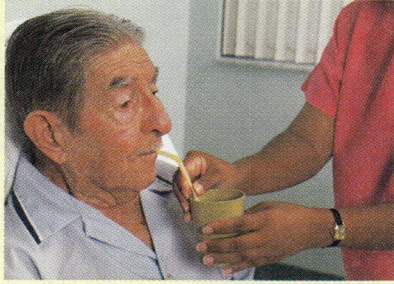

FIGURE 21–5
Use a straw when offering liquids

15. Feed the patient slowly. Remember that he may chew and swallow very slowly. Allow plenty of time between mouthfuls.

16. Encourage the patient to finish the meal, but do not use force.

17. When the patient has finished eating, help him to wipe his mouth with the napkin, or do this for the patient.

18. Note how much the patient has eaten and how much he has had to drink.

19. Record fluid intake on the intake and output sheet or as directed by your supervisor, when the patient is on intake and output.

20. Record how the patient has eaten his meal on the daily activity sheet or as directed by your supervisor. Record this information separately for breakfast, lunch, and supper:

a. Did the patient eat all the food served?

b. Did the patient eat about one-half the food served?

c. Did the patient eat very little food?

d. Did the patient refuse to eat anything?

21. As soon as you are sure the patient is finished with the tray, take it away. Put it in its proper place.

FOLLOW-UP

22. Adjust the backrest of the bed to make the patient comfortable, if this is allowed.

23. Brush crumbs from the bed, smooth the sheets, and straighten the bedding.

24. Assist the patient with oral care or provide oral care as needed.

25. Make the patient comfortable and replace the call light.

26. Lower the bed to a position of safety for the patient.

27. Raise the side rails when ordered or appropriate for patient safety.

28. Wash your hands.

29. Report the following to your immediate supervisor:

- That you have fed the patient.
- Your observations of anything unusual.

BETWEEN-MEAL NOURISHMENT

extra nourishment
Snacks

Extra **nourishment** in the form of food or drink is offered to patients during the day. This is a hospital "snack" given to patients to provide energy or to break the routine. Patients are often given extra nourishment as part of their medical care.

Examples of snacks are crackers and cheese, fruit and milk, and oral supplements such as a milkshake. In some institutions, extra nourishment is passed out to patients by workers from the food service department. However, you may be assigned this responsibility. If you are, your immediate supervisor will give you a list of which patients can have an extra nourishment and which have special restrictions. It is important to deliver the nourishment at the scheduled time that is ordered for patients on a special diet.

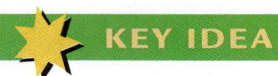

KEY IDEA

The nourishment or snacks provided must be acceptable within the therapeutic or special diet and will be included in the diet order.

PROCEDURE

SERVING BETWEEN-MEAL NOURISHMENT

PREPARATION

1. Wash your hands.
2. Assemble your equipment on a tray or a cart:
   a. Nourishment
   b. Cup, dish, and a spoon or straw
   c. Napkin

STEPS

3. Identify the patient by checking the identification bracelet.
4. If the patient has a choice of items, ask what the patient prefers.
5. Prepare the nourishment.
6. Take the nourishment to the patient on a tray or cart.
7. Encourage the patient to take the nourishment, assisting as needed. Offer a straw if this is more convenient.
8. After the patient has finished, collect the tray.
9. Discard the disposable equipment.
10. Record the intake for those patients who are on intake and output records or calorie counts. (See PROCEDURE: *Determining the Amounts Consumed* in Chapter 22.)

FOLLOW-UP

11. Make the patient comfortable and replace the call light.
12. Lower the bed to a position of safety for the patient.
13. Raise the side rails when ordered or appropriate for patient safety.
14. Wash your hands.
15. Report the following to your immediate supervisor:
    - That you have served the between-meal nourishment.
    - Your observations of anything unusual.

PASSING DRINKING WATER

Part of your job as a nursing assistant will be to see that the patients you are caring for have plenty of fresh water at their bedsides, unless a doctor orders otherwise. Some patients are not allowed to have more than a certain amount of water. Some, for brief periods, may not have water at all.

Fresh ice water is passed to patients at regular intervals during the day. Your instructor will tell you the schedule of your institution. Disposable pitchers and cups are used everywhere. Most patients like ice water. Others want water without ice, straight from the tap. You will be told which patients are allowed to have a choice. If a patient is not allowed to have ice, his water pitcher will be tagged "**Omit** Ice." Some patients are allowed ice chips only.

omit Leave out

PROCEDURE

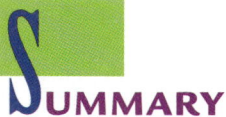

PASSING DRINKING WATER

PREPARATION

1. Assemble your equipment:
   a. Moving table (cart) with small ice chest and cover or disposable water pitcher liners
   b. Ice cubes
   c. Scoop
   d. Paper or disposable cups
   e. Disposable water pitchers
   f. Straws
   g. Paper towels
2. Wash your hands.

STEPS

3. Fill the disposable water pitcher liners or ice chest with ice cubes and cover it.
4. Put all the equipment on the table.
5. Before you pass drinking water, be sure you know:
   a. Which patients are NPO (nothing by mouth)
   b. Which patients are on restricted fluids and get only a measured amount of water
   c. Which patients get only tap water (**omit** ice)
   d. Which patients may have ice water
   e. Which patients may not have a straw
6. Roll the moving table into the hall outside the patient's room.
7. Go into the room and pick up one patient's water pitcher/container. Record the patient's intake. Empty it in the sink in the room.
8. Remove and discard the disposable liner.
9. Walk to the water table in the hall. Insert a new water pitcher liner into the pitcher/container. Fill it half full with tap water.
10. Fill the pitcher to the brim with ice cubes, *being sure the scoop does not touch the water pitcher.*
11. Replace the water pitcher on the same patient's table from which it was taken. If the pitcher is labeled with the patient's name, check it against the identification bracelet.
12. Throw away used paper cups.
13. Wipe the table with a clean paper towel. Discard the towel.
14. Place several clean paper cups next to the water pitcher.
15. Place several straws next to the water pitcher.
16. Be sure the patient can reach the water pitcher easily.
17. Offer to pour a fresh glass of water for the patient.

FOLLOW-UP

18. Wash your hands.
19. Report the following to your immediate supervisor:
    - That you have passed fresh drinking water to the patient.
    - Your observations of anything unusual.

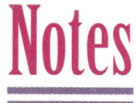

SUMMARY

Good nutrition is key to the recovery of many patients. Your role in providing that support includes observing the patient's needs, delivering food, water, and extra nourishment according to the order, and identifying any special circumstances that you encounter. Special diets are quite common and this chapter has provided an overview of many examples. A well-balanced diet containing the essential nutrients is important for all patients. Your knowledge of the food group pyramid can assist patients with their menu selections. As a nursing assistant, your role in providing good nutrition to the patient and identifying any patient nutrition problems is extremely important.

Notes

Patient Requests Fast Food—Case 1

THE NURSING ASSISTANT IN ACTION

You are assigned to Mr. Williams, who has hypertension and is on a low sodium diet. At mealtime he looks at his tray and says, "You call this food? This is not fit to eat! When you are on your lunch break, go get me some fried chicken or a Big Mac. Please do this for me, and I will treat you to lunch if you agree." You personally prefer any fast food over the cafeteria and were planning to go out anyway. Mr. Williams' family often brings him food when they visit.

What Is Your Response/Action?

1. What are the important pieces of information in this situation?

2. How will you respond to Mr. Williams' request?

3. What possible alternative choices could you offer Mr. Williams?

4. Would you accept his offer to buy your lunch? Why or why not?

5. What would you tell his family, if anything, about his request?

CHAPTER REVIEW

FILL IN THE BLANK

Read each sentence and fill in the blank line with a word that completes the sentence.

1. The process of counting or adding up all of the calories consumed in a 24-hour period is called a _____

   _____.

2. The food group guide to a well-balanced diet that is divided into six categories is the _____ _____.

3. Difficulty swallowing or chewing is called _____.

4. When feeding a patient, it is important not to _____ them while they eat.

5. A _____ or snack is given to patients to provide energy or as part of their medical care.

MULTIPLE CHOICE

Choose the best answer for each question or statement.

1. How many servings of breads, cereals, and pastas are recommended on the food pyramid?
   a. 2–3
   b. 3–5
   c. 5–6
   d. 6–11

2. How many servings of vegetables are recommended on the food pyramid?
   a. 2–3
   b. 3–5
   c. 5–6
   d. 6–11

3. Which of the following is generally not allowed on a clear liquid diet?
   a. apple juice
   b. jello
   c. tomato juice
   d. tea

4. When feeding a patient who has dysphasia, do all of the following except
   a. position the patient with his head up 90 degrees.
   b. offer dry foods such as crackers.
   c. encourage the patient to swallow twice after each bite.
   d. be patient and offer verbal cues.

5. When passing drinking water, do all of the following except
   a. wash your hands.
   b. note which patients are NPO.
   c. collect all the patient's pitchers and fill them from the ice machine.
   d. place a fresh glass of water within reach of the patient.

6. When preparing the patient to eat, you should try to make the environment as pleasant as possible.
   a. True
   b. False

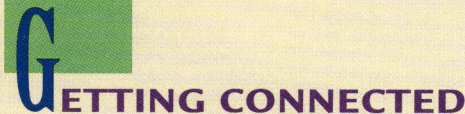

GETTING CONNECTED

MULTIMEDIA EXTENSION ACTIVITIES

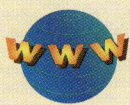

www.prenhall.com/wolgin

Use the above address to access the free, interactive Companion Website created for this textbook. Get hints, instant feedback, and textbook references to chapter-related multiple choice questions. Read and react to the "Nursing Assistants in Action." Link to other interesting sites.

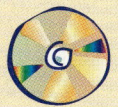

Audio Glossary

Use the CD-ROM disk enclosed with your textbook to hear the pronunciation of the key terms in the chapter.

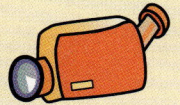

Video

Watch the "Transfer and Ambulation" video from the Care Provider Skills series.

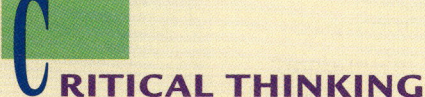

CRITICAL THINKING

USING KEY QUESTIONS

Read each question and think of what you might do in each situation.

1. A patient asks you "What is a food pyramid?" What would you tell her?

2. The RN tells you that your patient is on a calorie count. What should you do now?

3. How should the patient who is too weak or physically challenged be fed?

4. The RN asks you to note how the patient is doing with meals. What kinds of things will you look for?

5. Your patient has a poor appetite. What can you do to encourage your patient to eat?

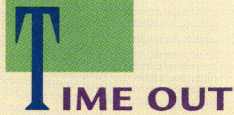

TIME OUT

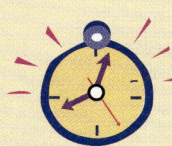

TIPS FOR TIME MANAGEMENT

SELF-DISCIPLINE TIP   Occasionally you may finish your work early and have time to spare. Avoid spending this extra time in the breakroom reading a magazine. Instead, use the time to restock supplies and talk with patients. Go back to the room of a patient who likes to chat or is lonely and sit with him or her. Visit a patient who does not have visitors very often.

The Urinary System and Related Care

22

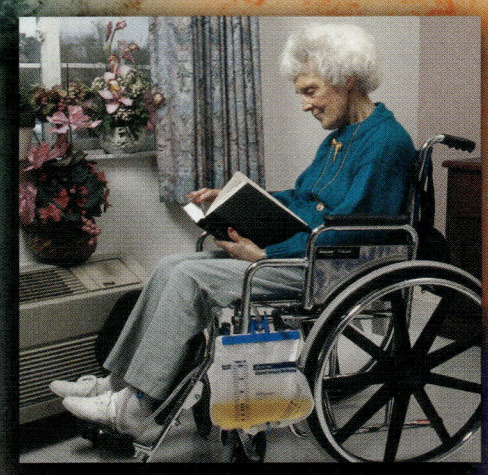

Several body systems participate in the elimination of waste products from the body. One such system is the urinary system. This vital body system plays a major role in maintaining homeostasis, the body's ability to maintain a steady state. Other systems that remove waste include the integumentary, respiratory, and digestive systems. Major organs of these systems include skin, lungs, and intestines, respectively. This chapter focuses on the four components of the urinary system—left and right kidneys, left and right ureters, bladder, and urethra—and the specific functions of these organs. The major function of this system is the formation and excretion of urine. The processes involved in the formation of urine and the significance of fluid balance in maintaining homeostasis are explained. A discussion of metric units of measurement required for monitoring and recording fluid intake and output are presented along with the concepts of force fluids, restrict fluids, and nothing by mouth (NPO). Your role is key in monitoring and recording fluid intake and output.

OBJECTIVES

When you have completed this chapter, you will be able to:

- State the main function of the urinary system.
- Label the four components of the urinary system and explain the function of each.
- Describe three processes by which urine is formed.
- Differentiate normal and abnormal urine.
- List common diseases and disorders of the urinary system.
- Explain fluid balance and imbalance.
- List the reasons for recording accurate measures of fluid intake and output.
- Accurately measure fluids using the metric system.
- Measure the capacity of serving containers.
- List ways to encourage a patient to increase fluid intake.
- Explain ways to restrict the patient's intake of fluid.
- List the ways in which the body loses fluid.
- Explain the function of urinary catheters.

KEY TERMS

absorb

balance of fluids

bladder distention

calibrated

convert

cubic centimeter

dehydration

discharge

edema

eliminate

evaporate

fluid

fluid balance

fluid imbalance

fluid intake

fluid output

force fluids

graduate

homeostasis

incontinent

indwelling urinary catheter

insensible fluid loss

nothing by mouth (NPO)

parenteral intake

peristaltic waves

perspiration

residual

restrict fluids

retain

tissue fluid

urinary system (excretory system)

urinate

urine

void

ANATOMY AND PHYSIOLOGY OF THE URINARY SYSTEM

urinary system (excretory system) The group of body components including the kidneys, ureters, bladder, and urethra that removes wastes from the blood and produces and eliminates urine

As nursing assistants you will have a major responsibility in helping other members of the health care team monitor the patient's urinary system function. The physician may order strict measurement of some patient's fluid intake and output. Since the **urinary system** is the system for excreting a large volume of fluid (urine), it is important that you understand some of the basic anatomy and physiology of the system (Figure 22–1). Descriptions of the four components that make up this system and the related function of each component follow.

■ Kidneys

The two kidneys are identical structures that look like lima beans. Fat and connective tissue surround the kidneys to provide support and help maintain the kidneys in normal position. The functional unit of the kidneys is called a *nephron*. Each kidney has more than one million nephrons. A nephron consists of a glomerulus, Bowman's capsule, and a tubular system. The glomerulus is a cluster of capillaries. This network of capillaries lies within a cupping of a tube known as Bowman's capsule. Extending from each Bowman's capsule is a renal tubule consisting of several sections. These different sections form the tubular system that consists of the proximal convoluted tubule, the descending limb of the loop of Henle, the ascending limb, the distal convoluted tubule, and a collecting tubule (see Figure 22–2).

FIGURE 22–1

The urinary system

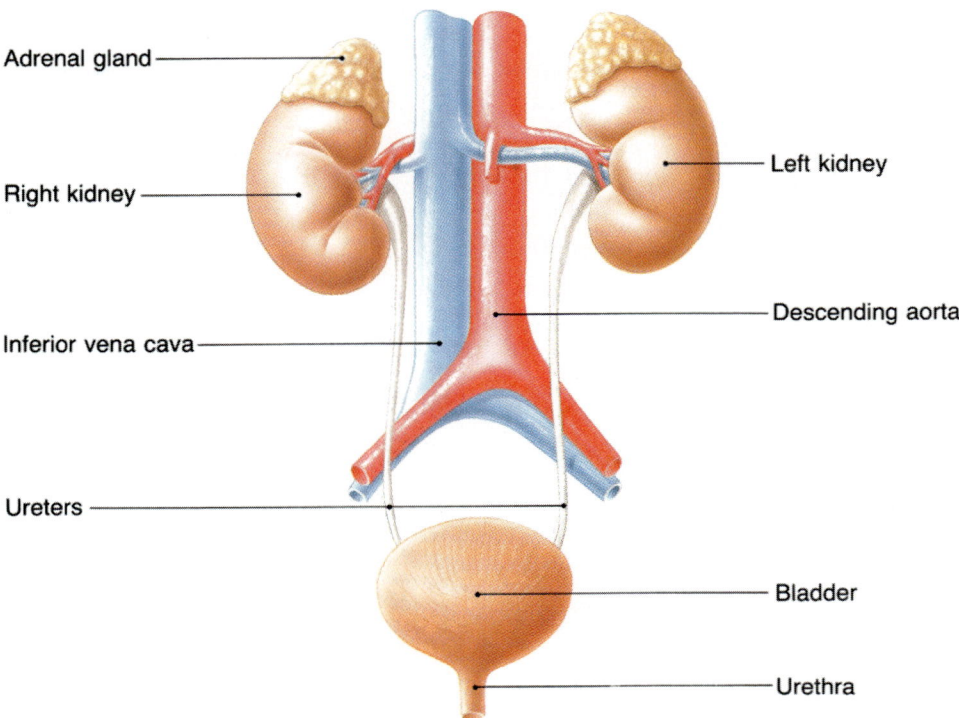

Adrenal gland

Right kidney

Inferior vena cava

Ureters

Left kidney

Descending aorta

Bladder

Urethra

FIGURE 22–2

The nephron unit

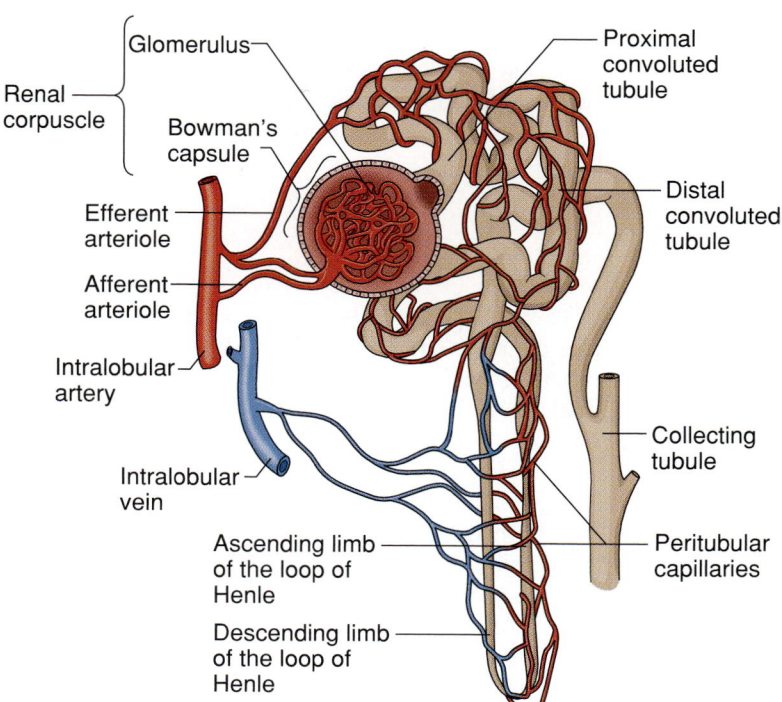

Formation of Urine

The main functions of the urinary system occur in the structural units (glomerulus, Bowman's capsule, and tubular system) of the nephrons. The three functions—glomerular filtration, tubular reabsorption, and tubular secretion—are the complex processes by which **urine** is formed and excreted by the kidney. Urine is the fluid secreted by the kidneys, stored in the bladder, and excreted through the urethra.

Step 1: Glomerular Filtration   Urine formation starts in the glomerulus with filtration of blood. The semipermeable membrane of the glomerulus allows free passage of water and certain solutes. This fluid is called glomerulus filtrate, and it flows into the Bowman's capsule. Glomerulus filtrate contains both essential and nonessential material.

Step 2: Tubular Reabsorption   Tubular reabsorption is the taking back of water and certain solutes—essential minerals dissolved in the water that the body needs. The process involves the movement of substances out of the filtrate into the blood. About 97–99 percent of the filtrate is reabsorbed by the tissues thereby restoring essential materials to the body.

Step 3: Tubular Secretion   Tubular secretion is the final step in the process of urine formation. It involves the movement of substances out of the blood into the filtrate for excretion thereby removing nonessential materials from the body.

urine The fluid secreted by the kidneys, stored in the bladder, and excreted through the urethra

Urine formation is the complex process that cleans blood plasma of unnecessary substances while selectively reabsorbing other essential materials. Specifically, waste products are removed and fluids, electrolytes, blood pressure, and pH are regulated to help the body maintain a normal state.

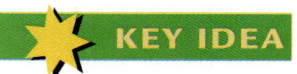

KEY IDEA

Ureters

Once urine is formed, it drips from the kidney into the ureter. The two ureters are tubes that help to form the renal pelvis at the end that connects to the kidney (see Figure 22–1).

peristaltic waves Waves
of involuntary contractions

These tubes are about 10–12 inches in length. The primary function of the ureters is to collect urine (in renal pelvis) and drain urine to the bladder. Urine flow through the ureters is aided by **peristaltic waves**, or involuntary contractions, similar to those of the digestive tract. Once urine drains from the ureters into the bladder, there are valves around the openings to prevent the back flow of urine when the bladder contracts. The urinary tract is sterile.

Bladder

void To urinate, pass
water

The bladder is the third component in the urinary system, and it serves as a reservoir for urine before it leaves the body. This collapsible organ is key to the excretion of urine. The muscular wall of the bladder contains stretch receptors. When these receptors are stimulated by as little as 300 cc to a completely full bladder, messages are sent to the brain that cause the person to urinate, or **void** (discharge urine from the body).

Urethra

The urethra, a small tube leading from the bladder floor to the external environment, serves to empty the bladder of collected urine. Because the urethra is open to the outside of the body, it may also provide a passageway for disease-causing organisms. The normal flow of urine will generally flush bacteria out. When organisms enter the bladder, a bladder infection (cystitis) may occur. The infection may also spread through the ureters to the kidney, causing a kidney infection (nephritis). Cystitis and nephritis are often called urinary-tract infections. Long-term nephritis may lead to kidney damage.

Women have shorter urethras than men. Therefore, women are at greater risk to acquire urinary tract infections.

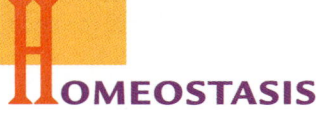

DISEASES AND DISORDERS OF THE URINARY SYSTEM

In a healthy person, fresh voided urine is a clear, straw color that turns cloudy upon standing. Painful urination, discoloration of urine, or failure to void are abnormal conditions that should be reported to appropriate members of the patient care team. Table 22–1 lists some common diseases and disorders of the urinary system and the causes, results, or symptoms associated with the disease or disorder.

HOMEOSTASIS

homeostasis Stability of
all body functions at
normal levels

Homeostasis is the body's attempt to keep its internal environment stable or in balance. Examples of the body's ability to maintain homeostasis are:

- The body temperature stays constant
- The blood pressure stays within specific limits
- The chemistry of the blood stays within certain normal limits

The urinary system is perhaps the most important system for maintaining homeostasis. This is because, as described above, the urinary system determines the content

TABLE 22–1

Diseases and Disorders of the Urinary System

DISEASE OR DISORDER	CAUSE, RESULT, OR SYMPTOM
Acute renal failure	Loss of kidney function
Anuria	No urine
Cancer of the urinary bladder	Malignant tumor
Chronic renal failure	Progressive deterioration of kidney function
Cystitis	Inflammation of the urinary bladder
Dysuria	Painful voiding
Hematuria	Blood in the urine
Hydronephrosis	Distention of the pelvis of one or both kidneys (urine is being made but cannot be excreted due to urinary back up)
Injury to the bladder	Due to trauma
Nocturia	Frequency of urination at night
Oliguria	Very small amount of urine in 24 hours
Polyuria	Unusually large volume of urine in 24 hours
Pyelonephritis	Infection of the kidney (acute or chronic)
Pyuria	Pus in the urine, an infection
Renal colic	Sharp, severe pain in lower back over kidney that accompanies forcible dilation of a ureter due to a stone or urinary calculus
Tuberculosis of the kidney	Caused by Mycobacterium tuberculosis in the kidney
Tumors of the kidney	Considered malignant until proven otherwise
Urethral stricture	Narrowing of the urethra caused by infection or instrumentation; results in frequent voiding, dysuria, and hematuria (blood in the urine)
Urethritis	Inflammation of the urethra, often by sexually transmitted diseases such as chlamydia or gonorrhea
Urinary retention	Inability to urinate
Urinary tract infection (UTI)	Presence of pathogenic microorganisms in the urinary tract
Urolithiasis (renal calculi)	Presence of stones in the urinary (excretory) system

(water and chemical) of the blood. The blood content, in turn, determines the content of the **tissue fluid**, which is the immediate environment of the cells. Many changes in kidney function, some normal, can be found in urine samples. Diagnostic studies of the urinary system include: urinalysis, creatinine clearance, urine culture, residual urine, protein determination, and glucose testing. You may be directly involved in collecting urine samples and performing certain tests (see Chapter 23). Changes in kidney function are also revealed in accurate measurement of intake and output. Sometimes in illness, especially after surgery, the patient is unable to void (**urinate**).

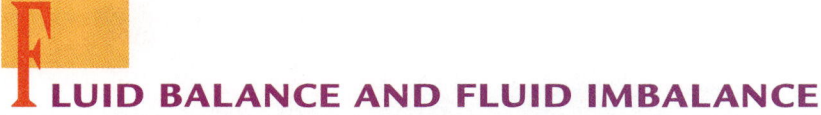

FLUID BALANCE AND FLUID IMBALANCE

Fluid balance means that the body eliminates just about the same amount that it takes in. An **imbalance of fluid** occurs when the body keeps, or **retains**, too much **fluid** or when the body loses too much fluid (Figure 22–3). In some medical conditions, fluid may be held in the body tissues and cause them to swell. This is called **edema**. When a patient experiences a fluid loss, or decrease in the amount of fluids in tissues, it is called **dehydration**. Inadequate fluid intake may be caused by vomiting, bleeding, wound drainage, severe diarrhea, or excessive sweating (**perspiration**). When a patient's body loses more fluid than is taken in or when the body retains fluid (puts out less fluid than it has taken in) the doctor can treat the condition in various ways. A

tissue fluid A watery environment around each cell that acts as a place of exchange for gases, food, and waste products between the cells and the blood

urinate To discharge urine from the body; other words for this function are void, micturate, and pass water

fluid balance The same amount of fluid that is taken in by the body is given out by the body

fluid imbalance When too much fluid is kept in the body or when too much fluid is lost

retain To keep or hold in

fluid Applies to liquid substances

edema Abnormal swelling of a part of the body caused by fluid collecting in that area; usually the swelling is in the ankles, legs, hands, or abdomen

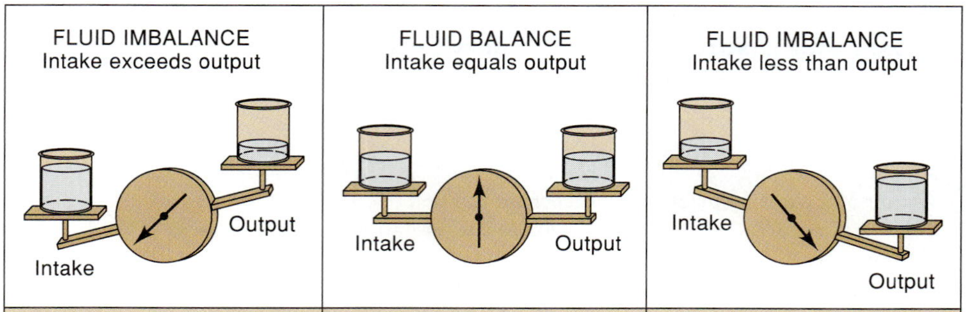

FIGURE 22–3

Fluid intake and output

FLUID IMBALANCE Intake exceeds output	FLUID BALANCE Intake equals output	FLUID IMBALANCE Intake less than output
Results from: Excessive intake . . . large amounts of • Liquids • Food or Restricted output . . . limited amounts of • Urine • Perspiration	**Results from:** Normal intake of • Liquids • Food • Breathing (inhaling) or Normal output • Breathing (exhaling) • Perspiration • Urine • Feces	**Results from:** Restricted intake . . . limited amounts of • Liquids • Food or Excessive output . . . large amounts of • Urine • Vomitus • Blood • Drainage • Perspiration • Stool (diarrhea)

dehydration A decrease in the amount of water in the tissues occurring when fluid output exceeds input or intake

perspiration Sweat

balance of fluids see *fluid balance*

specific method is prescribed to meet the needs of the individual patient. The only way a doctor can know when a patient's **balance of fluids** is not right is by knowing the patient's measurable intake and output.

KEY IDEA

A starving person can lose half of his body protein and almost half his body weight and still live, but losing only one-fifth of the body's fluid will result in death. This is why it is very important for the doctor to know the patient's balance of fluid.

Water is essential to human life (Figure 22–4). Next to oxygen, water is the most important thing for the body. About 50–60 percent of the adult human body is water. In an

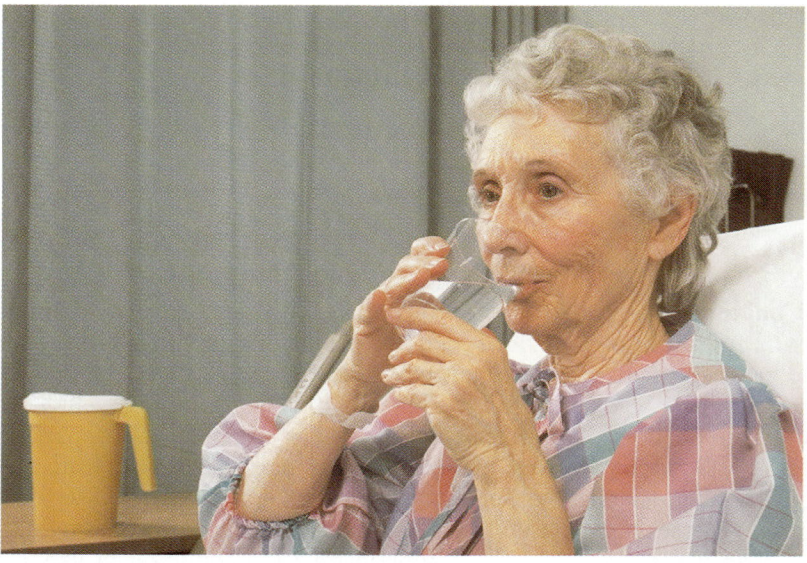

FIGURE 22–4

Water is essential to human life

infant 70–80 percent of the body composition is water; this places infants at high risk when fluid is lost. On the other hand, older adults are also at risk because of a decrease in the body's water content to about 45–50 percent.

◼ Fluid Intake

Through eating and drinking, the average healthy adult will take in about 3 quarts (3,312 cc) of fluid every day. This is his **fluid intake**. Although solid foods also contain some liquid, most of the fluids in the body are taken in when a person drinks liquids. Therefore, a patient's *fluid intake* includes everything the patient drinks: water, milk, milk drinks, fruit juices, soup, tea, coffee, or anything liquid. Ice cream and gelatin also are counted as liquids (Figure 22–5). Fluids taken in through an intravenous tube and/or nasogastrointestinal tube are also included in the patient's total fluid intake. Fluid taken in intravenously is referred to as **parenteral intake**. Fluid intake needs increase with high temperatures (weather), exercise, fever, illness, and excessive fluid loss.

◼ Fluid Output

Fluid output is the sum total of liquids that come out of the body. Most adults will eliminate the same amount of fluid taken in. Therefore, the adult above also will **eliminate** about 3 quarts (3,312 cc) of fluid every day. Fluid is discharged from the body of a healthy person in several ways:

- Most of the fluid passes through the kidneys and is discharged as urine

- Some of the fluid is lost from the body through perspiration

- Some fluid is **evaporated** from the lungs in breathing

- The rest is **absorbed** and **discharged** through the intestinal system

To urinate means to discharge urine from the body. Other terms for this body function are void and pass water. Fluid that is lost by breathing and perspiration is called **insensible fluid loss**. Approximately 100–200 cc of fluid is discharged from the body in feces. Output also includes emesis (vomitus), drainage from a wound or from the stomach, loss of blood, and diarrhea.

fluid intake The fluid taken into the body, from whatever source

parenteral intake Fluids taken in intravenously

fluid output The fluid passed or excreted out of the body; for example urine, vomit, diarrhea

eliminate To rid the body of waste products, to excrete, expel, remove, put out

evaporate To pass off as vapor, as water evaporating into the air

absorb To take or soak in, up, or through

discharge Flowing out of material (secretion or excretion) from any part of the body such as pus, feces, urine, or drainage from a wound

insensible fluid loss Fluid that is lost from the body without being noticed, such as in perspiration or air breathed out

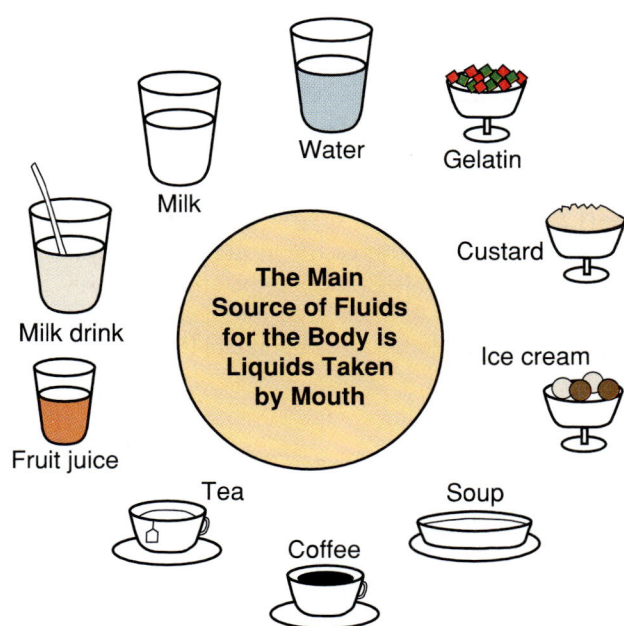

FIGURE 22–5

Although solid foods also contain some liquid, most of the fluids in the body are taken in when a person drinks liquids

It is difficult to measure accurately the amount of fluid discharged through evaporation and breathing. Therefore, a person may seem to have a greater fluid intake than output. There is, however, a fluid balance in the normally functioning body.

Many times the health care team will help with maintaining fluid balance by increasing or decreasing a patient's fluid intake or providing medical interventions to aid in the elimination of fluid. Therefore, it is very important for members of the nursing staff to keep accurate records of fluid intake and output. The record of the patient's intake and output is kept for a full 24-hour period. These records may be kept for any period of time (shift, days, or weeks) as prescribed by the physician. With some patients, the doctor is only interested in knowing the 24 hour totals. However, in sicker patients and patients with acute renal failure, he may want to know the fluid balance on an hour by hour basis. In some cases, the fluid balance may be monitored less frequently than every hour. The most important thing for you to remember is that the **records must be accurate**.

UNIT OF MEASUREMENT

The metric system of measurement is used in many countries of the world. In the United States, we normally use one system for measuring liquids (ounces, pints, quarts) and a different system for measuring lengths (inches, feet, yards, miles). You probably have already noticed that many quantities used in the health care field are measured in cubic centimeters or milliliters. Because most institutions use these terms for measuring intake and output, you should understand what they mean.

Scientists, engineers, and many health care institution personnel use the metric system for measuring liquids, lengths, and weight. The basic metric unit of measurement of length is the meter, which is a little longer than a yard. A centimeter [one one-hundredth (1/100) of a meter] is about four-tenths (4/10) of an inch.

■ Cubic Centimeters

cubic centimeter Having a volume equal to a cube whose edges are 1 centimeter long

The term cc is an abbreviation for **cubic centimeter**, a unit of measurement in the metric system. A cubic centimeter can be thought of as a square block with each edge of the block 1 centimeter long (Figure 22–6). If we filled this block with water, we would have 1 cubic centimeter (1 cc) of water.

The liter is the basic unit of liquid measure in the metric system. It is approximately the same as a quart. A milliliter (1/1000 liter) is the amount that would fill a cubic centimeter. Therefore the two units are often used interchangeably. The patient's liquid intake is measured in cubic centimeters (cc) or milliliters (ml).

■ Graduate Containers

graduate A measuring cup marked along its side to show various amounts so that the material placed in the cup can be measured accurately; the marks are called *calibrations*

calibrated Marked with lines and numbers for measuring

A container called a **graduate** (Figure 22–7) or a measuring cup is used to measure intake and output (I&O). The side of the graduate is marked (**calibrated**) with a row of short lines and numbers. These show the amount of liquid in both milliliters and ounces (see Table 22–2). This graduate is like the measuring cup you use at home to measure ingredients for cooking, only larger. Another calibrated graduate used in the home is a baby's milk bottle. This, too, is marked with a row of short lines and numbers. They

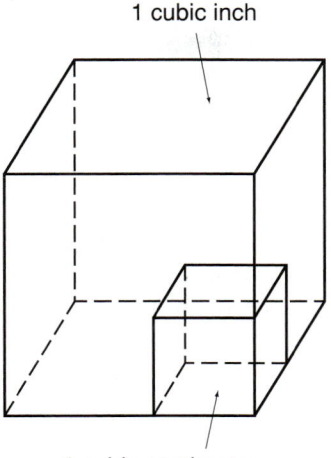

1 cubic inch

1 cubic centimeter

FIGURE 22–6

Actual size of cubic inch and cubic centimeter

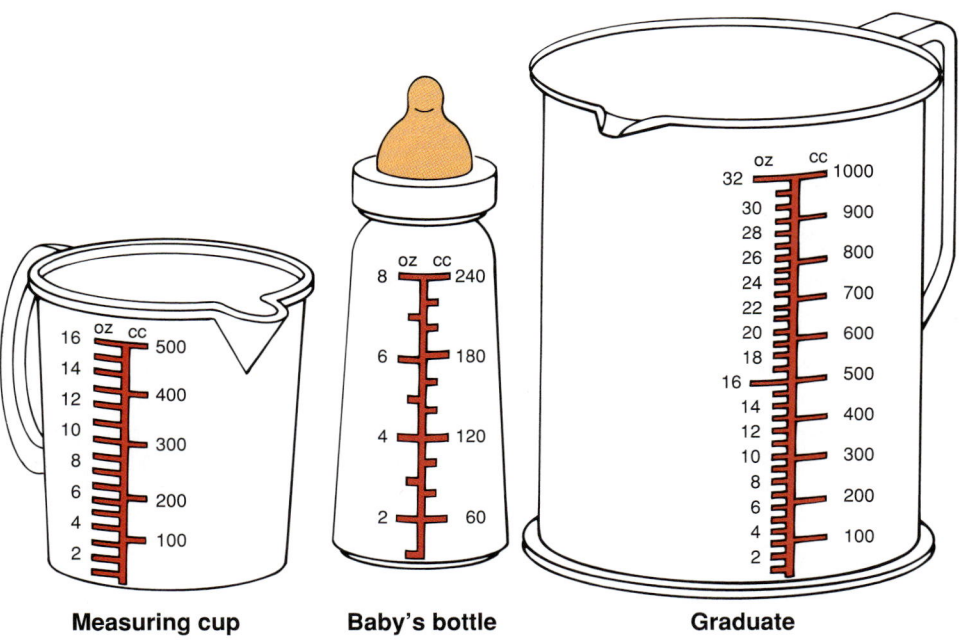

Measuring cup   **Baby's bottle**   **Graduate**

FIGURE 22–7

Examples of calibrated containers

TABLE 22–2

U.S. Customary Liquid Measure with Approximate Equivalent Apothecary and Metric Measurements

cc = cubic centimeter	150 cc = 5 oz
ml = milliliter	180 cc = 6 oz
oz = ounce	210 cc = 7 oz
1cc = 1 ml	240 cc = 8 oz
1/4 teaspoon = 1 cc	270 cc = 9 oz
1 teaspoon = 4 cc	300 cc = 10 oz
30 cc = 1 oz	500 cc = 1 pint
60 cc = 2 oz	1000 cc = 1 quart
90 cc = 3 oz	4000 cc = 1 gallon
120 cc = 4 oz	

TABLE 22–3

Capacities of Serving Containers

4-oz juice cup	120 cc
6-oz cup	180 cc
8-oz cup	240 cc
12-oz cup	360 cc
1-cup milk carton	240 cc
4-oz ice cream cup	120 cc
6-oz Jell-O cup	180 cc
6-oz coffee cup	180 cc
1-qt water pitcher	1000 cc

show the amount of milk in both ounces and milliliters. When full, most baby bottles contain 8 ounces, or 240 cubic centimeters (cc). To give the baby 4 ounces of milk, or 120 cc, you would fill it half-full or to the 4 ounce line.

Some things to remember about graduate containers are:

- They are all calibrated

- They are made of metal, glass, or plastic

- They are used for measuring liquids in cubic centimeters (cc)

- They are used for measuring liquids in ounces (oz)

- The measuring cup is used to measure liquids in the home

- The baby's bottle is used to measure liquids in the home

- The calibrated graduate is used to measure fluid

It is very important that you observe the exact amounts of fluids taken in by the patient and that you record them accurately. You will have to measure the amount of liquid contained in each serving container, bowl, glass, or cup used by the patient. If your institution does not have a list of the amounts contained in each container, bowl, glass, or cup, you will find it helpful to make such a list yourself (see Table 22–3).

MEASURING AND RECORDING FLUID INTAKE

Tell the patient that her fluid intake is being measured and recorded. Encourage her to help you, if she is not too ill, by asking her to keep track of how much liquid she drinks. This is your responsibility, however, not the patient's. Also, inform family members and visitors that patient's fluid intake is being recorded.

Fluids taken in by patients intravenously are recorded by the registered nurse. This record may also be kept on the intake and output sheet in a special column headed Parenteral Intake.

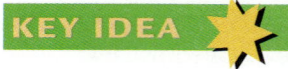

KEY IDEA

Regardless of how fluids are consumed, the important thing is that the doctor know as accurately as possible how much fluid the patient has taken in. *This is your responsibility, not the patient's.* You must monitor what your patients have on their meal trays and any fluids taken between meals.

The proper time for the nursing assistant to record the patient's fluids on the intake and output sheet is as soon as the patient has consumed the fluids. Before the end of each shift, the complete amount of intake should be totaled (added). Your task will be to remember to record all fluid taken each time the patient eats or drinks. Think about fluid intake every time you remove a tray, water pitcher, glass, or cup from a patient's bedside. Remember especially to check the water pitcher.

When measuring fluid intake, you will have to note the difference between the amount the patient actually drinks and the amount he leaves in the serving container. You will be required to **convert** (change) amounts such as a bowl of soup, glass of orange juice, or cup of tea into cc (cubic centimeters) when recording them.

convert Change

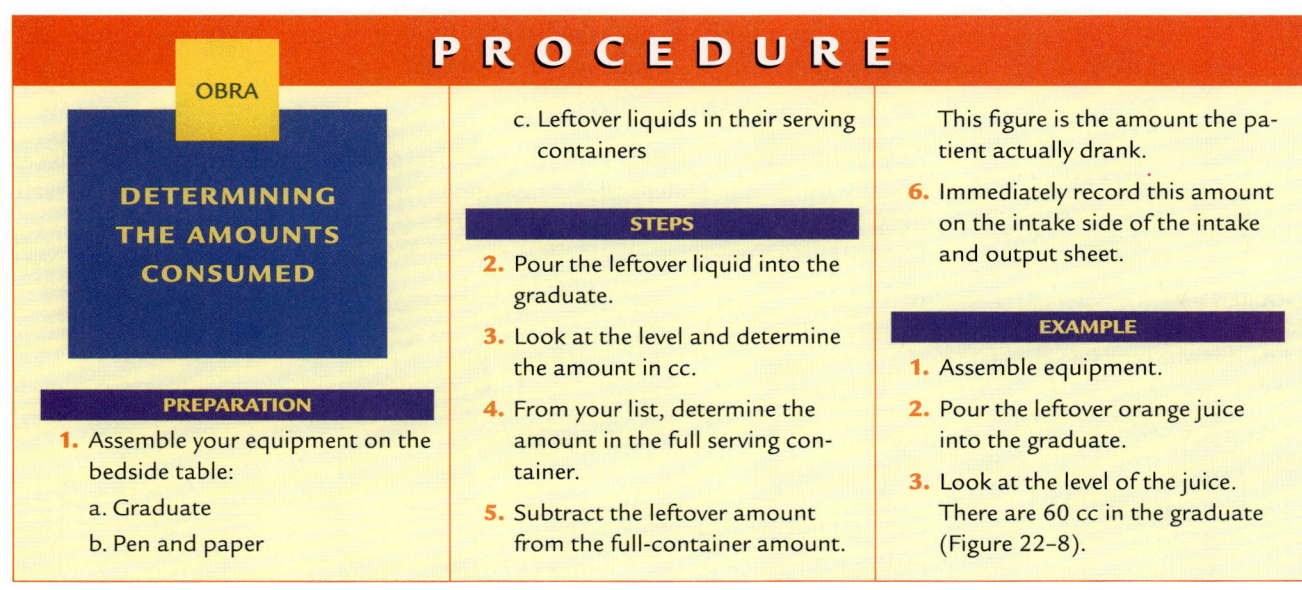

PROCEDURE

OBRA

MEASURING THE CAPACITY OF SERVING CONTAINERS

PREPARATION

1. Assemble your equipment in the utility room:

   a. Complete set of dishes, bowls, cups, and glasses used by the patients

   b. Graduate (measuring cup)

   c. Water

   d. Pen and paper

STEPS

2. Fill the first container with water.

3. Pour this water into the graduate.

4. Place the graduate on a flat surface for accuracy in measurement.

5. At eye level, carefully look at the level of the water and determine the amount in cc (cubic centimeters).

6. Write this information on the paper. For example, one carton of milk = 240 cc.

7. Repeat these steps for each dish, glass, bowl, or cup used by the patient.

FOLLOW-UP

8. You will have a complete list to use when measuring intake.

PROCEDURE

OBRA

DETERMINING THE AMOUNTS CONSUMED

PREPARATION

1. Assemble your equipment on the bedside table:

   a. Graduate

   b. Pen and paper

   c. Leftover liquids in their serving containers

STEPS

2. Pour the leftover liquid into the graduate.

3. Look at the level and determine the amount in cc.

4. From your list, determine the amount in the full serving container.

5. Subtract the leftover amount from the full-container amount. This figure is the amount the patient actually drank.

6. Immediately record this amount on the intake side of the intake and output sheet.

EXAMPLE

1. Assemble equipment.

2. Pour the leftover orange juice into the graduate.

3. Look at the level of the juice. There are 60 cc in the graduate (Figure 22–8).

PROCEDURE (CONTINUED)

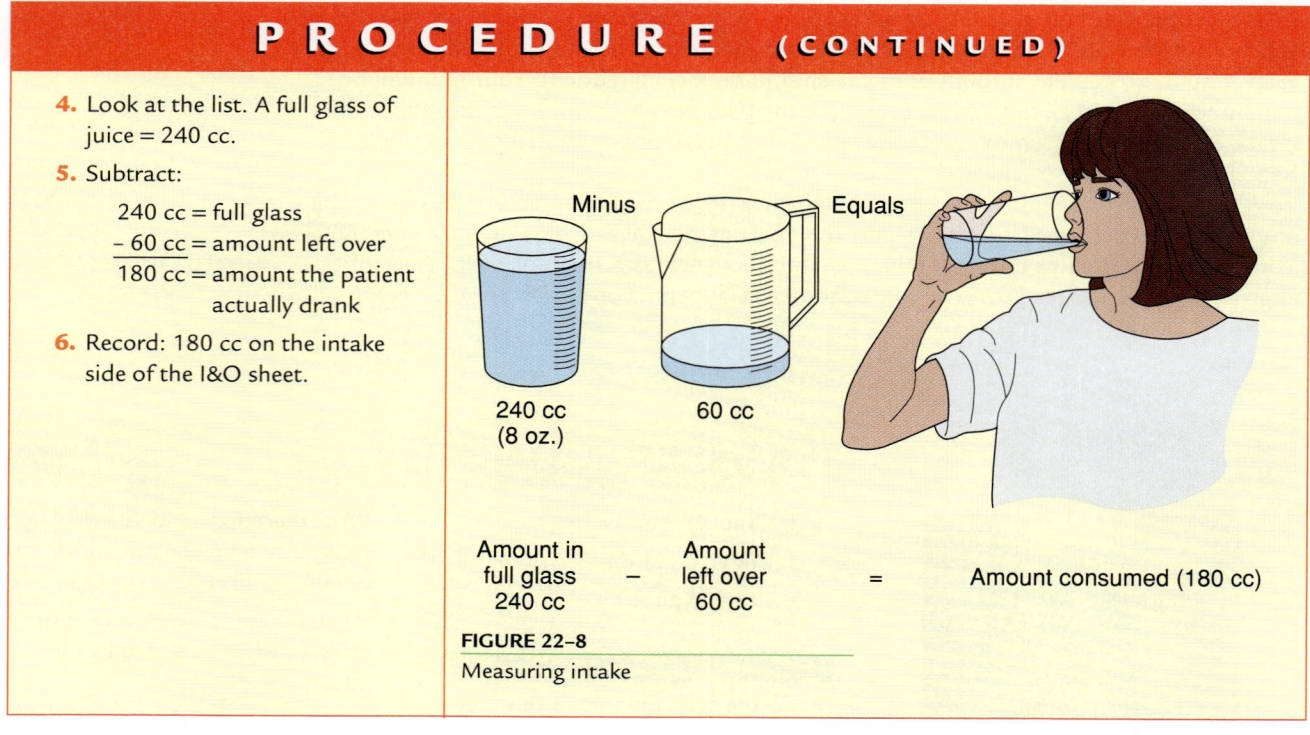

4. Look at the list. A full glass of juice = 240 cc.

5. Subtract:

240 cc = full glass
– 60 cc = amount left over
180 cc = amount the patient actually drank

6. Record: 180 cc on the intake side of the I&O sheet.

Minus   Equals

240 cc
(8 oz.)   60 cc

| Amount in full glass 240 cc | – | Amount left over 60 cc | = | Amount consumed (180 cc) |

FIGURE 22–8
Measuring intake

FORCE FLUIDS, RESTRICT FLUIDS, AND NPO

Force Fluids (FF)

force fluids Extra fluids to be taken in by a patient according to the doctor's orders (FF)

Patients who need to have more fluids added to their normal intake are put on **force fluids** and often need encouragement to drink more (Figure 22–9). FF is the abbreviation for force fluids. Patients may also be placed on FF when they fail to take in the normal amount of fluid that the body needs. A list of ways you can persuade the patient to drink more fluids and guidelines for patients on force fluids follow.

■ Offer fluids in small quantities

■ As permitted by the patient's therapeutic diet, provide different kinds of fluids, especially drinks the patient prefers; examples are hot tea, gelatin, soda, ice cream, milk, juice, broth, coffee, custard, and water

FIGURE 22–9

Sign placed on door or bed of patient who is on forced fluids

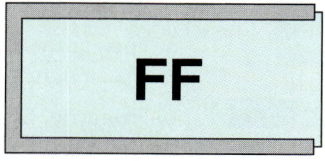

FF

■ Offer liquids without being asked

■ Remind patient of the importance of fluids in getting better

GUIDELINES

FORCE FLUIDS

- Verify that patient is on force fluids.
- Place a sign stating *force fluids* on the bed or door.
- Encourage the patient to drink the amount of fluids required. For example, 800 cc every 8 hours means the patient would have to drink 100 cc every hour. At the end of the 8-hour shift, the patient would have taken in 800 cc of fluids.
- Record the amount taken in by the patient in ccs on the intake side of the intake and output sheet.

Restrict Fluids

For some patients, the doctor writes orders to **restrict fluids** (Figure 22–10). This means that fluids may be limited to certain amounts. When you are caring for a patient on restrict fluids, it is important to follow orders exactly and to measure accurately. Your calm and reassuring attitude can make a big difference in how the patient feels and reacts. Usually, the water pitcher is removed from the bedside. Frequent oral hygiene is often necessary as it helps keep the mucous membranes of the mouth moist.

restrict fluids Fluids that are limited to certain amounts

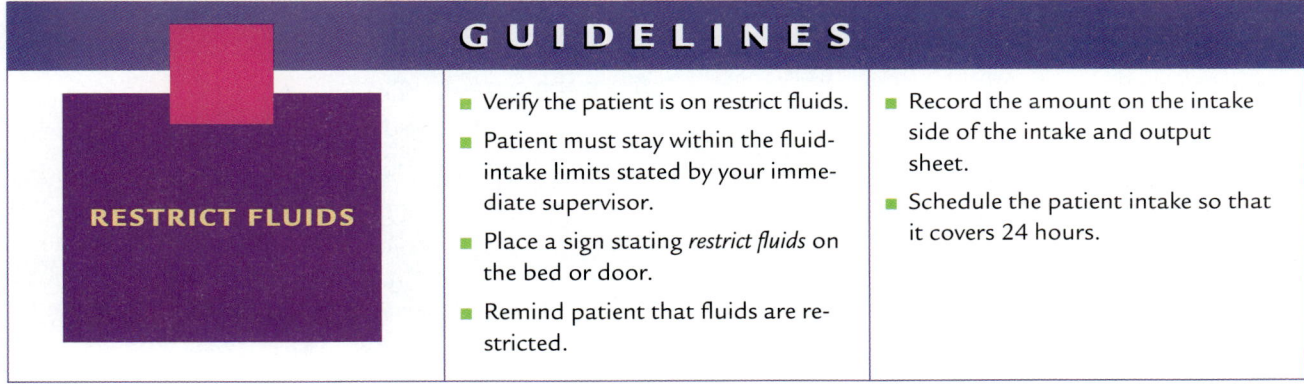

RESTRICT FLUIDS

FIGURE 22–10
Sign placed on door or bed of patient who is on restricted fluids

GUIDELINES

RESTRICT FLUIDS

- Verify the patient is on restrict fluids.
- Patient must stay within the fluid-intake limits stated by your immediate supervisor.
- Place a sign stating *restrict fluids* on the bed or door.
- Remind patient that fluids are restricted.
- Record the amount on the intake side of the intake and output sheet.
- Schedule the patient intake so that it covers 24 hours.

Nothing by Mouth (NPO)

For some patients, the doctor writes orders that the patient is to have **nothing by mouth**. This means that the patient cannot eat or drink anything at all. You may be asked to take away the patient's water pitcher and glass at midnight. You will post a sign saying NPO (Figure 22–11). NPO is taken from the Latin *nils per os,* which means nothing by mouth. Persons are usually NPO before and after surgery and before some lab tests or certain X-ray procedures. An NPO sign is put at the foot or the head of the bed or on the door of the patient's room. Some institutions do not allow a patient on NPO to have oral hygiene. Patients often become very irritable when they are not allowed to have anything to eat or drink. They may, therefore, be hard for you to deal with. Calm and reassuring behavior on your part can help the patient go through a very uncomfortable period. A smile and a few kind words will go a long way here.

nothing by mouth (NPO) Cannot eat or drink anything at all

FIGURE 22–11

Sign placed on door or bed of patient who is on nothing by mouth restriction

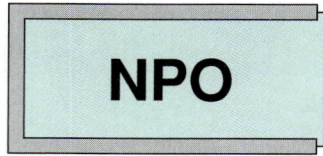

NPO

G U I D E L I N E S

OBRA

NOTHING BY MOUTH

- Verify the patient is on NPO.
- Explain to patient the NPO (nothing by mouth) restriction.
- Place a sign stating *NPO* on the bed or door.
- Remove the water pitcher and anything else with which the patient could take a drink or eat.

- Do not give any liquids or food to this patient.
- Make a note on the intake side of the intake and output sheet that the patient is NPO.

MEASURING AND RECORDING FLUID OUTPUT

A patient who is on intake and output must have both measured and recorded. This means that every time the patient uses the urinal, emesis basin, or bedpan, the urine and other liquids must be measured and recorded (Figure 22–12).

FIGURE 22–12

Intake and output sheet

INTAKE AND OUTPUT SHEET

Hospital # 125689400-2   Patient Name Mary Smith Jones

Date 1-2-XX   Room # 4011A

	INTAKE			OUTPUT			
				URINE		GASTRIC	
Time 11—7	BY MOUTH	TUBE	PARENTERAL	VOIDED	CATHETER	EMESIS	SUCTION
7:30a	120cc			250cc			
9:45	240cc						
10:30	60cc						
11:00				350cc			
11:20						200cc	
12:Noon	N.P.O.						
TOTAL	420cc	– – – –	– – – –	600cc	– – – –	200cc	– – – –
Time 7—3	NPO						
2:50p				450cc			
3:00			1000cc	200cc			300cc
TOTAL	– – –	– – – –	1000cc	650cc			300cc
Time 3—11	NPO						
5:00p				200cc			
11:00			1000cc	480cc			
							250cc
TOTAL	– – –	– – – –	1000cc	680cc	– – – –	– – –	250cc
24 HOUR TOTAL	320cc	– – – –	2000cc	1930cc	– – – –	– – – –	550cc

24 Hour Grand Total¥Intake 2320cc   24 Hour Grand Total¥Output 2480cc

You should tell the patient his output is being measured and ask him to cooperate. A female patient must urinate in a bedpan or specipan. The specipan is a disposable container that fits into the toilet bowl under the seat. The specipan can be placed in the patient's toilet bowl, if the patient is allowed out of bed. This pan covers only the front of the toilet, so stool can be expelled through the back of the toilet and toilet paper can be tossed. Ask the patient not to place toilet paper in the bedpan. Provide a wastepaper basket for her. Then discard tissue into the toilet or hopper. Female patients must also be asked not to let their bowels move while urinating into a bedpan. Male patients on output must be instructed to use a urinal.

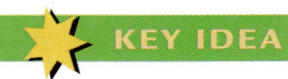

KEY IDEA

Provide each patient on output with a bedpan, specipan, or urinal. Any device used for measuring a patient's output must be used for that patient only and disposed of or sterilized when the patient is discharged. Be sure to follow Standard Precautions.

P R O C E D U R E

OBRA

MEASURING URINARY OUTPUT

PREPARATION

1. Assemble your equipment in the patient's bathroom:

   a. Bedpan, cover, urinal, or specipan

   b. Graduate (measuring container or calibrated container)

   c. Intake and output sheet

   d. Pencil or pen

   e. Disposable gloves

2. Wash your hands and put on gloves.

STEPS

3. Pour the urine from the bedpan or urinal into a graduate.

4. Place the graduate on a flat surface for accuracy in measurement.

5. At eye level, carefully look at the level of urine in the graduate to see the number reached by the level of the urine.

6. Record this amount in cc, as well as the time, on the output side of the intake and output sheet.

FOLLOW-UP

7. Wash, rinse, and return the graduate to its proper place.

8. Wash, rinse, and return the urinal or bedpan to its proper place.

9. Dispose of gloves and wash your hands.

10. Report to your immediate supervisor:

    ■ That you have measured the output for the patient.

    ■ Your observations of anything unusual.

■ Urinary Catheters

The urinary catheter is the most common kind of catheter used for draining urine out of the body (Figure 22–13). This catheter (made of plastic or silicon) is inserted through the patient's urethra into the bladder. This catheter may also be used when a patient is unable to void (urinate) naturally, or it may be used to measure the amount of urine left in the bladder after a patient has voided naturally (**residual** urine). When a patient is unable to void, the bladder may stretch out. The bladder is distended and the patient's symptom is described as urinary retention, or a **bladder distention**.

Sometimes a urinary catheter is used for only one withdrawal of urine. Sometimes, however, it is kept in place in the bladder for a number of days or even weeks.

Sometimes the bladder-drainage catheter is used to help keep an **incontinent** patient dry. An incontinent patient is one who cannot control his urine and/or feces. An **indwelling urinary catheter** is a tube inserted through the patient's urethra into the bladder to allow for urinary drainage. It really is two tubes, one inside the other. The inside tube is connected at one end to a kind of balloon. After the catheter has been inserted, the balloon is filled with water or air so the catheter will not slip out through the urethra. Urine drains out of the bladder through the outer tube. The urine collects in a container attached

residual Remaining or left over

bladder distention A stretching out of the bladder when urine produced is not excreted

incontinent Unable to control urine or feces

indwelling urinary catheter A bladder drainage tube that is allowed to remain in place within the bladder

FIGURE 22–13

Urinary catheter in the male

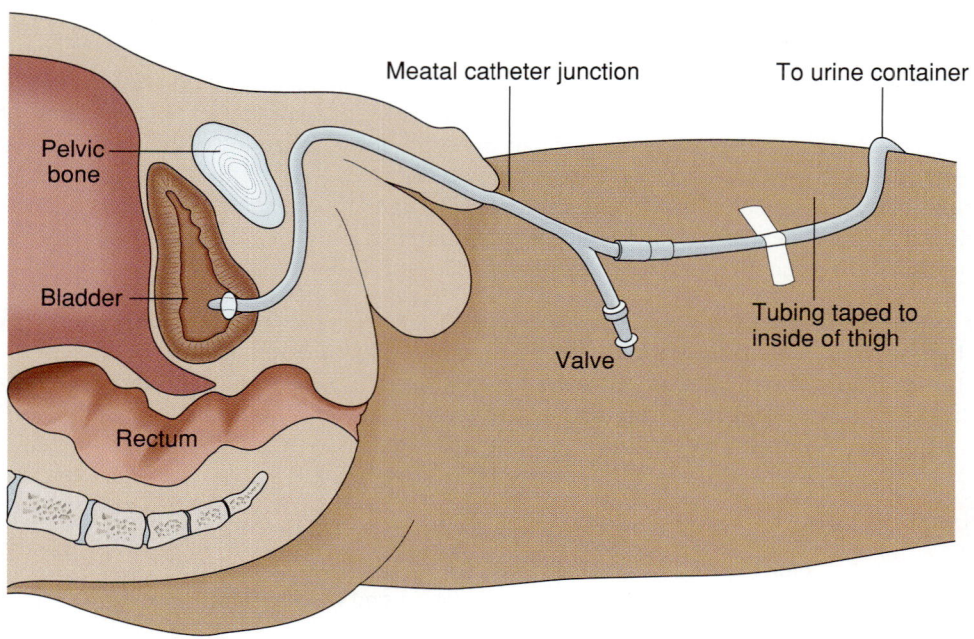

to the bed frame lower than the patient's urinary bladder. This is always maintained as a closed system, which means it is never opened except when emptying the urine collecting bag. A commercially prepared condom catheter is sometimes used for external drainage of urine from a male incontinent patient.

You will empty this container, measure the urine, and record the amount. This will always be done whenever it is full and always before the end of your working shift. The measurement is not taken from the soft expandable plastic urine collection container. A hard plastic graduate is always used as it is more accurate.

Figure 22–14 shows a drainage bag used for ambulatory patients and Figure 22–15 shows the plastic urine container for the nonambulatory patient.

GUIDELINES

OBRA

INDWELLING URINARY CATHETER

■ Check from time to time to make sure the level of urine has increased. If the level stays the same, report this to your immediate supervisor.

■ If the patient says he feels that his bladder is full or that he needs to urinate, report this to your immediate supervisor.

■ If the patient is allowed to get out of bed for short periods, the bag goes with the patient. It must be held lower than the patient's urinary bladder (below hip level) at all times to prevent the urine in the tubing and bag from draining back into the urinary bladder.

■ Check to make sure there are no kinks in the catheter and tubing. Be sure the patient is not lying on the catheter or the tubing. This would stop the flow of urine.

■ The catheter may be loosely taped or strapped at all times to the pa-

tient's inner thigh. This keeps it from being pulled on or being pulled out of the bladder.

■ Most patients with urinary drainage through a catheter are on output. You must keep a careful record of urinary output.

■ Keep tubing and drainage bag from touching the floor.

■ Catheter care should be done as ordered for these patients.

■ Report to your immediate supervisor any complaints the patient may have of burning, tenderness, or pain in the urethral area or any changes in the appearance of the urine.

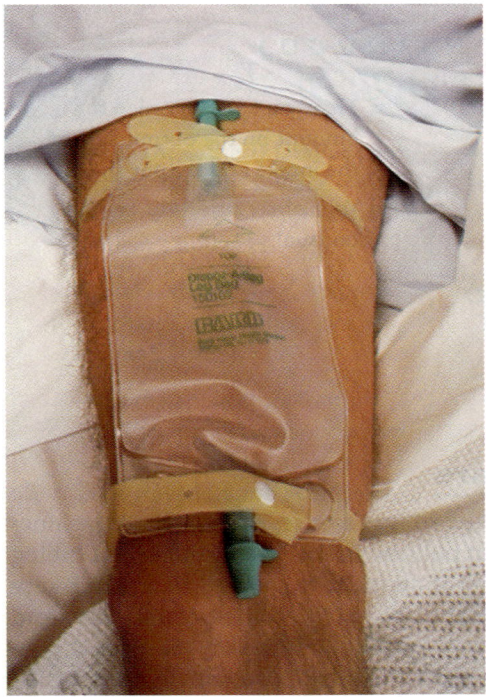

FIGURE 22–14

Leg drainage bag for ambulatory patient

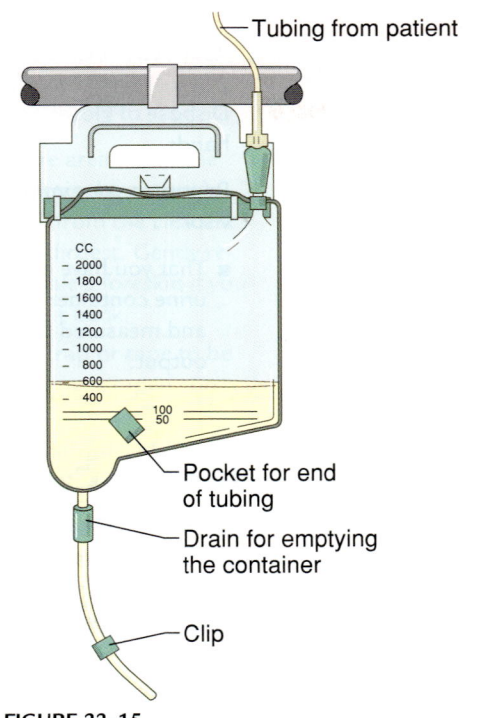

FIGURE 22–15

Plastic urine container for nonambulatory patient

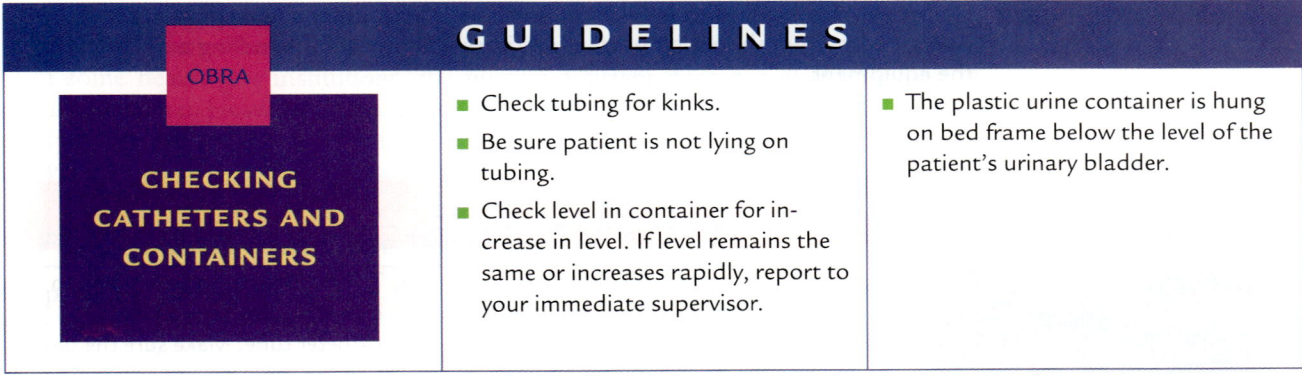

GUIDELINES

OBRA

CHECKING CATHETERS AND CONTAINERS

- Check tubing for kinks.
- Be sure patient is not lying on tubing.
- Check level in container for increase in level. If level remains the same or increases rapidly, report to your immediate supervisor.

- The plastic urine container is hung on bed frame below the level of the patient's urinary bladder.

PROCEDURE

OBRA

EMPTYING URINE FROM AN INDWELLING CATHETER CONTAINER

PREPARATION

1. Assemble your equipment:
   a. Calibrated graduate
   b. Alcohol swab
   c. Disposable gloves
2. Wash your hands and put on gloves.

STEPS

3. Open the drain at the bottom of the plastic urine container and let the urine run into the graduate; then close the drain, wipe with alcohol swab, and replace in the holder on the bag.

FIGURE 23–5

Write down the 24-hour period in which the urine is collected

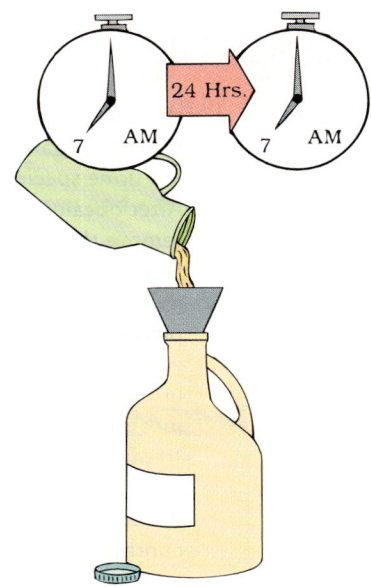

PROCEDURE

COLLECTING A 24-HOUR URINE SPECIMEN

PREPARATION

1. Assemble your equipment:

   a. Large container, usually a 1-liter plastic disposable bottle

   b. Funnel, if the neck of the bottle is small

   c. Graduate, used for measuring output, if the patient is on intake and output

   d. Patient's bedpan, urinal, or specipan

   e. Label for the container

   f. Laboratory request slip, which should be filled out by the nurse, team leader, or ward clerk

   g. Sign, to be placed over or on the patient's bed and in the patient's bathroom, to indi-

   cate that a 24-hour urine specimen is being collected

   h. Disposable gloves

2. Identify the patient by checking the identification bracelet.

STEPS

3. Tell the patient that a 24-hour urine specimen is needed.

4. Explain the procedure. Tell the patient you will be placing the large container in her bathroom.

5. Wash your hands.

6. Fill in the label for the large container. Copy all needed information from the patient's identification bracelet. Record the date and time of the first collection. Attach the label to the urine specimen container (the large, 1-liter, plastic disposable bottle). Place the container in the patient's bathroom. In many institutions specimens are refrigerated or kept on ice to control odor and the growth of bacteria.

7. Post the sign over or on the patient's bed and in the patient's bathroom. This is so all person-

nel will be aware that a 24-hour specimen is being collected.

8. Provide privacy each time the patient voids if she uses a bedpan or urinal at bedside rather than a specipan or urinal in the bathroom. Ask the patient to avoid placing tissue in the bedpan with the specimen, as tissue absorbs urine needed for testing. Provide the patient with a plastic-lined wastepaper basket to temporarily dispose of the toilet tissue. Then discard it in the toilet or hopper.

9. If the patient is on intake and output, measure all the urine each time the patient voids. Write the amount on the intake and output sheet.

10. When the collection starts, have the patient void. Throw away (discard) this first amount of urine. This is to be sure that the bladder is completely empty. This first voiding should not be included in the specimen. This is usually done in early A.M. per institutional policy. The test will continue until the same time the next day.

P R O C E D U R E (CONTINUED)

11. You may be instructed to refrigerate the urine or put it on ice. If so, fill a large bucket with ice cubes. Keep the large urine container in the ice in the patient's bathroom. All nursing assistants caring for this patient for the next 24 hours will be responsible for keeping the bucket filled with ice.

12. For the next 24 hours, save all urine voided by the patient. Pour the urine from each voiding into the large container.

13. At the end of the 24-hour period, have the patient void at the same time the test was started the day before. Add this to the collection of urine in the large container. This will be the last time you will collect the urine for this test.

14. The large labeled container with the 24-hour collection of urine is taken to the laboratory with a requisition or laboratory request slip that is made out by the head nurse, team leader, or ward clerk.

15. Clean the equipment and put it in its proper place. Discard disposable equipment.

16. Remove the 24-hour specimen sign from the patient's bed.

FOLLOW-UP

17. Make the patient comfortable and replace the call light.

18. Lower the bed to a position of safety.

19. Raise the side rails when ordered or appropriate for patient safety.

20. Wash your hands.

21. Report to your immediate supervisor:

- That a 24-hour urine specimen has been obtained.
- That the specimen has been sent to the laboratory.
- The date and time of collection.
- Your observations of anything unusual.

■ Straining the Urine

The urine is strained to determine if a patient has passed stones (calculi) or other matter from the kidneys. The doctor may order that all urine passed by the patient is to be strained.

The labeled specimen container must be taken to the laboratory with a requisition or laboratory request slip at the nurse's request.

P R O C E D U R E

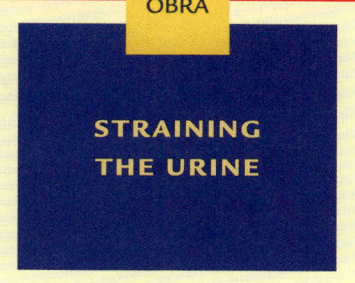

OBRA

STRAINING THE URINE

PREPARATION

1. Assemble your equipment in the patient's bathroom:

a. Disposable paper strainers or gauze squares

b. Specimen container with cover or a small plastic bag to be used as a specimen container

c. Label, if your institution's procedure is not to write on the cover

d. Patient's bedpan and cover, urinal, or specipan

e. Laboratory request slip, which should be filled out by the nurse, team leader, or ward clerk

f. Sign to be placed over or on the patient's bed indicating that all urine must be strained

g. Disposable gloves

2. Identify the patient by checking the identification bracelet.

STEPS

3. Tell the patient that each time she urinates it must be into a urinal, bedpan, or specipan, as all urine must be strained. Caution the patient not to put any tissue into the container. Provide the patient with a plastic-lined wastepaper basket to temporarily dispose of the toilet tissue. Then discard it in the toilet or hopper.

4. Provide privacy whenever the patient voids.

5. Wash your hands and put on gloves.

6. When the patient voids, take the bedpan or urinal to the patient's bathroom. Pour the urine through the strainer or gauze into the measuring container (Figure 23–6).

PROCEDURE (CONTINUED)

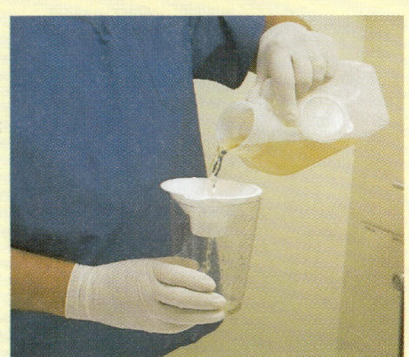

FIGURE 23–6

Pour urine through gauze or strainer into measuring container

7. If any particles show up on the gauze or the paper strainer, place the gauze or paper strainer with particles in a plastic bag or speci-

men container. Do not attempt to remove the particles because they may be lost or damaged.

8. Label the specimen container immediately. Copy all needed information from the patient's identification bracelet. Record the date and time of collection.

9. Measure the amount of the voiding and record it on the intake and output sheet, if the patient is on intake and output.

10. Discard the urine.

11. Clean and rinse the bedpan and graduate and put them in their proper places.

12. Dispose of gloves and wash your hands.

FOLLOW-UP

13. Make the patient comfortable and replace the call light.

14. Lower the bed to a position of safety.

15. Raise the side rails when ordered or appropriate for patient safety.

16. Report at once to your immediate supervisor:
    - That, in straining the urine, particles were obtained.
    - That a specimen was collected.
    - The date and time of collection.
    - Your observations of anything unusual.

SPUTUM SPECIMEN

sputum Waste material coughed up from the lungs or trachea

saliva The secretion of the salivary glands into the mouth; saliva moistens food and helps in swallowing

Sputum is a substance collected from a patient's lungs that contains saliva, mucus, and sometimes pus or blood. It is thicker than ordinary **saliva** (spit). Most of it is coughed up from the lungs and bronchial tubes. In some health care facilities, this procedure is carried out by the Respiratory Therapy Department (Pulmonary Medicine). Sputum specimens are studied to determine if a patient has pneumonia or tuberculosis.

Usually, early morning is the best time to obtain this specimen.

PROCEDURE

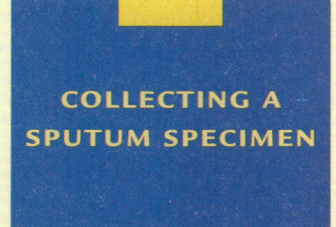

OBRA

COLLECTING A SPUTUM SPECIMEN

PREPARATION

1. Assemble your equipment:
   a. Sputum container with cover and tissues
   b. Label, if your institution's procedure is not to write on the cover

   c. Laboratory request slip, which should be filled out by the nurse, team leader, or ward clerk
   d. Disposable gloves

2. Identify the patient by checking the identification bracelet.

STEPS

3. Tell the patient that a sputum specimen is needed.

4. Wash your hands and put on gloves.

5. If the patient has eaten recently, have him rinse out his mouth. If he wants to have oral

hygiene at this time, help him as necessary.

6. Give the patient a sputum container (Figure 23–7a). Ask him to take three consecutive deep breaths and on the third exhalation to cough deep from within the lungs to bring up the thick sputum. Explain that saliva (spit) and nose secretions are not adequate for this test.

7. The patient may have to cough several times to bring up enough sputum for the specimen. One to two tablespoons is

PROCEDURE (CONTINUED)

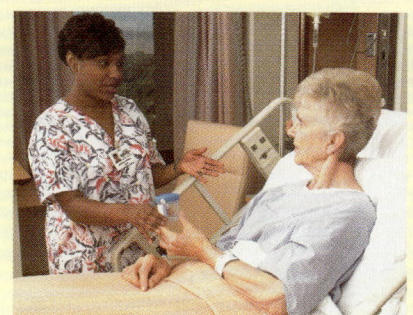

FIGURE 23–7a
Tell patient to cough deep within the lungs to bring up sputum for the specimen

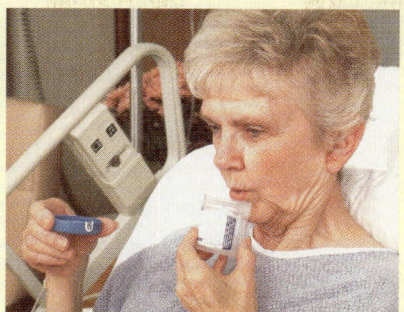

FIGURE 23–7b
Patient brings up sputum for the specimen

usually the required amount (Figure 23–7b).

8. Cover the container immediately. Be careful not to touch the inside of either the container or the cover to avoid contamination.

9. Label the container right away. Copy all needed information from the patient's identification bracelet. Record the time of collection and the date.

10. The labeled specimen container must be sent or taken immediately to the laboratory with a requisition or laboratory request slip. This should be filled out by the nurse or ward clerk. The test must be done in the laboratory before the sputum begins to dry.

FOLLOW-UP

11. Make the patient comfortable and replace the call light.

12. Lower the bed to a position of safety.

13. Raise the side rails when ordered or appropriate for patient safety.

14. Dispose of gloves and wash your hands.

15. Report at once to your immediate supervisor:
    - That a sputum specimen has been obtained.
    - The color, amount, odor, and consistency of the specimen.
    - That the specimen has been sent to the laboratory.
    - The date and time of collection.
    - How the patient tolerated the procedure.
    - Your observations of anything unusual.

STOOL SPECIMEN

Feces, **stool**, b.m., bowel movement, and fecal matter all mean the same thing—the solid waste from a patient's body. The doctor sometimes orders a stool specimen to help in the diagnosis of a patient's illness where blood or parasites are present in the patient's stool. Sometimes a warm specimen is ordered. This means that the specimen must be tested in the laboratory while the specimen is still warm from the patient's body. You will be told whether the specimen is to be warm.

In some institutions, you may be requested to prepare Hemoccult slides. The correct procedure follows.

feces Solid waste material discharged from the body through the rectum and anus; other names include excreta, excrement, bowel movement, and fecal matter

stool See feces

PROCEDURE

OBRA

COLLECTING A STOOL SPECIMEN

PREPARATION

1. Assemble your equipment (Figure 23–8):

   a. Patient's bedpan and cover

   b. Stool specimen container

   c. Wooden tongue depressor

   d. Label, if your institution's procedure is not to write on the cover

   e. Laboratory request slip, which should be filled out by the nurse, team leader, or ward clerk

PROCEDURE (CONTINUED)

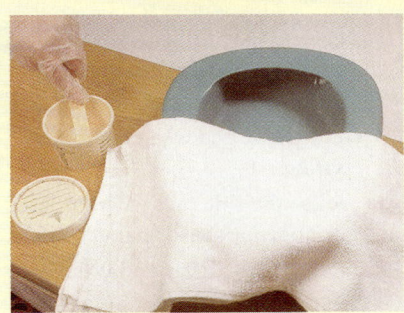

FIGURE 23–8

Equipment for collecting stool specimen

f. Plastic bag for warm specimen, if used by your institution

g. Disposable gloves

2. Identify the patient by checking the identification bracelet.

3. Wash your hands.

STEPS

4. Tell the patient that a stool specimen is needed. Explain that whenever he can move his bowels he is to call you so the specimen can be collected.

5. Provide privacy for the patient.

6. Have the patient move his bowels into the bedpan or into a specipan placed in the back half of the toilet.

7. Ask the patient *not to urinate into the bedpan* and not to put toilet tissue in the bedpan. Provide the patient with a plastic-lined wastepaper basket to temporarily dispose of the toilet tissue. Then discard it in the toilet or hopper.

8. Prepare the label immediately by copying all needed information from the patient's identification bracelet. Record the time of collection and the date.

9. Put on gloves.

10. After the patient has had a bowel movement, take the covered bedpan to the patient's bathroom or to the dirty utility room.

11. Using the wooden tongue depressor, take about 1 to 2 tablespoons of feces from different areas of the stool in the bedpan and place them in the stool specimen container. Label the specimen container.

12. Cover the container immediately. Be careful not to touch the inside of either the container or the cover to avoid contamination.

13. Wrap the tongue depressor in a paper towel and discard it.

14. Empty the remaining feces into the toilet or hopper.

15. Clean the bedpan and return it to its proper place.

16. Dispose of gloves and wash your hands.

17. If the nurse has told you this is a warm specimen, it must be taken to the laboratory for examination while it is still warm from the patient's body. Place the stool specimen container, fully labeled, in the plastic bag (if used by your institution). Attach the laboratory request slip to the bag. Carry it immediately to the laboratory.

FOLLOW-UP

18. Make the patient comfortable and replace the call light.

19. Lower the bed to a position of safety.

20. Raise the side rails when ordered or appropriate for patient safety.

21. Wash your hands.

22. Report at once to your immediate supervisor:

- That a stool specimen has been obtained.
- That the specimen has been sent to the laboratory.
- The date and time of collection.
- Your observations of anything unusual.

PROCEDURE

PREPARING A HEMOCCULT SLIDE

Note: Some states require that Hemoccult slides be collected by a nurse.

STEPS

1. Ask the patient to move her bowels into a bedpan or specipan, whenever this is possible.

2. Wash your hands and put on gloves.

3. Check the patient's identification bracelet.

4. Label the outside of the Hemoccult slide with the patient's name, address, hospital number, and the date this specimen is collected.

5. Collect a small amount of stool on a tongue depressor.

6. Apply small amount in box A on Hemoccult slide.

7. Open side 1.

8. From a different area of the stool, collect a small amount of stool on tongue depressor.

PROCEDURE (CONTINUED)

9. Apply small amount in box B.

10. Close cover of slide card and secure.

11. Check information with patient identification bracelet.

12. Dispose of gloves and wash your hands.

FOLLOW-UP

13. Send to the laboratory or give collected sample to the nurse if it is your institution's policy to check Hemoccult specimens on the unit.

14. Report to your immediate supervisor:

- That the Hemoccult specimen has been collected.

- The time and date it was collected.

- Your observations of anything unusual.

Summary

In collecting specimens for testing, it is important to remember to always explain to the patient what you are going to do before proceeding with the collection. This step helps to gain the patient's confidence and elicits cooperation in the procedure. Standard Precautions must be maintained while collecting specimens. Care must be taken to be accurate in all information related to obtaining and labeling the required specimens.

Notes

endocrine system System composed of endocrine glands; regulates body function by secreting hormones

gland An organ that is able to manufacture and discharge a chemical that will be used elsewhere in the body

secrete Produce and release into the body; glands secrete hormones

hormones Protein substances secreted by endocrine glands directly into the blood to stimulate increased activity

endocrine glands Ductless glands that produce hormones and secrete them directly into the blood or lymph

exocrine glands Glands that produce hormones and secrete them either directly or through a duct to epithelial tissue, such as a body cavity or the skin surface

ANATOMY AND PHYSIOLOGY OF THE ENDOCRINE SYSTEM

The **endocrine system** consists of several **glands** that **secrete** (produce and release) liquids called **hormones**. Through these hormones, the endocrine system helps the nervous system organize and direct the activities of the body. Figure 24–1 shows the locations of the **endocrine glands**. The endocrine glands secrete hormones directly into the bloodstream. In contrast, **exocrine glands**, such as the salivary glands, deliver their products through ducts into a body cavity or to the skin surface, as from sweat glands.

The pituitary gland is the master gland. Its hormones directly affect the other endocrine glands, stimulating them to produce their hormones. Hormones from the anterior and posterior portions of the pituitary gland regulate the metabolism of the body's billions of cells. The anterior portion manufactures and releases seven hormones. The pituitary hormones are especially important in reproduction and in all functions leading to puberty (the time at which a child takes on the physical characteristics of an adult man or woman). Hormones from the pituitary gland regulate the menstrual cycle in the female and sperm production in the male. Without these hormones, humans would be unable to reproduce.

The pituitary gland and its hormones are under the direct control of the hypothalamus, a tiny piece of tissue lying near the base of the brain. This structure seems to be the link between our thinking, our emotions, and our body functions.

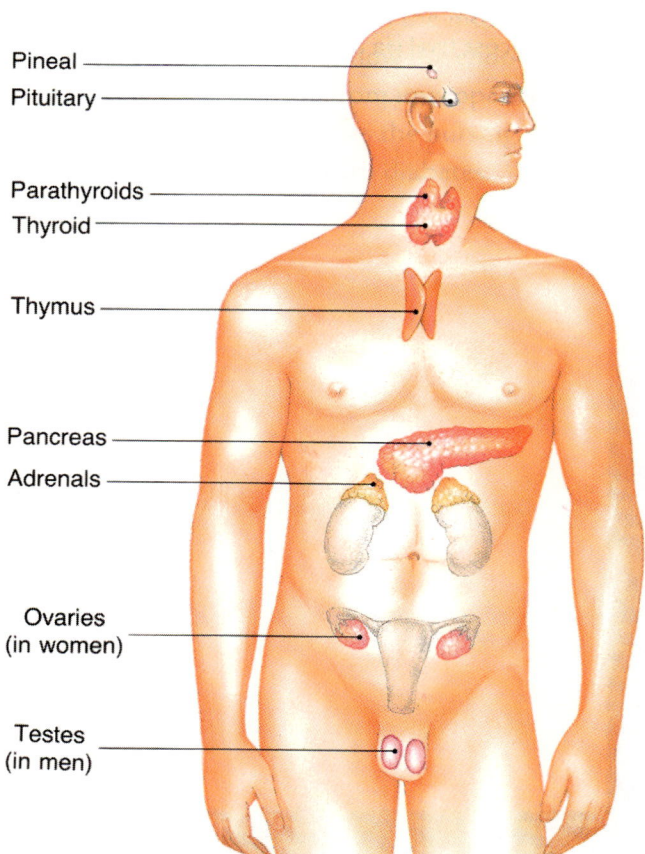

Pineal
Pituitary

Parathyroids
Thyroid

Thymus

Pancreas
Adrenals

Ovaries
(in women)

Testes
(in men)

FIGURE 24–1

Endocrine glands

The thyroid gland produces a hormone that regulates growth and general metabolism. The hormones secreted by the thyroid gland influence a person's energy level, skeletal growth, sexual development, skin texture, and hair luster.

The thymus gets smaller after puberty, but it plays an important part in the body's immune system. The immune system prevents us from getting many diseases.

The parathyroids are located within the capsule of the thyroid. They produce a hormone that, along with one of the hormones in the thyroid gland, regulates the level of calcium and potassium in the blood. Calcium is important for many functions of the body, such as muscle contraction and conduction of nerve impulses.

The pancreas is both an endocrine gland and an exocrine gland (a gland that has a duct). Its endocrine portion produces the hormone insulin. **Insulin** regulates the sugar content of the blood. If the body does not have enough insulin, the person develops hyperglycemia (high blood sugar) and becomes diabetic. The diabetic patient must be treated by reducing her carbohydrate or sugar intake and by regulating the balance between insulin and **glucose** (blood sugar).

The adrenal glands lie on top of the kidneys. They are very important in helping the body adapt to stress conditions by stimulating the autonomic nervous system. In an emergency, they produce adrenalin, which enables the body to quickly produce great amounts of energy.

In the female, the ovaries are responsible for secreting the hormones estrogen and progesterone. The rise and fall of the levels of these hormones in the blood determine the menstrual cycle. The hormones are also important in causing an ovum, or egg, to develop and in maintaining a pregnancy.

In the male, the testes produce testosterone, the primary sex hormone of the male. Testosterone is responsible for the masculine physical characteristics and causes the production of sperm.

insulin Hormone that regulates the sugar content of the blood

glucose A sugar formed during metabolism of carbohydrates; blood sugar

THE ENDOCRINE SYSTEM AND THE NORMAL AGING PROCESS

With age, some endocrine glands decrease their production of hormones. For example, secretion of thyroid, parathyroid, and adrenal hormones gradually diminishes. The production of estrogen and progesterone decreases as well.

Some hormones become less effective as the body ages. An example of such a hormone is insulin.

Together, changes in hormone levels and effectiveness decrease the endocrine system's ability to regulate activities of the body. In general, however, few age-related disorders are directly related to problems with the endocrine glands. Disorders of the endocrine system may occur at any age.

AGE-SPECIFIC CONSIDERATIONS

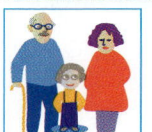

Diabetes is one of the most common endocrine diseases. It affects patients of all ages and has a major impact on patient's lives. For children, establish trust by being honest and answering questions truthfully. Use fantasy play or puppets to let children express how they feel. For adolescents, try to allow them options or choices in as many aspects of their care as possible. Take time to explain things, but do not argue. Teens need information as well as emotional support to make good decisions. Adults also need information to help them make lifestyle changes.

COMMON DISEASES AND DISORDERS OF THE ENDOCRINE SYSTEM

Diseases and disorders of the endocrine system generally involve production of too much or too little of some hormone. The most common diseases and disorders are as follows:

- *Hypothyroidism:* too little hormone secreted by the thyroid gland
- *Hyperthyroidism:* too much hormone secreted by the thyroid gland
- *Hyperparathyroidism:* overactivity of the parathyroid glands
- *Hypoparathyroidism:* absence of activity of the parathyroid glands
- *Diabetes mellitus:* abnormality of the insulin secretion of the pancreas, resulting in metabolic abnormalities
- *Cushing's syndrome:* hyperactivity of the adrenal glands
- *Addison's disease:* hypo-(less) function of the adrenal glands
- *Hyperpituitarism:* secretion of excessive amounts of growth hormone by the pituitary gland
- *Hypopituitarism:* pituitary insufficiency; secretion of too little hormone by the pituitary gland
- *Pituitary tumors:* cancer that causes changes in normal growth

DIABETES MELLITUS

The most common disorder arising from problems with the endocrine system is the chronic disease known as **diabetes mellitus**. Diabetes is a disturbance of carbohydrate metabolism. In other words, the body cannot change **carbohydrate** (starches and sugar) into energy and cannot store them, called **metabolism**, because of an imbalance of the hormone insulin.

There are two types of diabetes:

- *Insulin-dependent diabetes mellitus (IDDM), also known as Type I or juvenile-onset diabetes:* The body produces little or no insulin, so it must be given by injection.
- *Non-insulin-dependent diabetes mellitus (NIDDM), also known as Type II or adult-onset diabetes:* The body *may* produce a normal amount of insulin but cannot use it. Type II diabetes may be controlled with diet and exercise alone, or the patient may also need oral medication or insulin.

Most diabetics have Type II (NIDDM) diabetes.

Terms Often Used with Diabetes Mellitus

Many of the patients cared for by a nursing assistant have diabetes. Therefore, it is important to recognize terms often used in connection with this condition:

diabetes mellitus Disorder of carbohydrate metabolism caused by inability to convert sugar into energy because of inadequate production or utilization of insulin

carbohydrate Type of basic food element used by the body; composed of carbon, hydrogen, and oxygen; includes sugars and starches

metabolism The process through which food elements are converted into energy for use in the human body

- FBS: fasting blood sugar; a type of test to measure the amount of glucose in the patient's blood after the patient has not eaten for a given amount of time

- GTT: glucose tolerance test; a type of test that measures the amount of glucose in the patient's blood after the patient has consumed a specified amount of glucose

- **Hypoglycemia:** abnormally low blood sugar

- **Hyperglycemia:** abnormally high blood sugar

- Gangrene: necrosis (death) of a body part caused by lack of blood circulating to that part

- Pancreas: endocrine gland that produces insulin

- Islets of Langerhans: part of the pancreas that produces insulin

- PPBS: postprandial blood sugar; a type of test that measures the amount of glucose in the patient's blood after the patient has eaten

Signs and Symptoms of Diabetes Mellitus

The ability to recognize the signs and symptoms of diabetes also is very important. Although the nursing assistant does not diagnose illnesses, you can support the health care team by reporting any of the following signs to your supervisor:

- Fatigue, tiredness

- Loss of weight; hunger

- Vaginitis: inflammation of the vagina

- Skin erosions (lesions); sores healing poorly and slowly (a late sign)

- Hyperglycemia

- Glycosuria: sugar in the urine

- Polyuria: frequent and large amounts of urine

- Polydipsia: excessive thirst

- Poor vision: eyesight affected

Signs and Symptoms of Insulin Shock

One of the most common and serious complications related to diabetes is **insulin shock**, also called diabetic shock or insulin reaction. This condition occurs in patients with diabetes when they receive too much insulin, miss a meal, or have too much physical activity. Too much glucose leaves the blood, resulting in hypoglycemia (low blood sugar). Insulin shock has a sudden onset. The following signs and symptoms indicate that a patient may be experiencing insulin shock:

- Excessive sweating, perspiration

- Faintness, dizziness, weakness

- Hunger (polyphagia)

- Irritability, personality change, nervousness, anxious

- Numbness of tongue and lips

- Inability to awaken, coma, unconsciousness, stupor

- Headache

hypoglycemia
Abnormally low blood sugar

hyperglycemia
Abnormally high blood sugar

insulin shock Serious complication related to diabetes; occurs when the diabetic receives too much insulin, misses a meal, or has too much physical activity

- Tremors, trembling
- Blurred or impaired vision
- Upon examination: low blood sugar
- Blood sugar below 70 mg/dL.

■ Signs and Symptoms of Diabetic Coma

diabetic coma A coma (abnormal deep stupor) that can occur in a diabetic patient from lack of insulin

If the diabetic patient does not receive enough insulin to metabolize carbohydrates or when there is increased stress or infection, the patient may experience hyperglycemia (high blood sugar), resulting in **diabetic coma**, also called diabetic acidosis. A diabetic coma may have a gradual onset, but it can be life-threatening. Therefore, knowledge of its signs and symptoms is crucial:

- Air hunger, heavy labored breathing, increased respirations
- Loss of appetite
- Nausea and/or vomiting
- Weakness
- Abdominal pain or discomfort
- Generalized aches
- Increased thirst and parched tongue
- Sweet or fruity odor of the breath
- Flushed skin
- Dry skin
- Increased urination
- Dulled senses
- Loss of consciousness
- Upon examination: high blood sugar
- Blood sugar above 250 mg/dL

■ Caring for the Diabetic Patient: Reducing Pressure Points

Two conditions related to diabetes make pressure points a particular concern for the diabetic. First, a person with diabetes is more susceptible to arteriosclerosis, which involves narrowing of the arteries. Arteriosclerosis results in less blood flowing to the extremities, especially the legs and feet. Second, changes may occur in the nerves of the feet, causing less nerve sensation, a condition called neuropathy. When a person with diabetes has neuropathy, he is not aware when a pressure point is causing skin irritation. One extreme complication of such skin irritations is gangrene (no blood passes to a toe or to the foot). The body part with gangrene dies and must be surgically amputated.

To avoid skin irritation and its consequences, all patients with diabetes must reduce pressure points. Teaching the following guidelines will help patients do this.

GUIDELINES

OBRA

CARE OF THE FEET AND SKIN FOR DIABETICS

- Avoid standing or lying in one position for a long period of time. Change from sitting to walking or from lying to sitting and walking.

- Never walk barefoot or in stocking feet. Always wear shoes for protection. A cut will have difficulty healing.

- Never cross knees. Never wear rubber or elastic bands for garters, and never roll stockings or socks. This stops circulation in the lower extremities.

- Bathe every day, washing the feet very well.

- Never use very hot water for a shower or bath, as a burn will not heal readily.

- When drying the body after a shower or bath, do not rub hard; pat dry, especially between the toes.

- Use skin cream to prevent hard, dry skin areas.

- Follow the physician's instructions for cutting toenails.

- Do not use any nonprescription drugs, internally or externally, without the physician's permission.

- Tell every physician, dentist, eye doctor, and podiatrist who examines you that you have diabetes.

- Wear shoes and stockings that fit so that they do not cause pressure points by restricting movement in the toes.

- If you see any open skin, red area, scratched skin, sores, blisters, or any area of skin that looks different than normal, call and report this to your physician.

■ Testing of Blood Glucose

When a patient has diabetes, certain changes or adjustments in lifestyle are important. Some patients also need to use medication to keep their diabetes under control. The amounts of medication and food a diabetic needs are related to how high or low the blood sugar is. The symptoms listed previously can occur if the blood sugar is not at a desirable level. Testing procedures that can identify high or low blood sugar are therefore key in determining the correct amounts of medication and food.

In hospitals and nursing homes today, the most common method of testing the level of blood sugar is to use a blood glucose meter. In the past, urine testing was used to help monitor the diabetic's glucose levels. (Excess sugar in the blood is excreted in the urine.) However, doctors have found that routine urine testing is less accurate than testing blood samples with a blood glucose meter. Testing the blood reveals high or low blood sugar sooner than waiting until excess sugar has reached the urine.

Self-monitoring of blood glucose using meters can greatly improve the home patient's quality of life. It allows the patient to know whether the patient's diet, exercise, and medication protocol are working. Home testing of blood glucose enables the patient to have some control of the diabetes, rather than feeling that diabetes is controlling the patient's life.

There are many types of meters, each with different features. These meters are available at local pharmacies and medical supply stores. There are many manufacturers of battery-operated blood glucose meters (Figure 24–2). One new device allows the diabetic patient to obtain the blood sample from the forearm. This method is less painful than finger sticks. In addition, scientists are currently developing non-invasive methods of monitoring blood glucose, but these are not yet available.

FIGURE 24–2

This Accu Check meter measures the level of glucose in a blood sample

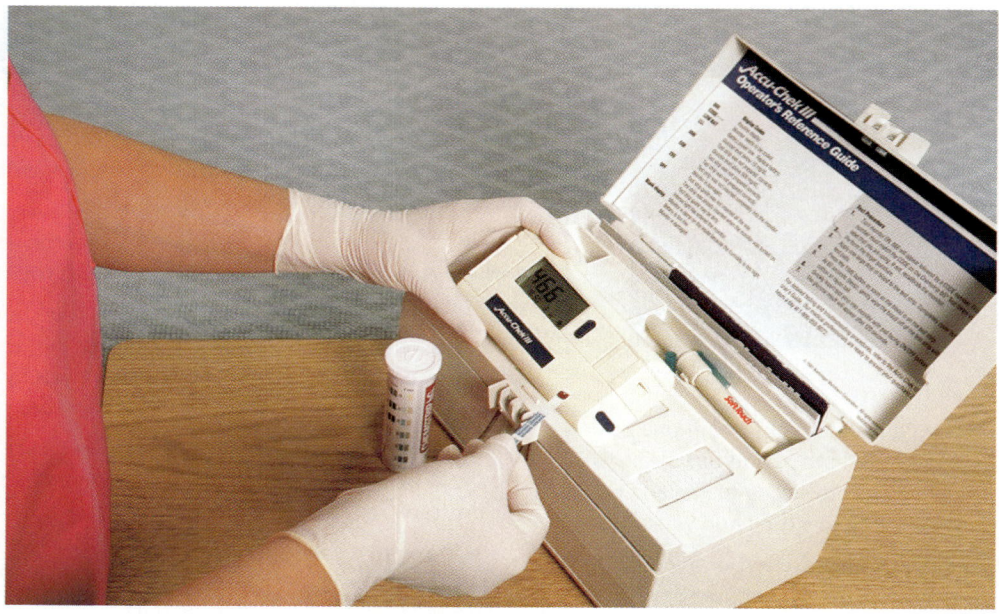

PROCEDURE

TESTING FOR GLUCOSE USING THE ONE-TOUCH PROFILE DIABETES TRACKING SYSTEM

PREPARATION

1. Wash your hands.
2. Explain to the patient that you are going to test his blood sugar.
3. Make the patient comfortable and wash his hands with soap and water.
4. Assemble your equipment:
   a. One-Touch Profile meter
   b. Test strips
   c. Penlet and lancet
   d. Disposable pipet
   e. Disposable gloves
   f. Band-Aid
5. Put on disposable gloves.

STEPS

6. Match the code on the test strips to the number on the meter. Check the expiration date on the test strips. Discard them if they have expired. The code number may have to be reset. Follow the manufacturer's instructions.
7. Remove test strip from container. Close the container. Do not touch the white area of the strip.
8. Press Power and insert the strip into the meter (Figure 24–3).
9. Insert the lancet into the Penlet according to the manufacturer's directions.
10. Place the end of the lancet firmly against the side of a fingertip of the patient.
11. Press the button on top of the Penlet.
12. Squeeze the finger gently to obtain a large drop of blood.
13. Using a disposable pipet, slowly draw up the drop of blood and apply the sample to the test

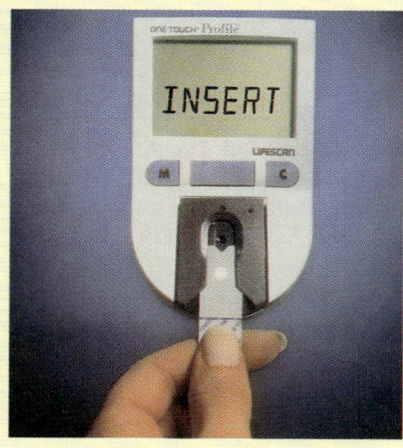

FIGURE 24–3

Press power and insert the strip into the meter (Photo Courtesy of Johnson & Johnson)

strip. This method prevents contamination of the patient and is preferred in a hospital or nursing home setting where several different patients use the same blood glucose meter. An alternative method for individual use (at home, for example) is to apply the blood sample directly to the strip (Figure 24–4).

P R O C E D U R E (CONTINUED)

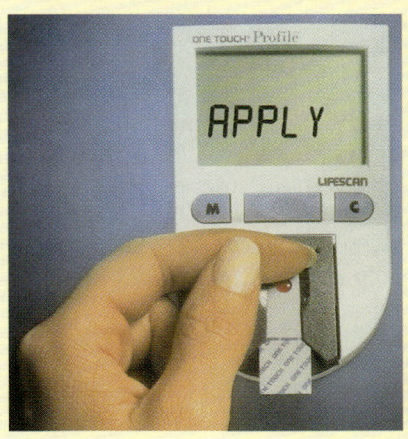

FIGURE 24–4

Apply the blood sample directly to the strip. (Photo courtesy of Johnson & Johnson)

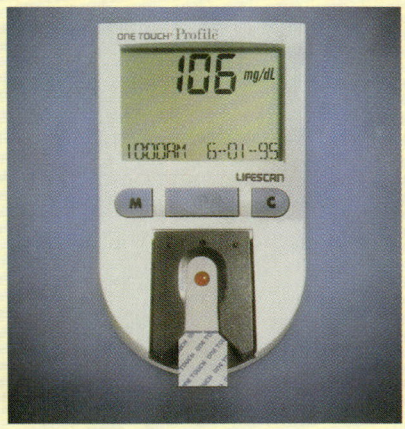

FIGURE 24–5

The results appear on the blood glucose meter. (Photo courtesy of Johnson & Johnson)

14. Wait a short time for the results to appear on the blood glucose meter (Figure 24–5).

15. Apply a bandage to the patient's finger.

FOLLOW-UP

16. Remove disposable gloves and wash your hands.

17. Record the results. Notify the supervisor if the results are above or below normal.

■ Urine Testing for Acetone

Very rarely, the nursing assistant may be asked to test a patient's urine. A fresh urine sample may be tested with test strips to measure for acetone, which can appear in the urine as a result of abnormal blood glucose levels (Figure 24–6). Follow your institution's guidelines.

Each bottle of test strips has pictures and instructions for using the specific product. Check the expiration date, and do not use any test strips past that date. Anytime you perform a urine test for acetone, use a fresh urine sample, wash your hands before and after the test, and wear disposable gloves (see Chapter 23).

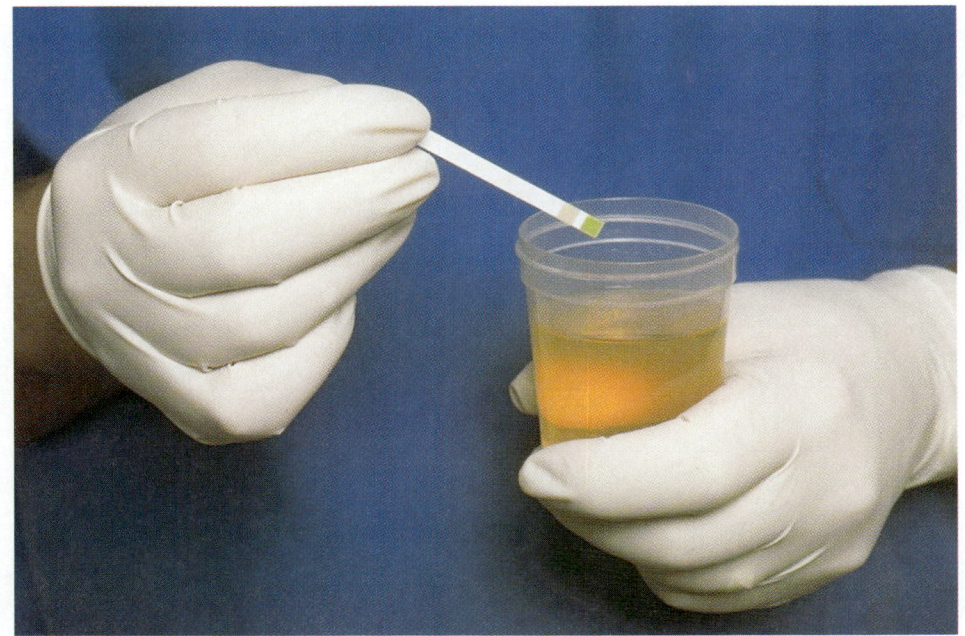

FIGURE 24–6

Test strips may be used to measure the acetone level in a urine sample

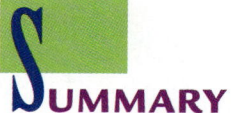

Summary

Understanding how the endocrine system regulates normal body metabolism is important for the caregiver. In particular, a nursing assistant can help correct problems and even save lives by identifying quickly any symptoms that indicate a patient's level of blood sugar is abnormal. The most common method of glucose monitoring for patients is the use of a blood glucose meter. This method can help the patient and the caregiver monitor the patient's blood glucose levels. At-home use of a blood glucose meter by the patient gives more independence and the ability to control daily activities and medication.

Notes

Family Brings Sugary Foods to a Diabetic

Mr. Tallchief is a newly diagnosed diabetic. He requires insulin injections to maintain his blood sugar at a normal level. When you walk into his room, you find him eating a big bowl of ice cream and cake brought in by his family to celebrate his fiftieth birthday. You know that Mr. Tallchief's blood sugar has been high and his insulin dose has had to be adjusted frequently. His wife says, "We know we are breaking your rules, but it is his birthday and we are celebrating!"

What Is Your Response/Action?

1. What are the important pieces of information in this situation?

2. What possible actions might you consider?

3. What action will you take?

4. What will you say, if anything, to Mr. Tallchief and his family about breaking the rules?

5. What have you learned that you can apply to other situations with patients and families?

The Reproductive System and Related Care

25

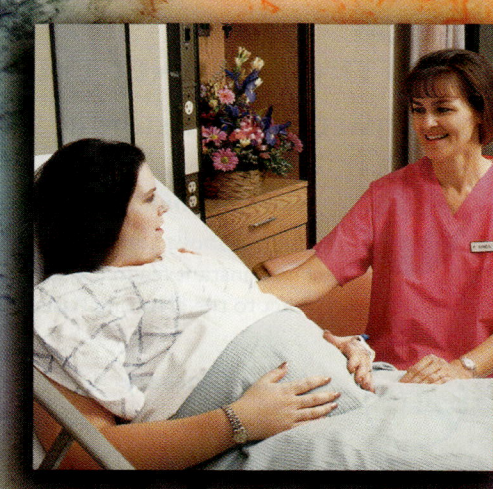

INTRODUCTION

To meet the needs of patients, the nursing assistant must have an understanding of the female and male reproductive systems. Because of misinformation or cultural values, patients may be sensitive to care they receive for this area of their bodies. Even if their own cultural identity differs from that of their patients, caregivers must maintain a compassionate and professional approach to patient care. This chapter provides guidance by discussing the male and female reproductive systems, sexuality, and patient care related to the reproductive system.

OBJECTIVES

When you have completed this chapter, you will be able to:

- Label a diagram with the female organs of the reproductive system and explain how each organ helps in the process of reproduction.

- Label a diagram with the male organs of the reproductive system and explain how each organ helps in the process of reproduction.

- Explain the meaning of sexuality and how the nursing assistant can appropriately respect the sexuality of patients.

- List the common disorders of the reproductive system.

- List the common sexually transmitted diseases (STDs).

- Explain HIV/AIDS precautions with all patients.

- Describe how to prepare a patient for a pelvic exam.

- Give a vaginal irrigation (douche).

- Identify important aspects of postpartum care.

KEY TERMS

AIDS

estrogen

fertile

fertilization

gynecological (GYN) patient

HIV

menopause

menstruation

ovulation

ova/ovum

perineal area

reproductive system

sexually transmitted diseases (STDs)

sperm

testosterone

vagina (vaginal canal)

vaginal irrigation (douche)

reproductive system The group of body organs that makes possible the creation of a new human life

ova/ovum The female reproductive cell(s) produced in the ovaries which is capable of uniting with a sperm cell and developing into a new organism

estrogen A female hormone that causes a buildup of the lining of the uterus to prepare it for possible pregnancy; also responsible for the development of secondary sexual characteristics

perineal area The area of the body between the thighs; includes the area of the anus and the external genital organs

vagina (vaginal canal) The canal leading from the cervix to the outside of the female body; serves as the organ for intercourse and the birth canal

ovulation Process whereby an ovum is released from one ovary into the opening of the fallopian tube and moves to the uterus

fertile Able to become pregnant; capable of reproduction

THE REPRODUCTIVE SYSTEM

The **reproductive system** is the group of body organs that makes possible the creation of a new human life. In the process of reproduction (creation of new life), the male and female each have an essential role.

Female Reproductive System

In the female, the primary reproductive organs are the two ovaries (Figure 25–1). The main task of the ovaries is the production of **ova** (eggs)/**ovum** (egg) and female hormones. The ovaries are the major sites of production of **estrogen** and progesterone in the amounts required for normal female growth, development, and function. The **perineal area** (the external genitalia and rectal area), has three openings:

1. The external urinary meatus, the end of the urethra

2. The **vagina** or **vaginal canal**, which serves as the organ for intercourse and the birth canal

3. The anus, the last portion of the gastrointestinal tract

The reproductive process begins with **ovulation**. During ovulation, an ovum is released from one ovary into the opening of the fallopian tube, through which it travels to the uterus (womb). Ovulation usually occurs once each month, and a woman normally is **fertile** (able to become pregnant) during this time. Also, estrogen is released, causing a buildup of the lining of the uterus (endometrium), preparing it for a possible pregnancy. The process of ovulation is controlled by hormones from the pituitary gland, under the

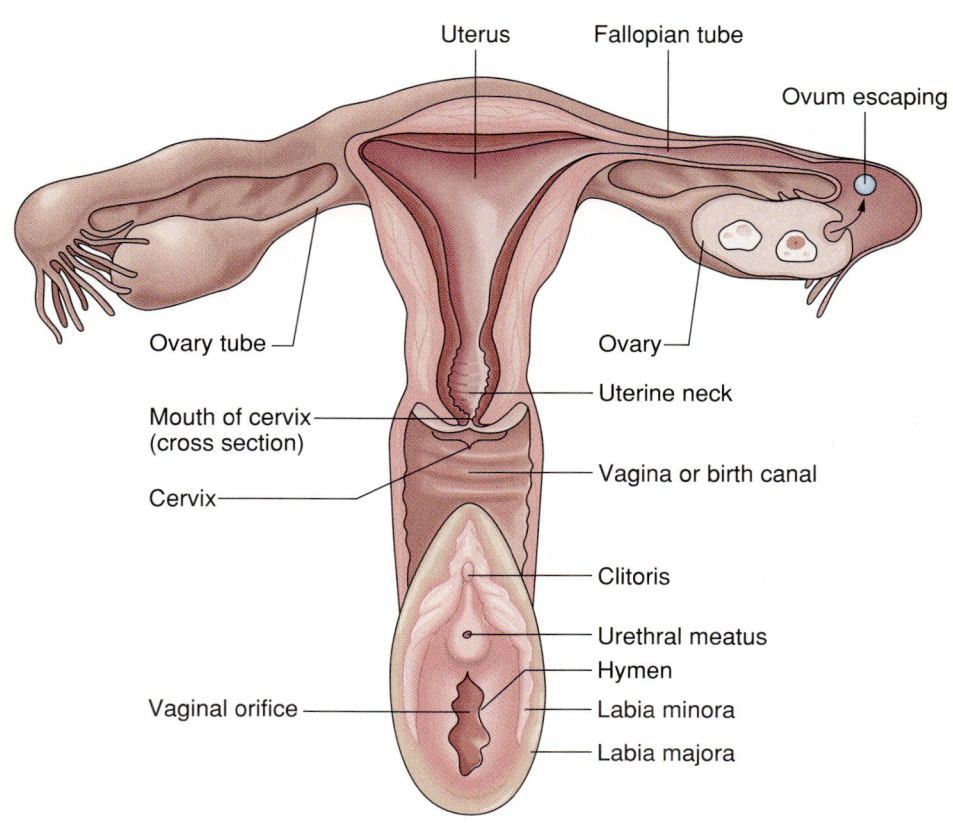

FIGURE 25–1

Female reproductive organs

FIGURE 25–2

Fertilization and cell division

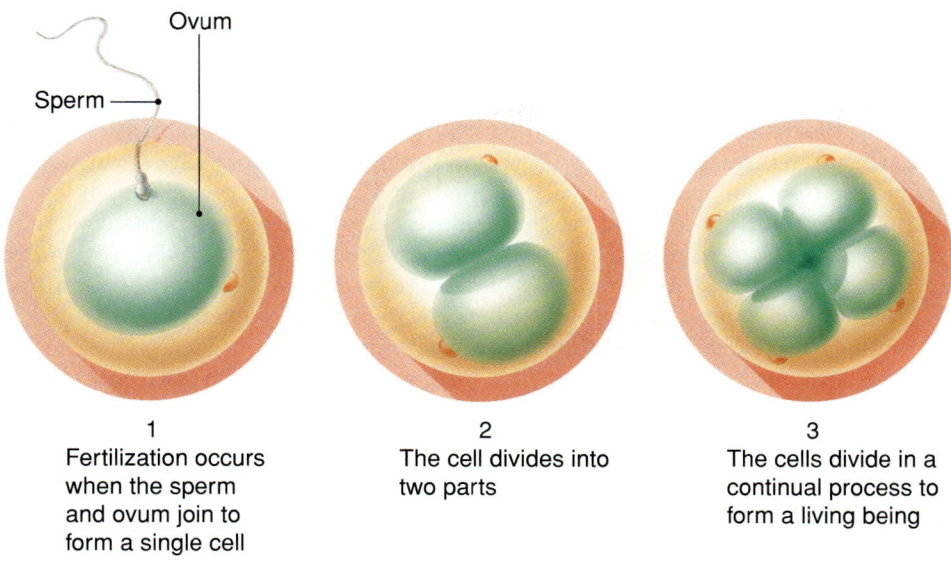

1
Fertilization occurs when the sperm and ovum join to form a single cell

2
The cell divides into two parts

3
The cells divide in a continual process to form a living being

fertilization Joining of a sperm and ovum to form a new cell

sperm The male reproductive cell produced in the testes, which is released from the male during intercourse

menstruation Periodic (monthly) loss of some blood and a small part of the lining of the uterus when a woman is not pregnant

menopause Time during which menstruation stops, resulting in decreased hormone production and an end of fertility

control of the hypothalamus. These hormones are involved in the development of the ovum and in maintaining pregnancy.

Fertilization occurs at this stage if an ovum unites with a **sperm** cell released from the male during intercourse. Artificial insemination is a process sometimes used to fertilize the ovum. After the egg is fertilized, it normally grows and develops in the uterus over a period of 40 weeks (Figure 25–2). Then the baby is born when the uterus contracts, gradually pushing the baby through the vagina (birth canal). In some cases, the baby is surgically removed from the uterus in an operation called a cesarean birth.

If the woman does not become pregnant, the next menstrual period begins about 14 days after ovulation. **Menstruation** is the periodic (monthly) loss of some blood and a small part of the lining of the uterus (Figure 25–3). The discharge flows out of the vagina for four to seven days. As the woman reaches age 45-55, menstruation gradually becomes less frequent, leading to the normal cessation of menstrual cycles, or **menopause**.

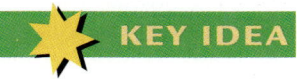

KEY IDEA

The reproductive cycle of a fertile woman begins with ovulation, during which the ovaries release an egg. The egg may be fertilized (joined by a sperm) so that it can develop into a fetus, or the egg may pass out of the body during menstruation.

FIGURE 25–3

The menstrual flow cycle, a physiological process in women of childbearing age

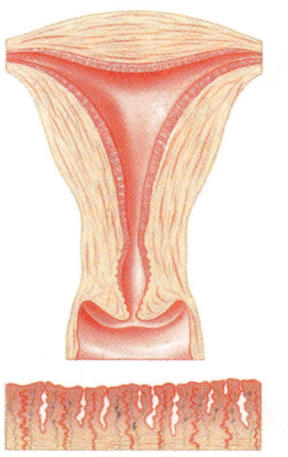
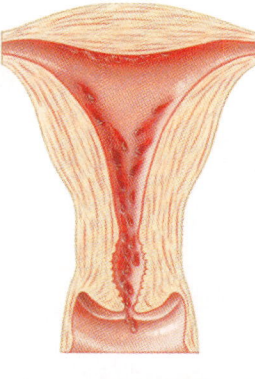
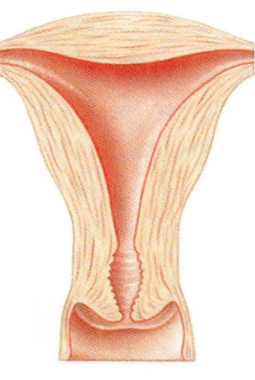

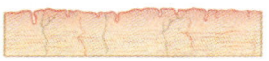

Premenstrual   Menstrual   Postmenstrual

■ Male Reproductive System

In the male, the primary reproductive organs are the testes (testicles), which produce sperm (Figure 25–4). The testes are paired glands that lie in a sac called the scrotum. The scrotum is located outside the body, posterior to the penis, which is the primary male sex organ.

The penis has three columns of spongy or cavernous tissue. During sexual excitement, blood rushes in through the penile artery and the veins constrict, trapping the blood so it fills these spaces. Then the penis becomes erect. This activity occurs under the influence of **testosterone**, the primary male sex hormone, which is also manufactured in the testes. It is secreted into the blood through the influence of the hormones from the anterior pituitary, which is under the control of the hypothalamus.

During intercourse, sperm travel up the vas deferens, or sperm duct, to the urethra. The sperm enter the urethra with secretions from other glands in the male reproductive system. These glands—the seminal vesicles, the prostate gland, and the bulbo-urethral gland (Cowper's gland)—contribute water, nutrients, and vitamins. Together, these secretions plus the sperm make up the semen. When the male has an orgasm, the semen is ejaculated (expelled) so that the sperm can travel up his partner's vagina, enabling a sperm to join with an ovum.

The penis has only one duct. It is used for the flow of urine and for the ejaculation of sperm in the semen. During intercourse, the internal sphincter of the male's urinary bladder closes tightly, so urine does not become mixed with the semen.

testosterone The primary male sex hormone; manufactured in the testes

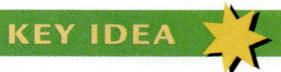

KEY IDEA

The male participates in the reproductive process by producing sperm in the testes. When a male ejaculates during intercourse, the semen carries many sperm up the vagina, where one sperm may fertilize an ovum.

FIGURE 25–4

Male reproductive organs

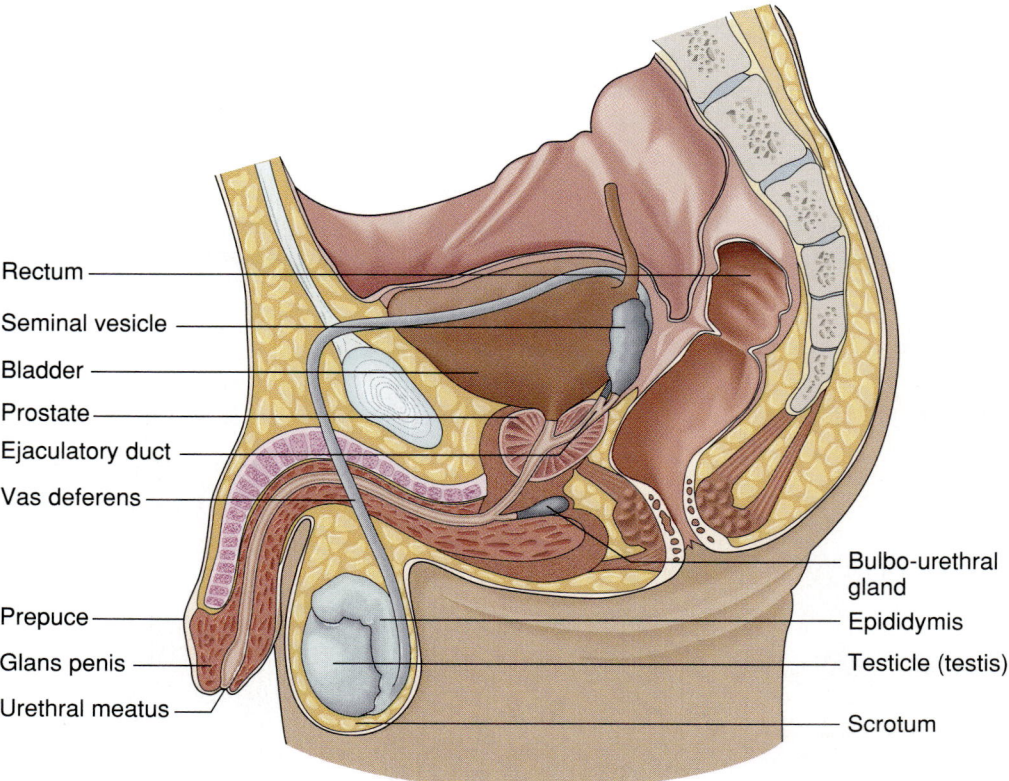

- Rectum
- Seminal vesicle
- Bladder
- Prostate
- Ejaculatory duct
- Vas deferens
- Prepuce
- Glans penis
- Urethral meatus
- Bulbo-urethral gland
- Epididymis
- Testicle (testis)
- Scrotum

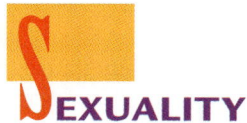

SEXUALITY

A person's reproductive system is just one part of that person's sexuality. Sexuality means the group of characteristics that identify the differences between male and female. During all the stages of growth and development, people are sexual beings. Their sexuality arises from their emotions, thoughts, and experiences related to warm, loving, and caring feelings shared between people, whether associated with the sex organs or not. Also, inherited sexual characteristics influence individual behavior patterns.

Because sexuality is a part of each person, the nursing assistant needs to care for patients in ways that respect their sexuality appropriately. Appropriate care is considerate of the patient's need for privacy. The nursing assistant should close doors and privacy curtains when providing patient care and should not talk in front of others about conditions the patient may find embarrassing. Also, the nursing assistant can show respect for the patient's sexuality by helping the patient look attractive. As needed, the nursing assistant can help the patient choose attractive clothing, care for the hair, and apply makeup, as appropriate.

The nursing assistant should expect that patients will have different views about sexuality and their reproductive systems. For example, cultural values may make some patients extremely concerned about privacy and reluctant to discuss problems related to sexual function or reproductive organs. Occasionally a patient may express his sexuality inappropriately by grabbing or touching the nursing assistant or other staff member. If this occurs, the nursing assistant should tell the patient calmly, "That is not appropriate behavior." If this response does not end the behavior, the nursing assistant should discuss the problem with her supervisor.

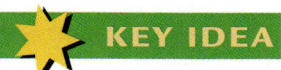

KEY IDEA

Sexuality describes a person's maleness or femaleness. It includes differences in male and female bodies, as well as the contrasting ways men and women learn to behave and their feelings about being a man or woman. Therefore, sexual behavior includes not only intercourse, but also many ways of touching and showing affection or attraction.

THE REPRODUCTIVE SYSTEM AND THE NORMAL AGING PROCESS

As a person ages, changes occur in hormone levels and in some parts of the reproductive system. Certain age-related problems are common in women, others in men.

AGE-SPECIFIC CONSIDERATIONS

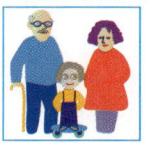

When caring for adolescents, keep in mind that they are beginning to develop sexual maturity. They may have a wide range of knowledge about their bodies and varying levels of comfort with their emerging sexuality. When caring for these patients, keep privacy concerns in mind as well as issues of confidentiality. Adolescents may or may not want to be examined and cared for with their parents present.

■Aging of the Female Reproductive System

A notable age-related change in the reproductive system of a woman is menopause, which typically occurs between ages 45 and 55. Besides the end of menstruation and fertility, menopause brings a decrease in the production of estrogen. The decline in estrogen production is thought to contribute to other age-related changes. Loss of elasticity of the vaginal tissues, decreased vaginal secretions, and other changes make the woman more susceptible to irritation and infection of the vulva and vagina. The decline in estrogen also can lead to a loss of calcium, causing the bones to become brittle.

As a woman ages, the pelvic muscles which support the structures in the perineal area can become weak. This can lead to stress incontinence; that is, involuntary urination when lifting, sneezing, or coughing. Exercise to strengthen the pelvic muscles helps to relieve this condition. Surgery is another option.

■Aging of the Male Reproductive System

When men grow older, their hormone levels also change, and the production of sperm decreases. Older men generally need more time to achieve an erection, and the erection is usually less firm but lasts longer. Perhaps the most significant age-related change affecting the male reproductive system is enlargement of the prostate gland. This firm, muscular gland encircles the urethra like a doughnut. When it expands, it squeezes the urethra and causes painful urination, decreased force of the urinary stream, and more frequent urination. If the condition remains untreated, it may lead to poor urinary control, dribbling, bleeding, obstruction, and kidney damage.

Among the most common treatments for an enlarged prostate is surgery to remove the prostate tissue surrounding the urethra. Many men fear surgery on their prostate gland (prostatectomy), because they believe it will end their sex life. The amount of semen ejaculated will be less, but, otherwise, 70 percent of the men who have had a prostatectomy are often capable of having the same sexual relations as before surgery. Some men, however, will experience a diminished ability to perform sexually after this surgery.

There have been recent advances yielding new drugs to take orally, by injection, or directly applied to the penis that offer men experiencing impotence for a variety of reasons the ability to achieve erections. Urologists have the most experience treating sexual problems. Cardiac work-ups are advised and usually required for men at risk. There can be complications or in rare cases deaths of men who take these drugs and exert themselves.

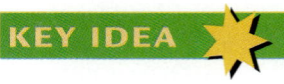

KEY IDEA

Aging alone does not cause an end of sexual desire. As people grow older, sexual desire may change, but sexuality and sexual needs continue.

COMMON DISEASES AND DISORDERS OF THE REPRODUCTIVE SYSTEM

A number of disorders may affect the female reproductive system:

- *Dysmenorrhea:* painful menstruation
- *Amenorrhea:* absence of menstruation

- *Menorrhagia:* excessive bleeding during menstruation

- *Pelvic inflammatory disease (PID):* infection that spreads to all structures in the pelvic cavity

- *Vaginitis:* inflammation of the vagina

- *Cystocele:* downward protrusion of the urinary bladder into the vagina

- *Rectocele:* protrusion of the rectum into the vagina

- *Cancer of the uterus:* malignancy of the uterus

- *Fibroids:* benign tumors of the uterus

- *Tumors of the breast:* new cell growth that may be benign or malignant

Male reproductive system disorders include the following:

- *Benign prostatic hyperplasia (BPH):* enlarged prostate gland

- *Cancer of the prostate gland:* malignant tumor

- *Prostatitis:* inflammation of the prostate gland

- *Hydrocele:* abnormal accumulation of fluid within the scrotum

- *Impotence:* inability to achieve or sustain an erection

- *Varicocele:* enlargement of the veins within the scrotum

- *Tumors of the testicle:* new cell growth that may be benign or malignant

- *Tumors of the breast:* new cell growth that may be benign or malignant

Sexually Transmitted Diseases

Diseases acquired as a result of sexual intercourse with a person who is infected are called **sexually transmitted diseases (STDs)**. Some of the most common STDs are as follows:

- *Chlamydia:* infection by Chlamydia bacteria (a type of rickettsia), whose incidence is on the rise

- *Gonorrhea:* contagious infection caused by gonococcus bacteria

- *AIDS (acquired immune deficiency syndrome):* group of signs and symptoms that characterizes a lethal disorder in T-cell immunity associated with either Karposi's sarcoma or opportunistic infections that impair immune function; caused by infection with a virus called **HIV**, which attacks white blood cells and impairs their response to infection

- *Syphilis:* an infectious, chronic, venereal disease characterized by lesions that may involve any organ or tissue; caused by *Treponema pallidum,* a spirochete

- *Genital herpes simplex (HSV):* a viral disease that may be recurrent and has no cure; open sores may be present in the genital area or inside the vagina, but most patients will not have visible signs of the disease; the sores do not need to be visible for the infection to be transmitted to another individual

- *Human papillomavirus (HPV) infection (genital warts):* genital and anal warts caused by infection with HPV; some forms can be cancerous; there is no cure or way to get rid of the virus (HPV), and treatment usually is aimed at treating the wart itself with medication

sexually transmitted diseases (STDs) Diseases acquired as a result of sexual intercourse with an infected person

HIV Human immunodeficiency virus; the microorganism that causes AIDS

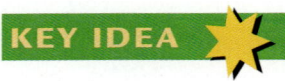

STDs can be prevented by sexual abstinence. Most STDs can be prevented by using barriers such as male or female condoms during intercourse, or using other methods of practicing safe sex.

■ Caring for Patients with AIDS

Measures to prevent HIV infection are especially important, according to current HIV/AIDS research. One reason is that AIDS frequently is a fatal syndrome. Many promising new drugs on the market can lessen the effect of HIV/AIDS, but no cure is available as of this writing. Currently, a combination of three drugs has been most useful to treat patients. Researchers are uncertain how effective this treatment will be as the AIDS virus mutates and may not continue to respond to the drugs. New cases continue as it is not always possible to know who may transmit the disease and because a person can carry the virus (HIV) for many years before developing AIDS.

AIDS Viral infection characterized by decreased immunity to opportunistic infections

Tests are available that indicate exposure to HIV, but these tests do not confirm a diagnosis of AIDS. To be diagnosed with **AIDS**, the patient must not only test positive for HIV but also meet at least one of the criteria set by the Centers for Disease Control (CDC). The CDC criteria include development of certain infections, cancers, wasting of the body, and dementia. A person infected with HIV can transmit the virus whether or not he has AIDS.

Both heterosexuals and homosexuals can be afflicted by HIV/AIDS. The following groups are most at risk for HIV/AIDS: IV drug users, people who engage in homosexual acts, people who have received contaminated blood, and anyone who has sexual intercourse with a person in these groups. At this time, the fastest growing numbers of new HIV infections are in the heterosexual group.

HIV/AIDS can be transmitted by blood and other body fluids or secretions that may contain blood. Gloves and protective eye gear are mandatory to protect the nursing assistant from exposure due to splashing when handling *any* patient's body fluids, such as blood, urine, feces, or saliva. If you as a nursing assistant come upon a needle and syringe, or any sharp object, you should immediately dispose of it in a puncture-proof container. Needles should never be bent, broken, or recapped.

The AIDS patient, too, requires protection. Because his immune system is suppressed, the patient needs to be protected from such normally routine illnesses as colds. The patient's privacy also may need to be protected, because many people are afraid of AIDS or have negative feelings about members of some major risk groups (homosexuals and IV drug users). Therefore, the nursing assistant should maintain confidentiality and follow the institution's policy and should not disclose that a patient has AIDS. However, a patient's condition needs to be known to the patient's caregivers.

The nursing assistant can also support the emotional well-being of the patient with AIDS. Having a terminal illness is distressing for any patient. And because this disease is widely feared, the patient's family and friends may be reluctant to touch or spend time with him. The nursing assistant can help by being sensitive and nonjudgmental with the patient. Also, when the nursing assistant works with the AIDS patient and touches him appropriately, her behavior can serve as a model to family members, helping them view the risks more realistically.

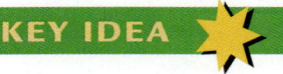

HIV is not spread by casual contact like hugging, coughing, or sharing a bathroom. The Standard Precautions (see Chapter 5, pages 78–108) provide protection against AIDS as well as other blood-borne diseases.

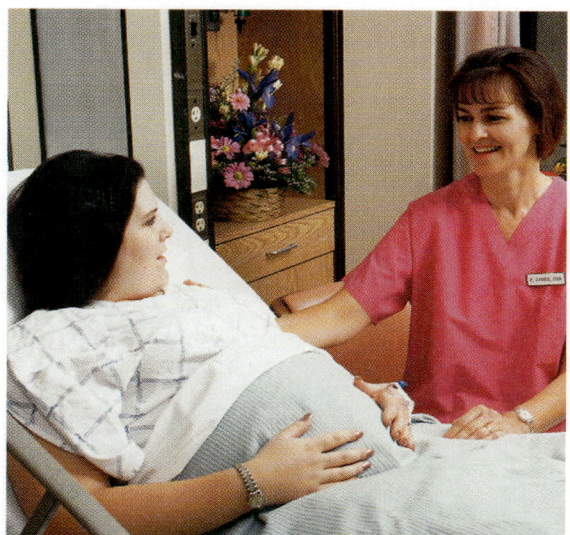

FIGURE 25–5
Many gynecological patients appreciate support and reassurance

CARE OF THE GYNECOLOGICAL PATIENT

A female patient receiving care of the reproductive system (including the breasts) is known as a **gynecological (GYN) patient** (Figure 25–5). Care of the gynecological patient often includes pelvic exams. Occasionally, the nursing assistant may also give a vaginal irrigation (also called a douche).

gynecological (GYN) patient Patient being treated for diseases or conditions of the female reproductive organs, including the breasts

Preparing the Patient for a Pelvic Exam

A pelvic examination is very important to assessing the condition of the female reproductive organs. However, patients often find the exam embarrassing or uncomfortable, so the nursing assistant should be especially careful to maintain privacy and comfort.

PROCEDURE

PREPARING THE PATIENT FOR A PELVIC EXAM

PREPARATION

1. Assemble the equipment (Figure 25–6):

   a. Disposable gloves
   b. Microscope slides
   c. Cotton applicators
   d. Cotton balls
   e. Pap smear fixative
   f. Vaginal speculum
   g. Uterine dressing forceps
   h. Lubricant
   i. Wooden tongue blade

2. Wash your hands and put on disposable gloves.

3. Provide privacy for the patient.

4. Tell the patient you are going to prepare her for a pelvic exam.

STEPS

5. Have the patient empty her bladder in the bathroom or assist with a bedpan.

6. Help the patient undress while providing coverage with a blanket.

7. Position the patient on her back with her knees separated and legs flexed (Figure 25–7). Stirrups

P R O C E D U R E   (CONTINUED)

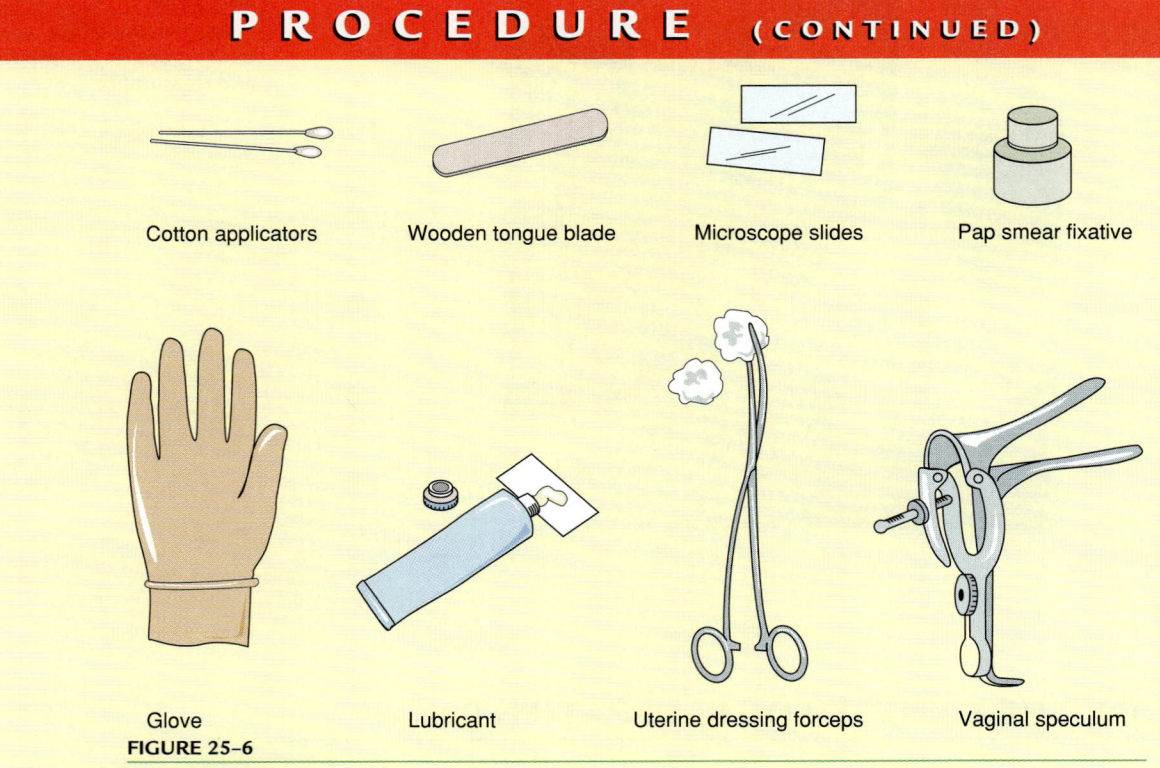

Cotton applicators   Wooden tongue blade   Microscope slides   Pap smear fixative

Glove   Lubricant   Uterine dressing forceps   Vaginal speculum

FIGURE 25–6

Assemble equipment for the pelvic exam

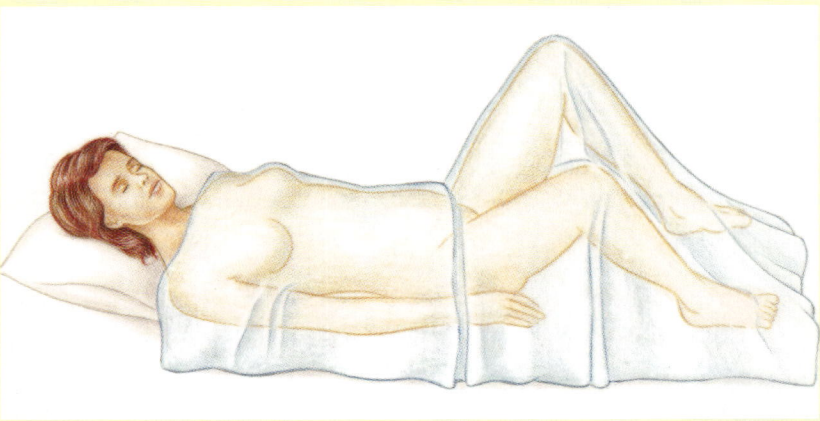

FIGURE 25–7

Position patient on her back with knees separated and legs flexed

---

may be used to position the legs and feet. An additional drape may be used to cover the legs.

8. If you leave the room before the exam, place the call light within easy reach of the patient. However, you may be asked to remain during the exam.

9. After the exam, assist the patient to dress or put on a gown.

FOLLOW-UP

10. Make sure the patient is comfortable.

11. Care for the equipment according to the institution's policy.

12. Remove your gloves and wash your hands.

13. Report to the supervisor:
    - That the exam was performed.
    - What time the exam was performed.

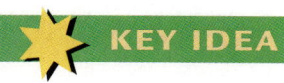

> When providing any type of gynecological care, the nursing assistant must be especially careful to protect the patient's privacy and to respect her ideas of modesty.

KEY IDEA

■ Vaginal Douche or Nonsterile Irrigation

The introduction of a solution into the vagina with an immediate return of the solution by gravity is called a **vaginal irrigation** or **douche**. This type of irrigation is usually used for cleansing the vaginal canal or relieving inflammation of the vaginal tract. A doctor may order this treatment to cleanse before surgery or an examination, in cases of severe discharge, to treat an inflammation, or to neutralize secretions in the vaginal canal.

When used to excess, vaginal irrigation can wash away normal protective secretions. This is one reason why such a procedure should never be done without a physician's order.

In carrying out a vaginal irrigation, follow the rules of medical asepsis. In some institutions this procedure is done while the patient is on the toilet. Follow the instructions of your immediate supervisor.

vaginal irrigation (douche) The introduction of a solution into the vagina with an immediate return of the solution by gravity; usually used for cleansing the vaginal canal or relieving inflammation of the vaginal tract

PROCEDURE

NONSTERILE VAGINAL IRRIGATION (DOUCHE)

PREPARATION

1. Assemble your equipment:
   a. Disposable douche
   b. Bedpan and cover (towel)
   c. Bath blanket
   d. Disposable waterproof bed protector
   e. Disposable gloves
2. Wash your hands and put on disposable gloves.
3. Identify the patient by checking the identification bracelet.
4. Ask visitors to step out of the room.
5. Tell the patient you are going to give her a vaginal douche.
6. Provide privacy for the patient.

STEPS

7. Offer the patient the bedpan, explaining that her bladder must be empty to ensure the desired results from the douche.
8. Remove the bedpan. Measure output if the patient is on intake and output. Record on the I&O sheet. Empty the contents of the bedpan; wash it and place it on a chair nearby.
9. Remove gloves and wash your hands. Put on clean gloves.
10. Wash the patient's hands.
11. Place the patient into the dorsal recumbent position. The head of the bed should be flat. Drape the patient with a small sheet.
12. Cover the patient with a bath blanket. Without exposing her, fanfold the top sheets to the foot of the bed. The patient holds the bath blanket while you do this. Leave the patient covered with only the bath blanket.
13. Place the disposable bed protector under the patient's hips (buttocks).

14. Raise the bed to a comfortable working position.
15. Open the douche kit.
16. Cleanse the perineum with soap and water, using a washcloth.
17. Place the bedpan under the patient's hips (buttocks).
18. With solution flowing, insert the douche nozzle tip into the vagina from 2 to 3 inches with an upward and then downward and backward gentle movement.
19. Allow the solution to flow.
20. Help the patient to sit up on the bedpan by raising the back of the bed, if allowed (Fowler's position). This will help the solution to drain from the vagina.
21. Dry the perineum with toilet tissue and discard into the bedpan.
22. Remove the bedpan and cover with towel.
23. Help the patient to turn on her side and dry the buttocks with toilet tissue.
24. Replace the bed protector with a dry one if wet.

PROCEDURE (CONTINUED)

25. Lower the bed to its lowest horizontal position.

26. Change any linen that has become damp.

27. Raise the top sheets over the bath blanket and then remove the bath blanket from under the top sheets.

FOLLOW-UP

28. Make the patient comfortable.

29. Lower the bed to a position of safety for the patient.

30. Raise the side rails where ordered, indicated, and appropriate for patient safety.

31. Place the call light within easy reach of the patient.

32. Observe the contents of the bedpan. Collect a specimen to show to your immediate supervisor if the returned solution is not as clear as when it was inserted.

33. Discard disposable supplies.

34. Clean the bedpan and return to its proper place.

35. Remove disposable gloves and wash your hands.

36. Report to your immediate supervisor:

- That the vaginal irrigation was done.
- The time the vaginal irrigation was done.
- Whether a specimen was collected, and why.
- How the patient tolerated the procedure.

POSTPARTUM CARE

During vaginal delivery of a baby, the vaginal canal stretches and sometimes tears through the perineal muscles. This can cause postpartum edema and tenderness. Sometimes during the birth the doctor will make a small cut (episiotomy) in the vagina to make the opening larger and to prevent tearing. This episiotomy will require stitches and will also be tender. Postpartum perineal care (cleansing of the perineum) promotes healing, cleanses, and gives comfort to that area.

Perineal care must be performed by the patient or caregiver after each elimination of urine or feces. It is generally performed by the patient on the toilet. The following procedure is for postpartum perineal care given in bed.

PROCEDURE

POSTPARTUM PERINEAL CARE

PREPARATION

1. Assemble your equipment:

a. Disposable bed protector

b. Bedpan and cover

c. Squirt bottle (peri bottle)

d. Toilet paper

e. Disposable gloves

2. Wash your hands.

3. Identify the patient by checking the identification bracelet.

4. Ask visitors to leave the room, if this is your hospital's policy.

5. Tell the patient you are going to clean the genital area.

6. Provide privacy for the patient.

7. Be sure there is plenty of light. Raise the bed to a comfortable working position.

STEPS

8. Cover the patient with a bath blanket. Without exposing her, fanfold the top sheets to the foot of the bed. Have the patient covered only with the blanket. Put on gloves.

9. Fill the squirt bottle with warm water at 100°F (37.7°C) or use the solution provided in your institution.

10. Place the disposable bed protector under the patient's hips (buttocks).

PROCEDURE (CONTINUED)

11. Help the patient to get on the bedpan.

12. Put on disposable gloves.

13. Spray the perineum with solution, working from anterior to posterior

14. Dry the patient gently with the toilet paper. Remove and discard the disposable gloves.

15. Remove the bedpan and disposable bed protector. Place them on a chair.

16. Cover the patient with the top sheets. Remove the bath blanket.

FOLLOW-UP

17. Make the patient comfortable.

18. Lower the bed to a position of safety for the patient.

19. Raise the side rails where ordered, indicated, and appropriate for patient safety.

20. Place the call light within easy reach of the patient.

21. Discard disposable equipment.

22. Empty, rinse, and put the equipment back where it belongs.

23. Remove your gloves and wash your hands.

24. Report to your immediate supervisor:
    - That postpartum perineal care was given.
    - Your observations of anything unusual.
    - How the patient tolerated the procedure.

Another important function of postpartum care is observation of the amount of blood that has accumulated on the perineal pads worn by the patient. Some institutions count the number of pads, and others also want a description of the amount of blood on the pad. In addition, the nursing assistant should observe the urine for blood clots (from the vagina) the first 24 hours after birth.

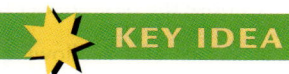

KEY IDEA

Never hand a baby to a mother who is sleepy and then leave her alone. You may need to put the side rails up for safety or remain with the mother while she feeds the baby. Follow the instructions of your immediate supervisor.

Another aspect of care for the postpartum patient is help with ambulation. The type of delivery—a vaginal or a cesarean birth—may influence her ability to ambulate without discomfort. It is very important that the patient have good feeling in her legs before attempting to walk. The legs may be numb from anesthesia she received for the birth. Some types of anesthesia require the patient to lie flat for several hours after birth until the anesthesia wears off to prevent developing a severe headache. Check with your supervisor if you are uncertain about the patient's ambulation orders or ability.

Finally, if the patient has had a cesarean section birth, she will require additional care. Follow the instructions in Chapter 18 for coughing and deep breathing and use of the incentive spirometer for patients who have had surgery.

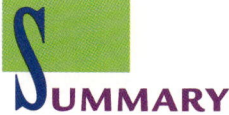

SUMMARY

The different reproductive structures in the female and male greatly influence the care provided by the nursing assistant. A basic understanding of the human reproductive anatomy and the common diseases and disorders is essential. Also important is a sensitivity to cultural differences that might affect the patient's expectations and reactions to care of the reproductive system. Providing privacy at all times is just as important as the physical care given to the patient. Because of the possibility of HIV/AIDS contamination, caregivers must wear protective gear where appropriate. Your immediate supervisor will assist you in identifying situations in which special protective gear must be worn.

The Nervous System and Related Care

26

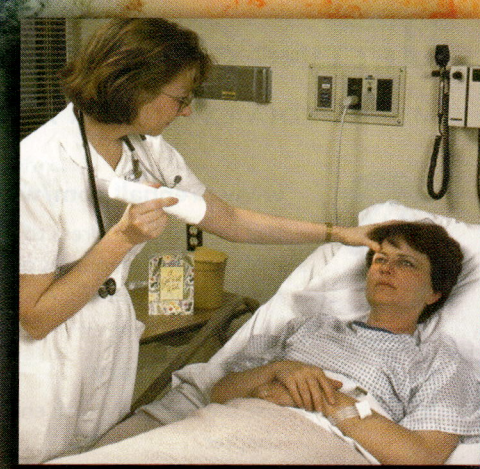

INTRODUCTION

Caring for a patient with a neurologic condition is challenging and rewarding. Neurologic conditions can involve any part of the nervous system and are very frightening for most patients and their families. Patients and their families often need both emotional and physical support. In the course of helping with the care of these patients, the nursing assistant has a chance to provide much of this support.

When you have completed this chapter, you will be able to:

- Describe the functions of the nervous system, the brain, and the spinal cord.
- List two divisions of the autonomic nervous system.
- List the five sense organs.
- Describe the care of a patient's artificial eye, eyeglasses, and hearing aid.
- Describe common age-related changes in the nervous system.
- List common diseases and disorders of the nervous system.
- Describe four types of seizures.
- Discuss five safety measures for the patient having a seizure.
- List four causes and results of a cerebrovascular accident (stroke).
- Describe the nursing assistant's role in care of a cerebrovascular accident patient.
- Describe the psychological aspects of caring for a patient who has had a cerebrovascular accident.
- Demonstrate how to communicate with an aphasic patient using correct technique.

aphasia

autonomic nervous system

canthus

cerebral spinal fluid

cerebrovascular accident (CVA)

complex partial seizure

contracture

convulsive

deficit

embolus

environment

hemiplegia

hemisphere

hemorrhage

hypothalamus

impulse

intervertebral discs

involuntary

meninges

myelin sheath

nervous system

neuron

normal pressure hydrocephalus

osteoporosis

plaque

respond

rupture

seizure

simple partial seizure

spasm

stimuli

thrombus

vascular

vertebral bodies

voluntary

nervous system The group of body organs consisting of the brain, spinal cord, and nerves that controls and regulates the activities of the body and the functions of the other body systems

voluntary Under control of the will; with conscious decision

involuntary Without conscious will, control, or decision

vascular Pertaining to blood vessels

neuron A type of nerve cell in the nervous system

environment All the surrounding conditions and influences affecting the life and development of an organism

impulse An electrical or chemical charge transmitted through certain tissues, especially nerve fibers and muscles

ANATOMY AND PHYSIOLOGY OF THE NERVOUS SYSTEM

The **nervous system** controls and organizes all body activity, both **voluntary** and **involuntary**. The nervous system is made up of the brain, the spinal cord, and the nerves. The nerves are spread throughout all areas of the body in an orderly way. The central nervous system is made up of the brain and spinal cord. The peripheral nervous system is made up of the nerves outside the brain and spinal cord.

The nervous system, and especially the brain, has a large **vascular** supply. That is, many blood vessels feed the brain so that it can carry out its many functions.

Nerve tissue is made up of cells called **neurons** and other supporting cells called neuroglia. A typical neuron consists of a cell body with one long column, called the axon, and many small outbranchings, called dendrites. Nerve impulses move from the dendrites through the cell body along the axon (Figure 26–1).

◼ Sensing and Responding to the Environment

Inside and outside our bodies, we have structures called receptor-end organs. Any change in our external or internal **environment** that is strong enough will set up a nervous **impulse** in these receptor-end organs. This impulse is carried by a sensory neuron

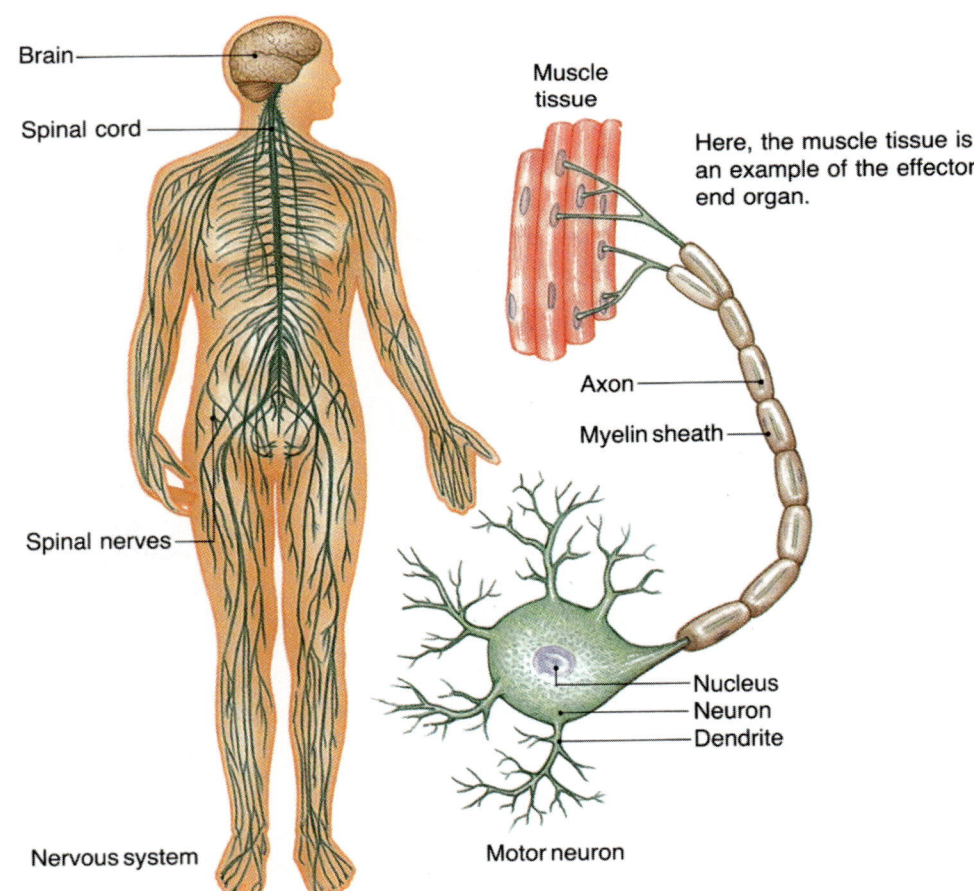

Brain

Spinal cord

Muscle tissue

Here, the muscle tissue is an example of the effector end organ.

Axon

Myelin sheath

Spinal nerves

Nucleus
Neuron
Dendrite

Nervous system

Motor neuron

FIGURE 26–1

The nervous system and a motor neuron

FIGURE 26–2

A synapse

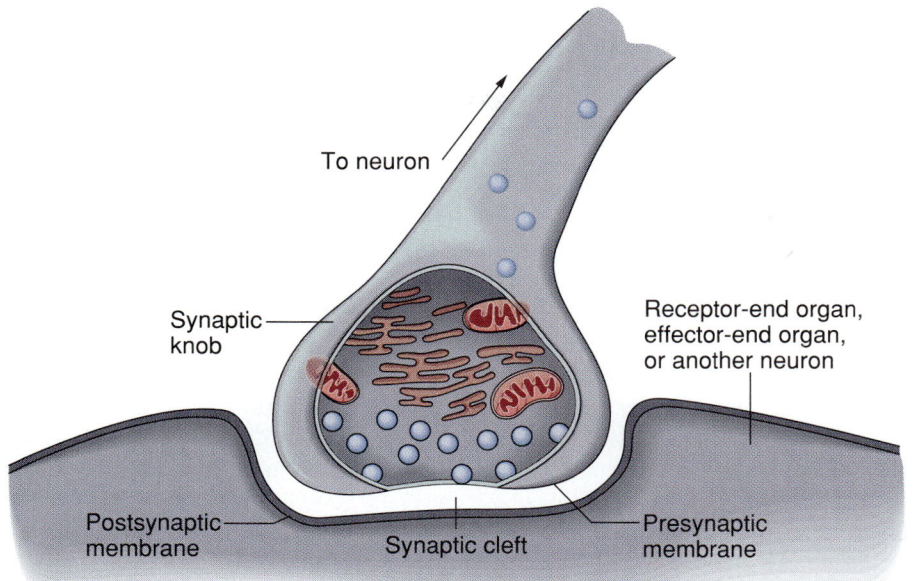

To neuron

Synaptic knob

Receptor-end organ, effector-end organ, or another neuron

Postsynaptic membrane

Synaptic cleft

Presynaptic membrane

to some part of the brain or spinal cord, where it connects with another neuron. The connection is called a synapse (Figure 26–2). Eventually the brain decides how to **respond** to the nerve impulse. This decision may come only after the interneuron has made hundreds of synapses (particularly in the cerebrum, the part of the brain in which we think). Once that happens, the proper impulses are sent down a motor neuron to the organ that will receive the impulse. When the organ (such as a muscle) receives the impulse, it responds. In the case of a muscle, it may contract or relax.

respond React; begin, end, or change activity in reaction to stimulation

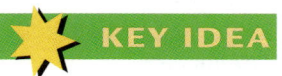   **KEY IDEA**

In the nervous system, when the body receives information, impulses travel from receptor-end organs through neurons to the brain. When the body responds to a stimulus, impulses travel from the brain through neurons to receiving organs, such as muscles.

■ Protection of the Nervous System

Most nerve cells outside the brain and spinal cord have a protective covering known as the **myelin sheath**. The task of the myelin sheath is to insulate the nerve cell. If you think of the nerve cell as an electrical wire, the myelin sheath is insulation that keeps the current in the correct pathway. This insulating sheath helps prevent damage to the cells and often helps the nerve return to healthy function, or regenerate, if it has been injured. Nerve cells with a myelin sheath also carry an impulse faster than those without myelin.

The neurons in the brain and spinal cord do not have this kind of protection and are not able to regrow. When nerve cells are injured, as they are by a stroke, or **cerebrovascular accident (CVA)**, another part of the brain must take over the function of the part that has been damaged. The rehabilitation department in your health care institution helps patients learn to do things again after such damage has been done.

The brain is well protected by bones, membranes, the **meninges**, and a cushion of fluid called **cerebral spinal fluid**. This fluid circulates outside and within the brain, as well as around the spinal cord.

myelin sheath Protective covering around most nerves

cerebrovascular accident (CVA) Stroke; blockage or bleeding of blood vessels in the brain, interrupting the blood supply to that part of the brain and damaging the surrounding area of the brain

meninges The covering of the brain and spinal cord. There are three layers: the dura mater, the arachnoid, and the pia mater

cerebral spinal fluid The fluid that circulates around and within the brain and spinal cord

The Brain

The brain coordinates and controls all of the functions of the central nervous system such as memory, sight, and walking (Figure 26–3). The brain is a very complicated organ made up of five components: the cerebrum, the cerebellum, the midbrain, the pons, and the medulla.

The cerebrum is divided into two halves, called **hemispheres**. These hemispheres make up the top portion of the brain. The right hemisphere of the cerebrum controls most of the activity on the left side of the body. The left hemisphere controls activity on the right side of the body.

The cerebrum is where all learning, memory, and associations are stored so that thought is possible. Also, decisions are made for voluntary action. Certain areas of the cerebrum seem to perform special organizing activities. For example, the occipital lobe is the place that interprets what you see. The frontal lobe is the primary area of thought and reason. The cerebellum is the part of the brain that coordinates voluntary motion. It works with part of the inner ear, the semicircular canals, to enable you to walk and move smoothly through your world.

The midbrain, pons, and medulla are primarily pathways through which nervous impulses reach the brain from the spinal cord. Nerves throughout the body send messages through the spinal cord. The impulses then travel up the spinal cord to the higher centers of the brain. There are 12 pairs of cranial nerves and 32 pairs of spinal nerves through which these nerve impulses can travel. These nerves have branches that go to all parts of the body. The nerve impulses travel down from the brain through the spinal cord and out to the body.

There are many small structures in the brain. They screen all nerve impulses going to the brain, either getting them there faster or slowing them down. One of these tiny structures is the **hypothalamus**, which in times of stress, emergency, excitement, or danger actually takes control of the body by controlling the pituitary gland, the body's master gland. We still know very little about the activity of the pituitary gland. We do know that it has tremendous control over most body activities. The hypothalamus seems to be the

hemisphere Half of a sphere; in the nervous system, one-half of the brain

hypothalamus Area of the brain responsible for control of the pituitary gland

FIGURE 26–3

The brain

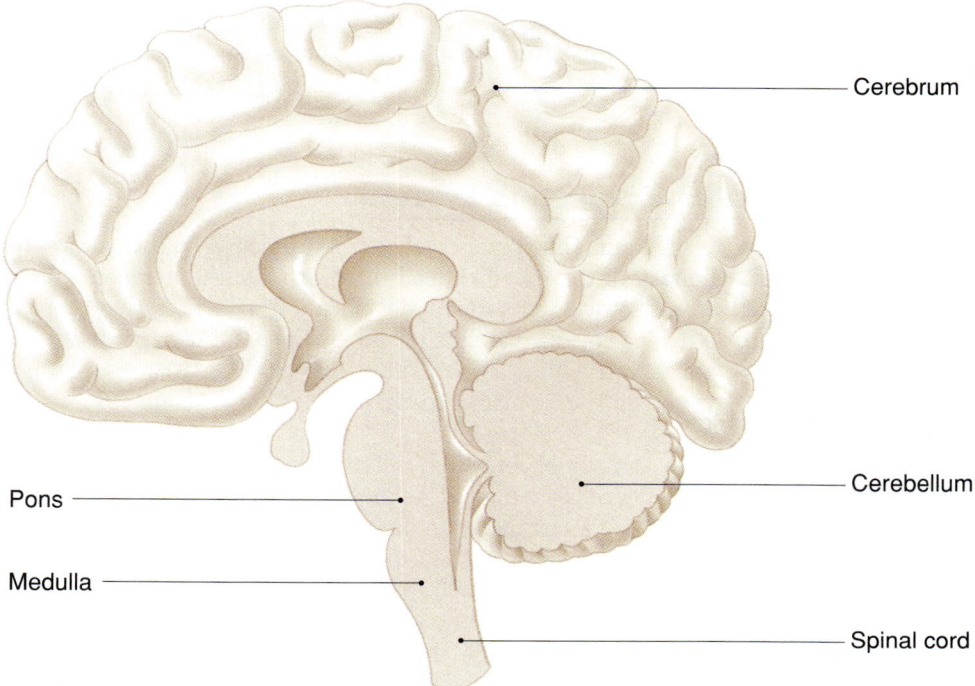

Cerebrum

Cerebellum

Pons

Medulla

Spinal cord

link between the mind and the body. It receives messages from the cerebrum, from the cerebellum, and from impulses coming up the spinal cord, and it has direct control over all the endocrine glands (glands that release hormones).

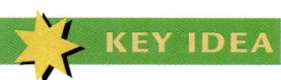

Among the activities of the cerebrum are learning, memory, and decision making. In general, the left hemisphere of the cerebrum controls the right side of the body, and the right hemisphere controls the left side. Thus, if the left side of the body were paralyzed, the right hemisphere is probably the affected side of the brain.

The Autonomic Nervous System

Much of the activity of the organs of the body is *involuntary*. In other words, we do not think about this activity, or we have little or no conscious control over it. The part of the nervous system that controls such involuntary activity as digestion and the functions of other visceral (abdominal) organs is the **autonomic nervous system**. This is really not separate from the brain and the spinal cord. The neurons that make up the autonomic nervous system use the same pathways as the neurons that control voluntary actions.

autonomic nervous system The part of the nervous system that carries messages without conscious thought

The autonomic nervous system has two divisions, which direct and control the activity of the internal organs. Each organ is supplied with neurons from each division of the autonomic nervous system.

One division is called the *sympathetic division*. The neurons that make up this division become active during stress, danger, excitement, or illness. These neurons cause the pupils of our eyes to become larger so that we can see more clearly and can see better at a distance. They also cause the heart to beat more strongly and to send more oxygen to the large muscles of the body in case it is necessary to fight or run. In today's fast-paced world, we are all subject to stress, and sometimes we cannot run away or fight. The action of the neurons from the sympathetic system responds by causing changes in the shape or activity of some of our organs. This action may also cause illness.

The *parasympathetic division* of the autonomic nervous system is in control when we are relaxed. It is known to conserve our energy.

Fortunately, a system of checks and balances operates between the two divisions. When one has been in action too long, the other automatically switches on. For example, during a stressful time when you may have been frightened, your heart rate increased. After you calmed down, your heart rate returned to normal. This is because stimulation of your sympathetic nervous system increases your heart rate and your parasympathetic nervous system causes your heart to return to normal functioning.

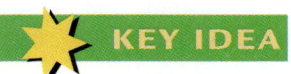

The body's response to stress comes from the sympathetic nervous system. A response from this division of the autonomic nervous system prepares the body to fight or run. When the parasympathetic nervous system is stimulated, it helps the body return to normal functioning.

The Sense Organs

We are aware of our environment through our sense organs: eyes, ears, nose, tongue, and skin. The sense organs contain specialized endings of the sensory neurons, which

FIGURE 26–4

Sensory and motor processes

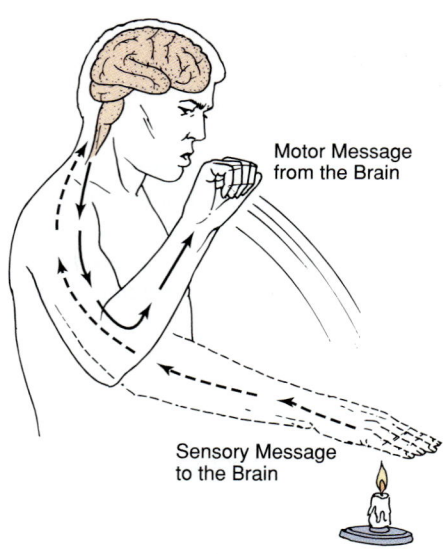

Motor Message from the Brain

Sensory Message to the Brain

stimuli Changes in the external or internal environment strong enough to set up a nervous impulse or other responses in an organism

are excited by changes in the outside environment. These changes are called **stimuli** (Figure 26–4). Each sense organ responds to a different category of stimuli:

- Eyes (Figure 26–5) respond to visual stimuli (what we see)

- Ears (Figure 26–6) respond mainly to sound stimuli (what we hear) and the body's position in space

- Membranes of the nose respond to smell

- Taste buds, located chiefly on the tongue, respond to taste sensations: sweet, sour, salty, and bitter

- Skin responds to heat, cold, touch, pressure, and pain (Figure 26–7)

KEY IDEA   The sense organs are a person's sources of information about the environment. Thus, proper care of the sense organs is essential to good health and a feeling of well-being.

FIGURE 26–5

The eye

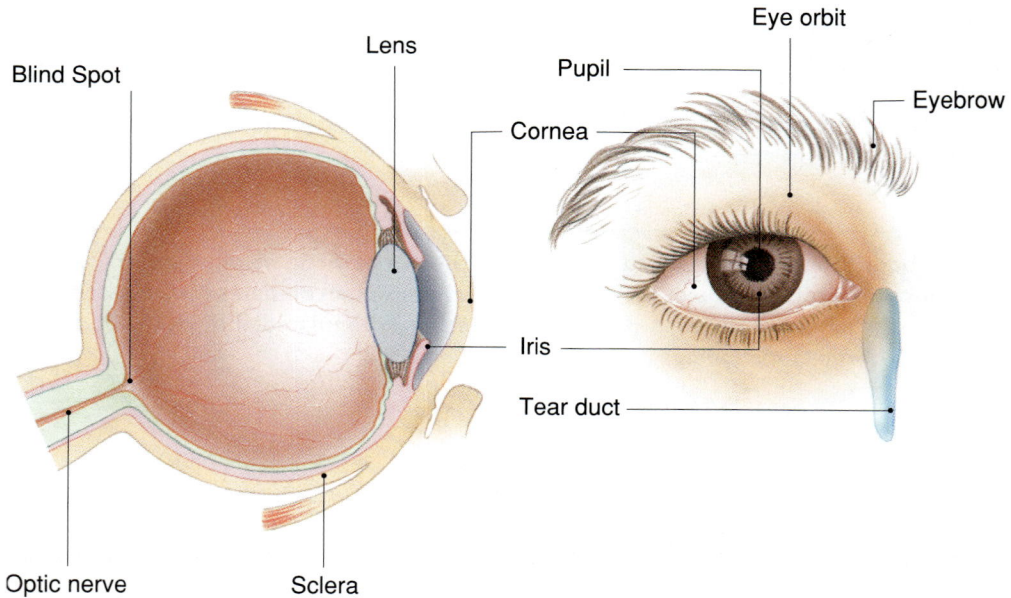

Blind Spot

Lens

Eye orbit

Pupil

Cornea

Eyebrow

Iris

Tear duct

Optic nerve

Sclera

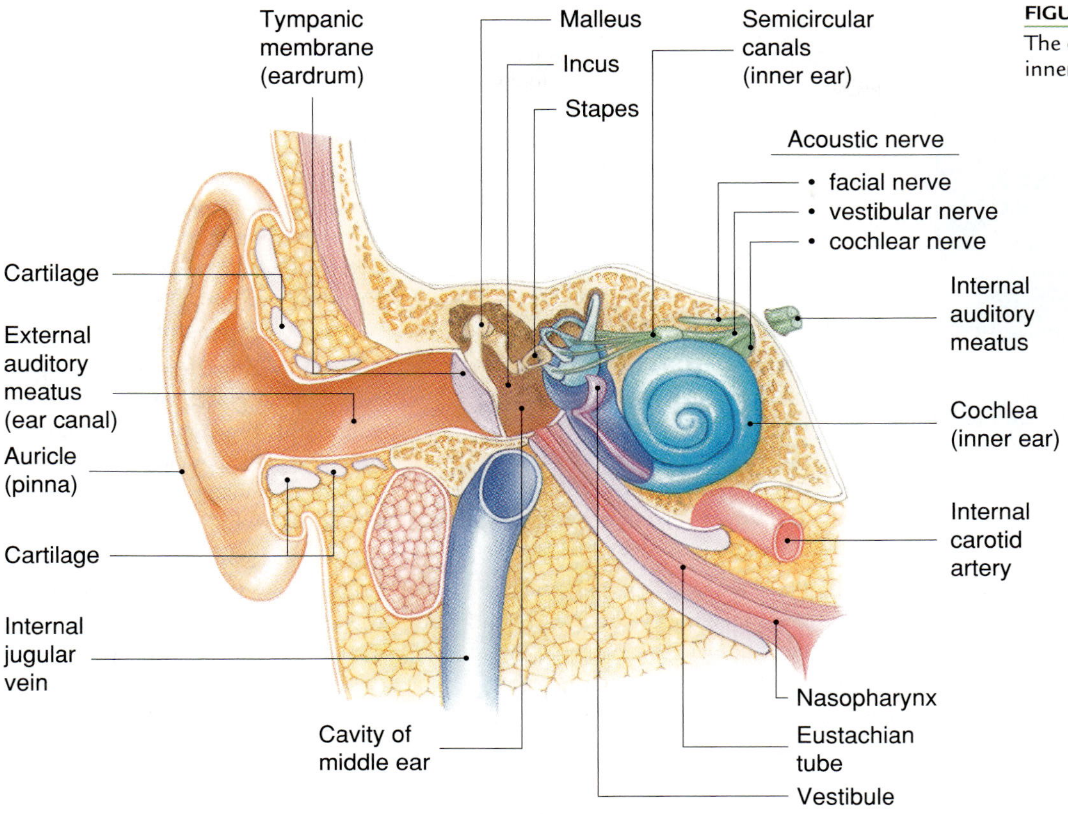

FIGURE 26–6
The outer, middle, and inner ear

Tympanic membrane (eardrum)

Malleus

Incus

Stapes

Semicircular canals (inner ear)

Acoustic nerve
• facial nerve
• vestibular nerve
• cochlear nerve

Internal auditory meatus

Cartilage

External auditory meatus (ear canal)

Auricle (pinna)

Cartilage

Internal jugular vein

Cavity of middle ear

Cochlea (inner ear)

Internal carotid artery

Nasopharynx

Eustachian tube

Vestibule

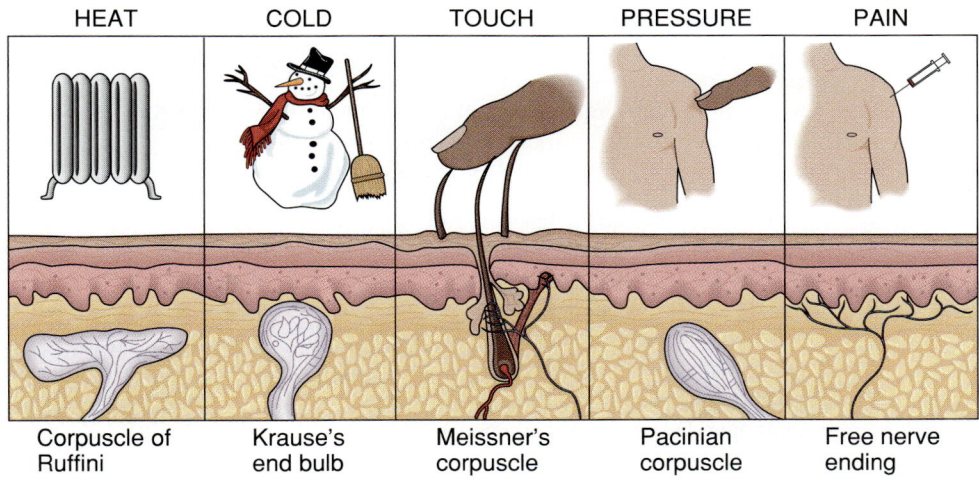

FIGURE 26–7
The skin responds to heat, cold, touch, pressure, and pain

HEAT	COLD	TOUCH	PRESSURE	PAIN
Corpuscle of Ruffini	Krause's end bulb	Meissner's corpuscle	Pacinian corpuscle	Free nerve ending

CARE OF THE ARTIFICIAL EYE

For a patient who has an artificial eye, cleaning the eye is part of daily personal hygiene. Proper care helps prevent infection and encrustation (formation of dried mucous material in the eye socket and around the artificial eye). Often a patient cannot care for his artificial eye himself. Encourage the patient to do as much as possible and assist as necessary.

PROCEDURE

CARING FOR THE ARTIFICIAL EYE

PREPARATION

1. Assemble your equipment on the bedside table:

   a. An eyecup half-filled with lukewarm water at 98° to 100°F (36.6° to 37.7°C) and labeled with the patient's name and room number (or, if no eyecup is available, use a clean denture cup)

   b. Gauze, 4″ × 4″ (3–4 pieces), for the bottom of the cup (or per your institution's policy)

   c. Small basin with lukewarm water

   d. Four cotton balls

   e. Special cleansing solution, if ordered by the doctor

2. Wash your hands.

3. Ask visitors to step out of the room, if this is your hospital's policy.

4. Identify the patient by checking the identification bracelet.

5. Tell the patient you are going to take care of his eye.

6. Pull the curtain around the bed for privacy.

STEPS

7. Help the patient lie down on the bed. This is to prevent accidental dropping of the artificial eye.

8. Put on gloves.

9. Have the patient close his eyes. Clean any external secretions from the patient's upper eyelid. Use cotton balls and warm water from the basin. Clean from the inner **canthus** to the outside of the eye area. This means you move from the nose to the outside of the eye. If you need to wipe more than once, use a clean (new) cotton ball each time. Use gentle strokes.

10. Remove the artificial eye. To do this, carefully depress the lower eyelid with your thumb. Lift the upper lid gently with your forefinger. The eye should slide out and down, into your hand. Have the patient do this, if he is able.

11. Place a 4″ × 4″ gauze in the cup and place the eye on the gauze. Let it soak in the water.

12. Wash off external matter and encrustations from the outside of the eye socket with cotton balls and warm water. Using gentle strokes, clean from the inner canthus to the outside of the eye.

13. Take the eyecup to the patient's bathroom. Close the drain in the sink. Fill the sink one-half full with water to prevent breakage if the eye is dropped.

14. Take the eye in your gloved hand and wash with running lukewarm water 98° to 100°F (36.6° to 37.7°C). Use plain water unless the doctor orders a special solution. Place the eye in the gauze from the eyecup and rub gently between your thumb and forefinger. *Do not use alcohol, ether, or acetone. These may dissolve the plastic of the artificial eye or dull the luster.*

15. Rinse the eye under running lukewarm water at 98° to 100°F (36.6° to 37.7°C), then dry it using the second 4″ × 4″ gauze. Discard the water from the eyecup. Place the slightly moistened eye on a dry gauze in the eyecup. A slightly moistened eye is easier to insert. Return to the patient's bedside.

16. If the patient cannot wear the eye immediately, store it by adding water to the eyecup and placing it in the bedside table drawer. Label the cup with the patient's name and room number.

17. Before inserting the artificial eye, remove your gloves and wash your hands thoroughly a second time. Put on clean gloves. If the patient is to insert the eye, have him wash his hands.

18. Insert the eye in the patient's eye socket. Have the notched edge toward the nose. Raise the upper lid with your forefinger. With your other hand, insert the eye. Place the eye under the upper lid. Then depress the lower lid. The eye should settle in place.

FOLLOW-UP

19. Make the patient comfortable.

20. Lower the bed to a position of safety for the patient.

21. Pull the curtains back to the open position.

22. Raise the side rails where ordered, indicated, and appropriate for patient safety.

23. Place the call light within easy reach of the patient.

24. Remove your gloves and wash your hands.

25. Report at once to your immediate supervisor:

   ■ That you have completed care of the artificial eye.

   ■ The time the procedure was done.

   ■ How the patient tolerated the procedure.

   ■ Your observations of anything unusual.

canthus The inner aspect of the eye closest to the nose

CARE OF EYEGLASSES

Proper care of a patient's eyeglasses is an essential task. Many patients find it difficult to function well without their eyeglasses because their vision is poor. Keeping the eyeglasses clean and scratch free is very important. Patients should always wear their glasses when they are walking or performing tasks if they cannot see well enough without them.

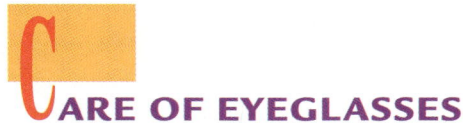

PROCEDURE

CARING FOR EYEGLASSES

PREPARATION

1. Knock or ask permission to enter the patient's room.
2. Assemble your equipment on the bedside table or in the bathroom:
   a. A soft cloth
   b. Cleaning solution if needed
3. Wash your hands.
4. Identify yourself.
5. Identify the patient.

STEPS

6. Explain what you are going to do. Remove the patient's eyeglasses from the case or take them off the patient's face with the patient's permission and assistance. Handle the glasses by the frame only.
7. Inspect the eyeglasses. Do this by holding them up to the light and looking for scratches, smears, or soiling. Look for any loose screws in the hinges of the frame.
8. Clean the eyeglasses by polishing them with a soft cloth. If more cleaning solution is needed, run them under warm water or use the cleaning solution provided by your institution. Dry the eyeglasses with a soft cloth.
9. Return the eyeglasses to the case or to the patient. Assist the pa-

tient with putting them on as needed.
10. Remember to always keep eyeglasses in the case when the patient is not wearing them to avoid breaking or scratching them.

FOLLOW-UP

11. Wash your hands.
12. Report at once to your immediate supervisor:
    - That you have completed care of the eyeglasses.
    - The time the procedure was done.
    - How the patient tolerated the procedure.
    - Your observations of anything unusual such as scratches on the eyeglasses or loose hinge screws.

HEARING AIDS

Even the best hearing aid cannot restore full, normal hearing ability. A patient who wears a hearing aid may still have trouble hearing. When talking to a patient who wears a hearing aid, face her and speak clearly. Speak in a normal tone of voice unless requested to speak louder by the patient.

Parts of the Hearing Aid

A hearing aid has several parts that a nursing assistant must recognize (Figure 26–8):

- *Microphone:* changes sound waves into electric signals and transmits sound

FIGURE 26–8

A hearing aid

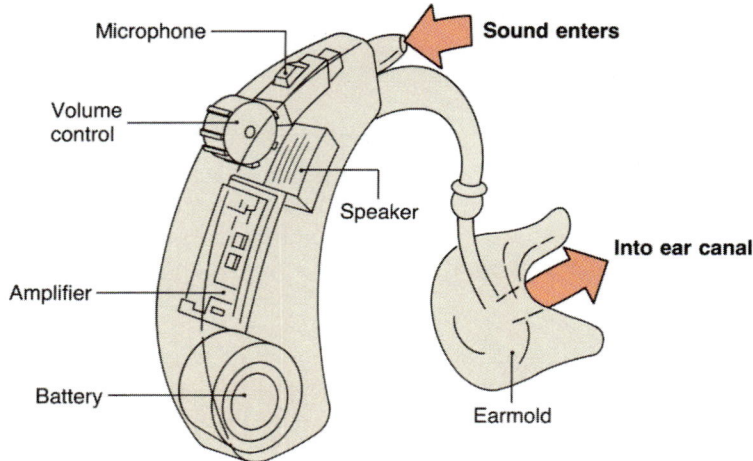

- *Amplifier:* uses battery energy to make the sound signals strong
- *Earmold:* channels the sound through the external ear canal to the eardrum (tympanic membrane)
- *Cord:* connects the amplifier to the earmold
- *Volume control:* adjusts the volume level

Placement of the Hearing Aid

- Turn down the volume to the lowest or Off position
- Place the hearing aid in the external ear canal; it should fit tightly but comfortably
- After the hearing aid is in place, turn it on and adjust the volume so the patient can hear in a normal tone; the patient will tell you when she can hear comfortably
- If the patient complains of an unpleasant whistle or squeal, check the placement in the ear and for a crack or break

Checking the Batteries

- Before applying a hearing aid, check the batteries. There are many styles of hearing aids (Figure 26–9). Be sure the batteries are the right size for the hearing aid. The battery case must close easily; if not, something is wrong.

FIGURE 26–9

Types of hearing aids (photo courtesy of SENSO by Widex)

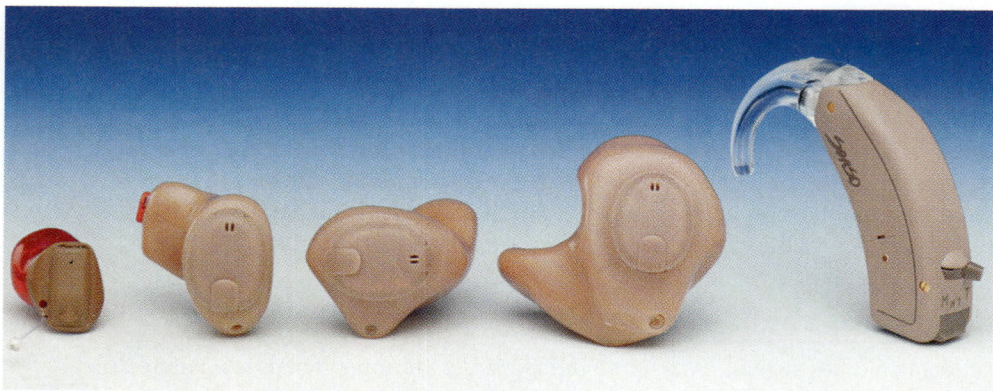

■ To test the batteries, place the volume control switch to On and turn up the volume. Cup your hand over the hearing aid; you should hear a whistle. If you do not hear the whistle, change the batteries.

■ If the patient complains that she cannot hear any sound, remove the hearing aid. Check the batteries and make sure the appliance is not broken.

■ If the patient complains of hearing only intermittent (not always occurring) sound, remove and check the batteries.

Caring for the Hearing Aid

■ Caution: Never wash a hearing aid; you will ruin it. When the hearing aid needs cleaning, it must go back to the dealer to be cleaned properly.

■ Never drop the hearing aid.

■ Do not expose the hearing aid to heat.

■ Do not let moisture get into the hearing aid. Do not use any kind of hair spray or medical spray on a patient while her hearing aid is in place. The spray can clog the microphone opening.

Storage of the Hearing Aid

■ Turn the hearing aid off when it is not in use

■ Remove the battery from the battery case and leave the case open when the hearing aid is not in use

■ Store the hearing aid in a container clearly marked with the patient's name and room number

THE NERVOUS SYSTEM AND THE NORMAL AGING PROCESS

As people age, the nervous system goes through changes. Age-related changes can be seen in the brain, the spinal cord, the peripheral nerves (the numerous nerves that send messages to the hands, feet, and throughout the body), and the senses. However, an inability to function is not considered a normal part of the aging process.

The weight and size of the brain decrease as a person ages. The ventricles, fluid-filled spaces in the brain, can enlarge and lead to a disorder called **normal pressure hydrocephalus**. People with this condition may have difficulty walking and become incontinent and confused.

Changes also occur in the chemicals of the brain that carry nerve impulses. If a patient is under stress, he may become confused because of these chemical changes. Nerve impulses are slower from the spinal cord to the brain and in the nerves outside the brain and spinal cord, which may lead to delayed responses.

Changes can occur in the **vertebral bodies**, the bones that surround the spinal cord, and the **intervertebral discs**, the material between the vertebral bodies that cushions the spinal column. There can be degeneration of the discs, and the bones can become thin and brittle (a condition known as **osteoporosis**). This may lead to fractures of these bones, causing pain.

normal pressure hydrocephalus A disorder caused by enlargement of the ventricles, fluid-filled spaces in the brain

vertebral bodies The bones around the spinal cord

intervertebral discs The material between the vertebral bodies that cushions the spinal column

osteoporosis Condition in which bones become brittle or thin and break easily

Some of the sensory changes include decreased or blurred vision and diminished hearing. Decreased hearing can be from wax in the ear or changes in the structure of the ear. The number of taste receptors on the tongue decreases. Nerve endings in fingers and toes may be decreased, leading to changes in the sensation of touch.

AGE-SPECIFIC CONSIDERATIONS

Diseases and conditions of the nervous system require age-related care. Adolescents who have seizure disorders may be concerned with being different. Paraplegia and quadriplegia as a result of accidents, most common in adolescents and the adult ages, have a profound affect on the patients' sense of development, body image, sexuality, and sense of identity. For the elderly, strokes, dementias, and disabling diseases like multiple sclerosis are fraught with fears of helplessness and loss. As a caregiver, allow the patient to help in any way possible with her care. Patience and understanding are very important as the patient learns and/or relearns how to perform self care and adjust to the progressions of their disease.

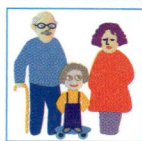

KEY IDEA

Being aware of possible changes in the nervous system helps the nursing assistant recognize opportunities to assist patients with self-care activities. Recognizing which age-related changes are usual and which are not helps the nursing assistant reassure patients and families and makes it easier to detect problems early.

Common Diseases and Disorders of the Nervous System

- *Bell's palsy:* paralysis or weakness of one side of the face

- *Stroke or cerebrovascular accident (CVA):* reduction of blood supply to the brain due to cerebral thrombosis, cerebral embolism, or intracerebral hemorrhage (see the later section on cerebrovascular accidents)

- *Aphasia:* impairment of the ability to speak and sometimes listen, read, and comprehend

- *Brain tumor:* may be a benign or malignant growth of cells

- *Epilepsy:* a group of neurological disorders with recurrent episodes of convulsions or seizures; an electrical dysfunction of the nerve cells of the brain; may be related to cerebral trauma, infection, tumor, vascular (blood vessel) disturbances, chemical imbalance, or unknown causes

- *Parkinson's disease:* progressive disorder with loss of control of movement; a person walks with a shuffling gait

- *Dementia:* a disorder characterized by confusion, disorientation, a decline in the ability to function, and impaired memory

- *Multiple sclerosis:* chronic progressive disease of the nervous system that begins slowly and progresses throughout the life span but may have periods of remission; it causes fatigue (tiredness) and weakness in legs and arms, which leads to difficulty with daily functioning

- *Shingles (Herpes zoster):* disease characterized by blisters along the course (path) of certain nerves

- *Hemiplegia:* paralysis (loss of motion and sensation) on one side of the body

- *Paraplegia:* paralysis (loss of motion and sensation) on lower part of the body

- *Quadriplegia:* paralysis (loss of motion and sensation) of all four extremities

- *Detached retina:* separation of the sensory retina from the pigment epithelium (layers of cells)

- *Cataracts:* condition in which the crystalline lens of the eye becomes opaque

- *Glaucoma:* increase of pressure within the eye

- *Chronic otitis media:* infection caused by breaks in the eardrum

- *Meniere's disease:* disease that involves the inner ear and causes dizziness

- *Alzheimer's disease:* a disease that is a type of dementia; a person becomes confused and has impaired memory; treatment is to help maintain nutritional status and assist with daily functioning (i.e., toileting, bathing, dressing)

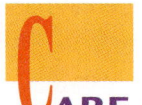

CARE OF THE SEIZURE PATIENT

A seizure is caused by an abnormality within the central nervous system thought to be an electrical problem or disturbance in the nerve cells or activity of the brain. Seizures can begin at the time of birth or may be the result of cancer (tumor), cerebral trauma (head injury), infection, vascular disturbances, imbalance or abnormality in brain chemistry, cerebrovascular accident (stroke), or unknown causes.

There are three major categories of seizures: partial seizures, generalized seizures, and unclassified epileptic seizures. Under each category there are different types of seizures. Four of the most common types are simple partial seizures, complex partial seizures, absence seizures, and generalized tonic clonic seizures. The length of time each of these seizures lasts can vary greatly.

Simple partial and **complex partial seizures** fall into the broad category of partial seizures. These may also be known as focal or local seizures. During a *simple partial seizure* a patient's level of consciousness is unchanged. The patient may have uncontrolled movements of a body part, hear unusual noises, or see things such as flashing lights. When experiencing a *complex partial seizure,* a patient's level of consciousness changes. The patient will be unaware of anyone's presence. The patient may also have the same type of motor symptoms that are seen in simple partial seizures. A complex partial seizure may start out as a simple partial seizure and become complex.

A generalized seizure can be **convulsive** or nonconvulsive. An absence seizure is a nonconvulsive seizure where a patient's level of consciousness is decreased. There may also be some muscle twitching. A generalized tonic clonic (GTC) seizure is the other major type of seizure in this category. With this type of seizure, a patient will have a loss of consciousness followed by convulsions. She may be incontinent of urine or stool.

In caring for a patient having a seizure, the major role of the nursing assistant is to prevent the patient from being injured. Wherever you are, help the patient lie down. If she is not in bed, carefully help her to the floor. Loosen the clothing and move any equipment or furniture that the patient might bump. Place a pillow or something soft under the head. *Turn the head to the side to promote drainage of saliva or vomitus. Never place anything in the mouth of a patient having a seizure. Objects can break and obstruct the patient's airway. Never try to move or restrain the patient.*

Stay with the patient and pull the emergency signal cord for help. **Observe carefully what the seizure looked like.** Give this information to the nurse. After the seizure, assist the patient to a comfortable position, if possible. The patient may be very sleepy. If she has been incontinent, assist her to clean herself or do this for her if she is unable.

seizure An episode, either partial or generalized, that may include altered consciousness, motor activity, or sensory phenomena or convulsions

simple partial seizure A seizure when the patient is aware of his surroundings but experiences either motor (muscle twitching or movement) or sensory changes (see or hear things not present)

complex partial seizure Seizure with motor and possible sensory symptoms (such as muscle twitching and smelling a foul odor) and a change in the level of consciousness

convulsive Involving convulsions—rhythmic, involuntary contraction of muscles

KEY IDEA

When a patient has a seizure, the nursing assistant's chief role is to protect the patient from injury. In addition, the nursing assistant should observe the patient and give these observations to the nurse.

THE CEREBROVASCULAR ACCIDENT (STROKE) PATIENT

A **cerebrovascular accident (CVA)**, or stroke, is a disease or disorder of the circulatory system, but the results affect the nervous system. The term is defined as follows:

- Cerebro: dealing with the brain

- Vascular: dealing with the blood vessels

- Accident: an unpredictable and unexpected occurrence

A cerebrovascular accident occurs when a blocked blood vessel interrupts the blood supply to a part of the brain. When the tissue of the brain is not supplied with blood, which carries oxygen and nutrients, it dies.

The blood supply may be interrupted due to a blood clot or rupture of a blood vessel in the brain. The four main causes of CVA are:

1. **Plaque**, which accumulates in a blood vessel and eventually closes it so that no blood can pass through

2. **Rupture**, meaning a blood vessel breaks open and causes a **hemorrhage** into the brain tissue

3. **Embolus**, that is, a clot that forms elsewhere in the body, travels to the brain through the circulatory system, lodges in a small blood vessel, and causes an obstruction

4. **Thrombus**, meaning a blood clot that remains at the site of its formation

High blood pressure and atherosclerosis increase the risk of cerebrovascular accidents.

Common Results of Cerebrovascular Accidents

The results of a cerebrovascular accident depend on which blood vessel is blocked and where it is located in the brain. Sometimes blood vessels surrounding the damaged area of the brain take over to supply the injured tissues. This is called collateral circulation.

Frequently, following a large stroke, the patient remains paralyzed on one side of the body. This is called **hemiplegia**. The terms *left hemiplegia* or *right hemiplegia* describe the side of the body that is paralyzed. Loss of sensation may also result from the cerebrovascular accident. This includes loss of the ability to feel heat, cold, pressure, and pain in the affected areas.

When the face is involved, an eyelid may droop, or the patient may be unable to close the eyelid. The eye may become dry and irritated because of decreased or absent tearing. The patient may have difficulty chewing and swallowing. There is often an inability to feel the food on the paralyzed side, increasing the risk of burns, choking, and accumulating food inside the cheek. Weakening of the muscles on one side of the face may cause drooling.

plaque Fatty deposits within blood vessels attached to vessel walls

rupture Break open

hemorrhage Excessive bleeding

embolus Blood clot or mass of other undissolved matter that travels through the circulatory system from its place of formation to another site, lodges in a small blood vessel, and causes an obstruction

thrombus A blood clot that remains at its site of formation

hemiplegia Paralysis of one-half of the body

GUIDELINES

OBRA

CARING FOR A CEREBROVASCULAR ACCIDENT PATIENT

- Encourage the patient. Point out the positive aspects of his progress.
- Always show *patience* and *understanding*. A patient can become easily frustrated if he cannot perform a task.
- Use techniques that provide a safe and secure environment.
- To prevent disability:
  - Position the patient in proper alignment.

- Provide good skin care and repositioning to prevent pressure areas that contribute to the cause of pressure ulcers.
- Do complete, passive range-of-motion exercises to strengthen muscles and prevent contractures, or assist the patient as he is able with active range-of-motion exercises.
- Encourage a well-balanced diet.
- Prevent withdrawal by treating the patient as a unique person with potential to improve.
- When feeding, place food on the unaffected (not paralyzed) side of the mouth.
- Assist with ambulation if permitted to prevent falls.

- When assisting with dressing, always dress the affected (paralyzed) side first.
- To move the patient from the bed to the wheelchair when one side of the body has been affected by the stroke, position the wheelchair on the unaffected side of the patient's body. This permits the patient to see the wheelchair and lead with the stronger leg.
- Encourage involvement in self-care, allowing the patient to do as much of the care as possible.
- Provide a climate or environment where independence is praised and encouraged. This will give hope and motivation toward rehabilitation and self-care.

Spasm, an involuntary contraction of muscles, may occur in paralyzed limbs. The stimulation of exercise, bathing, or dressing may cause the muscles to spasm into a position of flexion or extension. Spasms are increased by nervous tension, cold temperature, and pain. This greatly increases the risk of **contractures**, if the limb remains fixed in one position.

Paralysis of the arm and leg interferes with the ability to perform all activities of daily living. The inability to move increases the risk of contractures, pressure sores, pneumonia, constipation, blood clots, and urinary retention.

A patient may also develop difficulty speaking or understanding what is being said to them (aphasia). This will be discussed in a later section.

spasm An involuntary sudden movement or convulsive muscular contraction

contracture Drawing together, bunching up, or shortening of muscle tissue because of spasm or paralysis, either permanently or temporarily

◼ Psychological Aspects of Caring for a CVA Patient

When individuals experience a cerebrovascular accident, their lives change suddenly and drastically. The patient and family may grieve for the lost functions of paralyzed limbs, loss of ability to communicate, loss of independence, loss of control over his life, and lost hopes and dreams for the future.

The patient may experience multiple emotions, possibly including denial, anger, depression, acceptance, emotional instability, or overreaction to a stimulus. The patient may burst into tears or laughter for no apparent reason. This is frightening to both the patient and the family.

The loss of the ability to communicate also affects the patient in a variety of ways. Common responses include anger, fear, frustration, depression, and withdrawal.

Caring for someone who has experienced a stroke requires enormous patience. The patient and family may be grieving and experiencing difficult emotions. The nursing assistant should provide not only physical care but encouragement and praise, especially for efforts at self-care.

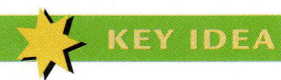

KEY IDEA

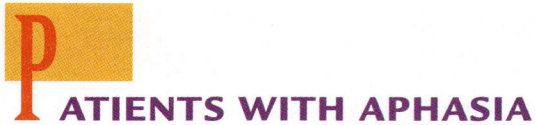

PATIENTS WITH APHASIA

aphasia Loss of language or speech

Many patients who have a cerebrovascular accident experience **aphasia**—a loss of language. Aphasia occurs most commonly with the right hemiplegic, because, for most people, the language area of the brain is on the left (the hemisphere that controls the right side of the body). The patient may have difficulties in understanding what is heard, using numbers, reading, writing, or speaking. Types of aphasia are receptive (words are not understood), expressive (a patient can't form or express words), or global (difficulty in all areas of speech).

Usually, automatic speech is retained. The patient may sing, swear, or use common phrases like "yes" or "no," even though not used correctly. Words are said automatically.

The most important quality in caring for the aphasic patient is patience. Do not avoid the patient or attempt to anticipate all her needs. Speech may return completely or partially. Use the following techniques for talking with an aphasic patient:

- If the patient is able to read, communicate through writing

- Allow enough time for a response

- Trigger the word by saying the first sound. For example, say, "Do you want cr— in your coffee?" If the patient cannot find the word, tell her

With patience and cooperation, communication may be established. Keys to communication with the aphasic patient should be written into the nursing plan of care or clinical pathway in order to maintain continuity of care on all shifts.

 KEY IDEA

> Aphasia involves a general loss of language. However, an aphasic patient may retain automatic speech, such as saying yes or no, singing, or cursing. These words and phrases are not used in a conscious way; that is why this speech is called "automatic."

Transient Ischemic Attacks (TIAs)

Transient ischemic attacks (TIAs) are sometimes called "mini strokes." They occur when there is a partial blockage of a blood vessel that sends blood to part of the brain. Symptoms of a TIA can include a change in vision, weakness in an arm or leg, or aphasia. A TIA generally lasts only 10 to 15 minutes, sometimes longer, but never more than 24 hours. There are no permanent **deficits** following a TIA.

deficit A temporary or permanent negative change in a patient's usual neurologic function

A TIA can alert nurses and physicians to a potential problem with the patient. Therefore, report unusual weakness or changes in a patient's vision or speech.

SUMMARY

This chapter has covered the anatomy and physiology of the nervous system and the care of patients with nervous system disorders. Patients with neurologic conditions have many concerns and needs. The type and amount of assistance necessary to meet these needs will depend on the patient's limitations. The patient and the family should be included in planning and delivering the patient's care whenever possible. Working with neurologic patients will be challenging and will provide a great deal of satisfaction.

THE
NURSING
ASSISTANT
IN ACTION

Aphasic Patient Confuses Family

You are caring for Mr. Morgan, who recently suffered a stroke, or CVA. His family asks you to come into the room. His wife and son are both very upset and are arguing. The son tells you that he asked Mr. Morgan if he could borrow some money, and Mr. Morgan replied, "Yes, yes." Mrs. Morgan says that the patient doesn't know what he is saying and can't understand what is being asked. Mr. Morgan then says, "No, no" in an agitated way. The son says, "See? That proves my point. He understands perfectly and wants me to have the money."

What Is Your Response/Action?

1. What are the important pieces of information in this situation?

2. What possible responses could you consider?

3. How will you respond and why?

4. What resources could you use to resolve this situation?

5. What have you learned from this situation that you could use in the future?

PRINCIPLES FOR WARM AND COLD APPLICATIONS

dilate Get bigger; expand

sitz bath A bath in which the patient sits in a specially designed chairtub or a regular bathtub with the hips and buttocks in water

inflammation A reaction of the tissues to disease or injury; there is usually pain, heat, redness, and swelling of the body part

constrict Get narrower

Blood vessels constrict in response to cold applications and dilate with heat applications (Figure 27–1). Heat may be applied to an area of the body to speed up the healing process. Heat **dilates** (expands) the blood vessels in the body and causes more blood to circulate to the injured tissues (Figure 27–2). Increased circulation can provide the body tissue with more food and oxygen which are needed for the repair (healing) of body tissue. Warm tub baths, sometimes with medication in the water, are often prescribed for this reason. A **sitz bath** is another example. In this procedure, warm water is applied to the patient's perineal or rectal area to speed healing after childbirth or surgery. Heat may also be applied to an area of the body to ease the pain caused by **inflammation** and congestion. When the blood vessels become dilated, the increased supply of blood may absorb and carry away the fluids that are causing the inflammation and pain. For example, people with certain bone and joint conditions often get relief from pain and can increase the movement of their body parts because of exercises in warm water.

Cold applications cause the blood vessels to **constrict** (Figure 27–3). This constriction may help to prevent or reduce swelling, as in the case of a sprained ankle or the beginning of a black eye. The constriction slows down the flow of blood, thereby reducing the amount of body fluids that are carried into the injured area. This may also reduce the pain that usually goes along with the swelling. Cold applications may be applied to control bleeding. When cold is applied, the blood flow becomes slower and less blood is able to seep out through a cut or other wounds. For example, when a patient has had a tonsillectomy, an ice collar or ice pack may be applied to the neck region. Cold may be applied to a patient's entire body. This is usually done to lower a

FIGURE 27–1

Blood vessels constrict in response to cold applications and dilate with heat applications

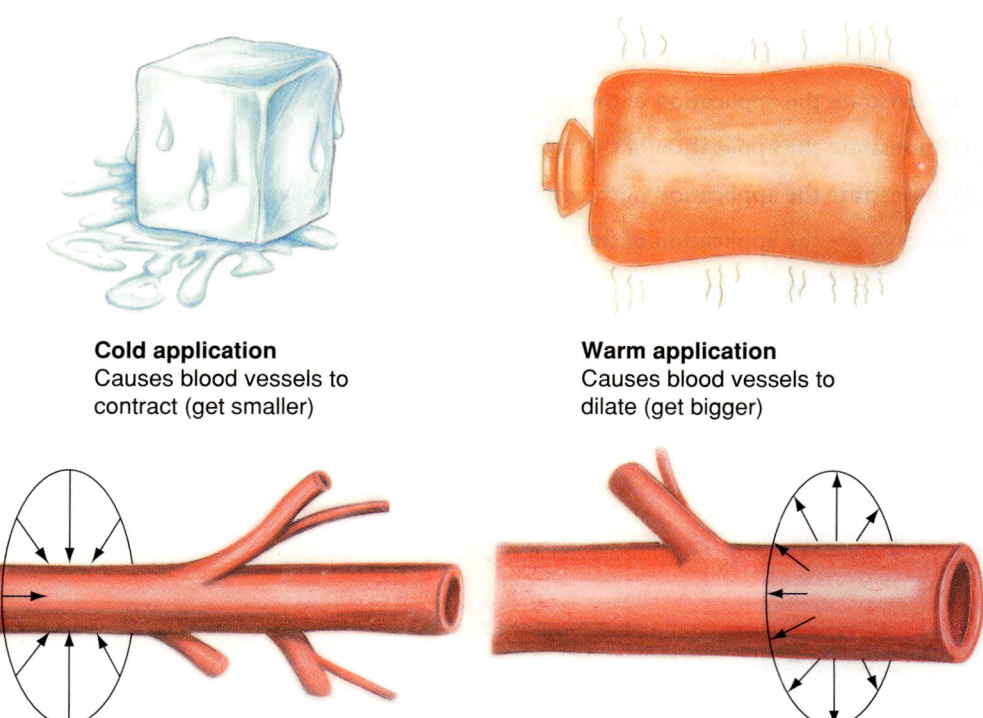

Cold application
Causes blood vessels to contract (get smaller)

Warm application
Causes blood vessels to dilate (get bigger)

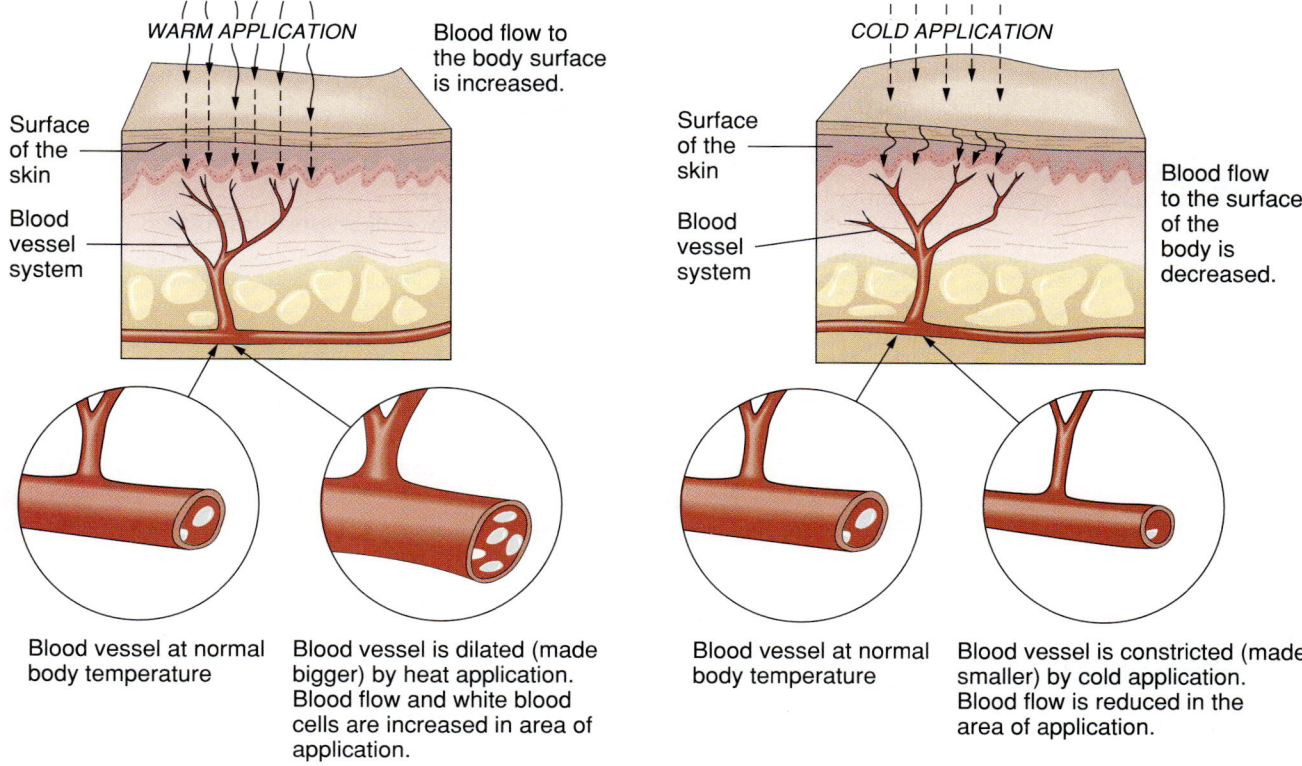

FIGURE 27–2

Principle of warm application

FIGURE 27–3

Principle of cold application

patient's body temperature when he or she has a fever. Special equipment such as a hypothermia blanket is used to help lower the body temperature.

Moist and Dry Applications

All applications are either moist or dry. A **moist application** is one in which water touches the skin. A **dry application** is one in which no water touches the skin. There are several types of both moist and dry applications listed in Table 27–1.

Compresses and soaks are both moist applications and can be either warm or cold. A **compress** is a localized application. A **soak** can be either localized or generalized. In applying a compress, a cloth is dipped into water, wrung out, and applied to the skin. To apply a soak, you immerse the body or body part completely in water. Warm-water

moist application A warm or cold application in which water touches the body

dry application A warm or cold application in which no water touches the skin

compress Folded piece of cloth used to apply pressure, moisture, heat, cold, or medication to a specific part of the body

soak Immerse the body or body part completely in water

TABLE 27–1

Types of Moist and Dry Applications

MOIST	DRY
Cool wet packs	Aquamatic K-pad
Compress: warm or cold	Commercial unit cold pack
Sitz bath	Commercial unit warm pack
Soak: warm or cold	Electric heat cradle
Tub bath	Heat lamp
	Hypothermia blankets
	Ice cap and ice collar
	Warm-water bottle

bottles, ice caps, and Aquamatic K-pads are considered dry applications because they have a dry surface. Water is used only inside the equipment and never touches the skin. Warm dry applications are sometimes used to keep warm moist applications at the correct temperature.

> **KEY IDEA**
>
> The length of time an application is applied is a serious issue. Skin damage may result with misuse of application. Follow your immediate supervisor's instructions as to the exact time to begin the application and how long the application is to stay in place.

◼ Keeping the Patient Safe and Comfortable

Be sure you know exactly where on the patient's body the warmth or cold is to be applied. A **generalized application** is one in which a warm or cold application is applied to a patient's whole body. A **localized application** is one that is applied to a specific part or area of a patient's body. Check the application often to keep it at the right temperature throughout the treatment. Suggested times for checking the temperatures of different kinds of applications are:

- Soaks and **intermittent** compresses: every 5 minutes
- Heat lamps: every 5 minutes

Keeping the Patient Safe

Avoid accidents. Be careful not to spill any water. Be sure electrical equipment does not come in contact with water. Be sure your hands are dry before touching electrical equipment. Be sure the bed is properly protected. Put the side rails in the upright position if needed.

Check the patient's skin under warm applications (Figure 27–4). Watch for too much redness. Look for a darker discoloration that might mean the patient is being burned. Listen when the patient complains. If you think a patient is being burned, remove the heat application and report to your immediate supervisor at once.

Check the patient's skin where cold is being applied. If the area appears to be blanched, very pale, white, or bluish, tell your immediate supervisor at once. Watch for changes in the color of parts of the patient's body. For example, if the patient's lips,

generalized Affecting, involving, or pertaining to the whole body

generalized application A warm or cold application applied to the entire body

localized Limited to one place or part; affecting, involving, or pertaining to a definite area

localized application A warm or cold application applied to a specific area or small part of the body

intermittent Alternating; stopping and beginning again

FIGURE 27–4

Check the patient's skin for redness or discoloration, signs the patient is being burned

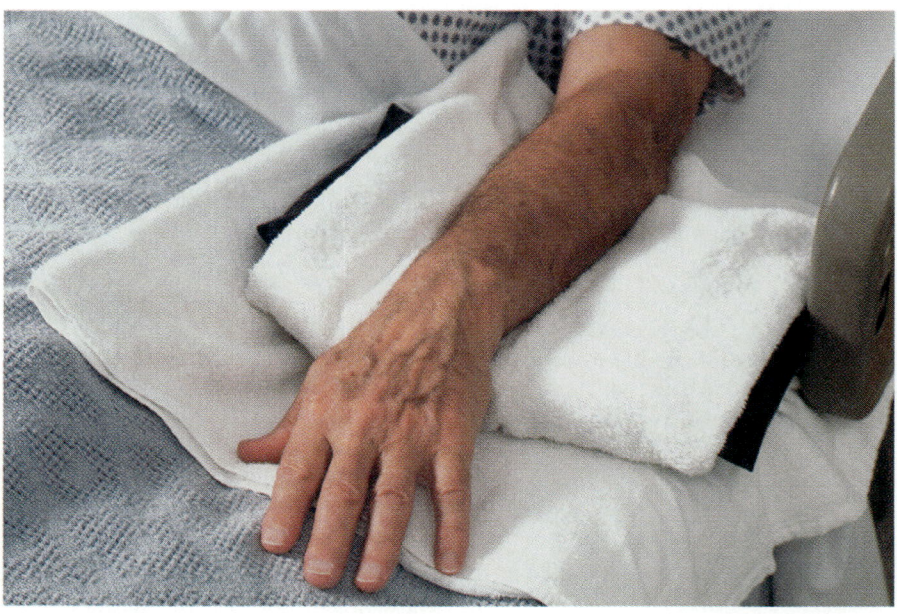

fingernails, and eyelids look blue or turn a dark color, this is **cyanosis**, which is a sign of less oxygen getting to that part of the body. Stop the treatment immediately and report to your immediate supervisor.

Some patients may not complain when being burned or frozen, because they have no feeling in the body area where the application is applied. Such a situation may be due to a disease process.

Always apply the ice cap and warm-water bottle with its metal or plastic stopper away from the patient's body. The stopper should never touch the patient's skin. It will be much warmer or colder than the application and could burn or freeze the patient's skin. You may be working with an unconscious patient. If so, you may be directed to protect him by putting a blanket between the skin and the warm water bottle or ice cap.

Keeping the Patient Comfortable

Make sure the patient is in a position that is comfortable for him and convenient for your work. Keep the patient covered and warm during the treatment. Otherwise, the patient might become chilled and uncomfortable. If a patient shivers during the cold application, stop the treatment. Cover him with a blanket. Then report this at once to your immediate supervisor who will tell you what to do.

Be aware that the weight of the ice bag/warm-water bottle may increase the pain of the injured area. Never fill a warm-water bottle or ice bag more than half full. It gets too heavy.

Always dry the bottle or bag. Check it for leaks by turning it upside down. Place it in a flannel cover or a cloth case. Never let the patient lie on an uncovered warm-water bottle or ice bag.

■ Heat Applications

In some institutions warm compresses are made by holding a cloth under running warm water or by microwaving a wet cloth. Sterile compresses are used in situations where there is an open wound or area of the body vulnerable to infection, for example, the eyes. If you are instructed to do this be careful to prevent too much heat. Follow the instructions of your immediate supervisor.

P R O C E D U R E

OBRA

APPLYING THE WARM COMPRESS (MOIST HEAT APPLICATIONS)

PREPARATION

1. Assemble your equipment:
   a. Disposable bed protector
   b. Basin
   c. Pitcher of water (115°F; 46.1°C)
   d. Washcloth, towel, or gauze pads (compress)
   e. Bath thermometer, if available
   f. Large sheet of plastic
   g. Bath towel
   h. Bath blanket
   i. Disposable gloves if any potential for exposure to body fluids
2. Identify the patient by checking the identification bracelet.
3. Wash your hands.
4. Tell the patient you are going to apply a warm compress.
5. Provide privacy for the patient.
6. Raise the bed to a comfortable working position.

STEPS

7. Help the patient into a comfortable, safe position. Have the body area exposed for application of a warm compress.
8. Place a disposable bed protector under the body area that is to be given the warm compress.
9. Fill the pitcher with warm water. Check the temperature of the

PROCEDURE (CONTINUED)

water with a bath thermometer (115°F or 46.1°C). Then pour the water into the basin.

10. Dip the compress into the water and wring it out thoroughly. Apply gloves if soaks will be applied to any area where exposure to body fluid could occur.

11. Apply the compress gently to the proper area (Figure 27–5).

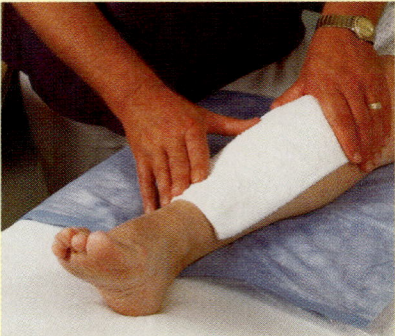

FIGURE 27–5
Apply the compress

12. Wrap the entire area with a large towel or a blue pad, covering the wet compress. Cover the entire area, compress, and towel with a plastic sheet (Figure 27–6a–b). Be sure the plastic does not touch the patient's skin. This will keep the compress warm.

13. If the patient is cold or chilly, cover him with a blanket.

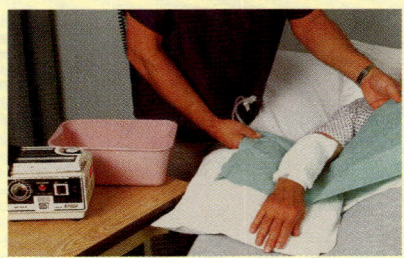

FIGURE 27–6a
Wrap entire area with a towel or blue pad

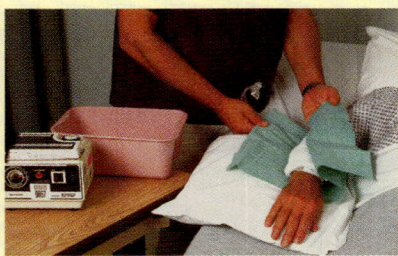

FIGURE 27–6b
Cover with a plastic sheet or blue pad

14. Change the compress and remoisten it, as necessary, to keep it warm. Sometimes a patient is able to apply the compress himself. If your immediate supervisor gives permission for this, position and assist the patient as necessary.

15. Check the skin under the application every 5 minutes. If the skin appears red, remove the compress. Cover the area with a towel or blanket. Report this to your immediate supervisor.

16. A warm compress is usually applied for 15 to 20 minutes. However, follow the instructions given to you by your immediate supervisor as to how long the warm compress is to be applied.

17. After the treatment is completed, remove the compress and gently pat the area dry with a towel.

FOLLOW-UP

18. Make the patient comfortable and replace the call light.

19. Lower the bed to a position of safety.

20. Raise the side rail when ordered or appropriate for patient safety.

21. Clean standard equipment and put it in its proper place. Discard disposable equipment and gloves if used.

22. Wash your hands.

23. Report to your immediate supervisor:

   ■ The time the warm compress was started.

   ■ How long the compress was in place.

   ■ The area of application.

   ■ How the patient tolerated the procedure.

   ■ Your observations of anything unusual.

PROCEDURE

OBRA

APPLYING THE WARM SOAK (MOIST WARM APPLICATION)

AGE-SPECIFIC CONSIDERATIONS

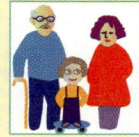

In adolescent patients, this is a time of concern over privacy. Be sure to take extra care to maintain an adolescent's privacy. This will increase their comfort and cooperation with the procedure. For geriatric patients, monitor the temperature of the soaks carefully. The aging process often results in a thinning of the skin, increasing the potential for burns. For patients of all ages, be very careful of treatments involving water. Leaking and melting bags, or bottles lead to an increased potential for slipping and falling.

PROCEDURE (CONTINUED)

PREPARATION

1. Assemble your equipment:

   a. Basin, foot tub, or arm basin

   b. Bath thermometer

   c. Disposable bed protector

   d. Bath towel

   e. Bath blanket

   f. Disposable gloves, if any potential for exposure to body fluids

2. Identify the patient by checking the identification bracelet.

3. Wash your hands.

4. Tell the patient you are going to apply a warm soak.

5. Provide privacy for the patient.

6. Raise the bed to a comfortable working position.

STEPS

7. Help the patient into a safe, comfortable position. Expose the area to be treated.

8. Fill the basin one-half full with warm water (100°F; 37.8°C). Check the temperature with a bath thermometer. Apply gloves if soaks will be applied to any area where exposure to body fluids could occur.

9. Place a disposable bed protector under the body area that is to receive the soak.

10. Place the basin in a position so the patient's arm, leg, foot, or hand can be dipped into the basin easily.

11. Place the patient's arm or leg into the water gradually.

12. Check the temperature of the water every 5 minutes. When you need to change the water, take the patient's arm, foot, or leg out of the basin. Wrap it with a bath blanket or bath towel to keep it warm.

13. If the patient says he feels weak or cold, stop the treatment. Cover the patient with extra blankets and report this to your immediate supervisor.

14. Check the skin every 5 minutes. If the skin is red, stop the treatment. Report this to your immediate supervisor.

15. When the treatment is finished, dry the patient's arm or leg by patting gently with a towel.

FOLLOW-UP

16. Make the patient comfortable and replace the call light.

17. Lower the bed to a position of safety.

18. Raise the side rails when ordered or appropriate for patient safety.

19. Clean standard equipment and put it in its proper place. Discard disposable equipment and gloves, if used.

20. Wash your hands.

21. Report to your immediate supervisor:

    ■ The time the warm soak was started.

    ■ The length of treatment.

    ■ The area of application.

    ■ How the patient tolerated the procedure.

    ■ Your observations of anything unusual.

PROCEDURE

OBRA

APPLYING THE WARM-WATER BOTTLE (DRY HEAT APPLICATION)

PREPARATION

1. Assemble your equipment:

   a. Warm-water bottle (may be disposable)

   b. Pitcher of warm water (120°F; 48.9°C). Note: Temperature for unresponsive adults and children is usually less (105°F; 40.5°C to 115°F; 46.1°C). If warm-water bottle is disposable, follow your institution's policies for the correct temperature of the water.

   c. Bath thermometer

   d. Flannel cover (or whatever type of cover is used in your institution)

2. Identify the patient by checking the identification bracelet.

3. Wash your hands.

4. Tell the patient you are going to apply a warm-water bottle.

5. Provide privacy for the patient.

6. Raise the bed to a comfortable working position.

STEPS

7. Fill the pitcher with water (120°F; 48.9°C). Check the

PROCEDURE (CONTINUED)

temperature with a bath thermometer.

8. Fill the warm-water bottle half full of water (Figure 27–7).

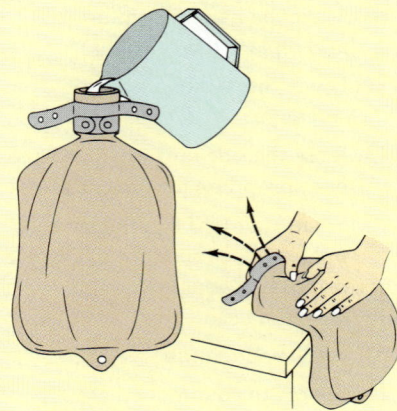

FIGURE 27–7
Fill bottle half full with warm water. Press excess air out of bag, then close the bag

9. Two methods of squeezing the air out of the bottle are:

- **Method A.** Place the bag on the edge of a counter. Have the part of the bag containing the water hanging down. Place the part of the bag without the water lying on the counter top. Put your hand on the top of the bag at the edge of the counter. Move your hand slowly toward the opening of the bag, pressing out the air. With the other hand, close the bag (see Figure 27–7).

- **Method B.** Place the warm-water bottle in a horizontal position on a flat surface. Hold the neck of the warm-water bottle upright until you can see water in the neck of the bottle. The water squeezes out the air.

10. Fasten the top tightly.

11. Dry the warm-water bottle. Check for leaks by turning it upside down.

12. Place the warm-water bottle in the type of cover used in your institution (Figure 27–8).

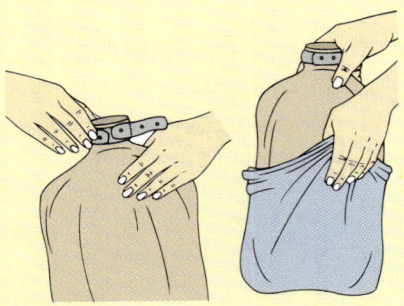

FIGURE 27–8
Place the warm water bottle in a cover

13. Help the patient into a safe, comfortable position. Expose the area to be treated. Apply the bottle gently to the proper body area (Figure 27–9). Use a pillow to support the bottle against the body area if necessary to keep it positioned.

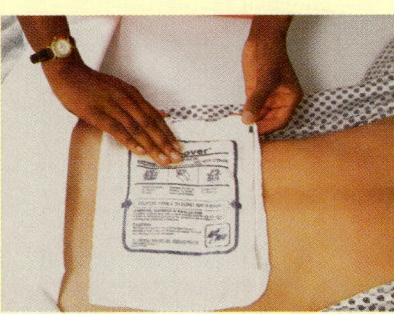

FIGURE 27–9
Apply the heat package or covered bottle to the proper area

14. Never place the warm-water bottle on top of a painful area. The weight will increase the pain. Place it on the side.

15. Check the warm-water bottle every hour to be sure the temperature is correct. Change the water in the bottle, when necessary, to continue the treatment at the same temperature.

16. Check the skin under the warm-water bottle after the first 5 minutes and then every hour. If the skin is red, remove the warm-water bottle and report to your immediate supervisor.

FOLLOW-UP

17. Clean standard equipment and put it in its proper place. Discard disposable equipment.

18. Make the patient comfortable and replace the call light.

19. Lower the bed to a position of safety.

20. Raise the side rails when ordered or appropriate for patient safety.

21. Wash your hands.

22. Report to your immediate supervisor:

- The time the warm-water bottle was applied.
- The length of treatment.
- The area of application.
- How the patient tolerated the procedure.
- Your observations of anything unusual.

PROCEDURE

APPLYING THE COMMERCIAL UNIT HEAT PACK (MOIST WARM APPLICATION)

PREPARATION

1. Assemble your equipment:
   a. Commercial unit, single-use heat pack that has been warmed in the heating lamp unit; Follow manufacturer's instructions
   b. Disposable bed protectors
   c. Large sheet of plastic or disposable bed protector
   d. Bath blanket
   e. Gloves, if indicated
2. Identify the patient by checking the identification bracelet.
3. Wash your hands.
4. Tell the patient you are going to apply a warm pack.
5. Provide privacy for the patient.
6. Raise the bed to a comfortable working position. Apply gloves if indicated.

STEPS

7. Help the patient into a safe, comfortable position. Expose the area to be treated.
8. Place the bed protector under the body part that is to receive the warm pack.
9. Tear the foil covering from the warm pack.
10. Place the moist warm pack on the proper body area.
11. Cover the pack with the sheet of plastic or the disposable bed protector. This will keep the pack warm.
12. Check the skin under the application every 5 minutes. If the skin appears red, remove the pack and cover the area with a blanket. Report this to your immediate supervisor.
13. Follow the instructions of your immediate supervisor as to the length of application. Replace with a new warm pack as necessary.

FOLLOW-UP

14. When the treatment is finished, discard disposable equipment and gloves, if used.
15. Make the patient comfortable and replace the call light.
16. Lower the bed to a position of safety.
17. Raise the side rails when ordered or appropriate for patient safety.
18. Wash your hands.
19. Report to your immediate supervisor:
    - The time the warm pack was applied.
    - The length of treatment.
    - The area of application.
    - How the patient tolerated the procedure.
    - Your observations of anything unusual.

PROCEDURE

OBRA

APPLYING A HEAT LAMP (DRY WARM APPLICATION)

PREPARATION

1. Assemble your equipment:
   a. Heat lamp
   b. Bath blanket
   c. Bath towel
   d. Tape measure
2. Identify the patient by checking the identification bracelet.
3. Wash your hands.
4. Tell the patient you are going to apply heat with a heat lamp.
5. Provide privacy for the patient.
6. Raise the bed to a comfortable working position.
7. Help the patient into a safe, comfortable position.
8. Expose only the body area that is to receive the heat. Drape the patient so that heat is directed to the proper area of the skin. Cover the rest of the patient's body with a bath blanket, sheet, or towel.
9. Check the electric cord to be sure it is in good condition and there are no frayed areas.

PROCEDURE (CONTINUED)

10. Plug in the lamp with the lamp turned off.

STEPS

11. Position the lamp so that heat will be directed to the proper skin area.

12. The part of the patient's body that is being treated should be at least 18 inches away from the heat lamp. Use a tape measure to check the distance.

13. Turn on the lamp. Be sure it is working properly.

14. Check the skin after 3 minutes. If the patient's skin becomes red, stop the treatment and report to your immediate supervisor.

15. There is a danger of fire when a heat lamp is being used. Therefore, keep all linen away from the lamp. Do not drape or cover the lamp. A cover on the lamp may catch fire. Tell patient to remain in position and not to touch the bulb of the heat lamp.

16. Leave the heat lamp on the patient from 5 to no more than 10 minutes, unless you have other instructions from your immediate supervisor.

FOLLOW-UP

17. After treatment is completed, unplug and remove the lamp.

18. Make the patient comfortable and replace the call light.

19. Lower the bed to a position of safety.

20. Raise the side rails when ordered or appropriate for patient safety.

21. Wipe the lamp with disinfectant solution and put it back in its proper place.

22. Wash your hands.

23. Report to your immediate supervisor:
    - The time the heat was applied.
    - The length of treatment.
    - The area of application.
    - How the patient tolerated the procedure.
    - Your observations of anything unusual.

PROCEDURE

OBRA

APPLYING THE AQUAMATIC HYDRO-THERMAL (K-PAD) (DRY HEAT APPLICATION)

PREPARATION

1. Assemble your equipment (Figure 27–10):

   a. Aquamatic Hydro-Thermal (K-pad) and control unit. (The temperature is preset by the central supply room. The container is filled with distilled water by central supply, or available in supply room.)

   b. Cover for pad (pillowcase, flannel cover, or cover from manufacturer)

2. Identify the patient by checking the identification bracelet.

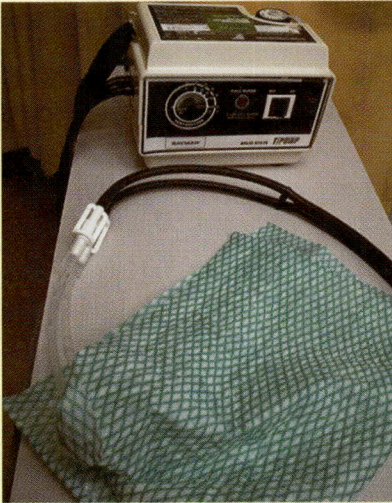

FIGURE 27–10
K-pad

3. Wash your hands.

4. Tell the patient you are going to apply the K-pad.

5. Provide privacy for the patient.

6. Raise the bed to a comfortable working position.

7. Help the patient into a safe, comfortable position. Expose the area to be treated.

8. Inspect the K-pad for leaks and make sure the cord and plug are in good condition.

9. Plug the cord into an electrical outlet.

10. Place the pad in the cover. *Do not use any pins!*

STEPS

11. Place the container on the bedside table. Arrange the tubing at the level of the pad. Do not allow the tubing to hang below the level of the bed.

12. Gently apply the pad in its cover to the proper dry body area.

13. Check the skin under the pad. Follow the instructions of your immediate supervisor as to how frequently to check the skin and the length of the application.

PROCEDURE (CONTINUED)

FOLLOW-UP

14. When the treatment is finished, return the equipment to its proper place.

15. Make the patient comfortable and replace the call light.

16. Lower the bed to a position of safety.

17. Raise the side rails when ordered or appropriate for patient safety.

18. Wash your hands.

19. Report to your immediate supervisor:
    - The time the K-pad was applied.
    - The length of treatment.
    - The area of application.
    - How the patient tolerated the procedure.
    - Your observations of anything unusual.

PROCEDURE

OBRA

USING THE DISPOSABLE SITZ BATH (MOIST WARM APPLICATION)

PREPARATION

1. Assemble your equipment:
   a. Disposable sitz bath kit (Figure 27–11):
      - Plastic bowl with a large brim
      - Water bag
      - Tubing and stopcock (clamp)

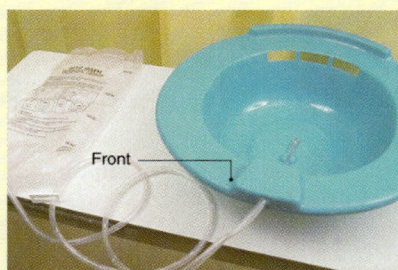

Front

FIGURE 27–11
Disposable sitz bath kit

   b. Plastic laundry bag
   c. Bath thermometer
   d. Bath towels
   e. Pitcher of warm water (105°F; 40.5°C)

2. Identify the patient by checking the identification bracelet.

3. Wash your hands.

4. Tell the patient you are going to give him a sitz bath.

5. Provide privacy for the patient.

6. Help the patient to put on his slippers and robe.

STEPS

7. Help the patient into the bathroom.

8. Raise the toilet seat.

9. Check the temperature of the water with the bath thermometer. It should be 105°F (40.5°C).

10. Put the plastic bowl into the toilet bowl. Be sure that the opening for overflow is toward the front of the toilet.

11. Pour the water into the bowl, filling it half full.

12. Close the stopcock on the tubing. Fill the water bag with water (105°F; 40.5°C) from the pitcher. Close the bag.

13. Hang the container for water 12 inches higher than the bowl.

14. Help the patient remove his robe and pajamas and sit down into the sitz bath. Be sure the patient can reach the signal cord.

15. Place the tubing inside the bowl with the opening of the tube under the water level. The tube fits into a little groove in the front of the basin.

16. Open the stopcock and adjust the flow if necessary.

17. Have the patient sit in the sitz bath with water running in for from 10 to 20 minutes, as instructed by your immediate supervisor.

18. If the patient says he feels weak or faint, stop the treatment. Turn on the signal light if you need help getting the patient out of the bathroom.

19. When the treatment is finished, remove the tubing. Help the patient out of the sitz bath.

20. Pat the patient's body gently with a towel to dry.

21. Help the patient back into bed.

FOLLOW-UP

22. Make the patient comfortable and replace the call light.

PROCEDURE (CONTINUED)

23. Lower the bed to a position of safety.

24. Raise the side rails when ordered or appropriate for patient safety.

25. Clean your equipment and return it to its proper place. Discard disposable equipment.

26. Bag and dispose of the dirty towels in the laundry hamper.

27. Wash your hands.

28. Report to your immediate supervisor:

- The time the sitz bath was started.

- The length of time the patient was in the sitz bath.

- How the patient tolerated the procedure.

- Your observations of anything unusual.

PROCEDURE

USING THE PORTABLE CHAIR-TYPE OR BUILT-IN SITZ BATH (MOIST WARM APPLICATION)

PREPARATION

1. Assemble your equipment:

   a. Portable chair or built-in sitz bath (Figure 27–12)

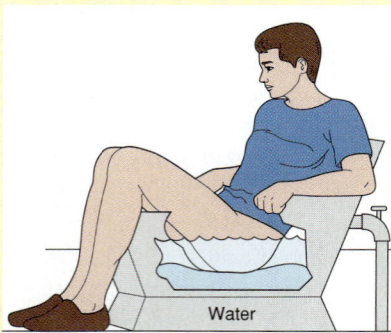

FIGURE 27–12
Patient using a built-in sitz bath

   b. Disinfectant cleaner

   c. Bath towels

   d. Bath blanket

   e. Bath thermometer

   f. Plastic laundry bag

   g. Disposable gloves

2. Clean the sitz bath with disinfectant cleanser and rinse it well.

3. Identify the patient by checking the identification bracelet.

4. Wash your hands.

5. Tell the patient you are going to give him a sitz bath.

6. Provide privacy for the patient.

STEPS

7. Bring the portable, chair-type sitz bath into the patient's room. Or help the patient (using a wheelchair if necessary) into the bathroom with the built-in chair-type sitz bath.

8. Fill it half full with water (105°F; 40.5°C).

9. Place a towel on the seat and on the front edge of the sitz bath. Apply gloves.

10. Help the patient undress, except for his gown and slippers.

11. Help the patient to sit down in the tub. Hold his gown up so it does not get wet.

12. Cover the patient's shoulders with a bath blanket if he complains of being cold.

13. Continue the treatment for 10 to 20 minutes, unless you have other instructions from your immediate supervisor.

14. Check the patient every 5 minutes.

15. If the patient feels weak or faint, stop the treatment. Turn on the signal light for help in getting the

patient out of the tub. Let the water out of the tub.

16. When the treatment is finished, help the patient out of the tub.

17. Pat his body gently with a towel to dry.

18. Help the patient back into bed.

FOLLOW-UP

19. Make the patient comfortable and replace the call light.

20. Lower the bed to a position of safety.

21. Raise the side rails when ordered or appropriate for patient safety.

22. Clean the sitz tub with disinfectant cleanser.

23. Put the portable, chair-type tub back in its proper place.

24. Bag and dispose of the dirty towels in the laundry hamper.

25. Dispose of gloves. Wash your hands.

26. Report to your immediate supervisor:

- The time the sitz bath was started.

- The length of time the patient was in the sitz bath.

- How the patient tolerated the procedure.

- Your observations of anything unusual.

Cold Applications

P R O C E D U R E

OBRA

APPLYING THE COLD COMPRESS (MOIST COLD APPLICATION)

PREPARATION

1. Assemble your equipment:

   a. Disposable bed protector

   b. Basin

   c. Washcloth, towel, or gauze pads (compress)

   d. Bath towel

   e. Bath blanket

   f. Pitcher of cold water (ice cubes, if ordered by your immediate supervisor)

2. Identify the patient by checking the identification bracelet.

3. Wash your hands.

4. Tell the patient you are going to apply a cold compress.

5. Provide privacy for the patient.

6. Raise the bed to a comfortable working position.

7. Help the patient into a comfortable, safe position. Expose the area to be treated.

STEPS

8. Place a disposable bed protector under the body area that is to be given the cold compress.

9. Put cold water in the basin (ice cubes only if ordered).

10. Dip the compress into the water and wring it out thoroughly.

11. Apply the compress gently to the proper area of the patient's body as quickly as possible. If you are slow, the compress will absorb heat from your hands and the air (Figure 27–13).

12. If the patient is cold or chilly, cover him with a blanket. Do not cover the compress or the area being treated.

13. Change the compress and re-moisten it, as necessary, to keep it cold. Sometimes a patient is able to apply the compress himself. If your immediate supervisor gives permission for this, position and assist the patient as necessary.

14. Check the skin under the application every 5 minutes. If the skin appears to be blanched or white, remove the compress. Cover the area with a towel or blanket. Report this to your head nurse or team leader.

15. A cold compress is usually applied for 15 to 20 minutes. However, follow the instructions of your immediate supervisor.

16. When the treatment is finished, remove the compress and gen-tly pat the area dry with a towel.

FOLLOW-UP

17. Make the patient comfortable and replace the call light.

18. Lower the bed to a position of safety.

19. Raise the side rails when ordered or appropriate for patient safety.

20. Clean your equipment and put it in its proper place. Discard disposable equipment.

21. Wash your hands.

22. Report to your immediate supervisor:

    ■ The time the cold compress was started.

    ■ How long it remained in place.

    ■ The area of application.

    ■ How the patient tolerated the procedure.

    ■ Your observations of anything unusual.

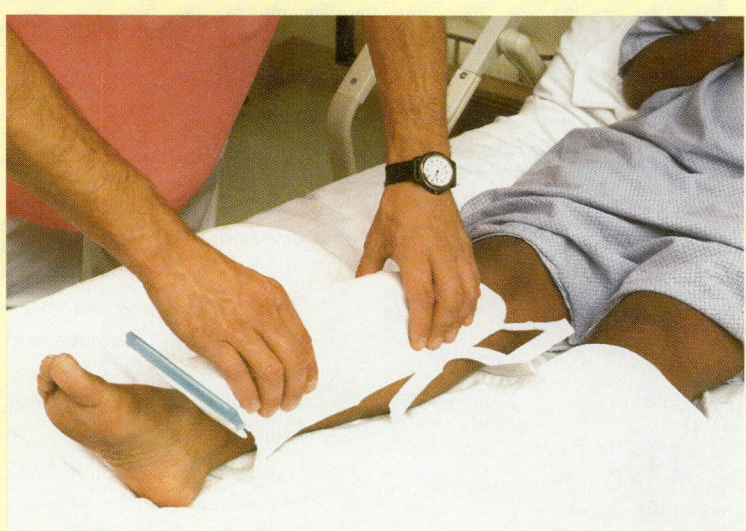

FIGURE 27–13

Apply compress to body area

PROCEDURE

OBRA

APPLYING THE COLD SOAK (MOIST COLD APPLICATION)

PREPARATION

1. Assemble your equipment:
   a. Basin, foot tub, or arm basin
   b. Disposable bed protector
   c. Washcloth, towel, or gauze pads (compress)
   d. Bath towel
   e. Bath blanket
   f. Gloves if indicated
2. Identify the patient by checking the identification bracelet.
3. Wash your hands and apply gloves if indicated.
4. Tell the patient you are going to apply a cold soak.
5. Provide privacy for the patient.
6. Raise the bed to a comfortable working position.
7. Help the patient into a safe, comfortable position. Expose the area to be treated.

STEPS

8. Fill the basin half full with cold water (Figure 27–14).

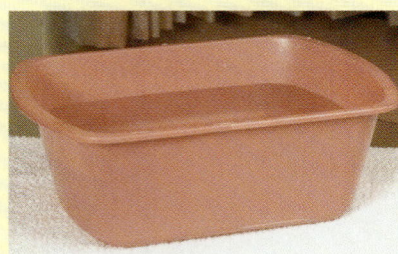

FIGURE 27–14
Fill the basin half full with water

9. Place a disposable bed protector under the body area that is to receive the cold soak.
10. Place the basin in a position so that the patient's arm, leg, foot, or hand can be dipped into the basin easily (Figure 27–15).

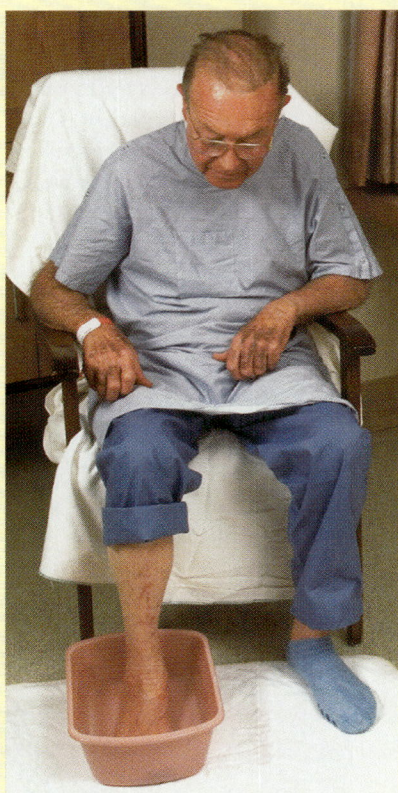

FIGURE 27–15
Place basin in position for patient to easily dip foot in it

11. Gradually place the patient's arm or leg into the water.
12. When you have to change the water, take the patient's arm or leg out of the basin. Wrap it with a bath towel or bath blanket to keep it warm.
13. If the patient says he feels weak or cold, stop the treatment. Cover the patient with extra blankets and report this to your immediate supervisor.
14. Check the skin every 5 minutes. If the skin is blanched or white, stop the treatment. Report to your immediate supervisor.
15. When the treatment is finished, dry the patient's arm or leg by gently patting with a towel.

FOLLOW-UP

16. Make the patient comfortable and replace the call light.
17. Lower the bed to a position of safety.
18. Raise the side rails when ordered or appropriate for patient safety.
19. Clean standard equipment and put it in its proper place. Discard disposable equipment and gloves, if used.
20. Wash your hands.
21. Report to your immediate supervisor:
    - The time the cold soak was started.
    - The length of treatment.
    - The area of application.
    - How the patient tolerated the procedure.
    - Your observations of anything unusual.

PROCEDURE

APPLYING THE ICE BAG, ICE CAP, OR ICE COLLAR (DRY COLD APPLICATION)

PREPARATION

1. Assemble your equipment:

   a. Ice bag, ice cap, or ice collar (may be disposable); Figure 27–16

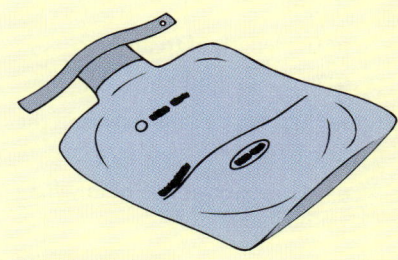

FIGURE 27–16

Ice bag

   b. Flannel cover (or whatever type of cover is used in your institution)

   c. Ice in a clean container

   d. Bath blanket

   e. Gloves, if indicated

2. Identify the patient by checking the identification bracelet.

3. Wash your hands. Apply gloves if indicated.

4. Tell the patient you are going to apply the ice bag, ice cap, or ice collar.

5. Provide privacy for the patient.

6. Raise the bed to a comfortable working position.

7. Help the patient into a safe, comfortable position. Expose the area to be treated.

8. Pour cold water over the ice to melt the sharp edges.

9. Fill the ice collar, ice bag, or ice cap one-half full of ice (Figure 27–17).

10. Squeeze the sides of the ice bag to force the air out of it.

11. Fasten the stopper tightly.

12. Dry the outside of the ice bag with a paper towel.

13. Invert the ice bag to test for leaking.

14. Place the ice bag into the type of cover used in your institution.

STEPS

15. Apply the ice bag to the proper area of the patient's body.

16. If the patient is cold or chilly, cover him with a blanket. Do not cover the ice bag or the area being treated.

17. Follow the instructions of your immediate supervisor as to the length of application. Replace the ice as necessary.

18. Check the skin under the application every 10 minutes. If the skin appears to be blanched or white, remove the ice bag. Cover the area with a towel and report to your head nurse or team leader.

FOLLOW-UP

19. Clean standard equipment and put it in its proper place. Discard disposable equipment and gloves, if used.

20. Make the patient comfortable and replace the call light.

21. Lower the bed to a position of safety for the patient.

22. Raise the side rails when ordered or appropriate for patient safety.

23. Wash your hands.

24. Report to your immediate supervisor:

    ■ The time the ice bag was applied.

    ■ The length of treatment.

    ■ The area of application.

    ■ How the patient tolerated the procedure.

    ■ Your observations of anything unusual.

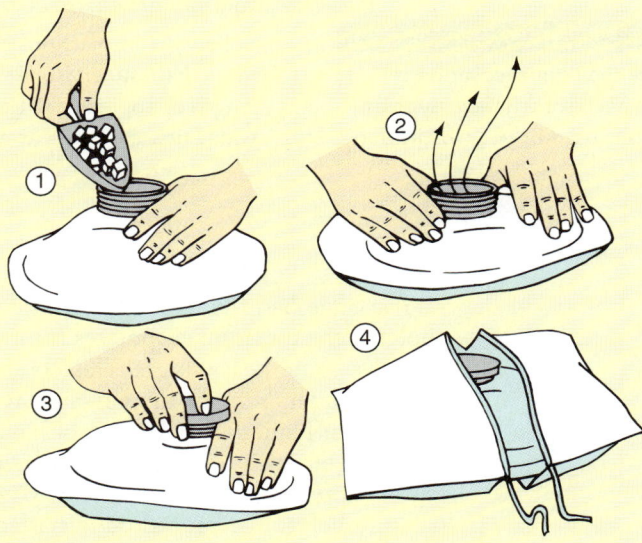

FIGURE 27–17

Preparing ice bag for use

PROCEDURE

OBRA

APPLYING THE COMMERCIAL UNIT COLD PACK (DRY COLD APPLICATION)

PREPARATION

1. Assemble your equipment:

   a. Commercial unit, single-use cold pack

   b. Cover used in your institution

   c. Bath blanket

   d. Gloves, if indicated

2. Identify the patient by checking the identification bracelet.

3. Wash your hands.

4. Tell the patient you are going to apply a cold pack.

5. Provide privacy for the patient.

6. Raise the bed to a comfortable working position.

7. Help the patient into a safe, comfortable position. Expose the area to be treated.

STEPS

8. Place the flannel cover on the cold pack (or whatever type of cover is used by your institution).

9. Hit or squeeze the cold pack to activate it according to the manufacturer's directions (Figure 27–18). Apply gloves, if indicated.

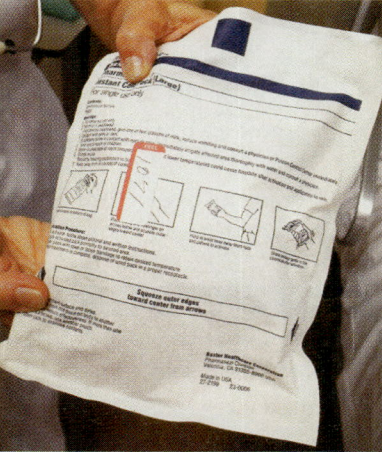

FIGURE 27–18
Disposable cold package

10. Apply the pack to the proper area of the patient's body.

11. Check the skin under the application every 10 minutes. If the skin appears blanched or white, remove the pack and cover the area with a blanket. Report this to your immediate supervisor.

12. Follow the instructions of your immediate supervisor as to the length of application. Replace with a new cold pack as necessary.

FOLLOW-UP

13. Discard disposable equipment and gloves, if used.

14. Make the patient comfortable and replace the call light.

15. Lower the bed to a position of safety for the patient.

16. Raise the side rails when ordered or appropriate for patient safety.

17. Wash your hands.

18. Report to your immediate supervisor:

    ■ The time the cold pack was applied.

    ■ The length of treatment.

    ■ The area of application.

    ■ How the patient tolerated the procedure.

    ■ Your observations of anything unusual.

The Cooling (Tepid) Sponge Bath

You have had the experience of perspiring on a warm summer day. You often feel cooler as the moisture evaporates from your skin. As perspiration evaporates into the air, it carries some heat with it. This cools the body. A tepid (slightly warm) sponge bath cools a patient's body in the same way. Patients who run temperatures near 105°F (40.5°C) or higher are in danger of having convulsions in some cases. A tepid bath can lower the temperature to one more desirable. Generally, the bath is ended if the patient's temperature reaches 101°–102°F (38.3°–38.8°C). It is important to take the patient's temperature before the procedure is started, and then every 10 minutes during the procedure. Cold water, ice, or alcohol is not used since this can cause chilling or irritation of the skin. Sponge baths are never used on infants, toddlers, or geriatric patients since such baths tend to cause chilling in these patients. Chilling can make them too cold too fast. Shivering can cause their temperatures to rise quickly.

All sponge baths require a doctor's order. The purpose of the tepid sponge bath is to lower the patient's body temperature.

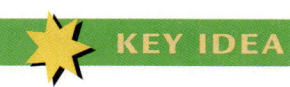
KEY IDEA

GUIDELINES

GIVING THE COOLING (TEPID) SPONGE BATH

- Place moist washcloths on the axillary area (armpits), the groin, the inner aspect of the elbows, and the back of the knees. These are places where many blood vessels are close to the surface of the body, and so evaporation can more quickly lower the body temperature at these places.

- Place a covered hot-water bottle at the patient's feet to prevent chilling.
- Use only tepid (slightly warm) water (70°–80°F; 21.1°–26.6°C).
- If the patient becomes chilled or starts to shiver, stop the treatment, dry the patient, and cover him with a light blanket. Call your immediate supervisor at once.
- Carefully monitor the patient's temperature before beginning the procedure, every 10 minutes during the procedure, and 10 minutes after the procedure. Stop the procedure at once if the temperature reaches a low of 102°F (38.8°C). Once the bathing begins, do not take the temperature in the axillary area (armpit) because the moist cloths will alter the correct readings. Also, take the oral temperature with care because chilling or shivering can cause the patient to bite down on the thermometer and break it, or injure his teeth. A rectal temperature is advised to prevent injury.
- To hasten the cooling a moist bath towel can be placed on the trunk (chest and abdomen) of the patient's body. Also, the use of a fan to move the room air is helpful in evaporation. *Do not direct the air flow at the patient.*

PROCEDURE

GIVING THE COOLING (TEPID) SPONGE BATH

PREPARATION

1. Assemble your equipment:
   a. Two hot-water bottles with covers
   b. Disposable gloves
   c. A waterproof sheet to protect the bed
   d. Two bath blankets
   e. One ice bag, covered
   f. Six washcloths
   g. One moist bath towel
   h. Two dry bath towels
   i. Oral or rectal thermometer (oral thermometer should not be glass)
   j. Basin with tepid water (70°–80°F; 21.1°–26.6°C)
   k. Bath thermometer
   l. Laundry bag
   m. Clock or wristwatch
2. Identify the patient by checking the identification bracelet.
3. Explain the procedure to the patient.
4. Provide privacy for the patient.
5. Wash your hands and put on gloves.
6. Raise the bed to a comfortable working position.

STEPS

7. Take the patient's temperature, pulse, and respirations. Record on a flowsheet.
8. Place protective waterproof sheet on the bed.
9. Cover patient with bath blanket. Slide top bed covers from under the bath blanket. Remove patient's gown and all other clothing without exposing the patient.
10. Place covered hot-water bottles at his feet to prevent chilling.
11. Place covered ice bag on his forehead.
12. Place moist washcloths on the axillary area (armpits), the groin, the inner aspect of the elbows, and the back of the knees.

PROCEDURE (CONTINUED)

13. A moist bath towel to hasten cooling can be placed on the trunk (chest and abdomen). This is optional.

14. Note the time on the clock or your wristwatch. Start by bathing (stroking the extremity with a washcloth moistened with tepid water from the basin) two extremities for 5 minutes each. *Take the temperature, pulse, and respirations. Record on flowsheet.*

15. Bathe two more extremities for 5 minutes each. *Take the temperature, pulse, and respirations. Record on flowsheet.*

16. Then bathe the chest and abdomen for 5 minutes if no moist towel has been used as stated in number 13.

17. Next bathe the back and buttocks for 5–10 minutes. *Take the*

temperature, pulse, and respirations. Record on flowsheet.

18. Notify your immediate supervisor if the temperature doesn't *start* to drop within 30 minutes of beginning the bathing.

19. Repeat the procedure until the desired temperature is reached.

20. Dry the patient and cover him with a bedsheet. Remove the protective sheet. Remove bath blanket. Assist patient to put on gown and replace other covers.

FOLLOW-UP

21. Make the patient comfortable and replace the call light.

22. Lower the bed to a position of safety.

23. Raise the side rails when ordered or appropriate for patient safety.

24. Clean reusable equipment and return to its proper place. Discard disposable equipment according to your institution's policy.

25. Bag and dispose of dirty linen in the laundry hamper.

26. Dispose of gloves and wash your hands.

27. Copy onto a permanent record the vital signs you have taken, or include the flowsheet in the patient's record according to your institution's policy.

28. Report to your immediate supervisor:
    - The time the procedure started.
    - The length of the procedure.
    - Your observations of anything unusual.

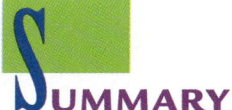

SUMMARY

This chapter has provided examples and procedures to safely apply warm and cold applications. You also learned that warm and cold applications may be either moist or dry and that they can be generalized or localized applications. The length of an application is always a serious issue since the misuse of an application may cause skin damage. You will follow the instructions of your supervisor as to the time to begin an application and how long the application should remain in place.

Notes

THE NURSING ASSISTANT IN ACTION

Cold Pack in Place an Unknown Length of Time

You are called into work early because Nancy, another nursing assistant, became ill and had to leave. When you check on each of your patients, you find a cold pack on Mr. Kenton's right knee. Nancy left about 10 minutes ago to go to the doctor, and she mentioned nothing to you about the cold pack. When you ask the nurse and the other nursing assistant, neither of them know how long the ice pack has been in place. Mr. Kenton is unaware of the ice pack and unable to tell you how his knee feels.

What Is Your Response/Action?

1. What are the important pieces of information in this situation?

2. What decision must you make?

3. What possible complications can occur because of your decision?

4. What resources can you use to make your decision?

5. What did you learn that can apply in other situations?

■ Preoperative Checklist

Your immediate supervisor will give you the preoperative checklist and instruct you as to:

- What each patient has been told about his operation
- What you are to tell the patient to prepare him for his surgery and postoperative care

FIGURE 28–2

Sample preoperative checklist to be completed by the nursing assistant

```
┌──────────────────────────────────────────────────────┐
│ IMMEDIATE PREOPERATIVE CHECKLIST                      │
│ Name                              Date                │
├──────────────────────────────────────────────────────┤
│ PATIENT IDENTIFICATION                                │
│   ID on and accurate (name and numbers)  ☐ Yes  ☐ No │
│   Comments _____           │
│                                                        │
│ PLANNED PROCEDURE                                      │
│   Patient's statement of: _____          │
│                                                        │
│ Patient verifies side:  ☐ Right   ☐ Left      ☐ N/A  │
│ ALLERGIES                                              │
│   any known allergies:      ☐ Yes   ☐ No              │
│   Specify if yes _____          │
│   _____            │
│                                                        │
│ NPO STATUS                                             │
│   NPO since midnight        ☐ Yes   ☐ No              │
│                                                        │
│ PREGNANCY                                              │
│   Patient   ☐ Denies  ☐ Confirms  ☐ Unsure  ☐ N/A    │
│   Comments _____            │
│ PERSONAL POSSESSIONS                                   │
│   Dental appliance      ☐ Yes   ☐ No _____        │
│   Prostheses/Implants   ☐ Yes   ☐ No _____        │
│                                       _____        │
│                                                        │
│   Valuables:        Item              Disposition      │
│   _____    _____     │
│   _____    _____     │
│   _____    _____     │
│                                                        │
│ HEIGHT_____ WEIGHT_____ lb/kg  ☐ Actual  ☐ Est.  │
│                                                        │
│ VITAL SIGNS  B/P___  T___  P___  R___  Time___        │
│                                                        │
│ PREOPERATIVE PREPARATION                               │
│   Physically prepared:      ☐ Yes   ☐ No              │
│     (personal clothes, glasses, contacts, nail polish, │
│     wigs, dentures, jewelry removed and hospital gown  │
│     applied)                                           │
│                          Yes   No      Comments        │
│   Med. sheets to OR      ☐     ☐   _____     │
│   Patient voided preop   ☐     ☐   _____     │
│   Preop meds given       ☐     ☐   _____     │
│   Meds/supplies to OR    ☐     ☐   _____     │
│   Side rails up          ☐     ☐   _____     │
│   Patient instructed     ☐     ☐   _____     │
│   to stay in bed                                       │
│   Preoperative treatments _____            │
│ PATIENT IDENTIFIED IN OR DEPT. BY DR. _____    │
│                                                        │
│ COMMENTS: _____            │
│   _____            │
│                                                        │
│ READY FOR OR            Date _____         │
│   Preoperative unit RN/LPN (initials) _____     │
│   Preoperative RN (initials)          _____     │
└──────────────────────────────────────────────────────┘
```

- How to handle and answer the patient's questions
- What care to give the patient the evening before surgery
- What care to give the patient the morning of surgery
- What portion, if any, of the preoperative checklist you are to complete

Figure 28–2 is an example of a preoperative checklist. By filling out this checklist, the nursing staff can be sure the patient has been prepared properly for surgery. Report to your supervisor when you have completed the activities you are responsible for on the checklist. Medications are given upon completion of the checklist.

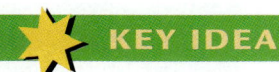
KEY IDEA

The patient signs a surgical consent form prior to surgery. Obtaining the patient's written consent for surgery is the doctor's responsibility. However, the doctor often delegates this responsibility to the nurse. You are never responsible for securing the patient's signature on this form.

You may be asked to take away the patient's water pitcher and glass at midnight and to post a sign saying **NPO** (Figure 28–3). NPO is taken from the Latin *nils per os,* which means "nothing by mouth." The sign is usually put at the head or foot of the bed; follow your immediate supervisor's instructions.

NPO (nothing by mouth) Cannot eat or drink anything at all, usually past midnight the night before surgery or a procedure

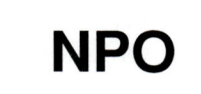

FIGURE 28–3
Nothing by mouth sign, usually posted at the head or foot of the patient's bed, if required

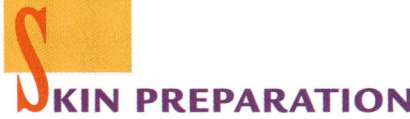

SKIN PREPARATION

Close to the time of an operation, the patient's skin in the operative area must be free of hair that would interfere with the operative or surgical procedure. The skin must be as clean as possible. Hair on the body is a breeding place for microorganisms. Because hair cannot be sterilized, it must be removed by shaving. The **skin prep** covers the area on the body where the operation is going to be done. When you are shaving a patient before an operation, watch for scratches, pimples, cuts, sores, or rashes on the skin. If you see anything on the skin that looks unusual, be sure to report this to your immediate supervisor. *For some procedures, shaving is no longer performed.* The nicks caused by shaving may actually harbor more microorganisms than the skin and hair.

In some hospitals, the patient is sent to the operating room suite one hour before he is scheduled for surgery. At that time, the nurses in the operating room will prep the patient (shave the skin in preparation for surgery). This is done in those hospitals that have holding areas in the operating room suite. In the holding area, each patient has his own cubicle (sometimes an anteroom) where preparation for surgery, including administration of medications, starting of intravenous infusions, and skin preps, are done.

In other hospitals, the staff does the prep the evening before surgery. The operating room staff does another complete prep after the patient is on the operating room table.

The prep is done with a special prep kit, which is obtained from the central supply room for each patient. After it is used, it is discarded in the dirty utility room. Each kit contains a safety razor and a sponge filled with soap. Most health care facilities have a

skin prep Shaving the area of the body where an operation is going to be performed in preparation for surgery

special place (usually a covered metal container) to dispose of razors. If your health care facility does not supply a disposable prep kit, get the individual items from central supply.

PROCEDURE

SHAVING A PATIENT IN PREPARATION FOR SURGERY

PREPARATION

1. Assemble your equipment:

   a. Disposable prep kit (Figure 28-4a–b) containing:
      - Razor and razor blades
      - Sponge filled with soap
      - Tissues

   b. Basin of warm water (115°F; 46.1°C)

   c. Bath blanket

   d. Towels

   e. Disposable gloves

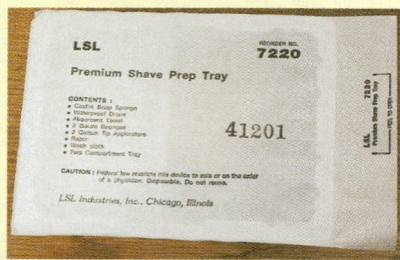

FIGURE 28–4a
Shave prep tray

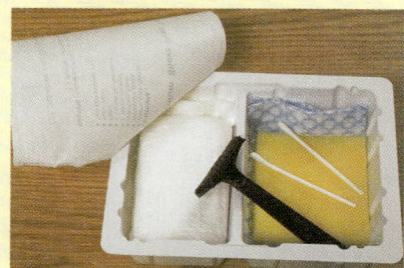

FIGURE 28–4b
Open shave prep tray

Note: Some health care institutions do a "dry prep;" they shave the skin without soap. Follow the policies of your institution.

2. Identify the patient by checking his identification bracelet.

3. Tell the patient that you are going to shave him.

4. Provide privacy for the patient.

5. Wash your hands and put on gloves.

6. Raise the bed to a comfortable working position.

STEPS

7. Place the bath blanket over the bedspread and top sheet. Ask the patient to hold the blanket in place. Fanfold the top sheets to the foot of the bed. Do this from underneath the blanket without exposing the patient.

8. Adjust the bedside lamp so that the area is well lighted. There should be no shadows where you will be working.

9. Open the disposable prep kit.

10. Wet the soap sponge in the basin of water. Next soap the area to be shaved. Work up a good lather with the sponge.

11. Check to be sure the razor blade is in the correct position in the razor.

12. Hold the skin taut with a dry tissue. Shave in the direction the hair grows. Rinse the razor often. Keep the razor and the patient's skin wet and soapy throughout the procedure.

13. Clean the patient's umbilicus (navel) if it is in the area to be shaved.

14. Rinse the soap off the patient's skin. Dry thoroughly with the towel.

15. Clean your equipment and put it in its proper place. Discard disposable equipment. Never throw razors in the garbage.

16. Cover the patient with the top sheet and bedspread. Ask him to hold them while you take the bath blanket from underneath without exposing the patient.

FOLLOW-UP

17. Make the patient comfortable and replace the call light.

18. Lower the bed to a position of safety.

19. Raise the side rails when ordered or appropriate for patient safety.

20. Dispose of gloves and wash your hands.

21. Report to your immediate supervisor:
    - The time at which you shaved the patient.
    - How the patient tolerated the procedure.
    - Your observations of anything unusual.

Areas to Be Shaved in Preparation for Surgery

The areas to be shaved in preparation for various types of surgery are shown in Figures 28–5 through 28–11. The area not being operated on is called the *unaffected side*. The area where the operation will be done is called the *affected side*. Clipping, a common alternative to shaving, is gaining preference, as there is a reduced chance of introducing infection (Figure 28–12).

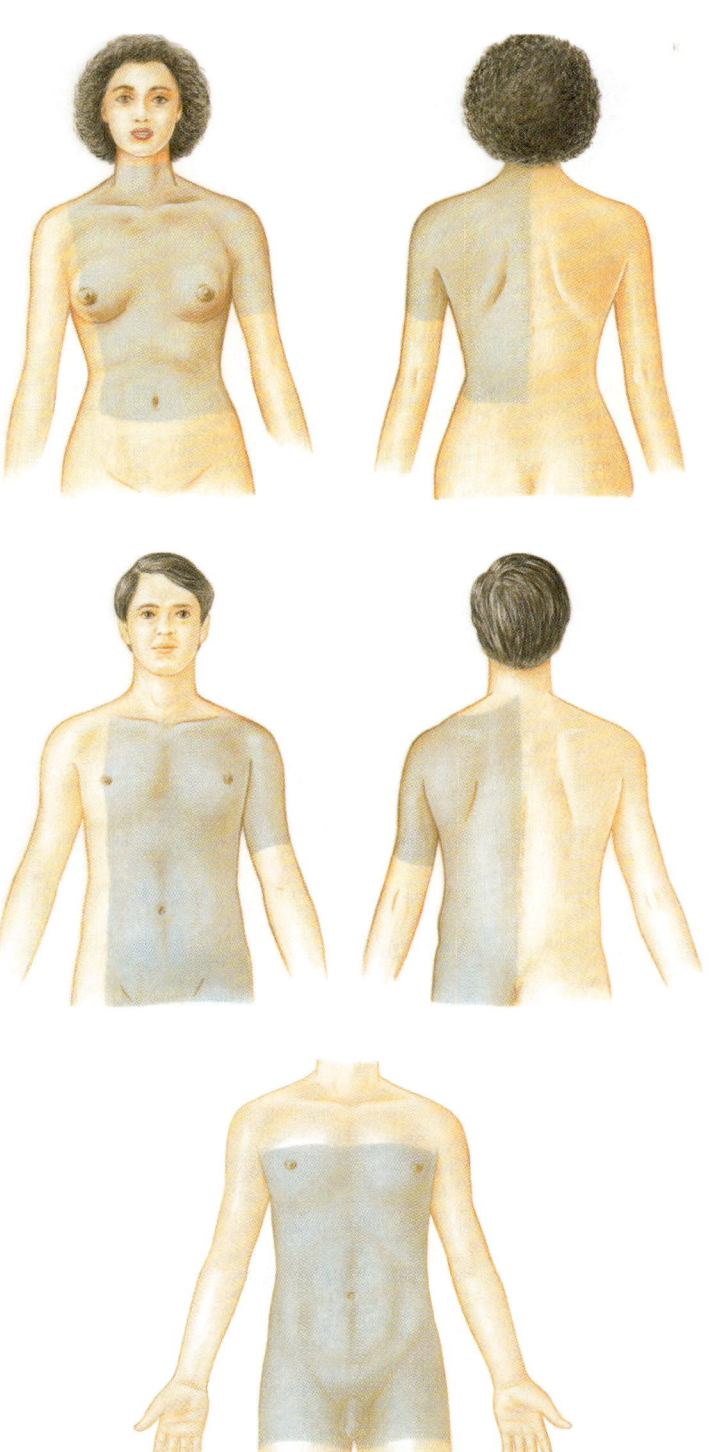

FIGURE 28–5

Prep for breast surgery. Shave from the nipple line of the unaffected side to the middle of the patient's back on the affected side. On the affected side, shave from the chin down to the umbilicus (navel), the axilla (armpit), and part of the upper arm.

FIGURE 28–6

Chest prep for thoracic surgery. Shave the area extending from the nipple of the unaffected side, across the chest area of the affected side, and across the back, from the top of the shoulders down to the pubic hair.

FIGURE 28–7

Abdominal prep. Shave from the nipple line on male patients and from below the breasts on female patients down to and including the pubic area. Shave the width of this area to each side of the body.

abdominal prep The procedure for making the patient's abdomen ready for surgery; includes thorough cleansing of the skin and careful shaving of body hair in the abdominal area

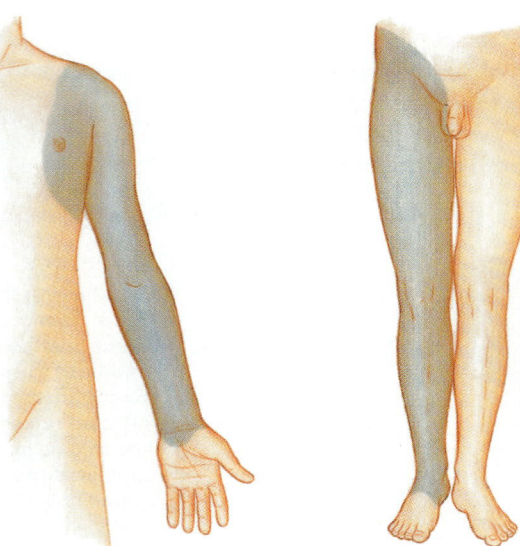

FIGURE 28–8

Prep for surgery of an extremity (arm or leg). If a joint such as an elbow or knee is going to be operated on, you will shave up to the next joint above and down to the next joint below. For example, if the patient's elbow is going to be operated on, you will shave the entire arm from the shoulder down to the wrist. If an area between joints is going to be operated on, you will shave the entire area, including the joints above and below. Shave all around an arm or a leg.

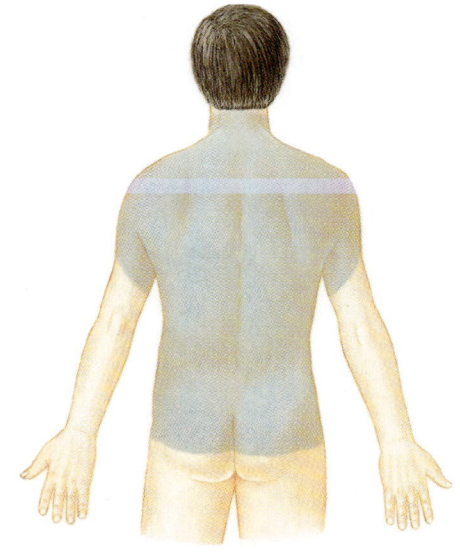

FIGURE 28–9

Back prep. Shave the patient's entire back, from the hairline on the neck down to the middle of the buttocks, including the axillary area.

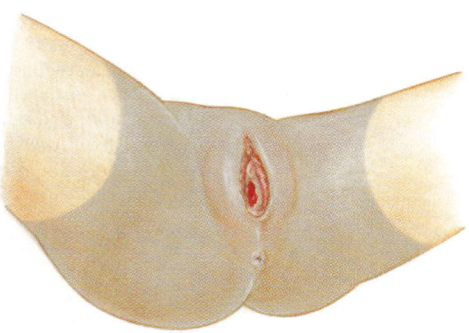

FIGURE 28–10

Vaginal prep, or the preparation of the genital area of female patients.

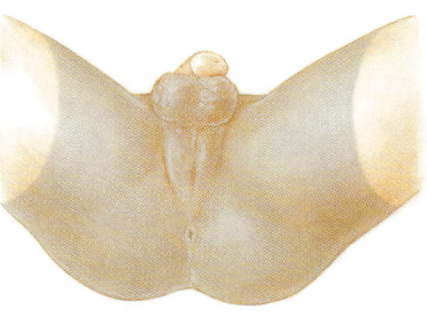

FIGURE 28–11

Scrotal prep, or the preparation of the genital area of male patients.

vaginal prep The procedures for making the genital area of a female patient ready for surgery; the preparation includes thoroughly cleansing the skin and carefully shaving the pubic hair; it may also include a cleansing douche

scrotal prep The procedures for making the genital area of a male patient ready for surgery; the preparation includes thoroughly cleansing the skin and carefully shaving the hair in the area

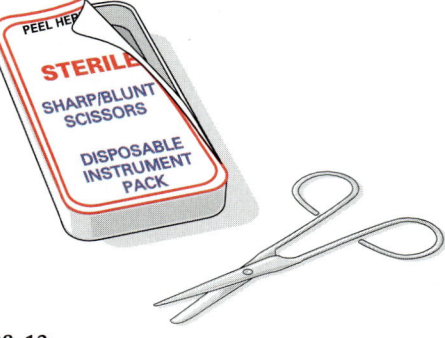

FIGURE 28–12

Clipping, a common alternative to shaving, is gaining preference as the chance of introducing infection is reduced.

THE MORNING OF SURGERY

After the patient has been given his preoperative medications by the medication nurse:

- Keep the side rails in the up position
- Remind the patient that he or she is not to smoke, eat, or get out of bed

The transportation attendant or the operating room assistant will come to the floor at the proper time to take the patient to the operating room suite. Move the furniture out of the way. Make the room ready for the stretcher to be brought into the room. Assist with moving the patient from the bed to the stretcher. Tell the patient that you or another nurse will see her in her room after the surgery.

The transportation assistant will then wheel the patient on the stretcher to the nurse's station (Figure 28–13). At this time, the nurse or unit clerk will give the attendant the patient's chart and check the name on the identification bracelet against the name on the chart. The attendant then takes the patient and chart to the operating room.

Readying the Postoperative Patient's Unit

Your next task is to strip the linen from the bed, make the OR or surgical bed, and prepare the unit to receive the patient postoperatively (Figure 28–14).

- Bring the IV pole to bedside
- Strip the linen from the bed; make the OR bed
- Place tissues and an emesis basin on the bedside table, along with any other equipment requested by the nurse
- Be sure to remove drinking water if so instructed

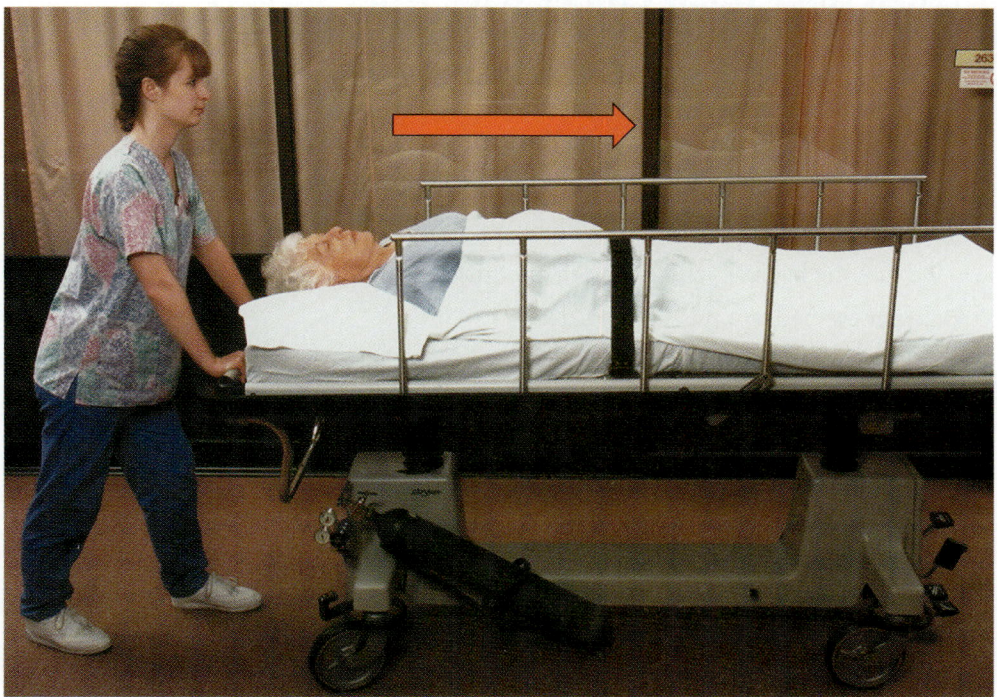

FIGURE 28–13

When transporting the patient to the operating room, cover the patient with a blanket or sheet, be sure the straps are secure, stand at the patient's head, and push the stretcher slowly

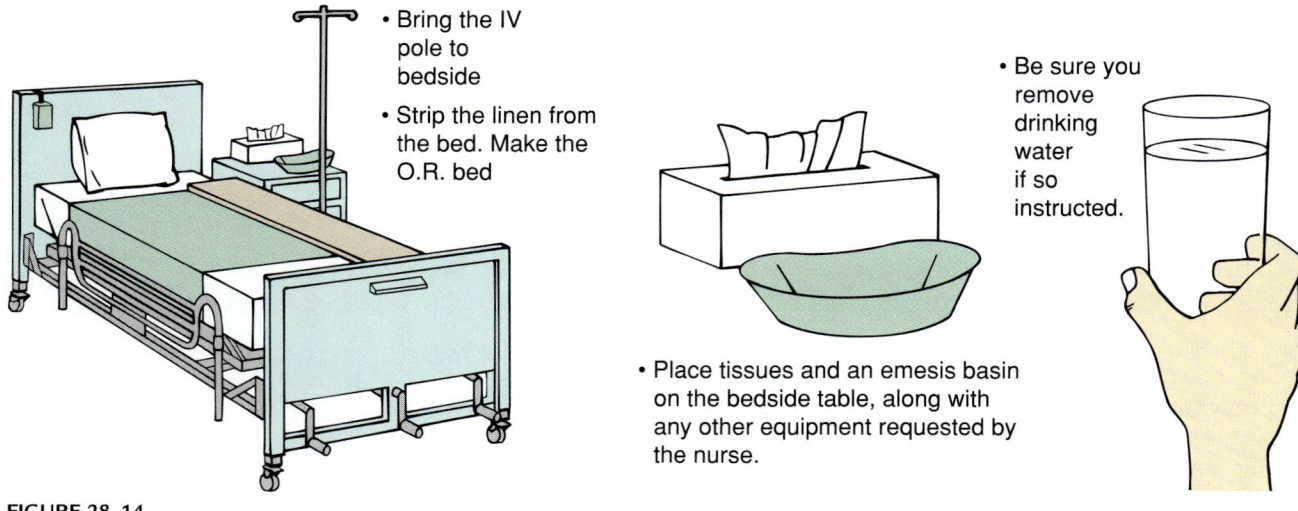

FIGURE 28–14

Responsibility list for preparing for the return of the postoperative patient

POSTOPERATIVE NURSING CARE

Postoperative care means taking care of a patient right after surgery. Most patients are taken to a surgical recovery room immediately following surgery. They remain in the recovery room until they begin to recover from the effects of anesthesia and vital signs have stabilized. When the patient returns to his room, you will begin assisting with postoperative nursing care. The patient must be watched closely for any complications such as fever, bleeding, extreme restlessness, choking, vomiting, or changes in vital signs. Report any such observations to your immediate supervisor immediately.

When the Patient Comes Back from Surgery

The patient will be coming back to his unit on a stretcher. Move the furniture out of the way and make sure the bedside area is clear. The stretcher can then be brought easily and quickly to its place next to the bed.

When the patient is brought back to the unit, you will do the following things:

- Help move the patient safely from the stretcher to the bed
- Be sure the patient is covered with blankets to keep warm
- Be sure the bedside rails are raised after the patient is in bed
- Lower the bed to a position of safety
- Measure the patient's vital signs (TPR and BP) as instructed by your immediate supervisor
- Place the call light within the patient's reach (Figure 28–15)
- Be sure all drinking water has been removed

Signal your immediate supervisor immediately if you observe any of the following signs or symptoms:

- Rise or fall of blood pressure
- Choking
- Pulse: fast (above 100), slow (below 60), or an irregular pulse beat

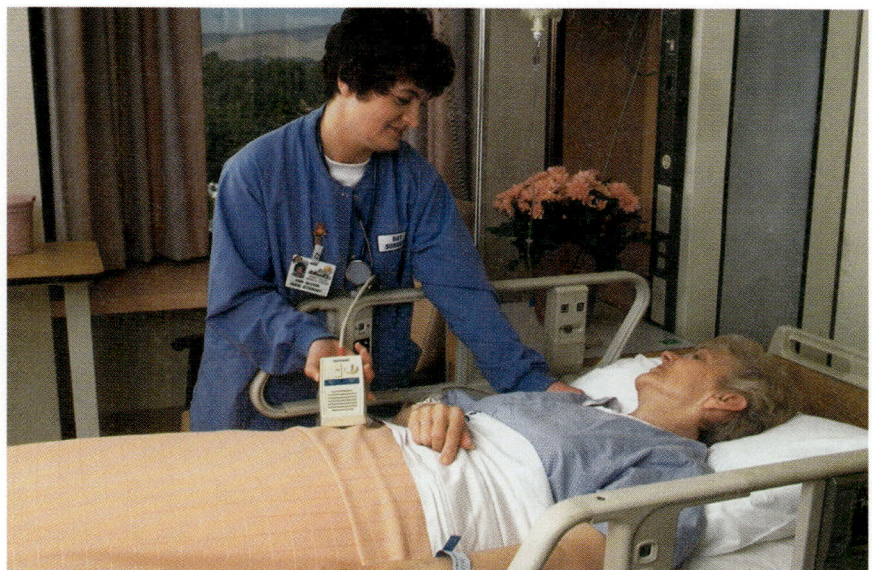

FIGURE 28–15
When the patient awakens from the anesthesia, call the patient by her preferred name; this reassures the patient that someone who knows her is present. Be sure the call light is within easy reach.

- Respirations: rapid (above 30), labored, very slow, or shallow
- Skin, lips, fingernails are very pale or turning blue (cyanosis)
- Thirst: patient asks for water often
- Unusual or extreme restlessness
- Moaning or complaining of pain
- Sudden, bright red bleeding
- Any other noticeable sudden changes
- Nausea or vomiting

The postoperative patient may appear to be unconscious, but not really be. He may be able to hear you. Say only those things you would want the patient to hear if he were fully conscious. Speak normally. Always tell the patient who you are and what you are doing. Figures 28–16 through 28–18 provide additional information on the techniques for postoperative care.

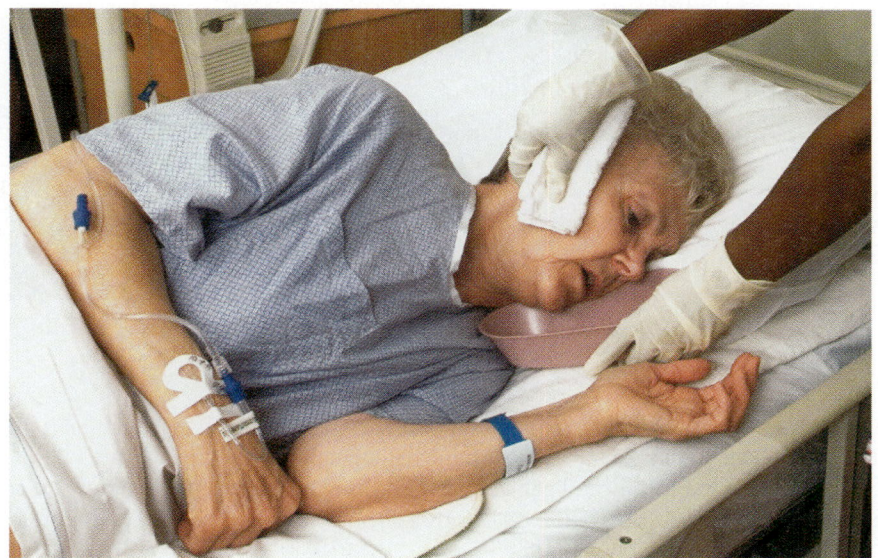

FIGURE 28–16
If the patient vomits, turn his head to one side to prevent vomitus from being drawn back into the lungs (aspiration); wipe the patient's mouth and chin. If the patient is conscious, rinse out his mouth with cold water. Caution: The patient is not to swallow the water.

FIGURE 28–17
The first voiding after surgery

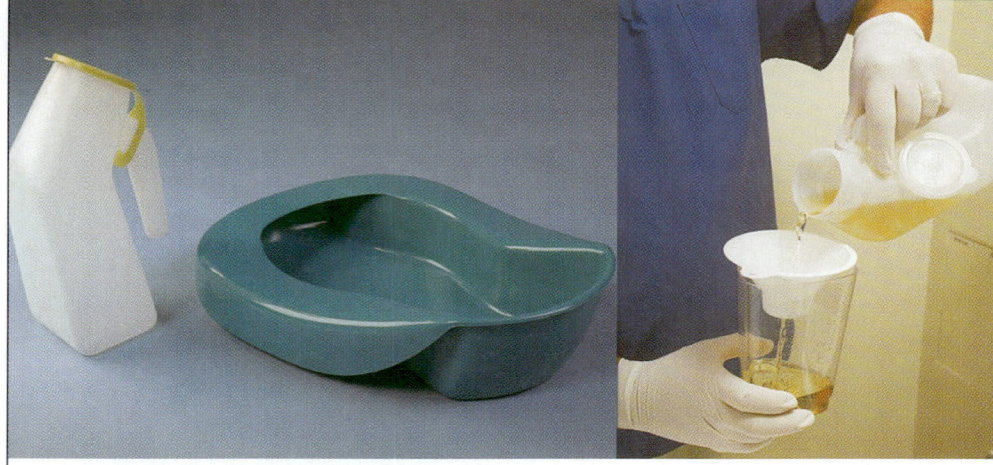

- Collect for a routine urine specimen
- Measure for amount
- Check for odor and color
- Record in a proper place on output side of I and O sheet
- Report if the patient has not yet **voided** on your shift
- Report if the patient voids only a few drops of urine
- If an indwelling urinary catheter is present:
  Be sure it is unclamped and draining
  Observe amount and color in the drainage bag

void To urinate, pass water

FIGURE 28–18
Keep side rails in the up position for patients who are coming out of an anesthetic

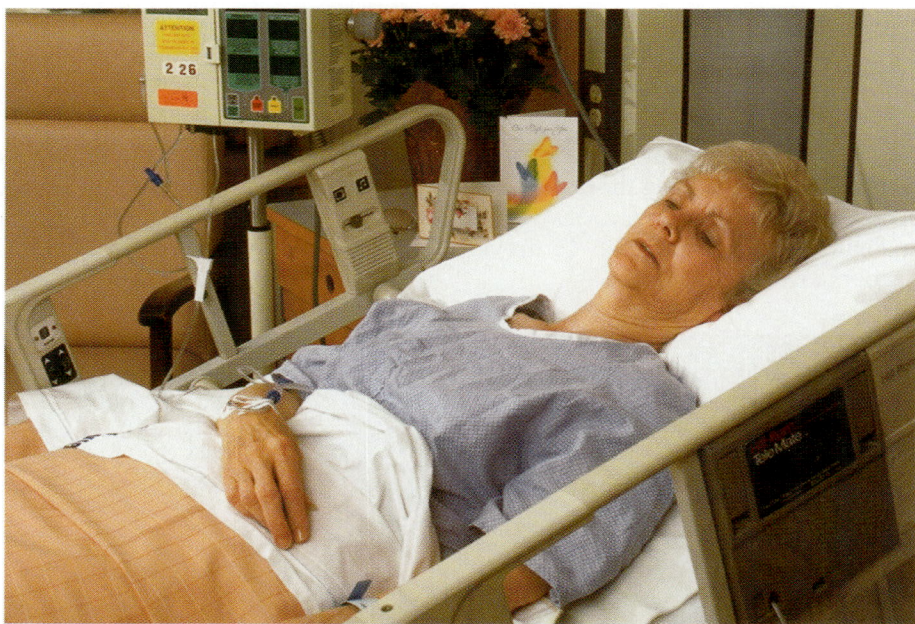

anesthetic A drug used to produce loss of feeling; can be given orally, rectally, by injection, or by inhalation; a person who has been given an anesthetic is anesthetized

anesthesia Loss of feeling or sensation in a part or all of the body

■ Anesthesia

Before surgery, the patient is given special medications that cause a loss of feeling in all or part of the body, which means the patient feels no pain. When the patient is under the influence of these special medications, called **anesthetics**, he is in a state of **anesthesia**. Some anesthetics cause the loss of sensation in the whole body. These are called

general anesthetics. Some anesthetics cause a numbness or loss of feeling in only a part of the body. These medications are called **local anesthetics**. A **spinal anesthetic** causes loss of feeling in a large area of the body, usually from the umbilicus down to and including the legs and feet.

The doctor who administers the anesthetic to the patient in the operating room is a medical doctor who is known as an **anesthesiologist**. The registered nurse who assists in administering the anesthetic to the patient in the operating room is known as an **anesthetist**.

Chest complications following anesthesia may happen for several reasons:

- The anesthetic may irritate the patient's respiratory passages (mouth, nose, trachea, lungs) and cause the secretions in these passages to increase. This might increase the chance of an infection in the lungs or other parts of the respiratory system.

- Smoking tends to irritate the whole respiratory system. Smoking may increase the secretion of mucus, which can also raise the chance of an infection.

- After surgery, many patients are so sore they cannot breathe deeply. They cannot cough up the increased amount of mucous material being secreted in the lungs. This can cause a respiratory infection, such as pneumonia. A patient might vomit while he is still **unconscious** after surgery. The vomitus (emesis, vomited material) might be **aspirated**, that is, drawn back into the lungs. This could very quickly cause an infection or even the patient's death. Saliva might also be drawn into the throat and block the air passages, which could cause an infection.

- Unconsciousness and inactivity during anesthesia allow mucus to accumulate in the patient's respiratory passages. If ordered by the physician, the head nurse or team leader will call the respiratory therapy department (pulmonary medicine). Staff persons from that department will treat the patient with chest complications.

Turning the Postoperative Patient

Unless you are instructed not to, you should move a postoperative patient into a new position every 2 hours (q2h). This protects his skin, promotes healing, prevents pneumonia, and increases blood circulation in the legs. Each time the patient is moved, he should be turned onto his opposite side so that he faces the other side of the bed (Figure 28–19). Move the patient's legs at the same time.

general anesthetics
General anesthetics cause loss of sensation in the entire body

local anesthetics Local anesthetics cause numbness or a loss of sensation in only a part of the body

spinal anesthetics Anesthetics that cause a loss of feeling in a large area of the body, usually from the umbilicus down to and including the legs and feet

anesthesiologist The medical doctor who administers the anesthetic to the patient in the operating room

anesthetist The registered nurse who assists the anesthesiologist

unconscious Unaware of the environment; occurs during sleep and in temporary episodes ranging from fainting or stupor to coma

aspirate Material (vomitus, food, or liquids) inhaled into the lungs

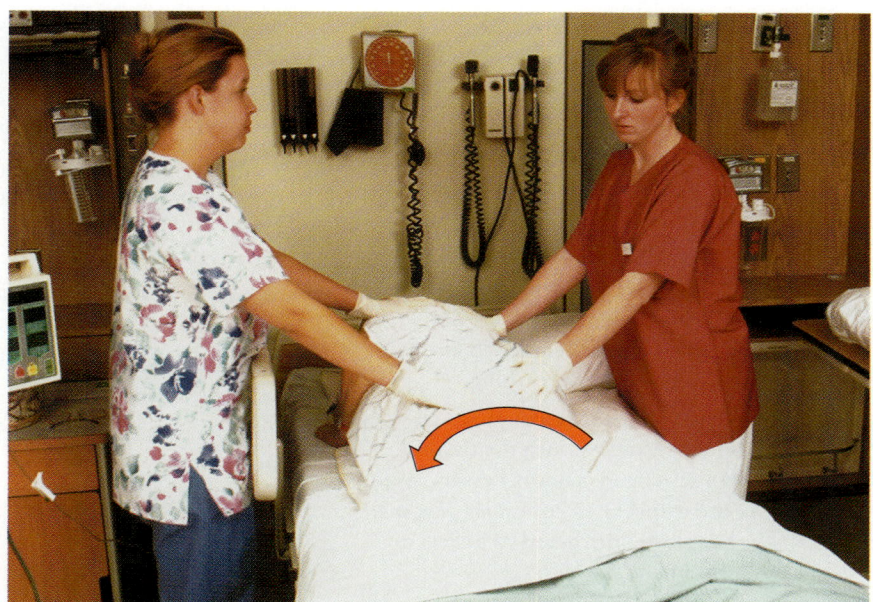

FIGURE 28–19

Turning the postoperative patient

If the patient's gown becomes wet, change it immediately. Change the bed linens whenever they become damp or soiled. Take the blankets off the bed if the patient complains of being too warm. Keep the side rails up at all times.

Check dressings when you turn the patient. Report to your immediate supervisor if there is new drainage (clear or red), or if the dressing is soaked.

▉ Deep-Breathing Exercises

Deep-breathing exercises expand the lungs by increasing lung movement and assist in bringing up lung secretions. These exercises will help prevent postoperative pneumonia, or pneumonitis. In many institutions, the patient will use a hand held spirometer to breathe into for expanding the lungs. If no spirometer is ordered, the following procedure may be used.

PROCEDURE

OBRA

ASSISTING THE PATIENT WITH DEEP-BREATHING EXERCISES

PREPARATION

1. Assemble your equipment:
   a. Pillow
   b. Specimen container, if a specimen is ordered
   c. Tissues
   d. Disposable gloves
2. Report to the medication nurse that you are ready to start deep-breathing exercises.
3. Identify the patient by checking her identification bracelet.
4. Tell the patient that you are going to help her with deep-breathing exercises.
5. Wash your hands and put on gloves.
6. Provide privacy for the patient.

STEPS

7. Raise the bed to a comfortable working position.
8. Offer the patient a bedpan or urinal.

9. Dangle the patient's legs over the side of the bed, if allowed. If not, place the patient in as much of a sitting position as possible.
10. If your patient had abdominal surgery, place the pillow on the patient's abdomen for support. Ask the patient to hold the pillow across the abdomen to splint the incision.
11. Ask her to breathe deeply 10 times. (Explain: Breathe slowly and evenly through your nose until your chest is fully expanded. Hold your breath 2–3 seconds and exhale through your mouth. Continue exhaling until your chest is deflated. Repeat.) Use an incentive spirometer if ordered.
12. Count the respirations out loud to the patient as she inhales and exhales. If the patient cannot breathe deeply, ask her to cough. Coughing is just another way of breathing deeply.
13. Ask the patient to feel her abdomen as she breathes to encourage deeper breathing.
14. Tell the patient to cough up all loose secretions into the tissues, if a specimen is not necessary, or into a specimen container, if you have been instructed to collect a specimen.

15. Assist the patient to a position of comfort and safety in bed.
16. If a specimen has been collected, label it and send it to the laboratory with a requisition slip.
17. Discard disposable equipment.
18. Dispose of gloves and wash your hands.

FOLLOW-UP

19. Replace the pillow under the patient's head.
20. Lower the bed to a position of safety and replace the call light.
21. Raise the side rails when ordered or appropriate for patient safety.
22. Report to your immediate supervisor:
    ■ That you have helped the patient with deep-breathing exercises.
    ■ The number of breathing exercises.
    ■ The color, amount, and consistency of the secretions the patient was able to cough up.
    ■ That a specimen was collected and sent to the laboratory.
    ■ How the patient tolerated the procedure.
    ■ Your observations of anything unusual.

SUMMARY

Preoperative care includes educating the patient about the routine activities before and after surgery. Psychological support means listening to any concerns of your patient and getting any questions answered. Being sure the patient does not get any water or food if NPO is ordered, giving a bath, and properly caring for dentures, glasses, and jewelry are only part of the care which must be done and marked on the preoperative checklist. Postoperatively, vital signs must be checked frequently and the patient watched closely for any complications such as fever, bleeding, extreme restlessness, choking, vomiting, or changes in vital signs. Any unusual observations must be reported at once. Turning the patient and assisting with deep breathing exercises as ordered can help prevent respiratory complications.

Notes

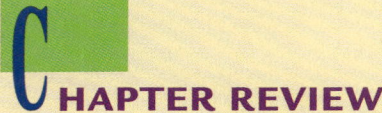CHAPTER REVIEW

FILL IN THE BLANK

Read each sentence and fill in each blank line with a word that completes the sentence.

1. A _____ is an unexpected condition, such as the development of an infection, in a patient who is already sick.

2. When a patient cannot eat or drink anything at all, it is called being _____.

3. Shaving the area of the body where surgery is to be performed is called a _____ _____.

4. Loss of feeling or sensation in a part or all of the body is called _____.

5. Exercises to expand the lungs after surgery are called _____ _____ exercises.

MULTIPLE CHOICE

Choose the best answer for each question or statement.

1. Things that might worry the patient going to surgery are
   a. how their hair will look.
   b. a possible disability or death because of the operation.
   c. who their roommate might be.
   d. None of the above.

2. You can give support to the patient and family by being there with them when they need assistance, by staying calm if they seem upset, and by being tactful.
   a. True
   b. False

3. Which of the following is not a type of surgical skin prep?
   a. Abdominal prep
   b. Vaginal prep
   c. Elbow prep
   d. Scrotal prep

4. All of the following is included in postoperative care except
   a. deep breathing exercises.
   b. measurement of intake and output.
   c. skin prep.
   d. measurement of vital signs.

5. Notify your supervisor immediately for all of the following except
   a. rise or fall of blood pressure.
   b. patient questions.
   c. bleeding.
   d. cyanosis.

6. All of the following are types of anesthetics except
   a. total body anesthetic.
   b. general anesthetic.
   c. spinal anesthetic.
   d. local anesthetic.

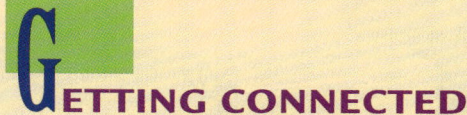

GETTING CONNECTED

MULTIMEDIA EXTENSION ACTIVITIES

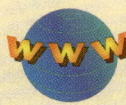

www.prenhall.com/wolgin

Use the above address to access the free, interactive Companion Website created for this textbook. Get hints, instant feedback, and textbook references to chapter-related multiple choice questions. Read and react to the "Nursing Assistants in Action." Link to other interesting sites.

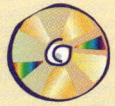

Audio Glossary

Use the CD-ROM disk enclosed with your textbook to hear the pronunciation of the key terms in the chapter.

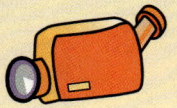

Video

Watch the patient privacy portion of the "Bed Bath" video from the Care Provider Skills series.

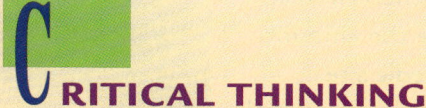

CRITICAL THINKING

USING KEY QUESTIONS

Read each question and think of what you might do in each situation.

1. Your patient is to go to surgery. What kind of things will you do to help get him ready?

2. What are your responsibilities when preparing the patient's room to receive her after surgery?

3. What are five reasons that chest complications might occur following surgery?

4. What types of conditions should you report to your supervisor immediately if you encounter them?

5. What should you do if a postoperative patient vomits?

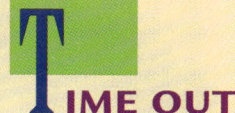

TIME OUT

TIPS FOR TIME MANAGEMENT

COMMUNICATION TIP   You may not always be told that you are doing a good job. Patients who are ill or unhappy do not often say thank you. Your supervisor and fellow workers may seem to take your work for granted. Give yourself compliments when you know you have done a good job. You may want to ask for feedback occasionally from your supervisor as well. You will work hardest and manage your time best when you feel rewarded for your work.

INTRAVENOUS INFUSION (IV) EQUIPMENT

intravenous infusion The injection of fluids, nutrients, or medication into a vein

An **intravenous infusion** is often used in the hospital to put fluids into the patient's body. A tube is connected to a bottle or plastic container. The container holds a fluid that could be a solution of salt or sugar, a prescribed medication, or blood (Figure 29–1).

The other end of the tube is connected to a needle. The needle is inserted by the doctor or the nurse into the patient's vein to give fluids, nourishment, or medications to the patient. It may be used to change the balance of certain chemicals in the patient's body. The solution flows from the container into the patient's vein and is circulated through the body.

The amount of fluid that can flow into the patient's body is controlled by a clamp on the tube. This clamp allows only a certain number of drops per minute to flow from the container. The IV flow may also be regulated by an IV pump. You have to move the patient in bed or change his position without interrupting the flow of the solution. The pump may be moved to assist the patient out of bed or to walk.

KEY IDEA

You, the nursing assistant, should never touch the IV clamp or change the IV pump controls. Only a doctor or a nurse may change or regulate the amount of flow of an IV solution.

FIGURE 29–1

Intravenous (IV) infusion equipment

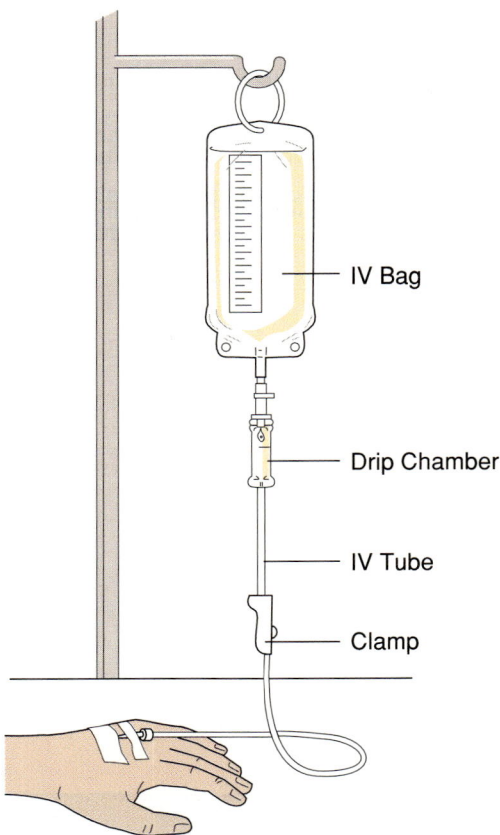

IV Bag

Drip Chamber

IV Tube

Clamp

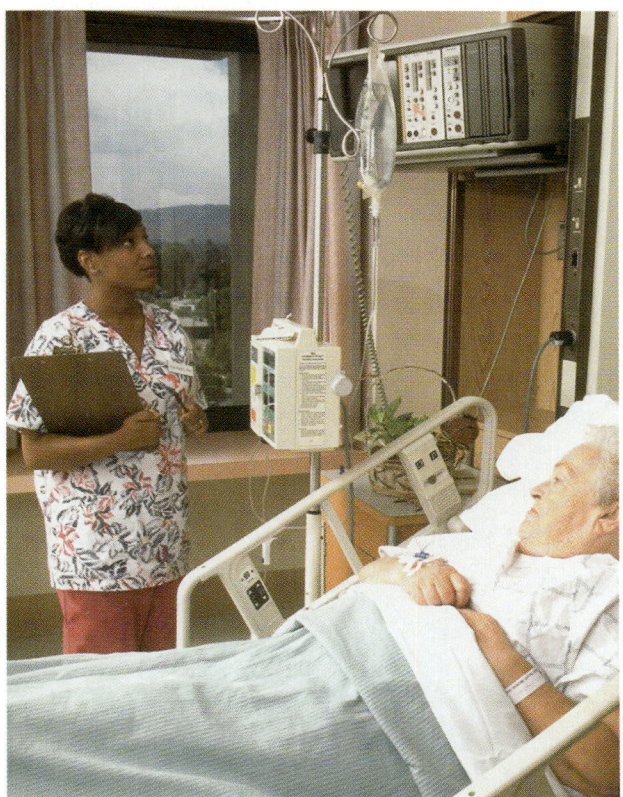

FIGURE 29–2
When a patient is receiving IV fluids, check the IV solution, drip chamber, and tubing

CARING FOR THE PATIENT WITH AN INTRAVENOUS INFUSION

Check the IV solution or blood transfusion to make sure it is flowing (Figure 29–2). Make sure the tubing is not kinked and that the patient is not lying on the tubing. Do not adjust the clamps or flow rate. Notify your supervisor immediately if the patient's skin around the needle is swollen or bleeding, if the fluid is not running properly, or if the patient complains of discomfort. It is possible that the solution is not running into the vein, but, instead, into the tissue nearby. This is called **infiltration** of an IV solution.

To change the patient's gown without disturbing the IV, use the following procedure.

infiltration Occurs when an IV solution runs into nearby tissue instead of into a vein

---

PROCEDURE

OBRA

CHANGING A PATIENT'S GOWN

PREPARATION
1. Place a clean gown and a laundry bag on the chair near the bed.
2. Untie the patient's gown.

STEPS
3. Remove the arm without the IV from the sleeve.

4. Remove the gown from the arm with the IV carefully, considering the tube and the container of fluid as part of the arm. Move the sleeve down the arm, over the tubing, and up to the bottle or container.

5. Remove the container or bottle from the hook, being careful not

PROCEDURE (CONTINUED)

to lower the bottle below the area on the patient's arm where the needle is inserted.

6. Slip the gown over the bottle and return the bottle or container to its hook.

7. Place the soiled gown in the laundry bag on the chair.

To put the clean gown on the patient, consider the bottle or container and tube as part of the patient's arm, and continue using these steps:

8. Lift the bottle from the hook carefully. Do not put the bottle or container below the area on the patient's arm where the needle has been inserted.

9. Slip the sleeve of the gown over the bottle or container quickly.

10. Replace the bottle on the hook.

11. Slip the gown down the tube and then over the patient's arm.

12. Slip the gown over the other arm without the IV.

13. Tie the back straps for the patient's comfort.

14. Make sure IV is running and the patient has no complaints.

FOLLOW-UP

15. Bag and dispose of soiled linen in the laundry hamper.

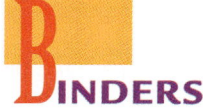

BINDERS

binder A type of bandage applied to a large body area (abdomen or chest) to secure a dressing in place or to put pressure on or support a body part

Binders are wide cloth bandages, usually made of cotton. They are applied mainly to the abdomen, chest, and perineal area of the patient for several reasons. Binders can be used postoperatively, or after childbirth, or whenever it is desirable to:

- Give support to a weakened body part
- Hold dressing and bandages in place
- Put pressure on parts of the body to make the patient more comfortable

Your immediate supervisor will tell you if a particular patient is to have a binder applied and what kind of binder is to be used. Remember, unless the binder is put on properly, it can be more uncomfortable for the patient than if it had not been used at all. Binders are obtained from central supply.

Straight abdominal binders are often ordered following lower back surgery. They provide needed support and can add to the patient's comfort. This binder is rectangular in shape, covers the area from the waist to the hips, and is fastened in the front.

GUIDELINES

BINDERS

- Keep the binder smooth and clean. Otherwise, it will be uncomfortable in the same way that crumbs or wrinkles in the patient's bed are uncomfortable. Bedsores (decubitus ulcers or pressure ulcers) can be caused by wrinkles or wetness of a binder.

- Watch for reddened areas on the patient's skin. Report these to your immediate supervisor.

- Use the correct type of binder. Be sure it is the correct size. Several different types of binders commonly used are:

  - Straight abdominal binder
  - T binder (Single T = female; Double T = male)
  - Breast binders

The *T binder* is used for males and females to keep dressings in place on the perineal (genital) area and rectal area. This binder is often used after a hemorrhoidectomy (an operation to remove hemorrhoids) or after the delivery of a baby. The binder is first wrapped around the patient's waist. Part of the binder then goes between the patient's legs and is brought back up to be fastened at the waist.

Breast binders are used for females following breast surgery.

ELASTIC STOCKINGS AND ELASTIC BANDAGES

Antiembolism elastic stockings and elastic bandages are applied to the body extremities (arms, hands, legs, feet). In postoperative care, they are most often used on the lower extremities or legs. They are used either as treatment for **thrombophlebitis** (blood clots in the veins) or for **phlebitis** (inflammation of the veins) or to prevent these conditions.

The purpose of antiembolism elastic stockings and elastic bandages is to compress the veins and, therefore, improve the return of venous blood to the heart, which improves circulation. In cases of sprain or strain at the joint, they are used to provide support and comfort.

thrombophlebitis
Inflammation and blood clots in a vein

phlebitis Inflammation of a vein

Applying Antiembolism Elastic Stockings

Antiembolism stockings are also called elastic support hose. These stockings can be either knee-length or full-length (Figure 29–3a and Figure 29–3b). ***Be careful to smooth out all the wrinkles***. ***Be sure the stocking is pulled up firmly***. Elastic stockings must be

antiembolism stockings
Designed to promote blood to flow and to prevent the formation of blood clots in the blood stream

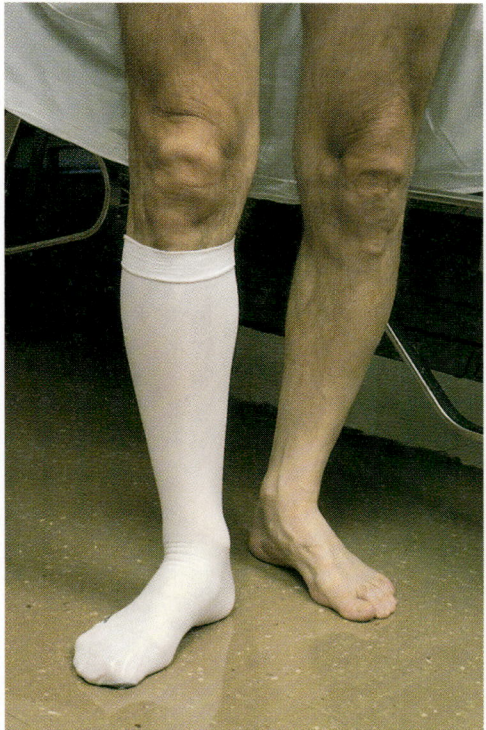

FIGURE 29–3a
Knee-length antiembolism stocking

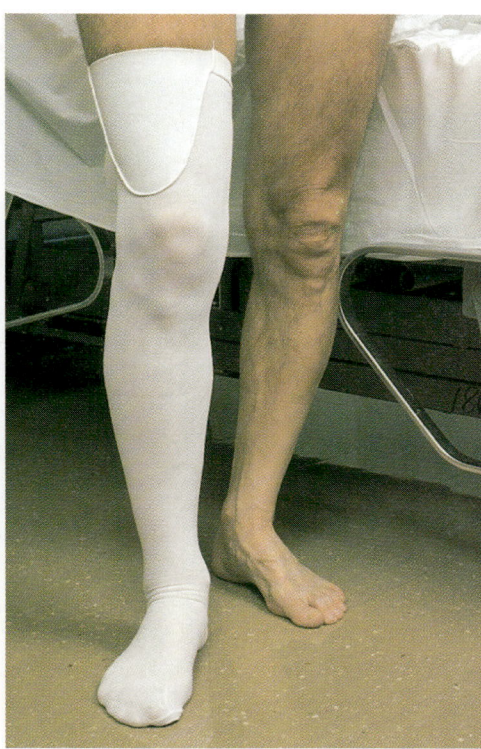

FIGURE 29–3b
Full-length antiembolism stocking

removed and reapplied at least once every 8 hours and more often if the doctor has so ordered. Always follow doctor's orders for application and removal. These stockings come in various sizes. When first ordered, the leg must be measured to be sure the stockings are the right size and fit the patient. They should be applied while the patient is lying down (not sitting in a chair) before getting out of bed. Elastic stockings should be applied only on the instructions of your immediate supervisor.

◼ Applying Elastic Bandages

Elastic bandages (sometimes called ACE® bandages) are long strips of elasticized cotton (Figure 29–4). They are wound neatly into rolls, with a metal clip or Velcro® to keep the end in place. They provide support, hold dressings in place, apply pressure to a body part, and improve return circulation. Bandages may be ordered toes to knees, toes to mid-thighs, toes to groin, or heel-free (heel-free means heel uncovered). Follow the instructions given to you by your immediate supervisor. Use as many bandages as necessary to cover the area as ordered.

If the bandage has been wrapped too tightly, circulation may be impaired and the patient may develop symptoms such as paleness, coldness, blueness (cyanosis), pain, swelling, or numbness in the extremities. Be very careful to wrap these bandages firmly but not too tightly. Check the patient's condition frequently. Elastic bandages should be removed and reapplied once per shift, unless otherwise ordered. Observe the condition, color, and sensation of the skin every hour (qh). Also, check for movement of fingers or toes if applicable.

FIGURE 29–4

Elastic stockings and bandages

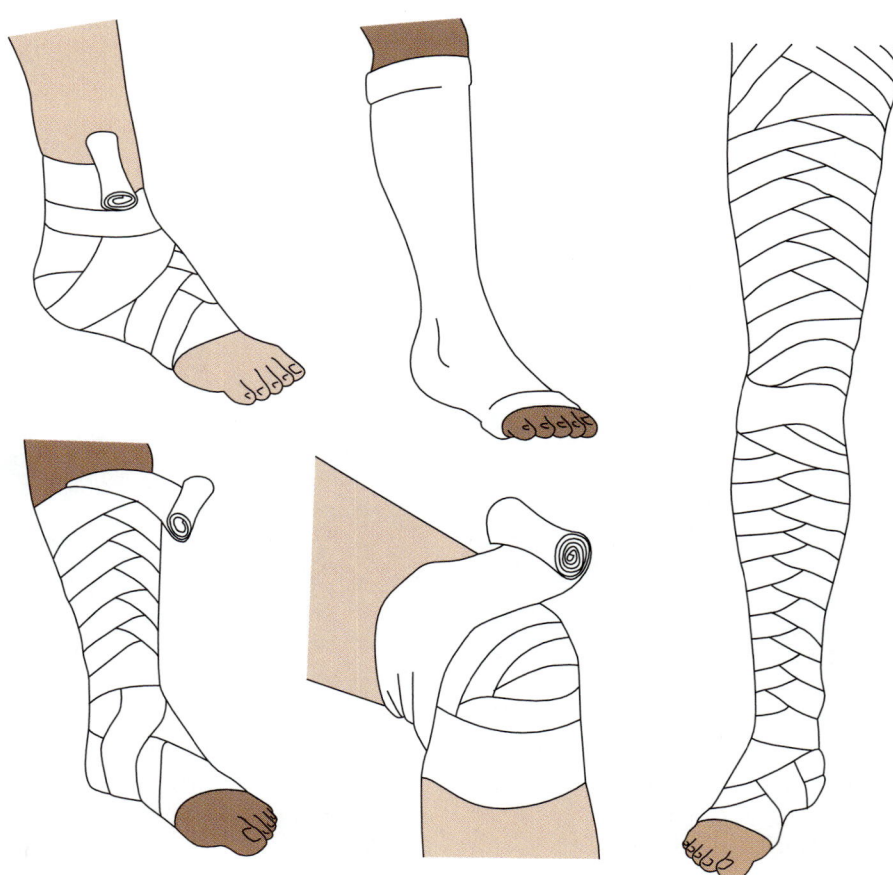

PROCEDURE

OBRA

APPLYING ELASTIC BANDAGES

PREPARATION

1. Assemble your equipment:
   a. Elastic bandages
   b. Clips or safety pins
   c. Disposable gloves
2. Identify the patient by checking the identification bracelet.
3. Explain to the patient that you are going to wrap his leg or arm (or whatever area is to be wrapped) with an elastic bandage.
4. Provide privacy for the patient.

STEPS

5. Wash your hands and put on gloves.
6. Raise the bed to a comfortable working position.
7. Place the patient in a comfortable position that is convenient for you to work. Expose the area to be wrapped.
8. Extend the part of the body to be bandaged. Support the patient's heel or wrist.
9. Stand directly in front of the patient or facing the part to be bandaged.
10. Hold the bandage with the loose end coming off the bottom of the roll.
11. Anchor the bandage by two circular turns around the body part at its smallest point. This usually is the ankle or the wrist.
12. Apply the bandage in the same direction as venous circulation, that is, toward the heart.
13. Roll the bandage smoothly and wrap it firmly but not too tightly.
14. Exert even pressure. Keep the bandage smooth. Be sure no skin areas show between the turns.
15. If possible, leave the toes or fingers exposed for observation of circulatory changes.
16. Continue wrapping upward with a spiral turn. Each turn should overlap the one before about one-half width of the bandage.
17. After applying the bandage, secure the terminal end by pinning it with a safety pin, applying bandage clips, or with Velcro®.
18. If more than one bandage is used, overlap them to prevent the bandages from slipping.
19. To remove the bandage, unwind it gently. Gather it into a loose mass, passing the mass from hand to hand as the bandage is unwound. Then roll the bandage smoothly so it is ready for the next application.

FOLLOW-UP

20. Make the patient comfortable and replace the call light.
21. Lower the bed to a position of safety for the patient.
22. Raise the side rails when ordered or appropriate for patient safety.
23. Dispose of gloves and wash your hands.
24. Report to your immediate supervisor:
    ■ That you have applied or removed the elastic bandages.
    ■ The area of application.
    ■ How the patient tolerated the procedure.
    ■ Your observations of anything unusual.

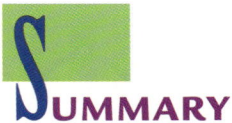

SUMMARY

In caring for a patient receiving an IV, the nursing assistant should check that the solution is dripping from the container, that the tubing is not kinked, and that there is no swelling or bleeding at the needle site. Straight, T, and breast binders are used to support or apply pressure to a body part or to hold a dressing in place. They must be applied without wrinkles. Antiembolism stockings and elastic bandages are two other types of binders and are frequently used to improve return circulation.

FIGURE 30–4

Signs of substance abuse

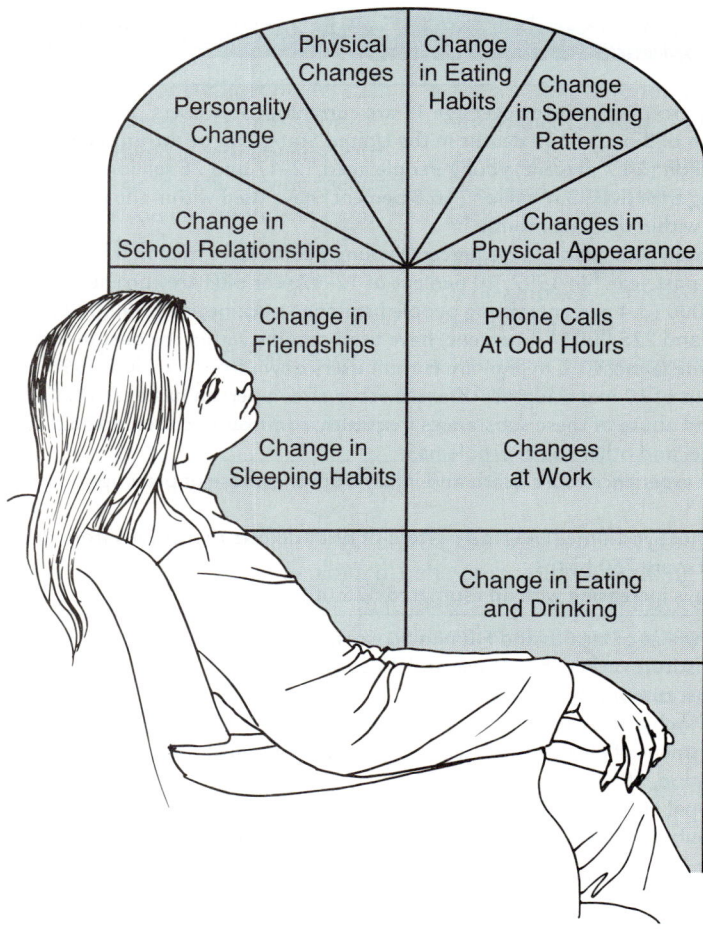

Such behavior changes can be observed at home, work, or school. Other signs that someone is under the influence of a mood-altering substance include:

- Missing liquor or pills
- Odor of alcohol
- Unsteady gait or problems with coordination
- Tremors of the hands
- Forgetfulness or lack of concentration
- Distorted mental perceptions

When you observe such behavior changes or signs in your patient or a coworker, report this to your supervisor. Treatment is available for persons with a substance abuse problem. Pretending that the problem does not exist can lead to physical problems, as well as loss of family and work.

Problem or binge drinking is common with high-school and college students as well as adults of all age groups. Review the Guidelines on the next page to help identify the signs and symptoms of a drinking problem. An understanding and non-judgmental approach to patients, families, and coworkers is very important for the nursing assistant. You need to recognize your own life experiences with substance use and abuse and be aware of how these experiences may influence your thoughts and feelings about caring for patients with substance abuse problems.

GUIDELINES

IDENTIFYING THE SIGNS AND SYMPTOMS OF A DRINKING PROBLEM

- Drinking to calm nerves, forget worries, or reduce depression
- Lack of interest in food or eating

- A tendency to gulp drinks
- Drinking alone, lying about or hiding drinks or alcohol
- Injuries from drinking or unexplained injuries
- Needing an increased amount of alcohol to get high
- Getting drunk more than 3–4 times per year
- Irritability, resentfulness, unreasonableness

- Medical, social, family, or financial problems caused by drinking
- Isolation or avoiding others who bring attention to the drinking

There are a variety of sources for help for both the drinker and those who live with or care for the problem drinker. Examples include counselors, clergy, Alcoholics Anonymous or other self-help groups, health-care providers, and social service agencies.

SUMMARY

This chapter has given you information about natural defense mechanisms of the human body. You will need to keep this information in mind when caring for individuals who are immunosuppressed. These patients have lost some of those natural defenses either due to medications they are taking, such as chemotherapy, or a condition or disease they have, such as AIDS or diabetes. Care for patients with cancer, including special considerations for patients who are undergoing chemotherapy and/or radiation therapy, was also discussed in this chapter. Information about mental health and illnesses with behavioral changes, for example mental illness and substance abuse, was also covered in this chapter.

Notes

_____

_____

_____

_____

_____

_____

_____

_____

_____

normal body temperature are placed into a warming device. Two kinds of warmers are incubators and radiant warmers. Care must be taken to monitor the temperature often to prevent overheating while the baby is in such a device. Ask your immediate supervisor for special instructions regarding these devices.

■ Infant Safety

You must take special precautions to protect an infant from preventable accidents. Reinforce to the mother or family caregivers the precautions for safe handling of the newborn (keeping a firm grip on the wet infant and never leaving the infant unattended on a table or couch). Even if an infant has not yet learned to roll over, she can wiggle and kick until she falls off beds, chairs, tables, or counters. Never leave an infant unattended on any of these surfaces. If you are far from the infant's crib and you must leave her unattended for a few seconds, put her on the floor. The safest place for an infant is in her crib, with the side rails up. Some people keep babies in a carriage because they do not have a crib. Other things you can do to prevent accidents when caring for an infant:

- Wash your hands before handling the infant or her supplies
- Place the infant on her side or back after eating to prevent aspiration
- Place the infant on her back or side to sleep, instead of her stomach
- Keep the crib rails in the up position when the infant is sleeping or playing
- Use only 1 or 2 inches of bath water and never leave the infant alone in the water
- Never place the infant who is in an infant seat on tables, chairs, beds, or counters
- Keep all medications and cleaning solutions out of the reach of all children (Figure 31–16)

FIGURE 31–16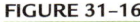

Keep hazards out of reach of all children

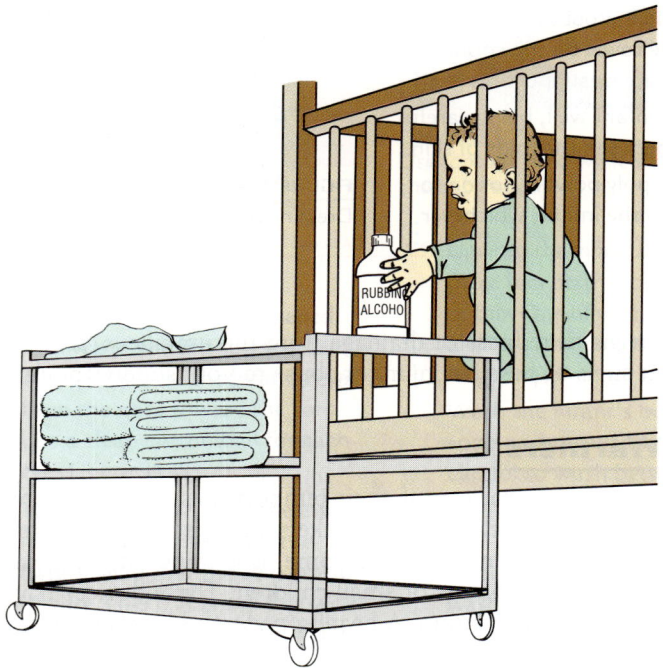

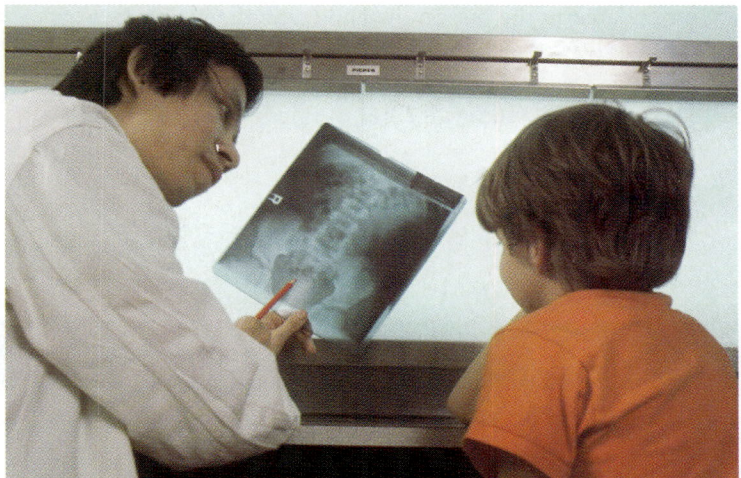

FIGURE 31–17
Communicating with a pediatric patient

PEDIATRIC CARE

Pediatric patients are children (Figure 31–17). In most hospitals, anyone under age 16 is called a pediatric patient. These patients may be grouped in several ways. For example, pediatric patients are sometimes grouped according to age because children of different ages need different kinds and amounts of care. Children also may be grouped according to their medical or surgical condition.

These developmental age groupings are often used in referring to pediatric patients.

- Premature babies are born before the completion of 37 weeks of gestation (pregnancy) or 3 weeks less than full term (the normal gestation period is 40 weeks). Low birth weight babies are under 2500 grams or 5.5 pounds in weight.

- Newborn babies (neonates) are full-term babies from birth until 1 month of age

- Infants are babies from 1 month to 1 year old

- Toddlers are children from 1 to 3 years of age

- Preschoolers are children from 3 to 5 years old

- School-age children are from 6 to 12 years old

- Adolescents are children from 12 to 19 years old

Pediatric patients are admitted to the health care facilities or require care at home for many reasons, for example, congenital defects, nutritional disorders, or accidents—falls, poisoning, fractures, or burns.

pediatric patient Any patient under the age of 16 years

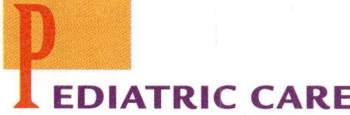

Nursing Care of Pediatric Patients

The nursing care of children is based on what is normal in terms of growth and development for a child of a certain age (see Chapter 15).

Three categories of nursing care for children:

1. The things one normally does for a child at a certain age, such as feeding, bathing, keeping the child safe, communicating with both the child and the family, or providing opportunities for play.

2. Nursing care related to the reason the child is in the health care institution, such as feeding a baby who has a cleft palate.

3. Regular nursing care procedures that have to be adapted to children, such as collecting a urine specimen or measuring vital signs.

■ Safety

There are several guidelines to follow to promote safety when caring for the child.

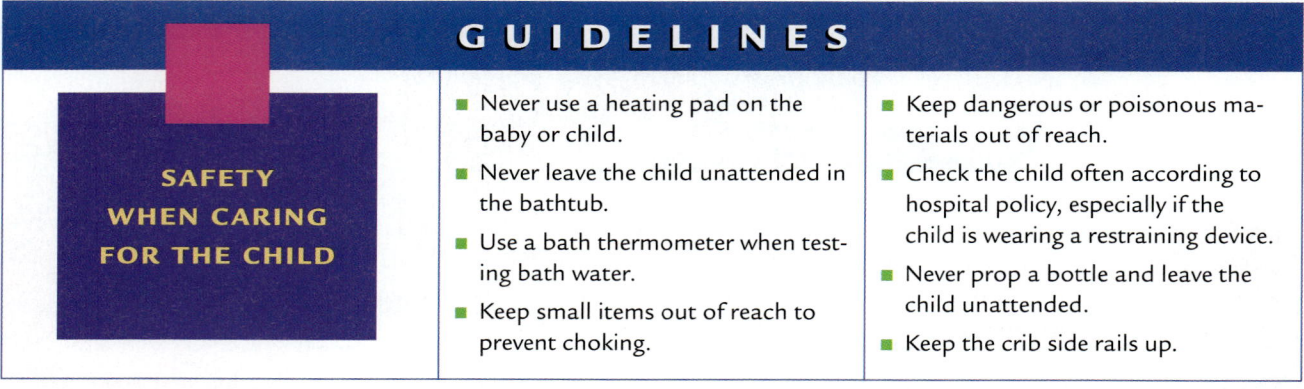

GUIDELINES

SAFETY WHEN CARING FOR THE CHILD

- Never use a heating pad on the baby or child.
- Never leave the child unattended in the bathtub.
- Use a bath thermometer when testing bath water.
- Keep small items out of reach to prevent choking.
- Keep dangerous or poisonous materials out of reach.
- Check the child often according to hospital policy, especially if the child is wearing a restraining device.
- Never prop a bottle and leave the child unattended.
- Keep the crib side rails up.

■ Measuring Vital Signs

Measuring vital signs (body temperature, pulse rate, respiratory rate, and blood pressure) may be a regular part of your duties as a nursing assistant, however, the pediatric patient requires special attention. Refer to Chapter 19 for more information about measuring vital signs. Be familiar with information that may be provided by your facility regarding the normal ranges for body temperature (see Table 31–1), pulse rate, respiratory rate, and blood pressure for the pediatric patient.

TABLE 31–1

Normal Temperature Readings

METHOD	CENTIGRADE	FAHRENHEIT
Oral	37.0	98.6
Axillary	36.4	97.6
Rectal	37.5	99.6

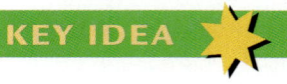

KEY IDEA   Always explain to the child and to the parent(s) or caregiver what you are going to do before providing care.

The *temperature* may be measured in the following ways:

- The *core (tympanic)* temperature is taken by placing an automatic device into the ear. Temperature is displayed within a few seconds. Read the result displayed on the device and record it. This has become a very popular method with the patient as well as the caregiver.

- The *rectal* temperature is taken by placing a lubricated thermometer into the rectum about 1/2 inch. The child may be on the back or stomach, but must be held securely to prevent movement. The thermometer should be shaken down before inserting, so that the reading is below 90 degrees. Leave in place for 4–5 minutes. Wipe off lubricant and read. Record the results. Remember to wear gloves and to wash your hands before and after the procedure.

- The *axillary* temperature is taken by shaking down the thermometer to below 90 degrees and placing it in the child's armpit. The arm is held close to the child's side or chest for about 10 minutes. Read the thermometer and record the results.

- The *oral* temperature is only taken if the child can understand and follow instructions to keep the thermometer under the tongue with the mouth closed for 4–7 minutes (above age 5) for glass thermometers. Remember to remain with the small child to prevent injury. The use of a digital thermometer requires the child to keep his mouth closed for 1 minute while the caregiver remains to hold the recording device.

In all of the above, handwashing and gloves are very important. Explain to the child and the child's parent(s) what you are going to do, and make sure to check the identification band before the procedure. After each use, clean and disinfect equipment (thermometer), and return it to the proper place. Discard disposable equipment in the place provided in your institution.

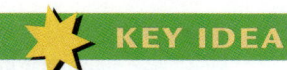

KEY IDEA

Remember to measure a child's pulse rate and respirations before you measure the temperature. Most children get upset when you measure the temperature, and this upset abnormally elevates the pulse and respirations.

Normal pulse rates (per minute) for different age groups:

- Before birth/birth: 120–160
- 4 weeks to 1 year: 80–160
- Childhood years: 80–115

Note: The radial pulse can be taken if the child is over 6 years old.

PROCEDURE

MEASURING THE CHILD'S PULSE RATE (HEARTBEAT)

PREPARATION

1. Assemble your equipment:
   a. Stethoscope and antiseptic swabs
   b. Watch with a second hand
   c. Pad and pencil
2. Wash your hands.
3. Identify the child by checking the identification bracelet.

STEPS

4. Explain to the child what you are going to do.
5. Place the diaphragm of the stethoscope over the heart.
6. Count the beats for one minute.
7. Immediately record the full-minute count.

FOLLOW-UP

8. Clean the earplugs of the stethoscope. Return equipment to its proper place.
9. Wash your hands.

PROCEDURE

MEASURING THE CHILD'S RESPIRATORY RATE

PREPARATION

1. Assemble your equipment:
   a. Watch with a second hand
   b. Pad and pencil
2. Wash your hands.
3. Verify the identification band.

STEPS

4. Do not tell child that you are going to count respirations. If the child is sleeping, count his respirations before he wakes up.
5. For infants and toddlers *watch the stomach and chest.*
6. For children over 4 years *watch the chest.*
7. Count the number of times the stomach and/or chest rises during one minute.
8. Immediately record the full-minute count.

FOLLOW-UP

9. Wash your hands.

PROCEDURE

MEASURING THE CHILD'S BLOOD PRESSURE

PREPARATION

1. Assemble your equipment:
   a. Blood pressure cuff (correct cuff size for size of child)
   b. Watch with a second hand
   c. Pad and pencil
2. Wash your hands.
3. Identify the child by checking the identification bracelet.

STEPS

4. Tell the child what you are going to do, explaining that he might feel a squeeze on his arm.
5. Wrap the cuff securely on the arm above the elbow area.
6. Feel for the brachial pulse on the inner aspect of the elbow below the cuff.
7. Place the stethoscope in your ears and the diaphragm over the area where you felt the pulse (Figure 31–18).

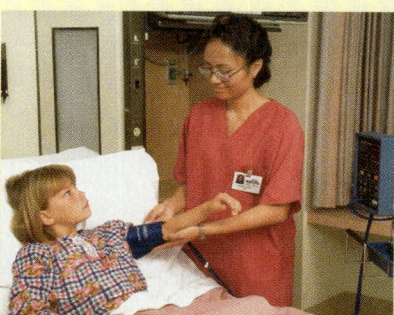

FIGURE 31–18
CNA taking child's blood pressure

8. Pump up the cuff until the pulse is no longer felt. If it is a manual blood pressure cuff, release the valve until you can hear the systolic and diastolic sounds. Count the beats for one minute. Many devices are automatic and will pump up the cuff, release the valve at the right time, and count and display the results.
9. Immediately record the results.

FOLLOW-UP

10. Clean the earplugs of the stethoscope. Return equipment to its proper place.
11. Wash your hands.

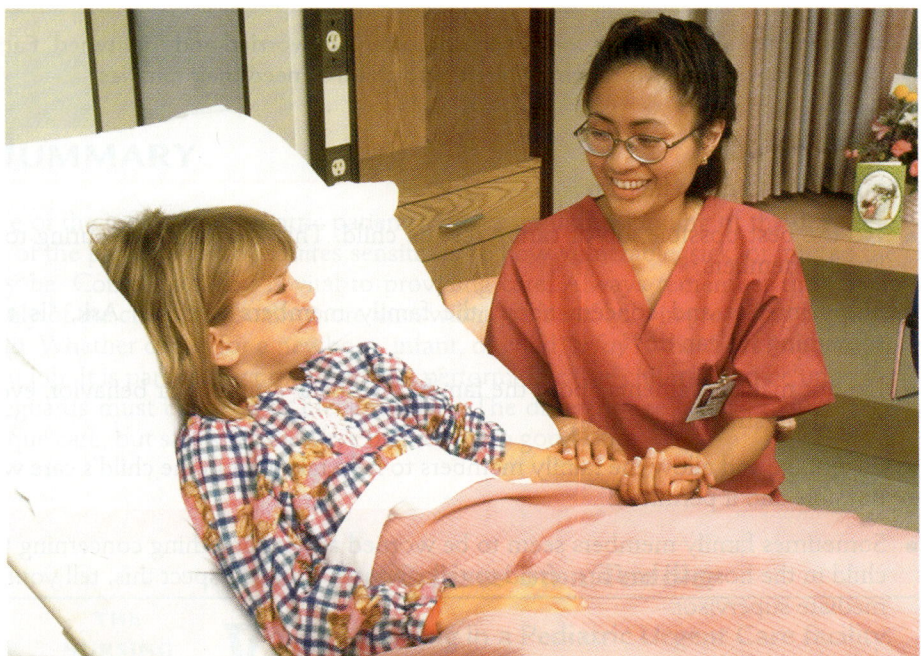

FIGURE 31–19
CNA communicating with a child

Communicating with Pediatric Patients

The child's parents are the primary care givers and as such play a key role in communicating with the child. The younger the child, the more important the family is in easing the child's fears. Many hospitals and pediatric patient care units have a policy of allowing a family member to stay with the child. *Most* facilities encourage such to happen. When this is not possible, it is important to make the child feel as safe and protected as possible (Figure 31–19).

Engage the child's parents and family members in supporting and calming the pediatric patient when possible and appropriate. It will be beneficial to the child, the parents, and you (Figure 31–20).

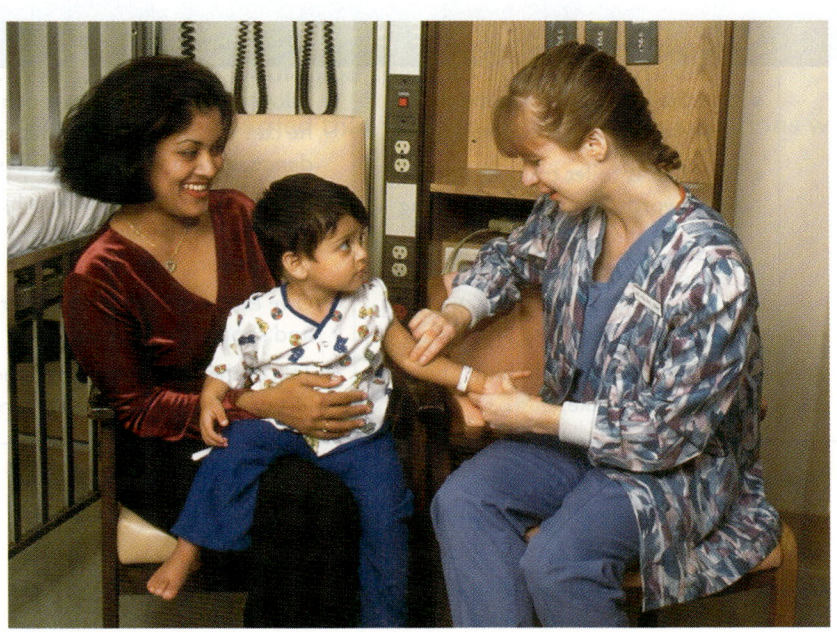

FIGURE 31–20
Encourage family members to take part in the child's care and provide comfort to the child

PHYSICAL CHANGES OF THE GERIATRIC PERSON

As we grow older, many physical changes take place that make functioning independently more and more difficult. The body's central nervous system slows down. This can create problems in detecting heat, pain, and cold, and cause slower reflexes. Thought processes may be slow and memory may become poor. All the senses (hearing, sight, taste, touch, and smell) may not be as sharp as they once were. Muscle tone may be poor due to lack of exercise and muscle atrophy. A disturbed sense of balance might make older adults unsteady on their feet or cause a change in walking patterns. The bones tend to become brittle and break easily. Quick changes in position can cause the blood pressure to drop and, as a result, the patient will feel dizzy or faint. Posture may become more stooped. Circulation becomes less efficient and bodily processes slow down. The skin loses elasticity and some fat. Because of decreased circulation, along with these skin changes, older patients will get cold quicker.

geriatric An aged person; elderly; over 65 years of age

Table 32–1 lists common physical changes experienced by and often observed in the older adult (**geriatric**) person. These changes may or may not occur in all persons.

TABLE 32–1

Common Physical Changes in the Older Adult Person

SYSTEM	PHYSICAL CHANGES
Skeletal	• Softening of the bones (osteoporosis), bones become more brittle and can break easily • Decreased flexibility of joints (arthritis) • Changes in vertebrae and feet (difficult ambulation) • Decreasing strength
Muscular	• Decrease in muscle mass and muscle tone • Decreased elasticity of tendons and ligaments
Cardiovascular	• Decreased cardiac output • Decreased elasticity of blood vessels (poor circulation; edema)
Respiratory	• Reduced tone of respiratory muscles and diaphragm • Decreased lung capacity • Increased risk of upper respiratory disease
Endocrine	• Increased incidence of metabolic disease (diabetes) • Decreased hormonal functioning (post menopause) • Decreased ability to heal
Nervous	• Decreased touch sensation (hot, cold, pain) • Decreased equilibrium or motor coordination (can cause dizziness) • Decreased reaction and response time • Decreased taste perception • Decreased sense of smell • Decreased visual perception (night vision, depth and color perceptions, drying of cornea) • Decreased elasticity of ear drum (alteration in hearing; delayed auditory impulse) • Shorter memory, forgetfulness
Integumentary	• Hair becomes more gray or white and thinner • Decreased fat cells • Decreased elasticity of skin • Decreased sweat and sebaceous gland secretions (loss of ability to regulate body temperature, therefore more tendency to be cold) • Increased pigmentation (aging spots) • Thinning of skin layers, dry skin develops • Nails become thick and tough

TABLE 32–1 (continued)

SYSTEM	PHYSICAL CHANGES
Urinary	▪ Decreased kidney function (urinary output) ▪ Decreased bladder tone (incontinence) ▪ Urine can become more concentrated
Gastrointestinal	▪ Alteration in metabolic rate ▪ Alteration in bowel habits, decreased peristalsis ▪ Decreased saliva production ▪ Difficulty swallowing ▪ Decreased appetite ▪ Loss of teeth
Mental Health	▪ Increased incidence of depression (loneliness, decrease in socialization, loss of friends or spouse) ▪ Changes in sleeping patterns

PSYCHOSOCIAL AND PSYCHOLOGICAL ASPECTS OF AGING

- *Psycho:* mental, spiritual, or emotional processes
- *Social:* interactions and relations among people

Social changes may be caused by physical problems, life crises, or the pressure of society. These may include:

- Retirement
- Change in income
- Fear of illness

Psychosocial changes

- Disruption of independence
- Increasing dependency
- Isolation from friends and family
- Death of a spouse, significant other, or close friends and family (Figure 32–1)
- Change in housing
- Increased dependence on others

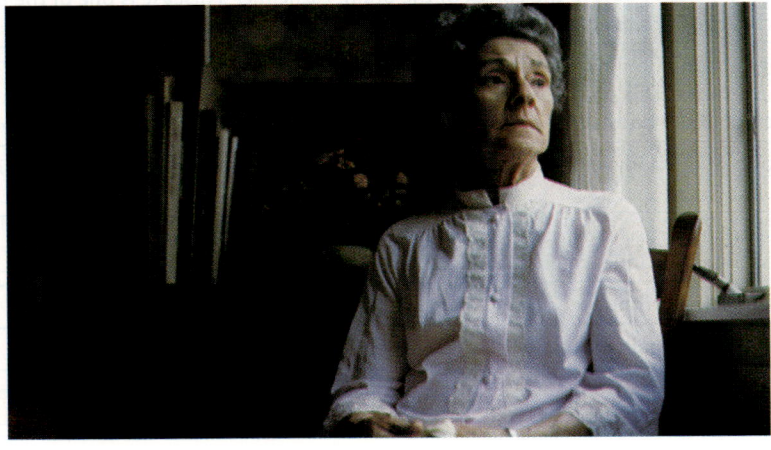

FIGURE 32–1

Losing one's spouse and friends occurs as one ages

EALITY ORIENTATION FOR THE CONFUSED PATIENT

Sometimes the older adult patient is confused for short or long periods. A patient may not know where he is. He may speak to people who are not in the room. Report any new episodes of or changes in confusion to your supervisor. They may be caused by any number of things, many of which are reversible. Make an effort to orient this kind of patient. Tell the patient the time of day and where he is. Tell him who you are and why you are there (Figure 32–3). Always make sure the patient is wearing his ID band.

KEY IDEA

Never pressure the disoriented person to respond correctly. This may increase the anxiety disorientation and lower self-esteem.

disoriented Unaware of or unable to remember, recognize, or describe people, places, or times; confused perception of reality

Patients who are **disoriented** may have difficulty remembering, recognizing, or describing people, places, or times. They may be unable to tell others who they are, where they are or the day, date, or time. These patients benefit from a consistent calm environment and routine. Display a clock and a calendar in a prominent place. Repetition is important. Remind the patient frequently of who he is, where he is, and the date and time. For example:

- Include the time when talking to the patient. "Good morning, it's 8 o'clock and breakfast is ready"
- Introduce yourself repeatedly

FIGURE 32–3

Reality boards are helpful in reality orientation

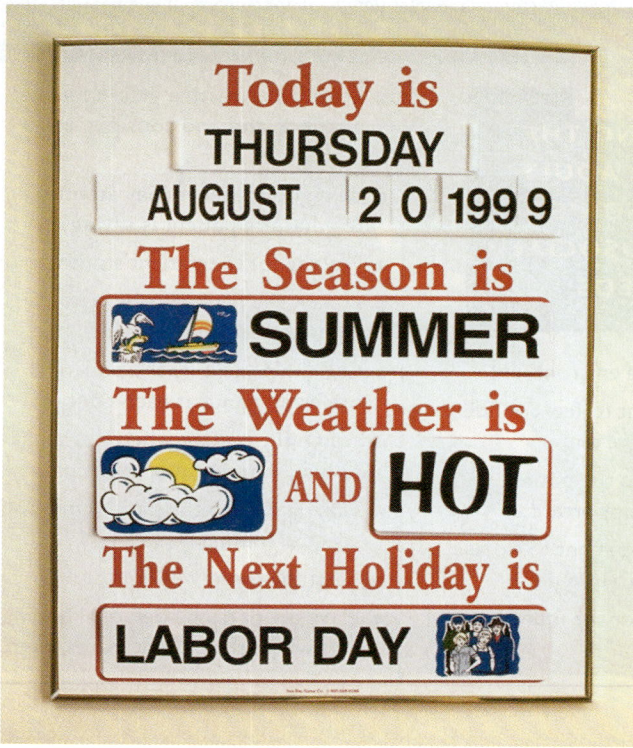

When a disoriented patient asks for or speaks to persons who are no longer living, gently remind him that this person has passed away. Going along with the patient may only increase his disorientation. However, do not pressure a disoriented person to respond correctly. This also may increase anxiety disorientation and lower self-esteem. If a calendar is displayed, the patient may find it helpful to mark off each day, to assist in remembering days. In your conversation with the patient, it may be of benefit to make reference to current events in order to continually orient the patient.

Sundowning syndrome is a term used to describe a state of increased confusion and disorientation that usually occurs in persons with cognitive dysfunction as evening approaches. It is characterized *by wandering, talking, or inappropriate behaviors at the usual evening bedtime.* Sundowning is a common problem encountered by many older adults. Sundowning is seen in older adults who become confused in the late afternoons or early evenings. Caregivers and family will notice that this is the only time when the older adult is likely to appear confused. The confused behavior is not seen in the mornings or during the night. The nursing assistant can play a key role in providing or recording observations about the behavior that occurs and how the older resident or patient responds. Risk factors that have been shown in the development of sundown syndrome include:

1. Recent changes in location or room within the facility.

2. Visual impairment

3. Low environmental light

4. Older age > 74 years

5. Disturbed sleep cycles

6. Dementia

The nursing assistant will need to be alert to these risk factors and observe if sundowning behavior occurs. If noted, record it if it continues on a daily basis or waxes and wanes intermittently. Some measures that can be used to help prevent the syndrome are:

- Avoiding relocation or changing rooms whenever possible
- Using soft music, singing or other social sensory stimulation in the late afternoons
- Offering fluids frequently
- Turning on lights before it is dark
- Providing environmental clues such as a large clock, a bright distinctive way to identify their door, or a large print calendar in the person's room

sundowning syndrome
A term used to describe a state of increased confusion and disorientation that usually occurs in persons with cognitive dysfunction as evening approaches

VALIDATION THERAPY

Validation therapy is a therapeutic approach based on the theory that confused residents have their own reality. It also teaches that as the thinking processes of confused residents become weaker, the strength of their feelings becomes stronger. The goal of validation therapy is to attempt to discover these feelings so meaningful contact can be made with the confused resident. In this way, we recognize and confirm—or validate—their feelings. Validation therapy does not restore mental functioning. However, people who have used this type of therapy with confused residents often find that these residents have less anxiety, are less hostile and exhibit fewer abusive behaviors. Validation therapy can also reduce the caregiver's stress. When we no longer try to convince confused residents of our reality but accept and validate their reality, a more trusting relationship develops, making giving more rewarding. Validation therapy reinforces the idea that it is never okay to argue with a resident or to lie to a resident.

Validation therapy is a way of communicating with confused people. It is based on the theory that the behavior of confused people is the result of an inner reality that makes sense to them—care providers do not know what that reality is. Validation therapy was pioneered by Naomi Fell, a social worker with extensive experience in working with the elderly. It is a program designed to be used to communicate with confused residents. Validation therapy does not restore mental functioning but it often reduces residents' anxiety and lessens disruptive behavior.

◼ Stages of Confusion—Helping Measures

Validation therapy describes four stages of confusion. There is no clear-cut division between the stages. Residents may show signs of more than one stage as their confusion progresses.

Stage One—Malorientation Description

In Stage One, called malorientation, the person knows the time, date, place, and who they are. However, they may have some degree of recent memory loss. Often they give a detailed description of an event that may or may not have happened in an attempt to cover the fact that they have forgotten what did happen. People in the Malorientation Stage often appear tense. They try to establish schedules and rules to follow in an attempt to maintain control because they are aware of their occasional confusion. They can do their own personal care although they may need some reminders. They can read and write and sing familiar songs. They walk with purpose. They are continent and make good eye contact. The people in this stage generally do not like to be around people who are less oriented than they are. They may also accuse others of taking their things when they cannot find them. ***Helping Measures:*** The best way to help people in this stage of confusion is to avoid confronting them. Use words that help them clarify what is happening. For instance, ask Who? What? Where? When? and How? Instead of saying "No, it didn't happen that way," ask "Why did it happen that way?" or "Who else was there when it happened?" This is less threatening to them. Listen to them vent their feelings, but do not try to explore the feelings.

Stage Two—Time Confusion Description

In Stage Two, time-confused residents give up trying to hang on to reality and no longer attempt to follow outside rules and schedules. They retreat inward. Their bodies become more relaxed, they walk more slowly, their eyes become unfocused, and their voices soften. They may be incontinent, but are aware when they are. Their speech may be garbled, although frequently they can still sing familiar songs. Often, early memories become their reality. Their speech and behavior reflect their inner reality. They are feeling sad because their mother just scolded them. They are trying to leave the facility because they have to get home to feed their baby. ***Helping Measures:*** The goal when working with someone in Stage Two is to build a trusting relationship rather than insisting that they recognize your version of reality. We should try to provide stimulation by touching them gently and responding to their emotional needs. It is best to approach these residents from the front to avoid startling them. Get close enough to make eye contact and let them hear you clearly. Bend down if necessary. Attract their attention by a gentle touch and a clear, nonharsh voice. Recognize their world and help them clarify it. Respond to the feelings they express and forget the facts as you see them. When the person states "I am gone, gone, gone," you might respond "Where have you gone?" If the person sounds frightened, the response might be "Is it frightening to be gone?" This type of response will help people in Stage Two more than "Mrs. Jones, you have not gone anywhere. You are sitting right here in this chair."

Stage Three—Repetitive Motion Description

In Stage Three, Repetitive Motion, residents usually pace restlessly or slump forward in their chair with their eyes closed. They do not listen or talk with others. They are unaware of being incontinent. In essence, they are unaware of their bodies. They may perform the same motions over and over, which has meaning to them although we do not know what it is. It is likely that these motions have a goal. ***Helping Measures:*** When working with residents in Stage Three, attempt to relate to them at some level. A gentle touch may result in a moment of recognition that another person is present. A reassuring voice may help reduce feelings of anxiety. Use a calm voice when you ask questions about what the person is doing, such as "Are you making a pie crust?" You may occasionally happen on the right action or feeling. If you do, the person may respond. If you do not, they will ignore you. When words do not work, try copying their motion. If they are rubbing their fingers, rub your fingers in the same way. This can let them know that you accept them and what they are doing. In this way, you validate their feelings. The resident may also respond well to having something like a ball, a towel, a pocketbook or a doll to hold.

Stage Four—Vegetation Description

In Stage Four, Vegetation, there is little movement. The eyes are usually closed, there is no facial expression and little body movement. There is little to indicate whether or not there is any thought process occurring. ***Helping Measures:*** Comforting touches, a reassuring tone of voice and good physical care are the most we can do at this stage.

The essence of Validation therapy is that for each confused person's behavior, there is a reason, although we may not know the reason. Confused residents, whether or not they understand what you say to them, will understand a caring touch and tone of voice.

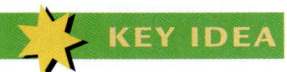

KEY IDEA

Validation therapy is generally used with residents who are confused with no hope of recovery from their confusion, as in dementia, organic brain syndrome, Alzheimer's disease, etc. In contrast, Reality Orientation is used with residents where some recovery may be realized, for example: head trauma, stroke, and postoperative.

SAFETY FOR THE OLDER ADULT PATIENT

In creating a safe environment for the older adult patient, be diligent in your efforts to protect your patient from accidents, especially falls. Every patient is an individual and has different needs. Some patients may need your assistance to get in and out of bed or to walk from room to room. If you notice that your patient is unsteady, report this to your supervisor. The unsteady patient may benefit from the use of a cane or a walker or regular exercise. A sturdy, hard chair placed beside the bed will give the patient something to hold on to when getting out of bed. Be sure the patient's clothing is not so long that it might cause the patient to trip and fall. If the height of the bed is adjustable, make sure it is in the lowest position at all times and the wheels are locked.

To keep the older adult patient safe, the nursing assistant must continually observe the patient and the environment. For example:

- Bed-bound older adult patients should be protected by side rails, when ordered, that are kept in the up position on both sides of the bed at all times. If the bed is adjustable, keep it at its lowest level in a position of safety for the patient at all times. With an agitated patient, side rails may make their state-of-mind worse. Check with your supervisor to see how this patient should be handled. Side rails are considered restraints and require orders and documentation. (See Chapter 6.)

dangling position Sitting up on the edge of the bed with the feet hanging down loosely

vertigo Dizziness

- Before the patient moves out of bed, she should come to a full sitting (**dangling position**) before standing. Patients who are weak or mentally confused may have **vertigo** dizziness or an inability to maintain normal balance when sitting or standing. Carefully lower the patient to a sitting or safe position if they become dizzy or appear unable to maintain their balance.

- When the patient gets out of bed, the nursing assistant must check to see that both of the patient's feet are firmly on the floor before the patient begins to stand. Assist the patient in securing shoes before walking whenever possible.

- The older adult patient who is permitted to smoke alone should be checked frequently. Provide a large ashtray to prevent ashes from falling on the bed or on any **flammable** article.

flammable Something that can be easily set on fire and burns quickly

- Remove harmful substances from the confused patient's reach, such as sharp equipment, Clinitest or Acetest supplies, matches, cigarette lighters, knives, and unauthorized medications.

- Monitor at all times any patient who may wander away. Some health care facilities use an alarm or security system with ankle bracelets to help monitor the whereabouts of patients who wander.

- Use a room closest to the nursing station and away from exits for the confused patient, so he can be monitored more frequently.

- Protect the patient from over exposure to sunlight.

- Keep frequently used articles within reach of the patient.

- Be alert at all times for any condition that might cause an accident or injury to the patient.

- Keep the patient's environment free from clutter. Keep the path from the bed and chair to the toilet clear.

Refer to Chapter 6 for more details on creating and maintaining a safe environment.

Ambulation Safety With and Without the Walker

- When a patient who is unsteady is using a walker the patient should be accompanied by the nursing assistant.

- A walker provides support for the unsteady patient (Figure 32–4). Make sure there are rubber tips on the legs of the walker so that it cannot slide. The patient is supported on both sides as he holds on to the walker with both hands and lifts it slightly ahead.

- When assisting the patient use an ambulation or gait belt on the patient and hold it lightly from behind (Figure 32–5).

- Some walkers have wheels and are used with patients who cannot lift the walker.

- If the walker is being moved, the patient's feet should be stationary. If the walker is stationary, the patient may move his feet forward.

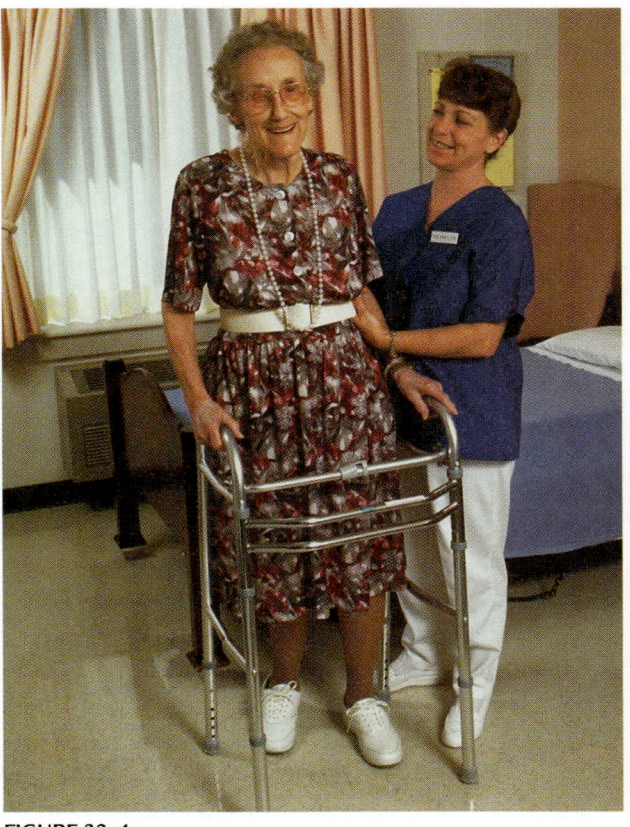

FIGURE 32–4
Using a walker for support

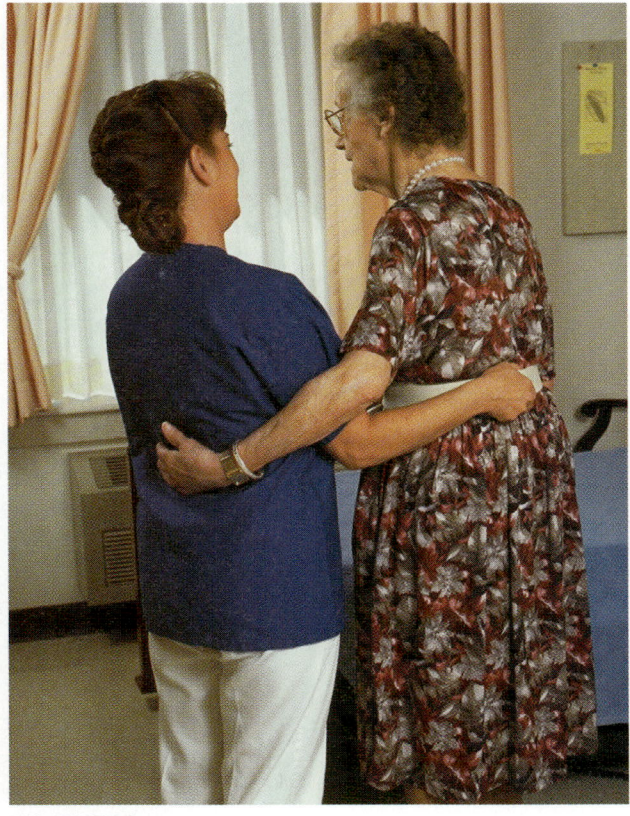

FIGURE 32–5
Steady the patient by holding the belt at the patient's back

■ Assisting the Older Adult Resident with Nutrition

Older adults, because of the physical changes they have experienced, may need the nursing assistant's help in meeting their nutritional needs. Make mealtime a positive experience and encourage the patient to eat (see Figure 32–6). Proper nutrition aids the healing process and maintenance of health. The box, *Tips for Improving the Older Adult Patient's Nutrition*, on page 642, provides some simple but effective tips for assisting the patient in getting proper nutrition.

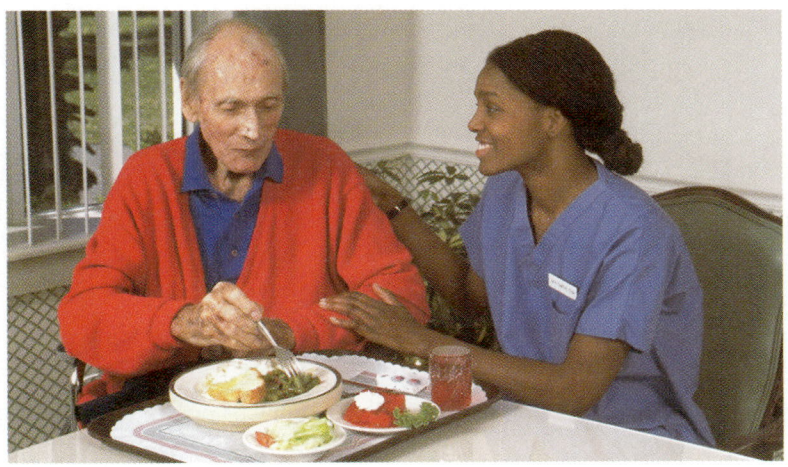

FIGURE 32–6
A positive or encouraging word may coax a reluctant patient to eat

dysphagia Difficulty in swallowing usually requiring evaluation by speech therapist to prescribe a certain diet and method of feeding

pouching Also known as pocketing of food; the retaining or holding of food in the mouth between the cheek and teeth

TIPS FOR IMPROVING THE OLDER ADULT PATIENT'S NUTRITION

- To reduce the risk or possibility of food aspiration, be sure the patient is sitting in an upright position. Offer fluids and solid food separately. (Refer to Guidelines: Feeding a Patient with **Dysphagia** in Chapter 21).

- Observe for difficulty in swallowing or for signs of possible food aspiration, watch for **pouching** of food, gurgly voice quality and cough. Discontinue feeding if any of these swallowing problems occur. Pouching, or pocketing of food, is the retaining of food between the cheek and teeth or holding in the mouth.

- Patients should always be fed with the nursing assistant seated at eye level to the patient.

- Set up the tray, remove wrappers and lids, cut up meat and large items.

- Identify the foods and tell visually impaired patients where in relation to a clock face to find them on the tray.

- Make sure dentures or dental work are in place.

- Verify that the diet served is appropriate to the patient's ability (soft foods, full thickened liquid, etc.)

- Be sure items are positioned within the patient's reach.

- Assist the patient, as needed. If the patient is to be totally fed, work at the patient's pace and do not rush. Offer liquids periodically between bites of solid food. Remind the patient to chew and swallow food.

- Report to your supervisor any change in appetite, food intake, nausea, or vomiting.

- If patient's appetite is poor, check with your supervisor to see if between meal nourishment, such as milkshakes or snacks, should be provided. It may be appropriate to offer small, more frequent meals instead of three large meals per day.

- Encourage socialization during mealtime to stimulate the patient's appetite. Eating in a dining room with other patient's or having the television news on are two ways to offer stimulation for mealtime.

- Acquaint yourself with special diets so you know what patients can and cannot have.

- Be aware of which patients are diabetic. Notify the supervisor of what amounts of food were eaten.

- Find out the patient's food preferences and favorites and have those available for meals.

- Check to see if foods can be seasoned to enhance flavor for patients whose smell or taste are diminished.

- Encourage fluids throughout the day, not just with meals.

NURSING CARE FOR THE OLDER ADULT PATIENT

Restoring or Fostering Independence

Nursing assistants can use the following guidelines to assist in restoring or fostering independence in the older adult.

1. Encourage the older adult or resident to do as much as possible for themselves.

2. Allow the patient to set the pace and avoid rushing him through his activities of daily living (ADLs).

3. When assisting with care for older adults, allow them some choices in the care they receive, clothes they wear, or their food or beverages.

4. Be alert to changes in function as the patient or resident performs his ADLs.

Skin Care

Use the following guidelines in providing skin care for the older adult.

- The older patient's skin may be extremely dry, flaky, and wrinkled. This is due to the decreased amounts of oils being produced by the oil glands and poor circulation.

- Dry skin is less elastic and more sensitive than normal skin.

- Circulation tends to slow down in the older patient. Lack of frequent movement and exercise can contribute to problems.

- Aging skin and circulation problems make the older adult patient especially susceptible to pressure ulcers.

- Give thorough skin care frequently and urge the patient to move about as often as he is able.

- Different patients will need varying amounts of assistance from you when changing position. You will need to turn the non-ambulatory patient many times each day. Practice good body mechanics and use a pull (turn) sheet to avoid friction.

- Sharpen your nursing skills concerning skin care by reviewing pressure ulcer care in Chapter 17.

- Use powder or lotion to protect the skin, depending on the patient's preference and skin condition. Note that powder has the tendency to cake on the skin, especially when used in combination with lotion. Lotion alone can effectively be used to protect the skin. Studies have shown that powder increases upper respiratory infections and increases the incidence of asthma as the dust is inhaled. When used in excess and inhaled, powder may cause calcification of the lungs.

- Report any skin tears, or reddened areas, bruises, rashes, and so on to your supervisor immediately.

The Bed-bound Older Adult Patient

The bed-bound patient has the same needs as the ambulatory patient, but will require more help in meeting those needs. Emotional support and encouragement can be very helpful. If family members are visiting the facility often, involve them in the care of the patient by permitting them to suggest the patient's favorite foods, feed the patient, shave the patient, comb the patient's hair, or do simple tasks.

Proper positioning in bed increases the patient's comfort. Be sure the back and joints are supported to prevent unnecessary strain. Changing the patient's position at least every 2 hours will promote circulation and help in preventing pressure ulcers. Support the patient's arms and legs. Pillows can be used for support, but never put the support behind the knees unless you have specific instructions to do so. At all times bed coverings should be smooth, clean, dry, and free from wrinkles.

Assist the bed-bound patient with the activities of daily living. Many facilities have schedules for moving bedbound patients to the bath or shower. Use available lifting equipment and practice good body mechanics when doing so. A daily bed bath will not only keep the patient clean, but also will help him to feel relaxed and refreshed. Oral hygiene, back rubs, and care of the hair and nails all help the patient look and feel better. The bed-bound patient may need less food than before illness due to a lack of physical activity. Meals should be well balanced and served attractively. Constipation may be aggravated by the lack of exercise.

MAINTAINING DIGNITY AND QUALITY OF LIFE

As you provide care to older adults, you will want to ensure privacy, dignity, and the same quality of care you would want for yourself. Geriatrics is a specialty within health care, with a specialized body of knowledge and patients who have very important needs. Over the years, there have been health care providers who have taken advantage of the elderly. If you witness this, or know of anyone who might be a party to unethical or inappropriate care of the older adult patient, report it immediately to the supervisor.

Long-term care (nursing-care) facilities are required by federal and state law to inform residents and their families of these rights orally and in writing at the time of admission. These rights are described in the 1987 Omnibus Budget Reconciliation Act (OBRA) which requires long-term care facilities to provide care and services that maintain, and in some cases improve, the quality of life, health, and safety of the residents in their facilities. Many health care institutions have a document known as a patient's bill of rights, which serves to protect all patients (see Chapter 2). Become familiar with this document, as well as its intent. Here are some of the residents' rights that long-term care facilities must protect and promote.

Residents have the right to:

1. A safe and clean living environment

2. Courteous and respectful treatment at all times

3. Adequate and appropriate medical treatment and nursing care

4. Prompt responses to all reasonable requests and inquiries

5. A change of clothes and bed sheets as needed

6. Communicate with the physician or other persons responsible for their care

7. A choice of doctors

8. Access to information in their medical records

9. Confidential treatment of personal and medical records

10. Withhold payment for physician visits if there were none

11. Privacy during medical examinations or treatment and in personal care

12. Refuse to participate (as a subject) in medical research

13. Be free from physical or chemical restraints or prolonged isolation unless medically indicated

14. Select a pharmacist of their choice

15. Vote and exercise all civil rights

16. Consume a reasonable amount of alcoholic beverages at their own expense unless medically contraindicated

17. Use tobacco at their own expense unless medically contraindicated

18. Retire and rise in accordance with reasonable requests

19. Observe religious obligations and participate in religious activities

20. Privacy in communications with family and other persons, in receiving and sending mail

21. Have access to private use of the telephone

22. Private visits at any reasonable hour

23. Privacy for visits by spouse or to share a room, if possible, if both are residents in the health care center

24. Have room doors closed

25. Retain and use personal clothing and possessions

26. Be fully informed of the facility's basic rates upon admission

27. Receipt of an itemized bill at least monthly by the person paying the bill

28. Manage personal financial affairs or to have an accounting if the facility manages the patients' finances

29. Be allowed unrestricted access at reasonable hours to property on deposit

30. Not be transferred or discharged from the home without cause

31. Voice grievances and recommend changes in policies and services

32. Be told of any significant change in health status or have reports sent to family or sponsor

Summary

This chapter focused on the care of older adults, known as the geriatric population. Changes in physiological and psychosocial needs were identified, along with conditions and diseases which can result from these changes. The nursing assistant should be aware of how the older person differs from younger adults and adapt care accordingly. Care of older adults may take more time and patience, but good care will be every bit as appreciated. This group of patients, who may be less able to care for themselves, will need the help of nursing assistants considerably.

Notes

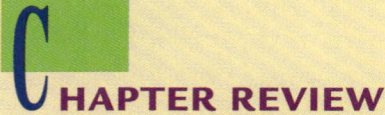

CHAPTER REVIEW

FILL IN THE BLANK

Read each sentence and fill in each blank line with a word that completes the sentence.

1. As patients age, there are many _____ changes that occur in the body.

2. _____ is an irreversible mental condition in which intellectual abilities are continuously reduced.

3. _____ is when a person is unable to remember, recognize or describe people, places, or times.

4. The specialty within health care that cares for the older adult is known as _____.

5. A patient _____ of _____ is a document that outlines ways the institution will protect the dignity and privacy of the older adult.

MULTIPLE CHOICE

Choose the best answer for each question or statement.

1. Which of the following is not generally a major life change for a geriatric patient?
   a. Isolation from friends and family
   b. Change in income
   c. Fear of illness
   d. Child care pressures

2. Which of the following is not a common disease of the elderly?
   a. Dementia
   b. Head injuries
   c. Emphysema
   d. Cataracts

3. Alzheimer's disease is a degenerative disorder that produces
   a. dementia.
   b. diabetes mellitus.
   c. delirium.
   d. double vision.

4. To meet the needs of the older adult, you should
   a. provide a variety of activities that are mentally stimulating.
   b. provide purposeful activities.
   c. encourage the patient to participate and interact with others.
   d. All of the above.

5. Reorienting the disoriented person includes all of the following except:
   a. telling the patient what day it is.
   b. telling the patient who you are.
   c. requiring the patient to verify the correct day, time, etc.
   d. making sure they have an accurate name band on.

6. All of the following are safety tips for caring for an older adult patient, except for one.
   a. Dangle the patient before they get out of bed.
   b. Let them smoke in bed.
   c. Make sure their feet are placed firmly on the floor before standing.
   d. Keep frequently used articles near the bed.

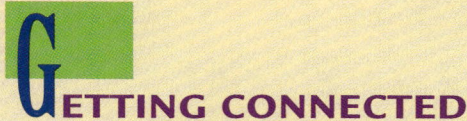

GETTING CONNECTED

MULTIMEDIA EXTENSION ACTIVITIES

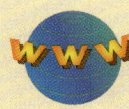

www.prenhall.com/wolgin

Use the above address to access the free, interactive Companion Website created for this textbook. Get hints, instant feedback, and textbook references to chapter-related multiple choice questions. Read and react to the "Nursing Assistants in Action." Link to other interesting sites.

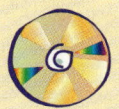

Audio Glossary

Use the CD-ROM disk enclosed with your textbook to hear the pronunciation of the key terms in the chapter.

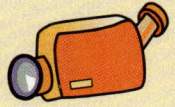

Video

Watch the "Dealing with Dementia" video and the "Transfer and Ambulation" video from the Care Provider Skills series.

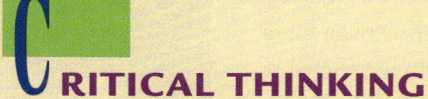

CRITICAL THINKING

USING KEY QUESTIONS

Read each question and think of what you might do in each situation.

1. You are caring for a patient with dementia. How can you weave in orientation factors while providing care?

2. Your patient is unsteady on her feet. What can you do to make her environment safer for her?

3. Your older adult patient is a diabetic. Why is good skin care so important for this patient?

4. Your patient is complaining about his care. What can he do about it within his rights?

5. A patient says to you, "All old people get diseases." Is this true?

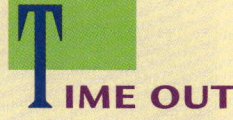

TIME OUT

TIPS FOR TIME MANAGEMENT

SELF-DISCIPLINE TIP   Allow patients to do as much as possible for themselves, even if you could do it faster and easier. You will rob a patient of independence if you do more for him or her than is needed. Take the time to encourage the patient to perform self-care when possible and praise all efforts. Helping a patient become more independent is worth the few extra minutes it requires.

Rehabilitation and Return to Self-Care

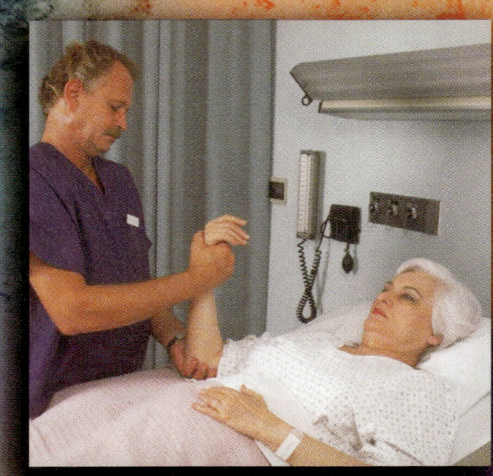

33

INTRODUCTION

In this chapter you will learn about the vital role of the nursing assistant as part of the rehabilitation team. As a nursing assistant, you help patients regain self-care abilities they may have lost through illness or injury. This chapter introduces the functions of the members of the rehabilitation team, emphasizing the functions of the nursing assistant. It details how you can help patients care for themselves, rebuild muscle strength, and stay motivated to participate in the rehabilitation process.

OBJECTIVES

When you have completed this chapter, you will be able to:

- Explain the goals of a holistic rehabilitation program.
- List key members of the rehabilitation team.
- Describe the roles of the rehabilitation nurse, occupational therapist, and physical therapist, as well as your role in helping them.
- Define your role in the rehabilitation process.
- Describe psychological aspects of rehabilitative care.
- Discuss how you can help address psychosocial concerns related to rehabilitation.
- Help the disabled patient bathe, dress, and groom.
- Assist the disabled patient with eating and drinking.
- Assist with bowel and bladder rehabilitation and retraining for the incontinent patient.
- Insert nonmedicated rectal suppositories.
- Explain the principles and rules of range of motion exercises.
- Perform active or passive range of motion exercises with a patient.
- Explain the difference between subacute and acute care settings and the reasons for growth in subacute care.

KEY TERMS

active motion

apathy

depression

fatigue

holistic

incontinence

mobility

mobilization

motivation

occupational therapist

orthotics

passive motion

physical therapist

prosthetics

psychological

psychosocial

range of motion (ROM) exercises

rehabilitation

rehabilitation nurse

restorative care

subacute care

suppository

unilateral neglect

rehabilitation The process by which people who have been disabled by injury or sickness are helped to recover as much as possible of their original abilities for the activities of daily living

restorative care Care given to help a patient attain and maintain the highest level of function and independence

holistic Intended to meet the needs of the whole patient; based on the belief that human beings function as complete units and cannot be effectively treated part by part

THE HOLISTIC APPROACH TO REHABILITATION

Rehabilitation means helping the patient regain a state of health. Its goal is to return the patient to the highest level of function while maintaining the abilities that have not been lost. The injury, illness, or condition that brings patients into the health care institution affects family relationships and patients' feelings about themselves, as well as their physical and medical needs. The rehabilitation team helps the patient and family set and reach realistic goals and enjoy any progress made toward regaining self-care skills. When planning for rehabilitative or **restorative care** (care given to help a patient attain and maintain the highest level of function and independence), the health care team must consider every aspect of the patient's life.

In the **holistic** approach, the health care team is concerned with every aspect of the patient, not just the injury or disease for which the patient was admitted to the health care institution. Thus, the holistic approach to rehabilitation requires meeting the total needs of the patient, including the following:

- Physical needs
- Emotional needs
- Social and economic needs
- Spiritual needs

This comprehensive effort seeks to restore patients to a medical, physical, psychological, psychosocial, and spiritual state of wellness. The goal is to help patients do as much as they can, as well as they can, for as long as they can.

KEY IDEA

Rehabilitation takes time and patience, and it often does not bring about a complete return to normal. A patient may have to accept a little progress at a time. The patient, as well as family members, must be aware that only minor gains may be possible. Rehabilitation therefore includes the patient's acceptance—and even enjoyment—of learning to accomplish small goals.

■ The Rehabilitation Program

Helping the patient return to the optimum level of wellness may require a rehabilitation program. This program is designed to lessen the effects of physical illness or trauma. It addresses the consequences of negative factors such as the following:

- Illness or trauma that has kept the patient inactive for a period of time and has resulted in weakness and lost function
- Surgery (for example, hip or knee replacement)
- Poor positioning for long periods of time
- Lack of weight bearing and disuse of muscle groups
- Catastrophic illness such as stroke
- Excessive stress
- Inability to perform activities of daily living

Rehabilitation begins when the acute phase of an illness or condition has passed. It follows the stage of illness when short- and long-term realistic goals are set for the patient.

The patient acquires or relearns skills and gains strength through repetition and practice. As the patient reaches goals and becomes more independent, the patient will feel more confident and will try to reach additional goals.

You, as a nursing assistant, help the patient gain skill in dressing, personal hygiene tasks, and feeding by making sure the patient has access to all needed supplies and by allowing enough time for the patient to accomplish tasks. You should encourage the patient, praise any accomplishments, remind the patient of what has been taught and accomplished, and report reactions to your immediate supervisor.

It is important that you praise all accomplishments, no matter how small, and handle failures by providing encouragement to try again or overlooking the failures. This helps to prevent **apathy**—a lack of feeling or interest in things.

apathy A lack of feeling or interest in things

OBRA REQUIREMENTS

Nursing facilities are required by OBRA to provide professional rehabilitative services. These services may be provided by facility staff members or an external provider may be contracted to provide these rehabilitative services. For example, the facility may collaborate or develop a shared services agreement with a partner or nearby hospital to obtain services from a physical therapist. The key requirement to be in compliance with OBRA rules is that those rehabilitative services identified and required in the resident's rehabilitation plan must be provided for the resident. This requirement holds true for physical therapy, speech therapy, recreational or activity services, and occupational therapy. A doctor's order is needed to provide rehabilitation services. Each facility is also required to maintain a rehabilitation/restorative nursing program to prevent deterioration and maintain optimal levels of functioning and independence.

To meet OBRA requirements, residents must receive the therapy outlined in their care plan.

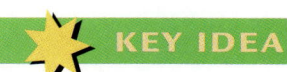
KEY IDEA

THE PROFESSIONAL REHABILITATION TEAM

In the holistic approach to rehabilitation, the professional rehabilitation team can have many members. Key team members are the following:

- Rehabilitation nurse
- Physical therapist
- Occupational therapist
- Nursing assistant
- Physician
- Speech therapist
- Social worker

Other rehabilitation team members may include:

- Rehabilitation psychologist
- Cardiac rehabilitation nurse
- Staff nurse
- Recreational therapist
- Case manager
- Vocational counselor
- Rehabilitation therapist
- Specialist(s)—orthopedist, neurologist, internist, and/or family practitioner
- Patient educator
- Physiatrist, or doctor of physical medicine and rehabilitation
- Spiritual counselor (priest, minister, or rabbi)
- Other professional personnel, where indicated

In keeping with the aim of holistic care (caring for all aspects of a person's needs), members of the rehabilitation team will provide a variety of services. As needed, their services may include medical care, surgical care, occupational therapy, rehabilitation nursing services, recreational activities, social services, remedial and continuing education, speech therapy, **prosthetics** (artificial limbs) and **orthotics** (braces to support body joints), psychological care, volunteer services, outpatient diagnostic and therapeutic services, inpatient diagnostic and therapeutic services, medical and paramedical services for acute and chronic rehabilitative care, vocational counseling, podiatry care, dental care, nutritional services, pastoral care, and beautician services.

The Role of the Rehabilitation Nurse

The **rehabilitation nurse** plays an important role in planning the care patients require. This member of the rehabilitation team establishes a routine for the patient, taking into consideration the following categories of patient needs:

- Physical
- Psychological
- Socioeconomic
- Spiritual
- Environmental

The rehabilitation nurse then writes a plan of care. This plan includes all the members of the rehabilitation team, the patient, and the patient's family or significant other. It can establish a length of time for each step of the rehabilitation process. In writing the plan, the nurse considers a patient's abilities, attitudes, and resources, such as the following:

- The degree of **active motion** (motion generated by the patient) or **passive motion** (motion applied to a patient's body part) the patient has
- The patient's sensory deficits in vision, hearing, speech, touch, and balance
- The patient's perception of the disability

prosthetics Artificial limbs or substitutes for missing body parts

orthotics The science concerned with making and fitting prosthetic devices

rehabilitation nurse A nurse with special training in the causes and treatment of disabilities; may be certified in this specialty with the title Certified Rehabilitation Registered Nurse (CRRN)

active motion Producing, involving, or participating in activity or movement

passive motion Not active, but acted upon; enduring with effort or resistance

- The patient's attitude, which includes:
  - Depression
  - Euphoria
  - Anger
  - Cooperation
  - Resentment
  - Frustration
  - Motivation
  - Acceptance of what has happened to him
- Other factors:
  - Activities the patient can do and will attempt to do for himself
  - Level of functioning before becoming disabled
  - Priorities
  - Barriers or obstacles to rehabilitation
  - Available support system

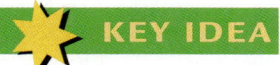

KEY IDEA

The rehabilitation nurse evaluates a multitude of factors about the patient and the patient's condition to develop a rehabilitation plan. Each plan is tailored to a particular patient's needs and abilities.

The Role of the Physical Therapist

The **physical therapist** is trained to assist patients with activities related to motion. The physical therapist and physical therapy assistants use special training and equipment to help the patient strengthen muscles and regain physical independence. Responsibilities of the physical therapist include the following:

- Evaluate muscle strength and **mobility** (ability to move).
- Help the patient regain muscle strength and mobility.
- Measure, fit, and help the patient to use a prosthesis (an artificial body part).
- Teach the use of canes, crutches, and walkers.

physical therapist Person trained to assist the patient with activities related to motion

mobility Ability to move

The Role of the Occupational Therapist

The **occupational therapist** focuses on increasing the functional ability of the patient within the environment. In other words, the occupational therapist helps the patient learn to carry out activities of daily living. The therapist will teach the patient to work with and learn to adapt to new skills. The occupational therapist generally works in several areas:

- **Mobilization**: teaching the patient techniques to use to change position or to reach, grasp, or turn while sitting, or to maintain balance during an activity
- Activities of daily living tasks: teaching the patient tasks to be performed each day, such as toileting, bathing, dressing, feeding, grooming, homemaking, and leisure activities

occupational therapist Person trained to assist the patient with performing activities of daily living

mobilization Making movable; putting into action

■ Coordination, strength, and activity tolerance: teaching the patient techniques to conserve energy, to perform the task to the patient's own satisfaction, and to use all physical resources to the fullest without tiring quickly

The nursing assistant should assist the occupational therapist. You can do this in several ways:

■ Completely understand what the patient is allowed to do

■ Help the patient perform activities of daily living as taught by the occupational therapist

■ Assist the patient to function independently following the occupational therapist's instructions

■ Keep the environment safe

■ Discuss the outside world with the patient with regard to:

　■ Change of seasons

　■ Events in the community

　■ Sports or other activity that the patient is interested in

　■ Other areas in which the patient can be involved with the whole world

■ Help the patient with daily needs by providing access to equipment and needed supplies

■ Report observations of the patient to the occupational therapist:

　■ Signs of pain

　■ Signs of being tired

　■ Signs of achievement of each task

　■ Tolerance of each procedure

　■ Any attempt at a newly taught procedure

KEY IDEA

The occupational therapist helps the patient learn to perform activities of daily living. The nursing assistant supports this effort by encouraging the patient to be actively engaged in the world.

■ The Nursing Assistant's Role in Rehabilitation

In addition to the previous examples of supporting the occupational therapist, the nursing assistant supports various members of the rehabilitation team. When other team members work with the patient, the nursing assistant's role is to help in the following ways:

■ Repeating exercises with the patient to achieve the best result possible

■ Maintaining a safe environment

■ Offering **psychological** support

■ Contributing information about the patient's condition and progress

■ Observing the patient

■ Listening to the patient

■ Establishing a relationship with the patient

psychological Involving aspects of the mind, such as feelings and thoughts

- Maintaining a positive attitude
- Allowing the patient to regain some degree of independent activity within the limitations of the disease or injury
- Motivating the patient to achieve the highest possible level of wellness

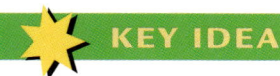

> Because nursing assistants interact closely with patients, they are in a good position to support the rehabilitation program through careful observation and the establishment of a therapeutic relationship.

PSYCHOLOGICAL ASPECTS OF REHABILITATIVE CARE

Rehabilitation is influenced by psychological factors, particularly depression and motivation. **Depression** is a persistent sad mood or feeling of low spirits. It can be a significant factor in the rehabilitation process. (See Chapter 30).

depression Low spirits that may or may not cause a change in activity

All members of the team must be alert to signs of depression in the patient. The following signs may indicate that a patient is depressed:

- Pessimism (a tendency to see or anticipate the worst)
- Unhappiness
- Persistent feelings of hopelessness
- Low self-esteem
- Withdrawal or isolation
- Loss of interest (apathy)
- Loss of appetite or excessive appetite with weight gain or significant weight loss
- Constant **fatigue** (a feeling of excessive tiredness or weariness)

fatigue A feeling of tiredness or weariness

- Slow movement or constant movement
- Excessive irritability
- Recurring thoughts of suicide or death

Another psychological factor influencing the outcome of a rehabilitation program is **motivation**—the reason, desire, or purpose that causes a person to do something. To be motivated, a person must understand what the goal is and have a sincere desire to reach it. In rehabilitation, the nursing assistant is in a unique position to support motivation by providing a safe, positive atmosphere in which the patient can gain confidence in developing self-care abilities.

motivation Reason, desire, need, or purpose that causes a person to do something

The Role of the Nursing Assistant

There are a number of specific ways in which you can support motivation:

- Involving the patient in recreational activities to provide a creative change of pace (Figure 33–1)
- Offering choices whenever possible and encouraging the patient to make decisions

PROCEDURE (CONTINUED)

10. When offering food on a spoon, touch the tip of the spoon on the patient's tongue and gently press down. If the patient has weakness on one side, place the food on the opposite side.

11. Allow the patient time to taste, chew, and swallow. If a patient doesn't drink a sufficient amount of fluids during the meal, tell the nurse so that additional fluids can be offered between meals.

12. Focus your attention on the patient you are feeding. Be alert for signs of choking.

FOLLOW-UP

13. Document or report patient's progress and any unusual observations.

Bowel and Bladder Rehabilitation for the Incontinent Patient

incontinence Inability to control the bowels or bladder; inability to control urination or defecation

Incontinent patients are those who have lost all or part of their control over their bowel and bladder functions. In some cases of **incontinence**, bladder or bowel training may be used to help the patient regain some or all of this control. Offering the patient the bedpan or urinal at regularly scheduled intervals may help the patient avoid incontinence.

A patient who is incontinent may suffer embarrassment and decreased self-image. It is vital for the rehabilitation team to work toward assisting the patient to regain control as much as possible. The process of retraining requires that everyone work toward that goal. The retraining program usually includes increased activity, adequate fluid intake, and a high-fiber diet.

Enlist the cooperation of the patient by explaining what can be accomplished with patience and commitment. Begin by keeping a log for three or four days, indicating what time the patient voided or has a bowel movement, whether it was during toileting or in between, in order to establish a voiding or evacuation pattern. If the patient is able to hold urine or stool for periods of time and to indicate the need to void or defecate, the patient may be a candidate for a retraining program.

The patient with an indwelling catheter (Foley) may also be on a restorative bladder program. In this case, the goal is to remove the catheter and prevent incontinence. The catheter may be clamped for a period of time, so that urine will not drain. The clamp is opened at specific times to allow the bladder to empty. The nursing assistant may be asked to clamp or unclamp the catheter. Report any complaints of pain or discomfort to the nurse. Remember, while the catheter is clamped, urine cannot drain from the bladder. Clamping and unclamping the catheter as scheduled will prevent injury to the bladder, which could occur from overfilling. Wear gloves and follow Standard Precautions when performing this procedure.

Some patients benefit from bowel movement programs, using rectal suppositories to cause the patient to evacuate bowel contents at predictable times, thereby helping to prevent accidents.

 KEY IDEA

Helping a patient learn to regain control over bladder and bowel functions not only allows the patient to perform a routine task but can boost self-esteem. The nursing assistant plays an important role in this aspect of rehabilitation by keeping records to establish a voiding or bowel pattern; helping the patient use the bedpan, bedside commode, or toilet; and inserting suppositories, if prescribed by the patient's physician.

PROCEDURE

BOWEL AND BLADDER REHABILITATION AND TRAINING

PREPARATION

1. Assemble your equipment:
   a. Urinal, if appropriate
   b. Bedpan or bedside commode
   c. Container of warm water at 105°F (40.5°C)
   d. Towel
   e. Suppositories, as ordered by the physician
2. Wash your hands.
3. Knock on the door and identify yourself to the patient. Explain your purpose.
4. Identify the patient by checking the identification bracelet.
5. Ask visitors to step out of the room, if this is your hospital's policy.
6. Tell the patient that you are going to assist with use of a bedpan, bedside commode, or toilet.
7. Pull the curtain for privacy.
8. Raise the bed to a comfortable working position.

STEPS

9. Place the patient on a bedpan or on the bedside commode, or walk the patient to the bathroom every 2 hours to stimulate evacuation of the bowel and bladder.
10. If the patient has difficulty in voiding, pour warm water at 105°F (40.5°C) over the genital area into the bedpan to stimulate elimination.
11. Dry the patient with toilet tissue when finished.
12. Remove the bedpan.
13. Help the patient back into bed from the bedside commode or toilet.
14. Wash the patient's hands.

FOLLOW-UP

15. Make the patient comfortable.
16. Lower the bed to a position of safety for the patient.
17. Pull the curtains back to the open position.
18. Raise the side rails where ordered, indicated, and appropriate for patient safety.
19. Place the call light within easy reach of the patient.
20. Wash your hands.
21. Report to your immediate supervisor:
    - That the patient was placed on the bedpan, commode, or toilet on a regular basis.
    - The time this was done.
    - Whether the patient urinated or had a bowel movement into the bedpan, commode, or toilet.
    - How the patient tolerated the procedure.
    - Your observations of anything unusual.

Rectal Suppositories

If prescribed by the physician, a rectal **suppository** ordered on a regular schedule can help train the patient to empty the rectum while on the bedpan. A single- or double-cone shape is used for adults; a long thin one is used for children. Simple, nonmedicinal suppositories are made of soap, glycerine, or cocoa butter. Medicinal suppositories that contain drugs are not administered by nursing assistants.

Rectal suppositories are inserted into the rectum to aid in elimination, to assist in healing, to relieve pain, or to re-toilet-train an incontinent patient (Figure 33–4). Typically,

suppository A semisolid preparation, sometimes medicated, that is inserted into the vagina or rectum

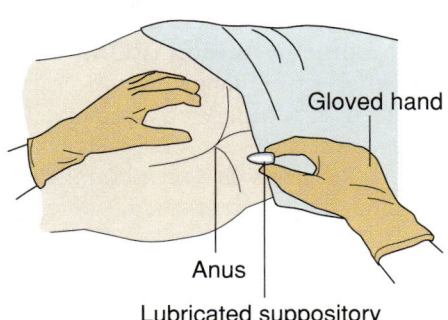

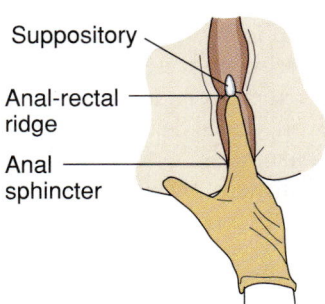

FIGURE 33–4

Inserting a rectal suppository

PROCEDURE

INSERTING A RECTAL SUPPOSITORY

PREPARATION

1. Assemble your equipment:
   a. A pair of disposable gloves
   b. Water-soluble lubricant such as K-Y jelly
   c. Bedpan and cover
   d. Protective covering for the bed
   e. Suppository
2. Check the physician's order to be certain you are giving the suppository that was ordered.
3. Wash your hands.
4. Identify the patient by checking the identification bracelet.
5. Ask visitors to step out of the room, if this is your hospital's policy.

STEPS

6. Tell the patient that you are going to insert a rectal suppository.
7. Pull the curtain for privacy.
8. Raise the bed to a comfortable working position.
9. Help the patient to roll to the left side and, if possible, raise the right knee toward the patient's chest. This is called the *left Sims's position*.
10. Put on the gloves and apply a small amount of lubricant to the tip of the suppository.
11. With one hand, hold the right buttock up to expose the anus. Insert the suppository with your free hand, gently pushing it up into the rectum about 2 inches, as far as your index finger will reach.
12. Keep the patient in the side-lying position for 5–10 minutes to allow the warmth of the body to melt the suppository. If you leave the room, place the call light within easy reach of the patient. It is best to leave siderails up for safety during this procedure.

13. Assist the patient onto the bedpan or to the toilet.
14. Remove the bedpan, cover it, and take it to the bathroom.
15. Assist the patient with hygiene if needed.
16. Remove your gloves and wash your hands.
17. If the patient was in the bathroom, assist the patient back to the bed or chair and make the patient comfortable.

FOLLOW-UP

18. Wash your hands again.
19. Report to your immediate supervisor:
    - The time the suppository was inserted.
    - The type of suppository used.
    - The patient's reaction, including any cramping or discomfort.
    - The results of the procedure—amount and color of stool.
    - Any unusual observations.

suppositories are considered a medication and are usually given by a nurse, except in home care situations. The nursing assistant should follow the instructions of the immediate supervisor for the time and type of suppository to be used.

■ Range of Motion

A patient who is confined to bed or is unable to move about freely will not be getting enough exercise. Therefore, the nursing assistant may have to help the patient exercise muscles and joints. This is accomplished through **range of motion (ROM) exercises**. These exercises move each muscle and joint through its full range of motion using the basic movements of adduction, abduction, extension, hyperextension, pronation, supination, flexion, dorsal flexion, and rotation (see also Chapter 16).

The nursing assistant's part in range of motion exercises will depend on the patient's level of ability and the physician's orders. According to these criteria, range of motion exercises will be one of the following types:

- *Active Range of Motion (AROM):* The patient is able to move limbs through their range of motion unassisted

range of motion (ROM) exercises Exercises that move each muscle and joint through its full range of motion and help a confined patient exercise the muscles and joints

- *Passive Range of Motion (PROM):* The nursing assistant moves the patient's limbs through the range of motion because the patient is unable, for whatever reason, to do it

- *Active Assist Range of Motion (AAROM):* The patient participates to the extent that the patient is able

---

GUIDELINES

OBRA

RANGE OF MOTION EXERCISES

- Do each exercise three times. (Follow the supervisor's instructions.)

- Follow a logical sequence so that each joint and muscle is exercised. For instance, start at the head and work your way down to the feet.

- If the patient is able to move some body parts, encourage the patient to do as much as possible.

- Be gentle. Never bend or extend a body part farther than it can go. Never exercise to the point of pain.

- If a patient complains of unusual pain or discomfort in a particular body part, be sure to report this to your immediate supervisor.

- Never exercise a reddened, swollen, or painful joint.

- Support all joints when exercising.

PROCEDURE

OBRA

RANGE OF MOTION EXERCISES

PREPARATION

1. Assemble your equipment:
   a. Blanket
   b. Extra lighting, if necessary
2. Wash your hands.
3. Knock on the door and identify yourself and your purpose.
4. Identify the patient by checking the identification bracelet.
5. Ask visitors to step out of the room, if this is your hospital's policy.
6. Explain to the patient that you are going to help him exercise his muscles and joints while he is in bed.
7. Pull the curtain around the bed for privacy.

8. Raise the bed to a comfortable working position.

STEPS

9. Place the patient in a supine position (on his back) with his knees extended and his arms at his side.
10. Loosen the top sheets, but don't expose the patient.
11. Raise the side rail on the far side of the bed.
12. Exercise the neck (Figures 33–5a and b, 33–6a and b, and 33–7a and b).

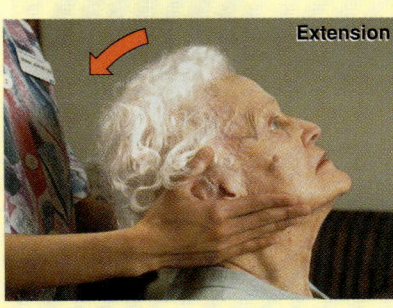

FIGURE 33–5a
Extension

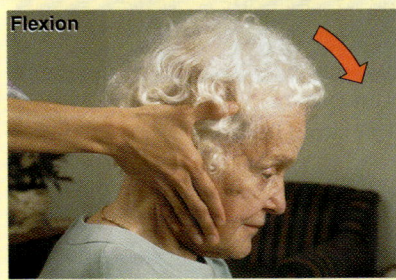

FIGURE 33–5b
Flexion

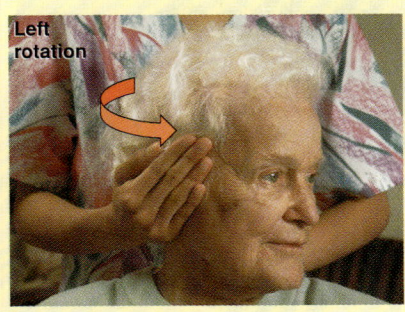

FIGURE 33–6a
Left rotation

PSYCHOLOGICAL/PSYCHOSOCIAL ASPECTS OF CARING FOR A TERMINALLY ILL PATIENT

Some patients who enter a health care institution are **terminally ill,** that is, dying. Sometimes death is sudden or unexpected. More often it is not. Your first responsibility to the terminally ill patient is to help make the patient as physically comfortable as possible. Your second responsibility is to assist in meeting the emotional needs of the patient and the patient's family or significant other.

The most important single fact to remember when you are caring for dying patients is that they are just as important as the patients who are going to recover. You will not have the satisfaction of contributing to recovery, but you will know that you have helped your patients face the end of their lives in peace, comfort, and dignity. Everyone must die. Surely we would all prefer to die in reassuring and comfortable surroundings.

Try to be very understanding. The patient may want to believe he will get well. He may want people around him to reassure him that he won't die. When a dying patient talks to you, listen. But don't give him false hopes. Don't tell him that he is getting better. Your supervisor can help you know what to say.

> **ALERT**
>
> For all patient contact, adhere to Standard Precautions (see Chapter 5, pages 78–108). Wear protective equipment as indicated.

terminally ill Having an illness that can be expected to cause death, usually within a predictable time

KEY IDEA

> People have different ideas about death and the hereafter. These ideas depend on their beliefs and background. You must show respect for patients' beliefs. Be careful not to impose your own beliefs on them, their families, or significant others.

When a patient suspects he is going to die, he may react in various ways. The patient may:

- Ask everyone about his chances for recovery
- Be afraid to be alone and want a lot of attention from you
- Ask a lot of questions
- Seem to complain constantly
- Signal members of the staff often
- Make many apparently unreasonable requests
- Rest and prefer to be left alone

When a patient is told that he has a terminal disease or condition, the patient enters a very difficult time of life. Death may be frightening and the patient's reactions reflect the quality of emotional support provided by everyone interacting with him, as well as his culturally determined attitudes. Feelings of isolation, hopelessness, despair, sorrow, and uselessness affect the coping mechanisms displayed by the patient and family members.

■ Stages of Dying

Elizabeth Kübler-Ross describes five "stages" of dying in her book, *Death and Dying* (Figure 34–1). These are not intended to be stages that the patient must go through. Rather, they are emotional experiences that are common to terminally ill patients. This is especially true for the newly diagnosed patient and much less so for the patient who has known he is dying for a while.

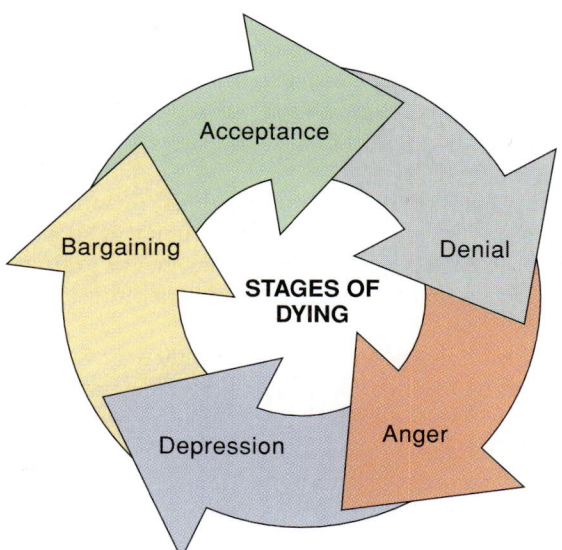

FIGURE 34–1
The five stages of dying

These "stages," or feelings common to terminally ill patients, are:

- **Denial:** This is a reaction to the shocking news. The patient may say, "No, this is not happening to me, this is something that happens to other people." This is sometimes the first reaction on the part of the patient.

- **Anger:** The patient resents what has happened—all the unfinished plans and the realization that he will be unable to finish or enjoy life's activities. It is at this point that the patient will begin to react to everything, making demands and asking for additional attention. The patient now is beginning to feel that soon he will be forgotten and that all is over.

- **Bargaining:** This is an attempt to make a bargain with God to postpone the inevitable. This bargaining may be connected with guilt for not having done what religious teachings tell us to do. It is here that the patient may request that a priest, minister, or rabbi be called.

- **Depression:** The patient reaches some acceptance of death. He may begin to grieve, to talk about his innermost feelings, and may want you to listen. By being a good listener at this point, you can help the patient.

- **Acceptance:** Communication often becomes difficult. Some patients become quiet and withdrawn, while others may become more talkative after accepting the inevitable. The patient may communicate his needs to you through body language or gestures. Your job as a nursing assistant is to make the patient as comfortable as possible.

denial Refusal to admit the truth or face reality

anger A strong emotional response of displeasure, irritation, and resentment

bargaining Trying to make a deal to change the situation

depression A state of sadness, grief, or low spirits that may or may not cause change of activity

acceptance Admitting, understanding, or facing the truth or reality of the situation, for example, one's death

THE PATIENT'S FAMILY OR SIGNIFICANT OTHER

When it is known that death is approaching, the dying patient's family may want to spend a lot of time with the patient. This should be encouraged and permitted as much as possible.

Everyone on the staff should respect the family's need for privacy during their visits. If a private room is not available, the patient's area should be screened so that they will have the privacy they need. When the patient is visited by his pastor, priest, rabbi, or minister, assure them that they will not be disturbed.

Don't stop doing your work just because the patient's family is present. Carry out your job quickly, quietly, and efficiently. Don't wait until the family has gone before taking care of the patient. They might think that, because the patient is dying, he is being neglected by the hospital staff.

The patient's family may ask you many questions. Respond to their questions. Answer any you can. Also, do whatever is asked of you, if it is allowed.

There will be some questions that you can't answer. For example, you may be asked, "What did the doctor say today about the patient's condition?" Refer the family to your immediate supervisor.

Even if the patient becomes unconscious, the family may want to stay with him. Family members may continue to hope for his recovery. They will watch you perform your patient care procedures. They will want you to make the patient comfortable, even if you cannot help him recover.

Unconscious patients require as thorough care as those who are conscious. Their needs must still be met. Sometimes you must ask the family to leave the bedside while you are giving care to the patient. Explain this to the family. Tell them that you will let them know when you have finished.

Some visitors stay with the patient for many hours at a time. Be as helpful to them as you can. You might suggest that they have some nourishment. Tell them where the cafeteria, vending machines, or coffee shop is located. Also, learn the policy in your institution on serving meals to visitors. You may be able to arrange for trays to be delivered to the patient's family at mealtimes. If this is not allowed, tell the visitors where they can find the cafeteria or a nearby restaurant. Make sure the visitors know the location of the washroom, lounge, and telephones.

Remember at all times to be quietly courteous, understanding, sympathetic, and willing to help (Figure 34–2). These are the marks of a competent nursing assistant.

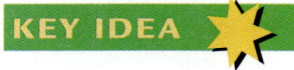

KEY IDEA

Don't feel helpless or guilty because you can't improve the patient's condition. You can help the patient and family most by maintaining a concerned and efficient approach to your work.

FIGURE 34–2

Supporting the family of the terminally ill patient is very important

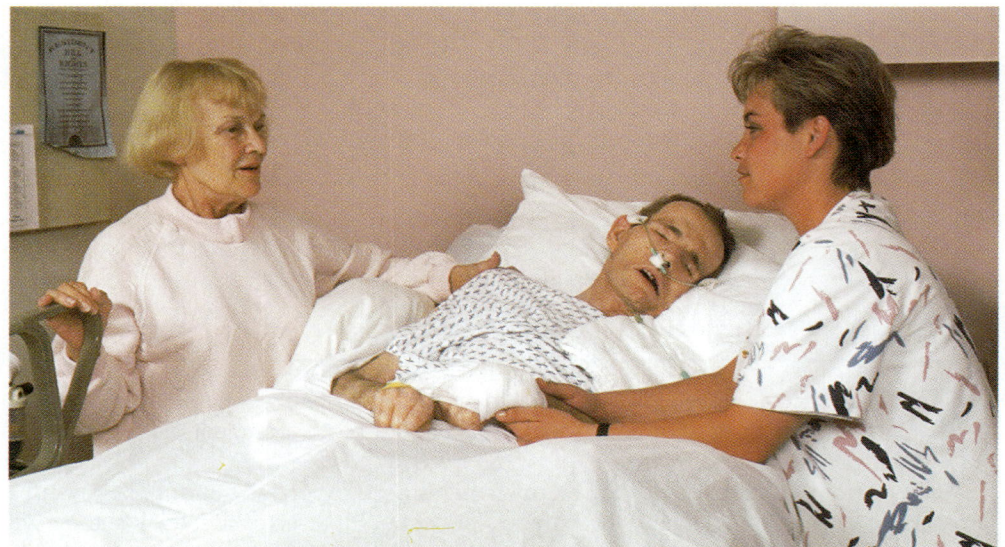

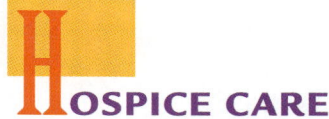OSPICE CARE

Hospice care is a method of health care delivery used to ensure individualized and humane care for the terminally ill. The philosophy of hospice stresses:

- Assisting with psychological, physiological, and spiritual problems
- Using a family-oriented approach
- Alleviating pain and other symptoms in the advanced stage of disease
- Offering professional and voluntary services to meet individual needs
- Making the patient as comfortable as possible

hospice Program that allows a dying patient to remain at home or in a nonhospital environment and die there while receiving professionally supervised care

Principles of Hospice Care

- To provide physical comfort
- To provide psychological counseling
- To assist the patient to maintain ability to participate in life
- To provide an environment that emphasizes the quality of life on a daily basis, rather than longevity
- To provide assurance that the patient and family will not be alone in a moment of crisis
- To provide the patient with evidence that family, friends, and staff care about what the patient thinks and feels
- To provide an environment that permits the patient to return to his own schedule of activities of daily living
- To encourage the patient to be surrounded by familiar belongings and people
- To provide assessment of changing needs
- To facilitate the grieving of the patient and family
- To provide the patient with the opportunity to die with dignity in familiar and caring surroundings

Characteristics of Hospice Programs

- Coordination of home and institutional care
- Patient and family regarded as one unit
- Physician and other health-care provider availability
- Care provided by an interdisciplinary team
- Control of symptoms and pain
- Availability of care 24 hours a day
- Volunteer involvement
- Follow-up care for bereaved families
- System of open communication between staff, volunteers, patient, and family

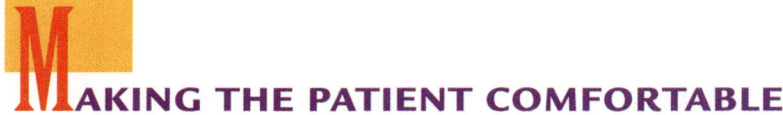

MAKING THE PATIENT COMFORTABLE

palliative Care designed to comfort, instead of cure, the patient

Remember that caring for the terminally ill patient is just as important as caring for a patient who is going to recover. Table 34–1 identifies the care needs of a terminally ill patient and gives a description of the care to be given. This care is often referred to as **palliative** care.

TABLE 34–1

Meeting the Terminally Ill Patient's Needs

PATIENT NEED	DESCRIPTION
Personal	A patient approaching death continues to be given routine personal care, such as baths and mouth care. That is, the patient receives the same care that would be given if she were expected to recover. Members of the nursing staff should stay calm and sympathetic. This may help to relieve some of the patient's fears and make this time easier. As the patient becomes weaker, her condition may require more of your time. You may need to do many things that the patient is no longer able to do for herself.
Positioning	The patient will tell you what position is most comfortable. It is important that the patient remain active as long as possible, and his position in bed be changed regularly to protect the skin (Figure 34–3).
Communication	Speak to the patient in your normal voice, even if she appears to be unconscious. You should still tell the patient who you are and what you are doing. The dying patient's hearing is usually one of the last senses to fail. We do not know how much an unconscious person hears or understands. It is guessed that this is a great deal. Encourage the family to continue to talk to the patient unless she is sleeping.
Visual	Adjust the light in the room to suit the patient. For some, bright lights are irritating; for others, a dark room is frightening.
Elimination	As death comes closer, the sphincters relax and the patient may lose control of the bowels and bladder. Your job is to keep the patient's body clean at all times. Change the bedding whenever necessary. This will keep the patient's skin from becoming irritated and will help to keep the patient comfortable. You may also be giving more back rubs than usual. The urine may become concentrated and strong smelling, and it is especially necessary to keep the skin clean. Foley catheters are rarely necessary with the use of incontinent pads and bed pads.
Nutrition	Usually the patient is allowed whatever foods he desires. However there is often a decreased appetite. Semisoft foods or semi-frozen liquid may be easier to handle than liquids.
Oral Hygiene	The patient approaching death needs special mouth care. The mouth may be dry because the patient is breathing through it. You might use an applicator with glycerin (or other lubricant) to swab the patient's mouth and lips. If the patient's mouth has a large amount of secretions in it, tell the nurse. The nurse may use suction to remove the secreted material. If the patient has dentures, ask your immediate supervisor if you should leave them in the patient's mouth or take them out. If you remove the dentures, place them in a denture cup half filled with water, with the patient's name on the cover. If the patient has cancer or AIDS, watch for and report sores in the mouth. Often persons near death have gums or lips that bleed. Using a dark-colored towel or washcloth may make this less frightening. A moist mouth will make it easier for the patient to eat.
Treatment: Oxygen Therapy	A patient may be receiving oxygen through a nasal catheter or mask. If so, check the nostrils from time to time. Tell your immediate supervisor if the nostrils are dry and encrusted. Check the tops of the ears or any other place the tubing contacts as it can cause skin irritation. A patient's nostrils also may become dry and encrusted because he has difficulty breathing. If you notice dryness, with your immediate supervisor's permission, clean the nostrils with cotton swabs moistened slightly with glycerin (or other lubricant).
Spiritual	Respect the patient's and family's need for spiritual support (Figure 34–4). Learn the policy in your institution concerning religious observances and requirements at the time of death. If the patient has particular beliefs or practices relative to death, such as the care of the body, it is important to know these before death occurs.

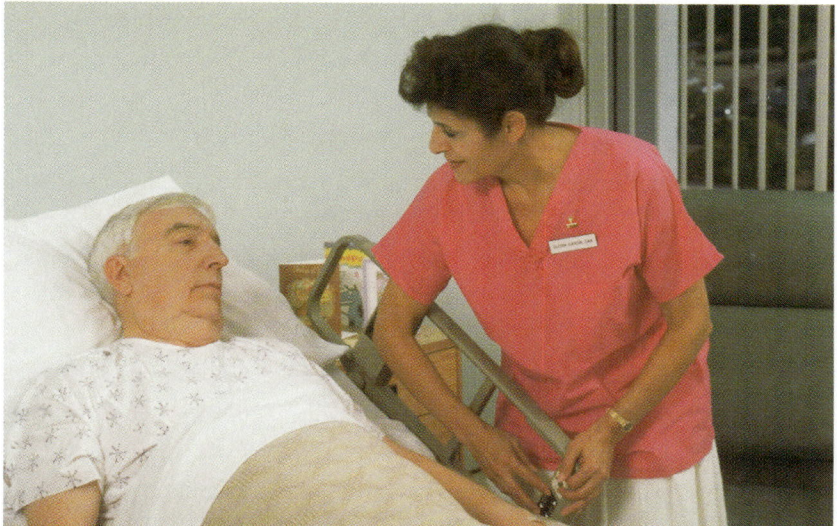

FIGURE 34–3
Changing the patient's position every 2 hours protects the patient's skin

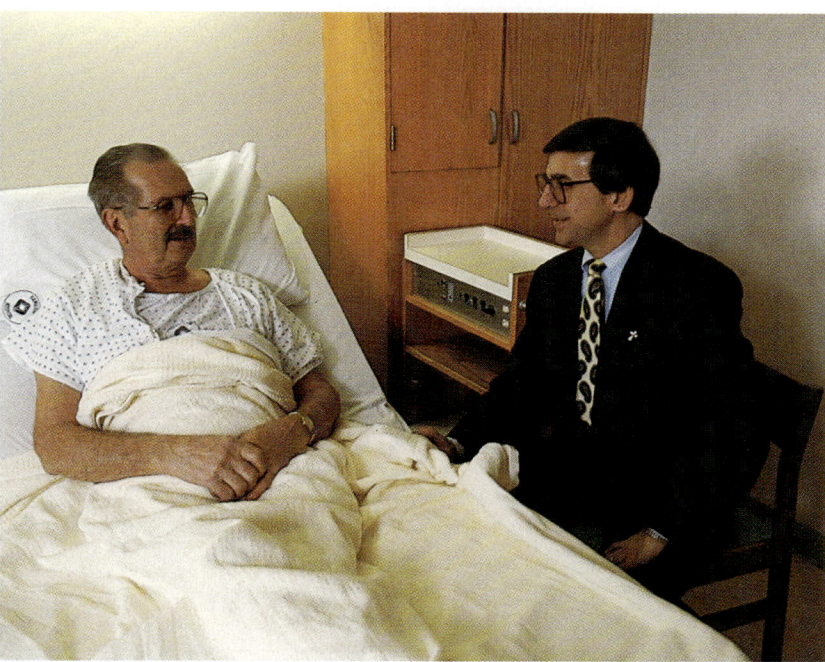

FIGURE 34–4
The dying patient may find spiritual comfort in a visit from the chaplain

SIGNS OF APPROACHING DEATH

Death comes in different ways. It may come quite suddenly. Or it may come after a long period during which there has been a steady decline of body functions. Death also may result from complications during convalescence. Here are some signs showing that death may be near:

- Blood circulation slows down. The patient's hands and feet are cold to the touch. If the patient is conscious, he may complain that he is cold. Keep the patient well covered. If possible adjust the room temperature as needed.

- The patient's face may become pale because of decreased circulation.

- The patient's eyes may be staring blankly into space. There may be no eye movement when you move your hand across her line of vision.

- The patient may perspire heavily, even though his body is cold.

- The patient loses muscle tone and her body becomes limp. The jaw may drop and the mouth may stay partly open. Eyes may not close in sleep.

- Respirations may become slower and more difficult or faster, or there may be brief periods of no breathing. Mucus collecting in the patient's throat and bronchial tubes may cause a sound that is sometimes called the "death rattle."

- The pulse may be rapid or may become weak and irregular.

- Just before death, respirations stop and the pulse gets very faint. You may not be able to feel the patient's pulse at all.

- Contrary to popular belief, a dying person is rarely in great pain. As the patient's condition gets worse, less blood may be flowing to the brain. Therefore, the patient may feel little or no pain.

- The patient may talk to persons who have died.

- The patient's urine output may decrease.

- The patient's swallowing ability may decrease.

- The patient may have periods of confusion and/or agitation.

If you notice any of these signs or any changes in the patient's condition, report them to your supervisor immediately. Sometimes the patient requests, and the physician orders, that no resuscitative measures be taken when the patient's lungs and heart cease to function. This is referred to as *DNR* (Do Not Resuscitate) *status*. Your immediate supervisor will be aware of this and will not initiate resuscitative procedures. Follow your supervisor's instructions.

Refer to Chapter 2 for information regarding living wills and other advance directives, for example the decision to refuse to be fed by artificial means such as a nasogastric or gastric feeding tube.

POSTMORTEM CARE (PMC)

If you observe any signs of approaching death, tell the nurse immediately. The nurse will examine the patient and confirm what you have found. In some health care institutions, a nurse, after confirming that a patient has no pulse or has stopped breathing, calls a "code." This code (Code Blue or some other term) is an emergency announcement to the entire staff. A preassigned team will come to help the patient and use every means available to keep the patient alive. Only when all efforts fail to keep the patient alive is the patient declared to be dead by a physician. In some cases, if it is known in advance that the patient may die, the physician may write a DNR (Do Not Resuscitate) order. In such cases the patient's death is not an emergency, and no code is called.

expired Deceased, dead

postmortem After death

When the patient has **expired**, **postmortem** care is given. The patient's body still must be treated with respect and must be given gentle care. The patient's family will be allowed to view the body again if they wish after you have completed postmortem care. Ask them if they would like to be alone with their loved one or if they would like you or another member of the health care team to stay with them.

Sometimes the family is not present when the patient dies. In this case, either the doctor or the nurse then notifies the family and finds out whether any family members wish to view the patient's body before it is sent to the **morgue**. If so, the body usually stays in the room until the family arrives.

When the family is present, they are given the patient's personal belongings. These items are checked against the admission valuables list to be sure that everything is accounted for. Jewelry remains on the patient unless the family requests its removal. Jewelry left on the body is taped in place and documented on the patient's record. Be specific describing the jewelry. You will learn the procedure in your health care institution for taking care of the deceased patient's clothes and belongings.

Postmortem care should be done before **rigor mortis** sets in. Each institution will have its own specific policies and procedures you must follow. Some general principles will apply in most institutions. For example, you may not remove some types of tubes, bandages, and so on from the body. Check with your immediate supervisor.

morgue A place for temporarily keeping dead bodies for identification, autopsy, retrieval by funeral home staff, and burial

rigor mortis The natural stiffening of a body and limbs shortly after death

PROCEDURE

OBRA

POSTMORTEM CARE

PREPARATION

1. Assemble your equipment:
   a. Soap
   b. Washcloth
   c. Towels
   d. Wash basin with warm water
   e. Bed protectors
   f. Clean gown
2. Wash your hands and put on gloves.

STEPS

3. Turn off oxygen, suction, or IVs at the nurse's or doctor's instructions.
4. Raise the bed to a comfortable working position.
5. Lower the head of the bed so the patient is lying flat with the pillow under the head. This will keep the blood from pooling in the face and neck.
6. Replace dentures if they are not in the patient's mouth.
7. Gently close the eyelids if they are open. If they do not remain closed, notify your supervisor before the family comes to be with the body.
8. If the body is soiled with urine or feces, clean gently to remove odor. Place clean bed protectors under the body.
9. Straighten the body in a dignified position.
10. Cover the body with clean bed linen, but do not cover the head.
11. Straighten the room and remove any emergency equipment.
12. Turn off the bright light over the bed.

FOLLOW-UP

13. Remove gloves and wash your hands.
14. Provide privacy and support for the family's visit.

SUMMARY

Terminally ill patients need psychological and psychosocial support as well as physical care. Being a good listener is the best way to provide psychological support. Recognizing the five stages of dying will help you be even more supportive of your patients, their families, and significant others. The patients may choose hospice care so they can remain at home. The signs of approaching death include changes in circulation, breathing, vital signs, and consciousness. Know which patients have a "do not resuscitate" order. Postmortem care should be given in a caring, respectful manner according to the policy and procedure of your institution.

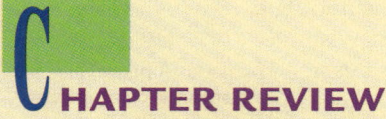

CHAPTER REVIEW

FILL IN THE BLANK

Read each sentence and fill in the blank line with a word that completes the sentence.

1. When a patient is _____ ill, they have an illness that is expected to cause death, usually within a predicted time.

2. When a patient is dying, respect the patient's and family's need for _____ as much as possible.

3. A program that allows a dying patient to remain at home is called _____.

4. Care designed to comfort rather than cure is called _____ care.

5. Rigor mortis is the natural _____ of the body after death.

MULTIPLE CHOICE

Choose the best answer for each question or statement.

1. People have different ideas about death and dying. As a nursing assistant, it is important that you do not impose your ideas on them.
   a. True
   b. False

2. Some common stages of dying are
   a. denial, anger, depression, bargaining, and acceptance.
   b. denial, depression, anger, bargaining, and acceptance.
   c. anger, denial, depression, repression and acceptance.
   d. anger, repression, denial, bargaining and acceptance.

3. Do all of the following for the family of the terminally ill patient except
   a. don't stop your work with the patient just because the family is present.
   b. answer the family's questions if you can.
   c. don't ever interrupt the family with the patient.
   d. let the family spend a lot of time with the patient.

4. All of the following are signs of approaching death except
   a. the hands and feet become cold to the touch.
   b. the patient's face may become pale.
   c. the arms and legs become stiff.
   d. the patient may perspire heavily even though his body is cold.

5. A DNR order is an order that states that emergency care must be given to the patient.
   a. True
   b. False

6. Postmortem care should be completed after rigor mortis sets in.
   a. True
   b. False

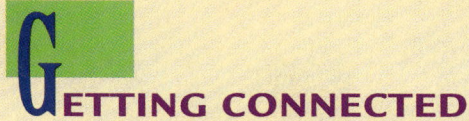

GETTING CONNECTED

MULTIMEDIA EXTENSION ACTIVITIES

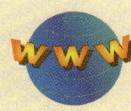

www.prenhall.com/wolgin

Use the above address to access the free, interactive Companion Website created for this textbook. Get hints, instant feedback, and textbook references to chapter-related multiple choice questions. Read and react to the "Nursing Assistants in Action." Link to other interesting sites.

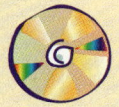

Audio Glossary

Use the CD-ROM disk enclosed with your textbook to hear the pronunciation of the key terms in the chapter.

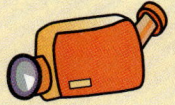

Video

Watch the "Communication" portion of the "Age-Specific Competency" video and the "Patient's Right to Refuse Care" portion of the "Patient's Rights" video from the Care Provider Skills series.

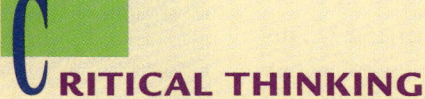

CRITICAL THINKING

USING KEY QUESTIONS

Read each question and think of what you might do in each situation.

1. Your patient, who is dying, is very depressed. Should you try and cheer him up?

2. What can you do to help the family of a patient who is dying?

3. Your patient is dying. What kinds of signs should you watch for?

4. Your patient has a DNR order. What does this mean?

5. Your patient dies. How will you provide postmortem care for your patient?

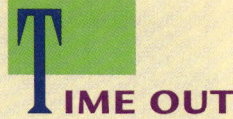

TIME OUT

TIPS FOR TIME MANAGEMENT

SELF-DISCIPLINE TIP   Keep personal phone calls and messages to a minimum while you are at work. Some facilities have policies prohibiting personal calls. Your family should contact you only if an urgent or emergency situation arises. Keep your work time focused on patients and their care.

Beginning Your Career as a Nursing Assistant

35

INTRODUCTION

In this chapter you will learn about the process of competency evaluation for nursing assistant candidates mandated by OBRA, the Omnibus Budget Reconciliation Act of 1987. This act requires nursing assistants employed in long-term care to demonstrate that they are capable of carrying out specific care-related tasks at the minimal level prior to having their name placed on the state's Nurse Aide Registry.

It is anticipated that all areas of health care will require a competency test for all nursing assistants in the future. Many institutions, including acute care hospitals, prefer to hire nursing assistants who have completed an approved training program and are competency tested at the time they apply for employment.

This chapter will also help you identify where to look for employment opportunities and describe the ways you can continue to develop and grow in your career.

OBJECTIVES

When you have completed this chapter, you will be able to:

- List the steps to be taken in completing competency evaluation and testing.

- Describe the function of the state Nurse Aide Registry.

- Select a method of preparing for competency testing.

- Successfully complete a model test.

- Identify job opportunities and be prepared for an interview.

- Write one or two possible career plans using the career options chart provided.

- Describe how your competencies can be assessed in an employment setting.

KEY TERMS

competency

continuing education

evaluation

staff development

PREPARING FOR THE COMPETENCY EVALUATION EXAM

competency A demonstrable skill or ability

evaluation Assessment of one's ability or skill to perform a given task

The Ominbus Budget Reconciliation Act of 1987 made many changes in the care and treatment of people who are cared for in long-term care and nursing facilities. OBRA regulations also require health care facilities to hire nursing assistants who hold certificates or licenses from state-approved training programs and have completed the Nursing Assistant Competency Evaluation as described in this chapter.

The Nursing Assistant **Competency Evaluation** is administered in two parts: a clinical/practical test and a written test. The candidate must successfully complete part one before progressing to the second test.

Candidates for the competency examination must have completed a state-approved training course consisting of a minimum of 75 hours of theory, lab practice, and supervised patient care. Based on written test scores, demonstration of skills learned, and observation of care given to assigned patients/residents during the required 75 hours, the student will be given a certificate or verification, indicating the satisfactory completion of the training course (Figure 35–1). Candidates may then begin the testing process.

Clinical Skills Examination

Usually, the first portion of the testing process is the skills demonstration, *Clinical Skills Examination* (CSE), *Nurse Aide State Examination,* or some similar examination. The CSE is administered in a skills lab or other area where needed supplies are at hand. The test-taker (you), a trained observer, and an actor (if one is used) are the only people present during testing. Any tasks that require the actor to be exposed in any way are performed on a mannequin. The care tasks the test-taker is required to perform are designed to demonstrate competencies you have acquired during training.

Remember this is not the time to ask questions! The observer will observe and document the steps you take in demonstrating your skills. No advice or prompting may be given during testing. Usually, the observer will not be able to tell you whether or not you have "passed." The test-scoring of the *Clinical Skills Examination* is done by an independent agency. Some national testing services, for example Vermont, have same day scoring and reporting.

FIGURE 35–1

Certificate received upon completion of Patient Care Assistant program

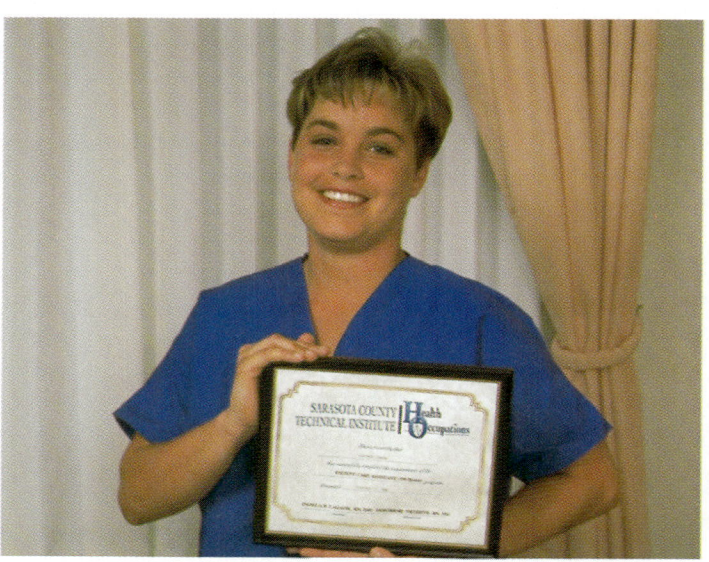

The actor may be a patient/resident or an employee of the facility where the test is being administered or someone else known to the test taker. The actor may NOT be anyone under the age of 18, unable to give informed consent or another nursing assistant student who has not yet taken the test. Do not bring an actor to the test site unless your instructor tells you to do so. The actor must remain impartial, giving no assistance or clues to the test taker.

Some of the tasks you may be asked to demonstrate are:

- Making an occupied or unoccupied bed
- Measuring and recording temperature, pulse, and respiration
- Toileting
- Transfer and positioning
- Applying a safety device
- Personal care and grooming tasks
  - Hair and nail care
  - Denture care and oral care
- Feeding or assisting with a meal
- Dressing
- Measuring and recording height and weight
- Giving a bed bath

Your training course provided you with demonstrations of these care skills and an opportunity to practice and demonstrate the skills yourself. It will help you to review the steps of each procedure in your textbook prior to taking the *Clinical Skills Examination/Skills Demonstration Examination.* In some states, the skills and written exams may be given at the same time, for example, the ASI test for long-term care facility competency evaluation program.

Written/Oral Examination

As previously mentioned, this part of the testing process takes place after you have successfully taken the *Clinical Skills Examination.* The written examination is also given in oral form in certain circumstances. Your instructor will provide you with information about the oral form of the test if necessary. The written test is administered by a national testing service, for example, the American Red Cross in some areas and by the State Board of Nursing in others. Your instructor will have specific information on how to register for the examination.

The test consists of 50 or more multiple choice questions. A sample test is provided following the section on Test Fees. These questions test your knowledge of care tasks and procedures you have learned as well as concepts like infection control, safety, ethics, and communicating with others. You may find it helpful to study with classmates in small groups, or have someone quiz you on topics in your textbook. Regardless of how you prepare for the written examination remember to review the medical terms and abbreviations included in the training course—many of them are included in the multiple choice test questions.

Some important terms to know:

abuse	elimination	Standard Precautions
ADL	ethics	therapeutic
ambulate	infection	transfer
body mechanics	isolation	void
dignity	privacy	
edema	pulse	

Test Fees and Time Requirements

Fees for the Clinical Skills/Skills Demonstration examination and the Written/Oral examination vary from state to state. Your instructor can advise you of the fee requirements in your area. Payment must be made by money order or cashier's check; no cash or personal checks are accepted. Test fees must be paid upon registration or at the time you take each test.

Both the Clinical Skills examination and the Written/Oral examination are given by appointment. It is important that you keep your appointments and arrive on time, and be prepared to take the examination. Upon completing your training course, you have a specified amount of time called a "window of opportunity" within which you must complete the testing process and register with the Nurse Aide Registry. Candidates who go past this "window" may be required to re-take the training course before being tested. Your instructor will provide you with information in your area.

When you have passed both portions of the competency examination your title will be Certified Nursing Assistant (CNA) or CENA. CENA stands for Competency Evaluated Nursing Assistant. You will be able to care for patients/residents at the basic level, providing personal care within your training (Figure 35–2). Some home health agencies will require you to "re-certify" within their organization by building on the skills you have learned to be able to provide care, usually without direct supervision in the home. The home health agency may require you to take a separate skills examination prior to working with patients in the home.

Nurse Aide Registry

All states are required to maintain a Nurse Aide Registry. After successfully completing the Nursing Assistant Competency Evaluation, your name may be placed on the Nurse Aide Registry. Employers can contact the agency to verify if you or anyone else they are considering for employment is properly certified/listed.

If a nursing assistant is involved in a situation involving the theft of a patient's property or suspected patient abuse, the employer reports this to the registry. The registry document of a nursing assistant who is convicted of misconduct is "flagged," and the individual is not permitted to work as a nursing assistant. Certain information is considered confidential and therefore is not given to prospective employers. However, the "flag" indicates that there is proof that a serious incident has occurred.

FIGURE 35–2

CNA receiving team player of the month award

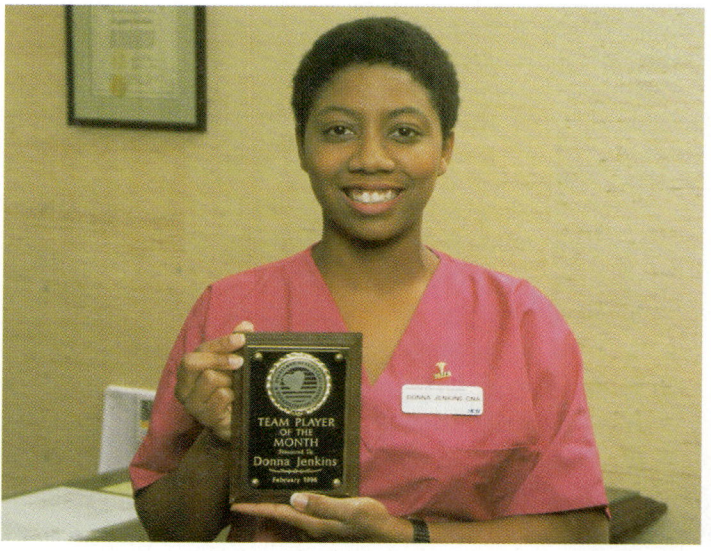

Some states have recently begun to require that registry documents be renewed every one to two years. A renewal form is mailed to your home and you will be instructed to complete a section indicating any changes such as your name, address, or telephone number. Your current or most recent health care employer may need to complete a section indicating that you meet the requirements for renewal.

Sample Test

This sample test contains questions similar to those that appear on the Nurse Assistant Competency test. Read carefully each question and all the possible answers before choosing the *one* correct answer.

1. Cyanosis means
   a. a bluish color to the skin.
   b. difficulty breathing.
   c. a colorless, odorless gas.
   d. abnormally high blood pressure.

2. Body temperature can be increased by
   a. dehydration.
   b. cold environment.
   c. medications.
   d. shock.

3. The first step in any procedure is to
   a. gather your supplies.
   b. wash your hands.
   c. explain what you will do.
   d. lower the side rail.

4. When moving and lifting a patient, the nurse assistant should
   a. plan all moves.
   b. be alert to safety.
   c. let the patient help if possible.
   d. All of the above.

5. The best definition of the word "emergency" is
   a. an unusual event or occurrence.
   b. a source of potential danger.
   c. an event that calls for immediate action.
   d. None of the above.

6. Pathogens can be destroyed by
   a. sterilization.
   b. handwashing.
   c. disinfection.
   d. careful handling.

7. You can maintain your own good health by
   a. getting enough rest and sleep.
   b. eating properly.
   c. washing your hands frequently.
   d. All of the above.

8. Select the example of a barrier to conversation.

   a. Speaking slowly and clearly.

   b. Avoiding eye contact.

   c. Identifying yourself.

   d. Calling the patient by name.

9. Elderly persons do not need a complete bath or shower every day because

   a. they might become chilled.

   b. their skin has less oil and is drier.

   c. they are too tired.

   d. None of the above.

10. You find a small blister on the buttock of your patient; your first action should be to

   a. apply a hot compress.

   b. report it to the nurse.

   c. massage the area.

   d. apply a bandage.

11. The brachial pulse is found

   a. inside the elbow.

   b. on the top of the foot.

   c. inside the wrist.

   d. behind the knee.

12. In caring for a hearing aid you should

   a. rinse with water daily.

   b. never remove it from the ear.

   c. avoid dropping it.

   d. keep the volume on high.

13. Your first action in case of a fire is to

   a. learn to use the fire extinguisher.

   b. rescue the patient.

   c. call for help.

   d. pull the fire alarm.

14. Which statement is true about physical restraints?

   a. They do not require a doctor's order.

   b. They must be removed every half hour.

   c. They can cause injury to a patient.

   d. They can be left on for up to four hours at a time.

15. The longest and strongest muscles in your body are

   a. in your buttocks.

   b. in your back.

   c. in your abdomen.

   d. in your thighs.

16. The proper positioning of a patient's body is called
   a. body mechanics.   c. body alignment.
   b. range of motion.   d. positioning.

17. Pressure ulcers are
   a. also called bedsores.
   b. always infected.
   c. prevented by frequent baths.
   d. only found in elderly people.

18. The term "ad lib" means
   a. immediately.   c. only once.
   b. as desired.   d. as necessary.

19. Miss Taylor's orders state "May have juice ac and hs"; You would give the juice
   a. morning and evening.   c. whenever she asked for it.
   b. before meals and at bedtime.   d. twice a day.

20. You find a resident who has fallen on the floor; your first action is to
   a. assist the resident to a chair.   c. find someone to help lift her.
   b. call for help.   d. call the doctor.

21. Another word for high blood pressure is
   a. hypotension.   c. hypertension.
   b. hypothyroid.   d. systolic pressure.

22. Elderly people may eat less because
   a. they have poorly fitting dentures.
   b. their sense of smell is decreased.
   c. they may be depressed.
   d. All of the above.

23. An example of an objective statement would be
   a. "Mr. Smith has a fever."
   b. "Miss Godfrey is in a bad mood."
   c. "Mr. Smith's temperature is 101."
   d. "Mrs. Davis is tired."

24. An example of meeting patients spiritual needs is
   a. taking them to church with you.
   b. providing privacy when their clergyman visits.
   c. talking to them about your religion.
   d. telling them their beliefs are old fashioned.

25. What equipment would you expect to find in a nursing home resident's unit?
   a. A bed, overbed table, and nightstand.
   b. A blood pressure cuff, oxygen tank, and sink.
   c. A clock, calendar, and bulletin board.
   d. A stretcher, bed, and mechanical lift.

■ Answer Key

1. a	6. a	11. a	16. c	21. c
2. a	7. d	12. c	17. a	22. d
3. b	8. b	13. b	18. b	23. c
4. d	9. b	14. c	19. b	24. b
5. c	10. b	15. d	20. b	25. a

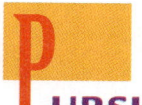

PURSUING EMPLOYMENT OPPORTUNITIES

Almost everyone has had the experience of pursuing employment opportunities once and perhaps several times during her lifetime. Some things are the same whether the person, a nursing assistant for example, is looking for that first job after course completion/certification, returning to work after several years' absence from the workplace, or looking for a position in another facility. Let's consider the situation of the nursing assistant looking for that first job after course completion/certification.

■ Where to Look for Jobs

Successful completion of your Patient Care Attendant (PCA)/Nursing Assistant (NA) training may be part of your orientation and career development. If not, you will need to find employment. There are several places to look, and it is best to try as many as possible. Here are some places to start your search for employment.

- Personal contacts:
  - Educational and professional contacts
  - Family and friends
- Want ads/Classifieds
- Employment agencies
- Local hospitals, nursing homes, other health care facilities; many post vacant positions on their Websites

Personal Contacts

Your instructor is an excellent place to start. Sometimes employers who have openings will contact training programs to alert the faculty and students that they are seeking applicants or have current open positions. Your instructor can tell you if there is a place where these requests are posted. You can also talk to your instructor about her willingness to provide a reference for you.

Family and friends are probably your best advocates since they know you personally and are aware that you have been preparing for a career in health care. Broadcast the fact that you will soon be available to work as a patient care attendant/nursing assistant. Let everyone you know, even casual acquaintances from your church, community group, or a day care center, that you are looking for employment. Leads may come from any of these sources. Be sure to thank anyone who helps you and let him know if you are interviewed or offered a position.

Want Ads/Classifieds

The Sunday papers are a good resource to check regularly. Many of the positions will be listed under health care or nursing. Some states have monthly publications with many health care positions or the names, addresses, and phone numbers of recruiters.

Employment Agencies

Most cities or towns have employment agencies or specialty placement agencies that routinely look for health care workers. These agencies may also hire and staff temporary placements or agency employees in positions. Most agencies prefer to hire people with experience. If there is a high demand for nursing assistants, you may be considered with little experience.

Local Hospitals/Nursing Homes/Facilities

Call the recruiters or personnel/human resources offices at local facilities and ask if they have or are expecting any openings for nursing assistants. Request an application be sent to you or ask when you may go to the office to complete an application. Be sure to ask directions if you are going to an unfamiliar place.

■Application Process

If you have not seen a health care facility application, refer to Figure 35–3. It is representative of many institutions' applications for employment. Once you have the application in hand, read it carefully and fill in the requested information. Most applications ask fairly common questions and request similar information. It is best to type or print the information on the application. Follow the instructions and complete the application as fully and accurately as you can. Return it in person or by mail as directed.

■Preparing a Résumé

Prepare a simple one-page résumé giving your name, address, and phone number; your objective, education, and previous jobs, especially those where you used people skills and had to work with others. It is best to type the résumé or have someone type it for you. The information should be presented as follows:

Name:

Address:

Phone:

Objective: To obtain a nursing assistant or patient care assistant position in a health care setting.

Education:

High school:

Training program:

Work experience:

References: Available upon request/or list one or two people who have supervised you, for example your instructor. Be sure to ask permission to use a person as a reference in advance of offering the person's name.

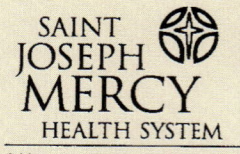

APPLICATION FOR EMPLOYMENT

SAINT JOSEPH MERCY HEALTH SYSTEM
A Member of Mercy Health Services

Please indicate Unit desired:
❏ St. Joseph Mercy Hospital, Ann Arbor
❏ McPherson Hospital, Howell
❏ Saline Community Hospital, Saline
❏ Other _____
please specify

We are an equal opportunity employer. Qualified applicants are considered for employment without regard to race, color, religion, sex, height, weight, national origin, age, marital or veteran status, or the presence of a non-job-related medical condition or disability. It is the applicant's responsibility to notify Saint Joseph Mercy Health System of any reasonable accommodation necessary to perform the essential duties of the position for which the applicant has applied.

Important - Please Type or Print Clearly in Ink

PERSONAL DATA

Date _____

Social Security Number _____

Last Name _____ First _____ Middle _____

Address _____ City _____ State _____ Zip Code _____

Home Telephone ( ) _____

Work or Alternate Telephone ( ) _____

Are you age 18 or older? ❏ Yes ❏ No

Are you currently authorized to work in the U.S.? ❏ Yes ❏ No

Have you ever been convicted of a crime other than a minor traffic violation? ❏ Yes ❏ No

If yes, give circumstances, place, and date: _____

Have you ever been employed at a Saint Joseph Mercy Health System Unit? ❏ Yes ❏ No

If yes, give date(s) and location(s): _____

Do you have any relative(s) working at Saint Joseph Mercy Health System? ❏ Yes ❏ No

List Name(s)/Relationship/Unit/Department _____

Have you ever been employed by Mercy Health Services? ❏ Yes ❏ No

If yes, give date(s) and location(s): _____

Have you ever worked or attended school under another name? ❏ Yes ❏ No

If yes, what name(s): _____

JOB INTEREST

Position Desired: _____

Department or Clinical Area Preferred (if applicable) _____

Indicate your availability to work (check all that apply) ❏ Full-time ❏ Part-time ❏ Contingent ❏ Temporary
❏ Days ❏ Afternoons ❏ Midnights ❏ Weekends ❏ Holidays ❏ Shift Rotations

If Part-time, specify days and hours available: _____

Earliest Date Available _____ Minimum Pay Required $ _____ Per Hour

How did you hear of this position? ❏ Newspaper/Journal* ❏ School* ❏ Recruitment visit/job fair*

❏ Employee ❏ Relative ❏ Friend ❏ Other*

*Please Specify _____

Are you currently employed? ❏ Yes ❏ No
May we contact your present employer? ❏ Yes ❏ No
01030R 8/97 (PC)D

*Contact must be made before an employment offer is finalized

FIGURE 35-3

Application for Employment (Courtesy of Saint Joseph Mercy Health System, Ann Arbor, MI)

EDUCATION AND TRAINING

	Date Started	Date Finished	School Name and Location	Major	Graduated	Degree/ Diploma	GPA
High School	████████				☐ Yes ☐ No Yrs. Completed _____		
College/ University					☐ Yes ☐ No Yrs. Completed _____		
College/ University					☐ Yes ☐ No Yrs. Completed _____		
Technical/ Vocational					☐ Yes ☐ No Yrs. Completed _____		
Other					☐ Yes ☐ No Yrs. Completed _____		

	Date Started	Date Finished	Name of Facility	Type of Clinical
Student Clinical Rotations, Internship Programs				

Describe work related skills, qualifications, achievements and contributions that you would bring to Saint Joseph Mercy Health System: _____

_____

_____

PROFESSIONAL CERTIFICATION REGISTRATION DATA

What profession(s) are you licensed, certified or registered to practice? _____

_____

By examination in: State _____ Number _____ Expiration date _____

By endorsement in (reciprocity): State _____ Number _____ Expiration date _____

Are there restrictions on your license? ☐ Yes ☐ No If yes, please explain: _____

Are you eligible for licensure, certification or registry? ☐ Yes ☐ No

Profession _____ Anticipated Date of Exam _____

List any current memberships in professional or technical associations. (Those which indicate race, color, religion, sex, or national origin may be excluded.)

_____

_____

_____

_____

_____

FIGURE 35–3 *(continued)*

Application for Employment

EMPLOYMENT HISTORY

Beginning with your CURRENT or most RECENT employer, list the last four positions held including Military Service in date order. (Should you choose to list volunteer activities, those which indicate race, color, religion, sex, national origin may be excluded.)

Name of Employer			Position Held	From (Month/Year) To (Month/Year)
Address			Name and Title of Supervisor	Hours Per Week
City	State	Zip	Telephone # ( )	Base Hourly Rate/Salary
Type of Business			Reason for Leaving	
Duties				

Name of Employer			Position Held	From (Month/Year) To (Month/Year)
Address			Name and Title of Supervisor	Hours Per Week
City	State	Zip	Telephone # ( )	Base Hourly Rate/Salary
Type of Business			Reason for Leaving	
Duties				

Name of Employer			Position Held	From (Month/Year) To (Month/Year)
Address			Name and Title of Supervisor	Hours Per Week
City	State	Zip	Telephone # ( )	Base Hourly Rate/Salary
Type of Business			Reason for Leaving	
Duties				

Name of Employer			Position Held	From (Month/Year) To (Month/Year)
Address			Name and Title of Supervisor	Hours Per Week
City	State	Zip	Telephone # ( )	Base Hourly Rate/Salary
Type of Business			Reason for Leaving	
Duties				

Please Read The Following Carefully And Sign Where Indicated Below:

I have read all the questions and answers, and certify that the information given by me in this application is correct to the best of my knowledge. I understand that any false statements or answers or omissions may be grounds for dismissal. I further understand that my employment is contingent upon the satisfactory completion of a physical examination, including a drug screen, to be conducted by Saint Joseph Mercy Health System. I specifically authorize Saint Joseph Mercy Health System and Mercy Health Services to release all records or other information pertaining to any disciplinary action taken against me during my employment. I hereby release Saint Joseph Mercy Health System and Mercy Health Services, and their agents and employees from any liability whatsoever resulting from the release of such records or information. I hereby waive my right to written notice from my present and/or former employers whenever a disciplinary report, letter or reprimand, or other disciplinary action regarding me is divulged by my present or former employers, including but not limited to reports of disciplinary action which by law must be disclosed pursuant to M.C.L. 333.20175(5).

Signature of Applicant _____ Date _____

FIGURE 35–3 (continued)

Application for Employment

TO BE COMPLETED BY HIRING DEPARTMENT

Position Title	Base Hourly Rate of Pay
Department Name	Position Code Pay Grade
Department/Cost Center Number	Hours/pay period

Employment Status
❒ New Hire   ❒ Rehire
Starting Date and Time _____

❒ Full-time   ❒ Non-Exempt   ❒ Hourly
❒ Part-time   ❒ Exempt   ❒ Salaried I
❒ Contingent   ❒ Salaried II
❒ Term   Expires ___/___/___
❒ Temporary   Expires ___/___/___

Shift Hours

_____ AM / PM   to   _____ AM / PM Days

_____ AM / PM   to   _____ AM / PM Afternoons

_____ AM / PM   to   _____ AM / PM Midnights

(Work hours and/or work days may change according to department needs.)

Special Conditions of Employment, If Any

(Weekends, holidays, shift rotation, etc.)

❒ Offer reviewed by Human Resources _____ (Specialist initials)

Authorized Management Signature _____ Date _____

I accept the above offer and in consideration of my employment I agree to conform to the rules, regulations and policies of Saint Joseph Mercy Health System. I understand the first 180 days of employment are designated as an orientation period.

New Employee Signature _____ Date _____

FIGURE 35–3 *(continued)*

Application for Employment

The Job Interview

If possible request a copy of the job description and review it before your interview. When you have an interview scheduled, check to be sure you know where to go and plan to arrive early. Write down the name and phone number of the person who will interview you, in case you get lost or need assistance finding the office when you arrive at the facility.

There is only one chance to make a good first impression. Dress conservatively in a suit or dress, if possible. Look as businesslike as you can. It is best to not wear jeans and casual clothes. Ask to see a job description if one has not already been provided. Discuss the duties listed, asking for clarification when necessary. Make notes on the job description, if appropriate.

If you have had very little experience, it is important to be as flexible as possible regarding what hours and days you are available to work. Health care systems need employees who are available to work on weekends, holidays, and over a 24-hour period. Usually, the open positions will be on the less desirable or rotating shifts. Experienced workers transfer to openings or positions that are more desirable or choose schedules with hours that are better suited to their life styles and personal needs.

After your interview, smile and shake the hand of the interviewer (Figure 35–4). Thank the person for the opportunity to interview for the position and in particular for the time the interviewer took to answer your questions and provide details and explanations you requested. If the person interviewing you would not be your supervisor, ask to meet that individual. Such meetings or interviews with possible supervisors are often part of the interview process in some institutions; other organizations plan such a meeting at the time of the second interview.

You may be told to call if you have questions, or in rare cases offered a position at the time of the interview. On the spot hiring is infrequent since there are usually several applicants for each position and employers require time to check references. You will probably be told that someone, possibly the interviewer, will get back to you. Ask for a time frame, for example 5–10 days or 2–3 weeks, within which you can expect to hear whether you will be offered the job.

Job Offer

The job offer may come in the form of a phone call or letter. It is best to get an offer in writing to be sure there are no misunderstandings about salary, hours or shifts you are to work, and the date you start. If the job offer is verbal or if the letter does not include these details, request that a letter covering these items be sent to you. Preferably, you

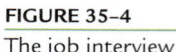

FIGURE 35–4

The job interview

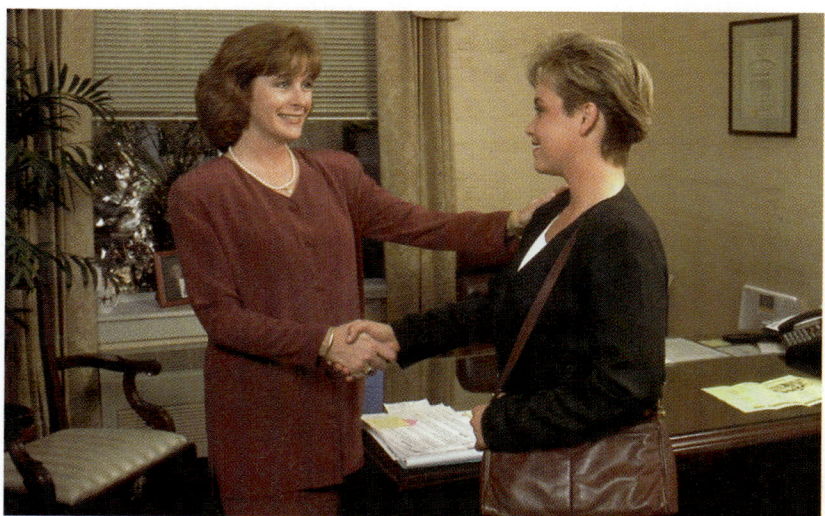

should accept the offer in writing. In some situations, a verbal acceptance is acceptable. The advantage of a written acceptance is that it provides you the opportunity of expressing your pleasure at receiving the job offer and restating the circumstances—salary, hours or shift you will work, and the date you are to start—of your acceptance as you understand it. This clarifies the issue for both you and the facility (personnel representative) hiring you. Some organizations do not require a written acceptance prior to hire.

◼ Orientation

When you begin work in a facility, move to a new position within your department, or take a position in another department, there is some form of orientation. *Orientation* refers to the period of time in which your employer orients or familiarizes you with your work environment, your benefits, organizational or facility policies, work rules, and your role and responsibilities in your new job. Usually, your immediate supervisor will discuss specific job expectations with you. Classroom or one-to-one sessions or a combination of both may be given by a staff development educator or trainer.

Most employers have a probationary period during which specific skills and competencies required for patient care in your setting are validated. Classroom and/or on the job performance during this probationary period are evaluated. Once you have successfully demonstrated your skills and competence to perform your job duties, you will have completed your orientation. During this period of orientation, ask questions and learn as much as you can about your role and responsibilities. Often someone is assigned to help you as you learn about and put into actual practice the policies and procedures in your new employment setting.

◼ Continuing to Learn

Continue your education! To keep up with new developments, all health care workers are expected to take refresher courses. As you continue to learn, your job will become more rewarding personally and professionally. Many agencies have a staff development or training person, group, or department. Services or training include orientation, inservice education, and ongoing **staff development**. Examples of inservice education include:

- learning a new procedure or technique

- learning to use new equipment

- learning about a change in a particular procedure that requires staff to do a task differently

- training in doing a new procedure

Every year there are required mandatory training classes in fire, safety, CPR, infection control, patients' rights, and confidentiality. There are some state to state variations in mandatory requirements.

Other examples of ongoing staff development training:

- communication

- computer training

- cultural diversity awareness

- domestic violence

- sensitivity training

The staff development specialist or human resources representative can tell you about other educational benefits or refer you to available training programs or other **continuing education** options. It is important that you share your career goals with those people in

staff development On the job training or classes provided to enhance or expand an employee's skills or abilities

continuing education Formal classes, courses, or training programs to develop new knowledge or qualify one for career advancement

your facility who can help you identify resources, support, and programs. Your supervisor may also offer you advice.

You can continue to learn while you are on the job. You can expand your knowledge of nursing care procedures, find better ways to do your work, and learn more about other aspects of health care. All this can make you a more effective nursing assistant, and you will become more secure in your job.

Planning Your Career Path

Figure 35–5 presents numerous career opportunities for the nursing assistant to consider in planning a career path. Some people know at an early age exactly what position or level they want to attain in the health care field. For others the path is not so clear. Take every opportunity to speak to friends, family, and coworkers in the health care field. Discuss the options and possibilities with education and career counselors at school or in the institution where you work. The opportunities are numerous.

If you enjoy your work as a nursing assistant, you may be interested in advancement where you are employed. Maybe you would like to be a multiskilled worker, advanced nursing assistant, or licensed practical (vocational) or registered nurse (Figure 35–6). The career path shown here can guide you in planning your advancement. You can modify your career path to meet your long-term and short-term *goals* or to address changing needs and new opportunities. Skills, time, hard work, and planning are needed to advance to the work and educational level you set for yourself. When you reach your work and educational goals, you may choose to set new goals requiring more education or training to further develop your skills and improve your nursing techniques, or you may choose to remain indefinitely at the level you have just reached.

If you do not have a high school diploma, attaining one should be your first goal. Adult education programs at local high schools offer basic education programs that lead to a high school equivalency diploma. Community colleges offer prerequisite courses necessary to enroll in licensed practical nurse or registered nurse programs. Education or

FIGURE 35–5

Health care options to consider as you chart your career path

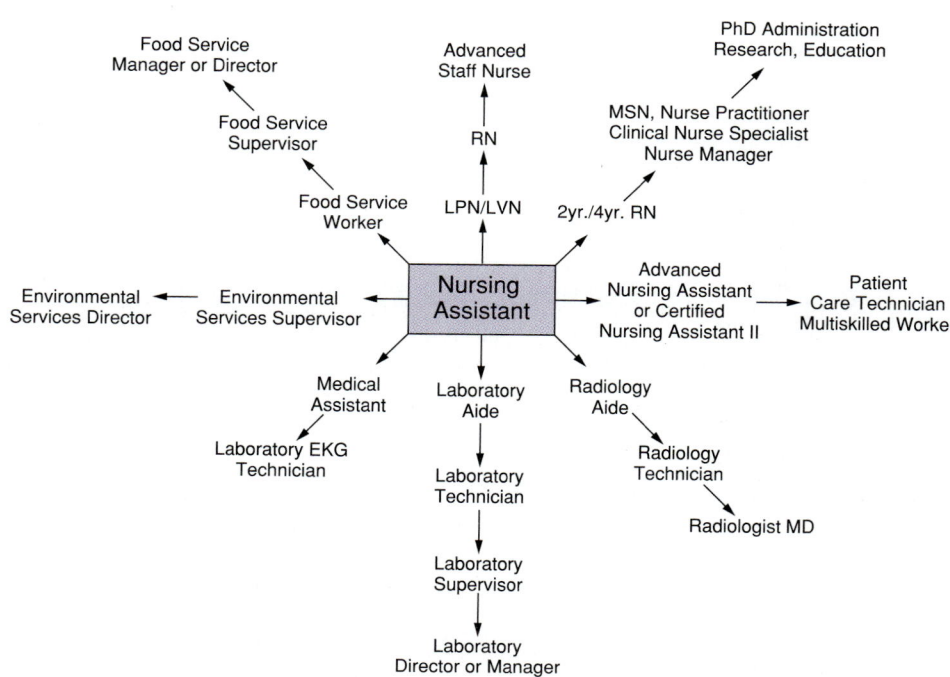

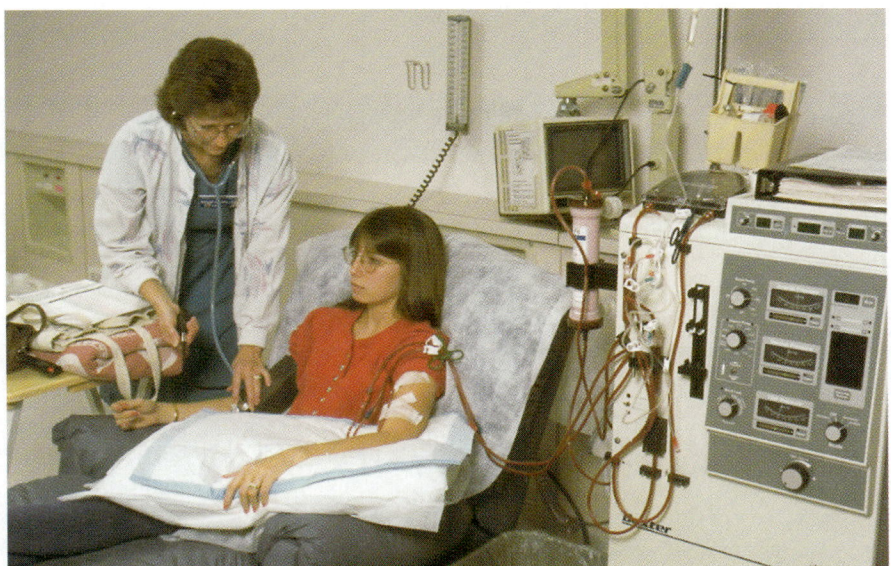

FIGURE 35–6
Work with a patient receiving kidney dialysis

career counselors are available at community colleges to advise you along the way. Take advantage of such resources.

The director of nursing education in your health care institution is the person to ask about planning your career path. You can find career satisfaction in your role as a nursing assistant or choose to continue your education and prepare yourself for an ever increasing number of health care career possibilities.

POSITIONING YOURSELF FOR PROMOTION

Changing Jobs

Gaining experience working as a nursing assistant will open many opportunities to you. Once you have demonstrated good work habits and have received positive evaluations from your employer, you will find there are many employers in a variety of work settings seeking to hire individuals into open positions. In many cases, better pay, improved benefits, closer proximity to your home, or more desirable hours motivate job searches.

There may be career opportunities within your place of initial employment. Some larger facilities have internal training and development staff who provide training to become advanced nursing assistants or patient care technicians. Entry into these programs requires a willingness to learn, the same good work habits and satisfactory attendance and no disciplinary actions in your record or file.

Many local community colleges offer courses or training programs that can lead to career advancement. Some employers have arrangements to pay or reimburse your tuition costs for attending programs. Your manager, staff development or human resource personnel usually know if such programs with tuition assistance are available. Colleges may be able to identify opportunities or programs where full or partial scholarships are available. If your supervisor is aware that you are interested in continuing your education, they are more likely to inform you of advanced training programs or other opportunities.

Keeping A Job

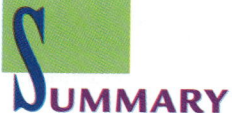

GUIDELINES

KEEPING A JOB

- Maintain at least a satisfactory or good work record.
- When you can, volunteer to work overtime or fill staffing needs.
- Problem solve using your best communication skills and the formal process within your work place.
- Be sure to call your employer when you are sick or unable to get to work for any reason.

- Recognize that most employers do not view accumulated "sick time" as an earned right for employees to use whenever needed for personal convenience. It is better to request time off in advance or trade with coworkers than to call in whenever your scheduled time to work conflicts with your personal life.

- Do not drink alcohol before work or come to work high. It is usually grounds for discipline or can be automatic dismissal. If you have a problem with substance abuse, seek help.

- Seek opportunities to learn new skills and keep up with the constant changes in health care.

- Ask for feedback from coworkers and your supervisor as to your performance and listen to suggestions or recommendations for improvement.

- Request and keep a copy of work rules. Ask questions about any rules or policies you do not understand. Many employers view stealing, lying on an application, and violating confidentiality of or abusing patients as automatic grounds for dismissal. Policies are usually reviewed in orientation but many employees forget them until there is a big problem.

Resignation Letters

Once you have a new job offer in writing or need to leave your job for any reason, it is best to give your current employer at least 2 weeks notice. Leaving a position with little or no notice is reflected in your employment records and can make getting a positive reference a problem. It is best to be as positive as possible in your resignation letter and briefly state the reason you are leaving, for another job, relocation or personal or family reasons.

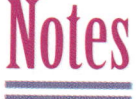

Summary

This chapter has presented information to help prepare you to take your competency evaluation and test to become a nursing assistant. It described how you can find and apply for job opportunities. The importance of continuing education was also discussed, along with career path or lattice possibilities. As you become involved in your career there will be increasing opportunities to learn and grow.

Notes

Lying on an Application

You are applying for a new job and need to fill out the application. On the form there is a question asking why you left your last job. While you performed well in your role while you were at work, there were several times that you called off or were late. Your previous employer dismissed you for attendance problems. Now you really need to get a new job.

What Is Your Response/Action

1. Explain why each of the following actions would be appropriate or inappropriate when filling out the job application:

   a. Be honest and explain that you were dismissed.

   b. Leave the section blank on the form and only discuss it if the interviewer asks.

   c. Make up a reason for leaving your last job.

   d. Do not list your last job; instead say that you have not been working this year.

   e. Explain that you were dismissed because of attendance problems, but they were not your fault; it was because of family illness, child-care problems, deaths of friends, bad weather, and lack of transportation.

2. What is your liability if your new employer finds out after hiring you that you were dismissed and did not say so?

3. If you are unsure what to do, who can you ask for advice?

Abbreviations Used in Charting, Reporting, and Keeping Notes

ABBREVIATION	MEANING
aa	Of each, equal parts
abd.	Abdomen
ac	Before meals
AD	Admitting diagnosis
A&D	Admission and discharge
ad lib	As desired, if the patient so desires
ADL	Activities of daily living
AIDS	Acquired Immune Deficiency Syndrome
AKA	Above Knee Amputation/Also Known As
A.M. or a.m., AM or am	Morning
amb.	Ambulation, walking, ambulatory, able to walk
amt.	Amount
AP or A.P.	Appendectomy
aqua	Water or H_2O
@	At
Approx.	Approximately
ASAP	As soon as possible
ATC	Around the Clock
bid or B.I.D. or b.i.d.	Twice a day
b.m. or B.M.	Bowel movement, feces
B.P. or BP	Blood pressure
BRP or B.R.P. or brp	Bathroom privileges
BR or br or B.R. or b.r.	Bedrest
BSC or bsc	Bedside commode
°C	Celsius degree (or centigrade)
c̄	With
Ca or CA	Cancer
Cal	Calorie
Cath.	Catheter
CBC or C.B.C.	Complete blood count
CBR or C.B.R. or cbr	Complete bed rest
cc or c.c.	Cubic centimeter
CCU or C.C.U.	Cardiac care unit/coronary care unit
Chol	Cholesterol
Cl liq	Clear liquids
CM or cm	Centimeter
C/O or c/o	Complaint of
CO_2	Carbon dioxide
CPR or C.P.R.	Cardiopulmonary resuscitation
CSR or csr and C.S.R.	Central supply room
CVA or C.V.A.	Cerebrovascular accident or stroke
DBP	Diastolic Blood Pressure
dc or d/c or D/C	Discontinue
D&I	Dry and intact
Disch. or dish or D/C	Discharge
D. & C. or D&C	Dilatation and curettage
DM	Diabetes Mellitus
DOA or D.O.A.	Dead on arrival
Dr. or Dr	Doctor
DRG	Diagnostic related group
drsg.	Dressing
DX	Diagnosis
E. or E	Enema
EBL	Estimated blood loss

ABBREVIATION	MEANING
ECG or EKG	Electrocardiogram
ED or E.D.	Emergency department
EEG or E.E.G.	Electroencephalogram
EENT or E.E.N.T.	Eye, ears, nose, and throat
ER or E.R.	Emergency room
ETOH	Alcohol
°F	Fahrenheit degree
F. or Fe. or F or Fe	Female
FBS or F. B. S.	Fasting blood sugar
FF or F.F.	Forced feeding or forced fluids
ft	Foot
Fx	Fracture
Fx urine	Fractional urine
gal	Gallon
GI or G.I.	Gastrointestinal
gt	One drop
gtt	Two or more drops
Gtt or G.T.T.	Glucose tolerance test
GU or G.U.	Genitourinary
Gyn or G.Y.N.	Gynecology
H/A	Headache
H_2O	Water or aqua
HMO	Health Maintenance Organization
HOB	Head of bed
HOH	Hard of Hearing
H & P	History and Physical
hr	Hour
HS or hs	Bedtime or hour of sleep
ht	Height
HTN	Hypertension
hyper	Above or high
hypo	Below or low
ICU or I.C.U.	Intensive care unit
I&O or I.&.O.	Intake and output
Irr	Irregular
Isol. or isol	Isolation
IV or I.V.	Intravenous
L	Liter
Ⓛ	Left
Lab. or lab	Laboratory
lb	Pound
Liq or liq.	Liquid
LPN or L.P.N.	Licensed practical nurse
LVN or L.V.N.	Licensed vocational nurse
M	Male
Mat	Maternity
MD or M.D.	Medical doctor
Meas	Measure
med	Medicine
MI	Myocardial Infarction
min	Minute
ml	Milliliter
Mn or mn or M/n	Midnight
N.A. or N/A	Nursing aide or nursing assistant
NAS	No added salt
N & V	Nausea and Vomiting

ABBREVIATION	MEANING
NKA	No known allergies
n/g tube or ng. tube or N.G.T.	Nasogastric tube
noct	At night
NP	Neuropsychiatric; or nursing procedure
NPO or N.P.O.	Nothing by mouth
nsy	Nursery
O₂	Oxygen
OB or O.B.	Obstetrics
Obt or obt.	Obtained
OJ or O.J.	Orange juice
Ord.	Orderly
OOB or O.O.B.	Out of bed
OPD or O.P.D.	Outpatient department
OR or O.R.	Operating room
Ortho	Orthopedics
OT or O.T.	Occupational therapy; or oral temperature
oz	Ounce
pc	After meals
Ped or Peds	Pediatrics
per	By, through
p.m. or P.M., pm or PM	Afternoon
PMC or P.M.C.	Postmortem care
PN or P.N.	Pneumonia
po	By mouth
post or p̄	After
postop or post op	Postoperative
PP	Postpartum (after delivery)
PPBS	Postprandial blood sugar
pre	Before
preop or pre op	Before surgery
prep	Prepare the patient for surgery by shaving the skin
prn or p.r.n.	Whenever necessary, when required
Pt or pt	Patient; pint
PT or P.T.	Physical therapy
q	Every
qam or q am or q.a.m.	Every morning
qd	Every day
qh	Every hour
q2h	Every 2 hours
q3h	Every 3 hours
q4h	Every 4 hours
QHS or qhs	Every night at bedtime/hour of sleep
QI	Quality Improvement
qid or Q.I.D.	Four times a day
qod or Q.O.D.	Every other day
qs	Quantity sufficient; as much as required
qt	Quart
r or R	rectal or Rectal
Ⓡ	Right
Reg	Regular
Rm or rm	Room
RN or R.N.	Registered nurse
R/O	Rule Out
rom or R.O.M.	Range of motion
RR or R.Rm.	Recovery room
Rx	Prescription or treatment ordered by a physician

ABBREVIATION	MEANING
s or s̄	Without
SCD	Sequential compression device
S&A or S.&A. Test	Sugar and acetone test
S&K or S.&K. Test	Sugar and ketone test
SO	Significant Other
SOB SOA	Shortness of breath (air)
sos	Whenever emergency arises; only if necessary
Spec or spec.	Specimen
ss or s̄s̄	One-half
SSE or S.S.E.	Soapsuds enema
stat	At once, immediately
STD	Sexually transmitted disease
Surg	Surgery
TB	Tuberculosis
TBI	Traumatic brain injury
tid or T.I.D.	Three times a day
TLC or tlc	Tender loving care
TPR	Temperature, pulse, respiration
TWE	Tap water enema
tx	Treatment
U/a or U/A or u/a	Urinalysis
VDRL	Test for syphilis
V.S. or VS	Vital signs
WBC or W.B.C.	White blood count
w/c	Wheelchair
wc or W.C.	Ward clerk
wt	Weight

Roman numerals are the letters used to represent numbers in the ancient Roman system. The dots or "eyes" are used to eliminate a margin of error:

$$1 = I \text{ or } \dot{I} \quad 2 = II \text{ or } \ddot{II} \quad 3 = III \text{ or } \dddot{III}$$

$$4 = IV \text{ or } \overline{IV} \quad 5 = V \text{ or } \overline{V}$$

$$10 = X \text{ or } \overline{X} \quad 50 = L \text{ or } \overline{L} \quad 100 = C \text{ or } \overline{C}$$

WORD ELEMENTS: ROOTS, PREFIXES, AND SUFFIXES

Many medical terms are composed of several smaller, simpler words or word elements. This discussion describes and shows how to use three primary word elements that are combined frequently to form medical terms. These three word elements are the prefix, the root, and the suffix:

- The **root** is the body or main part of the word. It denotes the primary meaning of the word as a whole.

- The **prefix** is a word element combined with the root. It changes or adds to the meaning of the words. A prefix is always added to the beginning of a root.

- The **suffix** is a word element used to change or add to the meaning of a root. It is always added to the end of the root.

Examples of Similarity Between Terms

WORD ELEMENT	EXAMPLE	MEANING
ante	antefebrile	**before** onset of fever
a	afebrile	**without** fever
cysto	cystogram	x-ray record of the **bladder**
cyto	cytogenesis	production (origin) **of the cell**
hyper	hypertension	**high** blood pressure
hypo	hypotension	**low** blood pressure
inter	interstitial	lying **between** spaces in tissue
intra	intracranial	**within** the skull
macro	macroscopy	seen **large,** as with the naked eye
micro	microscopy	seen **small,** as by microscope
pre	preclinical	**before** the onset of disease

The study of **medical terminology** can aid you in understanding the name of the specific disease for which the patient has been hospitalized. The suffix **itis** means inflammation. Almost every organ in the body is subject to infection by disease organisms that will cause an inflammatory reaction. The word to describe a diagnosis of this nature is formulated simply by adding the suffix *itis* to the word for the body organ affected.

Medical Terms with the Suffix –itis

MEDICAL TERM	DESCRIPTION
appendicitis	inflammation of the appendix
dermatitis	inflammation of the skin
hepatitis	inflammation of liver tissue
rhinitis	inflammation of nasal mucosa
stomatitis	inflammation of the mouth

The suffix **ectomy** means surgical removal. When used in combination with any word element denoting an organ or other body part, the term formed means that the organ or body part has been removed.

Medical Terms with the Suffix –ectomy

MEDICAL TERM	DESCRIPTION
gastrectomy	surgical removal of the stomach
thyroidectomy	surgical removal of the thyroid gland
colectomy	surgical removal of the large intestine

In many cases, an organ may be removed only partially. To indicate this procedure, other words are used to modify the medical term, for example:

- subtotal thyroidectomy

- partial cystectomy

Other modifying words may precede the medical term. This identifies the surgery performed even more accurately.

Detailed Medical Terms

MEDICAL TERM	DESCRIPTION
left salpingo-oophorectomy	removal of the left ovary and Fallopian tube
vaginal hysterectomy	removal of the uterus through the vagina
transurethral prostatectomy	removal of the prostate through the urethra
total abdominal hysterectomy	removal of the entire uterus through abdomen

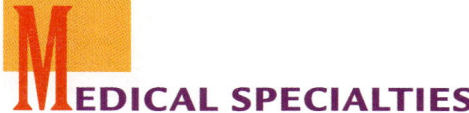

MEDICAL SPECIALTIES

Medical Specialty, Physician's Title, and Description of the Specialty

SPECIALTY	PHYSICIAN'S TITLE	DESCRIPTION
Allergy	Allergist	A subspecialty of internal medicine dealing with diagnosis and treatment of body reactions resulting from unusual sensitivity to foods, pollens, dust, medicine, or other substances.
Anesthesiology	Anesthesiologist	Administration of various forms of anesthesia in operations or procedures to cause loss of feeling or sensation.
Cardiology; cardiovascular diseases	Cardiologist	A subspecialty of internal medicine involving the diagnosis and treatment of diseases of the heart and blood vessels.
Dermatology	Dermatologist	The diagnosis and treatment of disorders of the skin.
Gastroenterology	Gastroenterologist	A subspecialty of internal medicine concerned with diagnosis and treatment of disorders of the digestive tract.
General practice: Family medicine	General practitioner	The diagnosis and treatment of disease by medical and surgical methods without limitations to organ systems or body regions and without restriction as to age of patients.
General surgery	Surgeon	The diagnosis and treatment of disease by surgical means without limitation to special organ or body regions.
Gynecology	Gynecologist	Diagnosis and treatment of diseases of the female reproductive system.
Internal medicine	Internist	The diagnosis and nonsurgical treatment of illness of adults.
Neurology	Neurosurgeon	Diagnosis and surgical treatment of brain, spinal cord, and nerve disorders.
	Neurologist	Diagnosis and treatment of disease of brain, spinal cord, and nerve disorders.
Obstetrics	Obstetrician	The care of women during pregnancy, childbirth, and immediately following.
Oncology	Oncologist	Diagnosis, study, and treatment of cancer, benign or cancer-related tumors.
Ophthalmology	Ophthalmologist	Diagnosis and treatment of diseases of the eye, including prescribing corrective lenses.

SPECIALTY	PHYSICIAN'S TITLE	DESCRIPTION
Orthopedics	Orthopedist	Diagnosis and treatment of disorders and diseases of muscular and skeletal systems.
Otolaryngology	Otolaryngologist	Diagnosis and treatment of diseases of the ear, nose, and throat.
Pathology	Pathologist	Study and interpretation of changes in organs, tissues, and cells and alterations in body chemistry to aid in diagnosing disease and determining treatment.
Pediatrics	Pediatrician	Prevention, diagnosis, and treatment of children's diseases.
Physical medicine and rehabilitation	Physiatrist	Diagnosis of disease and injury in the various systems and areas of the body and treatment by means of physical procedures, as well as treatment and restoration of the convalescent and physically handicapped patient.
Plastic surgery	Plastic surgeon	Cosmetic, corrective, or reparative surgery to restore deformed parts of the body.
Psychiatry	Psychiatrist	Medical branch concerned with diagnosis and treatment of mental disorders.
Radiology	Radiologist	Use of radiant energy, including x-rays, radioactive substances, and magnetic imagery in the diagnosis and treatment of diseases.
Thoracic surgery	Thoracic surgeon	Operative treatment of the lungs, heart, or the large blood vessels within the chest cavity.
Urology	Urologist	Diagnosis and treatment of diseases or disorders of the kidneys, bladder, ureters, urethra, and the male reproductive organs.

This appendix has introduced you to many of the abbreviations, medical terms, and specialists you will need to know to function successfully in the health care field. It is just the start. Be open to learning and seek out other medical reference materials in your health care facility. Your supervisor will assist you with explanations of specific terminology used in your work.

Glossary

abbreviation   A shortened form of a word or phrase used to represent the complete form (Appendix)

abdominal prep   The procedure for making the patient's abdomen ready for surgery; includes thorough cleansing of the skin and careful shaving of body hair in the abdominal area (28)*

abdominal respiration   Breathing in which the patient is using mostly the abdominal muscles (19)

abduction   Movement of an arm or leg away from the center of the body (16)

absorb   To take or soak in, up, or through (22)

absorption   Part of the digestive process in which digestive juices and enzymes break down food into useable parts (20)

acceptance   Admitting, understanding, or facing the truth or reality of the situation, for example, one's death (34)

accountable   To be answerable for one's behavior; legally or ethically responsible for the care of another (2)

accuracy   The quality of being exact or correct; exact conformity to truth and rules; free from errors or defects (2)

Acquired Immune Deficiency Syndrome (AIDS)   Condition caused by a virus that destroys a key part of the body's immune response system; viral infection characterized by decreased immunity to opportunistic infections (25, 30)

active motion   Producing, involving, or participating in activity or movement (33)

activities of daily living (ADL)   The activities or tasks usually performed every day, such as toileting, washing, eating, or dressing (12)

adduction   Movement of an arm or leg toward the center of the body (16)

admission   The administrative process that covers the period from the time the patient enters the institution door to the time the patient is settled (8)

AIDS   See *Acquired Immune Deficiency Syndrome*

*Following the definition of each term, the number(s) of the chapter(s) in which the term is defined appears in parentheses.

alternating-pressure mattress A pad similar to an air mattress that can be placed beneath the patient to reduce pressure on the head, shoulders, back, heels, elbows, and bony prominences (9)

ambulate To walk or move about (6)

ambulation To walk or move about in an upright position (6)

anatomy The study of the structure of an organism (14)

anemia A shortage of red blood cells (18)

aneroid sphygmomanometer Dial-type blood pressure equipment (19)

anesthesia Loss of feeling or sensation in a part or all of the body (28)

anesthesiologist The medical doctor who administers the anesthetic to the patient in the operating room (28)

anesthetic A drug used to produce loss of feeling; can be given orally, rectally, by injection, or by inhalation; a person who has been given an anesthetic is anesthetized (28)

anesthetist The registered nurse who assists the anesthesiologist (28)

anger A strong emotional response of displeasure, irritation, and resentment (34)

anterior Located in the front; opposite of posterior (14)

antiembolism stockings Designed to promote blood to flow and to prevent the formation of blood clots in the blood stream (29)

anus Muscular opening that controls elimination of stool from the rectum (20)

apathy A lack of feeling or interest in things (33)

aphasia Loss of language or speech (26)

apical pulse A measurement of the heartbeats at the apex of the heart, located just under the left breast (19)

apnea Periods of not breathing (19)

appendicitis Inflammation (swelling and irritation) and infection of the appendix, typically with pain in the right lower quadrant; surgery called appendectomy is usually performed to remove the appendix (20)

artery Blood vessel that carries oxygenated blood away from the heart (18)

asepsis The absence of microorganisms (germs); free of disease-causing organisms (5, 23)

aseptic Germ free, without disease-producing organisms (5)

aspirate Material (vomitus, food, or liquids) inhaled into the lungs (28)

assessing Gathering facts to identify needs and problems (8)

atrophic skin Thin, fragile, less elastic skin frequently associated with aging (17)

atrophy Wasting away of muscles; decrease in muscle size (16)

autoclave Device used to achieve sterility of an item through heat, pressure, and steam (5)

autonomic nervous system The part of the nervous system that carries messages without conscious thought (26)

axillary The area under the arms; the armpits (19)

bacteria Unicellular microorganism (5)

bargaining Trying to make a deal to change the situation (34)

bed cradle A frame shaped like a barrel cut in half lengthwise used to keep bed linens off a part of the patient's body (9)

bed-bound Unable to get out of bed (11)

bedpan A pan used by patients who must defecate or urinate while in bed (9, 12)

bedridden Unable to get out of bed (7)

benign tumor A tumor that stays at its site of origin and does not usually regrow once removed (30)

bile Substance manufactured by the liver that helps the food breakdown process (20)

binder A type of bandage applied to a large body area (abdomen or chest) to secure a dressing in place or to put pressure on or support a body part (29)

bladder distention A stretching out of the bladder when urine produced is not excreted (22)

blood and lymph tissue Tissue composed of singular cells that move within a fluid to every part of the body, circulating nutrients, oxygen, and antibodies and removing waste products (14)

blood pressure The force of the blood pushing against the walls of the blood vessels; the force of the blood exerted on the inner walls of the arteries, veins, and chambers of the heart as blood flows or circulates through the structures (18, 19)

body alignment The correct, or anatomical, positioning of a patient's body; also the arrangement of the body in a straight line (7)

body language Communication through hand movements (gestures), facial expressions, body movements, and touch (3)

bony prominences   Places where bones are close to the surface of the skin (17)

boot up   To start up the computer (3)

calibrated   Marked with lines and numbers for measuring (22)

calorie   Unit for measuring the energy produced when food is digested in the body (21)

calorie count   Counting or adding up a total of all calories consumed in a 24-hour period (21)

cancer   Refers to malignant neoplasms, or tumors (30)

cannula   A flexible tube that can be inserted into a body cavity and used to draw fluids out or give oxygen or fluids (6)

canthus   The inner aspect of the eye closest to the nose (26)

carbohydrate   Type of basic food element used by the body; composed of carbon, hydrogen, and oxygen; includes sugars and starches (24)

cardiac   Pertaining to the heart (18)

cardiac arrest   The unexpected stopping of the heartbeat and circulation (13)

cardiac muscle tissue   Involuntary muscle tissue found only in the heart (14)

cardiopulmonary resuscitation (CPR)   An emergency procedure used to reestablish effective circulation and respiration in order to prevent irreversible brain damage (13)

cardiovascular system   Circulatory system which includes heart, arteries, veins, and capillaries (13)

caregiver   The family member or significant other who is taking the major responsibility for the care of the patient (11)

cell   The basic unit of living matter (14)

centigrade   A system for measurement of temperature using a scale divided into 100 units or degrees; in this system, the freezing temperature of water is 0°C and water boils at 100°C; often referred to as Celsius (19)

central processing unit (CPU)   Central processing unit, the "computer brain" where information is stored or directed to appropriate pathways (3)

Central Supply Department   A central place for storing supplies and equipment, also called special purchasing department or central supply department (9)

cerebral spinal fluid   The fluid that circulates around and within the brain and spinal cord (26)

cerebrovascular accident (CVA)   Stroke; blockage or bleeding of blood vessels in the brain, interrupting the blood supply to that part of the brain and damaging the surrounding area of the brain (26)

chemotherapy   Refers to the use of drugs to treat cancer (30)

Cheyne-Stokes respiration   One kind of irregular breathing. At first the breathing is slow and shallow; then the respiration becomes faster and deeper until it reaches a peak. The respiration then slows down and becomes shallow again. The breathing may then stop completely for 10 seconds and then begin the pattern again; this type of respiration may be caused by certain cerebral (brain), cardiac (heart), or pulmonary (lung) diseases or conditions (19)

chronological age   Actual age in years and months (15)

circulation   The continuous movements of blood through the heart and blood vessels to all parts of the body (18)

circulatory system   The heart, blood vessels, blood, and all organs that pump and carry blood and other fluids throughout the body (18)

circumcise   Remove the foreskin of the penis by surgical procedure (31)

circumference   The distance around an object or body part, such as the head (15)

clean catch   Refers to the fact that the urine for this specimen is not contaminated by anything outside the patient's body (23)

client   An individual cared for by a home health agency or provider (4)

closed bed   Bed made with bedspread in place (10)

clove hitch   A type of knot that can be easily released in case of emergency (6)

cognitive   The mental processes by which knowledge is acquired (15)

commode   A movable chair enclosing a bedpan with an opening that can fit over a toilet (12)

communication   The exchange of thoughts, messages, or ideas by speech, signals, gestures, or writing between two or more people (3)

competency   A demonstrable skill or ability (2, 35)

complex partial seizure   Seizure with motor and possible sensory symptoms (such as muscle twitching and smelling a foul odor) and a change in the level of consciousness (26)

complication   An unexpected condition, such as the development of another illness in a patient who is already sick (28)

compress Folded piece of cloth used to apply pressure, moisture, heat, cold, or medication to a specific part of the body (27)

connective tissue Tissue that connects, supports, covers, lines, pads, or protects other body structures (14)

constipation Difficult, infrequent defecation with passage of unduly hard and dry fecal material (20, 31)

constrict Get narrower (27)

continuing education Formal classes, courses, or training programs to develop new knowledge or qualify one for career advancement (35)

continuous Uninterrupted, without a stop (20)

contract Get smaller; shortening the length of muscle, thereby making the angle formed by bones and muscles smaller (16)

contracture An abnormal shortening of a muscle (16); drawing together, bunching up, or shortening of muscle tissue because of spasm or paralysis, either permanently or temporarily (26)

convalescence The period of recovery after an illness or surgery (8)

convert Change (22)

convulsive Involving convulsions—rhythmic, involuntary contraction of muscles (26)

cooperation Working or acting together; uniting to produce an effect or to share an activity for mutual benefit (2)

courtesy Being polite and considerate (3)

cubic centimeter Having a volume equal to a cube whose edges are 1 centimeter long (22)

culture The thoughts, beliefs, and values of a social group (4)

cursor Flashing bar, or symbol, that indicates where the next character is to be placed or location on the computer screen (3)

customer-focused care Care designed to meet the needs of patients, residents, and clients (customers) (4)

cyanosis When the skin looks blue or gray, especially on the lips, nailbeds, and under the fingernails; in a black patient, it may appear as a darkening of color: This occurs when there is not enough oxygen in the blood (3, 27)

dangling position Sitting up on the edge of the bed with the feet hanging down loosely (32)

data Information that a user enters into a computer (3)

decubitus ulcers Tissue breakdown resulting from pressure or reduced blood flow (often called pressure sores or bed sores) (10)

deep Distant from the surface of the body (14)

deficit A temporary or permanent negative change in a patient's usual neurologic function (26)

dehydrate Loss of body fluids (31)

dehydration A decrease in the amount of water in the tissues occurring when fluid output exceeds input or intake (22)

dementia An irreversible mental condition in which intellectual abilities are continuously reduced (32)

denial Refusal to admit the truth or face reality (34)

dentures Artificial teeth. Dentures may replace some or all of a person's teeth; they are described as being partial or complete and upper or lower (12)

dependability A quality shown by coming to work every day on time and doing what is asked at the proper time and in the proper way (2)

depression A state of sadness, grief, or low spirits that may or may not cause change of activity (33, 34)

dermis The inner layer of skin (17)

deteriorate To make or grow worse; degenerate (32)

development The motor, language, cognitive, and social skills changes that occur in a person over the course of the life span (15)

diabetes mellitus Disorder of carbohydrate metabolism caused by inability to convert sugar into energy because of inadequate production or utilization of insulin (24)

diabetic coma A coma (abnormal deep stupor) that can occur in a diabetic patient from lack of insulin (24)

diagnosis Finding out what kind of disease or medical condition a patient has; a diagnosis is always made by a physician (1)

diaper Washable or disposable covering applied to the perineal area for the purpose of containing stool or urine (31)

diarrhea Frequent, watery stools; some causes of this problem are infection, certain particular foods, or complication from tube feedings; abnormally frequent discharge of fluid fecal material from the bowel (20, 31)

diastolic blood pressure In taking a patient's blood pressure, one records the bottom number as the reading for the diastolic pressure; this is the relaxing phase of the heartbeat (19)

digestion Breaking down the food that is eaten into a form that can be used by the body cells; this process is both mechanical and chemical (20)

dilate Get bigger; expand (27)

discharge The official procedure for helping patients to leave the health care institution, including teaching them how to care for themselves at home (8); flowing out of material (secretion or excretion) from any part of the body such as pus, feces, urine, or drainage from a wound (22)

disinfection The process of destroying as many harmful organisms as possible (5)

disoriented Unaware of or unable to remember, recognize, or describe people, places, or times; confused perception of reality (32)

disposable equipment Equipment that is used one time only or for one patient only and then thrown away (9)

dorsal Refers to the back or to the back part of an organ (14)

dorsal flexion Bending backward (33)

dorsal lithotomy position The position in which a patient lies on the back, with legs spread apart and knees bent (7)

dorsal recumbent position Lying down or reclining; refers to the back or the back part of an organ (7)

drape A covering used to provide privacy during an examination or operation (7)

draping Covering a patient or parts of a patient's body with a sheet, blanket, bath blanket, or other material during a physical examination or prior to surgery (7)

draw sheet Small sheet made of plastic, rubber, or cotton placed across the middle of the bed to cover and protect the bottom sheet and assist in moving the patient (10)

DRGs Diagnostically related groups of patients; a DRG includes patients whose diagnoses are related, usually by body system or broad disease type, such as heart disease (1)

dry application A warm or cold application in which no water touches the skin (27)

duodenum The first loop of the small intestine (20)

dysphagia Difficulty in swallowing usually requiring evaluation by speech therapist to prescribe a certain diet and method of feeding (32)

dyspnea Insufficient oxygenation of the blood resulting in labored or difficult breathing (19)

ectomy A suffix that means *surgical removal* (Appendix)

edema Abnormal swelling of a part of the body caused by fluid collecting in that area; usually the swelling is in the ankles, legs, hands, or abdomen (3, 22)

efficiency Getting all of one's duties completed in an organized fashion within a designated work period (11)

eliminate (defecate) To rid the body of waste products; to excrete, expel, remove, put out; (to have a bowel movement; to excrete waste matter from the bowels) (12, 22)

embolus Blood clot or mass of other undissolved matter that travels through the circulatory system from its place of formation to another site, lodges in a small blood vessel, and causes an obstruction (26)

emergency Events that call for immediate action (13)

emesis basin A pan used for catching material that a patient spits out, vomits, or expectorates (9)

empathy The ability to put yourself in another's place and to see things as they see them (3)

endocrine glands Ductless glands that produce hormones and secrete them directly into the blood or lymph (24)

endocrine system System composed of endocrine glands; regulates body function by secreting hormones (24)

enema Procedure of evacuation or washing out of waste materials (feces or stool) from a person's lower bowel (20)

enterally Delivery of a nutrition formula through a tube for patients with a functional GI tract who are unable to take in adequate calories or food by mouth (21)

environment All the surrounding conditions and influences affecting the life and development of an organism (26)

epidermis The outer layer or surface of the skin (17)

epithelial tissue Tissue that lines, protects, secretes, absorbs, and receives sensations (14)

equipment Materials, tools, devices, supplies, furnishings, necessary things used to perform a task (9)

essential nutrients Nutrients needed for the human body to function; they must be consumed in the diet every day (21)

estrogen A female hormone that causes a buildup of the lining of the uterus to prepare it for possible pregnancy; also responsible for the development of secondary sexual characteristics (25)

ethical behavior To keep promises and do what you should do; to act in accordance with the rules or standards for right conduct or practice (2)

ethnic diversity The variety of races, religions, and cultures in the world (4)

evacuation Discharge of the contents of the lower bowel through the rectum and anus (20)

evaluating Determining whether a plan (such as the patient care plan) has been effective (8)

evaluation Assessment of one's ability or skill to perform a given task (35)

evaporate To pass off as vapor, as water evaporating into the air (22)

exhaling The process of breathing out air in respiration (19)

exocrine glands Glands that produce hormones and secrete them either directly or through a duct to epithelial tissue, such as a body cavity or the skin surface (24)

expectorate To cough up matter from the lungs, trachea, or bronchial tubes and spit it out (23)

expired Deceased, dead (34)

extension Straightening or lengthening a muscle, thereby making the angle formed by bones and muscles greater (16)

extra nourishment Snacks (21)

Fahrenheit A system for measuring temperature. In the Fahrenheit system, the temperature of water at boiling is 212°. At freezing, it is 32°. These temperatures are usually written 212°F and 32°F (19)

family unit A group brought together by shared needs, interests, and mutual concern for the well-being of all its members (11)

fanfold Method of arranging bed linens so that the covers and bedspread are folded at the foot of the bed out of the way (10)

fatigue A feeling of tiredness or weariness (33)

feces Solid waste material discharged from the body through the rectum and anus; other names include excreta, excrement, bowel movement, stool, and fecal matter (23)

feedback Response of the receiver to the sender's message; the response, or feedback, lets the sender know if the message is acknowledged and clearly understood (3)

fertile Able to become pregnant; capable of reproduction (25)

fertilization Joining of a sperm and ovum to form a new cell (25)

fine motor Refers to the movement of small muscles, such as those in the hands and fingers (15)

first aid The first action taken to help a person who is in crisis (13)

flammable Capable of burning quickly and easily (9, 11, 32)

flatus Intestinal gas (20)

flex To bend; the act of bending a body part (16)

flexion Bending of a joint (elbow, wrist, knee) (16)

flow sheet A checklist or chart for recording the activities of daily living (12)

flowmeter A device used to control and regulate the flow of oxygen (6)

fluid Applies to liquid substances (22)

fluid balance The same amount of fluid that is taken in by the body is given out by the body (22)

fluid imbalance When too much fluid is kept in the body or when too much fluid is lost (22)

fluid intake The fluid taken into the body, from whatever source (22)

fluid output The fluid passed or excreted out of the body; for example urine, vomit, diarrhea (22)

force Strength or power; used to describe the beat of the pulse (19)

force fluids Extra fluids to be taken in by a patient according to the doctor's orders (FF) (22)

formula A liquid food prescribed for an infant containing most required nutrients (11)

Fowler's position The position in which the head of the patient's bed is at a 45°–90° angle (7)

fracture A break in a bone (16)

fracture pan A bedpan with a flat end that goes under the patient (12)

friction The process of rubbing two surfaces together, such as skin (5)

friction injuries Injuries resulting from the patient sliding against hard surfaces (17)

functional nursing A method of organizing the health care team in which the head nurse assigns and directs all patient care responsibilities for the nursing staff; this is sometimes called direct assignment (1)

gait training Rehabilitative exercise to help the patient improve walking ability (6)

gastrointestinal (GI) system The GI tract is about 30 feet long and consists primarily of the mouth, esophagus, stomach, small intestines, and large intestines (20)

gastrostomy An opening made through the abdomen to the stomach for the purpose of feeding (20)

gastrostomy tube (GT) Tube inserted into the abdomen for the introduction of fluids (20)

gavage Feeding through a nasogastric tube (20)

general anesthetics General anesthetics cause loss of sensation in the entire body (28)

generalized Affecting, involving, or pertaining to the whole body (27)

generalized application A warm or cold application applied to the entire body (27)

genital The external reproductive organs (23)

geriatric person Aging; elderly; over 65 years of age (32)

gland An organ that is able to manufacture and discharge a chemical that will be used elsewhere in the body (24)

glucose A sugar formed during metabolism of carbohydrates; blood sugar (24)

graduate A measuring cup marked along its side to show various amounts so that the material placed in the cup can be measured accurately; the marks are called *calibrations* (22)

gross motor Refers to the movement of large muscles, such as those used in walking or hitting a ball (15)

growth The physical changes that take place in a person's body over the life span (15)

gynecological (GYN) patient Patient being treated for diseases or conditions of the female reproductive organs, including the breasts (25)

hardware The actual physical equipment that is used by a computer to process data

hazard A source of danger; a possible cause of an accident (2)

health care institution (facility) Hospital, hospice, nursing home, convalescent home, or clinic where health care services are provided both on an inpatient and outpatient basis (1)

heart A four-chambered, hollow, muscular organ that lies in the chest cavity and pumps the blood through the lungs and into all parts of the body (18)

heart attack Interruption or damage to the blood supply to the heart muscle; myocardial infarction (13)

hemiplegia Paralysis of one-half of the body (26)

hemisphere Half of a sphere; in the nervous system, one-half of the brain (26)

hemorrhage The extreme or unexpected loss of blood; heavy/excessive bleeding (13, 26)

hepatitis B Blood borne disease, affects the liver and is easily transmitted within the health care setting following parenteral exposure (5)

hepatitis C Prior to 1988 known as non A-non B hepatitis. Transmitted best through needle sticks and may result in chronic liver disease (5)

HIV Human immunodeficiency virus; the microorganism that causes AIDS (25)

holistic An approach that reflects the four dimensions of a "whole" person: physiological, psychological, sociocultural, and spiritual (8); Intended to meet the needs of the whole patient; based on the belief that human beings function as complete units and cannot be effectively treated part by part (33)

homeostasis Stability of all body functions at normal levels (22)

hormones Protein substances secreted by endocrine glands directly into the blood to stimulate increased activity (24)

hospice An extended, or long term, care facility that provides health care services to terminally ill patients and their families (1); program that allows a dying patient to remain at home or in a nonhospital environment and die there while receiving professionally supervised care (34)

hospice care The care of patients with terminal conditions who choose to remain at home until their death (11)

hospital A short term, or emergency, care facility that provides health care services to patients (1)

hygiene The science that deals with the preservation of health; when used to describe an object or a person, it means clean and sanitary (2)

hyperglycemia Abnormally high blood sugar (24)

hypoglycemia Abnormally low blood sugar (24)

hypothalamus Area of the brain responsible for control of the pituitary gland (26)

immediate supervisor An individual responsible for providing direction, critiquing performance, and giving feedback related to that performance (1)

immunocompromised Means that the immune system is not functioning normally; immunocompromised and immunosuppressed mean the same and are used interchangeably (30)

implementing Carrying out or accomplishing a given plan (8)

impulse An electrical or chemical charge transmitted through certain tissues, especially nerve fibers and muscles (26)

incident An unforeseen event that occurs without intent (2)

incontinence Inability to control the bowels or bladder; inability to control urination or defecation (12, 33)

incontinent Unable to control the bowels or bladder; unable to control urine or feces (7, 17, 22)

indwelling urinary catheter A bladder drainage tube that is allowed to remain in place within the bladder (22)

infant A baby aged 1 month to 1 year (31)

infection Due to a pathogen producing a reaction that may cause soreness, tenderness, redness, and/or pus, fever, change in drainage, and so on (5)

infection control The effort to prevent the spread of pathogens; restraining or curbing the spread of microorganisms (5, 11)

inferior The lower portion of the body (14)

infiltration Occurs when an IV solution runs into nearby tissue instead of into a vein (29)

inflammation A reaction of the tissues to disease or injury; there is usually pain, heat, redness, and swelling of the body part (27)

inhaling The process of breathing in air in respiration (19)

insensible fluid loss Fluid that is lost from the body without being noticed, such as in perspiration or air breathed out (22)

insulin A hormone produced by the pancreas to help the body change sugar into energy; can be produced from an animal pancreas for use in the treatment of diabetes; hormone that regulates the sugar content of the blood (24)

insulin shock Serious complication related to diabetes; occurs when the diabetic receives too much insulin, misses a meal, or has too much physical activity (24)

integumentary system The body system that includes the skin, hair, nails, and sweat and oil glands, that provides the first line of defense against infection, maintains body temperature, provides fluids, and eliminates wastes (17)

intermittent Alternating; stopping and beginning again; procedure that is stopped from time to time (20, 27)

interpersonal skills Skills used in interacting with other persons, such as courtesy; good interpersonal skills enable people to interact or work together in a productive and satisfying manner (2)

intervertebral discs The material between the vertebral bodies that cushions the spinal column (26)

intravenous infusion The injection of fluids, nutrients, or medication into a vein (29)

intravenous pole A tall pole, also called IV pole, which attaches to a bed or is on rollers or casters; this pole is used to hold the containers or tubes needed, for example, during a blood transfusion (9)

involuntary Without conscious will, control, or decision (26)

irregular respiration The depth of breathing changes and the rate of the rise and fall of the chest is not steady (19)

isolation To separate or set apart (5)

itis A suffix that means *inflammation* (Appendix)

joint A part of the body where two bones come together (16)

keyboard An input device similar to a typewriter keyboard; has additional keys that allow the user to make selections to direct computer activity (3)

knee-chest position A bent posture with the knees and chest touching the examining table, sometimes used for examining the rectum or for women who have recently given birth, to allow the uterus to fall forward into its natural position (7)

labored respiration Working hard to breathe (19)

lamb's wool A wide strip of lamb's hide with the fleece attached or an imitation material used to increase patient comfort (9)

large intestine Distal colon that absorbs water from stool (20)

lavage The washing out of the stomach through a nasogastric tube, usually with normal saline (20)

left lateral position Lying on the left side (7)

lesion An abnormality, either benign or cancerous, of the tissues of the body, such as a wound, sore, rash, boil, tumors, or growths (17)

ligament Tough, white fibrous cord that connects bone to bone (16)

light pen A hand-held device shaped like a pen that has an electronic sensor for making selections on a computer screen (3)

liver Responsible for manufacturing bile and is a storage area for glucose; the liver also is the place where toxins, or poisons, are removed from the blood (20)

local anesthetics Local anesthetics cause numbness or a loss of sensation in only a part of the body (28)

localized Limited to one place or part; affecting, involving, or pertaining to a definite area (27)

localized application A warm or cold application applied to a specific area or small part of the body (27)

log on   To sign on to the computer using a password or personal identification number (3)

long-term supportive care   The care of chronically ill patients who are unable to care for themselves and live alone or have limited family support (11)

lumpectomy   Removal of a small part of the breast (30)

malignant (neoplasms)   New growths that spread, invade, and destroy organs (30)

malnutrition   Poor nutrition status (21)

malpractice   Negligence when applied to the performance of a professional (2)

mastectomy   Removal of the entire breast (30)

medical asepsis   Special practices and procedures for preventing the conditions that allow disease-producing bacteria to live, multiply, and spread (23)

medical terminology   The special vocabulary of words used in the health care professions (Appendix)

memory   The capacity of the computer to store data (3)

meninges   The covering of the brain and spinal cord. There are three layers: the dura mater, the arachnoid, and the pia mater (26)

menopause   Time during which menstruation stops, resulting in decreased hormone production and an end of fertility (25)

menstruation   Periodic (monthly) loss of some blood and a small part of the lining of the uterus when a woman is not pregnant (25)

mental health   Describes the best adjustment an individual can make at a given time, based on internal and external resources (30)

mental illness   Describes a number of chemical imbalances in the brain or genetically-based brain diseases that interfere significantly with people's abilities to live and work (30)

mercury sphygmomanometer   Blood pressure equipment containing a column of mercury (19)

metabolism   The total of all the physical and chemical changes that take place in living organisms and cells, including all the processes involved in the use of substances taken into the body; the process through which food elements are converted into energy for use in the human body (24)

metastasis   Refers to the spreading of cancer cells through the systems of the body (30)

microorganism   A living thing that is so small it cannot be seen with the naked eye but only through a microscope (5, 11)

midstream   Catching the urine specimen between the time the patient begins to void and the time he stops (23)

mobility   Ability to move (33)

mobilization   Making movable; putting into action (33)

moist application   A warm or cold application in which water touches the body (27)

monitor   A screen, similar to a television screen, that allows the user to see input and output (3)

morgue   A place for temporarily keeping dead bodies for identification, autopsy, retrieval by funeral home staff, and burial (34)

motivation   Reason, desire, need, or purpose that causes a person to do something (33)

mouse   A pointing and selecting device to input data; a small tabletop electronic pointing device used to make selections on a computer screen (3)

multidisciplinary team   A team of professionals and nonprofessionals from different disciplines that plans, makes decisions, and implements the delivery of patient care that is focused, or centered, on the patient's needs rather than any particular discipline's (department's) needs (1)

muscle tissue   Tissue that ensures movement; it is capable of stretching and contracting (14)

myelin sheath   Protective covering around most nerves (26)

nasal   Pertaining to the nose and nasal cavity (6)

nasogastric tube   A tube placed through one of the patient's nostrils (naso-), down the back of the throat, and through the esophagus into the patient's stomach (-gastric) (20)

need   A requirement for survival (4)

negligence   The commission of an act or failure to perform an act, where the respective performance or nonperformance deviates from the act that should have been done by a reasonably prudent person under the same or similar conditions (2)

neoplasm (tumor)   New growth; the words tumor and neoplasm are interchangeable (30)

nerve tissue   Tissue that carries nervous impulses between the brain, the spinal cord, and all parts of the body (14)

nervous system   The group of body organs consisting of the brain, spinal cord, and nerves that controls and regulates the activities of the body and the functions of the other body systems (26)

network   Several computers that are connected or wired together, having access to central computer programs; can interface to obtain information; located at different work stations (3)

neuron   A type of nerve cell in the nervous system (26)

nonambulatory   Unable to walk (7)

normal flora   Microorganisms that are necessary for health and usually live and grow in specific locations; they are nonpathogenic when in or on a natural reservoir (5)

normal pressure hydrocephalus   A disorder caused by enlargement of the ventricles, fluid-filled spaces in the brain (26)

nosocomial infection   Hospital acquired infection (5)

nothing by mouth (NPO)   Cannot eat or drink anything at all, usually past midnight the night before surgery or a procedure (22, 28)

nurse   A person educated and trained to provide health care for people and to help physicians and surgeons; nurses are licensed as registered nurses (RNs) and licensed practical nurses (LPNs) (1)

nurse manager   The RN leader responsible for the care delivery, personnel supervision, and operating budget of a unit, area, or facility (1)

nursing assistant   A person who helps the registered nurse to care for patients; nursing assistants work in hospitals, long-term care or other health care facilities, or in the patient's home (1)

nutrient   Chemical substances found in foods (21)

nutrition status assessment   Assessment by an RN or RD as to what a patient eats and how the body uses it; determination of any special nutritional needs (21)

obese   Very overweight (17)

objective observations   Signs that can be observed and reported exactly as they are seen (3)

objective reporting   Reporting exactly what you observe (3)

OBRA regulations   Federal rules and requirements established by the Omnibus Budget Reconciliation Act of 1987 (6)

observation   Gathering information about the patient by noticing any change (3)

occupational therapist   Person trained to assist the patient with performing activities of daily living (33)

occupied bed   One with a patient in it (10)

omit   Leave out (21)

open bed   Bed made with top sheet folded so as to give patient easy entrance (10)

oral   Anything to do with the mouth; examples are eating and speaking (19)

oral hygiene   Cleanliness of the mouth (12)

organ   A part of the body made of several types of tissue grouped together to perform a certain function; examples are the heart, stomach, and lungs (14)

orientation   An individual's ability to identify who she is, where she is, and some information about time (month, year, time of day) (30)

orthopedics   The medical specialty that covers the treatment of broken bones, deformities, or diseases that attack the bones, joints, and muscles (16)

orthotics   The science concerned with making and fitting prosthetic devices (33)

osteoporosis   Condition in which bones become brittle or thin and break easily (26)

ostomy   A surgical procedure (operation) in which a new opening, called a stoma, is created in the abdomen, usually for the discharge of wastes (urine or feces) from the body (20)

ostomy appliance   Collecting pouch usually attached to the skin around the stoma with adhesive (20)

ovulation   Process whereby an ovum is released from one ovary into the opening of the fallopian tube and moves to the uterus (25)

ovum   The female reproductive cell produced in the ovaries which is capable of uniting with a sperm cell and developing into a new organism (25)

oxygen   A colorless, odorless, tasteless gaseous element that is essential for respiration; air is 21 percent oxygen (6)

palliative   Care designed to comfort, instead of cure, the patient (34)

pancreas   Produces digestive juices and enzymes responsible for food breakdown in the small intestines (20)

parenteral intake   Fluids taken in intravenously (22)

parenteral nutrition   Nutrition therapy delivered by an IV catheter for patients with a nonfunctioning GI tract (21)

passive motion   Not active, but acted upon; enduring with effort or resistance (33)

password   A word or phrase that identifies a person and allows access to or entry to a program or record (3)

pathogen   Disease producing microorganism (5)

patient   An individual admitted to an inpatient or outpatient hospital, physician office, or clinic (4)

patient-focused care   A care delivery model in which multidisciplinary teams plan, make decisions, and deliver care with the patient's needs a focus rather than the needs or convenience of various departments or caregivers (1)

patient lift A mechanical device with a sling seat used for lifting a patient into and out of such equipment as the hospital bed, bathtub, or wheelchair (9)

patient plan of care A written plan stating the nursing diagnosis, the patient goals or expected outcomes, and the nursing orders, interventions, or actions to be taken (8)

patient unit The space for one patient, including the hospital bed, bedside table, chair, and other equipment (9)

pediatric patient Any patient under the age of 16 years (3, 31)

perineal area See *perineum* (25)

perineum (perineal area) The area of the body between the thighs; includes the area of the anus and the external genital organs; area between and around the urinary opening and the rectum (12, 17, 25)

peristalsis Rhythmic contractions of the muscle walls of the small and large intestines (20)

peristaltic waves Waves of involuntary contractions (22)

perspiration Sweat (22)

phlebitis Inflammation of a vein (29)

physical crisis management Methods for dealing with a dangerous situation involving a patient, resident, or client (4)

physical therapist Person trained to assist the patient with activities related to motion (33)

physiological Referring to a person's biological response to alterations in the body's structures and functions (8)

physiology The study of the functions of the body dealing with the physical and chemical processes of cells, tissues, and organs of living organisms (14)

PIN Personal identification number; password (3)

planning Deciding what to do and how to do it (8)

plaque Fatty deposits within blood vessels attached to vessel walls (26)

plasma The liquid portion of the blood (18)

poison Any substance ingested, inhaled, injected, or absorbed into the body that will interfere with normal physiological functions (13)

posterior Located in the back or toward the rear (14)

postmortem After death (34)

postoperative After surgery (28)

postoperative bed Bed made with top sheet folded lengthwise and positioned to one side, allowing transfer of the patient from the surgical stretcher to the bed without unnecessary movement (10)

pouching Also known as pocketing of food; the retaining or holding of food in the mouth between the cheek and teeth (32)

prefix A word element added to the beginning of a root (Appendix)

preoperative Before surgery (28)

pressure ulcers Also called bedsores; areas of the skin that become broken and painful; caused by continuous pressure on a body part and usually occur when a patient is kept in one position for a long period of time (17)

primary nursing A patient-oriented method of organizing the health care team in which the professional registered nurses are responsible for the total nursing care of the patient (1)

printer An output device for creating a hard copy (3)

prompt A reminder that the user must take some action so further processing of the data can continue (3)

prone position Lying on one's stomach (7)

proper/protective body mechanics Special ways of standing and moving one's body to make the best use of strength and to avoid fatigue (7)

prosthetics Artificial limbs or substitutes for missing body parts (33)

protective devices Measures taken to keep a patient safe or to prevent injury (6)

psychological Referring to a person's cognitive and emotional responses to the self and the surrounding environment (8); involving aspects of the mind, such as feelings and thoughts (33)

psychosocial Involving aspects of living together in a group of people (33)

pulmonary Pertaining to the lungs (18)

pulse The rhythmic expansion and contraction of the arteries caused by the beating of the heart; the expansion and contractions show how fast, how regular, and with what force the heart is beating (19)

pulse deficit A difference between the apical heartbeat and the radial pulse rate (19)

punctuality Arriving at one's planned destination on time (11)

radial pulse   This is the pulse felt at a person's wrist at the radial artery (19)

radiation therapy   The use of high doses of radiation, many times the dose used for x-ray exams, to treat the cancer (30)

range of motion exercises   Exercises that move each muscle and joint through its full range of motion and help a confined patient exercise the muscles and joints (33)

rate   Used to describe the number of pulse beats per minute (19)

rectal   Pertaining to the rectum (19)

rectal irrigation   Repeated washing out of the rectum; clean water runs into the rectum, gas (flatus) and water run out of the rectum, as in the Harris flush (20)

rectum   The lowest portion of the large intestine, which curves in an *S*-shape and stores fecal material (20)

registered dietitian (RD)   Person responsible for the preparation of well-balanced regular and therapeutic (special) diets to meet patients' nutritional needs (21)

regular diet   A basic, or well-balanced, diet containing appropriate amounts of foods from each of the food groups (21)

rehabilitation   The process by which people who have been disabled by injury or sickness are helped to recover as much as possible of their original abilities for the activities of daily living (33)

rehabilitation nurse   A nurse with special training in the causes and treatment of disabilities; may be certified in this specialty with the title Certified Rehabilitation Registered Nurse (CRRN) (33)

relax   To place in a resting position, in which muscle tension decreases and fibers lengthen (16)

reproductive system   The group of body organs that makes possible the creation of a new human life (25)

resident   An individual cared for in a nursing home or other long term/extended care facility (4)

residual   Remaining or left over (22)

respiratory system   The group of body organs that carries on the body function of respiration; the system brings oxygen into the body and eliminates carbon dioxide (18)

respond   React; begin, end, or change activity in reaction to stimulation (26)

responsibility   A duty or obligation; that for which one is accountable (11)

restorative care   Care given to help a patient attain or maintain their highest level of function and independence (32, 33)

restraint alternative   Protective measures such as a saddle or wedge cushion, self-releasing belt or lap tray that are used to help prevent falls but do not physically restrain an individual (6)

restraints   Protective measures ordered by a physician to prevent patients from harming themselves or others (6)

restrict fluids   Fluids that are limited to certain amounts (22)

retain   To keep or hold in (22)

retention   The patient keeps the enema fluid (oil) in the rectum for 20 minutes (20)

retrieval   To recall data stored in computer memory (3)

rhythm   Used to describe the regularity of the pulse beats (19)

Rickettsiae   An example of bacteria found in the tissues of fleas, lice, ticks, and other insects; Rickettsiae are transmitted to humans by insect bites (5)

rigor mortis   The natural stiffening of a body and limbs shortly after death (34)

Roman numerals   The letters used to represent numbers in the ancient Roman system (Appendix)

root   The body or main part of the word (Appendix)

rupture   Break open (26)

saliva   The secretion of the salivary glands into the mouth; saliva moistens food and helps in swallowing; substance containing chemicals that begin to digest the food being chewed (20, 23)

screen   A portion of data that is displayed at one time within the confined area of the computer monitor (3)

scrotal prep   The procedures for making the genital area of a male patient ready for surgery; the preparation includes thoroughly cleansing the skin and carefully shaving the hair in the area (28)

secrete   Produce and release into the body; glands secrete hormones (24)

secretions   The substances that flow out of or are produced by glandular organs; the process of producing this substance; for example: sweat, bile, lymph, saliva, or urine (3)

seizure   An episode, either partial or generalized, which may include altered consciousness, motor activity, or sensory phenomena and convulsions (13, 26)

self-care   Activities or care tasks performed by the patient (12)

semi-Fowler's position   The position in which the head of the patient's bed is at a 30°–45° angle (7)

service Factors such as attentiveness, quality of food, and cleanliness of environment that affect the care and comfort of the individual receiving health care (4)

sexually transmitted diseases (STDs) Diseases acquired as a result of sexual intercourse with an infected person (25)

shallow respiration Breathing with only the upper part of the lungs (19)

shear injuries Result from the skin remaining in place on top of a surface while the underlying structures, such as the bone, slide downward (17)

shock The failure of the cardiovascular system to provide sufficient blood circulation to every part of the body (13)

short-term intermittent skilled nursing care The care provided to acutely ill patients or those with an exacerbated illness with the purpose of educating the patients to become independent in self-care and functional ability (11)

side-lying positions Lying on one's side (7)

simple partial seizure A seizure when the patient is aware of their surroundings but experiences either motor (muscle twitching or movement) or sensory changes (see or hear things not present) (26)

Sims's position Position in which the patient lies on the left side with the right knee and thigh drawn up, often used for a rectal examination; often called the enema position (7, 20)

sitz bath A bath in which the patient sits in a specially designed chairtub or a regular bathtub with the hips and buttocks in water (27)

skin prep Shaving the area of the body where an operation is going to be performed in preparation for surgery (28)

small intestine The first, smaller portion of the bowel, including the duodenum, where most of digestion and food breakdown occurs; also known as the small bowel (20)

soak Immerse the body or body part completely in water (27)

sociocultural Referring to a person's interpersonal responses to socialization practices in the family and community (8)

software Set or sets of instructions that direct computer operations; computer programs (3)

spasm An involuntary sudden movement or convulsive muscular contraction (26)

special diet See *therapeutic diet* (21)

specialty bed A bed that constantly changes pressure under the patient. Used to minimize pressure points in the treatment or prevention of pressure ulcers (9)

specimen A sample of material taken from the patient's body; examples are urine specimens, feces specimens, and sputum specimens (23)

sperm The male reproductive cell produced in the testes, which is released from the male during intercourse (25)

sphincter Ring-shaped muscle that surrounds and controls a natural opening in the body, such as the anus (20)

sphygmomanometer An apparatus for measuring blood pressure (19)

spinal anesthetics Anesthetics that cause a loss of feeling in a large area of the body, usually from the umbilicus down to and including the legs and feet (28)

spiritual Referring to an individual's personal response to forces; inspirational (8)

spores Bacteria that have formed hard shells around themselves as a defense (5)

sputum Waste material coughed up from the lungs or trachea (23)

staff development On the job training or classes provided to enhance or expand an employee's skills or abilities (35)

sterilization The process of killing all microorganisms, including spores (5)

sterilize Destroying all microorganisms (11)

stertorous respiration The patient makes abnormal noises like snoring sounds when breathing (19)

stethoscope An instrument that allows one to listen to various sounds in the patient's body, such as the heartbeat or breathing sounds (19)

stimuli Changes in the external or internal environment strong enough to set up a nervous impulse or other responses in an organism (26)

stoma A surgically made opening connecting the urinary or intestinal tract with the outside, such as in an urostomy or colostomy (20)

stool Solid waste material discharged from the body through the rectum and anus; other names include feces, excreta, excrement, bowel movement, and fecal matter (23, 31)

stress A physical, mental, or emotional tension or strain triggered by a stimulus that requires some response or type of adjustment (2)

stretcher A narrow rolling table or cart with or without a mattress or simply a canvas stretched over a frame used to transport patients; the latter may also be called a litter or a gurney; a wheeled cart in which patients are moved from one place to another (7, 9)

stroke   Interruption or damage to the blood supply to the brain; a cerebrovascular accident (13)

subacute care   Ongoing medical, nursing, rehabilitative, or dietary care provided to patients who need a lower level of care than an acute care (i.e., hospital) setting provides; categories of subacute care are based on the patient's health status and the type of care and length of care needed (33)

subjective observations   Symptoms that can be felt and described only by the patient himself, such as pain, nausea, dizziness, ringing in the ears, and headaches (3)

subjective reporting   Giving your opinion about what you have observed; the nursing assistant should never use subjective reporting (3)

substance abuse   The excessive use of mood-altering drugs such as alcohol, cocaine, tobacco, or caffeine that results in negative changes to a person's life (30)

suction   Using negative pressure to remove material, usually fluid (20)

suffix   A word element used to change or add to the meaning of a root; it is always added to the end of a root (Appendix)

sundowning syndrome   A state of increased confusion and disorientation that usually occurs in persons with cognitive dysfunction as evening approaches (32)

superficial   On or near the surface of the body (14)

superior   The upper portion of the body (14)

supine position   Lying on one's back (7)

suppository   A semisolid preparation, sometimes medicated, that is inserted into the vagina or rectum (33)

system   A group of organs acting together to carry out one or more body functions (14)

systolic blood pressure   The force with which blood is pumped when the heart muscle is contracting; when taking a patient's blood pressure, the systolic blood pressure is recorded as the top number (19)

sterile field   An area created to work from when you are doing a sterile procedure (5)

tact   Doing or saying the right things at the right time (3)

task oriented   Nursing care that is arranged according to what must be done (1)

team leader   The nurse responsible for one area of a nursing unit, including patient care assignments (1)

team nursing   A task-oriented method of organizing the health care team in which the team leader gives patient care assignments to each team member (1)

terminal   A computer monitor that allows the computer operator to see input and output on a screen (3)

terminally ill   Having an illness that can be expected to cause death, usually within a predictable time (34)

testosterone   The primary male sex hormone manufactured in the testes, which is essential for normal sexual behavior and the development of secondary sexual characteristics (25)

therapeutic diet   Any special diet (21)

thermometer   An instrument used for measuring temperature (19)

thrombophlebitis   Inflammation and blood clots in a vein (29)

thrombus   A blood clot that remains at its site of formation (26)

time/travel record   Record or log describing how time is spent in a patient's home and/or account of travel time to and from the patient's home or running errands (11)

tissue   A group of cells of the same type (14)

tissue fluid   A watery environment around each cell that acts as a place of exchange for gases, food, and waste products between the cells and the blood (22)

traction   Exertion of pull by means of weights or pulleys, often used for realignment of bones or other limb tissues (16)

transfer   Moving a hospital patient from one room, unit, or facility to another (8)

transmission   The spread of microorganisms (5)

transporting   Moving something or someone from one place to another (7)

trapeze   A triangle-shaped bar attached to the overbed frame of a traction setup which enables the patient to pull himself up in bed (16)

Trendelenburg's position   Position in which the bed or operating table on which a patient is lying is tilted so that the patient's head is about one foot below the level of his or her knees, to allow more blood flow to the head and prevent shock; also called *shock position* (7)

tuberculosis (TB)   A highly infectious disease that usually affects the lungs (18)

umbilical cord   Rather long, flexible, rough organ that carries nourishment from the mother to the baby; it connects the umbilicus of the unborn baby in the mother's uterus to the placenta (31)

unconscious   Unaware of the environment; occurs during sleep and in temporary episodes ranging from fainting or stupor or coma (28)

unilateral neglect   Failure of a patient disabled on one side of the body to dress, bathe, or otherwise care for that side because the patient forgets the side exists (33)

urinal   A portable container given to male patients in bed so they can urinate without getting out of bed (9, 12)

urinary system (excretory system)   The group of body components including the kidneys, ureters, bladder, and urethra that remove wastes from the blood and produce and eliminates urine (22)

urinate   To discharge urine from the body; other words for this function are void, micturate, and pass water (12, 22)

urine   The fluid secreted by the kidneys, stored in the bladder, and excreted through the urethra (22)

vagina (vaginal canal)   The canal leading from the cervix to the outside of the female body; serves as the organ for intercourse and the birth canal (25)

vaginal irrigation (douche)   The introduction of a solution into the vagina with an immediate return of the solution by gravity; usually used for cleansing the vaginal canal or relieving inflammation of the vaginal tract (25)

vaginal prep   The procedures for making the genital area of a female patient ready for surgery; the preparation includes thoroughly cleansing the skin and carefully shaving the pubic hair; it may also include a cleansing douche (28)

validation therapy   A way of communicating with confused people (32)

vascular   Pertaining to blood vessels (26)

vein   Blood vessel that carries blood from parts of the body back to the heart (18)

ventral   On the abdominal, anterior, or front side of the body (14)

vertebral bodies   The bones around the spinal cord (26)

vertigo   Dizziness (32)

virus   A type of microorganism; much smaller than bacteria that can survive only in other living cells (5)

void   To urinate, pass water (22, 28)

voluntary   Under control of the will; with conscious decision (26)

walker   A metal frame device with handgrips and four legs that is open on one side; provides stability and security for the patient who is weak on one side or restricted in the amount of weight he can put on one foot; A stable frame made of metal tubing used to support the unsteady patient while walking; the patient holds the walker while taking a step, moves it forward, and takes another step (9, 16)

wheelchair   A chair on wheels used to transport patients (9)

Index

Note: A "t" following a page number indicates material within a table and an italicized page number indicates an illustration.

T

License Agreement

YOU SHOULD CAREFULLY READ THE FOLLOWING TERMS AND CONDITIONS BEFORE BREAKING THE SEAL ON THE PACKAGE. AMONG OTHER THINGS, THIS AGREEMENT LICENSES THE ENCLOSED SOFTWARE TO YOU AND CONTAINS WARRANTY AND LIABILITY DISCLAIMERS. BY BREAKING THE SEAL ON THE PACKAGE, YOU ARE ACCEPTING AND AGREEING TO THE TERMS AND CONDITIONS OF THIS AGREEMENT. IF YOU DO NOT AGREE TO THE TERMS OF THIS AGREEMENT, DO NOT BREAK THE SEAL. YOU SHOULD PROMPTLY RETURN THE PACKAGE UNOPENED.

■ LICENSE

Subject to the provisions contained herein, Prentice-Hall, Inc. ("PH") hereby grants to you a non-exclusive, non-transferable license to use the object code version of the computer software product ("Software") contained in the package on a single computer of the type identified on the package.

■ SOFTWARE AND DOCUMENTATION

PH shall furnish the Software to you on media in machine-readable object code form and may also provide the standard documentation ("Documentation") containing instructions for operation and use of the Software.

■ LICENSE TERM AND CHARGES

The term of this license commences upon delivery of the Software to you and is perpetual unless earlier terminated upon default or as otherwise set forth herein.

■ TITLE

Title, and ownership right, and intellectual property rights in and to the Software and Documentation shall remain in PH and/or in suppliers to PH of programs contained in the Software. The Software is provided for your own internal use under this license. This license does not include the right to sublicense and is personal to you and therefore may not be assigned (by operation of law or otherwise) or transferred without the prior written consent of PH. You acknowledge that the Software in source code form remains a confidential trade secret of PH and/or its suppliers and therefore you agree not to attempt to decipher or decompile, modify, disassemble, reverse engineer or prepare derivative works of the Software or develop source code for the Software or knowingly allow others to do so. Further, you may not copy the Documentation or other written materials accompanying the Software.

■ UPDATES

This license does not grant you any right, license, or interest in and to any improvements, modifications, enhancements, or updates to the Software and Documentation. Updates, if available, may be obtained by you at PH's then current standard pricing, terms, and conditions.

■ LIMITED WARRANTY AND DISCLAIMER

PH warrants that the media containing the Software, if provided by PH, is free from defects in material and workmanship under normal use for a period of sixty (60) days from the date you purchased a license to it.

THIS IS A LIMITED WARRANTY AND IT IS THE ONLY WARRANTY MADE BY PH. THE SOFTWARE IS PROVIDED 'AS IS' AND PH SPECIFICALLY DISCLAIMS ALL WARRANTIES OF ANY KIND, EITHER EXPRESS OR IMPLIED, INCLUDING, BUT NOT LIMITED TO, THE IMPLIED WARRANTY OF MERCHANTABILITY AND FITNESS FOR A PARTICULAR PURPOSE. FURTHER, COMPANY DOES NOT WARRANT, GUARANTY OR MAKE ANY REPRESENTATIONS REGARDING THE USE, OR THE RESULTS OF THE USE, OF THE SOFTWARE IN TERMS OF CORRECTNESS, ACCURACY, RELIABILITY, CURRENTNESS, OR OTHERWISE AND DOES NOT WARRANT THAT THE OPERATION OF ANY SOFTWARE WILL BE UNINTERRUPTED OR ERROR FREE. COMPANY EXPRESSLY DISCLAIMS ANY WARRANTIES NOT STATED HEREIN. NO ORAL OR WRITTEN INFORMATION OR ADVICE GIVEN BY PH, OR ANY PH DEALER, AGENT, EMPLOYEE OR OTHERS SHALL CREATE, MODIFY OR EXTEND A WARRANTY OR IN ANY WAY INCREASE THE SCOPE OF THE FOREGOING WARRANTY, AND NEITHER SUBLICENSEE OR PURCHASER MAY RELY ON ANY SUCH INFORMATION OR ADVICE. If the media is subjected to accident, abuse, or improper use; or if you violate the terms of this Agreement, then this warranty shall immediately be terminated. This warranty shall not apply if the Software is used on or in conjunction with hardware or programs other than the unmodified version of hardware and programs with which the Software was designed to be used as described in the Documentation.

■ LIMITATION OF LIABILITY

Your sole and exclusive remedies for any damage or loss in any way connected with the Software are set forth below. UNDER NO CIRCUMSTANCES AND UNDER NO LEGAL THEORY, TORT, CONTRACT, OR OTHERWISE, SHALL PH BE LIABLE TO YOU OR ANY OTHER PERSON FOR ANY INDIRECT, SPECIAL, INCIDENTAL, OR CONSEQUENTIAL DAMAGES OF ANY CHARACTER INCLUDING, WITHOUT LIMITATION, DAMAGES FOR LOSS OF GOODWILL, LOSS OF PROFIT, WORK STOPPAGE, COMPUTER FAILURE OR MALFUNCTION, OR ANY AND ALL OTHER COMMERCIAL DAMAGES OR LOSSES, OR FOR ANY OTHER DAMAGES EVEN IF PH SHALL HAVE BEEN INFORMED OF THE POSSIBILITY OF SUCH DAMAGES, OR FOR ANY CLAIM BY ANY OTHER PARTY. PH'S THIRD PARTY PROGRAM SUPPLIERS MAKE NO WARRANTY, AND HAVE NO LIABILITY WHATSOEVER, TO YOU. PH's sole and exclusive obligation and liability and your exclusive remedy shall be: upon PH's election, (i) the replacement of your defective media; or (ii) the repair or correction of your defective media if PH is able, so that it will conform to the above warranty; or (iii) if PH is unable to replace or repair, you may terminate this license by returning the Software. Only if you inform PH of your problem during the applicable warranty period will PH be obligated to honor this warranty. You may contact PH to inform PH of the problem as follows:

SOME STATES OR JURISDICTIONS DO NOT ALLOW THE EXCLUSION OF IMPLIED WARRANTIES OR LIMITATION OR EXCLUSION OF CONSEQUENTIAL DAMAGES, SO THE ABOVE LIMITATIONS OR EXCLUSIONS MAY NOT APPLY TO YOU. THIS WARRANTY GIVES YOU SPECIFIC LEGAL RIGHTS AND YOU MAY ALSO HAVE OTHER RIGHTS WHICH VARY BY STATE OR JURISDICTION.

■ MISCELLANEOUS

If any provision of this Agreement is held to be ineffective, unenforceable, or illegal under certain circumstances for any reason, such decision shall not affect the validity or enforceability (i) of such provision under other circumstances or (ii) of the remaining provisions hereof under all circumstances and such provision shall be reformed to and only to the extent necessary to make it effective, enforceable, and legal under such circumstances. All headings are solely for convenience and shall not be considered in interpreting this Agreement. This Agreement shall be governed by and construed under New York law as such law applies to agreements between New York residents entered into and to be performed entirely within New York, except as required by U.S. Government rules and regulations to be governed by Federal law.

YOU ACKNOWLEDGE THAT YOU HAVE READ THIS AGREEMENT, UNDERSTAND IT, AND AGREE TO BE BOUND BY ITS TERMS AND CONDITIONS. YOU FURTHER AGREE THAT IT IS THE COMPLETE AND EXCLUSIVE STATEMENT OF THE AGREEMENT BETWEEN US THAT SUPERSEDES ANY PROPOSAL OR PRIOR AGREEMENT, ORAL OR WRITTEN, AND ANY OTHER COMMUNICATIONS BETWEEN US RELATING TO THE SUBJECT MATTER OF THIS AGREEMENT.

■ U.S. GOVERNMENT RESTRICTED RIGHTS

Use, duplication or disclosure by the Government is subject to restrictions set forth in subparagraphs (a) through (d) of the Commercial Computer-Restricted Rights clause at FAR 52.227-19 when applicable, or in subparagraph (c) (1) (ii) of the Rights in Technical Data and Computer Software clause at DFARS 252.227-7013, and in similar clauses in the NASA FAR Supplement.